FIRST EDITION

PDR®

Concise
Drug Guide
for

OBSTETRICS &
GYNECOLOGY

P9-CST-932

PDR® CONCISE DRUG GUIDE FOR OBSTETRICS & GYNECOLOGY

FIRST EDITION

Senior Director, Editorial & Publishing: Bette LaGow
Director, Clinical Services: Michael DeLuca, PharmD, MBA
Manager, Clinical Services: Nermin Shenouda, PharmD
Drug Information Specialists: Anila Patel, PharmD; Greg Tallis, RPh
Manager, Editorial Services: Lori Murray
Project Editors: Sabina Borza, Kathleen Engel
Associate Editor: Jennifer Reed
Contributing Editors: Mariam Gerges; Majid Kerolous, PharmD; Cathy Kim, PharmD; Katie Rodgers, RPh
Senior Director, Client Services: Stephanie Struble
Project Manager: Christina Klinger
Manager, Production Purchasing: Thomas Westburgh
Manager, Art Department: Livio Udina
Electronic Publishing Designers: Deana DiVizio, Carrie Faeth
Production Associate: Joan K. Akerlind

Senior Director, Copy Sales: Bill Gaffney
Senior Product Manager: Richard Buchwald

PHYSICIANS' DESK REFERENCE

Executive Vice President, PDR: Thomas F. Rice
Vice President, Publishing & Operations: Valerie Berger
Vice President, Clinical Relations: Mukesh Mehta, RPh
Vice President: Product Management: Cy Caine
Vice President, Strategy and Business Development: Ray Zoeller
Vice President, Pharma Sales: Anthony Sorce
Vice President, Manufacturing & Vendor Management: Brian Holland

ISBN: 978-156363-727-8

Printed in the United States

Contents

iii

Drugs Commonly Prescribed by OB/GYNs

FOREWORD

The practicing Obstetrician Gynecologist of today is expected to function as a "Jack-of-All-Trades" in the healthcare of women. Not only does he or she serve their patients' obstetric and gynecologic needs, but are also frequently called upon to manage more traditional primary care issues such as hypertension, osteoporosis, disease screening and vaccination, in addition to attending to their patients' psychosocial concerns. Keeping up with all the new therapies and practice paradigms can be challenging for a busy clinician.

For decades, the *Physicians' Desk Reference*® has been a staple in the reference library of almost all physicians as a comprehensive source of drug prescribing information. The *PDR*® *Concise Drug Guide for Obstetrics/Gynecology* was designed as an easy-to-use source of information for the practicing OB/GYN. It contains a vast array of individual drug monographs outlining the pertinent information that a clinician would want to know about a particular drug, including Gardasil–the first HPV vaccine. Sorting through the various types of oral contraceptives with shorter hormone-free intervals, longer intervals between periodic bleeding and newer progestins can be confusing. To that end, one can also find a variety of customized tables that are relevant to the practice of Obstetrics and Gynecology. These include comparison tables on fertility drugs, oral contraceptives, and breast cancer treatment options as well as tables on topics such as risk factors for osteoporosis and breast cancer, just to name a few.

As you peruse the *PDR*® *Concise Drug Guide for Obstetrics/Gynecology*, you will be impressed, as I was, with the extensive and comprehensive nature of this easy-to-use, pocket-sized reference book. It would be a welcome addition to the reference library of any busy clinician involved in women's healthcare.

Fidel A. Valea, M.D.
Associate Professor
Residency Program Director
Department of Obstetrics and Gynecology
Duke University Health System

How to Use This Book

The *PDR® Concise Drug Guide for Obstetrics & Gynecology* allows you to quickly locate important drug information so you can care for patients with confidence. With over 1,700 monographs providing current, organized information, this handy reference is the perfect companion for the busy obstetrics & gynecology professional or student.

This compact guide is divided into four discrete sections. The first section consists of concise drug monographs based on FDA-approved prescribing information. These monographs are organized alphabetically by brand name. When a brand is no longer available, the generic name is used. Monographs may consist of:

- Brand Name
- Generic Name
- Manufacturer
- FDA/DEA Schedule
- Black Box Warnings
- Therapeutic Class
- Indications
- Dosage (adults, pediatrics, special populations)
- How Supplied (dosage form/strength)
- Contraindications
- Warnings/Precautions
- Interactions
- Adverse Reactions
- Pregnancy Category/Breastfeeding Precautions
- Mechanism of Action
- Pharmacokinetics

The second section contains two indices—one with drugs indexed by both brand and generic name, and the other organized by therapeutic class.

The third section comprises an extensive collection of tables and key references to help womens health professionals with decisions about prescribing medications and drug therapy. Tables provided include drug comparisons (both Rx and OTC), drug information centers, poison control centers, immunization schedules, and much more. The drug comparison tables, which are organized alphabetically by class, may include:

- Brand/Generic Name
- How Supplied (dosage form/strength)
- Indications
- Initial and Max Dosages
- Usual Dosage Range

The *PDR® Concise Drug Guide for Obstetrics & Gynecology* also contains a Visual Identification Guide featuring hundreds of product images listed by brand name. This section helps you quickly verify the identity of a capsule, tablet, or other solid oral medication. Each product image contains both the generic and brand name, strength, and the name of its supplier. Other strengths and dosage forms may be available; please check FDA-approved prescribing information for a complete listing of all strengths and dosage forms.

Important Information About Product Labeling

Entries in the *PDR® Concise Drug Guide for Obstetrics & Gynecology* are drawn from FDA-approved product labeling as published in *Physicians' Desk Reference®* or supplied by the manufacturer. The entries are compiled and updated on a regular basis by a staff of experienced pharmacists. While diligent efforts have been made to ensure the accuracy of each entry, it is essential to bear in mind that the information presented here is merely a synopsis of key points in the official labeling, and that the complete labeling contains additional precautionary information that may be of significance in specific cases. Similarly, please remember that only common and dangerous adverse reactions and interactions are included here, and that numerous less-prevalent adverse effects may be reported in the complete labeling. If an entry leaves any question unanswered, be sure to consult *Physicians' Desk Reference* or the manufacturer for additional information.

The function of the publisher is the compilation, organization, and distribution of this information. In organizing and presenting the material in the *PDR Concise Drug Guide for Obstetrics & Gynecology*, the publisher does not warrant or guarantee any of the products described, or perform any independent analysis in connection with any of the product information contained herein.

The *PDR® Concise Drug Guide for Obstetrics & Gynecology* assumes no obligation to obtain and include any information in these entries other than that provided by the manufacturer. The publisher does not warrant, guarantee, or advocate the use of any product described herein. The publisher and editors do not assume, and expressly disclaim, any liability for error, omissions, or typographical errors in the information contained herein or for misuse of any of the products listed.

DRUG MONOGRAPH KEY[1, 2]

BRAND NAME
FDA/DEA Class*
generic (Manufacturer)

> **Black Box Warning:** A brief description of the black box warning(s) that appear in the beginning of the official FDA-approved labeling for the drug.

OTHER BRAND NAMES: Brand name drugs that have the same generic components as the monograph drug.

THERAPEUTIC CLASS: Based on the active ingredients and their mechanism of action.

INDICATIONS: Only includes FDA-approved indications.

DOSAGE: Dosages for adults, pediatrics, and/or special populations as indicated in the official FDA-approved labeling.

HOW SUPPLIED: Product description including strength, formulation, [package size], and scored tablet information.

CONTRAINDICATIONS: Details harmful conditions related to the use of the drug and disease states or patient populations in which use of the monograph drug should be avoided.

WARNINGS/PRECAUTIONS: Details harmful conditions related to the use of the drug and disease states or patient populations where caution is dictated.

ADVERSE REACTIONS: Denotes side effects and adverse reactions listed in the official FDA-approved labeling as occurring with greater frequency (generally at a rate of ≥3%) or deemed significant based on the clinical judgment of the editors. Other side effects may be included if deemed serious or life-threatening. For a complete list of adverse reactions, please refer to the official FDA-approved labeling.

INTERACTIONS: Includes the effects and implications of other drugs and food on the monograph drug based on official FDA-approved labeling.

PREGNANCY: Indicated pregnancy and breastfeeding precautions and, when available, the FDA pregnancy rating system category.†

MECHANISM OF ACTION: Includes pharmacologic drug class and a brief description, or proposed mechanism, of how the drug produces its therapeutic effect.

PHARMACOKINETICS: Brief description of the important parameters described in the FDA-approved labeling related to the absorption, distribution, metabolism, and elimination of the drug. The majority of parameters included are an average or the approximate values provided in the FDA-approved labeling. Only a select group of parameters are included. Refer to the full prescribing information for more detailed pharmacokinetics information.

- **Absorption:** The process by which the drug enters the bloodstream and becomes bioavailable. Absorption parameters may include time to peak plasma concentration (T_{max}), area under the curve (AUC), peak plasma concentration (C_{max}), and absolute bioavailability.

- **Distribution:** Parameters related to the dispersion and dissemination of the monograph drug through bodily fluids and tissues. Distribution parameters may include plasma protein binding and volume of distribution (V_d).

- **Metabolism:** Summary of the biotransformation or detoxification of the parent compound into metabolites. Associated enzymes and active metabolites are included if applicable.

- **Elimination:** The parameters associated with the removal of the drug from the body. Elimination parameters may include elimination/terminal half-life ($T_{1/2}$) and percentage eliminated through urine or feces.

[1] Drug monographs contain concise information. Not all fields described in the Drug Monograph Key are included in every monograph. For more detailed information, please see the full FDA-approved labeling information for the drug.

[2] To identify abbreviated terms used within monographs, refer to the Abbreviations, Acronyms, and Symbols table in the appendix on page A1.

*FDA/DEA CLASS

OTC:	Available over-the-counter.
RX:	Requires a prescription.
CII:	Controlled substance; high potential for abuse.
CIII:	Controlled substance; some potential for abuse.
CIV:	Controlled substance; low potential for abuse.
CV:	Controlled substance; subject to state and local regulation.

†FDA USE-IN-PREGNANCY RATINGS

The FDA use-in-pregnancy rating system weighs the degree to which available information has ruled out risk to the fetus against the drug's potential benefit to the patient. The ratings, and the interpretation, are as follows:

CATEGORY	INTERPRETATION
A	**CONTROLLED STUDIES SHOW NO RISK.** Adequate, well-controlled studies in pregnant women have failed to demonstrate a risk to the fetus in any trimester of pregnancy.
B	**NO EVIDENCE OF RISK IN HUMANS.** Adequate, well controlled studies in pregnant women have not shown increased risk of fetal abnormalities despite adverse findings in animals, or, in the absence of adequate human studies, animal studies show no fetal risk. The chance of fetal harm is remote, but remains a possibility.
C	**RISK CANNOT BE RULED OUT.** Adequate, well-controlled human studies are lacking, and animal studies have shown a risk to the fetus or are lacking as well. There is a chance of fetal harm if the drug is administered during pregnancy; but the potential benefits may outweigh the potential risk.
D	**POSITIVE EVIDENCE OF RISK.** Studies in humans, or investigational or post-marketing data, have demonstrated fetal risk. Nevertheless, potential benefits from the use of the drug may outweigh the potential risk. For example, the drug may be acceptable if needed in a life-threatening situation or serious disease for which safer drugs cannot be used or are ineffective.
X	**CONTRAINDICATED IN PREGNANCY.** Studies in animals or humans, or investigational or post-marketing reports, have demonstrated positive evidence of fetal abnormalities or risk which clearly outweighs any possible benefit to the patient.

Concise Drug Monographs

ABBOKINASE

RX

urokinase (Abbott)

THERAPEUTIC CLASS: Thrombolytic agent

INDICATIONS: Lysis of acute massive pulmonary emboli (PE) and PE accompanied by unstable hemodynamics.

DOSAGE: *Adults:* LD: 4400 IU/kg IV at 90mL/hr over 10 min. Maint: 4400 IU/kg/hr IV at 15mL/hr for 12 hrs. Flush line after each cycle. For IV use only.

HOW SUPPLIED: Inj: 250,000 IU

CONTRAINDICATIONS: Active internal bleeding, intracranial neoplasm, arteriovenous malformation, aneurysm, bleeding diathesis, severe uncontrolled arterial HTN. Recent (within 2 months) CVA, intracranial or intraspinal surgery, trauma including resuscitation.

WARNINGS/PRECAUTIONS: Prior to use obtain Hct, platelet count, and aPTT. Increased risk of bleeding; fatalities due to hemorrhage, including intracranial and retroperitoneal, reported. Avoid IM injections, nonessential patient handling, frequent venipunctures. Use upper extremity vessels when performing arterial punctures. Increased risk of bleeding with recent (within 10 days) major surgery, obstetrical delivery, organ biopsy, previous puncture of noncompressible vessels, serious GI bleeding, high likelihood of left heart thrombus, subacute bacterial endocarditis, hemostatic defects including those secondary to severe hepatic or renal disease, pregnancy, cerebrovascular disease, diabetic hemorrhagic retinopathy, and any other condition in which bleeding may be a significant hazard or difficult to manage. May carry risk of transmitting infectious agents.

ADVERSE REACTIONS: Bleeding, fatal hemorrhage, anaphylaxis, allergic-type or infusion reactions.

INTERACTIONS: Increased risk of serious bleeding with other thrombolytic agents, anticoagulants, or agents inhibiting platelet function (eg, ASA, other NSAIDs, dipyridamole, GP IIb/IIIa inhibitors).

PREGNANCY: Category B, caution in nursing.

MECHANISM OF ACTION: Thrombolytic agent; acts on the endogenous fibrinolytic system. Converts plasminogen to the enzyme plasmin. Plasmin degrades fibrin clots, fibrinogen, and some plasma proteins.

PHARMACOKINETICS: Distribution: V_d=11.5L. **Metabolism:** Liver. **Elimination:** $T_{1/2}$=12.6 min; bile, urine.

ABELCET

RX

amphotericin B lipid complex (Enzon)

THERAPEUTIC CLASS: Polyene antifungal

INDICATIONS: Treatment of invasive fungal infections in patients refractory to or intolerant of conventional amphotericin B therapy.

DOSAGE: *Adults:* 5mg/kg IV at 2.5mg/kg/hr.
Pediatrics: ≥16 yrs: 5mg/kg IV at 2.5mg/kg/hr.

HOW SUPPLIED: Inj: 5mg/mL

WARNINGS/PRECAUTIONS: Anaphylaxis reported. D/C if respiratory distress occurs. Monitor SCr, LFTs, serum electrolytes, CBC during therapy.

ADVERSE REACTIONS: Chills, fever, increased SCr, multi-organ failure, nausea, hypotension, respiratory failure, vomiting, dyspnea, sepsis, diarrhea, headache, heart arrest, HTN, hypokalemia, infection, kidney failure, pain, thrombocytopenia.

INTERACTIONS: Antineoplastics may potentiate renal toxicity, bronchospasm, hypotension. Corticosteroids and corticotropin may potentiate hypokalemia predisposing patients to cardiac dysfunction. May potentiate digitalis toxicity. Increased risk of flucytosine toxicity. Acute pulmonary toxicity reported with leukocyte transfusions. Nephrotoxic drugs (eg, aminoglycosides, pentamidine) enhance potential for renal toxicity. Cyclosporine within several days of bone marrow ablation associated with nephrotoxicity. Hypokalemia effect may enhance curariform effect of skeletal muscle relaxants. May cause increased myelotoxicity and nephrotoxicity with concomitant zidovudine.

PREGNANCY: Category B, not for use in nursing.

MECHANISM OF ACTION: Acts by binding to sterols in cell membrane of susceptible fungi, with resultant change in membrane permeability.

PHARMACOKINETICS: Absorption: C_{max}=1.7mcg/mL, AUC=14mcg•h/mL. **Distribution:** V_d=131L/kg. **Elimination:** $T_{1/2}$=173.4 hrs.

ABILIFY RX
aripiprazole (Bristol-Myers Squibb/Otsuka America)

> Elderly patients with dementia-related psychosis treated with atypical antipsychotic drugs are at an increased risk of death; most appeared to be cardiovascular (eg, heart failure, sudden death) or infectious (eg, pneumonia) in nature. Aripiprazole is not approved for the treatment of patients with dementia-related psychosis. Children, adolescents, and young adults taking antidepressants for major depressive disorder and other psychiatric disorders are at increased risk of suicidal thinking and behavior.

OTHER BRAND NAMES: Abilify Discmelt (Bristol-Myers Squibb/Otsuka America)

THERAPEUTIC CLASS: Partial D_2/$5HT_{1A}$ agonist/$5HT_{2A}$ antagonist

INDICATIONS: (PO) Acute and maintenance treatment of schizophrenia in adults and adolescents aged 13-17 yrs. Acute and maintenance treatment of manic and mixed episodes associated with bipolar I disorder with or without psychotic features in adults and pediatrics aged 10-17 yrs. Adjunctive therapy to antidepressants for acute treatment of major depressive disorder (MDD) in adults. Adjunctive therapy to either lithium or valproate for the acute treatment of manic and mixed episodes associated with bipolar I disorder with or without psychotic features in adults and pediatrics aged 10-17 yrs. (Inj) Acute treatment of agitation associated with schizophrenia or bipolar disorder, manic or mixed, in adults.

DOSAGE: *Adults:* (PO) Schizophrenia: Initial/Target: 10-15mg qd. Titrate: Should not increase before 2 weeks. Max: 30mg/day. Bipolar Disorder (Monotherapy or Adjunct): Initial/Target: 15mg/day. Max: 30mg/day. MDD: Initial: 2-5mg/day. Titrate: May adjust dose at increments of ≤5mg/day at intervals ≥1 week. Range: 2-15mg/day. Max: 15mg/day. Periodically reassess need for maintenance therapy. Oral sol can be given on mg-per-mg basis up to 25mg. Patients receiving 30mg tabs should receive 25mg of oral sol. (Inj) Agitation: 9.75mg IM. Range: 5.25-15mg IM. Max: 30mg/day; initiate PO therapy as soon as possible. Concomitant Strong CYP3A4 Inhibitors (eg, ketoconazole, clarithromycin): Reduce usual aripiprazole dose by 50%. Concomitant CYP2D6 Inhibitors (eg, quinidine, fluoxetine, paroxetine): Reduce usual aripiprazole dose by 50%. Concomitant CYP3A4 Inducers (eg, carbamazepine): Double aripiprazole dose.
Pediatrics: Schizophrenia (13-17 yrs)/Bipolar Disorder (Monotherapy or Adjunct) (10-17 yrs): Initial: 2mg/day. Titrate: 5mg after 2 days. May adjust dose in 5mg/day increments. Recommended: 10mg/day. Max: 30mg/day. Periodically reassess need for maintenance therapy. Oral sol can be given on mg-per-mg basis up to 25mg. Patients receiving 30mg tabs should receive 25mg of oral sol. Concomitant Strong CYP3A4 Inhibitors (eg, ketoconazole, clarithromycin): Reduce usual aripiprazole dose by 50%. Concomitant CYP2D6 Inhibitors (eg, quinidine, fluoxetine, paroxetine): Reduce usual aripiprazole dose by 50%. Concomitant CYP3A4 Inducers (eg, carbamazepine): Double aripiprazole dose.

HOW SUPPLIED: Tab, Orally Disintegrating: (Discmelt) 10mg, 15mg; Tab: 2mg, 5mg, 10mg, 15mg, 20mg, 30mg; Sol: 1mg/mL [150mL]; Inj: 7.5mg/mL

WARNINGS/PRECAUTIONS: May develop tardive dyskinesia, NMS. Monitor for hyperglycemia, worsening of glucose control with DM, FBG levels with diabetes risk. Increased incidence of cerebrovascular adverse events (stroke) in elderly dementia patients. Orthostatic hypotension reported; caution with cardiovascular disease, conditions predisposed to hypotension (eg, dehydration, hypovolemia). May lower seizure threshold. Potential for cognitive and motor impairment. May disrupt body's temperature regulation. Possible esophageal dysmotility and aspiration; caution in patients at risk for aspiration pneumonia. Observe vigilance in treating psychosis associated with Alzheimer's.

ADVERSE REACTIONS: Headache, asthenia, rash, blurred vision, rhinitis, cough, tremor, anxiety, insomnia, nausea, vomiting, lightheadedness, somnolence, constipation, akathisia, extrapyramidal disorder, somnolence, oropharyngeal spasm, grand mal seizure, jaundice, nasopharyngitis, dizziness.

INTERACTIONS: May potentiate effect of antihypertensives. Caution with anticholinergic agents, other centrally acting drugs. Avoid alcohol. CYP3A4 inducers (eg, carbamazepine) may lower blood levels. CYP3A4 inhibitors (eg, ketoconazole, itraconazole) or 2D6 inhibitors (eg, quinidine, fluoxetine, paroxetine) can increase blood levels.

PREGNANCY: Category C, not for use in nursing.

MECHANISM OF ACTION: Not established; proposed that efficacy is mediated through a combination of partial agonist activity at D_2 and 5-HT_{1A} receptors and antagonist activity at 5-HT_{2A} receptors.

PHARMACOKINETICS: Absorption: Absolute bioavailability 87% (PO), 100% (IM); T_{max}=3-5 hrs (PO), 1-3 hrs (IM). **Distribution:** V_d=404L or 4.9L/kg (PO), plasma protein binding 99% (PO). **Metabolism:** Hepatic via dehydrogenation, hydroxylation, and N-dealkylation. Dehydro-aripiprazole (active metabolite) CYP3A4 and 2D6 enzymes (PO). Not systemically evaluated (IM). **Elimination:** Urine (25%), feces (55%); $T_{1/2}$=75-146 hrs.

ABRAXANE   RX
paclitaxel protein-bound particles (Abraxis)

> Do not administer to patients with metastatic breast cancer who have baseline neutrophil counts of less than 1,500 cells/mm³. Perform peripheral blood cell counts on all patients to monitor occurence of bone marrow suppression, primarily neutropenia. Should only be administered under the supervision of a physician experienced in the use of cancer chemotherapeutic agents. Do not substitute for or with other paclitaxel formulations.

THERAPEUTIC CLASS: Antimicrotubule agent

INDICATIONS: Treatment of breast cancer after failure of combination chemotherapy for metastatic disease or relapse within 6 months of adjuvant chemotherapy. Prior therapy should have included an anthracycline unless clinically contraindicated.

DOSAGE: *Adults:* 260mg/m² IV over 30 min every 3 weeks. Severe neutropenia (neutrophil <500 cells/mm³ for week or longer) or severe sensory neuropathy (Grade 3 or 4): Hold dose until neutrophil >1500 cells/mm³ or sensory neuropathy resolves to Grade 1 or 2. Reduce subsequent courses to 220mg/m², if recurrence reduce subsequent courses to 180mg/m².

HOW SUPPLIED: Inj: 100mg

CONTRAINDICATIONS: Patients with baseline neutrophil counts of < 1,500 cells/mm³.

WARNINGS/PRECAUTIONS: Perform frequent blood counts to monitor for bone marrow suppression. Men should be advised to not father a child while receiving treatment. Remote risk for transmission of viral diseases; theoretical risk for transmission of Creutzfeldt-Jacob disease. Sensory neuropathy occurs frequently. Reports of injection site reactions.

ADVERSE REACTIONS: Neutropenia, infectious episodes, anemia, hypotension, ECG abnormalities, dyspnea, cough, sensory neuropathy, ocular/visual disturbances, arthralgia, myalgia, nausea, vomiting, asthenia, abnormal liver function test.

PREGNANCY: Category D, not for use in nursing.

MECHANISM OF ACTION: Antimicrotubule agent; promotes assembly of microtubules from tubulin dimers and stabilizes microtubules by preventing depolymerization. This stability results in the inhibition of the normal dynamic reorganization of the microtubule network that is essential for vital interphase and mitotic cellular functions.

PHARMACOKINETICS: Absorption: C_{max}=18,741ng/mL. **Distribution:** V_d=632L/m^2, plasma protein binding (89-98%). **Metabolism:** Liver via CYP2C8 (6α, 3'-p-dihydroxypaclitaxel, major metabolite). **Elimination:** Urine (4%, unchanged), (≤1%, metabolite), feces (approximately 20%).

ABREVA   OTC
docosanol (GlaxoSmithKline Consumer)

THERAPEUTIC CLASS: Antiviral

INDICATIONS: To treat cold sore/fever blisters on the face or lips.

DOSAGE: *Adults:* Apply to affected area on face or lips at 1st sign of cold sore/fever blister (tingle). Use 5x/day until healed.
Pediatrics: ≥12 yrs: Apply to affected area on face or lips at 1st sign of cold sore/fever blister (tingle). Use 5x/day until healed.

HOW SUPPLIED: Cre: 10% [2g]

WARNINGS/PRECAUTIONS: Avoid in or near eyes, and inside mouth. D/C if sore worsens or does not heal in 10 days.

PREGNANCY: Safety in pregnancy and nursing is not known.

MECHANISM OF ACTION: Antiviral; works on the cell membrane to inhibit the ability of the virus to fuse with the cell membrane.

ACCOLATE   RX
zafirlukast (AstraZeneca)

THERAPEUTIC CLASS: Leukotriene receptor antagonist

INDICATIONS: Prophylaxis and chronic treatment of asthma.

DOSAGE: *Adults:* 20mg bid. Administer 1 hr ac or 2 hrs pc.
Pediatrics: ≥12 yrs: 20mg bid. 5-11 yrs: 10mg bid. Administer 1 hr ac or 2 hrs pc.

HOW SUPPLIED: Tab: 10mg, 20mg

WARNINGS/PRECAUTIONS: Not for treatment of acute asthma attacks. Bioavailability decreases with food. Hepatic dysfunction and systemic eosinophilia reported.

ADVERSE REACTIONS: Headache, infection, nausea, diarrhea, hypersensitivity reactions including angioedema.

INTERACTIONS: Potentiates warfarin. Caution with drugs metabolized by CYP2C9 (eg, tolbutamide, phenytoin, carbamazepine) or CYP3A4 (eg, dihydropyridine CCBs, cyclosporine, cisapride, astemizole). Increased levels with ASA. Decreased levels by erythromycin, theophylline. May increase theophylline levels.

PREGNANCY: Category B, not for use in nursing.

MECHANISM OF ACTION: Leukotriene receptor antagonist (LTRA); selective and competitive receptor antagonist of leukotriene D_4 and E_4 (LTD$_4$ and LTE$_4$), components of slow-reacting substance of anaphylaxis (SRSA); inhibits bronchoconstriction.

PHARMACOKINETICS: Absorption: Rapid. (Adult) C_{max}=326ng/mL; T_{max}=2 hrs; AUC=1137ng•h/mL. (7-11 yrs) C_{max}=601ng/mL; T_{max}=2.5 hrs; AUC=2027ng•h/mL. (5-6 yrs) C_{max}=756ng/mL; T_{max}=2.1 hrs; AUC=2458ng•h/mL. **Distribution**: V_d=approximately 70L; plasma protein binding (>99%). **Metabolism**: Liver, hydroxylation via CYP2C9. **Elimination**: $T_{1/2}$=10 hrs.

ACCUNEB
albuterol sulfate (Dey)

RX

THERAPEUTIC CLASS: Beta$_2$-agonist

INDICATIONS: Relief of bronchospasm with asthma.

DOSAGE: *Pediatrics:* 2-12 yrs: Initial: 0.63mg or 1.25mg tid-qid via nebulizer. 6-12 yrs with severe asthma, >40kg or 11-12 yrs: Initial: 1.25mg tid-qid.

HOW SUPPLIED: Sol: 1.25mg/3mL, 0.63mg/3mL [3mL, 25^s]

WARNINGS/PRECAUTIONS: Hypersensitivity reactions reported. Fatalities reported with excessive use. Caution with cardiovascular disorders, especially coronary insufficiency, arrhythmias and HTN. May need concomitant anti-inflammatory agents. Can produce paradoxical bronchospasm. Caution with DM. May cause hypokalemia.

ADVERSE REACTIONS: Asthma exacerbation, otitis media, allergic reaction, gastroenteritis, cold symptoms.

INTERACTIONS: Avoid other short-acting sympathomimetic bronchodilators and epinephrine. Extreme caution within 2 weeks of MAOI or TCA use. Monitor digoxin. ECG changes and/or hypokalemia with non-K$^+$-sparing diuretics may worsen. May be antagonized by β-blockers.

PREGNANCY: Category C, not for use in nursing.

MECHANISM OF ACTION: β$_2$ adrenergic agonist; stimulates adenyl cyclase, the enzyme that catalyzes the formation of ATP.

PHARMACOKINETICS: Absorption: (3mg): C_{max}=2.1ng/mL, T_{max}=0.5 hrs. **Elimination:** (4 mg): $T_{1/2}$=5-6 hrs.

ACCUPRIL
quinapril HCL (Parke-Davis)

RX

> ACE inhibitors can cause death/injury to developing fetus during 2nd and 3rd trimesters. Stop therapy if pregnancy detected.

THERAPEUTIC CLASS: ACE inhibitor

INDICATIONS: Treatment of hypertension. Adjunct therapy in heart failure with diuretics and/or digitalis.

DOSAGE: *Adults:* HTN: If possible, d/c diuretic 2-3 days prior to therapy. Initial: 10-20mg qd; 5mg qd with concomitant diuretic. Titrate at intervals of at least 2 weeks. Usual: 20-80mg/day given qd-bid. CrCl >60mL/min: Initial: 10mg/day. CrCl 30-60mL/min: Initial: 5mg/day. CrCl 10-30mL/min: Initial: 2.5mg/day. Heart Failure: Initial: 5mg bid. Titrate at weekly intervals. Usual: 10-20mg bid. CrCl >30mL/min: Initial: 5mg/day. CrCl 10-30mL/min: Initial: 2.5mg/day.

HOW SUPPLIED: Tab: 5mg*, 10mg, 20mg, 40mg *scored

CONTRAINDICATIONS: History of ACE inhibitor-associated angioedema.

WARNINGS/PRECAUTIONS: D/C if angioedema, jaundice, or if marked LFT elevation occurs. Risk of hyperkalemia with DM, renal dysfunction. Persistent nonproductive cough reported. Monitor WBCs in renal or collagen vascular disease. Anaphylactoid reactions reported. Fetal/neonatal morbidity and death reported. Monitor for hypotension in high risk patients (heart failure, surgery/anesthesia, hyponatremia, high-dose diuretic therapy, recent intensive diuresis, dialysis, or severe volume and/or salt depletion, etc). Caution with CHF, renal dysfunction, and renal artery stenosis. Less effective on BP in blacks and more reports of angioedema than nonblacks.

ADVERSE REACTIONS: Fatigue, headache, dizziness, cough, nausea, vomiting, hypotension, chest pain.

INTERACTIONS: Decreases tetracycline absorption (possibly due to magnesium content in quinapril); consider interaction with drugs that interact with magnesium. May increase lithium levels. Hypotension risk with diuretics.

Increased risk of hyperkalemia with K⁺-sparing diuretics, K⁺ supplements, or K⁺-containing salt substitutes.

PREGNANCY: Category C (1st trimester) and D (2nd and 3rd trimesters), not for use in nursing.

MECHANISM OF ACTION: Angiotensin-converting enzyme inhibitor; inhibits ACE activity, reducing angiotensin II formation.

PHARMACOKINETICS: Absorption: T_{max}=1hr. (Quinaprilat) T_{max}=2 hrs. **Distribution:** Plasma protein binding (97%). **Metabolism:** Deesterification. Quinaprilat (active metabolite). **Elimination:** (Quinaprilat) Renal; $T_{1/2}$= 2hrs.

Accuretic   RX
quinapril HCL - hydrochlorothiazide (Parke-Davis)

> ACE inhibitors can cause death/injury to developing fetus during 2nd and 3rd trimesters. Stop therapy if pregnancy detected.

THERAPEUTIC CLASS: ACE inhibitor/thiazide diuretic

INDICATIONS: Treatment of hypertension. Not for initial therapy.

DOSAGE: *Adults:* Initial (if not controlled on quinapril monotherapy): 10mg-12.5mg or 20mg-12.5mg tab qd. Titrate: May increase after 2-3 weeks. Initial (if controlled on HCTZ 25mg/day but significant K⁺ loss): 10mg-12.5mg or 20mg-12.5mg tab qd. If previously treated with 20mg quinapril and 25mg HCTZ, may switch to 20mg-25mg tab qd.

HOW SUPPLIED: Tab: (Quinapril-HCTZ) 10mg-12.5mg*, 20mg-12.5mg*, 20mg-25mg* *scored

CONTRAINDICATIONS: History of ACE inhibitor-associated angioedema, anuria, sulfonamide hypersensitivity.

WARNINGS/PRECAUTIONS: D/C if angioedema, jaundice, or marked LFT elevation occurs. Risk of hyperkalemia with DM, renal dysfunction. Persistent nonproductive cough reported. Monitor WBCs in renal or collagen vascular disease. Anaphylactoid reactions reported. Fetal/neonatal morbidity and death reported. Monitor for hypotension in high-risk patients (heart failure, surgery/anesthesia, hyponatremia, severe volume/salt depletion, etc). Caution with CHF, renal or hepatic dysfunction, and renal artery stenosis. Less effective on BP in blacks and more reports of angioedema than nonblacks. May exacerbate or activate SLE. Monitor serum electrolytes. Avoid if CrCl ≤30mL/min/1.73m². May increase cholesterol, TG, and uric acid levels and decrease glucose tolerance.

ADVERSE REACTIONS: Dizziness, headache, cough, myalgia.

INTERACTIONS: Decreases tetracycline absorption (possibly due to magnesium content in quinapril); consider interaction with drugs that interact with magnesium. Increase risk of hyperkalemia with K⁺-sparing diuretics, K⁺ supplements, or K⁺-containing salt substitutes. Potentiates orthostatic hypotension with alcohol, barbiturates, and narcotics. Adjust insulin and antidiabetic drugs. Impaired absorption with cholestyramine, colestipol. Corticosteroids and ACTH deplete electrolytes. May decrease response to pressor amines. Potentiates other antihypertensives. May increase responsiveness to skeletal muscle relaxants. Risk of lithium toxicity. NSAIDs decrease diuretic effects.

PREGNANCY: Category C (1st trimester) and D (2nd and 3rd trimesters), not for use in nursing.

MECHANISM OF ACTION: Quinapril: Angiotensin-converting enzyme inhibitor; inhibits ACE activity reducing angiotensin II formation. HCTZ: Thiazide diuretic; affects renal tubular mechanism of electrolyte reabsorption directly increasing excretion of Na⁺ and Cl⁻, and indirectly decreasing plasma volume.

PHARMACOKINETICS: Absorption: Quinapril: T_{max}=1 hr. (Quinaprilat) T_{max}=2 hrs. **Distribution:** Quinapril: Plasma protein binding (97%). HCTZ: V_d=3.6-7.8L/kg; plasma protein binding (67.9%); crosses placenta. **Metabolism:** Quinapril: Deesterification. Quinaprilat (metabolite). **Elimination:** Quinaprilat: Renal; $T_{1/2}$=2 hrs. HCTZ: Kidney (61%); $T_{1/2}$=4-15 hrs.

ACCUTANE   RX
isotretinoin (Roche Labs)

> Not for use by females who are or may become pregnant, or if breastfeeding. Birth defects have been documented. Increased risk of spontaneous abortion, and premature births reported. Approved for marketing only under special restricted distribution program called iPLEDGE™. Must have 2 negative pregnancy tests. Repeat pregnancy test monthly. Use 2 forms of contraception at least 1 month prior, during, and 1 month following discontinuation. Must fill written prescriptions within 7 days; refills require new prescriptions. May dispense maximum of 1 month supply. Prescriber, dispensing pharmacy, and patient must be registered with iPLEDGE.

OTHER BRAND NAMES: Sotret (Ranbaxy) - Claravis (Barr) - Amnesteem (Genpharm)

THERAPEUTIC CLASS: Retinoid

INDICATIONS: Severe recalcitrant nodular acne unresponsive to conventional therapy, including systemic antibiotics.

DOSAGE: *Adults:* Initial/Usual: 0.5-1mg/kg/day given bid for 15-20 weeks. Max: 2mg/kg/day (for very serious cases). Adjust for side effects and disease response. May discontinue if nodule count reduced by >70% prior to completion. Repeat only if necessary after 2 months off drug. Take with food.
Pediatrics: ≥12 yrs: Initial/Usual: 0.5-1mg/kg/day given bid for 15-20 weeks. Max: 2mg/kg/day (for very serious cases). Adjust for side effects and disease response. May discontinue if nodule count reduced by >70% prior to completion. Repeat only if necessary after 2 months off drug. Take with food.

HOW SUPPLIED: Cap: 10mg, 20mg, 40mg

CONTRAINDICATIONS: Pregnancy, paraben sensitivity (preservative in gelatin cap).

WARNINGS/PRECAUTIONS: Acute pancreatitis, impaired hearing, anaphylactic reactions, inflammatory bowel disease, elevated TG and LFTs, hepatotoxicity, premature epiphyseal closure, and hyperostosis reported. May cause depression, psychosis, aggressive and/or violent behaviors, rarely suicidal ideation/attempts and suicide; may need further evaluation after discontinuation. May cause decreased night vision, and corneal opacities. Associated with pseudotumor cerebri. Check lipids before therapy, and then at intervals until response established (within 4 weeks). D/C if significant decrease in WBC, hearing or visual impairment, abdominal pain, rectal bleeding, or severe diarrhea occurs. Monitor LFTs before therapy, weekly or biweekly until response established. May develop musculoskeletal symptoms. Avoid prolonged UV rays or sunlight, and donating blood up to 1 month after discontinuing therapy. Caution with genetic predisposition for age-related osteoporosis, history of childhood osteoporosis, osteomalacia, other bone metabolism disorders (eg, anorexia nervosa). Spontaneous osteoporosis, osteopenia, bone fractures, and delayed fracture healing reported; caution in sports with repetitive impact. Use 2 forms of effective contraception for 1 month. Female patients of childbearing potential must fill and pick up the prescription within 7 days of the date of specimen collection for the pregnancy test. Must only be dispensed in no more than 30-day supply and with a Medication Guide.

ADVERSE REACTIONS: Cheilitis, dry skin and mucous membranes, conjunctivitis, blood dyscrasias, epistaxis, decreased HDL, elevated cholesterol and TG, elevated blood sugar, arthralgias, back pain, hearing/vision impairment, rash, photosensitivity reactions, psychiatric disorders, abnormal menses, cardiovascular disorders.

INTERACTIONS: Avoid vitamin A. Limit alcohol consumption. Aoid use with tetracyclines; increased incidence of pseudotumor cerebri. Pregnancy reported with oral and injectable/implantable contraceptives. Avoid St. John's wort; may cause breakthrough bleeding with oral contraceptives. Caution with drugs that cause drug-induced osteoporosis/osteomalacia and affect vitamin D metabolism (eg, corticosteroids, phenytoin).

PREGNANCY: Category X, not for use in nursing.

MECHANISM OF ACTION: Retinoid; MOA not established. Suspected to inhibit sebaceous gland function and keratinization.

PHARMACOKINETICS: Absorption: C_{max}=862ng/mL (fed), 301ng/mL (fasted); T_{max}=5.3 hrs (fed), 3.2 hrs (fasted); AUC=10,004ng•hr/mL (fed), 3703ng•hr/mL (fasted). **Distribution:** Plasma protein binding (99.9%). **Metabolism:** Liver via CYP2C8, 2C9, 3A4, and 2B6; 4-*oxo*-isotretinoin, retinoic acid, and 4-*oxo*-retinoic acid (active metabolites). **Elimination:** Urine, feces; $T_{1/2}$=21 hrs (isotretinoin), 24 hrs (4-*oxo*-isotretinoin).

ACCUZYME   RX
papain - urea (Healthpoint)

THERAPEUTIC CLASS: Proteolytic enzyme (debriding agent)

INDICATIONS: Debridement of necrotic tissue and liquefaction of slough in acute and chronic lesions such as pressure ulcers, varicose and diabetic ulcers, burns, postoperative wounds, pilonidal cyst wounds, carbuncles and other traumatic or infected wounds.

DOSAGE: *Adults:* (Oint, Spray) Clean wound, then apply qd-bid. Cover with dressing. Irrigate wound at each re-dressing.

HOW SUPPLIED: (Papain-Urea) Oint: 830000 U/g-10% [6g, 30g]; Spray: 830000 U/g-10% [33mL]

WARNINGS/PRECAUTIONS: Avoid eyes.

ADVERSE REACTIONS: Transient burning, skin irritation.

INTERACTIONS: May be inactivated by hydrogen peroxide, and salts of heavy metals (eg, lead, silver, mercury).

PREGNANCY: Safety in pregnancy and nursing is not known.

MECHANISM OF ACTION: Papain: Proteolytic enzyme; potent digestant of nonviable protein matter. Urea: Denaturant of proteins. When both agents are combined, works to produce two chemical actions 1) to expose by solvent action the activators of papain 2) denature the nonviable protein matter in lesions, thereby rendering it more susceptible to enzymatic digestion.

ACEON   RX
perindopril erbumine (Solvay)

> **ACE inhibitors can cause death/injury to developing fetus during 2nd and 3rd trimesters. Stop therapy if pregnancy detected.**

THERAPEUTIC CLASS: ACE inhibitor

INDICATIONS: Treatment of hypertension (HTN). Risk reduction of cardiovascular mortality or nonfatal myocardial infarction in patients with stable coronary artery disease (CAD).

DOSAGE: *Adults:* HTN: If possible, d/c diuretic 2-3 days prior to therapy. Initial: 4mg qd; 2-4mg/day given qd-bid with concomitant diuretic. Maint: 4-8mg/day given qd-bid. Resume diuretic if BP not controlled. Max: 16mg/day. Elderly (>65 yrs): Initial: 4mg/day given qd-bid. Max (usual): 8mg/day. Renal Impairment: CrCl >30mL/min: Initial: 2mg/day. Max: 8mg/day. CAD: Initial: 4mg qd for 2 weeks. Maint: 8mg qd. Elderly (>70 yrs): Initial: 2mg qd for 1 week. Titrate: 4mg qd for Week 2. Maint: 8mg qd.

HOW SUPPLIED: Tab: 2mg*, 4mg*, 8mg* *scored

CONTRAINDICATIONS: History of ACE inhibitor-associated angioedema.

WARNINGS/PRECAUTIONS: D/C if angioedema, jaundice, or if marked LFT elevation occurs. Risk of hyperkalemia with DM, renal dysfunction. Persistent nonproductive cough reported. Monitor WBCs in renal and collagen vascular disease. Anaphylactoid reactions reported. Fetal/neonatal morbidity and death reported. Monitor for hypotension in high-risk patients (heart failure, surgery/anesthesia, hyponatremia, prolonged diuretic therapy, or volume and/or salt depletion). Caution with CHF, renal dysfunction, and renal artery stenosis. Less effective on BP in blacks and more reports of angioedema than nonblacks. Avoid if CrCl <30mL/min.

ADVERSE REACTIONS: Cough, headache, asthenia, dizziness, diarrhea, edema, respiratory infection, lower extremity pain.

INTERACTIONS: May increase lithium levels. Hypotension risk with diuretics. Increased risk of hyperkalemia with K$^+$-sparing diuretics, drugs that increase serum K$^+$, or K$^+$ supplements. Caution with gentamicin.

PREGNANCY: Category C (1st trimester) and D (2nd and 3rd trimesters), caution in nursing.

MECHANISM OF ACTION: Angiotensin-converting enzyme inhibitor; inhibits ACE activity, decreasing plasma angiotensin II, decreasing vasoconstriction, increasing plasma renin activity, and decreasing aldosterone secretion.

PHARMACOKINETICS: Absorption: Rapid; T_{max}=1 hr; absolute bioavailability (75%). Perindoprilat: Absolute bioavailability (25%); T_{max}=3-7 hrs. **Distribution:** Plasma protein binding (60%). Perindoprilat: Plasma protein binding (10-20%). **Metabolism:** Hepatic esterases (hydrolysis), glucuronidation, cyclization. Perindoprilat (active metabolite). **Elimination:** Urine (4-12%); $T_{1/2}$=0.8-1 hr. Perindoprilat: $T_{1/2}$=3-10 hrs.

ACETADOTE   RX
acetylcysteine (Cumberland)

THERAPEUTIC CLASS: Acetaminophen antidote

INDICATIONS: Prevent or lessen hepatic injury within 8-10 hrs of potentially hepatotoxic dose of APAP.

DOSAGE: *Adults:* LD: Infuse 150mg/kg IV over 60 min. Maint: 50mg/kg over 4 hrs followed by 100mg/kg over 16 hrs.

HOW SUPPLIED: Inj: 200mg/mL [30mL]

WARNINGS/PRECAUTIONS: Caution in patients with asthma or history of brochospasm; can cause serious anaphylactoid reactions. Acute flushing and erythema of skin may occur. Caution in patients <40kg; avoid fluid overload; adjust D5W volume.

ADVERSE REACTIONS: Rash, urticaria, pruritus, nausea, vomiting, bronchospasm, angioedema.

PREGNANCY: Category B, caution in nursing.

MECHANISM OF ACTION: Acetaminophen antidote; protects liver by maintaining or restoring gluthatione levels. Also acts as an alternate substrate for conjugation with, thus detoxification of the reactive metabolite.

PHARMACOKINETICS: Distribution: V_d=0.47L/kg; plasma protein binding (83%). **Metabolism:** Conjugation. **Elimination:** $T_{1/2}$=5.6 hrs.

ACETYLCYSTEINE   RX
acetylcysteine (Various)

THERAPEUTIC CLASS: Acetaminophen antidote/Mucolytic

INDICATIONS: Adjunctive mucolytic therapy in acute and chronic bronchopulmonary disease; pulmonary complications of cystic fibrosis and surgery; tracheostomy care; during anesthesia; post-traumatic chest conditions; atelectasis; diagnostic bronchial studies. Antidote for acute acetaminophen (APAP) toxicity.

DOSAGE: *Adults:* Antidote: Empty stomach by lavage or emesis before administration. Administer immediately, regardless of quantity, if APAP ingestion ≤24hrs. LD: 140mg/kg PO then 70mg/kg PO q4h for 17 doses starting 4 hrs after LD. D/C if predetoxification APAP level is in nontoxic range and overdose occurred at least 4 hrs before assay. Obtain 2nd plasma level if range is nontoxic and time of ingestion is unknown or <4 hrs. Mucolytic: Nebulization (face mask, mouth piece, tracheostomy): 1-10mL of 20% or 2-10mL of 10% q2-6h. Usual: 3-5mL of 20% or 6-10mL of 10% 3-4 times/day. Closed Tent or Croupette: Up to 300mL of 10% or 20%. Direct Instillation: 1-2 mL of 10% or 20% q1-4h. Percutaneous Intratracheal Catheter: 1-2mL of 20% or 2-4mL of

10% q1-4h. Diagnostic Bronchograms: Give before procedure. 2-3 doses of 1-2mL of 20% or 2-4mL of 10%.
Pediatrics: Antidote: Empty stomach by lavage or emesis before administration. Administer immediately, regardless of quantity, if APAP ingestion ≤24hrs. LD: 140mg/kg PO then 70mg/kg PO q4h for 17 doses starting 4 hours after LD. D/C if predetoxification APAP level is in nontoxic range and overdose occurred at least 4 hrs before assay. Obtain 2nd plasma level if range is nontoxic and time of ingestion is unknown or <4 hrs. Mucolytic: Nebulization (face mask, mouth piece, tracheostomy): 1-10mL of 20% or 2-10mL of 10% q2-6h. Usual: 3-5mL of 20% or 6-10mL of 10% 3-4 times/day. Closed Tent or Croupette: Up to 300mL of 10% or 20%. Direct Instillation: 1-2 mL of 10% or 20% q1-4h. Percutaneous Intratracheal Catheter: 1-2mL of 20% or 2-4mL of 10% q1-4h. Diagnostic Procedures: Give before procedure. 2-3 doses of 1-2mL of 20% or 2-4mL of 10%.

HOW SUPPLIED: Sol: 10%, 20%

WARNINGS/PRECAUTIONS: (Oral) D/C if generalized urticaria or encephalopathy due to hepatic failure develops. May aggravate vomiting; evaluate with risk of gastric hemorrhage. (Inhalation) Monitor asthmatics. D/C if bronchospasm progresses.

ADVERSE REACTIONS: (Oral) Nausea, vomiting, other GI symptoms. (Inhalation) Stomatitis, nausea, vomiting, fever, rhinorrhea, drowsiness, clamminess, chest tightness, bronchoconstriction.

PREGNANCY: Category B, caution in nursing.

MECHANISM OF ACTION: N-acetyl derivative. Mucolytic; opens disulfide linkages in mucus, thereby lowering viscosity. Antidote; protects liver by maintaining or restoring glutathione levels, or by acting as alternate substrate for conjugation with, and thus detoxification of reactive metabolites, reducing extent of liver injury.

PHARMACOKINETICS: Metabolism: Deacetylation, oxidation.

ACIPHEX   RX
rabeprazole sodium (Eisai/PRICARA)

THERAPEUTIC CLASS: Proton pump inhibitor

INDICATIONS: Short-term treatment in the healing and symptomatic relief of erosive or ulcerative gastroesophageal reflux disease (GERD). Maintenance of healing and reduction in relapse rates of heartburn symptoms in patients with erosive or ulcerative GERD. Treatment of daytime and nighttime heartburn and other symptoms associated with GERD. Short-term treatment in the healing and symptomatic relief of duodenal ulcers (DU). In combination with amoxicillin and clarithromycin as a 3-drug regimen for the treatment of patients with *H.pylori* infection and DU disease (active or history within the past 5 yrs) to eradicate *H.pylori* and reduce the risk of DU recurrence. Long-term treatment of pathological hypersecretory conditions, including Zollinger-Ellison syndrome.

DOSAGE: *Adults:* Erosive/Ulcerative GERD: Healing; 20mg qd for 4-8 weeks. May repeat for 8 weeks if needed. Maint: 20mg qd. Symptomatic GERD: 20mg qd for 4 weeks. May repeat for 4 weeks if needed. DU: 20mg qd after morning meal for up to 4 weeks. May need additional therapy. *H.pylori* Triple Therapy: 20mg + clarithromycin 500mg + amoxicillin 1g, all bid (qam and qpm) with food for 7 days. Pathological Hypersecretory Conditions: Initial: 60mg qd. Titrate: Adjust according to need. Maint: Up to 100mg qd or 60mg bid. May treat up to 1 yr. Swallow tabs whole; do not chew, crush, or split.

HOW SUPPLIED: Tab, Delayed-Release: 20mg

WARNINGS/PRECAUTIONS: Symptomatic response does not preclude the presence of gastric malignancy. Caution with severe hepatic impairment.

ADVERSE REACTIONS: Headache. Diarrhea and taste perversion with triple therapy.

INTERACTIONS: May alter absorption of pH-dependent drugs (eg, ketoconazole, digoxin). May inhibit cyclosporine metabolism. May increase digoxin plasma levels and decrease ketoconazole levels. Monitor PT/INR with warfarin. Increased rabeprazole and clarithromycin levels with triple therapy.

PREGNANCY: Category B, not for use in nursing.

MECHANISM OF ACTION: Proton pump inhibitor; suppresses gastric acid secretion by inhibiting the gastric (H^+, K^+)-ATPase enzyme at the secretory surface of the gastric parietal cell. Blocks the final step of gastric acid secretion.

PHARMACOKINETICS: Absorption: T_{max}=2-5 hrs; absolute bioavailability (52%). **Distribution:** Plasma protein binding (96.3%). **Metabolism:** Extensive. Liver via CYP3A4 to sulphone (primary metabolite) and CYP2C19 to desmethyl rabeprazole (primary metabolite). **Elimination:** Urine (90%), feces; $T_{1/2}$=1-2 hrs.

ACLOVATE
alclometasone dipropionate (GlaxoSmithKline)

RX

THERAPEUTIC CLASS: Corticosteroid

INDICATIONS: Relief of the inflammatory and pruritic manifestations of corticosteroid responsive dermatoses.

DOSAGE: *Adults:* Apply bid-tid. Reassess if no improvement after 2 weeks. *Pediatrics:* ≥1 yr: Apply bid-tid. Reassess if no improvement after 2 weeks.

HOW SUPPLIED: Cre, Oint: 0.05% [15g, 45g, 60g]

WARNINGS/PRECAUTIONS: May produce reversible HPA axis suppression, manifestations of Cushing's syndrome, hyperglycemia, and glucosuria. Use appropriate antifungal or antibacterial agent with dermatological infections. Peds may be more susceptible to systemic toxicity. Avoid occlusive dressings. Avoid diaper area. Not for use in diaper dermatitis. D/C if irritation occurs. Caution in peds.

ADVERSE REACTIONS: Itching, burning, erythema, dryness, irritation, papular rash, folliculitis, acneiform eruptions, hypopigmentation, perioral dermatitis, allergic contact dermatitis, secondary infection, skin atrophy, striae.

PREGNANCY: Category C, caution in nursing.

MECHANISM OF ACTION: Corticosteroid; has anti-inflammatory, antipruritic, and vasoconstrictive properties. Anti-inflammatory mechanism not established. Suspected to act by the induction of phospholipase A_2 inhibitory proteins (lipocortins), which may control the biosynthesis of potent mediators of inflammation (eg, prostaglandins, leukotrienes) by inhibiting the release of their common precursor, arachidonic acid. Arachidonic acid is released from membrane phospholipids by phospholipase A_2.

PHARMACOKINETICS: Distribution: Systemically administered corticosteroids are found in breast milk.

ACTHREL
corticorelin ovine triflutate (Ferring)

RX

THERAPEUTIC CLASS: CRH (human) peptide analogue

INDICATIONS: For use in differentiating pituitary and ectopic production of ACTH in patients with ACTH-dependent Cushing's syndrome.

DOSAGE: *Adults:* 1mcg/kg IV single dose. If repeated evaluation is needed, repeat test at the same time of day as the original test. Administer over 30 seconds and not as a bolus injection to decrease side effects. Doses >1mcg/kg are not recommended.

HOW SUPPLIED: Inj: 0.1mg

WARNINGS/PRECAUTIONS: Transient tachycardia, decreased BP, loss of consciousness, and asystole reported at higher than recommended doses.

ADVERSE REACTIONS: Flushing of the face, neck, and upper chest, the urge to take a deep breath.

INTERACTIONS: Pretreatment with dexamethasone inhibits or blunts plasma ACTH response. Major hypotensive reaction reported with heparin.

PREGNANCY: Category C, caution in nursing.

MECHANISM OF ACTION: CRH (human) peptide analogue; determines pituitary corticotroph responsiveness.

PHARMACOKINETICS: Distribution: V_d=6.2L. **Elimination:** $T_{1/2}$=11.6 min.

ACTICIN   RX
permethrin (Mylan Bertek)

THERAPEUTIC CLASS: Pyrethroid scabicidal agent

INDICATIONS: Treatment of scabies.

DOSAGE: *Adults:* Massage into skin from head to soles of feet. Wash off after 8-14 hrs. One treatment should be adequate. Retreat if living mites present after 14 days.
Pediatrics: ≥2 months: Massage into skin from head (scalp, temples and forehead) to soles of feet. Wash off after 8-14 hrs. One treatment should be adequate. Retreat if living mites present after 14 days.

HOW SUPPLIED: Cre: 5% [60g]

CONTRAINDICATIONS: Allergy to synthetic pyrethroid or pyrethrin.

WARNINGS/PRECAUTIONS: May temporarily exacerbate infection (eg pruritus, edema, erythema). Avoid eyes. D/C if hypersensitivity occurs.

ADVERSE REACTIONS: Burning, stinging, pruritus, erythema, numbness, tingling, rash.

PREGNANCY: Category B, not for use in nursing.

MECHANISM OF ACTION: Pyrethroid scabicidal agent; acts on the nerve cell membrane to disrupt the sodium channel current by which the polarization of the membrane is regulated. Results in depolarization and paralysis of pests. Active against a broad range of pests including lice, ticks, fleas, mites, and other arthropods.

PHARMACOKINETICS: Metabolism: Liver via ester hydrolysis. **Excretion:** Urine.

ACTIGALL   RX
ursodiol (Watson)

THERAPEUTIC CLASS: Bile acid

INDICATIONS: Treatment of radiolucent, noncalcified gallbladder stones <20mm in diameter in patients unable to undergo cholecystectomy. Prevention of gallstone formation in obese patients experiencing rapid weight loss.

DOSAGE: *Adults:* Treatment: 8-10mg/kg/day given bid-tid. Obtain ultrasound at 6 month intervals for 1 yr. Continue therapy after stones have dissolved and confirm with repeat ultrasound within 1-3 months. Prevention: 300mg bid.

HOW SUPPLIED: Cap: 300mg

CONTRAINDICATIONS: Calcified cholesterol stones, radiopaque stones, radiolucent bile pigment stones, unremitting acute cholecystitis, cholangitis, biliary obstruction, gallstone pancreatitis, biliary-gastrointestinal fistula, bile-acid hypersensitivity.

WARNINGS/PRECAUTIONS: Therapy is not associated with liver damage. Monitor LFTs at the initiation of therapy and periodically thereafter. Caution in elderly.

ADVERSE REACTIONS: Abdominal pain, constipation, diarrhea, dyspepsia, flatulence, nausea, arthralgia, coughing, viral infection, vomiting, bronchitis, pharyngitis, back pain, myalgia, headache, sinusitis, upper respiratory tract infection.

INTERACTIONS: Decreased absorption with bile acid sequestrants and aluminum based antacids. Estrogens, oral contraceptives, and clofibrate encourage gallstone formation.

PREGNANCY: Category B, caution in nursing.

MECHANISM OF ACTION: Bile acid; suppresses hepatic synthesis, cholesterol secretion, and inhibits intestinal cholesterol absorption; actions combine to change bile from cholesterol-precipitating to solubilizing, resulting in bile conducive to cholesterol stone dissolution.

PHARMACOKINETICS: Absorption: Small bowel (90%). **Metabolism:** Liver (1st pass, conjugation). **Elimination:** Feces.

ACTIQ   CII
fentanyl citrate (Cephalon)

> May cause life-threatening hypoventilation in opioid non-tolerant patients. Only for cancer pain in opioid tolerant patients with malignancies. Keep out of reach of children and discard properly. Concomitant use with moderate and strong CYP3A4 inhibitors may cause fatal respiratory depression.

THERAPEUTIC CLASS: Opioid analgesic

INDICATIONS: Management of breakthrough cancer pain in patients with malignancies who are already receiving and are tolerant to opioid therapy.

DOSAGE: *Adults:* Initial: 0.2mg (consume over 15 min). Titrate: Redose 15 min after previous dose is completed. No more than 2 units per breakthrough pain episode. May increase to next highest available strength if several breakthrough episodes (1-2 days) require more than 1 unit per pain episode. Repeat titration for each new dose. Max: 4 units/day. Prescribe 6 units with each new titration. The lozenge should be sucked, not chewed, and consumed over 15 min.
Pediatrics: ≥16 yrs: Initial: 0.2mg (consume over 15 min). Titrate: Redose 15 min after previous dose is completed. No more than 2 units per breakthrough pain episode. May increase to next highest available strength if several breakthrough episodes (1-2 days) require more than 1 unit per pain episode. Repeat titration for each new dose. Max: 4 units/day. Prescribe 6 units with each new titration. The lozenge should be sucked, not chewed, and consumed over 15 min.

HOW SUPPLIED: Loz: 0.2mg, 0.4mg, 0.6mg, 0.8mg, 1.2mg, 1.6mg

CONTRAINDICATIONS: Opioid non-tolerant patients and management of acute or postoperative pain.

WARNINGS/PRECAUTIONS: Caution with COPD, hepatic or renal dysfunction. Risk of clinically significant hypoventilation. Extreme caution with evidence of increased ICP or impaired consciousness. Can produce morphine-like dependence. Increased risk of dental decay; ensure proper oral hygiene. Caution with bradyarrhythmias, liver or kidney dysfunction. Patients on concomitant CNS depressants must be monitored for a change in opioid effects. May impair mental and/or physical status.

ADVERSE REACTIONS: Respiratory depression, circulatory depression, headache, hypotension, shock, nausea, vomiting, constipation, dizziness, dyspnea, anxiety, somnolence.

INTERACTIONS: Concomitant use with other CNS depressants, including opioids, sedatives, hypnotics, general anesthetics, phenothiazines, tranquilizers, skeletal muscle relaxants, sedating antihistamines, potent inhibitors of CYP3A4 (eg, erythromycin, ketoconazole, itraconazole, ritonavir, troleandomycin, clarithromycin, nelfinavir and nefazodone) or moderate inhibitors (eg, amprenavir, aprepitant, diltiazem, erythromycin, fluconazole, fosamprenavir, and verapamil) and alcohol may result in increased plasma concentrations. Avoid grapefruit juice. Avoid within 14 days of MAOIs.

PREGNANCY: Category C, not for use in nursing.

MECHANISM OF ACTION: Narcotic agonist analgesic: Principle therapeutic effect is analgesia. Not established. A μ-opioid receptor agonist. Specific CNS opioid receptors for endogenous compounds have been identified throughout brain and spinal cord and play a role in analgesic effects.

PHARMACOKINETICS: Absorption: Rapidly absorbed from buccal mucosa; slow absorption of swallowed fentanyl from GI tract. Absolute bioavailability (50%). C_{max}= 0.39-2.51ng/mL; T_{max}=20-40 min. **Distribution:** V_d=4L/kg; plasma protein binding (80-85%). Rapidly distributed to brain, heart, lungs, kidneys, spleen; slowly to muscles and fat. Readily crosses placenta; found in breast milk. . **Metabolism:** Liver, via CYP3A4; intestinal mucosa; norfentanyl (metabolite). **Elimination**: Urine (major), feces; $T_{1/2}$=7 hrs.

ACTIVASE   RX
alteplase (Genentech)

THERAPEUTIC CLASS: Thrombolytic agent

INDICATIONS: To improve ventricular function, reduce incidence of congestive heart failure, and reduce mortality with acute myocardial infarction (AMI). Management of acute ischemic stroke and acute massive pulmonary embolism (PE).

DOSAGE: *Adults:* AMI: Accelerated Infusion: >67kg: 15mg IV bolus, then 50mg over next 30 min, and then 35mg over next 60 min. ≤67kg: 15mg IV bolus, then 0.75mg/kg (max 50mg) over next 30 min, then 0.5mg/kg (max 35mg) over next 60 min. Max: 100mg total dose. 3-Hr Infusion: ≥65kg: 60mg in 1st hr (give 6-10mg as IV bolus), then 20mg over 2nd hr, then 20mg over 3rd hr. <65kg: 1.25mg/kg over 3 hrs as described above. Stroke: 0.9mg/kg IV over 1 hr (max 90mg total dose). Administer 10% of total dose as IV bolus over 1 min. PE: 100mg IV over 2 hrs. Start heparin at end or immediately after infusion when PTT or PT ≤2x normal.

HOW SUPPLIED: Inj: 50mg, 100mg

CONTRAINDICATIONS: (AMI, PE) Active internal bleeding, history of cerebrovascular accident (CVA), recent intracranial/intraspinal surgery or trauma, intracranial neoplasm, arteriovenous (AV) malformation, aneurysm, bleeding diathesis, severe uncontrolled HTN. (Stroke) Active internal bleeding, AV malformation, intracranial neoplasm or hemorrhage, aneurysm, bleeding diathesis, uncontrolled HTN, subarachnoid hemorrhage, seizure at stroke onset. Recent intracranial or intraspinal surgery, serious head trauma, previous stroke.

WARNINGS/PRECAUTIONS: Weigh benefits/risks with recent major surgery, cerebrovascular disease, recent GI or GU bleeding, recent trauma, HTN, left heart thrombus, acute pericarditis, subacute bacterial endocarditis, hemostatic defects, severe hepatic dysfunction, pregnancy, diabetic hemorrhagic retinopathy or other hemorrhagic ophthalmic conditions, septic thrombophlebitis or occluded AV cannula at a seriously infected site, elderly, any other bleeding condition that is difficult to manage. For stroke, also weigh benefits/risks with severe neurological deficit or major early infarct signs on CT. Cholesterol embolism and internal/superficial bleeding reported. Arrhythmias may occur with reperfusion. Avoid IM injection, noncompressible arterial puncture, and internal jugular or subclavian venous puncture. Caution with readministration.

ADVERSE REACTIONS: Bleeding.

INTERACTIONS: Increased risk of bleeding with heparin, vitamin K antagonists, drugs that alter platelets (eg, ASA, dipyridamole, abciximab) given before, during, or after alteplase therapy.

PREGNANCY: Category C, caution in nursing.

MECHANISM OF ACTION: Tissue plasminogen activator: has property of fibrin-enhanced conversion of plasminogen to plasmin. Produces limited conversion of plasminogen in absence of fibrin. Binds to fibrin in thrombus and converts entrapped plasminogen to plasmin. Initiates local fibrinolysis with limited systemic proteolysis.

PHARMACOKINETICS: Metabolism: Liver. **Elimination:** $T_{1/2}$=5 min (initial).

ACTIVELLA   RX
norethindrone - estradiol (Novo Nordisk)

> Estrogens and progestins, should not be used for the prevention of cardiovascular disease or dementia. Increased risks of MI, stroke, invasive breast cancer, PE, and DVT in postmenopausal women (50-79 yrs of age) reported. Increased risk of developing probable dementia in postmenopausal women ≥65 yrs of age reported.

THERAPEUTIC CLASS: Estrogen/progestogen combination

INDICATIONS: For women with intact uterus, treatment of moderate to severe vasomotor symptoms associated with menopause, vulvar/vaginal atrophy and prevention of postmenopausal osteoporosis

DOSAGE: *Adults:* 1 tab qd.

HOW SUPPLIED: Tab: (Estradiol-Norethindrone) 1mg-0.5mg, 0.5mg-1mg

CONTRAINDICATIONS: Pregnancy, breast cancer, abnormal genital bleeding, estrogen-dependent neoplasia, DVT, thromboembolic disorders, stroke, liver dysfunction or disease.

WARNINGS/PRECAUTIONS: Risk of gallbladder disease, endometrial and breast cancer, fetal congenital reproductive tract disorder, elevated BP, and hypercalcemia with breast cancer or bone metastases. Possible risk of cardiovascular disease. Increased risk of DVT, stroke, and PE; increased risk of endometrial, breast, and ovarian cancer with prolonged use. Risk of probable dementia-unknown risk in postmenopausal women under 65 years of age. Monitor for fluid retention with asthma, epilepsy, migraine, and cardiac/renal dysfunction. Avoid in post-menopausal women without a uterus. D/C if vision disturbances or thrombotic disorders occur. Caution with depression, DM, severe hypocalcemia. Acceleration of PT, PTT. Hypercoagulability effects. Impaired glucose tolerance. Increased triglycerides, fibrin/fibrinogen, and plasmin/plasminogen activity.

ADVERSE REACTIONS: Back pain, headache, nasopharyngitis, sinusitis, insomnia, upper respiratory tract infection, breast pain, postmenopausal bleeding/vaginal hemorrhage, endometrial thickening, uterine fibroid, pain in extremities, nausea, and diarrhea.

INTERACTIONS: CYP3A4 inducers (eg, St. John's wort, phenobarbital, carbamazepine, rifampin) may reduce estrogen levels. CYP3A4 inhibitors (eg, erythromycin, clarithromycin, ketoconazole, itraconazole, ritonavir, grapefruit juice) may increase estrogen levels.

PREGNANCY: Category X, caution in nursing.

MECHANISM OF ACTION: Estrogen/progestogen combination. Estradiol: Acts by binding to nuclear receptors in estrogen-responsive tissues and modulating pituitary secretion of gonadotropins, luteinizing hormone (LH), and follicle-stimulating hormone (FSH) through negative-feedback mechanism. Norethindrone: Exerts effect in target cells by binding to specific progesterone receptors that interact with progesterone-response elements in target genes. Responsible for enhancing cellular differentiation and opposing actions of estrogens by decreasing estrogen receptor levels, increasing local metabolism of estrogens to less active metabolites, and inducing gene products that blunt cellular responses to estrogen.

PHARMACOKINETICS: Absorption: Estradiol (E_2): Well-absorbed, T_{max}=5-8 hrs. Norethindrone (NET): Rapid. **Distribution:** Estrogens found in human breast milk. E_2: Sex-hormone-binding globulin (37%); albumin (61%); unbound (1-2%). NET: Sex-hormone-binding globulin (36%); albumin (61%). **Metabolism:** E_2: Liver to estrone, E_1 (metabolite); estriol (major urinary metabolite); enterohepatic recirculation via sulfate and glucuronide conjugation; biliary secretion of conjugates into the intestine, and hydrolysis in intestine; CYP3A4 (partial). NET: 5α-dihydro-norethindrone and tetrahydro-norethindrone (metabolites). **Elimination:** E_2: Urine; $T_{1/2}$=12-14 hrs. E_1: Urine; $T_{1/2}$=12-14 hrs; NET: $T_{1/2}$=8-11 hrs.

ACTONEL

risedronate sodium (Procter & Gamble)

RX

THERAPEUTIC CLASS: Bisphosphonate

INDICATIONS: Prevention and treatment of osteoporosis in postmenopausal women, glucocorticoid-induced osteoporosis in men and women. Increase bone mass in men with osteoporosis. Treatment of Paget's disease in men and women.

DOSAGE: *Adults:* Paget's Disease: 30mg qd for 2 months. May retreat after 2 months. Postmenopausal Osteoporosis Prevention/Treatment: 5mg qd or 35mg once weekly or 75mg on 2 consecutive days each month or 150mg once a month. Glucocorticoid-Induced Osteoporosis: 5mg qd. Increase Bone Mass in Men with Osteoporosis: 35mg once weekly. Take at least 30 min before the first food or drink of the day other than water. Swallow tab in upright position with 6-8 oz of plain water. Do not lie down for 30 min after dose.

HOW SUPPLIED: Tab: 5mg, 30mg, 35mg, 75mg, 150mg

CONTRAINDICATIONS: Hypocalcemia; inability to stand or sit upright for at least 30 min.

WARNINGS/PRECAUTIONS: May cause upper GI disorders (eg, dysphagia, esophagitis, esophageal or gastric ulcer). Treat hypocalcemia and other disturbances of bone and mineral metabolism before therapy. Give supplemental calcium and vitamin D if dietary intake is inadequate. Avoid with severe renal impairment (CrCl <30mL/min). Osteonecrosis, primarily in the jaw, has been reported. Postmarketing reports of severe and occasionally incapacitating bone, joint, and/or muscle pain, has been reported.

ADVERSE REACTIONS: Asthenia, diarrhea, abdominal pain, nausea, constipation, peripheral edema, arthralgia, leg cramps, headache, dizziness, sinusitis, rash, tinnitus.

INTERACTIONS: Calcium supplements and calcium-, aluminum-, and magnesium-containing agents may interfere with absorption; space doses.

PREGNANCY: Category C, not for use in nursing.

MECHANISM OF ACTION: Bisphosphonate; has an affinity for hydroxyapatite crystals in bone and acts as an antiresorptive agent. Inhibits osteoclast-mediated bone resorption and modulates bone metabolism.

PHARMACOKINETICS: Absorption: Relatively rapid; T_{max}=1 hr.; (30mg) absolute bioavailability (0.63%). **Distribution**: V_d=6.3L/kg, plasma protein binding (24%). **Elimination**: Urine, feces (unabsorbed dose); $T_{1/2}$=480 hrs.

ACTONEL WITH CALCIUM

risedronate sodium - calcium carbonate (Procter & Gamble)

RX

THERAPEUTIC CLASS: Bisphosphonate

INDICATIONS: Treatment and prevention of postmenopausal osteoporosis.

DOSAGE: *Adults:* Risedronate: 35mg once weekly (Day 1 of 7-day treatment cycle). Take at least 30 min before 1st food or drink of day other than water. Swallow tab in upright position with 6-8oz of plain water. Do not lie down for 30 min after dose. Calcium: 1250mg qd with food on each of remaining 6 days (Days 2-7 of the 7-day treatment cycle).

HOW SUPPLIED: Tab: (Risedronate Sodium) 35mg; Tab: (Calcium Carbonate) 1250mg

CONTRAINDICATIONS: (Risedronate) Hypocalcemia; inability to stand or sit upright for at least 30 min. (Calcium) Hypercalcemia from any cause (eg, hyperparathyroidism, hypercalcemia of malignancy, sarcoidosis).

WARNINGS/PRECAUTIONS: (Risedronate) May cause upper GI disorders (eg, dysphagia, esophagitis, esophageal or gastric ulcer). Treat hypocalcemia and other disturbances of bone and mineral metabolism before therapy. May cause osteonecrosis, primarily in jaw. Avoid with severe renal impairment

(CrCl <30mL/min). (Calcium) Should not be used to treat hypocalcemia. Daily intake above 2000mg has been associated with increased risk of adverse effects, including hypercalcemia and kidney stones. Patients with achlorhydria may have decreased absorption of calcium. Severe and occasionally incapacitating bone, joint, and/or muscle pain in patient taking bisphosphonates reported.

ADVERSE REACTIONS: Risedronate: Infection, pain, flu syndrome, abdominal pain, headache, asthenia, HTN, constipation, dyspepsia, nausea, arthralgia, nausea, diarrhea, dizziness, myalgia. Calcium: Constipation, flatulence, nausea, abdominal pain, and bloating.

INTERACTIONS: Risedronate: Calcium supplements, and calcium-, aluminum-, and magnesium-containing agents may interfere with absorption; space doses. Calcium: May reduce absorption of levothyroxine, fluoroquinolones, tetracycline. Calcium absorption reduced when taken with systemic glucocorticoids. Reduced urinary excretion of calcium with use of thiazide diuretics. Absorption of calcium increased with use of vitamin D and analogues. May interfere with absorption of iron. Take iron and calcium at different times of the day.

PREGNANCY: Category C, not for use in nursing.

MECHANISM OF ACTION: Risedronate: Bisphosphonate; inhibits osteoclast-mediated bone resorption and modulates bone metabolism. Calcium: Major substrate for mineralization, and has antiresorptive effect on bone. Suppresses PTH secretion and decreases bone turnover.

PHARMACOKINETICS: Absorption: Risedronate: Relatively rapid. T_{max}=1 hr; absolute bioavailability (30mg): (0.63%). **Distribution**: Risedronate: V_d=6.3L/kg, plasma protein binding (24%). Calcium: Plasma protein binding (40%). **Elimination**: Risedronate: Urine, feces (unabsorbed dose). $T_{1/2}$=480 hrs. Calcium: Renal, feces (unabsorbed dose).

ACTOPLUS MET   RX
pioglitazone HCL - metformin HCL (Takeda)

> Thiazolidinediones may cause or exacerbate CHF in some patients. Actoplus Met is not recommended in patients with symptomatic heart failure.

THERAPEUTIC CLASS: Thiazolidinedione/biguanide

INDICATIONS: Adjunct to diet and exercise, to improve glycemic control in type 2 diabetes mellitus in patients already treated with a combination of pioglitazone and metformin or whose diabetes is not adequately controlled with metformin alone, or for those patients who have initially responded to pioglitazone alone and require additional glycemic control.

DOSAGE: *Adults:* Individualize dose. Prior Pioglitazone/Metformin: Base on current regimen. Prior Metformin Monotherapy or Pioglitazone Monotherapy: Initial: 15mg-500mg or 15mg-850mg qd-bid. Titrate: Gradually increase after assessing adequacy of therapeutic response. Max: (Pioglitazone) 45mg, (Metformin) 2550mg. Elderly/Debilitated/Malnourished: Conservative dosing; do not titrate to max dose.

HOW SUPPLIED: Tab: (Pioglitazone-Metformin) 15mg-500mg, 15mg-850mg

CONTRAINDICATIONS: Established NYHA Class III or IV heart failure, renal disease or dysfunction (eg, SrCr ≥1.5mg/dL [males], ≥1.4mg/dL [females], or abnormal CrCl) and metabolic acidosis, including diabetic ketoacidosis. Temporarily d/c in patients undergoing radiologic studies involving intravascular iodinated contrast materials.

WARNINGS/PRECAUTIONS: (Metformin) Lactic acidosis reported (rare); increased risk with renal dysfunction, increased age, DM, CHF, and other conditions with risk of hypoperfusion and hypoxemia. Avoid in patients ≥80 yrs unless normal renal function. Monitor renal function and for ketoacidosis and metabolic acidosis. Avoid in renal/hepatic impairment. D/C in hypoxic states (eg, CHF, shock, acute MI), loss of blood glucose control due to stress (give insulin), acidosis, dehydration, sepsis. Temporarily d/c prior to surgery (due to restricted food intake) and procedures requiring IV iodinated contrast materials. May decrease serum B_{12} levels. Increased risk of hypoglycemia in elderly, debilitated/malnourished, adrenal or pituitary insufficiency, or alcohol intoxication. Monitor renal function. Alcohol known to potentiate effect of metformin on lactate metabolism. (Pioglitazone) May cause fluid retention and exacerbation/initiation of heart failure; d/c if cardiac status deteriorates. Avoid if NYHA Class III of IV cardiac status. Use lowest approved dose if systolic heart failure (NYHA Class II). Not for use in type 1 diabetes or for diabetic ketoacidosis treatment. Caution with edema. Dose-related weight gain reported. Ovulation in premenopausal anovulatory patients may occur; risk of pregnancy with inadequate contraception. May decrease Hgb and Hct. Avoid with active liver disease, if ALT levels >2.5x ULN. D/C if jaundice occurs or ALT >3x ULN on therapy. Macular edema reported.

ADVERSE REACTIONS: Upper respiratory tract infection, diarrhea, nausea, edema, headache, UTI, sinusitis, dizziness, weight increase, new onset or worsening diabetic macular edema.

INTERACTIONS: (Pioglitazone) Possible loss of contraception with ethinyl estradiol and norethindrone; caution when co-administering. Ketoconazole may inhibit pioglitazone metabolism; evaluate glycemic control more frequently. Risk for hypoglycemia with insulin or oral hypoglycemic agents. May cause reduction of midazolam levels. (Metformin) Furosemide, nifedipine, cimetidine, cationic drugs (eg, digoxin, amiloride, procainamide, quinidine, quinine, ranitidine, trimethoprim, vancomycin, triamterene, morphine) may increase metformin levels. Thiazides, other diuretics, corticosteroids, phenothiazines, thyroid products, estrogens, oral contraceptives, phenytoin, nicotinic acid, sympathomimetics, CCBs, or isoniazid may cause hyperglycemia. Risk of hypoglycemia with alcohol. Excess alcohol may increase potential for lactic acidosis. May decrease furosemide levels. An enzyme inhibitor of CYP2C8 (eg, gemfibrozil) may significantly increase AUC of pioglitazone and an enzyme inducer of CYP2C8 (eg, rifampin) may significantly decrease AUC of pioglitazone.

PREGNANCY: Category C, not for use in nursing.

MECHANISM OF ACTION: Pioglitazone: Thiazolidinedione; insulin sensitizing agent. Acts by enhancing peripheral glucose utilization. Metformin: Biguanide. Acts by decreasing endogenous hepatic glucose production.

PHARMACOKINETICS: Absorption: Pioglitazone: T_{max} =2-4 hrs; Metformin: Absolute bioavailability (50-60%), C_{max} =5µg/mL. **Distribution:** Pioglitazone: V_d =0.63L/kg, plasma protein binding (99%); Metformin: V_d =654L. **Metabolism:** Pioglitazone: Hydroxylation and oxidation (extensive); CYP450 2C8 and 3A4. Metformin: No hepatic metabolism. **Elimination:** Pioglitazone: Bile (unchanged), feces (metabolites), $T_{1/2}$ =3-7 hrs (pioglitazone), 16-24 hrs (total pioglitazone); Metformin: Urine (unchanged), $T_{1/2}$ =6.2 hrs.

ACTOS   RX
pioglitazone HCL (Takeda)

> Thiazolidinediones may cause or exacerbate CHF in some patients. Pioglitazone is not recommended in patients with symptomatic heart failure.

THERAPEUTIC CLASS: Thiazolidinedione

INDICATIONS: Adjunct to diet and exercise, to improve glycemic control in type 2 diabetes mellitus. May use in combination with a sulfonylurea, metformin, or insulin.

DOSAGE: *Adults:* Monotherapy: Initial: 15-30mg qd. Max: 45mg/day. Combination Therapy: Initial: 15-30mg qd. Max: 30mg/day. Decrease insulin dose by 10-25% if hypoglycemia occurs or if plasma glucose is <100mg/dL. Decrease sulfonylurea dose with hypoglycemia also.

HOW SUPPLIED: Tab: 15mg, 30mg, 45mg

CONTRAINDICATIONS: Established NYHA Class III or IV heart failure.

WARNINGS/PRECAUTIONS: May cause fluid retention and exacerbation/ initiation of heart failure; d/c if cardiac status deteriorates. Avoid if NYHA Class III or IV cardiac status. Use lowest approved dose if systolic heart failure

(NYHA Class II). Not for use in type 1 diabetes or for diabetic ketoacidosis treatment. Caution with edema. Dose-related weight gain reported. Ovulation in premenopausal anovulatory patients may occur; risk of pregnancy with inadequate contraception. May decrease Hgb and Hct. Avoid with active liver disease, if ALT levels >2.5x ULN, or if jaundice occurred with troglitazone. Check LFTs before therapy, every 2 months for 1 yr, and periodically thereafter, or if hepatic dysfunction symptoms occur. D/C if jaundice occurs or ALT >3x ULN on therapy. Macular edema reported. Increased incidence of bone fracture was noted in female patients.

ADVERSE REACTIONS: Upper respiratory tract infection, myalgia, tooth disorder, headache, sinusitis, pharyngitis, transient CPK level elevations, CHF, weight gain, aggravated DM, edema, dyspnea, new onset or worsening of diabetic macular edema.

INTERACTIONS: Possible loss of contraception with ethinyl estradiol and norethindrone; caution when co-administering. Ketoconazole may inhibit pioglitazone metabolism; evaluate glycemic control more frequently. Risk for hypoglycemia with insulin or oral hypoglycemic agents. May cause reduction of midazolam levels. An enzyme inhibitor of CYP2C8 (such as gemfibrozil) may significantly increase the AUC of pioglitazone and an enzyme inducer of CYP2C8 (such as rifampin) may significantly decrease the AUC of pioglitazone.

PREGNANCY: Category C, not for use in nursing.

MECHANISM OF ACTION: Thiazolidinedione, which decreases insulin resistance in the periphery and in the liver resulting in increased insulin-dependent glucose disposal and decreased hepatic glucose output.

PHARMACOKINETICS: Absorption: T_{max}= within 2 hrs (fasting), 3-4 hrs (with food). **Distribution:** V_d=0.63±0.41 L/kg. Plasma protein binding (>99%). **Metabolism:** Hydroxylation and oxidation; active metabolites: M-II and M-IV (hydroxy derivatives), M-III (keto derivative); CYP450 enzymes: 2C8, 3A4. **Elimination:** $T_{1/2}$=3-7 hrs (pioglitazone), 16-24 hrs (total pioglitazone). Bile (unchanged) and feces (metabolites).

ACULAR   RX
ketorolac tromethamine (Allergan)

THERAPEUTIC CLASS: NSAID

INDICATIONS: Ocular itching due to seasonal allergic conjunctivitis. Postoperative inflammation in cataract extraction.

DOSAGE: *Adults:* 1 drop qid. Post-op Inflammation: Begin 24 hrs post-op and continue for 2 weeks.
Pediatrics: ≥3 yrs: 1 drop qid. Post-op Inflammation: Begin 24 hrs post-op and continue for 2 weeks.

HOW SUPPLIED: Sol: 0.5% [3mL, 5mL, 10mL]

WARNINGS/PRECAUTIONS: May increase ocular tissue bleeding in conjunction with ocular surgery. Avoid use with contact lenses. D/C if corneal epithelium breakdown occurs. Caution in known bleeding tendencies, complicated ocular surgeries, corneal denervation, corneal epithelial defects, DM, ocular surface diseases (eg, dry eye syndrome), rheumatoid arthritis, or repeat ocular surgeries within a short period of time. Caution if used >24 hrs prior to surgery and use beyond 14 days post-surgery.

ADVERSE REACTIONS: Transient stinging/burning, superficial keratitis or infections, allergic reactions, ocular inflammation, corneal edema, iritis.

INTERACTIONS: Potential for cross-sensitivity to acetylsalicylic acid, phenylacetic acid derivatives, and other NSAIDs. Caution with agents that may prolong bleeding time. Increased potential for healing problems with topical steroids.

PREGNANCY: Category C, caution in nursing.

MECHANISM OF ACTION: NSAID; inhibits prostaglandin biosynthesis.

PHARMACOKINETICS: Absorption: C_{max} =95ng/mL; T_{max} =12hrs.

ADACEL

RX

diphtheria toxoid, reduced - pertussis vaccine acellular, adsorbed - tetanus toxoid (Sanofi Pasteur)

THERAPEUTIC CLASS: Vaccine

INDICATIONS: Active booster immunization against tetanus, diphtheria, and pertussis in persons 11-64 years of age.

DOSAGE: *Adults:* ≤64 yrs: 0.5mL IM (deltoid).
Pediatrics: ≥11 yrs: 0.5mL IM (deltoid).

HOW SUPPLIED: Inj: (Tetanus-Diphtheria-Pertussis) 5 LF- 2 LF-2.5mcg/0.5mL

CONTRAINDICATIONS: Encephalopathy not attributable to another identifiable cause within 7 days from initial vaccination. Progressive neurological disorder, uncontrolled epilepsy, or progressive encephalopathy.

WARNINGS/PRECAUTIONS: Evaluate risks/benefits of subsequent doses if temperature ≥105°F within 48 hrs not due to another identifiable cause; if collapse/shock occurs; persistent crying for ≥3 hrs within 48 hrs; and convulsions with or without fever within 3 days of vaccine. Continue with Td vaccine if pertussis must be withheld. Have epinephrine (1:1000) available. May not achieve expected immune response in immunosuppressed patients. Avoid injection into blood vessel. Should not be administered into the buttocks nor by the intradermal route.

ADVERSE REACTIONS: Injection site reactions, fever, headache, body aches, tiredness, chills, sore joints, nausea, lymph node swelling, diarrhea, and vomiting.

INTERACTIONS: Immunosuppressives (eg, irradiation, antimetabolites, alkylating agents, cytotoxic drugs, and corticosteroids) may reduce the immune response to vaccines.

PREGNANCY: Category C, caution in nursing

MECHANISM OF ACTION: Immunostimulant; elicits production of antibodies that may protect against tetanus, diphtheria, and pertussis.

ADALAT CC

RX

nifedipine (Schering)

OTHER BRAND NAMES: Afeditab CR (Watson)

THERAPEUTIC CLASS: Calcium channel blocker (dihydropyridine)

INDICATIONS: Treatment of hypertension.

DOSAGE: *Adults:* Initial: 30mg qd. Titrate over 7-14 days. Usual: 30-60mg qd. Max: 90mg/day. Take on empty stomach. Swallow tab whole.

HOW SUPPLIED: Tab, Extended-Release: (Adalat CC, Afeditab CR) 30mg, 60mg, (Adalat CC) 90mg

WARNINGS/PRECAUTIONS: May cause hypotension; monitor BP initially or with titration. May exacerbate angina from β-blocker withdrawal. CHF risk, especially with aortic stenosis or β-blockers. Peripheral edema reported. May increase angina or MI with severe obstructive CAD. Caution in elderly.

ADVERSE REACTIONS: Headache, flushing, heat sensation, dizziness, peripheral edema, fatigue, asthenia.

INTERACTIONS: β-blockers may increase risk of CHF, severe hypotension, or angina exacerbation. Possible hypotension with fentanyl. Monitor digoxin, quinidine, and coumarin levels. CYP3A4 inhibitors (eg, ketoconazole, erythromycin, protease inhibitors) may increase levels. Avoid grapefruit juice. Cimetidine may increase levels. CYP3A4 inducers (eg, phenytoin, St. John's wort) may decrease levels.

PREGNANCY: Category C, not for use in nursing.

MECHANISM OF ACTION: Calcium channel blocker; involved in peripheral arterial vasodilatation and consequently reduction in peripheral vascular resistance.

PHARMACOKINETICS: Absorption: Complete; Absolute bioavailability (84-89%); C_{max}=115ng/mL; T_{max}=2.5-5 hrs. **Distribution:** Plasma protein binding (92-98%); Found in breast milk. **Metabolism:** Liver (extensive). **Elimination:** $T_{1/2}$=7 hrs; Urine (60-80% as metabolite/unchanged), feces (metabolite).

ADDERALL
amphetamine salt combo (Shire)

`CII`

> High potential for abuse; avoid prolonged use. Misuse of amphetamine may cause sudden death and serious cardiovascular adverse events.

THERAPEUTIC CLASS: Sympathomimetic amine

INDICATIONS: Treatment of attention deficit disorder with hyperactivity (ADHD) and narcolepsy.

DOSAGE: *Adults:* Narcolepsy: Initial: 10mg/day. Titrate: May increase by 10mg/day every week. Usual: 5-60mg/day. Give 1st dose upon awakening, and additional doses q4-6h.
Pediatrics: ADHD: 3-5 yrs: Initial: 2.5mg qd. Titrate: May increase by 2.5mg weekly. ≥6 yrs: 5mg qd-bid. May increase by 5mg weekly. Max (usual): 40mg/day. Narcolepsy: 6-12 yrs: Initial: 5mg/day. May increase by 5mg weekly. ≥12 yrs: Initial: 10mg/day. Titrate: May increase by 10mg/day every week. Usual: 5-60mg/day. Give 1st dose upon awakening, and additional doses q4-6h.

HOW SUPPLIED: Tab: 5mg*, 7.5mg*, 10mg*, 12.5mg*, 15mg*, 20mg*, 30mg* *scored

CONTRAINDICATIONS: Advanced arteriosclerosis, symptomatic cardiovascular disease, moderate to severe HTN, hyperthyroidism, glaucoma, agitated states, history of drug abuse, during or within 14 days of MAOI use.

WARNINGS/PRECAUTIONS: May exacerbate symptoms of behavior disturbance and thought disorder in psychotic patients. Caution when using stimulants to treat patients with comorbid bipolar disorder because of concern for possible induction of mixed/manic episode in such patients. Stimulants at usual doses can cause treatment emergent psychotic or manic symptoms (eg, hallucinations, delusional thinking, mania) in children and adolescents without prior history of psychotic illness. Aggressive behavior or hostility reported in clinical trials and the postmarketing experience of some medications indicated for the treatment of ADHD. Monitor growth in children. May lower convulsive threshold; d/c in presence of seizures. Visual disturbances reported with stimulant treatment. May exacerbate Tourette's syndrome and phonic or motor tics. Caution with HTN and monitor BP. Interrupt occasionally to determine if patient requires continued therapy. Sudden death reported in children with structural cardiac abnormalities; avoid use in children or adults with structural cardiac abnormalities.

ADVERSE REACTIONS: HTN, tachycardia, palpitations, CNS overstimulation, dry mouth, GI disorders, anorexia, impotence, urticaria, rash, angioedema, anaphylaxis, Stevens-Johnson syndrome.

INTERACTIONS: GI acidifying agents (guanethidine, reserpine, glutamic acid, etc) and urinary acidifying agents (ammonium chloride, etc) decrease efficacy. MAOIs may cause hypertensive crisis. Potentiated by GI and urinary alkalinizers, propoxyphene overdose. Potentiated effects of both agents with TCAs. May delay absorption of phenytoin, ethosuximide, phenobarbital. Potentiates meperidine, norepinephrine, phenobarbital, phenytoin. Antagonized by haloperidol, chlorpromazine, lithium. Antagonizes adrenergic blockers, antihistamines, antihypertensives, veratrum alkaloids (antihypertensive). Avoid co-administration with alkalinizing agents (eg, antacids).

PREGNANCY: Category C, not for use in nursing.

MECHANISM OF ACTION: CNS stimulant; thought to block reuptake of nor-epinephrine and dopamine into presynaptic neuron and increase release of these monoamines into extraneuronal space.

PHARMACOKINETICS: Absorption: T_{max}=approximately 3 hrs (fasted). **Metabolism**: CYP2D6 (oxidation): 4-hydroxy-amphetamine and norephed-rine. **Elimination**: Urine, $T_{1/2}$=9.77-11 hrs (d-amphetamine), 11.5-13.8 hrs (l-amphetamine).

ADDERALL XR   CII
amphetamine salt combo (Shire)

> High potential for abuse; avoid prolonged use. Misuse of amphetamine may cause sudden death and serious cardiovascular adverse events.

THERAPEUTIC CLASS: Sympathomimetic amine

INDICATIONS: Treatment of attention deficit hyperactivity disorder (ADHD).

DOSAGE: *Adults:* Initial: 20mg qam. Currently Using Adderall: Switch to Adderall XR at the same total daily dose, taken once daily. Titrate at weekly intervals as needed. Swallow cap whole or open cap and sprinkle contents on applesauce; do not chew beads.
Pediatrics: ≥6 yrs: Initial: 10mg qam. Titrate: May increase weekly by 5-10mg/day. Max: 30mg/day. 13 to 17 yrs: Initial: 10mg/day. Titrate: May increase to 20mg/day after one week. Currently Using Adderall: Switch to Adderall XR at the same total daily dose, taken once daily. Titrate at weekly intervals as needed. Swallow cap whole or open cap and sprinkle contents on applesauce; do not chew beads.

HOW SUPPLIED: Cap, Extended-Release: 5mg, 10mg, 15mg, 20mg, 25mg, 30mg

CONTRAINDICATIONS: Advanced arteriosclerosis, symptomatic cardiovas-cular disease, moderate to severe HTN, hyperthyroidism, glaucoma, agitated states, history of drug abuse, during or within 14 days of MAOI use.

WARNINGS/PRECAUTIONS: May exacerbate symptoms of behavior distur-bance and thought disorder in psychotic patients. Caution when using stimu-lants to treat patients with comorbid bipolar disorder because of concern for possible induction of mixed/manic episode in such patients. Stimulants at usual doses can cause treatment emergent psychotic or manic symptoms (eg, hallucinations, delusional thinking, mania) in children and adolescents without prior history of psychotic illness. Aggressive behavior or hostility reported in clinical trials and postmarketing experience of some medications indicated for the treatment of ADHD. Monitor growth in children. May lower convulsive threshold; d/c in presence of seizures. Visual disturbances reported with stimulant treatment. May exacerbate Tourette's syndrome and phonic or mo-tor tics. Caution with HTN and monitor BP. Interrupt occasionally to determine if patient requires continued therapy. Sudden death reported in children with structural cardiac abnormalities; avoid use in children or adults with structural cardiac abnormalities. May decrease appetite.

ADVERSE REACTIONS: Abdominal pain, asthenia, fever, infection, viral infec-tion, loss of appetite, diarrhea, nausea, vomiting, emotional lability, insomnia, nervousness, weight loss, dry mouth, headache, urticaria, anaphylaxis.

INTERACTIONS: GI acidifying agents (guanethidine, reserpine, glutamic acid, etc) and urinary acidifying agents (ammonium chloride, etc) decrease efficacy. MAOIs may cause hypertensive crisis. Potentiated by GI and urinary alkalinizers, propoxyphene overdose. Potentiated effects of both agents with TCAs. May delay absorption of phenytoin, ethosuximide, phenobar-bital. Potentiates meperidine, norepinephrine, phenobarbital, phenytoin. Antagonized by haloperidol, chlorpromazine, lithium. Antagonizes adrenergic blockers, antihistamines, antihypertensives, veratrum alkaloids (antihyperten-sive). Avoid coadministration of alkalinizing agents (eg, antacid).

PREGNANCY: Category C, not for use in nursing.

MECHANISM OF ACTION: CNS stimulant; thought to block reuptake of nor-epinephrine and dopamine into presynaptic neuron and increase release of these monoamines into extraneuronal space.

ADENOCARD   RX
adenosine (Astellas)

THERAPEUTIC CLASS: Endogenous nucleoside

INDICATIONS: Conversion of paroxysmal supraventricular tachycardia (in-cluding Wolff-Parkinson-White syndrome) to sinus rhythm (SR).

DOSAGE: *Adults:* 6mg rapid IV bolus infusion over 1-2 sec. If not converted to SR within 1-2 min, give 12mg rapid IV bolus; may give 2nd 12mg dose if needed. Max: 12mg/dose.
Pediatrics: <50kg: 0.05-0.1mg/kg rapid IV bolus. If not converted to SR within 1-2 min, give additional bolus doses incrementally increasing amount by 0.05-0.1mg/kg. Follow each bolus with a saline flush. Continue process until SR or a maximum single dose of 0.3mg/kg is used. ≥50kg: 6mg rapid IV bolus infusion over 1-2 sec. If not converted to SR within 1-2 min, give 12mg rapid IV bolus; may give 2nd 12mg dose if needed. Max: 12mg/dose.

HOW SUPPLIED: Inj: 3mg/mL [2mL, 4mL]

CONTRAINDICATIONS: 2nd- or 3rd-degree AV block (except with pacemak-er), sinus node disease such as sick sinus syndrome or symptomatic bradycar-dia (except with pacemaker).

WARNINGS/PRECAUTIONS: May produce short-lasting heart block. Transient or prolonged asystole, respiratory alkalosis, ventricular fibrillation reported. Caution with obstructive lung disease (eg, emphysema, bronchitis). Avoid with bronchoconstriction/bronchospasm (eg, asthma). D/C if severe respiratory difficulties develop. New arrhythmias may appear on ECG at time of conver-sion. Caution in elderly.

ADVERSE REACTIONS: Facial flushing, dyspnea/SOB, chest pressure, nausea.

INTERACTIONS: Antagonized by methylxanthines (eg, theophylline, caffeine); may need larger adenosine dose. Potentiated by dipyridamole; use lower ad-enosine dose. Caution with digoxin, verapamil; ventricular fibrillation reported and potential for additive/synergistic depressant effects on SA and AV nodes. Possible higher degrees of heart block with carbamazepine.

PREGNANCY: Category C, safety in nursing not known.

MECHANISM OF ACTION: Endogenous nucleoside; slows conduction time through A-V node, can interrupt reentry pathways through the A-V node, and can restore normal sinus rhythm in patients with paroxysmal supraventricular tachycardia associated with Wolff-Parkinson-White syndrome.

PHARMACOKINETICS: Metabolism: Rapid (intracellular), through phosphory-lation and deamination. **Elimination:** $T_{1/2}$ <10 seconds.

ADENOSCAN   RX
adenosine (Astellas)

THERAPEUTIC CLASS: Vasodilator

INDICATIONS: Adjunct to thalium-201 myocardial perfusion scintigraphy in patients unable to exercise adequately.

DOSAGE: *Adults:* 140mcg/kg/min IV for 6 min (total dose 0.84mg/kg). Inject thallium-201 at midpoint of infusion.

HOW SUPPLIED: Inj: 3mg/mL

CONTRAINDICATIONS: 2nd-or 3rd-degree AV block (except with a pacemak-er), sinus node disease, bronchosconstrictive or bronchospastic lung disease.

WARNINGS/PRECAUTIONS: Fatal cardiac arrest, sustained ventricular tachy-cardia, MI reported. Exerts depressant effect on SA and AV nodes and may cause 1st-, 2nd-, 3rd-degree AV block or sinus bradycardia. May precipitate significant hypotension. Caution with autonomic dysfunction, stenotic valvular heart disease, pericarditis, stenotic carotid artery disease with CVA, uncorrected hypovolemia. Increase in BP reported. May cause bronchoconstriction in asthmatics.

ADVERSE REACTIONS: Flushing, chest discomfort, dyspnea, headache, throat, neck or jaw discomfort, GI disturbances, dizziness, ST segment depression, 1st and 2nd degree AV block, paresthesia, hypotension, nervousness, arrhythmia.

INTERACTIONS: Potential synergistic effects with other cardioactive drugs (eg, β-blockers, cardiac glycosides, and CCBs). Diminished effects with adenosine receptor antagonists (eg, theophylline, caffeine). Withold drugs that may inhibit or augment effects for at least 5 half-lives.

PREGNANCY: Category C, safety in nursing not known.

MECHANISM OF ACTION: Endogenous nucleoside: mechanism not established. Suspected to activate purine receptors, inhibiting slow inward calcium current, reducing calcium uptake and activating adenylate cyclase through A_2 receptors in smooth muscle cells; decreasing vascular tone by modulating sympathetic neurotransmission.

PHARMACOKINETICS: Metabolism: Phosphorylation, via adenosine kinase (adenosine monophosphate); Deamination, via adenosine deaminase (inosine).

ADIPEX-P
phentermine HCL (Gate)

THERAPEUTIC CLASS: Anorectic sympathomimetic amine

INDICATIONS: Short-term adjunct for exogenous obesity if initial BMI ≥30kg/m² or ≥27kg/m² with other risk factors (eg, HTN, diabetes, hyperlipidemia).

DOSAGE: *Adults:* Usual: 37.5mg before breakfast or 1-2 hrs after breakfast. Alternate Schedule: 18.75mg qd-bid. Avoid late evening dosing. *Pediatrics:* >16 yrs: Usual: 37.5mg before breakfast or 1-2 hrs after breakfast. Alternate Schedule: 18.75mg qd-bid. Avoid late evening dosing.

HOW SUPPLIED: Cap: 37.5mg; Tab: 37.5mg* *scored

CONTRAINDICATIONS: Advanced arteriosclerosis, cardiovascular disease, moderate to severe HTN, hyperthyroidism, glaucoma, agitated states, history of drug abuse, within 14 days of MAOI use.

WARNINGS/PRECAUTIONS: Only for short-term therapy. Primary pulmonary HTN and valvular heart disease reported. Abuse potential. Caution with mild HTN. Tolerance may develop.

ADVERSE REACTIONS: Primary pulmonary hypertension, regurgitant valvular heart disease, palpitation, tachycardia, BP elevation, CNS overstimulation, dry mouth, impotence, urticaria.

INTERACTIONS: May alter insulin requirements. Avoid alcohol and other weight loss products including SSRIs. Valvular heart disease and primary pulmonary hypertension reported with fenfluramine and dexfenfluramine. May decrease effects of guanethidine.

PREGNANCY: Category C, not for use in nursing.

MECHANISM OF ACTION: Anorectic sympathomimetic amine; not established as appetite suppressor; causes CNS stimulation and elevation of BP.

ADVAIR
salmeterol xinafoate - fluticasone propionate (GlaxoSmithKline)

RX

Long-acting β₂-adrenergic agonists, such as salmeterol, may increase risk of asthma-related deaths. Use of diskus should be reserved for patients not adequately controlled on other medications or whose disease severity warrants initiation with 2 maintenance therapies.

THERAPEUTIC CLASS: Corticosteroid/beta$_2$ agonist

INDICATIONS: Long-term, maintenance treatment of asthma in patients ≥4 yrs. (250/50 only): Maintenance treatment of airflow obstruction in patients with COPD, including chronic bronchitis and/or emphysema; to reduce exacerbations of COPD in patients with history of exacerbations.

DOSAGE: *Adults:* Asthma: 1 inh q12h. Without Prior Inhaled Corticosteroid (CS) Therapy/Inadequate Control on Current Inhaled CS: Initial: 100/50 or 250/50 bid. Max: 500/50 bid. If no response within 2 weeks, may increase to higher strength. COPD: (250/50 only): 1 inh q12h. Rinse mouth after use. *Pediatrics:* ≥12 yrs: Asthma: 1 inh q12h. Without Prior Inhaled Corticosteroid (CS)Therapy/Inadequate Control on Current Inhaled CS: Initial: 100/50 or 250/50 bid. Max: 500/50 bid. If no response within 2 weeks, may increase to higher strength. (100/50 only): 4-11 yrs: Symptomatic on Inhaled CS: 1 inh q12h. Rinse mouth after use.

HOW SUPPLIED: Disk (Inhalation): (Fluticasone-Salmeterol) (100/50) 0.1mg-0.05mg/inh, (250/50) 0.25mg-0.05mg/inh, (500/50) 0.5mg-0.05mg/inh [60 blisters]

CONTRAINDICATIONS: Status asthmaticus, other acute asthma or COPD episodes, and hypersensitivity to milk proteins.

WARNINGS/PRECAUTIONS: Deaths due to adrenal insufficiency have occurred with transfer from systemic corticosteroids to inhaled corticosteroids. Resume oral corticosteroids during stress or severe asthma attack. Observe for adrenal insufficiency, systemic corticosteroid withdrawal effects, hypercorticism, reduction in growth velocity (pediatrics). More susceptible to infection. Not for acute bronchospasm. D/C if bronchospasm occurs after dosing. Caution with TB; untreated systemic fungal, bacterial, viral, or parasitic infections; or ocular herpes simplex. *Candida* infection of mouth and pharynx, glaucoma, hypersensitivity reactions, increased IOP, cataracts reported. Monitor for increasing use of β$_2$ agonists. QTc interval prolongation reported with large doses. D/C if paradoxical bronchospasm occurs. Caution with cardiovascular or CNS disorders, convulsive disorders, thyrotoxicosis, DM, and keto-acidosis. May produce hypokalemia, hyperglycemia, and eosinophilic conditions.

ADVERSE REACTIONS: Upper respiratory tract inflammation, pharyngitis, sinusitis, cough, hoarseness, headaches, GI effects, musculoskeletal pain, palpitations.

INTERACTIONS: Extreme caution with TCAs or MAOIs during or within 14 days of use. Antagonized by β-blockers. Caution with non-potassium sparing diuretics; ECG changes, hypokalemia may develop. Concomitant use with strong CYP3A4 inhibitors (eg, ritonavir, atazanavir, indinavir, ketoconazole) is not recommended .

PREGNANCY: Category C, caution in nursing.

MECHANISM OF ACTION: Fluticasone: Corticosteroid with anti-inflammatory activity; inihibits multiple cell types (eg, mast cells, eosinophils, neutrophils, macrophages, lymphocytes) and mediators (eg, histamine, eicosanoids, leukotrienes and cytokines) involved in inflammation and asthmatic response. Salmeterol: Long-acting β$_2$-adrenergic agonist; stimulates intracellular adenyl cyclase, which catalyzes conversion of ATP to cAMP, producing relaxation of bronchial smooth muscle and inhibition of release of immediate hypersensitivity mediators from cells (eg, mast cells).

PHARMACOKINETICS: Absorption: Fluticasone: (Asthma, 500 bid) C_{max}=110pg/mL, (COPD, 250 bid) 53pg/mL. Salmeterol: C_{max}=167pg/mL, T_{max}=20 min. **Distribution:** Fluticasone: V_d=4.2L/kg; plasma protein binding (91%). Salmeterol: Plasma protein binding (96%). **Metabolism:** Fluticasone: Liver via CYP3A4. Salmeterol: Liver, via CYP3A4 to α-hydroxysalmeterol (metabolite). **Elimination:** Urine, feces; Fluticasone: $T_{1/2}$=7.8 hrs. Salmeterol: $T_{1/2}$=5.5 hrs.

ADVAIR HFA   RX
salmeterol xinafoate - fluticasone propionate (GlaxoSmithKline)

> Long-acting β₂-adrenergic agonists, such as salmeterol, may increase risk of asthma-related deaths.

THERAPEUTIC CLASS: Corticosteroid/beta₂ agonist

INDICATIONS: For long-term, maintenance treatment of asthma.

DOSAGE: *Adults:* Asthma: 2 inh q12h. Without Prior Inhaled Corticosteroid (CS): Initial: 2 inh of 45/21 bid or 1 inh of 115/21 bid. Max: 2 inh of 230/21 bid. Current Inhaled CS: Beclomethasone: ≤160mcg/day use 2 inh of 45/21 bid, 320mcg/day use 2 inh of 115/21 bid, 640mcg/day use 2 inh of 230/21 bid. Budesonide: ≤400mcg/day use 2 inh of 45/21 bid, 800-1200mcg/day use 2 inh of 115/21 bid, 1600mcg/day use 2 inh of 230/21 bid. Flunisolide: ≤1000mcg/day use 2 inh of 45/21 bid, 1250-2000mcg/day use 2 inh of 115/21 bid. Flunisolide HFA: ≤320mcg/day use 2 inh of 45/21 bid, 640mcg/day use 2 inh of 115/21 bid. Fluticasone Aerosol: ≤176mcg/day use 2 inh of 45/21 bid, 440mcg/day use 2 inh of 115/21 bid, 660-880mcg/day use 2 inh of 230/21 bid. Fluticasone Powder: ≤200mcg/day use 2 inh of 45/21 bid, 500mcg/day use 2 inh of 115/21 bid, 1000mcg/day use 2 inh of 230/21 bid. Mometasone Powder: 220mcg/day use 2 inh of 45/21 bid, 440mcg/day use 2 inh of 115/21 bid, 880mcg/day use 2 inh of 230/21 bid. Triamcinolone: ≤1000mcg/day use 2 inh of 45/21 bid, 1100-1600mcg/day use 2 inh of 115/21 bid. If no response within 2 weeks, increase to higher strength.

Pediatrics: ≥12 yrs: Asthma: 2 inh q12h. Without Prior Inhaled Corticosteroid (CS): Initial: 2 inh of 45/21 bid or 1 inh of 115/21 bid. Max: 2 inh of 230-21 bid. Current Inhaled CS: Beclomethasone: ≤160mcg/day use 2 inh of 45/21 bid, 320mcg/day use 2 inh of 115/21 bid, 640mcg/day use 2 inh of 230/21 bid. Budesonide: ≤400mcg/day use 2 inh of 45/21 bid, 800-1200mcg/day use 2 inh of 115/21 bid, 1600mcg/day use 2 inh of 230/21 bid. Flunisolide: ≤1000mcg/day use 2 inh of 45/21 bid, 1250-2000mcg/day use 2 inh of 115/21 bid. Flunisolide HFA: ≤320mcg/day use 2 inh of 45/21 bid, 640mcg/day use 2 inh of 115/21 bid. Fluticasone Aerosol: ≤176mcg/day use 2 inh of 45/21 bid, 440mcg/day use 2 inh of 115/21 bid, 660-880mcg/day use 2 inh of 230/21 bid. Fluticasone Powder: ≤200mcg/day use 2 inh of 45/21 bid, 500mcg/day use 2 inh of 115/21 bid, 1000mcg/day use 2 inh of 230/21 bid. Mometasone powder: 220mcg/day use 2 inh of 45/21 bid, 440mcg/day use 2 inh of 115/21 bid, 880mcg/day use 2 inh of 230/21 bid. Triamcinolone: ≤1000mcg/day use 2 inh of 45/21 bid, 1100-1600mcg/day use 2 inh of 115/21 bid. If no response within 2 weeks, increase to higher strength.

HOW SUPPLIED: MDI: (Fluticasone-Salmeterol) (45/21) 0.045mg-0.021mg/inh, (115/21) 0.115mg-0.021mg/inh, (230/21) 0.230mg-0.021mg/inh [120 inhalations]

CONTRAINDICATIONS: Status asthmaticus or other acute asthma.

WARNINGS/PRECAUTIONS: See Contraindications. Deaths due to adrenal insufficiency have occurred with transfer from systemic corticosteroids to inhaled corticosteroids. Resume oral corticosteroids during stress or severe asthma attack. Observe for adrenal insufficiency, systemic corticosteroid withdrawal effects, hypercorticism, reduction in growth velocity (pediatrics). More susceptible to infection. Not for acute bronchospasm. D/C if bronchospasm occurs after dosing. Caution with TB; untreated systemic fungal, bacterial, viral, or parasitic infections; or ocular herpes simplex. *Candida* infection of mouth and pharynx, glaucoma, hypersensitivity reactions, increased IOP, cataracts reported. Monitor for increasing use of β₂ agonists. QTc interval prolongation reported with large doses. D/C if paradoxical bronchospasm occurs. Caution with cardiovascular disorders.

ADVERSE REACTIONS: Upper respiratory tract infection, throat irritation, upper respiratory tract inflammation, headaches, nausea, vomiting, musculoskeletal pain, menstruation symptoms.

INTERACTIONS: Extreme caution with TCAs or MAOIs during or within 14 days of use. Antagonized by β-blockers. Caution with non-potassium sparing diuretics; ECG changes, hypokalemia may develop. Potentiated by ketoconazole, other CYP3A4 inhibitors.

PREGNANCY: Category C, caution in nursing.

MECHANISM OF ACTION: Fluticasone: Corticosteroid with anti-inflammatory activity. Inihibits multiple cell types (eg, mast cells, eosinophils, neutrophils, macrophages, lymphocytes) and mediators (eg, histamine, eicosanoids, leukotrienes and cytokines) involved in inflammation and asthmatic response. Salmeterol: β_2-adrenergic agonist; stimulates intracellular adenyl cyclase, which catalyzes conversion of ATP to cAMP, producing relaxation of bronchial smooth muscle and inhibition of release of immediate hypersensitivity mediators from cells (eg, mast cells).

PHARMACOKINETICS: Absorption: Salmeterol: C_{max}=150pg/mL. **Distribution**: Fluticasone: V_d=4.2 L/kg; plasma protein binding (99%). Salmeterol: Plasma protein binding (96%). **Metabolism**: Fluticasone: Liver, via CYP3A4. Salmeterol: Extensive by hydroxylation. **Elimination**: Fluticasone: Feces (major), urine (<5%); $T_{1/2}$=7.8 hrs. Salmeterol: Feces (60%), urine (25%); $T_{1/2}$=5.5 hrs.

ADVICOR   RX
lovastatin - niacin (Abbott)

THERAPEUTIC CLASS: B-complex vitamin/HMG-CoA reductase inhibitor

INDICATIONS: Treatment of hypercholesterolemia when use of both Niaspan® (niacin ER) and lovastatin is appropriate. (Niacin ER) Treatment of primary hypercholesterolemia and mixed dyslipidemia, hypertriglyceridemia, and secondary prevention of cardiovascular events. (Lovastatin) Treatment of primary hypercholesterolemia, primary and secondary prevention of cardiovascular events. See individual labeling for further details.

DOSAGE: *Adults:* ≥18 yrs: Initial: 500mg-20mg qhs. Titrate: Increase by no more than 500mg of niacin every 4 weeks. Max: 2000mg-40mg. Concomitant Cyclosporine/Danazol: Max Lovastatin: 20mg/day. Concomitant Amiodarone/Verapamil: Max Lovastatin: 40mg/day. Swallow tab whole. Take with low-fat snack. Pretreat 30 min prior with ASA to reduce flushing.

HOW SUPPLIED: Tab: (Extended-Release Niacin-Lovastatin) 500mg-20mg, 750mg-20mg, 1000mg-20mg, 1000mg-40mg

CONTRAINDICATIONS: Active liver disease, unexplained persistent elevations in serum transaminases, active PUD, arterial bleeding, pregnancy, nursing mothers.

WARNINGS/PRECAUTIONS: Do not substitute for equivalent dose of immediate-release niacin. Myopathy, rhabdomyolysis, severe hepatotoxicity reported. Caution with history of liver disease or jaundice, heavy alcohol use, hepatobilliary disease, peptic ulcer, diabetes, unstable angina, acute phase of MI, gout, renal dysfunction. Monitor LFTs prior to therapy, every 6-12 weeks for 1st 6 months, and periodically thereafter. May elevate PT, uric acid levels. D/C if AST or ALT ≥3x ULN persist, if myopathy diagnosed or suspected, and a few days before surgery. May reduce phosphorous levels. May disrupt therapy during a course of treatment with systemic antifungal azole, a macrolide antibiotic or ketolide antibiotic.

ADVERSE REACTIONS: Flushing, asthenia, flu syndrome, headache, infection, pain, GI effects, hyperglycemia, myalgia, pruritus, rash.

INTERACTIONS: May potentiate ganglionic blockers, vasoactive drugs. Decreased niacin clearance with ASA. Separate bile acid sequestrants by 4-6 hrs. Avoid concomitant alcohol and hot drinks; may increase flushing and pruritus. Antidiabetic agents may need adjustment. Caution with niacin-containing nutritional supplements. Increased risk of skeletal muscle disorders with CYP3A4 inhibitors (eg, cyclosporine, itraconazole, ketoconazole, erythromycin, clarithromycin, telithromycin, protease inhibitors, nefazodone, >1 quart/day of grapefruit juice), verapamil, fibrates (eg, gemfibrozil). Monitor warfarin. Caution with drugs that diminish levels or activity of steroid hormones (eg, ketoconazole, spironolactone, cimetidine). Caution with acute MI and nitrates, CCBs, and adrenergic blockers.

PREGNANCY: Category X, not for use in nursing.

MECHANISM OF ACTION: Niacin: Vitamin B complex; not completely understood and may include various actions, including partial inhibition of free fatty acids from adipose tissue and increased lipoprotein lipase activity. Decreases hepatic synthesis rate of VLDL-C and LDL-C. Lovastatin: Inhibits HMG-CoA reductase enzyme, which is needed for conversion of HMG-CoA to mevalonate. Has LDL-lowering effect by involving both reduction of VLDL-C concentration and induction of the LDL receptor, leading to reduction of production and/or increased catabolism of LDL-C.

PHARMACOKINETICS: Absorption: Niacin: C_{max}=18mcg/mL, T_{max}=5 hrs. Lovastatin: Incomplete, C_{max}=11ng/mL, T_{max}=2 hrs. **Distribution:** Niacin: serum protein binding (20%), found in breast milk. Lovastatin: plasma protein binding (95%), crosses blood-brain/placental barrier. **Metabolism:** Niacin: rapid and extensive. Through conjugation pathway. Lovastatin: liver (extensive) via CYP3A4. Lovastatin acid, 6'-hydroxy (active metabolites). **Elimination:** Niacin: urine (60%). $T_{1/2}$=20-48 min. Lovastatin: urine, bile. $T_{1/2}$=4.5 hrs, urine (10%), feces (83%).

AEROBID   RX
flunisolide (Forest)

OTHER BRAND NAMES: Aerobid-M (with menthol) (Forest)

THERAPEUTIC CLASS: Corticosteroid

INDICATIONS: Maintenance treatment of asthma as prophylactic therapy in patients ≥6 years and to reduce or eliminate the need for oral systemic corticosteroidal therapy.

DOSAGE: *Adults:* Initial: 2 inh bid. Max: 4 inh bid. Rinse mouth after use. *Pediatrics:* 6-15 yrs: 2 inh bid. Rinse mouth after use.

HOW SUPPLIED: MDI: 0.25mg/inh [7g]

CONTRAINDICATIONS: Primary treatment of status asthmaticus or other acute asthma attacks.

WARNINGS/PRECAUTIONS: Deaths due to adrenal insufficiency have occurred with transfer from systemic corticosteroids to inhaled corticosteroids. Resume oral corticosteroids during stress or severe asthma attack. Observe for adrenal insufficiency, systemic corticosteroid withdrawal effects, and growth suppression (children). More susceptible to infections. Not for acute bronchospasm. D/C if bronchospasm occurs after dosing. Caution with tuberculosis of the respiratory tract; untreated systemic fungal, bacterial, viral, or parasitic infections; or ocular herpes simplex. *Candida* infection of the mouth and pharynx reported.

ADVERSE REACTIONS: Upper respiratory infection, diarrhea, stomach upset, cold symptoms, nasal congestion, headache, nausea, vomiting, sore throat, unpleasant taste.

PREGNANCY: Category C, caution with nursing.

MECHANISM OF ACTION: Corticosteroid; demonstrated marked anti-inflammatory and anti-allergic activity in test systems.

PHARMACOKINETICS: Metabolism: Liver (1st pass). Metabolite (6β-OH). **Elimination:** $T_{1/2}$=1.8 hrs.

AFLURIA   RX
influenza virus vaccine (CSL Biotherapies)

THERAPEUTIC CLASS: Vaccine

INDICATIONS: Active immunization of individuals ≥18 yrs against influenza disease caused by influenza virus subtypes A and type B contained in the vaccine.

DOSAGE: Adults: ≥18 yrs: 0.5mL IM in deltoid region of upper arm.

HOW SUPPLIED: Inj: 0.5mL [10 syringes], MDV: 5mL [10 doses]

CONTRAINDICATIONS: Hypersensitivity to eggs or chicken protein, neomycin, or polymyxin, or life-threatening reaction to previous influenza vaccination.

WARNINGS/PRECAUTIONS: Caution if Guillain-Barre syndrome has occurred within 6 weeks of previous influenza vaccination. Caution in immunocompromised and those receiving immunosuppressive therapy. Have medical treatment and supervision to manage possible anaphylactic reaction. May not protect all individuals.

ADVERSE REACTIONS: Local: tenderness, pain, redness, swelling, bruising. Systemic: headache, malaise, muscle aches, nausea, chills/shivering.

INTERACTIONS: Do not mix with any other vaccine in the same syringe or vial. Administer at different injection sites if given at the same time as another injectable vaccine. Immunosuppressive therapies may diminish immune response.

PREGNANCY: Category C, caution in nursing.

MECHANISM OF ACTION: Stimulates the immune system to elicit an immune response that produces antibodies that may protect against influenza disease.

AGGRASTAT   RX
tirofiban HCL (Medicure)

THERAPEUTIC CLASS: Glycoprotein IIb/IIIa inhibitor

INDICATIONS: In combination with heparin, for treatment of acute coronary syndrome, in patients being medically managed or undergoing PTCA or atherectomy.

DOSAGE: *Adults:* Initial: 0.4mcg/kg/min IV for 30 min. Maint: 0.1mcg/kg/min IV. Continue through angiography and for 12-24 hrs after angioplasty or atherectomy. CrCl <30mL/min: Administer at half of usual rate of infusion.

HOW SUPPLIED: Inj: 0.05mg/mL, 0.25mg/mL

CONTRAINDICATIONS: Active internal bleeding, acute pericarditis, severe HTN, concomitant parenteral GP IIb/IIIa inhibitor, hemorrhagic stroke, aortic dissection, thrombocytopenia with prior exposure. Bleeding diathesis, stroke, major surgical procedure, or severe physical trauma within past 30 days. History of intracranial hemorrhage or neoplasm, arteriovenous malformation, aneurysm.

WARNINGS/PRECAUTIONS: Bleeding reported. Monitor platelets, Hgb, Hct before treatment, within 6 hrs after loading infusion, and daily during therapy. Monitor platelets earlier if previous GP IIb/IIIa inhibitor use. Determine APTT before and during therapy with heparin. Caution with platelets <150,000/mm^3, hemorrhagic retinopathy, chronic hemodialysis patients, femoral access site in percutaneous coronary intervention. Minimize vascular and other trauma. D/C if thrombocytopenia confirmed or if bleeding cannot be controlled by pressure.

ADVERSE REACTIONS: Bleeding, nausea, fever, headache, edema, anaphylaxis.

INTERACTIONS: Avoid other parenteral GP IIb/IIIa inhibitors. Increased bleeding with heparin and ASA. Caution with other drugs that affect hemostasis (eg, warfarin). Increased clearance with levothyroxine, omeprazole.

PREGNANCY: Category B, not for use in nursing.

MECHANISM OF ACTION: Glycoprotein IIB/IIIa inhibitor; reversible antagonist of fibrinogen binding to the GP IIb/IIIa receptor, the major platelet surface receptor involved in platelet aggregation. Inhibits platelet aggregation.

PHARMACOKINETICS: Absorption: C_{max}=0.01-25mcg/mL. **Distribution**: V_d=22-43L; Plasma protein bound (35%). **Metabolism:** Limited **Elimination**: Urine (65%), feces (25%); $T_{1/2}$=2 hrs.

AGGRENOX   RX
dipyridamole - aspirin (Boehringer Ingelheim)

THERAPEUTIC CLASS: Platelet aggregation inhibitor

INDICATIONS: Reduce risk of stroke in patients with transient brain ischemia or complete ischemic stroke due to thrombosis.

DOSAGE: *Adults:* 1 cap bid (am and pm).

HOW SUPPLIED: Cap: (Dipyridamole Extended-Release/ASA) 200mg-25mg

CONTRAINDICATIONS: NSAID allergy, children or teenagers with viral infections, syndrome of asthma, rhinitis, nasal polyps.

WARNINGS/PRECAUTIONS: Increased risk of bleeding with chronic, heavy alcohol use. Caution with inherited or acquired bleeding disorders, severe CAD, and hypotension. Monitor for signs of GI ulcers and bleeding. Avoid with history of peptic ulcer disease, severe renal failure (CrCl <10mL/min). Risk of hepatic dysfunction. Not interchangeable with individual components of ASA and Persantine tabs. Avoid in 3rd trimester of pregnancy.

ADVERSE REACTIONS: Headache, dyspepsia, abdominal pain, nausea, diarrhea, vomiting, fatigue, arthralgia, pain, hemorrhage.

INTERACTIONS: May decrease effects of ACE inhibitors, cholinesterase inhibitors, phenytoin, β-blockers. Potentiates adenosine, acetazolamide, methotrexate, oral hypoglycemics, valproic acid. Anticoagulants increase risk of bleeding. Decreased effects of diuretics in renal or cardiovascular disease. NSAIDs may increase risk of bleeding and decrease renal function. May antagonize uricosuric agents.

PREGNANCY: Category D, caution in nursing.

MECHANISM OF ACTION: Dipyridamole; platelet aggregation inhibitor. Inhibits uptake of adenosine into platelets, endothelial cells, and erythrocytes. Leads to increase in adenosine, which acts on platelet A_2-receptor to stimulate platelet adenylate cyclase and increase platelet cyclic-3',5'-adenosine monophosphate (cAMP) levels. Platelet aggregation is then inhibited in response to stimuli such as platelet activation factor (PAF), collagen, and adenosine diphosphate (ADP). Also responsible for inhibiting phosphodiesterase (PDE). Weakly inhibits cAMP-PDE. Therapeutic levels of dipyridamole inhibit cyclic-3',5'-guanosine monophosphate-PDE (cGMP-PDE), which helps to augment the increases in cGMP that are produced by endothelium-derived relaxing factor (EDRF). ASA: platelet aggregation inhibitor. Irreversibly inhibits platelet cyclooxygenase. Leads to inhibition in the generation of thromboxane A_2, a powerful inducer of platelet aggregation and vasoconstriction.

PHARMACOKINETICS: Absorption: Dipyridamole: C_{max}=1.98mcg/mL; T_{max}=2 hrs. ASA: C_{max}=319ng/mL; T_{max}=0.63 hrs. **Distribution:** Dipyridamole/ASA found in human breast milk. Dipyridamole: Plasma protein binding (99%); V_d=92L. ASA: Plasma protein binding (poor); V_d=10 L; salicyclic acid (ASA metabolite): highly protein bound (concentration dependent). **Metabolism:** Dipyridamole: Liver (conjugation); monoglucuronide (metabolite) (low activity). ASA: Liver (conjugation); salicyclic acid (metabolite). **Elimination:** Dipyridamole: Feces (95%) and urine (low), $T_{1/2}$=15.5 hrs. ASA: Urine; $T_{1/2}$=0.33 hrs, $T_{1/2}$=1.71 hrs. (metabolite).

AGRYLIN   RX
anagrelide HCL (Shire)

THERAPEUTIC CLASS: Platelet-reducing agent

INDICATIONS: Treatment of thrombocythemia secondary to myeloproliferative disorders.

DOSAGE: *Adults:* Initial: 0.5mg qid or 1mg bid for at least 1 week. Moderate Hepatic Impairment: Initial: 0.5mg qd for at least 1 week. Titrate: Increase by no more than 0.5mg/day per week. Max: 10mg/day or 2.5mg/dose. Adjust lowest effective dose to reduce and maintain platelets <600,000/mcL.

Monitor platelets every 2 days during first week, then weekly thereafter until reach maintenance dose.
Pediatrics: Initial: 0.5mg qd. Titrate: Increase by no more than 0.5mg/day per week. Max: 10mg/day or 2.5mg/dose. Adjust to lowest effective dose to reduce and maintain platelets <600,000/mcL. Monitor platelets every 2 days during first week, then weekly thereafter until reach maintenance dose.

HOW SUPPLIED: Cap: 0.5mg, 1mg

CONTRAINDICATIONS: Severe hepatic impairment.

WARNINGS/PRECAUTIONS: Caution with heart disease, renal or hepatic dysfunction. Perform pre-treatment cardiovascular exam and monitor during treatment; may cause cardiovascular effects (eg, vasodilation, tachycardia, palpitations, CHF). Monitor closely for renal toxicity if creatinine ≥2mg/dL or hepatic toxicity if bilirubin, SGOT, or LFTs >1.5x ULN. Monitor blood counts, renal and hepatic function while platelets are lowered. Increase in platelets after therapy interruption. Reduce dose in moderate hepatic impairment.

ADVERSE REACTIONS: Headache, palpitations, asthenia, edema, GI effects, dizziness, pain, dyspnea, fever, chest pain, rash, tachycardia, malaise, pharyngitis, cough, paresthesia.

INTERACTIONS: Sucralfate may interfere with absorption. Exacerbated effects of products that inhibit cyclic AMP PDE III (inotropes: milrinone, enoximone, amrinone, olparinone, cilostazol).

PREGNANCY: Category C, not for use in nursing.

MECHANISM OF ACTION: Platelet-reducing agent; not established. Suspected to reduce platelet production resulting from a decrease in megakaryocyte hypermaturation. Inhibits cyclic AMP phosphodiesterase III (PDEIII). PDEIII inhibitors can also inhibit platelet aggregation.

PHARMACOKINETICS: Metabolism: Liver, CYP1A2 (partial). RL603 and 3-hydroxy anagrelide (major metabolites). **Elimination**: Urine; $T_{1/2}$=1.3 hrs.

AK-FLUOR RX
fluorescein sodium (Akorn)

THERAPEUTIC CLASS: Diagnostic dye

INDICATIONS: Indicated in diagnostic fluorescein angiography or angioscopy of the fundus and iris vasculature.

DOSAGE: *Adults:* Perform intradermal skin test before IV use if suspect potential allergy. Inject contents of ampule rapidly into antecubital vein. A syringe with fluorescein is attached to transparent tubing and a 25 gauge scalp vein needle for injection. Insert needle and draw patient's blood to hub of syringe so small air bubble separates patient's blood in tubing from fluorescein. With room lights on, inject blood back into vein while watching skin over needle tip. If needle extravasated, patient's blood will bulge skin; stop injection before injecting fluorescein. When certain there is no extravasation, turn room light off and complete fluorescein injection. Luminescence appears in retina and choroidal vessels in 9-14 seconds.
Pediatrics: Perform intradermal skin test before IV use if suspect potential allergy. Dose is 35mg/10lbs. Inject contents of ampule/vial rapidly into antecubital vein. A syringe with fluorescein is attached to transparent tubing and a 25 gauge scalp vein needle for injection. Insert needle and draw patient's blood to hub of syringe so small air bubble separates patient's blood in tubing from fluorescein. With room lights on, inject blood back into vein while watching skin over needle tip. If needle extravasated, patient's blood will bulge skin; stop injection before injecting fluorescein. When certain there is no extravasation, turn room light off and complete fluorescein injection. Luminescence appears in retina and choroidal vessels in 9-14 seconds.

HOW SUPPLIED: Inj: 10% [5mL], 25% [2mL]

WARNINGS/PRECAUTIONS: Avoid extravasation; severe local tissue damage can occur. Caution with history of allergy or bronchial asthma. Have emergency tray (eg, 0.1% epinephrine IV/IM, antihistamine, soluble steroid, IV aminophylline) and oxygen available. Avoid angiography in pregnancy, especially 1st trimester. Skin attains temporary yellowish discoloration and urine attains bright yellow color.

ADVERSE REACTIONS: Nausea, vomiting, headache, GI distress, syncope, hypotension, cardiac arrest, basilar artery ischemia, severe shock, convulsions, thrombophlebitis.

PREGNANCY: Safety in pregnancy not known, caution in nursing.

MECHANISM OF ACTION: A diagnostic dye; demarcates the vascular area under observation, distinguishing it from adjacent areas.

Alamast   RX
pemirolast potassium (Vistakon)

THERAPEUTIC CLASS: Mast cell stabilizer

INDICATIONS: Prevention of ocular itching due to allergic conjunctivitis.

DOSAGE: *Adults:* 1-2 drops in affected eye qid.
Pediatrics: ≥3 yrs: 1-2 drops in affected eye qid.

HOW SUPPLIED: Sol: 0.1% [10mL]

WARNINGS/PRECAUTIONS: May reinsert soft contact lens after 10 min, if eyes are not red. Contains lauralkonium chloride; may be absorbed by soft contact lens.

ADVERSE REACTIONS: Headache, rhinitis, cold/flu symptoms, ocular burning/discomfort, dry eye, foreign body sensation.

PREGNANCY: Category C, caution in nursing.

MECHANISM OF ACTION: Mast cell stabilizer; inhibits type I immediate hypersensitivity reaction, antigen-induced release of inflammatory mediators (eg, histamine, leukotriene C_4, D_4, E_4) from human mast cell; also inhibits the chemotaxis of eosinophils into ocular tissue, blocks the release of mediators from human eosinophils, and prevents calcium influx into mast cells upon antigen stimulation (not established).

PHARMACOKINETICS: Absorption: C_{max}=4.7ng/mL, T_{max}=0.42 hrs. **Elimination:** Urine (10-15% unchanged); $T_{1/2}$=4.5 hrs.

Albalon   RX
naphazoline HCL (Allergan)

THERAPEUTIC CLASS: Decongestant

INDICATIONS: Topical ocular vasoconstrictor.

DOSAGE: *Adults:* 1-2 drops q3-4h prn.

HOW SUPPLIED: Sol: 0.1% [15mL]

CONTRAINDICATIONS: Anatomically narrow angle or narrow angle glaucoma.

WARNINGS/PRECAUTIONS: CNS depression leading to coma may occur in children and infants. Caution with HTN, cardiovascular abnormalities, DM, hyperthyroidism, infection, or injury.

ADVERSE REACTIONS: Mydriasis, increased redness, irritation, discomfort, blurring, punctate keratitis, lacrimation, increased IOP, dizziness, headache, nausea, sweating, nervousness, drowsiness, weakness, HTN, cardiac irregularities, hyperglycemia.

INTERACTIONS: Maprotiline, TCAs may potentiate pressor effects of naphazoline. Hypertensive crisis may occur with MAOIs.

PREGNANCY: Category C, caution in nursing.

MECHANISM OF ACTION: Ocular vasoconstrictor: Imidazole derivative of sympathomimetics; acts by direct stimulation upon the alpha-adrenergic receptors in the arterioles of the conjunctiva, resulting in decreased conjunctival congestion.

ALBENZA
albendazole (GlaxoSmithKline)

RX

THERAPEUTIC CLASS: Broad-spectrum anthelmintic

INDICATIONS: Treatment of parenchymal neurocysticercosis and cystic hydatid disease of the liver, lung, and peritoneum.

DOSAGE: *Adults:* Hydatid Disease: ≥60kg: 400mg bid. <60kg: 7.5mg/kg bid up to 800mg/day. Take with meals for 28 days, then 14 days drug-free, repeat for a total of 3 cycles. Neurocysticercosis: Same dose as Hydatid disease. Treat for 8-30 days.
Pediatrics: ≥6 yrs: Hydatid Disease: ≥60kg: 400mg bid. <60kg: 7.5mg/kg bid up to 800mg/day. Take with meals for 28 days, then 14 days drug-free, repeat for a total of 3 cycles. Neurocysticercosis: Same dose as Hydatid disease. Treat for 8-30 days.

HOW SUPPLIED: Tab: 200mg

WARNINGS/PRECAUTIONS: Monitor blood counts at the beginning of each 28-day cycle, and every 2 weeks during therapy; bone marrow suppression, aplastic anemia, and agranulocytosis have been reported. May continue if total WBC and absolute neutrophil count decrease are modest and do not progress. Not for use in pregnancy unless no other therapy is appropriate. Avoid pregnancy at least 1 month after discontinuing therapy. D/C immediately if become pregnant. Treatment for neurocysticercosis should include anticonvulsants and steroids. Examine for retinal lesions before therapy. Elevated LFTs reported. Can cause bone marrow suppression, aplastic anemia, and agranulocytosis in patients with and without underlying hepatic dysfunction.

ADVERSE REACTIONS: Abnormal LFTs, abdominal pain, nausea, vomiting, headache.

INTERACTIONS: Monitor theophylline levels during and after therapy. Increased levels with dexamethasone, praziquantel, and cimetidine.

PREGNANCY: Category C, caution in nursing.

MECHANISM OF ACTION: Broad spectrum anthelmintic; exerts action by inhibitory effect on tubulin polymerization, which results in loss of cytoplasmic microtubules.

PHARMACOKINETICS: Absorption: GI tract (poorly absorbed); C_{max}=1.31mcg/mL; T_{max}=2-5 hrs. **Distribution:** Plasma protein binding (70%). **Metabolism:** Liver; metabolite: Albendazole sulfoxide (major metabolite). **Elimination:** Bile, urine (<1%); $T_{1/2}$=8-12 hrs.

ALBUMINAR
albumin (CSL Behring)

RX

OTHER BRAND NAMES: Albuminar-25 (CSL Behring) - Albuminar-5 (CSL Behring)

THERAPEUTIC CLASS: Human albumin

INDICATIONS: (5%, 25%) Emergency treatment of shock and burns and in other similar conditions where the restoration of blood volume is urgent. (5%) Acute hypoproteinemia where sodium restriction is not a problem. (25%) Hypoproteinemia with or without edema.

DOSAGE: *Adults:* Shock: Initial: (5%) 500mL given as rapidly as tolerated. May repeat 30 min later if needed. Guide therapy by clinical response, BP, assessment of relative anemia. (25%) Dose dependent on BP, degree of pulmonary congestion, Hct. May repeat 15-30 min later if needed. Severe Burns: (5%) Large volumes of crystalloid with lesser amount of albumin 5%. May increase ratio of albumin to crystalloid after 24 hrs to maintain plasma albumin level 2.5g/100mL or total serum protein level 5.2g/100mL. Burns: (25%) Large volumes of crystalloid during 1st 24 hrs. More albumin than crystalloid after 24 hrs is required. Hypoproteinemia: (5%) Use to replace protein lost. (25%) 200-300mL to reduce edema and normalize serum protein.

ALBUTEROL

HOW SUPPLIED: Inj: 5%, 25%

CONTRAINDICATIONS: Severe anemia, cardiac failure, history of human albumin allergy.

WARNINGS/PRECAUTIONS: Avoid if turbid or sediment in bottle. Do not begin administration >4 hrs after container has been entered. Made from human plasma; risk of viral disease transmission. Supplement with RBCs or whole blood when administer large quantities. Slower administration with HTN. Observe for bleeding points due to quick response of BP. Caution with low cardiac reserve or with no albumin deficiency.

ADVERSE REACTIONS: Anaphylaxis, nausea, vomiting, increased salivation, chills, febrile reactions, urticaria, pruritus, edema, erythema, hypotension, bronchospasm, rash.

PREGNANCY: Category C, safety in nursing not known.

MECHANISM OF ACTION: Albumin: Osmotically active and regulates the volume of circulating blood.

ALBUTEROL   RX
albuterol sulfate (Various)

THERAPEUTIC CLASS: Beta$_2$-agonist

INDICATIONS: (Aerosol) Prevention and treatment of bronchospasm with reversible obstructive airway disease. Prevention of Exercise-Induced Bronchospasm (EIB). (Sol) Relief of bronchospasm with reversible obstructive airway disease and acute attacks of bronchospasm in patients ≥12 yrs. (Tab, Tab, Extended-Release) Relief of bronchospasm with reversible obstructive airway disease in patients ≥6 yrs. (Syrup) Relief of bronchospasm in patients ≥2 yrs with reversible obstructive airway disease.

DOSAGE: *Adults:* Bronchospasm: (Aerosol) 2 inh q4-6h or 1 inh q4h. (Repetabs) Initial: 4-8mg q12h. Max: 32mg/day. (Sol) 2.5mg tid-qid by nebulizer. (Syrup, Tabs) 2-4mg tid-qid. Max: 32mg/day (8mg qid). Elderly/β-Adrenergic Sensitivity: (Syrup, Tabs) Initial: 2mg tid-qid. Max: (Tabs) 8mg tid-qid. EIB: (Aerosol) 2 inh 15 min before activity.
Pediatrics: Bronchospasm: >14 yrs: (Syrup) Initial: 2-4mg tid-qid. Max: 8mg qid. ≥12 yrs: (Aerosol) 2 inh q4-6h or 1 inh q4h. (Sol) 2.5mg tid-qid by nebulizer. (Tabs) Initial: 2-4mg tid-qid. Max: 8mg qid. >12 yrs: (Repetabs) Initial: 4-8mg q12h. Max: 32mg/day. 6-14 yrs: (Syrup) Initial: 2mg tid-qid. Max: 24mg/day. 6-12 yrs: (Repetabs) Initial: 4mg q12h. Max: 24mg/day. (Tabs) Initial: 2mg tid-qid. Max: 24mg/day. 2-5 yrs: (Syrup) Initial: 0.1mg/kg tid (not to exceed 2mg tid). Titrate: May increase to 0.2mg/kg/day. Max: 4mg tid. EIB: ≥12 yrs: (Aerosol) 2 inh 15 min before activity.

HOW SUPPLIED: MDI: 0.09mg/inh [17g]; Sol (neb): 0.083% [3mL, 25's], 0.5% [20mL]; Syrup: 2mg/5mL; Tab: 2mg*, 4mg*; Tab, Extended-Release (Repetabs): 4mg *scored

WARNINGS/PRECAUTIONS: Hypersensitivity reactions reported. Monitor for worsening asthma. Fatalities reported with excessive use. Caution with cardiovascular disorders, especially coronary insufficiency, arrhythmias and HTN. May need concomitant corticosteroids. Can produce paradoxical bron-chospasm. Caution with DM, hyperthyroidism, seizures. May cause transient hypokalemia.

ADVERSE REACTIONS: Tachycardia, increased BP, tremor, nervousness, diz-ziness, nausea/vomiting, palpitations, paradoxical bronchospasm, heartburn, rhinitis, respiratory tract infection.

INTERACTIONS: Avoid other sympathomimetic agents. Extreme caution with MAOIs and TCAs. Monitor digoxin. May worsen ECG changes and/or hy-pokalemia with nonpotassium-sparing diuretics. Antagonized by β-blockers.

PREGNANCY: Category C, not for use in nursing.

MECHANISM OF ACTION: β$_2$-adrenergic agonist; stimulates intracellular adenyl cyclase, which catalyzes conversion of ATP to cAMP to produce relaxation of bronchial smooth muscle and inhibition of release of mediators of immediate hypersensitivity from cells (mast cells).

PHARMACOKINETICS: Absorption: (Aerosol) T_{max}=2-4 hrs. (Syrup, Tab) Rapid. C_{max}=18ng/mL; T_{max}=2 hrs. **Elimination:** (Aerosol) Urine (28%); $T_{1/2}$=3.8 hrs. (Syrup, Tab) $T_{1/2}$=5 hrs.

ALCORTIN   RX
iodoquinol - hydrocortisone (Primus)

THERAPEUTIC CLASS: Corticosteroid/Anti-infective

INDICATIONS: "Possibly" Effective: Contact or atopic dermatitis, impetig-inized eczema, nummular eczema, endogenous chronic infectious dermatitis, stasis dermatitis, pyoderma, nuchal eczema and chronic eczematoid otitis externa, acne urticata, localized or disseminated neurodermatitis, lichen simplex chronicus, anogenital pruritus (vulvae, scroti, ani), folliculitis, bacterial dermatoses, mycotic dermatoses such as tinea (capitis, cruris, corporis, pedis), monliasis, intertrigo.

DOSAGE: *Adults:* Apply to affected area(s) tid-qid.
Pediatrics: ≥12 yrs: Apply to affected area(s) tid-qid.

HOW SUPPLIED: Gel: (Hydrocortisone-Iodoquinol) 2%-1% [2g]

WARNINGS/PRECAUTIONS: For external use only. Avoid eyes. D/C if irrita-tion develops. May stain skin, hair, or fabrics. Risk of systemic absorption with treatment of extensive areas or use of occlusive dressings. Increased risk of systemic absorption in children. Iodoquinol may interfere with thyroid tests. False-positive phenylketonuria test reported. Prolonged use may result in overgrowth of nonsusceptible organisms.

ADVERSE REACTIONS: Burning, itching, irritation, dryness, folliculitis, hyper-trichosis, acneiform eruptions, hypopigmentation, perioral dermatitis, allergic dermatitis, skin maceration, secondary infection, skin atrophy, striae, miliaria.

PREGNANCY: Category C, caution in nursing.

MECHANISM OF ACTION: Corticosteroid/Anti-infective. Hydrocortisone: Corticosteroid; possesses anti-inflammatory, antipruritic, and vasoconstrictive properties. Anti-inflammatory effect unclear; however, there is a recogniz-able correlation between vasoconstrictor potency and therapeutic efficacy. Iodoquinol: Anti-infective; possesses both antifungal and antibacterial properties.

PHARMACOKINETICS: Absorption: Hydrocortisone: Absorbed from nor-mal intact skin. Inflammation of skin increases absorption. **Metabolism:** Hydrocortisone: Liver and most body tissues. Tetrahydrocortisone and tetra-hydrocortisol (metabolites). **Elimination:** Hydrocortisone: Urine (unchanged and glucuronides). Iodoquinol: Urine (3-5% glucuronide).

ALDACTAZIDE   RX
hydrochlorothiazide - spironolactone (Pharmacia & Upjohn)

> Tumorigenic in chronic toxicity animal studies; avoid unnecessary use. Not for initial therapy.

THERAPEUTIC CLASS: K⁺-sparing diuretic/thiazide diuretic

INDICATIONS: Management of edematous conditions (CHF, hepatic cirrhosis with edema/ascites, nephrotic syndrome) and hypertension.

DOSAGE: *Adults:* Edema: 100mg/day per component qd or in divided doses. Maint: 25-200mg/day per component. HTN: 50-100mg/day per component qd or in divided doses.

HOW SUPPLIED: Tab: (Spironolactone-HCTZ) 25mg-25mg, 50mg-50mg* *scored

CONTRAINDICATIONS: Acute renal impairment, significantly impaired renal excretory function, hyperkalemia, acute or severe hepatic dysfunction, anuria, sulfonamide hypersensitivity.

ALDACTONE

WARNINGS/PRECAUTIONS: Monitor for fluid/electrolyte imbalance. Caution with renal and hepatic dysfunction. Hyperchloremic metabolic acidosis reported with decompensated hepatic cirrhosis. Mild acidosis, gynecomastia, transient BUN elevation, hypercalcemia, hyperglycemia, hyperuricemia, hypomagnesemia, and sensitivity reactions may occur. D/C if hyperkalemia occurs. Risk of dilutional hyponatremia. Enhanced effects in post-sympathectomy patient. May increase cholesterol and TG levels. May manifest latent DM.

ADVERSE REACTIONS: Gastric bleeding, ulceration, gynecomastia, impotence, agranulocytosis, fever, urticaria, confusion, ataxia, renal dysfunction, blood dyscrasias, electrolyte disturbances, weakness, irregular menses, amenorrhea.

INTERACTIONS: Risk of hyperkalemia with K⁺-sparing diuretics, K⁺ supplements, NSAIDs, ACE inhibitors. Alcohol, barbiturates, or narcotics potentiate orthostatic hypotension. Corticosteroids, ACTH may intensify electrolyte depletion. Reduced vascular response to norepinephrine. Increased response to nondepolarizing skeletal muscle relaxants. Risk of digoxin, lithium toxicity. NSAIDs may reduce effects. Antidiabetic agents may need adjustment.

PREGNANCY: Category C, not for use in nursing.

MECHANISM OF ACTION: Spironolactone: Aldosterone antagonist; competitively binds to receptors at aldosterone-dependent sodium-potassium exchange site. HCTZ: Thiazide diuretic; promotes excretion of sodium and water by inhibiting reabsorption.

PHARMACOKINETICS: Absorption: Spironolactone: C_{max}=80ng/mL; T_{max}=2.6 hrs. HCTZ: Rapid; T_{max}=1-2 hrs. **Distribution:** Spironolactone: Plasma protein binding (90%). **Elimination:** Spironolactone: Urine (major), bile (minor). HCTZ: Urine.

ALDACTONE   RX

spironolactone (Pharmacia & Upjohn)

> Tumorigenic in chronic toxicity animal studies; avoid unnecessary use.

THERAPEUTIC CLASS: K⁺-sparing diuretic

INDICATIONS: Management of primary hyperaldosteronism (diagnosis, short-term preoperative, and long-term maintenance treatment); edematous conditions (CHF, hepatic cirrhosis with edema/ascites, nephrotic syndrome); hypertension. Treatment and prophylaxis of hypokalemia.

DOSAGE: *Adults:* Hyperaldosteronism: (Diagnostic) 400mg/day for 3-4 weeks or 400mg/day for 4 days. (Preoperative) 100-400mg/day. Maint: Lowest effective dose. Edema: Initial: 100mg/day given qd or in divided doses for at least 5 days. Maint: 25-200mg/day given qd-bid. HTN: Initial: 50-100mg/day given qd or in divided doses. Titrate: Adjust at 2-week intervals. Hypokalemia: 25-100mg/day.

HOW SUPPLIED: Tab: 25mg, 50mg*, 100mg* *scored

CONTRAINDICATIONS: Anuria, acute renal insufficiency, significantly impaired renal excretory function, hyperkalemia.

WARNINGS/PRECAUTIONS: Monitor for fluid/electrolyte imbalance. Caution with renal and hepatic dysfunction. Hyperchloremic metabolic acidosis reported with decompensated hepatic cirrhosis. Mild acidosis, gynecomastia, transient BUN elevation may occur. D/C and monitor ECG if hyperkalemia occurs. Risk of dilutional hyponatremia.

ADVERSE REACTIONS: Gastric bleeding, ulceration, gynecomastia, impotence, agranulocytosis, fever, urticaria, confusion, ataxia, renal dysfunction, irregular menses, amenorrhea.

INTERACTIONS: Risk of hyperkalemia with K⁺-sparing diuretics, K⁺ supplements, NSAIDs, ACE inhibitors. Alcohol, barbiturates, or narcotics potentiate orthostatic hypotension. Corticosteroids, ACTH may intensify electrolyte depletion. Reduced vascular response to norepinephrine. Increased response to nondepolarizing skeletal muscle relaxants. Risk of digoxin, lithium toxicity. NSAIDs may reduce effects.

PREGNANCY: Category C, not for use in nursing.

MECHANISM OF ACTION: Aldosterone antagonist; competitively binds to receptors at aldosterone-dependent Na$^+$-K$^+$ exchange site in distal convoluted renal tubule, causing increased Na$^+$ and water excretion and K$^+$ retention.

PHARMACOKINETICS: Absorption: C_{max}=80ng/mL; T_{max}=2.6 hrs. **Distribution:** Plasma protein binding (>90%). **Elimination:** Urine (major), bile (minor).

ALDARA RX
imiquimod (Graceway)

THERAPEUTIC CLASS: Immune response modifier

INDICATIONS: Actinic keratoses on face or scalp in immunocompetent adults. External genital and perianal warts/condyloma acuminata. Biopsy-confirmed, primary superficial basal cell carcinoma (sBCC) in immunocompetent adults, with a maximum tumor diameter of 2cm, located on trunk (excluding anogenital skin), neck, or extremities (excluding hands and feet), only when surgical methods are medically less appropriate and follow-up can be assured.

DOSAGE: *Adults:* Use before bedtime. Actinic Keratosis: Usual: Apply 2x/week to defined area on face or scalp (but not both concurrently). Wash off after 8 hrs with soap and water. Max: 16 weeks. External Genital and Perianal Warts/Condyloma: Usual: Apply 3x/week. Wash off after 6-10 hrs with soap and water. Use until warts are clear. Max: 16 weeks. May suspend use for several days to manage local reactions. Do not occlude treatment area. sBCC: Apply 5x/week for 6 weeks. If tumor diameter is 0.5 to <1cm, use 4mm (10mg) of cream. If tumor is ≥1 to <1.5cm, use 5mm (25mg) of cream. If tumor is ≥1.5 to 2cm, use 7mm (40mg) of cream. Max diameter of tumor: ≤2cm. Treatment area should include a 1cm margin of skin around the tumor. Wash off after 8 hrs with soap and water.
Pediatrics: ≥12 yrs: External Genital and Perianal Warts/Condyloma: Usual: Apply 3x/week before bedtime. Wash off after 6-10 hrs with soap and water. Use until warts are clear. Max: 16 weeks. May suspend use for several days to manage local reactions. Do not occlude treatment area.

HOW SUPPLIED: Cre: 5% [12 pkts]

WARNINGS/PRECAUTIONS: Not for urethral, intra-vaginal, cervical, rectal, or intra-anal human papilloma viral disease. Avoid sexual contact while cream is on skin. May weaken condoms and diaphragms; avoid concurrent use. Avoid or minimize exposure to sunlight. May exacerbate inflammatory skin conditions. Avoid contact with eyes, lips, nostrils. Avoid after surgery or with sunburn until tissue is healed.

ADVERSE REACTIONS: Wart (erythema, erosion, flaking, edema) and application site reactions (bleeding, burning, itching, pain), flu-like symptoms, headache.

INTERACTIONS: Avoid topical drugs immediately after treatment of warts.

PREGNANCY: Category C, safety in nursing not known.

MECHANISM OF ACTION: Immune response modifier; not established. In basal cell carcinoma, suspected to increase infiltration of lymphocytes, dendritic cells, and macrophages in the tumor lesion. In external genital warts, suspected to induce mRNA encoding cytokines, including interferon-α at the treatment site.

PHARMACOKINETICS: Absorption: C_{max}=0.1ng/mL (12.5mg, face), 0.2ng/mL (25mg, scalp), 3.5ng/mL (75mg, hands/arms). **Distribution:** Excreted in breast milk. **Elimination:** Urine: Male (0.11%), female (2.41%).

ALESSE RX
ethinyl estradiol - levonorgestrel (Wyeth)

OTHER BRAND NAMES: Lessina (Barr) - Aviane (Duramed)
THERAPEUTIC CLASS: Estrogen/progestogen combination

INDICATIONS: Prevention of pregnancy.

DOSAGE: *Adults:* 1 tab qd for 28 days, then repeat. Start 1st Sunday after menses begin or 1st day of menses.

HOW SUPPLIED: Tab: (Ethinyl Estradiol-Levonorgestrel) 0.02mg-0.1mg

CONTRAINDICATIONS: Thrombophlebitis, DVT or thromboembolic disorders, pregnancy, cerebrovascular or coronary artery disease, undiagnosed abnormal genital bleeding, cholestatic jaundice of pregnancy or jaundice with prior pill use, hepatic adenomas or carcinomas, active liver disease (as long as liver function has not returned to normal), breast cancer or other estrogen-dependent neoplasia, thrombogenic valvulopathies, thrombogenic rhythm disorders, diabetes with vascular involvement, uncontrolled HTN.

WARNINGS/PRECAUTIONS: Cigarette smoking increases risk of serious cardiovascular side effects; risk increases with age (especially >35 yrs) and heavy smoking. Increased risk of MI, vascular disease, thromboembolism, stroke and gallbladder disease. Retinal thrombosis, hepatic neoplasia, carcinoma of breast and reproductive organs reported. May cause glucose intolerance. May increase BP, elevate LDL levels or cause other lipid changes, fluid retention, breakthrough bleeding, and spotting. May cause or exacerbate migraine. May develop visual changes with contact lens. Diarrhea and/or vomiting may reduce absorption. Increased risk of MI with HTN, hyperlipidemia, obesity, and diabetes. D/C if jaundice, significant depression or ophthalmic irregularities develop. Perform annual physical exam. Use before menarche is not indicated. May affect certain endocrine, LFTs and blood components.

ADVERSE REACTIONS: Nausea, vomiting, breakthrough bleeding, spotting, amenorrhea, migraine, depression, vaginal candidiasis, edema, weight changes.

INTERACTIONS: Reduced effects, increased breakthrough bleeding, and menstrual irregularities with rifampin, barbiturates, phenylbutazone, phenytoin, griseofulvin, topiramate, some protease inhibitors, modafinil, ampicillin, tetracyclines, and possibly with St. John's wort. Troleandomycin may increase risk of intrahepatic cholestasis. Ascorbic acid, APAP, CYP3A4 inhibitors (eg, indinavir, fluconazole, troleandomycin), atorvastatin may increase plasma levels. Increased plasma levels of cyclosporine, theophylline, and corticosteroids.

PREGNANCY: Category X, not for use in nursing.

MECHANISM OF ACTION: Oral contraceptive: inhibits ovulation by suppression of gonadotropins. Causes changes in cervical mucus (increases difficulty of sperm entry into uterus) and in endometrium (reduces likelihood of implantation).

PHARMACOKINETICS: Absorption: Levonorgestrel: Rapid and complete, bioavailability (100%), $C_{max(mean)}$=2.8ng/mL (single dose), 6.0ng/mL (multiple doses), $T_{max(mean)}$=1.6 hrs (single dose), 1.5 hrs (multiple doses); Ethinyl Estradiol: Rapid, bioavailability; (38-48%); $C_{max(mean)}$=62 pg/mL (single dose), 77pg/mL (multiple doses), $T_{max(mean)}$=1.5 hrs (single dose), 1.3 hrs (multiple doses). **Distribution:** Levonogestrel: Primarily bound to SHBG. Ethinyl estradiol: Plasma protein binding (97%). **Metabolism:** Levonorgestrel: Reduction, hydroxylation, and conjugation. Ethinyl Estradiol: Hepatic, via CYP3A4 (hydroxylation), methylation, and glucuronidation. **Elimination:** Levonorgestrel: Urine (40-68%), feces (16-48%); $T_{1/2(mean)}$=36 hrs. Ethinyl Estradiol: $T_{1/2(mean)}$=18 hrs.

ALEVE   OTC
naproxen sodium (Bayer Healthcare)

THERAPEUTIC CLASS: NSAID

INDICATIONS: Relief of minor aches and pains. Reduction of fever.

DOSAGE: *Adults:* Initial: 1-2 tabs, then 1 tab q8-12h. Max: 660mg/24 hrs or 440mg/12 hrs. Elderly: >65 yrs: 1 tab q12h.
Pediatrics: ≥12 yrs: Initial: 1-2 tabs, then 1 tab q8-12h. Max: 660mg/24 hrs or 440mg/12 hrs.

HOW SUPPLIED: Tab: 220mg

WARNINGS/PRECAUTIONS: Avoid during last trimester of pregnancy. Do not use >10 days for pain or >3 days for fever.

INTERACTIONS: Increased risk of GI bleeding with alcohol.

PREGNANCY: Safety in pregnancy or nursing not known.

ALFENTANIL CII
alfentanil HCL (Various)

OTHER BRAND NAMES: Alfenta (Akorn)

THERAPEUTIC CLASS: Opioid analgesic

INDICATIONS: As an analgesic adjunct given in incremental doses in the maintenance of anesthesia with barbiturate/nitrous oxide/oxygen. As an analgesic administered by continuous infusion with nitrous oxide/oxygen in the maintenance of general anesthesia. As a primary anesthetic agent for the induction of anesthesia in patients undergoing general surgery in which endotracheal intubation and mechanical ventilation are required. As the analgesic component for monitored anesthesia care (MAC).

DOSAGE: *Adults:* Individualize dose. Spontaneous Breathing/Assisted Ventilation: Induction: 8-20mcg/kg. Maint: 3-5mcg/kg q 5-20 min or 0.5-1mcg/kg/min. Total: 8-40mcg/kg. Assisted or Controlled Ventilation: Incremental Injection: Induction: 20-50mcg/kg. Maint: 5-15mcg/kg q 5-20 min. Total: Up to 75mcg/kg. Continuous Infusion: Induction: 50-75mcg/kg. Maint: 0.5-3mcg/kg/min (average rate 1-1.5mcg/kg/min). Total: Dependent on duration of procedure. Anesthetic Induction: Induction: 130-245 mcg/kg. Maint: 0.5-1.5mcg/kg/min or general anesthetic. Total: dependent on duration of procedure. Monitored Anesthesia Care (MAC): Induction: 3-8mcg/kg. Maint: 3-5 mcg/kg q 5-20 min or 0.25-1mcg/kg/min. Total: 3-40mcg/kg.

HOW SUPPLIED: Inj: 500mcg/mL

WARNINGS/PRECAUTIONS: May cause delayed respiratory depression, respiratory arrest, bradycardia, asystole, arrhythmias, and hypotension; an opioid antagonist, resuscitative and intubation equipment and oxygen should be readily available. Use in caution with patients with head injury, increased ICP, pulmonary disease, and liver or kidney dysfunction. Initial dose of alfentanil should be appropriately reduced in elderly and debilitated patients.

ADVERSE REACTIONS: Respiratory depression, skeletal muscle rigidity, nausea, vomiting, HTN, hypotension, bradycardia, tachycardia, dizziness, skeletal muscle movements, apnea, chest wall rigidity.

INTERACTIONS: Coadministration with CNS depressants such as barbituates, tranquilizers, opioids, or inhalation general anesthetics may enhance CNS effects and postoperative respiratory depression. Erythromycin may significantly inhibit alfentanil clearance and increase the risk of prolonged or delayed respiratory depression. Cimetidine reduces clearance of alfentanil and may extend duration of action.

PREGNANCY: Category C, caution in nursing

MECHANISM OF ACTION: Opioid analgesic; attenuates the catecholamine response with more rapid recovery and reduced need for postoperative analgesics.

PHARMACOKINETICS: Distribution: V_d=0.4-1L/kg, plasma protein binding (Approximately 92%). **Metabolism:** Liver **Elimination:** $T_{1/2}$=90-111 min, urine (1%unchanged, drug).

ALIMTA RX
pemetrexed (Lilly)

THERAPEUTIC CLASS: Antifolate

INDICATIONS: In combination with cisplatin for the treatment of patients with unresectable malignant pleural mesothelioma who are not candidates for curative surgery. Monotherapy for the treatment of patients with locally advanced or metastatic non-small cell lung cancer (NSCLC) after prior chemotherapy.

DOSAGE: *Adults:* Premedication: Dexamethasone: 4mg po bid day before, day of, and day after pemetrexed. Folic Acid: At least 5 daily doses (350-1000mcg) during 7 days prior to pemetrexed. Continue for 21 days after last pemetrexed dose. Vitamin B$_{12}$: 1000mcg IM once during week preceding first pemetrexed dose and every 3 cycles thereafter. Treatment: Mesothelioma: 500mg/m^2 IV over 10 min on Day 1 of each 21-day cycle with cisplatin 75mg/m^2 infused over 2 hrs beginning 30 min after pemetrexed. NSCLC: 500mg/m^2 IV over 10 min on Day 1 of each 21-day cycle. Refer to PI for dose adjustments for hematologic, nonhematologic and neurotoxicities.

HOW SUPPLIED: Inj: 100mg, 500mg

WARNINGS/PRECAUTIONS: Avoid use if CrCl <45mL/min. May suppress bone marrow function. With pleural effusions, ascites, consider draining prior to therapy. Monitor CBCs, for nadir and recovery before each dose and on Days 8 and 15 of each cycle. Do not begin new cycle unless ANC ≥1500 cells/mm^3, platelets ≥100,000 cells/mm^3, CrCl ≥45mL/min.

ADVERSE REACTIONS: Nausea, fatigue, dyspnea, vomiting, hematologic effects, constipation, chest pain, anorexia, fever, infection, stomatitis, pharyngitis, rash/desquamation.

INTERACTIONS: Delayed clearance with nephrotoxic or tubularly secreted drugs (eg, probenecid). Reduced clearance with ibuprofen; caution with CrCl <80mL/min. In mild-moderate renal insufficiency, avoid NSAIDs with short elimination half-lives from 2 days prior to 2 days following therapy. Interrupt NSAID dosing with longer half-lives from at least 5 days before to 2 days following therapy.

PREGNANCY: Category D, not for use in nursing.

MECHANISM OF ACTION: Antifolate agent; disrupts folate-dependent metabolic processes essential for cell replication. Inhibits thymidylate synthase, dihydrofolate reductase, glycinamide ribonucleotide formyltransferase, and folate-dependent enzymes involved in the *de novo* biosynthesis of thymidine and purine nucleotides.

PHARMACOKINETICS: Distribution: Steady-state V$_d$=16.1L. Plasma protein binding (81%). **Elimination:** T$_{1/2}$=3.5 hrs; urine (70-90%).

ALINIA   RX
nitazoxanide (Romark)

THERAPEUTIC CLASS: Antiprotozoal agent

INDICATIONS: Treatment of diarrhea caused by *Cryptosporidium parvum* and *Giardia lamblia.*

DOSAGE: *Adults:* ≥12 yrs: *G.lamblia* Diarrhea: 500mg q12h for 3 days. Take with food.
Pediatrics: C.parvum/G.lamblia Diarrhea: 1-3 yrs: 100mg (5mL) q12h for 3 days. 4-11yrs: 200mg (10mL) q12h for 3 days. *G.lamblia* Diarrhea: ≥12 yrs: 500mg (1 tab or 25mL) q12h for 3 days. Take with food.

HOW SUPPLIED: Sus: 100mg/5mL [60mL]; Tab: 500mg [60^s, 3-Day Therapy Packs, 6^s]

WARNINGS/PRECAUTIONS: Caution with hepatic and biliary disease, renal disease. Contains 1.48g sucrose/5mL. Safety and effectiveness have not been established in HIV positive or immunodeficient patients.

ADVERSE REACTIONS: Abdominal pain, diarrhea, headache, nausea.

INTERACTIONS: Highly protein bound; caution with other highly plasma protein-bound drugs with narrow therapeutic indices.

PREGNANCY: Category B; caution in nursing.

MECHANISM OF ACTION: Antiprotozoal agent; interferes with the pyruvate, ferredoxin oxidoreductase enzyme-dependent electron transfer reaction, which is essential to anaerobic energy metabolism.

PHARMACOKINETICS: Absorption: Tizoxanide: (Tab, 500mg) 12-17 yrs: C_{max}=9.1mcg/mL, T_{max}=4 hrs, AUC=39.5mcg•hr/mL; ≥18 yrs: C_{max}=10.6mcg/mL, T_{max}=3 hrs, AUC=41.9mcg•hr/mL. (Sus, 100mg) 1-3 yrs: C_{max}=3.11mcg/mL, T_{max}=3.5 hrs, AUC=11.7mcg•hr/mL; 4-11 yrs: C_{max}=3mcg/mL, T_{max}=2 hrs, AUC=13.5mcg•hr/mL. **Distribution**: Tizoxanide: Plasma protein binding (>99%). **Metabolism**: Hydrolysis, glucuronidation: Tizoxanide and tizoxanide glucuronide (active). **Elimination**: Urine (33%), bile and feces (66%). Refer to PI for complete kinetics information.

ALKERAN RX
melphalan HCL (Celgene)

Severe bone marrow suppression resulting in bleeding or infection may occur. Potentially mutagenic and leukemogenic.

THERAPEUTIC CLASS: Nitrogen mustard alkylating agent

INDICATIONS: (Inj) Palliative treatment of multiple myeloma where oral therapy is not appropriate. (Tab) Palliative treatment of multiple myeloma and palliation of nonresectable epithelial carcinoma of the ovary.

DOSAGE: *Adults:* (Inj) Usual: 16mg/m² IV at 2-week intervals for 4 doses. After recover from toxicity, resume at 4-week intervals. Renal Impairment (BUN ≥ 30mg/dL): Reduce dose up to 50%. (Tab) Multiple Myeloma: 6mg qd. Adjust weekly based on blood counts. After 2-3 weeks, d/c for up to 4 weeks and monitor blood counts. Maint: 2mg qd. Epithelial Ovarian Cancer: 0.2mg/kg qd for 5 days. Repeat every 4-5 weeks depending on hematologic tolerance.

HOW SUPPLIED: Inj: 50mg; Tab: 2mg

CONTRAINDICATIONS: Prior resistance to agent.

WARNINGS/PRECAUTIONS: Marked bone marrow suppression with excessive doses. Monitor platelets, Hgb, WBCs, and differential before therapy and each dose. Use blood counts for dosing to avoid toxicity. Do not readminister if hypersensitivity occurs. Secondary malignancies reported. Ovary function suppression (eg, amenorrhea) may occur in premenopausal women. Reversible and irreversible testicular suppression reported. Extreme caution with compromised bone marrow reserve or if marrow function recovering from previous cytotoxic therapy. Caution in renal dysfunction; reduce IV dose. (Tab) If leukocytes <3000 cells/mcL or platelets <100,000 cells/mcL; d/c until peripheral blood counts recover. Avoid live vaccines in the immunocompromised.

ADVERSE REACTIONS: Bone marrow suppression, alopecia, hemolytic anemia, pulmonary fibrosis, interstitial pneumonitis, GI reactions (eg, nausea, vomiting, diarrhea, oral ulceration), hepatic disorders (eg, abnormal LFTs, hepatitis, jaundice). (Inj) Hypersensitivity reactions (eg, urticaria, pruritus, edema, tachycardia).

INTERACTIONS: (Inj) Severe renal failure reported with oral cyclosporine. Cisplatin may alter melphalan clearance by inducing renal dysfunction. May reduce the threshold for BCNU lung toxicity. Nalidixic acid may increase incidence of severe hemorrhagic necrotic enterocolitis in peds.

PREGNANCY: Category D, not for use in nursing.

MECHANISM OF ACTION: Nitrogen mustard (phenylalanine derivative); cytotoxic action appears related to the extent of its interstrand cross-linking with DNA by probable binding at N^7 position of guanine; active against both resting and rapidly dividing tumor cells.

PHARMACOKINETICS: Absorption: (Tab: 0.2-0.25 mg/kg); T_{max}=1 hr, C_{max}=212ng/mL, AUC=498ng•hr/mL. (IV: 10mg/m², 20mg/m²): C_{max}=1.2mcg/mL, 2.8mcg/mL. **Distribution**: Plasma protein binding (60-90%). V_d=0.5L/kg. **Elimination**: Hydrolysis. (IV) $T_{1/2}$=75 mins. (Tab: 0.6mg/kg): $T_{1/2}$=1.5 hrs, Urine (10%). (0.2-0.25mg/kg): $T_{1/2}$=1 hr.

ALLEGRA

RX

fexofenadine HCL (Sanofi-Aventis)

THERAPEUTIC CLASS: H₁-antagonist

INDICATIONS: (ODT) 6-11 yrs; (Sus) 2-11 yrs: Relief of symptoms associated with seasonal allergic rhinitis in children. (ODT) 6-11 yrs; (Sus) 6 months-11 yrs: Treatment of uncomplicated skin manifestations of chronic idiopathic urticaria in children. (Tab) Relief of symptoms associated with seasonal allergic rhinitis and treatment of uncomplicated skin manifestations of chronic idiopathic urticaria in adults and children ≥6 yrs.

DOSAGE: *Adults:* Tab: Rhinitis/Urticaria: 60mg bid or 180mg qd. Renal Dysfunction: Initial: 60mg qd.
Pediatrics: Tab: ≥12 yrs: Rhinitis/Urticaria: 60mg bid or 180mg qd. Renal Dysfunction: Initial: 60mg qd. 6-11 yrs: Rhinitis/Urticaria: 30mg bid. Renal Dysfunction: Initial: 30mg qd. ODT: Rhinitis/Urticaria: 6-11 yrs: 30mg bid. Renal Dysfunction: 30mg qd. Sus: Rhinitis: 2-11 yrs: 30mg (5mL) bid. Renal Dysfunction: 30mg (5mL) qd. Urticaria: 2-11 yrs: 30mg (5mL) bid. Renal Dysfunction: 30mg (5mL) qd. 6 months to <2 yrs: 15mg (2.5mL) bid. Renal Dysfunction: 15mg (2.5mL) qd.

HOW SUPPLIED: Tab: 30mg, 60mg, 180mg; Tab, Orally Disintegrating: 30mg; Sus: 30mg/5mL

ADVERSE REACTIONS: Headache, cough, upper respiratory tract infection, back pain, fever, pain, otitis media, vomiting, diarrhea.

INTERACTIONS: Increased plasma levels with erythromycin or ketoconazole. Avoid concomitant aluminum- and magnesium-containing antacids. Fruit juices (eg, grapefruit, orange, and apple) may decrease levels.

PREGNANCY: Category C, caution in nursing.

MECHANISM OF ACTION: Antihistamine with selective peripheral H₁-receptor antagonist activity; prevents antigen-induced bronchospasm and histamine release from periotoneal mast cells.

PHARMACOKINETICS: Absorption: Rapid; (Cap, 120mg) T_{max}=2.6 hrs; (Cap, 60mg) C_{max}=131ng/mL; (Tab, 60mg) C_{max}=142ng/mL; (Tab, 180mg) C_{max}=494ng/mL; (Sus, 30mg) C_{max}=118.0ng/mL, T_{max}=1.0 hrs. **Distribution:** Plasma protein binding (60-70%). **Metabolism:** Liver (5%). **Elimination:** Urine (80%), feces (11%); $T_{1/2}$=14.4 hrs.

ALLEGRA-D

RX

fexofenadine HCL - pseudoephedrine HCL (Sanofi-Aventis)

THERAPEUTIC CLASS: H₁-antagonist/sympathomimetic amine

INDICATIONS: Relief of symptoms of seasonal allergic rhinitis.

DOSAGE: *Adults:* 60mg-120mg tab bid or 180mg-240mg tab qd without food. Renal Dysfunction: Initial: 60mg-120mg tab qd; avoid 180mg-240mg tab. Do not crush or chew.
Pediatrics: ≥12 yrs: 60mg-120mg tab bid or 180mg-240mg tab qd without food. Renal Dysfunction: Initial: 60mg-120mg tab qd; avoid 180mg-240mg tab. Do not crush or chew.

HOW SUPPLIED: Tab, Extended-Release: (Fexofenadine-Pseudoephedrine) (12-Hour) 60mg-120mg, (24-Hour) 180mg-240mg

CONTRAINDICATIONS: Narrow-angle glaucoma, urinary retention, severe HTN, severe CAD, within 14 days of MAOI therapy.

WARNINGS/PRECAUTIONS: Caution with HTN, DM, ischemic heart disease, increased IOP, hyperthyroidism, renal impairment, or prostatic hypertrophy. May produce CNS stimulation with convulsions or cardiovascular collapse with hypotension.

ADVERSE REACTIONS: Headache, insomnia, nausea, dry mouth, dyspepsia, throat irritation.

INTERACTIONS: Increased plasma levels with erythromycin or ketoconazole. Avoid MAOIs. Increased ectopic pacemaker activity can occur with digitalis. Caution with other sympathomimetic amines. Reduced effects of antihypertensive drugs which interfere with sympathetic activity (eg, methyldopa, mecamylamine, reserpine).

PREGNANCY: Category C, caution with nursing.

MECHANISM OF ACTION: H_1-receptor antagonist/sympathomimetic amine. Fexofenadine: Selective peripheral H_1-receptor antagonist; inhibits antigen-induced bronchospasm and histamine release from peritoneal mast cells. Pseudoephedrine: Exerts a decongestant action on the nasal mucosa.

PHARMACOKINETICS: Absorption: Fexofenadine: Rapidly absorbed; C_{max}=634ng/mL (single dose), 674ng/mL (multiple doses); T_{max}=1.8-2 hrs. Pseudoephedrine: C_{max}=394ng/mL (single dose), 495ng/mL (multiple doses); T_{max}=12 hrs. **Distribution:** Fexofenadine: Plasma protein binding (60-70%). Pseudoephedrine: V_d=2.6-3.5L/kg. **Metabolism:** Fexofenadine and pseudoephedrine: Hepatic (5% of fexofenadine; <1% of pseudoephedrine). **Elimination:** Fexofenadine: Feces (80%), urine (11%); $T_{1/2}$=14.6 hrs. Pseudoephedrine: $T_{1/2}$=7 hrs.

ALLERX RX
pseudoephedrine HCL - chlorpheniramine maleate - methscopolamine nitrate (Cornerstone)

THERAPEUTIC CLASS: Antihistamine/anticholinergic/decongestant

INDICATIONS: Temporary relief of symptoms associated with allergic rhinitis, vasomotor rhinitis, sinusitis, and the common cold.

DOSAGE: *Adults:* 1 AM Dose tab in morning and 1 PM Dose tab in evening. *Pediatrics:* ≥12 yrs: 1 AM Dose tab in morning and 1 PM Dose tab in evening.

HOW SUPPLIED: Tab, Extended-Release: (AM Dose) (Methscopolamine-Pseudoephedrine) 2.5mg-120mg; (PM Dose) (Chlorpheniramine-Methscopolamine) 8mg-2.5mg

CONTRAINDICATIONS: Severe HTN or CAD, MAOI use or within 14 days of discontinuation, nursing mothers taking MAOIs, narrow-angle glaucoma, urinary retention, peptic ulcer, during asthma attack.

WARNINGS/PRECAUTIONS: Caution with elderly, HTN, DM, ischemic heart disease, hyperthyroidism, prostatic hypertrophy, CVD, increased IOP. May produce CNS stimulation with convulsions or cardiovascular collapse with hypotension. Excitability reported especially in children.

ADVERSE REACTIONS: Drowsiness, lassitude, nausea, giddiness, dry mouth, blurred vision, cardiac palpitations, flushing, increased irritability.

INTERACTIONS: May enhance effects of TCAs, barbiturates, alcohol, other CNS depressants. May diminish antihypertensive effects of reserpine, veratrum alkaloids, methyldopa, mecamylamine. Increased sympathomimetic effect with β-blockers and MAOIs. Contraindicated with or within 14 days of discontinuing MAOIs. Hypotension potentiated with sildenafil or other organic nitrates; avoid concomitant use. Caution with hyperactivity to sympathomimetics.

PREGNANCY: Category C, not for use in nursing.

MECHANISM OF ACTION: Pseudoephedrine: Antihistamine decongestant; indirect-acting sympathomimetic amine that exerts decongestant action on the nasal mucosa. Chlorpheniramine: Alkylamine-type antihistamine. Methscopolamine: Anticholinergic; quaternary ammonium derivative of the anticholinergic scopolamine which possesses the peripheral actions of the belladonna alkaloids. Causes inhibition of salivary secretions, reduction in vol and total acid content of gastric secretion and inhibition of GI motility.

PHARMACOKINETICS: Absorption: Pseudoephedrine: Rapidly and almost completely absorbed by GIT. Methscopolamine: Poorly absorbed. **Distribution:** Methscopolamine: Crosses blood-brain barrier. **Metabolism:** Pseudoephedrine: Liver via N-demethylation, parahydroxylation and oxidative deamination. **Elimination:** Pseudoephedrine: Urine (50-75% unchanged). Methscopolamine: Urine, bile, feces; T$_{1/2}$=4-6 hrs.

ALLI   OTC
orlistat (GlaxoSmithKline)

INDICATIONS: For weight loss in overweight adults in conjunction with a reduced-calorie, low-fat diet.

DOSAGE: *Adults:* ≥18 yrs: 1 cap qd with each meal containing fat. Max: 3 caps qd. Use with reduced-calorie, low-fat diet, and exercise program. Take a multi-vitamin qd at bedtime.

HOW SUPPLIED: Cap: 60mg

WARNINGS/PRECAUTIONS: Avoid use with organ transplant, cyclosporine, problems absorbing food or in patients not overweight. Caution with gallbladder problems, kidney stones, and pancreatitis.

ADVERSE REACTIONS: Gas with oily spotting, loose stools, hard-to-control frequent stools.

INTERACTIONS: Monitor dose of warfarin, thyroid medications, and antidiabetic agents; dose adjustment may be needed.

PREGNANCY: Not for use in pregnancy and nursing.

MECHANISM OF ACTION: Weight loss aid; prevents absorption of certain fats from food.

ALOCRIL   RX
nedocromil sodium (Allergan)

THERAPEUTIC CLASS: Mast cell stabilizer

INDICATIONS: Treatment of itching associated with allergic conjunctivitis.

DOSAGE: *Adults:* 1-2 drops bid. Continue throughout period of exposure. *Pediatrics:* ≥3 yrs: 1-2 drops bid. Continue throughout period of exposure.

HOW SUPPLIED: Sol: 2% [5mL]

WARNINGS/PRECAUTIONS: Avoid wearing contacts while symptoms of allergic conjunctivitis persist.

ADVERSE REACTIONS: Headache, ocular burning, irritation, stinging, unpleasant taste, nasal congestion, asthma, conjunctivitis, eye redness, photophobia, rhinitis.

PREGNANCY: Category B, caution in nursing.

MECHANISM OF ACTION: Mast cell stabilizer; inhibits release of mediators from cells involved in hypersensitivity reactions, decreases chemotaxis and activation of eosinophils.

PHARMACOKINETICS: Absorption: Low systemic absorption. **Metabolism:** Not metabolized. **Elimination:** Urine (70% unchanged), feces (30%).

ALOMIDE   RX
lodoxamide tromethamine (Alcon)

THERAPEUTIC CLASS: Mast cell stabilizer

INDICATIONS: Ocular disorders including vernal keratoconjunctivitis, vernal conjunctivitis, and vernal keratitis.

DOSAGE: *Adults:* 1-2 drops qid for up to 3 months. *Pediatrics:* >2 yrs: 1-2 drops qid for up to 3 months.

HOW SUPPLIED: Sol: 0.1% [10mL]

WARNINGS/PRECAUTIONS: Do not wear soft contacts during treatment. Transient burning and stinging upon instillation.

ADVERSE REACTIONS: Ocular pruritus, blurred vision, dry eye, tearing, discharge, hyperemia, crystalline deposits, foreign body sensation.

PREGNANCY: Category B, caution in nursing.

MECHANISM OF ACTION: Mast cell stabilizer; not established; suspected to inhibit the Type I immediate hypersensitivity reaction, decrease cutaneous vascular permeability associated with reagin or IgE and antigen-mediated reactions, and prevent calcium influx into mast cells upon stimulation.

PHARMACOKINETICS: Elimination: Urine; $T_{1/2}$=8.5 hrs.

Aloprim
allopurinol sodium (Nabi)   RX

THERAPEUTIC CLASS: Xanthine oxidase inhibitor

INDICATIONS: Management of elevated serum and urinary uric acid levels in patients with leukemia, lymphoma, and solid tumor malignancies receiving cancer therapy when oral therapy is not tolerated.

DOSAGE: *Adults:* Initial: 200-400mg/m²/day IV as qd or in divided doses every 6, 8, or 12 hrs. Max: 600mg/day. CrCl 10-20mL/min: 200mg/day. CrCl 3-10mL/min: 100mg/day. CrCl <3mL/min: 100mg/day at extended intervals.
Pediatrics: Initial: 200mg/m²/day IV as qd or in divided doses every 6, 8, or 12 hrs.

HOW SUPPLIED: Inj: 500mg

CONTRAINDICATIONS: Previous severe reaction to therapy.

WARNINGS/PRECAUTIONS: D/C at first appearance of hypersensitivity; increased risk in decreased renal function. Monitor LFTs during early stages of therapy in liver disease. Monitor renal function and uric acid levels; adjust dose if needed. Maintain sufficient fluid intake to yield a daily urinary output ≥2L. Drowsiness, hepatotoxicity, bone marrow suppression reported.

ADVERSE REACTIONS: Skin rash, eosinophilia, local injection site reaction, nausea, vomiting, diarrhea, renal failure/insufficiency.

INTERACTIONS: Decrease mercaptopurine and azathioprine dose to 1/3-1/4 of usual dose. Increased risk of skin rash with ampicillin, amoxicillin. Increased toxicity and risk of hypersensitivity with thiazide diuretics; monitor renal function. Caution with anticoagulants. Hypoglycemia reported with chlorpropamide. Enhanced myelosuppressive effects of cyclophosphamide, other cytotoxic agents. Increased cyclosporine levels. Increased urinary excretion of uric acid with uricosuric agents. Monitor PT with dicumarol.

PREGNANCY: Category C, caution in nursing.

MECHANISM OF ACTION: Xanthine oxidase inhibitor; reduces production of uric acid by inhibiting the biochemical reactions immediately preceding its formation.

PHARMACOKINETICS: Absorption: Absolute bioavailability (100%); C_{max}=1.58µg/mL (100mg), 5.12µg/mL (300mg); T_{max}=0.5 hrs; AUC=1.99 hr•µg/mL (100mg), 7.1 hr•µg/mL (300mg). **Metabolism:** Oxidative; oxypurinol (active metabolite). **Elimination:** Urine (12% unchanged); $T_{1/2}$=1 hr (parent), 24.1 hrs (oxypurinol).

Alora
estradiol (Watson)   RX

Estrogens increase risk of endometrial cancer. Estrogens, with or without progestins, should not be used for the prevention of cardiovascular disease or dementia. Increased risks of MI, stroke, invasive breast cancer, PE, and DVT in postmenopausal women (50-79 yrs of age) reported. Increased risk of developing probable dementia in postmenopausal women ≥65 yrs of age reported.

THERAPEUTIC CLASS: Estrogen

INDICATIONS: Treatment of moderate to severe vasomotor symptoms associated with menopause. Treatment of vulvar/vaginal atrophy. Treatment of hypoestrogenism due to hypogonadism, castration, or primary ovarian failure. Prevention of postmenopausal osteoporosis.

DOSAGE: *Adults:* Apply to lower abdomen, upper quadrant of the buttocks or the hip; avoid breasts and waistline. Rotate application sites. Vasomotor Symptoms/Vulvar/Vaginal Atrophy/Hypoestrogenism: Initial: Apply 0.05mg/day twice weekly. Titrate: Adjust dose to control symptoms. Use continuously without an intact uterus. Use cyclic schedule (3 weeks on, 1 week off) with an intact uterus without a progestin. Discontinue or taper at 3-6 month intervals. In women who are taking oral estrogens, initiate therapy 1 week after withdrawal of oral estrogens or sooner if menopausal symptoms reappear in less than 1 week. Osteoporosis Prevention: Apply 0.025mg/day twice weekly. Titrate: May increase depending on bone mineral density and adverse events.

HOW SUPPLIED: Patch: 0.025mg/24 hrs, 0.05mg/24 hrs [8^s 24^s], 0.075mg/24 hrs, 0.1mg/24 hrs [8^s]

CONTRAINDICATIONS: Pregnancy, undiagnosed abnormal genital bleeding, breast cancer unless being treated for metastatic disease, estrogen-dependent neoplasia, DVT/PE, active or recent (eg, within past year) arterial thromboembolic disease (eg, stroke, MI), liver dysfunction or disease.

WARNINGS/PRECAUTIONS: May increase risk of cardiovascular events (eg, MI, stroke), venous thrombosis, and PE; d/c immediately if any of these events occur or are suspected. May increase risk of breast/endometrial cancer, and gallbladder disease. May lead to severe hypercalcemia with breast cancer and bone metastases; monitor and d/c if hypercalcemia occurs. Retinal vascular thrombosis reported; monitor and d/c if papilledema or retinal vascular lesions occur. Consider addition of a progestin if no hysterectomy. May elevate BP; monitor at regular intervals. May cause elevations of plasma triglycerides with pre-existing hypertriglyceridemia. Caution with history of cholestatic jaundice associated with past estrogen use or with pregnancy; d/c with recurrence. May lead to increased thyroid-binding globulin levels; monitor thyroid function. May cause fluid retention; caution with cardiac/renal dysfunction. Caution with severe hypocalcemia. May increase risk of ovarian cancer. May exacerbate endometriosis, asthma, DM, epilepsy, migraine, porphyria; use with caution.

ADVERSE REACTIONS: Redness/irritation at application site, altered uterine/vaginal bleeding, vaginal candidiasis, breast tenderness/enlargement, GI effects, melasma, CNS effects, weight changes, edema, altered libido.

INTERACTIONS: CYP3A4 inducers (eg, St. John's wort, phenobarbital, carbamazepine, rifampin) may decrease levels which may decrease therapeutic effects and/or change uterine bleeding profile. CYP3A4 inhibitors (eg, erythromycin, clarithromycin, ketoconazole, itraconazole, ritonavir, grapefruit juice) may increase levels which may result in side effects.

PREGNANCY: Category X, caution in nursing.

MECHANISM OF ACTION: Estrogen: acts by binding to nuclear receptors in estrogen-responsive tissues. Modulates pituitary secretion of gonadotropins, luteinizing hormone (LH) and follicle stimulating hormone (FSH), through negative feedback mechanism.

PHARMACOKINETICS: Absorption: Transdermal administration of variable doses resulted in altered parameters. Absorbed through intact skin. **Distribution:** Widely. Bound to sex hormone binding globulin (SHBG) and albumin. Estrogen found in human breast milk. **Metabolism:** Liver to estrone (metabolite); estriol (major urinary metabolite). Undergoes enterohepatic recirculation via sulfate and glucuronide conjugation; biliary secretion of conjugates into the intestine; hydrolysis in gut; and reabsorption. CYP3A4 (partial). **Elimination:** Urine; $T_{1/2}$=1.75 hrs.

ALOXI   RX
palonosetron HCL (MGI Pharma)

THERAPEUTIC CLASS: 5-HT$_3$-antagonist

INDICATIONS: Prevention of acute nausea and vomiting associated with initial and repeat courses of moderately and highly emetogenic cancer chemotherapy. Prevention of delayed nausea and vomiting associated with initial and repeat courses of moderately emetogenic cancer chemotherapy. Prevention of postoperative nausea and vomiting (PONV) for up to 24 hrs following surgery.

DOSAGE: *Adults:* Chemotherapy-Induced Nausea/Vomiting: 0.25mg IV single dose 30 min before start of chemotherapy. Repeated dosing within a 7 day interval not recommended. PONV: 0.075mg IV single dose 10 sec before induction of anesthesia.

HOW SUPPLIED: Inj: 0.25mg/5mL, 0.075mg/1.5mL

WARNINGS/PRECAUTIONS: Hypersensitivity reaction may occur.

ADVERSE REACTIONS: Headache, constipation, diarrhea, dizziness.

PREGNANCY: Category B, not for use in nursing.

MECHANISM OF ACTION: 5-HT$_3$ receptor antagonist with antiemetic and antinauseant properties.

PHARMACOKINETICS: Absorption: C$_{max}$=5.6ng/ml, AUC=35.8ng•hr/mL. **Distribution:** V$_d$=8.3L/kg. Plasma protein binding (62%). **Metabolism:** 50% metabolized via CYP2D6; N-oxide-palonosetron and 6-S-hydroxy-palonosetron (primary metabolites). **Elimination:** Urine (40%), T$_{1/2}$=40 hrs.

ALPHAGAN P   RX
brimonidine tartrate (Allergan)

THERAPEUTIC CLASS: Selective alpha$_2$ agonist

INDICATIONS: Treatment of open-angle glaucoma and ocular hypertension.

DOSAGE: *Adults:* 1 drop tid, give q8h. Space dosing of other topical products that lower IOP by 5 min.
Pediatrics: ≥2 yrs: 1 drop tid, give q8h. Space dosing of other topical products that lower IOP by 5 min.

HOW SUPPLIED: Sol: 0.1% [5mL, 10mL, 15mL], 0.15% [5mL, 10mL, 15mL] (contains Purite)

CONTRAINDICATIONS: Concomitant MAOI therapy.

WARNINGS/PRECAUTIONS: Caution with severe CV disease, hepatic or renal dysfunction, depression, cerebral or coronary insufficiency, Raynaud's phenomenon, orthostatic hypotension, thromboangiitis obliterans. Wait 15 min before reinserting contacts with 0.2% solution. Monitor IOP.

ADVERSE REACTIONS: Oral dryness, ocular hyperemia, ocular pruritus, burning, stinging, ocular allergic reaction, blurred vision, foreign body sensation, fatigue, drowsiness, headache, conjunctival follicles.

INTERACTIONS: See Contraindications. May potentiate CNS depressants. May reduce BP; caution with β-blockers, antihypertensives, cardiac glycosides. Caution with TCAs. May be given with other topical products to lower IOP.

PREGNANCY: Category B, not for use in nursing.

MECHANISM OF ACTION: An α-2-adrenergic receptor agonist; reduces aqueous humor production and increases uveoscleral outflow.

PHARMACOKINETICS: Absorption: T$_{max}$=0.5-2.5 hrs. **Metabolism:** Liver (extensive). **Elimination:** Urine (74%).

ALREX   RX
loteprednol etabonate (Bausch & Lomb)

THERAPEUTIC CLASS: Corticosteroid

INDICATIONS: Relief of signs and symptoms of seasonal allergic conjunctivitis.

DOSAGE: *Adults:* 1 drop qid.

HOW SUPPLIED: Sus: 0.2% [5mL, 10mL]

CONTRAINDICATIONS: Viral diseases of the cornea and conjunctiva, including epithelial herpes simplex keratitis, vaccinia, and varicella. Mycobacterial infection and fungal diseases of the eye.

WARNINGS/PRECAUTIONS: Caution with glaucoma, herpes simplex, diseases causing thinning of cornea/sclera and other ocular viral infections. Prolonged use can cause glaucoma or secondary ocular infections (eg, fungal). Monitor IOP beyond 10 days of therapy. Wait 10 min after instillation before inserting soft contact lenses. Re-evaluate if no response after 2 days.

ADVERSE REACTIONS: Elevated IOP, foreign body sensation, itching, chemosis, epiphora, blurred vision, burning on instillation, discharge, dry eyes, photophobia.

PREGNANCY: Category C, caution in nursing.

MECHANISM OF ACTION: Corticosteroid; anti-inflammatory agent. MOA not established. Inhibits edema, fibrin deposition, capillary dilation, leukocyte migration, fibroblast proliferation, deposition of collagen, and scar formation associated with inflammation by induction of phospholipase A_2 inhibitory protein lipocortin.

PHARMACOKINETICS: Absorption: C_{max}<1ng/mL.

ALTABAX   RX
retapamulin (GlaxoSmithKline)

THERAPEUTIC CLASS: Pleuromutilin antibacterial

INDICATIONS: Topical treatment of impetigo caused by susceptible strains of microorganisms, in patients ≥9 months.

DOSAGE: *Adults:* Apply thin layer (up to 100 cm^2 in total area) bid for 5 days. May cover with sterile bandage or gauze.
Pediatrics: ≥9 months: Apply thin layer (up to 2% total BSA) bid for 5 days. May cover with sterile bandage or gauze.

HOW SUPPLIED: Oint: 1% [5g, 10g, 15g]

WARNINGS/PRECAUTIONS: D/C if sensitization or irritation occurs. Not intended for oral, intranasal, ophthalmic or intravaginal use. May cause superinfection during therapy.

ADVERSE REACTIONS: Application site reactions.

INTERACTIONS: Coadministration with ketoconazole may increase levels.

PREGNANCY: Category B, caution in nursing.

MECHANISM OF ACTION: Pleuromutilin antibacterial; selectively inhibits bacterial protein synthesis by interacting at a site on the 50S subunit of the bacterial ribosome. The binding site involves ribosomal protein L3 and is in the region of the ribosomal P site and peptidyl transferase center. By binding to this site, peptidyl transfer is inhibited, P-site interactions are blocked, and the formation of normal active 50S ribosomal subunits is prevented.

PHARMACOKINETICS: Absorption: Low systemic exposure. Following application to 800cm^2 of intact skin: C_{max}=3.5ng/mL (multiple doses). Following application to 200cm^2 of abraded skin: C_{max}=11.7ng/mL (single dose), 9.0ng/mL (multiple doses). **Distribution:** Plasma protein binding (94%). **Metabolism:** Liver via CYP3A4 (mono-oxygenation, N-demethylation). **Elimination:** Not investigated.

ALTACE RX
ramipril (King)

> ACE inhibitors can cause death/injury to developing fetus during 2nd and 3rd trimesters. Stop therapy if pregnancy detected.

THERAPEUTIC CLASS: ACE inhibitor

INDICATIONS: Hypertension, alone or with thiazide diuretics. To decrease hospitalization and mortality in stable post-MI patients that show signs of congestive heart failure. To reduce risk of MI, stroke, and cardiovascular (CV) death in patients ≥55 yrs who are at risk due to history of coronary artery disease, stroke, peripheral vascular disease, or diabetes with at least 1 other CV risk factor.

DOSAGE: *Adults:* HTN: Initial: 2.5mg qd. Maint: 2.5-20mg/day given qd or bid. Add diuretic if BP not controlled. CrCl <40mL/min: Initial: 1.25mg qd. Titrate/Max: 5mg/day. CHF Post-MI: Initial: 2.5mg bid, 1.25mg bid if hypotensive. Titrate: Increase to 5mg bid. CrCl <40mL/min: Initial: 1.25mg qd. Titrate: May increase to 1.25mg bid. Max: 2.5mg bid. Risk Reduction of MI, Stroke, Death (≥55 yrs): Initial: 2.5mg qd for 1 week. Increase to 5mg qd for next 3 weeks. Maint: 10mg qd. Reduce or d/c diuretic if possible. With Volume Depletion/Renal Artery Stenosis: Initial: 1.25mg qd.

HOW SUPPLIED: Cap: 1.25mg, 2.5mg, 5mg, 10mg

CONTRAINDICATIONS: History of ACE inhibitor-associated angioedema.

WARNINGS/PRECAUTIONS: D/C if angioedema, jaundice, or if marked LFT elevation occurs. Risk of hyperkalemia with DM, renal dysfunction. Persistent nonproductive cough and anaphylactoid reactions reported. Monitor WBCs in renal and collagen vascular disease. Fetal/neonatal morbidity and death reported. Monitor for hypotension in high-risk patients (heart failure, surgery/anesthesia, hyponatremia, high dose diuretic therapy, recent intensive diuresis, dialysis, or severe volume and/or salt depletion, etc). Caution with CHF, renal dysfunction, severe liver cirrhosis and/or ascites, and renal artery stenosis. Less effective on BP in blacks and more reports of angioedema than nonblacks. May reduce RBCs, Hgb, WBCs or platelets. May cause agranulocytosis, pancytopenia, and bone marrow depression.

ADVERSE REACTIONS: Hypotension, cough, dizziness, fatigue, angina, impotence, Stevens-Johnson syndrome.

INTERACTIONS: May increase lithium levels. Hypotension risk with diuretics. Increase risk of hyperkalemia with K+-sparing diuretics, K+ supplements, or K+-containing salt substitutes. NSAIDs may worsen renal failure and increase serum potassium.

PREGNANCY: Category C (1st trimester) and D (2nd and 3rd trimesters), not for use in nursing.

ALTOPREV RX
lovastatin (Sciele)

THERAPEUTIC CLASS: HMG-CoA reductase inhibitor

INDICATIONS: Adjunct to diet, to slow progression of coronary atherosclerosis in coronary heart disease. Adjunct to diet, for reduction of elevated total cholesterol (total-C), LDL-C, Apo B, and TG, and to increase HDL-C in patients with primary hypercholesterolemia (heterozygous familial and non-familial) and mixed dyslipidemia (Fredrickson types IIa and IIb). To reduce risk of MI, unstable angina and coronary revascularization procedures associated with asymptomatic cardiovascular disease with average to moderately elevated Total-C and LDL-C, and below average HDL-C.

DOSAGE: *Adults:* Initial: 20, 40, or 60mg qhs. Consider immediate-release lovastatin in patients requiring smaller reductions. May adjust at intervals of ≥4 weeks. Concomitant Fibrates/Niacin (≥1g/day): Try to avoid. Max: 20mg/day. Concomitant Amiodarone/Verapamil: Max: 20mg/day.

CrCl <30mL/min: Consider dose increase of >20mg/day carefully and implement cautiously. Swallow whole; do not chew or crush.

HOW SUPPLIED: Tab: Extended-Release: 20mg, 40mg, 60mg

CONTRAINDICATIONS: Active liver disease, unexplained persistent elevations of serum transaminases, pregnancy, nursing mothers.

WARNINGS/PRECAUTIONS: May increase serum transaminases and CPK levels; consider in differential diagnosis of chest pain. D/C if AST or ALT ≥3x ULN persist, if myopathy diagnosed or suspected, and a few days before major surgery. Monitor LFTs prior to therapy, at 6 weeks, 12 weeks, then periodically or with dose elevation. Caution with heavy alcohol use and/or history of hepatic disease. Caution with dose escalation in renal insufficiency. Lovastatin immediate-release found to be less effective with homozygous familial hypercholesterolemia. Rhabdomyolysis (rare), myopathy reported.

ADVERSE REACTIONS: Nausea, abdominal pain, insomnia, dyspepsia, headache, asthenia, myalgia.

INTERACTIONS: Due to increased risk of myopathy: suspend lovastatin if itraconazole, ketoconazole, erythromycin or clarithromycin must be used; avoid other CYP3A4 inhibitors (protease inhibitors, nefazodone, >1 quart/day of grapefruit juice); avoid gemfibrozil (reduce max lovastatin dose if must be used); reduce max lovastatin dose with amiodarone, verapamil, if must be used; caution with other fibrates, ≥1g/day of niacin. Avoid use with cyclosporine. Monitor warfarin. May blunt adrenal and/or gonadal steroid production; caution with steroid hormone suppressive drugs (eg, ketoconazole, spironolactone, cimetidine).

PREGNANCY: Category X, not for use in nursing.

MECHANISM OF ACTION: HMG-CoA reductase inhibitor; reduces LDL-C and total-C.

PHARMACOKINETICS: Absorption: Lovastatin: C_{max}=5.5ng/mL, T_{max}=14.2 hrs, AUC=77ng•h/mL. Lovastatine acid: C_{max}=5.8ng/mL, T_{max}=14.2 hr, AUC=87ng•h/mL. **Distribution:** Plasma protein binding (>95%). Cross blood brain/placental barriers. **Metabolism:** Liver (extensive), β-hydroxy acid (active inhibitor). **Elimination:** Urine, bile.

AMARYL   RX
glimepiride (Sanofi-Aventis)

THERAPEUTIC CLASS: Sulfonylurea (2nd generation)

INDICATIONS: Adjunct to diet and exercise, to improve glycemic control in type 2 diabetes mellitus. May use in combination with metformin or insulin.

DOSAGE: *Adults:* Initial: 1-2mg qd with breakfast or 1st main meal. Titrate: After 2mg, may increase by up to 2mg every 1-2 weeks. Maint: 1-4mg qd. Max: 8mg qd. Amaryl/Metformin: Add Metformin to 8mg qd for better glucose control. Amaryl/Insulin Therapy: If FBG >150mg/dL on 8mg qd, add low-dose insulin; increase insulin weekly as needed. Renal Insufficiency: Initial: 1mg qd. Elderly/Debilitated/Malnourished/Hepatic Insufficiency: Dose conservatively to avoid hypoglycemia.

HOW SUPPLIED: Tab: 1mg*, 2mg*, 4mg* *scored

CONTRAINDICATIONS: Diabetic ketoacidosis.

WARNINGS/PRECAUTIONS: Increased cardiovascular mortality. Hypoglycemia risk if debilitated, malnourished, or with adrenal, pituitary, renal or hepatic insufficiency. Hypoglycemia may be masked in elderly. May lose blood glucose control with stress. Secondary failure may occur. D/C if skin reactions persist or worsen.

ADVERSE REACTIONS: Dizziness, nausea, asthenia, headache, hypoglycemia.

INTERACTIONS: Potentiated hypoglycemia with alcohol, NSAIDs, highly protein-bound drugs, such as salicylates, sulfonamides, chloramphenicol, coumarins, probenecid, MAOIs, miconazole, and β-blockers. Risk of hyperglycemia with diuretics, corticosteroids, phenothiazines, thyroid products, estrogens, oral contraceptives, phenytoin, nicotinic acid, sympathomimetics, and isoniazid. Monitor for hypoglycemia when switching from long-acting sulfonylurea, and with combination therapy with insulin and metformin. Hypoglycemia may be masked with β-blockers/sympatholytic agents.

PREGNANCY: Category C, not for use in nursing.

MECHANISM OF ACTION: Sulfonylurea; lowers blood glucose by stimulating insulin release from functioning pancreatic beta cells.

PHARMACOKINETICS: Absorption: Complete (GI tract); T_{max}=2-3 hrs; (4mg PO) C_{max}=308ng/mL. **Distribution:** (IV) V_d=8.8L, (PO) 21.8L; plasma protein binding (99.5%). **Metabolism:** Complete (liver); CYP2C9; major metabolites: M1 & M2. **Elimination:** $T_{1/2}$=5.3 hrs; urine (60%) and feces (40%).

AMBIEN
zolpidem tartrate (Sanofi-Aventis) CIV

THERAPEUTIC CLASS: Imidazopyridine hypnotic

INDICATIONS: Short-term treatment of insomnia characterized by difficulties with sleep initiation.

DOSAGE: *Adults:* Tab: Usual: 10mg qhs. Elderly/Debilitated/Hepatic Insufficiency: Initial: 5mg. Decrease dose with other CNS depressants. Max: 10mg qd. Reevaluate if insomnia persists after 7-10 days.

HOW SUPPLIED: Tab: 5mg, 10mg

WARNINGS/PRECAUTIONS: Severe anaphylactic/anaphylactoid reactions reported. Abnormal thinking, behavior changes and complex behaviors (eg, sleep driving) reported. Worsening of depression or suicidal thinking may occur; use lowest feasible amount to avoid intentional overdose. Withdrawal symptoms may occur with rapid dose reduction or discontinuation. Potential impairment of activities requiring complete mental alertness (eg, operating machinery) after ingestion and following day. Avoid with alcohol. Monitor elderly and debilitated patients for impaired motor performance. Caution with hepatic impairment, mild to moderate COPD or sleep apnea, impaired drug metabolism or hemodynamic responses. Avoid if you cannot get a full night's sleep.

ADVERSE REACTIONS: Drowsiness, dizziness, headache, nausea, diarrhea, drugged feeling, dyspepsia, myalgia, lethargy, memory loss, anxiety, abnormal thoughts and behavior, tongue or throat swelling.

INTERACTIONS: Decreased alertness with imipramine. Impaired alertness and psychomotor performance with chlorpromazine. Additive psychomotor impairment with alcohol and other CNS depressants. Rifampin may decrease effects. Flumazenil may reverse effect.

PREGNANCY: Category B, not for use in nursing.

MECHANISM OF ACTION: Imidazopyridine, a non-benzodiazepine hypnotic; binds to $GABA_A$ receptor complex at the α-subunit/benzodiazepine receptor, the major modulatory site. GABA receptor complex modulation is hypothesized to be responsible for the sedative, anticonvulsant, anxiolytic, myorelaxant properties.

PHARMACOKINETICS: Absorption: Rapid. C_{max}=59ng/mL (5mg), 121ng/mL (10mg). T_{max}=1.6 (5mg, 10mg). **Distribution:** Plasma protein binding (92.5%). **Metabolism:** CYP450. **Elimination:** Renal; $T_{1/2}$=2.6 hrs (5mg), 2.5 hrs (10mg).

AMBIEN CR
zolpidem tartrate (Sanofi-Aventis) CIV

THERAPEUTIC CLASS: Imidazopyridine hypnotic

INDICATIONS: Treatment of insomnia, characterized by difficulties with sleep onset and/or sleep maintenance.

DOSAGE: *Adults:* 12.5mg qhs. Elderly/Debilitated/Hepatic Insufficiency: 6.25mg qhs. Swallow whole; do not divide, crush, or chew.

AMBISOME

HOW SUPPLIED: Tab, Extended-Release: 6.25mg, 12.5mg

WARNINGS/PRECAUTIONS: Use smallest possible effective dose, especially in elderly. Abnormal thinking and behavior changes reported with use of sedative/hypnotics. Caution with depression and conditions that could affect metabolism or hemodynamic responses. Signs and symptoms of withdrawal reported with abrupt discontinuation of sedative/hypnotics. Monitor elderly and debilitated patients for impaired motor and/or cognitive performance.

ADVERSE REACTIONS: Headache, somnolence, dizziness, nausea, hallucinations, back pain, myalgia, fatigue.

INTERACTIONS: Increased effect with alcohol and other CNS depressants. Rifampin may decrease effects. Flumazenil reverses effect.

PREGNANCY: Category C, not for use in nursing.

MECHANISM OF ACTION: Imidazopyridine, non-benzodiazepine hypnotic; binds to GABA$_A$ receptor complex at the α subunit/benzodiazepine receptor, the major modulatory site. GABA receptor complex modulation is hypothesized to be responsible for the sedative, anticonvulsant, anxiolytic, myorelaxant properties.

PHARMACOKINETICS: Absorption: Rapid; 12mg: C_{max}=134ng/mL, T_{max}=1.5 hrs, AUC=740ng•hr/mL. **Distribution:** Plasma protein binding (92.5%). **Metabolism**: CYP450. **Elimination:** Urine; $T_{1/2}$=2.8 hrs.

AMBISOME   RX
amphotericin B (Astellas)

THERAPEUTIC CLASS: Polyene antifungal

INDICATIONS: Empirical therapy for presumed fungal infection in febrile, neutropenic patients. Treatment of *Aspergillus, Candida,* or *Cryptococcus* infections refractory to amphotericin B deoxycholate or where renal impairment or unacceptable toxicity precludes its use. Treatment of cryptococcal meningitis in HIV-infected patients. Treatment of visceral leishmaniasis.

DOSAGE: *Adults:* Empiric Therapy: 3mg/kg/day IV. Systemic Infections (*Aspergillus, Candida, Cryptococcus*): 3-5mg/kg/day IV. Cryptococcal Meningitis in HIV: 6mg/kg/day IV. Visceral Leishmaniasis: Immunocompetent: 3mg/kg/day IV on Days 1-5, 14, 21. May repeat course if needed. Immunocompromised: 4mg/kg/day IV on Days 1-5, 10, 17, 24, 31, 38.
Pediatrics: 1 month-16 yrs: Empirical Therapy: 3mg/kg/day IV. Systemic Infections (*Aspergillus, Candida, Cryptococcus*): 3-5mg/kg/day IV. Cryptococcal Meningitis in HIV: 6mg/kg/day IV.Visceral Leishmaniasis: Immunocompetent: 3mg/kg/day IV on Days 1-5, 14, 21. May repeat course if needed. Immunocompromised: 4mg/kg/day IV on Days 1-5, 10, 17, 24, 31, 38.

HOW SUPPLIED: Inj: 50mg

WARNINGS/PRECAUTIONS: If anaphylaxis occurs, d/c all further infusions. Significantly less toxic than amphotericin B deoxycholate. Monitor renal, hepatic, hematopoietic function and electrolytes (especially K$^+$, Mg^{++}).

ADVERSE REACTIONS: Chills, asthenia, back pain, pain, infection, chest pain, HTN, hypotension, tachycardia, GI hemorrhage, diarrhea, nausea, vomiting, hyperglycemia, hypokalemia, dyspnea.

INTERACTIONS: Antineoplastic agents may potentiate renal toxicity, bronchospasm, hypotension. Corticosteroids and corticotropin may potentiate hypokalemia. May potentiate digitalis toxicity. May increase flucytosine toxicity. Acute pulmonary toxicity with leukocyte transfusions reported. Nephrotoxic drugs enhance potential for renal toxicity. May enhance curariform effect of skeletal muscle relaxants due to hypokalemia. Imidazoles (eg, ketocoazole, miconazole, clotrimazole, fluconazole) may induce fungal resistance; caution with combination therapy especially in immunocompromised patients.

PREGNANCY: Category B, not for use in nursing.

MECHANISM OF ACTION: Antifungal agent. Acts by binding to the sterol component of the cell membrane, which leads to changes in cell permeability and cell death in susceptible fungi. Also binds to the cholesterol component of the mammalian cell, leading to cytotoxicity.

PHARMACOKINETICS: Absorption: IV administration of variable doses resulted from different parameters. **Metabolism:** Not known.

AMCINONIDE RX
amcinonide (Various)

THERAPEUTIC CLASS: Corticosteroid

INDICATIONS: Corticosteroid responsive dermatoses.

DOSAGE: *Adults:* Apply bid-tid depending on severity.
Pediatrics: Apply bid-tid depending on severity.

HOW SUPPLIED: Cre, Oint: 0.1% [15g, 30g, 60g]; Lot: 0.1% [20mL, 60mL]

WARNINGS/PRECAUTIONS: Systemic absorption may produce reversible HPA axis suppression, manifestations of Cushing's syndrome, hyperglycemia, and glucosuria. D/C if irritation occurs. Use appropriate antifungal or antibacterial agent with dermatological infections. Pediatrics may be more susceptible to systemic toxicity. Caution when applied to large surface areas or with occlusive dressings.

ADVERSE REACTIONS: Itching, stinging, soreness, burning, irritation, folliculitis, hypertrichosis, hypopigmentation, perioral dermatitis, skin maceration, striae, miliaria, skin atrophy, secondary infection, contact dermatitis.

PREGNANCY: Category C, not for use in nursing.

MECHANISM OF ACTION: Corticosteroid: possesses anti-inflammatory, antipruritic and vasoconstrictive properties. Anti-inflammatory effects not established.

PHARMACOKINETICS: Absorption: Percutaneous; inflammation, other disease states, and use of occlusive dressings may increase absorption. **Distribution:** Systemically administered corticosteroids found in breast milk. **Metabolism:** Liver. **Elimination:** Renal, bile.

AMERGE RX
naratriptan HCL (GlaxoSmithKline)

THERAPEUTIC CLASS: 5-HT$_{1D 1B}$-agonist

INDICATIONS: Acute treatment of migraine with or without aura.

DOSAGE: *Adults:* ≥18 yrs: 1mg or 2.5mg taken with fluids; may repeat dose once after 4 hrs. Max: 5mg/24 hrs. Mild-Moderate Renal/Hepatic Impairment. Initial: Lower dose. Max: 2.5mg/24 hrs. Safety of treating >4 headaches/30 days not known.

HOW SUPPLIED: Tab: 1mg, 2.5mg

CONTRAINDICATIONS: Uncontrolled HTN, ischemic cardiac, cerebrovascular or peripheral vascular syndromes, other significant CVD, severe renal or hepatic impairment and basilar or hemiplegic migraine. Within 24 hrs of another 5-HT$_1$ agonist, ergotamine-containing or ergot-containing drug (dihydroergotamine or methysergide).

WARNINGS/PRECAUTIONS: Confirm diagnosis. Supervise 1st dose and monitor cardiac function in those at risk of CAD (eg, HTN, hypercholesterolemia, smoker, obesity, diabetes, CAD family history, postmenopausal women, males >40 yrs). Monitor cardiovascular function with long-term intermittent use. May cause vasospastic reactions or cerebrovascular events. Caution with renal or hepatic dysfunction. Avoid in elderly.

ADVERSE REACTIONS: Paresthesias, dizziness, drowsiness, malaise/fatigue, throat and neck symptoms (eg, pain/pressure sensation).

INTERACTIONS: Ergotamine-containing and ergot-type (dihydroergotamine or methysergide) drugs may cause prolonged vasospastic reactions. Avoid other 5-HT$_1$ agonist drugs within 24-hr period due to additive effects. SSRIs may cause weakness, hyperreflexia, and incoordination.

PREGNANCY: Category C, caution in nursing.

MECHANISM OF ACTION: Selective 5-HT$_1$ receptor agonist; binds with high affinity to 5-HT$_{1D/1B}$ receptors; two theories explain its efficacy in migraine. One theory suggests that activation of 5-HT$_{1D/1B}$ receptors located on intracranial blood vessels, including those on arteriovenous anastomoses, leads to vasoconstriction that correlates with relief of migraine. Another suggests that activation of 5-HT$_{1D/1B}$ receptors in trigeminal system results in inhibition of pro-inflammatory neuropeptide release.

PHARMACOKINETICS: Absorption: Well; bioavailability (70%); T$_{max}$=2-3 hr. **Metabolism:** Via CYP 450 isoenzymes. **Distribution:** V$_d$=170L, plasma protein binding (28-31%); found in breast milk. **Elimination:** Urine (50% unchanged, 30% metabolites); T$_{1/2}$=6 hrs.

AMEVIVE RX
alefacept (Astellas)

THERAPEUTIC CLASS: Immunosuppressive agent

INDICATIONS: Treatment of moderate to severe chronic plaque psoriasis for candidates of systemic therapy or phototherapy.

DOSAGE: *Adults:* 7.5mg IV bolus or 15mg IM once weekly for 12 weeks. May initiate retreatment with an additional 12-week course if CD4+ T-lymphocyte counts are within normal range and a 12-week minimum interval has passed since the previous course of treatment. CD4+ T-Lymphocyte Counts <250 cells/microliter: Withhold dose. D/C if counts remain below 250 cells/microliter for 1 month.

HOW SUPPLIED: Inj: (IV) 7.5mg, (IM) 15mg

CONTRAINDICATIONS: HIV.

WARNINGS/PRECAUTIONS: Do not initiate with CD4+ T-lymphocyte counts below normal; monitor weekly. Caution with history or risk of malignancy; d/c if malignancy develops. May increase risk of infection or reactivate latent, chronic infections; avoid with clinically important infections, caution with chronic or history of recurrent infections; d/c if serious infection develops. D/C if serious hypersensitivity reactions occur. Caution in elderly. Avoid concurrent phototherapy.

ADVERSE REACTIONS: Pharyngitis, dizziness, increased cough, nausea, pruritus, myalgia, chills, injection site pain/inflammation, lymphopenia, malignancies, serious infections, hypersensitivity reactions.

INTERACTIONS: Avoid with other immunosuppressive agents.

PREGNANCY: Category B, not for use in nursing.

MECHANISM OF ACTION: Immunosuppressive agent; interferes with lymphocyte activation by specifically binding to the lymphocyte antigen CD2, and inhibiting LFA-2/CD2 interaction. Causes reduction in subsets of CD2+ T lymphocytes (primarily CD45RO+), presumably by bridging between CD2 on target lymphocytes and immunoglobulin Fc receptors on cytotoxic cells, such as natural killer cells, which results in reduction of circulating total CD4+ and CD8+ T-lymphocyte counts.

PHARMACOKINETICS: Distribution: V$_d$=94mL/kg. **Elimination:** T$_{1/2}$=270 hrs.

AMICAR RX
aminocaproic acid (Xanodyne)

THERAPEUTIC CLASS: Monoamino carboxylic acid anti-fibrinolytic

INDICATIONS: To enhance hemostasis when fibrinolysis contributes to bleeding.

DOSAGE: *Adults:* IV: 16-20mL (4-5g) in 250mL diluent during 1st hr, then 4mL/hr (1g) in 50mL of diluent. PO: 5g during 1st hr, then 5mL (syr) or 1g (tabs) per hr. Continue therapy for 8 hrs or until bleeding is controlled.

HOW SUPPLIED: Inj: 250mg/mL [20mL]; Syrup: 1.25g/5mL; Tab: 500mg*, 1000mg* *scored

CONTRAINDICATIONS: Active intravascular clotting process, disseminated intravascular coagulation without concomitant heparin.

WARNINGS/PRECAUTIONS: Avoid in hematuria of upper urinary tract origin due to risk of intrarenal obstruction from glomerular capillary thrombosis or clots in renal pelvis and ureters. Skeletal muscle weakness with necrosis of muscle fibers reported after prolonged therapy. Consider cardiac muscle damage with skeletal myopathy. Avoid rapid IV infusion. Thrombophlebitis may occur. Contains benzyl alcohol; do not administer to neonates due to risk of fatal "gasping syndrome." Do not administer without a definite diagnosis of hyperfibrinolysis.

ADVERSE REACTIONS: Edema, headache, anaphylactoid reactions, injection site reactions, pain, bradycardia, hypotension, abdominal pain, diarrhea, nausea, vomiting, agranulocytosis, increased CPK, confusion, dyspnea, pruritus, tinnitus.

INTERACTIONS: Increased risk of thrombosis with Factor IX Complex concentrates, Anti-Inhibitor Coagulant concentrates.

PREGNANCY: Category C, caution in nursing.

MECHANISM OF ACTION: Monoamino carboxylic acid anti-fibrinolytic; fibrinolysis inhibitory effects are exerted principally by inhibition of plasminogen activators and to a lesser extent through antiplasmin activity.

PHARMACOKINETICS: Absorption: (PO) C_{max}=164mcg/mL; T_{max}=1.2 hrs. **Distribution:** (PO) V_d=23.1L; (IV) V_d=30L. **Metabolism:** Adipic acid (metabolite). **Elimination:** Renal: Urine 65% (unchanged), 11% (metabolite); $T_{1/2}$=2 hrs.

AMIKACIN   RX
amikacin sulfate (Various)

> Potential for ototoxicity and nephrotoxicity. Neuromuscular blockade, respiratory blockade reported. Avoid potent diuretics and other neurotoxic, nephrotoxic, and ototoxic drugs.

THERAPEUTIC CLASS: Aminoglycoside

INDICATIONS: Short-term treatment of serious infections due to susceptible strains of gram-negative bacteria. Shown to be effective in bacterial septicemia; respiratory tract, bone/joint, CNS (including meningitis), skin and soft tissue, and intra-abdominal infections; burns and postoperative infections; complicated and recurrent urinary tract infections (UTI) due to susceptible strains of microorganisms.

DOSAGE: *Adults:* (IM/IV) 15mg/kg/day given q8h or q12h. Max: 15mg/kg/day. Heavier Wt Patients: Max: 1.5g/day. Recurrent Uncomplicated UTI: 250mg bid. Usual Duration: 7-10 days. D/C therapy if no response after 3-5 days. D/C if azotemia increases or if progressive decrease in urinary output occurs. Renal Impairment: Reduce dose.
Pediatrics: 15mg/kg/day given q8h or q12h. Newborns: LD: 10mg/kg. Maint: 7.5mg/kg q12h. Usual Duration: 7-10 days. D/C if azotemia increases or if progressive decrease in urinary output occurs. Renal Impairment: Reduce dose.

HOW SUPPLIED: Inj: 50mg/mL, 250mg/mL

CONTRAINDICATIONS: History of serious toxic reactions to aminoglycosides.

WARNINGS/PRECAUTIONS: May aggravate muscle weakness; caution with muscular disorders (eg, myasthenia gravis, parkinsonism). May cause fetal harm in pregnancy. Contains sodium metabisulfite, allergic reactions may occur especially in asthmatics. Maintain adequate hydration. Assess kidney function before therapy, then daily.

ADVERSE REACTIONS: Ototoxicity, neuromuscular blockage, nephrotoxicity, skin rash, drug fever, headache, paresthesia, tremor, nausea, arthralgia, anemia, hypotension.

INTERACTIONS: Increased nephrotoxicity with cephalosporins. Significant mutual inactivation may occur with β-lactams (eg, penicillin, cephalosporins). Cross-allergenicity between aminoglycosides. Avoid potent diuretics (eg, ethacrynic acid, furosemide), bacitracin, cisplatin, amphotericin B, paromomycin, polymyxin B, colistin, vancomycin, other aminoglycosides, and other neurotoxic, nephrotoxic and ototoxic drugs. Increased risk of neuromuscular blockade and respiratory paralysis with anesthetics, neuromuscular blockers, or massive transfusions of citrate-anticoagulated blood.

PREGNANCY: Category D, not for use in nursing.

MECHANISM OF ACTION: Semi-synthetic aminoglycoside antibiotic derived from kanamycin.

PHARMACOKINETICS: Absorption: Rapidly absorbed after IM administration. (IV) C_{max}=38mcg/mL. **Distribution:** V_d=24L; crosses placenta; plasma protein binding (0-11%). **Elimination:** Urine; $T_{1/2}$≥2 hr; (IM) 91.9% at 8 hrs, 98.2% at 24 hrs; (IV) 84% at 9 hrs, 94% at 24 hrs.

AMILORIDE RX
amiloride HCL (Various)

THERAPEUTIC CLASS: K+-sparing diuretic

INDICATIONS: Adjunct therapy in CHF or hypertension to help restore normal serum K+ levels and to prevent hypokalemia.

DOSAGE: *Adults:* Initial: 5mg qd. Titrate: Increase to 10mg/day. If hyperkalemia persists, may increase to 15mg/day then to 20mg/day with careful monitoring. Take with food.

HOW SUPPLIED: Tab: 5mg

CONTRAINDICATIONS: Hyperkalemia, anuria, acute or chronic renal insufficiency, diabetic neuropathy, K+-sparing agents (eg, diuretics), and K+ supplements, K+ salt substitutes, K+-rich diet (except with severe hypokalemia).

WARNINGS/PRECAUTIONS: Risk of hyperkalemia (≥5.5mEq/L) especially with renal impairment, elderly, DM; monitor levels frequently. D/C if hyperkalemia occurs. Caution in severely ill in whom respiratory or metabolic acidosis may occur; monitor acid-base balance frequently. Hepatic encephalopathy reported with severe hepatic disease. Increased BUN reported. D/C at least 3 days before glucose tolerance test. Monitor electrolytes and renal function in DM.

ADVERSE REACTIONS: Headache, nausea, anorexia, vomiting, elevated serum potassium, diarrhea, muscle cramps, impotence.

INTERACTIONS: Increased risk of hyperkalemia with ACE inhibitors, angiotensin II receptor antagonists, indomethacin, cyclosporine, and tacrolimus. Risk of lithium toxicity. Decreased effects with NSAIDs. Hyponatremia and hypochloremia with other diuretics.

PREGNANCY: Category B, not for use in nursing.

MECHANISM OF ACTION: Antikaliuretic-diuretic; inhibits Na+ reabsorption at tubules and collecting duct, decreasing potential of tubular lumen, reducing K+ and H+ secretion and excretion.

PHARMACOKINETICS: Absorption: T_{max}=3-4 hrs. **Elimination:** $T_{1/2}$=6-9 hrs; Urine (50%), feces (40%).

AMILORIDE/HCTZ RX
amiloride HCL - hydrochlorothiazide (Various)

THERAPEUTIC CLASS: K+-sparing diuretic/thiazide diuretic

INDICATIONS: Treatment of hypertension or congestive heart failure if hypokalemia occurs on thiazides or kaliuretic diuretics alone, or if maintenance of normal serum K⁺ levels is clinically important.

DOSAGE: *Adults:* Initial: 1 tab qd. Titrate: May increase to 2 tabs qd or in divided doses. Max: 2 tabs/day. May give intermittently once diuresis is achieved. Take with food.

HOW SUPPLIED: Tab: (Amiloride-HCTZ) 5mg-50mg* *scored

CONTRAINDICATIONS: Hyperkalemia, anuria, sulfonamide hypersensitivity, acute or chronic renal insufficiency, diabetic neuropathy. Concomitant K⁺-sparing agents (eg, spironolactone, triamterene), K⁺ supplements, salt substitutes, K⁺-rich diet (except with severe hypokalemia).

WARNINGS/PRECAUTIONS: Risk of hyperkalemia (≥5.5mEq/L) especially with renal impairment or DM; d/c if hyperkalemia occurs. Monitor for fluid/electrolyte imbalance; hyponatremia and hypochloremia may occur. Caution in severely ill (risk of respiratory or metabolic acidosis). Increases BUN, cholesterol, and TG levels. D/C at least 3 days before glucose tolerance test. May precipitate gout or exacerbate SLE. May precipitate azotemia with renal disease.

ADVERSE REACTIONS: Nausea, anorexia, rash, headache, weakness, hyperkalemia, dizziness.

INTERACTIONS: May potentiate other antihypertensives. Risk of lithium toxicity. Increased risk of hyperkalemia with ACE inhibitors, angiotensin II receptor antagonists, indomethacin, cyclosporine, tacrolimus. May increase responsiveness to nondepolarizing muscle relaxants. May decrease response to norepinephrine. Antidiabetic agents may need adjustment. Alcohol, barbiturates, or narcotics may potentiate orthostatic hypotension. NSAIDs may decrease effects. Cholestyramine, colestipol impair absorption. ACTH, corticosteroids intensify electrolyte depletion. Increased response to nondepolarizing muscle relaxants.

PREGNANCY: Category B, not for use in nursing.

MECHANISM OF ACTION: Amiloride: Antikaliuretic diuretic; inhibits Na⁺ reabsorption at tubules and collecting duct, decreasing potential of tubular lumen, reducing K⁺ and H⁺ secretion and excretion. HCTZ: Thiazide diuretic; affects distal renal tubular mechanism of electrolyte reabsorption, increasing Na⁺ and Cl⁻ excretion.

PHARMACOKINETICS: Absorption: Amiloride: T_{max}=3-4 hrs. **Distribution:** HCTZ: Crosses placenta; excreted in breast milk. **Elimination:** Amiloride: Urine (50%), feces (40%); $T_{1/2}$=6-9 hrs. HCTZ: Kidney (61%); $T_{1/2}$=5.6-14.8 hrs.

AMITIZA   RX
lubiprostone (Sucampo/Takeda)

THERAPEUTIC CLASS: Chloride channel activator

INDICATIONS: Treatment of chronic idiopathic constipation in adults. Treatment of the irritable bowel syndrome with constipation (IBS-C) in women ≥18 yrs.

DOSAGE: *Adults:* Chronic Idiopathic Constipation: 24mcg bid with food. IBS-C: 8mcg bid with food.

HOW SUPPLIED: Cap: 8mcg, 24mcg

CONTRAINDICATIONS: History of mechanical gastrointestinal obstruction.

WARNINGS/PRECAUTIONS: Potential to cause fetal loss; women who could become pregnant should have a negative pregnancy test prior to initiation of therapy and comply with effective contraceptive measures. May cause nausea. Do not prescribe to patients with severe diarrhea. Dyspnea reported. Confirm absence of mechanical GI obstruction prior to initiating therapy.

ADVERSE REACTIONS: Nausea, diarrhea, abdominal distention/pain/discomfort, flatulence, vomiting, loose stools, sinusitis, urinary/upper respiratory tract infections, headache, dizziness, peripheral edema, arthralgia.

PREGNANCY: Category C, not for use in nursing.

MECHANISM OF ACTION: Chloride channel activator; enhances chloride-rich intestinal fluid secretion, increasing motility in the intestine, thereby facilitating the passage of stool.

PHARMACOKINETICS: Absorption: (M3): T_{max}=1.1 hrs, C_{max}=41.5pg/mL, AUC=57.1pg•hr/mL. **Distribution:** Plasma protein binding (94%). **Metabolism:** Stomach, jejunum (biotransformation via carbonyl reductase). (Metabolite): M3. **Elimination:** (M3) $T_{1/2}$=0.9-1.4hrs.

AMITRIPTYLINE   RX
amitriptyline HCL (Various)

> Antidepressants increased the risk of suicidal thinking and behavior (suicidality) in short-term studies in children, adolescents, and young adults with Major Depressive Disorder (MDD) and other psychiatric disorders.

THERAPEUTIC CLASS: Tricyclic antidepressant

INDICATIONS: Treatment of depression, especially endogenous depression.

DOSAGE: *Adults:* PO: Initial: (Outpatient) 75mg/day in divided doses or 50-100mg qhs. (Inpatient) 100mg/day. Titrate: (Outpatient) Increase by 25-50mg qhs. (Inpatient) Increase to 200mg/day. Maint: 50-100mg qhs. Max: (Outpatient) 150mg/day. (Inpatient) 300mg/day. IM: Initial: 20-30mg qid. Elderly: 10mg tid and 20mg qhs.

HOW SUPPLIED: Inj: 10mg/mL; Tab: 10mg, 25mg, 50mg, 75mg, 100mg, 150mg

CONTRAINDICATIONS: MAOI use or within 14 days; acute recovery period following MI; concurrent cisapride.

WARNINGS/PRECAUTIONS: Caution with history of seizures, urinary retention, angle-closure glaucoma, increased IOP, hyperthyroidism, cardiovascular disorders, liver dysfunction. Increases symptoms with schizophrenia and manic-depression. D/C several weeks before elective surgery. May alter blood glucose levels.

ADVERSE REACTIONS: MI, stroke, seizure, paralytic ileus, urinary retention, constipation, blurred vision, dry mouth, hyperpyrexia, rash, bone marrow depression, testicular swelling, gynecomastia (male), breast enlargement (female), alopecia, edema.

INTERACTIONS: See Contraindications. May block antihypertensive effects of guanethidine. Potentiates other CNS depressants, alcohol, barbiturates. Increased levels with CYP2D6 inhibitors (eg, quinidine, cimetidine, SSRIs) and enzyme substrates (eg, phenothiazines, propafenone, flecainide). Avoid within 5 weeks of fluoxetine use. Caution with thyroid drugs. Delirium reported with disulfiram and ethchlorvynol. Paralytic ileus and hyperpyrexia with anticholinergics. Monitor with sympathomimetics and neuroleptics. Increased plasma levels with cimetidine.

PREGNANCY: Category C, not for use in nursing.

MECHANISM OF ACTION: Dibenzocycloheptadiene derivative; suspected to inhibit the membrane pump mechanism responsible for uptake of norepinephrine and serotonin in adrenergic and serotonergic neurons.

PHARMACOKINETICS: Absorption: Rapid. **Distribution:** Excreted in breast milk. **Metabolism:** N-demethylation and hydroxylation.

AMITRIPTYLINE/PERPHENAZINE   RX
amitriptyline HCL - perphenazine (Various)

> Antidepressants increased the risk of suicidal thinking and behavior (suicidality) in short-term studies in children and adolescents with Major Depressive Disorder (MDD) and other psychiatric disorders.

THERAPEUTIC CLASS: Piperazine phenothiazine/tricyclic antidepressant

INDICATIONS: Treatment of depression and anxiety.

DOSAGE: *Adults:* Initial: 25mg-2mg tab or 25mg-4mg tab tid-qid or 50mg-4mg bid. Maint: 25mg-2mg tab or 25mg-4mg tab bid-qid or 50mg-4mg bid. Max: 4 tabs/day of 50mg-4mg or 8 tabs/day any other strength. Severe Illness with Schizophrenia: Initial: 2 tabs of 25mg-4mg tid and hs prn. Elderly/Adolescents: Initial: 10mg-4mg tab tid-qid.

HOW SUPPLIED: Tab: (Amitriptyline-Perphenazine) 10mg-2mg, 25mg-2mg, 25mg-4mg

CONTRAINDICATIONS: CNS depression from drugs, bone marrow depression, MAOI use within 14 days, acute recovery phase following MI.

WARNINGS/PRECAUTIONS: Tardive dyskinesia may develop. NMS reported. May alter blood glucose levels. D/C before elective surgery. Caution with urinary retention, angle-closure glaucoma, increased IOP, hyperthyroidism, convulsive disorders, hepatic dysfunction and cardiovascular disorders. May increase prolactin levels. May obscure diagnosis of brain tumor or intestinal obstruction due to antiemetic effects. D/C if significant increase in body temperature develops. May impair mental/physical abilities.

ADVERSE REACTIONS: Sedation, hypotension, HTN, neurological impairment, dry mouth.

INTERACTIONS: See Contraindications. May block antihypertensive effects of guanethidine. May enhance response to alcohol, opiates, analgesics, atropine, and barbiturates. Delirium reported with disulfiram. Monitor closely with thyroid agents, anticholinergics and sympathomimetics. Anticonvulsants may need dose increase. Antagonizes epinephrine. Caution with SSRIs, ethchlorvynol. May need dose reduction with CYP2D6 inhibitors (eg, quinidine, cimetidine, propafenone, flecainide). May potentiate phosphorous insecticides. Reduced metabolism with cimetidine.

PREGNANCY: Not for use in pregnancy or nursing.

AMOXAPINE   RX
amoxapine (Watson)

> Antidepressants increased the risk of suicidal thinking and behavior (suicidality) in short-term studies in children, adolescents, and young adults with Major Depressive Disorder (MDD) and other psychiatric disorders.

THERAPEUTIC CLASS: Tricyclic antidepressant

INDICATIONS: Treatment of neurotic or reactive depressive disorders, endogenous and psychotic depression, and depression accompanied by anxiety or agitation.

DOSAGE: *Adults:* Initial: 50mg bid-tid. Titrate: May increase to 100mg bid-tid by end of first week. Usual: 200-300mg/day. Max: Outpatients: 400mg/day; Inpatients: 600mg/day. Elderly: Initial: 25mg bid-tid. Titrate: May increase to 50mg bid-tid by end of first week. Max: 300mg/day. Doses ≤300mg/day may be given as single dose at bedtime.

HOW SUPPLIED: Tab: 25mg*, 50mg*, 100mg*, 150mg* *scored

CONTRAINDICATIONS: During or within 14 days of MAOIs; recent MI.

WARNINGS/PRECAUTIONS: D/C if NMS, TD, rash and/or drug fever occur. Caution with history of urinary retention, angle-closure glaucoma, or increased IOP, suicidal tendencies. May induce sinus tachycardia, changes in conduction time, arrhythmias. MI, stroke reported. Extreme caution with history of seizure disorders. Activation of mania, increased psychosis reported. May impair mental/physical abilities.

ADVERSE REACTIONS: Drowsiness, dry mouth, constipation, blurred vision.

INTERACTIONS: Avoid MAOIs (during or within 14 days of therapy). Additive effects with alcohol, barbiturates, other CNS depressants. Increased levels in poor metabolizers of CYP2D6, quinidine, cimetidine, other antidepressants, phenothiazines, propafenone, flecainide. Caution with SSRIs.

PREGNANCY: Category C, caution in nursing.

MECHANISM OF ACTION: Dibenzoxazepine; reduces uptake of NE and 5-HT and blocks response of dopamine receptors to dopamine (animal studies).

PHARMACOKINETICS: Absorption: Rapid. T_{max}=90 min. **Distribution:** Plasma protein binding (90%). **Metabolism:** Metabolite (8-hydroxyamoxapine). **Elimination:** Kidneys.

AMOXIL   RX
amoxicillin (GlaxoSmithKline)

THERAPEUTIC CLASS: Semisynthetic ampicillin derivative

INDICATIONS: Treatment of infections of the ear, nose, throat, genitourinary tract, skin and skin structure, lower respiratory tract (LRTI); acute, uncomplicated gonorrhea due to susceptible (β-lactamase negative) strains of microorganisms. Combination therapy for *H.pylori* eradication to reduce the risk of duodenal ulcer recurrence.

DOSAGE: *Adults:* Ear/Nose/Throat/SSSI/GU: (Mild/Moderate) 500mg q12h or 250mg q8h. (Severe) 875mg q12h or 500mg q8h. LRTI: 875mg q12h or 500mg q8h. Gonorrhea: 3g as single dose. *H.pylori:* (Dual Therapy) 1g + 30mg lansoprazole, both tid x 14 days. (Triple Therapy) 1g + 30mg lansoprazole + 500mg clarithromycin, all q12h x 14 days. (Amoxicillin) CrCl 10-30mL/min: 250-500mg q12h. CrCl <10mL/min: 250-500mg q24h. Hemodialysis: 250-500mg or 250mg q24h, additional dose during and at end of dialysis.
Pediatrics: Neonates: ≤12 weeks: Max: 30mg/kg/day divided q12h. >3 months: Ear/Nose/Throat/SSSI/GU: (Mild/Moderate) 25mg/kg/day given q12h or 20mg/kg/day given q8h. (Severe) 45mg/kg/day given q12h or 40mg/kg/day given q8h. LRTI: 45mg/kg/day given q12h or 40mg/kg/day given q8h. Gonorrhea: (Prepubertal) 50mg/kg with 25mg/kg probenecid as single dose. (Not for <2yrs). >40kg: Dose as adult.

HOW SUPPLIED: Cap: 500mg; Sus: 50mg/mL [30mL], 200mg/5mL [50mL, 75mL, 100mL], 250mg/5mL [100mL, 150mL], 400mg/5mL [50mL, 75mL, 100mL]; Tab: 500mg, 875mg; Tab, Chewable: 200mg, 400mg

WARNINGS/PRECAUTIONS: Serious, sometimes fatal, hypersensitivity reactions reported with PCN therapy. *Clostridium difficile*-associated diarrhea has been reported. Monitor renal, hepatic, and blood with prolonged use. The 200mg and 400mg chewable tabs contain phenylalanine.

ADVERSE REACTIONS: Nausea, vomiting, diarrhea, pseudomembranous colitis, hypersensitivity reactions, blood dyscrasias, superinfection (prolonged use).

INTERACTIONS: Increased levels with probenecid. Chloramphenicol, macrolides, sulfonamides, tetracyclines may interfere with bactericidal effects. False (+) for urine glucose with Clinitest®, Benedict's or Fehling's solution.

PREGNANCY: Category B, caution in nursing.

MECHANISM OF ACTION: Ampicillin analog; has a broad-spectrum bactericidal activity against susceptible organisms during active multiplication; acts through inhibition of biosynthesis of cell-wall mucopeptide.

PHARMACOKINETICS: Absorption: Rapid. Cap (500mg): T_{max}=1-2 hrs. Tab (875mg): C_{max}=13.8mcg/mL, AUC=35.4mcg•hr/mL. Oral suspension (400mg): C_{max}=5.92mcg/mL, AUC=17.1mcg•hr/mL. Chewable tab (400mg): C_{max}=5.18mcg/mL, AUC=17.9mcg•hr/mL. Oral suspension (125-250mg) T_{max}=1-2 hrs. **Distribution:** Plasma protein binding, (20%). Diffuses to spinal fluid and brain only if meninges inflamed. **Elimination:** Urine (unchanged); $T_{1/2}$=61.3 min.

AMPHOCIN
amphotericin B (Pharmacia & Upjohn)

RX

> Treatment primarily for progressive and potentially life-threatening fungal infections. Not for noninvasive fungal infections (eg, oral thrush, vaginal and esophageal candidiasis) in patients with normal neutrophil counts. Exercise caution to prevent inadvertent OD; verify product name and dose if dose >1.5mg/kg.

THERAPEUTIC CLASS: Polyene antifungal

INDICATIONS: Treatment of potentially life-threatening fungal infections including aspergillosis, cryptococcosis, North American blastomycosis, systemic candidiasis, coccidioidomycosis, histoplasmosis, zygomycosis, sporotrichosis, and infections due to susceptible species of *Conidiobolus* and *Basidiobolus*. May be useful for treatment of American mucocutaneous leishmaniasis.

DOSAGE: *Adults:* Administer by slow IV infusion. Test dose: 1mg in 20mL of D5W over 20-30 min. Treatment: Initial: 0.25mg/kg. Severe Infection: Initial: 0.3mg/kg. Give smaller initial dose if impaired cardio-renal function or severe reaction to test dose. Titrate: May increase by 5-10mg/day, depending on cardio-renal status, up to 0.5-0.7mg/kg/day. Max: 1mg/kg/day or 1.5mg/kg/day when given on alternate days. Sporotrichosis: Therapy has ranged up to 9 months with total dose up to 2.5g. Aspergillosis: Has been treated up to 11 months with total dose up to 3.6g. Rhinocerebral Phycomycosis: Cumulative dose of at least 3g is recommended. Whenever therapy is interrupted for >7 days, resume with lowest dose.

HOW SUPPLIED: Inj: 50mg

WARNINGS/PRECAUTIONS: Acute reactions (eg, fever, shaking chills, hypotension, anorexia, nausea, vomiting, tachypnea) 1-3 hrs after starting infusion may occur. Avoid rapid infusion. Caution with renal impairment. Decreased risk of nephrotoxicity with hydration and sodium repletion. Acute pulmonary reactions reported with leukocyte infusions; separate infusions and monitor pulmonary function. Leukoencephalopathy reported. Monitor renal function, LFTs, electrolytes, blood counts, Hgb.

ADVERSE REACTIONS: Fever, malaise, weight loss, hypotension, tachypnea, anorexia, nausea, vomiting, diarrhea, dyspepsia, normochromic normocytic anemia, injection site pain, renal dysfunction.

INTERACTIONS: Antineoplastics may potentiate renal toxicity, bronchospasm, hypotension. Corticosteroids and corticotropin may potentiate hypokalemia. May increase flucytosine toxicity. Caution with imidazoles (eg, ketoconazole, clotrimazole, miconazole, fluconazole). Increased risk of renal toxicity with nephrotoxic drugs (eg, aminoglycosides, cyclosporine, pentamidine). May enhance curariform effect of skeletal muscle relaxants (eg, tubocurarine) or digitalis toxicity with hypokalemia.

PREGNANCY: Category B, not for use in nursing.

MECHANISM OF ACTION: Fungistatic or fungicidal; binds to sterols in cell membranes of susceptible fungi, resulting in change in membrane permeability, allowing leakage of intracellular components.

PHARMACOKINETICS: Absorption: C_{max} = approximately 0.5-2mcg/mL. **Distribution:** Plasma protein binding (>90%). **Elimination:** Renal excretion. $T_{1/2}$ = approximately 15 days. Urine= approximately 40% (urinary output over 7-day period).

AMPHOTEC
amphotericin B cholesteryl sulfate (Three Rivers)

RX

THERAPEUTIC CLASS: Polyene antifungal

INDICATIONS: Treatment of invasive aspergillosis in patients with renal impairment, unacceptable toxicity, or previous failure to amphotericin deoxycholate.

DOSAGE: *Adults:* Test Dose: Infuse small amount over 15-30 min. Treatment: 3-4mg/kg/day IV at 1mg/kg/hr.
Pediatrics: Test Dose: Infuse small amount over 15-30 min. Treatment: 3-4mg/kg/day IV at 1mg/kg/hr.

HOW SUPPLIED: Inj: 50mg, 100mg

WARNINGS/PRECAUTIONS: Anaphylaxis may occur. D/C if severe respiratory distress occurs. Acute reactions (eg, fever, shaking chills, hypotension, nausea, tachypnea) 1-3 hrs after starting infusion. Monitor renal/hepatic function, electrolytes, CBC, PT during therapy.

ADVERSE REACTIONS: Chills, fever, headache, hypotension, tachycardia, HTN, nausea, vomiting, thrombocytopenia, increased creatinine, hypokalemia, dyspnea, hypoxia.

INTERACTIONS: Antineoplastics may potentiate renal toxicity, bronchospasm, hypotension. Corticosteroids and corticotropin may potentiate hypokalemia. May increase flucytosine toxicity. Caution with imidazoles (eg, ketoconazole, clotrimazole, miconazole, fluconazole). Increased risk of renal toxicity with nephrotoxic drugs (eg, aminoglycosides, cyclosporine, pentamidine). May enhance curariform effect of skeletal muscle relaxants (eg, tubocurarine) or digitalis toxicity with hypokalemia.

PREGNANCY: Category B, not for use in nursing.

MECHANISM OF ACTION: Polyene antibiotic; binds to sterols (primarily ergosterol) in cell membranes of sensitive fungi, with subsequent leakage of intracellular contents and cell death. Also binds to cholesterol in mammalian cell membranes, which may account for human toxicity.

PHARMACOKINETICS: Administration: Variable doses resulted in altered parameters. **Absorption:** 3mg/kg/day: AUC=29μg/mL•hr, C_{max}=2.6μg/mL. 4mg/kg/day: AUC=36μg/mL•hr, C_{max}=2.9μg/mL. **Distribution:** 3mg/kg/day: V_d=3.8L/kg. 4mg/kg/day: V_d=4.1L/kg. **Metabolism:** Unknown. **Elimination:** 3mg/kg/day: $T_{1/2}$=27.5 hrs. 4mg/kg/day: $T_{1/2}$=28.2 hrs.

AMPICILLIN INJECTION   RX
ampicillin sodium (Various)

THERAPEUTIC CLASS: Semisynthetic penicillin derivative

INDICATIONS: Treatment of respiratory tract, urinary tract, and GI infections, bacterial meningitis, septicemia, and endocarditis caused by susceptible strains of microorganisms.

DOSAGE: *Adults:* IM/IV: Respiratory Tract/Soft Tissues: ≥40kg: 250-500mg q6h. <40kg: 25-50mg/kg/day given q6-8h. GI/GU: ≥40kg: 500mg q6h. <40kg: 50mg/kg/day given q6-8h. Urethritis (Caused by *N.gonorrhea* in Males): 500mg q8-12h for 2 doses; may retreat if needed. Bacterial Meningitis: 150-200mg/kg/day given q3-4h. Septicemia: 150-200mg/kg/day IV for 3 days, continue with IM q3-4h. Treatment of all infections should be continued for a minimum of 48-72 hrs after becoming asymptomatic. Minimum of 10 days treatment recommended for Group A β-hemolytic streptococci.
Pediatrics: Bacterial Meningitis: 150-200mg/kg/day given q3-4h. Septicemia: 150-200mg/kg/day IV given q3-4h for 3 days, continue with IM q3-4h. Treatment of all infections should be continued for a minimum of 48-72 hrs after becoming asymptomatic. Minimum of 10 days treatment recommended for Group A β-hemolytic streptococci.

HOW SUPPLIED: Inj: 250mg, 500mg, 1g, 2g

WARNINGS/PRECAUTIONS: Serious, sometimes fatal, hypersensitivity reactions reported with PCN therapy. Caution with renal impairment. Cross-sensitivity with other β-lactams. May cause skin rash, especially in mononucleosis; avoid use. Pseudomembranous colitis reported. May result in overgrowth of nonsusceptible organisms.

ADVERSE REACTIONS: Headache, nausea, vomiting, oral and vaginal candidiasis, diarrhea, urticaria, allergic reactions, anaphylaxis, serum sickness-like reactions, exfoliative dermatitis.

INTERACTIONS: Potentiated by probenecid. May decrease effects of oral contraceptives. Allopurinol increases incidence of skin rash.

PREGNANCY: Category B, caution in nursing.

MECHANISM OF ACTION: Penicillin derivative; bactericidal against gram-positive and gram-negative organisms.

PHARMACOKINETICS: Distribution: Plasma protein binding (20%), found in breast milk. Penetrates to CSF and brain only if meninges are inflamed. **Elimination:** Urine (unchanged).

AMPICILLIN ORAL   RX
ampicillin (Various)

THERAPEUTIC CLASS: Semisynthetic penicillin derivative

INDICATIONS: Genitourinary tract (GU) infections, including gonorrhea, respiratory and GI tract infections, and meningitis.

DOSAGE: *Adults:* GI/GU: 500mg qid. Use larger doses in chronic or severe infections. Gonorrhea: 3.5g single dose with 1g probenecid. Respiratory: 250mg qid. Treat minimum 48-72 hrs after eradication. Treat minimum 10 days for hemolytic strains of strep.
Pediatrics: >20kg: GI/GU: 500mg qid. Respiratory: 250mg qid. ≤20kg: GI/GU: 25mg/kg qid. Respiratory: 50mg/kg/day given tid-qid. Do not exceed adult doses. Use larger doses in chronic or severe infections. Treat minimum 48-72 hrs after eradication. Treat minimum 10 days for hemolytic strains of strep.

HOW SUPPLIED: Cap: 250mg, 500mg; Sus: 125mg/5mL, 250mg/5mL [100mL, 200mL]

CONTRAINDICATIONS: Infections caused by penicillinase-producing organisms.

WARNINGS/PRECAUTIONS: Possible cross-sensitivity with cephalosporins. Pseudomembranous colitis and anaphylatic reactions may occur.

ADVERSE REACTIONS: Stomatitis, nausea, vomiting, diarrhea, rash, SGOT elevation, blood dyscrasias, eosinophilia, thrombocytopenic purpura, hypersensitivity reactions, superinfection (prolonged use).

INTERACTIONS: Increased risk of rash with allopurinol. Bacteriostatic antibiotics (eg, chloramphenicol, erythromycins, sulfonamides or tetracyclines) may interfere with bactericidal activity. May decrease the effectiveness of oral contraceptives. Increased blood levels with probenecid.

PREGNANCY: Category B, not for use in nursing.

MECHANISM OF ACTION: Penicillin derivative; bactericidal against gram-positive and gram-negative organisms.

PHARMACOKINETICS: Absorption: Well-absorbed; (500mg Cap) C_{max}=3mcg/mL; (250mg Sus) C_{max}=2.3mcg/mL. **Distribution:** Plasma protein binding (20%). **Elimination:** Urine (unchanged).

AMRIX   RX
cyclobenzaprine HCL (Cephalon)

THERAPEUTIC CLASS: Skeletal muscle relaxant (central-acting)

INDICATIONS: Adjunct to rest and physical therapy to relieve muscle spasm associated with acute, painful musculoskeletal conditions. Use for only short periods of time (up to 2-3 weeks).

DOSAGE: *Adults:* Usual: 15mg qd. Titrate: May increase to 30mg qd if needed. Use for longer than 2-3 weeks not recommended.

HOW SUPPLIED: Cap, Extended-Release: 15mg, 30mg

CONTRAINDICATIONS: MAOI use during or within 14 days. Hyperpyretic crisis seizures and deaths associated with concomitant use of cyclobenzaprine (or stucturally similar to TCAs) and MAOIs reported. Acute recovery phase of MI, arrhythmias, heart block conduction disturbances, CHF, hyperthyroidism.

AMVISC PLUS

WARNINGS/PRECAUTIONS: Avoid in hepatic impairment and elderly patients. Caution with history of urinary retention, angle-closure glaucoma, increased IOP, and use of anticholinergic medication. May impair mental and/or physical performance.

ADVERSE REACTIONS: Drowsiness, dry mouth, dizziness, somnolence, headache.

INTERACTIONS: Contraindicated with MAOIs. Enhances effects of alcohol, barbiturates and other CNS depressants. TCAs may block antihypertensive action of guanethidine and similar compounds and may enhance seizure risk with tramadol.

PREGNANCY: Category B, caution in nursing.

MECHANISM OF ACTION: Skeletal muscle relaxant; acts primarily within the CNS at brain stem as opposed to spinal cord level, although overlapping action on the latter may contribute to its overall skeletal muscle relaxant activity; suggested to reduce tonic somatic motor activity influencing both gamma and α motor systems.

PHARMACOKINETICS: Absorption: C_{max}=8.3ng/mL, T_{max}=8.1 hrs, AUC=354.1ng•h/mL; see Full Prescribing Information for more detailed information. **Metabolism:** Extensive; via CYP3A4, 1A2, and 2D6 through N-demethylation pathway. **Elimination:** Urine (glucuronides); $T_{1/2}$=33.4 hrs.

AMVISC PLUS   RX
sodium hyaluronate (Bausch & Lomb)

THERAPEUTIC CLASS: Surgical aid

INDICATIONS: Surgical aid in ophthalmic anterior and posterior segment procedures (eg, cataract extraction, intraocular lens (IOL) implantation, corneal transplant surgery, glaucoma filtering surgery, surgical procedures to reattach retina).

DOSAGE: *Adults:* Cataract Surgery/IOL Implant: Infuse required amount slowly through needle/cannula into anterior chamber. Perform prior to cataract extraction and IOL insertion. May apply to IOL prior to insertion. May inject prn during procedure. Corneal Transplant: Remove corneal button and fill anterior chamber until level with cornea surface. Place donor graft on top and suture into place. May use prn during procedures. Glaucoma Filtration: Inject through corneal paracentesis to restore and maintain anterior chamber volume during trabeculectomy. May use prn during procedures. Intraocular Injection With Scleral Buckling Procedures For Retina Reattachment: After release subretinal fluid and develop buckling by tying mattress sutures, inject air into vitreous cavity and exchange with sodium hyaluronate (2-4mL) injected with 22-30 gauge needle passed via pars plana epithelium.

HOW SUPPLIED: Sol: 16mg/mL [0.5mL, 0.8mL]

WARNINGS/PRECAUTIONS: Do not use excessive quantity. Remove from anterior chamber at end of surgery. Administer appropriate therapy if post-op IOP above expected levels. Avoid reuse of cannula. Diffuse particulates and haziness reported after injection.

ADVERSE REACTIONS: Transient post-op inflammation and increased IOP.

PREGNANCY: Safety in pregnancy or nursing not known.

ANAFRANIL   RX
clomipramine HCL (Mallinckrodt)

> Antidepressants increased the risk of suicidal thinking and behavior (suicidality) in short-term studies in children, adolescents, and young adults with Major Depressive Disorder (MDD) and other psychiatric disorders. Clomipramine is not approved for use in pediatric patients except for patients with OCD.

THERAPEUTIC CLASS: Tricyclic antidepressant

INDICATIONS: Treatment of OCD.

DOSAGE: *Adults:* Initial: 25mg/day with meals. Titrate: Increase within 2 weeks to 100mg/day. Increase further over several weeks. Max: 250mg/day. Maint: May give total daily dose at bedtime.
Pediatrics: >10 yrs: Initial: 25mg/day with meals. Titrate: Increase within 2 weeks to 3mg/kg or 100mg/day, whichever is smaller. Increase further over several weeks. Max: 3mg/kg/day or 200mg/day. Maint: May give total daily dose at bedtime.

HOW SUPPLIED: Cap: 25mg, 50mg, 75mg

CONTRAINDICATIONS: MAOI use within 14 days, acute recovery period following MI.

WARNINGS/PRECAUTIONS: Pooled analyses of short-term placebo-controlled trials of antidepressant drugs showed that these drugs increase the risk of suicidal thinking and behavior (suicidality) in children, adolescents, and young adults (ages 18-24) with major depressive disorder (MDD) and other psychiatric disorders. Increased risks with electroconvulsive therapy. D/C prior to elective surgery. Avoid abrupt withdrawal. Caution with seizure disorder, conditions predisposing to seizures (eg, brain damage, alcoholism), urinary retention, narrow-angle glaucoma, adrenal medulla tumors, increased IOP, hyperthyroidism, cardiovascular disorders, liver dysfunction, significant renal dysfunction. Monitor hepatic enzymes with liver dysfunction. Weight changes, sexual dysfunction, blood dyscrasias, elevated liver enzymes reported. Hypomania/mania reported with affective disorder. Psychosis reported with schizophrenia. All patients being treated with antidepressants for any indication should be monitored appropriately and observed closely for clinical worsening, suicidality, and unusual changes in behavior, especially during the initial few months of therapy or at times of dose changes.

ADVERSE REACTIONS: Dry mouth, constipation, nausea, dyspepsia, anorexia, weight gain, increased sweating, increased appetite, myoclonus, nervousness, libido change, dizziness, tremor, somnolence, impotence, visual changes.

INTERACTIONS: See Contraindications. Caution with anticholinergics, sympathomimetics, thyroid and CNS drugs. May block effects of clonidine, guanethidine. Increased levels with haloperidol, methyphenidate, highly protein bound drugs, CYP2D6 inhibitors (eg, quinidine, cimetidine, SSRIs) and enzyme substrates (eg, phenothiazines, propafenone, flecainide). At least 5 weeks must elapse before starting TCA therapy after fluoxetine discontinuation. Decreased levels with enzyme inducers (eg, barbiturates, phenytoin). Additive effects with CNS depressants, barbiturates, alcohol. NMS reported with neuroleptics. Increases phenobarbital and highly protein bound drugs (eg, warfarin, digoxin) plasma levels.

PREGNANCY: Category C, not for use in nursing.

MECHANISM OF ACTION: Dibenzazepine (TCA); unknown, capacity to inhibit reuptake of 5-HT.

PHARMACOKINETICS: Absorption: Administration of variable doses resulted in different parameters. **Distribution:** Plasma protein binding (97%); excreted in breast milk. **Metabolism:** Hepatic (biotransformation). Metabolite (desmethylclomipramine). **Elimination:** Biliary excretion. Clomipramine: $T_{1/2}$=32 hrs. Desmethylclomipramine: $T_{1/2}$=69 hrs.

ANALPRAM-HC   RX
pramoxine HCL - hydrocortisone acetate (Ferndale)

THERAPEUTIC CLASS: Corticosteroid/anesthetic

INDICATIONS: Corticosteroid responsive dermatoses of the anal region.

DOSAGE: *Adults:* Apply tid-qid. May use occlusive dressings in psoriasis or recalcitrant conditions. For cleansing anogenital area, spread lotion on cotton or tissue and wipe affected area.
Pediatrics: Apply tid-qid. May use occlusive dressings in psoriasis or recalcitrant conditions. For cleansing anogenital area, spread lotion on cotton or tissue and wipe affected area.

AnaMantle HC

HOW SUPPLIED: Cre: (Hydrocortisone-Pramoxine) 1%-1%, 2.5%-1% [30g]; Lot: 2.5%-1% [60mL]

WARNINGS/PRECAUTIONS: May produce reversible HPA axis suppression, manifestations of Cushing's syndrome, hyperglycemia, and glucosuria. D/C use if irritation occurs. Avoid eyes. Peds may be more susceptible to systemic toxicity. Use appropriate therapy with infections.

ADVERSE REACTIONS: Burning, itching, irritation, dryness, folliculitis, hyper-trichosis, acneiform eruptions, hypopigmentation, perioral dermatitis, allergic contact dermatitis, secondary infection, skin maceration, skin atrophy, striae, miliaria.

PREGNANCY: Category C, caution in nursing.

MECHANISM OF ACTION: Unknown. Hydrocortisone: Suspected to act as anti-inflammatory, anti-pruritic, and vasoconstrictor. Pramoxine: Anesthetic agent, suspected to stabilize neuronal membrane of nerve endings.

PHARMACOKINETICS: Absorption: Absorbed from normal intact skin. **Distribution:** Plasma protein binding in varying degrees. **Metabolism:** Liver. **Elimination:** Kidney, bile (metabolites).

AnaMantle HC RX
lidocaine HCL - hydrocortisone acetate (Kenwood Therapeutics)

THERAPEUTIC CLASS: Corticosteroid/local anesthetic

INDICATIONS: Relief of itching, pain, soreness, discomfort due to hemor-rhoids, anal fissures, pruritus ani.

DOSAGE: *Adults:* Apply rectally bid.

HOW SUPPLIED: Cre: (Hydrocortisone-Lidocaine): 0.5%-3% [7g]

CONTRAINDICATIONS: Tuberculosis, fungal lesions, skin vaccinia, varicella, acute herpes simplex.

WARNINGS/PRECAUTIONS: Caution with impaired liver function, debilitated, elderly. D/C if irritation occurs. Not for prolonged use. May cause adrenal sup-pression with systemic absorption.

ADVERSE REACTIONS: Transient stinging or burning, transient blanching, erythema.

INTERACTIONS: Additive adverse effects with Class I antiarrhythmics.

PREGNANCY: Category B, caution in nursing.

Anaprox DS RX
naproxen sodium (Roche Labs)

> NSAIDs may cause an increased risk of serious cardiovascular thrombotic events, MI, stroke, and serious GI adverse events including bleeding, ulceration, and perforation of the stomach or intestines. Contraindicated for the treatment of perioperative pain in the setting of coronary artery bypass graft (CABG) surgery.

OTHER BRAND NAMES: Anaprox (Roche Labs)

THERAPEUTIC CLASS: NSAID

INDICATIONS: Relief of signs and symptoms of rheumatoid arthritis (RA), osteoarthritis (OA), ankylosing spondylitis, juvenile arthritis (JA), tendinitis, bursitis, and acute gout. Management of pain and primary dysmenorrhea.

DOSAGE: *Adults:* RA/OA/AS: 275mg bid or 550mg bid. Max: 1650mg/day. Acute Gout: 825mg followed by 275mg q8h. Pain/Dysmenorrhea/Tendinitis/Bursitis: 550mg followed by 550mg q12h or 275mg q6-8h prn. Max: 1375mg on Day 1, then 1100mg/day.

HOW SUPPLIED: (Anaprox) Tab: 275mg; (Anaprox DS) Tab: 550mg* *scored

CONTRAINDICATIONS: History of ASA or NSAID allergy that caused symp-toms of asthma, rhinitis, nasal polyps, and hypotension. Treatment of periop-erative pain in the setting of CABG surgery.

WARNINGS/PRECAUTIONS: May lead to onset of new HTN or worsening of pre-existing HTN; monitor BP closely. Fluid retention, edema, and peripheral edema reported; caution with fluid retention, HTN, or heart failure. Renal papillary necrosis and other renal injury reported after long-term use. Not recommended for use with advanced renal disease; if therapy must be initiated, monitor renal function. Anaphylactoid reactions may occur. May cause serious skin adverse events (eg, exfoliative dermatitis, Stevens-Johnson syndrome, and toxic epidermal necrolysis). Avoid in late pregnancy; may cause premature closure of ductus arteriosis. Monitor Hgb levels with long-term therapy if initial Hgb ≤10g. Monitor for visual changes or disturbances. May cause elevations of LFTs; d/c if liver disease develops or systemic manifestations occur. Caution with high doses in chronic alcoholic liver disease and elderly. Anemia may occur; with long-term use, monitor Hgb/Hct if signs or symptoms of anemia develop. May inhibit platelet aggregation and prolong bleeding time; monitor with coagulation disorders. Caution with asthma and avoid with ASA-sensitive asthma.

ADVERSE REACTIONS: Edema, drowsiness, dizziness, constipation, heartburn, abdominal pain, nausea, headache, tinnitus, dyspnea, pruritus, skin eruptions, ecchymoses.

INTERACTIONS: Avoid other products containing naproxen. Decreased plasma levels with ASA. May reduce tubular secretion of methotrexate; monitor for toxicity. May diminish antihypertensive effect and potentiate renal disease with ACE inhibitors. May reduce natriuretic effect of furosemide and thiazides. May increase lithium levels; monitor for toxicity. Synergistic effects on GI bleeding with warfarin. Observe for dose adjustment with hydantoins, sulfonamides, or sulfonylureas. May reduce antihypertensive effects of propranolol and other β-blockers. Probenecid may increase half-life.

PREGNANCY: Category C, not for use in nursing.

MECHANISM OF ACTION: NSAIDs; unknown, suspected to inhibit prostaglandin synthetase.

PHARMACOKINETICS: Absorption: Rapid and complete. Bioavailability (95%). T_{max}=1-2 hrs. **Distribution:** Plasma protein binding (>99%). V_d=0.16 L/kg; excreted in breast milk. **Metabolism:** Hepatic, metabolite (6-O-desmethyl naproxen). **Elimination:** Kidneys, urine (95%), feces (≤3%), $T_{1/2}$=12-17 hrs.

ANCOBON RX
flucytosine (Valeant)

> Extreme caution with renal dysfunction. Monitor hematologic, renal, and hepatic status closely.

THERAPEUTIC CLASS: 5-fluorocytosine antifungal

INDICATIONS: Treatment of septicemia, endocarditis, and urinary tract infections caused by Candida. Treatment of meningitis and pulmonary infection caused by Cryptococcus.

DOSAGE: Adults: 50-150mg/kg/day given q6h. Renal Impairment: Reduce initial dose. Take a few caps over 15 min to reduce nausea/vomiting.

HOW SUPPLIED: Cap: 250mg, 500mg

WARNINGS/PRECAUTIONS: Caution with renal dysfunction and bone marrow depression. Bone marrow depression can be irreversible and fatal.

ADVERSE REACTIONS: Myocardial toxicity, chest pain, dyspnea, rash, pruritus, urticaria, photosensitivity, nausea, vomiting, jaundice, renal failure, pyrexia, crystalluria, anemia, leukopenia, eosinophilia, thrombocytopenia, ataxia, hearing loss, neuropathy.

INTERACTIONS: Antagonized by cytosine. Drugs that impair glomerular filtration may prolong half-life. Antifungal synergism with polyene antibiotics (eg, amphotericin B).

PREGNANCY: Category C, not for use in nursing.

MECHANISM OF ACTION: Antifungal agent not established. Is metabolized to 5-fluorouracil by entering the fungal organism via cytosine permease. The 5-fluorouracil is then incorporated into the fungal RNA where it inhibits the synthesis of both RNA and DNA, inhibiting fungal growth, leading to fungal death.

PHARMACOKINETICS: Administration: 78% to 89% absolute bioavailability; C_{max}=30-40µg/mL; T_{max}=2 hrs. **Distribution:** Penetrates blood-brain barrier. Clinically significant amounts found in CSF. **Metabolism:** Alpha-fluro-beta-ureido-propionic acid (metabolite). **Elimination:** Renal. Urine (90%), feces (small amount); $T_{1/2}$=2.4 to 4.8 hrs.

ANDRODERM
testosterone (Watson)

THERAPEUTIC CLASS: Androgen

INDICATIONS: Testosterone replacement therapy in males due to primary or secondary hypogonadism.

DOSAGE: *Adults:* Initial: 5mg/day. Maint: 2.5mg-7.5mg/day. Apply patch nightly to intact skin of back, abdomen, upper arm or thigh. Rotate sites; avoid same site for 7 days. Do not apply to scrotum or oily, damaged, irritated areas. May apply 2 patches at same time.
Pediatrics: ≥15 yrs: Initial: 5mg/day. Maint: 2.5mg-7.5mg/day. Apply patch nightly to intact skin of back, abdomen, upper arm or thigh. Rotate sites; avoid same site for 7 days. Do not apply to scrotum or oily, damaged, irritated areas. May apply 2 patches at same time.

HOW SUPPLIED: Patch: 2.5mg/24 hrs [60s], 5mg/24 hrs [30s]

CONTRAINDICATIONS: Breast or prostate cancer in men. Women.

WARNINGS/PRECAUTIONS: Prolonged use is associated with serious hepatic effects. Increased risk for prostatic hyperplasia/carcinoma in elderly. Risk of edema with pre-existing cardiac, renal, or hepatic disease; d/c if edema occurs. Risk of virilization of female sex partner. Monitor LFTs, Hgb, Hct, PSA, cholesterol, lipids.

ADVERSE REACTIONS: Gynecomastia, pruritus/erythema/vesicles/blister at application site, prostate abnormalities, headache, depression.

INTERACTIONS: May potentiate effects of anticoagulants, oxyphenbutazone. May decrease blood glucose and insulin requirements in diabetics. Pretreatment with ointments may reduce testosterone absorption.

PREGNANCY: Category X, not for use in nursing.

MECHANISM OF ACTION: Endogenous androgen; responsible for normal growth and development of male sex organs and for maintenance of secondary sex characteristics.

PHARMACOKINETICS: Absorption: C_{max}=753ng/dL, T_{max}=7.9 hrs. **Distribution:** SHBG and albumin binding. **Metabolism:** Liver, estradiol, and DHT (major metabolite). **Elimination:** (IM) Urine=90% (glucuronide and sulfate conjugates), feces=6% (unconjugated); $T_{1/2}$=71 min.

ANDROGEL
testosterone (Unimed)
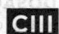

THERAPEUTIC CLASS: Androgen

INDICATIONS: Testosterone replacement in males with primary hypogonadism or hypogonadotrophic hypogonadism.

DOSAGE: *Adults:* Apply 5g qd to clean, dry, intact skin of shoulders and upper arms and/or abdomen. Allow to dry prior to dressing. Titrate: May increase to 7.5g qd, then 10g qd if response not achieved. Do not apply to scrotum/genitals. Pump: 4 actuations (5g), 6 actuations (7.5g), 8 actuations (10g).

HOW SUPPLIED: Gel: 1% [2.5g, 5g pkts; 75g pump]

CONTRAINDICATIONS: Breast or prostate carcinoma in men. Women. Pregnant women should avoid skin contact with application sites in men.

WARNINGS/PRECAUTIONS: Prolonged use is associated with serious hepatic effects. Increased risk for prostatic hyperplasia/carcinoma in elderly. Risk of edema with pre-existing cardiac, renal, or hepatic disease; d/c if edema occurs. Risk of virilization of female sex partner. Monitor LFTs, Hgb, Hct, PSA, cholesterol, lipids. May potentiate sleep apnea. Transfer of testosterone can occur with skin to skin contact. Gels are flammable; avoid fire, flame, or smoking during use.

ADVERSE REACTIONS: Acne, application site reaction, abnormal lab tests, prostatic disorders.

INTERACTIONS: May decrease blood glucose and insulin requirements. Concurrent use with ACTH or corticosteroids may enhance edema. Changes in anticoagulant activity may be seen with androgens, increase frequency of monitoring INR and PT with concomitant anticoagulants.

PREGNANCY: Category X, not for use in nursing.

MECHANISM OF ACTION: Endogenous androgen; responsible for normal growth and development of male sex organs and for maintenance of secondary sex characteristics.

PHARMACOKINETICS: Absorption: 10% absorbed systemically. **Distribution:** SHBG binding (40%), albumin binding (2%). **Metabolism:** Estradiol and DHT (active metabolites). **Elimination:** $T_{1/2}$=10-100 min, urine (90%, glucuronic and sulfuric acid conjugates), feces (6%, unconjugated).

ANECTINE   RX
succinylcholine chloride (Sandoz)

> Rare reports of acute rhabdomyolysis with hyperkalemia followed by ventricular dysrhythmias, cardiac arrest, and death in children with undiagnosed skeletal muscle myopathy. Reserve in children for emergency intubation where securing airway is necessary.

THERAPEUTIC CLASS: Skeletal muscle relaxant (depolarizing)

INDICATIONS: Adjunct to general anesthesia to facilitate tracheal intubation and to provide skeletal muscle relaxation during surgery or mechanical ventilation.

DOSAGE: *Adults:* Short Surgical Procedure: Average Dose: 0.6mg/kg IV. Range: 0.3-1.1mg/kg IV. Blockade develops in 1 min, may persist up to 2 min. Long Surgical Procedure: 2.5-4.3mg/min IV; or 0.3-1.1mg/kg initial IV inj, then 0.04-0.07mg/kg IV at appropriate intervals. IM (if vein not accessible): Up to 3-4mg/kg IM. Max: 150mg/total dose. Effect observed in 2-3 min. *Pediatrics:* Procedure to Secure Airway: Infants/Small Children: 2mg/kg IV. Older Children/Adolescents: 1mg/kg IV. IM (if vein not accessible): Infants/ Older Children: Up to 3-4mg/kg IM. Max: 150mg/total dose. Effect observed in 2-3 min.

HOW SUPPLIED: Inj: 20mg/mL

CONTRAINDICATIONS: Personal or familial history of malignant hyperthermia, skeletal muscle myopathies. Acute phase of injury following major burns, multiple trauma, extensive skeletal muscle denervation, upper motor neuron injury.

WARNINGS/PRECAUTIONS: Avoid administration before unconsciousness has been induced. May induce arrhythmias or cardiac arrest in electrolyte abnormalities or massive digitalis toxicity. Caution with chronic abdominal infection, subarachnoid hemorrhage, conditions causing degeneration of central and peripheral nervous system, fractures, muscle spasms, reduced plasma cholinesterase activity, and acute phase of injury following major burns, multiple trauma, extensive skeletal muscle denervation, upper motor neuron injury. Malignant hyperthermia reported. Higher incidence of bradycardia progressing to asystole with 2nd dose. May increase IOP, intracranial or intragastric pressure. With prolonged therapy, Phase I block will progress to Phase II block associated with prolonged respiratory paralysis and weakness. Confirm Phase II block before therapy. Hypokalemia or hypocalcemia prolong neuromuscular blockade.

ADVERSE REACTIONS: Respiratory depression, cardiac arrest, malignant hyperthermia, arrhythmia, bradycardia, tachycardia, HTN, hypotension, hyperkalemia, increased IOP, muscle fasciculation, jaw rigidity, post-op muscle pains.

INTERACTIONS: Enhanced effects with promazine, oxytocin, certain non-penicillin antibiotics, β-blockers, procainamide, lidocaine, trimethaphan, lithium carbonate, magnesium salts, quinine, aprotinin, chloroquine, diethylether, isoflurane, desflurane, metoclopramide, terbutaline, and drugs that reduce plasma cholinesterase activity (eg, chronically administered oral contraceptives, glucocorticoids, certain MAOIs) or inhibit plasma cholinesterase. Increased risk of malignant hyperthermia with volatile anesthetics.

PREGNANCY: Category C, caution in nursing.

MECHANISM OF ACTION: Depolarizing skeletal muscle relaxant; combines with the cholinergic receptors of motor end plate to produce depolarization, and subsequent neuromuscular transmission inhibition.

PHARMACOKINETICS: Metabolism: Rapid; via plasma cholinesterases through hydrolysis to succinylmonocholine and to succinic and choline. **Elimination:** Urine 10% (unchanged).

ANEXSIA   CIII
hydrocodone bitartrate - acetaminophen (Mallinckrodt)

THERAPEUTIC CLASS: Opioid analgesic

INDICATIONS: Relief of moderate to moderately severe pain.

DOSAGE: *Adults:* (5-500mg) Usual: 1-2 tabs q4-6h prn. Max: 8 tabs/day. (7.5-650mg) Usual: 1 tab q4-6h prn. Max: 6 tabs/day.

HOW SUPPLIED: Tab: (Hydrocodone-APAP) 5mg-325mg, 7.5mg-325mg, 5mg-500mg, 7.5mg-650mg

WARNINGS/PRECAUTIONS: Caution in elderly, debilitated, severe hepatic or renal dysfunction, hypothyroidism, Addison's disease, prostatic hypertrophy, urethral stricture, pulmonary disease, and postoperative use. Impairs mental/physical abilities. May obscure diagnosis or clinical course of acute abdominal conditions or head injuries. May produce dose-related respiratory depression. Monitor for tolerance. Suppresses cough reflex.

ADVERSE REACTIONS: Lightheadedness, dizziness, sedation, nausea, vomiting, constipation, rash, respiratory depression.

INTERACTIONS: Additive CNS depression with other narcotic analgesics, antihistamines, antipsychotics, antianxiety agents, alcohol and other CNS depressants. Increased effect of antidepressant or hydrocodone with MAOIs or TCAs.

PREGNANCY: Category C, not for use in nursing.

ANGELIQ   RX
drospirenone - estradiol (Bayer Healthcare)

> Estrogens and progestins should not be used for prevention of cardiovascular disease or dementia. Increased risk of MI, stroke, invasive breast cancer, PE, and DVT in postmenopausal women (50-79 yrs of age) reported. Increased risk of developing probable dementia in postmenopausal women ≥65 yrs of age reported.

THERAPEUTIC CLASS: Estrogen/progestogen combination

INDICATIONS: Treatment of moderate to severe vasomotor symptoms and/or vulvar/vaginal atrophy associated with menopause.

DOSAGE: *Adults:* 1 tab qd. Re-evaluate after 3-6 months.

HOW SUPPLIED: Tab: (Drospirenone-Estradiol) 0.5mg-1mg

CONTRAINDICATIONS: Pregnancy, undiagnosed abnormal genital bleeding, breast cancer, estrogen-dependent neoplasia, DVT/PE, active or recent (eg, within past year) arterial thromboembolic disease (eg, stroke, MI), liver dysfunction or disease, renal insufficiency, adrenal insufficiency.

WARNINGS/PRECAUTIONS: Not for use in renal insufficiency, hepatic dysfunction, and adrenal insufficiency due to increased risk of hyperkalemia. May increase risk of cardiovascular events (eg, MI, stroke), venous thrombosis, and PE; d/c immediately if any of these events occur or are suspected. May increase risk of breast/endometrial cancer, and gallbladder disease. May lead to severe hypercalcemia with breast cancer and bone metastases; monitor and d/c if hypercalcemia occurs. Retinal vascular thrombosis reported; monitor and d/c if papilledema or retinal vascular lesions occur. May elevate BP; monitor at regular intervals. May cause elevations of plasma triglycerides with pre-existing hypertriglyceridemia. Caution with history of cholestatic jaundice associated with past estrogen use or with pregnancy; d/c with recurrence. May lead to increased thyroid-binding globulin levels; monitor thyroid function. May cause fluid retention; caution with cardiac/renal dysfunction. Caution with severe hypocalcemia. May increase risk of ovarian cancer. May exacerbate endometriosis, asthma, DM, epilepsy, migraine, porphyria, SLE, and hepatic hemangiomas; use with caution.

ADVERSE REACTIONS: Abdominal pain, pain in extremity, back pain, flu syndrome, enlarged abdomen, headache, upper respiratory infection, sinusitis, breast pain, vaginal hemorrhage.

INTERACTIONS: CYP3A4 inducers (eg, St. John's wort, phenobarbital, carbamazepine, rifampin) may decrease levels which may decrease therapeutic effects and/or change uterine bleeding profile. CYP3A4 inhibitors (eg, erythromycin, clarithromycin, ketoconazole, itraconazole, ritonavir, grapefruit juice) may increase levels which may result in side effects. Increased risk of hyperkalemia with ACE inhibitors, angiotensin receptor blockers, NSAIDs, potassium-sparing diuretics, potassium supplements, and heparin.

PREGNANCY: Contraindicated in pregnancy, caution in nursing.

MECHANISM OF ACTION: Estrogen/progestogen combination. Estradiol: Acts through binding to nuclear receptors in estrogen-responsive tissues. Modulates pituitary secretion of gonadotropins, leutenizing hormone (LH) and follicle stimulating hormone (FSH), through a negative feedback mechanism. Drospirenone (DSRP): Synthetic progestin and spironolactone analog with antimineralocorticoid activity. Possesses anti-androgenic activity. Counters estrogenic effects by decreasing the number of nuclear estradiol receptors and suppressing epithelial DNA synthesis in endometrial tissue.

PHARMACOKINETICS: Absorption: DRSP: C_{max}=18.3ng/mL; T_{max}=1.0 hr; AUC_{0-24hr}=208ng•hr/mL. Absolute bioavailability (76-85%) Estradiol; C_{max}=43.8pg/mL; T_{max}=2.5 hrs; $AUC_{0-24 hr}$=665pg•hr/mL. Estrone (metabolite): C_{max}=245pg/mL; T_{max}=4 hrs; $AUC_{(0-24 hr}$=3814pg•hr/mL **Distribution:** Estrogens and DRSP found in breast milk. DRSP: V_d=4.2L/kg, serum protein binding (97%). Estradiol: Sex hormone binding globulin (SHBG) (37%); albumin binding (61%). **Metabolism:** DRSP: Extensive; CYP3A4 (minor). Estradiol: Liver to estrone (metabolite); estriol (major urinary metabolite); enterohepatic recirculation via sulfate and glucuronide conjugation in the liver; biliary secretion of conjugates in the intestine; hydrolysis in the gut; reabsorption. **Elimination:** DRSP: $T_{1/2}$=36-42 hrs; Urine (38-47%, glucuronide and sulfate conjugates), feces (17-20%, glucuronide and sulfate conjugates). Estradiol: Urine. Estrone: Urine; $T_{1/2}$=23 hrs.

ANGIOMAX   RX
bivalirudin (The Medicines Company)

THERAPEUTIC CLASS: Thrombin inhibitor

INDICATIONS: Adjunct to aspirin for anticoagulation in patients with unstable angina undergoing percutaneous transluminal coronary angioplasty (PTCA) or percutaneous coronary intervention (PCI). Patients with, or at risk of, HIT/HITTS undergoing PCI.

DOSAGE: *Adults:* Initial: 0.75mg/kg IV bolus, then 1.75mg/kg/hr for duration of PCI procedure. Additional bolus of 0.3mg/kg can be given if needed based on ACT. Continuation of infusion for up to 4 hrs post-procedure is optional. After 4 hrs, if needed, an additional 0.2mg/kg/hr IV for up to 20 hrs may be initiated. Renal Impairment: CrCl <30mL/min: 1mg/kg/hr infusion. Hemodialysis: 0.25mg/kg/hr infusion. Reduction in bolus dose not necessary; monitor anticoagulation.

HOW SUPPLIED: Inj: 250mg

CONTRAINDICATIONS: Active major bleeding.

WARNINGS/PRECAUTIONS: Not for IM administration. Hemorrhage can occur at any site. D/C with unexplained symptom, fall in BP or Hct. There is no known antidote to treatment, but can be hemodialyzable. Caution when used during brachytherapy procedures.

ADVERSE REACTIONS: Bleeding, back pain, pain, nausea, vomiting, headache, hypotension, HTN, bradycardia, dyspepsia, urinary retention, insomnia, anxiety, abdominal pain, fever, nervousness.

INTERACTIONS: Increased risk of major bleed with heparin, warfarin, thrombolytics, glycoprotein IIb/IIIa inhibitors.

PREGNANCY: Category B, caution in nursing.

MECHANISM OF ACTION: Reversible direct thrombin inhibitor; inhibits thrombin by specifically binding to catalytic site and to anion-binding exosite of circulating and clot-bound thrombin.

PHARMACOKINETICS: Metabolism: Renal mechanisms and proteolytic cleavage. **Elimination:** Urine; $T_{1/2}$=25 min.

ANSAID   RX
flurbiprofen (Pharmacia & Upjohn)

> NSAIDs may cause an increased risk of serious cardiovascular thrombotic events, MI, stroke, and serious GI adverse events including bleeding, ulceration, and perforation of the stomach or intestines. Contraindicated for the treatment of perioperative pain in the setting of coronary artery bypass graft (CABG) surgery.

THERAPEUTIC CLASS: NSAID

INDICATIONS: Relief of the signs and symptoms of rheumatoid arthritis or osteoarthritis.

DOSAGE: *Adults:* Initial: 200-300mg/day given bid, tid or qid. Max: 300mg/day or 100mg/dose.

HOW SUPPLIED: Tab: 50mg, 100mg

CONTRAINDICATIONS: ASA, with ASA triad, or other NSAID allergy that precipitates acute asthmatic attack, urticaria, or rhinitis. Treatment of perioperative pain in the setting of CABG surgery.

WARNINGS/PRECAUTIONS: May lead to onset of new HTN or worsening of pre-existing HTN; monitor BP closely. Fluid retention and edema reported; caution with fluid retention or heart failure. Renal papillary necrosis and other renal injury reported after long-term use. Not recommended for use with advanced renal disease; if therapy must be initiated, monitor renal function. Anaphylactoid reactions may occur. Avoid in late pregnancy; may cause premature closure of ductus arteriosis. May cause elevations of LFTs; d/c if liver disease develops or systemic manifestations occur. Caution in elderly. Anemia may occur; monitor Hgb/Hct with long-term use. May inhibit platelet aggregation and prolong bleeding time; monitor with coagulation disorders. Caution with asthma and avoid with ASA-sensitive asthma. Monitor for visual changes or disturbances. Risk of GI ulceration, bleeding, and perforation. May cause serious skin adverse events (eg, exfoliative dermatitis, Stevens-Johnson syndrome, toxic epidermal necrolysis).

ADVERSE REACTIONS: Dyspepsia, diarrhea, abdominal pain, constipation, headache, nausea, edema.

INTERACTIONS: Caution with anticoagulants; serious bleeding reported. Concomitant ASA is not recommended. May decrease hypotensive effects of β-blockers, decrease diuretic effects and diminish the antihypertensive effects of ACE inhibitors. May elevate plasma lithium levels and could enhance the toxicity of methotrexate.

PREGNANCY: Category C, not for use in nursing.

MECHANISM OF ACTION: NSAID; suspected to inhibit prostaglandin synthetase and exerts anti-inflammatory, analgesic and antipyretic actions.

PHARMACOKINETICS: Absorption: Rapid; Bioavailability 96%; T_{max} =2 hrs. **Distribution:** V_d=0.12L/kg; Plasma protein binding (99%); Found in breast milk. **Metabolism:** CYP2C9. 4'-hydroxy-flurbiprofen (major metabolite). **Elimination:** Urine ≤3% (unchanged) and 70% (parent drug and metabolites); $T_{1/2}$=4.7 hrs (R-flurbiprofen) and 5.7 hrs (S-flurbiprofen).

ANTABUSE   RX
disulfiram (Odyssey)

> Do not give if in a state of alcohol intoxication, or without full knowledge. Instruct relatives accordingly.

THERAPEUTIC CLASS: Alcohol oxidation inhibitor

INDICATIONS: Aid in the management of selected chronic alcoholics who want to remain sober for supportive and psychotherapeutic treatment.

DOSAGE: *Adults:* Initial: Up to 500mg/day as a single dose for 1-2 weeks. Maint: 125-500mg/day. Max: 500mg/day. Abstain from alcohol at least 12 hours prior to therapy.

HOW SUPPLIED: Tab: 250mg

CONTRAINDICATIONS: Severe myocardial disease, coronary occlusion, psychoses, hypersensitivity to thiuram derivatives in pesticides and rubber vulcanization, and if receiving or recently received metronidazole, paraldehyde, alcohol, or alcohol-containing preparations (eg, cough syrups).

WARNINGS/PRECAUTIONS: Avoid in alcohol intoxication or without patients full knowledge. Antabuse-alcohol reaction; can cause respiratory and cardiovascular problems. Avoid alcohol-containing products (eg, sauces, vinegars, cough mixtures, after shave lotions, back rubs) and ethylene dibromide or its vapors. Reactions with alcohol up to 14 days after ingestion. Evaluate for hypersensitivity if history of rubber contact dermatitis. Hepatic toxicity/failure has been reported. Perform baseline and follow-up LFTs (10-14 days) and monitor CBC and SMA-12. Caution with diabetes mellitus, hypothyroidism, epilepsy, cerebral damage, chronic and acute nephritis, hepatic cirrhosis or insufficiency.

ADVERSE REACTIONS: Optic neuritis, peripheral neuritis, polyneuritis peripheral neuropathy, hepatitis, skin eruptions, drowsiness, fatigability, impotence, headache, acneiform eruptions, allergic dermatitis, metallic or garlic-like aftertaste.

INTERACTIONS: Increases phenytoin level; monitor for toxicity. May prolong PT; adjust oral anticoagulants. Stop therapy if unsteady gait or marked changes in mental status with isoniazid.

PREGNANCY: Safety not known in pregnancy, not for use in nursing.

MECHANISM OF ACTION: Alcohol antagonist; blocks alcohol oxidation at the acetaldehyde stage.

PHARMACOKINETICS: Absorption/Elimination: Slow.

ANTARA   RX
fenofibrate (Oscient)

THERAPEUTIC CLASS: Fibric acid derivative

INDICATIONS: Adjunct to diet, for treatment of hypertriglyceridemia (Types IV and V) and to reduce elevated LDL-C, Total-C, TG, Apo B, and to increase HDL-C in primary hypercholesterolemia or mixed dyslipidemia (Types IIa and IIb).

ANTIVENIN

DOSAGE: *Adults:* Hypercholesterolemia/Mixed Dyslipidemia: Initial: 130mg qd. Hypertriglyceridemia: Initial: 43-130mg/day. Titrate: Adjust if needed after repeat lipid levels at 4-8 week intervals. Max: 130mg/day. Renal Dysfunction/Elderly: Initial: 43mg/day. Take with meals.

HOW SUPPLIED: Cap: 43mg, 130mg

CONTRAINDICATIONS: Hepatic or severe renal dysfunction (including primary cirrhosis), unexplained persistent hepatic function abnormality, pre-existing gallbladder disease.

WARNINGS/PRECAUTIONS: Monitor LFTs regularly; d/c if >3x ULN. May cause cholelithiasis; d/c if gallstones found. D/C if myopathy or marked CPK elevation occurs. Decreased Hgb, Hct, WBCs, thrombocytopenia, and agranulocytosis reported; monitor CBCs during first 12 months of therapy. Acute hypersensitivity reactions (rare) and pancreatitis reported. Rare cases of rhabdomyolysis. Evaluate for myopathy. Monitor lipids periodically initially, d/c if inadequate response after 2 months on 130mg/day. Minimize dose in severe renal impairment. Caution in elderly.

ADVERSE REACTIONS: Abdominal pain, back pain, headache, abnormal LFTs, respiratory disorder, increased creatinine phosphokinase, increased SGPT/SGOT.

INTERACTIONS: May potentiate coumarin anticoagulants; reduce anticoagulant dose and monitor PT/INR. Avoid HMG-CoA reductase inhibitors unless benefits outweigh risks. Bile acid sequestrants may impede absorption; take at least 1 hr before or 4-6 hrs after the resin. Evaluate benefits/risks with immunosuppressants (eg, cyclosporine) and other nephrotoxic agents.

PREGNANCY: Category C, not for use in nursing.

MECHANISM OF ACTION: Fenofabric acid; increases lipolysis and elimination of triglyceride-rich particles from plasma by activating lipoprotein lipase and reducing production of apoprotein C-III. Reduces serum uric acid levels in hyperuricemic and normal individuals by increasing urinary excretion of uric acid.

PHARMACOKINETICS: Absorption: Well. T_{max}=4.8 hrs. **Distribution:** Plasma protein binding (99%). **Metabolism:** Rapid, via esterase. Fenofibric acid (active metabolite). **Elimination:** Urine (60%), feces (25%), $T_{1/2}$=23 hrs.

ANTIVENIN   RX
black widow spider antivenin [lactrodectus mactans] (Merck)

THERAPEUTIC CLASS: Immunoglobulin

INDICATIONS: Treat symptoms due to black widow spider bites.

DOSAGE: *Adults:* 1 vial (2.5mL) IM, preferably given in anterolateral thigh. May repeat if necessary. Shock/Severe Cases: 1 vial (2.5mL) IV in 10-50mL saline solution over 15 min.
Pediatrics: <12 yrs: 1 vial (2.5mL) IV in 10-50mL saline solution over 15 min.

HOW SUPPLIED: Inj: 6000 U

WARNINGS/PRECAUTIONS: Serum sickness/death could result from the use of horse serum in sensitive patients. Perform skin test prior to treatment. Observe for serum sickness for 8-12 days following treatment. Attempt desensitization only to save life.

ADVERSE REACTIONS: Anaphylaxis, serum sickness.

PREGNANCY: Category C, caution in nursing.

MECHANISM OF ACTION: Venom neutralizing globulin; not established.

ANTIVERT   RX
meclizine HCL (Pfizer)

THERAPEUTIC CLASS: Antihistamine

A

INDICATIONS: Management of nausea, vomiting and dizziness associated with motion sickness. Management of vertigo associated with diseases affecting the vestibular system.

DOSAGE: *Adults:* Motion Sickness: 25-50mg 1 hr prior to trip/departure, repeat q24h prn. Vertigo: 25-100mg/day in divided doses.
Pediatrics: ≥12 yrs: Motion Sickness: 25-50mg 1 hr prior to trip/departure, repeat q24h prn. Vertigo: 25-100mg/day in divided doses.

HOW SUPPLIED: Tab: 12.5mg, 25mg, 50mg* *scored

WARNINGS/PRECAUTIONS: Caution with asthma, glaucoma, prostatic hypertrophy.

ADVERSE REACTIONS: Drowsiness, dry mouth, blurred vision (rare).

INTERACTIONS: Avoid alcoholic beverages.

PREGNANCY: Category B, safety in nursing is not known.

MECHANISM OF ACTION: Antihistaminic agent; blocks vasodepressor response to histamine; slight blocking against acetylcholine.

ANTIZOL RX
fomepizole (Orphan Medical)

THERAPEUTIC CLASS: Alcohol dehydrogenase inhibitor

INDICATIONS: Antidote for ethylene glycol or methanol poisoning either alone or with hemodialysis (HD).

DOSAGE: *Adults:* IV: LD: 15mg/kg. Maint: 10mg/kg q12h for 4 doses, then 15mg/kg q12h until levels are undetectable or <20mg/dL. Dose at Beginning of HD: If ≥6 hrs since last dose, give next scheduled dose. Dose During HD: Give q4h. Dose at time when HD is Complete: Give 50% of dose if 1-3 hrs between the last dose and the end of HD. If >3 hrs between last dose and end of HD, give next dose.

HOW SUPPLIED: Sol: 1g/mL

CONTRAINDICATIONS: Pyrazole hypersensitivity.

WARNINGS/PRECAUTIONS: Do not give undiluted or as a bolus injection. Monitor for allergic reactions (eg, mild rash, eosinophilia). Monitor LFTs, WBC during therapy.

ADVERSE REACTIONS: Headache, nausea, dizziness, increased drowsiness, bad/metallic taste.

INTERACTIONS: Reduced elimination of ethanol and fomepizole (PO).

PREGNANCY: Category C, caution in nursing.

MECHANISM OF ACTION: Alcohol dehydrogenase inhibitor; prevents the conversion of ethanol to acetaldehyde.

PHARMACOKINETICS: Distribution: Rapid distribution. V_d=0.6L/Kg-1.02L/Kg. **Metabolism:** Via CYP450. 4-carboxypyrazole (major metabolite). **Elimination:** Urine: 80-85%.

ANUSOL-HC CREAM RX
hydrocortisone (Salix)

OTHER BRAND NAMES: Proctozone-HC (Rising) - Proctocream HC (Schwarz Pharma) - Proctosol HC (NuCare)

THERAPEUTIC CLASS: Corticosteroid

INDICATIONS: Corticosteroid responsive dermatoses.

DOSAGE: *Adults:* Apply bid-qid. May use occlusive dressings for psoriasis or recalcitrant conditions; d/c dressings if infection develops.
Pediatrics: Apply bid-qid. May use occlusive dressings for psoriasis or recalcitrant conditions; d/c dressings if infection develops.

HOW SUPPLIED: Cre: 2.5% [30g]

WARNINGS/PRECAUTIONS: May cause reversible adrenal suppression, manifestations of Cushing's syndrome, hyperglycemia, glucosuria. Caution when applied to large surface areas or under occlusive dressings. Use appropriate therapy with infections. Pediatrics may be more susceptible to systemic toxicity. D/C if irritation occurs. Avoid eyes.

ADVERSE REACTIONS: Burning, itching, irritation, dryness, folliculitis, hypertrichosis, acneiform eruptions, hypopigmentation, perioral dermatitis, allergic contact dermatitis, maceration skin, secondary infection, skin atrophy, striae, miliaria.

PREGNANCY: Category C, caution in nursing.

MECHANISM OF ACTION: Topical corticosteroid, suspected to produce antiinflammatory, antipruritic, and vasoconstrictive actions.

PHARMACOKINETICS: Absorption: Absorbed from normal intact skin. **Distribution:** Plasma protein binding in varying degrees. **Metabolism:** Liver. **Elimination:** Kidneys, bile (metabolites). $T_{1/2}$=8-12 hr.

ANUSOL-HC SUPPOSITORY   RX
hydrocortisone acetate (Salix)

OTHER BRAND NAMES: Hemorrhoidal HC (Alpharma) - Anucort HC (G & W Labs)

THERAPEUTIC CLASS: Corticosteroid

INDICATIONS: For use in inflamed hemorrhoids and post irradiation (factitial) proctitis. Adjunct for chronic ulcerative colitis, cryptitis, other anorectum inflammation and pruritus ani.

DOSAGE: *Adults:* Nonspecific Proctitis: 1 sup rectally bid for 2 weeks. More Severe Cases: 1 sup rectally tid or 2 sup rectally bid. Factitial Proctitis: Use up to 6-8 weeks.

HOW SUPPLIED: Sup: (Anusol-HC) 25mg [12s 24s]

WARNINGS/PRECAUTIONS: D/C if irritation develops. D/C if infection develops that does not respond to appropriate therapy. May stain fabric. Only use after adequate proctologic exam.

ADVERSE REACTIONS: Burning, itching, irritation, dryness, folliculitis, hypopigmentation, allergic contact dermatitis, secondary infection.

PREGNANCY: Category C, not for use in nursing.

ANZEMET   RX
dolasetron mesylate (Sanofi-Aventis)

THERAPEUTIC CLASS: 5-HT$_3$-antagonist

INDICATIONS: (Inj) Prevention of nausea/vomiting associated with emetogenic cancer chemotherapy including high-dose cisplatin. Prevention and treatment of post-op nausea/vomiting. (Tab) Prevention of nausea/vomiting associated with moderately emetogenic cancer chemotherapy and prevention of post-op nausea/vomiting.

DOSAGE: *Adults:* (Inj) Prevention of Chemotherapy Nausea/Vomiting: 1.8mg/kg IV single dose or 100mg IV 30 min before chemotherapy. Prevention/Treatment of Post-op Nausea/Vomiting: 12.5mg IV single dose 15 min before cessation of anesthesia or as soon as nausea/vomiting presents. (Tab) Prevention of Chemotherapy-Induced Nausea/Vomiting: 100mg PO within 1 hr before chemotherapy. Prevention of Postoperative Nausea/Vomiting: 100mg PO within 2 hrs before surgery.
Pediatrics: 2-16 yrs: (Inj) Prevention of Chemotherapy Nausea/Vomiting: 1.8mg/kg IV single dose 30 min before chemotherapy. Max: 100mg. May mix inj in apple or grape juice and take orally within 1 hr before chemotherapy. Prevention/Treatment of Post-op Nausea/Vomiting: 0.35mg/kg IV single dose 15 min before cessation of anesthesia or as soon as nausea/vomiting presents. Max: 12.5mg single dose. May mix 1.2mg/kg inj in apple or grape juice and

take orally within 2 hrs before surgery. Max: 100mg/dose. (Tab) Prevention of Chemotherapy-Induced Nausea/Vomiting: 1.8mg/kg PO within 1 hr before chemotherapy. Max: 100mg. Prevention of Postoperative Nausea/Vomiting: 1.2mg/kg PO within 2 hrs before surgery. Max: 100mg.

HOW SUPPLIED: Inj: 20mg/mL; Tab: 50mg, 100mg

WARNINGS/PRECAUTIONS: Caution in patients with or who may develop cardiac conduction interval prolongation, especially those with congenital QT syndrome, hypokalemia and hypomagnesemia. Cross sensitivity may occur with other 5-HT$_3$ antagonists. Can cause ECG interval changes.

ADVERSE REACTIONS: Headache, diarrhea, fever, fatigue, dizziness, abnormal hepatic function, chills/shivering, urinary retention, abdominal pain, HTN, wide complex tachycardia or ventricular tachycardia, ventricular fibrillation.

INTERACTIONS: Increased risk of prolongation of cardiac conduction intervals with diuretics, antiarrhythmics, drugs that prolong QTc interval and cumulative high dose anthracycline therapy. Increased levels with cimetidine. Decreased levels with rifampin. Decreased clearance with IV atenolol.

PREGNANCY: Category B, caution in nursing.

MECHANISM OF ACTION: 5-HT$_3$ receptor antagonist.

PHARMACOKINETICS: Absorption: T_{max}=0.6 hr. **Distribution:** V_d=5.8L/Kg; plasma protein binding (77%). **Metabolism:** Complete. Via carbonyl reductase CYP2D6 and flavin monooxygenase through reduction, hydroxylation, and N-oxidation. **Elimination:** Urine 53% (unchanged), feces; $T_{1/2}$=7.3 hrs.

APHTHASOL   OTC
amlexanox (GlaxoSmithKline Consumer)

THERAPEUTIC CLASS: Inflammatory mediator inhibitor

INDICATIONS: Treatment of aphthous ulcers in people with normal immune systems.

DOSAGE: *Adults:* Begin at 1st sign of aphthous ulcer. Apply 1/4 inch qid, pc and qhs, following oral hygiene. Use until ulcer heals. Re-evaluate if healing or pain reduction has not occurred after 10 days of use.

HOW SUPPLIED: Paste: 5% [5g]

WARNINGS/PRECAUTIONS: Wash hands immediately after applying paste. D/C if rash or contact mucositis occurs. Avoid eyes.

ADVERSE REACTIONS: Transient pain, stinging, burning.

PREGNANCY: Category B, caution in nursing.

MECHANISM OF ACTION: Inflammatory mediator inhibitor. MOA not established. Suspected to inhibit formation and/or release of inflammatory mediators (histamine and leukotrienes) from mast cells, neutrophils, and mononuclear cells.

PHARMACOKINETICS: Absorption: Absorbed in gastrointestinal tract. C_{max}=approximately 120ng/mL, T_{max}=2.4 hrs. **Elimination:** $T_{1/2(mean)}$=3.5 hrs. Urine (approximately 17%).

APIDRA   RX
insulin glulisine, rdna (Sanofi-Aventis)

THERAPEUTIC CLASS: Insulin

INDICATIONS: Treatment of adults with DM for the control of hyperglycemia.

DOSAGE: *Adults:* Individualize dose. Inject SQ within 15 min before a meal or within 20 min after starting a meal. Rotate inj site (abdomen, thigh, or deltoid).

HOW SUPPLIED: Inj: 100 U/mL

CONTRAINDICATIONS: Episodes of hypoglycemia.

WARNINGS/PRECAUTIONS: Hypoglycemia and hypokalemia may occur; monitor glucose and potassium levels. Rapid onset and short duration of action; follow dosage directions. Adjust dose if change in physical activity or usual meal plan. Longer-acting insulin or insulin infusion pump may be required to maintain glucose control. When used in an external pump for SQ infusion, do not dilute or mix with any other insulin. Caution when changing insulin strength, manufacturer, type, or species. Concomitant antidiabetic therapy may need adjustment. As with other insulin therapy hypoglycemic reactions and local/systemic allergic reactions may occur. May be given IV under proper medical supervision. Caution in renal/hepatic impairment.

ADVERSE REACTIONS: Allergic reactions, injection site reactions, lipodystrophy, pruritus, rash, hypoglycemia.

INTERACTIONS: Decreased effect with corticosteroids, danazol, diazoxide, diuretics, sympathomimetic agents (eg, epinephrine, albuterol, terbutaline), glucagon, isoniazid, phenothiazine derivatives, somatropin, thyroid hormones, estrogens, progestogens (eg, in oral contraceptives), protease inhibitors, and atypical antipsychotic medications (eg, olanzepine and clozapine). Increased effect with ACEIs, MAOIs, oral antidiabetics, disopyramide, fibrates, fluoxetine, pentoxifylline, propoxyphene, salicylates, sulfonomide antibiotics. Decreased or increased effect with β-blockers, clonidine, lithium salts, and alcohol. Pentamidine may cause hypoglycemia followed by hyperglycemia. β-blockers, clonidine, guanethidine, and reserpine may reduce or mask signs of hypoglycemia.

PREGNANCY: Category C, caution in nursing.

MECHANISM OF ACTION: Insulin glulisine (rDNA origin); lowers blood glucose by stimulating peripheral glucose uptake by skeletal muscle and fat and by inhibiting hepatic glucose production.

PHARMACOKINETICS: Absorption: T_{max}=55, 89, 76 min (0.15, 0.2, 0.3 IU/kg); C_{max}=82, 81, 199µIU/mL (0.15, 0.2, 0.3 IU/kg). **Distribution:** V_d=13L. **Elimination:** Rapidly eliminated; $T_{1/2}$=42 min.

APOKYN   RX
apomorphine HCL (Mylan Bertek)

THERAPEUTIC CLASS: Non-ergoline dopamine agonist

INDICATIONS: Acute, intermittent treatment of hypomobility, "off" episodes ("end-of-dose wearing off" and unpredictable "on/off" episodes) associated with advanced Parkinson's disease.

DOSAGE: *Adults:* Initial: Test Dose: 2mg SC; closely monitor BP. Titrate: Increase by 1mg every few days; assess efficacy/tolerability. Max: 6mg/day. Renal Impairment: Initial: 1mg SC.

HOW SUPPLIED: Inj: 10mg/mL [2mL, 3mL]

CONTRAINDICATIONS: Concomitant use with $5HT_3$ antagonists (eg, ondansetron, granisetron, dolasetron, palonosetron, alosetron).

WARNINGS/PRECAUTIONS: Avoid IV administration; serious adverse events reported (thrombus formation and PE). Nausea, vomiting, syncope, symptomatic hypotension, falls, hallucinations, falling asleep during activities of daily living, coronary events (eg, angina, MI, cardiac arrest, suddden death) reported. May prolong QT interval; potential proarrhythmic effects; caution with drugs that prolong QT/QTc interval. Caution with sulfite sensitivity. May cause or worsen dyskinesias. Withdrawal-emergent hyperpyrexia and confusion reported with rapid dose reduction/withdrawal/changes in therapy. Fibrotic complications (eg, retroperitoneal fibrosis, pulmonary infiltrates, pleural effusion/thickening, cardiac valvulopathy) reported. May cause priapism. Caution with hepatic/renal impairment.

ADVERSE REACTIONS: Yawning, somnolence, dizziness, rhinorrhea, edema, chest pain, increased sweating, flushing, pallor.

INTERACTIONS: See Contraindications. Antihypertensives and vasodilators may increase risk of hypotension, MI, serious pneumonia/falls, bone and joint injuries. Dopamine antagonists (eg, phenothiazines, butyrophenones, thioxanthenes, metoclopramide) may diminish effectiveness.

PREGNANCY: Category C, not for use in nursing.

MECHANISM OF ACTION: Not established. Non-ergoline dopamine agonist, suspected to stimulate post-synaptic dopamine D2-type receptors within the caudate-putamen in the brain.

PHARMACOKINETICS: Absorption: Rapidly absorbed. T_{max}=10-60 min. **Distribution:** Mean V_d=218L. **Metabolism:** Sulfation, N-demethylation, glucuronidation and oxidation. **Elimination:** $T_{1/2}$=40 min.

APTIVUS RX
tipranavir (Boehringer Ingelheim)

> Both fatal and non-fatal intracranial hemorrhage, clinical hepatitis, and hepatic decompensation, including some fatalities, have been reported. Extra vigilance is warranted in patients with chronic hepatitis B or hepatitis C co-infection, as these patients have an increased risk of hepatotoxicity.

THERAPEUTIC CLASS: Protease inhibitor

INDICATIONS: Co-administered with 200mg of ritonavir for treatment of HIV-1 infected patients with evidence of viral replication, who are highly treatment-experienced or have HIV-1 strains resistant to multiple protease inhibitors.

DOSAGE: *Adults:* 500mg, with 200mg ritonavir, bid with food.

HOW SUPPLIED: Cap: 250mg

CONTRAINDICATIONS: Moderate to severe (Child-Pugh Class B and C) hepatic insufficiency. Concomitant administration with amiodarone, bepridil, flecainide, propafenone, quinidine, rifampin, dihydroergotamine, ergonovine, ergotamine, methylergonovine, cisapride, St. John's wort, lovastatin, simvastatin, pimozide, midazolam, and triazolam.

WARNINGS/PRECAUTIONS: Must be co-administered with ritonavir. Not recommended for use in treatment-naive patients. Caution with mild hepatic impairment (Child-Pugh Class A); monitor LFTs prior to therapy and during therapy. D/C for signs and symptoms of clinical hepatitis. D/C if asymptomatic elevations in AST or ALT >10 times the upper limit of normal or if asymptomatic elevations in AST or ALT between 5-10 times the upper limit of normal and increases in total bilirubin >2.5 times the upper limit of normal occurs. Caution in patients at risk of increased bleeding from trauma, surgery, or other medical conditions, or who are receiving medications known to increase risk of bleeding (eg, antiplatelet agents, anticoagulants, high doses of vitamin E). Reports of new-onset DM, exacerbation of pre-existing DM, hyperglycemia; rash (urticarial rash, maculopapular rash, and possible photosensitivity) and rash accompanied with joint pain/stiffness, throat tightness, generalized pruritus; increased bleeding with hemophilia Types A and B; and increased total cholesterol and triglycerides. Caution with known sulfonamide allergy. D/C with severe rash. Possible redistribution/accumulation of body fat. Immune reconstitution syndrome reported with combination therapy.

ADVERSE REACTIONS: Diarrhea, nausea, vomiting, abdominal pain, pyrexia, fatigue, asthenia, bronchitis, headache, depression, insomnia, cough, rash.

INTERACTIONS: See Contraindications. Do not use with rifampin, St. John's wort, lovastatin, simvastatin, amiodarone, bepridil, flecainide, propafenone, quinidine, ergot derivatives, cisapride, pimozide, midazolam, and triazolam. Decreased levels of abacavir, atazanavir, didanosine, zidovudine, amprenavir, lopinavir, saquinavir, valproic acid, methadone, meperidine, and omeprazole. Increased levels of fluoxetine, paroxetine, sertraline, tipranavir, rosuvastatin, tadalafil. Caution with carbamazepine, phenobarbital, phenytoin, valproic acid, trazodone, itraconazole, ketoconazole, voriconazole, diltiazem, felodipine, nicardipine, nisoldipine, verapamil, disulfiram/metronidazole, atorvastatin, rosuvastatin, fluticasone, omeprazole, cyclosporine, sirolimus, and tacrolimus. Starting dose of sildenafil should not exceed 25mg within 48 hours, tadalafil 10mg every 72 hours, and vardenafil 2.5mg every 72 hours. Decreased levels of ethinyl estradiol; use alternative forms of birth control.

Dosage reduction needed for clarithromycin by 50% if CrCl 30-60mL/min and 75% if <30mL/min; rifabutin by 75%; desipramine. Increased levels with fluconazole. Monitor glucose with glimepiride, glipizide, glyburide, pioglitazone, repaglinide, or tolbutamine. Monitor INR with warfarin.

PREGNANCY: Category C, not for use in nursing.

MECHANISM OF ACTION: HIV-1 protease inhibitor; inhibits processing of Gag and Gag-Pol polyproteins, preventing formation of mature virions.

PHARMACOKINETICS: Absorption: Tipranavir/Ritonavir: C_{max}=94.8μM (female), 77.6μM (male). T_{max}=2.9 hrs (female), 3.0 hrs (male). **Distribution:** Plasma protein binding (≥99.9%). **Metabolism:** Hepatic via CYP3A4. **Elimination:** Urine (0.5%), feces (79.9%). Tipranavir/Ritonavir: $T_{1/2}$=4.8 hrs (healthy), 6.0 hrs (HIV-infected).

ARALEN   RX
chloroquine phosphate (Sanofi-Aventis)

THERAPEUTIC CLASS: Aminoquinolone

INDICATIONS: Treatment of extraintestinal amebiasis and acute attacks of malaria. Suppression of malaria.

DOSAGE: *Adults:* Malaria: Initial: 1g, then 500mg 6-8 hrs later, then 500mg qd for 2 consecutive days (total of 2.5g in 3 days). Suppression: 500mg on the same day each week. Start 2 weeks before exposure (double initial dose if <2 weeks before exposure) and continue for 8 weeks after return. Extraintestinal Amebiasis: 1g qd for 2 days, then 500mg qd for at least 2-3 weeks. Treatment usually combined with intestinal amebicide.
Pediatrics: Malaria: Total dose of 25mg base/kg taken over 3 day, as follows: 1st Dose: 10mg base/kg (max 600mg base single dose). 2nd Dose: 5mg base/kg (300mg base single dose) 6 hrs after 1st dose. 3rd Dose: 5mg base/kg 18 hrs after 2nd dose. 4th Dose: 5mg base/kg 24 hrs after 3rd dose. Suppression: 5mg base/kg/week. Max: 300mg base/dose. Start 2 weeks before exposure (double initial dose if <2 weeks before exposure) and continue for 8 weeks after return.

HOW SUPPLIED: Tab: (Phosphate) 500mg (500mg tab=300mg base)

CONTRAINDICATIONS: Retinal or visual field changes.

WARNINGS/PRECAUTIONS: Caution with G6PD deficiency, pre-existing auditory damage, hepatic impairment, alcoholism, porphyria, psoriasis, elderly, and history of seizures. Monitor CBCs, vision, reflexes with prolonged use. D/C if visual or hematological disturbances, muscle weakness, hearing defects develop. Chloroquine resistance is widespread.

ADVERSE REACTIONS: Headache, pruritus, psychic stimulation, visual disturbances, pleomorphic skin eruptions, GI effects, convulsions, tinnitus, nerve type deafness.

INTERACTIONS: Caution with hepatotoxic drugs. Space dosing of antacids/kaolin by 4 hours. Increased levels with cimetidine; avoid concomitant use. Space dosing of ampicillin by at least 2 hours. May increase cyclosporine levels; monitor closely.

PREGNANCY: Avoid in pregnancy except for treatment of malaria if benefits outweigh risks. Not for use in nursing.

MECHANISM OF ACTION: Antimalarial aminoquinolone; unknown, suspected to inhibit certain enzymes, resulting from its interaction with DNA.

PHARMACOKINETICS: Absorption: Rapidly and completely absorbed (GIT). **Distribution:** Plasma protein binding (approximately 55%). Crosses placenta. **Metabolism:** Undergoes appreciable degradation. Desethylchloroquine (main metabolite). **Elimination:** Urine (unchanged).

ARAMINE RX
metaraminol bitartrate (Merck)

THERAPEUTIC CLASS: Sympathomimetic amine

INDICATIONS: Prevention and treatment of the acute hypotensive state occurring with spinal anesthesia. Adjunct treatment of hypotension due to hemorrhage, reactions to medications, surgical complications, and shock associated with brain damage due to trauma or tumor.

DOSAGE: *Adults:* Hypotension Prevention: 2-10mg IM/SC. Hypotension Adjunct Treatment: Adjust 15-100mg IV infusion to maintain desired BP. Severe Shock: 0.5-5mg direct IV injection, followed by 15-100mg IV infusion.

HOW SUPPLIED: Inj: 10mg/mL

CONTRAINDICATIONS: Cyclopropane or halothane anesthesia.

WARNINGS/PRECAUTIONS: Contains sodium bisulfate; may cause allergic reaction especially in asthmatics. Avoid excessive BP response. Possible prolonged BP elevation after discontinuation. Caution with cirrhosis, heart or thyroid disease, HTN, or diabetes. If used for long periods, the resulting vasoconstriction may prevent adequate expansion of circulating volume and cause perpetuation of shock. May provoke relapse in patients with history of malaria.

ADVERSE REACTIONS: Tachycardia, arrhythmia, abscess formation/tissue necrosis/sloughing at injection site.

INTERACTIONS: See Contraindications. Caution in digitalized patients; digitalis with sympathomimetic amines may cause ectopic arrhythmias. MAOIs or TCAs may potentiate pressor effect; lower initial dose of metaraminol.

PREGNANCY: Category C, caution in nursing.

MECHANISM OF ACTION: Sympathomimetic amine; has a positive inotropic effect on the heart and a peripheral vasoconstrictor action. It increases both systolic and diastolic blood pressure.

ARANESP RX
darbepoetin alfa (Amgen)

> Increased mortality, serious cardiovascular/thromboembolic events, and tumor progression. Erythropoiesis-stimulating agents (ESAs) may increase risk for death and/or serious cardiovascular events when administered to a target Hgb >12g/dL. Use lowest level sufficient to avoid need for RBC transfusion. When ESAs are used preoperatively for reduction of allogenic RBC transfusions, a higher incidence of DVT was reported in patients not receiving prophylactic anticoagulation; darbepoetin alfa is not approved for this indication. ESAs shortened overall survival in patients with breast, head and neck, lymphoid, non-small cell lung, and cervical cancers when dosed to target Hgb ≥ 12 g/dL. Use only for treatment of anemia due to concomitant myelosuppressive chemotherapy. D/C following completion of chemotherapy.

THERAPEUTIC CLASS: Erythropoiesis stimulator

INDICATIONS: Treatment of anemia associated with chronic renal failure (CRF), and anemia in patients with non-myeloid malignancies due to chemotherapy.

DOSAGE: *Adults:* CRF: Initial: 0.45mcg/kg IV/SQ weekly. Titrate: Adjust to target Hgb <12g/dL. If Hgb increases >1g/dL in a 2-week period or is approaching 12g/dL, decrease dose by 25%. If Hgb continues to increase, hold dose until Hgb begins to decrease, and reinitiate at 25% below previous dose. Do not increase more than once monthly. Conversion from Epoetin Alfa: Base dose on weekly epoetin dose. Give once weekly if receiving epoetin 2-3x/week. Give every 2 weeks if receiving epoetin once weekly. (See PI for details). Malignancy: Initial: 2.25mcg/kg SQ weekly or 500mcg once every 3 weeks. Titrate: Increase to 4.5mcg/kg if Hgb increases <1g/dL after 6 weeks of therapy. If Hgb increases by >1g/dL in a 2-week period or if Hgb >12g/dL, decrease dose by 40%. If Hgb >13g/dL, hold dose until Hgb falls to 12g/dL and reinitiate at 40% below previous dose.
Pediatrics: ≥1 years: CRF: Conversion from Epoetin Alfa: Base dose on weekly

epoetin dose. Give once weekly if receiving epoetin 2-3x/week. Give every 2 weeks if receiving epoetin once weekly. (See Full Prescribing Information for details).

HOW SUPPLIED: Inj: Syringe: 0.025mg/0.42mL, 0.04mg/0.4mL, 0.06mg/0.3mL, 0.1mg/0.5mL, 0.15mg/0.3mL, 0.2mg/0.4mL, 0.3mg/0.6mL, 0.5mg/mL; SDV: 0.025mg/mL, 0.04mg/mL, 0.06mg/mL, 0.1mg/mL, 0.15mg/0.75mL, 0.2mg/mL, 0.3mg/mL

CONTRAINDICATIONS: Uncontrolled HTN.

WARNINGS/PRECAUTIONS: Pure red cell aplasia and severe anemia (with or without other cytopenias) may occur. Due to increased Hgb, increased risk of cardiovascular events including death may occur. This includes MI, stroke, CHF, and hemodialysis vascular access thrombosis. Control BP before therapy. Seizures reported. Increased risk of thrombotic events. Evaluate etiology if lack/loss of response occurs. Permanently d/c if serious allergic reaction occurs. Monitor renal function, fluid, and electrolytes. Albumin solution carries risk of transmission of viral diseases. May need interval of 2-6 weeks between dose adjustment and response. Monitor Hgb weekly until stabilized and maintenance dose is established, and for at least 4 weeks after dosage change. Monitor iron status before and during therapy. Increases RBCs and decreases plasma volume. ESAs shortened time to tumor progression in patients with advanced head and neck cancer receiving radiation therapy.

ADVERSE REACTIONS: Thrombic events, infection, myalgia, HTN, hypotension, headache, diarrhea, fatigue, edema, nausea, vomiting, fever, dyspnea.

PREGNANCY: Category C, caution in nursing.

MECHANISM OF ACTION: Erythropoiesis stimulating protein; stimulates erythropoiesis (same mechanism as endogenous erythropoietin) in response to hypoxia by interacting with progenitor stem cells to increase RBC production.

PHARMACOKINETICS: Absorption: Adults: (SQ) Bioavailability (37%). (2.25mcg/kg; 6.75mcg/kg) T_{max}=90 hrs; 71 hrs. **Pediatrics:** Bioavailability (54%). **Elimination:** (IV, SQ): $T_{1/2}$=21 hrs; 74 hrs.

ARAVA RX
leflunomide (Sanofi-Aventis)

> Avoid pregnancy during treatment or before completion of drug elimination procedure after treatment.

THERAPEUTIC CLASS: Pyrimidine synthesis inhibitor

INDICATIONS: Treatment of active rheumatoid arthritis to reduce signs/symptoms, inhibit structural damage, or improve physical function.

DOSAGE: *Adults:* LD: 100mg qd for 3 days. Maint: 20mg qd. If not tolerated and/or ALT elevations >2 but ≤3x ULN: Reduce to 10mg qd. If elevations persist or >3x ULN, d/c and give cholestyramine or charcoal. Max: 20mg/day.

HOW SUPPLIED: Tab: 10mg, 20mg, 100mg

CONTRAINDICATIONS: Pregnancy.

WARNINGS/PRECAUTIONS: May cause immunosuppression. Avoid with severe immunodeficiency, bone marrow dysplasia, severe, uncontrolled infections, significant hepatic impairment, or evidence of hepatitis B or C. *Pneumocystis jiroveci* pneumonia, tuberculosis, aspergillosis, and sepsis reported. Rare reports of pancytopenia, agranulocytosis, thrombocytopenia, Stevens-Johnson syndrome, toxic epidermal necrolysis, and potentially fatal severe liver injury. Monitor WBCs, platelets, Hgb, Hct, LFTs (esp ALT) at baseline then monthly for 6 months, and every 6-8 weeks thereafter; monitor monthly with concomitant MTX and/or other immunosuppressive agents. D/C with evidence of bone marrow suppression. Women of childbearing potential must have negative pregnancy test. Interstitial lung disease reported. Caution with renal impairment.

ADVERSE REACTIONS: Diarrhea, respiratory infections, HTN, alopecia, rash, nausea, bronchitis, abdominal/back pain, abnormal liver enzymes, urinary tract infections, dyspepsia.

INTERACTIONS: Decreased levels with cholestyramine or activated charcoal. Increased side effects with hepatotoxic substances. Increased levels with rifampin; caution with concomitant use. May increase levels of diclofenac, ibuprofen, or tolbutamide. Avoid vaccination with live vaccines.

PREGNANCY: Category X, not for use in nursing.

MECHANISM OF ACTION: Pyrimidine synthesis inhibitor; immunomodulatory agent. Acts by inhibiting dihydroorotate dehydrogenase. Produces antiproliferative activity.

PHARMACOKINETICS: Absorption: A77 1726 (M1) (major active metabolite): T_{max}=6-12 hrs. Oral administration of various doses led to different parameters. **Distribution**: (M1) V_d=0.13L/kg; Plasma protein binding (>99.3%). **Metabolism**: M1 and many minor metabolites. **Elimination**: Urine (43%), feces (48%).

AREDIA   RX
pamidronate disodium (Novartis)

THERAPEUTIC CLASS: Bone resorption inhibitor

INDICATIONS: Treatment of moderate to severe hypercalcemia of malignancy, Paget's disease. Adjunct to standard antineoplastic therapy for treatment of osteolytic bone metastases of breast cancer and osteolytic lesions of multiple myeloma.

DOSAGE: *Adults:* Moderate Hypercalcemia: 60-90mg IV single dose over 2-24 hrs. Severe Hypercalcemia: 90mg IV single dose over 2-24 hrs. Retreatment: May repeat after 7 days. Paget's Disease: 30mg IV over 4 hrs for 3 consecutive days. Osteolytic Bone Lesions of Multiple Myeloma: 90mg IV over 4 hrs once a month. Osteolytic Bone Metastases of Breast Cancer: 90mg IV over 2 hrs every 3-4 weeks. Max: 90mg/single dose for all indications. Renal Dysfunction With Bone Metastases: Withhold dose if SrCr increases by 0.5mg/dL (normal baseline) or by 1mg/dL (abnormal baseline). Resume when SrCr returns to within 10% of baseline.

HOW SUPPLIED: Inj: 30mg, 90mg

WARNINGS/PRECAUTIONS: Associated with renal toxicity; monitor serum creatinine prior to each treatment. Monitor serum calcium, electrolytes, phosphate, magnesium, CBC with differential, Hct/Hgb closely. Monitor for 2 weeks post-treatment if pre-existing anemia, leukopenia, thrombocytopenia. Increased risk of renal adverse reactions with renal impairment; monitor renal function. Avoid treatment of bone metastases in severe renal impairment. Reports of osteonecrosis of jaw in cancer patients treated with bisphosphonates; avoid invasive dental procedures.

ADVERSE REACTIONS: Malaise, fever, convulsions, hypomagnesemia, hypocalcemia, hypokalemia, fluid overload, hypophosphatemia, nausea, diarrhea, constipation, anorexia, abnormal hepatic function, bone pain, dyspnea.

PREGNANCY: Category D, caution in nursing.

MECHANISM OF ACTION: Bone resorption inhibitor; mechanism of antiresorptive action not established. Absorbs to calcium phosphate crystals in bone and may directly block dissolution of this mineral component of bone. Inhibition of osteoclast activity contributes to inhibition of bone resorption.

PHARMACOKINETICS: Elimination: Urine (46% unchanged); $T_{1/2}$=28 hrs.

ARGATROBAN   RX
argatroban (GlaxoSmithKline)

THERAPEUTIC CLASS: Direct thrombin inhibitor

INDICATIONS: Prophylaxis or treatment of thrombosis in heparin-induced thrombocytopenia (HIT). As an anticoagulant in patients with or at risk for HIT undergoing percutaneous coronary intervention (PCI).

DOSAGE: *Adults:* Thrombosis: D/C heparin and obtain baseline aPTT. Initial: 2mcg/kg/min IV. Check aPTT after 2 hrs. Titrate: Increase dose until aPTT is 1.5-3x initial baseline. Max: 10mcg/kg/min. Moderate Hepatic Impairment: Initial: 0.5mcg/kg/min. PCI: Initial: 350mcg/kg bolus with 25mcg/kg/min IV. Check activated clotting time (ACT) 5-10 min after bolus. Proceed with PCI if ACT >300 sec. If ACT <300 sec, give additional 150mcg/kg bolus and increase infusion to 30mcg/kg/min. Check ACT 5-10 min later. If ACT >450 sec, decrease to 15mcg/kg/min and check ACT 5-10 min later. Continue infusion dose at therapeutic ACT (300-450 sec) during procedure. May give additional 150mcg/kg bolus and increase infusion to 40mcg/kg/min if dissection, impending abrupt closure, thrombus formation, or inability to achieve/maintain ACT >300 sec. After PCI, may use lower infusion rate if anticoagulation is needed.

HOW SUPPLIED: Inj: 100mg/mL

CONTRAINDICATIONS: Overt major bleeding.

WARNINGS/PRECAUTIONS: D/C all parenteral anticoagulants before administering. Extreme caution in conditions associated with an increased danger of hemorrhage (eg, severe HTN, immediately following lumbar puncture, bleeding disorder, GI lesions, spinal anesthesia, major surgery, etc). Caution in hepatic impairment. Avoid high doses in PCI patients with significant hepatic disease or AST/ALT ≥3x ULN. Monitor aPTT. For PCI, obtain ACT before dose, 5-10 min after bolus and infusion rate change, at the end of PCI, and every 20-30 min during prolonged procedures.

ADVERSE REACTIONS: GI bleed, GU bleed, Hct/Hgb decrease, hypotension, fever, diarrhea, sepsis, cardiac arrest, nausea, ventricular tachycardia, vomiting, allergic reactions, chest pain (in PCI).

INTERACTIONS: Initiate after cessation of heparin therapy; allow time for heparin's effect on the aPTT to decrease. Prolongation of PT/INR with warfarin. Antiplatelets, thrombolytics, and other anticoagulants may increase risk of bleeding. Discontinue all anticoagulants before argatroban administration.

PREGNANCY: Category B, not for use in nursing.

MECHANISM OF ACTION: Direct thrombin inhibitor; reversibly binds to thrombin active site. Exerts anticoagulant effects by inhibiting thrombin-catalyzed or thrombin-induced reactions, including fibrin formation; activation of coagulation factors V, VIII, XIII; activation of protein C; and platelet aggregation. Capable of inhibiting both free and clot-associated thrombin.

PHARMACOKINETICS: Distribution: V_d= 174mL/Kg; Plasma protein binding (54%). **Metabolism:** Liver, via hydroxylation and aromatization; CYP3A4/5; M1 (primary metabolite). **Elimination:** Feces (primary), urine; $T_{1/2}$=39-51 min.

ARICEPT   RX
donepezil HCL (Eisai/Pfizer)

OTHER BRAND NAMES: Aricept ODT (Eisai/Pfizer)

THERAPEUTIC CLASS: Acetylcholinesterase inhibitor

INDICATIONS: Treatment of dementia of the Alzheimer's type.

DOSAGE: *Adults:* Mild to Moderate Alzheimer's Disease: Initial: 5mg qd. Titrate: May increase to 10mg after 4-6 weeks. Severe Alzheimer's Disease: 10mg qd. Start with 5mg qd and increase to 10mg after 4-6 weeks.

HOW SUPPLIED: Tab: 5mg, 10mg; Tab, Disintegrating: 5mg, 10mg

CONTRAINDICATIONS: Hypersensitivity to piperidine derivatives.

WARNINGS/PRECAUTIONS: May exaggerate succinylcholine-type muscle relaxation during anesthesia. May have vagotonic effects on sinoatrial and atrioventricular node; may cause bradycardia or heart block. May increase gastric acid secretion; monitor for GI bleeding. May cause bladder outflow obstruction or seizures. Caution with asthma or COPD.

ADVERSE REACTIONS: Nausea, diarrhea, insomnia, vomiting, muscle cramps, fatigue, anorexia, dizziness, depression, weight decrease, infection, HTN, back pain, abnormal dreams, ecchymosis.

INTERACTIONS: Synergistic effect with neuromuscular blocking agents (eg, succinylcholine) and cholinergic agonists (eg, bethanechol). May interfere with anticholinergic medications. CYP2D6 and CYP3A4 inducers (eg, phenytoin, carbamazepine, dexamethasone, rifampin, phenobarbital) may increase elimination rate. Ketoconazole and quinidine inhibitors of CYP450, 3A4, and 2D6, respectively, inhibit donepezil metabolism.

PREGNANCY: Category C, not for use in nursing.

MECHANISM OF ACTION: Acetylcholinesterase inhibitor; postulated to exert effect by increasing acetylcholine concentrations through inhibition of its hydrolysis by AChE.

PHARMACOKINETICS: Absorption: Absolute bioavailability (complete) T_{max}=3-4 hrs. **Distribution:** plasma protein binding (96%) **Metabolism:** Hepatic (glucoronidation) via CYP2D6 and CYP3A4. **Elimination:** Urine (57%), feces (15%). $T_{1/2}$=70 hrs.

ARIMIDEX   RX
anastrozole (AstraZeneca)

THERAPEUTIC CLASS: Aromatase inhibitor (non-steroidal)

INDICATIONS: Adjuvant treatment of postmenopausal women with hormone-receptor positive early breast cancer. First-line treatment of postmenopausal women with hormone-receptor positive or hormone-receptor unknown locally advanced or metastatic breast cancer. Treatment of advanced breast cancer in postmenopausal women with disease progression following tamoxifen therapy. Patients with ER-negative disease and patients who did not respond to previous tamoxifen therapy rarely respond.

DOSAGE: *Adults:* 1mg qd. Continue until tumor progression with advanced breast cancer.

HOW SUPPLIED: Tab: 1mg

WARNINGS/PRECAUTIONS: May cause fetal harm during pregnancy. Avoid in premenopausal women. May cause reduction in bone mineral density. May elevate serum cholesterol.

ADVERSE REACTIONS: Joint disorders, mood disturbances, pharyngitis, depression, HTN, osteoporosis, peripheral edema, bone fractures, asthenia, headache, hot flushes, dyspnea, nausea, vomiting, cough, pain, edema.

INTERACTIONS: Avoid tamoxifen, estrogen-containing therapies.

PREGNANCY: Category D, caution in nursing.

MECHANISM OF ACTION: Nonsteroidal aromatase inhibitor; lowers estradiol concentrations and has no detectable effect on formation of adrenal cortico-steroids or aldosterone.

PHARMACOKINETICS: Distribution: Plasma protein binding (40%). **Metabolism:** Liver via N-dealkylation, hydroxylation, and glucuronidation. **Elimination:** Hepatic (major), renal (minor); $T_{1/2}$=50 hrs; urine (10%).

ARIXTRA   RX
fondaparinux sodium (GlaxoSmithKline)

> Risk of paralysis by spinal/epidural hematoma with neuraxial anesthesia or spinal puncture. Increased risk with indwelling epidural catheters for analgesia, drugs affecting hemostasis (eg, NSAIDs, platelet inhibitors, anticoagulants), and traumatic or repeated epidural or spinal puncture.

THERAPEUTIC CLASS: Specific factor Xa inhibitor

INDICATIONS: Prophylaxis of DVT in patients undergoing hip fracture surgery, including extended prophylaxis; hip replacement surgery; knee replacement surgery; abdominal surgery who are at risk of thromboembolic complications. With concomitant warfarin, treatment of acute PE when initial therapy is administered in hospital and acute DVT.

DOSAGE: *Adults:* DVT Prophylaxis: 2.5mg SQ qd, starting 6-8 hrs post-op for 5-9 days (up to 11 days). Hip Fracture Surgery: Extended prophylaxis up to 24 additional days is recommended. DVT/PE Treatment: <50kg: 5mg SQ qd. 50-100kg: 7.5mg SQ qd. >100kg: 10mg SQ qd. Add concomitant warfarin ASAP (usually within 72 hrs) and continue for 5-9 days (up to 26 days) until INR=2-3.

HOW SUPPLIED: Inj: (Syringe) 2.5mg/0.5mL, 5mg/0.4mL, 7.5mg/0.6mL, 10mg/0.8mL

CONTRAINDICATIONS: Severe renal impairment (CrCl <30mL/min), body weight <50kg undergoing hip fracture, hip/knee replacement or abdominal surgery, bacterial endocarditis, active major bleeding, thrombocytopenia with a positive *in vitro* test for anti-platelet antibody.

WARNINGS/PRECAUTIONS: Not for IM injection. Cannot use interchangeably unit for unit with heparin or other low molecular weight heparins. Risk of hemorrhage increases with renal impairment. Caution with moderate renal dysfunction, elderly, history of HIT, bleeding diathesis, uncontrolled arterial HTN, recent GI ulceration, diabetic retinopathy, hemorrhage. Monitor renal function periodically. Extreme caution in conditions with an increased risk of hemorrhage (eg, bleeding disorders, hemorrhagic stroke, etc). Perform routine CBC, SCr, stool occult blood tests. D/C if platelets <100,000/mm³. Thrombocytopenia reported. Major bleeding with abdominal surgery reported.

ADVERSE REACTIONS: Bleeding complications, thrombocytopenia, local reactions (eg, rash, pruritus), anemia, fever, nausea, edema, constipation, vomiting, insomnia, hypokalemia, UTI, dizziness, pupura, hypotension.

INTERACTIONS: Discontinue agents that may enhance risk of hemorrhage (eg, platelet inhibitors); monitor closely if co-administered.

PREGNANCY: Category B, caution in nursing.

MECHANISM OF ACTION: Specific factor Xa inhibitor; selectively binds to antithrombin III (ATIII). Potentiates the innate neutralization of Factor Xa by ATIII. Neutralization of Factor Xa interrupts the blood coagulation cascade and thus inhibits thrombin formation and thrombus development.

PHARMACOKINETICS: Absorption: Rapid, complete; Absolute bioavailability (100%); C_{max}=0.39-0.5 mg/L (2.5 mg QD); 1.2-1.26mg/L (5mg, 7.5mg, 10mg QD); T_{max}=3 hrs (2.5 mg QD). **Distribution:** V_d=7-11L; bound to ATIII (94%). **Metabolism:** Not investigated. **Elimination:** Urine (77%); $T_{1/2}$=17-21 hrs.

ARMOUR THYROID   RX
thyroid (Forest)

THERAPEUTIC CLASS: Thyroid replacement hormone

INDICATIONS: Treatment of hypothyroidism. As a pituitary TSH suppressant in the treatment or prevention of various types of euthyroid goiters. Diagnostic agent in suppression tests to differentiate suspected mild hyperthyroidism or thyroid gland autonomy. Management of thyroid cancer.

DOSAGE: *Adults:* Hypothyroidism: Initial: 30mg qd. Titrate: Increase by 15mg q2-3 weeks. Myxedema with Cardiovascular Disorder: 15mg qd. Maint: 60-120mg/day. Thyroid Cancer: Higher doses than replacement therapy are required. Myxedema Coma: Levothyroxine Sodium: Initial: 400mcg IV then 100-200mcg/day IV. Continue with oral therapy when stabilized. Thyroid Suppression: 1.56mg/kg/day for 7-10 days. Elderly: Initial: Use lower dose (eg, 15-30mg qd).
Pediatrics: Hypothyroidism: 0-6 months: 4.8-6mg/kg/day; 6-12 months: 3.6-4.8mg/kg/day; 1-5 yrs: 3-3.6mg/kg/day; 6-12 yrs: 2.4-3mg/kg/day; >12 yrs: 1.2-1.8mg/kg/day.

HOW SUPPLIED: Tab: 15mg, 30mg, 60mg, 90mg, 120mg, 180mg, 240mg, 300mg

CONTRAINDICATIONS: Untreated thyrotoxicosis; uncorrected adrenal cortical insufficiency.

WARNINGS/PRECAUTIONS: Do not use in the treatment of obesity; larger doses in euthyroid patients can cause serious or even life threatening toxicity. Caution with cardiovascular disease, DM, diabetes insipidus, elderly, and adrenal cortical insufficiency.

INTERACTIONS: May increase insulin or oral hypoglycemic requirements. Reduced absorption with cholestyramine and colestipol; space dosing by 4-5 hrs. Altered effect of oral anticoagulants; monitor PT/INR. Estrogens increase thyroxine-binding globulin; increase in thyroid dose may be needed. Serious or life-threatening side effects can occur with sympathomimetic amines. Androgens, corticosteroids, estrogens, iodine-containing preparations, and salicylates may interfere with thyroid lab tests.

PREGNANCY: Category A, caution in nursing.

MECHANISM OF ACTION: Thyroid hormone; not established, suspected to enhance oxygen consumption by most tissues of the body, increase the basal metabolic rate and metabolism of carbohydrates, lipids, and proteins.

PHARMACOKINETICS: Abosrption: (T_3) Completely absorbed; T_{max}=4 hrs; (T_4) partially absorbed. **Distribution:** Plasma protein binding (>99%), found in breast milk. **Metabolism:** Deiodination in liver, kidneys, other tissues.

AROMASIN   RX
exemestane (Pharmacia & Upjohn)

THERAPEUTIC CLASS: Aromatase inactivator

INDICATIONS: In postmenopausal women, treatment of advanced breast cancer that has progressed after tamoxifen therapy. Adjuvant treatment of postmenopausal women with estrogen-receptor positive early breast cancer who have received 2-3 years of tamoxifen and are switched to exemestane for a total completion of 5 consecutive years to adjuvant hormonal therapy.

DOSAGE: *Adults:* Early/Advanced: 25mg qd after a meal. Continue in the absence of recurrence of contralateral breast cancer until completion of 5 years of adjuvant endocrine therapy in postmenopausal women with early breast cancer treated with 2-3 years of tamoxifen. Continue until tumor progression is evident. Concomitant Potent CYP3A4 Inducers (eg, rifampicin, phenytoin): 50mg qd after a meal.

HOW SUPPLIED: Tab: 25mg

WARNINGS/PRECAUTIONS: Fetal harm in pregnancy. Avoid in premenopausal women.

ADVERSE REACTIONS: Fatigue, nausea, hot flashes, pain, depression, insomnia, anxiety, dyspnea, dizziness, headache, vomiting, increased sweating, edema, HTN, anorexia.

INTERACTIONS: Avoid coadministration with estrogen-containing agents. Potent CYP3A4 inducers (eg, rifampin, phenytoin, carbamazepine, phenobarbital, St. John's wort) may decrease plasma levels.

PREGNANCY: Category D, caution in nursing.

MECHANISM OF ACTION: Irreversible steroidal aromatase inactivator; acts as false substrate for aromatase enzyme; processed to intermediate that binds irreversibly to active site of enzyme, causing inactivation.

PHARMACOKINETICS: Absorption: Rapid. (Healthy) T_{max}=2.9 hrs; AUC=41.4ng•h/mL. (Breast cancer) T_{max}=1.2 hrs; AUC=75.4ng•h/mL. **Distribution:** Plasma protein binding (90%). **Metabolism:** Oxidation via CYP3A4; reduction. **Elimination:** Urine (<1%), $T_{1/2}$=24 hrs.

ARRANON   RX
nelarabine (GlaxoSmithKline)

> Severe neurologic events reported; close monitoring is strongly recommended. Discontinue for neurologic events of NCI Common Toxicity Criteria ≥ grade 2.

THERAPEUTIC CLASS: Deoxyguanosine analogue

INDICATIONS: Treatment of T-cell acute lymphoblastic leukemia and T-cell lymphoblastic lymphoma in patients whose disease has not responded to or has relapsed following treatment with at least two chemotherapy regimens.

DOSAGE: *Adults:* 1500mg/m² IV over 2 hrs on days 1, 3, and 5 repeated every 21 days. CrCl <50ml/min: Insufficient data to support dose recommendation. *Pediatrics:* 650mg/m²/day IV over 1 hr daily for 5 consecutive days. Repeat every 21 days. CrCl <50ml/min: Insufficient data to support dose recommendation.

HOW SUPPLIED: Inj: 5mg/mL

WARNINGS/PRECAUTIONS: Leukopenia, thrombocytopenia, anemia, neutropenia/febrile neutropenia reported; regularly monitor CBC including platelets. Intravenous hydration recommended for management of hyperuricemia with risk of tumor lysis syndrome; may also consider allopurinol. Avoid administration of live vaccines. Closely monitor toxicities with severe renal impairment (eg, CrCl <30mL/min) and/or severe hepatic impairment (eg, bilirubin >3mg/dL); increased risk of adverse reactions.

ADVERSE REACTIONS: See Black Box Warning, Warnings/Precautions. **Pediatrics:** headache, increased transaminases, decreased blood potassium, decreased/increased blood albumin, vomiting. **Adults:** fatigue, nausea, diarrhea, vomiting, constipation, cough, dyspnea, dizziness, pyrexia, blurred vision.

PREGNANCY: Category D, not for use in nursing.

MECHANISM OF ACTION: Deoxyguanosine analogue; inhibits DNA synthesis, causing cell death.

PHARMACOKINETICS: Absorption: Nelarabine: C_{max}=5µg/mL; AUC=162µg•h/mL. ara-G: C_{max}=31.4µg/mL; AUC=4.4µg•h/mL. **Distribution:** Plasma protein binding (<25%). Nelarabine: (Adults) V_{ss}=197L/m²; (Pediatrics) V_{ss}=213L/m². ara-G: (Adults) V_{ss}=50L/m²; (Pediatrics) V_{ss}=33L/m². **Metabolism:** O-demethylation via adenosine deaminase. (Metabolite): Ara-G. **Elimination:** Kidneys (partial). Nelarabine: Urine (6.6%); $T_{1/2}$=30 min. ara-G: Urine (27%); $T_{1/2}$=3 hrs.

ARTHROTEC   RX
diclofenac sodium - misoprostol (G.D. Searle)

> Contraindicated in pregnancy. Must have negative pregnancy test 2 weeks before therapy. Provide oral and written hazards of misoprostol. Begin on 2nd or 3rd day of the next normal menstrual period. Use reliable contraception. NSAIDs may cause an increased risk of serious cardiovascular thrombotic events, MI, stroke, and serious GI adverse events including bleeding, ulceration, and perforation of the stomach or intestines. Contraindicated for the treatment of perioperative pain in the setting of coronary artery bypass graft (CABG) surgery.

THERAPEUTIC CLASS: NSAID/prostaglandin E₁ analogue

INDICATIONS: Treatment of the signs and symptoms of osteoarthritis (OA) or rheumatoid arthritis (RA) in patients at high risk of developing NSAID-induced gastric and duodenal ulcers.

DOSAGE: *Adults:* OA: 50mg tid. RA: 50mg tid-qid. OA/RA: If not tolerable, give 50-75mg bid (less effective in preventing ulcers). Do not crush, chew, or divide.

HOW SUPPLIED: Tab: (Diclofenac-Misoprostol) 50mg-0.2mg, 75mg-0.2mg

CONTRAINDICATIONS: Pregnancy. ASA or other NSAID allergy that precipitates asthma, urticaria, or other allergic reactions. Treatment of perioperative pain in the setting of CABG surgery.

WARNINGS/PRECAUTIONS: May lead to onset of new HTN or worsening of pre-existing HTN; monitor BP closely. Fluid retention and edema reported; caution with fluid retention or heart failure. Renal papillary necrosis and other renal injury reported after long-term use. Not recommended for use with advanced renal disease; if therapy must be initiated, monitor renal function. May cause elevations of LFTs; d/c if abnormal LFTs persist/worsen, liver disease develops or systemic manifestations occur. Anaphylactoid reactions may occur. May cause serious skin adverse events (eg, exfoliative dermatitis, Stevens-Johnson syndrome, and toxic epidermal necrolysis). Avoid in late pregnancy; may cause premature closure of ductus arteriosus. Caution in elderly. Anemia may occur; with long-term use, monitor Hgb/Hct if signs or symptoms of anemia. May inhibit platelet aggregation and prolong bleeding time; monitor with coagulation disorders. Caution with asthma and avoid with ASA-sensitive asthma. Aseptic meningitis with fever and coma reported. Avoid with hepatic porphyria.

ADVERSE REACTIONS: Abdominal pain, diarrhea, dyspepsia, nausea, flatulence, GI disorders.

INTERACTIONS: Avoid magnesium-containing antacids, salicylates, ASA, other NSAIDs. Caution with anticoagulants; may have synergistic GI bleeding effects with warfarin. May decrease effects of antihypertensives, diuretics. Increased serum potassium with K⁺-sparing diuretics. May alter response to insulin or oral hypoglycemics. Monitor for digoxin, methotrexate, cyclosporine, phenobarbital, and lithium toxicities.

PREGNANCY: Category X, not for use in nursing.

MECHANISM OF ACTION: Diclofenac: NSAID; mechanism not established. May be related to prostaglandin synthetase inhibition. Possesses anti-inflammatory, analgesic, and antipyretic properties. Misoprostol: prostaglandin E_1 analog with gastric antisecretory and mucosal protective properties.

PHARMACOKINETICS: Absorption: Oral administration of a single dose or multiple doses of medication are similar to pharmacokinetics of two individual components. Refer to PI for further information. **Distribution:** Diclofenac: Albumin binding (99%); V_d=550mL/kg; found in breast milk. Misoprostol: Plasma protein binding (<90%). **Metabolism:** Diclofenac: Glucuronide and sulfate conjugation. Misoprostol: Rapidly, to misoprostol acid (active metabolite). **Elimination:** Diclofenac: Urine (65%), bile (35%); $T_{1/2}$=2 hrs. Misoprostol: Urine (70%); $T_{1/2}$=30 min.

ASACOL   RX
mesalamine (Procter & Gamble)

THERAPEUTIC CLASS: Anti-inflammatory Agent

INDICATIONS: Treatment of mild to moderately active ulcerative colitis and maintenance of remission of ulcerative colitis.

DOSAGE: *Adults:* Mild-Moderate Active Ulcerative Colitis: Usual: 800mg tid for 6 weeks. Maintenance of Remission: 1.6g/day in divided doses.

HOW SUPPLIED: Tab, Delayed-Release: 400mg

CONTRAINDICATIONS: Hypersensitivity to salicylates.

WARNINGS/PRECAUTIONS: Exacerbation of colitis reported upon initiation of therapy; symptoms abate with discontinuation. Caution with sulfasalazine hypersensitivity. Caution with renal dysfunction or history of renal disease. Monitor renal function prior to therapy and periodically after. Pyloric stenosis could delay mesalamine release in the colon.

ADVERSE REACTIONS: Diarrhea, headache, nausea, pharyngitis, abdominal pain, pain, eructation, dizziness, asthenia, fever, dysmenorrhea, arthralgia, dyspepsia, vomiting.

PREGNANCY: Category B, caution in nursing.

MECHANISM OF ACTION: Unknown, possibly diminishes inflammation by blocking cyclooxygenase and inhibiting prostaglandin production in the colon.

PHARMACOKINETICS: Absorption: T_{max}=4-12 hrs. **Metabolism:** Gut mucosal wall and liver via rapid acetylation. Metabolite (N-acetyl-5-aminosalicylic acid). **Elimination:** $T_{1/2}$=2-15 hrs. Renally excreted as metabolite.

ASMANEX   RX
mometasone furoate (Schering)

THERAPEUTIC CLASS: Corticosteroid

INDICATIONS: Maintenance treatment of asthma as prophylactic therapy in patients ≥4 yrs.

DOSAGE: *Adults:* Previous Therapy with Bronchodilators Alone or Inhaled Corticosteroids: Initial: 220mcg qpm. Max: 440mcg qpm or 220mcg bid. Previous Therapy with Oral Corticosteroids: Initial: 440mcg bid. Max: 880mcg/day. Titrate to lowest effective dose once asthma stability achieved. *Pediatrics:* ≥12 yrs: Previous Therapy with Bronchodilators Alone or Inhaled Corticosteroids (CS): Initial: 220mcg qpm. Max: 440mcg qpm or 220mcg bid. Previous Therapy with Oral CS: Initial: 440mcg bid. Max: 880mcg/day. 4-11 yrs: 110mcg qpm regardless of prior therapy. Titrate to lowest effective dose once asthma stability achieved.

HOW SUPPLIED: Twisthaler: 110mcg/inh, 220mcg/inh

CONTRAINDICATIONS: Primary treatment of status asthmaticus or other acute episodes of asthma where intensive measures are required.

WARNINGS/PRECAUTIONS: Deaths due to adrenal insufficiency have occurred with transfer from systemic corticosteroids to inhaled corticosteroids. Wean slowly from systemic corticosteroid therapy. Resume oral corticosteroids during stress or severe asthma attack. May unmask allergic conditions previously suppressed by systemic corticosteroid therapy. May increase susceptibility to infections. Not for rapid relief of bronchospasm or other acute episodes of asthma. D/C if bronchospasm occurs after dosing. Observe for systemic corticosteroid withdrawal effects, hypercorticism, reduced bone mineral density, and adrenal suppression; reduce dose slowly if needed. Decreased growth velocity may occur in pediatric patients. *Candida* infections in the mouth and pharynx reported. Caution with active or quiescent TB infection of respiratory tract; untreated systemic fungal, bacterial, viral, or parasitic infections; or ocular herpes simplex. Glaucoma, increased IOP, and cataracts reported.

ADVERSE REACTIONS: Headache, allergic rhinitis, pharyngitis, upper respiratory tract infection, sinusitis, oral candidiasis, dysmenorrhea, musculoskeletal pain, back pain, dyspepsia, myalgia, abdominal pain, nausea.

INTERACTIONS: Ketoconazole may increase plasma levels.

PREGNANCY: Category C, caution in nursing.

MECHANISM OF ACTION: Corticosteroid; shown to have inhibitory effects on multiple cell types (mast cells, eosinophils, neutrophils, macrophages, and lymphocytes) and mediators (histamine, eicosanoids, leukotrienes and cytokines), involved in inflammatory and asthmatic response.

PHARMACOKINETICS: Absorption: Absolute bioavailability (≤1%); C_{max}=94-114pcg/mL; T_{max}=1.0-2.5 hrs. **Distribution:** V_d=152L, plasma protein binding (98-99%). **Metabolism:** Liver, via CYP3A4. **Elimination:** $T_{1/2}$=5 hrs.

ASPIRIN WITH CODEINE   CIII
codeine - aspirin (Various)

THERAPEUTIC CLASS: Opioid analgesic

INDICATIONS: For relief of mild, moderate, and moderate to severe pain.

DOSAGE: *Adults:* 1-2 tabs of 325mg-30mg q4h prn. 1 tab of 325mg-60mg q4h prn.

HOW SUPPLIED: Tab: (ASA-Codeine) 325mg-30mg, 325mg-60mg

CONTRAINDICATIONS: Severe bleeding, disorders of coagulation or primary hemostasis (eg, hemophilia, hypoprothrombinemia, von Willebrand's disease, thrombocytopenia, thromboasthenia), ill defined hereditary platelet dysfunction, severe vitamin K deficiency, severe hepatic damage, anticoagulant therapy, peptic ulcer, serious GI lesions.

WARNINGS/PRECAUTIONS: May cause anaphylactic shock, severe allergic reactions. Serious bleeding can occur with peptic ulcer, GI lesions, and bleeding disorders. May prolong bleeding time if given preoperatively. Enhanced respiratory depression and CSF pressure with head injury or intracranial lesion. May obscure signs of acute abdominal conditions or head injury. Caution in children and teenagers with chickenpox or flu. Caution in elderly, debilitated, severe renal/hepatic impairment, gallbladder disease or gallstones, respiratory impairment, arrhythmias, inflammatory GI tract disorders, hypothyroidism, Addison's disease, prostatic hypertrophy, urethral stricture, coagulation disorders, head injuries, or acute abdominal conditions.

ADVERSE REACTIONS: Lightheadedness, dizziness, drowsiness, nausea, vomiting, constipation, hearing impairment, tinnitus, diminished vision, headache, respiratory depression, sweating.

INTERACTIONS: May enhance effects of MAOIs, oral anticoagulants, oral antidiabetic agents, insulin, 6-MP, methotrexate, penicillins, sulfonamides, NSAIDs, narcotic analgesics, alcohol, general anesthetics, tranquilizers, corticosteroids. May diminish effects of uricosurics. Accumulation to toxic levels can occur with para-aminosalicylic acid, furosemide, and vitamin C.

PREGNANCY: Category C, not for use in nursing.

ASTELIN   RX
azelastine HCL (MedPointe)

THERAPEUTIC CLASS: Antihistamine

INDICATIONS: Treatemnt of the symptoms of seasonal allergic rhinitis and vasomotor rhinitis.

DOSAGE: *Adults:* 2 sprays per nostril bid.
Pediatrics: Seasonal Allergic/Vasomotor Rhinitis: ≥12 yrs: 2 sprays per nostril bid. Seasonal Allergic Rhinitis: 5-11 yrs: 1 spray per nostril bid.

HOW SUPPLIED: Spray: 137mcg/spray [30mg]

ADVERSE REACTIONS: Bitter taste, somnolence, weight increase, headache, nasal burning, pharyngitis, paroxysmal sneezing, dry mouth, nausea, atrial fibrillation, palpitations.

INTERACTIONS: Avoid alcohol or other CNS depressants; additive CNS impairment may occur. Increased azelastine levels with cimetidine.

PREGNANCY: Category C, caution in nursing.

MECHANISM OF ACTION: Phthalazinone derivative; inhibits histamine H_1 receptor activity.

PHARMACOKINETICS: Absorption: T_{max}=2-3 hrs. **Distribution:** Azelastine: Plasma protein binding (88%); Desmethylazelastine: V_d=14.5L/kg; plasma protein binding (97%).

ASTRAMORPH PF   CII
morphine sulfate (Abraxis)

THERAPEUTIC CLASS: Opioid analgesic

INDICATIONS: Management of pain unresponsive to non-narcotic analgesics.

DOSAGE: *Adults:* IV: Initial: 2-10mg/70kg. Epidural Injection: Initial: 5mg in lumbar region. Titrate: If inadequate pain relief within 1 hr, increase by 1-2mg.

Max: 10mg/24hrs. Continuous Epidural: Initial: 2-4mg/24hrs. Give additional 1-2mg if needed. Intrathecal: 0.2-1mg single dose, do not repeat; may follow with 0.6mg/hr naloxone infusion to reduce incidence of side effects. Elderly/Debilitated: Epidural: <5mg/24hrs. Intrathecal: Lower dose.

HOW SUPPLIED: Inj: 0.5mg/mL, 1mg/mL

CONTRAINDICATIONS: Allergy to opiates, acute bronchial asthma, upper airway obstruction. Epidural/intrathecal routes with injection site infection, anticoagulants, bleeding diathesis, within 2 weeks of IV corticosteroids.

WARNINGS/PRECAUTIONS: Have resuscitation equipment, trained personnel and narcotic antagonists available; severe respiratory depression may occur. Avoid rapid administration. May be habit-forming. Caution with head injury, increased intracranial/intraocular pressure, decreased respiratory reserve, hepatic/renal dysfunction, elderly, debilitated. High doses may cause seizures. Smooth muscle hypertonicity may cause biliary colic, urinary difficulty or retention. Orthostatic hypotension may occur with hypovolemia or myocardial dysfunction. Acute respiratory failure reported with COPD or acute asthmatic attack. Limit epidural/intrathecal route to lumbar area.

ADVERSE REACTIONS: Respiratory depression, hypotension, pruritus, urinary retention, nausea, vomiting, constipation, anxiety, cough reflex depression, oliguria.

INTERACTIONS: CNS depressants (eg, alcohol, sedatives, antihistamines) and psychotropics (eg, MAOIs, phenothiazines, TCAs) potentiate CNS depression. Neuroleptics may increase respiratory depression.

PREGNANCY: Category C, safety in nursing not known.

MECHANISM OF ACTION: Opioid analgesic. Analgesic effect involves 3 areas of the CNS; the periaqueductal periventricular gray matter, the ventromedial medulla, and the spinal cord. Interacts predominantly with the μ-receptor to produce analgesic effects; μ-binding sites are found in the brain, spinal cord, and in the trigeminal nerve.

PHARMACOKINETICS: Absorption: (Epidural): C_{max}=33-40ng/mL; (intrathecal) C_{max}=<1-7.8ng/mL; (epidural, intrathecal) T_{max}=5-10 min. **Distribution:** Plasma protein binding (36%), muscle tissue binding (54%), (IV) V_d= 1-4.7L/kg; (intrathecal) V_d=22 mL. **Metabolism:** Hepatic glucuronidation. Found in breast milk. **Elimination:** Urine (major), feces (10%). (IV) $T_{1/2}$=1.5-2 hrs; (Epidural): $T_{1/2}$=39-249 min.

ATACAND   RX
candesartan cilexetil (AstraZeneca)

> Can cause death/injury to developing fetus during 2nd and 3rd trimesters. Stop therapy if pregnancy is detected.

THERAPEUTIC CLASS: Angiotensin II receptor antagonist

INDICATIONS: Treatment of hypertension, alone or with other antihypertensives. Treatment of heart failure (NYHA class II-IV, ejection fraction ≤40%) to reduce risk of death and hospitalizations.

DOSAGE: *Adults:* HTN: Monotherapy Without Volume Depletion: Initial: 16mg qd. Usual: 8-32mg/day given qd-bid. May add diuretic if BP not controlled. Intravascular Volume Depletion/Moderate Hepatic Impairment: Lower initial dose. Heart Failure: Initial: 4mg qd. Usual: 32mg qd. Titrate: Double dose every 2 weeks, as tolerated.

HOW SUPPLIED: Tab: 4mg, 8mg, 16mg, 32mg

WARNINGS/PRECAUTIONS: Can cause fetal injury/death. Correct volume or salt depletion before therapy or monitor closely. Changes in renal function may occur; caution with renal artery stenosis, CHF. Risk of hypotension; caution in major surgery and anesthesia, or when initiating therapy in heart failure. May cause hyperkalemia in heart failure patients; monitor serum potassium.

ADVERSE REACTIONS: Back pain, dizziness, upper respiratory infection.

INTERACTIONS: Increases lithium levels.

PREGNANCY: Category C (1st trimester) and D (2nd and 3rd trimesters), not for use in nursing.

MECHANISM OF ACTION: Angiotensin II receptor antagonist; selective for AT_1 receptors, with tight binding to and slow dissociation from receptor.

PHARMACOKINETICS: Absorption: Absolute bioavailability (14%); T_{max}=3-4 hrs. **Distribution:** Plasma protein binding (>99%); V_d=0.1L/kg. **Metabolism:** Ester hydrolysis (metabolite: candesartan); CYP2C9 (minor). **Elimination:** $T_{1/2}$=9 hrs; feces (56%), urine (26%).

ATACAND HCT   RX
candesartan cilexetil - hydrochlorothiazide (AstraZeneca)

> Can cause death/injury to developing fetus during 2nd and 3rd trimesters. Stop therapy if pregnancy detected.

THERAPEUTIC CLASS: Angiotensin II receptor antagonist/thiazide diuretic

INDICATIONS: Treatment of hypertension. Not for initial therapy.

DOSAGE: Initial: If BP not controlled on HCTZ 25mg/day or controlled but serum K+ decreased: 16mg-12.5mg tab qd. If BP not controlled on 32mg candesartan/day, give 32mg-12.5mg qd; may increase to 32mg-25mg qd.

HOW SUPPLIED: Tab: (Candesartan-HCTZ) 16mg-12.5mg, 32mg-12.5mg

CONTRAINDICATIONS: Anuria, sulfonamide hypersensitivity.

WARNINGS/PRECAUTIONS: Can cause fetal injury/death. Correct volume or salt depletion before therapy. Caution with hepatic or renal dysfunction, renal artery stenosis, severe CHF, history of allergies, and asthma. May exacerbate or activate SLE. Monitor serum electrolytes. Avoid if CrCl ≤30mL/min. Hyperuricemia, hyperglycemia, hypokalemia, hypomagnesemia, hypercalcemia may occur. Enhanced effects in post-sympathectomy patient. May increase cholesterol and triglyceride levels. Risk of hypotension; caution in major surgery or anesthesia.

ADVERSE REACTIONS: Upper respiratory infection, back pain, influenza-like symptoms, dizziness, headache.

INTERACTIONS: Potentiates orthostatic hypotension with alcohol, barbiturates, and narcotics. Adjust insulin and antidiabetic drugs. Impaired absorption with cholestyramine, colestipol. Corticosteroids and ACTH deplete electrolytes. May decrease response to pressor amines. Potentiates other antihypertensives. May increase responsiveness to skeletal muscle relaxants. Risk of lithium toxicity. NSAIDs decrease diuretic effects.

PREGNANCY: Category C (1st trimester) and D (2nd and 3rd trimesters), not for use in nursing.

MECHANISM OF ACTION: Candesartan: Angiotensin II receptor antagonist; blocks vasoconstrictor and aldosterone-secreting effects of angiotensin II by blocking binding of angiotensin II to AT_1 receptor. HCTZ: Thiazide diuretic; affects renal tubular mechanism of electrolyte reabsorption, directly increasing excretion of Na+ and Cl-, and indirectly reducing plasma volume.

PHARMACOKINETICS: Absorption: Candesartan: Rapid and complete; absolute bioavailability (15%); T_{max}=3-4 hrs. **Distribution:** Candesartan: Plasma protein binding (>99%); V_d=0.13 L/kg; crosses placenta. HCTZ: crosses placenta; excreted in breast milk. **Metabolism:** Candesartan: Ester hydrolysis (GIT); O-deethylation (liver). **Elimination:** Candesartan: Urine (26%), feces; $T_{1/2}$= 9 hrs. HCTZ: Kidney; Urine (61%); $T_{1/2}$=5.6-14.8 hrs.

ATGAM   RX
lymphocyte immune globulin, anti-thymocyte globulin (equine) (Pharmacia & Upjohn)

> Administer by experienced physician in immunosuppressive therapy in facility equipped and staffed with adequate lab and supportive medical resources.

THERAPEUTIC CLASS: Lymphocyte-selective immunosuppressant

INDICATIONS: Management of allograft rejection in renal transplantation. Treatment of moderate to severe aplastic anemia unsuitable for bone marrow transplantation.

DOSAGE: *Adults:* Renal Transplant: Delaying Rejection Onset: 15mg/kg/day for 14 days, then every other day for 14 days for total of 21 doses in 28 days. Give 1st dose 24 hrs before or after transplant. Rejection Treatment: 10-15mg/kg/day for 14 days. May give additional alternate day therapy up to total of 21 doses. May delay 1st dose until diagnosis of 1st rejection episode. Aplastic Anemia: 10-20mg/kg/day for 8-14 days. May give additional alternate day therapy up to total of 21 doses.
Pediatrics: Renal Transplant: Delaying Rejection Onset: 15mg/kg/day for 14 days, then every other day for 14 days for total of 21 doses in 28 days. Give 1st dose 24 hrs before or after transplant. Rejection Treatment: 10-15mg/kg/day for 14 days. May give additional alternate day therapy up to total of 21 doses. May delay 1st dose until diagnosis of 1st rejection episode. Aplastic Anemia: 10-20mg/kg/day for 8-14 days. May give additional alternate day therapy up to total of 21 doses.

HOW SUPPLIED: Inj: 50mg/mL [5mL]

CONTRAINDICATIONS: History of severe systemic reaction to this product or other equine gamma globulin agents.

WARNINGS/PRECAUTIONS: Potency of agent may vary from lot to lot. D/C if anaphylaxis (eg, respiratory distress, hypotension) occurs, or if severe and un-remitting thrombocytopenia or leukopenia occur in renal transplant patients. Risk of infectious transmission due to equine and human blood components. Monitor for leukopenia, thrombocytopenia, or infection (eg, CMV). Decide whether or not to continue therapy based on clinical circumstances (eg, infection).

ADVERSE REACTIONS: Fever, chills, leukopenia, thrombocytopenia, rash, pruritus, urticaria, wheal, flare, arthralgia, headache, phlebitis, chest/back pain, diarrhea, vomiting, nausea, dyspnea, hypotension, night sweats, stomatitis.

INTERACTIONS: Previously masked reactions may appear with corticosteroid or immunosuppressant dose reduction. Do not dilute with dextrose or use highly acidic infusions.

PREGNANCY: Category C, caution in nursing.

MECHANISM OF ACTION: Lymphocyte-selective immunosuppressant; re-duces the number of circulating, thymus-dependent lymphocytes.

ATIVAN   CIV
lorazepam (Biovail)

THERAPEUTIC CLASS: Benzodiazepine

INDICATIONS: Management of anxiety disorders or for short-term relief of the symptoms of anxiety or anxiety associated with depressive symptoms.

DOSAGE: *Adults:* Initial: 2-3mg/day given bid-tid. Usual: 2-6mg/day in divided doses. Insomnia: 2-4mg qhs. Elderly/Debilitated: 1-2mg/day in divided doses. *Pediatrics:* >12 yrs: Initial: 2-3mg/day given bid-tid. Usual: 2-6mg/day in di-vided doses. Insomnia: 2-4mg qhs.

HOW SUPPLIED: Tab: 0.5mg, 1mg*, 2mg* *scored

CONTRAINDICATIONS: Acute narrow-angle glaucoma.

WARNINGS/PRECAUTIONS: Avoid with primary depression or psychosis. Withdrawal symptoms with abrupt discontinuation. Careful supervision if addiction-prone. Caution in patients with compromised respiratory function. Caution with elderly, and renal or hepatic dysfunction. Monitor for GI disease with prolonged therapy. Periodic blood counts and LFTs with long-term therapy.

ADVERSE REACTIONS: Sedation, dizziness, weakness, unsteadiness, transient amnesia, memory impairment, visual disturbance, depression, respiratory depression, constipation, vertigo, change in appetite, headache.

INTERACTIONS: CNS-depressant effects with barbiturates, alcohol. Diminished tolerance to alcohol and other CNS depressants. Increased plasma levels with valproate and probenecid, decrease dose by 50%.

PREGNANCY: Not for use in pregnancy or nursing.

MECHANISM OF ACTION: Benzodiazepine; antianxiety agent, interacts with GABA-benzodiazepine receptor complex.

PHARMACOKINETICS: Absorption: Absolute bioavailability (90%); C_{max}=20ng/mL (2mg PO); T_{max}=2 hrs. **Distribution:** Plasma protein binding (85%). **Metabolism:** Glucuronidation. **Elimination:** Urine; $T_{1/2}$=12 hrs.

ATIVAN INJECTION
lorazepam (Baxter)

THERAPEUTIC CLASS: Benzodiazepine

INDICATIONS: Treatment of status epilepticus and preanesthetic medication in adults.

DOSAGE: *Adults:* ≥18 yrs: Status Epilepticus: 4mg IV (given slowly at 2mg/min); may repeat 1 dose after 10-15 min if seizures recur or fail to cease. Preanesthetic Sedation: Usual: 0.05mg/kg IM; 2mg or 0.044mg/kg IV (whichever is smaller). Max: 4mg IM/IV.

HOW SUPPLIED: Inj: 2mg/mL, 4mg/mL

CONTRAINDICATIONS: Acute narrow-angle glaucoma, sleep apnea syndrome, severe respiratory insufficiency. Not for intra-arterial injection.

WARNINGS/PRECAUTIONS: Monitor all parameters to maintain vital function. Risk of respiratory depression or airway obstruction in heavily sedated patients. May cause fetal damage during pregnancy. Increased risk of CNS and respiratory depression in elderly. Avoid with hepatic/renal failure. Caution with mild to moderate hepatic/renal disease. Avoid outpatient endoscopic procedures. Possible propylene glycol toxicity in renal impairment. Extreme caution when administering injections to elderly, very ill, or to patients with limited pulmonary reserve, hypoventilation and/or hypoxic cardiac arrest may occur. Gasping syndrome, characterized by CNS depression, metabolic acidosis, gasping respirations, and high levels of benzyl alcohol, may occur.

ADVERSE REACTIONS: Respiratory depression/failure, hypotension, somnolence, headache, hypoventilation.

INTERACTIONS: Additive CNS depression with other CNS depressants (eg, ethyl alcohol, phenothiazines, barbiturates, MAOIs). Increased sedation, hallucinations and irrational behavior with scopolamine. Decreased clearance with valproate, probenecid. Increased clearance with oral contraceptives. Severe adverse effects with clozapine and haloperidol reported.

PREGNANCY: Category D, not for use in nursing.

MECHANISM OF ACTION: Benzodiazepine; antianxiety, sedative and anticonvulsant effects. Interacts with GABA-benzodiazepine receptor complex in human brain. Exhibits relatively high and specific affinity for its recognition site but does not displace GABA. Attachment to the specific binding site enhances the affinity of GABA for its receptor site on the same receptor complex.

PHARMACOKINETICS: Absorption: Completely, rapidly absorbed, C_{max}=48ng/mL, T_{max}=within 3 hrs. **Distribution:** Plasma protein binding (91%),

V_d=approximately 1.3L/kg, crosses blood brain barrier. **Elimination:** Urine (88%), feces (7%), (0.3%, unchanged). $T_{1/2}$=14 hrs.

ATRALIN RX
tretinoin (DPT Laboratories)

THERAPEUTIC CLASS: Retinoid

INDICATIONS: Topical treatment of acne vulgaris.

DOSAGE: *Adults:* Cleanse area(s) thoroughly, then apply thin layer qd before bedtime.
Pediatrics: ≥10 yrs: Cleanse area(s) thoroughly, then apply thin layer qd before bedtime.

HOW SUPPLIED: Gel: 0.05% [45g]

WARNINGS/PRECAUTIONS: Avoid eyes, mouth, paranasal creases, and mucous membranes. Skin may become dry, red, or exfoliated. If degree of irritation warrants, temporarily reduce amount/frequency, or d/c use temporarily or altogether. May cause mild to moderate dryness; use appropriate moisturizer. Caution with eczematous or sunburned skin, with high levels of exposure to sun, wind, or cold, or with known sensitivity to fish allergy.

ADVERSE REACTIONS: Dry skin, peeling, scaling, flaking skin, burning sensation, erythema.

INTERACTIONS: Caution with topical medications, medicated or abrasive soaps and cleansers, products with strong drying effects, high concentrations of alcohol, astringents, spices, or lime. Caution with benzoyl peroxide, sulfur, resorcinol, or salicylic acid; allow effects of these agents to subside before use.

PREGNANCY: Category C, caution in nursing.

MECHANISM OF ACTION: Retinoic acid derivative: Binds with high affinity to three specific retinoic acid nuclear receptors (RARα, RARβ, and RAR$_y$) which are located in both the cytosol and nucleus. Acts to modify gene expression, subsequent protein synthesis, and epithelial cell growth and differentiation. Decreases the cohesiveness of follicular epithelial cells with decreased microcomedo formation. Stimulates mitotic activity and increases turnover of follicular epithelial cells causing extrusion of the comedones.

PHARMACOKINETICS: Absorption: Tretinoin: Baseline plasma concentrations=0.68ng/mL, Day 14 plasma concentrations=0.69-2.88ng/mL. **Metabolism:** Major metabolites: 13-cis-retinoic acid and 4-oxo-13-cis-retinoic acid.

ATRIPLA RX
tenofovir disoproxil fumarate - emtricitabine - efavirenz (Bristol-Myers Squibb/ Gilead Sciences)

> Lactic acidosis and severe hepatomegaly with steatosis, including fatal cases, have been reported with the use of nucleoside analogs alone or in combination with other antiretrovirals. Not indicated for the treatment of chronic hepatitis B virus (HBV) infection and the safety and efficacy have not been established in patients co-infected with HBV and HIV. Severe acute exacerbations of hepatitis B have been reported in patients who have discontinued Emtriva or Viread. Hepatic function should be monitored closely with both clinical and laboratory follow-up for at least several months in patients who discontinue Atripla and are co-infected with HIV and HBV. If appropriate, initiation of anti-hepatitis B therapy may be warranted.

THERAPEUTIC CLASS: Non-nucleoside reverse transcriptase inhibitor/nucleoside analog combination

INDICATIONS: For use alone as a complete regimen or in combination with other antiretroviral agents for the treatment of HIV-1 infection in adults.

DOSAGE: *Adults:* ≥18 yrs: 1 tab qd on empty stomach. Bedtime dosing may improve tolerability of nervous system effects.

HOW SUPPLIED: Tab: (Efavirenz-Emtricitabine-Tenofovir DF) 600mg-200mg-300mg

CONTRAINDICATIONS: Concomitant astemizole, cisapride, midazolam, triazolam, ergot derivatives, voriconazole, bepridil, pimozide.

WARNINGS/PRECAUTIONS: Obesity and prolonged nucleoside exposure may be risk factors for lactic acidosis and severe hepatomegaly with steatosis. Suspend treatment if clinical or laboratory findings suggestive of lactic acidosis or pronounced hepatotoxicity. Test for presence of HBV prior to initiation; post-treatment exacerbations reported. Monitor hepatic function for several months with discontinuation and with co-infection with HIV and HBV. Serious psychiatric adverse experiences reported. CNS symptoms reported. May cause renal impairment. Monitor SrCr and phosphorous with risk or with a history of renal dysfunction and with concomitant nephrotoxic agents. Avoid in pregnancy; use barrier contraception with other contraception methods and obtain negative pregnancy test before therapy. Severe skin rash reported. Monitoring of liver enzymes recommended with known or suspected history of hepatitis B or C infection and with other medications associated with liver toxicity. Bone monitoring should be considered for HIV infected patients with a history of pathologic bone fracture or are at risk for osteopenia. Caution with history of seizures. Possible redistribution/accumulation of body fat. Immune reconstitution syndrome reported.

ADVERSE REACTIONS: Diarrhea, nausea, fatigue, sinusitis, upper respiratory tract infections, drowsiness, headache, dizziness, depression, insomnia, abnormal dreams, rash, laboratory abnormalities.

INTERACTIONS: Efavirenz is a CYP3A4 inducer *in vivo*, increasing the biotransformation of some drugs metabolized by CYP3A4. Co-administration of efavirenz with drugs primarily metabolized by 2C9, 2C19, and 3A4 isozymes may result in altered plasma concentrations of the co-administered drug. Drugs which induce CYP3A4 activity (eg, phenobarbital, rifampin, rifabutin) may increase clearance of efavirenz resulting in lowered plasma concentrations. Levels of efavirenz may be decreased by lopinavir/ritonavir, nelfinavir, saquinavir (SGC), rifabutin, rifampin, carbamazepine. St. John's wort to suboptimal levels, leading to loss of virologic response and possible resistance. Levels of efavirenz are increased by ritonavir, clarithromycin, sertraline, voriconazole, diltiazem. Efavirenz decreased levels of atazanavir, indinavir, lopinavir/ritonavir, saquinavir (SGC), clarithromycin, rifabutin, carbamazepine, methadone, sertraline and significantly reduced levels of voriconazole, itraconazole, atorvastatin, pravastatin, simvastatin, diltiazem. Efavirenz increased levels of nelfinavir, ritonavir, ethinyl estradiol. Co-administration of emtricitabine and tenofovir DF with drugs that are eliminated by active tubular secretion may increase concentrations of emtricitabine, tenofovir, and/or the co-administered drug. Drugs that decrease renal function may increase concentrations of emtricitabine and/or tenofovir. Levels of tenofovir increased by atazanavir, lopinavir/ritonavir may potentiate tenofovir-associated adverse events, including renal disorders. Tenofovir decreased levels of atazanavir, atazanavir/ritonavir. Co-administration of tenofovir DF with didanosine buffered tablets or EC capsules significantly increases the C_{max} and AUC of didanosine; patients receiving this combination should be monitored closely for didanosine-associated adverse events. Related drugs not for co-administration include Emtriva, Viread, Truvada, and Sustiva. Should not be co-administered with drugs containing lamivudine, including Combivir, Epivir, Epivir-HBV, Epzicom, and Trizivir.

PREGNANCY: Category D, not for use in nursing.

MECHANISM OF ACTION: Efavirenz: Non-nucleoside reverse transcriptase inhibitor; noncompetitive inhibition of HIV-1 reverse transcriptase (RT). Emtricitabine: Nucleoside analog of cytidine; inhibits activity of HIV-1 RT by competing with natural substrate deoxycytidine 5'-triphosphate and incorporating into nascent viral DNA, resulting in chain termination. Tenofovir disoproxil: Acyclic nucleoside phosphonate diester analog of adenosine monophosphate; inhibits activity of HIV-1 RT by competing with natural substrate deoxyadenosine 5'-triphosphate and incorporating into DNA by DNA chain termination.

PHARMACOKINETICS: Absorption: Efavirenz: T_{max}=3-5 hrs. C_{max}=12.9μM. AUC=184μM•hr. Emtricitabine: Rapid; T_{max}=1-2 hrs; C_{max}=1.8μg/mL; AUC=10μg•hr/mL; absolute bioavailability (93%). Tenofovir disoproxil: T_{max}=1hr; C_{max}=296ng/mL; AUC= 2287ng•hr/mL; absolute bioavailability (25%). **Distribution:** Efavirenz: Plasma protein binding (99.5%-99.75%). Emtricitabine: Plasma protein binding (<4%). Tenofovir disoproxil: Plasma protein binding (<0.7%). **Metabolism:** Efavirenz: Hepatic via CYP3A4 and CYP2B6. **Elimination:** Efavirenz: $T_{1/2}$=52-76 hrs. Emtricitabine: Urine (86%); $T_{1/2}$=10 hrs. Tenofovir disoproxil: Urine (70-80%); $T_{1/2}$=17 hrs.

ATROPINE SULFATE   RX
atropine sulfate (Various)

THERAPEUTIC CLASS: Anticholinergic

INDICATIONS: Antisialagogue for preanesthetic medication to prevent or reduce secretions of the respiratory tract. To restore cardiac rate and arterial pressure during anesthesia when vagal stimulation produced by intra-abdominal surgical traction causes a sudden decrease in pulse rate and cardiac action. To lessen degree of AV heart block when increased vagal tone is a major factor in the conduction defect (possibly due to digitalis). To overcome severe bradycardia and syncope due to hyperactive carotid sinus reflex, as an antidote (with external cardiac massage) for cardiovascular collapse from the injudicious use of choline ester (cholinergic) drug. In the treatment of anticholinesterase poisoning from organophosphorus insecticides, and as an antidote for the "rapid" type of mushroom poisoning due to presence of the alkaloid muscarine, in certain species of fungus such as *Amanita muscaria*.

DOSAGE: *Adults:* Usual: 0.5mg IM/IV/SC. Range: 0.4-0.6mg. If used as an antisialagogue, inject IM prior to anesthesia induction. Bradyarrhythmias: 0.4-1mg every 1-2 hrs prn. Max: 2mg/dose. May be used as antidote for cardiovascular collapse resulting from injudicious administration of choline ester. When cardiac arrest has occurred, external cardiac massage or other method of resuscitation is required to distribute the drug after IV injection. Anticholinesterase Poisoning From Insecticide Poisoning: 2-3mg IV. Repeat until signs of atropine intoxication appear. Mushroom Poisoning: Administer sufficient doses to control parasympathomimetic signs before coma and cardiovascular collapse supervene.
Pediatrics: Range: 0.1mg (newborn) to 0.6mg (>12 yrs). Inject SC 30 min before surgery. Bradyarrhythmias: Range: 0.01-0.03mg/kg IV.

HOW SUPPLIED: Inj: 0.05mg/mL, 0.1mg/mL, 0.4mg/mL, 0.5mg/mL, 1mg/mL

CONTRAINDICATIONS: Glaucoma, pyloric stenosis, or prostatic hypertrophy except in doses used for preanesthetic medication.

WARNINGS/PRECAUTIONS: Avoid overdose in IV administration. Increased susceptibility to toxic effects in children. Caution in patients >40 yrs. Conventional doses may precipitate glaucoma in susceptible patients, convert partial organic pyloric stenosis into complete obstruction, lead to complete urinary retention in patients with prostatic hypertrophy or cause inspissation of bronchial secretions and formation of dangerous viscid plugs in patients with chronic lung disease.

ADVERSE REACTIONS: Dryness of the mouth, blurred vision, photophobia, tachycardia, anhidrosis.

PREGNANCY: Category C, safety in nursing not known.

MECHANISM OF ACTION: Anticholinergic; inhibits smooth muscle and glands innervated by postganglionic cholinergic nerves; stimulates/depresses CNS activity depending upon the dose.

PHARMACOKINETICS: Distribution: Plasma protein binding (44%), crosses placental barrier. **Metabolism:** Via enzymatic hydrolysis in liver. Noratropine, atropin-n-oxide, tropine, and tropic acid (major metabolites). **Elimination:** Urine (50% unchanged); $T_{1/2}$=2.5 hrs.

ATROVENT HFA RX
ipratropium bromide (Boehringer Ingelheim)

THERAPEUTIC CLASS: Anticholinergic bronchodilator

INDICATIONS: Maintenance treatment of bronchospasm associated with COPD, including chronic bronchitis and emphysema.

DOSAGE: *Adults:* Initial: 2 inh qid. Max: 12 inh/24hrs.

HOW SUPPLIED: MDI: 0.017mg/inh [12.9g]

CONTRAINDICATIONS: Hypersensitivity to atropine or its derivatives.

WARNINGS/PRECAUTIONS: Not for acute episodes. Immediate hypersensitivity reaction reported. Caution with narrow-angle glaucoma, prostatic hypertrophy or bladder-neck obstruction.

ADVERSE REACTIONS: Back pain, bronchitis, dyspnea, dizziness, headache, nausea, blurred vision, dry mouth, exacerbation of symptoms.

INTERACTIONS: Caution with anticholinergic-containing drugs.

PREGNANCY: Category B, caution in nursing.

MECHANISM OF ACTION: Anticholinergic; inhibits vagally-mediated refluxes by antagonizing the action of acetylcholine; prevents increase in intracellular concentration of cGMP caused by interaction of acetylcholine with muscarinic receptors on bronchial smooth muscle (animal studies).

PHARMACOKINETICS: Absorption: C_{max}=59pg/mL. **Distribution:** Plasma protein binding (0-9%). **Metabolism:** Partial. **Elimination:** $T_{1/2}$=2 hrs.

ATROVENT NASAL RX
ipratropium bromide (Boehringer Ingelheim)

THERAPEUTIC CLASS: Anticholinergic

INDICATIONS: (0.03%) Relief of rhinorrhea associated with allergic and nonallergic perennial rhinitis in adults and children ≥6 yrs. (0.06%) Relief of rhinorrhea associated with the common cold or seasonal allergic rhinitis in adults and children ≥5 yrs.

DOSAGE: *Adults:* Rhinorrhea w/Allergic/Nonallergic Perennial Rhinitis: (0.03%) 2 sprays per nostril bid-tid. Rhinorrhea w/Common Cold: (0.06%) 2 sprays per nostril tid-qid. Rhinorrhea w/Seasonal Allergic Rhinitis: (0.06%) 2 sprays per nostril qid.
Pediatrics: Rhinorrhea w/Allergic/Nonallergic Perennial Rhinitis: ≥6 yrs: (0.03%) 2 sprays per nostril bid-tid. Rhinorrhea w/Common Cold: ≥12 yrs: (0.06%) 2 sprays per nostril tid-qid. 5-11 yrs: (0.06%) 2 sprays per nostril tid. Rhinorrhea w/Seasonal Allergic Rhinitis: ≥5 yrs: (0.06%) 2 sprays per nostril qid.

HOW SUPPLIED: Spray: (0.03%) 21mcg/spray [31g], (0.06%) 42mcg/spray [16.6g]

CONTRAINDICATIONS: Hypersensitivity to atropine or its derivatives.

WARNINGS/PRECAUTIONS: Immediate hypersensitivity reaction reported. Caution with narrow-angle glaucoma, prostatic hyperplasia or bladder-neck obstruction.

ADVERSE REACTIONS: Epistaxis, nasal dryness, dry mouth, dry throat, headache, upper respiratory infection, pharyngitis.

INTERACTIONS: May produce additive effects with other anticholinergic agents.

PREGNANCY: Category B, caution in nursing.

MECHANISM OF ACTION: Anticholinergic; inhibits secretions from serous and seromucous glands lining the nasal mucosa.

PHARMACOKINETICS: Absorption: 6-18 yrs old: C_{max}=undetectable up to 0.49 ng/mL. **Distribution:** Plasma protein binding (0-9%). **Elimination:** 6-18 yrs old: Urine (8.6-11.1% unchanged). **Adults:** Urine (3.7-5.6% unchanged).

ATTENUVAX RX
measles vaccine live (Merck)

THERAPEUTIC CLASS: Vaccine

INDICATIONS: Vaccination against measles.

DOSAGE: *Pediatrics:* 0.5mL SQ in the upper arm at 12-15 months old. If vaccinated <12 months old, revaccinate at 12-15 months old. Revaccinate prior to school entry.

HOW SUPPLIED: Inj: 1000TCID$_{50}$/vial

CONTRAINDICATIONS: Pregnancy, anaphylactic reaction to neomycin, febrile respiratory illness or other active febrile infection, immunosuppressive therapy, blood dyscrasias, leukemia, lymphomas, malignant neoplasms affecting bone marrow or lymphatic systems, immunodeficiency states.

WARNINGS/PRECAUTIONS: Caution with egg hypersensitivity, history of cerebral injury, individual or family history of convulsions, and avoid conditions that cause stress due to fever. May potentiate thrombocytopenia. Defer for 3 months or longer after blood or plasma transfusions, or immune globulin administration. Have epinephrine injection (1:1000) available.

ADVERSE REACTIONS: Panniculitis, atypical measles, fever, syncope, headache, vasculitis, diarrhea, thrombocytopenia, lymphadenopathy, Guilliain-Barre syndrome, febrile convulsion, pneumonitis, cough, rhinitis, Stevens-Johnson syndrome, erythema multiforme, rash.

INTERACTIONS: Immune globulins may interfere with immune response. Temporary depression of tuberculin skin sensitivity.

PREGNANCY: Category C, caution in nursing.

MECHANISM OF ACTION: Stimulates immune response to produce antibodies that may protect against measles (rubeola).

AUGMENTIN RX
clavulanate potassium - amoxicillin (GlaxoSmithKline)

THERAPEUTIC CLASS: Aminopenicillin/beta lactamase inhibitor

INDICATIONS: Treatment of lower respiratory tract (LRTI), skin and skin structure (SSSI), and urinary tract infections (UTI), otitis media (OM), sinusitis caused by susceptible strains of microorganisms.

DOSAGE: *Adults:* (Dose based on amoxicillin) 500mg q12h or 250mg q8h. Severe Infections/RTI: 875mg q12h or 500mg q8h. May use 125mg/5mL or 250mg/5mL sus in place of 500mg tab and 200mg/5mL sus or 400mg/5mL sus in place of 875mg tab. CrCl <30mL/min: Do not use 875mg tab. CrCl 10-30mL/min: 250-500mg q12h. CrCl <10mL/min: 250-500mg q24h. Hemodialysis: 250-500mg q24h, give additional dose during and at end of dialysis.
Pediatrics: (Dose based on amoxicillin) >40kg: Use adult dose. ≥12 weeks: Sinusitis/Otitis Media/LRTI/Severe Infections: (Sus/Tab, Chewable) 45mg/kg/day given q12h or 40mg/kg/day given q8h. Treat otitis media for 10 days. Less Severe Infections: 25mg/kg/day given q12h or 20mg/kg/day given q8h. <12 weeks: 15mg/kg q12h (use 125mg/5mL sus).

HOW SUPPLIED: (Amoxicillin-Clavulanate) Sus: 125-31.25mg/5mL [75mL, 100mL, 150mL], 200-28.5mg/5mL [50mL, 75mL, 100mL], 250-62.5mg/5mL [75mL, 100mL, 150mL], 400-57mg/5mL [50mL, 75mL, 100mL]; Tab: 250-125mg, 500-125mg, 875-125mg*; Tab, Chewable: 200-28.5mg, 250-62.5mg, 400-57mg *scored

CONTRAINDICATIONS: History of PCN allergy or amoxicillin-clavulanate associated cholestatic jaundice/hepatic dysfunction.

WARNINGS/PRECAUTIONS: Serious, sometimes fatal, hypersensitivity reactions reported with PCN therapy. *Clostridium difficile*-associated diarrhea reported. Possibility of superinfection. Caution with hepatic dysfunction. Monitor renal, hepatic, and hematopoietic functions with prolonged use.

Avoid with mononucleosis. Take with food to reduce GI upset. The 200mg and 400mg chewable tabs and 200mg/5mL and 400mg/5mL sus contain phenylalanine. The 250mg tab and chewable tab are not interchangeable due to unequal clavulanic acid amounts. Only use 250mg tab in pediatrics ≥40kg. False (+) for urine glucose with Clinitest® and Benedict's or Fehling's solution.

ADVERSE REACTIONS: Diarrhea/loose stools, nausea, skin rashes, urticaria, vomiting, vaginitis.

INTERACTIONS: Increased and prolonged plasma levels with probenecid. May reduce effects of oral contraceptives. Allopurinol may increase incidence of rash. May increase PT with anticoagulant therapy.

PREGNANCY: Category B, caution in nursing.

MECHANISM OF ACTION: Amoxicillin: Semisynthetic antibiotic with broad spectrum of bactericidal activity against gram-positive and gram-negative organisms. Clavulanate: β-lactamase inhibitor; possesses ability to inactivate a wide range of β-lactamase enzymes commonly found in microorganisms resistant to PCN and cephalosporins.

PHARMACOKINETICS: Absorption: Well absorbed from GI tract. C_{max} and AUC varied according to dose and regimen; see Full Prescribing Information for more information. (Tab, Sol) T_{max}=1.5 hrs, 1 hr. **Distribution:** Found in breast milk. Amoxicillin: Diffuses readily in body tissues and fluids. Clavulanic: Well distributed in body tissues. Plasma protein binding: Amoxicillin (18%), clavulanic (25%). **Elimination:** Urine, amoxicillin (50-70% unchanged), clavulanic (25-40% unchanged). $T_{1/2}$=1.3 hrs (amoxicillin), 1 hr (clavulanic).

AUGMENTIN ES-600   RX
clavulanate potassium - amoxicillin (GlaxoSmithKline)

THERAPEUTIC CLASS: Aminopenicillin/beta lactamase inhibitor

INDICATIONS: Treatment of pediatric patients with recurrent or persistent acute otitis media due to susceptible strains of microorganisms.

DOSAGE: *Pediatrics:* 3 months-12 yrs: <40kg: (Dose based on amoxicillin content) 45mg/kg q12h for 10 days.

HOW SUPPLIED: Sus: (Amoxicillin-Clavulanate) 600mg-42.9mg/5mL [75mL, 125mL, 200mL]

CONTRAINDICATIONS: History of PCN allergy or amoxicillin-clavulanate associated cholestatic jaundice/hepatic dysfunction.

WARNINGS/PRECAUTIONS: Serious, sometimes fatal, hypersensitivity reactions reported with PCN therapy. *Clostridium difficile*-associated diarrhea reported. Possibility of superinfection. Caution with hepatic dysfunction. Monitor renal, hepatic, and hematopoietic functions with prolonged use. Avoid with mononucleosis. Contains phenylalanine. False (+) for urine glucose with Clinitest® and Benedict's or Fehling's solution.

ADVERSE REACTIONS: Diaper rash, diarrhea, vomiting, moniliasis, rash.

INTERACTIONS: Increased and prolonged plasma levels with probenecid. May reduce effects of oral contraceptives. Allopurinol may increase incidence of rash. May increase PT with anticoagulant therapy.

PREGNANCY: Category B, caution in nursing.

MECHANISM OF ACTION: Amoxicillin: Semisynthetic antibiotic with broad spectrum of bactericidal activity against gram-positive and gram-negative organisms. Clavulanate: β-lactamase inhibitor. Possesses ability to inactivate a wide range of β-lactamase enzymes commonly found in microorganisms resistant to PCN and cephalosporins.

PHARMACOKINETICS: Absorption: Amoxicillin: C_{max}=15.7mcg/mL; T_{max}=2.0 hr, AUC=59.8mcg•hr/mL. Clavulanic acid: C_{max}=1.7mcg/mL; T_{max}=1.1 hr, AUC=4.0mcg•hr/mL. **Distribution:** Plasma protein binding 18% (amoxicillin), 25% (clavulanic acid). Well distributed in bodily tissues except brain and spinal fluid. **Elimination:** Urine (unchanged) amoxicillin (50-70%); clavulanic acid (25-40%).

AUGMENTIN XR

RX

clavulanate potassium - amoxicillin (GlaxoSmithKline)

THERAPEUTIC CLASS: Aminopenicillin/beta lactamase inhibitor

INDICATIONS: Treatment of community-acquired pneumonia (CAP) or acute bacterial sinusitis due to confirmed or suspected β-lactamase producing pathogens and *S.pneumoniae* with reduced susceptibility to PCN.

DOSAGE: *Adults:* Sinusitis: 2 tabs q12h for 10 days. CAP: 2 tabs q12h for 7-10 days. Take at start of a meal.
Pediatrics: ≥16 yrs: Sinusitis: 2 tabs q12h for 10 days. CAP: 2 tabs q12h for 7-10 days. Take at the start of a meal.

HOW SUPPLIED: Tab, Extended-Release: (Amoxicillin-Clavulanate) 1000mg-62.5mg

CONTRAINDICATIONS: History of PCN allergy or amoxicillin-clavulanate associated cholestatic jaundice/hepatic dysfunction, severe renal impairment (CrCl <30mL/min), hemodialysis.

WARNINGS/PRECAUTIONS: Serious, sometimes fatal, hypersensitivity reactions reported with PCN therapy. *Clostridium difficile*-associated diarrhea reported. Possibility of superinfection. Caution with hepatic dysfunction. Monitor renal, hepatic, and hematopoietic functions with prolonged use. Avoid with mononucleosis. Not interchangeable with other Augmentin products due to unequal clavulanic acid amounts. False (+) for urine glucose with Clinitest® and Benedict's or Fehling's solution.

ADVERSE REACTIONS: Diarrhea, nausea, genital moniliasis, abdominal pain, vaginal mycosis.

INTERACTIONS: Increased and prolonged plasma levels with probenecid. May reduce effects of oral contraceptives. Allopurinol may increase incidence of rash. May increase PT with anticoagulant therapy.

PREGNANCY: Category B, caution in nursing.

MECHANISM OF ACTION: Amoxicillin: Semisynthetic antibiotic with broad spectrum of bactericidal activity against gram-positive and gram-negative organisms. Clavulanate: β-lactamase inhibitor; possesses ability to inactivate a wide range of β-lactamase enzymes commonly found in microorganisms resistant to PCN and cephalosporins.

PHARMACOKINETICS: Absorption: Well-absorbed. Amoxicillin: AUC=71.6mcg•hr/mL, C_{max}=17 mcg/mL. T_{max}=1.5 hrs. Clavulanate potassium: AUC=5.29mcg•hr/mL, C_{max}=2.05mcg/mL. T_{max}=1.03 hrs. **Distribution:** Plasma protein binding: Amoxicillin (18%); Clavulante potassium (25%). Found in breast milk. Well distributed to body tissues except brain and spinal fluid. **Elimination:** Urine: Amoxicillin: 60-80% (unchanged); $T_{1/2}$=1.27 hrs. Clavulanate potassium: 30-50% unchanged; $T_{1/2}$=1.03 hrs.

AUROTO

RX

glycerin - benzocaine - antipyrine (Alpharma)

OTHER BRAND NAMES: A/B Otic (Qualitest)

THERAPEUTIC CLASS: Analgesic/hygroscopic agent

INDICATIONS: To reduce pain in acute otitis media. For cerumen removal.

DOSAGE: *Adults:* Otitis Media: Fill ear canal and insert moistened cotton plug. Repeat q1-2h, until pain and congestion resolve. Cerumen Removal: Fill ear canal tid for 2-3 days before cerumen removal; insert moistened cotton plug. Use after removal to dry out canal and relieve discomfort.

HOW SUPPLIED: Sol: (Antipyrine-Benzocaine) 54mg-14mg/mL [15mL]

CONTRAINDICATIONS: Perforated tympanic membrane.

WARNINGS/PRECAUTIONS: D/C if irritation occurs.

PREGNANCY: Category C, caution in nursing.

AVAGE
RX

tazarotene (Allergan)

THERAPEUTIC CLASS: Retinoid

INDICATIONS: Adjunct to a comprehensive skin care and sunlight avoidance program, in the mitigation (palliation) of facial fine wrinkling, facial mottled hyper- and hypopigmentation, and benign facial lentigines.

DOSAGE: *Adults:* ≥17 yrs: Cleanse and dry skin. Apply a pea-sized (1/4 inch or 5mm diameter) amount to face (including eyelids, if desired) qhs.

HOW SUPPLIED: Cre: 0.1% [30g]

CONTRAINDICATIONS: Women who are or may become pregnant.

WARNINGS/PRECAUTIONS: Use adequate birth control measures. Obtain negative pregnancy test within 2 weeks before therapy. Begin therapy during normal menstrual period. Avoid mouth, eyes, sunlight exposure (including sunlamps), or sunburned or eczematous skin. Stop therapy or reduce dosing interval with pruritus, burning, skin redness, or peeling. Weather extremes (eg, wind, cold) may be irritating. Sunscreen (minimum SPF 15) and protective clothing should be used.

ADVERSE REACTIONS: Desquamation, erythema, burning sensation, dry skin, skin irritation, pruritus, irritant contact dermatitis.

INTERACTIONS: Avoid topical agents that have a strong drying effect. Caution with photosensitizers (eg, thiazides, tetracyclines, fluoroquinolones, phenothiazines, sulfonamides).

PREGNANCY: Category X; caution in nursing.

MECHANISM OF ACTION: Retinoic acid derivative; binds to all 3 members of the retinoic acid receptor (RAR family): RARα, RARβ, and RAR-gamma, but shows relative selectivity for RARβ and RAR-gamma and may modify gene expression. Its mechanism in amelioration of fine wrinkling, facial mottled hypo- and hyperpigmentation, and benign facial lentigines has not been established.

PHARMACOKINETICS: Distribution: Plasma protein binding (>99%). **Metabolism:** Undergoes esterase hydrolysis. Tazarotenic acid (active metabolite). Tazarotene and tazarotenic acid are metabolized to sulfoxides, sulfones, and other polar metabolites. **Elimination:** Urine and feces. $T_{1/2}$= approximately 18 hrs.

AVALIDE
RX

irbesartan - hydrochlorothiazide (Bristol-Myers Squibb/Sanofi-Aventis)

> Can cause death/injury to developing fetus during 2nd and 3rd trimesters. Stop therapy if pregnancy detected.

THERAPEUTIC CLASS: Angiotensin II receptor antagonist/thiazide diuretic

INDICATIONS: Treatment of hypertension in patients not adequately controlled with monotherapy. As initial therapy in patients likely to need multiple drugs.

DOSAGE: *Adults:* Not controlled on Monotherapy: 150mg/12.5mg qd. Titrate: May increase to 300mg/12.5mg, then 300mg/25mg qd if needed. Intial Therapy: Initiate with 150mg/12.5mg qd for 1 to 2 weeks. Titrate: As needed to maximum 300mg/25mg qd. Replacement Therapy: May substitute for titrated components. Elderly: Start at low end of dosing range. Avoid with CrCl ≤30mL/min.

HOW SUPPLIED: Tab: (Irbesartan-HCTZ) 150mg-12.5mg, 300mg-12.5mg, 300mg-25mg

CONTRAINDICATIONS: Anuria, sulfonamide hypersensitivity.

WARNINGS/PRECAUTIONS: Can cause fetal injury/death when administered to pregnant women. Correct volume or salt depletion before therapy. Caution with hepatic or renal dysfunction, renal artery stenosis, severe CHF, history

103

of allergies, elderly, and asthma. May exacerbate or activate SLE. Monitor serum electrolytes. Avoid if CrCl ≤30mL/min. Hyperuricemia, hyperglycemia, hypokalemia, hypomagnesemia, and hypercalcemia may occur. Enhanced effects in post-sympathectomy patient. May increase cholesterol and triglyceride levels. Caution in elderly.

ADVERSE REACTIONS: Dizziness, fatigue, musculoskeletal pain, influenza, edema, nausea, vomiting, fever, chills, flushing, HTN, pruritus, sexual dysfunction, diarrhea, anxiety, vision disturbance, pancreatitis, aplastic anemia.

INTERACTIONS: Potentiation of orthostatic hypotension may occur with alcohol, barbiturates, and narcotics. Dosage adjustment of insulin or oral hypoglycemic agents may be required. Impaired absorption with cholestyramine, colestipol. Corticosteroids and ACTH deplete electrolytes. May decrease response to pressor amines. Potentiates other antihypertensives. May increase responsiveness to skeletal muscle relaxants. Increased risk of lithium toxicity. NSAIDs may reduce diuretic effects.

PREGNANCY: Category D, not for use in nursing.

MECHANISM OF ACTION: Irbesartan: Angiotensin II receptor antagonist. Blocks vasoconstrictor and aldosterone-secreting effects of angiotensin II by selecting binding AT$_1$ angiotensin II receptor. HCTZ: Thiazide diuretic. Affects renal tubular mechanism of electrolyte reabsorption, directly increasing sodium and chloride and indirectly reducing plasma volume.

PHARMACOKINETICS: Irbesartan: Rapid, complete; Absolute bioavailability (60-80%); T$_{max}$=1.5-2 hrs. **Distribution:** Irbesartan: Plasma protein binding (90%), V$_d$=53-93L, crosses placenta, excreted in breast milk. HCTZ: Crosses placenta, excreted in breast milk. **Metabolism:** Irbesartan: CYP2C9 (oxidation), glucuronide conjugation. **Elimination:** Irbesartan: T$_{1/2}$=11-15 hrs. HCTZ: Kidney (61%); T$_{1/2}$=5.6-14.8 hrs

AVANDAMET RX
metformin HCL - rosiglitazone maleate (GlaxoSmithKline)

> Thiazolidinediones may cause or exacerbate CHF in some patients. Avandamet is not recommended in patients with symptomatic heart failure.

THERAPEUTIC CLASS: Thiazolidinedione/biguanide

INDICATIONS: Adjunct to diet and exercise, to improve glycemic control in type 2 diabetes mellitus when treatment with dual rosiglitazone and metformin therapy is appropriate.

DOSAGE: *Adults:* Prior Metformin Therapy of 1000mg/day: Initial: 2mg-500mg tab bid. Prior Metformin Therapy of 2000mg/day: Initial: 2mg-1000mg tab bid. Prior Rosiglitazone Therapy of 4mg/day: Initial: 2mg-500mg tab bid. Prior Rosiglitazone Therapy of 8mg/day: 4mg-500mg tab bid. Titrate: May increase by increments of 4mg rosiglitazone and/or 500mg metformin. Max: 8mg-2000mg/day. Drug-Naive Patients: Initial: 2mg-500mg qd-bid. If HbA1c >11% and FPG >270mg/dL: Initial: 2mg-500mg bid. Titrate: After 4 weeks, may increase by increments of 2mg-500mg per day. Max: 8mg-2000mg per day. Elderly/Debilitated/Malnourished: Conservative dosing; do not titrate to max dose. Take with meals.

HOW SUPPLIED: Tab: (Rosiglitazone-Metformin) 2mg-500mg, 4mg-500mg, 2mg-1000mg, 4mg-1000mg

CONTRAINDICATIONS: Established NYHA Class III or IV heart failure, renal disease/dysfunction (SrCr ≥1.5mg/dL [males], ≥1.4mg/dL [females], or abnormal CrCl), metabolic acidosis, including diabetic ketoacidosis. D/C temporarily (48 hrs) for radiologic studies with intravascular iodinated contrast materials.

WARNINGS/PRECAUTIONS: Lactic acidosis reported (rare); increased risk with renal dysfunction, increased age, DM, CHF, and other conditions with risk of hypoperfusion and hypoxemia. Avoid use in patients ≥80 yrs unless renal function is normal. Monitor renal function and for ketoacidosis and metabolic acidosis. D/C in hypoxic states (eg, CHF, shock, acute MI), loss of blood glucose control due to stress, acidosis and prior to surgical procedures (due to restricted food intake). May decrease serum vitamin B$_{12}$ levels. Increased risk of hypoglycemia with concomitant use with other hypoglycemic agents, elderly, debilitated/malnourished, adrenal or pituitary insufficiency, or alcohol intoxication. May cause fluid retention and exacerbation/initiation of heart failure; d/c if cardiac status deteriorates. Avoid with NYHA Class III or IV cardiac status. Not for use in type 1 diabetes or for diabetic ketoacidosis treatment. Caution with edema. Dose-related weight gain reported. Ovulation in premenopausal anovulatory patients may occur; risk of pregnancy with inadequate contraception. May decrease Hgb and Hct. Avoid with active liver disease, if ALT levels >2.5x ULN, or if jaundice occurred with troglitazone. Check LFTs before therapy, every 2 months for 1 year, and periodically thereafter, or if hepatic dysfunction symptoms occur. D/C if ALT >3x ULN on therapy. Not for use with insulin. Increased incidence of bone fracture was noted in female patients

ADVERSE REACTIONS: Upper respiratory tract infection, headache, back pain, hyperglycemia, fatigue, sinusitis, diarrhea, viral infection, arthralgia, anemia, dyspepsia, dizziness, abdominal pain, nausea, vomiting.

INTERACTIONS: Furosemide, nifedipine, cimetidine and cationic drugs (eg, digoxin, amiloride, procainamide, quinidine, quinine, ranitidine, trimethoprim, vancomycin, triamterene, morphine) may increase metformin levels. Thiazides and other diuretics, corticosteroids, phenothiazines, thyroid products, estrogens, oral contraceptives, phenytoin, nicotinic acid, sympathomimetics, CCBs, and isoniazid may cause hyperglycemia. Risk of hypoglycemia with alcohol. Excess alcohol may increase potential for lactic acidosis. May decrease furosemide levels. Inhibitors of CYP2C8 (eg, gemfibrozil) may increase rosiglitazone AUC. Inducers of CYP2C8 (eg, rifampin) may decrease rosiglitazone AUC.

PREGNANCY: Category C, not for use in nursing.

MECHANISM OF ACTION: Rosiglitazone: Thiazolidinedione; insulin sensitizing agent that acts by enhancing peripheral glucose utilization. Metformin: Biguanide; decreases hepatic glucose production, decreases intestinal absorption of glucose, and increases peripheral glucose uptake and utilization.

PHARMACOKINETICS: Absorption: Rosiglitazone: Absolute bioavailability (99%). (4mg) C_{max}=242ng/mL. T_{max}=1 hr. Metformin: Absolute bioavailability (50-60%). (500mg) C_{max}=1106ng/mL; T_{max}=3 hrs. **Distribution:** Rosiglitazone: V_d=17.6L; plasma protein binding (99.8%). Metformin: V_d=654L. **Metabolism:** Rosiglitazone: Liver (extensive); CYP2C8 (major), 2C9 (minor). Metformin: No hepatic metabolism. **Elimination:** Rosiglitazone: $T_{1/2}$=3-4 hrs; urine (64%) and feces (23%). Metformin: $T_{1/2}$=6.2 hrs (plasma); urine (unchanged).

AVANDARYL RX
rosiglitazone maleate - glimepiride (GlaxoSmithKline)

> Thiazolidinediones may cause or exacerbate CHF in some patients. Avandaryl is not recommended in patients with symptomatic heart failure.

THERAPEUTIC CLASS: Thiazolidinedione/sulfonylurea

INDICATIONS: Adjunct to diet and exercise to improve glycemic control in type 2 DM when treatment with dual rosiglitazone and glimepiride therapy is appropriate.

DOSAGE: *Adults:* Initial: 4mg-1mg qd with 1st meal of day. With Sulfonylurea or Thiazolidinedione: Initial: 4mg-2mg qd. Switching From Prior Combination Therapy: Same dose of each component already being taken. Prior Thiazolidinedione Monotherapy: Titrate dose. After 1-2 weeks with inadequate control, increase glimepiride component in no more than 2mg increments at 1-2 week intervals. Max: 8mg-4mg qd. Prior Sulfonylurea Monotherapy: May take 2-3 months for full effect of rosiglitazone; do not exceed 8mg of rosiglitazone daily. Titrate: May increase glimepiride component. Elderly/Debilitated/ Malnourished/Renal, Hepatic or Adrenal Insufficiency: Initial: 4mg-1mg qd. Titrate carefully.

HOW SUPPLIED: Tab: (Rosiglitazone-Glimepiride) 4mg-1mg, 4mg-2mg, 4mg-4mg, 8mg-2mg, 8mg-4mg

CONTRAINDICATIONS: Established NYHA Class III or IV heart failure, diabetic ketoacidosis.

WARNINGS/PRECAUTIONS: (Glimepiride) Increased cardiovascular mortality. Hypoglycemia risk if debilitated, malnourished, or with adrenal, pituitary, renal or hepatic insufficiency. Hypoglycemia may be masked in elderly. May lose blood glucose control with stress. Secondary failure may occur. D/C if skin reactions persist or worsen. (Rosiglitazone) May cause fluid retention and exacerbation/initiation of heart failure; d/c if cardiac status deteriorates. Increased risk of CV events with NYHA Class I and II heart failure. Not for use in type 1 DM or diabetic ketoacidosis treatment. Caution with edema. May cause macular edema. Dose-related weight gain reported. Ovulation in premenopausal anovulatory patient may occur; risk of pregnancy with inadequate contraception. May decrease Hgb and Hct. Avoid with active liver disease, if ALT levels >2.5x ULN, or if jaundice occurred with rosiglitazone. Check LFTs before therapy, every 2 months for 1 yr, and periodically thereafter, or if hepatic dysfunction symptoms occur. D/C if ALT >3x ULN on therapy. Increased incidence of bone fracture was noted in female patients. Combination use with insulin not recommended.

ADVERSE REACTIONS: Upper respiratory tract infection, injury, headache, hypoglycemia, anemia, edema.

INTERACTIONS: (Rosiglitazone): CYP2C8 inhibitors (eg, gemfibrozil) may increase the AUC. CYP2C8 inducers (eg, rifampin) may decrease the AUC. (Glimepiride): Risk of hyperglycemia with thiazides, corticosteroids, phenothiazines, thyroid products, estrogens, oral contraceptives, phenytoin, nicotinic acid, sympathomimetics, and isoniazid. Risk of severe hypoglycemia with oral miconazole. β-blockers may mask symptoms of hypoglycemia.

PREGNANCY: Category C, not for use in nursing.

MECHANISM OF ACTION: Rosiglitazone: Thiazolidinedione; insulin sensitizing agent which acts by enhancing peripheral glucose utilization. Glimepiride: Sulfonylurea; stimulate insulin release from functional pancreatic beta cells.

PHARMACOKINETICS: Absorption: Rosiglitazone: Absolute bioavailability (99%); T_{max}=1 hr; (4mg) C_{max}=257ng/mL. Glimepiride: Complete; T_{max}=2-3 hrs; (4mg) C_{max}=151ng/mL. **Distribution:** Rosiglitazone: V_d=17.6L; plasma protein binding (99.8%). Glimepiride: (IV) V_d=8.8L; protein binding (>99.5%). **Metabolism:** Rosiglitazone: N-demethylation & hydroxylation followed by conjugation; CYP2C8 (major), 2C9 (minor). Glimepiride: Liver (complete); major metabolites M1 & M2; CYP2C9. **Elimination:** Rosiglitazone: $T_{1/2}$=3-4 hrs; urine (64%), feces (23%). Glimepiride: $T_{1/2}$=5-7 hrs; urine (60%), feces (40%).

AVANDIA   RX
rosiglitazone maleate (GlaxoSmithKline)

> Thiazolidinediones may cause or exacerbate CHF in some patients. Rosiglitazone is not recommended in patients with symptomatic heart failure. Studies have shown rosiglitazone to be associated with an increased risk of myocardial ischemic events, such as angina or MI.

THERAPEUTIC CLASS: Thiazolidinedione

INDICATIONS: Adjunct to diet and exercise, to improve glycemic control in type 2 diabetes mellitus. May use in combination with metformin, insulin, or a sulfonylurea.

DOSAGE: *Adults:* ≥18 yrs: Initial: 2mg bid or 4mg qd. Titrate: May increase after 8-12 weeks to 4mg bid or 8mg qd. Max: 8mg/day as monotherapy or with metformin; 4mg/day in combination with sulfonylureas or insulin. Decrease insulin by 10-25% if hypoglycemic or FPG <100mg/dL; individualize further adjustments based on glucose-lowering response.

HOW SUPPLIED: Tab: 2mg, 4mg, 8mg

CONTRAINDICATIONS: Established NYHA Class III or IV heart failure. Coadministration with insulin or nitrates.

WARNINGS/PRECAUTIONS: May cause fluid retention and exacerbation/initiation of heart failure; d/c if cardiac status deteriorates. Increased risk of

CV events with NYHA Class I or II cardiac status; avoid with NYHA Class III or IV cardiac status. Not for use in type 1 diabetes or diabetic ketoacidosis treatment. Caution with edema. Macular edema reported. Dose-related weight gain reported. Ovulation in premenopausal anovulatory patients may occur; risk of pregnancy with inadequate contraception. May decrease Hgb and Hct. Avoid with active liver disease, if ALT levels >2.5x ULN, or if jaundice occurred with troglitazone. Check LFTs before therapy, every 2 months for 1 year, and periodically thereafter, or if hepatic dysfunction symptoms occur. D/C if ALT >3x ULN on therapy. Increased incidence of bone fracture in female patients. Increased risk of myocardial ischemic events observed. Risk for hypoglycemia. Monitor blood glucose and Hb_{A1c} measurements. CHF and MI during coadministration with insulin. Increased incidence of bone fractures in female patients.

ADVERSE REACTIONS: Upper respiratory tract infection, injury, headache, back pain, hyperglycemia, fatigue, sinusitis, anemia, edema.

INTERACTIONS: Risk of hypoglycemia when used in combination with other hypoglycemic agents. CYP2C8 inhibitors (eg, gemfibrozil) may increase AUC of rosiglitazone. CYP2C8 inducers (eg, rifampin) may decrease AUC of rosiglitazone.

PREGNANCY: Category C, not for use in nursing.

AVAPRO   RX
irbesartan (Bristol-Myers Squibb/Sanofi-Aventis)

> Can cause death/injury to developing fetus during 2nd and 3rd trimesters. Stop therapy if pregnancy detected.

THERAPEUTIC CLASS: Angiotensin II receptor antagonist

INDICATIONS: Hypertension, alone or with other antihypertensives. Diabetic nephropathy with an elevated serum creatinine and proteinuria (>300mg/day) in patients with type 2 diabetes and hypertension.

DOSAGE: *Adults:* HTN: Initial: 150mg qd. Titrate: May increase to 300mg qd. Intravascular Volume/Salt Depletion: Initial: 75mg qd. Nephropathy: Maint: 300mg qd.
Pediatrics: HTN: ≥17 yrs: Initial: 150mg qd. Titrate: May increase to 300mg qd. Intravascular Volume/Salt Depletion: Initial: 75mg qd.

HOW SUPPLIED: Tab: 75mg, 150mg, 300mg

WARNINGS/PRECAUTIONS: Can cause fetal injury/death. Correct volume or salt depletion before therapy. Changes in renal function may occur; caution with renal artery stenosis, severe CHF. Angioedema reported.

ADVERSE REACTIONS: Diarrhea, dyspepsia/heartburn, musculoskeletal trauma, fatigue, upper respiratory infection.

PREGNANCY: Category C (1st trimester) and D (2nd and 3rd trimesters), not for use in nursing.

AVASTIN   RX
bevacizumab (Genentech)

> Fatal pulmonary hemorrhage has occurred in patients with non-small cell lung cancer treated with chemotherapy and bevacizumab; avoid with recent hemoptysis. Avoid if GI perforation or wound dehiscence develops; may be fatal.

THERAPEUTIC CLASS: Vascular endothelial growth factor (VEGF) inhibitor

INDICATIONS: First- or second-line treatment of metastatic carcinoma of the colon or rectum, in combination with 5-fluorouracil-based chemotherapy. First-line treatment of unresectable, locally advanced, recurrent or metastatic non-squamous, non-small cell lung cancer, in combination with carboplatin and paclitaxel. Treatment of patients who have not received chemotherapy for metastatic HER2 negative breast cancer, in combination with paclitaxel.

DOSAGE: *Adults:* Colon/Rectum Metastatic Carcinoma: 5mg/kg (in combination with bolus IFL) or 10 mg/kg (in combination with FOLFOX4) given once every 14 days. Lung Cancer: 15mg/kg every 3 weeks. Breast Cancer: 10mg/kg every 2 weeks. Give as IV infusion over 90 min, if 1st infusion is well tolerated, give 2nd infusion over 60 min and subsequent doses over 30 min.

HOW SUPPLIED: Inj: 25mg/mL [4mL, 16mL]

WARNINGS/PRECAUTIONS: D/C with GI perforation, wound dehiscence, nephrotic syndrome, or serious hemorrhage and arterial thromboembolic events. Increased risk of HTN; permanently d/c if hypertensive crisis or hypertensive encephalopathy occurs. Monitor BP every 2-3 weeks during treatment. Increased incidence/severity of proteinuria. Potential for immunogenicity. CHF and neutropenia reported. Avoid initiation of therapy for at least 28 days following major surgery; surgical incision must be fully healed prior to start of therapy. Suspend treatment prior to elective surgery. Reversible posterior leukoencephalopathy syndrome reported; d/c and treat HTN if present. Non-GI fistula formation reported. May impair fertility.

ADVERSE REACTIONS: Asthenia, pain, abdominal pain, headache, HTN, diarrhea, nausea, vomiting, anorexia, stomatitis, constipation, upper respiratory infection, epistaxis, dyspnea, exfoliative dermatitis.

INTERACTIONS: Increased risk of thromboembolic events when coadministered with chemotherapy; d/c if severe arterial thromboembolic event occurs.

PREGNANCY: Category C, not for use in nursing.

MECHANISM OF ACTION: Vascular endothelial growth factor (VEGF) inhibitor; monoclonal IgG$_1$ antibody that binds to VEGF and prevents interaction with receptors (Flt-1, KDR) on surface of endothelial cells, inhibiting endothelial cell proliferation and new blood vessel formation.

PHARMACOKINETICS: Distribution: V_d=3.25L (males), 2.66L (females). **Elimination:** $T_{1/2}$=20 days.

AVC   RX
sulfanilamide (Novavax)

THERAPEUTIC CLASS: Antifungal agent

INDICATIONS: Treatment of vulvovaginitis caused by *Candida albicans.*

DOSAGE: *Adults:* 1 applicatorful intravaginally qd-bid. Continue for 30 days.

HOW SUPPLIED: Cre: 15% [120g]

CONTRAINDICATIONS: Sulfonamide sensitivity.

WARNINGS/PRECAUTIONS: Observe for skin rash or evidence of systemic toxicity. Goiter, diuresis, hypoglycemia, and deaths from hypersensitivity reactions, agranulocytosis, aplastic anemia, and blood dyscrasias reported with oral sulfonamides. Caution after 7th month of pregnancy.

ADVERSE REACTIONS: Local sensitivity reaction (eg, discomfort, burning).

PREGNANCY: Category C, not for use in nursing.

AVELOX   RX
moxifloxacin HCL (Schering)

THERAPEUTIC CLASS: Fluoroquinolone

INDICATIONS: Treatment of acute bacterial sinusitis, acute bacterial exacerbation of chronic bronchitis (ABECB), uncomplicated skin and skin structure infections (SSSI), complicated skin and skin structure infections (cSSSI), complicated intra-abdominal infections (cIAI), and community-acquired pneumonia (CAP) caused by susceptible strains of microorganisms.

DOSAGE: *Adults:* ≥18 yrs: Sinusitis: 400mg PO/IV q24h for 10 days. ABECB: 400mg PO/IV q24h for 5 days. SSSI: 400mg PO/IV q24h for 7 days. cSSSI: 400mg PO/IV q24h for 7-21 days. cIAI: 400mg IV q24h for 5-14 days. CAP: 400mg PO/IV q24h for 7-14 days.

HOW SUPPLIED: Inj: 400mg/250mL; Tab: 400mg [ABC Pack, 5 tabs]

WARNINGS/PRECAUTIONS: Avoid in pregnancy, nursing, and patients <18 yrs. QT prolongation risk may increase if >65 yrs and may be dose or infusion-rate dependent; do not exceed recommended dose. Avoid with known QT interval prolongation, and uncorrected hypokalemia. Caution with ongoing proarrhythmic conditions (eg, significant bradycardia, acute MI). *Clostridium difficile*-associated diarrhea reported. Caution with CNS disorders (eg, severe cerebral arteriosclerosis, epilepsy). Tendon ruptures reported. D/C if convulsions, CNS effects, hypersensitivity reaction, or tendon rupture occurs.

ADVERSE REACTIONS: Nausea, diarrhea, dizziness.

INTERACTIONS: Take oral formulation at least 4 hrs before or 8 hrs after aluminum-, magnesium-, or calcium-containing antacids, sucralfate, multivitamins with iron or zinc, and didanosine chewable/buffered tablets or oral solution. Avoid Class IA (eg, quinidine, procainamide) or Class III (eg, amiodarone, sotalol) antiarrhythmics. Caution with drugs that prolong the QT interval (eg, cisapride, erythromycin, antipsychotics, TCAs). NSAIDs may increase risk of CNS stimulation and convulsions. Monitor PT with warfarin. Corticosteroids in elderly may increase risk of tendon rupture. Do not add other substances, additives, or medications to injection or infuse simultaneously through same IV line.

PREGNANCY: Category C, not for use in nursing.

MECHANISM OF ACTION: Fluoroquinolone: synthetic broad-spectrum antibiotic with activity against gram-positive and gram-negative microorganisms. Inhibits topoisomerase II (DNA gyrase) and topoisomerase IV, which are required for bacterial DNA replication, transcription, repair, and recombination.

PHARMACOKINETICS: Absorption: Well-absorbed; Absolute bioavailability (90%). Single dose: (Oral) C_{max}=3.1mg/L, AUC=36.1mg•hr/L; (IV) C_{max}=3.9mg/L, AUC=39.3mg•hr/L. Refer to PI for further info. **Distribution:** Plasma protein binding (30-50%); V_d=1.7-2.7L/kg; Widely distributed. **Metabolism:** Glucuronide and sulfate conjugation. **Elimination:** 45% unchanged; urine (20%), feces (25%); $T_{1/2}$=11.5-15.6 hrs (oral), 8.2-15.4 hrs (IV).

AVINZA   CII
morphine sulfate (King)

> Swallow capsules whole or sprinkle contents on applesauce. Do not crush, chew, or dissolve capsule beads. Avoid alcohol and alcohol-containing medications; consumption of alcohol may result in the rapid release and absorption of potentially fatal dose of morphine.

THERAPEUTIC CLASS: Opioid analgesic

INDICATIONS: Relief of moderate to severe pain requiring continuous opioid therapy for an extended period of time.

DOSAGE: *Adults:* ≥18 yrs: Conversion from Other Oral Morphine Products: Give total daily morphine dose as a single dose q24h. Conversion from Parenteral Morphine: Initial: Give about 3x the previous daily parenteral morphine requirement. Conversion from Other Parenteral or Oral Non-Morphine Opioids: Initial: Give 1/2 of estimated daily morphine requirement q24h. Supplement with immediate-release morphine or short-acting analgesics if needed. Titrate: Adjust dose as frequently as every other day. Non-Opioid Tolerant: 30mg q24h. Titrate: Increase by increments ≤30mg every 4 days. The 60, 90, and 120mg caps are for opioid-tolerant patients. Max: 1600mg/day. Doses >1600mg/day contain a quantity of fumaric acid, which may cause renal toxicity.

HOW SUPPLIED: Cap, Extended-Release: 30mg, 60mg, 90mg, 120mg

CONTRAINDICATIONS: Respiratory depression in the absence of resuscitative equipment, acute or severe bronchial asthma, paralytic ileus.

WARNINGS/PRECAUTIONS: Abuse potential. Extreme caution with COPD, cor pulmonale, decreased respiratory reserve (eg, severe kyphoscoliosis), hypoxia, hypercapnia, pre-existing respiratory depression, increased ICP, head injury. May cause orthostatic hypotension, syncope, severe hypotension with depleted blood volume. Caution with circulatory shock, biliary tract disease, severe renal/hepatic insufficiency, Addison's disease, hypothyroidism, prostatic hypertrophy, urethral stricture, elderly or debilitated, CNS depression, toxic psychosis, acute alcoholism, delirium tremens, seizure disorders. Avoid with GI obstruction. Withdrawal symptoms with abrupt discontinuation. Tolerance and physical dependence may develop. Potential for severe constipation; use laxatives, stool softeners at onset of therapy.

ADVERSE REACTIONS: Constipation, nausea, somnolence, vomiting, dehydration, headache, peripheral edema, diarrhea, abdominal pain, infection, UTI, flu syndrome, back pain, rash, sweating, fever, insomnia, depression, paresthesia, anorexia, dry mouth, asthenia, dyspnea.

INTERACTIONS: See Black Box Warning. Additive effects with alcohol, other opioids, illicit drugs that cause CNS depression. Reduce dose with other CNS depressants (eg, sedatives, hypnotics, general anesthetics, antiemetics, phenothiazines, tranquilizers, alcohol). May enhance neuromuscular blocking action of skeletal muscle relaxants. Avoid with mixed agonist/antagonists (eg, pentazocine, nalbuphine, butorphanol) and within 14 days of MAOI use. Monitor for increased respiratory and CNS depression with cimetidine.

PREGNANCY: Category C, not for use in nursing.

MECHANISM OF ACTION: Opioid analgesic: pure opioid agonist that is relatively selective for μ-receptor but may interact with other opioid receptors at higher doses. Mechanism of analgesic effects not established. Specific CNS opiate receptors (eg, μ-receptors) and endogenous compounds with morphine-like activity are found throughout brain and spinal cord and are likely to play a role in analgesic effects.

PHARMACOKINETICS: Absorption: AUC=273.25ng/mL•h; C_{max}=18.65ng/mL. **Distribution:** Plasma protein binding (20-35%), V_d=1-6L/kg, distributed to skeletal muscle, kidneys, liver, GI tract, lung, spleen and brain. Small quantities cross the blood-brain barrier. Found in placental membranes and human breast milk. **Metabolism:** Hepatic conjugation; 3-glucuronide (M3G) (metabolite); 6-glucuronide (M6G) (active metabolite). **Elimination:** Urine (major); bile (small), feces (7-10%); (IV) $T_{1/2}$=2 hrs.

AVITA   RX
tretinoin (Mylan Bertek)

INDICATIONS: Acne vulgaris.

DOSAGE: *Adults:* Apply qpm to cleansed skin. May reduce dosing frequency if irritation occurs.

HOW SUPPLIED: Cre: 0.025% [20g, 45g]; Gel: 0.025% [20g, 45g]

WARNINGS/PRECAUTIONS: Avoid eyes, lips, paranasal creases, mucous membranes, and sunburned skin. May exacerbate acne during 1st weeks of therapy. Severe irritation with eczematous skin. Extreme weather may increase skin irritatation. Gel is flammable.

ADVERSE REACTIONS: Local skin reactions (red, edematous, blistered, crusted), photosensitivity, temporary skin pigmentation changes.

INTERACTIONS: Caution with other topicals with strong drying effects, high concentration of alcohol, astringents, spices, or lime. Caution with sulfur, resorcinol, or salicylic acid, allow effects of these agents to subside before application of tretinoin.

PREGNANCY: Category C, caution in nursing.

AVODART   RX
dutasteride (GlaxoSmithKline)

THERAPEUTIC CLASS: Type I and II 5 alpha-reductase inhibitor (2nd generation)

INDICATIONS: Benign prostatic hyperplasia (BPH). To reduce risk of acute urinary retention and need for BPH-related surgery.

DOSAGE: *Adults:* 0.5mg qd. Swallow caps whole.

HOW SUPPLIED: Cap: 0.5mg

CONTRAINDICATIONS: Women and children.

WARNINGS/PRECAUTIONS: Risk to male fetus; should not be handled by pregnant women. Monitor for obstructive uropathy with large residual urinary volume and/or severely diminished urinary flow. Avoid donating blood until 6 months after last dose. Caution with liver disease. Decreases serum PSA levels by about 40%-50%; adjust (double) PSA results after 6 months or more of therapy to compare with normal values.

ADVERSE REACTIONS: Impotence, decreased libido.

INTERACTIONS: CYP3A4 inhibitors (eg, ritonavir, ketoconazole, verapamil, diltiazem, cimetidine, ciprofloxacin) may increase blood levels.

PREGNANCY: Category X, not for use in nursing.

MECHANISM OF ACTION: Type I, II 5α-reductase inhibitor; inhibits conversion of testosterone to 5α-dihydrotestosterone, androgen responsible for development and enlargement of prostate gland.

PHARMACOKINETICS: Absorption: T_{max}=2-3 hrs; Absolute bioavailability (60%). **Distribution:** V_d=300-500L; Plasma protein binding (99%) **Metabolism:** CYP3A4, 3A5. **Elimination:** Feces (5%), urine (<1%); $T_{1/2}$=5 weeks.

AVONEX   RX
interferon beta-1a (Biogen Idec)

THERAPEUTIC CLASS: Biological response modifier

INDICATIONS: Treatment of relapsing forms of multiple sclerosis (MS) including patients who experienced a first clinical episode and have MRI features consistent with MS.

DOSAGE: *Adults:* 30mcg IM once a week.

HOW SUPPLIED: Kit: 33mcg

CONTRAINDICATIONS: Hypersensitivity to human albumin.

WARNINGS/PRECAUTIONS: Caution with depression, mood disorders, pre-existing seizure disorders. Depression, suicidal ideation, and development of new or worsening pre-existing other psychiatric disorders reported. Anaphylaxis (rare), suicidal ideation, psychosis, decreased peripheral blood counts, autoimmune disorders (eg, thrombocytopenia, hyper- and hypothyroidism), hepatic injury including hepatitis reported. Rare reports of severe hepatic injury, including cases of hepatic failure; monitor for signs of hepatic injury. Monitor closely with cardiac disease (eg, angina, CHF, arrhythmia). Risk of transmission of viral diseases. Abortifacient potential. Perform TFTs, LFTs, CBCs, differential WBCs, and platelets during therapy.

ADVERSE REACTIONS: Flu-like symptoms, myalgia, depression, fever, chills, asthenia, headache, pain, dizziness, nausea, sinusitis, upper respiratory tract infection, UTI.

INTERACTIONS: Caution with other drugs associated with hepatic injury.

PREGNANCY: Category C, not for use in nursing.

MECHANISM OF ACTION: Human interferon β; not established (MS), exerts biological effects by binding to specific receptors on surface of human cells, initiating complex cascade of intracellular events that leads to expression of numerous interferon-induced gene products and markers.

PHARMACOKINETICS: Absorption: T_{max}=3-15 hrs. **Elimination:** $T_{1/2}$=10 hrs.

AXERT   RX
almotriptan malate (Ortho-McNeil)

THERAPEUTIC CLASS: 5-HT$_{1D 1B}$-agonist

INDICATIONS: Acute treatment of migraine with or without aura.

DOSAGE: *Adults:* ≥18 yrs: Initial: 6.25-12.5mg at onset of headache. May repeat after 2 hrs. Max: 2 doses/24 hrs. Hepatic/Renal Impairment: 6.25mg at onset of headache. Max: 12.5mg/24 hrs. Safety of treating >4 headaches/30 days not known.

HOW SUPPLIED: Tab: 6.25mg, 12.5mg

CONTRAINDICATIONS: Ischemic heart disease, coronary artery vasospasm, other significant CVD, uncontrolled HTN, within 24 hrs of another 5-HT$_1$ agonist or ergot type agent, hemiplegic or basilar migraine.

WARNINGS/PRECAUTIONS: Confirm diagnosis. Supervise first dose and monitor cardiac function in those at risk of CAD (eg, HTN, hypercholesterolemia, smoker, obesity, diabetes, CAD family history, postmenopausal women, males >40 yrs). Monitor cardiovascular function with long-term intermittent use. May cause vasospastic reactions or cerebrovascular events. Caution with renal or hepatic dysfunction. Avoid in elderly.

ADVERSE REACTIONS: Nausea, somnolence, headache, paresthesia, dry mouth, coronary artery vasospasm, MI, ventricular tachycardia, fibrillation.

INTERACTIONS: Additive vasospastic reactions with ergotamines. SSRIs may cause weakness, hyperreflexia, and incoordination. Avoid other 5-HT$_1$ agonist drugs within 24-hr period. Clearance may be decreased by MAOIs. Increased levels possible with CYP3A4 inhibitors (eg, ketoconazole).

PREGNANCY: Category C, caution in nursing.

MECHANISM OF ACTION: Selective 5-HT$_{1B/1D}$-receptor agonist; binds with high affinity to 5-HT$_{1B/1D/1F}$ receptors and weak affinity to 5-HT$_{1A/7}$ receptors. Attributed to agonist effects at 5-HT$_{1B/1D}$ receptors on extracerebral, intracranial blood vessels that become dilated during migraine attack and on nerve terminal in trigeminal system. Activation of these receptors results in cranial nerve constriction, inhibition of neuropeptide release, and reduced transmission in trigeminal pain pathways.

PHARMACOKINETICS: Absorption: Well-absorbed; absolute bioavailabiliy (70%); T_{max}=1-3 hrs. **Distribution:** V_d=180-200L; plasma protein binding (35%). **Metabolism:** Monoamine oxidase (MAO)-mediated oxidative deamination and CYP450-mediated oxidation (major pathways); Indoleacetic acid, gamma-aminobutyric acid (inactive metabolites). **Elimination:** Urine (40% unchanged), feces (13%, unchanged and metabolized); $T_{1/2}$=3-4 hrs.

AXID   RX
nizatidine (GlaxoSmithKline)

OTHER BRAND NAMES: Axid Oral Solution (Reliant)

THERAPEUTIC CLASS: H$_2$-blocker

INDICATIONS: Short term treatment of active duodenal ulcer (DU) and benign gastric ulcer (GU). Maintenance therapy for duodenal ulcers. Treatment of endoscopically diagnosed esophagitis, including erosive and ulcerative esophagitis, and heartburn due to GERD.

DOSAGE: *Adults:* Active DU/Active Benign GU: Usual: 300mg qhs or 150mg bid up to 8 weeks. Healed DU: Maint: 150mg qhs, up to 1 year. GERD: 150mg bid up to 12 weeks. Renal Impairment: Treatment: CrCl 20-50mL/min: 150mg/day. CrCl <20mL/min: 150mg every other day. Maint: CrCl 20-50mL/min: 150mg every other day. CrCl <20mL/min: 150mg every 3 days.
Pediatrics: ≥12 yrs: (Sol) Erosive Esophagitis/GERD: 150mg bid up to 8 weeks. Max: 300mg/day. Renal Impairment: Treatment: CrCl 20-50mL/min: 150mg/day. CrCl <20mL/min: 150mg every other day. Maint: CrCl 20-50mL/min: 150mg every other day. CrCl <20mL/min: 150mg every 3 days.

HOW SUPPLIED: Cap: 150mg, 300mg; Sol: 15mg/mL

WARNINGS/PRECAUTIONS: Caution with renal dysfunction; reduce dose. Symptomatic response does not preclude the presence of gastric malignancy. False positive tests for urobilinogen with Multistix.

ADVERSE REACTIONS: Headache, abdominal pain, pain, asthenia, diarrhea, nausea, flatulence, vomiting, dyspepsia, rhinitis, pharyngitis, dizziness, headache.

INTERACTIONS: May elevate serum salicylate levels with high dose ASA.

PREGNANCY: Category B, not for use in nursing.

MECHANISM OF ACTION: H_2 receptor antagonist; competitive, reversible inhibitor of histamine at the histamine H_2 receptors, particularly those in gastroparietal cells.

PHARMACOKINETICS: Absorption: Absolute bioavailability (>70%); (150mg, 300mg) C_{max}=700-1800mcg/L, 1400-3600mcg/L; T_{max}=0.5-3 hrs. (12-18 yrs, 150mg) C_{max}=1422.9ng/mL; T_{max}=1.3 hrs; AUC=3764ng•hr/mL. **Distribution:** (Adult) V_d=0.8-1.5L/kg; (12-18 yrs) V_d=71.4L. Plasma protein binding (35%); found in breast milk. **Metabolism:** N_2-monodesmethylnizatidine (major). **Excretion:** Urine (90%, 60% unchanged); feces (6%). (Adult) $T_{1/2}$=1-2 hrs; (12-18 yrs) $T_{1/2}$=1.2 hrs.

AYGESTIN RX
norethindrone acetate (Duramed)

THERAPEUTIC CLASS: Progestogen

INDICATIONS: Treatment of secondary amenorrhea, endometriosis, and abnormal uterine bleeding due to hormonal imbalance in the absence of organic pathology.

DOSAGE: *Adults:* Assume interval between menses is 28 days. Secondary Amenorrhea/Abnormal Uterine Bleeding: 2.5-10mg qd for 5-10 days during second half of menstrual cycle. Endometriosis: Initial: 5mg qd for 2 weeks. Titrate: Increase by 2.5mg qd every 2 weeks until 15mg/day. Continue for 6-9 months or until breakthrough bleeding demands temporary termination.

HOW SUPPLIED: Tab: 5mg* *scored

CONTRAINDICATIONS: Pregnancy, thrombophlebitis, thromboembolic disorders, cerebral apoplexy, liver impairment, breast carcinoma, undiagnosed vaginal bleeding, missed abortion, use as a pregnancy diagnostic test.

WARNINGS/PRECAUTIONS: D/C with migraine, vision loss, proptosis, diplopia, papilledema, or retinal vascular lesions. May cause thrombophlebitis, pulmonary embolism, and fluid retention. Caution with epilepsy, migraine, psychic depression, asthma, cardiac or renal dysfunction, depression, DM, and hyperlipidemia. May mask onset of climacteric. Not for use during the first trimester of pregnancy; risk to the fetus.

ADVERSE REACTIONS: Breakthrough bleeding, spotting, change in menstrual flow, amenorrhea, edema, weight changes, cervical changes, cholestatic jaundice, rash, melasma, chloasma, depression.

PREGNANCY: Category X, safety in nursing is not known.

MECHANISM OF ACTION: Progestogen; induces secretory changes in estrogen-primed endometrium.

PHARMACOKINETICS: Absorption: Rapid; T_{max}=1.83 hrs; C_{max}=26.19ng/mL; AUC=166.9ng/mL•hr. **Distribution:** Found in breast milk. Sex hormone binding globulin (SHBG) (36%); albumin binding (61%); V_d=4L/kg. **Metabolism:** Extensive, via reduction; sulfate and glucuronide conjugation. **Elimination:** Urine, feces (metabolites); $T_{1/2}$=9 hrs.

AZACTAM

RX

aztreonam (Elan)

THERAPEUTIC CLASS: Monobactam

INDICATIONS: Treatment of septicemia and lower respiratory tract (eg, pneumonia, bronchitis), skin and skin-structure, urinary tract (UTI), gynecologic (eg, endometritis), and intra-abdominal (eg, peritonitis) infections caused by susceptible microorganisms. Adjunct therapy to surgery for management of infections caused by susceptible microorganisms.

DOSAGE: *Adults:* UTI: 500mg-1g IM/IV q8-12h. Moderately Severe Systemic Infections: 1-2g IM/IV q8-12h. Severe Systemic/Life-Threatening Infections/ *Pseudomonas aeruginosa:* 2g IV q6-8h. Max: 8g/day. CrCl 10-30mL/ min/1.73m^2: Initial: LD: 1 or 2g. Maint: 50% of usual dose. CrCl <10mL/ min/1.73m^2: Initial: LD: 500mg, 1g or 2g. Maint: 25% of usual initial dose at usual intervals. Serious/Life-Threatening Infections: In addition to maint dose, give 1/8 initial dose after each hemodialysis session. IV route recommended for single doses >1g or for bacterial septicemia, localized parenchymal abscess (eg, intra-abdominal abscess), peritonitis, or other severe systemic or life-threatening infections. Continue for at least 48 hrs after patient is asymptomatic or evidence of bacterial eradication.
Pediatrics: 9 months-16 yrs: Mild-Moderate Infections: 30mg/kg IV q8h. Moderate-Severe Infections: 30mg/kg IV q6-8h. Max: 120mg/kg/day. IV route is recommended for single doses >1g or for bacterial septicemia, localized parenchymal abscess (eg, intra-abdominal abscess), peritonitis, or other severe systemic or life-threatening infections. Continue for at least 48 hrs after patient is asymptomatic or evidence of bacterial eradication.

HOW SUPPLIED: Inj: 1g, 2g, 1g/50mL, 2g/50mL

WARNINGS/PRECAUTIONS: Caution with hypersensitivity to other β-lactams or allergens. *Clostridium difficile*-associated diarrhea reported. May promote overgrowth of nonsusceptible organisms. Monitor with renal or hepatic impairment. Toxic epidermal necrolysis reported (rarely) in bone marrow transplant with multiple risk factors including sepsis.

ADVERSE REACTIONS: Diarrhea, nausea, vomiting, rash, abdominal cramps, vaginal candidiasis, discomfort/swelling at injection site, hypersensitivity reaction.

INTERACTIONS: Monitor renal function with aminoglycosides; increased risk of nephrotoxicity, ototoxicity. Toxic epidermal necrolysis reported (rarely) in bone marrow transplant with radiation therapy and other drugs associated with toxic epidermal necrolysis.

PREGNANCY: Category B, not for use in nursing.

MECHANISM OF ACTION: Monobactam, synthetic bactericidal antibiotic. Inhibits bacterial cell wall synthesis due to high affinity of aztreonam for penicillin-binding protein 3 (PBP3).

PHARMACOKINETICS: Absorption: C_{max}=90μ/ml (1g dose), 204μ/ml (2g dose); T_{max}=1 hr. **Distribution:** V_d=12.6L; found in breast milk. **Elimination:** Urine. $T_{1/2}$=1.7 hr.

AZASAN

RX

azathioprine (Salix)

> Increased risk of neoplasia with chronic therapy. Mutagenic potential and possible hematological toxicities.

THERAPEUTIC CLASS: Purine antagonist antimetabolite

INDICATIONS: Adjunct therapy for prevention of rejection in renal homotransplantation. Management of severe, active rheumatoid arthritis (RA) unresponsive to rest, ASA, NSAIDs, or gold.

DOSAGE: *Adults:* Renal Homotransplantation: Initial: 3-5mg/kg/day, start at time of transplant. Maint: 1-3mg/kg/day. Rheumatoid Arthritis: Initial:

1mg/kg/day given qd-bid. Titrate: Increase by 0.5mg/kg/day after 6-8 weeks, then at 4 week intervals. Max: 2.5mg/kg/day. Maint: Lowest effective dose. Decrease by 0.5mg/kg/day or 25mg/day every 4 weeks. If no response by week 12, then considered refractory. Renal Dysfunction: Lower dose

HOW SUPPLIED: Tab: 25mg*, 50mg*, 75mg*, 100mg* *scored

CONTRAINDICATIONS: Pregnancy in RA treatment. Previous treatment of RA with alkylating agents (eg, cyclophosphamide, chlorambucil, melphalan) may increase risk of neoplasia.

WARNINGS/PRECAUTIONS: Dose-related leukopenia, thrombocytopenia, macrocytic anemia, and severe bone marrow suppression may occur. Monitor CBCs, including platelets, weekly during the 1st month, twice monthly for the 2nd and 3rd months, then monthly or more frequently if dose/therapy changes. Monitor for infections.

ADVERSE REACTIONS: Leukopenia, thrombocytopenia, infections, nausea, vomiting, hepatotoxicity.

INTERACTIONS: Reduce dose by 1/3-1/4 with allopurinol. Drugs affecting leukocyte production (eg, co-trimazole) may exaggerate leukopenia. ACE inhibitors may induce severe leukopenia.

PREGNANCY: Category D, not for use in nursing.

MECHANISM OF ACTION: Imidazole derivative; immunosuppression antime-tabolite, mechanism of action is obscure in homograft survival; it suppresses hypersensitivities of the cell-mediated type and causes variable alterations in antibody production and in immuno-inflammatory response eg, autoimmune diseases. Immuno-inflammatory response not established; believed that it supresses disease manifestations and underlying pathology.

PHARMACOKINETICS: Absorption: Well absorbed. T_{max}=1-2 hrs. **Distribution:** (30%) bound to plasma protein. Crosses the placenta and found in breast milk. **Metabolism:** Liver and erythrocytes through oxidation and methylation pathways to 6-mercaptopurine (6-MP). Activation of 6-MP via hypoxanthine-guanine-phosphoribosyl-transferase to form 6-thioguanine nucleotides (6-TGNs) (major metabolite). **Elimination:** Urine, $T_{1/2}$=8 hrs.

AZASITE   RX
azithromycin (Inspire)

THERAPEUTIC CLASS: Macrolide

INDICATIONS: Treatment of bacterial conjunctivitis caused by susceptible strains of microorganisms.

DOSAGE: *Adults:* Initial: 1 drop bid, 8 to 12 hrs apart, for first 2 days. Maint: 1 drop qd for next 5 days.
Pediatrics: ≥1 yr: Initial: 1 drop bid, 8 to 12 hrs apart, for first 2 days. Maint: 1 drop qd for next 5 days.

HOW SUPPLIED: Sol: 1% [2.5mL]

WARNINGS/PRECAUTIONS: Not for injection; do not give systemically, inject subconjunctivally or into chamber of eye. Caution may cause hypersensitivity reactions. Growth of resistant organisms including fungi may occur with prolonged use. Avoid contact lens use.

ADVERSE REACTIONS: Eye irritation, burning, stinging and irritation upon instillation, contact dermatitis, corneal erosion, dry eye, dysgeusia, nasal congestion, ocular discharge, punctate keratitis, sinusitis.

PREGNANCY: Category B, caution in nursing.

MECHANISM OF ACTION: Macrolide; binds to the 50S ribosomal subunit of susceptible microorganisms and interferes with microbial protein synthesis.

PHARMACOKINETICS: Absorption: C_{max}≤10ng/mL

AZELEX

RX

azelaic acid (Allergan)

THERAPEUTIC CLASS: Dicarboxylic acid antimicrobial

INDICATIONS: Mild to moderate inflammatory acne vulgaris.

DOSAGE: *Adults:* Wash and dry skin. Massage gently into affected area bid (am and pm).
Pediatrics: ≥12 yrs: Wash and dry skin. Massage gently into affected area bid (am and pm).

HOW SUPPLIED: Cre: 20% [30g, 50g]

WARNINGS/PRECAUTIONS: Avoid mouth, eyes, mucous membranes, and occlusive dressings.

ADVERSE REACTIONS: Pruritus, burning, stinging, tingling, hypopigmentation.

PREGNANCY: Category B, caution in nursing.

MECHANISM OF ACTION: Dicarboxylic acid antimicrobial; not established. Possesses antimicrobial activity that may be attributable to inhibition of microbial cellular protein synthesis. A normalization of keratinization leading to an anticomedonal effect of azelaic acid may also contribute to clinical activity.

PHARMACOKINETICS: Absorption: Penetrates stratum corneum (3-5%), up to 10% of dose found in dermis and epidermis; systemic absorption (4%); C_{max}=20-80ng/mL. **Metabolism:** Cutaneous (negligible), beta-oxidation. **Elimination:** Urine (mainly unchanged); $T_{1/2}$=12 hrs (after topical dosing).

AZILECT

RX

rasagiline mesylate (Teva)

THERAPEUTIC CLASS: Monoamine oxidase inhibitor (Type B)

INDICATIONS: Treatment of signs and symptoms of idiopathic Parkinson's disease as initial monotherapy and adjunct therapy to levodopa.

DOSAGE: *Adults:* Monotherapy: 1mg qd. Adjunctive Therapy: Initial: 0.5mg qd. Titrate: May increase to 1mg qd. Adjust dose of levodopa with concomitant use. Concomitant Ciprofloxacin or Other CYP1A2 Inhibitors/Hepatic Impairment: 0.5mg qd.

HOW SUPPLIED: Tab: 0.5mg, 1mg

CONTRAINDICATIONS: Pheochromocytoma. Concomitant use with meperidine, tramadol, methadone, propoxyphene, dextromethorphan, St. John's wort, mirtazapine, cyclobenzaprine, sympathomimetic amines (eg, amphetamines, cold products containing pseudoephedrine, phenylephrine, phenylpropanolamine, and ephedrine), other MAOIs, cocaine, general anesthesia, local anesthesia containing vasoconstrictors.

WARNINGS/PRECAUTIONS: May increase incidence of melanoma. Concomitant use with levodopa may potentiate dopaminergic side effects and exacerbate pre-existing dyskinesia. Postural hypotension reported. Patients should be warned to restrict dietary tyramines and avoid amine-containing medications for 2 weeks after discontinuation.

ADVERSE REACTIONS: Headache, arthralgia, depression, fall, flu syndrome, dyskinesia, accidental injury, nausea, weight loss, constipation, postural hypotension, vomiting, dry mouth, rash, somnolence.

INTERACTIONS: See Contraindications. Concomitant use with SSRIs, SNRIs, tricyclic and tetracyclic antidepressants is not recommended due to severe CNS toxicity. Increased plasma concentrations up to 2-fold with concomitant ciprofloxacin and other CYP1A2. Severe hypertensive reactions reported with concomitant use of sympathomimetics.

PREGNANCY: Category C, caution in nursing.

MECHANISM OF ACTION: MAO-B inhibitor: Suspected to inhibit MAO type B, which causes an increase in extracellular dopamine levels in the striatum and increases dopaminergic activity.

PHARMACOKINETICS: Absorption: Rapid. T_{max}= approximately 1 hr. Absolute bioavailability (36%). **Distribution**: V_d=87L. Plasma protein binding (88-94%). **Metabolism**: N-dealkylation, hydroxylation; CYP1A2: 1-aminoindan (AI), 3-hydroxy-N-propargyl-1 aminoindan (1-OH-PAI) and 3-hydroxy-1-aminoindan (3-OH-AI). **Elimination**: $T_{1/2}$=3 hrs. Urine (62% over 7 days), (84% over 38 days), (<1% unchanged), feces (7%).

AZMACORT RX
triamcinolone acetonide (Abbott)

THERAPEUTIC CLASS: Corticosteroid

INDICATIONS: Maintenance treatment of asthma as prophylactic therapy in patients ≥6 yrs; to reduce or eliminate the need for oral corticosteroidal therapy.

DOSAGE: *Adults:* 2 inh (150mcg) tid-qid or 4 inh (300mcg) bid. Severe Asthma: Initial: 12-16 inh/day. Max: 16 inh/day (1200mcg). Rinse mouth after use.
Pediatrics: >12 yrs: 2 inh (150mcg) tid-qid or 4 inh (300mcg) bid. Severe Asthma: Initial: 12-16 inh/day. Max: 16 inh/day (1200mcg). 6-12 yrs: 1-2 inh (75-150mcg) tid-qid or 2-4 (150-300mcg) inh bid. Max: 12 inh/day (900mcg). Rinse mouth after use.

HOW SUPPLIED: MDI: 75mcg/inh [20g]

CONTRAINDICATIONS: Primary treatment of status asthmaticus or other acute asthma attacks.

WARNINGS/PRECAUTIONS: Deaths due to adrenal insufficiency have occurred with transfer from systemic corticosteroids to inhaled corticosteroids. Resume oral corticosteroids during stress or severe asthma attack. Observe for adrenal insufficiency, systemic corticosteroid withdrawal effects, hypercorticism and growth suppression (children). More susceptible to infections. Not for acute bronchospasm. D/C if bronchospasm occurs after dosing. Caution with TB of respiratory tract; untreated systemic fungal, bacterial, viral or parasitic infections; or ocular herpes simplex. *Candida* infection of mouth and pharynx reported.

ADVERSE REACTIONS: Pharyngitis, sinusitis, headache, flu syndrome.

INTERACTIONS: Caution with prednisone.

PREGNANCY: Category C, caution in nursing.

MECHANISM OF ACTION: Corticosteroid; not established. Inhaled route makes possible to provide local anti-inflammatory activity.

PHARMACOKINETICS: Absorption: T_{max}=1.5-2 hrs. **Distribution:** V_d=99.5L; plasma protein binding (68%). **Elimination:** Urine (40%), feces (60%); $T_{1/2}$=88 min.

AZOPT RX
brinzolamide (Alcon)

THERAPEUTIC CLASS: Carbonic anhydrase inhibitor

INDICATIONS: Open-angle glaucoma. Ocular hypertension.

DOSAGE: *Adults:* 1 drop tid. Space dosing other ophthalmic drugs by 10 min.

HOW SUPPLIED: Sus: 1% [5mL, 10mL, 15mL]

WARNINGS/PRECAUTIONS: Systemically absorbed. Avoid with sulfonamide allergy or severe renal impairment. Caution with hepatic impairment. Not studied in acute angle-closure glaucoma.

ADVERSE REACTIONS: Blurred vision, taste disturbances, blepharitis, dermatitis, dry eye, foreign body sensation, headache, hyperemia, ocular discharge, ocular discomfort, ocular keratitis, ocular pain, ocular pruritus, rhinitis.

INTERACTIONS: Caution with high-dose salicylates. Acid-base disturbances with oral carbonic anhydrase inhibitors. Avoid oral carbonic anhydrase inhibitors due to additive effects. Wait 10 min before using another ophthalmic drug.

PREGNANCY: Category C, not for use in nursing.

MECHANISM OF ACTION: Carbonic anhydrase II inhibitor: Inhibits aqueous humor formation and reduces elevated intraocular pressure.

PHARMACOKINETICS: Distribution: Plasma protein binding (approximately 60%). **Elimination:** Urine (unchanged).

Azor RX
amlodipine besylate - olmesartan medoxomil (Daiichi Sankyo)

> When used in pregnancy during 2nd and 3rd trimesters, drugs that act directly on the renin-angiotensin system can cause injury and even death to developing fetus. When pregnancy is detected, d/c therapy asap.

THERAPEUTIC CLASS: ARB/Calcium channel blocker (dihydropyridine)

INDICATIONS: Treatment of hypertension, alone or with other antihypertensive agents.

DOSAGE: *Adults:* Replacement Therapy: May substitute for individually titrated components for patients on amlodipine and olmesartan. When substituting for individual components, the dose of 1 or both components may be increased if needed. Add-On Therapy: May use as add-on therapy when not adequately controlled on amlodipine or olmesartan. May increase dose after 2 weeks to maximum dose of 10mg-40mg qd.

HOW SUPPLIED: Tab: (Amlodipine-Olmesartan) 5mg-20mg, 10mg-20mg, 5mg-40mg, 10mg-40mg

WARNINGS/PRECAUTIONS: Hypotension, especially in volume- or salt-depleted patients, may occur with treatment initiation; monitor closely. Caution with severe aortic stenosis, heart failure, or severe hepatic impairment. Increased angina or MI with CCBs may occur with dosage initiation or increase. Changes in renal function, oliguria, progressive azotemia, or acute renal failure may occur.

ADVERSE REACTIONS: Edema.

PREGNANCY: Category C (1st trimester) and D (2nd and 3rd trimester), not for use in nursing.

MECHANISM OF ACTION: Amlodipine: Calcium channel receptor blocker (dihydropyridine); inhibits transmembrane influx of calcium ions. Olmesartan: Angiotensin II receptor blocker; blocks vasoconstrictor effect of angiotensin II.

PHARMACOKINETICS: Absorption: Amlodipine: T_{max}=6-12 hrs, absolute bioavailability (64-90%). Olmesartan: Rapid and complete, absolute bioavailability (26%), T_{max}=1-2 hrs. **Distribution:** Amlodipine: Plasma protein binding (93%). Olmesartan: V_d=17L, plasma protein binding (99%), crosses placenta and excreted in breast milk. **Metabolism:** Amlodipine: Liver. Olmesartan: Ester hydrolysis. **Elimination:** Amlodipine: Urine (10%), $T_{1/2}$=30-50 hrs. Olmesartan: Urine (35-50%), feces, $T_{1/2}$=13 hrs.

Azulfidine RX
sulfasalazine (Pharmacia & Upjohn)

THERAPEUTIC CLASS: 5-Aminosalicylic acid derivative/sulfapyridine

INDICATIONS: Treatment of mild to moderate ulcerative colitis. Adjunct therapy in severe ulcerative colitis. To prolong remission period between acute attacks of ulcerative colitis.

DOSAGE: *Adults:* Initial: 3-4g/day in divided doses. May initiate at 1-2g/day to reduce GI intolerance. Maint: 2g/day.
Pediatrics: ≥2 yrs: 40-60mg/kg/day divided into 3-6 doses. Maint: 7.5mg/kg qid.

HOW SUPPLIED: Tab: 500mg* *scored

CONTRAINDICATIONS: <2 yrs, intestinal or urinary obstruction, porphyria, hypersensitivity to sulfonamides, salicylates.

WARNINGS/PRECAUTIONS: Caution with hepatic/renal impairment, blood dyscrasias, severe allergy, bronchial asthma, G6PD deficiency. Monitor CBC, WBC, LFTs, at baseline, every 2nd week for 1st 3 months, monthly for next 3 months, and every 3 months thereafter. Monitor renal function periodically. Maintain adequate fluid intake to prevent crystalluria and stone formation. D/C if hypersensitivity or toxic reaction occurs.

ADVERSE REACTIONS: Anorexia, headache, nausea, vomiting, gastric distress, reversible oligospermia.

INTERACTIONS: Reduces absorption of folic acid, digoxin.

PREGNANCY: Category B, caution in nursing.

MECHANISM OF ACTION: 5-aminosalicylic acid (5-ASA) derivative/sulfapyridine (SP); not established, may be related to anti-inflammatory and/or immunodulatory properties of sulfasalazine (SSZ) or its metabolites (5-ASA and SP), its affinity for connective tissue, and/or to relatively high concentration reached in serous fluids, liver, and intestinal wall.

PHARMACOKINETICS: Absorption: SSZ: C_{max}=6mcg/mL, T_{max}=6 hrs; 5-ASA; SP: T_{max}=10 hrs. SSZ: Absolute bioavailability <15%; SP: Well absorbed from colon, estimated bioavailability 60%. 5-ASA: Much less well absorbed from GI tract, estimated bioavailability 10-30%. **Distribution:** SSZ: V_d=7.5L; plasma protein binding >99.3%. SP: Plasma protein binding 70%. **Metabolism:** Intestinal bacteria to 5-ASA and SP; liver (acetylation). **Elimination:** Urine (37%), feces. SSZ: $T_{1/2}$=7.6 hrs; SP: $T_{1/2}$=10.4 hrs (slow acetylators), 14.8 hrs (fast acetylators).

AZULFIDINE EN   RX
sulfasalazine (Pharmacia & Upjohn)

THERAPEUTIC CLASS: 5-Aminosalicylic acid derivative/sulfapyridine

INDICATIONS: Mild to moderate ulcerative colitis, as an adjunct treatment of severe ulcerative colitis, and for the prolongation of the remission period between acute attacks of ulcerative colitis. Rheumatoid arthritis and polyarticular-course juvenile rheumatoid arthritis that has responded inadequately to salicylates or other NSAIDs.

DOSAGE: *Adults:* Ulcerative Colitis: Initial: 1-4g/day in divided doses at intervals not exceeding 8 hrs. Maint: 2g/day. Rheumatoid Arthritis: Initial: 0.5-1g/day. Maint: 2g/day given bid. Swallow tabs whole after meals.
Pediatrics: ≥6 yrs: Ulcerative Colitis: Initial: 40-60mg/kg/24 hrs in 3-6 divided doses. Maint: 7.5mg/kg qid. Juvenile Rheumatoid Arthritis: 30-50mg/kg/day given bid. To reduce GI effects give 1/4 to 1/3 initial dose; increase weekly for 1 month. Max: 2g/day. Swallow tabs whole after meals.

HOW SUPPLIED: Tab, Delayed-Release: 500mg

CONTRAINDICATIONS: Intestinal or urinary obstruction, porphyria, hypersensitivity to sulfonamides or salicylates.

WARNINGS/PRECAUTIONS: Caution with hepatic or renal impairment, blood dyscrasias, severe allergy, bronchial asthma or G6PD deficiency. Monitor CBC, WBC, and LFTs prior to therapy and every other week for the 1st 3 months, once monthly for next 3 months, then every 3 months. Monitor renal function periodically. Maintain adequate fluid intake. Fatal hypersensitivity reactions reported. D/C if tabs pass undisintegrated or if hypersensitivity reactions occur.

ADVERSE REACTIONS: Anorexia, headache, nausea, vomiting, gastric distress, oligospermia, rash, pruritus, urticaria, fever, orange-yellow urine or skin.

INTERACTIONS: Reduces absorption of folic acid and digoxin. Increased incidence of GI adverse events with combination of sulfasalazine (2g/day) and MTX (7.5mg/week).

PREGNANCY: Category B, caution in nursing.

MECHANISM OF ACTION: 5-aminosalicylic acid (5-ASA) derivative/sulfapyridine (SP); not established, may be related to the anti-inflammatory and/or immunodulatory properties of sulfasalazine (SSZ) or its metabolites (5-ASA and SP), its affinity for connective tissue, and/or to relatively high concentration reached in serous fluids, liver and intestinal wall.

PHARMACOKINETICS: Absorption: SSZ: C_{max}=6mcg/mL, T_{max}=6 hrs; 5-ASA. SP: T_{max}=10 hrs. SSZ: Absolute bioavailability <15%; SP: Well absorbed from colon, estimated bioavailability 60%. 5-ASA: Much less well absorbed from GI tract, estimated bioavailability 10-30%. **Distribution:** SSZ: V_d=7.5L; plasma protein binding >99.3%. SP: Plasma protein binding 70%. **Metabolism:** Intestinal bacteria to 5-ASA and SP; liver (acetylation). **Elimination:** Urine (37%), feces. SSZ: $T_{1/2}$=7.6 hrs, SP: $T_{1/2}$=10.4 hrs (slow acetylators), 14.8 hrs (fast acetylators).

BACITRACIN INJECTION   RX
bacitracin (Pharmacia & Upjohn)

> May cause renal failure due to tubular and glomerular necrosis. Monitor renal function prior to, and daily during therapy. Fluid intake and urinary output should be maintained at proper levels to avoid kidney toxicity. Discontinue if renal toxicity occurs. Avoid other nephrotoxic drugs.

THERAPEUTIC CLASS: Antibiotic

INDICATIONS: Treatment of pneumonia and empyema caused by staphylococci.

DOSAGE: Pediatrics: <2500g: 900U/kg/24h IM. >2500g: 1000U/kg/24h IM. Administer in 2-3 divided doses. Inject in upper outer quadrant of buttocks.

HOW SUPPLIED: Inj: 50,000U

WARNINGS/PRECAUTIONS: Use appropriate therapy if superinfection occurs.

ADVERSE REACTIONS: Albuminuria, cylindruria, azotemia, nausea, vomiting, pain at injection site, skin rashes, rising blood levels without increase in dosage.

INTERACTIONS: Avoid with other nephrotoxic drugs (eg, streptomycin, kanamycin, polymyxin B, polymyxin E, neomycin).

PREGNANCY: Safety in pregnancy or nursing not known.

MECHANISM OF ACTION: Exerts antibacterial action *in vitro* against variety of gram-positive and some gram-negative organisms.

PHARMACOKINETICS: Absorption: Rapid and complete. **Distribution:** Widely distributed in all body organs; found in ascitic and pleural fluid.

BACITRACIN/POLYMYXIN B OPHTHALMIC   RX
bacitracin zinc - polymyxin B sulfate (Various)

THERAPEUTIC CLASS: Antibacterial combination

INDICATIONS: Superficial ocular infections involving the conjunctiva and/or cornea caused by susceptible organisms.

DOSAGE: *Adults:* Apply q3-4h for 7-10 days, depending on severity.

HOW SUPPLIED: Oint: (Bacitracin-Polymyxin B) 500U-10,000U/g [3.5g]

WARNINGS/PRECAUTIONS: May retard corneal wound healing or cause cutaneous sensitization.

ADVERSE REACTIONS: Allergic reactions (eg, itching, swelling, conjunctival erythema), local irritation upon instillation, superinfection (prolonged use).

PREGNANCY: Category C, caution in nursing.

BACLOFEN   RX
baclofen (Various)

OTHER BRAND NAMES: Kemstro (Schwarz)

THERAPEUTIC CLASS: GABA analog

INDICATIONS: Treatment of spasticity associated with multiple sclerosis. May be effective in spinal cord injuries and other spinal cord diseases.

DOSAGE: *Adults:* Initial: 5mg tid for 3 days. Titrate: May increase dose by 5mg tid every 3 days. Usual: 40-80mg/day. Max: 80 mg/day (20mg qid). Renal Impairment: Reduce dose.
Pediatrics: ≥12 yrs: Initial: 5mg tid for 3 days. Titrate: May increase dose by 5mg tid every 3 days. Usual: 40-80mg/day. Max: 80 mg/day (20mg qid). Renal Impairment: Reduce dose.

HOW SUPPLIED: Tab: (Generic) 10mg, 20mg; Tab, Disintegrating (ODT): (Kemstro) 10mg, 20mg

WARNINGS/PRECAUTIONS: Caution with psychosis, schizophrenia, confusional states; may exacerbate conditions. Caution with bladder sphincter hypertonia, peptic ulceration, seizures, elderly, cerebrovascular disorder, respiratory failure, hepatic or renal failure. Abnormal AST, alkaline phosphatase and blood glucose reported. Caution when used to maintain locomotion or to obtain increased function. Decreased alertness with operating machinery. Has not significantly benefited stroke patients. Avoid abrupt discontinuation; reduce dose slowly over 1-2 weeks.

ADVERSE REACTIONS: Drowsiness, dizziness, weakness, fatigue, confusion, daytime sedation, headache, insomnia, hypotension, nausea, constipation, urinary frequency.

INTERACTIONS: May potentiate antihypertensives. May increase CNS depressant effects with MAO inhibitors. Potentiated by TCAs. Mental confusion, hallucinations and agitation with levodopa plus carbidopa therapy. May increase blood glucose and require dosage adjustment of antidiabetic agents. Synergistic effects with magnesium sulfate and other neuromuscular blockers. Additive CNS effects with alcohol and other CNS depressants.

PREGNANCY: Category C, caution in nursing.

MECHANISM OF ACTION: A GABA analog; muscle relaxant/antispastic agent; not fully known; capable of inhibiting both monosynaptic and polysynaptic reflexes at the spinal level, possibly by hyperpolarization of afferent terminals, although actions at supraspinal sites may also occur and contribute to its clinical effect.

BACTRIM   RX
sulfamethoxazole - trimethoprim (AR Scientific)

OTHER BRAND NAMES: Bactrim DS (AR Scientific)

THERAPEUTIC CLASS: Sulfonamide/tetrahydrofolic acid inhibitor

INDICATIONS: Treatment of urinary tract infection (UTI), acute otitis media, acute exacerbation of chronic bronchitis (AECB), traveler's diarrhea, shigellosis, and *Pneumocystis carinii* pneumonia (PCP).

DOSAGE: *Adults:* UTI: 800mg SMX-160mg TMP or 2 tabs of 400mg SMX-80mg TMP q12h for 10-14 days. Shigellosis: 800mg SMX-160mg TMP or 2 tabs of 400mg SMX-80mg TMP q12h for 5 days. AECB: 800mg SMX-160mg TMP or 2 tabs of 400mg SMX-80mg TMP q12h for 14 days. PCP Treatment: 15-20mg/kg TMP and 75-100mg/kg SMX per 24 hrs given q6h for 14-21 days.

PCP Prophylaxis: 800mg SMX-160mg TMP qd. Traveler's Diarrhea: 800mg SMX-160mg TMP q12h for 5 days. CrCl: 15-30mL/min: 50% usual dose. CrCl: <15mL/min: Not recommended.

Pediatrics: ≥2 months: UTI/Otitis Media: 4mg/kg TMP and 20mg/kg SMX q12h for 10 days. Shigellosis: 8mg/kg TMP and 40mg/kg SMX per 24 hrs given q12h for 5 days. PCP Treatment: 15-20mg/kg TMP and 75-100mg/kg SMX per 24 hrs given q6h for 14-21 days. PCP Prophylaxis: 150mg/m²/day TMP with 750mg/m²/day SMX given bid, on 3 consecutive days/week. Max: 320mg TMP/1600mg SMX/day. CrCl: 15-30mL/min: 50% usual dose. CrCl: <15mL/min: Not recommended.

HOW SUPPLIED: (Sulfamethoxazole [SMX]-Trimethoprim [TMP]) Tab: 400mg-80mg*; Tab, DS: 800mg-160mg* *scored

CONTRAINDICATIONS: Megaloblastic anemia due to folate deficiency, pregnancy, nursing, infants <2 months, marked hepatic damage, severe renal insufficiency if cannot monitor renal status.

WARNINGS/PRECAUTIONS: Fatal hypersensitivity reactions (eg, Stevens-Johnson syndrome, toxic epidermal necrolysis, fulminant hepatic necrosis, agranulocytosis, aplastic anemia) may occur. Pseudomembranous colitis, cough, SOB, and pulmonary infiltrates reported. Avoid with group A β-hemolytic streptococcal infections. Caution with hepatic/renal impairment, elderly, folate deficiency (eg, chronic alcoholics, anticonvulsants, malabsorption, malnutrition), bronchial asthma, and other allergies. In G6PD deficiency, hemolysis may occur. Increased incidence of adverse events with AIDS. Ensure adequate fluid intake and urinary output. Caution with porphyria, thyroid dysfunction.

ADVERSE REACTIONS: Nausea, vomiting, anorexia, rash, urticaria.

INTERACTIONS: Diuretics (especially thiazides) may increase risk of thrombocytopenia with purpura in elderly patients. Caution with warfarin, may prolong PT. Increased effects of phenytoin, oral hypoglycemics. Increased plasma levels of methotrexate, digoxin (especially in elderly). Marked but reversible nephrotoxicity reported with cyclosporine. May develop megaloblastic anemia with pyrimethamine >25mg/week. Increased levels with indomethacin. May decrease effects of TCAs. Single case of toxic delirium with amantadine.

PREGNANCY: Category C, contraindicated in nursing.

MECHANISM OF ACTION: Sulfamethoxazole: Inhibits bacterial synthesis of dyhydrofolic acid by competing with PABA. Trimethoprim: Blocks the production of tetrahydrofolic acid from dihydrofolic acid by binding to and reversibly inhibiting the required enzyme, dihydrofolate reductase.

PHARMACOKINETICS: Absorption: Rapid; T_{max}=1-4 hrs; Sulfamethoxazole: C_{max}=57.4mcg/mL (free), 68.0mcg/mL (total); Trimethoprim: C_{max}=1.72mcg/mL. **Distribution:** Sulfamethoxazole: Plasma protein binding (70%); Trimethoprim: Plasme protein binding (44%). Both pass placental barrier and excreted in breast milk. **Metabolism:** Sulfamethoxazole: N_4-acetylation; Trimethoprim: 1- and 3-oxides, 3'-4'-hydroxy derivatives (principal metabolites). **Elimination:** Sulfamethoxazole: $T_{1/2}$=0.72 hrs. Urine: Total sulfonamide (84.5%), 30% (free), and the remaining (N_4-acetylated metabolite); 66.8% (trimethoprim); $T_{1/2}$=10 hrs (sulfamethoxazole), 8-10 hrs (trimethoprim).

BACTROBAN   RX
mupirocin (GlaxoSmithKline)

THERAPEUTIC CLASS: Bacterial protein synthesis inhibitor

INDICATIONS: (Oint) Topical treatment of impetigo due to *S.aureus* and *S.pyogenes*. (Cre) Treatment of secondarily infected traumatic skin lesions (up to 10cm in length or 100cm²) due to *S.aureus* and *S.pyogenes*.

DOSAGE: *Adults:* (Oint) Apply tid. (Cre) Apply tid for 10 days. May cover with gauze. Re-evaluate if no response within 3-5 days.
Pediatrics: (Oint) 2 months -16 yrs: Apply tid. (Cre) 3 months-16 yrs: Apply tid for 10 days. May cover with gauze. Re-evaluate if no response within 3-5 days.

HOW SUPPLIED: Cre: 2% [15g, 30g]; Oint: 2% [22g]

WARNINGS/PRECAUTIONS: Avoid eyes. D/C if sensitization or irritation occurs. May cause superinfection with prolonged use. Caution with oint in renal dysfunction. Avoid mucosal surfaces. Avoid open wounds or damaged skin with oint.

ADVERSE REACTIONS: Burning, pain, pruritus, headache, rash, nausea.

PREGNANCY: Category B, caution in nursing.

MECHANISM OF ACTION: Bacterial protein synthesis inhibitor; inhibits bacterial protein synthesis by reversibly and specifically binding to bacterial isoleucyl transfer-RNA synthetase. Active against a wide range of gram-positive bacteria including methicillin-resistant *Staphylococcus aureus* (MRSA). Also active against certain gram-negative bacteria.

PHARMACOKINETICS: Absorption: Minimal percutaneous absorption. **Metabolism:** Rapid. Monic acid (inactive metabolite). **Elimination:** Renal (metabolite).

BACTROBAN NASAL   RX
mupirocin calcium (GlaxoSmithKline)

THERAPEUTIC CLASS: Antibacterial agent

INDICATIONS: Eradication of nasal colonization of MRSA in adults and healthcare workers in certain institutional settings during outbreaks of MRSA.

DOSAGE: *Adults:* Apply 1/2 of the single-use tube into each nostril bid for 5 days. Spread oint by pressing together and releasing the sides of the nose repetitively for 1 min. Do not re-use tube.
Pediatrics: ≥12 yrs: Apply 1/2 of the single-use tube into each nostril bid for 5 days. Spread oint by pressing together and releasing the sides of the nose repetitively for 1 min. Do not re-use tube.

HOW SUPPLIED: Oint: 2% [1g pkt]

WARNINGS/PRECAUTIONS: Avoid eyes. D/C if sensitization or irritation occurs. May cause superinfection with prolonged use.

ADVERSE REACTIONS: Headache, rhinitis, respiratory disorder, pharyngitis, taste perversion.

INTERACTIONS: Avoid use with other intranasal products.

PREGNANCY: Category B, caution in nursing.

MECHANISM OF ACTION: Antibacterial agent; inhibits protein synthesis by reversibly and specifically binding to bacterial isoleucyl transfer-RNA synthetase.

PHARMACOKINETICS: Absorption: Significant in neonates and premature infants. **Elimination:** Urine.

BARACLUDE   RX
entecavir (Bristol-Myers Squibb)

> Lactic acidosis and severe, possibly fatal, hepatomegaly with steatosis reported. Reports of severe acute exacerbations of hepatitis B upon discontinuation of therapy. Follow-up liver function monitoring required. Limited clinical experience suggests there is a potential for the development of resistance to HIV nucleoside reverse transcriptase inhibitors if Baraclude is used to treat chronic hepatitis B virus infection in patients with HIV infection that is not being treated. Not recommended for HIV/HBV coinfected patients who are not receiving highly active antiretroviral therapy (HAART).

THERAPEUTIC CLASS: Guanosine nucleoside analogue

INDICATIONS: Treatment of chronic hepatitis B virus (HBV) infection with active viral replication and persistent elevations in serum aminotransferases (ALT or AST) or histologically active disease.

DOSAGE: *Adults:* Nucleoside-Treatment-Naive: 0.5mg qd. CrCl 30 to <50mL/min: 0.25mg qd or 0.5mg q48h. CrCl 10 to <30mL/min: 0.15mg qd or 0.5mg q72h. CrCl <10mL/min: 0.05mg qd or 0.5mg q7 days. Receiving Lamivudine

or Known Lamivudine Resistance Mutation: 1mg qd. CrCl 30 to <50mL/min: 0.5mg qd or 1mg q48h. CrCl 10 to <30mL/min: 0.3mg qd or 1mg q72h. CrCl <10mL/min: 0.1mg qd or 1mg q7 days. Take on empty stomach.
Pediatrics: ≥16 yrs: Nucleoside-Treatment-Naive:0.5mg qd. CrCl 30 to <50mL/min: 0.25mg qd or 0.5mg q48h. CrCl 10 to <30mL/min: 0.15mg qd or 0.5mg q72h. CrCl <10mL/min: 0.05mg qd or 0.5mg q7 days. Receiving Lamivudine or Known Lamivudine Resistance Mutation: 1mg qd. CrCl 30 to <50mL/min: 0.5mg qd or 1mg q48h. CrCl 10 to <30mL/min: 0.3mg qd or 1mg q72h. CrCl <10mL/min: 0.1mg qd or 1mg q7 days. Take on empty stomach.

HOW SUPPLIED: Sol: 0.05mg/mL; Tab: 0.5mg, 1mg

WARNINGS/PRECAUTIONS: See BlackBox Warning. Reduce dose in renal dysfunction (CrCl <50mL/min) including patients on hemodialysis or CAPD (continuous ambulatory peritoneal dialysis). Exacerbations of hepatitis after discontinuation of treatment.

ADVERSE REACTIONS: Headache, fatigue, dizziness, nausea, hyperglycemia, lipase ≥2.1 X ULN, glycosuria, hematuria and increase in total bilirubin.

INTERACTIONS: May increase serum concentrations of entecavir or coad-ministered drug with drugs that reduce renal function or compete for active tubular secretion.

PREGNANCY: Category C, not for use in nursing.

MECHANISM OF ACTION: Guanosine nucleoside analogue; inhibits base priming, reverse transcription of negative strand from pregenomic mRNA, and synthesis of positive strand of HBV DNA.

PHARMACOKINETICS: Absorption: (0.5mg) C_{max}=4.2ng/mL; T_{max}=0.5-1.5 hrs. (1.0mg) C_{max}=8.2ng/mL. Bioavailability (100%). **Distribution:** Plasma protein binding (13%). **Metabolism:** Hepatic. **Elimination:** Kidneys; urine (62-73%); $T_{1/2}$=128-149 hrs.

BAYER ASPIRIN   OTC
aspirin (Bayer Healthcare)

OTHER BRAND NAMES: Bayer Aspirin Children's (Bayer Healthcare) - Bayer Aspirin Regimen with Calcium (Bayer Healthcare) - Bayer Aspirin Regimen (Bayer Healthcare) - Genuine Bayer Aspirin (Bayer Healthcare)

THERAPEUTIC CLASS: Salicylate

INDICATIONS: To reduce the risk of death and nonfatal stroke with previous ischemic stroke or transient ischemia of the brain. To reduce risk of vascular mortality with suspected acute MI. To reduce risk of death and nonfatal MI with previous MI or unstable angina. To reduce risk of MI and sudden death in chronic stable angina pectoris. For patients who have undergone revascular-ization procedures with a pre-existing condition for which ASA is indicated. Relief of signs of rheumatoid arthritis (RA), juvenile rheumatoid arthritis (JRA), osteoarthritis (OA), spondyloarthropathies, arthritis, and pleurisy asso-ciated with systemic lupus erythematosus (SLE). For minor aches and pains.

DOSAGE: *Adults:* Ischemic Stroke/TIA: 50-325mg qd. Suspected Acute MI: Initial: 160-162.5mg qd as soon as suspect MI. Maint: 160-162.5mg qd for 30 days post-infarction, consider further therapy for prevention/recurrent MI. Prevention or Recurrent MI/Unstable Angina/Chronic Stable Angina: 75-325mg qd. CABG: 325mg qd, start 6 hrs post-surgery. Continue for 1 yr. PTCA: Initial: 325mg, 2 hrs pre-surgery. Maint: 160-325mg qd. Carotid Endarterectomy: 80mg qd to 650mg bid, start pre-surgery. RA: Initial: 3g qd in divided doses. Increase for anti-inflammatory efficacy to 150-300mcg/mL plasma salicylate level. Spondyloarthropathies: Up to 4g/day in divided doses. OA: Up to 3g/day in divided doses. Arthritis/SLE Pleurisy: Initial: 3g/day in divided doses. Increase for anti-inflammatory efficacy to 150-300mcg/mL plasma salicylate level. Pain: 325-650mg q4-6h. Max: 4g/day.
Pediatrics: JRA: Initial: 90-130mg/kg/day in divided doses. Increase for anti-inflammatory efficacy to 150-300mcg/mL plasma salicylate level. Pain: ≥12 yrs: 325-650mg q4-6h. Max: 4g/day.

HOW SUPPLIED: Tab: (Genuine Bayer Aspirin) 325mg; Tab: (Bayer Aspirin Regimen with Calcium) 81mg; Tab, Chewable: (Bayer Aspirin Children's) 81mg; Tab, Delayed-Release: (Bayer Aspirin Regimen) 81mg, 325mg

CONTRAINDICATIONS: NSAID allergy, viral infections in children or teenagers, syndrome of asthma, rhinitis, and nasal polyps.

WARNINGS/PRECAUTIONS: Increased risk of bleeding with heavy alcohol use (≥3 drinks/day). May inhibit platelet function; can adversely affect inherited (hemophilia) or acquired (hepatic disease, vitamin K deficiency) bleeding disorders. Monitor for bleeding and ulceration. Avoid in history of active peptic ulcer, severe renal failure, severe hepatic insufficiency, and sodium restricted diets. Associated with elevated LFTs, BUN, and serum creatinine; hyperkalemia; proteinuria; and prolonged bleeding time. Avoid 1 week before and during labor.

ADVERSE REACTIONS: Fever, hypothermia, dysrhythmias, hypotension, agitation, cerebral edema, dehydration, hyperkalemia, dyspepsia, GI bleed, hearing loss, tinnitus, problems in pregnancy.

INTERACTIONS: Diminished hypotensive and hyponatremic effects of ACE inhibitors. May increase levels of acetazolamide, valproic acid. Increased bleeding risk with heparin, warfarin. Decreased levels of phenytoin. Decreased hypotensive effects of β-blockers. Decreased diuretic effects with renal or cardiovascular disease. Decreased methotrexate clearance; increased risk of bone marrow toxicity. Avoid NSAIDs. Increased effects of hypoglycemic agents. Antagonizes uricosuric agents.

PREGNANCY: Avoid in 3rd trimester of pregnancy and nursing.

MECHANISM OF ACTION: Provides temporary relief from arthritis pain and arthritis inflammation.

BAYER ASPIRIN EXTRA STRENGTH   OTC
aspirin (Bayer Healthcare)

THERAPEUTIC CLASS: Salicylate

INDICATIONS: Temporary relief of headache, pain and fever of colds, muscle aches and pains, menstrual pain, toothache pain, minor aches and arthritis pain.

DOSAGE: *Adults:* 500-1000mg q4-6h prn. Max: 4g/24hrs.
Pediatrics: ≥12 yrs: 500-1000mg q4-6h prn. Max: 4g/24hrs.

HOW SUPPLIED: Tab: 500mg

WARNINGS/PRECAUTIONS: Avoid in children or teenagers for chickenpox or flu symptoms; Reye's syndrome may occur. Do not take >10 days for pain or >3 days for fever. Avoid in asthma, stomach problems that persist or recur, gastric ulcers, or bleeding problems. Stop therapy if ringing in the ears or loss of hearing occurs.

INTERACTIONS: Avoid with drugs for anticoagulation, diabetes, gout, or arthritis. Increased risk of stomach bleeding with alcohol use (≥3 drinks/day).

PREGNANCY: Avoid in 3rd trimester of pregnancy; safety in nursing not known.

BECONASE AQ   RX
beclomethasone dipropionate (GlaxoSmithKline)

THERAPEUTIC CLASS: Corticosteroid

INDICATIONS: Relief of symptoms of seasonal or perennial allergic and nonallergic rhinitis. Prevention of nasal polyp recurrence following surgical removal.

DOSAGE: *Adults:* 1-2 sprays per nostril bid. Max: 2 sprays per nostril bid.
Pediatrics: ≥6 yrs: 1-2 sprays per nostril bid. Max: 2 sprays per nostril bid.

HOW SUPPLIED: Spray: 42mcg/spray [25g]

WARNINGS/PRECAUTIONS: Risk of adrenal insufficiency and withdrawal symptoms when replacing systemic corticosteroids with topical corticosteroids. Caution with active or quiescent TB, ocular herpes simplex, or untreated bacterial, fungal and systemic viral infections. Avoid with recent nasal trauma/surgery or septum ulcers. Risk for more severe/fatal course of infections (eg, chickenpox, measles) and for *Candida* infection of the nose and pharynx. Potential for growth velocity reduction in pediatrics.

ADVERSE REACTIONS: Nasopharyngeal irritation, sneezing, headache, nausea, lightheadedness, irritated/dry nose and throat, unpleasant taste/smell.

INTERACTIONS: Concomitant systemic corticosteroids increase risk of hypercorticism and/or HPA axis suppression.

PREGNANCY: Category C, caution in nursing.

MECHANISM OF ACTION: Corticosteroid; not established; anti-inflammatory and vasoconstrictor effects.

PHARMACOKINETICS: Absorption: Absolute bioavailability (44%) (for the active metabolite B-17-MP). $C_{max} \leq 50pg/mL$. **Distribution:** $V_d=20L$ (parent drug); $V_d=424L$ (B-17-MP). Plasma protein binding (87%). **Metabolism:** B-17-MP (active metabolite) via esterase enzymes.

BENADRYL ALLERGY   OTC
diphenhydramine HCL (McNeil)

THERAPEUTIC CLASS: Antihistamine

INDICATIONS: Relief of hay fever or upper respiratory allergies, and rhinorrhea/sneezing due to the common cold.

DOSAGE: *Adults:* 25-50mg q4-6h. Max: 300mg/24hrs.
Pediatrics: ≥12 yrs: 25-50mg q4-6h. Max: 300mg/24 hrs. 6-11 yrs: 12.5-25mg q4-6h. Max: 150mg/24hrs.

HOW SUPPLIED: Cap: 25mg; Sol: 12.5mg/5mL; Tab: 25mg; Tab, Chewable: 12.5mg

WARNINGS/PRECAUTIONS: Caution with emphysema, chronic bronchitis, glaucoma, or difficulty in urination due to prostate gland enlargement. May impair mental/physical abilities.

ADVERSE REACTIONS: Drowsiness, excitability (especially in children).

INTERACTIONS: Increased drowsiness with alcohol, sedatives, tranquilizers.

PREGNANCY: Safety in pregnancy and nursing not known.

BENICAR   RX
olmesartan medoxomil (Daiichi Sankyo)

> Can cause death/injury to developing fetus during 2nd and 3rd trimesters. Stop therapy if pregnancy detected.

THERAPEUTIC CLASS: Angiotensin II receptor antagonist

INDICATIONS: Hypertension, alone or with other antihypertensives.

DOSAGE: *Adults:* Monotherapy Without Volume Depletion: Initial: 20mg qd. Titrate: May increase to 40mg qd after 2 weeks if needed. May add diuretic if BP not controlled. Intravascular Volume Depletion (eg, with diuretics, impaired renal function): Lower initial dose; monitor closely.

HOW SUPPLIED: Tab: 5mg, 20mg, 40mg

WARNINGS/PRECAUTIONS: Can cause fetal injury/death. Symptomatic hypotension may occur in volume- and/or salt-depleted patients; monitor closely. Changes in renal function may occur; caution with severe CHF. Increases in serum creatinine or BUN reported with renal artery stenosis.

ADVERSE REACTIONS: Dizziness, transient hypotension, hyperkalemia.

INTERACTIONS: Risk of hypotension with high-dose diuretics.

PREGNANCY: Category C (1st trimester) and D (2nd and 3rd trimesters), not for use in nursing.

MECHANISM OF ACTION: Angiotensin II receptor antagonist; blocks vasoconstrictor effects of angiotensin II by selectively blocking binding of angiotensin II to AT_1 receptor in vascular smooth muscle.

PHARMACOKINETICS: Absorption: Rapid, complete. Absolute bioavailability (26%); T_{max}=1-2 hrs. **Distribution:** V_d=17L; Plasma protein binding (99%). Crosses placenta, excreted in breast milk. **Metabolism:** Ester hydrolysis. **Elimination:** $T_{1/2}$=13 hrs; urine (35-50%), feces.

BENICAR HCT
olmesartan medoxomil - hydrochlorothiazide (Daiichi Sankyo)

RX

> Can cause death/injury to developing fetus during 2nd and 3rd trimesters. Stop therapy if pregnancy detected.

THERAPEUTIC CLASS: Angiotensin II receptor antagonist/thiazide diuretic

INDICATIONS: Hypertension. Not for initial therapy.

DOSAGE: *Adults:* If BP not controlled with olmesartan alone: Add HCTZ 12.5mg qd. May titrate to 25mg qd if BP uncontrolled after 2-4 weeks. If BP not controlled with HCTZ alone: Add olmesartan 20mg qd. May titrate to 40mg qd if BP uncontrolled after 2-4 weeks. Intravascular Volume Depletion (eg, with diuretics, impaired renal function): Lower initial dose; monitor closely. Elderly: Start at lower end of dosing range.

HOW SUPPLIED: Tab: (Olmesartan-HCTZ) 20mg-12.5mg, 40mg-12.5mg, 40mg-25mg

CONTRAINDICATIONS: Sulfonamide hypersensitivity.

WARNINGS/PRECAUTIONS: Can cause fetal injury/death. Correct volume or salt depletion before therapy or monitor closely. Caution with hepatic or severe renal dysfunction, progressive liver disease, history of allergies or asthma, renal artery stenosis, severe CHF. Avoid if CrCl ≤30mL/min. May exacerbate or activate SLE. Monitor serum electrolytes. Hyperuricemia, hyperglycemia, hypercalcemia, hypomagnesemia may occur. May increase cholesterol and triglyceride levels.

ADVERSE REACTIONS: Dizziness, upper respiratory tract infection, hyperuricemia, nausea, asthenia, angioedema, vomiting, hyperkalemia, rhabdomyolysis, ARF, alopecia, urticaria.

INTERACTIONS: Potentiates orthostatic hypotension with alcohol, barbiturates, or narcotics. May need to adjust antidiabetics. Potentiates other antihypertensives. Impaired absorption with cholestyramine, colestipol. Corticosteroids, ACTH deplete electrolytes. May decrease response to pressor amines. May potentiate non-depolarizing skeletal muscle relaxants. Risk of lithium toxicity. NSAIDs decrease diuretic effects.

PREGNANCY: Category C (1st trimester) and D (2nd and 3rd trimesters), not for use in nursing.

MECHANISM OF ACTION: Olmesartan: Angiotensin II receptor antagonist; blocks vasoconstrictor effects of angiotensin II by selectively blocking binding of angiotensin II to AT_1 receptor in vascular smooth muscle. HCTZ: Thiazide diuretic; affects renal tubular mechanism of electrolyte reabsorption, directly increasing excretion of sodium and chloride and indirectly reducing plasma volume.

PHARMACOKINETICS: Absorption: Olmesartan: Rapid, complete. Absolute bioavailability (26%); T_{max}=1-2 hrs. **Distribution:** Olmesartan: V_d=17 L; plasma protein binding (99%). Crosses placenta and excreted in breast milk. HCTZ: Crosses placenta and excreted in breast milk. **Metabolism:** Olmesartan: Ester hydrolysis. **Elimination:** Olmesartan: Urine (35-50%), feces; $T_{1/2}$=13 hrs. HCTZ: Kidney (61%); $T_{1/2}$=5.6-14.8 hrs.

B

BENTYL

RX

dicyclomine HCL (Axcan Scandipharm)

THERAPEUTIC CLASS: Anticholinergic

INDICATIONS: Treatment of functional bowel/irritable bowel syndrome.

DOSAGE: *Adults:* (Tab/Syrup) Initial: 20mg qid. Usual: 40mg qid if tolerated. Discontinue if no improvement after 2 weeks or if doses ≥80mg/day are not tolerated. (Inj) 20mg IM qid for 1-2 days, followed by oral dicyclomine. Not for IV use.

HOW SUPPLIED: Cap: 10mg; Inj: 10mg/mL; Syrup: 10mg/5mL; Tab: 20mg

CONTRAINDICATIONS: GI tract obstruction, obstructive uropathy, severe ulcerative colitis, reflux esophagitis, myasthenia gravis, unstable cardiovascular status and in acute hemorrhage, nursing mothers, infants <6 months of age.

WARNINGS/PRECAUTIONS: Caution in autonomic neuropathy, hepatic/renal impairment, ulcerative colitis, hyperthyroidism, HTN, CHF, cardiac tachyarrhythmia, coronary heart disease, hiatal hernia, and prostatic hypertrophy. Heat prostration may occur in high environmental temperature. Monitor for diarrhea, may be the early symptom of intestinal obstruction. Psychosis reported. Serious respiratory symptoms, seizures, syncope and death reported in infants.

ADVERSE REACTIONS: Dry mouth, nausea, vomiting, blurred vision, dizziness, drowsiness, nervousness, mental confusion/excitement (especially in the elderly), mydriasis, increased ocular tension, urinary retention, dyspnea, apnea, tachycardia, decreased sweating, lactation suppression, impotence.

INTERACTIONS: Potentiated by amantadine, Class I antiarrhythmics (eg, quinidine), antihistamines, antipsychotics (eg, phenothiazines), benzodiazepines, MAOIs, narcotic analgesics (eg, meperidine), nitrates/nitrites, sympathomimetics, TCAs. Antagonizes the effects of antiglaucoma agents; do not give with corticosteroid eye drops. Antagonizes the effect of metoclopramide. May effect the GI absorption of delayed release digoxin. Decreased absorption with antacids. Antagonized by drugs treating achlorhydria and those used to test gastric secretion.

PREGNANCY: Category B, contraindicated in nursing.

MECHANISM OF ACTION: Dicyclomine anticholinergic and antispasmodic agent; relieves smooth muscle spasm of the GI tract, and antagonizes bradykinin- and histamine-induced spasms.

PHARMACOKINETICS: Absorption: Rapidly absorbed. T_{max}=60-90 mins. **Distribution:** V_d=approx.3.65L/Kg (extensive). Excreted in breast milk **Elimination:** Urine (79.5%), feces (8.4%). $T_{1/2}$=1.8 hrs.

BENZAC AC

RX

benzoyl peroxide (Galderma)

THERAPEUTIC CLASS: Antibacterial/keratolytic

INDICATIONS: Topical treatment of acne vulgaris.

DOSAGE: *Adults:* (Sol) Wash area qd-bid. Rinse and dry area. (Gel) Apply qd-bid to clean affected area.

HOW SUPPLIED: Gel: 5%, 10% [60g]; Sol (Wash): 5%, 10% [240mL]

WARNINGS/PRECAUTIONS: External use only. Avoid contact with eyes, lips, mucous membranes. D/C if severe irritation occurs.

ADVERSE REACTIONS: Allergic contact dermatitis, dryness.

PREGNANCY: Category C, caution in nursing.

BENZACLIN
clindamycin - benzoyl peroxide (Dermik)

RX

THERAPEUTIC CLASS: Antibacterial/keratolytic

INDICATIONS: Topical treatment of acne vulgaris.

DOSAGE: *Adults:* Wash face and pat dry. Apply bid (am and pm).
Pediatrics: ≥12 yrs: Wash face and pat dry. Apply bid (am and pm).

HOW SUPPLIED: Gel: (Clindamycin-Benzoyl Peroxide) 1%-5% [25g, 50g]

CONTRAINDICATIONS: Hypersensitivity to lincomycin. History of regional enteritis, ulcerative colitis, and antibiotic-associated colitis.

WARNINGS/PRECAUTIONS: Severe colitis reported with oral and parenteral clindamycin. D/C if severe diarrhea occurs. Avoid contact with eyes and mucous membranes.

ADVERSE REACTIONS: Dry skin, pruritus, peeling, erythema, sunburn.

INTERACTIONS: Cumulative irritancy possible with other topical acne agents. Avoid erythromycin agents.

PREGNANCY: Category C, not for use in nursing.

MECHANISM OF ACTION: Antibacterial/keratolytic; acts against *Propionibacterium acnes*.

PHARMACOKINETICS: Absorption: Benzoyl peroxide: Systemic bioavailability (<2%). Clindamycin: Systemic bioavailability (≤1%).

BENZAGEL
benzoyl peroxide (Dermik)

RX

THERAPEUTIC CLASS: Antibacterial/keratolytic

INDICATIONS: Treatment of mild to moderate acne, used alone or as an adjunct.

DOSAGE: *Adults:* Apply qd or more often to clean affected area. Very fair patients should start with single application qhs.
Pediatrics: ≥12 yrs: Apply qd or more often to clean affected area. Very fair patients should start with single application qhs.

HOW SUPPLIED: Gel: 5%, 10% [42.5g]

WARNINGS/PRECAUTIONS: D/C if itching, redness, burning, swelling, or undue dryness occurs. Avoid contact with eyes and mucous membranes. May bleach colored fabrics or hair.

ADVERSE REACTIONS: Irritation, contact dermatitis.

PREGNANCY: Category C, caution in nursing.

MECHANISM OF ACTION: Antibacterial/keratolytic agent. Effective against *Propionibacterium acnes*.

BENZAMYCIN
erythromycin - benzoyl peroxide (Dermik)

RX

THERAPEUTIC CLASS: Antibacterial/keratolytic

INDICATIONS: Topical treatment of acne vulgaris.

DOSAGE: *Adults:* Wash skin and dry. Apply bid (am and pm).
Pediatrics: ≥12 yrs: Wash skin and dry. Apply bid (am and pm).

HOW SUPPLIED: Gel: (Benzoyl Peroxide-Erythromycin) 5%-3% [0.8g/pkt, 60ᵍ]

WARNINGS/PRECAUTIONS: D/C if severe irritation occurs. Avoid eyes, mouth, and mucous membranes. Keep refrigerated after reconstitution and discard after 3 months.

ADVERSE REACTIONS: Dryness, urticaria, skin irritation, skin discoloration, oiliness, tenderness.

INTERACTIONS: Additive irritation with peeling, desquamating, or abrasive agents.

PREGNANCY: Category C, caution in nursing.

MECHANISM OF ACTION: Antibacterial/keratolytic agent; mechanism not fully known. Erythromycin: Antibacterial agent; inhibits protein synthesis by reversibly binding to 50S ribosomal subunits, thereby inhibiting transloca-tion of aminoacyl transfer-RNA and inhibiting polypeptide synthesis. Benzoyl peroxide: Believed to act by releasing active oxygen.

PHARMACOKINETICS: Absorption: Benzoyl peroxide shown to be absorbed by skin, where it is converted to benzoic acid. **Distribution:** Orally and paren-terally administered erythromycin found in breast milk.

BENZTROPINE   RX
benztropine mesylate (Various)

OTHER BRAND NAMES: Cogentin (Merck)

THERAPEUTIC CLASS: Anticholinergic

INDICATIONS: Adjunct in all forms of parkinsonism. Control of drug-induced extrapyramidal disorders.

DOSAGE: *Adults:* Parkinsonism: Initial: 0.5-1mg PO/IV/IM qhs. Titrate: May increase every 5-6 days by 0.5mg. Usual: 1-2mg PO/IV/IM qhs. Max: 6mg/day. Extrapyramidal Disorders: 1-4mg PO/IV/IM qd-bid. Acute Dystonic Reactions: 1-2mg IM/IV, then 1-2mg PO bid.

HOW SUPPLIED: Inj: 1mg/mL; Tab: 0.5mg, 1mg, 2mg

CONTRAINDICATIONS: Patients <3 yrs.

WARNINGS/PRECAUTIONS: May produce anhidrosis, caution in hot weather. Muscle weakness and dysuria may occur. Caution in pediatrics >3 years of age. Not recommended for tardive dyskinesia. Avoid with angle-closure glaucoma. Caution with CNS disease, mental disorders, tachycardia, prostatic hypertro-phy, alcoholics, chronically ill, those exposed to hot environments.

ADVERSE REACTIONS: Tachycardia, paralytic ileus, constipation, vomiting, nausea, dry mouth, confusion, blurred vision, urinary retention, heat stroke, hyperthermia, fever.

INTERACTIONS: Paralytic ileus, hyperthermia and heat stroke reported with phenothiazines and TCAs. Caution with other atropine-like agents.

PREGNANCY: Safety in pregnancy and nursing not known.

MECHANISM OF ACTION: Anticholinergic agent; controls extrapyramidal symptoms in parkinsonism.

BETAGAN   RX
levobunolol HCL (Allergan)

THERAPEUTIC CLASS: Nonselective beta-blocker

INDICATIONS: Treatment of elevated IOP in chronic open-angle glaucoma and ocular hypertension.

DOSAGE: *Adults:* (0.5%) 1-2 drops qd; bid for more severe or uncontrolled glaucoma. (0.25%): 1-2 drops bid.

HOW SUPPLIED: Sol: 0.25% [5mL, 10mL], 0.5% [2mL, 5mL, 10mL, 15mL]

CONTRAINDICATIONS: Bronchial asthma, COPD, overt cardiac failure, sinus bradycardia, 2nd- and 3rd-degree AV block, cardiogenic shock.

WARNINGS/PRECAUTIONS: Caution with cardiac failure, DM, COPD, cere-bral insufficiency, pulmonary disease, bronchospastic disease, surgery and hepatic impairment. May mask symptoms of hypoglycemia and thyrotoxicosis. Contains sodium metabisulfite. Follow with a miotic in angle-closure glau-coma. Potentiates muscle weakness (eg, diplopia, ptosis).

ADVERSE REACTIONS: Ocular burning, ocular stinging, decreased heart rate, decreased blood pressure.

INTERACTIONS: Mydriasis with epinephrine. Additive effects with catecholamine-depleting drugs (eg, reserpine) and systemic β-blockers. AV conduction disturbance with calcium antagonists and digitalis. Left ventricular failure and hypotension with calcium antagonists also. Additive hypotensive effects with phenothiazine-related drugs. Risk of hypoglycemia with insulin and oral hypoglycemic agents.

PREGNANCY: Category C, caution in nursing.

MECHANISM OF ACTION: Noncardioselective β-adrenoceptor blocking agent. Equipotent at both β_1 and β_2 receptors. Responsible for reducing cardiac output, increasing airway resistance, and lowering elevated as well as normal intraocular pressure. Presumed to lower IOP through decreasing production of aqueous humor.

PHARMACOKINETICS: Absorption: T_{max}=2 and 6 hrs.

BETAMETHASONE DIPROPIONATE   RX
betamethasone dipropionate (Various)

THERAPEUTIC CLASS: Corticosteroid

INDICATIONS: Corticosteroid-responsive dermatoses.

DOSAGE: *Adults:* (Cre, Oint) Apply qd-bid. (Lot) Apply a few drops bid, am and pm.
Pediatrics: (Cre, Oint) Apply qd-bid. (Lot) Apply a few drops bid, am and pm.

HOW SUPPLIED: Cre, Oint: 0.05% [15g, 45g]; Lot: 0.05% [60mL]

WARNINGS/PRECAUTIONS: May produce reversible HPA axis suppression, manifestations of Cushing's syndrome, hyperglycemia, and glucosuria. Avoid occlusive dressings. Pediatrics are more prone to systemic toxicity. D/C if irritation occurs. Avoid eyes.

ADVERSE REACTIONS: Burning, itching, irritation, dryness, folliculitis, hypertrichosis, acneiform eruptions, hypopigmentation, perioral dermatitis, allergic contact dermatitis, skin maceration, secondary infection, skin atrophy, striae, miliaria.

PREGNANCY: Category C, caution in nursing.

MECHANISM OF ACTION: Corticosteroid: Not established. Possesses anti-inflammatory, anti-pruritic, and vasoconstrictive actions. Effective in treating corticosteroid-responsive dermatoses.

PHARMACOKINETICS: Absorption: Percutaneous; inflammation, other disease states, and occlusive dressings increase absorption. **Metabolism**: Liver. **Elimination**: Kidney, bile.

BETAPACE   RX
sotalol HCL (Bayer Healthcare)

> To minimize risk of arrhythmia, place patients initiated or reinitiated on therapy for minimum of 3 days in a facility that can provide ECG monitoring and cardiac resuscitation. Perform CrCl before therapy. Do not substitute Betapace® for Betapace AF®.

THERAPEUTIC CLASS: Beta-blocker (group II/III antiarrhythmic)

INDICATIONS: Treatment of documented life-threatening ventricular arrhythmias.

DOSAGE: *Adults:* Initial: 80mg bid. Titrate: Increase to 120-160mg bid if needed. Allow 3 days between dose increments. Usual: 160-320mg/day given bid-tid. Refractory Patients: 480-640mg/day. CrCl 30-59mL/min: Dose q24h. CrCl 10-29mL/min: Dose q36-48h. CrCl <10mL/min: Individualize dose. May increase dose with renal impairment after at least 5-6 doses.
Pediatrics: ≥2 yrs: Initial: 30mg/m² tid. Titrate: Wait at least 36 hrs between dose increases. Guide dose by response, HR, and QTc. Max: 60mg/m².

B

<2 yrs: See dosing chart in PI. Reduce dose or d/c if QTc >550msec. Renal Impairment: Reduce dose or increase interval. Preparation of 5mg/mL Oral Solution: Add five 120mg tabs to 120mL simple syrup in a 6oz plastic, amber bottle. Shake bottle to wet all tabs. Allow tabs to hydrate for 2 hrs then shake bottle intermittently over 2 hrs until tabs are completely disintegrated. Shake before administration. Store at room temp for 3 months.

HOW SUPPLIED: Tab: 80mg*, 120mg*, 160mg* *scored

CONTRAINDICATIONS: Bronchial asthma, sinus bradycardia, 2nd- and 3rd-degree AV block (unless a functioning pacemaker is present), long QT syndromes, cardiogenic shock, uncontrolled CHF.

WARNINGS/PRECAUTIONS: Caution with heart failure controlled by digitalis and/or diuretics, DM, left ventricular dysfunction, non-allergic bronchospasm, sick sinus syndrome, renal impairment, 2-weeks post-MI. Avoid with hypokalemia, hypomagnesemia, excessive QT interval prolongation (>550msec). Correct electrolyte imbalances before therapy. May provoke new or worsen ventricular arrhythmias. Avoid abrupt withdrawal. Use in surgery is controversial. May mask hypoglycemia, hyperthyroidism symptoms. Proarrhythmic events reported.

ADVERSE REACTIONS: Dyspnea, fatigue, dizziness, bradycardia, chest pain, palpitation, asthenia, abnormal ECG, hypotension, headache, lightheadedness, edema.

INTERACTIONS: May block epinephrine effects. Caution with drugs that prolong the QT interval (eg, Class I and III antiarrhythmics, phenothiazines, TCAs, bepridil, certain quinolones and oral macrolides, astemizole). Avoid within 2 hrs of aluminum- or magnesium-containing antacids. Potentiates rebound HTN with clonidine withdrawal. May potentiate bradycardia or hypotension with catecholamine-depleting drugs (eg, reserpine). Antidiabetic agents may need adjustment. Avoid Class IA and Class III antiarrhythmics; potential to prolong refractoriness. β_2-agonists (eg, terbutaline) may need dose increase. Additive Class II effects with β-blockers. Additive conduction abnormalities with digoxin and CCBs. Caution with diuretics.

PREGNANCY: Category B, not for use in nursing.

MECHANISM OF ACTION: Has both β-adrenoceptor blocking and cardiac action potential duration prolongation antiarrhythmic property. It prolongs the plateau phase of the cardiac action potential.

PHARMACOKINETICS: Absorption: T_{max}=2.5-4 hrs. **Distribution:** Crosses blood-brain barrier (poor); found in breast milk. **Elimination:** Urine (unchanged); $T_{1/2}$=12 hrs.

BETAPACE AF   RX
sotalol HCL (Bayer Healthcare)

> To minimize risk of arrhythmia, place patients initiated or reinitiated on therapy for minimum of 3 days in a facility that can provide CrCl, ECG monitoring, and cardiac resuscitation. Do not substitute Betapace® for Betapace AF®.

THERAPEUTIC CLASS: Beta-blocker (group II/III antiarrhythmic)

INDICATIONS: Maintenance of normal sinus rhythm with symptomatic atrial fibrillation/atrial flutter (AFIB/AFL) in patients who are currently in sinus rhythm.

DOSAGE: *Adults:* Initiate with continuous ECG monitoring. Give dose qd for CrCl 40-60mL/min and bid for CrCl >60mL/min. Initial: 80mg. Monitor QT 2-4hrs after each dose. Reduce dose or d/c if QT ≥500msec. If QT <500msec after 3 days (after 5th or 6th dose if receiving qd dosing), discharge on current treatment. Alternately, may increase dose to 120mg during hospitalization, and follow for 3 days with bid dose and for 5 or 6 doses if receiving qd dose. Max: 160mg qd or bid depending on CrCl.
Pediatrics: ≥2 yrs: Initial: 30mg/m² tid. Titrate: Wait at least 36 hrs between dose increases. Guide dose by response, heart rate and QTc. Max: 60mg/m².
<2 yrs: See dosing chart in PI. Reduce dose or d/c if QTc >550msec. Renal Impairment: Reduce dose or increase interval. Preparation of 5mg/mL Oral

Solution: Add five 120mg tabs to 120mL simple syrup in a 6oz plastic, amber bottle. Shake bottle to wet all tabs. Allow tabs to hydrate for 2 hrs then shake bottle intermittently over 2 hrs until tabs are completely disintegrated. Shake before administration. Store at room temp for 3 months.

HOW SUPPLIED: Tab: 80mg*, 120mg*, 160mg* *scored

CONTRAINDICATIONS: Sinus bradycardia (<50bpm during waking hrs), sick sinus syndrome or 2nd- or 3rd-degree AV block (unless a functioning pacemaker is present), long QT syndromes, baseline QT interval >450msec, cardiogenic shock, uncontrolled heart failure, hypokalemia (<4meq/L), CrCl <40mL/min, bronchial asthma.

WARNINGS/PRECAUTIONS: Can cause serious ventricular arrhythmias. Avoid with hypokalemia, hypomagnesemia. Correct electrolyte imbalances before therapy. Bradycardia reported. Caution with heart failure controlled by digitalis and/or diuretics, non-allergic bronchospasm, sick sinus syndrome, left ventricular dysfunction, DM, renal dysfunction, post-MI. Avoid abrupt withdrawal. Use in surgery is controversial. May mask hypoglycemia, hyperthyroidism symptoms.

ADVERSE REACTIONS: Bradycardia, dyspnea, fatigue, dose-related QT interval prolongation, abnormal ECG, chest pain, diarrhea, nausea, vomiting, hyperhidrosis, dizziness.

INTERACTIONS: May block epinephrine effects. Avoid drugs that prolong the QT interval (eg, antiarrhythmics, phenothiazines, TCAs, bepridil, certain oral macrolides). Avoid within 2 hrs of aluminum- or magnesium-containing antacids. Potentiates rebound HTN with clonidine withdrawal. May potentiate bradycardia or hypotension with catecholamine-depleting drugs (eg, reserpine). Antidiabetic agents may need adjustment. β$_2$-agonists (eg, terbutaline) may need dose increase. Additive conduction abnormalities with digoxin and CCBs. Caution with diuretics.

PREGNANCY: Category B, not for use in nursing.

MECHANISM OF ACTION: Antiarrhythmic drug (Class II and III properties); has both β-adrenoceptor blocking and cardiac action potential duration prolongation property.

PHARMACOKINETICS: Absorption: T$_{max}$ =2.5-4 hrs. **Distribution:** Crosses blood brain barrier (poor); found in breast milk. **Elimination:** Urine (unchanged); T$_{1/2}$=12 hrs.

BETASERON   RX
interferon beta-1b (Bayer Healthcare)

THERAPEUTIC CLASS: Biological response modifier

INDICATIONS: Treatment in patients who have experienced a first clinical episode and have MRI features consistent with Multiple Sclerosis (MS). To reduce frequency of clinical exacerbations in patients with relapsing-remitting MS.

DOSAGE: *Adults:* Initial: 0.0625mg SQ every other day. Titrate: Increase over 6 wks to 0.25mg SQ every other day.

HOW SUPPLIED: Inj: 0.3mg

CONTRAINDICATIONS: Hypersensitivity to human albumin.

WARNINGS/PRECAUTIONS: Caution with depression. Injection site necrosis reported; d/c if multiple lesions occur. Perform Hgb, LFTs, CBC, differential WBC and platelet count before therapy and periodically thereafter.

ADVERSE REACTIONS: Injection site reactions/necrosis, flu-like symptoms, headache, lymphopenia, liver enzyme elevations, pain, fever, chills, diarrhea, abdominal pain, vomiting, constipation, nausea, myalgia, asthenia, malaise, hypertonia, sinusitis, sweating, dizziness, menstrual disorders.

INTERACTIONS: May inhibit antipyrine elimination.

PREGNANCY: Category C, not for use in nursing.

MECHANISM OF ACTION: Interferon beta-1b; not established; it is believed that interferon beta-1b receptor binding induces the expression of proteins that are responsible for pleiotropic bioactivities. Immunomodulatory effects include the enhancement of suppressor T cell activity, reduction of pro-imflammatory cytokine production, down-regulation of antigen presentation, and inhibition of lymphocyte trafficking into the CNS.

PHARMACOKINETICS: Absorption: T_{max}=1-8 hrs., C_{max}=40IU/mL. **Distribution:** V_d=(0.25-2.88)L/kg. **Elimination:** $T_{1/2}$=8.0 min.-4.3 hrs.

BETAXOLOL HCL   RX
betaxolol HCL (Various)

OTHER BRAND NAMES: Kerlone (Sanofi-Aventis)

THERAPEUTIC CLASS: Selective beta₁-blocker

INDICATIONS: Management of hypertension.

DOSAGE: *Adults:* Initial: 10mg qd. Titrate: May increase to 20mg qd after 7-14 days. Max (usual): 20mg/day. Severe Renal Impairment/Dialysis: Initial: 5mg qd. Titrate: May increase by 5mg/day every 2 weeks. Max: 20mg/day. Elderly: Initial: 5mg qd.

HOW SUPPLIED: Tab: 10mg, 20mg

CONTRAINDICATIONS: Sinus bradycardia, >1st-degree heart block, cardiogenic shock, overt cardiac failure.

WARNINGS/PRECAUTIONS: Caution in CHF controlled by digitalis and diuretics, bronchospastic disease, renal or hepatic dysfunction. Can cause cardiac failure. Avoid abrupt withdrawal. Withdrawal before surgery is controversial. May mask hypoglycemia and hyperthyroidism symptoms. May decrease IOP and interfere with glaucoma-screening test. Bradycardia may occur more often in elderly. May develop antinuclear antibodies (ANA).

ADVERSE REACTIONS: Bradycardia, fatigue, dyspnea, lethargy, impotence, dyspepsia, arthralgia, headache, dizziness, insomnia.

INTERACTIONS: May block epinephrine effects. Possible additive effects with catecholamine-depleting drugs (eg, reserpine). D/C gradually before clonidine withdrawal. Avoid oral CCBs with cardiac dysfunction; may increase cardiac adverse effects.

PREGNANCY: Category C, caution in nursing.

MECHANISM OF ACTION: β₁-selective adrenergic receptor blocking agent; not established, proposed to competitively antagonize catecholamines at peripheral adrenergic-neuronal sites, have central effect leading to reduced sympathetic outflow to periphery, and suppression of renin activity.

PHARMACOKINETICS: Absorption: Complete; absolute bioavailability (89%); C_{max}=21.6ng/mL; T_{max}=1.5-6 hrs. **Distribution:** Plasma protein binding (50%). **Metabolism:** Liver. **Elimination:** Urine (15%).

BETAXOLOL HCL OPHTHALMIC   RX
betaxolol HCL (Alcon)

THERAPEUTIC CLASS: Selective beta₁-blocker

INDICATIONS: Treatment of ocular HTN and chronic open-angle glaucoma. May be used alone or in combination with other anti-glaucoma drugs.

DOSAGE: *Adults:* 1-2 drops in the affected eye(s) bid.

HOW SUPPLIED: Sol: 5mL, 10mL, 15mL

CONTRAINDICATIONS: Sinus bradycardia, heart block >1st degree, cardiogenic shock, overt cardiac failure.

WARNINGS/PRECAUTIONS: Caution with history of cardiac failure or heart block; d/c at first signs of cardiac failure. May mask signs/symptoms of hypoglycemia or hyperthyroidism. Abrupt withdrawal may also exacerbate symptoms of hyperthyroidism or precipitate a thyroid storm. May potentiate muscle weakness consistent with certain myasthenic symptoms. Withdrawal before surgery is controversial. Caution with glaucoma patients; asthmatic attacks and pulmonary distress reported. Caution with history of atopy or severe anaphylactic reactions.

ADVERSE REACTIONS: Eye discomfort, blurred vision, foreign body sensation, dryness of the eyes, eye inflammation, discharge, ocular pain, decreased visual acuity, crusty lashes.

INTERACTIONS: May block epinephrine effects. Possible additive effects with oral beta-adrenergic blocking agents and catecholamine-depleting drugs (eg, reserpine). Caution with concomitant adrenergic psychotropic drugs.

PREGNANCY: Category C, caution in nursing.

MECHANISM OF ACTION: Selective β-1-adrenergic receptor blocking agent; reduces IOP.

BETIMOL   RX
timolol (Vistakon)

THERAPEUTIC CLASS: Nonselective beta-blocker

INDICATIONS: Treatment of elevated IOP in patients with open-angle glaucoma or ocular hypertension.

DOSAGE: *Adults:* Initial: 1 drop 0.25% bid. May increase to max of 1 drop 0.5% bid. Maint: If adequate control, may try 1 drop 0.25-0.5% qd.

HOW SUPPLIED: Sol: 0.25%, 0.5% [2.5mL, 5mL, 10mL, 15mL]

CONTRAINDICATIONS: Bronchial asthma, history of bronchial asthma, severe COPD, sinus bradycardia, 2nd- or 3rd-degree AV block, overt cardiac failure, cardiogenic shock.

WARNINGS/PRECAUTIONS: Caution with cardiac failure, DM, cerebrovascular insufficiency. Severe cardiac and respiratory reactions reported. May mask symptoms of hypoglycemia and hyperthyroidism. Bacterial keratitis reported with contaminated containers. May reinsert contacts 5 min after applying drops. Avoid with COPD, bronchospastic disease. Not for use alone in angle-closure glaucoma. May potentiate muscle weakness. D/C if cardiac failure develops. Withdrawal before surgery is controversial.

ADVERSE REACTIONS: Burning/stinging on instillation, dry eyes, itching, foreign body sensation, eye discomfort, eyelid erythema, conjunctival injection, headache.

INTERACTIONS: May potentiate systemic β-blockers and catecholamine-depleting drugs (eg, reserpine). Oral/IV calcium antagonists can cause AV conduction disturbances, left ventricular failure, or hypotension. Digitalis can cause additive effects in prolonging AV conduction time. May antagonize epinephrine.

PREGNANCY: Category C, not for use in nursing.

MECHANISM OF ACTION: A nonselective β-adrenergic antagonist. Blocks both β$_1$- and β$_2$-adrenergic receptors. Thought to reduce intraocular pressure through reducing production of aqueous humor.

PHARMACOKINETICS: Elimination: Urine (metabolites); T$_{1/2}$=4 hrs

BETOPTIC S   RX
betaxolol HCL (Alcon)

THERAPEUTIC CLASS: Selective beta$_1$-blocker

INDICATIONS: Chronic open-angle glaucoma. Ocular hypertension.

DOSAGE: *Adults:* 1-2 drops bid.

HOW SUPPLIED: Sus: 0.25% [2.5mL, 5mL, 10mL, 15mL]

CONTRAINDICATIONS: Sinus bradycardia, greater than 1st-degree AV block, cardiogenic shock or overt cardiac failure.

WARNINGS/PRECAUTIONS: May be absorbed systemically. Caution with cardiac failure, heart block, DM, asthma. May mask hypoglycemic symptoms and signs of hyperthyroidism. May potentiate muscle weakness. D/C before general anesthesia. Avoid abrupt withdrawal. Caution in patients with cerebrovascular insufficiency.

ADVERSE REACTIONS: Transient ocular discomfort, blurred vision, corneal punctate keratitis, foreign body sensation, tearing, photophobia, tearing, itching, dryness of eye, erythema, inflammation, discharge, ocular pain, decreased visual acuity, crusty lashes.

INTERACTIONS: May potentiate systemic β-blockers and catecholamine-depleting drugs (eg, reserpine). May be potentiated by systemic β-blockers. May antagonize adrenergic psychotropics. May increase risk of hypoglycemia with insulin or oral hypoglycemic drugs.

PREGNANCY: Category C, caution with nursing.

MECHANISM OF ACTION: It is a cardioselective (β-1-adrenergic) receptor inhibitor. Responsible for reducing intraocular pressure through a reduction of aqueous production.

PHARMACOKINETICS: Absorption: T_{max}=2 hrs.

BEXXAR   RX
iodine I 131 tositumomab - tositumomab (GlaxoSmithKline)

> Hypersensitivity reactions, including anaphylaxis, and prolonged and severe cytopenias reported. Can cause fetal harm if given during pregnancy. Contains radioactive component.

THERAPEUTIC CLASS: Monoclonal antibody/CD20-blocker

INDICATIONS: Treatment of CD20-positive, follicular, non-Hodgkin's lymphoma (NHL), with and without transformation, in patients refractory to rituximab and who have relapsed following chemotherapy.

DOSAGE: *Adults:* Premedication: Day 1: Begin thyro-protective regimen of either SSKI (4 drops po tid), Lugol's sol (20 drops po tid), or potassium iodide (130mg po qd). Continue until 14 days post-therapeutic dose. Day 0: APAP 650mg and diphenhydramine 50mg. Dosimetric Step: IV: 450mg tositumomab over 60 min followed by 5mCi Iodine I 131 tositumomab (35mg) over 20 min. Day 0 + Day 2, 3, or 4 + Day 6 or 7: Whole body dosimetry and biodistribution. Day 6 or 7: Calculation of patient-specific activity of iodine I 131 tositumomab to deliver 75cGy total body irradiation or 65cGy if platelets ≥100,000 but <150,000 platelets/mm³. Day 7 (up to Day 14): Premedicate with APAP and diphenhydramine. Therapeutic Step: IV: Do not administer if biodistribution is altered. 450mg tositumomab over 60 min followed by prescribed therapeutic dose of iodine I 131 tositumomab (35mg) over 20 min.

HOW SUPPLIED: Inj: For Dosimetric Dosing: Tositumomab: 225mg [2 single-use vials], 35mg [1 single-use vial]; Iodine I 131 Tositumomab: 1 single-use vial. For Therapeutic Dosing: Tositumomab: 225mg [2 single-use vials], 35mg [1 single-use vial]; Iodine I 131 Tositumomab: 1 or 2 single-use vials.

CONTRAINDICATIONS: Pregnant women.

WARNINGS/PRECAUTIONS: Obtain CBCs weekly for 10-12 weeks. Safety not established with >25% lymphoma marrow involvement, platelet <100,000 cells/mm³, or neutrophil count <1500 cells/mm³. Secondary malignancies reported. May cause hypothyroidism; monitor TSH prior to initiation and then annually. Thyroid blocking agents must be used; initiate at least 24 hrs before dosimetric dose and continue until 14 days after therapeutic dose. Caution with impaired renal function. Effective contraceptive methods should be used during, and for 12 months following treatment. Increased risk of serious allergic reactions if positive for human anti-murine antibodies (HAMA).

ADVERSE REACTIONS: Neutropenia, thrombocytopenia, anemia, asthenia, fever, infection, cough, pain, chills, headache, GI effects, myalgia, arthralgia, pharyngitis, dyspnea, rash.

INTERACTIONS: Weigh risks vs benefits of concomitant agents that interfere with platelet function and/or anticoagulation.

PREGNANCY: Category X, not for use in nursing.

MECHANISM OF ACTION: Monoclonal antibody; possibly induces apoptosis, complement-dependent cytotoxicity, antibody-dependent cellular cytotoxicity mediated by the antibody; cell death associated with ionizing radiation from radioisotope. Tositumomab; murine IgG2a lambda monoclonal antibody directed against CD20 antigen found on surface of B lymphocytes. Iodine I 131 Tositumomab; radio-iodinated derivative of Tositumomab, covalently linked to Iodine-131.

PHARMACOKINETICS: Elimination: (Iodine-131): Decay (β and gamma emissions). Physical $T_{1/2}$=8.04 days. Excreted in urine; (Iodine I 131 Tositumonab): Urine, $T_{1/2}$=67 hrs.

BIAXIN   RX
clarithromycin (Abbott)

THERAPEUTIC CLASS: Macrolide

INDICATIONS: Treatment of the following infections caused by susceptible strains of microorganisms: (Adults): Pharyngitis/tonsillitis, acute maxillary sinusitis, acute bacterial exacerbation of chronic bronchitis (ABECB), community-aquired pneumonia (CAP), uncomplicated skin and skin structure infections (SSSI), and disseminated mycobacterial infections. Combination therapy for *H.pylori* infection with duodenal ulcers. MAC prophylaxis in advanced HIV. (Pediatrics): Pharyngitis/tonsillitis, CAP, acute maxillary sinusitis, acute otitis media, uncomplicated SSSI, disseminated mycobacterial infections. MAC prophylaxis in advanced HIV.

DOSAGE: *Adults:* Pharyngitis/Tonsillitis: 250mg q12h for 10 days. Sinusitis: 500mg q12h for 14 days. ABECB: 250-500mg q12h for 7-14 days. SSSI/ CAP: 250mg q12h for 7-14 days. MAC Prophylaxis/Treatment: 500mg bid. CrCl <30mL/min: Give 50% dose or double interval. *H.pylori:* Triple Therapy: 500mg + amoxicillin 1g + omeprazole 20mg, all q12h for 10 days; or 500mg + amoxicillin 1g + lansoprazole 30mg, all q12h for 10-14 days. Give additional omeprazole 20mg qd for 18 days with active ulcer. Dual Therapy: 500mg q8h + omeprazole 40mg qd for 14 days (give additional omeprazole 20mg qd for 14 days with active ulcer); or 500mg q8h or q12h + ranitidine bismuth citrate 400mg q12h for 14 days (give additional ranitidine bismuth citrate 400mg bid for 14 days with active ulcer). Avoid combination with ranitidine bismuth citrate if CrCl<25mL/min.
Pediatrics: ≥6 months: Usual: 7.5mg/kg q12h for 10 days. MAC Prophylaxis/ Treatment: ≥20 months: 7.5mg/kg bid, up to 500mg bid. CrCl <30mL/min: Give 50% dose or double interval.

HOW SUPPLIED: Sus: 125mg/5mL, 250mg/5mL [50mL, 100mL]; Tab: 250mg, 500mg

CONTRAINDICATIONS: Concomitant cisapride, pimozide, astemizole, terfenadine, ergotamine or dihydroergotamine, or other macrolide antibiotics.

WARNINGS/PRECAUTIONS: Avoid in pregnancy. *Clostridium difficile*-associated diarrhea reported. Adjust dose with severe renal impairment. Colchicine toxicity reported; avoid concomitant use especially in elderly.

ADVERSE REACTIONS: Diarrhea, nausea, abnormal taste, dyspepsia, abdominal pain, headache, vomiting, rash.

INTERACTIONS: See Contraindications. Increases serum levels of theophylline, digoxin, HMG-CoA reductase inhibitors, omeprazole, carbamazepine, drugs metabolized by CYP450. Decreases zidovudine plasma levels. Potentiates oral anticoagulant effects. Decreased clearance of triazolam. Avoid ranitidine, bismuth citrate if CrCl <25mL/min or history of porphyria. Reduce dose with ritonavir if CrCl <60mL/min. Increased levels with fluconazole. Caution with concomitant colchicine use.

PREGNANCY: Category C, caution in nursing.

MECHANISM OF ACTION: Macrolide antibiotic; exerts antibacterial action by binding to the 50S ribosomal subunit of susceptible microorganisms, resulting in inhibition of protein synthesis. Active against aerobic and anaerobic gram-positive and gram-negative microorganisms.

PHARMACOKINETICS: Absorption: Rapid; absolute bioavailability 50%; C_{max}=1-2mcg/mL (250mg tab); 3-4mcg/mL (500mg tab), 2mcg/mL (sus); T_{max}=2-3 hrs. **Metabolism:** 14-OH clarithromycin (principal metabolite). **Elimination:** Urine: 20% (250mg tab), 40% (500mg tab), 10-15% (14-OH). Parent drug; $T_{1/2}$=3-4 hrs (250mg tab, sus), 5-7 hrs (500mg tab). 14-OH: $T_{1/2}$=5-6 hrs (250mg tab, sus), 7-9 hrs (500mg tab).

BIAXIN XL   RX
clarithromycin (Abbott)

THERAPEUTIC CLASS: Macrolide

INDICATIONS: Treatment of acute maxillary sinusitis, community-acquired pneumonia (CAP), and acute bacterial exacerbation of chronic bronchitis (ABECB).

DOSAGE: *Adults:* Sinusitis: 1000mg qd for 14 days. ABECB/CAP: 1000mg qd for 7 days. CrCl <30mL/min: Give 50% dose or double interval. Take with food.

HOW SUPPLIED: Tab, Extended-Release: 500mg [PAC 14s]

CONTRAINDICATIONS: Concomitant cisapride, pimozide, astemizole, ter-fenadine, ergotamine or dihydroergotamine, or other macrolide antibiotics.

WARNINGS/PRECAUTIONS: Avoid in pregnancy. *Clostridium difficile*-associ-ated diarrhea reported. Adjust dose with severe renal impairment. Colchicine toxicity reported, avoid concomitant use especially in the elderly.

ADVERSE REACTIONS: Diarrhea, nausea, abnormal taste, dyspepsia, abdomi-nal pain, headache, vomiting, rash.

INTERACTIONS: See Contraindications. May increase serum levels of theophylline, digoxin, HMG-CoA reductase inhibitors, omeprazole, carbam-azepine and drugs metabolized by CYP450. May decrease zidovudine plasma levels. May potentiate oral anticoagulant effects. May decrease clearance of triazolam. Avoid ranitidine bismuth citrate if CrCl <25mL/min or history of porphyria. Reduce dose with ritonavir if CrCl <60mL/min. Increased levels with fluconazole. Caution with concomitant colchicine use.

PREGNANCY: Category C, caution in nursing.

MECHANISM OF ACTION: Macrolide antibiotic: exerts antibacterial action by binding to 50S ribosomal subunit of susceptible microorganisms resulting in inhibition of protein synthesis. Active against aerobic and anaerobic gram-positive and gram-negativie microorganisms.

PHARMACOKINETICS: Absorption: Rapid. (2 x 500mg dose): (parent drug) C_{max}=2-3μg/mL, T_{max}=5-8 hrs.(14-OH); C_{max}=0.8μg/mL, T_{max}=6-9 hrs. (1 x 500mg dose): (parent drug) C_{max}=1-2μg/mL, T_{max}=5-6 hr; (14-OH) C_{max}=0.6μ/mL, T_{max}=6 hrs. **Distribution:** Body tissues, fluids. **Metabolism:** 14-OH clarithro-mycin (principal metabolite). **Elimination:** Urine; (40%).

BICILLIN C-R   RX
penicillin G procaine - penicillin G benzathine (King)

> Not for IV use nor for admix with other IV solutions. Cardiorespiratory arrest and death reported with inadvertent IV administration.

THERAPEUTIC CLASS: Penicillin

INDICATIONS: Treatment of moderately severe to severe upper-respiratory tract (URTI) and skin and soft-tissue infections (SSTI), scarlet fever and ery-sipelas due to streptococci. Treatment of moderately severe pneumonia and otitis media due to pneumococci.

DOSAGE: *Adults:* Group A Strep: URTI/SSTI/Scarlet Fever/Erysipelas: 2.4MU IM. Treat at a single session using multiple IM sites, or use an alter-native schedule and give 1/2 of the total dose on Day 1 and 1/2 on Day 3. Pneumococcal Infections (Except Meningitis): 1.2MU IM, repeat every 2-3 days until temperature is normal for 48 hrs. Administer IM into upper, outer quadrant of buttock.

Pediatrics: Group A Strep: URTI/SSTI/Scarlet Fever/Erysipelas: >60 lbs: 2.4MU IM. 30-60 lbs: 900,000U-1.2MU IM. <30 lbs: 600,000U IM. Treat at a single session using multiple IM sites, or use an alternative schedule and give 1/2 of the total dose on Day 1 and 1/2 on Day 3. Pneumococcal Infections (Except Meningitis): 600,000U IM, repeat every 2-3 days until temperature is normal for 48 hrs. Administer IM into upper, outer quadrant of buttock. Use the mid-lateral aspect of thigh in neonates, infants, and small children.

HOW SUPPLIED: Inj: (Penicillin G Benzathine-Penicillin G Procaine) 300,000-300,000U/mL [2mL]

CONTRAINDICATIONS: Do not inject into or near an artery or nerve.

WARNINGS/PRECAUTIONS: Serious, fatal anaphylactic reactions reported; increased risk with hypersensitivity to PCN, cephalosporins, and other allergens. *Clostridium difficile* associated with diarrhea reported. reported. Avoid IV, intra-arterial administration, or injection into/near major peripheral nerves or blood vessels may cause severe neurovascular and neurological damage. IM administration into anterolateral thigh may cause quadriceps femoris fibrosis and atrophy. Caution with asthma. Avoid with procaine sensitivity. May result in overgrowth of nonsusceptible organisms. Monitor culture after therapy completion to determine eradication. Monitor renal and hematopoietic systems periodically with prolonged and high-dose therapy.

ADVERSE REACTIONS: Maculopapular/exfoliative dermatitis, urticaria, laryngeal edema, fever, pseudomembranous colitis, hemolytic anemia, leukopenia, thrombocytopenia, neuropathy, nephropathy.

INTERACTIONS: Increased and prolonged levels with probenecid. Tetracycline may antagonize bacterial effect; avoid concomitant use.

PREGNANCY: Category B, caution in nursing.

MECHANISM OF ACTION: Penicillin; exerts bactericidal action against susceptible organisms during the active multiplication stage. Acts through inhibition of biosynthesis of cell-wall mucopeptide.

PHARMACOKINETICS: Absorption: Slow; C_{max}=1-3 U/mL (600,000 U), 2.1-2.6 units/mL (1,200,000 U); T_{max}=3 hrs. **Distribution:** Plasma protein binding (60%). Found in breast milk, high cocentration in kidney, lesser extent in liver, skin, and intestines. **Metabolism:** Hydrolysis. **Elimination:** Urine.

BICILLIN C-R 900/300   RX
penicillin G procaine - penicillin G benzathine (King)

> Not for IV use nor for admix with other IV solutions. Cardiorespiratory arrest and death reported with inadvertent IV administration.

THERAPEUTIC CLASS: Penicillin

INDICATIONS: Treatment of moderately severe to severe upper-respiratory tract (URTI) and skin and soft-tissue infections (SSTI), scarlet fever and erysipelas due to streptococcus. Treatment of moderately severe pneumonia and otitis media due to pneumococci. Not for treatment of venereal diseases.

DOSAGE: *Pediatrics:* Group A Strep: URTI/SSTI/Scarlet Fever/Erysipelas: 1.2MU IM single dose. Pneumococcal Infections (Except Meningitis): 1.2MU IM every 2-3 days until temperature is normal for 48 hrs. Administer IM into upper, outer quadrant of buttock. Use midlateral aspect of thigh in neonates, infants, and small children.

HOW SUPPLIED: Inj: (Penicillin G Benzathine-Penicillin G Procaine) 900,000-300,000U/2mL

CONTRAINDICATIONS: Do not inject into or near an artery or nerve.

WARNINGS/PRECAUTIONS: Serious, fatal anaphylactic reactions reported; increased risk with hypersensitivity to penicillin, cephalosporins, and other allergens. *Clostridium difficile* associated with diarrhea reported. Avoid IV, intra-arterial administration, or injection into/near major peripheral nerves or blood vessels may cause severe neurovascular and neurological damage. IM administration into anterolateral thigh may cause quadriceps femoris fibrosis and atrophy. Caution with asthma. Avoid with procaine sensitivity. May result in overgrowth of nonsusceptible organisms. Monitor culture after therapy completion to determine eradication. Monitor renal and hematopoietic systems periodically with prolonged and high-dose therapy.

ADVERSE REACTIONS: Maculopapular/exfoliative dermatitis, urticaria, laryngeal edema, fever, pseudomembranous colitis, hemolytic anemia, leukopenia, thrombocytopenia, neuropathy, nephropathy.

INTERACTIONS: Increased and prolonged levels with probenecid. Tetracycline may antagonize bactericidal effect; avoid concurrent use.

PREGNANCY: Category B, caution in nursing.

MECHANISM OF ACTION: Penicillin G; exerts bactericidal action against susceptible organisms during the active multiplication stage. Acts through inhibition of biosynthesis of cell-wall mucopepetide.

PHARMACOKINETICS: Absorption: Slow. **Distribution:** Plasma protein binding (60%). Found in breast milk, high concentration in kidney, lesser extent in liver, skin, and intestines. **Metabolism :** Hyrolysis. **Elimination**: Urine.

BICILLIN L-A   RX
penicillin G benzathine (King)

> Not for IV use nor for admix with other IV solutions. Cardiorespiratory arrest and death reported with inadvertent IV administration.

THERAPEUTIC CLASS: Penicillin

INDICATIONS: Treatment of mild to moderate upper respiratory tract infections (URTI) due to streptococci and venereal infections (eg, syphilis, yaws, bejel, pinta). Prophylaxis to prevent recurrence of rheumatic fever or chorea.

DOSAGE: *Adults:* Group A Strep: URTI: 1.2MU IM single dose. Primary/Secondary/Latent Syphilis: 2.4MU IM single dose. Late Syphilis (Tertiary/Neurosyphilis): 2.4MU IM every 7 days for 3 doses. Yaws/Bejel/Pinta: 1.2MU IM single dose. Rheumatic Fever/Glomerulonephritis Prophylaxis: 1.2MU IM once a month or 600,000U IM every 2 weeks. Administer IM into upper, outer quadrant of buttock.
Pediatrics: Group A Strep: URTI: Older **Pediatrics:** 900,000U IM single dose. <60 lbs: 300,000-600,000U IM single dose. Congenital Syphilis: 2-12 yrs: Adjust dose based on adult schedule. <2 yrs: 50,000U/kg IM single dose. Rheumatic Fever/Glomerulonephritis Prophylaxis: 1.2MU IM once a month or 600,000U every 2 weeks. Administer IM into upper, outer quadrant of buttock. Use the midlateral aspect of thigh in neonates, infants, and small children.

HOW SUPPLIED: Inj: 600,000U/mL

CONTRAINDICATIONS: Do not inject into or near an artery or nerve.

WARNINGS/PRECAUTIONS: Serious, fatal anaphylactic reactions reported; increased risk with hypersensitivity to PCNs, cephalosporins, and other allergens. Pseudomembranous colitis reported. Avoid IV, intra-arterial administration, or injection into/near major peripheral nerves or blood vessels may cause severe neurovascular and neurological damage. IM administration into anterolateral thigh may cause quadriceps femoris fibrosis and atrophy. Caution with asthma. May result in overgrowth of nonsusceptible organisms. Monitor culture after therapy completion to determine eradication.

ADVERSE REACTIONS: Maculopapular/exfoliative dermatitis, urticaria, laryngeal edema, fever, pseudomembranous colitis, hemolytic anemia, leukopenia, thrombocytopenia, neuropathy, nephropathy.

INTERACTIONS: Increased and prolonged levels with probenecid. Tetracycline may antagonize bactericidal effect.

PREGNANCY: Category B, caution in nursing.

MECHANISM OF ACTION: Penicillin G exerts a bactericidal action against susceptible organisms during the active multiplication stage. Acts through inhibition of biosynthesis of cell-wall mucopepetide.

PHARMACOKINETICS: Absorption: Slow. **Distribution:** Plasma protein binding (60%). **Metabolism:** Hydrolysis. **Elimination:** Urine.

BıCNU   RX
carmustine (Bristol-Myers Squibb)

> Bone marrow suppression, thrombocytopenia, leukopenia reported. Monitor blood counts weekly for at least 6 weeks after dose. Base dose adjustments on nadir blood counts from prior dose. Pulmonary toxicity may be dose related (>1400 mg/m² at greater risk) and can occur years after treatment. Administer only under supervision of a physician experienced in the use of antineoplastic agents.

THERAPEUTIC CLASS: Nitrosourea alkylating agent

INDICATIONS: Palliative therapy as single or adjunct agent for treatment of brain tumors, multiple myeloma, Hodgkin's disease, and non-Hodgkin's lymphomas.

DOSAGE: *Adults:* Single Agent in Untreated Patients: 150-200mg/m² IV every 6 weeks, as a single dose or divide into daily injections (75-100mg/m² for 2 days). Adjust subsequent doses according to hematologic response. If leukocytes 2000-2999 and platelets 25,000-74,999, give 70% of dose. If leukocytes <2000 and platelets <25,000, then give 50% of dose.

HOW SUPPLIED: Inj: 100mg

WARNINGS/PRECAUTIONS: Long-term use may be associated with secondary malignancies. Monitor hepatic/renal function. Conduct baseline and periodic pulmonary function tests during treatment. Caution in elderly; monitor renal function.

ADVERSE REACTIONS: Delayed myelosuppression, pulmonary infiltrates/fibrosis, nausea, vomiting, hepatic toxicity, azotemia, renal failure, neuroretinitis, chest pain, headache, allergic reaction, hypotension, tachycardia.

INTERACTIONS: Greater myelotoxicity when combined with cimetidine.

PREGNANCY: Category D, not for use in nursing.

MECHANISM OF ACTION: Nitrosureas; alkylates DNA and RNA; may inhibit several key enzymatic processes by carbamoylation of amino acids in proteins.

PHARMACOKINETICS: Absorption: Rapid. **Elimination:** Urine and respiration.

BıDıL   RX
hydralazine HCL - isosorbide dinitrate (NitroMed)

THERAPEUTIC CLASS: Vasodilator combination

INDICATIONS: Treatment of heart failure as an adjunct to standard therapy in self-identified black patients to improve survival, prolong time to hospitalization for heart failure, and improve patient-reported functional status.

DOSAGE: *Adults:* Initial: 1 tab tid. Max: 2 tabs tid.

HOW SUPPLIED: Tab: (Hydralazine-Isosorbide) 37.5mg-20mg

CONTRAINDICATIONS: Allergies to organic nitrates.

WARNINGS/PRECAUTIONS: May produce a clinical picture simulating systemic lupus erythematosus including glomerulonephritis. May cause symptomatic hypotension, tachycardia, peripheral neuritis. Caution in patients with acute MI, hemodynamic and clinical monitoring recommended. May aggravate angina associated with hypertrophic cardiomyopathy.

ADVERSE REACTIONS: Headache, dizziness, chest pain, asthenia, nausea, bronchitis, hypotension, sinusitis, ventricular tachycardia, palpitations, hyperglycemia, rhinitis, paresthesia, vomiting, amblyopia, hyperlipidemia.

INTERACTIONS: Increased vasodilatory effects with phosphodiesterase inhibitors (sildenafil, vardenafil, tadalafil). Increased risk of hypotension with potent parenteral antihypertensive agents. Caution with MAOIs.

PREGNANCY: Category C, caution in nursing.

MECHANISM OF ACTION: Isosorbide: Vasodilator; not established, exhibits dilator properties from release of nitric oxide and subsequent activation of guanyl cyclase and relaxation of vascular smooth muscle. Hydralazine: Vasodilator; selective dilator of arterial smooth muscle.

PHARMACOKINETICS: Absorption: Isosorbide: Absolute bioavailability (25%). Hydralazine: Absolute bioavailability (10-26%). **Distribution:** Isosorbide: V_d=2-4 L/kg; plasma protein binding (28%). Hydralazine: V_d=2.2 L/kg. **Metabolism:** Isosorbide: Denitration. 2-mononitrate, 5-mononitrate (active metabolites). Hydralazine: Acetylation, ring oxidation and conjugation. **Elimination:** Isosorbide: Renal, $T_{1/2}$=1 hr, 5 hrs (5-mononitrate). Hydralazine: Urine.

BILTRICIDE   RX
praziquantel (Schering)

INDICATIONS: Treatment of infections due to all species of schistosoma and due to liver flukes.

DOSAGE: *Adults:* Schistosomiasis: 20mg/kg tid for 1 day. Clonorchiasis/Opisthorchiasis: 25mg/kg tid for 1 day. Take with fluids during meals; do not chew. Dosage interval should not be <4 hrs or >6 hrs.
Pediatrics: ≥4 yrs: Schistosomiasis: 20mg/kg tid for 1 day. Clonorchiasis/Opisthorchiasis: 25mg/kg tid for 1 day. Take with fluids during meals; do not chew. Dosage interval should not be <4 hrs or >6 hrs.

HOW SUPPLIED: Tab: 600mg [6^s]

CONTRAINDICATIONS: Ocular cysticercosis.

WARNINGS/PRECAUTIONS: Avoid driving or operating machinery until one day after treatment. Minimal increases in liver enzymes reported. Hospitalize if schistosomiasis or fluke infection is associated with cerebral cysticercosis. Monitor during treatment with cardiac irregularities.

ADVERSE REACTIONS: Malaise, headache, dizziness, abdominal discomfort, nausea, rise in temperature.

INTERACTIONS: CYP450 inducers, eg antiepileptic drugs (phenytoin, phenobarbital, carbamazepine), dexamethasone, may reduce plasma levels. Avoid concomitant rifampin. CYP450 inhibitors, eg cimetidine, ketoconazole, itraconazole, erythromycin may increase plasma levels. Chloroquine, may lead to lower concentrations of praziquantel in blood. Grapefruit juice can increase Cmax and AUC.

PREGNANCY: Category B, not for use in nursing.

MECHANISM OF ACTION: Praziquantel; antihelminthic that induces rapid contraction of schistosomes by a specific effect on permeability of the cell membrane. Drug further causes vacuolisation and disintegration of the schistosome tegument.

PHARMACOKINETICS: Absorption: Rapid. PO administration in different groups of people with varying degrees of hepatic dysfunction resulted in different pharmacokinetic parameters. **Distribution:** Appears in breast milk. **Elimination:** Urine (approximately 80%, drug), >99% (metabolites); $T_{1/2}$=0.8-1.5 hrs.

BIOLON   RX
sodium hyaluronate (Akorn)

THERAPEUTIC CLASS: Surgical aid

INDICATIONS: Surgical aid to protect corneal endothelium during cataract extraction (extra-capsular) procedures, intraocular lens (IOL) implantation, and anterior segment surgery.

DOSAGE: *Adults:* Cataract Surgery/IOL Implantation: Introduce 0.2-0.5mL slowly into anterior chamber by using cannula. Inject before or after delivery of the lens. May use to coat lens and surgical instruments prior to lens insertion. Can inject during surgery to replace any of the drug lost during surgery.

HOW SUPPLIED: Inj: 1% [0.5mL, 1mL]

WARNINGS/PRECAUTIONS: Precipitate will form with quaternary ammonium salts (eg, benzalkonium chloride). Use only with single-use cannula provided in package. Do not use excessive quantity. Remove all solution by irrigation or aspiration at end of surgery. Administer appropriate therapy if post-op IOP significantly rises. Cannulas are for single patient use only. Remove any cloudy or precipitated material by irrigation or aspiration. Injection of biological substances carry immunological, allergic, and other potential risks. Avoid trapping eye bubbles behind the agent.

ADVERSE REACTIONS: Increased IOP, superficial/conjunctival punctate keratitis, cystoid macular edema, posterior capsule opacity.

INTERACTIONS: Do not irrigate with solution containing quaternary ammonium salts (eg, benzalkonium chloride); precipitate will form.

PREGNANCY: Safety in pregnancy or nursing not known.

BIOTHRAX   RX
anthrax vaccine adsorbed (Bioport)

THERAPEUTIC CLASS: Vaccine

INDICATIONS: Active immunization against Bacillus anthracis in individuals who come in contact with animal products (eg, hides, hairs, bones) that come from anthrax endemic areas and that may be contaminated with spores. Also for individuals at high risk of exposure to these spores (eg, veterinarians, laboratory workers).

DOSAGE: *Adults:* 18-65 yrs: 0.5mL SQ for 3 doses given 2 weeks apart, followed by 3 additional doses of 0.5mL given at 6, 12, 18 months. Booster injections of 0.5mL recommended at 1-year intervals.

HOW SUPPLIED: Inj: 5mL

WARNINGS/PRECAUTIONS: May cause birth defects if given during pregnancy. Review history for vaccine sensitivities. Avoid with history of Guillain-Barre syndrome. Increased risk of local adverse reaction with history of anthrax disease. Possible inadequate immunization with impaired immune responsiveness (eg, congenital/acquired immunodeficiency). Postpone vaccination with moderate to severe illness. Caution with latex sensitivity.

ADVERSE REACTIONS: (Local) tenderness, erythema, SQ nodule, induration, warmth, pruritus, arm motion limitation. (Systemic) headache, respiratory difficulty, fever, malaise, myalgia, fever, anorexia, nausea, vomiting.

INTERACTIONS: Possible inadequate immunization with immunosuppressives. Chemotherapy, high-dose corticosteroid therapy >2 week duration, or radiation therapy may cause suboptimal vaccine response; defer vaccination until 3 months after completion of therapy.

PREGNANCY: Category D, safety in nursing not known.

MECHANISM OF ACTION: Not established; producing of antibodies that are raised against protective antigen, which may contribute to protection by neutralizing the activities of the toxin.

BLENOXANE   RX
bleomycin sulfate (Bristol-Myers Squibb)

> Pulmonary fibrosis is the most severe toxicity reported (usually presents as pneumonitis occasionally progressing to pulmonary fibrosis); higher occurrence in elderly and if receiving >400 units total dose. A severe idiosyncratic reaction including hypotension, mental confusion, fever, chills, and wheezing reported in lymphoma patients. Administer only under supervision of a physician experienced in the use of antineoplastic agents.

THERAPEUTIC CLASS: Cytotoxic glycopeptide antibiotic

Bleph-10

INDICATIONS: Palliative treatment of squamous cell carcinoma (eg, head and neck, penis, cervix, vulva), Hodgkin's Disease, non-Hodgkin's lymphoma, testicular carcinoma (embryonal cell, choriocarcinoma, teratocarcinoma). As a sclerosing agent for treatment of malignant pleural effusion and prevention of recurrent pleural effusions.

DOSAGE: *Adults:* Squamous Cell Carcinoma/Non-Hodgkin's Lymphoma/Testicular Carcinoma: 0.25-0.5U/kg IV/IM/SQ weekly or twice weekly. For lymphoma patients, give ≤2U for the 1st two doses; continue with regular dosage schedule if no acute reaction occurs. Hodgkin's Disease: 0.25-0.5U/kg IV/IM/SQ weekly or twice weekly. Maint: After 50% response, give 1U/day or 5U weekly IV/IM. Malignant Pleural Effusion: 60U as a single dose bolus intrapleural injection.

HOW SUPPLIED: Inj: 15 U, 30 U

WARNINGS/PRECAUTIONS: Extreme caution with significant renal impairment or compromised pulmonary function. Pulmonary toxicity (dose and age related) may occur; frequent roentgenograms are recommended. Monitor for severe idiosyncratic reactions, especially after 1st and 2nd doses. Renal and hepatic toxicity reported. Can cause fetal harm during pregnancy. Risk of pulmonary toxicity with total dose >400 U. Caution with dose selection in elderly.

ADVERSE REACTIONS: Pneumonitis, erythema, rash, striae, vesiculation, hyperpigmentation, skin tenderness, hyperkeratosis, nail changes, alopecia, pruritus, stomatitis, pulmonary toxicity.

INTERACTIONS: In combination with other antineoplastics, pulmonary toxicities may occur at lower doses.

PREGNANCY: Category D, not for use in nursing.

MECHANISM OF ACTION: Cytotoxic glycopeptide antibiotic; not established, suspected to inhibit DNA, RNA, and protein synthesis.

PHARMACOKINETICS: Absorption: Rapid, T_{max}=30-60min. (IM): Systemic bioavailability (100%). (SC): Systemic bioavailability (70%). [Intraperitoneal (IP), intrapleural (IPL)]: Systemic bioavailability (45%). **Distribution:** V_d=17.5L/m². **Metabolism:** Inactivated by bleomycin hydrolase. **Elimination:** Kidney. (IV): $T_{1/2}$=2 hrs. (IV): Urine (65%). (IPL): Urine (40%).

Bleph-10   RX

sulfacetamide sodium (Allergan)

OTHER BRAND NAMES: AK-Sulf (Akorn)

THERAPEUTIC CLASS: Sulfonamide

INDICATIONS: (Oint, Sol) Treatment of conjunctivitis and other superficial ocular infections. (Sol) Adjunct to systemic sulfonamide therapy of trachoma.

DOSAGE: *Adults:* Conjunctivitis/Superficial Infections: (Sol) 1-2 drops q2-3h initially. (Oint) Apply 1/2 inch q3-4h and hs. Taper dose by decreasing frequency with improvement. Treat for 7-10 days. Trachoma: (Sol) 2 drops q2h with systemic therapy.
Pediatrics: ≥2 months: Conjunctivitis/Superficial Infections: (Sol) 1-2 drops q2-3h initially. (Oint) Apply 1/2 inch q3-4h and hs. Taper dose by decreasing frequency with improvement. Treat for 7-10 days. Trachoma: (Sol) 2 drops q2h with systemic therapy.

HOW SUPPLIED: Oint: (AK-Sulf) 10% [3.5g]; Sol: (Bleph-10) 10% [5mL, 15mL]

WARNINGS/PRECAUTIONS: Fatalities reported from severe reactions to sulfonamides. D/C if develop sign of hypersensitivity. Ointments may retard corneal wound healing.

ADVERSE REACTIONS: Local irritation, stinging, burning.

INTERACTIONS: Incompatible with silver preparations.

PREGNANCY: Category C, not for use in nursing.

MECHANISM OF ACTION: Sulfonamide; inhibits bacterial synthesis of dihydrofolic acid by preventing the condensation of the pteridine with aminobenzoic acid through competitive inhibition of the enzyme dihydropteroate synthetase.

BLEPHAMIDE RX

sulfacetamide sodium - prednisolone acetate (Allergan)

OTHER BRAND NAMES: Blephamide S.O.P. (Allergan)

THERAPEUTIC CLASS: Sulfonamide/corticosteroid

INDICATIONS: For steroid-responsive inflammatory ocular conditions associated with bacterial infection or risks of bacterial infection (eg, corneal injury).

DOSAGE: *Adults:* (Sus) 2 drops into conjunctival sac q4h and qhs. (Oint) Apply 1/2 inch into conjunctival sac tid-qid and qd-bid at night. Re-evaluate if no improvement after 2 days. Decrease dose as condition improves. Max: 20mL or 8g prescribed initially.
Pediatrics: ≥6 yrs: (Sus) 2 drops into conjunctival sac q4h and qhs. (Oint) Apply 1/2 inch into conjunctival sac tid-qid and qd-bid at night. Re-evaluate if no improvement after 2 days. Decrease dose as condition improves. Max: 20mL or 8g prescribed initially.

HOW SUPPLIED: (Sulfacetamide-Prednisolone) Oint: 10%-0.2% [3.5g]; Sus: 10%-0.2% [5mL, 10mL]

CONTRAINDICATIONS: Most viral diseases of the cornea and conjunctiva (eg, epithelial herpes simplex keratitis, vaccinia, and varicella), mycobacterial infection of the eye, fungal diseases of ocular structures.

WARNINGS/PRECAUTIONS: Not for injection. Ocular HTN, glaucoma, secondary infections may occur with prolonged use. Acute anterior uveitis may occur. May mask or enhance infection with acute purulent conditions. Caution with glaucoma, treatment of herpes simplex. Monitor IOP. Staphylococcal isolates may be resistant to sulfonamides. Not effective in mustard gas keratitis and Sjogren's keratoconjunctivitis. Sensitization may recur with sulfonamides. May delay healing after cataract surgery. Fatalities reported due to adverse effects.

ADVERSE REACTIONS: Local irritation, intraocular pressure elevation, acute anterior uveitis, mydriasis, allergic sensitization (Stevens-Johnson syndrome, toxic epidermal necrolysis, fulminant hepatic necrosis, etc.).

INTERACTIONS: Incompatible with silver preparations. Local anesthetics related to p-amino benzoic acid may antagonize sulfonamides.

PREGNANCY: Category C, not for use in nursing.

MECHANISM OF ACTION: Prednisolone: Corticosteroid; suppresses inflammatory response and probably delays or slows healing. Sulfacetamide: Antibacterial; exerts bacteriostatic effect by restricting synthesis of folic acid required for growth through competition with p-aminobenzoic acid.

BONIVA RX

ibandronate sodium (Roche)

THERAPEUTIC CLASS: Bisphosphonate

INDICATIONS: (Inj) Treatment of osteoporosis in postmenopausal women. (PO) Treatment and prevention of postmenopausal osteoporosis.

DOSAGE: *Adults:* Inj: 3mg IV over 15-30 sec every 3 months. PO: 2.5mg qd or 150mg once monthly. Swallow whole with 6-8oz. of water. Do not lie down for 60 min after dose. Take at least 60 min before 1st food, drink (other than water), medication, or supplementation.

HOW SUPPLIED: Inj: 3mg/3mL; Tab: 2.5mg, 150mg

CONTRAINDICATIONS: (Inj, PO) Hypocalcemia. (PO) Inability to stand or sit upright for at least 60 min.

WARNINGS/PRECAUTIONS: (Inj, PO) Not recommended in severe renal impairment (CrCl <30mL/min). Reports of osteonecrosis, primarily in the jaw, and severe, incapacitating bone, joint, and/or muscle pain. (PO) May cause upper GI disorders (eg, dysphagia, esophagitis, esophageal or gastric ulcer).

ADVERSE REACTIONS: (Inj) Influenza, nasopharyngitis, cystitis, gastroenteritis, UTI, abdominal pain, dysepsia, nausea, constipation, arthralgia, back pain, HTN. (PO) Back pain, extremity pain, infection, dyspepsia, diarrhea, hypercholesterolemia, myalgia, headache, dizziness, upper respiratory infection, bronchitis, pneumonia, UTI.

INTERACTIONS: (PO) Calcium and other multivalent cations may interfere with absorption.

PREGNANCY: Category C, caution in nursing.

MECHANISM OF ACTION: Bisphosphonate; has affinity for hydroxyapatite, a component of the mineral matrix of the bone. Inhibits osteoclast activity and reduces bone resorption and turnover.

PHARMACOKINETICS: Absorption: (PO): T_{max}=0.5-2 hrs. **Distribution:** V_d=90L. Serum protein binding (85.7-99.5%). **Elimination:** (IV, PO): Kidney (50-60%); (PO): feces (unabsorbed dose); (PO)(150mg): $T_{1/2}$=37-157 hrs; (IV, 2mg): $T_{1/2}$=6.6-15.3 hrs; (IV, 4mg): $T_{1/2}$=5-25.5 hrs.

BONTRIL SLOW-RELEASE

phendimetrazine tartrate (Valeant)

OTHER BRAND NAMES: Bontril PDM (Valeant)

THERAPEUTIC CLASS: Anorectic sympathomimetic amine

INDICATIONS: Short-term adjunct treatment of exogenous obesity.

DOSAGE: *Adults:* (Slow-Release) 105mg qam, 30-60 min before breakfast. (PDM) 35mg bid-tid, 1 hr before meals; may reduce to 17.5mg/dose. Max: 70mg tid.
Pediatrics: ≥12 yrs: (Slow-Release) 105mg qam, 30-60 min before breakfast. (PDM) 35mg bid-tid, 1 hr before meals; may reduce to 17.5mg/dose. Max: 70mg tabs tid.

HOW SUPPLIED: Cap, Extended-Release: (Slow-Release) 105mg; Tab: (PDM) 35mg* *scored

CONTRAINDICATIONS: Advanced arteriosclerosis, symptomatic cardiovascular disease, moderate and severe HTN, hyperthyroidism, glaucoma, agitated states, history of drug abuse, concomitant CNS stimulants including MAOIs.

WARNINGS/PRECAUTIONS: Tolerance to anorectic effect develops within a few weeks, d/c if this occurs. Fatigue and depression with abrupt withdrawal after prolonged high dose therapy. Caution with mild HTN.

ADVERSE REACTIONS: Palpitation, tachycardia, BP elevation, overstimulation, restlessness, dizziness, dry mouth, diarrhea, constipation, nausea, libido changes, dysuria, insomnia.

INTERACTIONS: Hypertensive crisis if used within 14 days of MAOIs. May decrease hypotensive effects of guanethidine. May alter insulin requirements.

PREGNANCY: Not for use in pregnancy, safety in nursing not known.

MECHANISM OF ACTION: Anorectic sympathomimetic amine; CNS stimulant, elevates BP. As anorectic, appetite suppression as primary action not established.

PHARMACOKINETICS: Elimination: Urine; $T_{1/2}$=9.8 hrs (slow release), 3.7 hrs (PDM).

BOOSTRIX
RX

pertussis vaccine, acellular - diphtheria toxoid - tetanus toxoid
(GlaxoSmithKline)

THERAPEUTIC CLASS: Vaccine/toxoid combination

INDICATIONS: Active booster immunization against tetanus, diphtheria, and pertussis as a single dose in individuals 10-18 yrs of age.

DOSAGE: *Pediatrics:* 10-18 yrs: 0.5mL IM into the deltoid muscle.

HOW SUPPLIED: Inj: (Tetanus-Diphtheria-Pertussis) 5LF-2.5LF-8mcg/0.5mL.

CONTRAINDICATIONS: Hypersensitivity to any component; serious allergic reaction (eg, anaphylaxis) associated with previous dose. Encephalopathy not due to an identifiable cause within 7 days prior to pertussis immunization and progressive neurologic disorder, uncontrolled epilepsy, or progressive encephalopathy.

WARNINGS/PRECAUTIONS: May cause allergic reactions in latex sensitive patients. Caution if within 48 hrs of fever ≥105°F not due to another identifiable cause; collapse or shock-like state; persistent, inconsolable crying lasting ≥3 hrs. Caution if within 3 days of seizure with or without fever. Do not administer in patients with bleeding disorders such as hemophilia or thrombocytopenia, or patients on anticoagulant therapy unless potential benefit outweighs risk. Caution if Guillain-Barre syndrome within 6 weeks of tetanus toxoid vaccine. Do not give Td, Tdap, or emergency dose of Td more frequently then every 10 yrs if patient has experienced Arthus-type reaction. Hypersensitivity reaction possible; epinephrine injection (1:1000) should be readily available.

ADVERSE REACTIONS: Local: pain, redness, swelling. Systemic: headache, fatigue, fever, nausea, vomiting, diarrhea, abdominal pain.

INTERACTIONS: Immunosuppressive therapies, including irradiation, antimetabolites, alkylating agents, cytotoxic drugs, and corticosteroids may reduce the immune response to vaccines.

PREGNANCY: Category C, caution in nursing.

MECHANISM OF ACTION: Stimulates immune system to elicit immune response, which produces antibodies that may protect against tetanus, diphtheria, and pertussis.

Bravelle
urofollitropin (Ferring)

RX

THERAPEUTIC CLASS: Follicle stimulating hormone

INDICATIONS: With hCG, to induce ovulation in patients who previously received pituitary suppression. With hCG, for multiple follicular development (controlled ovarian stimulation) during assisted reproductive technologies (ART) cycles in patients who previously received pituitary suppression.

DOSAGE: *Adults:* Ovulation Induction: Initial: 150 IU SQ/IM qd for 1st 5 days. Adjust subsequent dose to individual response at intervals no less than every 2 days and not exceeding 75-150 IU/adjustment. Max: 450 IU/day. Dosing >12 days is not recommended. If adequate response, give 5000-10,000 U hCG 1 day following last dose. May repeat course if inadequate follicle development or ovulation without pregnancy occurs. ART: 225 IU SQ qd for 1st 5 days. Adjust subsequent dose to individual response at intervals no less than every 2 days and not exceeding 75-150 IU/adjustment. Max: 450 IU/day. Dosing >12 days is not recommended. If adequate follicular development, give 5000-10,000 U hCG to induce final follicular maturation in preparation for oocyte retrieval.

HOW SUPPLIED: Inj: 75 IU

CONTRAINDICATIONS: High FSH levels indicating primary ovarian failure, uncontrolled thyroid or adrenal dysfunction, organic intracranial lesions (eg, pituitary tumor), any cause of infertility other than anovulation, abnormal bleeding of undetermined origin, ovarian cysts or enlargement not due to polycystic ovary syndrome, pregnancy.

WARNINGS/PRECAUTIONS: Exclude primary ovarian failure. Ovarian enlargement may occur; monitor ovarian response. Ovarian hyperstimulation syndrome (OHSS), multiple births, hypersensitivity/anaphylactic reactions, serious pulmonary and vascular complications reported. Avoid hCG if ovaries

B

are abnormally enlarged on last day of therapy. Monitor follicle growth and maturation with estradiol levels and ultrasonography.

ADVERSE REACTIONS: OHSS, vaginal hemorrhage, pelvic pain, nausea, headache, pain, UTI, respiratory disorder, hot flashes, abdominal enlargement or pain.

PREGNANCY: Category X, not for use in nursing.

MECHANISM OF ACTION: Follicle stimulating hormone; produces ovarian follicular growth.

PHARMACOKINETICS: Absorption: C_{max}=6.0mIU/mL (SC); 8.8mIU/mL (IM). T_{max}=20.5 hrs (SC); 17.4 hrs (IM). AUC=379mIU•hr/mL (SC); 331mIU•hr/mL (IM). **Elimination:** $T_{1/2}$=31.8 hrs (SC); 37 hrs (IM).

BREVIBLOC   RX
esmolol HCL (Baxter)

THERAPEUTIC CLASS: Selective beta$_1$-blocker

INDICATIONS: For rapid control of ventricular rate in atrial fibrillation or atrial flutter in perioperative, postoperative, or other emergent circumstances. For noncompensatory sinus tachycardia. Treatment of tachycardia and hypertension that occur during induction and tracheal intubation, during surgery, on emergence from anesthesia, and in the postoperative period.

DOSAGE: *Adults:* Supraventricular Tachycardia: Titrate dose based on ventricular rate. Load: 0.5mg/kg over 1 min. Maint: 0.05mg/kg/min for next 4 min. May increase by 0.05mg/kg/min at intervals of 4 min or more up to 0.2mg/kg/min. Rapid slowing of ventricular response: Repeat 0.5mg/kg load over 1 min, then 0.1mg/kg/min for 4 min. If needed, another (final) load of 0.5mg/kg over 1 min, then 0.15mg/kg/min for 4 min up to 0.2mg/kg/min. May continue infusions for 24-48hrs. Intraoperative/Postoperative Tachycardia and/or HTN: Immediate Control: Initial: 80mg bolus over 30 sec. Maint: 0.15mg/kg/min. May titrate up to 0.3mg/kg/min. Gradual Control: Initial: 0.5mg/kg over 1 min. Maint: 0.05mg/kg/min for 4 min. Then, if needed, may repeat load and increase to 0.1mg/kg/min.

HOW SUPPLIED: Inj: 10mg/mL [10mL, 250mL], 20mg/mL [5mL, 100mL]

CONTRAINDICATIONS: Sinus bradycardia, heart block greater than first degree, cardiogenic shock or overt heart failure.

WARNINGS/PRECAUTIONS: Hypotension may occur; monitor BP and reduce dose or d/c if needed. May cause cardiac failure; withdraw at 1st sign of impending cardiac failure. Caution with supraventricular arrhythmias when patient is compromised hemodynamically or is taking other drugs that decrease peripheral resistance, myocardial filling/contractility, and/or electrical impulse propagation in the myocardium. Not for HTN associated with hypothermia. Caution in bronchospastic diseases; titrate to lowest possible effective dose and terminate immediately in the event of bronchospasm. Caution in diabetics; may mask tachycardia occurring with hypoglycemia. Caution in impaired renal function. Avoid concentrations >10mg/mL and infusions into small veins or through butterfly catheters. Sloughing of skin and necrosis reported with infiltration and extravasation. Use caution when discontinuing infusion in CAD patients.

ADVERSE REACTIONS: Hypotension, dizziness, diaphoresis, somnolence, confusion, headache, agitation, bronchospasm, nausea, infusion site reactions.

INTERACTIONS: Additive effects with catecholamine-depleting agents (eg, reserpine); monitor for hypotension or bradycardia. Levels increased by warfarin or morphine; titrate with caution. May increase digoxin levels; titrate with caution. May prolong effects of succinylcholine; titrate with caution. Caution when using with verapamil in depressed myocardial function; fatal cardiac arrest may occur. Do not use to control supraventricular tachycardia with vasoconstrictive and inotropic agents (eg, dopamine, epinephrine, norepinephrine) because of the danger of blocking cardiac contractility when systemic vascular resistance is high. Patients with a history of severe anaphylactic reaction may be more reactive to repeated challenge and unresponsive to the usual doses of epinephrine used to treat allergic reaction.

PREGNANCY: Category C, caution in nursing.

MECHANISM OF ACTION: Selective β_1 blocker: inhibits β_1 receptors located chiefly in cardiac muscle, and at higher doses begins to inhibit β_2 receptors located chiefly in the bronchial and vascular musculature.

PHARMACOKINETICS: Distribution: Plasma protein bound (55%). **Metabolism:** Rapid. Through hydrolysis of the ester linkage in red blood cells to methanol and free acid. **Elimination:** Urine (73-88%, unchanged). $T_{1/2}$ = 9 min. (Brevibloc), and 3.7 hrs. (acid metabolites).

BREVITAL
methohexital sodium (King)
CIV

> Should be used only in hospital or ambulatory care settings that provide for continuous monitoring of respiratory and cardiac function. Immediate availability of resuscitative drugs and age- and size-appropriate equipment for bag/valve/mask ventilation and intubation and personnel trained in their use and skilled in airway management should be assured. For deeply sedated patients, a designated individual other than practitioner performing procedure should be present to continuously monitor patient.

THERAPEUTIC CLASS: Barbiturate

INDICATIONS: IV induction of anesthesia prior to the use of other general anesthetic agents. IV induction of anesthesia and as adjunct to subpotent inhalational anesthetic agents (such as nitrous oxide in oxygen) for short surgical procedures. For use along with other parenteral agents, usually narcotic analgesics, to supplement subpotent inhalational anesthetic agents (such as nitrous oxide in oxygen) for longer surgical procedures. IV anesthesia for short surgical, diagnostic, or therapeutic procedures associated with minimal painful stimuli. Agent for inducing a hypnotic state. Pediatrics (>1 month): Rectal or IM induction of anesthesia prior to the use of other general anesthetic agents; rectal or IM induction of anesthesia and as adjunct to subpotent inhalational anesthetic agents for surgical procedures; rectal or IM anesthesia for short surgical, diagnostic, or therapeutic procedures associated with minimal painful stimuli.

DOSAGE: *Adults:* Individualize dose. Induction: 1% sol administered at rate of 1mL/5 sec. Range: 50-120mg or more (average: 70mg). Usual dose: 1-1.5mg/kg. Maint: Intermittent: 20-40mg (2-4mL of 1% sol) q 4-7 min. Continuous drip: Average rate of administration is 3mL of a 0.2% sol/min (1 drop/sec).
Pediatrics: ≥1 month: Individualize dose: Induction: IM: 6.6 to 10mg/kg IM of 5% concentration. Rectal: 25mg/kg rectally of the 1% sol.

HOW SUPPLIED: Inj: 500mg, 2.5g

CONTRAINDICATIONS: Patients with latent or manifest porphyria.

WARNINGS/PRECAUTIONS: Seizures may be elicited in patients with previous history of convulsive activity. Caution in severe hepatic dysfunction, severe cardiovascular instability, shock-like condition, asthma, COPD, severe HTN or hypotension, MI, CHF, severe anemia, status asthmaticus, extreme obesity, debilitated patients or those with impaired function of respiratory, circulatory, renal, hepatic, or endocrine system. Unintended intra-arterial injection may produce platelet aggregates and thrombosis at site of injection.

ADVERSE REACTIONS: Circulatory depression, thrombophlebitis, hypotension, tachycardia, respiratory depression, skeletal muscle hypersensitivity (twitching), emergence delirium.

INTERACTIONS: May influence metabolism of other concomitantly used drugs, such as phenytoin, halothane, anticoagulants, corticosteroids, ethyl alcohol, and propylene glycol-containing solutions. Prior chronic administration of barbituates or phenytoin may reduce effectiveness of methohexital. Additive CNS effects with other CNS depressants, including ethyl alcohol and propylene alcohol.

PREGNANCY: Category B, caution in nursing.

B

MECHANISM OF ACTION: Ultra-short acting barbiturate anesthetic; rapid uptake by the brain and rapid induction of sleep.

PHARMACOKINETICS: Absorption: Pediatrics: (IM) C_{max}=3mcg/mL; T_{max}=15 min. (PR) C_{max}=6.9-7.9mcg/mL; T_{max}=15 min; absolute bioavailability (17%). **Metabolism:** Liver; (demethylation and oxidation). **Elimination:** Urine.

BREVOXYL RX
benzoyl peroxide (Stiefel)

THERAPEUTIC CLASS: Antibacterial/keratolytic

INDICATIONS: Topical treatment of mild to moderate acne vulgaris.

DOSAGE: *Adults:* (Gel) Apply qd-bid to clean affected area. (Lot) Shake well. Wet affected area and wash qd for 1st week, then bid thereafter if tolerated. *Pediatrics:* ≥12 yrs: (Gel) Apply qd-bid to clean affected area. (Lot) Shake well. Wet affected area and wash qd for 1st week, then bid thereafter if tolerated.

HOW SUPPLIED: Gel: 4%, 8% [42.5g, 90g]; Lot: (Cleanser) 4%, 8% [297g]; Lot: (Creamy Wash) 4%, 8% [170g]

WARNINGS/PRECAUTIONS: Avoid contact with hair, eyes, mucous membranes, carpeting, and fabrics.

ADVERSE REACTIONS: Erythema, peeling.

PREGNANCY: Category C, caution in nursing.

MECHANISM OF ACTION: Antibacterial/keratolytic agent; not established; demonstrated activity against *Propionibacterium acnes*. Has also shown to have a mild keratolytic effect.

PHARMACOKINETICS: Absorption: Absorbed by skin. **Metabolism:** Metabolized in skin to benzoic acid. **Elimination:** Urine (benzoate; metabolite).

BROMFED RX
pseudoephedrine HCL - brompheniramine maleate (Muro)

OTHER BRAND NAMES: Bromfenex-PD (Ethex) - Bromfenex (Ethex) - Bromfed-PD (Muro)

THERAPEUTIC CLASS: Antihistamine/decongestant

INDICATIONS: Treatment of symptoms of seasonal and perennial allergic rhinitis, and vasomotor rhinitis, including nasal congestion.

DOSAGE: *Adults:* (12mg-120mg) 1 cap q12h. (6mg-60mg) 1-2 caps q12h. *Pediatrics:* ≥12 yrs: (12mg-120mg) 1 cap q12h. (6mg-60mg) 1-2 caps q12h. 6-11 yrs: (6mg-60mg) 1 cap q12h.

HOW SUPPLIED: (Brompheniramine-Pseudoephedrine) Cap, Extended-Release: (PD) 6mg- 60mg, (Bromfed, Bromfenex) 12mg-120mg

CONTRAINDICATIONS: Severe HTN, CAD, narrow-angle glaucoma, MAOI therapy, urinary retention, peptic ulcer, during an asthmatic attack.

WARNINGS/PRECAUTIONS: Caution with HTN, DM, ischemic heart disease, hyperthyroidism, increased IOP, prostatic hypertrophy, and elderly. Caution while operating machinery.

ADVERSE REACTIONS: Drowsiness, lassitude, nausea, giddiness, dryness of the mouth, blurred vision, palpitations, flushing, increased irritability or excitement.

INTERACTIONS: Potentiated by MAOIs and β-blockers. Reduced antihypertensive effects of methyldopa, mecamylamine, reserpine, and veratrum alkaloids. Additive effects with alcohol and other CNS depressants.

PREGNANCY: Safety in pregnancy and nursing not known.

MECHANISM OF ACTION: Brompheniramine: Histamine antagonist; specifically an H₁-receptor blocking agent, also has anticholinergic and sedative effects and antagonizes the allergic response of nasal tissues. Pseudoephedrine: Sympathomimetic; acts predominantly on α-receptor, has a little action on β-receptor. Functions as an oral nasal decongestant with minimal CNS stimulation.

BROVANA
arformoterol tartrate (Sepracor)

RX

> Long-acting β₂-adrenergic agonists may increase the risk of asthma-related death.

THERAPEUTIC CLASS: Beta₂-agonist

INDICATIONS: Long-term maintenance treatment of bronchoconstriction in patients with COPD, including chronic bronchitis and emphysema.

DOSAGE: *Adults:* Usual: 15mcg bid (am and pm). Max: 30mcg/day. Administer via nebulizer.

HOW SUPPLIED: Sol, Inhalation: 15mcg/2mL [30ˢ, 60ˢ]

CONTRAINDICATIONS: Hypersensitivity to racemic formoterol

WARNINGS/PRECAUTIONS: Not indicated for treatment of acute episodes of bronchospasm. Should not be initiated or used in children or patients with acutely deteriorating COPD. Fatalities reported with excessive use of inhaled sympathomimetics, avoid use with other long-acting β₂-agonists. D/C regular use of short acting β₂-agonists (eg, qid) before initiating therapy. May produce life-threatening paradoxical bronchospasm. Caution in patients with convulsive disorders, thyrotoxicosis, cardiovascular disorders especially coronary insufficiency, cardiac arrhythmias, and HTN. Immediate hypersensitivity reactions may occur.

ADVERSE REACTIONS: Pain, chest pain, back pain , diarrhea, sinusitis, leg cramps, dyspnea, rash, flu syndrome, peripheral edema.

INTERACTIONS: Sympathetic effects may be potentiated with concomitant use of additional adrenergic agonists. Concomitant use with methylxanthines, steroids, or diuretics may potentiate hypokalemia. Caution with co-administration with non-potassium sparing diuretics may cause ECG changes. Use extreme caution in patients being treated with MAOIs, TCAs, or any drugs known to prolong the QTc interval. Caution with β-blockers.

PREGNANCY: Category C, caution in nursing.

MECHANISM OF ACTION: β₂-adrenergic agonist. Stimulates intracellular adenyl cyclase, which catalyzes conversion of ATP to cAMP to produce relaxation of bronchial smooth muscle and inhibition of release of mediators of immediate hypersensitivity from cells (mast cells).

PHARMACOKINETICS: Absorption: C_{max}=4.3pg/mL, AUC=34.5pg•hr/mL, T_{max}=30 min. **Distribution:** Plasma protein binding (52-65%). **Metabolism:** Glucoronidation (major) via uridine diphosphoglucuronosyltransferase (UGT) isoenzymes, O-demethylation (minor) via CYP2D6, CYP2C19. **Elimination:** Urine (1%); $T_{1/2}$=26 hrs.

BUMETANIDE
bumetanide (Various)

RX

> Can lead to profound water and electrolyte depletion with excessive use.

OTHER BRAND NAMES: Bumex (Roche Labs)

THERAPEUTIC CLASS: Loop diuretic

INDICATIONS: Treatment of edema associated with CHF, hepatic disease, and renal disease including nephrotic syndrome.

DOSAGE: *Adults:* ≥18 yrs: PO: Usual: 0.5-2mg qd. Maint: May give every other day or every 3-4 days. Max: 10mg/day. IV/IM: Initial: 0.5-1mg over 1-2 min, may repeat every 2-3 hrs for 2-3 doses. Max: 10mg/day. Elderly: Start at low end of dosing range.

HOW SUPPLIED: Inj: 0.25mg/mL; Tab: 0.5mg*, 1mg*, 2mg* *scored

CONTRAINDICATIONS: Anuria, hepatic coma, severe electrolyte depletion.

WARNINGS/PRECAUTIONS: Monitor for volume/electrolyte depletion, hypokalemia, blood dyscrasias, hepatic damage. Elderly are prone to volume/electrolyte depletion. Caution in elderly, hepatic cirrhosis and ascites. Associated with ototoxicity, hypocalcemia, thrombocytopenia, hypomagnesemia, hypokalemia, and hyperuricemia. Hypersensitivity with sulfonamide allergy. D/C if marked increase in BUN or creatinine or if develop oliguria with progressive renal disease.

ADVERSE REACTIONS: Muscle cramps, dizziness, hypotension, headache, nausea, hyperuricemia, hypokalemia, hyponatremia, hyperglycemia, azotemia, increase serum creatinine.

INTERACTIONS: Avoid aminoglycosides, ototoxic and nephrotoxic drugs, indomethacin. Lithium toxicity. Probenecid reduces effects. Potentiates antihypertensives.

PREGNANCY: Category C, not for use in nursing.

MECHANISM OF ACTION: Loop diuretic; inhibits sodium reabsorption in ascending loop of Henle.

PHARMACOKINETICS: Absorption: (IV) T_{max}=15-30 min. (Tab) T_{max}=1-2 hrs. **Distribution:** Plasma protein binding (94-96%). **Metabolism:** Oxidation. **Elimination:** Urine, bile (2%); $T_{1/2}$=1-1.5 hrs.

BUPRENEX CIII
buprenorphine HCL (Reckitt Benckiser)

THERAPEUTIC CLASS: Opioid analgesic

INDICATIONS: Relief of moderate to severe pain.

DOSAGE: *Adults:* 0.3mg IM/IV q6h prn. Repeat if needed, 30-60 min after initial dose and then prn. High Risk Patients/Concomitant CNS depressants: Reduce dose by approximately 50%. May use single doses ≤0.6mg IM if not at high-risk.
Pediatrics: ≥13 yrs: 0.3mg IM/IV q6h prn. Repeat if needed, 30-60 min after initial dose and then prn. High Risk Patients/Concomitant CNS depressants: Reduce dose by approximately 50%. May use single doses ≤0.6mg IM if not at high-risk. 2-12 yrs: 2-6mcg/kg IM/IV q4-6h.

HOW SUPPLIED: Inj: 0.3mg/mL

WARNINGS/PRECAUTIONS: Significant respiratory depression reported; caution with compromised respiratory function. May increase CSF pressure; caution with head injury, intracranial lesions. Caution with debilitated, BPH, biliary tract dysfunction, myxedema, hypothyroidism, urethral stricture, acute alcoholism, Addison's disease, CNS disease, coma, toxic psychoses, delirium tremens, elderly, pediatrics, kyphoscoliosis or hepatic/renal/pulmonary impairment. May impair mental or physical abilities. May precipitate withdrawal in narcotic-dependence. May lead to psychological dependence.

ADVERSE REACTIONS: Sedation, nausea, dizziness, sweating, hypotension, vomiting, headache, miosis, hypoventilation.

INTERACTIONS: Caution with MAOIs, CNS and respiratory depressants. Respiratory and cardiovascular collapse reported with diazepam. Increased CNS depression with other narcotic analgesics, general anesthetics, antihistamines, benzodiazepines, phenothiazines, other tranquilizers, sedative-hypnotics. Decreased clearance with CYP3A4 inhibitors (eg, macrolides, azole antifungals, protease inhibitors). Increased clearance with CYP3A4 inducers (eg, rifampin, carbamazepine, phenytoin).

PREGNANCY: Category C, not for use in nursing.

MECHANISM OF ACTION: Opioid analgesic; high affinity binding to μ opiate receptors in CNS. Possesses slow rate of dissociation from its receptor. Also possesses narcotic antagonist activity.

PHARMACOKINETICS: Absorption: T_{max}=1 hr. **Distribution:** Found in breast milk. **Metabolism:** Liver. **Elimination:** $T_{1/2}$=1.2-7.2 hrs.

BuSpar RX
buspirone HCL (Bristol-Myers Squibb)

THERAPEUTIC CLASS: Atypical anxiolytic

INDICATIONS: Management of anxiety disorders, short-term relief of anxiety symptoms.

DOSAGE: *Adults:* Usual: 7.5mg bid. Titrate: May increase by 5mg/day every 2-3 days. Usual: 20-30mg/day. Max: 60mg/day. Use low dose with potent CYP450 3A4 inhibitors (eg, 2.5mg qd with nefazodone). Take consistently with or without food; bioavailability increased with food.

HOW SUPPLIED: Tab: 5mg*, 10mg*, 15mg*, 30mg* *scored

WARNINGS/PRECAUTIONS: Avoid with hepatic or renal impairment.

ADVERSE REACTIONS: Dizziness, nausea, headache, nervousness, lightheadedness, excitement, dystonia, fatigue, parkinsonism, akathisia, restless leg syndrome, restlessness.

INTERACTIONS: Avoid MAOIs and alcohol. Withdraw other CNS depressants gradually before therapy. Caution with psychotropics. Elevated liver transaminases reported with trazodone. Increases haloperidol levels. Verapamil, diltiazem, grapefruit juice, nefazodone, itraconazole, cimetidine, erythromycin increase plasma levels. May increase levels of both drugs with nefazodone; decrease dose of buspirone. Decreased plasma levels and effects with rifampin; may need to adjust buspirone dose. CYP3A4 inhibitors may increase plasma levels and CYP3A4 inducers may increase metabolism of buspirone; may need dose adjustment. Presystemic clearance may be decreased with food. May displace digoxin.

PREGNANCY: Category B, not for use in nursing.

MECHANISM OF ACTION: Atypical antianxiety agent; not fully established. Binds with high affinity to serotonin receptors (5-HT$_{1A}$) and moderate affinity to dopamine receptors (D$_2$); may have indirect effects on other neurotransmitter systems.

PHARMACOKINETICS: Absorption: Rapid. C$_{max}$=1-6ng/mL; T$_{max}$=40-90 min. **Distribution:** Plasma protein binding (86%). **Metabolism:** CYP3A4; oxidation and hyroxylation; 1-pyrimidinylpiperazine (active metabolite). **Elimination:** Urine (29-63%), feces (18-38%); T$_{1/2}$=2-3 hrs.

Byetta RX
exenatide (Amylin/Lilly)

THERAPEUTIC CLASS: Incretin mimetic

INDICATIONS: Adjunctive therapy to improve glycemic control in patients with type 2 DM who are taking metformin, a sulfonylurea, a thiazolidinedione, a combination of metformin/sulfonylurea or metformin/thiazolidinedione, but have not achieved adequate glycemic control.

DOSAGE: *Adults:* 5mcg SQ bid, 60 min before am & pm meals. Titrate: May increase to 10mcg bid after 1 month. Reduction of sulfonylurea dose may be considered to reduce risk of hypoglycemia.

HOW SUPPLIED: Inj: 5mcg/dose, 10mcg/dose [60-dose prefilled pen]

WARNINGS/PRECAUTIONS: Not a substitute for insulin. Avoid with type 1 DM, treatment of diabetic ketoacidosis, ESRD, severe renal impairment (CrCl <30mL/min), or severe GI disease. Acute pancreatitis reported. Increased incidence of hypoglycemia with sulfonylureas. Observe for signs and symptoms of hypersensitivity reactions; patients with abdominal pain should be investigated. When used with thiazolidinediones possible CP and/or chronic hypersensitivity pneumonitis.

ADVERSE REACTIONS: Nausea, vomiting, diarrhea, feeling jittery, dizziness, headache, dyspepsia, injection-site reactions; dysgeusia, somnolence, generalized pruritus and/or urticaria, macular or papular rash, angioedema, rare reports of anaphylactic reaction, abdominal pain, hypoglycemia.

INTERACTIONS: Caution with drugs that require rapid GI absorption. Drugs dependent on threshold concentrations for efficacy (eg, contraceptives, antibiotics) should be taken 1 hr before. Caution with concomitant use of warfarin; may lead to increased INR and possible bleeding.

PREGNANCY: Category C, caution in nursing.

MECHANISM OF ACTION: Antihyperglycemic, incretin-mimetic agent; enhances glucose-dependent insulin secretion by the pancreatic β-cell, suppresses inappropriately elevated glucagon secretion and slows gastric emptying.

PHARMACOKINETICS: Absorption: (SC administration) mean C_{max}=211pg/mL, T_{max}=2.1 hrs. **Distribution:** V_d=28.3L. **Elimination:** mean $T_{1/2}$=2.4 hrs.

BYSTOLIC   RX
nebivolol (Forest)

THERAPEUTIC CLASS: Selective beta$_1$-blocker

INDICATIONS: Treatment of hypertension. May be used alone or in combination with other antihypertensive agents.

DOSAGE: *Adults:* Monotherapy/Combination Therapy: Initial: 5mg qd. Titrate: May increase dose if needed at 2-week intervals. Max: 40mg. Hepatic Impairment/CrCl <30mL/min: 2.5mg qd; upward titration may be performed cautiously.

HOW SUPPLIED: Tab: 2.5mg, 5mg, 10mg

CONTRAINDICATIONS: Severe bradycardia, heart block >1st degree, cardiogenic shock, decompensated cardiac failure, sick sinus syndrome (unless permanent pacemaker in place), severe hepatic impairment (Child-Pugh >B).

WARNINGS/PRECAUTIONS: Exacerbation of angina, and occurrence of MI and ventricular arrhythmias reported in patients with CAD following abrupt withdrawal; taper over 1-2 weeks when possible. Avoid with bronchospastic disease. Caution with compensated CHF; consider d/c if heart failure worsens. Caution with PVD, severe renal/moderate hepatic impairment. May mask signs/symptoms of hypoglycemia or hyperthyroidism. Abrupt withdrawal may also exacerbate symptoms of hyperthyroidism or precipitate a thyroid storm. Caution with history of severe anaphylactic reactions. Patients with known/suspected pheochromocytoma should initially receive an α-blocker prior to use of any β-blocker. No studies done in patients with angina pectoris, recent MI, or severe hepatic impairment.

ADVERSE REACTIONS: Headache, fatigue, dizziness, diarrhea, nausea.

INTERACTIONS: CYP2D6 inhibitors (eg, fluoxetine, quinidine, propafenone, paroxetine) may increase nebivolol levels; monitor and consider dosage adjustment. Sildenafil may decrease nebivolol levels. May depress myocardial function with anesthetic agents (eg, ether, cyclopropane, trichloroethylene); monitor closely. May potentiate hypoglycemic effect of glucose-lowering agents (eg, insulin, oral hypoglycemic agents); use with caution. Caution with calcium antagonists (particularly verapamil and diltiazem type) or antiarrhythmic agents (eg, disopyramide). Excessive reduction of sympathetic activity may occur with catecholamine-depleting drugs (eg, reserpine, guanethidine); monitor closely. D/C for several days before gradually tapering clonidine.

PREGNANCY: Category C, not for use in nursing.

MECHANISM OF ACTION: A β-adrenergic receptor blocking agent.

PHARMACOKINETICS: Administration: Bioavailability has not yet determined, mean C_{max} = 2mg, mean T_{max} = 1-4 hrs. **Distribution:** Plasma protein bound 98%. **Metabolism**: N-dealkylation and oxidation via P450 2D6. **Elimination**: 38% urine, 44% feces.

CADUET RX
atorvastatin calcium - amlodipine besylate (Pfizer)

THERAPEUTIC CLASS: Calcium channel blocker/HMG-CoA reductase inhibitor

INDICATIONS: When treatment with both amlodipine and atorvastatin is appropriate. (Amlodipine) Treatment of hypertension, chronic stable or vasospastic angina (Prinzmetal's or Variant Angina). (Atorvastatin) Adjunct to diet to reduce total cholesterol (total-C), LDL-C, TG, and Apo B levels, and to increase HDL-C in primary hypercholesterolemia (heterozygous familial and nonfamilial) and mixed dyslipidemia (Types IIa and IIb). Adjunct to diet for elevated serum TG levels (Type IV). Treatment of primary dysbetalipoproteinemia (Type III) inadequately responding to diet. Adjunct to other lipid-lowering treatments or if treatments are unavailable, to reduce total-C and LDL-C in homozygous familial hypercholesterolemia. Adjunct to diet to lower total-C, LDL-C and Apo B in boys and postmenarchal girls with heterozygous familial hypercholesterolemia.

DOSAGE: *Adults:* Dosing should be individualized and based on the appropriate combination of recommendations for the monotherapies. (Amlodipine): HTN: Initial: 5mg qd. Titrate over 7-14 days. Max: 10mg qd. Small, Fragile, or Elderly/Hepatic Dysfunction/Concomitant Antihypertensive: Initial: 2.5mg qd. Angina: 5-10mg qd. Elderly/Hepatic Dysfunction: 5mg qd. (Atorvastatin): Hypercholesterolemia/Mixed Dyslipidemia: Initial: 10-20mg qd (or 40mg qd for LDL-C reduction >45%). Titrate: Adjust dose if needed at 2-4 week intervals. Usual: 10-80mg qd. Homozygous Familial Hypercholesterolemia: 10-80mg qd.
Pediatrics: ≥10 yrs (postmenarchal): (Amlodipine): HTN: 2.5-5mg qd. 10-17 yrs (postmenarchal): (Atorvastatin): Heterozygous Familial Hypercholesterolemia: Initial: 10mg/day. Titrate: Adjust dose if needed at intervals of ≥4 weeks. Max: 20mg/day.

HOW SUPPLIED: Tab: (Amlodipine-Atorvastatin) 2.5mg-10mg, 2.5mg-20mg, 2.5mg-40mg, 5mg-10mg, 5mg-20mg, 5mg-40mg, 5mg-80mg, 10mg-10mg, 10mg-20mg, 10mg-40mg, 10mg-80mg

CONTRAINDICATIONS: Active liver disease, unexplained persistent elevations of serum transaminases, pregnancy, nursing mothers.

WARNINGS/PRECAUTIONS: May rarely increase angina or MI with severe obstructive CAD. Monitor LFTs prior to therapy, at 12 weeks after initiation, with dose elevation, and periodically thereafter. Reduce dose or withdraw if AST or ALT >3x ULN persist. Caution with heavy alcohol use and/or history of hepatic disease, severe aortic stenosis, CHF. D/C if markedly elevated CPK levels occur, if myopathy is diagnosed or suspected, or if predisposition to renal failure secondary to rhabdomyolysis. Increased risk of hemorrhagic stroke in patients with recent stroke or TIA.

ADVERSE REACTIONS: Headache, edema, palpitation, dizziness, fatigue, constipation, flatulence, dyspepsia, abdominal pain.

INTERACTIONS: Increases levels with erythromycin. Increases levels of oral contraceptives (norethindrone, ethinyl estradiol), digoxin. Cyclosporine, fibric acid derivatives, niacin, erythromycin, azole antifungals may increase risk of myopathy. Caution with drugs that decrease levels or activity of endogenous steroid hormones (eg, ketoconazole, spironolactone, cimetidine). Decreased levels with Maalox® TC, but LDL-C reduction not altered. Colestipol decreases levels when coadministered, but greater LDL-C reduction with coadministration than when each given alone. Avoid fibrates.

PREGNANCY: Category X, not for use in nursing

CAFCIT RX
caffeine citrate (Mead Johnson)

THERAPEUTIC CLASS: Methylxanthine

C

INDICATIONS: Short-term treatment of apnea of prematurity in infants.

DOSAGE: *Pediatrics:* 28-<33 weeks: LD: 1mL/kg (20mg/kg) IV over 30 min. Maint: 0.25mL/kg (5mg/kg) IV over 30 min or PO q24h beginning 24 hrs after LD.

HOW SUPPLIED: Inj: 20mg/mL [3mL]; Sol: 20mg/mL [3mL]

WARNINGS/PRECAUTIONS: Necrotizing enterocolitis, seizures reported. Rule out other possible causes of apnea before initiating therapy. Caution with CVD, seizure disorder, renal/hepatic impairment. Monitor baseline caffeine levels if previously exposed to theophylline.

ADVERSE REACTIONS: Feeding intolerance, sepsis, hemorrhage, necrotizing enterocolitis, gastritis, GI hemorrhage, DIC, acidosis, abnormal healing, dyspnea, cerebral hemorrhage, dyspnea, lung edema, dry skin, rash, skin breakdown, retinopathy of prematurity.

INTERACTIONS: Potential for interaction with CYP450 1A2 substrates, inducers, inhibitors. May need lower dose with cimetidine, ketoconazole. May need dose increase with phenobarbital, phenytoin.

PREGNANCY: Category C, safety in nursing not known.

MECHANISM OF ACTION: Bronchial smooth muscle relaxant, CNS stimulant, cardiac muscle stimulant, and diuretic. Preventing apnea in prematurity not established; believed it has been attributed to antagonism of adenosine receptors, both A_1 and A_2 subtypes.

PHARMACOKINETICS: Absorption: C_{max}=6-10mg/L, T_{max}=30 min-2 hrs. **Distribution:** V_d=0.8-0.9L/kg (infants), V_d=0.6L/kg (adults); plasma protein binding (approximately 36%); crosses placental barrier. **Metabolism:** Liver via CYP1A2. **Elimination:** Urine, (neonates) $T_{1/2}$=approximately 3-4 days, (86%) unchanged, (>9months, adults) $T_{1/2}$=5 hrs, (1%) unchanged.

CAFERGOT TABLETS   RX
ergotamine tartrate - caffeine (Sandoz)

> Serious and/or life-threatening peripheral ischemia has been associated with coadministration of Cafergot® with potent CYP3A4 inhibitors (eg, protease inhibitors, macrolide antibiotics). Because CYP3A4 inhibition elevates serum levels of Cafergot®, the risk for vasospasm leading to cerebral ischemia and/or ischemia of the extremities is increased. Concomitant use of these medications is contraindicated.

THERAPEUTIC CLASS: Ergot alkaloid

INDICATIONS: To abort or prevent vascular headaches.

DOSAGE: *Adults:* 2 tabs at start of attack. Repeat 1 tab every 1/2 hr prn. Max: 6 tabs/attack, 10 tabs/week. May give at bedtime as short-term preventive measure.

HOW SUPPLIED: Tab: (Ergotamine-Caffeine) 1mg-100mg

CONTRAINDICATIONS: Pregnancy, peripheral vascular disease, CHD, HTN, hepatic/renal dysfunction, coadministration with potent CYP3A4 inhibitors (eg, ritonavir, nelfinavir, erythromycin, clarithromycin, troleandomycin, ketoconazole, itraonazole).

WARNINGS/PRECAUTIONS: Do not exceed recommended dosage; ergotism may develop. Fibrotic complications (eg, retroperitoneal and/or pleuropulmonary fibrosis) reported.

ADVERSE REACTIONS: Precordial distress, transient tachycardia or bradycardia, nausea, vomiting, localized edema, itching, numbness/tingling of fingers/toes, muscle pain, leg weakness.

INTERACTIONS: See Black Box Warning. Avoid coadministration with potent CYP3A4 inhibitors (eg, protease inhibitors, macrolide anitbiotics). Coadministration with less potent CYP3A4 inhibitors (eg, saquinavir, nefazodone, fluconazole, fluoxetine, grapefruit juice, fluvoxamine, zileuton, metronidazole, clotrimazole) may lead to potential risk for serious toxicity, including vasospasm. Avoid coadministration with other vasoconstrictors. Use with sympathomimetics (pressor agents) may cause extreme BP elevation.

Propranolol may potentiate vasoconstrictive action. Nicotine may provoke vasoconstriction, predisposing to greater ischemic response.

PREGNANCY: Category X, not for use in nursing.

MECHANISM OF ACTION: Ergotamine: α-adrenergic blocker; directly stimulates smooth muscle of peripheral and cranial blood vessels and produces depression of central vasomotor center. Caffeine: Cranial vasodilator; enhances vasoconstrictive effect.

CALAN   RX
verapamil HCL (Pharmacia & Upjohn)

THERAPEUTIC CLASS: Calcium channel blocker (nondihydropyridine)

INDICATIONS: Treatment of hypertension and vasospastic, unstable and chronic stable angina. With digitalis, for control of ventricular rate at rest and during stress in patients with chronic atrial flutter and/or atrial fibrillation. Prophylaxis of repetitive paroxysmal supraventricular tachycardia.

DOSAGE: *Adults:* HTN: Initial: 80mg tid. Usual: 360-480mg/day. Elderly/Small Stature: Initial: 40mg tid. Angina: Usual: 80-120mg tid. Elderly/Small Stature: Initial: 40mg tid. Titrate: Increase daily or weekly. A-Fib (Digitalized): Usual: 240-320mg/day given tid-qid. PSVT Prophylaxis (Non-Digitalized): 240-480mg/day given tid-qid. Max: 480mg/day. Severe Hepatic Dysfunction: Give 30% of normal dose.

HOW SUPPLIED: Tab: 40mg, 80mg*, 120mg* *scored

CONTRAINDICATIONS: Severe ventricular dysfunction, hypotension, cardiogenic shock, sick sinus syndrome or 2nd- or 3rd-degree AV block (except with functioning ventricular pacemaker), A-Fib/Flutter with an accessory bypass tract.

WARNINGS/PRECAUTIONS: Avoid with moderate to severe cardiac failure, and ventricular dysfunction if taking a β-blocker. May cause hypotension, AV block, transient bradycardia, PR interval prolongation. Monitor LFTs periodically; hepatocellular injury reported. Caution with hypertrophic cardiomyopathy, renal or hepatic dysfunction. Decrease dose with decreased neuromuscular transmission.

ADVERSE REACTIONS: Constipation, dizziness, nausea, hypotension, headache, edema, CHF, fatigue, elevated liver enzymes, dyspnea, bradycardia, AV block, rash, flushing.

INTERACTIONS: Additive effects on HR, AV conduction, and contractility with β-blockers. Potentiates other antihypertensives. May increase digoxin, carbamazepine, theophylline, cyclosporine and alcohol levels. Avoid disopyramide within 48 hrs before or 24 hrs after verapamil. Additive negative inotropic effects and AV conduction prolongation with flecainide. Avoid quinidine with hypertrophic cardiomyopathy. Monitor lithium. Increased clearance with phenobarbital. Rifampin may reduce oral bioavailability. May potentiate neuromuscular blockers; both agents may need dose reduction.

PREGNANCY: Category C, not for use in nursing.

MECHANISM OF ACTION: Calcium channel blocker; modulates influx of ionic calcium across cell membrane of arterial smooth muscle, conductile and contractile myocardial cells.

PHARMACOKINETICS: Absorption: Bioavailability (20-35%), T_{max}=1-2 hrs. **Distribution:** Plasma protein binding (90%). **Metabolism:** Biotransformation. Norverapamil (metabolite). **Elimination:** Urine (3-4%), feces, $T_{1/2}$=4.5-12 hrs.

CALAN SR   RX
verapamil HCL (Pharmacia & Upjohn)

THERAPEUTIC CLASS: Calcium channel blocker (nondihydropyridine)

INDICATIONS: Treatment of hypertension.

DOSAGE: *Adults:* ≥18 yrs: Initial: 180mg qam. Titrate: If inadequate response, increase to 240mg qam, then 180mg bid; or 240mg qam plus 120mg qpm, then 240mg q12h. Elderly/Small Stature: Initial: 120mg qam. Take with food.

HOW SUPPLIED: Tab, Extended-Release: 120mg, 180mg*, 240mg* *scored

CONTRAINDICATIONS: Severe ventricular dysfunction, hypotension, cardiogenic shock, sick sinus syndrome or 2nd- or 3rd-degree AV block (except with functioning ventricular pacemaker), A-Fib/Flutter with an accessory bypass tract.

WARNINGS/PRECAUTIONS: Avoid with moderate to severe cardiac failure, and ventricular dysfunction if taking a β-blocker. May cause hypotension, AV block, transient bradycardia, PR interval prolongation. Monitor LFTs periodically; hepatocellular injury reported. Caution with hypertrophic cardiomyopathy, renal or hepatic dysfunction. Decrease dose with decreased neuromuscular transmission.

ADVERSE REACTIONS: Constipation, dizziness, nausea, hypotension, headache, edema, CHF, fatigue, elevated liver enzymes, dyspnea, bradycardia, AV block, rash, flushing.

INTERACTIONS: Additive effects on HR, AV conduction, and contractility with β-blockers. Potentiates other antihypertensives. May increase digoxin, carbamazepine, theophylline, cyclosporine, and alcohol levels. Avoid disopyramide within 48 hrs before or 24 hrs after verapamil. Additive negative inotropic effects and AV conduction prolongation with flecainide. Avoid quinidine with hypertrophic cardiomyopathy. Monitor lithium. Increased clearance with phenobarbital. Rifampin may reduce oral bioavailability. May potentiate neuromuscular blockers; both agents may need dose reduction.

PREGNANCY: Category C, not for use in nursing.

MECHANISM OF ACTION: Calcium channel blocker; modulates influx of ionic calcium across cell membrane of arterial smooth muscle and in conductile and contractile myocardial cells.

PHARMACOKINETICS: Absorption: Absolute bioavailability (20-35%); T_{max}=7.7 hrs; C_{max}=79ng/mL; AUC=841ng•h/mL. **Distribution:** Plasma protein binding (90%). **Metabolism:** Biotransformation; norverapamil (metabolite). **Elimination:** $T_{1/2}$=4.5-12 hrs; urine (3-4%), feces.

CAMPATH   RX
alemtuzumab (Bayer Healthcare)

> Cytopenias such as serious, including fatal, pancytopenia/marrow hypoplasia, autoimmune idiopathic thrombocytopenia, and autoimmune hemolytic anemia may occur; avoid single doses >30mg or cumulative doses >90mg/week. Serious, including fatal, infusion reactions can result; gradually escalate dose to prevent. Serious, including fatal, bacterial, viral, fungal, and protozoan infections can occur; administer prophylaxis against PCP and herpes virus infections.

THERAPEUTIC CLASS: Monoclonal antibody/CD52-blocker

INDICATIONS: As a single agent for the treatment of B-cell chronic lymphocytic leukemia (B-CLL).

DOSAGE: *Adults:* Administer as IV infusion over 2 hours. Initial: 3mg IV qd until tolerated, then increase to 10mg IV qd. Continue until tolerated, then increase to maint dose of 30mg (escalation to 30mg usually takes 3-7 days). Maint: 30mg/day IV 3x/week on alternate days up to 12 weeks. Max: 30mg single dose or 90mg/week. Refer to prescribing information for dose modifications for neutropenia or thrombocytopenia.

HOW SUPPLIED: Inj: 30mg/mL

WARNINGS/PRECAUTIONS: Premedicate with oral antihistamine, APAP to avoid infusion reactions. Monitor BP, hypotensive symptoms in ischemic heart disease, with antihypertensives. If serious infection occurs, withhold treatment until infection resolves. Monitor CBC, platelets weekly during therapy and CD4 counts after therapy. D/C for autoimmune or severe hematologic adverse reactions. Severe, including fatal, autoimmune anemia and thrombocytopenia, and prolonged myelosuppression reported. Hemolytic anemia, pure red cell aplasia, bone marrow aplasia, and hypoplasia reported. D/C for autoimmune cytopenias. Severe and prolonged lymphopenias with increased incidence of opportunistic infections reported. Administer PCP and herpes viral prophylaxis for a minimum of 2 months after completion or until CD4+ count is ≥200 cells/µL and monitor for CMV infection during and for at least 2 months after completion of treatment.

ADVERSE REACTIONS: Cytopenias, infusion reactions, cytomegalovirus (CMV) and other infections, nausea, emesis, diarrhea, insomnia.

INTERACTIONS: Avoid live viral vaccines.

PREGNANCY: Category C, not for use in nursing.

MECHANISM OF ACTION: Monoclonal antibody/CD52-blocker; binds to CD52 on surfaces of B and T lymphocytes, monocytes, macrophages, NK cells, granulocytes and bone marrow cells, causing antibody-dependent cellular-mediated cell death.

PHARMACOKINETICS: Distribution: V_d=0.18L/kg. **Elimination:** (1st dose): $T_{1/2}$=11 hrs. (Last dose): $T_{1/2}$=6 days.

CAMPRAL RX
acamprosate calcium (Forest)

THERAPEUTIC CLASS: GABA analog

INDICATIONS: Maintenance of abstinence from alcohol in patients with alcohol dependence who are abstinent at treatment initiation.

DOSAGE: *Adults:* 2 tabs tid. CrCl 30-50mL/min: 1 tab tid.

HOW SUPPLIED: Tab: 333mg

CONTRAINDICATIONS: Severe renal impairment (CrCl ≤30mL/min).

WARNINGS/PRECAUTIONS: Use does not eliminate or diminish withdrawal symptoms. Dose reduction required with renal impairment (CrCl ≤30-50mL/min). Suicidal events reported.

ADVERSE REACTIONS: Accidental injury, asthenia, pain, anorexia, diarrhea, flatulence, nausea, anxiety, depression, dizziness, dry mouth, insomnia, paresthesia, pruritus, sweating.

INTERACTIONS: Naltrexone may increase levels. Weight gain/weight loss may occur with antidepressants.

PREGNANCY: Category C, caution in nursing.

MECHANISM OF ACTION: GABA analogue; not completely understood; suspected to interact with glutamate and GABA neurotransmitter systems centrally, hypothesized that the drug restores this balance.

PHARMACOKINETICS: Absorption: Absolute bioavailability (11%). C_{max}=350ng/mL; T_{max}=3-8 hrs. **Distribution:** V_d=72-109L. **Elimination:** Urine. $T_{1/2}$=20-33 hrs.

CAMPTOSAR RX
irinotecan HCL (Pharmacia & Upjohn)

> Early and/or late forms of diarrhea, severe myelosuppression may occur. Interrupt and reduce subsequent doses if severe diarrhea occurs. Carefully monitor with diarrhea; give fluid/electrolyte replacement if dehydrated or give antibiotics if ileus, fever, or severe neutropenia develops.

THERAPEUTIC CLASS: Topoisomerase I inhibitor

INDICATIONS: First-line therapy in combination with 5-fluorouracil (5-FU) and leucovorin (LV) for metastatic colon or rectal carcinomas, and for disease that has progressed or recurred following initial 5-FU therapy.

DOSAGE: *Adults:* Combination Therapy (5-FU/LV, see PI for dosage): 125mg/m² IV over 90 min on days 1, 8, 15, 22 for 6 weeks; or 180mg/m² IV over 90 min on days 1, 15, and 29 for 6 weeks. Both regimens: Begin next cycle on Day 43. Single Therapy: 125mg/m² IV over 90 min on days 1, 8, 15, 22 followed by a 2 week rest; or 350mg/m² IV over 90 min once every 3 weeks. Premedicate with antiemetics at least 30 min prior to therapy. Dose modifications for reduced UGT1A1 activity, neutropenia, diarrhea, and other toxicities: See PI. All dose modifications should be based on worst preceding toxicity.

HOW SUPPLIED: Inj: 20mg/mL

CONTRAINDICATIONS: Concomitant ketoconazole or St. John's wort.

WARNINGS/PRECAUTIONS: Due to increased toxicity, avoid use of irinotecan with the "Mayo Clinic" regimen of 5-FU/LV (given 4-5 days every 4 weeks). Treat/prevent early diarrhea with atropine IV/SQ and late diarrhea (occurring >24 hrs after dose) with loperamide PO. If late diarrhea occurs, delay therapy until return of pretreatment bowel function for at least 24 hrs without antidiarrheals; decrease subsequent doses if late diarrhea is Grade 2, 3 or 4. Deaths due to sepsis reported following severe neutropenia. Temporarily hold therapy if neutropenic fever occurs or if neutrophils <1000/mm³. Increased risk for neutropenia in patients homozygous for the UGT1A1 28 allele. Consider reduced initial dose. Heterozygous patients may also have increased risk. Hypersensitivity reactions, colitis, ileus, and renal impairment/failure, thromboembolic events reported. May cause fetal harm during pregnancy. Monitor for extravasation at infusion site. Consider atropine for cholinergic symptoms. Caution with modestly elevated baseline bilirubin levels (eg, 1-2mg/dL), abnormal glucuronidation of bilirubin, hepatic insufficiency, elderly with comorbidities, previous pelvic/abdominal irradiation. Careful monitoring of WBC with differential, Hgb, and platelets is recommended before each dose. Avoid in severe bone marrow failure, and fructose intolerant patients.

ADVERSE REACTIONS: Nausea, vomiting, diarrhea, abdominal pain, blood dyscrasias, asthenia, muscositis, anorexia, alopecia, fever, pain, constipation, infection, dyspnea, increased bilirubin.

INTERACTIONS: Exacerbated myelosuppression and diarrhea with antineoplastic agents having similar adverse effects. Avoid concurrent irradiation therapy. Possible hyperglycemia and lymphocytopenia with dexamethasone. Akathisia reported with prochlorperazine. Laxatives may worsen diarrhea. Consider withholding diuretics with irinotecan therapy. Decreased levels with CYP3A4 inducing anticonvulsants and St. John's wort. Consider substituting non-enzyme inducing anticonvulsants 2 weeks prior to and during treatment. Increased levels with ketoconazole. Discontinue ketoconazole at least 1 week prior to and during therapy.

PREGNANCY: Category D, not for use in nursing.

MECHANISM OF ACTION: Topoisomerase I inhibitor; binds to topoisomerase I-DNA complex and prevents religation of single-strand breaks induced by the enzyme to relieve torsional strain in DNA.

PHARMACOKINETICS: Absorption: Irinotecan: (125mg/m²); C_{max}=1660ng/ml; AUC_{0-24}=10200ng•h/mL. (340mg/m²); C_{max}=3392ng/ml; AUC_{0-24}=20604ng•h/mL; SN-38: (125mg/m²) C_{max}=26.3ng/ml; AUC_{0-24}=229ng•h/mL. (340mg/m²) C_{max}=56ng/ml; AUC_{0-24}=474ng•h/mL. **Distribution:** Irinotecan: (125mg/m²) V_d=110L/m². (340mg/m²) V_d=234L/m². Plasma protein binding (30-68%). SN-38: Plasma protein binding (95%). **Metabolism:** Liver via carboxyl esterase. Metabolite (SN-38). **Elimination:** Irinotecan: Urine (11-20%). (125mg/m²) $T_{1/2}$=5.8 hrs. (340mg/m²) $T_{1/2}$=11.7 hrs. SN-38: Urine (<1%). (125mg/m²) $T_{1/2}$=10.4 hrs. (340mg/m²) $T_{1/2}$=21 hrs

CANASA   RX
mesalamine (Axcan Scandipharm)

THERAPEUTIC CLASS: Anti-inflammatory Agent

INDICATIONS: Treatment of active ulcerative proctitis.

DOSAGE: *Adults:* 1000mg rectally qhs. Retain suppository for at least 1-3 hrs.

HOW SUPPLIED: Sup: 1000mg

CONTRAINDICATIONS: Hypersensitivity to suppository vehicle (eg, saturated vegetable fatty acid esters) or salicylates.

WARNINGS/PRECAUTIONS: D/C if acute intolerance syndrome develops (eg, cramping, bloody diarrhea, abdominal pain, headache); consider sulfasalazine hypersensitivity. If rechallenge is considered, perform under careful observation. Caution with sulfasalazine hypersensitivity. Carefully monitor with renal dysfunction. Pancolitis, pericarditis (rare) reported.

ADVERSE REACTIONS: Dizziness, rectal pain, fever, acne, colitis, rash, hair loss.

PREGNANCY: Category B, caution in nursing.

MECHANISM OF ACTION: Not fully established; anti-inflammatory drug appears to act topically rather than systemically. Postulated to have a role as free radical scavenger or inhibitor of tumor necrosis factor.

PHARMACOKINETICS: Absorption: Variable; C_{max}=361ng/mL. **Metabolism:** Extensively metabolized to N-acetyl-5-ASA. **Elimination:** Urine; $T_{1/2}$=7 hrs.

CANCIDAS   RX
caspofungin acetate (Merck)

THERAPEUTIC CLASS: Glucan synthesis inhibitor

INDICATIONS: Empirical therapy for presumed fungal infections in febrile, neutropenic patients. Treatment of candidemia and the following *Candida* infections: intra-abdominal abscesses, peritonitis, and pleural space infections. Treatment of esophageal candidiasis. Treatment of invasive aspergillosis in patients refractory to or intolerant of other therapies (eg, amphotericin B, itraconazole).

DOSAGE: *Adults:* Empirical Therapy: LD: 70mg IV on Day 1. Maint: 50mg IV qd. If 50mg is well tolerated but does not provide adequate clinical response, daily dose can be increased to 70mg. Fungal infections should be treated for a minimum of 14 days. Continue treatment 7 days after neutropenia and clinical symptoms are resolved. Candidemia/*Candida* Infections: LD: 70mg IV on Day 1. Maint: 50mg IV qd. Esophageal Candidiasis: 50mg IV qd. Consider PO suppressive therapy with HIV. Invasive Aspergillosis: LD: 70mg IV on Day 1. Maint: 50mg IV qd. Moderate Hepatic Insufficiency (Child-Pugh Score 7-9): LD: 70mg IV on Day 1. Maint: 35mg IV qd. Concomitant Rifampin: 70mg IV qd. Concomitant Nevirapine/Efavirenz/Carbamazepine/Dexamethasone/ Phenytoin: May need to increase dose to 70mg IV qd. Base duration of treatment on severity of disease, clinical response, microbiological response, and recovery from immunosuppression.

HOW SUPPLIED: Inj: 50mg, 70mg

WARNINGS/PRECAUTIONS: LFT abnormalities may be seen; if abnormal LFTs develop, monitor for evidence of worsening hepatic function and re-evaluate.

ADVERSE REACTIONS: Fever, chills, infused vein complications, nausea, vomiting, hypokalemia, headache, rash, anaphylaxis.

INTERACTIONS: Reduces blood levels of tacrolimus. Efavirenz, nevirapine, phenytoin, rifampin, dexamethasone, carbamazepine may decrease levels. Increased levels with cyclosporine; use only when benefits outweigh risks. Do not mix or co-infuse with other medications. Do not use with dextrose-containing diluents.

PREGNANCY: Category C, caution in nursing.

MECHANISM OF ACTION: Antifungal. Inhibits the synthesis of β (1,3)-D-glucan, a primary component responsible for cell wall synthesis in susceptible fungi.

PHARMACOKINETICS: Distribution: 97% Plasma protein binding. Found in breast milk. **Metabolism:** Hydrolysis and N-acetylation (slowly). **Elimination:** Urine (41%), feces (35%).

CAPEX RX
fluocinolone acetonide (Galderma)

THERAPEUTIC CLASS: Corticosteroid

INDICATIONS: Treatment of seborrheic dermatitis of the scalp.

DOSAGE: *Adults:* Apply up to 1oz to scalp qd. Work into lather, rinse after 5 min.

HOW SUPPLIED: Shampoo: 0.01% [120mL]

WARNINGS/PRECAUTIONS: May produce reversible HPA axis suppression, manifestations of Cushing's syndrome, hyperglycemia, and glucosuria. Evaluate periodically for HPA axis suppression if applied to large surface area or with occlusive dressings. D/C if irritation occurs. Pediatrics may be more susceptible to systemic toxicity. Use appropriate therapy with infections.

ADVERSE REACTIONS: Allergic contact dermatitis, secondary infection, skin atrophy, striae, miliaria, burning, itching, irritation, hypopigmentation, perioral dermatitis, dryness, folliculitis, acneiform eruptions.

PREGNANCY: Category C, caution in nursing.

MECHANISM OF ACTION: Corticosteroid; possesses anti-inflammatory, antipruritic, and vasoconstrictive properties. Mechanism of anti-inflammatory effects not established. Suspected to act by induction of phospholipase A_2 inhibitory proteins, lipocortins. Lipocortins control biosynthesis of potent mediators of inflammation (eg, prostaglandins, leukotrienes) by inhibiting release of their common precursor, arachidonic acid.

PHARMACOKINETICS: Absorption: Percutaneous. Inflammation, other disease states, and use of occlusive dressings may increase absorption. **Distribution:** Systemically administered corticosteroids appear in breast milk.

CAPOZIDE RX
hydrochlorothiazide - captopril (Par)

> ACE inhibitors can cause death/injury to developing fetus during 2nd and 3rd trimesters. Stop therapy if pregnancy detected.

THERAPEUTIC CLASS: ACE inhibitor/thiazide diuretic

INDICATIONS: Treatment of hypertension.

DOSAGE: *Adults:* Initial: 25mg-15mg tab qd. Titrate: Adjust dose at 6-week intervals. Max: 150mg captopril/50mg HCTZ per day. Replacement Therapy: Substitute combination for titrated components. Renal Impairment: Decrease dose or increase interval. Take 1 hr before meals.

HOW SUPPLIED: Tab: (Captopril-HCTZ) 25mg-15mg*, 25mg-25mg*, 50mg-15mg*, 50mg-25mg* *scored

CONTRAINDICATIONS: History of ACE inhibitor-associated angioedema, anuria, sulfonamide hypersensitivity.

WARNINGS/PRECAUTIONS: D/C if angioedema, jaundice, or if marked LFT elevation occurs. Risk of hyperkalemia with DM, renal dysfunction. Monitor WBCs in renal and collagen vascular disease. Fetal/neonatal morbidity and death reported. Monitor for hypotension in high-risk patients (eg, surgery/anesthesia, volume/salt depletion). Caution with renal or hepatic dysfunction. More reports of angioedema in blacks than nonblacks. May exacerbate or activate Systemic lupus erythematosus. Monitor electrolytes. Hypercalcemia, hypomagnesemia, hyperuricemia may occur. With renal impairment, monitor WBCs and differential before therapy, every 2 weeks for 3 months, then periodically. Neutropenia with myeloid hypoplasia, persistent nonproductive cough, anaphylactoid reactions, proteinuria reported.

ADVERSE REACTIONS: Cough, hypotension, rash, pruritus, fever, arthralgia, eosinophilia, dysgeusia, neutropenia/thrombocytopenia.

INTERACTIONS: Increased risk of hyperkalemia with K⁺-sparing diuretics, K⁺ supplements, or K⁺-containing salt substitutes. Potentiates orthostatic hypotension with alcohol, barbiturates, and narcotics. Adjust other antihypertensives, anticoagulants, antidiabetic, or antigout drugs. Reduced absorption with cholestyramine, colestipol. Amphotericin B, corticosteroids, ACTH deplete electrolytes. May decrease methenamine effects. May decrease response to pressor amines. May potentiate non-depolarizing skeletal muscle relaxants, anesthetics. Risk of lithium toxicity. NSAIDs (eg, indomethacin) reduce effects. Enhanced hypotensive effects with MAOIs. Probenecid, sulfinpyrazone may need dose increase. Diazoxide enhances hyperglycemic, hyperuricemic and antihypertensive effects. Monitor serum calcium levels with calcium salts. Monitor potassium levels with cardiac glycosides. Caution with agents affecting sympathetic activity. D/C vasodilators before therapy. Caution and decrease vasodilator dose if resumed during therapy.

PREGNANCY: Category C (1st trimester) and D (2nd and 3rd trimesters), not for use in nursing.

MECHANISM OF ACTION: Captopril: ACE inhibitor; mechanism not established. Effects appear to result from suppression of renin-angiotensin-aldosterone system. HCTZ: Thiazide diuretic.Affects renal tubular mechanism of electrolyte reabsorption.

PHARMACOKINETICS: Absorption: Captopril: Rapid; T_{max}=1 hr. **Distribution:** Captopril: Plasma protein binding (25-30%). **Elimination:** Captopril: Urine (40-50%); $T_{1/2}$=<2 hrs. HCTZ: Kidney; $T_{1/2}$=2.5 hrs.

CAPTOPRIL
RX

captopril (Various)

> ACE inhibitors can cause death/injury to developing fetus during 2nd and 3rd trimesters. Stop therapy if pregnancy detected.

OTHER BRAND NAMES: Capoten (Par)

THERAPEUTIC CLASS: ACE inhibitor

INDICATIONS: Treatment of hypertension and/or CHF. To decrease hospitalization and mortality in stable post-MI patients with left ventricular dysfunction. Diabetic nephropathy (proteinuria >500mg/day) and slows progression of renal insufficiency in type I diabetes.

DOSAGE: *Adults:* Take 1 hour before meals. HTN: If possible, d/c recent antihypertensive drug for 1 week prior to therapy. Initial: 25mg bid-tid. Titrate: May increase to 50mg bid-tid after 1-2 weeks. Usual: 25-150mg bid-tid. Max: 450mg/day. CHF: Initial: 25mg tid; 6.25-12.5mg tid with risk of hypotension or salt/volume depletion. Usual: 50-100mg tid. Max: 450mg/day. Left Ventricular Dysfunction Post-MI: Initial: 6.25mg single dose, then 12.5mg tid. Titrate: Increase to 25mg tid over next several days, then to 50mg tid over next several weeks. Usual: 50mg tid. Diabetic Nephropathy: 25mg tid. Significant Renal Dysfunction: Decrease initial dose and titrate slowly.

HOW SUPPLIED: Tab: 12.5mg*, 25mg*, 50mg*, 100mg* *scored

CONTRAINDICATIONS: History of ACE inhibitor associated angioedema.

WARNINGS/PRECAUTIONS: D/C if jaundice or marked LFT elevation occurs. Risk of hyperkalemia with DM, renal dysfunction. Persistent nonproductive cough, anaphylactoid reactions, neutropenia with myeloid hypoplasia reported. Fetal/neonatal morbidity and death reported. Monitor for hypotension in high-risk patients (surgery/anesthesia, dialysis, heart failure, volume/salt depletion, etc). Caution with CHF, renal dysfunction, renal artery stenosis, collagen vascular disease (especially with renal dysfunction). Monitor WBC before therapy, then every 2 weeks for 3 months, then periodically. Less effective on BP in blacks and more reports of angioedema than nonblacks.

ADVERSE REACTIONS: Proteinuria, rash, hypotension, dysgeusia, cough, MI, CHF.

INTERACTIONS: May increase lithium levels. NSAIDs may decrease antihypertensive effects. Hypotension risk with diuretics. Increased risk of hyperkalemia with K+-sparing diuretics, K+-containing salt substitutes, or K+ supplements. Caution with vasodilators or agents affecting sympathetic activity. Augmented effect by antihypertensives that cause renin release (eg, thiazides).

PREGNANCY: Category C (1st trimester) and D (2nd and 3rd trimesters), not for use in nursing.

MECHANISM OF ACTION: ACE inhibitor; mechanism not established. Effects appear to result from suppression of renin-angiotensin-aldosterone system.

PHARMACOKINETICS: Absorption: Rapid; T_{max}=1 hr. **Distribution:** Plasma protein binding (25-30%). **Elimination:** $T_{1/2}$=<2 hrs; urine (40-50%).

CARAC   RX
fluorouracil (Dermik)

THERAPEUTIC CLASS: Antimetabolite

INDICATIONS: Topical treatment of multiple actinic or solar keratosis of the face and anterior scalp.

DOSAGE: *Adults:* ≥18 yrs: Apply thin film qd to lesions for up to 4 weeks. Apply 10 min after washing and drying area.

HOW SUPPLIED: Cre: 0.5% [30g]

CONTRAINDICATIONS: Pregnancy, dihydropyrimidine dehydrogenase (DPD) enzyme deficiency.

WARNINGS/PRECAUTIONS: D/C if symptoms of DPD enzyme deficiency develop. Avoid contact with eyes, eyelids, nostrils, mouth, and sun/UV light. Increased absorption with ulcerated or inflamed skin. Wash hands after application.

ADVERSE REACTIONS: Application site reaction (eg, erythema, dryness, burning, erosion, pain, edema), eye irritation.

PREGNANCY: Category X, not for use in nursing.

MECHANISM OF ACTION: Antimetabolite; interferes with synthesis of DNA and to a lesser extent inhibits formation of RNA, to create a thymine deficiency, which provokes unbalanced growth and cell death.

PHARMACOKINETICS: Absorption: C_{max}=0.77ng/mL; T_{max}=1 hr; AUC=2.8ng•hr/mL.

CARAFATE   RX
sucralfate (Axcan Scandipharm)

THERAPEUTIC CLASS: Duodenal ulcer adherent complex

INDICATIONS: (Sus/Tab) Short-term treatment of active duodenal ulcer. (Tab) Maintenance therapy of healed duodenal ulcers.

DOSAGE: *Adults:* Active Ulcer: (Sus/Tab) 1g qid for 4-8 weeks. Maint: (Tab) 1g bid. Take on empty stomach.

HOW SUPPLIED: Sus: 1g/10mL [414mL]; Tab: 1g* *scored

WARNINGS/PRECAUTIONS: Caution with chronic renal failure and dialysis.

ADVERSE REACTIONS: Constipation, diarrhea, nausea, vomiting, pruritus, rash, dizziness, insomnia, back pain, headache.

INTERACTIONS: Reduced absorption of cimetidine, digoxin, fluoroquinolones, ketoconazole, levothyroxine, phenytoin, quinidine, ranitidine, tetracycline, and theophylline; dose concomitant drugs 2 hrs before sucralfate. Monitor warfarin. Additive aluminum absorption with aluminum-containing products. Antacids should not be taken within 1/2 hr before or after sucralfate.

PREGNANCY: Category B, caution with nursing.

MECHANISM OF ACTION: Duodenal ulcer adherent complex; not fully established. Forms ulcer-adherent complex that covers ulcer site and protects it against further attack by acid, pepsin, and bile salts.

PHARMACOKINETICS: Absorption: Minimally absorbed. **Elimination:** Urine.

CARBATROL
RX
carbamazepine (Shire)

> Serious and fatal dermatologic reactions, including toxic epidermal necrolysis (TEN), Stevens-Johnson syndrome (SJS) and presence of HLA-B*1502 allele reported. Aplastic anemia and agranulocytosis reported. Obtain complete pretreatment hematological testing as a baseline. D/C if evidence of bone marrow depression develops.

THERAPEUTIC CLASS: Carboxamide

INDICATIONS: Treatment of partial seizures with complex symptomatology, generalized tonic-clonic seizures, and mixed seizure patterns of these or other partial or generalized seizures. Treatment of trigeminal neuralgia pain.

DOSAGE: *Adults:* Epilepsy: Initial: 200mg bid. Titrate: May increase weekly by 200mg/day. Maint: 800-1200mg/day. Max: 1200mg/day. Trigeminal Neuralgia: Initial (Day 1): 200mg qd. Titrate: May increase by 200mg/day q12h. Maint: 400-800mg/day. Max: 1200mg/day. Re-evaluate every 3 months. *Pediatrics:* Epilepsy: >12 yrs: Initial: 200mg bid. Titrate: May increase weekly by 200mg/day. Max: 12-15 yrs: 1000mg/day. >15 yrs: 1200mg/day. 6 months-12 yrs: May convert immediate-release dose ≥400mg/day to equal daily dose using bid regimen. Usual/Max: ≤35mg/kg/day.

HOW SUPPLIED: Cap, Extended-Release:100mg, 200mg, 300mg

CONTRAINDICATIONS: History of bone marrow depression, MAOI use within 14 days, sensitivity to TCAs.

WARNINGS/PRECAUTIONS: Toxic epidermal necrolysis (Lyell's syndrome), Stevens-Johnson syndrome (SJS), multi-organ hypersensitivity reactions, and presence of HLA-B*1502 reported. Caution with history of adverse hematologic reaction to any drug, increased IOP, the elderly, mixed seizure with atypical absence seizure. Fetal harm with pregnancy. May activate latent psychosis. Caution with cardiac, hepatic, or renal damage. Perform eye exam and monitor LFTs and renal function at baseline and periodically.

ADVERSE REACTIONS: Dizziness, drowsiness, unsteadiness, nausea, vomiting, bone marrow depression, rash, urticaria, hypersensitivity reactions, photosensitivity reactions, CHF, edema, HTN, hypotension.

INTERACTIONS: See Contraindications. Metabolism is inhibited by CYP3A4 inhibitors (eg, cimetidine, macrolides, etc.) and induced by CYP3A4 inducers (eg, rifampin, phenytoin, trazodone, etc.). Decreases oral contraceptive effectiveness. Increases plasma levels of clomipramine, phenytoin, and primidone. Decreases levels of APAP, alprazolam, clonazepam, clozapine, dicumarol, doxycycline, ethosuximide, haloperidol, methsuximide, phensuximide, phenytoin, theophylline, valproate, warfarin. Increased risk of neurotoxic side effects with lithium.

PREGNANCY: Category D, not for use in nursing.

MECHANISM OF ACTION: Carboxamide anticonvulsant; suspected to reduce polysynaptic responses and blocks post-tetanic potentiation.

PHARMACOKINETICS: Absorption: C_{max}=1.9mcg/mL (200mg); T_{max}=19 hrs (200mg). Distribution: Plasma protein binding (76%). Metabolism: Liver, via CYP3A4 to carbamazepine-10,11-epoxide (metabolite). Elimination: Urine (72%), feces (28%); $T_{1/2}$=35-40 hrs.

CARBOPLATIN
RX
carboplatin (Various)

> Bone marrow suppression, resulting in infection or bleeding reported. Anemia and anaphylactic-like reactions reported.

THERAPEUTIC CLASS: Platinum coordination compound

INDICATIONS: Initial treatment of advanced ovarian carcinoma. Palliative treatment of advanced ovarian carcinoma recurrent after prior chemotherapy.

DOSAGE: *Adults:* Monotherapy: 360mg/m² IV on Day 1 every 4 weeks. Concomitant Cyclophosphamide: 300mg/m² IV on Day 1 every 4 weeks for 6 cycles, with cyclophosphamide 600mg/m² IV on Day 1 every 4 weeks for 6 cycles. If platelets >100,000 or neutrophils >2000: Give 125% of dose. If platelets <50,000 or neutrophils <500: Give 75% of dose. Renal Impairment: Initial: CrCl 41-59mL/min: 250mg/m². CrCl 16-40mL/min: 200mg/m². Subsequent dose adjustments based on the degree of bone marrow suppression.

HOW SUPPLIED: Inj: 10mg/mL

CONTRAINDICATIONS: Severe bone marrow depression, significant bleeding. History of severe allergic reactions to cisplatin, platinum-containing compounds, or mannitol.

WARNINGS/PRECAUTIONS: Bone marrow suppression is dose-dependent and is the dose-limiting toxicity. May need transfusion for anemia. Bone marrow suppression increased in patients who received prior therapy. Neurotoxicity increased if ≥65 yrs and previous cisplatin treatment. LFT abnormalities and temporary loss of vision with high doses. Emesis reported.

ADVERSE REACTIONS: Blood dyscrasias, infection, bleeding, nausea, vomiting, peripheral neuropathies, ototoxicity, central neurotoxicity, elevated LFTs/bilirubin/serum creatinine, electrolyte loss, allergic reactions, alopecia, mucositis.

INTERACTIONS: Nephrotoxic compounds may potentiate renal adverse effects. Aminoglycosides may increase ototoxic or nephrotoxic effects.

PREGNANCY: Category D, not for use in nursing.

MECHANISM OF ACTION: Platinum coordination compound; exerts its action by interstranding DNA cross links.

PHARMACOKINETICS: Distribution: V_d=16L. **Elimination:** Urine. Carboplatin: Initial $T_{1/2}$=1.1-2 hrs, post-distribution $T_{1/2}$=2.6-5.9 hrs. Platinum: Irreversibly bound to plasma proteins; $T_{1/2}$=5 days.

CARDENE IV   RX
nicardipine HCL (PDL)

THERAPEUTIC CLASS: Calcium channel blocker (dihydropyridine)

INDICATIONS: Short-term treatment of hypertension when oral therapy is not feasible or desirable.

DOSAGE: *Adults:* IV: Individualized dose; Administer by slow continuous infusion at a concentration of 0.1mg/mL. Gradual Reduction: Initial: 50mL/hr (5mg/hr). Titrate: May increase by 25mL/hr (2.5mg/hr) q15 min. Max: 150mL/hr (15mg/hr). Rapid BP Reduction: Initial 50mL/hr (5mg/hr). Titrate: 25mL/hr(2.5mg/hr) q5 min. Max 150mL/hr (15mg/hr). Decrease rate to 30mL/hr (3mg/hr) after BP reduction is achieved. Equiv. PO/IV Dose: 20mg q8h=0.5mg/hr, 30mg q8h=1.2mg/hr, 40mg q8h=2.2mg/hr.

HOW SUPPLIED: Inj: 2.5mg/mL

CONTRAINDICATIONS: Advanced aortic stenosis.

WARNINGS/PRECAUTIONS: May induce or exacerbate angina. Caution with CHF, significant left ventricular dysfunction, or pheochromocytoma. Change IV site every 12 hrs to minimize risk of peripheral venous irritation. Monitor BP during administration. Caution in hepatic/renal impairment or reduced hepatic blood flow.

ADVERSE REACTIONS: Headache, hypotension, tachycardia, nausea/vomiting.

INTERACTIONS: Monitor with other antihypertensive agents. Caution with β-blockers in CHF. Increased levels with cimetidine. Monitor digoxin levels. Caution with fentanyl anesthesia. May increase cyclosporine levels.

PREGNANCY: Category C, not for use in nursing.

MECHANISM OF ACTION: Ca^{2+} channel blocker; inhibits transmembrane influx of Ca^{2+} ions into cardiac muscle and smooth muscles without changing serum Ca^{2+} concentration.

PHARMACOKINETICS: Distribution: Plasma protein binding (>95%); V_d=8.3L/kg. **Metabolism:** Liver. **Elimination:** Urine, feces; $T_{1/2}$=14.4 hrs.

CARDENE SR
nicardipine HCL (PDL)

RX

C

THERAPEUTIC CLASS: Calcium channel blocker (dihydropyridine)

INDICATIONS: Treatment of hypertension.

DOSAGE: *Adults:* Initial: 30mg bid. Usual: 30-60mg bid.

HOW SUPPLIED: Cap, Extended-Release: 30mg, 45mg, 60mg

CONTRAINDICATIONS: Advanced aortic stenosis.

WARNINGS/PRECAUTIONS: Increased angina reported in patients with angina. Caution when titrating dose. Caution in hepatic/renal impairment, or reduced hepatic blood flow. May cause symptomatic hypotension. Measure BP 2-4 hrs after 1st dose or dose increase.

ADVERSE REACTIONS: Headache, pedal edema, vasodilation, palpitations, nausea, dizziness, asthenia, flushing, increased angina.

INTERACTIONS: Increased levels with cimetidine. Elevates cyclosporine levels. With β-blocker withdrawal, gradually reduce over 8-10 days. Monitor digoxin levels. Caution with fentanyl anesthesia.

PREGNANCY: Category C, not for use in nursing.

MECHANISM OF ACTION: Ca^{2+} channel blocker; inhibits transmembrane influx of Ca^{2+} ions into cardiac muscle and smooth muscle without changing serum Ca^{2+} concentration.

PHARMACOKINETICS: Absorption: Complete; Bioavailability (35%). T_{max}=1-4 hrs. C_{max}=13.4ng/mL (30mg), 34.0ng/mL (45mg), 58.4ng/mL (60mg). **Distribution:** Plasma protein binding (>95%). **Metabolism:** Liver. **Elimination:** Urine (<1%), feces; $T_{1/2}$=8.6 hrs.

CARDIZEM
diltiazem HCL (Biovail)

RX

THERAPEUTIC CLASS: Calcium channel blocker (nondihydropyridine)

INDICATIONS: Management of chronic stable angina or angina due to coronary artery spasm.

DOSAGE: *Adults:* Initial: 30mg qid (before meals and qhs). Adjust at 1-2 day intervals. Usual: 180-360mg/day.

HOW SUPPLIED: Tab: 30mg, 60mg*, 90mg*, 120mg* *scored

CONTRAINDICATIONS: Sick sinus syndrome and 2nd- or 3rd-degree AV block (except with functioning pacemaker), hypotension (<90mmHg systolic), acute MI, pulmonary congestion.

WARNINGS/PRECAUTIONS: Caution in renal, hepatic, or ventricular dysfunction. Monitor LFTs and renal function with prolonged use. D/C if persistent rash occurs. Symptomatic hypotension may occur. Acute hepatic injury reported.

ADVERSE REACTIONS: Headache, dizziness, asthenia, flushing, 1st-degree AV block, edema, nausea, bradycardia, rash.

INTERACTIONS: Increased levels of propranolol, digoxin, carbamazepine, cyclosporine, lovastatin, quinidine; monitor closely. Increased levels of diltiazem with cimetidine. Potentiates depression of cardiac contractility, conductivity, automaticity and vascular dilation with anesthetics. Additive cardiac conduction effects with digitalis or β-blockers. Potential additive effects with agents known to affect cardiac contractility and/or conduction. May increase levels of midazolam/triazolam. Avoid with CYP3A4 inducers (eg, rifampin). Enhanced effects and increased toxicity of buspirone.

PREGNANCY: Category C, not for use in nursing.

MECHANISM OF ACTION: Calcium channel blocker; still being delineated; believed to be potent dilator of coronary arteries both epicardial and subendocardial. It inhibits spontaneous and ergonovine-induced coronary artery spasm. It increases exercise tolerance by its ability to reduce myocardial oxygen demand; this is accomplished via reduction in heart rate and systemic BP.

PHARMACOKINETICS: Absorption: Well absorbed, absolute bioavailability (40%). T_{max}=2-4 hrs. **Distribution:** Plasma protein bound (70-80%); found in breast milk. **Metabolism:** Liver (extensive). **Elimination:** Urine (2-4%); unchanged, and bile.

CARDIZEM CD RX
diltiazem HCL (Biovail)

OTHER BRAND NAMES: Cardizem LA (Abbott) - Cartia XT (Andrx)

THERAPEUTIC CLASS: Calcium channel blocker (nondihydropyridine)

INDICATIONS: Treatment of hypertension. Management of chronic stable angina (LA) or angina due to coronary artery spasm.

DOSAGE: *Adults:* HTN: (CD, Cartia XT) Initial (monotherapy): 180-240mg qd. Titrate: Adjust at 2-week intervals. Usual: 240-360mg qd. Max: 480mg qd. (LA) Initial: 180-240mg qd. Adjust at 2-week intervals. Max: 540mg qd. Angina: (CD, Cartia XT) Initial: 120-180mg qd. Adjust at 1-2 week intervals. Max: 480mg/day. (LA) Initial: 180mg qd. Adjust at 1-2 week intervals.

HOW SUPPLIED: Cap, Extended-Release: (Cardizem CD, Cartia XT) 120mg, 180mg, 240mg, 300mg, (Cardizem CD) 360mg; Tab, Extended-Release: (Cardizem LA) 120mg, 180mg, 240mg, 300mg, 360mg, 420mg

CONTRAINDICATIONS: Sick sinus syndrome and 2nd- or 3rd-degree AV block (except with functioning pacemaker), hypotension (<90mmHg systolic), acute MI, pulmonary congestion.

WARNINGS/PRECAUTIONS: Caution in renal, hepatic, or ventricular dysfunction. Monitor LFTs and renal function with prolonged use. D/C if persistent rash occurs. Symptomatic hypotension may occur. Acute hepatic injury reported.

ADVERSE REACTIONS: Headache, dizziness, asthenia, flushing, 1st-degree AV block, edema, nausea, bradycardia, rash.

INTERACTIONS: May require dosage adjustment with concomitant CYP3A4 substrates. Increased levels of propranolol, digoxin, carbamazepine, lovastatin. Increased levels of diltiazem with cimetidine. May increase effects of benzodiazepines. Monitor digoxin, cyclosporine. Potentiates the depression of cardiac contractility, conductivity, automaticity and vascular dilation with anesthetics. Avoid concurrent use with CYP3A4 inducers (eg, rifampin). Additive cardiac conduction effects with digitalis or β-blockers. Potential additive effects with agents known to affect cardiac contractility and/or conduction.

PREGNANCY: Category C, not for use in nursing.

MECHANISM OF ACTION: Calcium channel blocker; inhibits influx of Ca^{2+} ions during membrane depolarization of cardiac and vascular smooth muscle.

PHARMACOKINETICS: Absorption: CD: T_{max}=10-14 hrs; absolute bioavailability (40%). LA: T_{max}=11-18 hrs. **Distribution:** Plasma protein binding (70-80%). **Elimination:** CD: $T_{1/2}$=5-8 hrs; urine (2-4%). LA: $T_{1/2}$=6-9 hrs.

CARDURA RX
doxazosin mesylate (Pfizer)

THERAPEUTIC CLASS: Alpha$_1$-blocker (quinazoline)

INDICATIONS: Treatment of hypertension and/or benign prostatic hyperplasia (BPH).

DOSAGE: *Adults:* HTN: Initial: 1mg qd (am or pm). Monitor BP 2-6 hrs and 24 hrs after 1st dose. Titrate: Increase to 2mg qd then upwards as needed. Max:

16mg/day. BPH: Initial: 1mg qd (am or pm). Titrate: May double the dose every 1-2 weeks. Max: 8mg/day.

HOW SUPPLIED: Tab: 1mg*, 2mg*, 4mg*, 8mg* *scored

WARNINGS/PRECAUTIONS: Monitor for orthostatic hypotension and syncope with 1st dose and dose increase. Caution with hepatic dysfunction. Rule out prostate cancer. Priapism (rare), leukopenia/neutropenia reported.

ADVERSE REACTIONS: Fatigue/malaise, hypotension, edema, dizziness, dyspnea, weight gain.

PREGNANCY: Category C, caution with nursing.

MECHANISM OF ACTION: alpha-adrenergic receptor inhibitor: (BPH) antagonizes phenylephrine induced contractions in prostate; (HTN) competitively antagonizes pressor effects of phenylephrine and systolic pressor effect of norepinephrine.

PHARMACOKINETICS: Absorption: Absolute bioavailability (65%); T_{max}=2-3 hrs. **Distribution:** Plasma protein binding (98%). **Metabolism:** O-demethylation or hydroxylation. **Elimination:** Feces (4.8%), urine (trace); $T_{1/2}$=22 hrs.

CARDURA XL   RX
doxazosin mesylate (Pfizer)

THERAPEUTIC CLASS: Alpha$_1$-blocker (quinazoline)

INDICATIONS: Treatment of the signs and symptoms of benign prostatic hyperplasia.

DOSAGE: *Adults:* Initial: 4mg qd with breakfast. Titrate: May increase to 8mg after 3-4 weeks. Max: 8mg. Swallow whole; do not chew, divide, cut, or crush.

HOW SUPPLIED: Tab, Extended-Release: 4mg, 8mg

WARNINGS/PRECAUTIONS: Postural hypotension with or without symptoms (eg, dizziness) may develop; caution with symptomatic hypotension or hypotensive response to other medications. Rule out prostate cancer. Intraoperative Floppy Iris Syndrome has been observed during cataract surgery in some patients on or previously treated with alpha$_1$ blockers. Caution with preexisting severe GI narrowing (pathologic or iatrogenic). Caution with mild or moderate hepatic dysfunction; avoid with severe hepatic dysfunction. D/C with worsening of or new-onset angina pectoris symptoms.

ADVERSE REACTIONS: Dizziness, dyspnea, asthenia, headache, hypotension, postural hypotension, somnolence, respiratory tract infection, backache.

INTERACTIONS: Caution with potent CYP3A4 inhibitors (eg, atanazavir, clarithromycin, indinavir, itraconazole, ketoconazole, nefazodone, nelfinavir, ritonavir, saquinavir, telithromycin, voriconazole).

PREGNANCY: Category C, not for use in nursing.

MECHANISM OF ACTION: Quinazoline; selectively inhibits α$_1$-subtype of α adrenergic receptors decreasing urethral resistance, which may relieve BPH symptoms and improve urine flow.

PHARMACOKINETICS: Absorption: (4mg) C_{max}=10.1ng/mL, AUC=183ng•hr/mL, T_{max}=8 hrs. (8mg) C_{max}=25.8ng/mL, AUC=472ng-hr/mL, T_{max}=9 hrs. **Distribution**: Plasma protein binding (98%). **Metabolism**: CYP3A4 (major); 2D6, 2C19 (minor). **Elimination**: $T_{1/2}$=15-19 hrs.

CARMOL 40   RX
urea (Doak)

THERAPEUTIC CLASS: Debriding/Healing Agent

INDICATIONS: Debridement and promotion of normal healing of hyperkeratotic surface lesions, particularly where healing is retarded by local infection, necrotic tissue, fibrinous or prurient debris or eschar. Treatment of hyperkeratotic conditions such as dry, rough skin, dermatitis, psoriasis, xerosis, ichthyosis, eczema, keratosis, corns and calluses, damaged ingrown and devitalized nails.

DOSAGE: *Adults:* Apply bid. Rub until absorbed.

HOW SUPPLIED: Cre: 40% [28.35g, 85g, 198.6g]; Gel: 40% [15mL]; Lot: 40% [236.6mL]

WARNINGS/PRECAUTIONS: Avoid contact with eyes, lips, or mucous membranes.

ADVERSE REACTIONS: Transient stinging, burning, itching, or irritation.

PREGNANCY: Category C, caution in nursing.

MECHANISM OF ACTION: Keratolytic emollient; urea gently dissolves the intercellular matrix which results in loosening the horny layer of skin and shedding scaly skin at regular intervals, thereby softening hyperkeratotic areas.

CARNITOR   RX
levocarnitine (Sigma-Tau)

OTHER BRAND NAMES: Carnitor SF (Sigma-Tau)

THERAPEUTIC CLASS: Carnitine supplement

INDICATIONS: (Tab) Primary carnitine deficiency. (Inj/Tab) Acute and chronic treatment of inborn error of metabolism in secondary carnitine deficiency. (Inj) Prevention and treatment of carnitine deficiency in dialysis patients with end stage renal disease (ESRD).

DOSAGE: *Adults:* (Inj) Usual: 50mg/kg/day IV bolus or infusion. Max: 300mg/kg/day. Severe Metabolic Crisis: LD: 50mg/kg, then 50mg/kg over the next 24 hrs given q3-4h, and never less than q6h by infusion or IV injection. ESRD: Initial: 10-20mg/kg bolus into venous return line after dialysis. Adjust dose based on trough (pre-dialysis) levocarnitine levels. Can make downward dose adjustments the 3rd or 4th week of therapy. (Tab) 990mg PO bid-tid. (Sol) Initial: 1g/day. Usual: 1-3g/day per 50kg. Take after meals. May dissolve solution in fluids/liquid foods; drink slowly.
Pediatrics: (Inj) Usual: 50mg/kg/day IV bolus or infusion. Max: 300mg/kg/day. Severe Metabolic Crisis: LD: 50mg/kg, then 50mg/kg over the next 24 hrs given q3-4h, and never less than q6h by infusion or IV injection. ESRD: Initial: 10-20mg/kg bolus into venous return line after dialysis. Adjust dose based on trough (pre-dialysis) levocarnitine levels. Can make downward dose adjustments the 3rd or 4th week of therapy. (Sol/Tab) Infants/Children: Initial: 50mg/kg/day. Maint: 50-100mg/kg/day in divided doses. Max: 3g/day. Take after meals. May dissolve solution in fluids/liquid foods; drink slowly.

HOW SUPPLIED: Inj: 200mg/mL; Sol: 100mg/mL [118mL]; Tab: 330mg; Sol: (Carnitor SF) 100mg/mL [118mL]

WARNINGS/PRECAUTIONS: Avoid long term, high oral dose therapy with severely compromised renal function or ESRD with dialysis. Monitor carnitine levels periodically.

ADVERSE REACTIONS: Nausea, vomiting, abdominal cramps, diarrhea, gastritis, seizures.

PREGNANCY: Category B, not for use in nursing.

MECHANISM OF ACTION: Carnitine supplement; facilitates long-chain fatty acid entry into cellular mitochondria, thereby delivering substrate for oxidation and subsequent energy production.

PHARMACOKINETICS: Absorption: Absolute bioavailability: 15.1% (Tab), 15.9% (Oral Sol); C_{max}=80µmol/L, T_{max}=3.3 hrs. **Distribution:** Not bound to plasma protein. **Metabolism:** Trimethylamine N-oxide and [hydrogen-3]-gamma-butyrobetaine (major metabolites). **Elimination:** Urine (approximately 4-8% of dose); feces (<1%, total drug); $T_{1/2}$=17.4 hrs.

CARTEOLOL   RX
carteolol HCL (Bausch & Lomb)

THERAPEUTIC CLASS: Nonselective beta-blocker

INDICATIONS: Reduction of IOP in chronic open-angle glaucoma and in-traocular hypertension.

DOSAGE: *Adults:* 1 drop bid.

HOW SUPPLIED: Sol: 1% [5mL, 10mL, 15mL]

CONTRAINDICATIONS: Bronchial asthma, severe COPD, sinus bradycardia, 2nd- and 3rd-degree AV block, overt cardiac failure, cardiogenic shock.

WARNINGS/PRECAUTIONS: May be absorbed systemically. Caution with cardiac failure, bronchospasm, diminished pulmonary function, and DM. May mask symptoms of hypoglycemia and hyperthyroidism. Not for use alone in angle-closure glaucoma. May potentiate muscle weakness. D/C if cardiac failure develops. Withdrawal before surgery is controversial.

ADVERSE REACTIONS: Eye irritation, burning, tearing, conjunctival hyper-emia, conjunctival edema, photophobia, decreased night vision, ptosis.

INTERACTIONS: May potentiate systemic effects with oral β-blockers. Possible hypotension and bradycardia with catecholamine-depleting drugs (eg, reserpine). May antagonize epinephrine.

PREGNANCY: Category C, caution in nursing.

MECHANISM OF ACTION: Nonselective β-adrenergic blocking agent: re-sponsible for reducing IOP. Reduces cardiac output and may increase airway resistance in the bronchi and bronchioles.

CASODEX   RX
bicalutamide (AstraZeneca)

THERAPEUTIC CLASS: Nonsteroidal antiandrogen

INDICATIONS: Treatment of stage D_2 metastatic carcinoma of the prostate in combination with a luteinizing hormone-releasing hormone (LHRH) analogue.

DOSAGE: *Adults:* 50mg qd at the same time each day. Initiate with LHRH analogue therapy.

HOW SUPPLIED: Tab: 50mg

CONTRAINDICATIONS: Women, pregnancy.

WARNINGS/PRECAUTIONS: Rare cases of death or hospitalization due to severe liver injury reported. Hepatitis and marked increases in liver enzymes leading to drug discontinuation have occured. Caution with moderate-severe hepatic impairment; serum transamine levels should be measured prior to starting treatment, at regular intervals for 1st four months, then periodically. Monitor PSA regularly to assess therapy. For patients who have objective progression of disease together with elevated PSA, a treatment-free period of anti-androgen, while continuing LHRH analogue, may be considered. Gynecomastia, breast pain reported with single agent.

ADVERSE REACTIONS: Hot flushes, pain, back pain, asthenia, constipation, pelvic pain, infection, nausea, dyspnea, peripheral edema, diarrhea, hematu-ria, nocturia.

INTERACTIONS: Can displace coumarin anticoagulants, such as warfarin, from their protein-binding sites; monitor PT.

PREGNANCY: Category X, caution in nursing.

MECHANISM OF ACTION: Nonsteroidal antiandrogen; inhibits the action of androgens by binding to cytosol androgen receptors in target tissue.

PHARMACOKINETICS: Absorption: Well-absorbed, mean C_{max}=0.768mcg/mL, mean T_{max}=31.3 hrs. **Distribution:** Plasma protein binding (96%). **Metabolism:** Liver via oxidation and glucoronidation. **Elimination:** Urine and feces. $T_{1/2}$=5.8 days.

C

CATAFLAM   RX
diclofenac potassium (Novartis)

NSAIDs may cause an increased risk of serious cardiovascular thrombotic events, MI, stroke, and serious GI adverse events including bleeding, ulceration, and perforation of the stomach or intestines. Contraindicated for the treatment of perioperative pain in the setting of coronary artery bypass graft (CABG) surgery.

THERAPEUTIC CLASS: NSAID (benzeneacetic acid derivative)

INDICATIONS: Relief of signs and symptoms of osteoarthritis (OA) and rheumatoid arthritis (RA). Treatment of primary dysmenorrhea and relief of mild to moderate pain.

DOSAGE: *Adults:* OA: 50mg bid-tid. Max: 150mg/day. RA: 50mg tid-qid. Max: 200mg/day. Pain/Primary Dysmenorrhea: Initial: 50mg tid or 100mg on 1st dose, then 50mg on subsequent doses.

HOW SUPPLIED: Tab: 50mg

CONTRAINDICATIONS: ASA or other NSAID allergy that precipitates asthma, urticaria, or allergic reactions. Treatment of perioperative pain in the setting of CABG surgery.

WARNINGS/PRECAUTIONS: May lead to onset of new HTN or worsening of pre-existing HTN; monitor BP closely. Fluid retention and edema reported; caution with fluid retention or heart failure. Renal papillary necrosis and other renal injury reported after long-term use. Not recommended for use with advanced renal disease; if therapy must be initiated, monitor renal function. Anaphylactoid reactions may occur. May cause serious skin adverse events (eg, exfoliative dermatitis, Stevens-Johnson syndrome, and toxic epidermal necrolysis). Avoid in late pregnancy; may cause premature closure of ductus arteriosus. May cause elevations of LFTs; d/c if liver disease develops or systemic manifestations occur. Caution in elderly. Anemia may occur; with long-term use, monitor Hgb/Hct if signs or symptoms of anemia develop. May inhibit platelet aggregation and prolong bleeding time; monitor with coagulation disorders. Caution with asthma and avoid with ASA-sensitive asthma.

ADVERSE REACTIONS: Fluid retention, dizziness, rash, nausea, abdominal cramps, LFT abnormalities, constipation, diarrhea, heartburn, tinnitus, GI ulceration, HTN, insomnia, stomatitis, pruritus.

INTERACTIONS: Avoid with other diclofenac products. Increased adverse effects with ASA; avoid use. May enhance methotrexate toxicity; caution when co-administering. May increase nephrotoxicity of cyclosporine; caution when co-administering. May diminish antihypertensive effect of ACE-inhibitors. May reduce natriuretic effect of furosemide and thiazides; monitor for renal failure. May increase lithium levels; monitor for toxicity. Synergistic effects on GI bleeding with warfarin.

PREGNANCY: Category C, not for use in nursing.

MECHANISM OF ACTION: NSAID (benzeneacetic acid derivative); suspected to inhibit prostaglandin synthetase, exerts anti-inflammatory, analgesic, and antipyretic actions.

PHARMACOKINETICS: Absorption: Mean absolute bioavailabilty (55%), T_{max}=1 hr. **Distribution**: V_d=1.3L/kg. Serum protein binding (>99%). **Metabolism**: Metabolites: 4-hydroxy-, 5-hydroxy-, 3-hydroxy-, 4,'5-dihydroxy-, and 3'-hydroxy-4'-methoxy diclofenac. **Elimination:** Urine (65%.) Bile (35%) $T_{1/2}$= approximately 2 hrs.

CATAPRES   RX
clonidine (Boehringer Ingelheim)

OTHER BRAND NAMES: Catapres-TTS (Boehringer Ingelheim)
THERAPEUTIC CLASS: Central alpha-adrenergic agonist
INDICATIONS: Treatment of hypertension.

DOSAGE: *Adults:* (Patch) Apply to hairless, intact area of upper arm or chest weekly. Taper withdrawal of previous antihypertensive. Initial: 0.1mg/24 hr patch weekly. Titrate: May increase after 1-2 weeks. Max: 0.6mg/24 hr. (Tab) Initial: 0.1mg bid. Titrate: May increase by 0.1mg weekly. Usual: 0.2-0.6mg/day in divided doses. Max: 2.4mg/day. (Patch, Tab) Renal Impairment: Adjust according to degree of impairment.

HOW SUPPLIED: Patch, Extended-Release (TTS): 0.1mg/24 hr [4^s], 0.2mg/24 hr [4^s], 0.3mg/24 hr [4^s]; Tab: 0.1mg*, 0.2mg*, 0.3mg* *scored

WARNINGS/PRECAUTIONS: Avoid abrupt discontinuation. Tabs may cause rash if have allergic reaction to patch. Continue tabs to within 4 hrs of surgery resume and as soon as possible thereafter. Do not remove patch for surgery. Caution with severe coronary insufficiency, conduction disturbances, recent MI, cerebrovascular disease or chronic renal failure. Remove patch before defibrillation or cardioversion due to the potential risk of altered electrical conductivity or MRI due to the ocurrence of burns.

ADVERSE REACTIONS: Dry mouth, drowsiness, dizziness, constipation, sedation, impotence/sexual dysfunction, nausea, vomiting, alopecia, weakness, orthostatic symptoms, nervousness, localized skin reactions (patch).

INTERACTIONS: May potentiate CNS depression with alcohol, barbiturates, or other sedatives. Additive bradycardia and AV block with agents that affect sinus node function or AV nodal conduction (eg, digitalis, CCBs, and β-blockers). Hypotensive effect reduced by TCAs.

PREGNANCY: Category C, caution in nursing.

MECHANISM OF ACTION: Central acting α-agonist; stimulates α-adrenoreceptor in brain stem, reducing sympathetic outflow from CNS and decreasing HR, BP, peripheral and renal vascular resistance.

PHARMACOKINETICS: Absorption: T_{max} = 3-5 hrs. **Metabolism:** Liver. **Elimination:** $T_{1/2}$=12-16 hrs.; Urine (40-60%).

CATHFLO ACTIVASE RX

alteplase (Genentech)

THERAPEUTIC CLASS: Thrombolytic agent

INDICATIONS: To restore function to central venous access devices as assessed by ability to withdraw blood.

DOSAGE: *Adults:* ≥30kg: 2mg in 2mL. <30kg: 110% of catheter internal lumen volume, not to exceed 2mg in 2mL. If function not restored after 120 min, may instill 2nd dose. Max: 2mg/dose. Reconstitute to final concentration of 1mg/mL.
Pediatrics: ≥2 yrs: ≥30kg: 2mg in 2mL. 10 to <30kg: 110% of catheter internal lumen volume, not to exceed 2mg in 2mL. If function not restored after 120 min, may instill 2nd dose. Max: 2mg/dose. Reconstitute to final concentration of 1mg/mL.

HOW SUPPLIED: Inj: 2mg

WARNINGS/PRECAUTIONS: Before therapy, consider catheter dysfunction due to causes other than thrombus formation. Avoid excessive pressure when instilling alteplase into catheter. D/C and withdraw drug from catheter if serious bleeding in critical location occurs. Caution if active internal bleeding, infection in the catheter, any bleeding condition that is difficult to manage, thrombocytopenia, hemostatic defects, or if high risk for embolic complications. Caution if any of the following occurred within 48 hrs: surgery, OB delivery, percutaneous biopsy of viscera or deep tissues, or puncture of non-compressible vessels.

ADVERSE REACTIONS: Sepsis, GI bleeding, venous thrombosis.

PREGNANCY: Category C, caution in nursing.

MECHANISM OF ACTION: Thrombolytic agent; enzyme produces fibrin-enhanced conversion of plasminogen to plasmin. Produces limited conversion of plasminogen in the absence of fibrin. Binds to fibrin in thrombus and converts the entrapped plasminogen to plasmin, thereby initiating local fibrinolysis.

PHARMACOKINETICS: Metabolism: Liver. **Elimination:** $T_{1/2}$=5 min (initial); $T_{1/2}$=72 minutes (terminal).

CEDAX
ceftibuten (Shionogi)

RX

THERAPEUTIC CLASS: Cephalosporin (3rd generation)

INDICATIONS: Acute bacterial exacerbations of chronic bronchitis (ABECB), acute bacterial otitis media, pharyngitis and tonsillitis.

DOSAGE: *Adults:* ABECB/Otitis Media/Pharyngitis/Tonsillitis: 400mg qd for 10 days. Max: 400mg/day. CrCl 30-49mL/min: 4.5mg/kg or 200mg qd. CrCl 5-29mL/min: 2.25mg/kg or 100mg qd. Take 2 hrs before or at least 1 hr after a meal.
Pediatrics: ≥6 months: Pharyngitis/Tonsillitis/Otitis Media: 9mg/kg qd for 10 days. Max: 400mg. ABECB/Otitis Media/Pharyngitis/Tonsillitis: ≥12 yrs: 400mg qd for 10 days. Max: 400mg/day. CrCl 30-49mL/min: 4.5mg/kg or 200mg qd. CrCl 5-29mL/min: 2.25mg/kg or 100mg qd. Take 2 hrs before or at least 1 hr after a meal.

HOW SUPPLIED: Cap: 400mg; Sus: 90mg/5mL [30mL, 60mL, 90mL, 120mL]

WARNINGS/PRECAUTIONS: Pseudomembranous colitis (toxin produced by *Clostridium difficile* is the primary cause) reported. Caution with history of GI disease. Cross-sensitivity with cephalosporins and penicillins.

ADVERSE REACTIONS: Diarrhea, vomiting, nausea, abdominal pain, anorexia, dizziness, dyspepsia, dry mouth, dyspnea, dysuria, fatigue, flatulence, loose stools, headache, pruritus, rash, rigors, urticaria, superinfection (prolonged use).

PREGNANCY: Category B, caution in nursing.

MECHANISM OF ACTION: 3rd generation cephalosporin; binds to essential target proteins of bacterial cell wall, leading to inhibition of cell-wall synthesis.

PHARMACOKINETICS: Absorption: Rapid. C_{max}=15.0(3.3)mcg/mL (Cap), 13.3mcg/mL (Sus). AUC=73.7mcg•hr/mL (Cap), 56.0mcg•hr/mL (Sus). T_{max}=2.6 hrs. (Cap), 2 hrs. (Sus). **Distribution:** Vd=0.21L/kg (Cap), 0.5L/kg (Sus); plasma protein binding (65%). **Metabolism:** Cis-ceftibuten (metabolite). **Elimination:** Urine (56%), feces (39%).

CEENU
lomustine (Bristol-Myers Squibb)

RX

> Bone-marrow suppression (eg, thrombocytopenia, leukopenia) may contribute to bleeding and infections in compromised patients. Monitor blood counts weekly for 6 weeks after each dose. Adjust dose based on nadir blood counts from prior dose.

THERAPEUTIC CLASS: Nitrosourea alkylating agent

INDICATIONS: Single or adjunct treatment in primary/metastatic brain tumors in patients who already received surgical and/or radiation therapy. Secondary combination therapy of Hodgkin's disease in patients who relapse/ fail primary therapy.

DOSAGE: *Adults:* Single Regimen/Previously Untreated: 130mg/m² PO single dose every 6 weeks. Compromised Bone Marrow: 100mg/m² PO single dose every 6 weeks. Subsequent Doses: Adjust according to hematologic response. Leukocytes 2000-2999, platelets 25,000-74,999: Give 70% of dose. Leukocytes <2000, platelets <25,000: Give 50% of dose.
Pediatrics: Single Regimen/Previously Untreated: 130mg/m² PO single dose every 6 weeks. Compromised Bone Marrow: 100mg/m² PO single dose every 6 weeks. Subsequent Doses: Adjust according to hematologic response. Leukocytes 2000-2999, platelets 25,000-74,999: Give 70% of dose. Leukocytes <2000, platelets <25,000: Give 50% of dose.

HOW SUPPLIED: Cap: 10mg, 40mg, 100mg

WARNINGS/PRECAUTIONS: Pulmonary toxicity is dose-related. May develop secondary malignancies with long-term use. Monitor hepatic and renal function. Caution in elderly.

ADVERSE REACTIONS: Delayed myleosuppression, pulmonary infiltrates/fibrosis, nausea, vomiting, hepatotoxicity, azotemia, renal failure, stomatitis, alopecia, optic atrophy, visual disturbances, lethargy, ataxia.

PREGNANCY: Category D, not for use in nursing.

MECHANISM OF ACTION: Nitrosourea alkylating agent; alkylates DNA and RNA. Inhibits several key enzymatic processes by carbamyolation of amino acids in proteins.

PHARMACOKINETICS: Elimination: Urine, $T_{1/2}$=16 hrs-2 days.

CEFACLOR RX
cefaclor (Various)

THERAPEUTIC CLASS: Cephalosporin (2nd generation)

INDICATIONS: Treatment of otitis media, pharyngitis, tonsillitis, lower respiratory tract, urinary tract, and skin and skin structure infections caused by susceptible strains of microorganisms.

DOSAGE: *Adults:* Usual: 250mg q8h. Severe Infections/Pneumonia: 500mg q8h. Treat β-hemolytic strep for 10 days.
Pediatrics: ≥1 month: Usual: 20mg/kg/day given q8h. Otitis Media/Serious Infections/Infections Caused by Less Susceptible Organisms: 40mg/kg/day. Max: 1g/day. May administer q12h for otitis media and pharyngitis. Treat β-hemolytic strep for 10 days.

HOW SUPPLIED: Cap: 250mg, 500mg; Sus: 125mg/5mL [75mL, 150mL], 187mg/5mL [50mL, 100mL], 250mg/5mL [75mL, 150mL], 375mg/5mL [50mL, 100mL]

WARNINGS/PRECAUTIONS: Cross-sensitivity to PCNs and other cephalosporins may occur. *Clostridium difficile*-associated diarrhea reported. Positive direct Coombs' test reported. Caution with markedly impaired renal function, history of GI disease. False (+) for urine glucose with Benedict's, Fehling's solution, and Clinitest® tablets.

ADVERSE REACTIONS: Hypersensitivity reactions, diarrhea, eosinophilia, genital pruritus and vaginitis, serum-sickness-like reactions, superinfection.

INTERACTIONS: Renal excretion inhibited by probenecid. May potentiate warfarin and other anticoagulants; monitor PT/INR.

PREGNANCY: Category B, caution in nursing.

MECHANISM OF ACTION: Cephalosporin; bactericidal agent, inhibits cell-wall synthesis.

PHARMACOKINETICS: Absorption: Well-absorbed; (Fasting): C_{max}=7mcg/mL (250mg), 13mcg (500mg), 23mcg (1g); T_{max}=30-60 min. **Elimination:** Urine; 60-85% (unchanged); $T_{1/2}$= 0.6-0.9 hrs.

CEFACLOR ER RX
cefaclor (Various)

THERAPEUTIC CLASS: Cephalosporin (2nd generation)

INDICATIONS: Treatment of acute bacterial exacerbation of chronic bronchitis (ABECB), secondary bacterial infections of acute bronchitis, pharyngitis, tonsillitis, and uncomplicated skin and skin structure infections (SSSI) caused by susceptible strains of microorganisms.

DOSAGE: *Adults:* ABECB/Acute Bronchitis: 500mg q12h for 7 days. Pharyngitis/Tonsillitis: 375mg q12h for 10 days. SSSI: 375mg q12h for 7-10 days. Take with meals. Do not crush, cut, or chew tab.
Pediatrics: ≥16 yrs: ABECB/Acute Bronchitis: 500mg q12h for 7 days.

Pharyngitis/Tonsillitis: 375mg q12h for 10 days. SSSI: 375mg q12h for 7-10 days. Take with meals. Do not crush, cut, or chew tab.

HOW SUPPLIED: Tab, Extended-Release: 500mg

WARNINGS/PRECAUTIONS: Cross-sensitivity to PCNs and other cephalosporins may occur. *Clostridium difficile*-associated diarrhea reported. Positive direct Coombs' test reported. Caution with markedly impaired renal function, history of GI disease. False (+) for urine glucose with Benedict's, Fehling's solution, and Clinitest® tablets.

ADVERSE REACTIONS: Headache, rhinitis, diarrhea, nausea, vaginitis, abdominal pain, pharyngitis, increased cough, pruritus, back pain, serum-sickness-like reactions, superinfection (prolonged use).

INTERACTIONS: Decreased absorption with aluminum or magnesium hydroxide-containing antacids; space dose by 1 hr. Potentiated by probenecid. May potentiate warfarin, and other anticoagulants; monitor PT/INR.

PREGNANCY: Category B, caution in nursing.

MECHANISM OF ACTION: Cephalosporin; bactericidal, inhibits cell-wall synthesis.

PHARMACOKINETICS: Absorption: Fed: (375mg) C_{max}=3.7mcg/ml, T_{max}=2.7 hr, AUC=9.9mcg•hr/mL. (500mg) C_{max}=4.2mcg/ml, T_{max}=2.5 hr, AUC=18.1mcg•hr/ml. Fasting: C_{max}=5.4, T_{max}=1.5 hrs, AUC=14.8mcg•hr/mL.

CEFADROXIL   RX
cefadroxil monohydrate (Various)

THERAPEUTIC CLASS: Cephalosporin (1st generation)

INDICATIONS: Treatment of skin and skin structure (SSSI) and urinary tract infections (UTI), pharyngitis, and tonsillitis caused by susceptible strains of microorganisms.

DOSAGE: *Adults:* Uncomplicated Lower UTI: 1-2g/day given qd or bid. Other UTI: 1g bid. SSSI: 1g qd or 500mg bid. Group A β-hemolytic Strep Pharyngitis/Tonsillitis: 1g qd or 500mg bid for 10 days. CrCl ≤50mL/min: Initial: 1g. Maint: CrCl 25-50mL/min: 500mg q12h; CrCl 10-25mL/min: 500mg q24h; CrCl 0-10mL/min: 500mg q36h.
Pediatrics: UTI/SSSI: 15mg/kg q12h. Pharyngitis/Tonsillitis/Impetigo: 30mg/kg qd or 15mg/kg q12h. Treat β-hemolytic strep infections for at least 10 days.

HOW SUPPLIED: Cap: 500mg; Sus: 250mg/5mL [100mL], 500mg/5mL [75mL, 100mL]; Tab: 1g* *scored

WARNINGS/PRECAUTIONS: Caution with markedly impaired renal function, history of GI disease. Cross-sensitivity with cephalosporins and PCNs. False (+) direct Coombs' tests, colitis, and *Clostridium difficile*-associated diarrhea (CDAD) reported.

ADVERSE REACTIONS: Diarrhea, rash, hypersensitivity reactions, pruritus, hepatic dysfunction, genital moniliasis, vaginitis, fever, superinfection (prolonged use).

PREGNANCY: Category B, caution in nursing.

CEFAZOLIN   RX
cefazolin (Various)

THERAPEUTIC CLASS: Cephalosporin (1st generation)

INDICATIONS: Treatment of respiratory tract, urinary tract (UTI), skin and skin structure, biliary tract, bone and joint, and genital infections, septicemia, and endocarditis caused by susceptible strains of microorganisms. Perioperative prophylaxis for surgical procedures classified as contaminated or potentially contaminated.

DOSAGE: *Adults:* Moderate-Severe Infections: 500mg-1g q6-8h. Mild Gram-Positive Cocci Infection: 250-500mg q8h. Acute, Uncomplicated UTI: 1g q12h.

Pneumococcal Pneumonia: 500mg q12h. Severe Life-Threatening Infection (eg, Endocarditis, Septicemia): 1-1.5g q6h; Max: 12g/day (rare). Perioperative Prophylaxis: 1g IM/IV 0.5-1 hr before surgery. For Procedures ≥2 hrs: 500mg-1g IM/IV during surgery. Maint: 500mg-1g IM/IV q6-8h for 24 hrs post-op. Continue for 3-5 days post-op for devastating procedures (eg, open-heart surgery and prosthetic arthroplasty). Renal Impairment: CrCl 35-54mL/min: Full dose q8h. CrCl 11-34mL/min: 1/2 usual dose q12h. CrCl <10mL/min: 1/2 usual dose q18-24h. Apply reduced dosage recommendations after initial LD is given.

Pediatrics: Mild-Moderately Severe Infection: 25-50mg/kg/day in 3-4 equal doses. Severe Infection: 100mg/kg/day in divided doses. Renal Impairment: CrCl 40-70mL/min: 60% of normal daily dose in equally divided doses q12h. CrCl 20-40mL/min: 25% of normal daily dose in equally divided doses q12h. CrCl 5-20mL/min: 10% of normal daily dose q24h. Apply reduced dosage recommendations after initial LD is given.

HOW SUPPLIED: Inj: 500mg, 1g, 10g, 20g

WARNINGS/PRECAUTIONS: Prolonged use may result in overgrowth of nonsusceptible organisms. Possible cross-sensitivity between PCNs, cephalosporins, and other β-lactam antibiotics. Pseudomembranous colitis reported. Elevated levels with renal insufficiency can lead to seizures. Caution with colitis and other GI diseases. Safety in premature infants and neonates not established.

ADVERSE REACTIONS: Diarrhea, oral candidiasis, vomiting, nausea, stomach cramps, anorexia, allergic reactions, blood dyscrasias, renal failure, transient rise in SGOT/SGPT/BUN/SCr/alkaline phosphatase, local reactions.

INTERACTIONS: Decreased renal tubular secretion with probenecid.

PREGNANCY: Category B, caution in nursing.

MECHANISM OF ACTION: Cephalosporin; inhibits cell wall synthesis.

PHARMACOKINETICS: Absorption: C_{max}=185mcg/mL. **Distribution:** Crosses placenta; found in breast milk. **Elimination:** Urine (unchanged); $T_{1/2}$=1.8 hrs.

CEFIZOX   RX
ceftizoxime (Astellas)

THERAPEUTIC CLASS: Cephalosporin (3rd generation)

INDICATIONS: Treatment of lower respiratory tract, skin and skin structure, intra-abdominal, bone and joint, and urinary tract infections (UTI), gonorrhea, pelvic inflammatory disease (PID), meningitis, and septicemia.

DOSAGE: *Adults:* Uncomplicated UTI: 500mg q12h IM/IV. Other Sites: 1g q8-12h IM/IV. Severe/Refractory Infections: 1-2g IM/IV q8-12h. PID: 2g IV q8h. Life Threatening Infections: 3-4g IV q8h. Uncomplicated Gonorrhea: 1g IM as single dose. Renal Impairment: LD: 500mg-1g IM/IV. Less Severe Infection: Maint: CrCl 50-79mL/min: 500mg q8h. CrCl 5-49mL/min: 250-500mg q12h. CrCl 0-4mL/min (Dialysis): 500mg q48h or 250mg q24h. Life-Threatening Infection: Maint: CrCl 50-79mL/min: 0.75-1.5g q8h. CrCl 5-49mL/min: 0.5-1g q12h. CrCl 0-4mL/min (Dialysis): 0.5-1g q48h or 0.5g q24h. *Pediatrics:* ≥6 months: 50mg/kg IM/IV q6-8h, up to 200mg/kg/day. Max: 6g/day for serious infections.

HOW SUPPLIED: Inj: 500mg, 1g, 2g

WARNINGS/PRECAUTIONS: *Clostridium difficile*-associated diarrhea reported. Caution with history of GI disease. Cross-sensitivity with cephalosporins and PCNs may occur. Prolonged use may result in overgrowth of superinfection, (+) Coombs test.

ADVERSE REACTIONS: Rash, pruritus, fever, BUN elevation, injection site reactions (eg, burning, cellulitis, phlebitis, pain, induration, tenderness), eosinophilia, thrombocytosis, elevated liver enzymes, GI effects.

INTERACTIONS: Risk of nephrotoxicity with aminoglycosides and other cephalosporins.

PREGNANCY: Category B, caution in nursing.

C

MECHANISM OF ACTION: 3rd-generation cephalosporin; inhibits cell wall systhesis.

PHARMACOKINETICS: Absorption: IV administration of variable doses resulted in different parameters. **Distribution:** Plasma protein binding (30%); found in various bodily fluids and tissues and breast milk; CSF only if meninges inflamed. **Elimination:** Urine (unchanged); $T_{1/2}$=1.7 hrs.

CEFOL RX
multiple vitamin (Abbott)

THERAPEUTIC CLASS: Vitamin supplement

INDICATIONS: Vitamin C deficiency associated with deficient intake or increased need for Vitamin B-Complex, Folic Acid, and Vitamin E in non-pregnant patients.

DOSAGE: *Adults:* 1 tab qd.

HOW SUPPLIED: Tab: Calcium Pantothenate 20mg-Folic Acid 0.5mg-Niacinamide 100mg-Vitamin B_1 15mg-Vitamin B_2 10mg-Vitamin B_6 5mg-Vitamin B_{12} 6mcg-Vitamin C 750mg-Vitamin E 30 IU

WARNINGS/PRECAUTIONS: Folic acid alone is improper treatment of pernicious anemia and other megaloblastic anemias with Vitamin B_{12}-deficiency. Folic acid >0.1mg/day may obscure pernicious anemia.

ADVERSE REACTIONS: Allergic sensitization.

PREGNANCY: Safety in pregnancy and nursing not known.

CEFOXITIN RX
cefoxitin sodium (Various)

OTHER BRAND NAMES: Mefoxin (Merck)

THERAPEUTIC CLASS: Cephalosporin (2nd generation)

INDICATIONS: Treatment of lower respiratory tract, urinary tract, intra-abdominal, gynecological, skin and skin structure, and bone and joint infections, and septicemia caused by susceptible strains of microorganisms. Prophylaxis of infection in patients undergoing uncontaminated GI surgery, abdominal/vaginal hysterectomy, or cesarean section.

DOSAGE: *Adults:* Usual: 1-2g IV q6-8h. Uncomplicated Infections: 1g IV q6-8h. Moderate-Severe: 1g IV q4h or 2g IV q6-8h. Gas Gangrene/Other Infections Requiring Higher Dose: 2g IV q4h or 3g IV q6h. Renal Insufficiency: LD: 1-2g IV. Maint: CrCl 30-50mL/min: 1-2g IV q8-12h. CrCl 10-29mL/min: 1-2g IV q12-24h. CrCl 5-9mL/min: 0.5-1g IV q12-24h. CrCl <5mL/min: 0.5-1g IV q24-48h. Hemodialysis: LD: 1-2g IV after dialysis. Maint: See renal insufficiency doses above. Prophylaxis: Uncontaminated GI Surgery/Hysterectomy: 2g IV 0.5-1 hr prior to surgery (1/2-1 hr before initial incision), then 2g IV q6h after 1st dose up to 24 hrs. C-Section: 2g IV single dose as soon as umbilical cord is clamped, or 2g IV as soon as umbilical cord is clamped, followed by 2g IV at 4 and 8 hrs after initial dose.
Pediatrics: ≥3 months: 80-160mg/kg/day divided into 4-6 equal doses. Max: 12g/day. Prophylaxis: Uncontaminated GI Surgery/Hysterectomy: 30-40mg/kg IV 0.5-1 hr prior to surgery, then 30-40mg/kg IV q6h after first dose for up to 24 hrs.

HOW SUPPLIED: Inj: 1g, 1g/50mL, 2g, 2g/50mL, 10g

WARNINGS/PRECAUTIONS: Possible cross-sensitivity between PCNs and cephalosporins. *Clostridium difficile*-associated diarrhea reported. Caution with allergies, GI disease, particularly colitis. Prolonged use may result in overgrowth of nonsusceptible organisms. Monitor renal, hepatic, hematopoietic functions, especially with prolonged therapy. False (+) for urine glucose with Clinitest® tabs.

ADVERSE REACTIONS: Thrombophlebitis, rash, pseudomembranous colitis, pruritus, fever, dyspnea, hypotension, diarrhea, blood dyscrasias, elevated LFTs, changes in renal function tests, exacerbation of myasthenia gravis.

INTERACTIONS: Increased nephrotoxicity with concomitant aminoglycosides.

PREGNANCY: Category B, caution use in nursing.

MECHANISM OF ACTION: 2nd generation cephalosporin; inhibits bacterial cell wall synthesis.

PHARMACOKINETICS: Metabolism: Passes pleural and joint fluids; found in bile and breast milk. **Elimination:** Urine (85% unchanged); $T_{1/2}$=41-59 min.

CEFTAZIDIME   RX
ceftazidime (Various)

THERAPEUTIC CLASS: Cephalosporin (3rd generation)

INDICATIONS: Treatment of lower respiratory tract (eg, pneumonia), skin and skin structure (SSSI), bone and joint, gynecologic, CNS (eg, meningitis), intra-abdominal, and urinary tract infections (UTI), and septicemia caused by susceptible strains of microorganisms. For use in sepsis.

DOSAGE: *Adults:* Usual: 1g IM/IV q8-12h. Uncomplicated UTI: 250mg IM/IV q12h. Complicated UTI: 500mg IM/IV q8-12h. Bone and Joint Infection: 2g IV q12h. Uncomplicated Pneumonia/SSSI: 500mg-1g IM/IV q8h. Gynecological/ Intra-Abdominal/Meningitis/Severe Life-Threatening Infection: 2g IV q8h. Lung Infection caused by Pseudomonas spp. in Cystic Fibrosis (normal renal function): 30-50mg/kg IV q8h. Max: 6g/day. CrCl 31-50mL/min: 1g q12h. CrCl 16-30mL/min: 1g q24h. CrCl 6-15mL/min: 500mg q24h. CrCl <5mL/min: 500mg q48h. For severe infections (6g/day), increase renal impairment dose by 50% or increase dosing interval. Apply reduced dosage recommendations after initial 1g LD is given. Hemodialysis: Give 1g before then 1g after each hemodialysis. Intra-Peritoneal Dialysis/Continuous Ambulatory Peritoneal Dialysis: Give 1g followed by 500mg q24h.
Pediatrics: ≥12 yrs: Usual: 1g IM/IV q8-12h. Uncomplicated UTI: 250mg IM/IV q12h. Complicated UTI: 500mg IM/IV q8-12h. Bone and Joint Infection: 2g IV q12h. Uncomplicated Pneumonia/SSSI: 500mg-1g IM/IV q8h. Gynecological/ Intra-Abdominal/Meningitis/Severe Life-Threatening Infection: 2g IV q8h. Lung Infection caused by Pseudomonas spp. in Cystic Fibrosis (normal renal function): 30-50mg/kg IV q8h. Max: 6g/day. CrCl 31-50mL/min: 1g q12h. CrCl 16-30mL/min: 1g q24h. CrCl 6-15mL/min: 500mg q24h. CrCl <5mL/min: 500mg q48h. For severe infections (6g/day), increase renal impairment dose by 50% or increase dosing interval. Apply reduced dosage recommendations after initial 1g LD is given. Hemodialysis: Give 1g before then 1g after each hemodialysis. Intra-Peritoneal Dialysis/Continuous Ambulatory Peritoneal Dialysis: Give 1g followed by 500mg q24h.

HOW SUPPLIED: Inj: 1g, 2g, 6g

WARNINGS/PRECAUTIONS: Monitor renal function; potential for nephrotox-icity. Prolonged use may result in overgrowth of nonsusceptible organisms. Possible cross-sensitivity between PCNs, cephalosporins, and other β-lactam antibiotics. Pseudomembranous colitis reported. Elevated levels with renal insufficiency can lead to seizures, encephalopathy, asterixis, coma, and neu-romuscular excitability. Possible decrease in PT; caution with renal or hepatic impairment, poor nutritional state; monitor PT and give vitamin K if needed. Caution with colitis and other GI diseases. Distal necrosis can occur after inadvertent intra-arterial administration. Continue therapy for 2 days after the signs and symptoms of infection have disappeared, but in complicated infec-tions longer therapy may be required. False positive for urine glucose with Benedict's, Fehling's solution, and Clinitest® tablets.

ADVERSE REACTIONS: Phlebitis and inflammation at injection site, pruritus, rash, fever, diarrhea.

INTERACTIONS: Nephrotoxicity reported with aminoglycosides or potent diuretics (eg, furosemide). Avoid with chloramphenicol; may decrease effect of β-lactam antibiotics.

C

PREGNANCY: Category B, not for use in nursing.

MECHANISM OF ACTION: Broad spectrum, β-lactam antibiotic; exerts effects by inhibiting enzymes responsible for cell-wall synthesis.

PHARMACOKINETICS: Absorption: (IV) C_{max}=45mcg/mL (500mg), 90mcg/mL (1g). (IM) C_{max}=17mcg/mL (500mg), 39mcg/mL (1g), T_{max}=1 hr. **Distribution:** Plasma protein binding (<10%); found in breast milk. **Elimination:** Urine, (80-90%, unchanged). $T_{1/2}$=1.9 hrs (IV), 2 hrs (IM).

Ceftin RX
cefuroxime axetil (GlaxoSmithKline)

THERAPEUTIC CLASS: Cephalosporin (2nd generation)

INDICATIONS: Treatment of the following infections caused by susceptible strains of microorganisms: (Sus/Tab) Pharyngitis/tonsillitis, acute otitis media, and impetigo. (Tab) Uncomplicated skin and skin structure (SSSI), and urinary tract infection (UTI), gonorrhea, early Lyme disease, acute bacterial maxillary sinusitis, acute bacterial exacerbations of chronic bronchitis (ABECB) and secondary bacterial infections of acute bronchitis.

DOSAGE: *Adults:* (Tab) Pharyngitis/Tonsillitis/Sinusitis: 250mg bid for 10 days. ABECB/SSSI: 250-500mg bid for 10 days. Acute Bronchitis: 250-500mg bid for 5-10 days. UTI: 250mg bid for 7-10 days. Gonorrhea: 1000mg single dose. Lyme Disease: 500mg bid for 20 days.
Pediatrics: ≥13 yrs: (Tab) Pharyngitis/Tonsillitis/Sinusitis: 250mg bid for 10 days. ABECB/SSSI: 250-500mg bid for 10 days. Acute Bronchitis: 250-500mg bid for 5-10 days. UTI: 250mg bid for 7-10 days. Gonorrhea: 1000mg single dose. Lyme Disease: 500mg bid for 20 days. 3 months-12 yrs: (Sus) Pharyngitis/Tonsillitis: 10mg/kg bid for 10 days. Max: 500mg/day. Otitis Media/Sinusitis/Impetigo: 15mg/kg bid for 10 days. Max: 1000mg/day. (Tab-if can swallow whole) Otitis Media/Sinusitis: 250mg bid for 10 days.

HOW SUPPLIED: Sus: 125mg/5mL [100mL], 250mg/5mL [50mL, 100mL]; Tab: 250mg, 500mg

WARNINGS/PRECAUTIONS: Tabs are not bioequivalent to sus. Caution with colitis, renal impairment. Cross-sensitivity with cephalosporins and PCNs. False (+) for urine glucose with Benedict's, Fehling's solution, and Clinitest® tablets. May cause fall in PT; risk in patients stable on anticoagulants, if receiving a protracted course of antibiotics, renal/hepatic impairment, or a poor nutritional state; give vitamin K as needed. Watery, bloody stools (with or without stomach cramps and fever) may develop after starting treatment; notify physician. *Clostridium difficile*-associated diarrhea (CDAD) reported.

ADVERSE REACTIONS: Diarrhea, nausea, vomiting, vaginitis, (suspension in peds) taste aversion, superinfection (prolonged use).

INTERACTIONS: Probenecid increases plasma levels. Lower bioavailability with drugs that lower gastric acidity. Caution with agents causing adverse effects on renal function (diuretics). Reduced efficacy of combined oral estrogen/progesterone contraceptives.

PREGNANCY: Category B, not for use in nursing.

MECHANISM OF ACTION: 2nd-generation cephalosporin; binds to essential target proteins and inhibits cell-wall synthesis.

PHARMACOKINETICS: Absorption: Absolute bioavailability (52%, with food). PO administration of variable doses resulted in different parameters. **Distribution:** Plasma protein binding (50%). **Metabolism:** Rapid hydrolysis, via nonspecific esterases in the intestinal mucosa and blood. **Elimination:** Urine (50% unchanged).

Cefzil RX
cefprozil (Bristol-Myers Squibb)

THERAPEUTIC CLASS: Cephalosporin (2nd generation)

INDICATIONS: Treatment of mild to moderate pharyngitis/tonsillitis, otitis media, acute sinusitis, secondary bacterial infection of acute bronchitis, acute bacterial exacerbation of chronic bronchitis (ABECB), and uncomplicated skin and skin structure infections (SSSI) caused by susceptible strains of microorganisms.

DOSAGE: *Adults:* Pharyngitis/Tonsillitis: 500mg q24h for 10 days. Acute Sinusitis: 250-500mg q12h for 10 days. ABECB/Acute Bronchitis: 500mg q12h for 10 days. SSSI: 250-500mg q12h or 500mg q24h for 10 days. CrCl <30mL/min: 50% of standard dose.
Pediatrics: ≥13 yrs: Use adult dose. 2-12 yrs: Pharyngitis/Tonsillitis: 7.5mg/kg q12h for 10 days. SSSI: 20mg/kg q24h for 10 days. 6 months-12 yrs: Otitis Media: 15mg/kg q12h for 10 days. Acute Sinusitis: 7.5-15mg/kg q12h for 10 days. Do not exceed adult dose. CrCl <30mL/min: 50% of standard dose.

HOW SUPPLIED: Sus: 125mg/5mL [50mL, 75mL, 100mL], 250mg/5mL [50mL, 75mL, 100mL]; Tab: 250mg, 500mg

WARNINGS/PRECAUTIONS: Cross-sensitivity with cephalosporins and PCNs. False (+) direct Coombs' tests reported. *Clostridium difficile*-associated diarrhea reported. Caution with GI disease, renal impairment, elderly. False (+) for urine glucose with Benedict's, Fehling's solution, and Clinitest® tablets. Sus contains phenylalanine.

ADVERSE REACTIONS: Diarrhea, nausea, hepatic enzyme elevations, eosinophilia, genital pruritus, vaginitis, superinfection (prolonged use).

INTERACTIONS: Nephrotoxicity with aminoglycosides reported. Probenecid may increase plasma levels. Caution with agents causing adverse effects on renal function (diuretics).

PREGNANCY: Category B, caution in nursing.

MECHANISM OF ACTION: 2nd-generation cephalosporin; inhibits bacterial cell-wall synthesis.

PHARMACOKINETICS: Absorption: C_{max}=6.1mcg/mL (250mg), 10.5mcg/mL (500mg), 18.3mcg/mL(1g); T_{max}=1.5 hrs (adults), 1-2 hrs (peds). Plasma concentration (peds) at 7.5, 15, and 30mg/kg doses similar to those observed within same time frame in normal adults at 250, 500, and 1000mg doses, respectively. **Distribution:** V_d=0.23L/kg; plasma protein binding (36%); found in breast milk. **Elimination:** Urine (60%); $T_{1/2}$=1.3 hrs (adults), 1.5 hrs (peds).

CELEBREX
RX

celecoxib (G.D. Searle)

> NSAIDs may cause an increased risk of serious cardiovascular thrombotic events, MI, stroke and serious GI adverse events including bleeding, ulceration, and perforation of the stomach or intestines. Contraindicated for the treatment of perioperative pain in the setting of coronary artery bypass graft (CABG) surgery.

THERAPEUTIC CLASS: COX-2 inhibitor

INDICATIONS: Relief of signs and symtoms of rheumatoid arthritis (RA) in adults, osteoarthritis (OA), and ankylosing spondylitis (AS). Management of acute pain in adults. Treatment of primary dysmenorrhea. To reduce the number of adematous colorectal polyps in familial adenomatous polyposis (FAP). Relief of signs and symptoms of juvenile rheumatoid arithis (JRA) in patients ≥2 yrs.

DOSAGE: *Adults:* ≥18 yrs: OA: 200mg qd or 100mg bid. RA: 100-200mg bid. AS: 200mg qd or 100mg bid. Titrate: May increase to 400mg/day after 6 weeks. FAP: 400mg bid with food. Acute Pain/Primary Dysmenorrhea: Day 1: 400mg, then 200mg if needed. Maint: 200mg bid prn. Moderate Hepatic Insufficiency: Reduce daily dose by 50%.
Pediatrics: JRA: ≥2 yrs: 10-25kg: 50mg bid. >25kg: 100mg bid.

HOW SUPPLIED: Cap: 50mg, 100mg, 200mg, 400mg

CONTRAINDICATIONS: Sulfonamide hypersensitivity. Asthma, urticaria, or allergic type reactions after ASA or NSAID use. Treatment of perioperative pain in the setting of CABG surgery.

C

WARNINGS/PRECAUTIONS: Increased risk of serious adverse cardiovascular thrombotic events, MI, and stroke. May lead to onset of new HTN or worsening of pre-existing HTN; monitor BP closely. Fluid retention and edema reported; caution with fluid retention or heart failure. Renal papillary necrosis and other renal injury reported after long-term use. Not recommended for use with advanced renal disease; if therapy must be initiated, monitor renal function. Greatest risk with those taking diuretics and ACE-inhibitors. Anaphylactoid reactions may occur. May cause serious skin adverse events (eg, exfoliative dermatitis, Stevens-Johnson syndrome, and toxic epidermal necrolysis). Avoid in late pregnancy; may cause premature closure of ductus arteriosus. May cause elevations of LFTs; d/c if liver disease develops or systemic manifestations occur. Caution in elderly. Anemia may occur; with long-term use, monitor Hgb/Hct if signs or symptoms of anemia or blood loss develop. May inhibit platelet aggregation and prolong bleeding time (prolonged APTT); monitor with coagulation disorders. Caution with asthma and avoid with ASA-sensitive asthma. Caution in pediatric patients with systemic onset JRA due to increased possibly of DIC.

ADVERSE REACTIONS: Dyspepsia, diarrhea, abdominal pain, nausea, dizziness, headache, sinusitis, upper respiratory infection, rash, fever, cough, arthralgia, HTN, insomnia, pharyngitis.

INTERACTIONS: Monitor oral anticoagulants; reports of serious bleeding, some fatal, with warfarin. Decrease effects of ACE-inhibitors, furosemide, and thiazides. Increased levels with fluconazole. Monitor lithium. Caution with CYP2C9 inhibitors and drugs metabolized by CYP2D6. Celecoxib is not a substitute for ASA for cardiovascular prophylaxis; may use with low-dose ASA but may increase GI complications.

PREGNANCY: Category C, not for use in nursing.

MECHANISM OF ACTION: NSAID; inhibits prostaglandin synthesis primarily via inhibition of COX-2.

PHARMACOKINETICS: Absorption: C_{max}=705ng/mL, T_{max}=2.8 hrs. **Distribution:** V_d=429L; plasma protein binding (97%). **Metabolism:** CYP2C9. Primary alcohol, carboxylic acid, glucuronide conjugate (metabolites). **Elimination:** Urine (27%), feces (57%); $T_{1/2}$=11.2 hrs.

CELESTONE RX
betamethasone (Schering)

THERAPEUTIC CLASS: Glucocorticoid

INDICATIONS: Steroid responsive disorders.

DOSAGE: *Adults:* Initial: 0.6-7.2mg/day depending on disease. Maintain until sufficient response. Maint: Decrease dose by small amounts to lowest effective dose. D/C gradually.
Pediatrics: Initial: 0.6-7.2mg/day depending on disease. Maintain until sufficient response. Maint: Decrease dose by small amounts to lowest effective dose. D/C gradually.

HOW SUPPLIED: Syrup: 0.6mg/5mL [118mL]

CONTRAINDICATIONS: Systemic fungal infections.

WARNINGS/PRECAUTIONS: May need to increase dose before, during, and after stressful situations. May mask signs of infection or cause new infections. Prolonged use may produce posterior subcapsular cataracts, glaucoma, optic nerve damage, secondary ocular infections. Increases BP, salt/water retention, potassium and calcium excretion. More severe/fatal course of infections reported with chickenpox, measles. Caution with threadworm infestation, latent TB, hypothyroidism, cirrhosis, ocular herpes simplex, HTN, diverticulitis, fresh intestinal anastomosis, ulcerative colitis, osteoporosis, myasthenia gravis, renal insufficiency, peptic ulcer disease. Growth and development of children on prolonged therapy should be monitored. Monitor for psychic disturbances. Avoid abrupt withdrawal.

ADVERSE REACTIONS: Sodium retention, fluid retention, potassium loss, muscle weakness, myopathy, peptic ulcer, impaired wound healing, thin fragile skin, convulsions, menstrual irregularities, cataracts.

INTERACTIONS: Caution with ASA in hypoprothrombinemia. Increased susceptibility to infections with immunosuppressives. Avoid smallpox vaccines and other immunization procedures at high doses. Increased requirements of insulin or oral hypoglycemic agents.

PREGNANCY: Safety in pregnancy and nursing not known.

MECHANISM OF ACTION: Glucocorticoid; has16β-methyl group that enhaces anti-inflammatory action and reduces sodium- and water-retaining properties of fluorine atom bound at carbon 9.

PHARMACOKINETICS: Absorption: Readily absorbed. **Distribution:** Found in breast milk. **Metabolism:** Liver.

CELESTONE SOLUSPAN RX
betamethasone acetate - betamethasone (augmented) sodium phosphate
(Schering)

THERAPEUTIC CLASS: Glucocorticoid

INDICATIONS: When oral therapy is not feasible, use IM route for steroid-responsive treatment of endocrine, rheumatic, collagen, dermatologic, respiratory, ophthalmic, neoplastic, hematologic, and GI disorders, allergic and edematous states and Tuberculous meningitis with subarachnoid block and trichinosis with neurologic/myocardial involvement. Intra-articular or soft tissue administration for short-term adjunct treatment of synovitis, osteoarthritis (OA), rheumatoid arthritis (RA), bursitis, acute gouty arthritis, epicondylitis, acute nonspecific tenosynovitis. Intralesional injection for keloids, discoid lupus erythematosus, necrobiosis lipoidica diabeticorum, alopecia areata, lesions of: lichen planus, psoriatic plaques, granuloma, annulare, lichen simplex chronicus.

DOSAGE: *Adults:* Initial: 0.5-9mg/day IM. Parenteral dose is usually 1/2-1/3 the oral dose given q12h. Maintain until sufficient response occurs. Maint: Decrease in small increments at appropriate time intervals until lowest effective dose. D/C gradually. Bursitis/Tenosynovitis/Peritendinitis: 1mL intrabursal injection. Tenosynovitis/Tendinitis: Give 3-4 injections every 1-2 weeks. Chronic Bursitis: Reduce initial dose. Ganglion Cysts: 0.5mL into cyst. RA/OA: 0.5-2mL intra-articularly. Dermatologic Conditions: 0.2mL/sq cm intradermally. Max: 1mL/week.
Pediatrics: Initial: 0.5-9mg/day IM. Parenteral dose is usually 1/2-1/3 the oral dose given q12h. Maintain until sufficient response. Maint: Decrease in small increments at appropriate time intervals until reach lowest dose that sustains response. D/C gradually.

HOW SUPPLIED: Inj: (Betamethasone Acetate-Betamethasone Sodium Phosphate) 3mg-3mg/mL

CONTRAINDICATIONS: Systemic fungal infections.

WARNINGS/PRECAUTIONS: May need to increase dose before, during, and after stressful situations. May mask signs of infection or cause new infections. Prolonged use may produce posterior subcapsular cataracts, glaucoma, optic nerve damage, secondary ocular infections. Increases BP, salt/water retention, potassium and calcium excretion. More severe/fatal course of infections reported with chickenpox, measles. Caution with threadworm infestation, latent TB, hypothyroidism, cirrhosis, ocular herpes simplex, HTN, diverticulitis, fresh intestinal anastomosis, ulcerative colitis, osteoporosis, myasthenia gravis, renal insufficiency, peptic ulcer disease. Growth and development of children on prolonged therapy should be monitored. Monitor for psychic disturbances. Avoid abrupt withdrawal. (Intra-articular) Examine joint fluid to rule out a septic process. Avoid injection into previously infected joint.

ADVERSE REACTIONS: Sodium retention, fluid retention, potassium loss, muscle weakness, myopathy, peptic ulcer, impaired wound healing, thin fragile skin, convulsions, menstrual irregularities, cataracts.

INTERACTIONS: Caution with ASA in hypoprothrombinemia. Increased susceptibility to infections with immunosuppressives. Avoid smallpox vaccines and other immunization procedures at high doses. Increased requirements of insulin or oral hypoglycemic agents. Avoid diluents containing methylparaben, phenol, propylparaben; may cause flocculation of steroid.

PREGNANCY: Safety in pregnancy and nursing not known.

MECHANISM OF ACTION: Glucocorticoid; has 16β-methyl group that enhances anti-inflammatory action and reduces sodium- and water-retaining properties of flourine atom bound at carbon 9.

PHARMACOKINETICS: Absorption: GI tract (Readily absorbed). **Distribution:** Found in breast milk. **Metabolism:** Liver.

CELEXA   RX
citalopram hydrobromide (Forest)

> Antidepressants increased the risk of suicidal thinking and behavior (suicidality) in short-term studies in children, adolescents, and young adults with Major Depressive Disorder (MDD) and other psychiatric disorders. Citalopram is not approved for use in pediatric patients.

THERAPEUTIC CLASS: Selective serotonin reuptake inhibitor

INDICATIONS: Treatment of depression.

DOSAGE: *Adults:* Initial: 20mg qd, in the am or pm. Titrate: Increase by 20mg at intervals of no less than 1 week. Max: 40mg/day (non-responders may require 60mg/day). Elderly/Hepatic Impairment: 20mg/day; titrate to 40mg/day in nonresponders.

HOW SUPPLIED: Sol: 10mg/5mL [240mL]; Tab: 10mg, 20mg*, 40mg* *scored

CONTRAINDICATIONS: Concomitant MAOI or pimozide therapy.

WARNINGS/PRECAUTIONS: Activation of mania/hypomania, SIADH, hyponatremia reported. Close supervision with high risk suicide patients. Caution with history of mania or seizures, hepatic impairment, severe renal impairment, conditions that alter metabolism or hemodynamic responses. May impair judgment, thinking, or motor skills.

ADVERSE REACTIONS: Nausea, dyspepsia, vomiting, diarrhea, dry mouth, somnolence, insomnia, increased sweating, ejaculation disorder, rhinitis, anxiety, anorexia, skeletal pain, agitation.

INTERACTIONS: See Contraindications. Avoid alcohol. Caution with other CNS drugs, TCAs, lithium, carbamazepine, cimetidine. Increased risk of bleeding with warfarin, ASA, NSAIDs. Rare reports of weakness, hyperreflexia, incoordination with SSRI's and sumatriptan. Clearance may be decreased with potent CYP3A4 (eg, ketoconazole, itraconazole, fluconazole, erythromycin) and CYP2C19 (eg, omeprazole) inhibitors. May increase metoprolol levels which leads to decreased cardioselectivity.

PREGNANCY: Category C, not for use in nursing.

MECHANISM OF ACTION: Selective serotonin reuptake inhibitor; inhibits CNS neuronal reuptake of serotonin.

PHARMACOKINETICS: Absorption: T_{max}=4 hrs, absolute bioavailability (80%). **Distribution:** V_d=12L/kg. **Metabolism:** Hepatic (biotransformation: N-demethylation) via CYP3A4 and CYP2C19 . **Elimination:** Mean $T_{1/2}$=35 hrs; urine (10%).

CELLCEPT   RX
mycophenolate mofetil (Roche Labs)

> Immunosuppression may lead to increased susceptibility to infection and possible development of lymphoma. Female users of childbearing potential must use contraception. Use of CellCept during pregnancy is associated with increased risk of pregnancy loss and congenital malformations.

THERAPEUTIC CLASS: Inosine monophosphate dehydrogenase inhibitor

INDICATIONS: Prophylaxis of organ rejection in allogeneic renal, cardiac, or hepatic transplants. Use with cyclosporine and corticosteroids.

DOSAGE: *Adults:* Renal Transplant: 1g IV/PO bid. Cardiac Transplant: 1.5g IV/PO bid. Hepatic Transplant: 1g IV bid or 1.5g PO bid. Start PO as soon as possible after transplant. Start IV within 24 hrs after transplant; can continue for up to 14 days. Switch to oral when tolerated. Give on an empty stomach. *Pediatrics:* Renal Transplant: (Sus) 600mg/m² PO bid. Max: 2g/day (10 mL/day). (Cap) BSA 1.25m² to 1.5m²: 750mg PO bid. (Cap/Tab) BSA >1.5m²: 1g bid.

HOW SUPPLIED: Cap: 250mg; Inj: 500mg; Sus: 200mg/mL [175mL]; Tab: 500mg

CONTRAINDICATIONS: (Inj) Hypersensitivity to Polysorbate 80 (TWEEN).

WARNINGS/PRECAUTIONS: Risk of lymphomas and other malignancies, especially of the skin. Avoid sunlight to decrease risk of skin cancer. May cause fetal harm during pregnancy. Must have negative serum/urine pregnancy test within 1 week before therapy. Two reliable forms of contraception required before and during therapy, and 6 weeks following discontinuation. Monitor for bone marrow suppression. Risk of GI ulceration, hemorrhage, and perforation; caution with active digestive system disease. Caution with delayed renal graft function post-transplant. Oral suspension contains phenylalanine; caution with phenylketonurics. Monitor CBC weekly during the 1st month, twice monthly for the 2nd and 3rd months, and then monthly through 1st year. Avoid with rare hereditary deficiency of hypoxanthine-guanine phosphoribosyl-transferase (eg, Lesch-Nyhan and Kelley-Seegmiller syndrome). Increased susceptibility infections/ sepsis.

ADVERSE REACTIONS: Infections, diarrhea, leukopenia, sepsis, vomiting, GI bleeding, pain, abdominal pain, fever, headache, asthenia, chest pain, back pain, anemia, leukopenia, thrombocytopenia.

INTERACTIONS: Additive bone marrow suppression with azathioprine; avoid use. Reduced efficacy with drugs that interfere with enterohepatic recirculation (eg, cholestyramine). Efficacy/safety with other immunosuppressive agents not determined. Avoid live attenuated vaccines. Increased levels of both drugs with acyclovir, ganciclovir. Decreased levels with magnesium- and aluminum-containing antacids; space dosing. Decreased effects of oral contraceptives. Increased levels with probenecid. Other drugs that compete for renal tubular secretion may raise levels of both drugs.

PREGNANCY: Category D, not for use in nursing.

MECHANISM OF ACTION: Prolongs the survival of allogeneic transplants (kidney, heart, liver, intestine, limb, small bowel, pancreatic islets, and bone marrow). Inhibits proliferative arteriopathy in experimental models of aortic and cardiac allografts in rats as well as in primate cardiac xenografts. Inhibits immunologically mediated inflammatory responses and tumor development and prolongs survival in tumor transplant models.

PHARMACOKINETICS: Absorption: Oral; rapid and complete, absolute bioavailability (94%). MPA C_{max} decreased by 40% with food. **Distribution**: V_d=3.6L/kg (IV), 4L/kg (oral); plasma protein binding of MPA (97%), MPAG (82%). **Metabolism**: MPA (active metabolite) metabolized by glucuronyl transferase to MPAG, which is converted to MPA via entrohepatic recirculation. **Elimination**: Oral: Urine (93%), feces (6%). Urine: MPA (<1%) and MPAG (87%). MPA: (Oral) $T_{1/2}$=17.9 hrs. (Oral) and (IV) $T_{1/2}$=16.6 hrs. In pediatrics: Oral administarion in different age groups ranging between 1-18 years results in different pharmacokinetics.

CELONTIN   RX
methsuximide (Parke-Davis)

THERAPEUTIC CLASS: Succinimide

INDICATIONS: Management of absence (petit mal) seizures refractory to other drugs.

DOSAGE: *Adults:* Initial: 300mg qd for 7 days. Titrate: Increase weekly by 300mg/day for 3 weeks if needed. Max: 1.2g/day.

Pediatrics: Initial: 300mg qd for 7 days. Titrate: Increase weekly by 300mg/day 3 weeks if needed. Max: 1.2g/day. Use 150mg caps in small children.

HOW SUPPLIED: Cap: 150mg, 300mg

WARNINGS/PRECAUTIONS: Fatal blood dyscrasias reported; monitor blood counts periodically or if signs of infection. SLE reported. Withdraw slowly if altered behavior appears. May increase frequency of grand mal seizures if given alone in mixed type of seizures. Avoid abrupt withdrawal. Caution with renal/hepatic disease. May impair mental/physical abilities.

ADVERSE REACTIONS: GI effects, blood dyscrasias, dermatologic manifestations, drowsiness, ataxia, dizziness, hyperemia, proteinuria, periorbital edema.

INTERACTIONS: May interact with other anticonvulsants; monitor serum levels periodically.

PREGNANCY: Safety in pregnancy and nursing not known.

MECHANISM OF ACTION: Anticonvulsant succinamide; supresses the paroxysmal three cycle/second spike and wave activity associated with lapses of conciousness. Also depresses the motor cortex and elevation of the CNS threshold to convulsive stimuli.

CENESTIN   RX
conjugated estrogens (Duramed)

> Estrogens increase risk of endometrial cancer. Estrogens, with or without progestins, should not be used for the prevention of cardiovascular disease. Increased risks of MI, stroke, invasive breast cancer, PE, and DVT in postmenopausal women reported.

THERAPEUTIC CLASS: Estrogen

INDICATIONS: (0.45mg, 0.625mg, 0.9mg, 1.25mg) Treatment of moderate to severe vasomotor symptoms associated with menopause. (0.3mg) Treatment of vulvar and vaginal atrophy.

DOSAGE: *Adults:* Vasomotor Symptoms: Initial: 0.45mg/day. Adjust dose based on response. Discontinue or taper at 3-6 month intervals. Vulvar/Vaginal Atrophy: 0.3mg qd.

HOW SUPPLIED: Tab: 0.3mg, 0.45mg, 0.625mg, 0.9mg, 1.25mg

CONTRAINDICATIONS: Pregnancy, undiagnosed abnormal genital bleeding, breast cancer, estrogen-dependent neoplasia, DVT/PE, active or recent (eg, within past year) arterial thromboembolic disease (eg, stroke, MI), liver dysfunction or disease.

WARNINGS/PRECAUTIONS: May increase risk of cardiovascular events (eg, MI, stroke), venous thrombosis, and PE; d/c immediately if any of these events occur or are suspected. May increase risk of breast/endometrial cancer, and gallbladder disease. May lead to severe hypercalcemia with breast cancer and bone metastases; monitor and d/c if hypercalcemia occurs. Retinal vascular thrombosis reported; monitor and d/c if papilledema or retinal vascular lesions occur. Consider addition of a progestin if no hysterectomy. May elevate BP; monitor at regular intervals. May cause elevations of plasma triglycerides with pre-existing hypertriglyceridemia. Caution with history of cholestatic jaundice associated with past estrogen use or with pregnancy; d/c with recurrence. May lead to increased thyroid-binding globulin levels; monitor thyroid function. May cause fluid retention; caution with cardiac/renal dysfunction. Caution with severe hypocalcemia. May increase risk of ovarian cancer. May exacerbate endometriosis, asthma, DM, epilepsy, migraine, porphyria, SLE, and hepatic hemangiomas; use with caution.

ADVERSE REACTIONS: Abdominal pain, back pain, pain, headache, infection, vomiting, leg cramps, paresthesia, breast pain, metrorrhagia, endometrial thickening, vaginitis.

INTERACTIONS: CYP3A4 inducers (eg, St. John's wort, phenobarbital, carbamazepine, rifampin) may decrease levels which may decrease therapeutic effects and/or change uterine bleeding profile. CYP3A4 inhibitors (eg, erythromycin, clarithromycin, ketoconazole, itraconazole, ritonavir, grapefruit juice) may increase levels which may result in side effects.

PREGNANCY: Contraindicated in pregnancy; caution in nursing.

MECHANISM OF ACTION: Estrogen; binds to nuclear receptor in estrogen-responsive tissues. Modulates the pituitary secretion of gonadotrophins, luteinizing hormone (LH) and follicle stimulating hormone (FSH), through a negative feedback mechanism.

PHARMACOKINETICS: Absorption: Well-absorbed; conjugated and unconjugated estrogens had altered parameters. **Distribution:** Estrogens found in human breast milk; Largely bound to sex hormone binding globulin (SHBG) and albumin. **Metabolism:** Liver, to estrone (metabolite); estriol (major urinary metabolite); enterohepatic recirculation, via sulfate and glucuronide conjugation; biliary secretion of conjugates into the intestine; hydrolysis in gut; reabsorption; CYP3A4 (partial). **Elimination:** Urine.

CENOGEN ULTRA   RX
folic acid - multiple vitamin - minerals (US Pharmaceutical)

THERAPEUTIC CLASS: Prenatal vitamin

INDICATIONS: Vitamin and mineral supplementation for before, during, and after pregnancy.

DOSAGE: *Adults:* 1 cap qd between meals.

HOW SUPPLIED: Cap: Copper 0.8mg-Ferrous Fumarate 324mg-Folic Acid 1mg-Manganese 1.3mg-Niacinamide 30mg-Pantothenic Acid 10mg-Vitamin B_1 10mg-Vitamin B_2 6mg-Vitamin B_6 5mg-Vitamin B_{12} 0.015mg-Vitamin C 200mg

CONTRAINDICATIONS: Hemochromatosis, hemosiderosis, hemolytic or pernicious anemias.

WARNINGS/PRECAUTIONS: Accidental overdose of iron-containing products is a leading cause of fatal poisoning in children <6 yrs. Not for the treatment of pernicious anemia and other megaloblastic anemias where vitamin B_{12} is deficient. Folic acid >0.1mg-0.4mg/day may obscure pernicious anemia.

ADVERSE REACTIONS: GI disturbances.

MECHANISM OF ACTION: Vitamin and mineral supplement.

CEREBYX   RX
fosphenytoin sodium (Parke-Davis)

THERAPEUTIC CLASS: Hydantoin

INDICATIONS: Short-term (up to 5 days) parenteral administration when other means of phenytoin administration are unavailable, inappropriate, or less advantageous, including to control general convulsive status epilepticus, prevent or treat seizures during neurosurgery, as a short-term substitute for oral phenytoin.

DOSAGE: *Adults:* Doses, concentration in dosing solutions, and infusion rates are expressed as phenytoin sodium equivalents (PE). Status Epilepticus: LD: 15-20 PE/kg IV at 100-150mg PE/min then switch to maintenance dose. Non-Emergent Cases: LD: 10-20mg PE/kg IV (max 150mg PE/min) or IM. Maint: Initial: 4-6mg PE/kg/day. May substitute for oral phenytoin sodium at the same total daily dose.

HOW SUPPLIED: Inj: 50mg PE/mL (2mL, 10mL)

CONTRAINDICATIONS: Sinus bradycardia, sino-atrial block, 2nd- and 3rd-degree AV block, Adams-Stokes syndrome.

WARNINGS/PRECAUTIONS: Avoid abrupt discontinuation. Not for use in absence seizures. Hypotension and severe cardiovascular reactions and fatalities reported; continuously monitor ECG, BP, and respiration during and for at least 20 min after IV infusion and monitor phenytoin levels at least 2 hrs after IV infusion or 4 hrs after IM injection. Caution with severe myocardial

C

insufficiency, porphyria, hepatic/renal dysfunction, hypoalbuminemia, elderly, and diabetes. Acute hepatotoxicity, lymphadenopathy, hemopoietic complications, hyperglycemia reported. D/C if rash or acute hepatotoxicity occurs. Neonatal postpartum bleeding disorder, congenital malformations, and increased seizure frequency reported with use during pregnancy. Avoid use with seizures due to hypoglycemia or other metabolic causes. Caution with phosphate restriction because of phosphate load (0.0037mmol phosphate/mg PE). May lower folate levels.

ADVERSE REACTIONS: Nystagmus, dizziness, pruritus, paresthesia, headache, somnolence, ataxia, tinnitus, stupor, nausea, hypotension, vasodilation, tremor, incoordination, dry mouth.

INTERACTIONS: Increased levels with acute alcohol intake, amiodarone, chloramphenicol, chlordiazepoxide, cimetidine, diazepam, dicumarol, disulfiram, estrogens, ethosuximide, fluoxetine, H_2-antagonists, halothane, isoniazid, methylphenidate, phenothiazines, phenylbutazone, salicylates, succinimides, sulfonamides, tolbutamide, trazodone. Decreased levels with carbamazepine, chronic alcohol abuse, reserpine. Decreases efficacy of anticoagulants, corticosteroids, coumarin, digitoxin, doxycycline, estrogens, furosemide, oral contraceptives, rifampin, quinidine, theophylline, vitamin D. Variable effects (increase or decrease levels) with phenobarbital, valproic acid, and sodium valproate. Caution with drugs highly bound to serum albumin. TCAs may precipitate seizures.

PREGNANCY: Category D, not for use in nursing.

MECHANISM OF ACTION: Anticonvulsant; prodrug of phenytoin. Modulates voltage-dependent sodium and calcium channels of neurons, inhibits calcium flux across neuronal membranes, and enhances sodium-potassium ATPase activity of neurons and glial cells.

PHARMACOKINETICS: Absorption: Fosphenytoin is completely converted to phenytoin. (IM) T_{max}=30 min. **Distribution:** Plasma protein binding (95-99%); V_d=4.3-10.8L. **Metabolism:** Phosphatases (conversion to phenytoin); liver (phenytoin metabolism). **Elimination:** Urine (1-5% phenytoin and metabolites); $T_{1/2}$=15 min (fosphenytoin), 12-28.9 hrs (phenytoin).

CEREZYME   RX
imiglucerase (Genzyme)

THERAPEUTIC CLASS: Beta-glucocerebrosidase

INDICATIONS: Long-term enzyme replacement therapy in Type 1 Gaucher disease.

DOSAGE: *Adults:* Initial: 2.5U/kg TIW to 60U/kg once every 2 weeks IV infusion over 1-2 hours. Adjust dose based on therapeutic goals.
Pediatrics: ≥2 yrs: Initial: 2.5U/kg TIW to 60U/kg once every 2 weeks IV infusion over 1-2 hours. Adjust dose based on therapeutic goals.

HOW SUPPLIED: Inj: 200U, 400U

WARNINGS/PRECAUTIONS: Monitor for IgG antibody formation during the 1st year of therapy. Reduce rate of infusion and pretreat with antihistamines and/or corticosteroids if anaphylactoid reactions occur. Caution in patients who developed antibodies or hypersensitivity reactions to alglucerase.

ADVERSE REACTIONS: Injection site reactions, pruritus, flushing, urticaria, angioedema, chest discomfort, dyspnea, coughing, cyanosis, hypotension, nausea, vomiting, rash, headache, fever.

PREGNANCY: Category C, caution in nursing.

MECHANISM OF ACTION: β-glucocerebrosidase; catalyzes hydrolysis of the glycolipid glucocerebroside to glucose and ceramide.

PHARMACOKINETICS: Distribution: V_d=0.09-0.15L/kg. **Elimination:** $T_{1/2}$=3.6-10.4 min.

CERUBIDINE RX
daunorubicin HCL (Bedford)

> Avoid IM/SQ route. Severe local tissue necrosis with extravasation. Myocardial toxicity may occur during or after terminate therapy; increased risk if cumulative dose >400-550mg/m² in adults, >300mg/m² in pediatrics >2 yrs, or >10mg/m² in pediatrics <2 yrs. Severe myelosuppression may occur. Reduce dose with impaired hepatic or renal function.

THERAPEUTIC CLASS: Anthracycline

INDICATIONS: In combination with other anticancer drugs, for remission induction in acute nonlymphocytic leukemia (ANLL) in adults, and for remission induction in acute lymphocytic leukemia (ALL) in children and adults.

DOSAGE: *Adults:* ANLL: Combination Therapy: <60 yrs: 45mg/m²/day IV on Days 1, 2, 3 of 1st course and on Days 1, 2 of subsequent courses. ≥60 yrs: 30mg/m²/day IV on Days 1, 2, 3 of 1st course and on Days 1, 2 of subsequent courses. ALL: Combination Therapy: 45mg/m²/day IV on Days 1, 2, 3. Renal Impairment: If SCr >3mg%, reduce dose by 50%. Hepatic Impairment: If serum bilirubin 1.2-3mg%, reduce dose by 25%. If >3mg%, reduce dose by 50%. *Pediatrics:* ALL: Combination Therapy: 25mg/m² IV on Day 1 every week. If complete remission not obtained after 4 courses, may give additional 1-2 courses. If <2 yrs or <0.5m² BSA, calculate dose based on weight (1mg/kg) instead of BSA.

HOW SUPPLIED: Inj: 20mg

WARNINGS/PRECAUTIONS: Avoid if pre-existing drug-induced bone-marrow suppression occurs unless benefit warrants the risk. May cause fetal harm during pregnancy. May impart red color to urine. Monitor blood uric acid levels. Determine CBC frequently. Evaluate cardiac, renal, and hepatic function before each course.

ADVERSE REACTIONS: Cardiotoxicity, myelosuppression, alopecia, nausea, vomiting, diarrhea, abdominal pain, hyperuricemia, mucositis (3-7 days after therapy).

INTERACTIONS: Possible secondary leukemias with other antineoplastics or radiation therapy. Increased risk of cardiotoxicity with previous doxorubicin therapy or with concomitant cyclophosphamide. May need dose reduction with other myelosuppressants. Hepatotoxic agents (eg, high dose MTX) may increase risk of toxicity.

PREGNANCY: Category D, not for use in nursing.

MECHANISM OF ACTION: Anthracycline antineoplastic agent; inhibits topoisomerase II activity by stabilizing the DNA-topoisomerase II complex, preventing the religation portion of the ligation-religation reaction that topoisomerase II catalyzes, and resulting in single-strand and double-strand DNA breaks.

PHARMACOKINETICS: Distribution: Widely distributed in tissues. **Metabolism:** Liver (extensively), via cytoplasmic aldo-keto reductases, 4-O demethylation, conjugation. Daunorubicinol (major metabolite). **Elimination:** Urine and bile (40%). $T_{1/2}$(daunorubicinol)=26.7 hrs.

CERUMENEX RX
triethanolamine polypeptide oleate (Purdue Frederick)

THERAPEUTIC CLASS: Ceruminolytic

INDICATIONS: Removal of impacted cerumen.

DOSAGE: *Adults:* Fill ear canal and insert cotton plug for 15-30 min. Flush with warm water. Repeat if needed.

HOW SUPPLIED: Sol: 10% [6mL, 12mL]

CONTRAINDICATIONS: Perforated tympanic membrane, otitis media.

C

WARNINGS/PRECAUTIONS: D/C if sensitization or irritation occurs. Extreme caution with allergies. Limit exposure of ear canal to 15-30 min. Avoid undue exposure of skin outside ear. Caution with external otitis.

ADVERSE REACTIONS: Mild erythema, pruritus of external ear, contact dermatitis, skin ulcerations, burning/pain at application site, skin rash.

PREGNANCY: Category C, caution in nursing.

MECHANISM OF ACTION: Surfactant; emulsifies and disperses excess or impacted ear wax to facilitate removal by subsequent water irrigation.

CERVIDIL   RX
dinoprostone (Forest)

THERAPEUTIC CLASS: Oxytocic agent

INDICATIONS: For cervical ripening initiation and/or continuation in patients at or near term with a medical or obstetrical need for labor induction.

DOSAGE: *Adults:* 10mg to release 0.3mg/hr over 12 hrs. Place one unit transversely in posterior fornix of the vagina immediately after removal from its foil package. Remove at onset of active labor or 12 hrs after insertion.

HOW SUPPLIED: Insert: 0.3mg/hr

CONTRAINDICATIONS: Fetal distress where delivery is not imminent, marked cephalopelvic disproportion, unexplained vaginal bleeding during this pregnancy, when oxytocic drugs are contraindicated, when prolonged uterus contraction may be detrimental to fetal safety or uterine integrity, concomitant IV oxytocic drugs, multipara with 6 or more previous term pregnancies.

WARNINGS/PRECAUTIONS: Avoid with history of cesarean section or uterine surgery. Caution with ruptured membranes, history of uterine hypertony, glaucoma, childhood asthma (even if no attacks in adulthood). Monitor uterine activity, fetal status, progression of cervical dilation and effacement. Remove if hyperstimulation occurs and before amniotomy.

ADVERSE REACTIONS: Uterine hyperstimulation, fetal distress.

INTERACTIONS: May augment activity of other oxytocic drugs; avoid concomitant use. Wait 30 minutes after removal of dinoprostone before useing oxytocin.

PREGNANCY: Category C, safety in nursing not known.

MECHANISM OF ACTION: PGE$_2$; stimulates production of PGF$_{2a}$ (sensitizes myometrium to oxytocin), capable of initiating uterine contractions, important role in cervical ripening without affecting uterine contractions.

CESAMET   CII
nabilone (Valeant)

THERAPEUTIC CLASS: Cannabinoid

INDICATIONS: Treatment of the nausea and vomiting associated with chemotherapy when conventional treatment has failed.

DOSAGE: *Adults:* Initial: 1 or 2mg bid; given 1-3 hrs before chemotherapy. A dose of 1 or 2mg the night before may be useful. Max: 6mg/day given in divided doses tid.

HOW SUPPLIED: Cap: 1mg

WARNINGS/PRECAUTIONS: Patients should remain under the supervision of a responsible adult during treatment, especially during initial use and dose adjustments. Caution when initiating therapy with HTN, heart disease, current or previous psychiatric disorders and with history of substance abuse. Avoid driving, operating heavy machinery, or engaging in any hazardous activity during treatment. May cause dizziness, euphoria, ataxia, anxiety, disorientation, depression, hallucinations, and psychosis. Adverse psychiatric reactions can persist for 48-72 hrs following cessation of treatment. Avoid with alcohol, sedatives, hypnotics, or other psychoactive substances. May cause tachycardia and orthostatic hypotension.

ADVERSE REACTIONS: Drowsiness, vertigo, dry mouth, euphoria, ataxia, headache, concentration difficulties, nausea, dysphoria, sleep/visual disturbance, asthenia, anorexia.

INTERACTIONS: Additive HTN, tachycardia, possibly cardiotoxicity may occur with amphetamines, cocaine, other sympathomimetics. Additive or super-additive tachycardia, drowsiness may occur with atropine, scopolamine, antihistamines, other anticholinergics. Additive tachycardia, HTN, drowsiness may occur with TCAs. Additive drowsiness and CNS depression may occur with barbiturates, benzodiazepines, ethanol, lithium, opioids, buspirone, antihistamines, muscle relaxants, other CNS depressants. Hypomanic reaction reported with disulfiram, fluoxetine. May decrease clearance of antipyrine, barbiturates. May increase metabolism of theophylline. Cross-tolerance and mutual potentiation with opioids. Effects may be enhanced by opioid receptor blockade. Alcohol may increase the positive subjective mood effects.

PREGNANCY: Category C, not for use in nursing.

MECHANISM OF ACTION: Cannabinoid; interacts with the cannabinoid receptor system (CB (1) receptor that has been discovered in neural tissues).

PHARMACOKINETICS: Absorption: Complete, C_{max}=2ng/mL, T_{max}=2.0 hrs. **Distribution:** V_d=12.5L/kg **Metabolism:** Liver (extensive), via stereospecific enzymes and multiple P450 enzyme isoforms. Isomeric carbinol (metabolite). **Elimination:** Feces (60%), urine (24%); $T_{1/2}$=2 hrs (identified metabolite), 35 hrs (unidentified metabolite).

CETROTIDE RX
cetrorelix acetate (EMD Serono)

THERAPEUTIC CLASS: GnRH antagonist

INDICATIONS: For inhibition of premature LH surges in women undergoing controlled ovarian stimulation.

DOSAGE: *Adults:* Multiple-Dose Regimen: 0.25mg SQ qd; start on day 5 (AM or PM) or day 6 (AM). Continue until HCG administration. Single-Dose Regimen: 3mg SQ single dose when estradiol level indicates appropriate stimulation response, usually on Day 7. If HCG not given within 4 days, then give 0.25mg SQ qd until day of HCG administration.

HOW SUPPLIED: Inj: 0.25mg, 3mg

CONTRAINDICATIONS: Pregnancy, nursing, hypersensitivity to extrinsic peptide hormones or mannitol, severe renal impairment.

WARNINGS/PRECAUTIONS: Exclude pregnancy before initiating therapy.

ADVERSE REACTIONS: Ovarian hyperstimulation syndrome, nausea, headache.

PREGNANCY: Category X, not for use in nursing.

MECHANISM OF ACTION: GnRH antagonist; controls the release of FSH and LH.

PHARMACOKINETICS: Absorption: Rapid. T_{max} (3mg, 2.5mg)=(1.5, 1 hr). **Distribution:** V_d=1L/Kg. Plasma protein binding (86%). **Elimination:** Urine (unchanged); $T_{1/2}$(3mg, 2.5mg)=(62.8, 5 hrs)

CHANTIX RX
varenicline tartrate (Pfizer)

THERAPEUTIC CLASS: Nicotinic Acetylcholine Receptor Agonist

INDICATIONS: Aid to smoking cessation treatment.

DOSAGE: *Adults:* ≥18 yrs: Days 1-3: 0.5mg qd. Days 4-7: 0.5mg bid. Day 8 to End of Treatment: 1mg bid. Duration: 12 weeks with additional 12 weeks after successful completion to ensure long-term abstinence. Severe Renal

Impairment: Initial: 0.5mg qd. Titrate: Max: 0.5mg bid. End-Stage Renal Disease: Max: 0.5mg qd.

HOW SUPPLIED: Tab: 0.5mg, 1mg

WARNINGS/PRECAUTIONS: Serious neuropsychiatric symptoms (eg, changes in behavior, agitation, depressed mood, suicidal ideation, suicidal behavior) reported. Physiological changes resulting from smoking cessation may alter pharmacokinetics or pharmacodynamics of some drugs (eg, theophylline, warfarin, insulin). Use caution driving or operating machinery in patients until they know how quitting smoking with varenicline may affect them.

ADVERSE REACTIONS: Nausea, sleep disturbance, constipation, flatulence, vomiting.

INTERACTIONS: Reduced renal clearance with cimetidine. Increased incidence of side effects (eg, vomiting, headache, nausea) with nicotine replacement therapy.

PREGNANCY: Category C, not for use in nursing.

MECHANISM OF ACTION: Nicotinic acetylcholine receptor agonist; binds with high affinity and selectivity at α4β2 neuronal nicotinic acetylcholine receptors, blocking ability of nicotine to activate these receptors, and thus stimulating central nervous mesolimbic dopamine system.

PHARMACOKINETICS: Absorption: T_{max}=3-4 hrs. **Distribution:** Plasma protein binding (≤20%). **Metabolism:** Minimal. **Elimination:** Urine (92%, unchanged). $T_{1/2}$=24 hrs.

CHERACOL W/CODEINE
codeine phosphate - guaifenesin (Lee Pharmaceuticals)

OTHER BRAND NAMES: Mytussin AC (Morton Grove) - Halotussin AC (Watson) - Guaituss AC (Alpharma) - Cheratussin AC (Vintage)

THERAPEUTIC CLASS: Cough suppressant/expectorant

INDICATIONS: Relief of cough due to minor throat and bronchial irritation from a cold or inhaled irritants. Loosens phlegm and thins bronchial secretions to make coughs more productive.

DOSAGE: *Adults:* 10mL q4h. Max: 60mL/24 hrs.
Pediatrics: ≥12 yrs: 10mL q4h. Max: 60mL/24 hrs. 6 to <12 yrs: 5mL q4h. Max: 30mL/24 hrs.

HOW SUPPLIED: Syrup: (Codeine-Guaifenesin) 10-100mg/5mL [120mL]

WARNINGS/PRECAUTIONS: Use caution with persistant/chronic cough, cough with excessive phlegm, chronic pulmonary disease, or shortness of breath. May cause or aggravate constipation.

ADVERSE REACTIONS: Constipation, sedation.

INTERACTIONS: Increased sedation with sedatives, tranquilizers and antidepressants, especially MAOIs.

PREGNANCY: Safety in pregnancy and nursing not known.

CHLORAL HYDRATE
chloral hydrate (Pharmaceutical Associates)

THERAPEUTIC CLASS: Trichloroacetaldehyde monohydrate

INDICATIONS: Short-term sedative/hypnotic (<2 weeks). To allay anxiety or induce sedation preoperatively or prior to EEG evaluations. Alone or with paraldehyde to prevent or suppress alcohol withdrawal syndrome. To reduce anxiety associated with withdrawal of other drugs such as narcotics or barbiturates.

DOSAGE: *Adults:* Dilute in half glass of water, fruit juice, or ginger ale. Hypnotic: Usual: 500mg-1g 15-30 min before bedtime. Sedative: Usual: 250mg tid pc. Alcohol Withdrawal: Usual: 500mg-1g q6h prn. Max: 2g/day.

Pediatrics: Hypnotic: 50mg/kg. Max: 1g/dose. Sedative: 8mg/kg tid. Max: 500mg tid. Prior to EEG: 20-25mg/kg.

HOW SUPPLIED: Syrup: 500mg/5mL

CONTRAINDICATIONS: Marked hepatic or renal impairment.

WARNINGS/PRECAUTIONS: May be habit forming. Caution with depression, suicidal tendencies, history of drug abuse. Avoid with esophagitis, gastritis or gastric or duodenal ulcers, large doses with severe cardiac disease. May impair mental/physical abilities. Risk of gastritis, skin eruptions, parenchymatous renal damage with prolonged use. Withdraw gradually with chronic use.

ADVERSE REACTIONS: Nausea, vomiting, diarrhea, ataxia, dizziness.

INTERACTIONS: Reduces effectiveness of coumarin anticoagulants. May result in transient potentiation of warfarin-induced hypoprothrombinemia. Additive CNS effects with other CNS depressants (eg, paraldehyde, barbiturates, alcohol). Use with IV furosemide may cause diaphoresis, flushes, variable BP; use alternative hypnotic.

PREGNANCY: Category C, caution in nursing.

MECHANISM OF ACTION: Sedative/hypnotic agent, confined to cerebral hemispheres.

PHARMACOKINETICS: Distribution: Found in breast milk. **Metabolism:** Liver. **Elimination:** Kidneys.

CHLORPROMAZINE   RX
chlorpromazine (Various)

THERAPEUTIC CLASS: Phenothiazine

INDICATIONS: Treatment of schizophrenia. Control of nausea and vomiting. Relief of restlessness and apprehension before surgery. Treatment of acute intermittent porphyria. Adjunct treatment of tetanus. To control the manic type of manic-depressive illness. Relief of intractable hiccups. Treatment of severe behavioral problems in children. Short-term treatment of hyperactivity in children.

DOSAGE: *Adults:* Severe Behavioral Problems: Inpatient: Acute Schizophrenic/Manic State: 25mg IM, then 25-50mg IM in 1 hr if needed. Titrate: Increase over several days up to 400mg q4-6h until controlled then switch to PO. Usual: 500mg/day PO. Max: 1000mg/day PO. Less Acutely Disturbed: 25mg PO tid. Titrate: Increase gradually to 400mg/day. Outpatient: 10mg PO tid-qid or 25mg PO bid-tid. More Severe: 25mg PO tid. Titrate: After 1-2 days, increase by 20-50mg twice weekly until calm. Prompt Control of Severe Symptoms: 25mg IM, may repeat in 1 hr then 25-50mg PO tid. Nausea/ Vomiting: Usual: 10-25mg PO q4-6h prn; 25mg IM then, if no hypotension, 25-50mg q3-4h prn until vomiting stops then switch to PO; 100mg rectally q6-8h prn. Nausea/Vomiting in Surgery: 12.5mg IM, may repeat in 1/2 hr; 2mg IV per fractional injection at 2 min intervals. Max: 25mg. Presurgical Apprehension: 25-50mg PO 2-3 hrs pre-op; 12.5-25mg IM 1-2 hrs pre-op. Intractable Hiccups: 25-50mg PO tid-qid; if symptoms persist after 2-3 days, give 25-50mg IM; if symptoms still persist, give 25-50mg slow IV. Porphyria: 25-50mg PO tid-qid; 25mg IM tid-qid until PO therapy. Tetanus: 25-50mg IM tid-qid; 25-50mg IV. Elderly: Use lower doses, increase dose more gradually, monitor closely. *Pediatrics:* 6 months-12 yrs: Severe Behavioral Problems: Outpatient: 0.25mg/ lb PO q4-6h prn; 0.5mg/lb sup rectally q6-8h prn; 0.25mg/lb IM q6-8h prn. Inpatient: Start low and increase gradually to 50-100mg/day; ≥200mg/day in older children. Max: 500mg/day. <5 yrs (<50lbs): Max: ≤40mg/day IM; 5-12 yrs (50-100lbs): Max: ≤75mg/day IM. Nausea/Vomiting: 0.25mg/lb PO q4-6h; 0.5mg/lb sup rectally q6-8h prn. Max: 6 months-5 yrs (or 50 lbs): <40mg/day. 5-12 yrs (or 50-100lbs): <75mg/day except in severe cases. During Surgery: 0.125mg/lb IM repeat in 1/2 hr if needed; 1mg IV per fractional injection at 2 min intervals and not exceeding recommended IM dosage. Presurgical Apprehension: 0.25mg/lb PO 2-3 hrs (or IM 1-2 hrs) before operation. Tetanus: 0.25mg/lb IM/IV q6-8h. <50lbs: Max: ≤40mg/day; 50-100lbs: Max: ≤75mg/day.

HOW SUPPLIED: Cap, Extended-Release: 30mg, 75mg, 150mg; Inj: 25mg/mL; Sup: 25mg, 100mg; Syrup: 10mg/5mL [120mL]; Tab: 10mg, 25mg, 50mg, 100mg, 200mg

CONTRAINDICATIONS: Comatose states, or with large amounts of CNS depressants. Hypersensitivity to phenothiazines.

WARNINGS/PRECAUTIONS: Tardive dyskinesia, NMS may occur. Caution with chronic respiratory disorders, acute respiratory infections (especially in children), glaucoma, cardiovascular, hepatic, or renal disease, history of hepatic encephalopathy due to cirrhosis. Suppresses cough reflex; aspiration of vomitus possible. Caution if exposed to extreme heat or organophosphates. Avoid in children/adolescents with signs of Reye's syndrome. Lowers seizure threshold. Reduce dose gradually to prevent side effects. May mask signs of overdoses to other drugs and obscure diagnosis of other conditions (eg, intestinal obstruction, brain tumor, Reye's syndrome). May produce false-positive PKU test. May elevate prolactin levels. Injection contains sulfites.

ADVERSE REACTIONS: Drowsiness, jaundice, agranulocytosis, hypotensive effects, EKG changes, dystonias, motor restlessness, pseudo-parkinsonism, tardive dyskinesia, anticholinergic effects, NMS, ocular changes.

INTERACTIONS: See Contraindications. May decrease effects of oral anticoagulants, guanethidine. Propranolol increases plasma levels of both agents. Thiazide diuretics may potentiate orthostatic hypotension. Potentiates effects of CNS depressants (eg, anesthetic, barbiturates, narcotics); reduce doses of these drugs by 1/4 to 1/2. Anticonvulsants may need adjustment; phenytoin toxicity reported. Do not use with Amipaque®; discontinue at least 48 hrs before myelography and resume at least 24 hrs after. Can cause α-adrenergic blockade. Caution with atropine or related drugs. Encephalopathic syndrome reported with lithium.

PREGNANCY: Safety in pregnancy not known. Not for use in nursing.

MECHANISM OF ACTION: Phenothiazine; not established. Suspected to act at all levels of CNS, primarily at subcortical levels as well as on multiple organ systems. Exerts psychotropic, sedative, and antiemetic activity. Has strong antiadrenergic and weaker peripheral anticholinergic activity and ganglionic blocking action.

CHROMAGEN   RX
ferrous fumarate - vitamin B12 - dessicated stomach substance - vitamin C
(Savage)

OTHER BRAND NAMES: Anemagen (Ethex)

THERAPEUTIC CLASS: Iron/vitamin

INDICATIONS: Treatment of all anemias responsive to oral iron therapy.

DOSAGE: *Adults:* 1 cap qd.

HOW SUPPLIED: Cap: Dessicated Stomach Substance 100mg-Ferrous Fumarate 200mg-Vitamin B$_{12}$ 0.01mg-Vitamin C 250mg

CONTRAINDICATIONS: Hemochromatosis, hemosiderosis.

ADVERSE REACTIONS: Nausea, rash, vomiting, diarrhea, precordial pain, flushing.

PREGNANCY: Safety in pregnancy and nursing not known.

CHROMAGEN FA   RX
ferrous fumarate - vitamin B12 - folic acid - vitamin C (Savage)

THERAPEUTIC CLASS: Iron/vitamin

INDICATIONS: Treatment of all anemias responsive to oral iron therapy.

DOSAGE: *Adults:* 1 cap qd.

HOW SUPPLIED: (Ferrous Fumarate-Folic Acid-Vitamin B$_{12}$-Vitamin C) Cap: 200mg-1mg-0.01mg-250mg

CONTRAINDICATIONS: Hemochromatosis, hemosiderosis. Folic acid is contraindicated in pernicious anemia.

WARNINGS/PRECAUTIONS: Accidental overdose of iron-containing products is a leading cause of fatal poisoning in children <6 yrs. Avoid folic acid unless the diagnosis of pernicious anemia has been excluded.

ADVERSE REACTIONS: Nausea, rash, vomiting, diarrhea, precordial pain, flushing.

PREGNANCY: Safety in pregnancy and nursing is not known.

CHROMAGEN FORTE RX
ferrous fumarate - vitamin B12 - folic acid - vitamin C (Savage)

THERAPEUTIC CLASS: Iron/vitamin

INDICATIONS: Treatment of all anemias responsive to oral iron therapy.

DOSAGE: *Adults:* 1-2 caps qd.

HOW SUPPLIED: Cap: Ferrous Fumarate 460mg-Folic Acid 1mg-Vitamin B$_{12}$ 0.01mg-Vitamin C 60mg

CONTRAINDICATIONS: Hemochromatosis, hemosiderosis, pernicious anemia.

WARNINGS/PRECAUTIONS: Accidental overdose of iron-containing products is a leading cause of fatal poisoning in children <6 yrs. Avoid folic acid unless the diagnosis of pernicious anemia has been excluded.

ADVERSE REACTIONS: Nausea, rash, vomiting, diarrhea, precordial pain, flushing.

PREGNANCY: Safety in pregnancy and nursing not known.

CIALIS RX
tadalafil (Lilly ICOS)

THERAPEUTIC CLASS: Phosphodiesterase type 5 inhibitor

INDICATIONS: Treatment of erectile dysfunction (ED).

DOSAGE: *Adults:* Prn Use: Take prior to sexual activity. Initial: 10mg. Range: 5-20mg. Renal Impairment: CrCl 31-50mL/min: Initial: 5mg. Max: 10mg/48 hrs. CrCl <30mL/min/Hemodialysis: Max: 5mg/72 hrs. Mild/Moderate Hepatic Impairment: Max: 10mg. Severe Hepatic Impairment: Avoid use. With Potent CYP3A4 Inhibitors (eg, Ketoconazole, Itraconazole, Ritonavir): Max: 10mg/72 hrs. Once Daily Use: Initial: 2.5mg qd without regard to timing of sexual activity. Titrate: May increase to 5mg qd based on efficacy and tolerability. CrCl <30mL/min/Hemodialysis/Severe Hepatic Impairment: Avoid use. Mild/Moderate Hepatic Impairment: Use with caution. With Potent CYP3A4 Inhibitors (eg, Ketoconazole, Itraconazole, Ritonavir): Max: 2.5mg.

HOW SUPPLIED: Tab: 2.5mg, 5mg, 10mg, 20mg

CONTRAINDICATIONS: Concomitant nitrates.

WARNINGS/PRECAUTIONS: Avoid in men for whom sexual activity is inadvisable due to underlying CV status. Increased sensitivity to vasodilatory effect with left ventricular outflow obstruction. Avoid with MI (within last 90 days); unstable angina or angina occurring during sexual intercourse; NYHA Class 2 or greater heart failure (in the last 6 months); uncontrolled arrhythmias, hypotension (<90/50mmHg); or uncontrolled HTN (>170/100mmHg); stroke within the last 6 months; severe hepatic impairment (Childs-Pugh Class C); degenerative retinal disorders, including retinitis pigmentosa. Prolonged erection reported. Substantial consumption of alcohol with tadalafil can increase HR, decrease BP, dizziness, and headache. Caution with predisposition to priapism (eg, sickle cell anemia, multiple myeloma, leukemia), anatomical deformation of the penis, bleeding disorders, or active peptic ulceration. May cause transient decrease in BP. Caution with coadministration of PDE5 inhibitors and α-blockers. May cause additive hypotensive effect. Initiate at lowest dose once patient is stable on either therapy. Rare reports of nonarteritic anterior ischemic optic neuropathy (NAION) with PDE5 inhibitors. Sudden decrease or loss of hearing, tinnitus, and dizziness reported. D/C if experienced these symptoms.

ADVERSE REACTIONS: Headache, dyspepsia, back pain, myalgia, nasal congestion, flushing, limb pain, urticaria, Stevens-Johnson syndrome, exoliative dermatitis, migraine, visual field defect, retinal vein occlusion, retinal artery occlusion, sudden decrease or loss of hearing, tinnitus.

INTERACTIONS: See Contraindications. Increased levels with CYP3A4 inhibitors (eg, ketoconazole, HIV-protease inhibitors, erythromycin, itraconazole, grapefruit juice). Decreased levels with CYP3A4 inducers (eg, rifampin, carbamazepine, phenytoin, phenobarbital). Additive hypotensive effects with alcohol, α-blockers (eg, tamsulosin, doxazosin, alfuzosin), antihypertensives (eg, amlodipine, metoprolol, bendrofluazide, enalapril, angiotensin-II receptor blockers).

PREGNANCY: Category B, not for use in nursing.

MECHANISM OF ACTION: Phosphodiesterase type 5 inhibitor; enhances the effect of nitric oxide by inhibiting phosphodiesterase type 5, which is responsible for the degradation of cGMP in the corpus cavernosum.

PHARMACOKINETICS: Absorption: C_{max}=2hrs. **Distribution:** Plasma protein binding (94%); V_d=63L. **Metabolism:** Via CYP3A4 to a catechol metabolite which undergoes extensive methylation and glucuronidation; methylcatechol glucuronide (major metabolite). **Elimination:** $T_{1/2}$=17.5 hrs.; urine (36%), feces (61%).

CILOXAN   RX
ciprofloxacin HCL (Alcon)

THERAPEUTIC CLASS: Fluoroquinolone

INDICATIONS: Bacterial conjunctivitis and corneal ulcers.

DOSAGE: *Adults:* Bacterial Conjunctivitis: Sol: 1-2 drops q2h while awake for 2 days, then 1-2 drops q4h while awake for 5 days. Oint: 1/2 inch tid for 2 days, then bid for 5 days. Corneal Ulcer: Sol: 2 drops every 15 min for 1st 6 hrs, then 2 drops every 30 min for rest of Day 1, then 2 drops every hr on Day 2, then 2 drops q4h on Days 3-14. May continue if re-epithelialization has not occurred. *Pediatrics:* Bacterial Conjunctivitis: ≥1 yr: Sol: 1-2 drops q2h while awake for 2 days, then 1-2 drops q4h while awake for 5 days. ≥2 yrs: Oint: 1/2 inch tid for 2 days, then bid for 5 days. Corneal Ulcer: Sol: ≥1 yr: 2 drops every 15 min for 1st 6 hrs, then 2 drops every 30 min for rest of Day 1, then 2 drops every hr on Day 2, then 2 drops q4h on Days 3-14. May continue if re-epithelialization has not occurred.

HOW SUPPLIED: Oint: 0.3% [3.5g]; Sol: 0.3% [2.5mL, 5mL, 10mL]

WARNINGS/PRECAUTIONS: Not for injection into eye. Superinfection may result with prolonged use. Fatal hypersensitivity reactions reported after 1st dose of systemic quinolone therapy. Avoid allowing tip of container to contact eye or surrounding structures. Avoid contact lenses with conjunctivitis. Risk of crystalline precipitate in cornea. Ointment may slow corneal healing and cause visual blurring.

ADVERSE REACTIONS: Local burning, white crystalline precipitants, lid margin crusting, crystals/scales, foreign body sensation, itching, conjunctival hyperemia, bad taste.

INTERACTIONS: Systemic quinolone therapy may increase theophylline levels, interfere with caffeine metabolism, enhance warfarin effects, and elevate serum creatinine with cyclosporine.

PREGNANCY: Category C, caution in nursing.

MECHANISM OF ACTION: Fluoroquinolone antibacterial agent. Bactericidal; interferes with the enzyme DNA gyrase which is needed for synthesis of bacterial DNA.

PHARMACOKINETICS: Absorption: $C_{max} \leq 5ng/mL$.

CIMETIDINE   RX
cimetidine (Various)

OTHER BRAND NAMES: Tagamet (GlaxoSmithKline)

THERAPEUTIC CLASS: H_2-blocker

INDICATIONS: Short-term treatment of active duodenal ulcer (DU), active benign gastric ulcer (GU). Maintenance of healed duodenal ulcer. Treatment of GERD and/or pathological hypersecretory conditions (eg, Zollinger-Ellison syndrome). Prevention of upper GI bleeding in critically ill patients.

DOSAGE: *Adults:* (PO) Active DU: 800mg qhs or 300mg qid or 400mg bid for 4-8 weeks. Maint: 400mg qhs. Active Benign GU: 800mg qhs or 300mg qid for 6 weeks. GERD: 800mg bid or 400mg qid for 12 weeks. Hypersecretory Conditions: 300mg qid. Max: 2400mg/day. (Inj) 300mg IM/IV q6-8h. Max: 2400mg/day. Rapid Gastric pH Elevation: LD: 150mg IV, then 37.5mg/hr IV. Upper GI Bleed Prevention: Continuous IV infusion of 50mg/hr for 7 days. CrCl <30mL/min: Give half the recommended dose.
Pediatrics: ≥16 yrs: (PO) Active DU: 800mg qhs or 300mg qid or 400mg bid for 4-8 weeks. Maint: 400mg qhs. Active Benign GU: 800mg qhs or 300mg qid for 6 weeks. GERD: 800mg bid or 400mg qid for 12 weeks. Hypersecretory Conditions: 300mg qid. Max: 2400mg/day. (Inj) 300mg IM/IV q6-8h. Max: 2400mg/day. Rapid Gastric pH Elevation: LD: 150mg IV, then 37.5mg/hr IV. Upper GI Bleed Prevention: Continuous IV infusion of 50mg/hr for 7 days. CrCl <30mL/min: Give half the recommended dose.

HOW SUPPLIED: Inj: (HCl) 150mg/mL, 300mg/5mL; Sol: (HCl) 300mg/5mL; Tab: 200mg, 300mg, 400mg*, 800mg* *scored

WARNINGS/PRECAUTIONS: Cardiac arrhythmias and hypotension reported following rapid IV administration (rare). Symptomatic response does not preclude the presence of gastric malignancy. Reversible confusional states reported, especially in severely ill patients. Elderly, renal and/or hepatic impairment are risk factors for confusional states. Risk of hyperinfection of strongyloidiasis in immunocompromised patients.

ADVERSE REACTIONS: Diarrhea, headache, dizziness, somnolence, reversible confusional states, impotence, increased serum transaminases, rash, gynecomastia, blood dyscrasias.

INTERACTIONS: Reduces metabolism of warfarin-type anticoagulants, phenytoin, propranolol, nifedipine, chlordiazepoxide, diazepam, certain TCAs, lidocaine, theophylline and metronidazole. Monitor PT/INR. Adverse effects reported with phenytoin, lidocaine and theophylline; monitor levels. May affect absorption of drugs (eg, ketoconazole) affected by gastric pH; give 2 hrs before cimetidine. Antacids may interfer with absorption of cimetidine; space the dosing.

PREGNANCY: Category B, not for use in nursing.

MECHANISM OF ACTION: H_2-receptor antagonist; competitively inhibits the action of histamine at the histamine H_2 receptors of the parietal cells.

PHARMACOKINETICS: Absorption: (PO) Rapid. T_{max}=45-90 mins. (IV) C_{max}=0.9mcg/mL. **Metabolism:** Sulfoxide (major metabolite). **Elimination:** Urine, (PO 48%); (IV/IM 75%); $T_{1/2}$=2 hrs.

CIMZIA   RX
certolizumab pegol (UCB)

> Tuberculosis (TB), invasive fungal infections, and other opportunistic infections have occured. Evaluate for latent TB and treat if necessary prior to therapy. Monitor all patients for active TB during treatment, even if initial tuberculin skin test is negative.

THERAPEUTIC CLASS: TNF-receptor blocker

INDICATIONS: For reducing signs and symptoms of Crohn's disease and maintaining clinical response in adults with moderately to severely active disease who have had an inadequate response to conventional therapy.

DOSAGE: *Adults:* Initial: 400mg SQ at Weeks 2 and 4. Maint: 400mg SQ every 4 weeks

HOW SUPPLIED: Inj: 200mg

WARNINGS/PRECAUTIONS: Serious infections, sepsis, and cases of opportunistic infections, including fatalities reported. Caution with history of recurrent infection, concomitant immunosuppressive therapy, or underlying conditions that may predispose to infections. May increase risk of reactivation of hepatitis B virus; monitor HBV carriers during and several months after therapy. Lymphoma and other malignancies have occurred with TNF-blockers. Anaphylaxis or serious allergic reactions may occur. Caution with pre-existing or recent onset CNS demyelinating disorders. Rare cases of pancytopenia, including aplastic anemia, reported; d/c if significant hematologic abnormalities occur.Caution with heart failure; monitor closely. May cause autoimmune antibodies; d/c if lupus-like syndrome develops.

ADVERSE REACTIONS: Upper respiratory tract infection, UTI, arthralgia.

INTERACTIONS: Avoid combination treatment with anakinra. Do not give live vaccines concurrently.

PREGNANCY: Category B, not for use in nursing

MECHANISM OF ACTION: TNF-blocker; binds to TNF-α and selectively neutralizes and inhibits its central role in inflammatory processes.

PHARMACOKINETICS: Absorption: Bioavailability (80%) **Distribution:** V_d= 6.4L **Elimination:** $T_{1/2}$ = 14 days.

CIPRO HC   RX
ciprofloxacin HCL - hydrocortisone (Alcon)

THERAPEUTIC CLASS: Antibacterial/corticosteroid combination

INDICATIONS: Acute otitis externa in adults and pediatric patients ≥1 year.

DOSAGE: *Adults:* 3 drops into affected ear bid for 7 days. Warm bottle in hand for 1-2 min to avoid dizziness. Shake well before use.
Pediatrics: ≥1 yr: 3 drops into affected ear bid for 7 days. Warm bottle in hand for 1-2 min to avoid dizziness. Shake well before use.

HOW SUPPLIED: Sus: (Ciprofloxacin-Hydrocortisone) 0.2%-1% [10mL]

CONTRAINDICATIONS: Perforated tympanic membrane, viral infections of external ear canal (eg, varicella and herpes simplex infections).

WARNINGS/PRECAUTIONS: D/C if hypersensitivity reaction occurs. Re-evaluate if no improvement after one week.

ADVERSE REACTIONS: Headache, pruritus.

PREGNANCY: Category C, not for use in nursing.

MECHANISM OF ACTION: Broad-spectrum anti-inflammatory antibiotic; exerts antimicrobial activity against gram-positive and gram-negative bacteria.

CIPRO IV   RX
ciprofloxacin (Bayer/Schering)

THERAPEUTIC CLASS: Fluoroquinolone

INDICATIONS: Treatment of skin and skin structure (SSSI), bone and joint, complicated intra-abdominal infections, lower respiratory tract infections (LRTI), urinary tract infections (UTI), nosocomial pneumonia, acute sinusitis, chronic bacterial prostatitis, postexposure inhalational anthrax, empirical therapy for febrile neutropenia, complicated UTI and pyelonephritis in pediatrics.

DOSAGE: *Adults:* ≥18 yrs: IV: UTI: Mild-Moderate: 200mg q12h for 7-14 days. Complicated/Severe: 400mg q12h for 7-14 days. LRTI/SSSI: Mild-Moderate:

400mg q12h for 7-14 days. Complicated/Severe: 400mg q8h for 7-14 days. Bone and Joint: Mild-Moderate: 400mg q12h for ≥4-6 weeks. Complicated/ Severe: 400mg q8h for ≥4-6 weeks. Nosocomial Pneumonia: 400mg q8h for 10-14 days. Complicated Intra-Abdominal: 400mg q12h (w/metronidazole) for 7-14 days. Acute Sinusitis: 400mg q12h for 10 days. Chronic Bacterial Prostatitis: 400mg q12h for 28 days. Febrile Neutropenia: 400mg q8h (w/ piperacillin 50mg/kg q4h) for 7-14 days. Max: 24g/day. Inhalational Anthrax: 400mg q12h for 60 days. Administer over 60 min. CrCl 5-29mL/min: 200-400mg q18-24h.
Pediatrics: <18 yrs: Inhalational Anthrax: 10mg/kg q12h for 60 days. Max: 400mg/dose; 800mg/day. 1-17 yrs: Complicated UTI/Pyleonephritis: 6-10mg/kg q8h for 10-21 days. Max: 400mg/dose.

HOW SUPPLIED: Inj: 10mg/mL, 200mg/100mL, 400mg/200mL

CONTRAINDICATIONS: Concomitant administration with tizanidine.

WARNINGS/PRECAUTIONS: Convulsions, increased ICP, and toxic psychosis reported. Caution with CNS disorders or if predisposed to seizures. Severe, fatal hypersensitivity reactions may occur. *Clostridium difficile*-associated diarrhea, achilles and other tendon ruptures reported. D/C at first sign of rash/ hypersensitivity or if pain, inflammation, or ruptured tendon occur. May permit overgrowth of clostridia. Maintain hydration; avoid alkaline urine. Avoid excessive sunlight and UV light. Do not give via feeding tube. Monitor renal, hepatic and hematopoietic function with prolonged use. Adust dose with renal dysfunction. Caution with concomitant drugs that may result in prolongation of QT interval or in patients with risk factors for torsade de pointes.

ADVERSE REACTIONS: Nausea, diarrhea, CNS disturbances, local IV site reactions, hepatic enzyme abnormalities, eosinophilia, headache, restlessness, rash.

INTERACTIONS: See Contraindications. Increases theophylline and caffeine levels and prolongs effects. Altered serum levels of phenytoin. Severe hypoglycemia with glyburide (rare). Potentiated by probenecid. Transient serum creatinine elevations with cyclosporine. Enhances oral anticoagulant effects. Caution with drugs that lower seizure threshold. Severe tendon disorder risks are increased with concomitant corticosteroid therapy. Caution with concomitant drugs that may result in prolongation of QT interval.

PREGNANCY: Category C, not for use in nursing.

MECHANISM OF ACTION: Synthetic broad-spectrum antimicrobial agent. Inhibits the enzymes topoisomerase II (DNA gyrase) and topoisomerase IV, which are required for bacterial DNA replication, transcription, repair, and recombination.

PHARMACOKINETICS: Absorption: Absolute bioavailability (70-80%); C_{max}=0.1, 002µg/mL (200mg, 400mg, after 12 hrs). **Distribution:** Plasma protein binding (20-40%). **Metabolism:** CYP1A2. **Elimination:** Urine (unchanged), feces (15%). $T_{1/2}$=5-6 hrs.

CIPRO ORAL   RX
ciprofloxacin HCL (Bayer/Schering)

THERAPEUTIC CLASS: Fluoroquinolone

INDICATIONS: Treatment of lower respiratory tract (LRTI), complicated intra-abdominal, skin and skin structure (SSSI), bone and joint, and urinary tract infections (UTI), acute exacerbations of chronic bronchitis, acute sinusitis, acute uncomplicated cystitis in females, chronic bacterial prostatitis, infectious diarrhea, typhoid fever, postexposure inhalational anthrax, uncomplicated cervical and urethral gonorrhea, complicated UTI and pyelonephritis in pediatrics.

DOSAGE: *Adults:* ≥18 yrs: Acute Sinusitis/Typhoid Fever: 500mg q12h for 10 days. LRTI/SSSI: Mild-Moderate: 500mg q12h for 7-14 days. Severe/ Complicated: 750mg q12h for 7-14 days. Cystitis/Acute Uncomplicated UTI: 250mg q12h for 3 days. Mild-Moderate UTI: 250mg q12h for 7-14 days. Severe/ Complicated UTI: 500mg q12h for 7-14 days. Chronic Bacterial Prostatitis:

500mg q12h for 28 days. Intra-Abdominal: 500mg q12h (w/ metronidazole) for 7-14 days. Bone and Joint: Mild-Moderate: 500mg q12h for ≥4-6 weeks. Severe/Complicated: 750mg q12h for ≥4-6 weeks. Infectious Diarrhea: 500mg q12h for 5-7 days. Uncomplicated Urethral/Cervical Gonococcal Infections: 250mg single dose. Inhalational Anthrax: 500mg q12h for 60 days. CrCl 30-50mL/min: 250-500mg q12h. CrCl 5-29mL/min: 250-500mg q18h. Hemodialysis/Peritoneal Dialysis: 250-500mg q24h (after dialysis). Administer at least 2 hrs before or 6 hrs after magnesium- or aluminum-containing antacids, sucralfate, Videx (didanosine) chewable/buffered tablets or pediatric powder, or other products containing calcium, iron, or zinc. *Pediatrics:* <18 yrs: Inhalational Anthrax: 15mg/kg q12h for 60 days. Max: 500mg/dose. 1-17 yrs: Complicated UTI/Pyelonephritis: 10-20mg/kg q12h for 10-21 days. Max: 750mg/dose.

HOW SUPPLIED: Sus: 250mg/5mL, 500mg/5mL [100mL]; Tab: 250mg, 500mg, 750mg

CONTRAINDICATIONS: Concomitant administration with tizanidine.

WARNINGS/PRECAUTIONS: Convulsions, increased ICP, and toxic psychosis reported. Caution with CNS disorders or if predisposed to seizures. Severe, fatal hypersensitivity reactions may occur. *Clostridium difficile*-associated diarrhea, colitis, achilles and other tendon ruptures reported. D/C at first sign of rash or if pain, inflammation, or ruptured tendon occurs. Maintain hydration; avoid alkaline urine. Avoid excessive sunlight and UV light. Do not give via feeding tube. Monitor renal, hepatic, and hematopoietic function with prolonged use. Adjust dose with renal dysfunction. Caution with concomitant drugs that may result in prolongation of the QT interval or in patients with risk factors for torsade de pointes.

ADVERSE REACTIONS: Nausea, dizziness, headache, CNS disturbances, vomiting, diarrhea, rash, abdominal pain/discomfort, pain, swelling, tendon tears.

INTERACTIONS: See Contraindications. Increases theophylline and caffeine levels and prolongs effects. Fatal reactions have occurred with theophylline. Magnesium- or aluminum-containing antacids, sucralfate, Videx (didanosine) chewable/buffered tablets or pediatric powder, and products containing calcium, iron, or zinc decrease serum and urine levels; space doses at least 2 hrs before or 6 hrs after administration. Altered serum levels of phenytoin. Severe hypoglycemia with glyburide (rare). Potentiated by probenecid. Transient serum creatinine elevations with cyclosporine. Enhances oral anticoagulant effects. Monitor PT. Caution with drugs that lower seizure threshold. Severe tendon disorder risks increased with concomitant corticosteroid therapy. Caution with concomitant drugs that may result in prolongation of the QT interval.

PREGNANCY: Category C, not for use in nursing.

MECHANISM OF ACTION: Synthetic broad-spectrum antimicrobial agent; inhibits enzymes topoisomerase II (DNA gyrase) and topoisomerase IV, which are required for bacterial DNA replication.

PHARMACOKINETICS: Absorption: Absolute bioavailability (70%); C_{max}=0.1, 0.2, 0.4mcg/mL (250mg, 500mg, 750mg, after 12 hrs); T_{max}=1-2 hrs. **Distribution:** Plasma protein binding (20-40%). **Metabolism:** CYP1A2. **Elimination:** Urine (40-50%); $T_{1/2}$=4 hrs.

Cipro XR   RX

ciprofloxacin (Bayer/Schering)

THERAPEUTIC CLASS: Fluoroquinolone

INDICATIONS: Uncomplicated (acute cystitis) and complicated urinary tract infections (UTI), and acute uncomplicated pyelonephritis due to *E.coli*.

DOSAGE: *Adults:* ≥18 yrs: Uncomplicated UTI: 500mg qd for 3 days. Complicated UTI: 1000mg qd for 7-14 days. CrCl <30mL/min: 500 mg qd. Acute Uncomplicated Pyelonephritis: 1000mg qd for 7-14 days. CrCl <30mL/min: 500mg qd. Take with fluids. Administer at least 2 hrs before or 6 hrs after magnesium or aluminum containing antacids, sucralfate, Videx (didanosine) chewable/buffered tablets or pediatric powder, metal cations (eg, iron), multivitamins with zinc. Avoid concomitant administration with dairy products alone, or with calcium-fortified products. Space concomitant calcium intake (>800mg) by at least 2 hrs. Do not split, crush, or chew. Swallow tab whole. Dialysis: Give after procedure is completed.

HOW SUPPLIED: Tab, Extended-Release: 500mg, 1000mg

CONTRAINDICATIONS: Concomitant administration with tizanidine.

WARNINGS/PRECAUTIONS: Convulsions, increased ICP and toxic psychosis reported. Caution with CNS disorders or if predisposed to seizures. Severe, sometimes fatal, hypersensitivity reactions may occur. *Clostridium difficile*-associated diarrhea, colitis, achilles, and other tendon ruptures reported. D/C at first sign of rash or if pain, inflammation, or ruptured tendon occurs. Maintain hydration; avoid alkaline urine. Avoid excessive sunlight and UV light. Not interchangeable with immediate-release tablets. To d/c treatment, rest and refrain from exercise. Caution with concomitant drugs that may result in prolongation of the QT interval or in patients with risk factors for torsade de pointes.

ADVERSE REACTIONS: Nausea, headache, diarrhea, pain, swelling, tendon tears.

INTERACTIONS: See Contraindications. Increases theophylline and caffeine levels and prolongs effects. Serious/fatal reactions have occurred with theophylline. Magnesium or aluminum containing antacids, sucralfate, Videx (didanosine) chewable/buffered tablets or pediatric powder, and products containing calcium, iron, or zinc decrease serum and urine levels; space doses at least 2 hrs before or 6 hrs after administration. Altered serum levels of phenytoin. Severe hypoglycemia with glyburide (rare). Potentiated by probenecid. Transient serum creatinine elevations with cyclosporine. Enhances oral anticoagulant effects. Caution with drugs that lower seizure threshold. Severe tendon disorder risks increased with concomitant corticosteroid thereapy. Caution with concomitant drugs that may result in prolongation of the QT interval.

PREGNANCY: Category C, not for use in nursing.

MECHANISM OF ACTION: Synthetic broad-spectrum antimicrobial agent. Inhibits topoisomearase II (DNA gyrase) and topoisomerase IV, which are required for bacterial DNA replication, transcription, repair and recombination.

PHARMACOKINETICS: Absorption: Oral administration of variable doses resulted in different parameters. T_{max}=1-4 hrs. **Distribution:** (IV) V_d= approximately 2.1-2.7L/Kg, plasma protein binding (20-40%). **Metabolism:** Primary metabolites: oxociprofloxacin and sulfociprofloxacin. **Elimination:** Urine (approximately 35%, unchanged).

CIPRODEX   RX
dexamethasone - ciprofloxacin (Alcon)

THERAPEUTIC CLASS: Antibacterial/corticosteroid combination

INDICATIONS: Acute otitis media in pediatric patients with tympanostomy tubes. Acute otitis externa.

DOSAGE: *Adults:* Acute Otitis Externa: 4 drops in affected ear(s) bid for 7 days. Warm bottle in hand for 1-2 min to avoid dizziness. Shake well before use.
Pediatrics: ≥6 months: 4 drops in affected ear(s) bid for 7 days. Warm bottle in hand for 1-2 min to avoid dizziness. Shake well before use.

HOW SUPPLIED: Sus: (Ciprofloxacin-Dexamethasone) 0.3%-0.1% [5mL, 7.5mL]

CONTRAINDICATIONS: Viral infections of external ear canal including herpes simplex infections.

WARNINGS/PRECAUTIONS: D/C if hypersensitivity reaction occurs. Re-evaluate if no improvement after one week.

ADVERSE REACTIONS: Ear pain/discomfort/pruritus.

PREGNANCY: Category C, not for use in nursing.

MECHANISM OF ACTION: Fluoroquinolone, corticosteroid; antibacterial/anti-inflammatory; bactericidal action results from interference with the enzyme (DNA gyrase), which is needed for the synthesis of bacterial DNA.

PHARMACOKINETICS: Absorption: Ciprofloxacin: C_{max}=1.39ng/mL, T_{max}=15 min-2 hrs. Dexamethasone: C_{max}=1.14ng/mL, T_{max}=15 min-2 hrs.

CitraNatal DHA RX
docusate sodium - folic acid - multiple vitamin - minerals - iron (Mission)

OTHER BRAND NAMES: CitraNatal 90 DHA (Mission)

THERAPEUTIC CLASS: Prenatal vitamin

INDICATIONS: Vitamin and mineral supplementation for before, during, and after pregnancy.

DOSAGE: *Adults:* 1 tab and 1 cap qd.

HOW SUPPLIED: Tab: (CitraNatal DHA) Calcium 125mg-Copper 2mg-Docusate Sodium 50mg-Folic Acid 1mg-Iodine 150mcg-Iron 27mg-Niacinamide 20mg-Vitamin B_1 3mg-Vitamin B_2 3.4mg-Vitamin B_6 20mg-Vitamin C 120mg-Vitamin D 400IU-Vitamin E 30IU-Zinc 25mg*; (CitraNatal 90 DHA) Calcium 200mg-Copper 2mg-Docusate Sodium 50mg-Folic Acid 1mg-Iodine 150mcg-Iron 90mg-Niacinamide 20mg-Vitamin B_1 3mg-Vitamin B_2 3.4mg-Vitamin B_6 20mg-Vitamin C 120mg-Vitamin D 400IU-Vitamin E 30IU-Zinc 25mg*; Cap: (CitraNatal DHA/CitraNatal 90 DHA) DHA 250mg *scored

WARNINGS/PRECAUTIONS: Accidental overdose of iron-containing products is a leading cause of fatal poisoning in children <6 yrs. Not for the treatment of pernicious anemia and other megaloblastic anemias where vitamin B_{12} is deficient. Folic acid >0.1mg/day may obscure pernicious anemia. Omega-3 fatty acids may increase bleeding time and INR; avoid with anticoagulants and with inherited or acquired bleeding diathesis.

ADVERSE REACTIONS: Allergic sensitization.

INTERACTIONS: Avoid omega-3 fatty acids with anticoagulants.

MECHANISM OF ACTION: Multivitamin/mineral supplement.

Claforan RX
cefotaxime sodium (Sanofi-Aventis)

THERAPEUTIC CLASS: Cephalosporin (3rd generation)

INDICATIONS: Treatment of lower respiratory tract, genitourinary, gynecologic, intra-abdominal, skin and skin structure, bone and joint, and CNS infections (eg, meningitis), bacteremia, and septicemia caused by susceptible strains of microorganisms. For surgical prophylaxis of certain infections.

DOSAGE: *Adults:* Gonococcal Urethritis/Cervicitis (Males/Females): 500mg single dose IM. Rectal Gonorrhea: 0.5g (females) or 1g (males) single dose IM. Uncomplicated Infections: 1g IM/IV q12h. Moderate-Severe Infections: 1-2g IM/IV q8h. Septicemia: 2g IV q6-8h. Life-Threatening Infections: 2g IV q4h. Max: 12g/day. Surgical Prophylaxis: 1g IM/IV 30-90 min before surgery. Cesarean Section: 1g IV when umbilical cord is clamped, then 1g IV at 6 and 12 hrs after 1st dose. CrCl <20mL/min/1.73m²: Give 1/2 of usual dose.
Pediatrics: ≥50kg: Use adult dose. Max: 12g/day. 1 month-12 yrs and ≤50kg: 50-180mg/kg/day IM/IV divided in 4-6 doses. 1-4 weeks: 50mg/kg IV q8h. 0-1 week: 50mg/kg IV q12h. CrCl <20mL/min/1.73m²: Give 1/2 of usual dose.

HOW SUPPLIED: Inj: 500mg, 1g, 2g, 10g

WARNINGS/PRECAUTIONS: Cross sensitivity to PCNs and other cephalosporins may occur. *Clostridium difficile*-associated diarrhea reported. May result in overgrowth of nonsusceptible organisms. Caution with history of GI disease. Reduce dose with renal dysfunction. Granulocytopenia may occur with long-term use. Monitor blood counts if therapy >10 days. Monitor injection site for tissue inflammation. False (+) direct Coombs' tests reported.

ADVERSE REACTIONS: Injection site reactions, rash, pruritus, fever, eosinophilia, colitis, diarrhea.

INTERACTIONS: Increased nephrotoxicity with aminoglycosides.

PREGNANCY: Category B, caution in nursing.

MECHANISM OF ACTION: 3rd-generation cephalosporin; inhibits cell wall synthesis.

PHARMACOKINETICS: Absorption: IM: C_{max} (500mg, 1g)=11.7, 20.5mcg/mL; T_{max}=30min. **Elimination:** Unchanged, cefotaxime and desacetyl derivative (major metabolite) are excreted by kidneys; $T_{1/2}$=1 hr.

CLARINEX   RX
desloratadine (Schering)

OTHER BRAND NAMES: Clarinex Syrup (Schering) - Clarinex RediTabs (Schering)

THERAPEUTIC CLASS: H_1-antagonist

INDICATIONS: Relief of perennial allergic rhinitis and chronic idiopathic urticaria in patients ≥6 months. Relief of seasonal allergic rhinitis in patients ≥2 yrs.

DOSAGE: *Adults:* 5mg qd. Hepatic/Renal Impairment: 5mg every other day. Dissolve RediTabs on tongue with or without water.
Pediatrics: Tabs: ≥12 yrs: 5mg qd. 6-11 yrs: 2.5mg qd. Syrup: ≥12 yrs: 10mL (5mg) qd. 6-11 yrs: 5mL (2.5mg) qd. 12 months-5 yrs: 2.5mL (1.25mg) qd. 6-11 months: 2mL (1mg) qd. Dissolve RediTabs on tongue with or without water.

HOW SUPPLIED: Tab: 5mg; Tab, Disintegrating: (RediTabs) 2.5mg, 5mg; Syrup: 0.5mg/mL

WARNINGS/PRECAUTIONS: Adjust dose with renal or hepatic impairment. Caution in elderly.

ADVERSE REACTIONS: Pharyngitis, dry mouth, headache, fever, diarrhea, cough, upper respiratory tract infection, cough, irritability, somnolence, bronchitis, otitis media, vomiting, nausea, fatigue.

INTERACTIONS: Erythromycin, ketoconazole increase plasma levels.

PREGNANCY: Category C, not for use in nursing.

MECHANISM OF ACTION: Long-acting tricyclic histamine antagonist with selective H_1-receptor histamine antagonist activity; inhibits histamine release from human mast cells.

PHARMACOKINETICS: Absorption: T_{max}=3 hrs., C_{max}=4ng/mL, AUC=56.9ng•hr/mL. **Distribution:** Found in breast milk; plasma protein binding (82-87% of desloratadine), (85-89% of 3-hydroxydesloratidine). **Metabolism:** Extensive. Desloratadine (major metabolite), 3-hydroxydesloratadine (active metabolite): **Elimination:** Urine and feces (metabolites); $T_{1/2}$=27 hrs.

CLARINEX-D   RX
pseudoephedrine sulfate - desloratadine (Schering)

THERAPEUTIC CLASS: H_1-antagonist/sympathomimetic amine

INDICATIONS: Relief of nasal and non-nasal symptoms of seasonal allergic rhinitis including nasal congestion.

DOSAGE: *Adults:* 2.5mg-120mg tab bid or 5mg-240mg tab qd w/ or w/o food. Hepatic Impairment: 12-Hour/24-Hour: Avoid use. Renal Impairment: 12-Hour: Avoid use. 24-Hour: 1 tab qod.
Pediatrics: ≥12 yrs: 2.5mg-120mg tab bid or 5mg-240mg tab qd w/ or w/o food. Hepatic Impairment: 12-Hour/24-Hour: Avoid use. Renal Impairment: 12-Hour: Avoid use. 24-Hour: 1 tab qod.

HOW SUPPLIED: Tab, Extended-Release: (Desloratadine-Pseudoephedrine) (12-Hour) 2.5mg-120mg, (24-Hour) 5mg-240mg

CONTRAINDICATIONS: Narrow-angle glaucoma, urinary retention, MAOI therapy or within 14 days of discontinuation, severe HTN, severe CAD, hypersensitivity or idiosyncrasy to adrenergic agents, or to other drugs of similar chemical structures.

WARNINGS/PRECAUTIONS: Caution with HTN, DM, ischemic heart disease, increased intraocular pressure, hyperthyroidism, renal impairment, or prostatic hypertrophy. CNS stimulation with convulsions or cardiovascular collapse with accompanying hypotension may be produced by sympathomimetic amines. Avoid with hepatic insufficiency.

ADVERSE REACTIONS: Dry mouth, headache, insomnia, fatigue, pharyngitis, somnolence

INTERACTIONS: Do not use with MAOIs or within 14 days of discontinuation. Antihypertensive effects of β-adrenergic blocking agents, methyldopa, mecamylamine, reserpine, and veratrum alkaloids may be reduced by sympathomimetics (eg, pseudoephedrine). Increased ectopic pacemaker activity with digitalis.

PREGNANCY: Category C, not for use in nursing.

MECHANISM OF ACTION: Desloratadine: Long acting tricyclic histamine antagonist with selective H_1-receptor antagonist activity. Inhibits histamine release from human mast cells *in vitro*. Pseudoephedrine: Orally active sympathomimetic amine, which exerts a decongestant action on nasal mucosa.

PHARMACOKINETICS: Absorption: Desloratadine: (24 hr) C_{max}=approximately 1.79ng/mL; T_{max}=approximately 6-7 hrs, AUC=approximately 61.1ng•hr/mL. (12 hr) C_{max}=approximately 1.09ng/ml; T_{max}=approximately 4-5 hrs, AUC=31.6ng•hr/ml. Pseudoephedrine: (24 hr) C_{max}=approximately 328ng/mL, T_{max}=8-9 hrs, AUC=6438ng•hr/mL. (12 hr) C_{max}=263ng/ml, T_{max}=approximately 6-7 hr, AUC=approximately 4588ng•hr/ml. **Distribution:** Desloratadine: Found in breast milk, plasma protein binding (approximately 82-87%), 3-hydroxydesloratadine (85%-89%). **Metabolism:** Desloratadine (major metabolite): Extensive, 3-hydroxydesloratadine (active metabolite) and glucuronidation pathway. Pseudoephedrine: Liver (incomplete), through N-demethylation. **Elimination:** Desloratadine: (24 hr) $T_{1/2}$=approximately 24 hrs, (12 hr) $T_{1/2}$=27 hrs. Pseudoephedrine: Urine (55-96%, unchanged). If urinary pH=5, ($T_{1/2}$=3-6 hrs); if urinary pH=8, ($T_{1/2}$ =9-16 hrs).

CLARIPEL RX
hydroquinone (Stiefel)

THERAPEUTIC CLASS: Depigmenting agent

INDICATIONS: Gradual treatment of ultraviolet induced dyschromia and discoloration resulting from use of oral contraceptives, pregnancy, hormone replacement therapy, or skin trauma.

DOSAGE: *Adults:* Apply bid.
Pediatrics: ≥12 yrs: Apply bid.

HOW SUPPLIED: Cre: 4% [28g, 45g]

WARNINGS/PRECAUTIONS: Avoid sun exposure on bleached skin. Claripel contains sunscreen. May produce unwanted cosmetic effects if not used as directed. Test for skin sensitivity. D/C if no lightening effect after 2 months of therapy, if blue-black skin discoloration occurs, or if itching, vesicle formation, or excessive inflammatory reactions occur. Contains sodium metabisulfite; may cause serious allergic type reactions. Avoid contact with eyes.

ADVERSE REACTIONS: Cutaneous hypersensitivity (contact dermatitis).

PREGNANCY: Category C, caution in nursing.

MECHANISM OF ACTION: Produces a reversible depigmentation of the skin by inhibition of the enzymatic oxidation of tyrosine to 3-(3,4-dihydroxyphenyl) alanine (dopa)[1] and suppression of other melanocyte metabolic processes.

CLARITIN OTC
loratadine (Schering)

OTC

OTHER BRAND NAMES: Claritin Reditab OTC (Schering)

THERAPEUTIC CLASS: H_1-antagonist

INDICATIONS: Relief of symptoms due to hay fever or other upper respiratory allergies.

DOSAGE: *Adults:* (Reditab, Syrup, Tab) 10mg qd. Max: 10mg/d. Dissolve Reditab on tongue. Hepatic/Renal Impairment: May need to adjust dose.
Pediatrics: ≥6 yrs: (Reditab, Syr, Tab) 10mg qd. Max: 10mg/d. 2-5 yrs: (Syr) 5mg qd. Max: 5mg/d. Dissolve Reditab on tongue. Hepatic/Renal Impairment: May need to adjust dose.

HOW SUPPLIED: Syrup: 1mg/mL; Tab, Extended-Release: (24 hr) 10mg; Tab, Disintegrating: (Reditab) 10mg

WARNINGS/PRECAUTIONS: Caution with hepatic or renal impairment.

PREGNANCY: Safety in pregnancy and nursing is not known.

CLARITIN-D OTC
pseudoephedrine sulfate - loratadine (Schering)

OTC

THERAPEUTIC CLASS: H_1-antagonist/sympathomimetic amine

INDICATIONS: Relief of symptoms due to hay fever or other upper respiratory allergies. Reduces swelling of nasal passages. Relief of sinus congestion and pressure.

DOSAGE: *Adults:* 5-120mg tab q12h or 10-240mg tab qd (with full glass of water). Max: 10-240mg/24 hrs. Hepatic/Renal Impairment: May need to adjust dose. Do not divide, crush, chew or dissolve tabs.
Pediatrics: ≥12 yrs: 5-120mg tab q12h, or 10-240mg tab qd (with full glass of water). Max: 10-240mg/24 hrs. Hepatic/Renal Impairment: May need to adjust dose. Do not divide, crush, chew or dissolve tabs.

HOW SUPPLIED: Tab, Extended-Release: (Loratadine-Pseudoephedrine) (12-Hour) 5-120mg, (24-Hour) 10-240mg

WARNINGS/PRECAUTIONS: Caution with hepatic or renal impairment, heart disease, thyroid disease, high BP, diabetes, enlarged prostate.

ADVERSE REACTIONS: Dizziness, insomnia, nervousness.

INTERACTIONS: Avoid during or within 14 days MAOIs.

PREGNANCY: Safety in pregnancy and nursing is not known.

CLENIA
sulfacetamide sodium - sulfur (Upsher-Smith)

RX

THERAPEUTIC CLASS: Sulfonamide/sulfur combination

INDICATIONS: Topical treatment of acne vulgaris, acne rosacea, and seborrheic dermatitis.

DOSAGE: *Adults:* (Cleanser) Wash qd-bid. Massage into skin for 10-20 seconds, then rinse and dry. (Cre) Initial: Apply qd. Titrate: Increase up to bid-tid prn.
Pediatrics: ≥12 yrs: (Cleanser) Wash qd-bid. Massage into skin for 10-20 seconds, then rinse and dry. (Cre) Initial: Apply qd. Titrate: Increase up to bid-tid prn.

HOW SUPPLIED: Cleanser: (Sulfacetamide-Sulfur) 10%-5% [170g, 340g]; Cre: 10%-5% [28g]

CONTRAINDICATIONS: Kidney disease.

C

WARNINGS/PRECAUTIONS: D/C if excessive irritation occurs. Avoid contact with eyes, eyelid, lips, or mucous membranes. Caution with denuded or abraded skin. Can cause reddening and scaling of epidermis.

ADVERSE REACTIONS: Dryness, erythema, itching, edema.

PREGNANCY: Category C, caution in nursing.

MECHANISM OF ACTION: Sulfacetamide: Believed to block bacterial growth by acting as a competitive antagonist of para-aminobenzoic acid (PABA). Sulfur: Not established. Keratolytic activity reported to result from the interaction with the cysteine content of keratinocytes. In combination with sulfacetamide, it inhibits *Propionibacterium acnes*, thereby reducing associated inflammation.

PHARMACOKINETICS: Absorption: 1% of topically applied sulfur is absorbed through intact skin. **Distribution:** Small amounts of orally administered sulfonamides have been found in breast milk.

CLEOCIN   RX
clindamycin HCL (Pharmacia & Upjohn)

> *Clostridium difficile*-associated diarrhea (CDAD) reported with use of nearly all antibacterial agents, including clindamycin, and may range in severity from mild diarrhea to fatal colitis. If CDAD is suspected or confirmed, ongoing antibiotic use not directed against *C.difficile* may need to be discontinued.

THERAPEUTIC CLASS: Lincomycin derivative

INDICATIONS: Serious infections caused by anaerobes, streptococci, pneumococci, and staphylococci.

DOSAGE: *Adults:* Serious Infection: 150-300mg PO q6h or 600-1200mg/day IM/IV given bid-qid. More Severe Infection: 300-450mg PO q6h or 1200-2700mg/day IM/IV given bid-qid. Life-Threatening Infections: Up to 4800mg/day IV. Max: 600mg per IM injection. Take caps with full glass of water. Treat β-hemolytic strep for at least 10 days.
Pediatrics: Give tid or qid. Cap: Serious Infections: 8-16mg/kg/day. More Severe Infections: 16-20mg/kg/day. Sol: Serious Infections: 8-12mg/kg/day. Severe Infections: 13-16mg/kg/day. More Severe Infections: 17-25mg/kg/day. IM/IV: 1 month-16 yrs: 20-40mg/kg/day; use the higher dose for more severe infections. <1 month: 15-20mg/kg/day. Take caps with full glass of water. Treat β-hemolytic strep for at least 10 days.

HOW SUPPLIED: Cap: (HCl) 75mg, 150mg, 300mg; Inj: (Phosphate) 150mg/mL, 300mg/50mL, 600mg/50mL, 900mg/50mL; Sol: (Palmitate HCl) 75mg/5mL [100mL]

WARNINGS/PRECAUTIONS: May permit overgrowth of clostridia. Not for treatment of meningitis. Caution with atopic patients, GI disease (eg, colitis), hepatic disease, and the elderly. Monitor blood, hepatic and renal function with long-term use. Do not give injection undiluted as bolus. The 75mg and 100mg caps contain tartrazine.

ADVERSE REACTIONS: Abdominal pain, colitis, esophagitis, nausea, vomiting, diarrhea, hypersensitivity reactions, jaundice, blood dyscrasias, pruritus, vaginitis, superinfection (prolonged use).

INTERACTIONS: Antagonism may occur with erythromycin. May potentiate neuromuscular blockers.

PREGNANCY: Category B, not for use in nursing.

MECHANISM OF ACTION: Clindamycin: Inhibits bacterial protein synthesis at the level of the bacterial ribosome and binds preferentially to the 50S ribosomal subunit affecting process of peptide chain initiation.

PHARMACOKINETICS: Absorption: Cap: Rapid, complete; C_{max}=2.5mcg/mL, T_{max}=45 min. Inj: C_{max}=10.8mcg/mL (adults, IV 600mg q8h), 9mcg/mL (adults, IM q12h), 10mcg/ml (peds, IV), 8mcg/mL (peds, IM); T_{max}=3 hrs (adults), 1 hr (peds). Oral Sol: C_{max}=1.24mcg/mL (peds, 8mg/kg/day), 2.25mcg/mL (12mg/kg/day). **Distribution:** Wide; body fluids, tissues, and bones; found in breast milk. **Elimination:** Cap: Urine (10% unchanged), feces (3.6%

unchanged); T$_{1/2}$=3.2 hr. Inj: T$_{1/2}$=3 hrs (adults), 2.5 hrs (peds). Oral Sol: T$_{1/2}$=2 hrs (peds).

CLEOCIN T   RX
clindamycin phosphate (Pharmacia & Upjohn)

THERAPEUTIC CLASS: Lincomycin derivative

INDICATIONS: Acne vulgaris.

DOSAGE: *Adults:* Apply thin film bid.
Pediatrics: ≥12 yrs: Apply thin film bid. May use more than 1 pledget.

HOW SUPPLIED: Gel: 1% [30g, 60g]; Lot: 1% [60mL]; Sol: 1% [30mL, 60mL]; Swab (Pledgets): 1% [60^s]

CONTRAINDICATIONS: Hypersensitivity to lincomycin. History of regional enteritis, ulcerative colitis, or antibiotic-associated colitis.

WARNINGS/PRECAUTIONS: Avoid eyes, abraded skin, mucous membranes, and mouth. Caution in atopic patients. D/C if significant diarrhea occurs.

ADVERSE REACTIONS: Dryness, oily skin, erythema, peeling, burning, itching, pseudomembranous colitis (rare).

INTERACTIONS: May potentiate neuromuscular blockers.

PREGNANCY: Category B, not for use in nursing.

MECHANISM OF ACTION: Inhibits growth of *Propionibacterium acnes* and decreases free fatty acids on the skin surface.

PHARMACOKINETICS: Absorption: Following topical administration of multiple doses, serum levels of clindamycin were measured at 0-3ng/mL. **Distribution:** Orally and parenterally administered clindamycin has been found in breast milk. **Metabolism:** Hydrolysis. **Elimination:** Urine (≤0.2% found as clindamycin).

CLEOCIN VAGINAL   RX
clindamycin phosphate (Pharmacia & Upjohn)

OTHER BRAND NAMES: Clindamax Vaginal (PharmaDerm) - Cleocin Vaginal Ovules (Pharmacia & Upjohn)

THERAPEUTIC CLASS: Lincomycin derivative

INDICATIONS: (Cream) Treatment of bacterial vaginosis in non-pregnant women and pregnant women during the 2nd and 3rd trimester. (Sup) Treatment of bacterial vaginosis in non-pregnant women.

DOSAGE: *Adults:* (Cream) 1 applicatorful intravaginally qhs. Treat non-pregnant females for 3 or 7 days. Treat pregnant females (2nd and 3rd trimester) for 7 days. (Sup) 1 suppository intravaginally qhs for 3 days.
Pediatrics: Post-Menarchal: (Sup) 1 suppository intravaginally qhs for 3 days.

HOW SUPPLIED: Cre: 2% [40g]; Sup, Vaginal: (Ovules) 100mg [3^s]

CONTRAINDICATIONS: Hypersensitivity to lincomycin. History of regional enteritis, ulcerative colitis, or antibiotic-associated colitis.

WARNINGS/PRECAUTIONS: Do not use condoms or contraceptive diaphragms within 72 hrs following treatment. Monitor for pseudomembranous colitis. Avoid eye contact. Do not engage in vaginal intercourse or use other vaginal products (such as tampons or douches) during treatment. Monitor for pseudomembranous colitis. May result in overgrowth of nonsusceptible organisms in vagina.

ADVERSE REACTIONS: Vaginitis, vulvovaginal disorder, candidiasis, moniliasis, pruritus, abnormal labor.

INTERACTIONS: May potentiate neuromuscular blockers.

PREGNANCY: Category B, not for use in nursing.

MECHANISM OF ACTION: Antibiotic; inhibits bacterial protein synthesis at the level of the bacterial ribosome and binds preferentially to the 50S ribosomal subunit affecting peptide chain initiation.

PHARMACOKINETICS: Absorption: (Day 1) C_{max} =13ng/ml; (Day 7) C_{max} =16ng/mL, T_{max} =14 hrs. **Elimination:** $T_{1/2}$ =1.5-2.6 hrs.

CLIMARA   RX
estradiol (Bayer Healthcare)

> Estrogens increase risk of endometrial cancer. Estrogens, with or without progestins, should not be used for the prevention of cardiovascular disease or dementia. Increased risks of MI, stroke, invasive breast cancer, PE, and DVT in postmenopausal women (50-79 yrs of age) reported. Increased risk of developing probable dementia in postmenopausal women ≥65 yrs of age reported.

THERAPEUTIC CLASS: Estrogen

INDICATIONS: Treatment of moderate to severe vasomotor symptoms and/or vulvar/vaginal atrophy associated with menopause. Treatment of hypoestrogenism due to hypogonadism, castration, or primary ovarian failure. Prevention of postmenopausal osteoporosis.

DOSAGE: *Adults:* Apply 1 patch weekly to lower abdomen or upper area of buttocks (avoid breasts and waistline). Rotate application sites. Vasomotor Symptoms: Initial: 0.025mg/day patch once weekly. Titrate: Adjust dose as needed. Wait 1 week after withdrawal of oral therapy before initiating patch. Discontinue or taper at 3-6 month intervals. Osteoporosis Prevention: Minimum Effective Dose: 0.025mg/day once weekly.

HOW SUPPLIED: Patch: 0.025mg/day, 0.0375mg/day, 0.05mg/day, 0.06mg/day, 0.075mg/day, 0.1mg/day [4ˢ]

CONTRAINDICATIONS: Pregnancy, undiagnosed abnormal genital bleeding, breast cancer, estrogen-dependent neoplasia, DVT/PE, active or recent (eg, within 1 year) thromboembolic disease (eg, stroke, MI), liver dysfunction or disease.

WARNINGS/PRECAUTIONS: May increase risk of cardiovascular events (eg, MI, stroke), venous thrombosis, and PE; d/c immediately if any of these events occur or are suspected. May increase risk of breast/endometrial cancer, and gallbladder disease. Retinal vascular thrombosis reported; monitor and d/c if papilledema or retinal vascular lesions occur. Consider addition of a progestin if no hysterectomy. May elevate BP; monitor at regular intervals. May cause elevations of plasma triglycerides with pre-existing hypertriglyceridemia. Caution with history of cholestatic jaundice associated with past estrogen use or with pregnancy; d/c with recurrence. May lead to increased thyroid-binding globulin levels; monitor thyroid function. May cause fluid retention; caution with cardiac/renal dysfunction. Caution with severe hypocalcemia. May increase risk of ovarian cancer. May exacerbate endometriosis, asthma, DM, epilepsy, migraine, porphyria, systemic lupus erythematosus, hepatic hemangiomas; use with caution.

ADVERSE REACTIONS: Skin irritation, headache, arthralgia, depression, breast pain, leukorrhea, upper respiratory tract infection, sinusitis.

INTERACTIONS: CYP3A4 inducers (eg, St. John's wort, phenobarbital, carbamazepine, rifampin) may decrease levels which may decrease therapeutic effects and/or change uterine bleeding profile. CYP3A4 inhibitors (eg, erythromycin, clarithromycin, ketoconazole, itraconazole, ritonavir, grapefruit juice) may increase levels which may result in side effects.

PREGNANCY: Contraindicated in pregnancy, caution in nursing.

MECHANISM OF ACTION: Estrogen; acts by binding to nuclear receptors in estrogen-responsive tissues. Modulates the pituitary secretion of gonadotrophins, luteinizing hormone (LH) and follicle stimulating hormone (FSH), through a negative feedback mechanism.

PHARMACOKINETICS: Absorption: Transdermal administration of different doses resulted in different parameters. **Distribution**: Estrogens are found in human breast milk. Widely; largely bound to sex hormone binding globulin

(SHBG) and albumin. **Metabolism:** Liver to estrone (metabolite); estriol (major urinary metabolite); enterohepatic recirculation via sulfate and glucuronide conjugation; biliary secretion of conjugates into the intestine; hydrolysis in the gut; and reabsorbtion. CYP3A4 (partial). **Elimination:** Urine.

CLIMARA PRO RX
levonorgestrel - estradiol (Bayer Healthcare)

> Estrogens and progestins should not be used for the prevention of cardiovascular disease or dementia. Increased risks of MI, stroke, invasive breast cancer, PE, and DVT in postmenopausal women (50-79 yrs of age) reported. Increased risk of developing probable dementia in postmenopausal women ≥65 yrs of age reported.

THERAPEUTIC CLASS: Estrogen/progestogen combination

INDICATIONS: Treatment of moderate to severe vasomotor symptoms associated with menopause. Prevention of postmenopausal osteoporosis.

DOSAGE: *Adults:* Apply 1 patch weekly to lower abdomen (avoid breasts and waistline). Rotate application site; allow 1 week between same site. Reevaluate periodically (3-6 month intervals).

HOW SUPPLIED: Patch: (Estradiol-Levonorgestrel): 0.045mg-0.015mg/day [4^s]

CONTRAINDICATIONS: Pregnancy, undiagnosed abnormal genital bleeding, breast cancer, estrogen-dependent neoplasia, DVT/PE, active or recent (eg, within 1 year) thromboembolic disease (eg, stroke, MI), liver dysfunction or disease.

WARNINGS/PRECAUTIONS: May increase risk of cardiovascular events (eg, MI, stroke), venous thrombosis, and PE; d/c immediately if any of these events occur or are suspected. May increase risk of breast/endometrial cancer, and gallbladder disease. Retinal vascular thrombosis reported; monitor and d/c if papilledema or retinal vascular lesions occur. Consider addition of a progestin if no hysterectomy. May elevate BP; monitor at regular intervals. May cause elevations of plasma triglycerides with pre-existing hypertriglyceridemia. Caution with history of cholestatic jaundice associated with past estrogen use or with pregnancy; d/c with recurrence. May lead to increased thyroid-binding globulin levels; monitor thyroid function. May cause fluid retention; caution with cardiac/renal dysfunction. Caution with severe hypocalcemia. May increase risk of ovarian cancer. May exacerbate endometriosis, asthma, DM, epilepsy, migraine, porphyria; use with caution.

ADVERSE REACTIONS: Application site reaction, vaginal bleeding, breast pain, upper respiratory infection, back pain, headache, depression, arthralgia, flu syndrome, abdominal pain.

INTERACTIONS: CYP3A4 inducers (eg, St. John's wort, phenobarbital, carbamazepine, rifampin) may decrease levels which may decrease therapeutic effects and/or change uterine bleeding profile. CYP3A4 inhibitors (eg, erythromycin, clarithromycin, ketoconazole, itraconazole, ritonavir, grapefruit juice) may increase levels which may result in side effects.

PREGNANCY: Contraindicated in pregnancy, caution in nursing.

MECHANISM OF ACTION: Estradiol: estrogen. Binds to nuclear receptors in estrogen-responsive tissue. Modulates pituitary secretion of gonadotrophins, luteinizing hormone (LH) and follicle stimulating hormone, through negative feedback mechanism. Levonorgestrel: progestogen. Inhibits gonadotropin production resulting in retardation of follicular growth and inhibition of ovulation. Counteracts proliferative effects of estrogens in endometrium.

PHARMACOKINETICS: Absorption:(Single dose): Estradiol: C_{max}=54.3pg/mL, T_{max}=42 hrs, AUC=6340pg•hr/mL; Estrone (metabolite): C_{max}=43.9pg/mL, T_{max}=84 hrs, AUC=6890pg•hr/ mL; Levonorgestrel: C_{max}=138pg/mL, T_{max}=90 hrs, AUC=22900pg•hr/mL. **Distribution:** Estrogens and progestin found in breast milk. Estradiol: Widely distributed; largely bound to sex hormone binding globulin (SHBG) and albumin. Levonorgestrel: Bound to SHBG and albumin. **Metabolism:** Estradiol: Hepatic, to estrone (metabolite); estriol (major urinary metabolite); enterohepatic recirculation, via sulfate and glucuronide conjugation; biliary secretion of conjugates into intestine; hydrolysis in gut, reabsorption. CYP3A4 (partial). Levonorgestrel: Reduction, hydroxylation, conjugation. **Elimination:** Estradiol, estrone, estriol: Urine. Estradiol: $T_{1/2}$=3 hrs. Levonorgestrel: Urine; $T_{1/2}$=28 hrs.

CLINDAGEL   RX
clindamycin phosphate (Galderma)

THERAPEUTIC CLASS: Lincomycin derivative

INDICATIONS: Acne vulgaris.

DOSAGE: *Adults:* Apply thin film once daily.
Pediatrics: ≥12 yrs: Apply thin film once daily.

HOW SUPPLIED: Gel: 1% [40mL, 75mL]

CONTRAINDICATIONS: Hypersensitivity to lincomycin. History of regional enteritis, ulcerative colitis, or antibiotic-associated colitis.

WARNINGS/PRECAUTIONS: D/C if significant diarrhea occurs. Caution in atopic individuals.

ADVERSE REACTIONS: Peeling, pruritus, pseudomembranous colitis (rare).

INTERACTIONS: May potentiate neuromuscular blockers.

PREGNANCY: Category B, not for use in nursing.

MECHANISM OF ACTION: Lincomycin derivative; inhibits bacteria protein synthesis at ribosomal level by binding to the 50S ribosomal subunit and affecting the process of peptide chain initiation.

PHARMACOKINETICS: Absorption: C_{max}≤5.5ng/mL. **Distribution:** Orally and parenterally administered clindamycin appears in breast milk. **Excretion:** Urine (<0.4% of total dose).

CLINDAMYCIN PHOSPHATE   RX
clindamycin phosphate (Various)

THERAPEUTIC CLASS: Lincomycin derivative

INDICATIONS: Treatment of acne vulgaris.

DOSAGE: *Adults:* Apply thin film bid.
Pediatrics: ≥12 yrs: Apply thin film bid.

HOW SUPPLIED: Swab: 1% [69 pads]

CONTRAINDICATIONS: History of regional enteritis, ulcerative colitis, or antibiotic-associated colitis.

WARNINGS/PRECAUTIONS: Avoid eyes, abraded skin, mucous membranes and mouth. Caution in atopic patients. Diarrhea, bloody diarrhea and colitis reported with systemic and topical use. D/C if significant diarrhea occurs.

ADVERSE REACTIONS: Burning, itching, dryness, erythema, oily skin, peeling.

INTERACTIONS: May potentiate neuromuscular blockers.

PREGNANCY: Category B, not for use in nursing.

CLINDESSE   RX
clindamycin phosphate (Ther-Rx)

THERAPEUTIC CLASS: Lincomycin derivative

INDICATIONS: Treatment of bacterial vaginosis in non-pregnant women.

DOSAGE: *Adults:* 1 applicatorful administered intravaginally any time of day.

HOW SUPPLIED: Cre: 2% [5g]

CONTRAINDICATIONS: Hypersensitivity to lincomycin. History of regional enteritis, ulcerative colitis, or antibiotic-associated colitis.

WARNINGS/PRECAUTIONS: Do not use condoms or contraceptive diaphragms within 5 days following treatment. Monitor for pseudomembranous colitis. Avoid eye contact. Do not engage in vaginal intercourse or use other vaginal products (such as tampons or douches) during treatment. May result in overgrowth of nonsusceptible organisms in vagina.

ADVERSE REACTIONS: Fungal vaginosis, vulvovaginal pruritus.

INTERACTIONS: May potentiate neuromuscular blockers.

PREGNANCY: Category B, not for use in nursing

MECHANISM OF ACTION: Inhibits bacterial protein synthesis at the level of the bacterial ribosome. Binds preferentially to the 50S ribosomal subunit and effects the process of peptide chain initiation.

PHARMACOKINETICS: Absorption: AUC=175ng.mL•hr, C_{max}=6.6ng/mL, T_{max}=20hrs.

CLOBEVATE RX
clobetasol propionate (Stiefel)

THERAPEUTIC CLASS: Corticosteroid

INDICATIONS: Inflammatory and pruritic manifestations of corticosteroid-responsive dermatoses.

DOSAGE: *Adults:* Apply thin layer bid. Limit treatment to 2 consecutive weeks. Max: 50g/week. Avoid with occlusive dressings.
Pediatrics: ≥12 yrs: Apply thin layer bid. Limit treatment to 2 consecutive weeks. Max: 50g/week. Avoid with occlusive dressings.

HOW SUPPLIED: Gel: 0.05% [45g]

WARNINGS/PRECAUTIONS: May produce reversible HPA axis suppression, manifestations of Cushing's syndrome, hyperglycemia, and glucosuria. Pediatrics may be more susceptible to systemic toxicity. D/C if irritation occurs. Use appropriate antifungal or antibacterial with concomitant skin infections; d/c if infection does not clear. Should not be used to treat rosacea or perioral dermatitis. Avoid use on face, groin, or axillae.

ADVERSE REACTIONS: Burning, stinging, irritation, pruritus, erythema, folliculitis, cracking and fissuring of the skin, numbness of fingers, skin atrophy, telangiectasia.

PREGNANCY: Category C, caution in nursing.

MECHANISM OF ACTION: Corticosteroid; not established. Has anti-inflammatory, antipruritic, and vasoconstrictive properties. Anti-inflammatory not established; thought to induct phospholipase A_2 inhibitory proteins called lipocortins. Lipocortins control the biosynthesis of potent mediators of inflammation (eg, prostaglandins, leukotrienes) through inhibition of their common precursor, arachidonic acid. Arachidonic acid is released from membrane phospholipids by phospholipase A_2.

PHARMACOKINETICS: Absorption: Absorbed through skin. Occlusive dressings ≤24 hrs, no effect. Occlusive dressings at 96 hrs, markedly enhances penetration. **Distribution:** Systemically administered corticosteroids appear in human breast milk.

CLOBEX RX
clobetasol propionate (Galderma)

THERAPEUTIC CLASS: Corticosteroid

INDICATIONS: (Lot) Relief of corticosteroid responsive dermatoses. Treatment of moderate to severe plaque psoriasis (<10% BSA). (Shampoo) Treatment of moderate to severe scalp psoriasis. (Spray) Treatment of moderate to severe plaque psoriasis affecting up to 20% BSA.

DOSAGE: *Adults:* ≥18 yrs: (Lot) Apply bid for up to 2 consecutive weeks. Psoriasis: Reassess after 2 weeks; may repeat for additional 2 weeks. Max:

50g/week or 50mL/week. (Shampoo) Apply thin film daily to dry scalp for up to 4 consecutive weeks. Leave in place for 15 mins before lathering and rinsing. (Spray) Spray on affected area(s) bid. Rub in gently and completely. Reassess after 2 weeks; may repeat for additional 2 weeks. Limit treatment to 4 weeks. Max: 50g/week.

HOW SUPPLIED: Lot: 0.05% [30mL, 59mL]; Shampoo: 0.05% [118mL]; Spray: 0.05% [2oz]

WARNINGS/PRECAUTIONS: Not for use on the face, groin, axillae, eyes, lips, or for the treatment of rosacea or perioral dermatitis. May produce reversible HPA axis suppression, manifestations of Cushing's syndrome, hyperglycemia, and glucosuria. D/C if irritation occurs. Use appropriate antifungal or antibacterial agent with dermatological infections.

ADVERSE REACTIONS: Burning/stinging, pruritus, folliculitis, skin dryness, skin atrophy, telangiectasia.

PREGNANCY: Category C, caution in nursing.

MECHANISM OF ACTION: Corticosteroid; MOA not fully established. Contains anti-inflammatory, antipruritic, and vasoconstrictive properties. Corticosteroids thought to act by induction of phospholipase A_2 inhibitory proteins, called lipocortins. Lipocortins control the biosynthesis of potent mediators of inflammation (eg, prostaglandins, leukotrienes) through inhibiting the release of their precursor, arachidonic acid. Arachidonic acid is released from membrane phospholipids by phospholipase A_2.

PHARMACOKINETICS: Absorption: Use of occlusive dressings ≥24 hrs, no change in drug penetration; use of occlusive dressings for up to 96 hrs, markedly increased drug penetration. **Distribution:** Systemically administered corticosteroids are found in breast milk. **Metabolism:** Liver **Elimination:** Kidneys, bile.

CLODERM   RX
clocortolone pivalate (Healthpoint)

THERAPEUTIC CLASS: Topical corticosteroid

INDICATIONS: Corticosteroid-responsive dermatoses.

DOSAGE: *Adults:* Apply tid. Use with occlusive dressing for management of psoriasis or recalcitrant conditions.
Pediatrics: Apply TID. Use with occlusive dressing for management of psoriasis or recalcitrant conditions.

HOW SUPPLIED: Cre: 0.1% [15g, 45g, 90g]

WARNINGS/PRECAUTIONS: May produce reversible HPA axis suppression, manifestations of Cushing's syndrome, hyperglycemia, glucosuria. Caution when applied to large surface areas or under occlusive dressings. Use appropriate antifungal or antibacterial agent with dermatological infections. D/C if infection is not adequately controlled or if irritation develops.

ADVERSE REACTIONS: Burning, itching, irritation, dryness, folliculitis, hypertrichosis, acneform eruptions, hypopigmentation, perioral/allergic contact dermatitis, secondary infection, skin atrophy.

PREGNANCY: Category C, caution in nursing.

MECHANISM OF ACTION: Topical corticosteroid; not established. Possesses anti-inflammatory, anti-pruritic, and vasoconstrictive actions.

PHARMACOKINETICS: Absorption: Percutaneous; occlusion, inflammation, and other skin diseases, increase absorption. **Distribution:** Bound to plasma protein to varying degrees. Systemically administered corticosteroids found in breast milk. **Metabolism:** Liver. **Elimination:** Kidney and bile.

CLOLAR   RX
clofarabine (Genzyme)

THERAPEUTIC CLASS: Antimetabolite

INDICATIONS: Treatment of pediatric patients 1-21 years old with relapsed or refractory acute lymphoblastic leukemia after at least two prior regimens.

DOSAGE: *Pediatrics:* 1-21 yrs: 52mg/m² IV over 2 hours daily for 5 consecutive days. Treatment cycles are repeated following recovery or return to baseline organ function, approximately 2-6 weeks. Continuous IV fluids throughout 5 days of clofarabine therapy is recommended. The use of prophylactic steroids (eg, 100mg/m² hydrocortisone on Days 1-3) may be of benefit in preventing signs and symptoms of systemic inflammatory response syndrome (SIRS) or capillary leak. If patient develops signs and symptoms of SIRS or capillary leak, clofarabine therapy should be discontinued and appropriate supportive measures should be provided. Close monitoring of renal and hepatic function is required. If substantial increases in creatine or bilirubin occur, clofarabine therapy should be discontinued.

HOW SUPPLIED: Inj: 1mg/mL

WARNINGS/PRECAUTIONS: Suppression of bone marrow function should be anticipated. Increased risk of infection, including severe sepsis is possible. Monitor for signs and symptoms of tumor lysis syndrome, as well as cytokine release that could develop into SIRS/capillary leak syndrome and organ dysfunction. D/C immediately if SIRS or capillary leak syndrome develop. Severe bone marrow suppression, including neutropenia, anemia and thrombocytopenia have been observed. Dehydration may occur due to vomiting and diarrhea. Clofarabine should be discontinued if patient develops hypotension for any reason during the 5 days of administration. Since clofarabine is excreted primarily by the kidneys, drugs with known renal toxicity should be avoided during the 5 days of administration. Since the liver is a known target of clofarabine, concomitant use of medications known to induce hepatic toxicity should also be avoided. Patients taking medications known to affect BP or cardiac function should be closely monitored during administration.

ADVERSE REACTIONS: Vomiting, nausea, diarrhea, anemia, leukopenia, thrombocytopenia, neutropenia, febrile neutropenia, and infection.

PREGNANCY: Category D, not for use in nursing.

MECHANISM OF ACTION: Antimetabolite; inhibits DNA synthesis by decreasing cellular deoxynucleotide triphosphate pools through an inhibitory action on ribonucleotide reductase, and by terminating DNA chain elongation and inhibiting repair through incorporation into DNA chain by competitive inhibition of DNA polymerases.

PHARMACOKINETICS: Distribution: V_d=172L/m²; plasma protein binding (47%). **Elimination:** Urine (unchanged); $T_{1/2}$=5.2 hrs.

CLOMID   RX
clomiphene citrate (Sanofi-Aventis)

THERAPEUTIC CLASS: Ovulatory stimulant

INDICATIONS: Treatment of ovulatory dysfunction in women desiring pregnancy.

DOSAGE: *Adults:* Initial: 50mg/day for 5 days. Start any time if no recent uterine bleeding. If progestin-induced bleeding is intended, or if spontaneous uterine bleeding occurs, start on the 5th day of the cycle. If ovulation does not occur, increase to 100mg qd for 5 days, 30 days after the 1st course. Max: 100mg qd for 5 days and 3 courses of therapy.

HOW SUPPLIED: Tab: 50mg* *scored

CONTRAINDICATIONS: Pregnancy, liver disease or history of liver dysfunction, abnormal uterine bleeding of undetermined origin, ovarian cysts or enlargement not due to polycystic ovarian syndrome, uncontrolled thyroid or adrenal dysfunction, organic intracranial lesion (eg, pituitary tumor).

WARNINGS/PRECAUTIONS: Increased incidence of visual symptoms with increasing total dose or therapy duration; d/c treatment and perform complete ophthalmological evaluation. Ovarian hyperstimulation syndrome reported; monitor for abdominal pain, nausea, vomiting, diarrhea, weight gain. Increased chance of multiple pregnancy. Perform pelvic exam before initiating therapy and before each course. Prolonged use may increase risk of border-line/invasive ovarian tumor.

ADVERSE REACTIONS: Ovarian enlargement, vasomotor flushes, nausea, vomiting, breast discomfort, abdominal-pelvic discomfort/distention/bloating, visual symptoms, headache, abnormal uterine bleeding.

PREGNANCY: Category X, caution in nursing.

MECHANISM OF ACTION: Ovulatory stimulant; acts to increase release of pituitary gonadotropins; initiates steroidogenesis and folliculogenesis, resulting in growth of ovarian follicle and increase in circulating levels of estradiol, thus culminating in a preovulatory gonadotropin surge and subsequent follicular rupture. Following ovulation, plasma progesterone and estradiol rise and fall as they would in normal ovulatory cycle.

PHARMACOKINETICS: Absorption: Readily absorbed. **Elimination:** Feces, urine.

CLORPRES   RX
clonidine HCL - chlorthalidone (Mylan Bertek)

THERAPEUTIC CLASS: Central alpha-agonist/monosulfamyl diuretic

INDICATIONS: Treatment of hypertension. Not for initial therapy.

DOSAGE: *Adults:* Determine dose by individual titration. 0.1mg clonidine-15mg chlorthalidone tab qd-bid. Max: 0.6mg clonidine-30mg chlorthalidone/day.

HOW SUPPLIED: Tab: (Clonidine-Chlorthalidone) 0.1mg-15mg*, 0.2mg-15mg*, 0.3mg-15mg* *scored

CONTRAINDICATIONS: Anuria, sulfonamide hypersensitivity.

WARNINGS/PRECAUTIONS: Caution with severe renal disease, hepatic dysfunction, asthma, severe coronary insufficiency, recent MI, cerebrovascular disease. May develop allergic reaction to oral clonidine if sensitive to clonidine patch. Avoid abrupt withdrawal. Continue therapy to within 4 hrs of surgery and resume after. Monitor for fluid/electrolyte imbalance. Hyperuricemia, hypokalemia, hyponatremia, hypochloremic alkalosis, and hyperglycemia may occur.

ADVERSE REACTIONS: Drowsiness, dizziness, constipation, sedation, nausea, vomiting, blood dyscrasias, hypersensitivity reactions, orthostatic symptoms, impotence.

INTERACTIONS: Potentiates other antihypertensives. May increase response to tubocurarine. May decrease arterial response to norepinephrine. Antidiabetic agents may need adjustment. Risk of lithium toxicity. TCAs may reduce effects of clonidine. Amitriptyline may enhance ocular toxicity. Enhanced CNS-depressive effects of alcohol, barbiturates or other sedatives. Orthostatic hypotension aggravated by alcohol, barbiturates, narcotics.

PREGNANCY: (Clonidine) Category C, caution in nursing. (Chlorthalidone) Category B, not for use in nursing.

MECHANISM OF ACTION: Clonidine: Imidazoline derivative; stimulates α-adrenoceptor in brain stem, resulting in reduced sympathetic outflow from CNS and decrease in peripheral resistance, renal vascular resistance, heart rate, and BP. Chlorthalidone: Monosulfamyl diuretic; increases excretion of sodium and chloride; decreases extracellular fluid volume, plasma volume, cardiac output, total exchangeable sodium, glomerular filtration rate, and renal plasma flow.

PHARMACOKINETICS: Absorption: Clonidine: T_{max}=3-5 hrs. **Distribution:** Chlorthalidone: Plasma protein binding (75%). **Metabolism:** Clonidine: Liver. **Elimination:** Clonidine: Urine (40-60%); $T_{1/2}$=12-16 hrs. Chlorthalidone: urine; $T_{1/2}$=40-60 hrs.

CLOTRIMAZOLE TOPICAL   RX
clotrimazole (Various)

THERAPEUTIC CLASS: Azole antifungal

INDICATIONS: Topical treatment of candidiasis caused by *Candida albicans* and tinea versicolor caused by *Malassezia furfur*.

DOSAGE: *Adults:* Apply bid (am and pm). Re-evaluate if no improvement after 4 weeks.
Pediatrics: Apply bid (am and pm). Re-evaluate if no improvement after 4 weeks.

HOW SUPPLIED: Cre: 1% [15g, 30g]; Sol: 1% [10mL]

WARNINGS/PRECAUTIONS: D/C if irritation or sensitivity occurs. Not for ophthalmic use.

ADVERSE REACTIONS: Erythema, stinging, blistering, peeling, edema, pruritus, urticaria, burning, irritation.

PREGNANCY: Category B, caution in nursing.

MECHANISM OF ACTION: Broad spectrum antifungal agent; primary action is against dividing and growing organisms. Causes leakage of intracellular phosphorus compounds into the ambient medium with concomitant breakdown of cellular nucleic acids and accelerated potassium efflux.

PHARMACOKINETICS: Absorption: Minimally absorbed. **Elimination:** Urine (≤0.5%).

CLOZAPINE   RX
clozapine (Various)

> Risk of agranulocytosis, seizures, myocarditis, and other cardiovascular and respiratory effects. Conduct baseline WBC and differential before therapy, then regularly, and 4 weeks after discontinuation. Elderly patients with dementia-related psychosis treated with atypical antipsychotic drugs are at an increased risk of death; most appeared to be cardiovascular (eg, heart failure, sudden death) or infectious (eg, pneumonia) in nature. Clozapine is not approved for the treatment of patients with dementia-related psychosis.

OTHER BRAND NAMES: Clozaril (Novartis)

THERAPEUTIC CLASS: Dibenzapine derivative

INDICATIONS: Management of severe schizophrenia when response to standard schizophrenia treatment fails. To reduce the risk of recurrent suicidal behavior with schizophrenia or schizoaffective disorder.

DOSAGE: *Adults:* Initial: 12.5mg qd-bid. Titrate: Increase by 25-50mg/day, up to 300-450mg/day by end of 2nd week, then increase weekly or bi-weekly by up to 100mg. Usual: 100-900mg/day given tid. Max: 900mg/day. If at risk of suicidal behavior then treat for at least 2 yrs then assess; reassess thereafter at regular intervals. To d/c, gradually reduce dose over 1-2 weeks. Monitor for psychotic symptoms if abrupt discontinuation warranted (eg, leukopenia).

HOW SUPPLIED: Tab: (Clozapine) 12.5mg, 25mg, 100mg; (Clozaril) 25mg*, 100mg* *scored

CONTRAINDICATIONS: Myeloproliferative disorders, uncontrolled epilepsy, paralytic ileus, history of clozapine induced agranulocytosis or severe granulocytopenia, severe CNS depression, coma, with agents with potential to cause agranulocytosis or suppress bone marrow function.

WARNINGS/PRECAUTIONS: Reserve treatment for severely ill patients unresponsive to other schizophrenia therapies. Monitor for hyperglycemia, worsening of glucose control with DM, FBG levels with diabetes risk. Significant risk of orthostatic hypotension, and tachycardia. May impair alertness with initial doses. May cause high fever, hyperglycemia, or pulmonary embolism. Cardiomyopathy reported; d/c unless benefit outweighs risk. Caution with prostatic enlargement, narrow angle glaucoma, and renal, hepatic, or cardiac/pulmonary disease. NMS and tardive dyskinesia reported. Acquire WBC and

ANC at baseline, then weekly for 1st 6 months of therapy, then every 2 weeks for 6 months, and then every 4 weeks thereafter if WBCs and ANC are acceptable. Avoid initiation of treatment if WBCs <3500/mm³, ANC <2000/mm³, history of myeloproliferative disorder, previous clozapine-induced agranulocytosis or granulocytopenia. D/C treatment if WBCs <3000/mm³, ANC <1500/mm³, eosinophils >4000/mm³, or if myocarditis develops. D/C over 1-2 weeks. Varying degrees of intestinal peristalsis impairment (eg, constipation, intestinal obstruction, paralytic ileus), ECG changes reported.

ADVERSE REACTIONS: Drowsiness, vertigo, headache, tremor, salivation, sweating, dry mouth, visual disturbances, tachycardia, hypotension, syncope, constipation, nausea, blood dyscrasias, fever.

INTERACTIONS: See Contraindications. Avoid with bone-marrow suppressants, epinephrine, and carbamazepine. Caution with CNS-active drugs, anesthesia, alcohol, paroxetine, sertraline, fluvoxamine, benzodiazepines, other psychotropics, inhibitors/inducers of CYP1A2, 2D6, 3A4. Potentiates hypotensive effects of antihypertensives and anticholinergic effects of atropine-type drugs. Decrease dose with drugs metabolized by CYP2D6. Caution with general anesthesia. CYP450 inducers (eg, phenytoin, nicotine, rifampin) decrease plasma levels. CYP450 inhibitors (eg, cimetidine, caffeine, erythromycin, citalopram) increase plasma levels.

PREGNANCY: Category B, not for use in nursing.

MECHANISM OF ACTION: Atypical antipsychotic agent: interferes with binding of dopamine at D_1, D_2, D_3, and D_5 receptors. Has high affinity for D_4 receptor. Also acts as antagonist at adrenergic, cholinergic, histaminergic, and serotonergic receptors.

PHARMACOKINETICS: Absorption: C_{max}=319ng/mL; T_{max}=2.5 hrs. **Distribution:** Plasma protein binding (97%). **Elimination:** $T_{1/2}$=8 hrs (after single dose), $T_{1/2}$=12 hrs (after multiple doses); urine (50%), feces (30%).

COGNEX RX
tacrine HCL (Sciele)

THERAPEUTIC CLASS: Reversible cholinesterase inhibitor

INDICATIONS: Treatment of mild to moderate dementia of the Alzheimer's type.

DOSAGE: *Adults:* Initial: 10mg qid. Titrate: Increase to 20mg qid after 4 weeks, then increase at 4-week intervals to 30mg qid then to 40mg qid. ALT/SGPT: >3 to ≤5x ULN: Reduce dose by 40mg/day and resume dose titration when levels are normal. >5x ULN: Stop therapy and monitor; may rechallenge when ALT/SGPT levels are normal. D/C and do not rechallenge if jaundice and/or signs of hypersensitivity. Rechallenge: 10mg qid, may titrate if normal ALT/SGPT after 6 weeks. Monitor weekly for 16 weeks, then monthly for 2 months, and every 3 months thereafter. Take between meals.

HOW SUPPLIED: Cap: 10mg, 20mg, 30mg, 40mg

CONTRAINDICATIONS: Hypersensitivity to acridine derivatives, history of tacrine-associated jaundice (bilirubin >3mg/dL) or signs of hypersensitivity associated with ALT/SGPT elevations.

WARNINGS/PRECAUTIONS: Vagotonic effects; caution with conduction abnormalities, bradyarrhythmia, sick sinus syndrome. May increase risk of developing ulcers. Monitor LFTs every other week from weeks 4-16 from start of therapy, then every 3 months. Modify LFT monitoring based on LFTs (see dosage). Higher incidence of LFTs elevation in females. May cause seizures, bladder outflow obstruction, neutrophil abnormalities. May worsen cognitive function with abrupt withdrawal. Caution with liver disease, ulcers, asthma. D/C with clinical jaundice or hypersensitivity with ALT/SGPT elevations.

ADVERSE REACTIONS: Elevated LFTs, nausea, vomiting, diarrhea, dyspepsia, myalgia, anorexia, ataxia, dizziness.

INTERACTIONS: May potentiate succinylcholine, cholinesterase inhibitors, cholinergic agonists, and theophylline. May interact with drugs metabolized by CYP450. Fluvoxamine increases levels. May antagonize anticholinergics. Monitor for GI disease with NSAIDs. Increased levels with cimetidine.

PREGNANCY: Category C, caution in nursing.

MECHANISM OF ACTION: Reversible cholinesterase inhibitor: Suspected to increase acetylcholine concentration through inhibition of its hydrolysis by cholinesterase.

PHARMACOKINETICS: Absorption: Rapid. Absolute bioavailability (17%). T_{max}=1-2 hrs. **Distribution:** mean V_d=349L. Plasma protein binding (55%). **Metabolism:** Liver (glucuronidation) via CYP450. **Elimination:** $T_{1/2}$=2-4 hrs.

COLACE   OTC
docusate sodium (Purdue Products)

THERAPEUTIC CLASS: Stool softener

INDICATIONS: (PO) Stool softener for constipation, painful anorectal conditions and in cardiac conditions.

DOSAGE: *Adults:* 50-200mg/day. (Retention or Flushing Enema) Add 5-10mL of liquid to enema fluid. Mix Liq/Syr into 6-8 oz of milk or juice.
Pediatrics: ≥12 yrs: 50-200mg/day. 6-12 yrs: 40-120mg/day Liq. 3-6 yrs: 2mL Liq tid. Mix Liq/Syr into 6-8 oz of milk, juice or formula. (Retention/Flushing Enema) Add 5-10mL of liquid to enema fluid.

HOW SUPPLIED: Cap: 50mg, 100mg; Liq: 10mg/mL; Syrup: 20mg/5mL

WARNINGS/PRECAUTIONS: Avoid with abdominal pain, nausea, or vomiting. D/C enema if rectal bleeding occurs or fail to have a bowel movement.

ADVERSE REACTIONS: Bitter taste, throat irritation, nausea, rash.

PREGNANCY: Safety in pregnancy and nursing not known.

COLAZAL   RX
balsalazide disodium (Salix)

THERAPEUTIC CLASS: Anti-inflammatory Agent

INDICATIONS: Treatment of mild-to-moderate active ulcerative colitis in patients ≥5 yrs.

DOSAGE: *Adults:* 3 caps tid for up to 8 weeks (or 12 weeks if needed). May open cap and sprinkle on applesauce.
Pediatrics: 5-17 yrs: 1 or 3 caps tid for 8 weeks. May open cap and sprinkle on applesauce.

HOW SUPPLIED: Cap: 750mg

CONTRAINDICATIONS: Hypersensitivity to salicylates.

WARNINGS/PRECAUTIONS: May exacerbate symptoms of colitis. Prolonged gastric retention with pyloric stenosis. Caution with renal dysfunction or history of renal disease.

ADVERSE REACTIONS: Headache, abdominal pain, diarrhea, nausea, vomiting, respiratory problems, arthralgia, rhinitis, insomnia, fatigue, rectal bleeding, flatulence, fever, dyspepsia.

INTERACTIONS: Oral antibiotics may interfere with the release of mesalamine in the colon.

PREGNANCY: Category B, caution in nursing.

MECHANISM OF ACTION: Not established; a prodrug enzymatically cleaved in colon to produce mesalamine (5-ASA), an anti-inflammatory drug that acts locally to block production of arachidonic acid metabolites in the colon.

PHARMACOKINETICS: Absorption: Different dosing conditions (fasted, fed, sprinkled) resulted in variable parameters. **Distribution:** Plasma protein binding (≥99%). **Metabolism:** Key metabolites: 5-ASA and N-acetyl-5-ASA. **Elimination:** Urine, feces.

COLCHICINE
colchicine (Various)

RX

THERAPEUTIC CLASS: Miscellaneous gout agent

INDICATIONS: Treatment and prophylaxis of acute gouty arthritis.

DOSAGE: *Adults:* Acute Treatment: Initial: 1-1.2mg, followed by 0.5-0.6mg q1h, or 1-1.2mg q2h or 0.5-0.6mg q2-3h until pain relief, GI discomfort or diarrhea ensues. Usual: 4-8mg/attack. Wait 3 days before retreatment. Prophylaxis: <1 attack/yr: 0.5-0.6mg/day given 3-4x/week. >1 attack/yr: 0.5-0.6mg qd. Severe Cases: 2-3 tabs of 0.5mg or 0.6mg daily. Surgical Gout Prophylaxis: 0.5-0.6mg tid 3 days before and 3 days after surgery.

HOW SUPPLIED: Tab: 0.5mg, 0.6mg

CONTRAINDICATIONS: Serious GI, renal, hepatic or cardiac disorders, and blood dyscrasias.

WARNINGS/PRECAUTIONS: Caution in elderly, debilitated, or with GI, renal, hepatic, cardiac and hematologic disorders. D/C if nausea, vomiting, or diarrhea occurs. Monitor blood counts periodically with long-term therapy. May adversely affect spermatogenesis. Elevates SGOT and alkaline phosphatase. May cause false (+) for urine RBC and Hgb.

ADVERSE REACTIONS: Bone marrow depression, peripheral neuritis, purpura, myopathy, alopecia, dermatoses, reversible azoospermia, nausea, vomiting, diarrhea.

INTERACTIONS: Inhibited by acidifying agents. Potentiated by alkalinizing agents. Potentiates sympathomimetics and CNS depressants.

PREGNANCY: Category C, caution in nursing.

MECHANISM OF ACTION: Colchicum alkaloid; MOA not established, but involves reduction in lactic acid production by leukocytes, resulting in a decrease in uric acid deposition and reduction in phagocytosis, abating inflammatory response.

PHARMACOKINETICS: Absorption: Rapid. **Elimination:** Biliary and renal excretion.

COLCHICINE/PROBENECID
probenecid - colchicine (Various)

RX

THERAPEUTIC CLASS: Uricosuric

INDICATIONS: Chronic gouty arthritis complicated by frequent, recurrent acute gout attacks.

DOSAGE: *Adults:* Initial: 1 tab qd for 1 week, then 1 tab bid. Titrate: May increase by 1 tab/day every 4 weeks. Max: 4 tabs/day. May reduce dose by 1 tab every 6 months if acute attacks have been absent ≥6 months. Decrease dose with gastric intolerance. Renal Impairment: May need to increase dose. May not be effective if CrCl ≤30mL/min.

HOW SUPPLIED: Tab: (Colchicine-Probenecid) 0.5mg-500mg

CONTRAINDICATIONS: Blood dyscrasias, uric acid kidney stones, children <2 yrs and pregnancy. Do not use in acute gout attack.

WARNINGS/PRECAUTIONS: Exacerbation of gout may occur. Use APAP if analgesic needed. Severe allergic reaction and anaphylaxis reported (rare). D/C if hypersensitivity occurs. Caution with peptic ulcer. Monitor for glycosuria. Determine benefit/risk ratio with long-term therapy. Maintain liberal fluid intake and alkalization of urine.

ADVERSE REACTIONS: Headache, dizziness, hepatic necrosis, vomiting, nausea, anorexia, sore gums, uric acid stones, renal colic, anaphylaxis, fever, pruritus, blood dyscrasias, peripheral neuritis, muscular weakness, abdominal pain, diarrhea, alopecia, dermatitis.

INTERACTIONS: Probenecid increases plasma levels of penicillin and other β-lactams; psychic disturbances reported. Salicylates and pyrazinamide antagonize uricosuric effects. Increased plasma levels of methotrexate, sulfonamides, sulfonylureas, thiopental or ketamine-induced anesthesia, some NSAIDs (eg, indomethacin, naproxen), lorazepam, APAP, and rifampin. Possible false high plasma levels of theophylline.

PREGNANCY: Contraindicated in pregnancy; safety in nursing not known.

MECHANISM OF ACTION: Probenecid: Uricosuric/renal tubular blocking agent; inhibits tubular reabsorption of urate, increasing urinary excretion of uric acid and decreasing serum urate levels. Colchicine: Colchicum alkaloid; not been established, has prophylactic, suppressive effect helping to reduce incidence of acute attacks and relieve residual pain and mild discomfort.

COLESTID   RX
colestipol HCL (Pharmacia & Upjohn)

THERAPEUTIC CLASS: Bile acid sequestrant

INDICATIONS: Adjunct to diet, to reduce elevated serum total and LDL-C in primary hypercholesterolemia.

DOSAGE: *Adults:* Initial: 2g, 1 pkt or 1 scoopful qd-bid. Titrate: Increase by 2g qd or bid at 1-2 month intervals. Usual: 2-16g/day (tab) or 1-6 pkts or scoopfuls qd or in divided doses. Always mix granules with liquid. Swallow tabs whole with plenty of liquid.

HOW SUPPLIED: Granules: 5g/pkt [30^s 90^s], 5g/scoopful [300g, 500g]; Tab: 1g

WARNINGS/PRECAUTIONS: Exclude secondary causes of hypercholesterolemia and perform a lipid profile. May produce hyperchloremic acidosis with prolonged use. Monitor cholesterol and TG based on NCEP guidelines. May cause hypothyroidism. May interfere with normal fat absorption. Chronic use may produce or worsen constipation. Avoid constipation with symptomatic CAD. May increase bleeding tendency due to vitamin K deficiency.

ADVERSE REACTIONS: Constipation, musculoskeletal pain, headache, migraine headache, sinus headache.

INTERACTIONS: May interfere with absorption of folic acid, fat-soluble vitamins (eg, A, D, K), oral phosphate supplements, hydrocortisone. May delay or reduce absorption of concomitant oral medication; take other drugs 1 hr before or 4 hrs after colestipol. Reduces absorption of chlorothiazide, tetracycline, furosemide, penicillin G, hydrochlorothiazide, and gemfibrozil. Caution with digitalis agents, propranolol.

PREGNANCY: Safety in pregnancy not known, caution in nursing.

MECHANISM OF ACTION: Binds to bile acids in the intestine, forming a complex that is excreted in the feces, leading to increased fecal loss of bile acids and increased oxidation of cholesterol to bile acids, a decrease in β lipoprotein or LDL, and a decrease in serum cholesterol levels.

PHARMACOKINETICS: Elimination: Feces.

COLLYRIUM   OTC
sodium borate - sodium chloride - boric acid (Bausch & Lomb)

THERAPEUTIC CLASS: Eye wash

INDICATIONS: To cleanse the eye to help relieve irritation by removing loose foreign material, air pollutants or chlorinated water.

DOSAGE: *Adults:* Fill eye cup with sol and apply cup to affected eye. Press tightly to prevent escape of liquid and tilt head backwards. Open eyelids wide and rotate eyeball to ensure thorough bathing with the wash. If not using cup, flush affected eye prn, controlling rate of solution flow by pressure on bottle.

HOW SUPPLIED: Sol: [120mL]

WARNINGS/PRECAUTIONS: Do not touch container tip to any surface to avoid contamination. D/C if eye pain or vision changes occur, if redness or irritation continues, or if condition worsens or persists.

PREGNANCY: Safety in pregnancy or nursing not known.

COLOCORT
hydrocortisone (Paddock)

RX

THERAPEUTIC CLASS: Corticosteroid

INDICATIONS: Adjunct treatment of ulcerative colitis, ulcerative proctitis, and ulcerative proctosigmoiditis.

DOSAGE: *Adults:* 1 enema qhs for 21 days or until remission. After 21 days, decrease to every other night for 2-3 weeks. D/C if no clinical improvement after 2-3 weeks. Difficult cases may require 2-3 months of therapy. Retain for 1 hr minimum, preferably all night.

HOW SUPPLIED: Enema: 100mg/60mL

CONTRAINDICATIONS: Systemic fungal infections, ileocolostomy during the immediate or early postoperative.

WARNINGS/PRECAUTIONS: Rectal wall damage with improper insertion. May mask signs of infection and cause new infections; avoid exposure to chickenpox and measles. Prolonged use may cause adrenocortical insufficiency, cataracts, glaucoma, optic nerve damage, and may enhance secondary ocular infections. May cause elevated BP, salt and water retention, increased potassium and calcium excretion and reactivation of TB. Caution with perforation, abscess, obstruction, fistulas, sinus tracts, peptic ulcer, diverticulitis, renal impairment, HTN, osteoporosis, ocular herpes simplex, and myasthenia gravis. Enhanced effects in hypothyroidism and cirrhosis. May need increased dose in stressful situation. Do not vaccinate against smallpox or perform other immunization procedure; risk of neurological complications and lack of antibody response. Observe growth in pediatrics. Psychic derangement may appear; caution with emotional instability or psychotic tendencies.

ADVERSE REACTIONS: Local pain/burning/bleeding, fluid retention, HTN, muscle weakness, osteoporosis, peptic ulcer, abdominal distention, impaired wound healing, ecchymosis, facial erythema, sweating, menstrual disorders, Cushingoid state, decreased glucose tolerance.

INTERACTIONS: Caution with ASA in hypoprothrombinemia. Avoid vaccinations.

PREGNANCY: Safety in pregnancy and nursing is not known.

MECHANISM OF ACTION: Glucocorticoid; provides potent anti-inflammatory effect.

COLY-MYCIN M
colistimethate sodium (King)

RX

THERAPEUTIC CLASS: Antibacterial agent

INDICATIONS: Treatment of acute or chronic infections due to certain gram-negative bacilli (eg, *Pseudomonas aeruginosa, Enterobacter aerogenes, E. coli, Klebsiella pneumoniae*).

DOSAGE: *Adults:* Usual: 2.5-5mg/kg/day IV/IM in 2-4 divided doses. Max: 5mg/kg/day. SCr 1.3-1.5mg/dL: 2.5-3.8mg/kg/day IV/IM in 2 divided doses. SCr 1.6-2.5mg/dL: 2.5mg/kg/day IV/IM in 1-2 divided doses. SCr 2.6-4mg/dL: 1.5mg/kg/day IV/IM q36h. Obesity: Base dose on IBW.
Pediatrics: Usual: 2.5-5mg/kg/day IV/IM in 2-4 divided doses. Max: 5mg/kg/day. SCr 1.3-1.5mg/dL: 2.5-3.8mg/kg/day IV/IM in 2 divided doses. SCr 1.6-2.5mg/dL: 2.5mg/kg/day IV/IM in 1-2 divided doses. SCr 2.6-4mg/dL: 1.5mg/kg/day IV/IM q36h. Obesity: Base dose on IBW.

HOW SUPPLIED: Inj: 150mg

WARNINGS/PRECAUTIONS: Transient neurological disturbances may occur; dose reduction may alleviate symptoms. Respiratory arrest reported after IM administration. Increased risk of apnea and neuromuscular blockade with renal impairment. Reversible dose-dependent nephrotoxicity reported. Pseudomembranous colitis reported. May permit overgrowth of clostridia. Use extreme caution with renal impairment; d/c with further impairment.

ADVERSE REACTIONS: GI upset, tingling of extremities and tongue, slurred speech, dizziness, vertigo, paresthesia, itching, urticaria, rash, fever, increased BUN and creatinine, decreased creatinine clearance, respiratory distress, apnea, nephrotoxicity, decreased urine output.

INTERACTIONS: Avoid certain antibiotics (eg, aminoglycosides, polymyxin); may interfere with nerve transmission at neuromuscular junction. Extreme caution with curariform muscle relaxants (eg, tubocurarine), succinylcholine, gallamine, decamethonium and sodium citrate; may potentiate neuromuscular blocking effect. Avoid sodium cephalothin; may enhance nephrotoxicity.

PREGNANCY: Category C, caution in nursing.

MECHANISM OF ACTION: Antibacterial agent; penetrates into and disrupts the bacterial cell membrane.

PHARMACOKINETICS: Elimination: $T_{1/2}$=2-3 hrs.

COLYTE   RX

polyethylene glycol 3350 - sodium bicarbonate - potassium chloride - sodium chloride - sodium sulfate (Schwarz)

OTHER BRAND NAMES: Colyte w/ Flavor Packs (Schwarz) - Colyte-Flavored (Schwarz)

THERAPEUTIC CLASS: Bowel cleanser

INDICATIONS: Bowel cleansing prior to colonoscopy or barium enema X-ray.

DOSAGE: *Adults:* Oral: 240mL every 10 min until fecal discharge is clear. NG-Tube: 20-30mL/min (1.2-1.8L/hr). Patient should fast at least 3 hrs before administration, except for clear liquids.

HOW SUPPLIED: Sol: (Polyethylene Glycol-Potassium Chloride-Sodium Bicarbonate-Sodium Chloride-Sodium Sulfate) 60g-0.745g-1.68g-1.46g-5.68g/L [3754mL, 4000mL]

CONTRAINDICATIONS: Ileus, gastric retention, GI obstruction, bowel perforation, toxic colitis, toxic megacolon.

WARNINGS/PRECAUTIONS: Caution with severe ulcerative colitis. Monitor therapy with impaired gag reflex, semi- or unconsciousness, and risk of regurgitation or aspiration especially with NG tube.

ADVERSE REACTIONS: Nausea, abdominal fullness/cramps, bloating, anal irritation, vomiting.

INTERACTIONS: Medications taken within 1 hr of start of administration may not be absorbed.

PREGNANCY: Category C, safety in nursing is unkown.

MECHANISM OF ACTION: Osmotic laxative; cleanses the bowel by induction of diarrhea.

COMBIGAN   RX

timolol maleate - brimonidine tartrate (Allergan)

THERAPEUTIC CLASS: Alpha$_2$-agonist/beta-blocker

INDICATIONS: Reduction of elevated intraocular pressure (IOP) in patients with glaucoma or ocular hypertension who require adjunctive or replacement therapy due to inadequately controlled IOP.

DOSAGE: *Adults:* 1 drop in affected eye(s) bid approximately 12 hrs apart. Instill other topical ophthalmic products at least 5 min apart.

Pediatrics: ≥2 yrs: 1 drop in affected eye(s) bid approximately 12 hrs apart. Instill other topical ophthalmic products at least 5 min apart.

HOW SUPPLIED: Sol: (Brimonidine-Timolol) 2mg-5mg/mL

CONTRAINDICATIONS: Bronchial asthma, history of bronchial asthma, severe COPD, sinus bradycardia, second or third degree AV block, overt cardiac failure, cardiogenic shock.

WARNINGS/PRECAUTIONS: Systemic absorption, leading to adverse reactions (including severe respiratory reactions) may occur. Caution with cardiac failure; d/c if cardiac failure develops. Avoid with bronchospastic disease and/or mild-to-moderate COPD. May potentiate syndromes associated with vascular insufficiency; caution with depression, cerebral or coronary insufficiency, Raynaud's phenomenon, orthostatic hypotension, or thromboangiitis obliterans. May increase reactivity to allergens. May potentiate muscle weakness consistent with certain myasthenic symptoms. May mask signs/symptoms of acute hypoglycemia; caution in patients subject to spontaneous hypoglycemia or diabetic patients receiving insulin or hypoglycemic agents. May mask signs of hyperthyroidism. Bacterial keratitis reported with use of multuple dose containers of topical ophthalmic products. May need to gradually withdraw β-blocking agents in patients undergoing elective surgery.

ADVERSE REACTIONS: Allergic conjunctivitis, conjunctival folliculosis, conjunctival hyperemia, eye pruritus, ocular burning/stinging.

INTERACTIONS: May reduce BP; caution with antihypertensives and/or cardiac glycosides. Monitor with concomitant oral β-blockers; avoid concomitant use of 2 topical β-blocking agents. Caution with concomitant oral or IV calcium antagonists; avoid concomitant use with impaired cardiac function. Monitor closely with concomitant catecholamine-depleting drugs (eg, reserpine). Possibility of additive or potentiating effect with CNS depressants (eg, alcohol, barbiturates, opiates, sedatives, anesthetics). Concomitant use of β-blockers with digitalis and/or calcium antagonists may have additive effects in prolonging AV-conduction time. Potentiated systemic β-blockade reported with CYP2D6 inhibitors and timolol. Caution with TCAs and/or MAOIs.

PREGNANCY: Category C, not for use in nursing.

MECHANISM OF ACTION: Decreases elevated IOP. Brimonidine: Selective α-2 adrenergic receptor. Timolol: Non selective β-blocker.

PHARMACOKINETICS: Absorption: Brimonidine: C_{max}=30pg/mL; T_{max}= 1-4 hrs. Timolol: C_{max}=400pg/mL; T_{max}=1-3 hrs. **Distribution:** Timolol: Plasma protein binding (60%). **Metabolism:** Brimonidine: Liver (extensive). Timolol: Liver (partial). **Elimination:** Brimonidine: Urine (74%); $T_{1/2}$=3 hrs. Timolol: Excreted mainly by kidney; $T_{1/2}$=7 hrs.

COMBIPATCH RX
norethindrone acetate - estradiol (Novartis)

> Estrogens and progestins should not be used for prevention of cardiovascular disease or dementia. Increased risks of MI, stroke, invasive breast cancer, PE, and DVT in postmenopausal women (50-79 yrs of age) reported. Increased risk of developing probable dementia in postmenopausal women ≥65 yrs of age reported.

THERAPEUTIC CLASS: Estrogen/progestogen combination

INDICATIONS: In women with an intact uterus, for the treatment of moderate to severe vasomotor symptoms associated with menopause, vulvar/vaginal atrophy. Treatment of hypoestrogenism due to hypogonadism, castration, or primary ovarian failure.

DOSAGE: *Adults:* Continuous Combined Regimen: Apply 0.05mg/0.14mg patch on lower abdomen (avoid breasts and waistline). Apply twice weekly during 28-day cycle. Continuous Sequential Regimen: Wear estradiol-only patch for 1st 14 days of 28-day cycle, replace twice weekly. Apply 0.05mg/0.14mg patch for remaining 14 days, replace twice weekly. For both regimens, use 0.05mg/0.25mg patch if additional progestin required. Re-evaluate at 3-6 month intervals. Rotate sites; allow 1 week between same site.

HOW SUPPLIED: Patch: (Estradiol-Norethindrone) 0.05-0.14mg/day, 0.05-0.25mg/day [8[s], 24[s]]

CONTRAINDICATIONS: Undiagnosed abnormal genital bleeding, breast cancer, estrogen-dependent neoplasia, DVT, PE, arterial thromboembolic disorder (eg, stroke, MI), liver dysfunction or disease.

WARNINGS/PRECAUTIONS: May increase risk of cardiovascular events (eg, MI, stroke), venous thrombosis, and PE; d/c immediately if any of these events occur or are suspected. May increase risk of breast/endometrial cancer, and gallbladder disease. May lead to severe hypercalcemia with breast cancer and bone metastases; monitor and d/c if hypercalcemia occurs. Retinal vascular thrombosis reported; monitor and d/c if papilledema or retinal vascular lesions occur. May elevate BP; monitor at regular intervals. May cause elevations of plasma triglycerides with pre-existing hypertriglyceridemia. Caution with history of cholestatic jaundice associated with past estrogen use or with pregnancy; d/c with recurrence. May lead to increased thyroid-binding globulin levels; monitor thyroid function. May cause fluid retention; caution with cardiac/renal dysfunction. Caution with severe hypocalcemia. May increase risk of ovarian cancer. May exacerbate endometriosis, asthma, DM, epilepsy, migraine, porphyria, SLE, and hepatic hemangiomas; use with caution.

ADVERSE REACTIONS: Abdominal pain, back pain, asthenia, flu syndrome, application site reaction, nausea, nervousness, pharyngitis, respiratory disorder, breast pain, dysmenorrhea, menstrual disorder, vaginitis.

INTERACTIONS: CYP3A4 inducers (eg, St. John's wort, phenobarbital, carbamazepine, rifampin) may decrease levels which may decrease therapeutic effects and/or change uterine bleeding profile. CYP3A4 inhibitors (eg, erythromycin, clarithromycin, ketoconazole, itraconazole, ritonavir, grapefruit juice) may increase levels which may result in side effects.

PREGNANCY: Contraindicated in pregnancy, caution in nursing.

MECHANISM OF ACTION: Estrogen/progestogen. Estradiol: Acts by binding to nuclear receptors in estrogen-responsive tissues. Modulates pituitary secretion of gonadotropins, luteinizing hormone, and follicle stimulating hormone, through negative feedback mechanism.

PHARMACOKINETICS: Absorption: Estradiol: Well-absorbed. Administration of various doses led to altered parameters; Norethindrone: Well-absorbed. Administration of various doses led to altered parameters. **Distribution:** Estrogens and progestins found in breast milk. Estradiol: Largely bound to sex hormone binding globulin (SHBG) and albumin. Norethindrone: 90% to SHBG and albumin. **Metabolism:** Liver, to estrone (metabolite); estriol (major urinary metabolite); enterohepatic recirculation, via sulfate and glucuronide conjugation; biliary secretion of conjugates in the intestine; hydrolysis in gut; reabsorption; CYP 3A4 (partial). Norethindrone: Liver. **Elimination:** Estradiol, estrone, estriol: Urine; $T_{1/2}$=2-3 hrs. Norethindrone: $T_{1/2}$=6-8 hrs.

COMBIVENT RX
ipratropium bromide - albuterol sulfate (Boehringer Ingelheim)

THERAPEUTIC CLASS: Beta$_2$-agonist/anticholinergic

INDICATIONS: Adjunct therapy for bronchospasm in COPD if currently on a regular aerosol bronchodilator and require a second bronchodilator.

DOSAGE: *Adults:* 2 inh qid. Max: 12 inh/24 hrs.

HOW SUPPLIED: MDI: (Albuterol-Ipratropium) 0.09mg-0.018mg/inh [14.7g]

CONTRAINDICATIONS: History of hypersensitivity to soya lecithin or related food products (eg, soybeans, peanuts).

WARNINGS/PRECAUTIONS: Paradoxical bronchospasm reported. Hypersensitivity reactions reported. Caution with coronary insufficiency, arrhythmias, narrow-angle glaucoma, prostatic hypertrophy, bladder-neck obstruction, HTN, DM, hyperthyroidism, seizures, renal or hepatic dysfunction, and in those unusually responsive to sympathomimetic amines. May produce transient hypokalemia. Fatalities reported with excessive use.

C

ADVERSE REACTIONS: Headache, cough, respiratory disorders, pain, dyspnea, bronchitis.

INTERACTIONS: Potential additive interactions with other anticholinergic drugs. Increased risk of cardiovascular effects with other sympathomimetics. β-blockers and albuterol inhibit effects of each other. ECG changes and/or hypokalemia may occur with non-K⁺ sparing diuretics. Avoid MAOIs and TCAs.

PREGNANCY: Category C, not for use in nursing.

MECHANISM OF ACTION: Ipratropium: Anticholinergic bronchodilator; inhibits vagally mediated reflexes by antagonizing the action of acetylcholine. Albuterol: Selective β_2-adrenergic bronchodilator; activates β_2-receptors on airway smooth muscle, leading to activation of adenylyl cyclase and increase of intracellular cyclic AMP concentrations. This leads to activation of protein kinase A, which inhibits phosphorylation of myosin and lowers intracellular ionic calcium concentrations, resulting in relaxation.

PHARMACOKINETICS: Absorption: Ipratropium: Not readily absorbed. Albuterol: Rapid, complete; C_{max}=492pg/mL; T_{max}=3 hrs. **Distribution:** Ipratropium: Plasma protein binding (0-9%). **Metabolism:** Ipratropium: Partial; ester hydrolysis. Albuterol: Conjugation; albuterol 4'-O-sulfate (metabolite). **Elimination:** Ipratropiuim: Urine (50% unchanged); $T_{1/2}$=2 hrs. Albuterol: Urine (unchanged); $T_{1/2}$=3.9 hrs.

COMBIVIR   RX
zidovudine - lamivudine (GlaxoSmithKline)

> Zidovudine has been associated with hematologic toxicity (eg, granulocytopenia, severe anemia), especially with advanced HIV disease, and symptomatic myopathy reported with prolonged use. Lactic acidosis and severe, fatal hepatomegaly with steatosis reported with nucleoside analogues. Severe acute exacerbations of hepatitis B reported in patients coinfected with hepatitis B virus and HIV who discontinued lamivudine (a component of Combivir); monitor hepatic function closely after discontinuation.

THERAPEUTIC CLASS: Nucleoside analog combination

INDICATIONS: Treatment of HIV infection in combination with other antiretrovirals.

DOSAGE: *Adults:* 1 tab bid. Do not give if CrCl ≤50mL/min or with dose-limiting adverse events.
Pediatrics: ≥12 yrs: 1 tab bid. Do not give if CrCl ≤50mL/min or with dose-limiting adverse events.

HOW SUPPLIED: Tab: (Lamivudine-Zidovudine) 150mg-300mg

WARNINGS/PRECAUTIONS: Caution with granulocyte count <1000cells/mm³ or Hgb <9.5g/dL; monitor blood counts frequently with advanced HIV and periodically with asymptomatic or early HIV. Hepatic decompensation occured when used with interferon alfa w/ or w/o ribavirin. Avoid with CrCl ≤50mL/min, and hepatic impairment. Myopathy, myositis may occur. Posttreatment exacerbation of hepatitis reported. Lamivudine-resistant hepatitis B virus reported. Caution in elderly. Possible redistribution or accumulation of body fat. Immune reconstitution syndrome reported.

ADVERSE REACTIONS: Headache, malaise, fatigue, fever, chills, nausea, diarrhea, anorexia, abdominal pain/cramps, neuropathy, insomnia, dizziness, neutropenia, musculoskeletal pain, myalgia, rash, cough, aplastic anemia, gynecomastia, oral mucosal pigmentation.

INTERACTIONS: Ganciclovir, interferon-α, other bone marrow suppressives and cytotoxic agents may increase the hematologic toxicity of zidovudine. Increased lamivudine exposure with trimethoprim 160mg/sulfamethoxazole 800mg. Avoid with zalcitabine, stavudine, doxorubicin, ribavirin, zidovudine, lamivudine, and fixed-dose combinations of abacavir, lamivudine, and zidovudine.

PREGNANCY: Category C, not for use in nursing.

MECHANISM OF ACTION: Nucleoside analogue; inhibits reverse transcriptase via DNA chain termination.

PHARMACOKINETICS: Absorption: Lamivudine: Rapid. Absolute bioavail-abilty (86%). Zidovudine: Rapid. Absolute bioavialiabilty (64%). **Distribution:** Lamivudine: V_d=1.3L/kg; plasma protein binding (<36%). Zidovudine: V_d=1.6L/kg; plasma protein binding (<38%). **Metabolism:** Lamivudine: Trans-sulfoxide (metabolite). Zidovudine: Hepatic. 3'-azido-3'-deoxy-5'-O-β-D-glucopyranurosylthymidine (metabolite). **Elimination:** Lamivudine: Urine (70%, unchanged), $T_{1/2}$=5-7 hrs. Zidovudine: Urine (14-74%); $T_{1/2}$=0.5-3 hrs.

COMBUNOX
oxycodone HCL - ibuprofen (Forest)

CII

> NSAIDs may cause an increased risk of serious cardiovascular thrombotic events, MI, stroke and serious GI adverse events including bleeding, ulceration, and perforation of the stomach or intestines. Contraindicated for the treatment of perioperative pain in the setting of coronary artery bypass graft (CABG) surgery.

THERAPEUTIC CLASS: Opioid analgesic

INDICATIONS: Short term (<7 days) management of acute, moderate to severe pain.

DOSAGE: *Adults:* 1 tab/dose. Do not exceed 4 tabs/day and 7 days.

HOW SUPPLIED: Tab: (Oxycodone-Ibuprofen) 5mg-400mg

CONTRAINDICATIONS: Significant respiratory depression, acute or severe bronchial asthma, hypercarbia, paralytic ileus, or in patients who have experienced acute asthma, urticaria, allergic-type reactions after taking ASA or NSAIDs. Treatment of perioperative pain in the setting of CABG surgery.

WARNINGS/PRECAUTIONS: May cause drug dependence and tolerance; potential for abuse. Risk of dose-related respiratory depression. May cause severe hypotension. Can lead to HTN or worsening of pre-existing HTN. Fluid retention and edema reported. Capacity to elevate CSF pressure may be ex-aggerated with head injury, other intracranial lesions or pre-existing increase in ICP. May obscure diagnosis or clinical course with head injuries or acute abdominal conditions. Risk of GI ulceration, bleeding, and perforation. Risk of anaphylactoid reactions. NSAIDs can cause exfoliative dermatitis, Stevens-Johnson syndrome, and toxic epidermal necrolysis (TEN). Caution with severe hepatic impairment, pulmonary or renal dysfunction, hypothyroidism, Addison's disease, acute alcoholism, convulsive disorders, CNS depression or coma, delirium tremens, kyphoscoliosis associated with respiratory depression, toxic psychosis, prostatic hypertrophy, urethral stricture, biliary tract disease, anemia, pre-existing asthma, elderly or debilitated, aseptic meningitis.

ADVERSE REACTIONS: Nausea, vomiting, somnolence, dizziness, asthenia, fever, headache, vasodilation, constipation.

INTERACTIONS: (Oxycodone) Respiratory depression, hypotension and profound sedation with other CNS depressants (eg, narcotics, tranquilizers, sedatives, anesthetics, phenothiazines, alcohol). Concurrent use with anticho-linergics may produce paralytic ileus. Mixed agonist/antagonist analgesics may reduce the analgesic effect and/or cause withdrawal. Do not use with or within 14 days of discontinuing MAOIs. May enhance skeletal muscle relax-ant effects and increase respiratory depression. (Ibuprofen) May diminish antihypertensive effect of ACEIs. Use caution with anticoagulants, such as warfarin. May enhance methotrexate toxicity. May decrease natriuretic effect of furosemide and thiazides. Avoid with ASA. May decrease lithium clearance; monitor for toxicity.

PREGNANCY: Category C, caution in nursing.

MECHANISM OF ACTION: Oxycodone: Opioid analgesic; mechanism not fully established. Suspected to be related to binding to opiate receptors in the CNS. Also may produce sedation and respiratory depression. Ibuprofen: Nonsteroidal anti-inflammatory agent; mechanism not fully established. Possesses analgesic and antipyretic activity. Inhibits cyclooxygenase activity and prostaglandin synthesis, and is a peripherally acting analgesic.

PHARMACOKINETICS: Absorption: Oxycodone: Rapid; C_{max}=9.8-11.7ng/mL; T_{max}=1.3-2.1 hrs. Ibuprofen: Rapid; C_{max}=18.5-34.3mcg/mL; T_{max}=1.6-3.1

C

hrs. **Distribution:** Oxycodone: Plasma protein binding (45%). Ibuprofen: Plasma protein binding (99%). **Metabolism:** Oxycodone: Liver via CYP2D6 (N-demethylation, O-demethylation, 6-ketoreduction, glucuronidation); oxymorphone (active metabolite). Ibuprofen: Undergoes interconversion in plasma from R- to S-isomer: (+)-2-4'-(2-hydroxy-2-methyl-propyl) phenyl propionic acid, (+)-2-4'-(carboxypropyl) phenylpropionic acid (primary metabolites). **Elimination:** Oxycodone: Urine (4%, unchanged); $T_{1/2}$=3.1-3.7 hrs. Ibuprofen: Urine (≤0.2%, unchanged); $T_{1/2}$=1.8-2.6 hrs.

COMMIT   OTC
nicotine polacrilex (GlaxoSmithKline Consumer)

THERAPEUTIC CLASS: Nicotine

INDICATIONS: To reduce withdrawal symptoms associated with smoking cessation.

DOSAGE: *Adults:* Stop smoking completely before use. Use 4mg loz if time to 1st cigarette is within 30 min of waking. Use 2mg loz if your time to 1st cigarette is >30 min after waking. Weeks 1-6: 1 loz q1-2h. Weeks 7-9: 1 loz q2-4h. Weeks 10-12: 1 loz q4-8h. Use at least 9 loz/day for first 6 weeks. Max: 5 loz/6 hrs or 20 loz/day. Dissolve loz in mouth for 20-30 min (minimize swallowing) moving it from 1 side of mouth to the other; do not chew or swallow whole. Do not eat/drink for 15 min before or during use.

HOW SUPPLIED: Loz: 2mg, 4mg

WARNINGS/PRECAUTIONS: Do not use if continue to smoke, chew tobacco, use snuff, use a nicotine patch, or other nicotine products. Caution with heart disease, recent MI, irregular heartbeat, HTN, stomach ulcers or diabetes. May increase BP and HR. D/C with mouth problems, persistent indigestion, severe sore throat, palpitations, irregular heartbeat, or with symptoms of nicotine overdose (nausea, vomiting, dizziness, weakness, palpitations). Contains phenylalanine. Use 1 loz at a time. Do not continuously use one after another. Use under medical supervision if <18 yrs of age.

INTERACTIONS: Antidepressants and antiasthmatic agents may need adjustment.

PREGNANCY: Safety in pregnancy and nursing is not known.

COMTAN   RX
entacapone (Novartis)

THERAPEUTIC CLASS: COMT inhibitor

INDICATIONS: Adjunct to levodopa/carbidopa for treatment of idiopathic Parkinson's disease if experience signs of end-of-dose "wearing-off."

DOSAGE: *Adults:* 200mg with each levodopa/carbidopa dose. Max: 1600mg/day. Withdraw slowly for discontinuation.

HOW SUPPLIED: Tab: 200mg

WARNINGS/PRECAUTIONS: Hypotension/syncope, diarrhea, hallucinations, dyskinesia, rhabdomyolysis, hyperpyrexia, confusion, and fibrotic complications may occur due to increased dopaminergic activity. Caution with hepatic impairment, biliary obstruction. Avoid rapid withdrawal or abrupt dose reduction. May impair mental and/or motor performance.

ADVERSE REACTIONS: Sweating, back pain, dyskinesia, hyperkinesia, hypokinesia, nausea, diarrhea, abdominal pain, urine discoloration.

INTERACTIONS: Avoid non-selective MAOIs (eg, phenelzine, tranylcypromine). Caution with drugs metabolized by COMT (eg, isoproterenol, epinephrine, norepinephrine, dopamine, dobutamine, α-methyldopa, apomorphine, isoetherine, bitolterol); increased HR, arrhythmias, and BP changes may occur. Additive sedative effects with CNS depressants. Probenecid, cholestyramine, and some antibiotics (eg, erythromycin, rifamipicin, ampicillin, chloramphenicol) may interfere with biliary excretion.

PREGNANCY: Category C, caution with nursing.

MECHANISM OF ACTION: COMT inhibitor; selectively and reversibly inhibits catechol-O-methyltransferase, increasing levodopa levels.

PHARMACOKINETICS: Absorption: (PO) Rapid; absolute bioavailability (35%); C_{max}=1.2mcg/mL; T_{max}=1 hr. **Distribution:** Plasma protein binding (98%); V_d=20L. **Metabolism:** Isomerization to *cis*-isomer, and direct glucuronidation. **Elimination:** $T_{1/2}$=2.4 hrs (levodopa); urine 10% (0.2% unchanged), feces (90%).

COMVAX RX
hepatitis B (recombinant) - haemophilus B conjugate (Merck)

THERAPEUTIC CLASS: Vaccine

INDICATIONS: Vaccination against diseases caused by *Haemophilus influenza* type b and hepatitis B virus in infants born to HBsAg negative mothers.

DOSAGE: *Pediatrics:* ≥6 weeks: 0.5mL IM at 2, 4, and 12-15 months of age. If schedule cannot be followed, wait at least 6 weeks between 1st 2 doses. 2nd and 3rd dose should be close to 8-11 months apart.

HOW SUPPLIED: Inj: (Haemophilus B Conjugate Vaccine-Hepatitis B Recombinant Vaccine) 7.5mcg-5mcg-125mcg/0.5mL

WARNINGS/PRECAUTIONS: Possible suboptimal response with malignancy, immunosuppression, or immunocompromised patients. Delay vaccine in acute febrile illness. Have epinephrine injection (1:1000) available.

ADVERSE REACTIONS: Injection site pain, irritability, somnolence, anorexia, fever, seizures, febrile seizures.

INTERACTIONS: Immunosuppressive therapies may reduce effectiveness.

PREGNANCY: Category C, safety in nursing not known.

MECHANISM OF ACTION: Vaccine; elicits the formation of antibodies that may protect against *H.influenzae* type b and hepatitis B infections.

CONCERTA CII
methylphenidate HCL (McNeil Pediatrics)

THERAPEUTIC CLASS: Sympathomimetic amine

INDICATIONS: Treatment of attention deficit hyperactivity disorder (ADHD) in patients ≥6 yrs.

DOSAGE: *Adults:* Methylphenidate-Naive or Receiving Other Stimulant: Initial: 18mg qam. Titrate: Adjust dose at weekly intervals. Previous Methylphenidate Use: Initial: 18mg qam if previous dose 10-15mg/day; 36mg qam if previous dose 20-30mg/day; 54mg qam if previous dose 30-45mg/day. Initial conversion should not exceed 54mg/day. Titrate: Adjust dose at weekly intervals. Max: 72mg/day. Reduce dose or discontinue if paradoxical aggravation of symptoms occurs. Discontinue if no improvement after appropriate dosage adjustments over 1 month. Swallow whole with liquids. Do not crush, chew, or divide.
Pediatrics: ≥6 yrs: Methylphenidate-Naive or Receiving Other Stimulant: Initial: 18mg qam. Titrate: Adjust dose at weekly intervals. Max: 6-12 yrs: 54mg/day; 13-17 yrs: 72mg/day not to exceed 2mg/kg/day. Previous Methylphenidate Use: Initial: 18mg qam if previous dose 10-15mg/day; 36mg qam if previous dose 20-30mg/day; 54mg qam if previous dose 30-45mg/day. Initial conversion should not exceed 54mg/day. Titrate: Adjust dose at weekly intervals. Max: 72mg/day. Reduce dose or discontinue if paradoxical aggravation of symptoms occurs. Discontinue if no improvement after appropriate dosage adjustments over 1 month. Swallow whole with liquids. Do not crush, chew, or divide.

HOW SUPPLIED: Tab, Extended-Release: 18mg, 27mg, 36mg, 54mg

CONTRAINDICATIONS: Marked anxiety, tension, and agitation; glaucoma; motor tics or family history or diagnosis of Tourette's syndrome, during or within 14 days of MAOI use.

WARNINGS/PRECAUTIONS: Monitor growth during treatment in children. Not for severe depression or fatigue. May exacerbate symptoms of behavior disturbance and thought disorder in psychotic patients. Avoid with severe GI narrowing (eg, esophageal motility disorders, small bowel inflammatory disease, short-gut syndrome). May lower seizure threshold, especially in known EEG abnormalities. Caution with HTN, conditions affected by BP or HR elevation, history of drug abuse or alcoholism. Monitor during withdrawal from abusive use. Visual disturbances may occur (rare). Monitor CBC, differential, and platelets with prolonged use. Caution when using stimulants to treat patients with comorbid bipolar disorder because of concern for possible induction of mixed/manic episode in such patients. Stimulants at usual dose can cause treatment emergent psychotic or manic symptoms (eg, hallucinations, delusional thinking, mania) in children and adolescents without prior history of psychotic illness. Aggressive behavior or hostility reported in clinical trials and postmarketing experience of some medications indicated for the treatment of ADHD. Avoid with known structural cardiac abnormalities or other serious cardiac problems.

ADVERSE REACTIONS: Headache, abdominal pain, anorexia, insomnia, upper respiratory tract infection, vomiting, rhinitis, fever, cough, pharyngitis, sinusitis.

INTERACTIONS: Avoid MAOIs. Potentiates anticoagulants, anticonvulsants (eg, phenobarbital, phenytoin, primidone), TCAs, and SSRIs. Caution with α$_2$-agonists (eg, clonidine) and pressor agents.

PREGNANCY: Category C, caution in nursing.

MECHANISM OF ACTION: Sympathomimetic amine; blocks reuptake of norepinephrine and dopamine into presynaptic neuron and increases release of these monoamines into extraneuronal space.

PHARMACOKINETICS: Absorption: (PO) Readily absorbed; T_{max}=6-10 hrs. **Metabolism:** De-esterification; α-phenyl-piperidine acetic acid (metabolite). **Elimination:** Urine (90%); $T_{1/2}$=3.5 hrs.

CONDYLOX   RX
podofilox (Oclassen)

THERAPEUTIC CLASS: Antimitotic

INDICATIONS: (Gel) Topical treatment of external genital warts and perianal warts. (Sol) Topical treatment of external genital warts.

DOSAGE: *Adults:* Apply q12h for 3 days then discontinue for 4 days. May repeat for up to 4 treatment cycles. Max: 0.5g/day or 0.5mL/day and <10cm² of wart tissue.

HOW SUPPLIED: Gel: 0.5% [3.5g]; Sol: 0.5% [3.5mL]

WARNINGS/PRECAUTIONS: Confirm diagnosis before therapy. Avoid eyes. For cutaneous use only. Avoid use on the mucous membranes of genital area (eg, urethra, rectum, vagina).

ADVERSE REACTIONS: Inflammation, burning, erosion, pain, itching, bleeding.

PREGNANCY: Category C, not for use in nursing.

MECHANISM OF ACTION: Podofilox; an antimitotic agent; not established; necrosis of visible wart.

PHARMACOKINETICS: Absorption: Dose: (0.1-1.5mL); C_{max}=1-17ng/mL, T_{max}=1-2 hrs. **Elimination:** $T_{1/2}$=1-4.5 hrs.

COPAXONE   RX
glatiramer acetate (Teva Neuroscience)

THERAPEUTIC CLASS: Immunomodulatory agent

INDICATIONS: To reduce the frequency of relapses with relapsing-remitting multiple sclerosis.

DOSAGE: *Adults:* Usual: 20mg SQ qd.

HOW SUPPLIED: Inj: 20mg/mL

CONTRAINDICATIONS: Hypersensitivity to mannitol.

WARNINGS/PRECAUTIONS: Do not administer IV. May interfere with normal functioning of immune system. Rotate sites; do not use any site more than once a week. Administer first injection under professional supervision.

ADVERSE REACTIONS: Flushing, chest pain, palpitations, anxiety, dyspnea, constriction of throat, pruritus, rash, asthenia, back pain, infection, flu, nausea, arthralgia, injection site reactions.

PREGNANCY: Category B, caution in nursing.

MECHANISM OF ACTION: Immunomodulatory agent; not fully established. Thought to act by modifying immune processes that are currently responsible for the pathogenesis of MS.

COPEGUS   RX
ribavirin (Roche Labs)

> Not for monotherapy treatment of chronic hepatitis C. Primary toxicity is hemolytic anemia. Avoid with significant or unstable cardiac disease. Contraindicated in pregnancy and male partners of pregnant women. Use 2 forms of contraception during therapy and for 6 months after discontinuation.

THERAPEUTIC CLASS: Nucleoside analogue

INDICATIONS: Treatment of chronic hepatitis C, in combination with Pegasys®, in adults with compensated liver disease not previously treated with interferon alpha. Patients in whom efficacy was demonstrated included patients with compensated liver disease and histological evidence of cirrhosis (Child-Pugh class A) and patients with HIV disease that is clinically stable.

DOSAGE: *Adults:* HCV: Give bid in divided doses. Treat for 24-48 weeks with Pegasys 180mcg. Genotypes 1 and 4: <75kg: 1000mg/day for 48 weeks. ≥75kg: 1200mg/day for 48 weeks. Genotypes 2 and 3: 800mg/day for 24 weeks. HCV/HIV: 800mg qd. Treat for 48 weeks with Pegasys 180mcg. Dose Modifications: Reduce to 600mg/day if Hgb <10g/dL with no cardiac history, or if Hgb decreases by ≥2g/dL during a 4-week period with stable cardiac disease. D/C if Hgb <8.5g/dL with no cardiac history or if Hgb <12g/dL after 4 weeks of dose reduction with stable cardiac disease. After dose modification, may restart at 600mg/day, then may increase to 800mg/day. CrCl <50mL/min: Avoid use.

HOW SUPPLIED: Tab: 200mg

CONTRAINDICATIONS: Pregnancy, male partners of pregnant women, hemoglobinopathies (eg, thalassemia major, sickle cell anemia). Autoimmune hepatitis, and hepatic decompensation (Child-Pugh score greater than 6, Class B and C) in cirrhotic CHC patients, and in cirrhotic CHC patients coinfected with HIV before or during treatment when used in combination with Pegasys.

WARNINGS/PRECAUTIONS: D/C with hepatic decompensation, confirmed pancreatitis, and hypersensitivity reaction. Severe depression, suicidal ideation, hemolytic anemia, bone marrow suppression, autoimmune and infectious disorders, pancreatitis, and diabetes reported. Pulmonary symptoms reported; monitor closely with evidence of pulmonary infiltrates or pulmonary function impairment and d/c if appropriate. Assess for underlying cardiac disease (obtain EKG); fatal and nonfatal MI reported with anemia. Caution with cardiac disease, d/c if cardiovascular status deteriorates. Hemolytic anemia reported; monitor Hgb or Hct initially then at week 2 and 4 (or more if needed) of therapy. Suspend therapy if symptoms of pancreatitis arise. Avoid if CrCl <50mL/min. Obtain negative pregnancy test prior to initiation then monthly, and for 6 months post-therapy.

ADVERSE REACTIONS: Injection site reaction, fatigue/asthenia, pyrexia, rigors, nausea/vomiting, neutropenia, anorexia, myalgia, headache, irritability/anxiety/nervousness, insomnia, alopecia.

INTERACTIONS: Avoid concomitant use with didanosine and zidovudine. Hepatic decompensation can occur with concomitant use of NRTIs and Pegasys/Copegus.

PREGNANCY: Category X, not for use in nursing.

MECHANISM OF ACTION: Nucleotide analogue; unknown.

PHARMACOKINETICS: Absorption: AUC=25361ng•hr/mL; C_{max}=2748ng/mL; T_{max}=2 hrs. **Elimination:** $T_{1/2}$=120-170 hrs.

CORDARONE   RX
amiodarone HCL (Wyeth)

THERAPEUTIC CLASS: Class III antiarrhythmic

INDICATIONS: Treatment of documented, life-threatening recurrent ventricular fibrillation and recurrent hemodynamically unstable ventricular tachycardia.

DOSAGE: *Adults:* Give LD in hospital. LD: 800-1600mg/day in divided doses for 1-3 weeks. After control is achieved, then 600-800mg/day for 1 month. Maint: 400mg/day; up to 600mg/day if needed. Use lowest effective dose. Take with meals. Elderly: Start at low end of dosing range.

HOW SUPPLIED: Tab: 200mg* *scored

CONTRAINDICATIONS: Severe sinus-node dysfunction causing marked sinus bradycardia; 2nd- and 3rd-degree AV block; when episodes of bradycardia have caused syncope (except when used with a pacemaker); cardiogenic shock. Hypersensitivity to iodine.

WARNINGS/PRECAUTIONS: Only for life-threatening arrhythmias due to its substantial toxicity (eg, pulmonary toxicity including pulmonary alveolar hemorrhage, hepatic injury, arrhythmia exacerbation). Hospitalize when giving LD. May cause a clinical syndrome of cough and progressive dyspnea. D/C if LFTs are 3x ULN or if elevated baseline doubles; monitor LFTs regularly. Optic neuropathy, optic neuritis reported. Fetal harm in pregnancy. May develop reversible corneal micro deposits (eg, visual halos, blurred vision), photosensitivity, peripheral neuropathy (rare). May decrease T_3 levels, increase thyroxine levels, increase inactive reverse T_3 levels and can cause hypo- or hyperthyroidism. Hyperthyroidism may result in thyrotoxicosis and/or the possibility of arrhythmia breakthrough or aggravation. ARDS reported with surgery. Correct K^+ or magnesium deficiency before therapy. Caution in elderly.

ADVERSE REACTIONS: Pulmonary toxicity (eg, inflammation, fibrosis), arrhythmia exacerbation, hepatic injury, malaise, fatigue, tremor, poor coordination, paresthesis, nausea, vomiting, constipation, anorexia, ophthalmic abnormalities, photosensitivity, akinesia, bradykinesia.

INTERACTIONS: Risk of interactions after discontinuation due to its long half-life. May increase sensitivity to myocardial depressant and conduction effects of halogenated inhalation anesthetics. Elevates cyclosporine plasma levels. D/C or reduce digoxin dose by 50%. D/C or decrease warfarin dose by 1/3-1/2. Avoid grapefruit juice. Caution with β-blockers, CCBs, lidocaine, methotrexate. May increase levels of quinidine, procainamide, phenytoin, flecainide. Initiate added antiarrhythmic drug at lower than usual dose. D/C or decrease quinidine dose by 1/3-1/2. D/C or decrease procainamide dose by 1/3. Caution with loratadine, trazadone, disopyramide, fluoroquinolones, macrolides, azoles; QT prolongation reported. Decreased levels with cholestyramine, rifampin, phenytoin, St. John's wort. Rhabdomyolysis/myopathy reported with HMG-CoA reductase inhibitors (simvastatin and atorvastatin). Ineffective inhibition of platelet aggregation with clopidogrel. Fentanyl may cause hypotension, bradycardia, and decreased cardiac output. Increased levels with protease inhibitors; monitor for toxicity. Increased levels of CYP1A2, CYP2C9, CYP2D6, CYP3A4 substrates reported. Interactions reported with CYP3A4 inducers. CYP2C8 and CYP3A4 inhibitors may increase amiodarone levels.

PREGNANCY: Category D, not for use in nursing.

MECHANISM OF ACTION: Class III antiarrhythmic; prolongs myocardial cell-action potential duration and refractory period, and causes noncompetitive α- and β-adrenergic inhibition.

PHARMACOKINETICS: Absorption: Slow and variable; T_{max}=3-7 hrs. **Distribution:** V_d=60L/kg; plasma protein binding (96%); found in breast milk. **Metabolism:** CYP3A4, 2C8; desethylamiodarone (major metabolite). **Elimination:** Bile, urine; $T_{1/2}$=58 days, 36 days (metabolite).

CORDARONE IV   RX
amiodarone HCL (Wyeth)

THERAPEUTIC CLASS: Class III antiarrhythmic

INDICATIONS: Initiation of treatment and prophylaxis of frequently recurring ventricular fibrillation and hemodynamically unstable ventricular tachycardia refractory to other therapies.

DOSAGE: *Adults:* LD: 150mg over 1st 10 min (15mg/min), then 360mg over next 6 hrs (1mg/min), then 540mg over remaining 18 hrs (0.5mg/min). Maint: 0.5mg/min for 2-3 weeks. Breakthrough Ventricular Tachycardia/Ventricular Fibrillation: 150mg supplement IV over 10 min. Increase rate to achieve suppression. Elderly: Start at low end of dosing range. Administer infusions >2 hrs in a glass or polyolefin bottle containing D_5W. Amiodarone leaches out plasticizers (eg, DEHP from IV tubing) especially at higher infusion concentrations, and lower flow rates.

HOW SUPPLIED: Inj: 50mg/mL [3mL]

CONTRAINDICATIONS: Cardiogenic shock, marked sinus bradycardia, 2nd- or 3rd-degree AV block (unless a functioning pacemaker is available). Hypersensitivity to iodine.

WARNINGS/PRECAUTIONS: Bradycardia and AV block reported. Hypotension reported; do not exceed initial rate of infusion. Correct hypokalemia or hypomagnesemia before therapy to prevent exaggeration of QT_c prolongation. Congenital goiter/hypothyroidism, hyperthyroidism, post-operative ARDS reported with oral therapy. Hyperthyroidism may result in thyrotoxicosis and/or the possibility of arrhythmia breakthrough or aggravation. Elevations of hepatic enzymes reported. May worsen or precipitate a new arrhythmia; monitor for QT_c prolongation. Adult respiratory distress syndrome (ARDS) reported. Pulmonary toxicity with long-term use. Contains benzyl alcohol. Caution in elderly.

ADVERSE REACTIONS: Hypotension, fever, bradycardia, CHF, heart arrest, ventricular tachycardia, abnormal LFTs, nausea.

INTERACTIONS: Risk of interactions may persist after discontinuation due to long half-life. May increase PT with warfarin. May elevate plasma levels of cyclosporine, digoxin, quinidine, procainamide, phenytoin, disopyramide, HMG-CoA reductase inhibitors. May increase QT prolongation with disopyramide. Reduce flecainide dose to maintain therapeutic plasma levels. Cholestyramine may decrease levels and half-life. Decreased levels with phenytoin. Risk of bradycardia, hypotension with β-blockers, fentanyl. Increased risk of AV block with verapamil or diltiazem and hypotension with CCBs. May increase sensitivity to myocardial depressant and conduction defects of halogenated inhalational anesthetics. CYP3A4 inhibitors (eg, protease inhibitors, cimetidine, grapefruite juice) may increase levels. QT prolongation and torsade de pointes with H_1 antagonists (eg, loratadine) and antidepressants (eg, trazodone) reported. Concomitant use with clopidogrel may result in ineffective inhibition of platelet aggregation. CYP3A4 inducers (eg, rifampin, St. John's wort) may decrease levels. Concomitant use with fentanyl may cause hypotension, bradycardia, and decreased cardiac output. QT_c prolongation reported with fluoroquinolones, macrolides, and azoles. Concomitant administration with propranolol, diltiazem, and verapamil may result in hemodynamic and electrophysiologic interactions.

PREGNANCY: Category D, not for use in nursing.

MECHANISM OF ACTION: Class III antiarrhythmic; blocks sodium, calcium, and potassium channels, exerts noncompetitive antisympathetic action, and negative chronotropic and dromotropic effects; lengthens cardiac action potential, decreases cardiac workload and myocardial oxygen consumption.

PHARMACOKINETICS: Absorption: C_{max}=5-41mg/L. **Distribution:** Plasma protein binding (>96%). **Metabolism:** CYP3A4, 2C8; N-desethylamiodarone (major active metabolite). **Elimination:** Urine; bile; $T_{1/2}$=20-47 days.

CORDRAN   RX
flurandrenolide (Watson)

OTHER BRAND NAMES: Cordran SP (Watson)

THERAPEUTIC CLASS: Corticosteroid

INDICATIONS: Treatment of corticosteroid responsive dermatoses.

DOSAGE: *Adults:* (Cre, Lot) Apply qd-qid depending on severity. For moist lesions, apply cream bid-tid. Apply lotion bid-tid. (Tape) Clean and dry skin. Shave or clip hair. Apply tape q12-24h.
Pediatrics: (Cre, Lot) Apply qd-qid depending on severity. For moist lesions, apply cream bid-tid. Apply lotion bid-tid. (Tape) Clean and dry skin. Shave or clip hair. Apply tape q12-24h.

HOW SUPPLIED: Cre (SP): 0.05% [15g, 30g, 60g]; Lot: 0.05% [15mL, 60mL]; Tape: 4mcg/cm²

CONTRAINDICATIONS: (Tape) Not for lesions exuding serum or in intertriginous areas.

WARNINGS/PRECAUTIONS: Systemic absorption may produce reversible HPA axis suppression, manifestations of Cushing's syndrome, hyperglycemia, and glucosuria. Application of more potent steroids, use on large surfaces, prolonged use, or occlusive dressings may augment systemic absorption. Evaluate periodically for HPA suppression if large dose applied to large area or with occlusive dressings. Pediatrics are more susceptible to toxicity. D/C if irritation develops. May use occlusive dressing for psoriasis or recalcitrant conditions.

ADVERSE REACTIONS: Burning, itching, irritation, dryness, folliculitis, hypertrichosis, acneform eruptions, hypopigmentation, dermatitis. Occlusive dressing may cause skin maceration, secondary infection, skin atrophy, miliaria.

PREGNANCY: Category C, caution in nursing.

MECHANISM OF ACTION: Corticosteroid; possesses anti-inflammatory, antipruritic, and vasoconstrictive properties. Suspected to stabilize cellular and lysosomal membranes, thereby preventing release of proteolytic enzymes, and consequently reducing inflammation.

PHARMACOKINETICS: Absorption: Extent of percutaneous absorption depends on integrity of skin, vehicle, and use of occlusive dressings. **Distribution:** Plasma protein binding (variable). **Metabolism:** Liver. **Elimination:** Kidney (major), bile.

COREG CR   RX
carvedilol (GlaxoSmithKline)

OTHER BRAND NAMES: Coreg (GlaxoSmithKline)

THERAPEUTIC CLASS: Alpha₁/Beta-blocker

INDICATIONS: Treatment of mild to severe heart failure of ischemic or cardiomypathic origin; left ventricular dysfunction (LVD) following MI; essential hypertension.

DOSAGE: *Adults:* Individualize dose. Take with food. Monitor dose increases. Take extended-release capsules in am and swallow whole. CHF: Tab: Initial: 3.125mg bid for 2 weeks. Titrate: May double dose every 2 weeks as tolerated. Max: 50mg bid if >85kg. Reduce dose if HR <55 beats/min. Cap, Extended-Release: Initial: 10mg qd for 2 weeks. Titrate: May double dose every 2 weeks as tolerated. Max: 80mg/day. Reduce dose if HR <55 beats/min. HTN: Tab: Initial: 6.25mg bid for 7-14 days. Titrate: May double dose at 7-14 day intervals. Max: 50mg/day. Cap, Extended-Release: Initial: 20mg qd for 7-14 days. Titrate: May double dose every 7-14 days as tolerated. Max: 80mg/day. LVD Post-MI: Tab: Initial: 6.25mg bid for 3-10 days. Titrate: May double dose every 3-10 days to target of 25mg bid. May begin with 3.125mg bid and slow up-titration rate if clinically indicated. Cap, Extended-Release: Initial: 20mg qd for 3-10 days. Titrate: May double dose every 3-10 days to target of 80mg qd.

HOW SUPPLIED: Tab: 3.125mg, 6.25mg, 12.5mg, 25mg; Cap, Extended-Release: 10mg, 20mg, 40mg, 80mg

CONTRAINDICATIONS: Bronchial asthma or related bronchospastic conditions, 2nd- or 3rd-degree AV block, sick sinus syndrome, severe bradycardia (without permanent pacemaker), cardiogenic shock, decompensated heart failure requiring IV inotropic therapy, severe hepatic impairment.

WARNINGS/PRECAUTIONS: Avoid abrupt discontinuation; taper over 1-2 weeks. Hepatic injury reported; d/c and do not restart if develop hepatic injury. Hypotension and syncope reported, most commonly during up-titration period; avoid driving or hazardous tasks during initiation period. May mask hypoglycemia and hyperthyroidism. May potentiate insulin-induced hypoglycemia and delay recovery of serum glucose levels. Decrease dose if pulse <55 beats/min. Monitor renal function during uptitration with low BP (SBP <100mmHg), ischemic heart disease, diffuse vascular disease and/or renal insufficiency. Worsening heart failure or fluid retention may occur with uptitration. Caution in pheochromocytoma, peripheral vascular disease, major surgery with anesthesia, Prinzmetal's variant angina, and bronchospastic disease. Effectiveness of carvedilol in patients younger than 18 years of age has not been established.

ADVERSE REACTIONS: Bradycardia, fatigue, edema, hypotension, dizziness, headache, diarrhea, nausea, vomiting, hyperglycemia, weight increase, dyspnea, anemia, increased cough, arthralgia.

INTERACTIONS: CYP2D6 inhibitors (eg, quinidine, fluoxetine, paroxetine, and propafenone) may increase levels. Monitor for hypotension and bradycardia with catecholamine-depleting agents (eg, reserpine, MAOIs). Clonidine may potentiate BP and HR lowering effects. Rifampin may reduce plasma levels. Cimetidine may increase AUC. Monitor ECG and BP with CCBs (eg, verapamil, diltiazem). Monitor with insulin, oral hypoglycemics, cyclosporin, and digoxin. Caution with anesthetic agents which may depress myocardial function (eg, cyclopropane, trichloroethylene). Alcohol may affect release properties of extended release caps; separate administration by ≥2 hrs. Digitalis glycosides and β-blockers slow atrioventricular conduction and decrease heart rate. Concomitant use can increase the risk of bradycardia.

PREGNANCY: Category C, not for use in nursing.

MECHANISM OF ACTION: Nonselective β-adrenergic and α_1 blocker.

PHARMACOKINETICS: Absorption: Rapid; absolute bioavailability (25-35%). Cap: T_{max}=5 hrs. **Distribution:** Plasma protein binding (>98%); V_d=115L. **Metabolism**: Oxidation and glucuronidation; CYP2D6, 2C9 (primary); CYP3A4, 2C19, 1A2, 2E1 (minor). **Elimination**: Urine (<2% unchanged); $T_{1/2}$=7-10 hrs.

CORGARD   RX
nadolol (King)

THERAPEUTIC CLASS: Nonselective beta-blocker

INDICATIONS: Long-term management of angina pectoris. Treatment of hypertension.

DOSAGE: *Adults:* Angina Pectoris: Initial: 40mg qd. Titrate: Increase by 40-80mg every 3-7 days. Usual: 40-80mg qd. Max: 240mg/day. HTN: Initial: 40mg qd. Titrate: Increase by 40-80mg. Max: 320mg/day. CrCl 31-50mL/min: Dose q24-36h. CrCl 10-30mL/min: Dose q24-48h. CrCl <10mL/min: Dose q40-60h.

HOW SUPPLIED: Tab: 20mg*, 40mg*, 80mg*, 120mg*, 160mg* *scored

CONTRAINDICATIONS: Bronchial asthma, sinus bradycardia and >1st-degree conduction block, cardiogenic shock, overt cardiac failure.

WARNINGS/PRECAUTIONS: Caution in well-compensated cardiac failure, nonallergic bronchospasm, renal dysfunction. Exacerbation of ischemic heart disease with abrupt withdrawal. Withdrawal before surgery is controversial. May mask hyperthyroidism or hypoglycemia symptoms. Can cause cardiac failure.

ADVERSE REACTIONS: Bradycardia, peripheral vascular insufficiency, dizziness, fatigue.

INTERACTIONS: Additive hypotension and/or bradycardia with catecholamine-depleting drugs. Antidiabetic agents may need adjustment. General anesthetics may exaggerate hypotension. May block epinephrine effects.

PREGNANCY: Category C, not for use in nursing.

MECHANISM OF ACTION: Nonselective β-adrenergic receptor blocker; inhibits β_1 and β_2 receptors inhibiting chronotrophic, inotropic, and vasodilator responses to β-adrenergic stimulation.

PHARMACOKINETICS: Absorption: T_{max}=3-4 hrs. **Distribution:** Plasma protein binding (30%). **Elimination:** Kidney; $T_{1/2}$=20-40 hrs.

CORLOPAM   RX
fenoldopam mesylate (Hospira)

THERAPEUTIC CLASS: Dopamine D_1-like receptor agonist

INDICATIONS: (Adults) For short-term (up to 48 hrs), in-hospital management of severe hypertension when rapid, but quickly reversible, emergency reduction of BP is clinically indicated, including malignant hypertension with deteriorating end-organ function. (Pediatrics) For in-hospital, short-term (up to 4 hours) reduction in BP.

DOSAGE: *Adults:* Range: Initial: 0.01-0.8 mcg/kg/min IV. Titrate: Increase/decrease by 0.05-0.1mcg/kg/min no more frequently than every 15 min. May use for up to 48 hrs. Refer to PI for detailed dosing info.
Pediatrics: <1 month-12 years: Initial: 0.2mcg/kg/min. May increase dose every 20-30 min up to 0.3-0.5 mcg/kg/min. Refer to PI for detailed dosing info.

HOW SUPPLIED: Inj: 10mg/mL

WARNINGS/PRECAUTIONS: Contains sodium metabisulfite; may cause allergic-type reactions especially in asthmatics. Caution in glaucoma or intraocular HTN. Dose-related tachycardia reported. Symptomatic hypotension may occur; monitor BP. Avoid hypotension with acute cerebral infarction or hemorrhage. Hypokalemia reported; monitor serum electrolytes.

ADVERSE REACTIONS: Headache, nausea, flushing, extrasystoles, palpitations, bradycardia, heart failure, elevated BUN/glucose/transaminase, chest pain, leukocytosis, bleeding, dyspnea.

INTERACTIONS: Avoid β-blockers; unexpected hypotension may occur.

PREGNANCY: Category B, caution in nursing.

MECHANISM OF ACTION: Dopamine D_1-like receptor agonist; rapid-acting vasodilator.

PHARMACOKINETICS: Metabolism: Conjugation. **Elimination:** (Adults) Urine (4%), feces; $T_{1/2}$=5 min. (Pediatrics) $T_{1/2}$=3-5 min.

CORMAX
clobetasol propionate (Watson)

RX

OTHER BRAND NAMES: Cormax Scalp (Watson)

THERAPEUTIC CLASS: Corticosteroid

INDICATIONS: Corticosteroid-responsive dermatoses.

DOSAGE: *Adults:* Apply bid. Limit treatment to 2 consecutive weeks. Max: 50g/week or 50mL/week.
Pediatrics: ≥12 yrs: (Cre, Sol) Apply bid. Limit treatment to 2 consecutive weeks. Max: 50g/week or 50mL/week.

HOW SUPPLIED: Cre: 0.05% [15g, 30g, 45g]; Sol (Scalp): 0.05% [25mL, 50mL]

CONTRAINDICATIONS: Primary infections of the scalp with solution.

WARNINGS/PRECAUTIONS: Not for treatment of rosacea or perioral dermatitis. May produce reversible HPA axis suppression, manifestations of Cushing's syndrome, hyperglycemia, and glucosuria. Reassess diagnosis if no improvement after 2 weeks. D/C if irritation occurs. Pediatrics may be more susceptible to systemic toxicity. Use appropriate antifungal or antibacterial agent with dermatological infections. Avoid occlusive dressings.

ADVERSE REACTIONS: Burning, stinging, pruritus, skin atrophy, cracking/fissuring of skin, irritation, (sol) tingling, (sol) folliculitis.

PREGNANCY: Category C, caution in nursing.

MECHANISM OF ACTION: Corticosteroid; possesses anti-inflammatory, anti-pruritic, and vasoconstrictive properties. Suspected to stabilize cellular and lysosomal membranes, thereby preventing release of proteolytic enzymes, and consequently reducing inflammation.

PHARMACOKINETICS: Absorption: Extent of percutaneous absorption depends on integrity of skin, vehicle, and use of occlusive dressings. **Distribution:** Plasma protein binding (variable). **Metabolism:** Liver. **Elimination:** Kidney (major), bile.

CORTANE-B
pramoxine HCL - hydrocortisone - chloroxylenol (Blansett)

RX

OTHER BRAND NAMES: Zoto HC (Sciele)

THERAPEUTIC CLASS: Antimicrobial/Corticosteroid/Topical anesthetic

INDICATIONS: Treatment of superficial infections of the external ear and to control inflammation and itching.

DOSAGE: *Adults:* Instill 4-5 drops tid-qid. Gauze or wick may be inserted into ear canal after 1st administration. Add additional drops to saturate wick q4h. Remove wick after 24 hrs and continue to instill. Do not treat for >10 days.
Pediatrics: Instill 3 drops tid-qid. Gauze or wick may be inserted into ear canal after 1st administration. Add additional drops to saturate wick q4h. Remove wick after 24 hrs and continue to instill. Do not treat for >10 days.

HOW SUPPLIED: Sol: (Chloroxylenol-Hydrocortisone-Pramoxine) 1mg-10mg-10mg/mL [10mL]

CONTRAINDICATIONS: Varicella, vaccinia, perforated ear drum or when medication can reach the middle ear.

WARNINGS/PRECAUTIONS: Caution in long-standing otitis media. D/C if local irritation or sensitization occur. Systemic absorption has produced HPA axis, manifestations of Cushing's syndrome, hyperglycemia, and glucosuria.

ADVERSE REACTIONS: Itching, burning, irritation, dryness, folliculitis, hypertrichosis, acneform eruptions, hypopigmentations.

PREGNANCY: Category C, caution in nursing.

MECHANISM OF ACTION: Chloroxylenol: Bactericidal agent. Hydrocortisone: Glucocorticoid, anti-inflammatory, and antipruritic agent. Pramoxine: Topical anesthetic.

PHARMACOKINETICS: Distribution: Secreted in breast milk.

CORTEF RX
hydrocortisone (Pharmacia & Upjohn)

THERAPEUTIC CLASS: Corticosteroid

INDICATIONS: Steroid-responsive disorders.

DOSAGE: *Adults:* Initial: 20-240mg/day depending on disease. Adjust until a satisfactory response. Maint: Decrease in small amounts to lowest effective dose. Acute Exacerbations of Multiple Sclerosis: Initial: (Tab) 200mg/day of prednisolone for 1 week, then 80mg every other day for 1 month (20mg hydrocortisone=5mg prednisolone).
Pediatrics: Initial: 20-240mg/day depending on disease. Adjust until a satisfactory response. Maint: After favorable response, decrease in small amounts to lowest effective dose. Acute Exacerbations of Multiple Sclerosis: Initial: (Tab) 200mg/day of prednisolone for 1 week, then 80mg every other day for 1 month (20mg hydrocortisone=5mg prednisolone).

HOW SUPPLIED: Sus: (Hydrocortisone Cypionate) 10mg/5mL [120mL]; Tab: (Hydrocortisone) 5mg, 10mg, 20mg

CONTRAINDICATIONS: Systemic fungal infections.

WARNINGS/PRECAUTIONS: May need to increase dose before, during, and after stressful situations. May mask signs of infections. Avoid abrupt withdrawal. Prolonged use may produce glaucoma, optic nerve damage, secondary ocular infections. Increases BP, salt/water retention, potassium excretion. More severe/fatal course of infections reported with chickenpox, measles. Caution with TB, hypothyroidism, cirrhosis, ocular herpes simplex, HTN, diverticulitis, fresh intestinal anastomosis, ulcerative colitis, osteoporosis, myasthenia gravis, renal insufficiency, peptic ulcer disease. Growth and development of children on prolonged therapy should be monitored. Monitor for psychic disturbances. Kaposi's sarcoma reported.

ADVERSE REACTIONS: Fluid and electrolyte disturbances, HTN, osteoporosis, muscle weakness, cushingoid state, menstrual irregularities, nervousness, insomnia, impaired wound healing, DM, ulcerative esophagitis, excessive sweating, increases intracranial pressure, carbohydrate intolerance, glaucoma, cataracts.

INTERACTIONS: Reduced efficacy and increased clearance with hepatic enzyme inducers (eg, phenobarbital, phenytoin, and rifampin). Decreased clearance with ketoconazole and troleandomycin. Increases clearance of chronic high dose ASA; caution with hypoprothrombinemia. Effects on oral anticoagulants are variable; monitor PT. Increased insulin and oral hypoglycemic requirements in DM. Avoid live vaccines with immunosuppressive doses. Possible decreased vaccine response with killed or inactivated vaccines with immunosuppressive doses.

PREGNANCY: Safety in pregnancy and nursing not known.

MECHANISM OF ACTION: Anti-inflammatory glucocorticoid; causes profound and varied metabolic effects and modifies the body's immune responses to diverse stimuli.

CORTIFOAM RX
hydrocortisone acetate (Schwarz)

THERAPEUTIC CLASS: Corticosteroid

INDICATIONS: Adjunct therapy in ulcerative proctitis of the distal part of the rectum for patients who cannot retain corticosteroid enemas.

DOSAGE: *Adults:* 1 applicatorful rectally qd-bid for 2-3 weeks, and every 2nd day thereafter. Maint: Decrease in small amounts to lowest effective dose. D/C if no improvement within 2-3 weeks.

HOW SUPPLIED: Foam: 10% [15g]

CONTRAINDICATIONS: Obstruction, abscess, perforation, peritonitis, fresh intestinal anastomoses, extensive fistulas and sinus tracts.

WARNINGS/PRECAUTIONS: Absorption may be greater than from other corticosteroid enemas. May elevate BP, cause salt and water retention, IOP, or increase potassium and calcium excretion. Caution with recent MI, hypo- or hyperthyroidism, Strongyloides infestation, TB, CHF, HTN, renal insufficiency, peptic ulcers, diverticulitis, nonspecific ulcerative colitis, cirrhosis, risk of osteoporosis. May produce reversible HPA axis suppression, posterior subcapsular cataracts, glaucoma with possible optic nerve damage. May mask signs of infection or cause new infections. Kaposi's sarcoma reported with chronic use. Avoid with cerebral malaria, systemic fungal infections, active ocular herpes simplex, postoperative ileorectostomy. Rule out latent or active amebiasis. Avoid exposure to chickenpox and/or measles. Observe growth in pediatrics. Withdraw gradually. Acute myopathy observed with high steroid doses. May aggravate existing emotional instability or psychosis. D/C if severe reaction occurs.

ADVERSE REACTIONS: Bradycardia, acne, abdominal distention, convulsions, depression, abnormal fat deposits, fluid/electrolyte disturbances, muscle weakness, osteoporosis, peptic ulcer, pancreatitis, impaired wound healing, headache, psychic disturbances, suppression of growth in children, glaucoma, hyperglycemia, weight gain, thromboembolism, malaise, hypersensitivity reactions.

INTERACTIONS: Avoid live vaccines with immunosuppressive doses. Risk of hypokalemia with amphotericin B injection, potassium depleting agents, digitalis glycosides. Caution with aminoglutethimide or neuromuscular blockers. Decreased clearance or metabolism with macrolide antibiotics, estrogens, ketoconazole. Increased metabolism with hepatic enzyme inducers (eg, barbiturates, phenytoin, carbamazepine, rifampin). Withdraw anticholinesterase agents 24 hrs prior to initiation. Inhibits response to warfarin; monitor PT/INR. May increase blood glucose levels; may need to adjust antidiabetic agents. May decrease isoniazid and salicylate levels. Caution with ASA in hypoprothrombinemia. Cyclosporine may increase activity of both drugs; convulsions reported with concomitant use. Increased clearance with cholestyramine. Increased risk for gastrointestinal side effects with ASA and other NSAIDs.

PREGNANCY: Category C, caution in nursing.

MECHANISM OF ACTION: Adrenocortical steroid; anti-inflammatory.

CORTISPORIN   RX
bacitracin zinc - hydrocortisone acetate - polymyxin B sulfate - neomycin sulfate (King)

THERAPEUTIC CLASS: Antibacterial/corticosteroid

INDICATIONS: Corticosteroid responsive dermatoses with secondary infection.

DOSAGE: *Adults:* Apply bid-qid for maximum of 7 days.

HOW SUPPLIED: Cre: (Neomycin-Polymyxin-Hydrocortisone) 0.35%-10,000 U/g-0.5% [7.5g]; Oint: (Bacitracin-Neomycin-Polymyxin-Hydrocortisone) 400 U-0.35%-5,000 U/g-1% [15g]

CONTRAINDICATIONS: Use in eyes or external ear canal if eardrum is perforated. Tuberculous, fungal, or viral skin lesions.

WARNINGS/PRECAUTIONS: Avoid prolonged use or use over a large area. Prolonged use may result in secondary infection. May encourage spread of infection. Occlusive dressings will increase systemic absorption. Percutaneous absorption may cause growth cessation in pediatrics. D/C if redness, irritation, swelling, or pain persists.

ADVERSE REACTIONS: Allergic sensitization, burning, itching, irritation, dryness, folliculitis, hypertrichosis, acneiform eruptions, secondary infection, skin maceration, striae.

PREGNANCY: Category C, caution with nursing.

MECHANISM OF ACTION: Neomycin, polymyxin B, bacitracin: Antibacterials; provide action against specific susceptible organisms. Hydrocortisone: Corticosteroid; suppresses the inflammatory response and may delay healing.

PHARMACOKINETICS: Distribution: Hydrocortisone appears in breast milk following oral administration.

CORTROSYN   RX
cosyntropin (Amphastar)

THERAPEUTIC CLASS: Synthetic ACTH

INDICATIONS: Diagnostic agent used to screen for adrenocortical insufficiency.

DOSAGE: *Adults:* 0.25-0.75mg IM/IV injection or 0.25-0.75mg IV over 4-8 hrs. (See PI for method details).
Pediatrics: >2 yrs: 0.25-0.75mg IM/IV injection or 0.25-0.75mg IV over 4-8 hrs. ≤2 yrs: 0.125mg IM/IV injection or IV over 4-8 hrs. (See PI for method details).

HOW SUPPLIED: Inj: 0.25mg

WARNINGS/PRECAUTIONS: Exhibits slight immunologic activity. Patients known to be sensitized to natural ACTH with markedly positive skin tests will, with few exceptions, react negatively when tested intradermally. Falsely high fluorescence measurements with high plasma bilirubin or if plasma contains free Hgb.

ADVERSE REACTIONS: Hypersensitivity/anaphylactic reactions (rare), bradycardia, tachycardia, HTN, peripheral edema, rash.

INTERACTIONS: May potentiate electrolyte loss associated with diuretics.

PREGNANCY: Category C, caution in nursing.

MECHANISM OF ACTION: Synthetic ACTH; a diagnostic agent used to screen for adrenocortical insufficiency.

CORVERT   RX
ibutilide fumarate (Pharmacia & Upjohn)

THERAPEUTIC CLASS: Class III antiarrhythmic

INDICATIONS: For rapid conversion of atrial fibrillation or flutter (A-Fib/Flutter) of recent onset to sinus rhythm.

DOSAGE: *Adults:* ≥60kg: 1mg over 10 min. <60kg: 0.01mg/kg over 10 min. If arrhythmia still present within 10 min after the end of the initial infusion, repeat infusion 10 min after completion of 1st infusion.

HOW SUPPLIED: Inj: 0.1mg/mL

WARNINGS/PRECAUTIONS: Proarrhythmic; can cause potentially fatal arrhythmias. Administer in setting with continuous ECG monitoring and person able to treat acute ventricular arrhythmia. Adequately anticoagulate if A-Fib >2-3 days. Correct hypokalemia and hypomagnesemia before therapy. Caution in elderly.

ADVERSE REACTIONS: Sustained and nonsustained polymorphic ventricular tachycardia, sustained and nonsustained monomorphic ventricular tachycardia, bundle branch and AV block, ventricular and supraventricular extrasystoles, hypotension, bradycardia.

INTERACTIONS: Avoid Class IA (eg, disopyramide, quinidine, procainamide) and other Class III (eg, amiodarone, sotalol) antiarrhythmics with or within 4 hrs postinfusion of ibutilide. Increase proarrhythmia potential with drugs that prolong the QT interval (eg, phenothiazines, TCAs). Supraventricular arrhythmias may mask cardiotoxicity associated with excessive digoxin levels.

PREGNANCY: Category C, not for use in nursing.

MECHANISM OF ACTION: Class III antiarrhythmic agent; prolongs atrial and ventricular action potential duration and refractoriness. Delays repolarization by activation of a slow, inward current, rather than blocking outward potassium currents.

PHARMACOKINETICS: Distribution: V_d=11 L/kg; plasma protein binding (40%). **Metabolism:** Omega-oxidation and β-oxidation; omega-hydroxy metabolite (active). **Elimination:** Urine 82% (7% unchanged); feces (19%); $T_{1/2}$=6 hrs.

CORZIDE   RX
bendroflumethiazide - nadolol (King)

THERAPEUTIC CLASS: Nonselective beta-blocker/thiazide diuretic

INDICATIONS: Management of hypertension. Not for initial therapy.

DOSAGE: *Adults:* Initial: 40mg-5mg tab qd. Max: 80mg-5mg tab qd. CrCl >50mL/min: Dose q24h. CrCl 31-50mL/min: Dose q24-36h. CrCl 10-30mL/min: Dose q24-48h. CrCl <10mL/min: Dose q40-60h.

HOW SUPPLIED: Tab: (Nadolol-Bendroflumethiazide) 40mg-5mg*, 80mg-5mg* *scored

CONTRAINDICATIONS: Bronchial asthma, sinus bradycardia and >1st-degree conduction block, cardiogenic shock, overt cardiac failure, anuria, sulfonamide hypersensitivity.

WARNINGS/PRECAUTIONS: Caution in well-compensated cardiac failure, nonallergic bronchospasm, progressive hepatic disease, and renal or hepatic dysfunction. Exacerbation of ischemic heart disease with abrupt withdrawal. Withdrawal before surgery is controversial. May mask hyperthyroidism or hypoglycemia symptoms. Can cause cardiac failure, sensitivity reactions, hypokalemia, hyperuricemia, hypomagnesemia, hypophosphatemia. May activate or exacerbate SLE. Monitor for fluid/electrolyte imbalance. Enhanced effects in postsympathectomy patient. May manifest latent DM. May decrease PBI levels.

ADVERSE REACTIONS: Bradycardia, peripheral vascular insufficiency, dizziness, fatigue, nausea, vomiting, blood dyscrasias, hypersensitivity reactions.

INTERACTIONS: Additive hypotension and/or bradycardia with catecholamine-depleting drugs. Antidiabetic agents, anticoagulants, other antihypertensives, antigout agents may need adjustment. General anesthetics may exaggerate hypotension. May block epinephrine effects. Lithium toxicity. Alcohol, barbiturates, narcotics potentiate orthostatic hypotension. Amphotericin B, ACTH, corticosteroids intensify electrolyte imbalance. Monitor calcium levels with calcium salts. Monitor digoxin. Cholestyramine and colestipol may delay or decrease absorption. Enhanced hyperglycemic, hyperuricemic, and antihypertensive effects with diazoxide. Enhanced hypotensive effects with MAOIs. Possible decreased effectiveness with methenamine. Decreased arterial responsiveness with pressor amines. Probenecid, sulfinpyrazone may need dose increase. May potentiate nondepolarizing muscle relaxants, preanesthetics, and anesthetics. NSAIDs may decrease effects.

PREGNANCY: Category C, not for use in nursing.

MECHANISM OF ACTION: Nadolol: Nonselective beta-adrenergic blocking agent; inhibits β_1 and β_2 receptors, inhibiting chronotropic, inotropic, and vasodilator responses to β-adrenergic stimulation. Bendroflumethiazide: Thiazide diuretic; interferes with renal tubular mechanism of electrolyte reabsorption, increasing excretion of Na^+ and Cl^-.

PHARMACOKINETICS: Absorption: Nadolol: T_{max}=3-4 hrs. **Distribution:** Nadolol: Plasma protein binding (30%). **Elimination:** Nadolol: Kidney; $T_{1/2}$=20-24 hrs. Bendroflumethiazide: Kidney.

COSMEGEN

RX

dactinomycin (Ovation)

> Administer only under supervision of physician experienced in the use of cancer chemothera-
> peutic agents. Drug is highly toxic; handle and administer with care. Avoid inhalation of dust
> or vapors and contact with skin or mucous membranes. Avoid exposure during pregnancy.
> Extremely corrosive to soft tissue. Severe damage to soft tissue will occur with extravasation
> during IV use.

THERAPEUTIC CLASS: Actinomycin antibiotic

INDICATIONS: Concomitant treatment of Wilms' tumor, childhood rhabdomyosarcoma, Ewing's sarcoma, and metastatic nonseminomatous testicular
carcinoma. Monotherapy for gestational trophoblastic neoplasia, and as palliative and/or adjunctive treatment of solid malignancies.

DOSAGE: *Adults:* Wilms' Tumor/Childhood Rhabdomyosarcoma/Ewing's
Sarcoma: 15mcg/kg IV daily for 5 days. Testicular Cancer: 1000mcg/m^2
IV on Day 1 of combination therapy. Gestational Trophoblastic Neoplasia:
Monotherapy: 12mcg/kg IV daily for 5 days. Combination Therapy:
500mcg/m^2 IV on Days 1 and 2. Solid Malignancies: 50mcg/kg IV for lower extremity or pelvis. 35mcg/kg IV for upper extremity. May need lower dose with
obese patients, or with previous chemotherapy or radiation use. Dose intensity per 2-week cycle should not exceed 15mcg/kg/day or 400-600mcg/m^2
daily for 5 days. Calculate dose for obese or edematous patients based on
BSA. Elderly: Start at low end of dosing range.
Pediatrics: >6-12 months: Wilms' Tumor, Childhood Rhabdomyosarcoma/
Ewing's Sarcoma: 15mcg/kg IV daily for 5 days. Testicular Carcinoma:
1000mcg/m^2 IV on Day 1 of combination therapy. Gestational Trophoblastic
Neoplasia: Monotherapy: 12mcg/kg IV daily for 5 days. Combination Therapy:
500mcg/m^2 IV on Days 1 and 2. Solid Malignancies: 50mcg/kg IV for lower extremity or pelvis. 35mcg/kg IV for upper extremity. May need lower dose with
obese patients, or with previous chemotherapy or radiation use. Dose intensity per 2-week cycle should not exceed 15mcg/kg/day or 400-600mcg/m^2
daily for 5 days. Calculate dose for obese or edematous patients based on
BSA.

HOW SUPPLIED: Inj: 0.5mg

CONTRAINDICATIONS: At or about the time of infection with chickenpox or
herpes zoster.

WARNINGS/PRECAUTIONS: Monitor renal, hepatic, and bone marrow functions frequently. Can cause fetal harm during pregnancy. Possible anaphylactoid reactions. If stomatitis, diarrhea, or severe hematopoietic depression
occurs; d/c until recovery. Caution in elderly; increased risk of myelosuppression. Veno-occlusive disease (primarily hepatic) reported. Not for oral
administration.

ADVERSE REACTIONS: Nausea, vomiting, fatigue, lethargy, fever, cheilitis,
esophagitis, abdominal pain, liver toxicity, anemia, blood dyscrasias, skin
eruptions, acne, alopecia.

INTERACTIONS: Increased GI toxicity, marrow suppression, and incidence
of secondary tumors with radiation. May reactivate erythema from previous
radiation therapy. Caution if used within 2 months of irradiation for treatment
of right-sided Wilms' tumor; hepatomegaly and elevated AST levels reported.
Only use with radiotherapy for Wilms' tumor if benefit outweighs risks.

PREGNANCY: Category D, not for use in nursing.

MECHANISM OF ACTION: Actinomycin antibiotic; bindd to DNA and inhibits
RNA synthesis.

PHARMACOKINETICS: Metabolism: Minimally metabolized. **Elimination:**
Feces (30%), urine; T$_{1/2}$=36 hrs.

COSOPT   RX
dorzolamide HCL - timolol maleate (Merck)

THERAPEUTIC CLASS: Carbonic anhydrase inhibitor/nonselective beta-blocker

INDICATIONS: Treatment of ocular hypertension and open-angle glaucoma insufficiently responsive to β-blockers.

DOSAGE: *Adults:* 1 drop bid. Space dosing of other ophthalmic drugs by 10 min.
Pediatrics: ≥2 yrs: 1 drop bid. Space dosing of other ophthalmic drugs by 10 min.

HOW SUPPLIED: Sol: (Dorzolamide-Timolol) 2%-0.5% [5mL, 10mL]

CONTRAINDICATIONS: Bronchial asthma, history of bronchial asthma, severe COPD, sinus bradycardia, 2nd- or 3rd-degree AV block, overt cardiac failure, cardiogenic shock.

WARNINGS/PRECAUTIONS: Caution with sulfonamide allergy, cardiac failure, DM, COPD, bronchospastic disease, surgery and hepatic impairment. May mask symptoms of hypoglycemia and thyrotoxicosis. Bacterial keratitis reported with contaminated containers. Avoid in severe renal impairment. D/C if hypersensitivity or ocular reaction occur. Reinsert contact lenses 15 minutes after applying drops.

ADVERSE REACTIONS: Taste perversion, ocular burning, conjunctival hyperemia, blurred vision, superficial punctate keratitis, eye itching.

INTERACTIONS: Avoid oral carbonic anhydrase inhibitors, oral β-blockers, or topical β-blockers due to potential additive effects. Oral/IV calcium antagonists can cause AV-conduction disturbances, left ventricular failure or hypotension. Potentiated systemic β-blockade with concomitant CYP2D6 inhibitors. Reserpine can cause additive effects, hypotension and/or bradycardia. AV conduction time prolonged with digitalis. Quinidine may potentiate β-blockade. Increased risk of hypoglycemia with insulin or oral hypoglycemic agents. Wait 10 minutes before using another ophthalmic drug.

PREGNANCY: Category C, not for use in nursing.

MECHANISM OF ACTION: Dorzolamide: Inhibitor of human carbonic anhydrase II; decreases aqueous humor secretion, presumably by slowing formation of bicarbonate ions with subsequent reduction in Na^+ and fluid transport. Timolol: β_1 and β_2 (non-selective) adrenergic receptor blocking agent; decrease elevated IOP by reducing aqueous humor secretion.

PHARMACOKINETICS: Absorption: Timolol: C_{max}=0.46ng/mL. **Distribution:** Dorzolamide: Plasma protein binding (33%). **Elimination:** Dorzolamide: Urine (unchanged).

COUMADIN   RX
warfarin sodium (Bristol-Myers Squibb)

> May cause major or fatal bleeding; monitor INR regularly.

OTHER BRAND NAMES: Jantoven (USL Pharma)

THERAPEUTIC CLASS: Vitamin K-dependent coagulation factor inhibitor

INDICATIONS: Prophylaxis and treatment of venous thrombosis, PE, and thromboembolic disorders associated with atrial fibrillation and/or cardiac valve replacement. To reduce risk of death, recurrent MI, and thromboembolic events after MI.

DOSAGE: *Adults:* ≥18 yrs: Adjust dose based on PT/INR. Give IV as alternate to PO. Initial: 2-5mg qd. Usual: 2-10mg qd. Venous Thromboembolism (including pulmonary embolism): INR 2-3. Atrial Fibrillation: INR 2-3. Post-MI: Initiate 2-4 weeks post-infarct and maintain INR 2.5-3.5. Mechanical/Bioprosthetic Heart Valve: INR 2-3 for 12 weeks after valve insertion, then INR 2.5-3.5 long term.

HOW SUPPLIED: Inj: (Coumadin) 5mg; Tab: (Coumadin, Jantoven) 1mg*, 2mg*, 2.5mg*, 3mg*, 4mg*, 5mg*, 6mg*, 7.5mg*, 10mg* *scored

CONTRAINDICATIONS: Hemorrhagic tendencies, blood dyscrasias, CNS surgery, ophthalmic or traumatic surgery, inadequate lab facility, threatened abortion, eclampsia, preeclampsia, major regional lumbar block anesthesia, malignant HTN, pregnancy and unsupervised senile, alcoholic or psychotic patients. Bleeding of GI, GU or respiratory tract, aneurysms, pericarditis and pericardial effusion, bacterial endocarditis, cerebrovascular hemorrhage, spinal puncture, procedures with potential for uncontrollable bleeding.

WARNINGS/PRECAUTIONS: Monitor PT/INR; many endogenous and exogenous factors may affect PT/INR. Weigh benefits/risks with severe-moderate hepatic or renal insufficiency, infectious disease, intestinal flora disturbance, lactation, surgery, trauma, severe-moderate HTN, protein C deficiency, polycythemia vera, vasculitis, severe DM, indwelling catheters. D/C if tissue necrosis, systemic cholesterol microembolization ("purple toe syndrome") occurs. Caution with HIT, DVT, elderly. Warfarin resistance, allergic reactions reported.

ADVERSE REACTIONS: Tissue or organ hemorrhage/necrosis, paresthesia, vasculitis, fever, rash, abdominal pain, hepatic disorders, fatigue, headache, alopecia.

INTERACTIONS: Interacts with protein bound drugs, hepatic enzyme inducers and inhibitors. Avoid streptokinase and urokinase. Caution with drugs that may cause hemorrhage (eg, NSAIDs, ASA). Potentiates hypoglycemic, anticonvulsant drugs, and antihyperlipidemic drugs like ezetimibe. See PI for extensive list.

PREGNANCY: Category X, weigh benefits/risks with nursing.

MECHANISM OF ACTION: Vitamin K-dependent coagulation factor inhibitor; interferes with clotting factor synthesis by inhibition of the C1 subunit of the vitamin K epoxide enzyme complex, thereby reducing the regeneration of vitamin K_1 epoxide.

PHARMACOKINETICS: Absorption: (PO) Complete; T_{max}=4 hrs. **Distribution:** V_d=0.14 L/kg; plasma protein binding (99%); found in fetal plasma. **Metabolism:** Hepatic via CYP2C9, 2C19, 2C8, 2C18, 1A2, 3A4. **Elimination:** Urine (major), bile; $T_{1/2}$=1 week.

COVERA-HS   RX
verapamil HCL (G.D. Searle)

THERAPEUTIC CLASS: Calcium channel blocker (nondihydropyridine)

INDICATIONS: Management of hypertension and angina.

DOSAGE: *Adults:* Initial: 180mg qhs. Titrate: May increase to 240mg qhs, then 360mg qhs, then 480mg qhs, if needed. Swallow tab whole. Elderly: Start at the low end of the dosing range.

HOW SUPPLIED: Tab, Extended-Release: 180mg, 240mg

CONTRAINDICATIONS: Severe ventricular dysfunction, hypotension, cardiogenic shock, sick sinus syndrome or 2nd- or 3rd-degree AV block (except with functioning ventricular pacemaker), A-Fib/Flutter with an accessory bypass tract.

WARNINGS/PRECAUTIONS: Avoid with moderate to severe cardiac failure, and ventricular dysfunction if taking a β-blocker. May cause hypotension, AV block, transient bradycardia, PR interval prolongation. Monitor LFTs periodically; hepatocellular injury reported. Give 30% of normal dose with severe hepatic dysfunction. Caution with hypertrophic cardiomyopathy, renal or hepatic dysfunction. Decrease dose with decreased neuromuscular transmission.

ADVERSE REACTIONS: Constipation, dizziness, nausea, hypotension, headache, edema, CHF, pulmonary edema, fatigue, dyspnea, bradycardia, AV block, rash, flushing.

INTERACTIONS: Additive effects on HR, AV conduction, and contractility with β-blockers. Potentiates other antihypertensives. May increase digoxin, carbamazepine, theophylline, cyclosporine, and alcohol levels. Avoid disopyramide within 48 hrs before or 24 hrs after verapamil. Additive negative inotropic effects and AV conduction prolongation with flecainide. Avoid quinidine with hypertrophic cardiomyopathy. Monitor lithium. CYP3A4 inhibitors (eg, erythromycin, ritonavir) and grapefruit juice may increase levels. CYP3A4 inducers (eg, rifampin, phenobarbital) may decrease levels. Increased bleeding time with ASA. May potentiate neuromuscular blockers; both agents may need dose reduction. Caution with inhalation anesthetics.

PREGNANCY: Category C, not for use in nursing.

MECHANISM OF ACTION: Calcium channel blocker; inhibits transmembrane influx of calcium ions into arterial smooth muscle, and conductile and contractile myocardial cells.

PHARMACOKINETICS: Absorption: T_{max}=11 hrs. R-Enantiomer: Bioavailability (33-65%). S-Enantiomer: Bioavailability (13-34%). Oral administration of variable doses resulted in different parameters. **Distribution:** R: Plasma protein binding (94%). S: Plasma protein binding (88%). **Metabolism:** Liver; norverapamil (active metabolite). **Elimination:** Urine 70% (3-4% unchanged).

COZAAR RX
losartan potassium (Merck)

> Can cause death/injury to developing fetus during 2nd and 3rd trimesters. Stop therapy if pregnancy detected.

THERAPEUTIC CLASS: Angiotensin II receptor antagonist

INDICATIONS: Treatment of hypertension (HTN), alone or with other antihypertensives. To reduce the risk of stroke in patients with HTN and left ventricular hypertrophy (LVH), but evidence shows this does not apply to black patients. Diabetic nephropathy with an elevated serum creatinine and proteinuria (urinary albumin to creatinine ratio ≥300mg/g) in patients with type 2 diabetes and HTN.

DOSAGE: *Adults:* HTN: Initial: 50mg qd. Usual: 25-100mg/day given qd-bid. Intravascular Volume Depletion/Hepatic Impairment: Initial: 25mg qd. HTN with LVH: Initial: 50mg qd. Add hydrochlorothiazide (HCTZ) 12.5mg qd and/or increase losartan to 100mg qd, followed by an increase in HCTZ to 25mg qd based on BP response. Nephropathy: Initial: 50 mg qd. Titrate: Increase to 100mg qd based on BP response.
Pediatrics: ≥6 yrs: HTN: Initial: 0.7mg/kg qd (up to 50mg/day). Max: 1.4mg/kg/day (100mg/day).

HOW SUPPLIED: Tab: 25mg, 50mg, 100mg

WARNINGS/PRECAUTIONS: Can cause fetal injury/death. Correct volume or salt depletion before therapy. Changes in renal function may occur; caution with renal artery stenosis, severe CHF. Angioedema reported. Consider dose adjustment with hepatic dysfunction.

ADVERSE REACTIONS: Dizziness, cough, upper respiratory infection, diarrhea.

INTERACTIONS: K^+-sparing diuretics (eg, spironolactone, triamterene, amiloride), K^+ supplements, or K^+-containing salt substitutes may increase serum K^+. May reduce excretion of lithium; monitor lithium levels. Combination with NSAIDs, including COX-2 inhibitors, may lead to further deterioration of renal function and diminish antihypertensive effect.

PREGNANCY: Category C (1st trimester) and D (2nd and 3rd trimesters), not for use in nursing.

MECHANISM OF ACTION: Angiotensin II receptor antagonist; blocks vasocontrictor and aldosterone-secreting effects of angiontensin II by selectively blocking binding of angiotensin II to AT_1 receptor.

PHARMACOKINETICS: Absorption: Bioavailability (33%). **Adults:** C_{max}=224ng/mL, T_{max}=0.9 hrs, AUC=442ng•h/mL. (Metabolite) C_{max}=212ng/mL, T_{max}=3.5 hrs, AUC= 1685 ng•h/mL. **Pediatrics:** C_{max}=141ng/mL, T_{max}=2 hrs, AUC=368ng•h/mL. (Metabolite) C_{max}=222ng/mL, T_{max}=4.1 hrs, AUC=1866ng•h/

mL. **Distribution:** V$_d$=34L, 12L (metabolite). **Metabolism:** Liver via CYP2C9, 3A4; carboxylic acid (active metabolite). **Elimination:** Urine (4% unchanged; 6% metabolite). **Adults:** T$_{1/2}$=2.1 hrs, 7.4 hrs (metabolite). **Pediatrics:** T$_{1/2}$=2.3 hrs, 5.6 hrs (metabolite).

CREON RX
protease - amylase - lipase (Solvay)

THERAPEUTIC CLASS: Pancreatic enzyme supplement

INDICATIONS: Treatment of pancreatic exocrine insufficiency, often associated with cystic fibrosis (CF), chronic pancreatitis, post-pancreatectomy, post-GI bypass surgery, and ductal obstruction from neoplasm.

DOSAGE: *Adults:* Initial: (Creon 5) 2-4 caps per meal/snack. (Creon 10) 1-2 caps per meal/snack. (Creon 20) 1 cap per meal/snack. CF: Usual: 1500-3000 U lipase/kg/meal. Adjust dose to disease severity, control of steatorrhea, and maintenance of good nutritional status. Do not chew/crush caps. May add capsule contents to soft food (pH <5.5) and swallow immediately without chewing; take with water.
Pediatrics: <6 yrs: Initial: (Creon 5) 1-2 caps per meal/snack. (Creon 10) 1 cap per meal/snack. (Creon 20) Dose based on clinical experience for age group. >6 yrs: Initial: (Creon 5) 2-4 caps per meal/snack. (Creon 10) 1-2 caps per meal/snack. (Creon 20) 1 cap per meal/snack. CF: Usual: 1500-3000 U lipase/kg/meal. Adjust dose to disease severity, control of steatorrhea, and maintenance of good nutritional status. Max: 6000 U lipase/kg/meal. Do not chew/crush caps. May add capsule contents to soft food (pH <5.5) and swallow immediately without chewing; take with water.

HOW SUPPLIED: Cap, Delayed-Release: (Amylase-Lipase-Protease) (Creon 5) 16,600 U-5000 U-18,750 U, (Creon 10) 33,200 U-10,000 U-37,500 U, (Creon 20) 66,400 U-20,000 U-75,000 U

CONTRAINDICATIONS: Pork protein hypersensitivity and early stages of acute pancreatitis.

WARNINGS/PRECAUTIONS: Strictures in the ileo-cecal region and/or ascending colon reported with ≥20,000 U lipase/cap in CF patients. Caution if >6000 U lipase/kg/meal fails to resolve symptoms especially with history of intestinal complications. Maintain adequate fluid intake. D/C if hypersensitivity occurs.

ADVERSE REACTIONS: Nausea, vomiting, bloating, cramping, constipation, diarrhea.

INTERACTIONS: Do not add capsule contents to food with pH >5.5.

PREGNANCY: Category C, caution in nursing.

MECHANISM OF ACTION: Pancreatic enzyme; catalyzes the hydrolysis of fats to glycerol and fatty acids, proteins into proteoses, and derived substances and starch into dextrins and short chain sugars.

CRESTOR RX
rosuvastatin calcium (AstraZeneca)

THERAPEUTIC CLASS: HMG-CoA reductase inhibitor

INDICATIONS: Adjunct to diet in primary hyperlipidemia (heterozygous familial and nonfamilial) and mixed dyslipidemia (Types IIa and IIb) to reduce elevated total-C, LDL-C, Apo B, non-HDL-C, and triglyceride (TG) levels and to increase HDL-C. Adjunct to diet for elevated serum TG levels (Type IV), Adjunct to other lipid-lowering agents or if these are unavailable, to reduce LDL-C, total-C, and Apo B in homozygous familial hypercholesterolemia. Adjunct to diet in slowing the progression of atherosclerosis as part of a treatment strategy to lower total-C and LDL-C.

DOSAGE: *Adults:* Hypercholesterolemia/Mixed Dyslipidemia/ Hypertriglyceridemia/Slowing Progression of Atherosclerosis: Initial: 10mg qd.

(20mg qd with LDL-C >190mg/dL). Titrate: Adjust dose if needed at 2-4 week intervals. Range: 5-40mg qd. Homozygous Familial Hypercholesterolemia: 20mg qd. Max: 40mg qd. Asian Patients: 5mg qd. Concomitant Cyclosporine: Max: 5mg qd. Concomitant Lopinavir/Ritonavir: Max 10mg qd. Concomitant Gemfibrozil: Max: 10mg qd. Severe Renal Impairment: CrCl <30mL/min (not on hemodialysis): Initial: 5mg qd. Max: 10mg qd.

HOW SUPPLIED: Tab: 5mg, 10mg, 20mg, 40mg

CONTRAINDICATIONS: Rash, pruritus, urticaria, angioedema, active liver disease, unexplained persistent elevations of serum transaminases, pregnancy, nursing mothers.

WARNINGS/PRECAUTIONS: Increased risk of myopathy with other lipid-lowering therapies, cyclosporine, or lopinavir/ritonavir. Rare cases of rhabdomyolysis with acute renal failure secondary to myoglobinuria reported. Monitor LFTs prior to therapy, at 12 weeks or with dose elevation, and periodically thereafter. Reduce dose or d/c if AST/ALT ≥3x ULN persist. Caution with heavy alcohol use, history of hepatic disease, renal impairment, hypothyroidism, elderly. D/C if markedly elevated CPK levels occur, if myopathy is diagnosed or suspected, or if predisposition to renal failure secondary to rhabdomyolysis. Approximately 2-fold elevation in median exposure in Asian subjects. Persistent elevations in hepatic transaminase occured. Monitor liver enzymes.

ADVERSE REACTIONS: Headache, myalgia, abdominal pain, asthenia, diarrhea, dyspepsia, nausea, rhabdomyolysis with myoglobinuria and ARF and myopathy, liver enzyme abnormalities.

INTERACTIONS: Increased levels and risk of myopathy with cyclosporine, fibrates, niacin, and lopinavir/ritonavir. Avoid gemfibrozil. Caution with drugs that decrease levels or activity of endogenous steroid hormones (eg, ketoconazole, spironolactone, cimetidine). Increases levels of oral contraceptives (norgestrel, ethinyl estradiol). Increases INR with warfarin. Space antacid dosing by 2 hrs.

PREGNANCY: Category X, not for use in nursing.

MECHANISM OF ACTION: HMG-CoA reductase inhibitor; increases the number of hepatic LDL receptors on the cell-surface and inhibits hepatic synthesis of VLDL which reduces the total number of VLDL and LDL particles.

PHARMACOKINETICS: Absorption: Absolute biovailability (20%). T_{max}=3-5 hrs. **Distribution:** V_d=134L, plasma protein binding (88%). **Metabolism:** CYP2C9; N-desmethyl rosuvastatin (active metabolite). **Elimination:** Feces (90%); $T_{1/2}$=19 hrs.

CRIXIVAN RX
indinavir sulfate (Merck)

THERAPEUTIC CLASS: Protease inhibitor

INDICATIONS: Treatment of HIV infection in combination with other antiretrovirals.

DOSAGE: *Adults:* 800mg q8h on empty stomach. Hepatic Insufficiency or Concomitant Delavirdine, Itraconazole, Ketoconazole: 600mg every 8 hrs. Concomitant Efavirenz or Rifabutin: 1g every 8 hrs (reduce rifabutin dose by 1/2). Maintain adequate hydration (1.5L fluid/24 hrs).

HOW SUPPLIED: Cap: 100mg, 200mg, 333mg, 400mg

CONTRAINDICATIONS: Concomitant terfenadine, cisapride, astemizole, triazolam, midazolam, alprazolam, ergot derivatives.

WARNINGS/PRECAUTIONS: D/C or suspend during acute nephrolithiasis/urolithiasis. Tubulointerstitial nephritis seen with asymptomatic severe leukocyturia; monitor frequently with urinalyses. Consider discontinuation with severe leukocyturia. Immune reconstitution syndrome, hemolytic anemia, hyperglycemia, hyperbilirubinemia, hepatitis and liver failure reported. Spontaneous bleeding may occur with hemophilia A and B. Monitor hepatic function. Maintain adequate hydration. Possible redistribution or accumulation of body fat. Caution in elderly.

ADVERSE REACTIONS: Nephrolithiasis, GI discomfort, headache, fatigue, insomnia, hyperbilirubinemia, hyperglycemia, hemolytic anemia, renal failure, hematuria, nausea.

INTERACTIONS: See Contraindications. Increased risk of myopathy with HMG-CoA reductase inhibitors metabolized by CYP3A4. Increased levels with delavirdine, itraconazole, ketoconazole; reduce dose. Decreased levels with efavirenz, rifabutin, St. John's wort, rifampin. Avoid coadministration with atazanavir. May increase rifabutin and CCB levels. Administer didanosine 1 hr apart on empty stomach. Caution with phenobarbital, phenytoin, carbamazepine, and dexamethasone. Substantially increases sildenafil plasma levels; increased risk of sildenafil adverse events (eg, hypotension, visual changes, priapism). Decreases metabolism of alprazolam; increased risk of alprazolam adverse effects (eg, sedation, respiratory depression)

PREGNANCY: Category C, not for use in nursing.

MECHANISM OF ACTION: HIV protease inhibitor: prevents cleavage of viral polyproteins, forming immature, non-infectious viral particles.

PHARMACOKINETICS: Absorption: Rapid; T_{max}=0.8 hrs; C_{max}=12617nM; AUC=30691nM•hr. **Distribution:** Plasma protein binding (60%). **Metabolism:** Hepatic via CYP3A4. **Elimination:** Urine (<20%), feces (83%); $T_{1/2}$=1.8 hrs.

CROFAB   RX
crotalidae polyvalent immune fab (ovine) (Savage)

THERAPEUTIC CLASS: Venom specific immunoglobulin Fab fragment

INDICATIONS: Management of minimal to moderate North American crotalid envenomation. Use within 6 hrs to prevent clinical deterioration and systemic coagulation abnormalities.

DOSAGE: *Adults:* Initial: 4-6 vials IV over 60 min. Observe patient for 1 hr following dose to determine if envenomation is controlled. If needed, administer additional 4-6 vials until envenomation controlled. Once control is achieved, give 2 vials q6h for up to 18 hrs (3 doses). Additional 2-vial doses may be given based on clinical course.
Pediatrics: Initial: 4-6 vials IV over 60 min. Observe patient for 1 hr following dose to determine if envenomation is controlled. If needed, administer additional 4-6 vials until envenomation controlled. Once control is achieved, give 2 vials q6h for up to 18 hrs (3 doses). Additional 2-vial doses may be given based on clinical course.

HOW SUPPLIED: Inj: 1g/vial

CONTRAINDICATIONS: Hypersensitivity to papaya or papain.

WARNINGS/PRECAUTIONS: Recurrent coagulopathy may persist for 1-2 weeks; monitor for symptoms. Risk of anaphylactic reaction. Sensitization may occur; caution with a repeat course of treatment for subsequent envenomation episode. Contains ethyl mercury; use with caution in children. Use caution with conditions that cause coagulation defects (eg, cancer, collagen disease, CHF, diarrhea, elevated temperature, hepatic disorders, hyperthyroidism, poor nutritional state, steatorrhea, vitamin K deficiency.

ADVERSE REACTIONS: Urticaria, rash.

PREGNANCY: Category C, caution in nursing.

MECHANISM OF ACTION: Venom-specific immunoglobulin Fab fragment; acts by binding and neutralizing venom toxins, facilitating their redistribution away from target tissues and their elimination from the body.

PHARMACOKINETICS: Distribution: V_d=0.3L/kg. **Elimination**: $T_{1/2}$=approximately 12-23 hrs.

CROLOM   RX
cromolyn sodium (Bausch & Lomb)

THERAPEUTIC CLASS: Mast cell stabilizer

INDICATIONS: Treatment of vernal keratoconjunctivitis, vernal conjunctivitis, and vernal keratitis.

DOSAGE: *Adults:* 1-2 drops 4-6x/day at regular intervals.
Pediatrics: ≥4 yrs: 1-2 drops 4-6x/day at regular intervals.

HOW SUPPLIED: Sol: 4% [10mL]

WARNINGS/PRECAUTIONS: Do not wear contacts during therapy. Do not exceed recommended frequency.

ADVERSE REACTIONS: Transient burning or stinging.

PREGNANCY: Category B, caution in nursing.

MECHANISM OF ACTION: Mast cell stabilizer; inhibits degranulation of sensitized mast cells which occur after exposure to specific antigens; inhibits release of histamine and SRS-A mast cells.

CROMOLYN   RX
cromolyn sodium (Various)

THERAPEUTIC CLASS: Mast cell stabilizer

INDICATIONS: Treatment of vernal keratoconjunctivitis, vernal conjunctivitis, and vernal keratitis.

DOSAGE: *Adults:* 1-2 drops 4-6x/day at regular intervals.
Pediatrics: ≥4 yrs: 1-2 drops 4-6x/day at regular intervals.

HOW SUPPLIED: Sol: 4% [10mL]

WARNINGS/PRECAUTIONS: Do not wear contacts during therapy. Do not exceed recommended frequency.

ADVERSE REACTIONS: Transient burning or stinging.

PREGNANCY: Category B, caution in nursing.

CROMOLYN SODIUM INHALATION   RX
cromolyn sodium (Various)

OTHER BRAND NAMES: Intal (King)

THERAPEUTIC CLASS: Mast cell stabilizer

INDICATIONS: Prophylactic treatment of bronchial asthma and of acute bronchoconstriction due to exercise, environmental agents, and known antigens.

DOSAGE: *Adults:* Asthma: (Inhaler) Usual/Max: 2 inh qid. (Sol) 20mg nebulized qid. Acute Bonchospasm Prevention: (Inhaler) Usual: 2 inh 10-60 min before exposure to precipitant. (Sol) 20mg nebulized shortly before exposure to precipitant. Renal/Hepatic Dysfunction: Decrease inhaler dose.
Pediatrics: Asthma: (Inhaler) ≥5 yrs: Usual/Max: 2 inh qid. (Sol) ≥2 yrs: 20mg nebulized qid. Acute Bronchospasm Prevention: (Inhaler) ≥5 yrs: Usual: 2 inh 10-60 min before exposure to precipitant. (Sol) ≥2 yrs: 20mg nebulized shortly before exposure to precipitant. Renal/Hepatic Dysfunction: Decrease inhaler dose.

HOW SUPPLIED: MDI: (Intal) 0.8mg/inh [8.1g, 14.2g]; Sol: (Cromolyn, neb) 10mg/mL [2mL, 10ˢ 60ˢ]

WARNINGS/PRECAUTIONS: Not for treatment of acute attack. Severe anaphylaxis may occur. D/C if eosinophilic pneumonia or pulmonary infiltrates with eosinophilia develop. May experience cough and/or bronchospasm. Caution with inhaler in CAD or history of cardiac arrhythmias. Decrease dose or d/c with renal/hepatic dysfunction.

ADVERSE REACTIONS: Throat irritation/dryness, bad taste, cough, nausea, bronchospasm, sneezing, wheezing.

INTERACTIONS: Avoid with isoproterenol during pregnancy.

PREGNANCY: Category B, caution in nursing.

MECHANISM OF ACTION: Mast cell stabilizer; inhibits sensitized mast cell degranulation, release of mediators from mast cells, and both immediate and non-immediate bronchoconstrictive reactions to inhaled antigen.

PHARMACOKINETICS: Absorption: 8% absorbed. **Elimination:** Urine, bile.

CUBICIN RX
daptomycin (Cubist)

THERAPEUTIC CLASS: Cyclic lipopeptide

INDICATIONS: Susceptible complicated skin and skin structure infections (cSSSI). *Staphylococcus aureus* bloodstream infections (bacteremia).

DOSAGE: *Adults:* ≥18 yrs: Administer as IV infusion over 30 min. cSSSI: 4mg/kg q24h for 7-14 days. *S.aureus* Bacteremia: 6mg/kg q24h for minimum 2-6 weeks. Renal impairment: CrCl <30mL/min, HD, or CAPD: 4mg/kg (cSSSI) or 6mg/kg (*S.aureus* bacteremia) once q48h.

HOW SUPPLIED: Inj: 500mg

WARNINGS/PRECAUTIONS: *Clostridium difficile*-associated diarrhea reported. D/C if CDAD confirmed. Monitor CPK levels weekly; d/c with unexplained signs and symptoms of myopathy and CPK elevation >1000 U/L (-5x ULN), or with CPK levels ≥10x ULN. Persisting or relapsing *S.aureus* infection or poor clinical response should have repeat blood cultures.

ADVERSE REACTIONS: Constipation, nausea, injection site reactions, headache, diarrhea, insomnia, rash, vomiting, abnormal LFTs, superinfection, pharyngolaryngeal pain, pain in extremity and pulmonary eosinophilia.

INTERACTIONS: Caution with tobramycin; may affect levels. Monitor PT/INR for first several days with warfarin. Consider temporarily suspending statins. HMG-CoA reductase inhibitors may cause myopathy; consider suspending these agents with concomitant therapy.

PREGNANCY: Category B, caution in nursing.

MECHANISM OF ACTION: Cyclic lipopeptide; binds to bacterial membranes and causes a rapid depolarization of membrane potential, causing inhibition of protein, DNA, RNA synthesis, which results in bacterial cell death.

PHARMACOKINETICS: Absorption: (6mg/kg) C_{max}=93.9µg/mL, AUC=632µg•h/mL. **Distribution:** Plasma protein binding (90-93%); V_d=0.1L/kg. **Elimination:** Urine (78%), feces (5.7%); $T_{1/2}$=7.7-8.3 hrs.

CUPRIMINE RX
penicillamine (Aton)

Supervise closely due to toxicity, special dosage considerations, and therapeutic benefits.

OTHER BRAND NAMES: Depen (Wallace)

THERAPEUTIC CLASS: Copper chelating agent

INDICATIONS: Treatment of Wilson's disease, cystinuria, and severe, active rheumatoid arthritis (RA) when conventional therapy has failed.

DOSAGE: *Adults:* Wilson's Disease: Determine dosage by 24-hr urinary copper excretion. Maint: 0.75-1.5g/day for 3 months. Max: Up to 2g/day, based on serum free copper. Cystinuria: Initial: 250mg qd. Usual: 250mg-1g qid. RA: Initial: 125-250mg/day. Titrate: May increase by 125-250mg/day every 1-3 months. If needed after 2-3 months, increase by 250mg/day every 2-3 months. D/C if no improvement after 3-4 months at dose of 1-1.5g/day. Maint: 500-750mg/day. Max: 1.5g/day. Give on empty stomach, 1 hr before or 2 hrs after meals, and 1 hr apart from any other drug, food or milk. Supplemental pyridoxine

25mg/day recommended.
Pediatrics: Cystinuria: 30mg/kg/day given qid.

HOW SUPPLIED: Cap: (Cuprimine): 250mg; Tab: (Depen) 250mg* *scored

CONTRAINDICATIONS: Pregnancy (except for treatment of Wilson's disease or certain cases of cystinuria), nursing, RA patients with renal insufficiency, history of penicillamine-related aplastic anemia or agranulocytosis.

WARNINGS/PRECAUTIONS: Aplastic anemia, agranulocytosis, drug fever, thrombocytopenia, Goodpasture's syndrome, myasthenia gravis, pemphigus foliaceus/vulgaris, obliterative bronchiolitis, proteinuria and hematuria reported. Routine urinalysis, CBC with differentials, Hgb and platelet count every 2 weeks for 6 months, then monthly.

ADVERSE REACTIONS: Rash, urticaria, anorexia, epigastric pain, nausea, vomiting, diarrhea, leukopenia, thrombocytopenia, proteinuria.

INTERACTIONS: Hematologic and renal adverse reactions increase with gold therapy, antimalarial or cytotoxic drugs, oxyphenbutazone and phenylbutazone. Systemic levels lowered by iron; separate doses by 2 hrs. Mineral supplements may block response to therapy.

PREGNANCY: Category D, not for use in nursing.

MECHANISM OF ACTION: Chelator: (Wilson's disease) removes excess copper; (cystinuria) reduces excess cystine excretion by disulfide interchange; interferes with formation of cross-links between tropocollagen molecules; (RA) not established, appears to suppress disease activity.

PHARMACOKINETICS: Absorption: Rapid, incomplete; C_{max}=1-2mg/mL (250mg); T_{max}=1-3 hrs. **Distribution:** Plasma protein binding (80%). **Metabolism:** Liver. **Elimination:** Renal; elimination phase=4-6 days.

CUTIVATE   RX
fluticasone propionate (PharmaDerm)

THERAPEUTIC CLASS: Corticosteroid

INDICATIONS: (Cre, Oint) Relief of the inflammatory and pruritic manifestations of corticosteroid-responsive dermatoses. Cre may be used with caution in pediatric patients ≥3 months of age. (Lot) Relief of the inflammatory and pruritic manifestations of atopic dermatitis in patients ≥1 yr of age.

DOSAGE: *Adults:* Atopic Dermatitis: (Cre) Apply qd-bid. (Lot) Apply qd. Other Dermatoses: (Cre) Apply bid. (Oint) Apply bid. (Cre, Lot, Oint) Avoid occlusive dressings and re-evaluate if no improvement after 2 weeks.
Pediatrics: ≥3 months: Atopic Dermatitis: (Cre) Apply qd-bid. Other Dermatoses: (Cre) Apply bid. Avoid in diaper area. ≥1 yr: Atopic Dermatitis: (Lot) Apply qd. (Cre, Lot) Avoid occlusive dressings and re-evaluate if no improvement after 2 weeks. Oint not approved in peds.

HOW SUPPLIED: Cre: 0.05% [30g, 60g]; Lot: 0.05% [120mL]; Oint: 0.005% [30g, 60g]

WARNINGS/PRECAUTIONS: Caution with cre in peds. May produce reversible HPA axis suppression, manifestations of Cushing's syndrome, hyperglycemia, and glucosuria. D/C if irritation occurs. Use appropriate antifungal or antibacterial agent with dermatological infections. Peds may be more susceptible to systemic toxicity. Caution when applied to large surface areas. Avoid with pre-existing skin atrophy. Not for use in rosacea or perioral dermatitis.

ADVERSE REACTIONS: (Cre) Pruritus, dryness, numbness of fingers, burning. (Oint) Pruritus, burning, hypertrichosis, increased erythema, hives, irritation, light-headedness. (Lot) Burning, stinging, dryness, common cold, upper respiratory tract infection, cough, fever.

PREGNANCY: Category C, caution in nursing.

MECHANISM OF ACTION: Corticosteroid; not fully established. Possesses anti-inflammatory, antipruritic, and vasoconstrictive properties. Suspected to act by the induction of phospholipase A_2 inhibitory proteins, called lipocortins. Lipocortins control biosynthesis of potent mediators of inflammation (eg, prostaglandins, leukotrienes) by inhibiting release of common precursor, arachidonic acid. Arachidonic acid is released from membrane phospholipids by phospholipase A$_2$.

PHARMACOKINETICS: Absorption: Extent of percutaneous absorption depends on skin integrity, vehicle, and use of occlusive dressings. **Distribution**: (IV) V$_d$=4.2L/kg; plasma protein binding (91%). **Metabolism**: Liver via CYP3A4 (hydrolysis). **Elimination**: (IV) T$_{1/2}$=7.2 hrs.

CYANIDE ANTIDOTE PACKAGE RX
amyl nitrite - sodium nitrite - sodium thiosulfate (Akorn)

THERAPEUTIC CLASS: Antidote

INDICATIONS: Treatment of cyanide poisoning.

DOSAGE: *Adults:* Apply 1 amp of Amyl Nitrite to handkerchief and hold in front of patient's mouth for 15 sec followed by rest for 15 sec. Then reapply until Sodium Nitrite can be administered. D/C Amyl Nitrite and give Sodium Nitrite IV 300mg at rate of 2.5-5mL/min. Immediately after, inject 12.5g of Sodium Thiosulfate. If poison taken by mouth, gastric lavage should be performed as soon as possible. If signs of poisoning reappear, repeat Sodium Nitrite and Sodium Thiosulfate at one-half original dose.
Pediatrics: Apply 1 amp of Amyl Nitrite to handkerchief and hold in front of patient's mouth for 15 sec followed by rest for 15 sec. Then reapply until Sodium Nitrite can be administered. D/C Amyl Nitrite and give 6-8mL/m^2 of Sodium Nitrite IV; Max: 10mL. Immediately after, inject 7g/m^2 of Sodium Thiosulfate; max: 12.5g. If poison taken by mouth, gastric lavage should be performed as soon as possible. If signs of poisoning reappear, repeat Sodium Nitrite and Sodium Thiosulfate at one-half original dose.

HOW SUPPLIED: Sodium Nitrite: 300mg/10mL [2 amps]; Sodium Thiosulfate: 12.5mg/50mL [2 vials]; Amyl Nitrite Inhalant: 0.3mL [12 amps]

WARNINGS/PRECAUTIONS: Sodium Nitrite and Amyl Nitrite in high doses induce methemoglobinemia and can cause death.

PREGNANCY: Safety in pregnancy and nursing is not known.

MECHANISM OF ACTION: Sodium nitrate: Reacts with Hgb to form methemoglobin. Sodium thiosulfate: Converts cyanide to thiocyanate, probably by rhodanese.

CYCLESSA RX
desogestrel - ethinyl estradiol (Organon)

OTHER BRAND NAMES: Velivet (Duramed Pharms Barr)

THERAPEUTIC CLASS: Estrogen/progestogen combination

INDICATIONS: Prevention of pregnancy.

DOSAGE: *Adults:* 1 tab qd for 28 days, then repeat. Start 1st Sunday after menses begin or 1st day of menses.

HOW SUPPLIED: Tab: (Ethinyl Estradiol-Desogesterol) 0.025mg-0.1mg, 0.025mg-0.125mg, 0.025mg-0.15mg

CONTRAINDICATIONS: Thrombophlebitis, DVT or thromboembolic disorders, pregnancy, cerebrovascular or coronary artery disease, undiagnosed abnormal genital bleeding, cholestatic jaundice of pregnancy or jaundice with prior pill use, hepatic adenomas or carcinomas, breast cancer or other estrogen-dependent neoplasia, hepatic tumors, active liver disease, and heavy smoking (≥15 cigarettes/day) and over age 35.

WARNINGS/PRECAUTIONS: Cigarette smoking increases risk of serious cardiovascular side effects; risk increases with age (especially >35 yrs) and heavy smoking. Increased risk of MI, vascular disease, thromboembolism, stroke and gallbladder disease. Retinal thrombosis, hepatic neoplasia, carcinoma of breast and reproductive organs reported. May cause glucose intolerance. May increase BP, elevate LDL levels or cause other lipid changes, fluid retention, breakthrough bleeding, and spotting. May cause or exacerbate migraine.

May develop visual changes with contact lens. Increased risk of MI with HTN, hyperlipidemia, obesity, and diabetes. Increased risk of stroke with thrombophilias, hyperlipidemias, obesity, and migraine (especially with aura). D/C if jaundice, significant depression or ophthalmic irregularities develop. Perform annual physical exam. Use before menarche is not indicated. May affect certain endocrine, LFTs and blood components. Should not be used if pregnant. Does not protect against STD's. Caution in nursing mothers and those who have lipid disorders.

ADVERSE REACTIONS: Nausea, vomiting, breakthrough bleeding, spotting, amenorrhea, migraine headache, mood changes including depression, vaginal candidiasis, edema, weight or appetite changes, and fluid retention.

INTERACTIONS: Reduced effects, increased breakthrough bleeding, and menstrual irregularities with some antibiotics, antifungals, anticonvulsants. Anti-HIV protease inhibitors may affect safety and efficacy. St. John's wort may induce hepatic enzymes and reduce effectiveness as well as resulting in breakthrough bleeding. Increased plasma concentrations of cyclosporine, prednisolone, and theophylline.

PREGNANCY: Category X, not for use in nursing.

MECHANISM OF ACTION: Triphasic oral contraceptive; acts by suppression of gonatropins, and inhibition of ovulation. Also causes changes in the cervical mucus and in the endometrium.

PHARMACOKINETICS: Absorption: Desogestrel and Ethinyl estradiol: Rapid and complete. **Distribution:** Etonogestrel: Plasma protein binding (98%). **Metabolism:** Desogestrel: Liver; hydroxylation in intestinal mucosa; CYP3A4, 2C9; etonogestrel (active metabolite). Ethinyl estradiol: Hepatic conjugation. **Elimination:** Urine, bile, feces. Etonogestrel: $T_{1/2}$=37.1 hrs. Ethinyl estradiol: $T_{1/2}$=28.2 hrs.

CYMBALTA   RX
duloxetine HCL (Lilly)

> Antidepressants increased the risk of suicidal thinking and behavior (suicidality) in short-term studies in children, adolescents, and young adults with major depressive disorder (MDD) and other psychiatric disorders. Not approved for use in pediatric patients.

THERAPEUTIC CLASS: Serotonin and norepinephrine reuptake inhibitor

INDICATIONS: Acute and maintenance treatment of MDD in adults. Management of neuropathic pain associated with diabetic peripheral neuropathy. Acute treatment of generalized anxiety disorder (GAD). Management of fibromyalgia (FM).

DOSAGE: *Adults:* MDD: Initial: 40mg/day (given as 20mg bid) to 60mg/day (given qd or as 30mg bid) or 30mg qd for 1 week before increasing to 60mg qd. Max:120mg. Re-evaluate periodically. Diabetic Peripheral Neuropathic Pain: 60mg/day given qd. May lower starting dose if tolerability a concern. Renal Impairment: Consider lower starting dose with gradual increase. GAD: Initial: 60mg qd or 30mg qd for 1 week to adjust before increasing to 60mg qd. Titrate: May increase by increments of 30mg qd if needed. Max: 120 mg qd. FM: Initial: 30mg qd for 1 week to adjust before increasing to 60mg qd. Max: 60mg qd. Do not chew or crush.

HOW SUPPLIED: Cap, Delayed-Release: 20mg, 30mg, 60mg

CONTRAINDICATIONS: Concomitant use of MAOIs, uncontrolled narrow-angle glaucoma.

WARNINGS/PRECAUTIONS: Monitor for clinical worsening and/or suicidality. May cause hepatotoxicity. Avoid with chronic liver disease. May increase BP; obtain baseline and monitor periodically. Orthostatic hypotension and syncope reported. Avoid abrupt cessation and with severe renal impairment/ESRD or hepatic insufficiency. Caution with conditions that may slow gastric emptying, history of mania or seizures. May increase risk of mydriasis; caution in patients with controlled narrow-angle glaucoma. Serotonin syndrome may occur; caution with concomitant use of serotonergic drugs. Hyponatremia reported. May affect urethral resistance. May increase risk of abnormal bleeding;

C

caution with aspirin, NSAIDs, warfarin. May increase risk of serum transaminase elevations.

ADVERSE REACTIONS: Nausea, dry mouth, constipation, diarrhea, vomiting, decreased appetite, fatigue, dizziness, somnolence, increased sweating, blurred vision, insomnia, agitation, erectile dysfunction.

INTERACTIONS: See Contraindications. Avoid within 14 days of MAOI therapy. Upon discontinuation, wait at least 5 days before starting MAOI therapy. Avoid thioridazine, CYP1A2 inhibitors (eg, fluvoxamine, some quinolone antibiotics), substantial alcohol use. Increased levels with potent CYP2D6 inhibitors (eg, paroxetine, fluoxetine, quinidine). Caution with drugs metabolized by CYP2D6 having a narrow therapeutic index (eg, TCAs, phenothiazines, type 1C antiarrhythmics), and CNS-active drugs. May increase free concentration levels of highly protein-bound drugs. Potential for interaction with drugs that affect gastric acidity. Caution with serotonergic drugs (including triptans, tramadol, SNRIs).

PREGNANCY: Category C, not for use in nursing.

MECHANISM OF ACTION: Selective serotonin and norepinephrine reuptake inhibitor; actions may be related to potentiation of serotonergic and noradrenergic activity in the CNS.

PHARMACOKINETICS: Absorption: T_{max}=6 hrs. **Distribution:** V_d=1640L; plasma protein binding (>90%). **Metabolism:** Hepatic via CYP1A2, 2D6; oxidation and conjugation. **Elimination:** Urine 70% (<1% unchanged), feces (20%); $T_{1/2}$=12 hrs.

CYPROHEPTADINE   RX
cyproheptadine HCL (Various)

THERAPEUTIC CLASS: Serotonin/histamine antagonist

INDICATIONS: Perennial and seasonal rhinitis, vasomotor rhinitis, allergic conjunctivitis, uncomplicated allergic skin manifestations, blood or plasma allergic reactions, cold urticaria, and dermatographism. Adjunct to anaphylaxis.

DOSAGE: *Adults:* Initial: 4mg tid. Usual: 4-20mg/day. Max: 0.5mg/kg/day. *Pediatrics:* 7-14 yrs: Usual: 4mg bid-tid. Max: 16mg/day. 2-6 yrs: Usual: 2mg bid-tid or 0.25mg/kg/day. Max: 12mg/day.

HOW SUPPLIED: Syrup: 2mg/5mL; Tab: 4mg* *scored

CONTRAINDICATIONS: Newborn or premature infants, nursing mothers, concomitant MAOIs, angle-closure glaucoma, stenosing peptic ulcer, symptomatic prostatic hypertrophy, bladder neck obstruction, pyloroduodenal obstruction, elderly, debilitated.

WARNINGS/PRECAUTIONS: Caution with bronchial asthma, increased IOP, hyperthyroidism, CVD, HTN, and elderly. May impair mental/physical abilities.

ADVERSE REACTIONS: Drowsiness, somnolence, sedation, dizziness, confusion, restlessness, excitation, nervousness, insomnia, blurred vision, hypotension, palpitation, dry mouth, urinary frequency and retention.

INTERACTIONS: Avoid MAOIs. Additive effects with alcohol and other CNS depressants.

PREGNANCY: Category B, not for use in nursing.

MECHANISM OF ACTION: Serotonin and histamine antagonist.

PHARMACOKINETICS: Metabolism: Quaternary ammonium glucuronide conjugate (principal metabolite). **Elimination**: Feces, urine.

CYTADREN   RX
aminoglutethimide (Novartis)

THERAPEUTIC CLASS: Adrenocortical steroid synthesis inhibitor

INDICATIONS: Suppression of adrenal function in selected patients with Cushing's syndrome.

DOSAGE: *Adults:* Initial: 250mg PO q6h. Titrate: May increase by 250mg/day q1-2 wks. Max: 2000mg. Discontinue if skin rash persists for >5-8 days or becomes severe. If glucocorticoid replacement therapy is needed, give 20-30mg of hydrocortisone PO in the morning.

HOW SUPPLIED: Tab: 250mg* *scored

WARNINGS/PRECAUTIONS: May cause adrenocortical hypofunction, especially under conditions of stress; monitor closely. May suppress aldosterone production by the adrenal cortex and may cause orthostatic or persistent hypotension; monitor BP. May cause fetal harm. Therapy should be initiated in a hospital. May impair mental/physical abilities.

ADVERSE REACTIONS: Drowsiness, morbilliform skin rash, nausea, anorexia, dizziness.

INTERACTIONS: Alcohol may potentiate effects. May accelerate metabolism of dexamethasone; if glucocorticoid replacement is needed, hydrocortisone should be prescribed. May diminish the effects of coumarin and warfarin.

PREGNANCY: Category D, not for use in nursing.

MECHANISM OF ACTION: Adrenocortical steroid synthesis inhibitor; inhibits the enzymatic conversion of cholesterol to delta^5-pregnenolone, resulting in a decrease in the production of adrenal glucocorticoids, mineralocorticoids, estrogens, and androgens. It also blocks C-11, C-18, and C-21 hydroxylations and the hydroxylations required for the aromatization of androgens to estrogens by binding to CYP450 enzymes.

PHARMACOKINETICS: Absorption: Rapid and complete. C_{max}=5.9µg/mL. T_{max}=1.5 hrs. **Metabolism:** Acetylation, N-acetyl derivative (metabolite). **Elimination:** Urine (34-54%; unchanged and metabolite). $T_{1/2}$=12.5 hrs.

CYTARABINE   RX
cytarabine (Various)

Associated with bone marrow suppression, nausea, vomiting, oral ulceration, hepatic dysfunction, diarrhea, and abdominal pain. For induction therapy, treat in a facility able to monitor drug tolerance and toxicity.

THERAPEUTIC CLASS: Antimetabolite

INDICATIONS: Adjunct therapy for remission induction in acute non-lymphocytic leukemia (ANLL). Found useful in the treatment of acute lymphocytic leukemia (ALL) and blast phase of chronic myelocytic leukemia (CML). Prophylaxis and treatment of meningeal lymphoma.

DOSAGE: *Adults:* ANLL: Induction: 100mg/m^2/day continuous infusion or 100mg/m^2 IV q12h for Days 1-7. Meningeal Leukemia: Give intrathecally. Range: 5-75mg/m^2 given qd to every 4 days. Usual: 30mg/m^2 every 4 days until CSF normal, followed by 1 additional treatment.
Pediatrics: ANLL: Induction: 100mg/m^2/day continuous infusion or 100mg/m^2 IV q12h for Days 1-7. Meningeal Leukemia: Give intrathecally. Range: 5-75mg/m^2 given qd to every 4 days. Usual: 30mg/m^2 every 4 days until CSF normal, followed by 1 additional treatment.

HOW SUPPLIED: Inj: 100mg, 500mg, 1g, 2g

WARNINGS/PRECAUTIONS: Caution with pre-existing drug-induced bone marrow suppression, hepatic or renal dysfunction. Perform leukocyte and platelet counts daily during induction therapy. Monitor bone marrow, hepatic and renal functions, platelets, and leukocytes frequently. Sudden respiratory distress, cardiomyopathy, alopecia reported with high dose therapy. Severe and fatal CNS, GI, and pulmonary toxicity reported. Contains benzyl alcohol; fatal "Gasping Syndrome" in premature infants reported. Acute pancreatitis, hyperuricemia reported.

ADVERSE REACTIONS: Anorexia, nausea, vomiting, diarrhea, oral/anal inflammation or ulceration, hepatic dysfunction, fever, rash, thrombophlebitis, bleeding (all sites).

INTERACTIONS: Antagonizes susceptibility of gentamicin for *K.pneumoniae*. May inhibit efficacy of flucytosine. Monitor digoxin. Acute

C

pancreatitis reported in patients receiving prior L-asparaginase treatment. Cardiomyopathy and death reported during high dose therapy with cyclophosphamide.

PREGNANCY: Category D, not for use in nursing.

MECHANISM OF ACTION: Antineoplastic; not established. Appears to act through inhibition of DNA polymerase. Also incorporates into both RNA and DNA.

PHARMACOKINETICS: Absorption: (SQ/IM) T_{max} =20-60 min. **Metabolism:** Rapid metabolism; 1-β-D-arabinofuranosyluracil (inactive metabolite). **Excretion:** Urine (80%); $T_{1/2}$=1-3 hrs.

CYTOGAM   RX
cytomegalovirus immune globulin (human) (MedImmune)

THERAPEUTIC CLASS: Immunoglobulin

INDICATIONS: Prophylaxis of cytomegalovirus (CMV) disease associated with kidney, lung, liver, pancreas and heart transplantation.

DOSAGE: *Adults:* Initial: 150mg/kg 72 hrs post-transplant. Maint: Kidney Transplant: Weeks 2,4,6, and 8: 100mg/kg IV. Week 12 and Week 16: 50mg/kg IV. Liver/Pancreas/Lung/Heart Transplant: Week 2, 4, 6, and 8: 150mg/kg IV. Week 12 and Week 16: 100mg/kg IV. Administration: Initial: 15mg/kg/hr IV; may increase to 30mg/kg/hr if no adverse reactions after 30 min (after 15 min for subsequent doses), then increased to 60mg/kg/hr. Max: 150mg/kg/dose.

HOW SUPPLIED: Inj: 50mg/mL

CONTRAINDICATIONS: Selective immunoglobulin A deficiency.

WARNINGS/PRECAUTIONS: Consider use with ganciclovir for transplantation other than kidney from CMV seropositive donors into seronegative recipients. Risk of transmission of blood-borne viral agents. Renal dysfunction, acute renal failure, osmotic nephrosis and death reported; caution in pre-existing renal impairment, DM, ≥65 yrs, volume depletion, sepsis, or paraproteinemia. Confirm patient is not volume depleted prior to therapy. Monitor vital signs continuously. Monitor renal function before and during therapy, and urine output. D/C if renal function deteriorates, anaphylaxis occurs, or aseptic meningitis syndrome.

ADVERSE REACTIONS: Flushing, chills, muscle cramps, back pain, fever, nausea, vomiting, arthralgia, wheezing, increased BUN and serum creatinine, angioneurotic edema.

INTERACTIONS: Defer live virus vaccines (eg, measles, mumps, rubella) for 3 months; may interfere with immune response. Caution with nephrotoxic drugs.

PREGNANCY: Category C, safety in nursing not known.

MECHANISM OF ACTION: Immune globulin: contains relatively high concentration of antibodies directed against CMV diseases.

CYTOMEL   RX
liothyronine sodium (King)

THERAPEUTIC CLASS: Thyroid replacement hormone

INDICATIONS: Hypothyroidism. As a pituitary TSH suppressant in the treatment and prevention of euthyroid goiters, including thyroid nodules, and Hashimoto's and multinodular goiter. Diagnostic agent in suppression tests to differentiate mild hyperthyroidism or thyroid gland autonomy.

DOSAGE: *Adults:* Mild Hypothyroidism: Initial: 25mcg qd. Titrate: May increase by up to 25mcg qd every 1-2 weeks. Maint: 25-75mcg qd. Myxedema: Initial: 5mcg qd. Titrate: May increase by 5-10mcg qd every 1-2 weeks up to 25mcg qd, then increase by 5-25mcg qd every 1-2 weeks. Maint: 50-100mcg/day. Goiter: Initial: 5mcg/day. Titrate: May increase by 5-10mcg qd every 1-2 weeks up to 25mcg qd, then by 12.5-25mcg qd every 1-2 weeks. Maint: 75mcg qd.

Elderly/Coronary Artery Disease: Initial: 5mcg qd. Titrate: Increase by no more than 5mcg qd every 2 weeks. Thyroid Suppression Therapy: 75-100mcg qd for 7 days. Radioactive iodine uptake is determined before and after administration of hormone.
Pediatrics: Congenital Hypothyroidism: Initial: 5mcg qd. Titrate: Increase by 5mcg qd every 3-4 days until desired response. Maint: <1 yr: 20mcg qd. 1-3 yrs: 50mcg qd. >3 yrs: 25-75mcg/day.

HOW SUPPLIED: Tab: 5mcg, 25mcg*, 50mcg* *scored

CONTRAINDICATIONS: Uncorrected adrenal cortical insufficiency and untreated thyrotoxicosis.

WARNINGS/PRECAUTIONS: Do not use in the treatment of obesity; larger doses in euthyroid patients can cause serious or even life threatening toxicity. Caution with angina pectoris and elderly; use lower doses. Rule out hypogonadism and nephrosis prior to therapy. With prolonged and severe hypothyroidism supplement with adrenocortical steroids. May aggravate diabetes mellitus or insipidus and adrenal cortical insufficiency. Add glucocorticoid with myxedema coma. Excessive doses may cause craniosynostosis in infants.

ADVERSE REACTIONS: Allergic skin reactions (rare).

INTERACTIONS: Hypothyroidism decreases and hyperthyroidism increases sensitivity to oral anticoagulants; monitor PT/INR. Monitor insulin and oral hypoglycemic requirements. Decreased absorption with cholestyramine; space dosing by 4-5 hrs. Large dose may cause life-threatening toxicities with sympathomimetic amines. Estrogens increase thyroxine-binding globulin; increase in thyroid dose may be needed. Additive effects of both agents with TCAs. HTN and tachycardia with ketamine. May potentiate digitalis toxicity. Increased adrenergic effects of catecholamines; caution with CAD.

PREGNANCY: Category A, caution in nursing.

MECHANISM OF ACTION: Synthetic thyroid hormone; not established, suspected to enhance oxygen consumption by tissues, increases the basal metabolic rate and metabolism of carbohydrates, lipids, and proteins.

PHARMACOKINETICS: Elimination: $T_{1/2}$=2.5 days.

CYTOTEC   RX
misoprostol (G.D. Searle)

> Can cause abortion, premature birth, or birth defects. Uterine rupture reported when used to induce labor or induce abortion beyond 8th week of pregnancy. Not for use by pregnant women to reduce risk of NSAID-induced ulcers. Only use in women of childbearing age if at high risk of GI ulcers or complications with NSAID therapy; patient must then have negative serum pregnancy test within 2 weeks before therapy, maintain contraceptive measures, and begin therapy on 2nd or 3rd day of menstrual period.

THERAPEUTIC CLASS: Prostaglandin E₁ analogue

INDICATIONS: Prevention of NSAID-induced gastric ulcers in patients at high risk of developing gastric ulcers.

DOSAGE: *Adults:* 200mcg qid, or if not tolerated, 100mcg qid. Take for the duration of NSAID therapy. Take with meals; last dose at bedtime.

HOW SUPPLIED: Tab: 100mcg, 200mcg* *scored

CONTRAINDICATIONS: Pregnant women to reduce risk of NSAID-induced ulcers, prostaglandin allergy.

ADVERSE REACTIONS: Diarrhea, abdominal pain, nausea, flatulence, headache, dyspepsia.

INTERACTIONS: Avoid with magnesium-containing antacids to decrease incidence of diarrhea.

PREGNANCY: Category X, not for use in nursing.

MECHANISM OF ACTION: Synthetic prostaglandin E₁ analog; has both antisecretory and mucosal protective properties. Inhibits basal and nocturnal gastric acid secretion and acid secretion in response to stimuli (meals, histamine, pentagastrin).

PHARMACOKINETICS: Absorption: Extensively absorbed. (Fed) C_{max}=303pg/mL, AUC=373pg•hr/mL, T_{max}=64 min.; (Fasting) C_{max}=811pg/mL, AUC=417pg•hr/mL, T_{max}=14 min. **Distribution:** Plasma protein binding (<90%). **Metabolism:** De-esterification to its free acid (active metabolite); β oxidation, omega oxidation. **Elimination:** $T_{1/2}$=20-40 min.

CYTOVENE   RX
ganciclovir (Roche Labs)

> Risk of granulocytopenia, anemia, and thrombocytopenia. More rapid rate of CMV retinitis progression with caps; only use as maintenance treatment when the risk is balanced by the benefit of avoiding daily IV infusions.

THERAPEUTIC CLASS: Synthetic guanine derivative

INDICATIONS: (Caps) Prevention of cytomegalovirus (CMV) in solid organ transplants and in advanced HIV patients at risk for CMV disease. Alternative to IV for maintenance treatment of CMV retinitis in immunocompromised patients, in whom retinitis is stable. (IV) Treatment of CMV retinitis in immuno-compromised patients. Prevention of CMV disease in transplant recipients at risk for CMV disease.

DOSAGE: *Adults:* CMV Retinitis Treatment: Initial: 5mg/kg IV q12h for 14-21 days. Maint: 5mg/kg IV qd for 7 days or 6mg/kg IV qd for 5 days/week or 1000mg PO tid or 500mg PO 6 times daily q3h, while awake. CMV Retinitis Prevention in HIV Patients: 1000mg PO tid. CMV Retinitis Prevention in Transplant Patients: Initial: 5mg/kg IV q12h for 7-14 days. Maint: 5mg/kg IV qd for 7 days or 6mg/kg IV for 5 days/week or 1000mg PO tid. Renal Impairment: See PI for details. Take caps with food.

HOW SUPPLIED: Cap: 250mg; Inj: 500mg

CONTRAINDICATIONS: Hypersensitivity to acyclovir.

WARNINGS/PRECAUTIONS: Avoid if ANC <500 cells/microliter, or platelets <25,000 cells/microliter. Caution in pre-existing cytopenias and history of cytopenic reactions to drugs, chemicals, and irradiation. Reduce dose in renal impairment. High frequency of renal dysfunction in transplant recipients. Women of childbearing potential should use effective contraception during treatment due to fetal mutagenic/teratogenic potential. Men should practice barrier contraception during and ≥90 days after therapy.

ADVERSE REACTIONS: Fever, diarrhea, anorexia, vomiting, leukopenia, anemia, sweating.

INTERACTIONS: Decreased effects with zidovudine; combination may potentiate zidovudine and cause severe neutropenia. Potentiated by probenecid. Avoid imipenem-cilastatin; may precipitate seizures. Extreme caution with other nucleoside analogues, dapsone, pentamidine, flucytosine, vincristine, vinblastine, adriamycin, cyclosporine, amphotericin B, bactrim; potential additive toxicity. Increased didanosine serum levels.

PREGNANCY: Category C, not for use in nursing.

MECHANISM OF ACTION: Guanine derivative; inhibits viral DNA synthesis by inhibiting viral DNA polymerase, incorporating into viral DNA, resulting in eventual termination of viral DNA elongation.

PHARMACOKINETICS: Absorption: AUC=22.1-26.8mcg•hr/mL; C_{max}=8.27-9mcg/mL. **Distribution:** Plasma protein binding (1-2%); V_d=0.74L/kg. **Elimination:** $T_{1/2}$=3.5 hrs (IV), 4.8 hrs (PO); urine (91.3%)

CYTOXAN   RX
cyclophosphamide (Bristol-Myers Squibb)

THERAPEUTIC CLASS: Nitrogen mustard alkylating agent

INDICATIONS: Treatment of malignant lymphomas, Hodgkin's disease, lymphocytic lymphoma, mixed-cell type or histiocytic lymphoma, Burkitt's lymphoma, multiple myeloma, chronic lymphocytic leukemia, chronic granulocytic leukemia, acute myelogenous and monocytic leukemia, acute lymphoblastic leukemia in children, mycosis fungoides, neuroblastoma, ovary adenocarcinoma, retinoblastoma, breast carcinoma. Treatment of biopsy proven "minimal change" nephrotic syndrome in children, but not as primary therapy.

DOSAGE: *Adults:* Malignant Diseases (Without Hematologic Deficiency): Monotherapy: Initial: 40-50mg/kg IV in divided doses over 2-5 days, or 10-15mg/kg IV given every 7-10 days, or 3-5mg/kg twice weekly. Oral Dosing: Initial/Maint: 1-5mg/kg/day PO. Adjust dose according to antitumor activity and/or leukopenia. May need to reduce dose when combined with other cytotoxic drugs.
Pediatrics: Malignant Diseases (Without Hematologic Deficiency): Monotherapy: Initial: 40-50mg/kg IV in divided doses over 2-5 days, or 10-15mg/kg IV given every 7-10 days, or 3-5mg/kg twice weekly. Oral Dosing: Initial/Maint: 1-5mg/kg/day PO. Adjust dose according to antitumor activity and/or leukopenia. May need to reduce dose when combined with other cyto-toxic drugs. Nephrotic Syndrome: 2.5-3mg/kg/day PO for 60-90 days.

HOW SUPPLIED: Inj (Lyophilized): 500mg, 1g, 2g; Tab: 25mg, 50mg

CONTRAINDICATIONS: Severely depressed bone marrow function.

WARNINGS/PRECAUTIONS: Second malignancies, cardiac dysfunction, and hemorrhagic cystitis reported. May cause fetal harm in pregnancy. Serious, fatal infections may develop if severely immunosuppressed. Monitor for toxicity with leukopenia, thrombocytopenia, tumor cell infiltration of bone marrow, previous x-ray therapy or cytotoxic therapy, and impaired hepatic and/or renal function. Monitor hematologic profile for hematopoietic sup-pression. Examine urine for red blood cells. Anaphylactic reactions reported. Possible cross-sensitivity with other alkylating agents. May cause sterility. May interfere with normal wound healing. Consider dose adjustment with adrenalectomy.

ADVERSE REACTIONS: Impairment of fertility, amenorrhea, nausea, vomiting, anorexia, abdominal discomfort, diarrhea, alopecia, leukopenia, thrombocy-topenia, hemorrhagic ureteritis, interstitial pneumonitis, malaise, asthenia, renal tubular necrosis.

INTERACTIONS: Chronic, high doses of phenobarbital increase metabolism and leukopenic activity. Potentiates succinylcholine chloride effects and doxorubicin-induced cardiotoxicity. Alert anesthesiologist if treated within 10 days of general anesthesia.

PREGNANCY: Category D, not for use in nursing.

MECHANISM OF ACTION: Nitrogen mustard alkylating agent; exerts action by cross linking of tumor cell DNA.

PHARMACOKINETICS: Absorption: Well absorbed; bioavailability (≥75%). **Distribution:** Plasma protein binding (≥60% as metabolites). **Metabolism:** Liver; active metabolites. **Elimination:** Urine (5-25% unchanged); $T_{1/2}$=3-12 hrs.

D.H.E. 45   RX
dihydroergotamine mesylate (Valeant)

> Serious and life-threatening peripheral ischemia reported with potent CYP450 3A4 inhibitors (eg, protease inhibitors, macrolides). Elevated levels of dihydroergotamine increases risk of vasospasm leading to cerebral ischemia or ischemia of the extremities. Concomitant use with CYP450 3A4 inhibitors is contraindicated.

THERAPEUTIC CLASS: Ergot alkaloid

INDICATIONS: Acute treatment of migraine with or without aura. Acute treat-ment of cluster headache episodes.

DOSAGE: *Adults:* 1mL IV/IM/SQ. May repeat at 1 hr intervals. Max: 3mL/24hrs IM/SC or 2mL/24hrs IV and 6mL/week.

HOW SUPPLIED: Inj: 1mg/mL

CONTRAINDICATIONS: Ergot alkaloids hypersensitivity, ischemic heart disease, coronary artery vasospasm (eg, Prinzmetal's variant angina), uncontrolled HTN, hemiplegic or basilar migraine, peripheral artery disease, sepsis, following vascular surgery, severe renal/hepatic dysfunction, pregnancy, nursing, with potent CYP3A4 inhibitors (eg, ritonavir, nelfinavir, indinavir, erythromycin, clarithromycin, troleandomycin, ketoconazole, itraconazole), concomitant peripheral and central vasoconstrictors, and within 24 hrs after taking 5-HT$_1$ agonists, methysergide, ergotamine-containing, or ergot-type agents.

WARNINGS/PRECAUTIONS: Confirm migraine diagnosis. Risk of adverse cardiac, cerebrovascular, and vasospastic events and fatalities. Avoid with cardiac risk factors (eg, HTN, hypercholesterolemia, smoker, obesity, DM, strong family history of CAD, females who are surgically/physiologically postmenopausal, or males >40 yrs) unless cardiovascular evaluation is done. Perform cardiovascular monitoring with long-term use. Significant BP elevations reported.

ADVERSE REACTIONS: Vasospasm, angina, paraesthesia, HTN, dizziness, anxiety, dyspnea, headache, flushing, diarrhea, rash, increased sweating.

INTERACTIONS: Potentiated BP elevation with peripheral and central vasoconstrictors. Additive coronary vasospastic effect with sumatriptan; avoid within 24 hrs of each other. Propranolol and nicotine may potentiate the vasoconstrictive action. Increased plasma levels and peripheral vasoconstriction with macrolides. Contraindicated with CYP3A4 inhibitors (eg, macrolides, protease inhibitors). Caution with less potent CYP3A4 inhibitors (eg, saquinavir, nefazodone, fluconazole, grapefruit juice, fluoxetine, fluvoxamine, zileuton, clotrimazole).

PREGNANCY: Category X, contraindicated in nursing.

MECHANISM OF ACTION: Ergotamine; binds with high affinity to 5-HT$_{1D}$ receptors on intracranial blood vessels, causing vasoconstriction, or activates 5-HT$_{1D}$ receptors on sensory nerve endings of trigeminal system, resulting in inhibition of proinflammatory neuropeptide release.

PHARMACOKINETICS: Distribution: Plasma protein binding (93%); V$_d$=800L. **Metabolism:** Liver; 8'-β-hydroxydihydroergotamine (major metabolite). **Elimination:** Feces (major), urine (6-7%); T$_{1/2}$=9 hrs.

DACOGEN   RX
decitabine (MGI Pharma)

THERAPEUTIC CLASS: DNA methyltransferase inhibitor

INDICATIONS: Treatment of myelodysplastic syndromes.

DOSAGE: *Adults*: Initial: 15mg/m² IV over 3 hrs q8h for 3 days. Repeat cycle every 6 weeks. Treat for ≥4 cycles. Adjust dose based on hematology lab values, renal function, and serum electrolytes.

HOW SUPPLIED: Inj: 50mg

WARNINGS/PRECAUTIONS: May cause fetal harm. Avoid pregnancy in women of childbearing potential. Men should be advised not to father a child while receiving treatment and for 2 months afterwards. Neutropenia and thrombocytopenia may occur; monitor CBC and platelets periodically (at minimum, before each cycle). Caution with renal and hepatic dysfunction. Avoid with serum creatinine >2mg/dL, transaminase >2 times normal, or serum bilirubin >1.5mg/dL.

ADVERSE REACTIONS: Neutropenia, thrombocytopenia, anemia, fatigue, pyrexia, nausea, cough, petechiae, constipation, diarrhea, hyperglycemia, febrile neutropenia, leukopenia, headache, insomnia.

PREGNANCY: Category D, not for use in nursing.

MECHANISM OF ACTION: DNA methyltransferase inhibitor. Inhibition of methyltransferase causes hypomethylation of DNA and cellular differentiation or apoptosis.

PHARMACOKINETICS: Distribution: Plasma protein binding (<1%). **Metabolism:** Deamination in liver, granulocytes, intestinal epithelium, and blood. **Elimination:** T$_{1/2}$=0.51 hrs.

DALMANE

flurazepam HCL (Valeant)

CIV

THERAPEUTIC CLASS: Benzodiazepine

INDICATIONS: Treatment of insomnia.

DOSAGE: *Adults:* Usual: 15-30mg at bedtime. Elderly/Debilitated: Initial: 15mg at bedtime.
Pediatrics: ≥15 yrs: Usual: 15-30mg at bedtime.

HOW SUPPLIED: Cap: 15mg, 30mg

CONTRAINDICATIONS: Pregnancy.

WARNINGS/PRECAUTIONS: Caution in elderly, debilitated, severely depressed, those with suicidal tendencies, hepatic/renal impairment, respiratory disease. Ataxia and falls reported in elderly and debilitated.Withdrawal symptoms after discontinuation; avoid abrupt discontinuation. Rare cases of angioedema involving the tongue, glottis, or larynx reported. Complex behaviors such as sleep driving, and other complex behaviors (eg, preparing and eating food, making phone calls, and having sex) reported.

ADVERSE REACTIONS: Confusion, dizziness, drowsiness, lightheadedness, ataxia.

INTERACTIONS: Additive effects with alcohol and other CNS depressants.

PREGNANCY: Not for use in pregnancy or nursing.

MECHANISM OF ACTION: Benzodiazepine; hypnotic.

PHARMACOKINETICS: Absorption: Rapid; C_{max}=4.0ng/mL; T_{max}=1 hr.
Metabolism: N_1-desalkyl-flurazepam (active metabolite); conjugation.
Elimination: Urine; $T_{1/2}$=2.3 hrs, 47-100 hrs (active metabolite).

DANTRIUM

dantrolene sodium (Procter & Gamble Pharmaceuticals)

RX

> Associated with hepatotoxicity; monitor hepatic function. Discontinue if no benefit after 45 days.

THERAPEUTIC CLASS: Direct acting skeletal muscle relaxant

INDICATIONS: To control manifestations of clinical spasticity from upper motor neuron disorders (eg, spinal cord injury, stroke, cerebral palsy, multiple sclerosis). Preoperatively to prevent or attenuate development of malignant hyperthermia, and after a malignant hyperthermia crisis.

DOSAGE: *Adults:* Chronic Spasticity: Initial: 25mg qd for 7 days. Titrate: Increase to 25mg tid for 7 days, then 50mg tid for 7 days, then 100mg tid. Max: 100mg qid. If no further benefit at next higher dose, decrease to previous lower dose. Malignant Hyperthermia: Pre-Op: 4-8mg/kg/day given tid-qid for 1-2 days before surgery, with last dose given 3-4 hrs before surgery. Post-Op Following Malignant Hyperthermia Crisis: 4-8mg/kg/day given qid for 1-3 days.
Pediatrics: ≥5 yrs: Chronic Spasticity: Initial: 0.5mg/kg qd for 7 days. Titrate: Increase to 0.5mg/kg tid for 7 days, then 1mg/kg tid for 7 days, then 2mg/kg tid. Max: 100mg qid. If no further benefit at next higher dose, decrease to previous lower dose.

HOW SUPPLIED: Cap: 25mg, 50mg, 100mg

CONTRAINDICATIONS: Active hepatic disease, where spasticity is utilized to sustain upright posture and balance in locomotion, when spasticity is utilized to obtain or maintain increased function.

WARNINGS/PRECAUTIONS: Monitor LFTs at baseline, then periodically. Increased risk of hepatocellular disease in females and patients >35 yrs. Caution with pulmonary, cardiac, and liver dysfunction. Photosensitivity reaction may occur; limit sunlight exposure.

ADVERSE REACTIONS: Drowsiness, dizziness, weakness, malaise, fatigue, diarrhea, hepatitis, tachycardia, aplastic anemia, thrombocytopenia, depression, seizure.

INTERACTIONS: Increased drowsiness with CNS depressants. Caution with estrogens; risk of hepatotoxicity. Avoid with CCBs; risk of cardiovascular collapse. May potentiate vecuronium-induced neuromuscular block.

PREGNANCY: Safety in nursing not known. Not for use in nursing.

MECHANISM OF ACTION: Direct acting skeletal muscle relaxant; interferes with the release of calcium ions from the sarcoplasmic reticulum.

PHARMACOKINETICS: Absorption: Incomplete/slow but consistent. **Metabolism:** Hepatic microsomal enzymes; 5-hydroxy and acetamido analog (major metabolites). **Elimination:** Urine; $T_{1/2}$=8.7 hrs.

DANTRIUM IV RX
dantrolene sodium (Procter & Gamble Pharmaceuticals)

THERAPEUTIC CLASS: Direct acting skeletal muscle relaxant

INDICATIONS: Adjunct management of fulminant hypermetabolism of skeletal muscle characteristic of malignant hyperthermia crises. For pre- and post-operative use to prevent or attenuate development of malignant hyperthermia.

DOSAGE: *Adults:* Malignant Hyperthermia: Initial: Minimum 1mg/kg IV push. Continue until symptoms subside or max cumulative dose 10mg/kg. Pre-Op Malignant Hyperthermia Prophylaxis: 2.5mg/kg 1.25 hrs before anesthesia and infuse over 1 hr. May need additional therapy during anesthesia/surgery if symptoms arise. Post-Op Prophylaxis: Initial: 1mg/kg or more as clinical situation dictates.
Pediatrics: Malignant Hyperthermia: Initial: Minimum 1mg/kg IV push. Continue until symptoms subside or max cumulative dose 10mg/kg.

HOW SUPPLIED: Inj: 20mg

WARNINGS/PRECAUTIONS: Use with supportive therapies to treat malignant hyperthermia. Take steps to prevent extravasation. Fatal and non-fatal hepatic disorders reported. Do not operate automobile or engage hazardous activity for 48 hrs after therapy. Caution at meals on day of administration because difficulty in swallowing/choking reported. Monitor vital signs if receive preoperatively.

ADVERSE REACTIONS: Loss of grip strength, weakness in legs, drowsiness, dizziness, pulmonary edema, thrombophlebitis, urticaria, erythema.

INTERACTIONS: Plasma protein-binding reduced by warfarin and clofibrate, and increased by tolbutamide. Avoid with CCBs; possible risk of cardiovascular collapse. Caution with tranquilizers. Possible increased metabolism by drugs known to induce hepatic microsomal enzymes. May potentiate vecuronium-induced neuromuscular block.

PREGNANCY: Category C, safety in nursing not known.

MECHANISM OF ACTION: Direct acting skeletal muscle relaxant; interferes with release of calcium ions from sarcoplasmic reticulum.

PHARMACOKINETICS: Distribution: Found in breast milk. **Metabolism:** Hydrolysis and oxidation; 5-hydroxy dantrolene and acetylamino analog (major metabolites). **Elimination:** Urine; $T_{1/2}$=4-8 hrs.

DAPSONE RX
dapsone (Jacobus)

THERAPEUTIC CLASS: Leprostatic agent

INDICATIONS: Treatment of dermatitis herpetiformis and leprosy.

DOSAGE: *Adults:* Dermatitis Herpetiformis: Initial: 50mg/day. Usual: 50-300mg/day, may increase dose if needed. Reduce to minimum maintenance dose. Leprosy: Give with 1 or more antileprosy drugs. Maint: 100mg/day. *Pediatrics:* Same schedule as adults but with correspondingly smaller doses.

HOW SUPPLIED: Tab: 25mg*, 100mg* *scored

WARNINGS/PRECAUTIONS: Agranulocytosis, aplastic anemia and other blood dyscrasias reported. CBC weekly for the 1st month, monthly for 6 months and semi-annually thereafter. D/C if significant reduction in leukocytes, platelets or hemopoiesis occurs. Treat severe anemia prior to therapy. D/C if sensitivity occurs. Caution in those with G6PD deficiency, methemoglobin reductase deficiency, or hemoglobin M. Toxic hepatitis and cholestatic jaundice reported. Monitor LFT's.

ADVERSE REACTIONS: Hemolysis, peripheral neuropathy, nausea, vomiting, abdominal pain, pancreatitis, vertigo, blurred vision, tinnitus, insomnia, fever, headache, psychosis, phototoxicity, pulmonary eosinophilia, tachycardia, albuminuria, renal papillary necrosis, male infertility.

INTERACTIONS: Rifampin lowers plasma levels. Folic acid antagonists (eg, pyrimethamine) may increase hematologic reactions. Dapsone and trimethoprim each raise the level of the other.

PREGNANCY: Category C, not for use in nursing.

MECHANISM OF ACTION: Antibacterial agent; not established.

PHARMACOKINETICS: Absorption: Rapid, almost complete. T_{max}=4-8 hrs. **Elimination:** $T_{1/2}$=28 hrs.

DAPTACEL   RX
pertussis vaccine acellular, adsorbed - diphtheria toxoid - tetanus toxoid
(Sanofi Pasteur)

THERAPEUTIC CLASS: Vaccine

INDICATIONS: Active immunization against diphtheria, tetanus, and pertussis as a five-dose series in infants and children 6 weeks through 6 years of age (prior to seventh birthday).

DOSAGE: *Pediatrics:* 6 weeks-up to 7 yrs: 0.5mL IM at 2, 4, 6 months (at intervals of 6-8 weeks), at 15-20 months, and at 4-6 years of age. The interval between 3rd and 4th dose should be at least 6 months. May use to complete series in infants who received ≥1 dose of whole-cell pertussis (DTP). First dose given early as 6 weeks of age.

HOW SUPPLIED: Inj: (Diphtheria-Pertussis-Tetanus-) 15Lf U-23mcg-5Lf U/0.5mL

CONTRAINDICATIONS: Adults and pediatrics ≥7yrs. Administration after immediate anaphylactic reaction, or encephalopathy not attributable to another identifiable cause within 7 days from initial vaccination. Moderate or serious illness. Outbreak of poliomyelitis.

WARNINGS/PRECAUTIONS: Stopper contains dry natural latex rubber. Evaluate risks/benefits of subsequent doses if temperature ≥105°F, or if collapse/shock occurs, or persistent crying for ≥3 hrs within 48 hrs, and convulsions with or without fever within 3 days of vaccine. Continue with DT vaccine if pertussis must be withheld. Caution if Guillain-Barre syndrome occurred within 6 weeks of recipt of prior vaccine containing tetanus toxoid. Increased risk of neurological events with family history of convulsions; administer antipyretic at time of and for 24 hrs after immunization. Enhanced risk of manifestation of underlying neurological within 2-3 days following vaccine. May not achieve expected immune response in immunosuppressed patients. Avoid injection into blood vessel.

ADVERSE REACTIONS: Local tenderness, fever, fretfulness, anorexia, drowsiness, vomiting.

INTERACTIONS: Immunosuppressives (eg, irradiation, antimetabolites, alkylating agents, cytotoxic drugs, corticosteroids) may reduce immune response to vaccine. Adequate immune response may not occur after recent immune globulin injection.

PREGNANCY: Category C, safety in nursing not known.

MECHANISM OF ACTION: Develops neutralizing antibodies against diphtheria, tetanus, and pertussis.

DARAPRIM   RX
pyrimethamine (GlaxoSmithKline)

THERAPEUTIC CLASS: Folic acid antagonist

INDICATIONS: Adjunct treatment of toxoplasmosis and acute malaria. Chemoprophylaxis of malaria.

DOSAGE: *Adults:* Toxoplasmosis: Initial: 50-75mg qd with 1-4g/day of sulfonamide. After 1-3 weeks, reduce dose of each drug to 1/2 of previous dose for additional 4-5 weeks. Acute Malaria: 25mg qd for 2 days with sulfonamide. As monotherapy in semi-immune persons, 50mg for 2 days. Follow with prophylaxis dose through periods of early recrudescence and late relapse. Malaria Prophylaxis: 25mg once weekly.
Pediatrics: Toxoplasmosis: 0.5mg/kg bid. After 2-4 days, reduce to 0.25mg/kg bid for 1 month. Use with usual pediatric sulfonamide dose. Acute Malaria: 4-10 yrs: As monotherapy in semi-immune persons, 25mg for 2 days. Follow with prophylaxis dose through periods of early recrudescence and late relapse. Malaria Prophylaxis: >10 yrs: 25mg once weekly. 4-10 yrs: 12.5 once weekly. <4 yrs: 6.25mg once weekly.

HOW SUPPLIED: Tab: 25mg* *scored

CONTRAINDICATIONS: Megaloblastic anemia due to folate deficiency.

WARNINGS/PRECAUTIONS: Dose for toxoplasmosis approaches toxic levels; reduce dose or d/c if develop folate deficiency. Administer leucovorin 5-15mg qd (po, IV, or IM) until normal hematopoiesis. May be carcinogenic. Pediatric deaths reported with accidental ingestion. Use small initial dose with convulsive disorders to avoid nervous system toxicity. Caution with renal or hepatic dysfunction or if possible folate deficiency (eg, pregnancy, malabsorption syndrome, alcoholism). Perform semiweekly blood counts, including platelets with high doses.

ADVERSE REACTIONS: Hypersensitivity reactions (eg, Stevens-Johnson syndrome, toxic epidermal necrolysis) hyperphenylalinemia (with sulfonamides), anorexia, vomiting, blood dyscrasias, cardiac rhythm disorders.

INTERACTIONS: Concurrent phenytoin may affect folate levels. Increased risk of bone marrow suppression with antifolic drugs (eg, sulfonamides or trimethoprim-sulfamethoxazole). Mild hepatotoxicity reported with lorazepam.

PREGNANCY: Category C, not for use in nursing.

MECHANISM OF ACTION: Folic acid antagonist highly selective against Toxoplasma gondii and plasmodia.

PHARMACOKINETICS: Absorption: Well absorbed. T_{max}=2-6hrs. **Distribution:** Plasma protein binding (87%). **Elimination:** $T_{1/2}$=96 hrs.

DARVOCET A500   CIV
propoxyphene napsylate - acetaminophen (Xanodyne)

THERAPEUTIC CLASS: Opioid analgesic

INDICATIONS: Relief of mild to moderate pain.

DOSAGE: *Adults:* Usual: 1 tab q4h prn for pain. Max: 6 tabs/24 hrs. Elderly: Increase dosing interval. Hepatic/Renal Impairment: Reduce daily dose.

HOW SUPPLIED: Tab: (Propoxyphene-APAP) 100mg-500mg

WARNINGS/PRECAUTIONS: Drug dependence potential. Not for suicidal or addiction-prone patients. Caution with hepatic or renal impairment, elderly.

ADVERSE REACTIONS: Dizziness, sedation, nausea, vomiting, liver dysfunction.

INTERACTIONS: Additive CNS-depressant effects with alcohol, sedatives, tranquilizers, muscle relaxants, antidepressants. Increases plasma levels of antidepressants, anticonvulsants, coumarins. Severe neurologic signs, including coma reported with carbamazepine.

PREGNANCY: Not for use in pregnancy, safety not known in nursing.

MECHANISM OF ACTION: Propoxyphene: Centrally acting narcotic analgesic. Acetaminophen: Produces antipyretic and analgesic activity.

PHARMACOKINETICS: Absorption: T_{max}=2-2.5 hrs; (100mg) C_{max}=0.05-0.1mcg/mL. **Distribution:** Found in human breast milk. **Metabolism:** Liver; norpropoxyphene (active metabolite). **Elimination:** $T_{1/2}$=6-12 hrs, 30-36 hrs (active metabolite).

DARVOCET-N
propoxyphene napsylate - acetaminophen (Xanodyne)

CIV

THERAPEUTIC CLASS: Opioid analgesic

INDICATIONS: Relief of mild to moderate pain.

DOSAGE: *Adults:* Usual: 100mg propoxyphene napsylate and 650mg APAP q4h prn for pain. Max: 600mg propoxyphene napsylate/day. Elderly: Increase dosing interval. Hepatic/Renal Impairment: Reduce daily dose.

HOW SUPPLIED: Tab: (Propoxyphene-APAP) 50mg-325mg, 100mg-650mg

WARNINGS/PRECAUTIONS: Drug dependence potential. Not for suicidal or addiction-prone patients. Caution with hepatic/renal impairment, elderly. May impair mental/physical abilities.

ADVERSE REACTIONS: Dizziness, sedation, nausea, vomiting, liver dysfunction.

INTERACTIONS: Additive CNS-depressant effects with alcohol, sedatives, tranquilizers, muscle relaxants, antidepressants. Increases plasma levels of antidepressants, anticonvulsants, coumarins. Severe neurologic signs, including coma reported with carbamazepine.

PREGNANCY: Not for use in pregnancy, safety not known in nursing.

MECHANISM OF ACTION: Propoxyphene; centrally acting narcotic analgesic agent. Acetaminophen; produces antipyretic-analgesic activity.

PHARMACOKINETICS: Absorption: T_{max}=2-2.5 hrs; C_{max}=0.05-0.1mcg/mL. **Distribution:** Found in human breast milk. **Metabolism:** Liver; norpropoxyphene (active metabolite). **Elimination:** $T_{1/2}$=6-12 hrs, 30-36 hrs (norpropoxyphene).

DARVON
propoxyphene HCL (Xanodyne)

CIV

THERAPEUTIC CLASS: Opioid analgesic

INDICATIONS: Relief of mild to moderate pain.

DOSAGE: *Adults:* Usual: 65mg q4h as needed for pain. Max: 390mg/day. Elderly: Increase dose interval. Hepatic/Renal Impairment: Reduce daily dose.

HOW SUPPLIED: Cap: 65mg

WARNINGS/PRECAUTIONS: Drug dependence potential. May impair mental/physical ability for operating machinery. Caution with hepatic or renal impairment and the elderly. Not for suicidal or addiction-prone patients. Do not exceed recommended dose.

ADVERSE REACTIONS: Dizziness, sedation, nausea, vomiting, liver dysfunction.

INTERACTIONS: Additive CNS-depressant effect with other CNS depressants, including alcohol. Increases plasma levels of antidepressants, anticonvulsants, and coumarins. Severe neurologic signs, including coma reported with carbamazepine. Caution with tranquilizers, antidepressants, and with excessive alcohol use.

PREGNANCY: Not for use in pregnancy, unknown use in nursing.
MECHANISM OF ACTION: Centrally acting narcotic analgesic agent.
PHARMACOKINETICS: Absorption: T_{max}=2-2.5 hrs; C_{max}=0.05-0.1mcg/mL.
Distribution: Found in human breast milk. **Metabolism:** Liver; norpropoxyphene (active metabolite). **Elimination:** $T_{1/2}$=6-12 hrs, 30-36 hrs (norpropoxyphene).

DARVON-N
propoxyphene napsylate (Xanodyne)

CIV

THERAPEUTIC CLASS: Opioid analgesic

INDICATIONS: Relief of mild to moderate pain.

DOSAGE: *Adults:* Usual: 100mg q4h prn pain. Max: 600mg/day. Elderly: Increase dose interval. Hepatic/Renal Impairment: Reduce daily dose.

HOW SUPPLIED: Tab: 100mg

WARNINGS/PRECAUTIONS: Avoid in suicidal or addiction-prone patients. May produce drug dependence in higher than recommended doses. May impair mental/physical ability. Caution with hepatic or renal impairment. Do not exceed recommended dose and limit alcohol intake.

ADVERSE REACTIONS: Dizziness, sedation, nausea, vomiting, constipation, abdominal pain, skin rashes, lightheadedness, headache, weakness, euphoria, dysphoria, hallucination.

INTERACTIONS: Additive CNS-depressant effect with other CNS depressants, including alcohol. Increases plasma levels of antidepressants, anticonvulsants and warfarin-like drugs. Severe neurologic signs, including coma reported with carbamazepine. Caution with tranquilizers, antidepressants, and excessive alcohol use.

PREGNANCY: Safety in pregnancy and nursing not known.

MECHANISM OF ACTION: Opioid analgesic; centrally acting narcotic analgesic.

PHARMACOKINETICS: Absorption: C_{max}=0.05-0.1mcg/mL; T_{max}=2-2.5 hrs.
Distribution: Found in human breast milk. **Metabolism:** Liver; norpropoxyphene (active metabolite). **Elimination:** $T_{1/2}$=6-12 hrs, 30-36 hrs (active metabolite).

DAUNORUBICIN
daunorubicin citrate liposome (Various)

RX

> Monitor for cardiac toxicity. Severe myelosuppression may occur. Reduce dose with hepatic dysfunction. A triad of back pain, flushing, and chest tightness reported during 1st 5 minutes of infusion; resume infusion at slower rate. Administer only under supervision of a physician experienced in the use of antineoplastic agents.

OTHER BRAND NAMES: DaunoXome (Gilead)

THERAPEUTIC CLASS: Anthracycline

INDICATIONS: First line cytotoxic therapy for advanced HIV-associated Kaposi's sarcoma.

DOSAGE: *Adults:* 40mg/m² IV infusion; repeat every 2 weeks until evidence of progressive disease or until other complications of HIV preclude continuation.

HOW SUPPLIED: Inj: 2mg/mL

WARNINGS/PRECAUTIONS: Primary toxicity is myelosuppression; careful hematologic monitoring (prior to each dose) required. Evaluate cardiac function before each course and determine left ventricular ejection fraction (LVEF) at total cumulative dose of 320mg/m², and every 160mg/m² thereafter. Monitor LVEF at cumulative doses prior to therapy and every 160mg/m² in those with prior anthracycline therapy, pre-existing cardiac disease, or previous radiotherapy. Avoid extravasation. Can cause fetal harm during pregnancy.

ADVERSE REACTIONS: Myelosuppression, alopecia, cardiomyopathy with CHF, nausea, vomiting, fatigue, fever, diarrhea, cough, dyspnea, abdominal pain, anorexia, rigors, back pain, increased sweating, rhinitis, neuropathy.

PREGNANCY: Category D, safety in nursing not known.

MECHANISM OF ACTION: Anthracycline antibiotic; produces antineoplastic activity. Liposomal preparation helps to maximize selectivity for solid tumors. Specific mechanism not established. Believed to be a function of increased permeability of the tumor neovasculature to particles in the size range of the medication.

PHARMACOKINETICS: Distribution: V_d=6.4L. **Metabolism:** Daunorubicinol (major active metabolite). **Elimination:** $T_{1/2}$=4.4 hrs.

DAYPRO   RX
oxaprozin (Pharmacia & Upjohn)

> NSAIDs may cause an increased risk of serious cardiovascular thrombotic events, MI, stroke and serious GI adverse events including bleeding, ulceration, and perforation of the stomach or intestines. Contraindicated for the treatment of perioperative pain in the setting of coronary artery bypass graft (CABG) surgery.

THERAPEUTIC CLASS: NSAID (propionic acid derivative)

INDICATIONS: Relief of signs and symptoms of osteoarthritis (OA), rheumatoid arthritis (RA), and juvenile rheumatoid arthritis (JRA).

DOSAGE: *Adults:* RA: 1200mg qd. Max: 1800mg/day in divided doses (not to exceed 26mg/kg/day). OA: 1200mg qd, give 600mg qd for low weight or milder disease. Max: 1800mg/day in divided doses (not to exceed 26mg/kg/day). Renal Dysfunction/Hemodialysis: Initial: 600mg qd. *Pediatrics:* 6-16yrs: JRA: ≥55kg: 1200mg qd. 32-54kg: 900mg qd. 22-31kg: 600mg qd.

HOW SUPPLIED: Tab: 600mg* *scored

CONTRAINDICATIONS: Complete or partial syndrome of nasal polyps, angioedema and bronchospastic reactivity to ASA or other NSAIDs. Treatment of perioperative pain in the setting of CABG surgery.

WARNINGS/PRECAUTIONS: May lead to onset of new HTN or worsening of pre-existing HTN; monitor BP closely. Fluid retention and edema reported; caution with fluid retention or heart failure. Renal papillary necrosis and other renal injury reported after long-term use. Not recommended for use with advanced renal disease; if therapy must be initiated, monitor renal function. Anaphylactoid reactions may occur. May cause serious skin adverse events (eg, exfoliative dermatitis, Stevens-Johnson syndrome, and toxic epidermal necrolysis). Avoid in late pregnancy; may cause premature closure of ductus arteriosus. May cause elevations of LFTs; d/c if liver disease develops or systemic manifestations occur. Caution in elderly. Anemia may occur; with long-term use, monitor Hgb/Hct if signs or symptoms of anemia develop. May inhibit platelet aggregation and prolong bleeding time; monitor with coagulation disorders. Caution with asthma and avoid with ASA-sensitive asthma. Rash and/or mild photosensitivity reactions reported.

ADVERSE REACTIONS: Constipation, diarrhea, dyspepsia, flatulence, nausea, rash.

INTERACTIONS: Avoid with ASA. Caution with oral anticoagulants. Reduces effects of ACE-inhibitors, furosemide, and thiazides. Increases lithium levels and toxicity of methotrexate. Monitor BP with β-blockers.

PREGNANCY: Category C, not for use in nursing.

MECHANISM OF ACTION: NSAIDs; unknown, suspected to inhibit prostaglandin synthetase.

PHARMACOKINETICS: Absorption: 95% absorbed. **Distribution:** V_d/F=11-17L/70kg; Plasma protein binding (99%); Exreted in human milk. **Metabolism:** Liver via oxidation (65%) and glucuronic acid conjugation (35%). **Elimination:** Feces (35%), urine (5% unchanged, 65% as metabolite); $T_{1/2}$=22 hrs.

DAYTRANA
methylphenidate (Shire)

`CII`

THERAPEUTIC CLASS: Sympathomimetic amine

INDICATIONS: Treatment of attention deficit hyperactivity disorder (ADHD).

DOSAGE: *Adults:* Individualize dose. Apply to hip area 2 hrs before effect is needed and remove 9 hrs after application. Recommended Titration Schedule: Week 1: 10mg/9 hrs. Week 2: 15mg/9 hrs. Week 3: 20mg/9 hrs. Week 4: 30mg/9 hrs.
Pediatrics: ≥6 yrs: Individualize dose. Apply to hip area 2 hrs before effect is needed and remove 9 hrs after application. Recommended Titration Schedule: Week 1: 10mg/9 hrs. Week 2: 15mg/9 hrs. Week 3: 20mg/9 hrs. Week 4: 30mg/9 hrs.

HOW SUPPLIED: Patch: 10mg/9 hrs, 15mg/9 hrs, 20mg/9 hrs, 30mg/9 hrs [10^s, 30^s]

CONTRAINDICATIONS: Marked anxiety, tension, and agitation; glaucoma; motor tics or family history or diagnosis of Tourette's syndrome; treatment with MAOIs and within minimum of 14 days following discontinuation.

WARNINGS/PRECAUTIONS: Avoid use with known structural cardiac abnormalities; sudden death reported. D/C if contact sensitization is suspected. Monitor growth during treatment. May exacerbate symptoms of behavior disturbance and thought disorder in psychotic patients. Caution when using stimulants to treat patients with comorbid bipolar disorder because of concern for possible induction of mixed/manic episode in such patients. Stimulants at usual doses can cause treatment emergent psychotic or manic symptoms (eg, hallucinations, delusional thinking, mania) in children and adolescents without prior history of psychotic illness. Aggressive behavior or hostility reported in clinical trials and postmarketing experience of some medications indicated for the treatment of ADHD. May lower convulsive threshold; d/c in the presence of seizures. Caution with HTN; monitor BP. Caution when underlying medical conditions might be compromised by increases in BP or HR (eg, pre-existing HTN, heart failure, recent MI, or hyperthyroidism). Visual disturbances reported. Caution with history of drug dependence or alcoholism. Avoid exposing application site to external heat sources (eg, heating pads, electric blankets, heated water beds, etc). Monitor CBC, differential, and platelet counts during prolonged therapy.

ADVERSE REACTIONS: Nausea, vomiting, nasopharyngitis, weight decrease, anorexia, decreased appetite, affect lability, insomnia, tic, nasal congestion.

INTERACTIONS: See Contraindications. Caution with pressor agents. May decrease effectiveness of antihypertensive agents. May inhibit metabolism of coumarin anticoagulants, anticonvulsants (eg, phenobarbital, phenytoin, primidone), some tricyclic drugs (eg, imipramine, clomipramine, desipramine), and SSRIs. Monitor drug levels (or coagulation times with coumarin) and consider dose adjustments with concomitant use. Serious adverse events reported with concomitant clonidine use.

PREGNANCY: Category C, caution in nursing.

MECHANISM OF ACTION: Sympathomimetic amine; CNS stimulant. Suspected to block reuptake of norepinephrine and dopamine into presynaptic neuron; increases release of monoamines into neuronal spaces.

PHARMACOKINETICS: Absorption: C_{max}=39ng/mL; T_{max}=7.5-10.5 hrs.
Distribution: Plasma concentrations decline in biexponential manner due to continued distribution from skin after patch removal. **Metabolism:** De-esterification; ritalinic acid (metabolite). **Elimination:** $T_{1/2}$=3-4 hrs (*d*-methylphenidate); $T_{1/2}$=1.4-2.9 hrs (*l*-methylphenidate).

DDAVP
RX
desmopressin acetate (Sanofi-Aventis)

OTHER BRAND NAMES: DDAVP Nasal Spray (Sanofi-Aventis) - DDAVP Rhinal Tube (Sanofi-Aventis)

THERAPEUTIC CLASS: Synthetic vasopressin analog

INDICATIONS: (Tab) Management of primary nocturnal enuresis. (Inj/Nasal Spray/Rhinal Tube/Tab) As antidiuretic replacement therapy in management of central (cranial) diabetes insipidus. Management of temporary polyuria and polydipsia following head trauma or surgery in pituitary region. (Inj) Hemophilia A with factor VIII coagulant activity levels >5% and mild to moderate classic von Willebrand's disease (Type I) with factor VIII levels >5%.

DOSAGE: *Adults:* Diabetes Insipidus: (Tab) Initial: 0.05mg bid. Titrate: May increase/decrease by 0.1-1.2mg/day given bid-tid. Maint: 0.1-0.8mg/day in divided doses. (Spray/Tube) Usual: 0.1-4mL/day given qd-tid. (Inj) 0.5-1mL/day IV/SQ given bid. Hemophilia A/von Willebrand's Disease: (Inj) 0.3mcg/kg IV over 15-30 min. Add 50mL diluent. If used pre-op, give 30 min before procedure.
Pediatrics: Diabetes Insipidus: (Tab) ≥4 yrs: Initial: 0.05mg bid. Titrate: May increase/decrease by 0.1-1.2mg/day given bid-tid. Maint: 0.1-0.8mg/day in divided doses. (Spray/Tube) 3 months-12 yrs: Usual: 0.05-0.3mL/day given qd-bid. (Inj) ≥12 yrs: 0.5-1mL/day IV/SQ given bid. Hemophilia A/von Willebrand's Disease: (Inj) ≥3 months: 0.3mcg/kg IV over 15-30 min. Add 50mL diluent (>10kg) or 10mL diluent (≤10kg). If used pre-op, give 30 min before procedure.

HOW SUPPLIED: Inj: 4mcg/mL; Nasal Spray: 10mcg/inh [5mL]; Tab: 0.1mg*, 0.2mg*; Rhinal Tube: 0.01% [2.5mL] *scored

CONTRAINDICATIONS: Moderate to severe renal impairment (CrCL<50mL/min), hyponatremia, or history of hyponatremia.

WARNINGS/PRECAUTIONS: Mucosal changes with nasal forms may occur; d/c until resolved. Decrease fluid intake in pediatrics and elderly to decrease risk of water intoxication and hyponatremia; monitor osmolality. Caution with coronary artery insufficiency, hypertensive cardiovascular disease, fluid and electrolyte imbalance (eg, cystic fibrosis). Anaphylaxis reported with IV use. Caution with IV use if history of thrombus formation. For diabetes insipidus, dosage must be adjusted according to diurnal pattern of response; estimate response by adequate duration of sleep and adequate, not excessive, water turnover.

ADVERSE REACTIONS: Inj: Headache, nausea, abdominal cramps, vulval pain, injection site reactions, facial flushing, BP changes. Spray: Headache, dizziness, rhinitis, nausea, nasal congestion, sore throat, cough, respiratory infection, epistaxis. Tab: Nausea, flushing, abdominal cramps, headache, increased SGOT, water intoxication, hyponatremia.

INTERACTIONS: Caution with other pressor agents.

PREGNANCY: Category B, caution in nursing.

MECHANISM OF ACTION: Synthetic vasopressin analog; antidiuretic affecting renal water conservation.

PHARMACOKINETICS: Absorption: (Inj) Rapid, T_{max}=90 min-2 hrs; (Tab, Nasal) Rapid, T_{max}=0.9-1.5 hrs. **Elimination:** Urine; (Inj, Nasal) $T_{1/2}$=3 hrs; (Tab) 1.5-2.5 hrs.

DECLOMYCIN
RX
demeclocycline HCL (Wyeth)

THERAPEUTIC CLASS: Tetracycline derivative

INDICATIONS: Treatment of infections due to rickettsiae, *Mycoplasma pneumoniae, B.recurrentis*, agents of psittacosis, ornithosis, lymphomagranuloma venereum or granuloma inguinale. Treatment of gram-negative infections (eg, respiratory, urinary tract), gram-positive infections (eg, respiratory tract, skin and soft tissue), trachoma, inclusion conjunctivitis. When PCN is contraindicated, treatment of gonorrhea, syphilis, listeriosis, anthrax, *Clostridium* species, and others. Adjunct therapy for amebicides.

DOSAGE: *Adults:* Usual: 150mg qid or 300mg bid. Gonorrhea: 600mg followed by 300mg q12h for 4 days to a total of 3g. Renal/Hepatic Impairment: Reduce dose and/or extend dose intervals. Continue therapy for at least 24-48 hrs after symptoms subside. Treat strep infections for at least 10 days. Take at least 1 hr before or 2 hrs after meals with plenty of fluids.
Pediatrics: >8 yrs: Usual: 7-13mg/kg/day divided bid-qid. Max: 600mg/day. Renal/Hepatic Impairment: Reduce dose and/or extend dose intervals. Continue therapy for at least 24-48 hrs after symptoms subside. Treat strep infections for at least 10 days. Take at least 1 hr before or 2 hrs after meals with plenty of fluids.

HOW SUPPLIED: Tab: 150mg, 300mg

CONTRAINDICATIONS: Hypersensitivity to any of the tetracyclines.

WARNINGS/PRECAUTIONS: May cause fetal harm during pregnancy. Use during tooth development (last half of pregnancy, infancy, <8 yrs), or long-term use, or repeated short-term use may cause permanent discoloration of the teeth. Pseudotumor cerebri (adults), bulging fontanels (infants) reported. Caution with renal or hepatic impairment. Long-term use may cause reversible, nephrogenic diabetes insipidus syndrome. May result in overgrowth of nonsusceptible organisms; d/c if superinfection develops. CNS symptoms may occur; caution when operating machinery. May decrease bone growth in premature infants. Monitor hematopoietic, renal, and hepatic function with long-term use. D/C at first evidence of skin erythema after sun/UV light exposure.

ADVERSE REACTIONS: GI problems, rash, esophageal ulceration, hypersensitivity reactions, dizziness, headache, tinnitus, blood dyscrasias, photosensitivity reactions, enamel hypoplasia, elevated BUN, acute renal failure.

INTERACTIONS: Decreases PT; may need to decrease dose of anticoagulants. May interfere with bactericidal action of PCN; avoid concomitant use. May decrease efficacy of oral contraceptives; use alternate method. Decreased absorption with antacids and iron-containing products. Fatal renal toxicity with methoxyflurane reported. Foods/dairy products interfere with absorption.

PREGNANCY: Category D, not for use in nursing.

MECHANISM OF ACTION: Tetracycline; thought to inhibit protein synthesis.

PHARMACOKINETICS: Absorption: T_{max}=4 hrs. **Distribution:** Plasma protein binding (40%), found in breast milk. **Elimination:** Feces (13 and 46%); active drug and urine (44%); $T_{1/2}$=10-16 hrs.

DELATESTRYL
testosterone enanthate (Indevus)

CIII

THERAPEUTIC CLASS: Androgen

INDICATIONS: Testosterone replacement in males with primary hypogonadism and hypogonadotropic hypogonadism. To stimulate puberty in males with delayed puberty. May also be used secondarily in females with advancing inoperable metastatic (skeletal) mammary cancer who are 1-5 years postmenopausal.

DOSAGE: *Adults:* Dose based on age, sex, and diagnosis. Adjust dose according to response and adverse reactions. Male Hypogonadism: 50-400mg IM every 2-4 weeks. Delayed Puberty: 50-200mg every 2-4 weeks for a limited duration (eg, 4-6 months). Breast Cancer: 200-400mg every 2-4 weeks.
Pediatrics: Dose based on age, sex, and diagnosis. Adjust dose according to response and adverse reactions. Male Hypogonadism: 50-400mg IM every 2-4 weeks. Delayed Puberty: 50-200mg every 2-4 weeks for a limited duration (eg, 4-6 months). Caution in children.

HOW SUPPLIED: Inj: 200mg/mL

CONTRAINDICATIONS: Breast or prostate carcinoma in men. Pregnancy.

WARNINGS/PRECAUTIONS: D/C if hypercalcemia occurs in breast cancer or immobilized patients; monitor calcium levels. Risk of hepatic adenomas, hepatocellular carcinoma, and peliosis hepatitis with prolonged high doses. D/C if jaundice, cholestatic hepatitis, or abnormal LFTs occur. Avoid use in elderly who has age related hypogonadism. D/C if edema occurs in patients with pre-existing cardiac, renal, or hepatic disease; restart at lower dose. Risk of compromised stature in children; monitor bone growth every 6 months. Monitor for virilization in females. Caution with a history of MI or CAD due to altered serum cholesterol levels. Monitor cholesterol, LFTs, Hct, Hgb periodically.

ADVERSE REACTIONS: Amenorrhea, virilization, menstrual irregularities, gynecomastia, excessive frequency/duration of penile erections, male pattern baldness, increased/decreased libido, oligospermia, hirsutism, acne, fluid and electrolyte disturbances, nausea, hypercholesterolemia, clotting factor suppression, polycythemia, altered LFTs, oligospermia, anxiety, depression.

INTERACTIONS: Potentiates oral anticoagulants and oxyphenbutazone. May decrease blood glucose and insulin requirements. ACTH and corticosteroids may enhance edema.

PREGNANCY: Category X, not for use in nursing.

MECHANISM OF ACTION: Endogenous androgen; responsible for normal growth and development of male sex organs and for maintenance of secondary sex characteristics.

PHARMACOKINETICS: Absorption: Slow. **Distribution:** Plasma protein binding (98%). **Metabolism:** Liver. **Elimination:** Urine (90%), feces (6%); $T_{1/2}$=10-100 minutes.

DELESTROGEN   RX
estradiol valerate (King)

> Estrogens increase the risk of endometrial cancer. Estrogens and progestins should not be used for the prevention of CVD. Increased risks of MI, stroke, invasive breast cancer, PE, and DVT in postmenopausal women (50-79 yrs of age) reported. Increased risk of developing probable dementia in postmenopausal women ≥65 yrs of age reported.

THERAPEUTIC CLASS: Estrogen

INDICATIONS: Treatment of moderate to severe vasomotor symptoms and vulvar/vaginal atrophy associated with menopause. Treatment of hypoestrogenism due to hypogonadism, castration, or primary ovarian failure. Palliative treatment of advanced androgen-dependent prostate carcinoma.

DOSAGE: *Adults:* Vasomotor Symptoms/Vaginal/Vulval Atrophy: 10-20mg IM every 4 weeks. Discontinue or taper at 3-6 month intervals. Hypoestrogenism: 10-20mg IM every 4 weeks. Prostate Carcinoma: 30mg or more every 1 or 2 weeks.

HOW SUPPLIED: Inj: 10mg/mL, 20mg/mL, 40mg/mL

CONTRAINDICATIONS: Pregnancy, undiagnosed abnormal genital bleeding, breast cancer, estrogen-dependent neoplasia, thrombophlebitis, thromboembolic disorders.

WARNINGS/PRECAUTIONS: May increase risk of cardiovascular events (eg, MI, stroke), venous thrombosis, and PE; d/c immediately if any of these events occur or are suspected. May increase risk of breast/endometrial cancer, and gallbladder disease. May lead to severe hypercalcemia with breast cancer and bone metastases; monitor and d/c if hypercalcemia occurs. Retinal vascular thrombosis reported; monitor and d/c if papilledema or retinal vascular lesions occur. Consider addition of a progestin if no hysterectomy. May elevate BP; monitor at regular intervals. May cause elevations of plasma triglycerides with pre-existing hypertriglyceridemia. Caution with history of cholestatic jaundice associated with past estrogen use or with pregnancy; d/c with recurrence. May lead to increased thyroid-binding globulin levels; monitor thyroid function. May cause fluid retention; caution with cardiac/renal dysfunction. Caution with severe hypocalcemia. May increase risk of ovarian cancer. May exacerbate endometriosis, asthma, DM, epilepsy, migraine, porphyria, SLE, and hepatic hemangiomas; use with caution. May cause hypercoagulability. May develop uterine bleeding and mastodynia.

ADVERSE REACTIONS: Altered vaginal bleeding, vaginal candidiasis, breast tenderness/enlargement, GI effects, CNS effects, chloasma, melasma, weight changes, edema, altered libido.

PREGNANCY: Contraindicated in pregnancy, caution in nursing.

MECHANISM OF ACTION: Estrogen; acts by binding to nuclear receptors in estrogen-responsive tissues. Modulates pituitary secretion of gonadotrophins, luteinizing hormone (LH) and follicle stimulating hormone (FSH), through negative feedback mechanism.

PHARMACOKINETICS: Absorption: Well-absorbed. **Distribution:** Widely-distributed; primarily bound to sex hormone binding globulin (SHBG) and albumin. Estrogens found in breast milk. **Metabolism:** Liver, to estrone (metabolite); estriol (major urinary metabolite); enterohepatic recirculation via sulfate and glucuronide conjugation; biliary secretion into intestine; hydrolysis in gut; CYP3A4 (partial). **Excretion:** Urine (estradiol, estrone, estriol).

DEMADEX RX
torsemide (Roche Labs)

THERAPEUTIC CLASS: Loop diuretic

INDICATIONS: Treatment of edema associated with CHF, renal disease, chronic renal failure or hepatic disease. Treatment of hypertension.

DOSAGE: *Adults:* PO/IV (bolus over 2 min or continuous): CHF: Initial: 10-20mg qd. Max: 200mg single dose. Chronic Renal Failure: Initial: 20mg qd. Max: 200mg single dose. Hepatic Cirrhosis: Initial: 5-10mg qd with aldosterone antagonist or K⁺-sparing diuretic. Titrate: Double dose. Max: 40mg single dose. HTN: Initial: 5mg qd. Titrate: May increase to 10mg qd in 4-6 weeks, then may add additional antihypertensive agent.

HOW SUPPLIED: Inj: 10mg/mL; Tab: 5mg*, 10mg*, 20mg*, 100mg* *scored

CONTRAINDICATIONS: Anuria, sulfonamide hypersensitivity.

WARNINGS/PRECAUTIONS: Caution with cirrhosis and ascites in hepatic disease. Tinnitus and hearing loss (usually reversible) reported. Avoid excessive diuresis, especially in elderly. Caution with brisk diuresis, inadequate oral intake of electrolytes, and cardiovascular disease, especially with digitalis glycosides. Monitor for electrolyte/volume depletion. Hyperglycemia, hypokalemia, hypermagnesemia, hypercalcemia, gout reported. May increase cholesterol and TG.

ADVERSE REACTIONS: Headache, excessive urination, dizziness, cough, ECG abnormality, asthenia, rhinitis, diarrhea.

INTERACTIONS: Caution with high-dose salicylates, aminoglycosides. Lithium toxicity. Indomethacin partially inhibits natriuretic effect. Avoid simultaneous cholestyramine administration. Probenecid decreases effects. Reduces spironolactone clearance. Risk of hypokalemia with ACTH, corticosteroids. Possible renal dysfunction with NSAIDs.

PREGNANCY: Category B, caution in nursing.

MECHANISM OF ACTION: Pyridine-sulfonylurea diuretic; acts within lumen of thick ascending part of loop of Henle, inhibiting Na⁺/K⁺/2 Cl⁻ carrier system.

PHARMACOKINETICS: Absorption: Absolute bioavailability (80%); T_{max}=1 hr. **Distribution:** Plasma protein binding (>99%); V_d=12-15L. **Metabolism:** Carboxylic acid (major metabolite). **Elimination:** Urine; $T_{1/2}$=3.5 hrs.

DEMEROL INJECTION CII
meperidine HCL (Hospira)

THERAPEUTIC CLASS: Opioid analgesic

INDICATIONS: For relief of moderate to severe pain. For preoperative medication, anesthesia support, and obstetrical analgesia.

DOSAGE: *Adults:* Pain: Usual: 50-150mg IM/SQ q3-4h prn. Preoperative: Usual: 50-100mg IM/SQ 30-90 min before anesthesia. Anesthesia Support: Use repeated slow IV inj of fractional doses (eg, 10mg/mL) or continuous IV infusion of a more dilute solution (eg, 1mg/mL). Titrate as needed. Obstetrical Analgesia: Usual: 50-100mg IM/SQ when pain is regular, may repeat at 1- to 3-hr intervals. Elderly: Start at lower end of dosage range and observe. With Phenothiazines/Other Tranquilizers: Reduce dose by 25 to 50%). IM method preferred with repeated use. For IV inj: Reduce dose and administer slowly, preferably using diluted solution.
Pediatrics: Pain: Usual: 0.5-0.8mg/lb IM/SQ, up to 50-150mg, q3-4h prn. Preoperative: Usual: 0.5-1mg/lb IM/SQ, up to 50-100mg, 30-90 min before anesthesia. With Phenothiazines/Other Tranquilizers: Reduce dose by 25 to 50%). IM method preferred with repeated use. For IV inj: Reduce dose and administer slowly, preferably using diluted solution.

HOW SUPPLIED: Inj: 25mg/mL, 50mg/mL, 75mg/mL, 100mg/mL

CONTRAINDICATIONS: MAOIs during or within 14 days of use.

WARNINGS/PRECAUTIONS: May develop tolerance and dependence; abuse potential. Extreme caution with head injury, increased ICP, intracranial lesions, acute asthmatic attack, chronic COPD or cor pulmonale, decreased respiratory reserve, respiratory depression, hypoxia, and hypercapnia. Rapid IV infusion may result in increased adverse reactions. Caution with acute abdominal conditions, atrial flutter, supraventricular tachycardias. May aggravate convulsive disorders. Caution and reduce initial dose with elderly or debilitated, renal/hepatic impairment, hypothyroidism, Addison's disease, prostatic hypertrophy or urethral stricture. Severe hypotension may occur post-op or if depleted blood volume. Orthostatic hypotension may occur. May impair mental/physical abilities. Not for use in pregnancy prior to labor. May produce depression of respiration and psychophysiologic functions in the newborn when used as an obstetrical analgesic.

ADVERSE REACTIONS: Lightheadedness, dizziness, sedation, nausea, vomiting, sweating, respiratory/circulatory depression.

INTERACTIONS: See Contraindications. Caution and reduce dose with other CNS depressants (eg, narcotics, anesthetics, phenothiazines, tranquilizers, sedative-hypnotics, TCAs, alcohol).

PREGNANCY: Safety in pregnancy and nursing not known.

MECHANISM OF ACTION: Narcotic analgesic; produces actions similiar to morphine. Principle actions involve the CNS and organs composed of smooth muscle. Produces analgesic and sedative effects.

PHARMACOKINETICS: Distribution: Crosses placental barrier; found in breast milk.

DEMEROL ORAL
meperidine HCL (Sanofi-Aventis)   CII

THERAPEUTIC CLASS: Opioid analgesic

INDICATIONS: Moderate to severe pain.

DOSAGE: *Adults:* Usual: 50-150mg q3-4h prn. Concomitant Phenothiazines/Other Tranquilizers: Reduce dose by 25-50%. Dilute syrup in 1/2 glass of water. *Pediatrics:* Usual: 1.1-1.8mg/kg up to 50-150mg q3-4h prn. Concomitant Phenothiazines/Other Tranquilizers: Reduce dose by 25-50%. Dilute syrup in 1/2 glass of water.

HOW SUPPLIED: Syrup: 50mg/5mL; Tab: 50mg*, 100mg *scored

CONTRAINDICATIONS: MAOI during or within 14 days of use.

WARNINGS/PRECAUTIONS: May develop tolerance and dependence; abuse potential. Extreme caution with head injury, increased ICP, intracranial lesions, acute asthma attack, chronic COPD, cor pulmonale, decreased respiratory reserve, respiratory depression, hypoxia, and hypercapnia. Caution with sickle cell anemia, pheochromocytoma, acute alcoholism, Addison's disease, CNS depression or coma, delirium tremens, elderly or debilitated, kyphoscoliosis associated with respiratory depression, myxedema, hypothyroidism, acute abdominal conditions, epilepsy, atrial flutter, other supraventricular tachycardias, renal or hepatic impairment, prostatic hypertrophy, urethral stricture, drug dependencies, neonates, and young infants. Severe hypotension may occur post-op or if depleted blood volume. Orthostatic hypotension may occur. Not for use in pregnancy prior to labor.

ADVERSE REACTIONS: Lightheadedness, dizziness, sedation, nausea, vomiting, sweating, respiratory depression.

INTERACTIONS: See Contraindications. Reduce dose with other CNS depressants (eg, narcotics, anesthetics, phenothiazines, tranquilizers, sedative-hypnotics, TCAs, alcohol). Mixed agonist/antagonist analgesics (eg, pentazocine, nalbuphine, butorphanol, buprenorphine) may reduce analgesic effects and/or precipitate withdrawal symptoms. Caution with acyclovir, cimetidine. Phenytoin may enhance hepatic metabolism. May enhance neuroblocking action of skeletal muscle relaxants. Increased levels with ritonavir; avoid concurrent administration.

PREGNANCY: Category C, not for use in nursing.

MECHANISM OF ACTION: Narcotic analgesic; produces actions similiar to morphine. Principle actions involve the CNS and organs composed of smooth muscle. Produces analgesic and sedative effects.

PHARMACOKINETICS: Distribution: Crosses placental barrier; found in breast milk.

DEMSER   RX
metyrosine (Aton)

THERAPEUTIC CLASS: Tyrosine hydroxylase inhibitor

INDICATIONS: Treatment of pheochromocytoma for preoperative preparation and when surgery is contraindicated. Chronic treatment with malignant pheochromocytoma.

DOSAGE: *Adults:* Initial: 250mg qid. Titrate: May increase by 250-500mg/day. Max: 4g/day. Titrate based on clinical symptoms and catecholamine excretion. Usual: 2-3g/day. Preoperative Preparation: Take 5-7 days before surgery. *Pediatrics:* ≥12 yrs: Initial: 250mg qid. Titrate: May increase by 250-500mg/day. Max: 4g/day. Titrate based on clinical symptoms and catecholamine excretion. Usual: 2-3g/day. Preoperative Preparation: Take 5-7 days before surgery.

HOW SUPPLIED: Cap: 250mg

WARNINGS/PRECAUTIONS: When used preoperatively or with α-adrenergic blockers, maintain intravascular volume intra- and post-operatively to avoid hypotension and decreased perfusion. Maintain adequate water intake to achieve urine volume of ≥2000mL to prevent crystalluria. Risk of hypertensive crisis or arrhythmias during tumor manipulation. Monitor BP and ECG continuously during surgery.

ADVERSE REACTIONS: Sedation, EPS, anxiety, depression, hallucinations, disorientation, confusion, diarrhea.

INTERACTIONS: Additive sedative effects with alcohol and other CNS depressants (eg, hypnotics, sedatives, tranquilizers). May potentiate EPS with phenothiazines and haloperidol.

PREGNANCY: Category C, caution in nursing.

MECHANISM OF ACTION: Tyrosine hydroxylase inhibitor; inhibits conversion of tyrosine to dihydroxyphenylalanine (DOPA), resulting in decreased catecholamines.

PHARMACOKINETICS: Elimination: Urine (69%); T$_{1/2}$=3-3.7 hrs.

DEMULEN   RX
ethynodiol diacetate - ethinyl estradiol (Pharmacia & Upjohn)

OTHER BRAND NAMES: Zovia (Watson)

THERAPEUTIC CLASS: Estrogen/progestogen combination

INDICATIONS: Prevention of pregnancy.

DOSAGE: *Adults:* Start 1st Sunday after menses begin or 1st day of menses. *21-day:* 1 tab qd for 21 days, stop 7 days, then repeat. *28-day:* 1 tab qd for 28 days, then repeat.

HOW SUPPLIED: (Ethinyl Estradiol-Ethynodiol Diacetate) Tab: (1/35) 0.035mg-1mg; (1/50) 0.05mg-1mg

CONTRAINDICATIONS: Thrombophlebitis, DVT or thromboembolic disorders, pregnancy, cerebrovascular or coronary artery disease, undiagnosed abnormal genital bleeding, cholestatic jaundice of pregnancy or jaundice with prior pill use, hepatic adenomas or carcinomas, breast cancer or other estrogen-dependent neoplasia.

WARNINGS/PRECAUTIONS: Cigarette smoking increases risk of serious cardiovascular side effects. This risk increases with age (especially >35 yrs) and heavy smoking. Increased risk of MI, vascular disease, thromboembolism, stroke and gallbladder disease. Retinal thrombosis, hepatic neoplasia, carcinoma of breast and reproductive organs reported. May cause glucose intolerance. May increase BP, elevate LDL levels or cause other lipid changes, fluid retention, breakthrough bleeding, and spotting. May cause or exacerbate migraine. May develop visual changes with contact lens. Increased risk of MI with HTN, hyperlipidemia, obesity, and diabetes. D/C if develop jaundice, significant depression or ophthalmic irregularities. Perform annual physical exam. Use before menarche is not indicated. May affect certain endocrine, LFTs and blood components.

ADVERSE REACTIONS: Nausea, vomiting, breakthrough bleeding, spotting, amenorrhea, migraine, depression, vaginal candidiasis, edema, weight changes.

INTERACTIONS: Reduced effects, increased breakthrough bleeding, and menstrual irregularities with rifampin, barbiturates, phenylbutazone, phenytoin, and possibly with griseofulvin, ampicillin, and tetracyclines. Troglitazone reduces plasma levels of hormones.

PREGNANCY: Category X, not for use in nursing.

DENAVIR   RX
penciclovir (Novartis)

THERAPEUTIC CLASS: Nucleoside analogue

INDICATIONS: Treatment of recurrent herpes labialis (cold sores) in adults and children ≥12 yrs.

DOSAGE: *Adults:* Apply q2h while awake for 4 days. Start with earliest sign or symptom.
Pediatrics: ≥12 yrs: Apply q2h while awake for 4 days. Start with earliest sign or symptom.

HOW SUPPLIED: Cre: 1% [1.5g]

WARNINGS/PRECAUTIONS: Only use on herpes labialis on the lips and face. Avoid mucous membranes or near the eyes. Effectiveness not established in immunocompromised patients.

ADVERSE REACTIONS: Headache, application site reaction, local anesthesia, taste perversion, rash.

PREGNANCY: Category B, not for use in nursing.

MECHANISM OF ACTION: Antiviral agent. Active against herpes simplex virus types 1 (HSV-1) and 2 (HSV-2). Inhibits HSV polymerase competitively with deoxyguanosine triphosphate. Consequently, herpes viral DNA synthesis and replication are selectively inhibited.

DEPACON RX

valproate sodium (Abbott)

> Fatal hepatic failure (<2 yrs at considerable risk), teratogenic effects (eg, neural tube defects), and life-threatening pancreatitis reported.

THERAPEUTIC CLASS: Carboxylic acid derivative

INDICATIONS: Monotherapy and adjunctive therapy for treatment of simple and complex absence seizures, and complex partial seizures. Adjunct therapy for multiple seizure types.

DOSAGE: *Adults:* Simplex/Complex Absence Seizure: Initial: 15mg/kg/day. Titrate: Increase weekly by 5-10mg/kg/day until optimal response. Max: 60mg/kg/day. Complex Partial Seizure: Initial: 10-15mg/kg/day. Titrate: Increase weekly by 5-10mg/kg/day until optimal response. Max: 60mg/kg/day. Elderly: Reduce initial dose and titrate slowly. If dose >250mg/day, give in divided doses. Administer as 60 min IV infusion, not >20mg/min. Not for use >14 days; switch to oral route as soon as clinically feasible. Decrease dose or d/c if decreased food or fluid intake or if excessive somnolence occurs.
Pediatrics: ≥2 yrs: Simplex/Complex Absence Seizure: Initial: 15mg/kg/day. Titrate: Increase weekly by 5-10mg/kg/day until optimal response. Max: 60mg/kg/day. ≥10 yrs: Complex Partial Seizure: Initial: 10-15mg/kg/day. Titrate: Increase weekly by 5-10mg/kg/day until optimal response. Max: 60mg/kg/day. If dose >250mg/day, give in divided doses. Administer as 60 min IV infusion, not >20mg/min. Not for use >14 days; switch to oral route as soon as clinically feasible. Decrease dose or d/c with decreased food or fluid intake and if excessive somnolence.

HOW SUPPLIED: Inj: 100mg/mL

CONTRAINDICATIONS: Hepatic disease, significant hepatic dysfunction, known urea cycle disorders (UCD).

WARNINGS/PRECAUTIONS: Hyperammonemic encephalopathy in UCD patients; d/c if this occurs. Prior to therapy, evaluate for UCD in high risk patients (eg, history of unexplained encephalopathy, coma, etc). Measure ammonia levels if develop unexplained lethargy, vomiting, or mental status changes. Caution in elderly; monitor for fluid/nutritional intake, dehydration, somnolence. Monitor LFTs before therapy and during 1st 6 months. D/C if develop hepatic dysfunction, pancreatitis. Increased risk of hepatotoxicity with multiple anticonvulsants, congenital metabolic disorders, severe seizure disorder with mental retardation, organic brain disease, children <2 yrs. Avoid abrupt withdrawal. Monitor platelets and coagulation tests before therapy and periodically thereafter. Elevated liver enzymes and thrombocytopenia may be dose-related. Not for prophylaxis of post-traumatic seizures in acute head trauma. May interfere with urine ketone and thyroid function tests.

ADVERSE REACTIONS: Dizziness, headache, nausea, local reactions.

INTERACTIONS: Clonazepam may induce absence status in patients with absence seizures. Potentiates amitriptyline, nortriptyline, carbamazepine, diazepam, ethosuximide, lamotrigine, phenobarbital, primidone, phenytoin, tolbutamide, warfarin, zidovudine. Potentiated by ASA and felbamate. Antagonized by rifampin, carbamazepine, phenobarbital, phenytoin. Additive CNS depression with other CNS depressants (eg, alcohol).

PREGNANCY: Category D, not for use in nursing.

MECHANISM OF ACTION: Anticonvulsant; increases GABA concentrations in the brain.

PHARMACOKINETICS: Absorption: T_{max}=1 hr. **Distribution:** Plasma protein binding (10%-18.5%). **Metabolism:** Liver; glucuronidation, mitochondrial β-oxidation. **Elimination:** Urine (<3% unchanged); $T_{1/2}$=16 hrs.

DEPAKENE RX
valproic acid (Abbott)

> Fatal hepatic failure (<2 yrs at considerable risk), teratogenic effects (eg, neural tube defects), and life-threatening pancreatitis reported.

THERAPEUTIC CLASS: Carboxylic acid derivative

INDICATIONS: Monotherapy and adjunctive therapy for treatment of simple and complex absence seizures, and complex partial seizures. Adjunct therapy for multiple seizure types.

DOSAGE: *Adults:* Simplex/Complex Absence Seizure: Initial: 15mg/kg/day. Titrate: Increase weekly by 5-10mg/kg/day until optimal response. Max: 60mg/kg/day. Complex Partial Seizure: Initial: 10-15mg/kg/day. Titrate: Increase weekly by 5-10mg/kg/day until optimal response. Max: 60mg/kg/day. If dose >250mg/day, give in divided doses. Elderly: Reduce initial dose. Swallow caps whole, do not chew.
Pediatrics: ≥10 yrs: Complex Partial Seizure: Initial: 10-15mg/kg/day. Titrate: Increase weekly by 5-10mg/kg/day until optimal response. Max: 60mg/kg/day. If dose >250mg/day, give in divided doses. Swallow caps whole, do not chew.

HOW SUPPLIED: Cap: 250mg; Syrup: 250mg/5mL

CONTRAINDICATIONS: Hepatic disease, significant hepatic dysfunction, known urea cycle disorders (UCD).

WARNINGS/PRECAUTIONS: Hyperammonemic encephalopathy in UCD patients; d/c if this occurs. Prior to therapy, evaluate for UCD in high risk patients (eg, history of unexplained encephalopathy, coma, etc). Measure ammonia levels if develop unexplained lethargy, vomiting, or mental status changes. Caution in elderly; monitor for fluid/nutritional intake, dehydration, somnolence. Monitor LFTs before therapy and during 1st 6 months. D/C if develop hepatic dysfunction, pancreatitis. Increased risk of hepatotoxicity with multiple anticonvulsants, congenital metabolic disorders, severe seizure disorder with mental retardation, organic brain disease, children <2 yrs. Avoid abrupt withdrawal. Hyperammonemia reported. Monitor platelets and coagulation tests before therapy and periodically thereafter. Elevated liver enzymes and thrombocytopenia may be dose-related. May interfere with urine ketone and thyroid function tests.

ADVERSE REACTIONS: Headache, asthenia, nausea, vomiting, diarrhea, abdominal pain, somnolence, tremor, dizziness, thrombocytopenia, ecchymosis, nystagmus, alopecia.

INTERACTIONS: Clonazepam may induce absence status in patients with absence seizures. Potentiates amitriptyline, nortriptyline, carbamazepine, diazepam, ethosuximide, lamotrigine, phenobarbital, primidone, phenytoin, tolbutamide, warfarin, zidovudine. Potentiated by ASA and felbamate. Antagonized by rifampin, carbamazepine, phenobarbital, phenytoin. Additive CNS depression with other CNS depressants (eg, alcohol).

PREGNANCY: Category D, not for use in nursing.

MECHANISM OF ACTION: Anticonvulsant; increases GABA concentration in the brain.

PHARMACOKINETICS: Absorption: T_{max}=4-8 hrs (tab), T_{max}=3.3-4.8 hrs (caps). **Distribution:** V_d=11L/1.73m²; plasma protein binding (10%-18.5%). **Metabolism:** Liver; glucuronidation, mitochondrial β-oxidation. **Elimination:** Urine (<3% unchanged); $T_{1/2}$=9-16 hrs.

DEPAKOTE RX
divalproex sodium (Abbott)

> Fatal hepatic failure (<2 yrs at considerable risk), teratogenic effects (eg, neural tube defects), and life-threatening pancreatitis reported.

THERAPEUTIC CLASS: Valproate compound

INDICATIONS: (Tab, Cap) Management of simple and complex absence seizures; complex partial seizures; and adjunctively with multiple seizure types including absence seizures. (Tab) Treatment of mania associated with bipolar disorder and migraine prophylaxis.

DOSAGE: *Adults:* (Cap/Tab) Complex Partial Seizures: Initial: 10-15mg/kg/day. Titrate: Increase by 5-10mg/kg/week. Max: 60mg/kg/day. Absence Seizures: Initial: 15mg/kg/day. Titrate: Increase weekly by 5-10mg/kg/day. Max: 60mg/kg/day. Give in divided doses if >250mg/day. (Tab) Migraine: Initial: ≥16 yrs: 250mg bid. Max: 1000mg/day. Mania: 750mg daily in divided doses. Titrate: Increase dose rapidly to clinical effect. Max: 60mg/kg/day. Elderly: Reduce initial dose and titrate slowly. Decrease dose or d/c if decreased food or fluid intake or if excessive somnolence occurs.
Pediatrics: ≥10 yrs: (Cap/Tab) Complex Partial Seizures: Initial: 10-15mg/kg/day. Titrate: Increase by 5-10mg/kg/week. Max: 60mg/kg/day. Absence Seizures: Initial: 15mg/kg/day. Titrate: Increase weekly by 5-10mg/kg/day. Max: 60mg/kg/day. Give in divided doses if >250mg/day.

HOW SUPPLIED: Cap, Delayed-Release: (Sprinkle) 125mg; Tab, Delayed-Release: 125mg, 250mg, 500mg

CONTRAINDICATIONS: Hepatic disease, significant hepatic dysfunction, known urea cycle disorders (UCD).

WARNINGS/PRECAUTIONS: Hyperammonemic encephalopathy in UCD patients; d/c if this occurs. Prior to therapy, evaluate for UCD in high risk patients (eg, history of unexplained encephalopathy, coma, etc). Measure ammonia levels if develop unexplained lethargy, vomiting, or mental status changes. Caution with hepatic disease. Check LFTs prior to therapy, then frequently during 1st six months. Dose-related thrombocytopenia and elevated liver enzymes reported. Monitor platelet and coagulation tests prior to therapy, then periodically. Altered thyroid function tests and urine ketone test. May stimulate replication of HIV and CMV viruses. Avoid abrupt discontinuation.

ADVERSE REACTIONS: Nausea, vomiting, diarrhea, somnolence, dyspepsia, thrombocytopenia, asthenia, abdominal pain, tremor, headache, anorexia, diplopia, blurred vision, weight gain, ataxia, nystagmus.

INTERACTIONS: Potentiates carbamazepine, amitriptyline, nortriptyline, diazepam, ethosuximide, primidone, lamotrigine, phenobarbital, phenytoin, tolbutamide, zidovudine, lorazepam. Efficacy potentiated by ASA, felbamate. Efficacy reduced by rifampin, carbamazepine, phenobarbital, phenytoin, primidone. Clonazepam may induce absence status in patients with absence type seizures. CNS depression with alcohol and other CNS depressants. Monitor PT/INR with warfarin.

PREGNANCY: Category D, not for use in nursing.

MECHANISM OF ACTION: Anticonvulsant; increases GABA concentrations in the brain.

PHARMACOKINETICS: Absorption: T_{max}=4-8 hrs (tab), T_{max}=3.3-4.8 hrs (cap). **Distribution:** Plasma protein binding (10%-18.5%). **Metabolism:** Liver; glucuronidation, mitochondrial β-oxidation. **Elimination:** Urine (<3% unchanged); $T_{1/2}$=9-16 hrs.

DEPAKOTE ER   RX
divalproex sodium (Abbott)

Fatal hepatic failure (<2 yrs at considerable risk), teratogenic effects (eg, neural tube defects), and life-threatening pancreatitis reported.

THERAPEUTIC CLASS: Valproate compound

INDICATIONS: Migraine prophylaxis. Monotherapy and adjunct therapy for treatment of complex partial seizures, and simple and complex absence seizures. Adjunct for multiple seizure types that include absence seizures. Acute manic or mixed episodes associated with bipolar disorder.

DOSAGE: *Adults:* For qd dosing. Migraine: Initial: 500mg qd for 1 week. Titrate: Increase to 1000mg qd. Max: 1000mg/day. Complex Partial Seizures: Monotherapy/Adjunct Therapy: Initial: 10-15mg/kg/day. Titrate: Increase by 5-10mg/kg/week to optimal response. Usual: Less than 60mg/kg/day (accepted therapeutic range 50-100mcg/mL). When converting to monotherapy, reduce concomitant antiepilepsy drug by 25% every 2 weeks starting at initiation or delay 1-2 weeks after start of therapy. Simple and Complex Absence Seizures: Initial: 15mg/kg/day. Titrate: Increase weekly by 5-10mg/kg/day to optimal response. Max: 60mg/kg/day. Bipolar Disorder: Initial: 25mg/kg/day given once daily. Titrate: Increase dose rapidly to clinical effect. Max: 60mg/kg/day. Conversion from Depakote: Administer Depakote ER qd using a dose 8-20% higher than the total daily dose of Depakote. If cannot directly convert to Depakote ER, consider increasing to next higher Depakote total daily dose before converting to appropriate total daily Depakote ER dose. Elderly: Give lower initial dose and titrate slowly. Decrease dose or d/c if decreased food or fluid intake or if excessive somnolence occurs. Swallow whole; do not crush or chew.
Pediatrics: ≥10yrs: For qd dosing. Complex Partial Seizures: Monotherapy/Adjunct Therapy: Initial: 10-15mg/kg/day. Titrate: Increase by 5-10mg/kg/week to optimal response. Usual: Less than 60mg/kg/day (accepted therapeutic range 50-100mcg/mL). When converting to monotherapy, reduce concomitant antiepilepsy drug by 25% every 2 weeks starting at initiation or delay 1-2 weeks after start of therapy. Simple and Complex Absence Seizures: Initial: 15mg/kg/day. Titrate: Increase weekly by 5-10mg/kg/day to optimal response. Max: 60mg/kg/day. Conversion from Depakote: Administer Depakote ER qd using a dose 8-20% higher than the total daily dose of Depakote. If cannot directly convert to Depakote ER, consider increasing to next higher Depakote total daily dose before converting to appropriate total daily Depakote ER dose. Swallow whole; do not crush or chew.

HOW SUPPLIED: Tab, Extended-Release: 250mg, 500mg

CONTRAINDICATIONS: Hepatic disease, significant hepatic dysfunction, known urea cycle disorders (UCD).

WARNINGS/PRECAUTIONS: Hyperammonemic encephalopathy in UCD patients; d/c if this occurs. Prior to therapy, evaluate for UCD in high risk patients (eg, history of unexplained encephalopathy, coma, etc). If unexplained lethargy, vomiting, or mental status changes occur measure ammonia levels. Caution with hepatic disease and elderly. Check LFTs prior to therapy, then frequently during 1st 6 months. Dose-related thrombocytopenia and elevated liver enzymes reported. Thrombocytopenia significantly increases with plasma trough levels >110mcg/mL in females and >135mcg/mL in males. Monitor platelet and coagulation tests prior to therapy, then periodically. Altered thyroid function tests and urine ketone test. May stimulate replication of HIV and CMV viruses. Avoid abrupt discontinuation.

ADVERSE REACTIONS: Nausea, dyspepsia, diarrhea, vomiting, abdominal pain, increased appetite, asthenia, somnolence, infection, dizziness, tremor, weight gain, back pain, alopecia.

INTERACTIONS: Potentiates carbamazepine, amitriptyline, nortriptyline, diazepam, ethosuximide, primidone, lamotrigine, phenobarbital, phenytoin, tolbutamide, zidovudine, lorazepam. Efficacy potentiated by ASA, felbamate. Efficacy reduced by rifampin, carbamazepine, phenobarbital, phenytoin, primidone. Clonazepam may induce absence status in patients with history of absence type seizures. CNS depression with alcohol and other CNS depressants. Monitor PT/INR with warfarin.

PREGNANCY: Category D, not for use in nursing.

MECHANISM OF ACTION: Anti-convulsant; increases GABA concentrations in the brain.

PHARMACOKINETICS: Absorption: Bioavailability (90%); T_{max}=4-17 hrs. **Distribution:** Plasma protein binding (10-18.5%). **Metabolism:** Liver; glucuronidation, mitochondrial β-oxidation. **Elimination:** Urine (<3% unchanged); $T_{1/2}$=9-16 hrs.

DepoCyt
cytarabine liposome (Enzon)

RX

> Chemical arachnoiditis (eg, nausea, vomiting, headache, fever), a common adverse event, can be fatal if untreated. Treat concurrently with dexamethasone to reduce incidence and severity.

THERAPEUTIC CLASS: Antimetabolite

INDICATIONS: Intrathecal treatment of lymphomatous meningitis.

DOSAGE: *Adults:* Induction: 50mg intrathecally every 14 days for 2 doses (weeks 1 and 3). Consolidation: 50mg intrathecally every 14 days for 3 doses (weeks 5, 7, and 9) followed by 1 additional dose at week 13. Maint: 50mg intrathecally every 28 days for 4 doses (weeks 17, 21, 25, and 29). Reduce to 25mg if drug-related neurotoxicity develops. Discontinue if toxicity persists.

HOW SUPPLIED: Inj: 10mg/mL

CONTRAINDICATIONS: Active meningeal infection.

WARNINGS/PRECAUTIONS: Intrathecal use of free cytarabine may cause myelopathy and other neurotoxicity. CSF blockage may increase free cytarabine levels and increase risk of neurotoxicity. Can cause fetal harm during pregnancy. Monitor for neurotoxicity. Anaphylactic reactions with IV free cytarabine. Transient elevations of CSF protein and WBC reported. Monitor hematopoietic system carefully.

ADVERSE REACTIONS: Chemical arachnoiditis (headache, fever, back pain, nausea, vomiting), confusion, somnolence, abnormal gait, peripheral edema, neutropenia, thrombocytopenia, urinary incontinence, convulsions, weakness.

INTERACTIONS: Intrathecal cytarabine in combination with other chemotherapeutic agents or with cranial/spinal irradiation may increase risk of neurotoxicity and other adverse events.

PREGNANCY: Category D, not for use in nursing.

MECHANISM OF ACTION: Antimetabolite; cell cycle phase-specific antineoplastic, affecting cells only during the S-phase of cell division. Intracellularly, it is converted into cytarabine-5'-triphosphate which inhibits DNA polymerase.

PHARMACOKINETICS: Absorption: C_{max}=30-50mcg, T_{max}=1 hr. **Metabolism:** Intracellular to ara-CTP. **Elimination:** Urine; $T_{1/2}$=5.9-82.4 hrs.

Depo-Estradiol
estradiol cypionate (Pharmacia & Upjohn)

RX

> Estrogens increase the risk of endometrial cancer. Estrogens, with or without progestins, should not be used for the prevention of cardiovascular disease or dementia. Increased risks of MI, stroke, invasive breast cancer, PE, and DVT in postmenopausal women (50-79 yrs of age) reported. Increased risk of developing probable dementia in postmenopausal women ≥65 yrs of age reported.

THERAPEUTIC CLASS: Estrogen

INDICATIONS: Treatment of moderate to severe vasomotor symptoms associated with menopause and hypoestrogenism due to hypogonadism.

DOSAGE: *Adults:* Vasomotor Symptoms/Vaginal/Vulval Atrophy: 1-5mg IM every 3-4 weeks cyclically. Discontinue or taper at 3-6 month intervals. Hypoestrogenism: 1.5-2mg IM every month.

HOW SUPPLIED: Inj: 5mg/mL

CONTRAINDICATIONS: Pregnancy, undiagnosed abnormal genital bleeding, breast cancer, estrogen-dependent neoplasia, DVT/PE, active or recent (eg, within past year) arterial thromboembolic disease (eg, stroke, MI), liver dysfunction or disease.

WARNINGS/PRECAUTIONS: May increase risk of cardiovascular events (eg, MI, stroke), venous thrombosis, and PE; d/c immediately if any of these events occur or are suspected. May increase risk of breast/endometrial cancer, and gallbladder disease. May lead to severe hypercalcemia with breast cancer and bone metastases; monitor and d/c if hypercalcemia occurs. Retinal vascular thrombosis reported; monitor and d/c if papilledema or retinal vascular lesions occur. Consider addition of a progestin if no hysterectomy. May elevate BP; monitor at regular intervals. May cause elevations of plasma triglycerides with pre-existing hypertriglyceridemia. Caution with history of cholestatic jaundice associated with past estrogen use or with pregnancy; d/c with recurrence. May lead to increased thyroid-binding globulin levels; monitor thyroid function. May cause fluid retention; caution with cardiac/renal dysfunction. Caution with severe hypocalcemia. May increase risk of ovarian cancer. May exacerbate endometriosis, asthma, DM, epilepsy, migraine, porphyria, SLE, and hepatic hemangiomas; use with caution.

ADVERSE REACTIONS: Changes in vaginal bleeding pattern, breakthrough bleeding, vaginal candidiasis, breast tenderness/enlargement, nausea, vomiting, abdominal cramps, headache, migraine, dizziness, increase/decrease in weight.

INTERACTIONS: CYP3A4 inducers (eg, St. John's wort, phenobarbital, carbamazepine, rifampin) may decrease levels which may decrease therapeutic effects and/or change uterine bleeding profile. CYP3A4 inhibitors (eg, erythromycin, clarithromycin, ketoconazole, itraconazole, ritonavir, grapefruit juice) may increase levels which may result in side effects.

PREGNANCY: Contraindicated in pregnancy, caution in nursing.

MECHANISM OF ACTION: Estrogen; binds to nuclear receptors in estrogen-responsive tissues. Modulates pituitary secretion of gonadotrophins, luteinizing hormone (LH) and follicle stimulating hormone (FSH), through negative feedback mechanism.

PHARMACOKINETICS: Absorption: Slow. **Distribution:** Wide; bound to sex hormone-binding globulin and albumin; found in human breast milk. **Metabolism:** Liver via CYP3A4 (partial); estrone (active metabolite); estriol (major urinary metabolite); enterohepatic recirculation via sulfate and glucuronide conjugation. **Elimination:** Urine (estradiol, estrone, estriol, conjugates).

DEPO-MEDROL   RX
methylprednisolone acetate (Pharmacia & Upjohn)

THERAPEUTIC CLASS: Glucocorticoid

INDICATIONS: Steroid-responsive disorders.

DOSAGE: *Adults:* Local Effect: Rheumatoid/Osteoarthritis: Large Joint: 20-80mg. Medium Joint: 10-40mg. Small Joint: 4-10mg. Administer intra-articularly into synovial space every 1-5 weeks or more depending on relief. Ganglion/Tendinitis/Epicondylitis: 4-30mg into cyst/area of greatest tenderness. May repeat if necessary. Dermatologic Conditions: Inject 20-60mg into lesion. Distribute 20-40mg doses by repeated injections into large lesions. Usual: 1-4 injections. Systemic Effect: Substitute for Oral Therapy: IM dose should equal total daily PO methylprednisolone dose q24h. Prolonged Therapy: Administer weekly PO dose as single IM injection. Androgenital Syndrome: 40mg IM every 2 weeks. Rheumatoid Arthritis: 40-120mg IM weekly. Dermatologic Lesions: 40-120mg IM weekly for 1-4 weeks. Acute Severe Dermatitis (Poison Ivy): 80-120mg IM single dose. Chronic Contact Dermatitis: May repeat injections every 5-10 days. Seborrheic Dermatitis: 80mg IM weekly. Multiple Sclerosis: 200mg/day prednisolone for 1 week, then 80mg every other day for 1 month (4mg methylprednisolone=5mg prednisolone). Asthma/Allergic Rhinitis: 80-120mg IM.
Pediatrics: Use lower adult doses. Determine dose by severity of condition and response.

HOW SUPPLIED: Inj: 20mg/mL, 40mg/mL, 80mg/mL

CONTRAINDICATIONS: Intrathecal administration, systemic fungal infections.

WARNINGS/PRECAUTIONS: Dermal and subdermal atrophy reported; do not exceed recommended doses. May need to increase dose before, during, and after stressful situations. May mask signs of infection or cause new infections.

D

Prolonged use may produce cataracts, glaucoma, secondary ocular infections. Increases BP, salt/water retention, potassium and calcium excretion. More severe/fatal course of infections reported with chickenpox, measles. Caution with Strongyloides, latent TB, hypothyroidism, cirrhosis, ocular herpes simplex, HTN, diverticulitis, fresh intestinal anastomoses, ulcerative colitis, osteoporosis, myasthenia gravis, renal insufficiency, peptic ulcer disease. Kaposi's sarcoma reported. Growth and development of children on prolonged therapy should be monitored. Monitor for psychic disturbances. Avoid abrupt withdrawal. Do not use intra-articularly, intrabursally, or for intratendinous administration in acute infection. Avoid injection into unstable and previously infected joints. Monitor urinalysis, blood sugar, BP, weight, chest X-ray, and upper GI x-ray (if ulcer history) regularly during prolonged therapy.

ADVERSE REACTIONS: Fluid and electrolyte disturbances, HTN, osteoporosis, muscle weakness, cushingoid state, menstrual irregularities, impaired wound healing, DM, ulcerative esophagitis, excessive sweating, increases intracranial pressure, carbohydrate intolerance, glaucoma, cataracts, urticaria, subcutaneous/cutaneous atrophy.

INTERACTIONS: Reduced efficacy with hepatic enzyme inducers (eg, phenobarbital, phenytoin, and rifampin). Increases clearance of chronic high dose ASA. Caution with ASA in hypoprothrombinemia. Effects on oral anticoagulants are variable; monitor PT. Increased insulin and oral hypoglycemic requirements in DM. Avoid live vaccines with immunosuppressive doses. Possible decreased vaccine response with killed or inactivated vaccines with immunosuppressive doses. Mutual inhibition of metabolism with cyclosporine; convulsions reported. Potentiated by ketoconazole and troleandomycin. Do not dilute or mix with other solutions.

PREGNANCY: Safety in pregnancy and nursing not known.

MECHANISM OF ACTION: Anti-inflammatory glucocorticoid; causes profound and varied metabolic effects and modifies the body's immune responses to diverse stimuli.

PHARMACOKINETICS: Absorption: C_{max}=11.8ng/mL; AUC=1286ng•hr/mL. **Elimination:** 139 hrs.

DEPO-PROVERA   RX
medroxyprogesterone acetate (Pharmacia & Upjohn)

THERAPEUTIC CLASS: Progestogen

INDICATIONS: Adjunct and palliative treatment of inoperable, recurrent, and metastatic endometrial or renal carcinoma.

DOSAGE: *Adults:* Initial: 400-1000mg IM weekly. Maint: 400mg/month if disease stabilizes and/or improves within a few weeks or months.

HOW SUPPLIED: Inj: 400mg/mL [2.5mL]

CONTRAINDICATIONS: Pregnancy, undiagnosed vaginal bleeding, breast malignancy, thrombophlebitis, thromboembolic disorders, cerebral vascular disease, liver dysfunction.

WARNINGS/PRECAUTIONS: Avoid during 1st 4 months of pregnancy. May cause thromboembolic disorders, ocular disorders, fluid retention. Caution with depression, family history of breast cancer or patients with breast nodules. May mask the onset of climacteric.

ADVERSE REACTIONS: Menstrual irregularities, nervousness, dizziness, edema, weight changes, cervical changes, cholestatic jaundice, breast tenderness, galactorrhea, rash, acne, alopecia, hirsutism, depression, pyrexia, fatigue, insomnia, nausea.

INTERACTIONS: Aminoglutethimide may decrease serum levels. Caution with estrogen.

PREGNANCY: Safety in pregnancy and nursing not known.

MECHANISM OF ACTION: Progestogen; inhibits secretion of gonadotropins which prevents follicular maturation and ovulation resulting in endometrial thinning thus produces its contraceptive effect.

PHARMACOKINETICS: Absorption: C$_{max}$=1-7ng/mL; T$_{max}$=3 weeks.
Distribution: Found in breast milk. **Elimination**: T$_{1/2}$=50 days.

DEPO-PROVERA CONTRACEPTIVE   RX
medroxyprogesterone acetate (Pharmacia & Upjohn)

> May cause significant loss of bone mineral density (BMD); greater with increasing duration of use and may not be completely reversible. Should be used as long-term birth control (>2yrs) only if other birth control methods are inadequate. Unknown if use during adolescence or early adulthood will reduce peak bone mass and increase risk of osteoporotic fractures in later life.

THERAPEUTIC CLASS: Progestogen

INDICATIONS: Prevention of pregnancy.

DOSAGE: *Adults:* 150mg IM every 3 months (13 weeks) in gluteal or deltoid muscle. Give 1st injection during 1st 5 days of menses; within 1st 5 days postpartum if not nursing; or 6 weeks postpartum if nursing.

HOW SUPPLIED: Inj: 150mg/mL

CONTRAINDICATIONS: Pregnancy, undiagnosed vaginal bleeding, breast malignancy, thrombophlebitis, thromboembolic disorders, cerebral vascular disease, liver dysfunction.

WARNINGS/PRECAUTIONS: Loss of BMD, may cause bleeding irregularities, cancer risk, thromboembolic disorders, ocular disorders, unexpected pregnancies, ectopic pregnancy, anaphylaxis and anaphylactoid reaction, fluid retention, return of fertility, decrease in glucose metabolism. Caution with CNS or convulsive disorders. D/C if jaundice develops.

ADVERSE REACTIONS: Menstrual irregularities, weight changes, abdominal pain, dizziness, headache, asthenia, nervousness, decreased libido, depression, nausea, insomnia, leukorrhea, acne, vaginitis, pelvic pain.

INTERACTIONS: Aminoglutethimide may decrease serum levels.

PREGNANCY: Category X, safety in nursing not known.

MECHANISM OF ACTION: Progestogen; inhibits secretion of gonadotropins, preventing follicular maturation and ovulation, resulting in endometrial thinning and producing its contraceptive effect.

PHARMACOKINETICS: Absorption: C$_{max}$=1-7ng/mL; T$_{max}$=3 weeks.
Distribution: Found in breast milk. **Elimination**: T$_{1/2}$=50 days.

DEPO-SUBQ PROVERA 104   RX
medroxyprogesterone acetate (Pharmacia & Upjohn)

> May cause significant loss of bone mineral density (BMD); greater with increasing duration of use and may not be completely reversible. Should be used as long-term birth control (>2yrs) only if other birth control methods are inadequate. Unknown if use during adolescence or early adulthood will reduce peak bone mass and increase risk of osteoporotic fractures in later life.

THERAPEUTIC CLASS: Progestogen

INDICATIONS: Prevention of pregnancy. Management of endometriosis-associated pain.

DOSAGE: *Adults:* 104mg SQ once every 3 months in the anterior thigh or abdomen. Give 1st injection during 1st 5 days of menses or 6 weeks postpartum if nursing.

HOW SUPPLIED: Inj: 104mg/0.65mL

CONTRAINDICATIONS: Pregnancy, undiagnosed vaginal bleeding, breast malignancy, thrombophlebitis, thromboembolic disorders, cerebral vascular disease, liver dysfunction.

WARNINGS/PRECAUTIONS: Loss of BMD, may cause bleeding irregularities, cancer risk, thromboembolic disorders, ocular disorders, unexpected pregnancies, ectopic pregnancy, anaphylaxis and anaphylactoid reaction, fluid retention, return of fertility, decrease in glucose metabolism. Caution with CNS or convulsive disorders. D/C if jaundice develops.

ADVERSE REACTIONS: Uterine bleeding irregularities, increased weight, decreased libido, acne, injection site reactions, headache, amenorrhea.

INTERACTIONS: Amioglutethimide may decrease serum levels.

PREGNANCY: Not for use in pregnancy, safety in nursing not known.

MECHANISM OF ACTION: Progestogen; inhibits secretion of gonadotropins, which prevents follicular maturation and ovulation, resulting in endometrial thinning and producing a contraceptive effect.

PHARMACOKINETICS: Absorption: C_{max}=1.56ng/mL; T_{max}=8.8 days; AUC=66.98ng•day/mL. **Distribution:** Plasma protein binding (86%); found in breast milk. **Metabolism:** Liver (extensive); reduction and hydroxylation. **Elimination:** Urine; $T_{1/2}$=43 days.

DEPO-TESTOSTERONE
testosterone cypionate (Pharmacia & Upjohn)

THERAPEUTIC CLASS: Androgen

INDICATIONS: Testosterone replacement in males with primary hypogonadism and hypogonadotropic hypogonadism.

DOSAGE: *Adults:* Male Hypogonadism: 50-400mg IM every 2-4 weeks. Dose based on age, sex, and diagnosis. Adjust dose according to response and adverse reactions.
Pediatrics: ≥12 yrs: Male Hypogonadism: 50-400mg IM every 2-4 weeks. Dose based on age, sex, and diagnosis. Adjust dose according to response and adverse reactions.

HOW SUPPLIED: Inj: 100mg/mL, 200mg/mL

CONTRAINDICATIONS: Severe renal, hepatic and cardiac disease. Males with carcinoma of the breast or prostate gland. Pregnancy.

WARNINGS/PRECAUTIONS: May accelerate bone maturation without linear growth; monitor bone growth every 6 months. Risk of hepatic damage with long-term use. D/C if hypercalcemia occurs in immobilized patients. D/C with acute urethral obstruction, priapism, excessive sexual stimulation, or oligospermia; restart at lower doses. Risk of edema; caution with pre-existing cardiac, renal or hepatic disease. Caution in the elderly; increased risk of prostatic hypertrophy and prostatic carcinoma. Caution with BPH. Should not be used for enhancement of athletic performance. Do not administer IV. Monitor Hct, Hgb, cholesterol periodically.

ADVERSE REACTIONS: Gynecomastia, excessive frequency/duration of penile erections, male pattern baldness, increased/decreased libido, oligospermia, hirsutism, acne, fluid and electrolyte disturbances, nausea, hypercholesterolemia, clotting factor suppression, polycythemia, altered LFTs, priapism, anxiety, depression.

INTERACTIONS: May potentiate oral anticoagulants (eg, warfarin) and oxyphenbutazone. May decrease blood glucose and insulin requirements in diabetics.

PREGNANCY: Category X, not for use in nursing.

MECHANISM OF ACTION: Endogenous androgen; responsible for normal growth and development of male sex organs and for maintenance of secondary sex characteristics.

PHARMACOKINETICS: Distribution: Plasma protein binding (98%). **Elimination:** Urine (90%), feces (6%). $T_{1/2}$=8 days.

DERMA-SMOOTHE/FS RX
fluocinolone acetonide (Hill Dermaceuticals)

THERAPEUTIC CLASS: Topical corticosteroid

INDICATIONS: Treatment of atopic dermatitis in adults and pediatrics ≥3 months.

DOSAGE: *Adults:* Atopic Dermatitis: Apply to affected area(s) tid.
Pediatrics: 3 months-17 yrs: Atopic Dermatitis: Moisten skin and apply bid for up to 4 weeks.

HOW SUPPLIED: Oil: 0.01% [120mL]

WARNINGS/PRECAUTIONS: May produce reversible hypothalamic-pituitary-adrenal (HPA) axis suppression, manifestations of Cushing's syndrome, hyperglycemia, and glucosuria. Children may be more susceptible to systemic toxicity. Use appropriate antifungal or antibacterial agent with dermatological infections. Contains refined peanut oil. D/C if hypersensitivity develops and treat accordingly. Avoid face, diaper area, and intertriginous areas with pediatrics.

ADVERSE REACTIONS: Atrophy, striae, telangiectasias, burning, itching, irritation, dryness, folliculitis, acneiform eruptions, hypopigmentation, perioral dermatitis, allergic contact dermatitis, secondary infections, miliaria.

PREGNANCY: Category C, caution in nursing.

MECHANISM OF ACTION: Corticosteroid; possesses anti-inflammatory, antipruritic, and vasoconstrictive properties. Anti-inflammatory action not established. Suspected to act by induction of phospholipase A_2 inhibitory proteins, lipocortins. Lipocortins control biosynthesis of prostaglandins and leukotrienes by inhibiting release of arachidonic acid. Arachidonic acid is released from membrane phospholipids by phospholipase A_2.

PHARMACOKINETICS: Absorption: Percutaneous; occlusion, inflammation, and other disease states may increase absorption. **Distribution:** Systemically administered corticosteroids found in breast milk.

DERMATOP RX
prednicarbate (Dermik)

THERAPEUTIC CLASS: Corticosteroid (medium-potency)

INDICATIONS: Corticosteroid responsive dermatoses.

DOSAGE: *Adults:* (Cre, Oint) Apply bid.
Pediatrics: ≥1 yr: (Cre) Apply bid. Max: 3 weeks of therapy. ≥10 yrs: (Oint) Apply bid.

HOW SUPPLIED: Cre, Oint: 0.1% [15g, 60g]

WARNINGS/PRECAUTIONS: May produce reversible HPA axis suppression, manifestations of Cushing's syndrome, hyperglycemia, and glucosuria. D/C if irritation occurs. Use appropriate antifungal or antibacterial agent with dermatological infections. Pediatrics may be more susceptible to systemic toxicity. Re-evaluate if no improvement after 2 weeks. Avoid eyes, occlusive dressings. Not for treatment of diaper dermatitis.

ADVERSE REACTIONS: Stinging, burning, dry skin, pruritus, urticaria, allergic contact dermatitis, edema, paresthesia, rash, skin atrophy.

PREGNANCY: Category C, caution in nursing.

MECHANISM OF ACTION: Corticosteroid; not established. Possesses anti-inflammatory, anti-pruritic, and vasoconstrictive properties. Suspected to act by induction of phospholipase A_2 inhibitory proteins, called lipocortins. Lipocortins control synthesis of potent inflammation mediators (eg, prostaglandins, leukotrienes) through inhibiting release of their common precursor, arachidonic acid. Arachidonic acid is released from membrane phospholipids by phospholipase A_2.

PHARMACOKINETICS: Absorption: Percutaneous; inflammation and/or other disease states increase absorption. Occlusive dressings for <24 hrs not shown to increase drug penetration; for 96 hrs markedly enhances penetration. **Distribution:** Systemically administered corticosteroids found in breast milk.

DESFERAL   RX
deferoxamine mesylate (Novartis)

THERAPEUTIC CLASS: Iron-chelating agent

INDICATIONS: Treatment of acute iron intoxication and of chronic iron overload due to transfusion-dependent anemias.

DOSAGE: *Adults:* See PI for solution preparation. Iron Intoxication: IM preferred for all patients not in shock. Only use IV slow infusion with cardiovascular collapse, and do not exceed 15mg/kg/hr for 1st 1g. Subsequent IV dosing should not exceed 125mg/hr. IM: Initial: 1g, then 500mg q4h for 2 doses. Give subsequent 500mg doses q4-12h depending upon clinical response. Max: 6g/24 hrs. IV: 1g, then 500mg over 4 hrs for 2 doses. Give subsequent 500mg doses over 4-12 hrs depending upon clinical response. Max: 6g/24 hrs. Iron Overload: IM: 500mg-1g/day IM. In addition, 2g IV per unit of blood transfused; not to exceed 15mg/kg/hr. Max: 1g without transfusion or 6g even with ≥3 units of blood or PRBC. SQ: 1-2g (20-40mg/kg/day) SQ over 8-24 hrs using small pump for continuous infusion. Individualize duration.
Pediatrics: ≥3 yrs: See PI for solution preparation. Iron Intoxication: IM preferred for all patients not in shock. Only use IV slow infusion with cardiovascular collapse, and do not exceed 15mg/kg/hr for 1st 1g. Subsequent IV dosing should not exceed 125mg/hr. IM: Initial: 1g, then 500mg q4h for 2 doses. Give subsequent 500mg doses q4-12h depending upon clinical response. Max: 6g/24 hrs. IV: 1g, then 500mg over 4 hrs for 2 doses. Give subsequent 500mg doses over 4-12 hrs depending upon clinical response. Max: 6g/24 hrs. Iron Overload: IM: 500mg-1g/day IM. In addition, 2g IV per unit of blood transfused; not to exceed 15mg/kg/hr. Max: 1g without transfusion or 6g even with ≥3 units of blood or PRBC. SQ: 1-2g (20-40mg/kg/day) SQ over 8-24 hrs using small pump for continuous infusion. Individualize duration.

HOW SUPPLIED: Inj: 500mg, 2g

CONTRAINDICATIONS: Severe renal disease, anuria.

WARNINGS/PRECAUTIONS: Ocular and auditory disturbances reported with prolonged use, high doses, or low ferritin levels. Periodic visual acuity tests, slit-lamp exams, funduscopy, and audiometry with prolonged treatment. High doses with low ferritin levels associated with growth retardation. Adult respiratory distress syndrome, also in children, reported after high IV doses in acute iron intoxication or thalassemia. Give IM, slow SQ, or IV infusion; skin flushing, urticaria, hypotension, and shock reported with rapid IV injection. High dose may exacerbate neurological dysfunction in aluminum-related encephalopathy. May precipitate onset of dialysis dementia. Aluminum overload with deferoxamine may decrease serum calcium and aggravate hyperparathyroidism. D/C with mucormycosis, *Yersinia enterocolitica* or *Yersinia pseudotuberculosis* infections. Monitor pediatrics body weight and growth every 3 months. Caution in elderly patients.

ADVERSE REACTIONS: Injection site reactions, hypersensitivity reactions, tachycardia, hypotension, shock, abdominal discomfort, diarrhea, nausea, vomiting, blood dyscrasia, leg cramps, growth retardation, bone changes, reddish urine.

INTERACTIONS: Cardiac dysfunction reported with high dose vitamin C (>500mg/day in adults) in patients with severe chronic iron overload; avoid vitamin C supplements in cardiac failure patients. Only give vitamin C after 1 month of deferoxamine therapy and monitor cardiac function. Do not exceed vitamin C 200mg/day in adults; 50mg/day for pediatrics <10 yrs and 100mg/day for older children usually suffices. Concurrent prochlorperazine may lead to temporary impairment of consciousness. May distort imaging results with gallium-67; discontinue deferoxamine 48 hrs before scintigraphy.

PREGNANCY: Category C, caution in nursing.

MECHANISM OF ACTION: Iron chelating agent; chelates iron by forming a stable complex that prevents iron from entering into further chemical reactions.

PHARMACOKINETICS: Metabolism: Metabolized primarily by plasma enzymes. **Elimination:** Urine, feces, bile.

DESOGEN

RX

desogestrel - ethinyl estradiol (Organon)

OTHER BRAND NAMES: Apri (Barr)

THERAPEUTIC CLASS: Estrogen/progestogen combination

INDICATIONS: Prevention of pregnancy.

DOSAGE: *Adults:* Start 1st Sunday after onset of menstruation or 1st day of menstruation. 1 tab qd for 28 days continuously, then repeat.

HOW SUPPLIED: Tab: (Ethinyl Estradiol-Desogestrel) 0.03mg-0.15mg

CONTRAINDICATIONS: Thrombophlebitis, DVT or thromboembolic disorders, pregnancy, cerebrovascular or coronary artery disease (current or history), undiagnosed abnormal genital bleeding, cholestatic jaundice of pregnancy or jaundice with prior hormonal contraceptive use, hepatic adenomas or carcinomas, breast cancer or other estrogen-dependent neoplasia, valvular heart disease with thrombogenic complications, hepatic tumors (benign or malignant) or active liver disease, heavy smoking (≥ 15 cigarettes per day) and over age 35.

WARNINGS/PRECAUTIONS: Cigarette smoking increases risk of serious cardiovascular side effects. This risk increases with age (especially >35 yrs) and heavy smoking. Increased risk of MI, vascular disease, thromboembolism, stroke and gallbladder disease. Retinal thrombosis, hepatic neoplasia, carcinoma of breast and reproductive organs reported. May cause glucose intolerance. May increase BP, elevate LDL levels or cause other lipid changes, fluid retention, breakthrough bleeding, and spotting. May cause or exacerbate migraine. May develop visual changes with contact lenses. Increased risk of MI with HTN, hyperlipidemia, certain inherited or acquired thrombophilias, obesity, and diabetes. D/C if jaundice, significant depression or ophthalmic irregularities develop. Perform annual physical exam. Use before menarche is not indicated. May affect certain endocrine, LFTs and blood components. D/C if pregnancy is confirmed.

ADVERSE REACTIONS: Nausea, vomiting, breakthrough bleeding, spotting, amenorrhea, migraine, mood changes including depression, vaginitis including candidiasis, edema, weight changes.

INTERACTIONS: Reduced effects, increased breakthrough bleeding, and menstrual irregularities with rifampin, barbiturates, phenylbutazone, phenytoin, and possibly with griseofulvin, ampicillin, and tetracyclines. Possible interaction with CYP2C9 substrates or inhibitors. St. John's wort may reduce the effectiveness of contraceptive steroids.

PREGNANCY: Category X, not for use in nursing.

MECHANISM OF ACTION: Estrogen/progestogen combination oral contraceptive: acts by suppression of gonadotropins. Also inhibits ovulation and causes changes in cervical mucus, which increases difficulty of sperm entry into uterus, and changes in endometrium, which reduces likelihood of implantation.

PHARMACOKINETICS: Absorption: Desogestrel: Rapid, complete; Etonogestrel: C_{max}=2805pg/mL (single dose), 5840pg/mL (multiple doses), T_{max}=1.4 hrs, AUC=33858pg/mL•hr (single dose), 52299pg/mL•hr (multiple doses). Ethinyl Estradiol: Rapid and complete, C_{max}=95pg/mL (single dose), 141pg/mL (multiple doses), T_{max}=1.5 hrs; AUC=1471pg/mL•hr (single dose), 1117pg/mL•hr (multiple doses). **Distribution:** Etonogestrel: Protein binding (98%). **Metabolism:** Desogestrel: Hepatic, hydroxylation in intestinal mucosa; CYP2C9, 3A4; Etonogestrel (major active metabolite). Ethinyl estradiol: Hepatic conjugation. **Elimination:** Urine, bile, feces. Desogestrel: $T_{1/2}$=38 hrs. Ethinyl Estradiol: $T_{1/2}$=26 hrs.

DESONATE
desonide (SkinMedica)

RX

THERAPEUTIC CLASS: Corticosteroid

INDICATIONS: Mild to moderate atopic dermatitis.

DOSAGE: *Adults*: Apply thin layer bid to affected area(s) and rub in gently. Not recommended beyond 4 consecutive weeks.
Pediatrics: ≥3 months: Apply a thin layer bid to the affected area(s) and rub in gently. Not recommended beyond 4 consecutive weeks.

HOW SUPPLIED: Gel: 0.05% [15g, 30g, 60g]

WARNINGS/PRECAUTIONS: May produce reversible HPA axis suppression, manifestations of Cushing's syndrome, hyperglycemia, and glucosuria. D/C if irritation occurs. Pediatrics may be more susceptible to systemic toxicity. Caution when applied to large surface areas. Avoid occlusive dressings. Avoid use beyond 4 wks.

ADVERSE REACTIONS: Burning, rash, application site pruritus.

PREGNANCY: Category C, caution in nursing.

MECHANISM OF ACTION: Corticosteroid; not established. Possesses anti-inflammatory, antipruritic, and vasoconstrictive properties. Suspected to act by the induction of phospholipase A_2 inhibitory proteins called lipocortins. Lipocortins control the biosynthesis of potent mediators of inflammation (eg, prostaglandins, leukotrienes) by inhibiting the release of their common precursor, arachidonic acid. Arachidonic acid is released from membrane phospholipids by phospholipase A_2.

PHARMACOKINETICS: Absorption: Percutaneous. Occlusion, inflammation and/or other disease processes may increase absorption. **Distribution:** Systemically administered corticosteroids appear in breast milk. **Metabolism:** Liver. **Elimination:** Kidneys and bile.

DESOWEN
desonide (Galderma)

RX

THERAPEUTIC CLASS: Corticosteroid

INDICATIONS: Corticosteroid responsive dermatoses.

DOSAGE: *Adults:* Apply bid-tid, depending on severity. Reassess if no improvement after 2 weeks.

HOW SUPPLIED: Cre, Oint: 0.05% [15g, 60g]; Lot: 0.05% [60mL, 120mL]

WARNINGS/PRECAUTIONS: May produce reversible HPA axis suppression, manifestations of Cushing's syndrome, hyperglycemia, and glucosuria. D/C if irritation occurs. Use appropriate antifungal or antibacterial agent with dermatological infections. Peds may be more susceptible to systemic toxicity. Caution when applied to large surface areas. Avoid occlusive dressings.

ADVERSE REACTIONS: Stinging, burning, irritation, erythema, contact dermatitis, worsening condition, skin peeling, dryness/scaliness.

PREGNANCY: Category C, caution in nursing.

MECHANISM OF ACTION: Corticosteroid; possesses anti-inflammatory, antipruritic, and vasoconstrictive properties. Suspected to act by induction of phospholipase A_2 inhibitory proteins called lipocortins. Lipocortins control biosynthesis of potent mediators of inflammation (eg, prostaglandins, leukotrienes) by inhibiting the release of their common precursor arachidonic acid.

PHARMACOKINETICS: Absorption: Extent of percutaneous absorption depends on skin integrity, vehicle, and use of occlusive dressings.

DESOXYN   CII
methamphetamine HCL (Ovation)

| High potential for abuse. Avoid prolonged therapy in obesity. |

THERAPEUTIC CLASS: Sympathomimetic amine

INDICATIONS: Attention deficit disorder with hyperactivity. Short-term adjunct to treat exogenous obesity.

DOSAGE: *Adults:* Obesity: 5mg, 1/2 hr before each meal. Do not exceed a few weeks of treatment.
Pediatrics: ADHD: ≥6 yrs: Initial: 5mg qd-bid. Titrate: Increase weekly by 5mg/day until optimum response. Usual: 20-25mg/day given bid. Obesity: ≥12 yrs: 5mg, 1/2 hr before each meal. Do not exceed a few weeks of treatment.

HOW SUPPLIED: Tab: 5mg

CONTRAINDICATIONS: Advanced arteriosclerosis, symptomatic cardiovascular disease, moderate to severe HTN, hyperthyroidism, glaucoma, agitated states, history of drug abuse, during or within 14 days of MAOI use.

WARNINGS/PRECAUTIONS: Tolerance to anorectic effect develops within a few weeks, do not exceed recommended dose to increase effect. Monitor growth in children. Caution with HTN. Do not use to combat fatigue or replace rest. Exacerbation of motor and phonic tics and Tourette's syndrome. May exacerbate behavior disturbance and thought disorder in psychotic pediatrics. Emergence of new psychotic symptoms may warrant discontinuation of therapy. Monitor for the appearance or worsening of aggressive behavior in children. Therapy may lower the convulsive threshold and cause blurred vision and difficulty with accommodation. Interrupt occasionally to determine if patient requires continued therapy. Misuse may cause sudden death and serious cardiovascular adverse events. Caution in patients with underlying cardiovascular conditions and comorbid bipolar disorder.

ADVERSE REACTIONS: BP elevation, tachycardia, palpitation, dizziness, insomnia, tremor, diarrhea, constipation, dry mouth, urticaria, impotence, changes in libido.

INTERACTIONS: May alter insulin requirements. May decrease hypotensive effect of guanethidine. Avoid MAOIs. Caution with TCAs and indirect acting sympathomimetic amines. Antagonized by phenothiazines.

PREGNANCY: Category C, not for use in nursing.

MECHANISM OF ACTION: Sympathomimetic amine; CNS stimulant. Peripheral actions involve elevation of BP, weak bronchodilation, and respiratory stimulant actions.

PHARMACOKINETICS: Absorption: Rapid. **Metabolism:** Liver; aromatic hydroxylation, N-dealkylation and deamination. **Elimination:** Urine (62%); $T_{1/2}$=4-5 hrs.

DETROL LA   RX
tolterodine tartrate (Pharmacia & Upjohn)

OTHER BRAND NAMES: Detrol (Pharmacia & Upjohn)

THERAPEUTIC CLASS: Muscarinic antagonist

INDICATIONS: Treatment of overactive bladder with symptoms of urinary frequency, urgency or urge incontinence.

DOSAGE: *Adults:* (LA Cap) Usual: 4mg qd, may lower to 2mg. (Tab) Initial: 2mg bid, may lower to 1mg bid. (LA Cap, Tab) Significant Hepatic/Renal Dysfunction/Concomitant CYP3A4 Inhibitors: 1mg bid or 2mg LA cap qd.

HOW SUPPLIED: Cap, Extended-Release: 2mg, 4mg; Tab: 1mg, 2mg

CONTRAINDICATIONS: Urinary retention, gastric retention, uncontrolled narrow-angle glaucoma.

WARNINGS/PRECAUTIONS: Risk of urinary retention with significant bladder outflow obstruction and risk of gastric retention with GI obstructive disorders. Caution with renal impairment and narrow-angle glaucoma. Reduce dose with significant hepatic or renal dysfunction. May cause blurred vision, drowsiness, or dizziness.

ADVERSE REACTIONS: Dry mouth, dizziness, headache, abdominal pain, constipation, diarrhea, dyspepsia, fatigue, somnolence, aggravation of symptoms of dementia reported.

INTERACTIONS: Reduce dose with concomitant CYP3A4 inhibitors (eg, erythromycin, clarithromycin, ketoconazole, itraconazole, and miconazole).

PREGNANCY: Category C, not for use in nursing.

MECHANISM OF ACTION: Muscarinic receptor antagonist; inhibits cholinergic muscarinic receptors mediating urinary bladder contraction and salivation.

PHARMACOKINETICS: Absorption: (Tab) Extensive metabolizers (EM) T_{max}=1.2 hrs, C_{max}=2.6mcg/L. Poor metabolizers (PM) T_{max}=1.9 hrs, C_{max}=19mcg/L. (Cap, Extended-Release) EM: T_{max}=4 hrs, C_{max}=3.4mcg/L. PM: T_{max}=4 hrs, C_{max}=19mcg/L. **Distribution:** High plasma protein binding; V_d=113 L. **Metabolism:** EM: CYP2D6 (oxidation); 5-hydroxymethyl (active metabolite). PM: CYP3A4 (dealkylation). **Elimination:** Urine (<1% unchanged), feces. (Tab) EM: $T_{1/2}$=2.2 hrs. PM: $T_{1/2}$=9.6 hrs. (Cap, Extended-Release) EM: $T_{1/2}$=6.9 hrs. PM: $T_{1/2}$= 18 hrs.

DEXAMETHASONE RX
dexamethasone (Various)

OTHER BRAND NAMES: Decadron (Merck)

THERAPEUTIC CLASS: Glucocorticoid

INDICATIONS: (PO) Treatment of steroid-responsive disorders. (Inj) Treatment of steroid responsive disorders when oral therapy not feasible.

DOSAGE: *Adults:* Individualize for disease and patient response. Withdraw gradually. (Tab) Initial: 0.75-9mg/day PO. Maint: Decrease in small amounts to lowest effective dose. Cushing's Syndrome Test: 1mg PO at 11pm; draw blood at 8am next morning. Or, 0.5mg PO q6h for 48 hrs; or 2mg (to distinguish if excess pituitary ACTH or other causes) PO q6h for 48 hrs; obtain 24-hr urine collections. (Inj) Initial: 0.5-9mg/day IV/IM. Cerebral Edema: Initial: 10mg IV, then 4mg IM q6h until edema subsides. Reduce dose after 2-4 days and gradually d/c over 5-7 days. Palliative Management of Recurrent/Inoperable Brain Tumors: Maint: 2mg IV/PO bid-tid. Acute Allergic Disorders: 4-8mg IM on 1st day, then 1.5mg PO bid for 2 days, then 0.75mg PO bid for 1 day, then 0.75mg PO qd for 2 days. (Inj) Usual: 0.2-9mg. Maint: Decrease in small amounts to lowest effective dose. Intra-Articular/Intralesional/Soft Tissue Injection: Usual: 0.2-6mg once every 3-5 days to once every 2-3 weeks. See PI for Shock Treatment. Take with meals and antacids to prevent peptic ulcer.
Pediatrics: Individualize for disease and patient response. Withdraw gradually. (Tab) Initial: 0.75-9mg/day PO. Maint: Decrease in small amounts to lowest effective dose. Cushing's Syndrome Test: 1mg PO at 11pm; draw blood at 8am next morning. Or, 0.5mg PO q6h for 48 hrs; or 2mg (to distinguish if excess pituitary ATCH or other causes) PO q6h for 48 hrs; obtain 24-hr urine collections. (Inj) Initial: 0.5-9mg/day IV/IM. Cerebral Edema: Initial: 10mg IV, then 4mg IM q6h until edema subsides. Reduce dose after 2-4 days and gradually d/c over 5-7 days. Palliative Management of Recurrent/Inoperable Brain Tumors: Maint: 2mg IV/PO bid-tid. Acute Allergic Disorders: 4-8mg IM on 1st day, then 1.5mg PO bid for 2 days, then 0.75mg PO bid for 1 day, then 0.75mg PO qd for 2 days. (Inj) Usual: 0.2-9mg. Maint: Decrease in small amounts to lowest effective dose. Intra-Articular/Intralesional/Soft Tissue Injection: Usual: 0.2-6mg once every 3-5 days to once every 2-3 weeks. See PI for shock treatment. Take with meals and antacids to prevent peptic ulcer.

HOW SUPPLIED: Inj: (Dexamethasone Sodium Phosphate) 4mg/mL, 10mg/mL; Sol: (Dexamethasone) 0.5mg/5mL, 1mg/mL; Tab: (Dexamethasone) 0.5mg*, 0.75mg*, 1mg*, 1.5mg*, 2mg*, 4mg*, 6mg* *scored

CONTRAINDICATIONS: Systemic fungal infections.

WARNINGS/PRECAUTIONS: Increase dose before, during, and after stressful situations. Avoid abrupt withdrawal. May mask signs of infection, activate latent amebiasis, elevate BP, cause salt/water retention, increase excretion of potassium and calcium. Prolonged use may produce cataracts, glaucoma, secondary ocular infections. Caution with recent MI, ocular herpes simplex, emotional instability, nonspecific ulcerative colitis, diverticulitis, peptic ulcer, renal insufficiency, HTN, osteoporosis, myasthenia gravis, threadworm infection, active tuberculosis. Enhanced effect with hypothyroidism, cirrhosis. Consider prophylactic therapy if exposed to measles or chickenpox. Risk of glaucoma, cataracts, and eye infections. False negative dexamethasone suppression test with indomethacin.

ADVERSE REACTIONS: Fluid/electrolyte disturbances, muscle weakness, osteoporosis, peptic ulcer, pancreatitis, ulcerative esophagitis, impaired wound healing, headache, psychic disturbances, growth suppression (pediatrics), glaucoma, hyperglycemia, weight gain, nausea, malaise.

INTERACTIONS: Caution with ASA. Inducers of CYP3A4 (eg, phenytoin, phenobarbital, carbamazepine, rifampin) and ephedrine enhance clearance; increase steroid dose. Inhibitors of CYP3A4 (ketoconazole, macrolides) may increase plasma levels. Drugs that affect metabolism may interfere with dexamethasone suppression tests. Increased clearance of drugs metabolized by CYP3A4 (eg, indinavir, erythromycin). May increase or decrease phenytoin levels. Ketoconazole may inhibit adrenal corticosteroid synthesis and cause adrenal insufficiency during corticosteroid withdrawal. Antagonizes or potentiates coumarins. Hypokalemia with potassium-depleting diuretics. Live virus vaccines are contraindicated with immunosuppressive doses.

PREGNANCY: Category C, not for use in nursing.

MECHANISM OF ACTION: Adrenocortical steroid; produces anti-inflammatory effects.

PHARMACOKINETICS: Distribution: Found in breast milk. **Metabolism**: Liver; CYP3A4.

DEXEDRINE
dextroamphetamine sulfate (GlaxoSmithKline)

CII

> High potential for abuse. Avoid prolonged use. Misuse may cause sudden death and serious CV adverse events.

OTHER BRAND NAMES: Dexedrine Spansules (GlaxoSmithKline)

THERAPEUTIC CLASS: Sympathomimetic amine

INDICATIONS: Treatment of attention deficit disorder with hyperactivity (ADHD) and narcolepsy.

DOSAGE: *Adults:* Narcolepsy: Initial: 10mg/day. Titrate: May increase by 10mg/day every week. Usual: 5-60mg/day. For tabs, give 1st dose upon awakening and additional every 4-6 hrs. May give caps once daily.
Pediatrics: Narcolepsy: 6-12 yrs: Initial: 5mg qd. Titrate: Increase weekly by 5mg/day. ≥12 yrs: Initial: 10mg qd. Titrate: Increase weekly by 10mg/day. Usual: 5-60mg/day in divided doses. ADHD: Initial: 3-5 yrs: 2.5mg qd. Titrate: Increase weekly by 2.5mg/day. ≥6 yrs: 5mg qd-bid. Titrate: Increase weekly by 5mg/day. Max: 40mg/day. For tabs, give 1st dose upon awakening and additional every 4-6 hrs. May give caps once daily.

HOW SUPPLIED: Cap, Extended-Release: (Spansules) 5mg, 10mg, 15mg; Tab: 5mg* *scored

CONTRAINDICATIONS: Advanced arteriosclerosis, symptomatic cardiovascular disease, moderate to severe HTN, hyperthyroidism, glaucoma, agitated states, history of drug abuse, during or within 14 days of MAOI use.

WARNINGS/PRECAUTIONS: May exacerbate symptoms of behavior disturbance and thought disorder in psychotic patients. Caution when using stimulants to treat patients with comorbid bipolar disorder because of concern for possible induction of mixed/manic episode in such patients. Stimulants at usual doses can cause treatment emergent psychotic or manic symptoms (eg, hallucinations, delusional thinking, mania) in children and adolescents without prior history of psychotic illness. Aggressive behavior or hostility reported in clinical trials and the postmarketing experience of some medications indicated for the treatment of ADHD. Caution with HTN. Tablets contain tartrazine; may cause allergy reactions. Exacerbation of motor and phonic tics and Tourette's syndrome. Monitor growth in children. Avoid with serious structural cardiac abnormalities, cardiomyopathy, serious heart rhythm abnormalities, CAD, or other serious cardiac problems. Avoid use in the presence of seizure. Visual disturbances reported with stimulant treatment.

ADVERSE REACTIONS: Palpitations, tachycardia, BP elevation, CNS overstimulation, restlessness, insomnia, dry mouth, GI disturbances, anorexia, urticaria, impotence.

INTERACTIONS: GI acidifying agents (guanethidine, reserpine, glutamic acid, etc.) and urinary acidifying agents (ammonium chloride, etc) decrease efficacy. MAOIs may cause hypertensive crisis. Potentiated by GI and urinary alkalinizers, propoxyphene overdose. Potentiated effects of both agents with TCAs. May delay absorption of phenytoin, ethosuximide, phenobarbital. Potentiates meperidine, norepinephrine, phenobarbital, phenytoin. Antagonized by haloperidol, chlorpromazine, lithium. Antagonizes adrenergic blockers, antihistamines, antihypertensives, veratrum alkaloids (antihypertensive).

PREGNANCY: Category C, not for use in nursing.

MECHANISM OF ACTION: Amphetamine; noncatecholamine sympathomimetic amine with CNS stimulant activity. Peripheral actions involve elevation of BP, weak bronchodilation, and respiratory stimulant actions.

PHARMACOKINETICS: Absorption: (15mg Tab) C_{max}=36.6ng/mL, T_{max}=3 hrs. (15mg Cap-ER) C_{max}=23.5ng/mL, T_{max}=8 hrs. **Elimination:** $T_{1/2}$=12 hrs.

DextroStat   CII
dextroamphetamine sulfate (Shire)

High potential for abuse. Avoid prolonged use.

THERAPEUTIC CLASS: Sympathomimetic amine

INDICATIONS: Treatment of narcolepsy and attention deficit disorder with hyperactivity (ADHD).

DOSAGE: *Adults:* Narcolepsy: Initial: 10mg/day. Titrate: May increase by 10mg/day every week. Usual: 5-60mg/day. Give 1st dose upon awakening, and additional doses every 4-6 hrs.
Pediatrics: Narcolepsy: 6-12 yrs: Initial: 5mg/day. Titrate: Increase weekly by 5mg/day. ≥12 yrs: Initial: 10mg/day. Titrate: Increase weekly by 10mg/day. Usual: 5-60mg/day in divided doses. ADHD: 3-5 yrs: Initial: 2.5mg/day. Titrate: Increase weekly by 2.5mg/day until optimum response. 6-16 yrs: Initial 5mg qd-bid. Titrate: Increase weekly by 5mg/day until optimum response. Give 1st dose upon awakening, and additional doses q4-6h.

HOW SUPPLIED: Tab: 5mg*, 10mg* *scored

CONTRAINDICATIONS: Advanced arteriosclerosis, symptomatic cardiovascular disease, moderate to severe HTN, hyperthyroidism, glaucoma, agitated states, history of drug abuse, during or within 14 days of MAOI use.

WARNINGS/PRECAUTIONS: Caution in HTN. Contains tartrazine, may cause allergic reactions. Exacerbation of motor and phonic tics and Tourette's syndrome. May exacerbate behavior disturbance and thought disorder in psychotic pediatrics. Interrupt occasionally to determine if patient requires continued therapy. Monitor growth in children.

ADVERSE REACTIONS: BP elevation, tachycardia, palpitation, dizziness, insomnia, tremor, diarrhea, constipation, dry mouth, urticaria, impotence, changes in libido.

INTERACTIONS: GI acidifying agents (guanethidine, reserpine, glutamic acid, etc.) and urinary acidifying agents (ammonium chloride, etc.) decrease efficacy. MAOIs may cause hypertensive crisis. Potentiated by GI and urinary alkalinizers, propoxyphene overdose. Potentiated effects of both agents with TCAs. May delay absorption of phenytoin, ethosuximide, phenobarbital. Potentiates meperidine, norepinephrine, phenobarbital, phenytoin. Antagonized by haloperidol, chlorpromazine, lithium. Antagonizes adrenergic blockers, antihistamines, antihypertensives, veratrum alkaloids (antihypertensive).

PREGNANCY: Category C, not for use in nursing.

MECHANISM OF ACTION: Sympathomimetic amine; CNS stimulant activity. Peripheral actions involve elevation of BP, weak bronchodilation, and respiratory stimulant actions.

PHARMACOKINETICS: Absorption: C_{max}=29.2ng/mL, T_{max}=2 hrs. **Elimination:** Urine (45%); $T_{1/2}$=10.25 hrs.

DiaBeta RX
glyburide (Sanofi-Aventis)

THERAPEUTIC CLASS: Sulfonylurea (2nd generation)

INDICATIONS: Adjunct to diet and exercise, to improve glycemic control in type 2 diabetes mellitus.

DOSAGE: *Adults:* Initial: 2.5-5mg qd with breakfast or first main meal; give 1.25mg if sensitive to hypoglycemia. Titrate: Increase by no more than 2.5mg/day at weekly intervals. Maint: 1.25-20mg given qd or in divided doses. Max: 20mg/day. May give bid with >10mg/day. Renal/Hepatic Disease, Elderly, Debilitated, Malnourished, Adrenal or Pituitary Insufficiency: Initial: 1.25mg qd. Transfer From Other Oral Antidiabetic Agents: Initial: 2.5-5mg/day. Switch From Insulin: If <20 U/day: 2.5-5mg qd. If 20-40 U/day: 5mg qd. If >40 U/day: Decrease insulin dose by 50% and give 5mg qd. Titrate: Progressive withdrawal of insulin and increase by 1.25-2.5mg/day every 2-10 days.

HOW SUPPLIED: Tab: 1.25mg*, 2.5mg*, 5mg* *scored

CONTRAINDICATIONS: Diabetic ketoacidosis.

WARNINGS/PRECAUTIONS: Increased risk of cardiovascular mortality. Risk of hypoglycemia, especially with renal and hepatic disease, elderly, debilitated or malnourished patients, and those with adrenal or pituitary insufficiency. May need to d/c and give insulin with stress (eg, fever, trauma). Secondary failure may occur. D/C if jaundice, hepatitis, or persistent skin reaction occur. Hematologic reactions and hyponatremia reported.

ADVERSE REACTIONS: Hypoglycemia, nausea, epigastric fullness, heartburn, allergic skin reactions, disulfiram-like reactions (rarely), hyponatremia, liver function abnormalities, photosensitivity reactions.

INTERACTIONS: Potentiated hypoglycemia with alcohol, NSAIDs, miconazole, fluoroquinolones, highly protein-bound drugs, salicylates, sulfonamides, chloramphenicol, probenecid, coumarins, MAOIs, and β-blockers. Risk of hyperglycemia with diuretics, corticosteroids, phenothiazines, thyroid products, estrogens, oral contraceptives, phenytoin, nicotinic acid, sympathomimetics, CCBs, and INH. β-blockers may mask hypoglycemia. Increased or decreased coumarin effects. Disulfiram-like reactions (rarely) with alcohol.

PREGNANCY: Category C, not for use in nursing.

MECHANISM OF ACTION: Sulfonylurea; acts by stimulating the release of insulin from functioning β-cell in pancreas.

PHARMACOKINETICS: Absorption: T_{max}=4 hrs. **Distribution:** Plasma protein binding (extensive). **Metabolism**: Hydroxylation. **Elimination:** Bile (50%), urine (50%); $T_{1/2}$=10 hrs.

Diabinese RX
chlorpropamide (Pfizer)

THERAPEUTIC CLASS: Sulfonylurea (1st generation)

INDICATIONS: Adjunct to diet and exercise, to improve glycemic control in type 2 diabetes mellitus.

DOSAGE: *Adults:* Initial: 250mg qd. Titrate: After 5-7 days, adjust by 50-125mg/day every 3-5 days for control. Maint: 100-500 qd. Max: 750mg qd. Elderly/Debilitated/Malnourished/Renal or Hepatic Dysfunction: Initial: 100-125mg qd. Maint: Conservative dosing. Take with breakfast. Divide dose with GI intolerance. If <40U/day insulin, discontinue therapy. If ≥40 U/day insulin, decrease dose by 50% and start chlorpropamide therapy. Adjust insulin dose depending on response.

HOW SUPPLIED: Tab: 100mg*, 250mg* *scored

CONTRAINDICATIONS: Diabetic ketoacidosis and Type I diabetes.

WARNINGS/PRECAUTIONS: Increased risk of cardiovascular mortality. Hypoglycemia risk especially with renal/hepatic insufficiency, elderly, debilitated, malnourished, and adrenal/pituitary insufficiency. Loss of blood glucose control when exposed to stress (fever, trauma, infection or surgery); d/c therapy and start insulin. Secondary failure can occur over a period of time.

ADVERSE REACTIONS: Hypoglycemia, cholestatic jaundice, diarrhea, nausea, vomiting, anorexia, pruritus, photosensitivity reactions, skin eruptions, blood dyscrasias, hepatic porphyria, disulfiram-like reactions.

INTERACTIONS: Potentiated hypoglycemia with NSAIDs, highly protein bound drugs, salicylates, sulfonamides, chloramphenicol, probenecid, coumarins, MAOIs, and β-blockers. Risk of hyperglycemia with diuretics, corticosteroids, phenothiazines, thyroid products, estrogens, oral contraceptives, phenytoin, nicotinic acid, sympathomimetics, CCBs, and isoniazid. Alcohol may produce disulfiram-like reaction. β-blockers may mask signs of hypoglycemia. Caution with barbiturates and miconazole.

PREGNANCY: Category C, not for use in nursing.

MECHANISM OF ACTION: Sulfonylurea; acts by stimulating release of insulin from functional β-cells in the pancreas.

PHARMACOKINETICS: Absorption: Rapid. T_{max}=2-4 hrs. **Metabolism:** Extensive via hydroxylation. **Elimination:** Urine (80-90%); $T_{1/2}$=36 hrs.

DIAMOX SEQUELS   RX
acetazolamide (Duramed)

THERAPEUTIC CLASS: Carbonic anhydrase inhibitor

INDICATIONS: Adjunct therapy for chronic open-angle glaucoma, secondary glaucoma and preoperatively in acute angle-closure glaucoma to lower IOP. Prophylaxis and amelioration of symptoms in acute mountain sickness.

DOSAGE: *Adults:* Glaucoma: 500mg bid. Acute Mountain Sickness: 500mg-1g/day in divided doses; 1g for rapid ascent. Initiate 24-48 hrs before ascent and continue for 48 hrs while at high altitude or longer as needed.

HOW SUPPLIED: Cap, Extended-Release: 500mg

CONTRAINDICATIONS: In sodium or potassium depleted patients, marked hepatic or kidney impairment, cirrhosis, suprarenal gland failure, hyperchloremic acidosis, (with long-term therapy) chronic noncongestive angle-closure glaucoma.

WARNINGS/PRECAUTIONS: Rare reports of fatal sulfonamide hypersensitivity reactions (eg, Stevens-Johnson syndrome, toxic epidermal necrolysis, fulminant hepatic necrosis, anaphylaxis, agranulocytosis, aplastic anemia, other blood dyscrasias) have occurred. D/C drug if this occurs. Sensitizations may recur despite route of administration. Dose increase does not increase diuresis and may result in decreased diuresis and increased drowsiness. Use with caution if patient predisposed to acid/base imbalances (elderly with renal impairment), DM, or impaired alveolar ventilation. Monitor serum electrolytes. Obtain CBC and platelet count before therapy and at regular intervals during therapy.

ADVERSE REACTIONS: Paresthesia, hearing dysfunction, tinnitus, loss of appetite, taste alteration, GI disturbances, polyuria, drowsiness, confusion, metabolic acidosis, electrolyte imbalance, transient myopia.

INTERACTIONS: Caution with high-dose ASA. May increase phenytoin levels; may increase occurrence of osteomalacia. May decrease levels of primidone, lithium. May increase effects of other carbonic anhydrase inhibitors, folic acid antagonists, quinidine, amphetamine. May prevent urinary antiseptic effect of methenamine. Increased risk of renal calculus formation with sodium bicarbonate. May increase levels of cyclosporine.

PREGNANCY: Category C, not for use in nursing.

MECHANISM OF ACTION: Carbonic anhydrase inhibitor. In eye, decreases secretion of aqueous humor, reducing IOP. In CNS, appears to retard abnormal, paroxysmal excessive discharge from CNS neurons. Diuretic effect is due to action in kidney, which produces reversible reaction involving hydration of carbon dioxide and dehydration of carbonic acid.

PHARMACOKINETICS: Absorption: T_{max}= 3-6 hrs.

DIASTAT
diazepam (Valeant)

 CIV

THERAPEUTIC CLASS: Benzodiazepine

INDICATIONS: Management of refractory patients with epilepsy, on stable regimens of anti-epileptic drugs, who require intermittent use to control bouts of increased seizure activity.

DOSAGE: *Adults:* 0.2mg/kg rectally. Calculate amount and round upwards to next available dose. May give 2nd dose 4-12 hrs later. Max: 5 episodes/month or 1 episode every 5 days.
Pediatrics: ≥12 yrs: 0.2mg/kg. 6-11yrs: 0.3mg/kg. 2-5 yrs: 0.5mg/kg. Calculate amount and round upwards to next available dose. May give 2nd dose 4-12 hrs later. For rectal administration. Max: 5 episodes/month and 1 episode every 5 days.

HOW SUPPLIED: Kit: 2.5mg, 5mg, 10mg, 15mg, 20mg

CONTRAINDICATIONS: Acute narrow angle glaucoma, untreated open angle glaucoma.

WARNINGS/PRECAUTIONS: Produces CNS depression. Avoid abrupt withdrawal. Caution with elderly, hepatic/renal dysfunction, compromised respiratory function, neurologic damage. Not for daily chronic use. Withdrawal symptoms reported with discontinuation.

ADVERSE REACTIONS: Somnolence, dizziness, headache, pain, abdominal pain, nervousness, vasodilation, diarrhea, ataxia, euphoria, incoordination, asthma, rhinitis, rash.

INTERACTIONS: Potentiated by phenothiazines, narcotics, barbiturates, valproate, MAOIs, and other antidepressants. Potential inhibitors of CYP450 2C19 (eg, cimetidine, quinidine, tranylcypromine) and CYP450 3A4 (eg, ketoconazole, troleandomycin, clotrimazole) may decrease elimination. CYP450 2C19 (eg, rifampin) and CYP450 3A4 (eg, carbamazepine, phenytoin, dexamethasone, phenobarbital) inducers could increase elimination. May interfere with metabolism of substrates for CYP450 2C19 (eg, omeprazole, propranolol, imipramine) and CYP450 3A4 (eg, cyclosporine, paclitaxel, terfenadine, theophylline, warfarin).

PREGNANCY: Category D, not for use in nursing.

MECHANISM OF ACTION: Benzodiazepine; unknown, suspected to suppress seizures through an interaction with GABA receptors (A-type). GABA acts at this receptor to allow entry of chloride ions, which causes an inhibitory potential that reduces the ability of neurons to depolarize to the threshold potential necessary to produce action potentials.

PHARMACOKINETICS: Absorption: Absolute bioavailability (90%); T_{max}=1.5 hrs. **Distribution:** V_d=1L/kg; plasma protein binding (95-98%). **Metabolism:** Hepatic (CYP3A4, CYP2C19) to form desmethyldiazepam (major active

metabolite), temazepam and oxazepam (minor active metabolites).
Elimination: $T_{1/2}$=46 hrs (15mg rectal).

DIAZEPAM INJECTION

diazepam (Various)

`CIV`

THERAPEUTIC CLASS: Benzodiazepine

INDICATIONS: Management of anxiety disorders and short-term relief of anxi-ety symptoms. Symptomatic relief of acute alcohol withdrawal. Adjunct prior to endoscopic procedures, surgical procedures and cardioversion. Adjunct therapy in skeletal muscle spasm (eg, tetanus, etc), status epilepticus and severe recurrent convulsive disorders.

DOSAGE: *Adults:* Anxiety (moderate): 2-5mg IM/IV, may repeat in 3-4 hrs. Anxiety (severe): 5-10mg IM/IV, may repeat in 3-4 hrs. Alcohol Withdrawal (acute): 10mg IM/IV, then 5-10mg in 3-4 hrs if needed. Endoscopic Procedures: Usual: ≤10mg IV (up to 20mg) or 5-10mg IM 30 min prior to pro-cedure. Muscle Spasm: 5-10mg IM/IV, then 5-10mg in 3-4 hrs if needed. Status Epilepticus/Severe Seizures: Initial: 5-10mg IV. Maint: May repeat at 10-15 min intervals. Max: 30mg. Preoperative: 10mg IM. Cardioversion: 5-15mg IV, 5-10 min prior to procedure. Elderly/Debilitated: Usual: 2-5mg.
Pediatrics: Tetanus: 30 days-5 yrs: 1-2mg IM/IV (slowly), may repeat every 3-4 hrs prn. ≥5 yrs: 5-10mg IM/IV, may repeat every 3-4 hrs. Status Epilepticus/Severe Seizures: 30 days-5 yrs: 0.2-0.5mg IV (slowly) every 2-5 min up to 5mg. ≥5 yrs: 1mg IV (slowly) every 2-5 min up to 10mg, may repeat in 2-4 hrs.

HOW SUPPLIED: Inj: 5mg/mL

CONTRAINDICATIONS: Acute narrow angle glaucoma, untreated open angle glaucoma.

WARNINGS/PRECAUTIONS: Inject slowly and avoid small veins with IV. Do not mix or dilute with other products in syringe or infusion flask. Extreme cau-tion in elderly, severely ill and those with limited pulmonary reserve. Avoid if in shock, coma or acute alcohol intoxication with depressed vital signs. May im-pair mental/physical abilities. Increase in grand mal seizures reported. Caution with kidney or hepatic dysfunction. Not for obstetrical use. Withdrawal symptoms may occur. Hypotension and muscular weakness reported. Monitor blood counts and LFTs. Not for maintenance of seizures once controlled.

ADVERSE REACTIONS: Drowsiness, fatigue, ataxia, venous thrombosis and phlebitis (injection site).

INTERACTIONS: Phenothiazines, narcotics, barbiturates, MAOIs, and other antidepressants may potentiate effects. Delayed clearance with cimetidine. Reduce narcotic dose by at least one-third. Risk of apnea with concomitant barbiturates, alcohol, or other CNS depressants.

PREGNANCY: Not for use during pregnancy, safety in nursing unknown.

MECHANISM OF ACTION: Antianxiety/hypnotic agent; induces calming effect on parts of the limbic system, the thalamus and the hypothalamus (animal study).

DIBENZYLINE

phenoxybenzamine HCL (WellSpring)

`RX`

THERAPEUTIC CLASS: Alpha blocker

INDICATIONS: To control episodes of hypertension and sweating associated with pheochromocytoma.

DOSAGE: *Adults:* Initial: 10mg bid. Titrate: Increase every other day to 20-40mg bid-tid, until BP is controlled.

HOW SUPPLIED: Cap: 10mg

CONTRAINDICATIONS: Conditions where fall in BP may be undesirable.

WARNINGS/PRECAUTIONS: Caution with marked cerebral or coronary arteriosclerosis, or renal damage. May aggravate symptoms of respiratory infections.

ADVERSE REACTIONS: Postural hypotension, tachycardia, ejaculation inhibition, nasal congestion, miosis, GI irritation, drowsiness, fatigue.

INTERACTIONS: Exaggerated hypotensive response and tachycardia with agents that stimulate both α and β-adrenergic receptors (eg, epinephrine). Blocks hyperthermia production by levarterenol, and blocks hypothermia production by reserpine.

PREGNANCY: Category C, not for use in nursing.

MECHANISM OF ACTION: α-receptor blocker; increases blood flow to skin, mucosa, abdominal viscera, and lowers both supine and erect BP.

PHARMACOKINETICS: Elimination: (IV) $T_{1/2}$=24 hrs.

DICLOXACILLIN   RX
dicloxacillin sodium (Various)

THERAPEUTIC CLASS: Penicillin (penicillinase-resistant)

INDICATIONS: Infections caused by penicillinase-producing staphylococci.

DOSAGE: *Adults:* Mild-Moderate Infection: 125mg q6h. Severe Infection: 250mg q6h for at least 14 days.
Pediatrics: <40kg: Mild-Moderate Infection: 12.5mg/kg/day in divided doses q6h. Severe Infection: 25mg/kg/day in divided doses q6h for at least 14 days.

HOW SUPPLIED: Cap: 250mg, 500mg

WARNINGS/PRECAUTIONS: Serious, fatal hypersensitivity reactions reported. Pseudomembranous colitis has been reported; toxin produced by *Clostridium difficile* is the primary cause. Caution with history of allergy and/or asthma. Monitor renal, hepatic, and hematopoietic function with prolonged use. Not for use as initial therapy with serious, life-threatening infections, or with nausea, vomiting, gastric dilation, cardiospasm, or intestinal hypermotility.

ADVERSE REACTIONS: Allergic reactions, nausea, vomiting, diarrhea, stomatitis, black or hairy tongue, superinfection (prolonged use), hepatotoxicity.

INTERACTIONS: Tetracycline may antagonize the bactericidal effects. Potentiated by probenecid.

PREGNANCY: Category B, caution in nursing.

MECHANISM OF ACTION: Penicillin (penicillinase-resistant); bactericidal against penicillin-susceptible microorganisms during state of active multiplication. Inhibits biosynthesis of bacterial cell-wall.

PHARMACOKINETICS: Absorption: Rapid/incomplete; C_{max}=1-1.5 hrs; T_{max}=10-17mcg/mL. **Distribution:** Serum protein binding (95%-99%); found in breast milk. **Elimination:** Urine (unchanged); $T_{1/2}$=0.7 hrs.

DIDREX   CIII
benzphetamine HCL (Pharmacia & Upjohn)

THERAPEUTIC CLASS: Anorectic sympathomimetic amine

INDICATIONS: Short-term adjunct treatment of exogenous obesity.

DOSAGE: *Adults:* Initial: 25-50mg qd. Usual: 25-50mg qd-tid.
Pediatrics: ≥12 yrs: Initial: 25-50mg qd. Usual: 25-50mg qd-tid.

HOW SUPPLIED: Tab: 50mg* *scored

CONTRAINDICATIONS: Advanced arteriosclerosis, symptomatic cardiovascular disease, moderate to severe HTN, agitated states, hyperthyroidism, glaucoma, history of drug abuse, concomitant CNS stimulants, MAOI use within 14 days, pregnancy.

WARNINGS/PRECAUTIONS: Caution with mild HTN. D/C if tolerance develops. Psychological disturbances reported with restrictive dietary regimen.

ADVERSE REACTIONS: Palpitations, tachycardia, BP elevation, restlessness, dizziness, insomnia, headache, tremor, sweating, dry mouth, nausea, diarrhea, unpleasant tastes, urticaria, altered libido.

INTERACTIONS: Hypertensive crisis risk if used within 14 days of MAOIs. Potentiates TCAs. Avoid with other CNS stimulants. Decreases effects of antihypertensives. Potentiated by urinary alkalinizing agents and reduced effect with urinary acidifying agents. May alter insulin requirements.

PREGNANCY: Category X, not for use in nursing.

MECHANISM OF ACTION: Anorectic sympathomimetic amine; CNS stimulant, elevates BP. As anorectic, appetite suppression as primary action not established.

DIDRONEL RX
etidronate disodium (Procter & Gamble)

THERAPEUTIC CLASS: Bone metabolism regulator

INDICATIONS: Treatment of Paget's disease. Treatment and prevention of heterotopic ossification following total hip replacement or due to spinal cord injury.

DOSAGE: *Adults:* Give as single dose (preferred) or in divided doses. Paget's disease: Initial: 5-10mg/kg/day up to 6 months or 11-20mg/kg/day up to 3 months. May retreat after drug free period of 90 days only if evidence of active disease process. Heterotopic Ossification: Hip Replacement: 20mg/kg/day 1 month before and 3 months after surgery. Spinal Cord: 20mg/kg/day for 2 weeks, followed by 10mg/kg/day for 10 weeks.

HOW SUPPLIED: Tab: 200mg, 400mg* *scored

CONTRAINDICATIONS: Overt osteomalacia.

WARNINGS/PRECAUTIONS: Therapy response in Paget's Disease may be of slow onset and continue for months after stopping. Maintain adequate dietary intake of calcium and vitamin D. Diarrhea reported with enterocolitis. Monitor with renal impairment. Reduce dose with decreased GFR. Max dose (20mg/day) or long-term therapy (>6 months) may increase fracture risk. Rachitic syndrome reported in children at doses of 10mg/kg/day for prolonged periods (approaching or exceeding 1 year).

ADVERSE REACTIONS: Diarrhea, nausea, increased bone pain in Paget's, alopecia, arthropathy, esophagitis, hypersensitivity reactions, osteomalacia, amnesia, confusion.

INTERACTIONS: Vitamins with mineral supplements or antacids that contain calcium, iron, aluminum, or magnesium reduce absorption (separate dosing by 2 hours). Monitor PT with warfarin.

PREGNANCY: Category C, caution with nursing.

MECHANISM OF ACTION: Bone metabolism regulator; inhibits the formation, growth, and dissolution of hydroxyapatite crystals and their amorphous precursors by chemisorption to calcium phosphate surfaces.

PHARMACOKINETICS: Metabolism: Not metabolized. **Elimination:** Urine (50% of absorbed drug) and feces (unabsorbed drug).

DIETHYLPROPION CIV
diethylpropion HCL (Various)

THERAPEUTIC CLASS: Sympathomimetic amine

INDICATIONS: Short-term adjunct for exogenous obesity in patients with initial BMI ≥30kg/m².

DOSAGE: *Adults:* (Tab) 25mg tid 1 hour before meals, and mid-evening if needed for night hunger. (Tab, ER): 75mg at qd in mid-morning, swallowed whole.

Pediatrics: ≥16 yrs: (Tab) 25mg tid 1 hour before meals, and mid-evening if needed for night hunger. (Tab, ER): 75mg at qd in mid-morning, swallowed whole.

HOW SUPPLIED: Tab: 25mg; Tab, Extended-Release: 75mg

CONTRAINDICATIONS: Advanced arteriosclerosis, hyperthyroidism, glaucoma, pulmonary HTN, severe HTN, within 14 days of MAOI use, agitated states, history of drug abuse, other concomitant anorectics.

WARNINGS/PRECAUTIONS: Possible risk of pulmonary HTN and valvular heart disease. Caution with HTN, symptomatic cardiovascular disease. Avoid with heart murmur, valvular heart disease, severe HTN. May increase convulsions with epilepsy. Prolonged use may induce dependence with withdrawal symptoms. D/C if tolerance develops or insignificant weight loss after 4 weeks of therapy.

ADVERSE REACTIONS: Palpitations, tachycardia, arrhythmias, blurred vision, dizziness, anxiety, insomnia, depression, urticaria, gynecomastia, nausea, vomiting, GI disturbances, bone marrow depression, impotence.

INTERACTIONS: See Contraindications. MAOIs may cause hypertensive crisis. Avoid with other anorectic agents (prescription, OTC, herbal products) or if used within prior year. Phenothiazines may antagonize anorectic effects. Potential for arrhythmias with general anesthetics. May interfere with antihypertensives (eg, guanethidine, methyldopa). Adverse reactions with alcohol. Antidiabetic drug requirements may be altered. Valvular heart disease reported with fenfluramine or dexfenfluramine.

PREGNANCY: Category B, caution in nursing.

MECHANISM OF ACTION: Anorectic sympathomimetic amine; not established as appetite suppressor; causes CNS stimulation and elevation of BP.

PHARMACOKINETICS: Absorption: Rapid. **Distribution**: Crosses placenta; found in breast milk. **Metabolism**: N-dealkylation, reduction; aminoketone (metabolites). **Elimination**: Urine; $T_{1/2}$=4-6 hrs (aminoketone).

DIFFERIN RX
adapalene (Galderma)

THERAPEUTIC CLASS: Naphthoic acid derivative (retinoid-like)

INDICATIONS: Topical treatment of acne vulgaris.

DOSAGE: *Adults:* Apply qhs after washing.
Pediatrics: ≥12 yrs: Apply qhs after washing.

HOW SUPPLIED: Cre: 0.1% [45g]; Gel: 0.1%, 0.3% [45g, 75g]

WARNINGS/PRECAUTIONS: Avoid contact with eyes, lips, paranasal creases, mucous membranes, cuts, abrasions, eczematous or sunburned skin. Minimize sun exposure. Extreme weather may increase skin irritation.

ADVERSE REACTIONS: Erythema, scaling, dryness, pruritus, burning, sunburn, acne flares.

INTERACTIONS: Caution with other topicals with strong drying effects, high concentration of alcohol, astringents, spices, or lime. Allow effects of sulfur, resorcinol, or salicylic acid to subside before use.

PREGNANCY: Category C, caution in nursing.

MECHANISM OF ACTION: Naphthoic acid derivative; not established. Suspected to normalize differentiation of follicular epithelial cells resulting in decreased microcomedone formation.

PHARMACOKINETICS: Absorption: Low. **Elimination:** Bile.

DIFLUCAN RX
fluconazole (Pfizer)

THERAPEUTIC CLASS: Azole antifungal

D

INDICATIONS: Treatment of vaginal, oropharyngeal, and esophageal candidiasis. Treatment of systemic *Candida* infections. Treatment of peritonitis and UTI caused by *Candida*. Treatment of cryptococcal meningitis. Prophylaxis in patients undergoing BMT.

DOSAGE: *Adults:* Vaginal Candidiasis: 150mg PO single dose. IV/PO: Oropharyngeal Candidiasis: 200mg on 1st day, then 100mg qd for at least 2 weeks. Esophageal Candidiasis: 200mg on 1st day, then 100mg qd for at least 3 weeks and for at least 2 weeks following resolution of symptoms. Max: 400mg/day. Systemic *Candida* Infections: Up to 400mg/day. UTI/Peritonitis: 50-200mg/day. Cryptococcal Meningitis: 400mg on 1st day, then 200mg qd for 10-12 weeks after negative CSF culture. Suppression of Cryptococcal Meningitis Relapse in AIDS: 200mg qd. Prophylaxis in BMT: 400mg qd. Renal Impairment: CrCl ≤50mL/min (no dialysis): Initial: LD 50-400mg. Maint: Give 50% of recommended dose. Dialysis: Give 100% of dose after each dialysis. *Pediatrics:* IV/PO: Oropharyngeal Candidiasis: 6mg/kg on 1st day, then 3mg/kg/day for at least 2 weeks. Esophageal Candidiasis: 6mg/kg on 1st day, then 3mg/kg/day for at least 3 weeks and for at least 2 weeks following resolution of symptoms. Max: 12mg/kg/day. Systemic *Candida* Infections: 6-12mg/kg/day. Cryptococcal Meningitis: 12mg/kg 1st day, then 6mg/kg/day for 10-12 weeks after negative CSF culture. Suppression of Cryptococcal Meningitis Relapse in AIDS: 6mg/kg qd. Renal Impairment: CrCl <50mL/min (no dialysis): Initial: LD: 50-400mg. Maint: Give 50% of recommended dose. Dialysis: Give 100% of dose after each dialysis.

HOW SUPPLIED: Inj: 200mg/100mL, 400mg/200mL; Sus: 50mg/5mL, 200mg/5mL [35mL]; Tab: 50mg, 100mg, 150mg, 200mg

CONTRAINDICATIONS: Coadministration with cisapride or terfenadine (with multiple Diflucan doses of ≥400mg). Caution if hypersensitive to other azoles.

WARNINGS/PRECAUTIONS: Monitor LFTs. D/C if hepatic dysfunction develops or exfoliative skin disorder progresses. Anaphylaxis reported.

ADVERSE REACTIONS: Headache, nausea, abdominal pain, diarrhea, skin rash, vomiting.

INTERACTIONS: See Contraindications. Severe hypoglycemia with oral hypoglycemics. May increase PT with coumarin-type drugs. Increases levels of phenytoin, cyclosporine, cisapride, astemizole, zidovudine and theophylline. Rifampin enhances metabolism of fluconazole. Cimetidine may decrease levels. HCTZ may increase levels. Contraindicated with terfenadine and cisapride due to prolongation of QTc interval. Cardiac events (torsade de pointes) reported with cisapride. Uveitis reported with rifabutin. Nephrotoxicity reported with tacrolimus. May increase or decrease levels of ethinyl estradiol- and levonorgestrel-containing oral contraceptives.

PREGNANCY: Category C, not for use in nursing.

MECHANISM OF ACTION: Antifungal; inhibits fungal CYP450 sterol C-14 α-demethylation. Subsequent loss of normal sterol correlates with accumulation of 14 α-methyl sterols in fungi and may be responsible for its fungistatic activity.

PHARMACOKINETICS: Absorption: Oral: Absolute bioavailability (90%); C_{max}=6.72mcg/mL (50-400mg), T_{max}=1-2 hrs (fasted). **Distribution:** Plasma protein binding (11-12%). **Elimination:** Urine (80% unchanged and 11% metabolites); $T_{1/2}$=30 hrs. Refer to PI for pediatric pharmacokinetic parameters.

DIGIBIND   RX
digoxin immune fab (ovine) (GlaxoSmithKline)

THERAPEUTIC CLASS: Antidote, digoxin toxicity

INDICATIONS: Treatment of life-threatening digoxin intoxication. Also has been successfully used to treat digitoxin overdose.

DOSAGE: *Adults:* Acute Ingestion of Unknown Amount: Usual: Administer 10 vials, observe response, then additional 10 vials if clinically indicated. Calculation: # vials = total digitalis body load (mg)/0.5mg of digitalis bound per vial. 1 vial will bind approximately 0.5mg of digoxin (or digitoxin). Steady-

State Serum Digoxin Concentrations: # of vials = (serum dig conc in ng/mL) x (wt in kg)/100. Steady-State Digitoxin Concentrations: # of vials = (serum digitoxin conc in ng/mL) x (wt in kg)/1000. If toxicity not adequately reversed after several hrs or appears to recur, may need readministration. See PI for details.

Pediatrics: Acute Ingestion of Unknown Amount: Usual: Administer 10 vials, observe response, then additional 10 vials if clinically indicated. Calculation: # vials = total digitalis body load (mg)/0.5mg of digitalis bound per vial. 1 vial will bind approximately 0.5mg of digoxin (or digitoxin). Steady-State Serum Digoxin Concentrations: Dose (mg) = (# vials) (38mg/vial). Steady-State Digitoxin Concentrations: # of vials = (serum digitoxin conc in ng/mL) x (wt in kg)/1000. If toxicity not adequately reversed after several hrs or appears to recur, may need readministration. See PI for details.

HOW SUPPLIED: Inj: 38mg

WARNINGS/PRECAUTIONS: Obtain digoxin level before initiation. Do not overlook possibility of multiple drug overdose. Risk of hypersensitivity is greater with allergies to papain, chymopapain, or other papaya extracts; skin testing may be appropriate for high-risk individuals. K^+ levels may drop rapidly after administration; monitor closely. Digitalis toxicity may recur with renal dysfunction; caution and monitor closely. Caution with cardiac dysfunction, further deterioration may occur from digoxin withdrawal. Consider additional support with inotropes or vasodilators. Monitor for volume overload in children. D/C if anaphylactoid reaction occurs and treat appropriately.

ADVERSE REACTIONS: Allergic reactions, exacerbation of low cardiac output, CHF, hypokalemia.

PREGNANCY: Category C, caution in nursing.

MECHANISM OF ACTION: Antidote; digoxin toxicity. Binds to molecules of digoxin, making them unavailable for binding at their site of action on cells.

PHARMACOKINETICS: Elimination: Urine. $T_{1/2}$=15-20 hrs.

DILACOR XR   RX
diltiazem HCL (Watson)

OTHER BRAND NAMES: Diltia XT (Andrx)

THERAPEUTIC CLASS: Calcium channel blocker (nondihydropyridine)

INDICATIONS: Treatment of hypertension and management of chronic stable angina.

DOSAGE: *Adults:* HTN: Initial: 180-240mg qd. Usual: 180-480mg qd. Max: 540mg qd. ≥60 yrs: Initial: 120mg qd. Angina: Initial: 120mg qd. Titrate: Adjust at 1-2 week intervals. Max: 480mg/day. Swallow whole on an empty stomach in the am.

HOW SUPPLIED: Cap, Extended-Release: 120mg, 180mg, 240mg

CONTRAINDICATIONS: Sick sinus syndrome, 2nd- or 3rd-degree AV block (except with functioning pacemaker), hypotension (<90mmHg systolic), acute MI, pulmonary congestion.

WARNINGS/PRECAUTIONS: Caution in renal, hepatic, or ventricular dysfunction. Monitor LFTs and renal function with prolonged use. D/C if persistent rash occurs. Symptomatic hypotension may occur. Acute hepatic injury reported.

ADVERSE REACTIONS: Rhinitis, pharyngitis, cough, flu syndrome, peripheral edema, myalgia, vomiting, sinusitis, asthenia, nausea, vasodilation, headache, constipation, diarrhea.

INTERACTIONS: Increased levels of propranolol. Increased levels of diltiazem with cimetidine. Monitor digoxin, cyclosporine. Potentiates cardiac contractility, conductivity, and automaticity; and vascular dilation with anesthetics. Additive cardiac conduction effects with digitalis or β-blockers. Potential additive effects with agents known to affect cardiac contractility and/or conduction.

PREGNANCY: Category C, not for use in nursing.

DILANTIN

MECHANISM OF ACTION: Ca^{2+} channel blocker; inhibits influx of calcium ion during membrane depolarization of cardiac and vascular smooth muscle with resultant decrease in peripheral vascular resistance.

PHARMACOKINETICS: Absorption: Absolute bioavailability (41%). T_{max}=4-6 hrs. **Distribution:** Plasma protein binding (70-80%). **Metabolism:** Liver. Desacetyldiltiazem (major metabolite). **Elimination:** Urine (2-4%); $T_{1/2}$=5-10 hrs.

DILANTIN RX
phenytoin (Parke-Davis)

THERAPEUTIC CLASS: Hydantoin

INDICATIONS: (CER, CTB) Control of generalized tonic-clonic (grand mal) and complex partial (psychomotor, temporal lobe) seizures. Prevention and treatment of neurosurgically induced seizures. (Sus) Control of tonic-clonic (grand mal) and psychomotor (temporal lobe) seizures.

DOSAGE: *Adults:* (CER) Initial: 100mg tid. Titrate: May increase at 7-10 day intervals. Max: 200mg tid. May give once daily with extended-release if controlled on 300mg daily. LD (clinic/hospital): 1g in 3 divided doses (400mg, 300mg, 300mg) given 2 hrs apart. Start maintenance 24 hrs later. (CTB) Initial: 100mg tid. Titrate: May increase at 7-10 day intervals. Usual: 300-400mg/day. Max: 600mg/day. May chew or swallow tab whole. Not for once daily dosing. (Sus) Initial: 125mg tid. Titrate: May increase at 7-10 day intervals. Max: 625mg/day.
Pediatrics: (CER, CTB, Sus) Initial: 5mg/kg/day given bid-tid. Titrate: May increase at 7-10 day intervals. Maint: 4-8mg/kg/day. Max: 300mg/day. >6 yrs: May require the minimum adult dose (300mg/day).

HOW SUPPLIED: Cap, Extended-Release (CER): 30mg, 100mg; Sus: 125mg/5mL [237mL]; Tab, Chewable (CTB): 50mg* *scored

WARNINGS/PRECAUTIONS: Avoid abrupt discontinuation. Caution with porphyria, hepatic dysfunction, elderly, diabetes, debilitated. D/C if rash occurs. Lymphadenopathy reported. Serum sickness may occur with lymph node involvement. Gingival hyperplasia reported; maintain proper dental hygiene. Hyperglycemia, birth defects and osteomalacia reported. Monitor levels. Confusional states reported with increased levels. Increased seizure frequency during pregnancy. Neonatal coagulation defects reported within first 24 hrs of birth. Give vitamin K to mother before delivery and to neonate after birth. Avoid use with seizures due to hypoglycemia or other metabolic causes.

ADVERSE REACTIONS: Nystagmus, ataxia, slurred speech, decreased coordination, confusion, dizziness, insomnia, transient nervousness, motor twitchings, headaches, nausea, vomiting, constipation, rash, hypersensitivity reactions.

INTERACTIONS: Increased levels with acute alcohol intake, amiodarone, chloramphenicol, chlordiazepoxide, diazepam, dicumarol, disulfiram, estrogens, H$_2$-antagonists, halothane, isoniazid, methylphenidate, phenothiazines, phenylbutazone, salicylates, succinamides, sulfonamides, tolbutamide, trazodone. Decreased levels with chronic alcohol abuse, carbamazepine, reserpine, sucralfate. Decreases effects of corticosteroids, coumarin anticoagulants, digitoxin, doxycycline, estrogens, furosemide, oral contraceptives, quinidine, rifampin, theophylline, vitamin D. Phenobarbital, sodium valproate, valproic acid may increase or decrease levels. May increase or decrease levels of phenobarbital, sodium valproate, valproic acid. Calcium antacids decrease absorption; space dosing. Moban® contains calcium ions that interfere with absorption. TCAs may precipitate seizures. Increased risk of phenytoin hypersensitivity with barbiturates, succinamides, oxazolidinediones.

PREGNANCY: Possibly teratogenic, weigh benefits versus risk; not for use in nursing.

MECHANISM OF ACTION: Anticonvulsant; inhibits seizure activity by promoting sodium efflux from neurons, stabilizing threshold against hyperexcitability caused by excessive stimulation of environmental changes capable of reducing membrane sodium gradient.

300 PDR® Concise Drug Guide

PHARMACOKINETICS: Absorption: T_{max}=1.5-3 hrs. **Distribution:** Highly protein bound. **Metabolism:** Liver (hydroxylation). **Elimination:** Bile, urine; $T_{1/2}$=22 hrs.

DILATRATE-SR   RX
isosorbide dinitrate (Schwarz)

THERAPEUTIC CLASS: Nitrate vasodilator

INDICATIONS: Prevention of angina pectoris.

DOSAGE: *Adults:* 40mg bid (separate doses by 6 hrs). Max: 160mg/day. Should have >18 hr nitrate-free interval.

HOW SUPPLIED: Cap, Extended-Release: 40mg

WARNINGS/PRECAUTIONS: Severe hypotension may occur; caution with volume depletion and hypotension. Hypotension may cause paradoxical bradycardia and increased angina pectoris. May aggravate angina caused by hypertrophic cardiomyopathy. Monitor for tolerance. Caution with CHF and acute MI.

ADVERSE REACTIONS: Headache, lightheadedness, hypotension, syncope, rebound HTN.

INTERACTIONS: Potentiates effects of other vasodilators such as alcohol. Severe hypotension with sildenafil.

PREGNANCY: Category C, caution in nursing.

MECHANISM OF ACTION: Nitrate vasodilator; relaxes vascular smooth muscle, and consequent dilatation of peripheral arteries and veins, especially the latter. Dilatation of the veins leads to reducing the left ventricular end-di-astolic pressure and pulmonary capillary wedge pressure (preload). Arteriolar relaxation reduces systemic vascular resistance, systolic arterial pressure and mean arterial pressure (afterload). It also dilates the coronary artery.

PHARMACOKINETICS: Distribution: V_d=2-4L/kg. **Metabolism:** Liver (extensive first-pass metabolism). Metabolites (2-mononitrate and 5-mononitrate) have biological activity. Both metabolites are cleared from serum through denitration, glucouronidation, and denitration/hydration pathways.

DILAUDID   CII
hydromorphone HCL (Abbott)

> Contains hydromorphone, a potent Schedule II opioid agonist which has the highest potential for abuse and risk of producing respiratory depression. HP formulation is a highly concentrated solution of hydromorphone; do not confuse with standard parenteral formulations of hydromorphone or other opioids as overdose and death could result. Alcohol, other opioids, CNS depressants potentiate respiratory depressant effects, increasing risk of respiratory depression which may result in death.

OTHER BRAND NAMES: Dilaudid-HP (Abbott)

THERAPEUTIC CLASS: Opioid analgesic

INDICATIONS: Management of pain. (HP) Relief of moderate to severe pain in opioid-tolerant patients who require larger than usual doses of opioids to provide adequate pain relief.

DOSAGE: *Adults:* Individualize dose. Initial: 1-2mg SQ/IM/IV q4-6h prn. (HP) Range: 1-14mg IM/SQ; adjust dose based on response. (Sol) 2.5-10mg PO q3-6h prn. (Tab) 2-4mg PO q4-6h prn. (Sup) Insert 1 PR q6-8h prn. Titrate: Increase dose as needed. Elderly: Start at lower end of dosing range.

HOW SUPPLIED: Inj: 1mg/mL, 2mg/mL, 4mg/mL, (HP) 10mg/mL, 250mg; Sol: 1mg/mL; Sup: 3mg; Tab: 2mg, 4mg, 8mg* *scored

CONTRAINDICATIONS: Intracranial lesions associated with increased ICP, COPD, cor pulmonale, emphysema, kyphoscoliosis, and in status asthmaticus. (HP-Inj) Obstetrical analgesia.

WARNINGS/PRECAUTIONS: Increased respiratory depression with head in-jury and/or increased ICP. May mask acute abdominal conditions. Caution with elderly/debilitated, seizures, biliary tract surgery, renal/hepatic impairment, hypothyroidism, Addison's disease, BPH, and urethral stricture; initial dose should be reduced in these patients. May suppress cough reflex. Potential for physical/psychological tolerance or dependence, especially in patients with alcoholism and drug dependencies; monitor closely. Seizures reported in compromised patients receiving high doses. Dilaudid-HP should only be used in patients already receiving large doses of narcotics. 8mg tab and sol contains sulfites.

ADVERSE REACTIONS: Excessive sedation, lethargy, mental clouding, anxiety, dysphoria, nausea, vomiting, constipation, urinary retention, respiratory depression. Orthostatic hypotension and fainting reported with injection.

INTERACTIONS: Additive CNS depression with other narcotic analgesics, neuromuscular blocking agents, general anesthetics, phenothiazines, tranquilizers, sedative hypnotics, TCAs, alcohol, or other CNS depressants. Mixed agonist/antagonist analgesics (eg, pentazocine, nalbuphine, butorphanol, bupernorphine) may reduce the analgesic effect of hydromorphone and/or may precipitate withdrawal symptoms.

PREGNANCY: Category C, not for use in nursing.

MECHANISM OF ACTION: Opiod analgesic; mechanism of analgesic effects not established. Suspected to bind to specific opiate receptors in the CNS to produce analgesia.

PHARMACOKINETICS: Absorption: (PO) Rapid; (Tab) C_{max}=5.5ng, T_{max}=0.74 hrs; (Sol) C_{max}=5.7ng, T_{max}=0.73 hrs. **Distribution**: Plasma protein binding (8-19%); (IV Bolus) V_d=302.9 L; crosses placenta, found in human breast milk. **Metabolism**: Liver; glucuronidation (extensive); hydromorphone-3-glucuronide (metabolite). **Elimination:** Urine; (IV) $T_{1/2}$=2.3 hrs; (Tab) $T_{1/2}$=2.6 hrs; (Sol) $T_{1/2}$=2.8 hrs.

DILTIAZEM INJECTION   RX
diltiazem HCL (Biovail)

THERAPEUTIC CLASS: Calcium channel blocker (nondihydropyridine)

INDICATIONS: Temporary control of rapid ventricular rate in atrial fibrillation/flutter (A-Fib/Flutter). Rapid conversion of paroxysmal supraventricular tachycardia (PSVT) to sinus rhythm.

DOSAGE: *Adults:* Bolus: (Injection/Lyo-Ject) 0.25mg/kg IV over 2 min. If no response after 15 min, may give 2nd dose of 0.35mg/kg over 2 min. Continuous Infusion: (Injection/Lyo-Ject/Monovial) 0.25-0.35mg/kg IV bolus, then 10mg/hr. Titrate: Increase by 5mg/hr. Max: 15mg/hr and duration up to 24 hrs.

HOW SUPPLIED: Inj: 5mg/mL

CONTRAINDICATIONS: Sick sinus syndrome and 2nd- or 3rd-degree AV block (except with functioning pacemaker), severe hypotension, cardiogenic shock, concomitant IV β-blockers or within a few hrs of use, A-Fib/Flutter associated with accessory bypass tract (eg, Wolff-Parkinson-White syndrome, short PR syndrome), ventricular tachycardia, (Lyo-Ject) neonates due to benzyl alcohol.

WARNINGS/PRECAUTIONS: Initiate in setting with resuscitation capabilities. Caution if hemodynamically compromised, and renal, hepatic, or ventricular dysfunction. Monitor ECG continuously and BP frequently. Symptomatic hypotension, acute hepatic injury reported. D/C if high-degree AV block occurs in sinus rhythm or if persistent rash occurs. Ventricular premature beats may be present on conversion of PSVT to sinus rhythm.

ADVERSE REACTIONS: Hypotension, injection site reactions (eg, itching, burning), vasodilation (flushing), arrhythmias.

INTERACTIONS: Caution with drugs that decrease peripheral resistance, intravascular volume, myocardial contractility or conduction. Increased AUC of midazolam, triazolam, buspirone, quinidine, and lovastatin; which may require a dose adjustment due to increased clinical effects or increased adverse events. Elevates carbamazepine levels, which may result in toxicity.

Cyclosporine may need dose adjustment. Potentiates the depression of cardiac contractility, conductivity, automaticity and vascular dilation with anesthetics. Possible bradycardia, AV block, and contractility depression with oral β-blockers. Possible competitive inhibition of metabolism with drugs metabolized by CYP450. Avoid IV β-blockers and rifampin. Monitor for excessive slowing of HR and/or AV block with digoxin. Cimetidine increases peak diltiazem plasma levels and AUC.

PREGNANCY: Category C, not for use in nursing.

MECHANISM OF ACTION: Calcium channel blocker; inhibits influx of Ca^{2+} ions during membrane depolarization of cardiac and vascular smooth muscle. Has ability to slow AV nodal conduction time and prolong AV nodal refractoriness, which has therapeutic benefits on supraventricular tachycardia. Decreases peripheral resistance, resulting in decreased systolic and diastolic BP.

PHARMACOKINETICS: Distribution: Plasma protein binding (70-80%); V_d=305-391L; found in breast milk. **Metabolism:**Liver (extensive) via CYP450; deacetylation, N-demethylation, O-demethylation, and conjugation; N-monodesmethyldiltiazem and desacetyldiltiazem (major metabolites). **Elimination:** Urine and bile; $T_{1/2}$=3.4 hrs (single IV inj); $T_{1/2}$=4.1-4.9 hrs (constant IV infusion).

DIOVAN
valsartan (Novartis)

RX

> When used in pregnancy, drugs that act directly on the renin-angiotensin system can cause injury and even death to the developing fetus. D/C therapy when pregnancy is detected.

THERAPEUTIC CLASS: Angiotensin II receptor antagonist

INDICATIONS: Treatment of hypertension, alone or with other antihypertensives. Treatment of heart failure (NYHA Class II-IV). Reduction of cardiovascular mortality in clinically stable patients with left ventricular failure or dysfunction following MI.

DOSAGE: *Adults:* HTN: Monotherapy Without Volume Depletion: Initial: 80mg or 160mg qd. Titrate: May increase to 320mg qd or add diuretic (greater effect than increasing dose >80mg). Hepatic/Severe Renal Dysfunction: Use with caution. Heart Failure: Initial: 40mg bid. Titrate: May increase to 80mg or 160mg bid (use highest dose tolerated). Max: 320mg/day in divided doses. Post-MI: Initial: 20mg bid. Titrate: May increase to 40mg bid within 7 days, with subsequent titrations up to 160mg bid.
Pediatrics: 6-16 yrs: HTN: Initial: 1.3mg/kg qd (up to 40mg total). Adjust dose according to BP response. Max: 2.7mg/kg (up to 160mg) qd. Use of a sus recommended for children who cannot swallow tabs, or children for whom calculated dosage (mg/kg) does not correspond to available tab strengths. Adjust dose accordingly when switching dosage forms. Hepatic/Severe Renal Impairment: Use with caution. Avoid use in pediatrics with GFR <30mL/min/1.73m².

HOW SUPPLIED: Tab: 40mg*, 80mg, 160mg, 320mg *scored

WARNINGS/PRECAUTIONS: Changes in renal function may occur; caution with renal artery stenosis, severe CHF. Caution with hepatic dysfunction, renal dysfunction, and obstructive biliary disorder. Risk of hypotension; caution when initiating therapy in heart failure or post-MI. Correct volume or salt depletion before therapy. Avoid use in pediatric patients with GFR <30mL/min/1.73m². May cause fetal harm when administered to pregnant women.

ADVERSE REACTIONS: (HTN) Headache, dizziness, viral infection, fatigue, abdominal pain. (Heart Failure) dizziness, hypotension, diarrhea, arthralgia, fatigue, back pain, hyperkalemia. (Post-MI) hypotension, cough, increased blood creatinine.

INTERACTIONS: Concomitant use of K+-sparing diuretics, K+ supplements, or salt substitutes containing K+ may increase serum K+ levels, and in heart failure patients increase SrCr.

PREGNANCY: Category D, not for use in nursing.

MECHANISM OF ACTION: Angiotensin II receptor antagonist; blocks vasoconstrictor and aldosterone-secreting effects of angiotensin II by selectively blocking binding of angiotensin II to AT_1 receptor.

PHARMACOKINETICS: Absorption: T_{max}=2-4 hrs, absolute bioavailability (25%). **Distribution:** (IV) V_d=17L, plasma protein binding (95%). **Metabolism:** Valeryl 4-hydroxy valsartan (metabolite). **Elimination:** Feces, urine; $T_{1/2}$=6 hrs.

DIOVAN HCT RX
hydrochlorothiazide - valsartan (Novartis)

When used in pregnancy, drugs that act directly on the renin-angiotensin system can cause injury and even death to the developing fetus. D/C therapy when pregnancy is detected.

THERAPEUTIC CLASS: Angiotensin II receptor antagonist/thiazide diuretic

INDICATIONS: Treatment of hypertension. Not for initial therapy.

DOSAGE: *Adults:* Initial: Uncontrolled on Valsartan Monotherapy: Switch to 80mg-12.5mg, 160mg-12.5mg, or 320mg-12.5mg qd. May increase dose if uncontrolled after 3-4 weeks. Max: 320mg-25mg/day. Uncontrolled on 25mg HCTZ/day or Controlled on 25mg HCTZ/day with Hypokalemia: Switch to 80mg-12.5mg or 160mg-12.5mg qd. May titrate if uncontrolled after 3-4 weeks. Max: 320mg-25mg/day. CrCl ≤30mL/min: Use not recommended.

HOW SUPPLIED: Tab: (Valsartan-HCTZ) 80mg-12.5mg, 160mg-12.5mg, 160mg-25mg, 320mg-12.5mg, 320mg-25mg

CONTRAINDICATIONS: Anuria, sulfonamide hypersensitivity.

WARNINGS/PRECAUTIONS: Correct volume or salt depletion before therapy. Caution with hepatic or renal dysfunction, biliary obstructive disorders, renal artery stenosis, severe CHF, history of allergies, and asthma. May exacerbate or activate SLE. Monitor serum electrolytes. Avoid if CrCl ≤30mL/min. Hyperuricemia, hyperglycemia, hypokalemia, hypomagnesemia, hypercalcemia may occur. Enhanced effects in post-sympathectomy patient. May increase cholesterol and triglyceride levels. May cause fetal and neonatal morbidity and death when given to pregnant women.

ADVERSE REACTIONS: Cough, headache, dizziness, fatigue, viral infection, pharyngitis, diarrhea.

INTERACTIONS: Alcohol, barbiturates, and narcotics may potentiate orthostatic hypotension. Insulin and oral antidiabetic agents may require dosage adjustment. Impaired absorption with cholestyramine, colestipol. Corticosteroids and ACTH deplete electrolytes. May decrease response to pressor amines. Potentiates other antihypertensives. May increase responsiveness to skeletal muscle relaxants. Risk of lithium toxicity; avoid concurrent use. NSAIDs may decrease diuretic effects; monitor closely.

PREGNANCY: Category C (1st trimester) and D (2nd and 3rd trimesters), not for use in nursing.

MECHANISM OF ACTION: Valsartan: Angiotensin II receptor antagonist; blocks vasoconstrictor and aldosterone-secreting effects of angiotensin II by selectively blocking binding of angiotensin II to AT_1 receptor. HCTZ: Thiazide diuretic; affects renal tubular mechanisms of electrolyte reabsorption, directly increasing excretion of sodium and chloride and indirectly reduces plasma volume.

PHARMACOKINETICS: Absorption: Valsartan: Absolute bioavailability (25%). T_{max}=2-4 hrs. **Distribution:** Valsartan: V_d=17L (IV). Plasma protein binding (95%). HCTZ: Crosses placenta; found in breast milk. **Metabolism:** Valsartan: valeryl 4-hydroxy valsartan (metabolite). **Elimination:** Valsartan: Feces, urine. $T_{1/2}$=6 hrs. HCTZ: Urine (61%). $T_{1/2}$=5.8-18.9 hrs.

DIPENTUM RX
olsalazine sodium (Celltech)

THERAPEUTIC CLASS: Anti-inflammatory Agent

INDICATIONS: Maintenance of ulcerative colitis in patients intolerant to sulfasalazine.

DOSAGE: *Adults:* 500mg bid with food.

HOW SUPPLIED: Cap: 250mg

CONTRAINDICATIONS: Salicylate hypersensitivity.

WARNINGS/PRECAUTIONS: May exacerbate colitis symptoms. Diarrhea may be dose related, or an underlying symptom of the disease. Caution with renal dysfunction; monitor urinalysis, BUN, creatinine levels. Monitor patients with severe allergies or asthma and impaired hepatic function.

ADVERSE REACTIONS: Diarrhea, abdominal pain, nausea, dyspepsia, headache, rash/itching, arthralgia.

INTERACTIONS: Increased risk of bleeding when co-administered with salicylates and LMW heparins. with Increased PT time with warfarin. May increase risk of myelosuppression with 6-mercaptopurine or thioguanine. Avoid salucylates for 6 weeks after varicella vaccine.

PREGNANCY: Category C, caution with nursing.

MECHANISM OF ACTION: Not fully established; bioconverted to 5-aminosalicylic acid (5-ASA), an anti-inflammatory drug that acts locally by blocking cyclooxygenase and inhibiting prostaglandin production in the colon.

PHARMACOKINETICS: Absorption: T_{max}=1 hr. **Distribution**: Plasma protein binding (>99%). **Metabolism**: Converted to 5-ASA (active), N-acetyl-5-ASA, olsalazine-O-sulfate. **Elimination**: $T_{1/2}$=0.9 hrs.

DIPHENHYDRAMINE HCL INJECTION   RX
diphenhydramine HCL (Various)

THERAPEUTIC CLASS: Antihistamine

INDICATIONS: Amelioration of allergic reactions to blood or plasma. Adjunct to epinephrine in anaphylaxis. For other uncomplicated immediate type allergic conditions when oral therapy is contraindicated. Treatment of motion sickness. For parkinsonism when oral therapy is not possible or contraindicated.

DOSAGE: *Adults:* Usual: 10-50mg IV or up to 100mg IM if needed. Max: 400mg/day.
Pediatrics: Usual: 5mg/kg/24hrs or 150mg/m²/24hrs IV/IM in 4 divided doses. Max: 300mg/day.

HOW SUPPLIED: Inj: 50mg/mL

CONTRAINDICATIONS: Neonates, premature infants, nursing, as a local anesthetic.

WARNINGS/PRECAUTIONS: Caution with narrow-angle glaucoma, stenosing peptic ulcer, pyloroduodenal obstruction, symptomatic prostatic hypertrophy, or bladder-neck obstruction. May cause excitation in pediatrics. Increased risk of dizziness, sedation, and hypotension in elderly. Caution with lower respiratory diseases, bronchial asthma, increased IOP, hyperthyroidism, cardiovascular disease, or HTN. Local necrosis with SQ or intradermal use.

ADVERSE REACTIONS: Sedation, drowsiness, dizziness, disturbed coordination, epigastric distress, thickening of bronchial secretions.

INTERACTIONS: Additive effects with alcohol, CNS depressants. MAOIs prolong and intensify anticholinergic effects.

PREGNANCY: Category B, contraindicated in nursing.

MECHANISM OF ACTION: Antihistamine; competes with histamine for cell receptor sites on effector cells.

PHARMACOKINETICS: Metabolism: Liver. **Elimination:** Urine.

DIPRIVAN   RX
propofol (Abraxis)

THERAPEUTIC CLASS: General anesthetic

INDICATIONS: Sedative-hypnotic agent used for both induction and maintenance of anesthesia. For initiation and maintenance of monitored anesthesia
care (MAC) sedation during diagnostic procedures and in conjunction with
local/regional anesthesia in patients undergoing surgical procedures. To
provide continuous sedation and control of stress responses in intubated,
mechanically ventilated adult patients in ICU.

DOSAGE: *Adults:* General Anesthesia: <55 yrs: 40mg IV every 10 seconds until
induction onset. Maint: 100-200mcg/kg/min IV or 20-50mg intermittently
byIV bolus prn. Elderly/Debilitated/ASA III & IV: 20mg IV every 10 seconds
until induction onset. Maint: 50-100mcg/kg/min IV. Cardiac Anesthesia:
20mg IV every 10 seconds until induction onset. Maint: 100-150mcg/kg/min
IV with secondary opioid or 50-100mcg/kg/min IV with primary opioid.
Neurosurgical Patients: 20mg IV every 10 seconds until induction onset. Maint:
100-200mcg/kg/min IV. MAC Sedation: 100-150mcg/kg/min IV infusion or
0.5mg/kg slow IV injection over 3-5 min followed immediately by maintenance infusion. Maint: 25-75mcg/kg/min IV infusion or 10-20mg incremental
IV boluses. Elderly/Debilitated/ASA III & IV: Use doses similar to healthy
adults. Avoid rapid boluses. Maint: 80% of the usual adult dose. ICU Sedation:
Initial: 5mcg/kg/min IV infusion for 5 min. Increase 5-10mcg/kg/min IV over
5-10 min. Maint: 5-50mcg/kg/min IV or higher may be required.
Pediatrics: 3-16 yrs: General Anesthesia: 2.5-3.5mg/kg IV over 20-30 seconds.
Maint: 2 months-16 yrs: 125-300mcg/kg/min IV.

HOW SUPPLIED: Inj: 10mg/mL

WARNINGS/PRECAUTIONS: Avoid rapid bolus administration in elderly, debilitated or ASA III/IV patients. Monitor oxygen saturation and for signs of significant hypotension, bradycardia, cardiovascular depression, apnea or airway
obstruction. Caution with hyperlipoproteinemia, diabetic hyperlipemia, pancreatitis, epilepsy. Rare reports of anaphylaxis reactions, pulmonary edema,
perioperative myoclonia, postoperative pancreatitis, bradycardia, asystole,
cardiac arrest, rhabdomyolysis. Minimize transient local pain by using larger
veins of forearm or antecubital fossa and/or prior lidocaine injection. May
elevate serum TG. Do not infuse for >5 days without drug holiday to replace
zinc losses; consider supplemental zinc with chronic use in those predisposed
to zinc deficiency. In renal impairment, perform baseline urinalysis/urinary
sediment then monitor on alternate days during sedation. (Neurosurgical
Anesthesia) Use infusion or slow bolus to avoid significant hypotension and
decreases in cerebral perfusion pressure. (Cardiac Anesthesia) Use slower
rates of administration in premedicated and geriatric patients, patients with
recent fluid shifts or those hemodynamically unstable. Correct fluid deficits
prior to use.

ADVERSE REACTIONS: Bradycardia, arrhythmia, hypotension, HTN, tachycardia nodal, decreased cardiac output, CNS movement, injection site burning/
stinging/pain, hyperlipemia, apnea, rash, pruritus, respiratory acidosis during
weaning.

INTERACTIONS: Increased effects with narcotics (eg, morphine, meperidine, fentanyl), combinations of opioids and sedatives (eg, benzodiazepines,
barbiturates, chloral hydrate, droperidol) and potent inhalational agents (eg,
isoflurane, enflurane, halothane). Concomitant fentanyl may cause bradycardia in pediatrics.

PREGNANCY: Category B, not for use in nursing.

MECHANISM OF ACTION: Sedative-hypnotic agent; uses in induction and
maintenance of anesthesia or sedation.

PHARMACOKINETICS: Distribution: Crosses placenta; found in breast milk.

DIPROLENE RX
betamethasone (augmented) dipropionate (Schering)

OTHER BRAND NAMES: Diprolene AF (Schering)

THERAPEUTIC CLASS: Corticosteroid

INDICATIONS: Relief of inflammatory and pruritic manifestations of corticos-teroid-responsive dermatoses.

DOSAGE: *Adults:* (Lot) Apply qd-bid for no more than 2 weeks. Max: 50mL/week. (Cre, Oint) Apply qd-bid, up to 45g/week.
Pediatrics: ≥13 yrs: (Cre) Apply qd-bid for no more than 2 weeks. Limit to 45g/week. ≥12 yrs: (Lot) Apply qd-bid for no more than 2 weeks. Limit to 50mL/week. (Oint) Apply qd-bid, up to 45g/week.

HOW SUPPLIED: Cre (AF), Oint: 0.05% [15g, 50g]; Lot: 0.05% [30mL, 60mL]

WARNINGS/PRECAUTIONS: May produce reversible HPA axis suppression, manifestations of Cushing's syndrome, hyperglycemia and glucosuria. D/C if irritation occurs. Use appropriate antifungal or antibacterial agent with dermatological infections. Pediatrics may be more susceptible to systemic toxicity. Caution when applied to large surface areas. Not for use with oc-clusive dressings. Gel is not for use in rosacea or perioral dermatitis or on the face, groin, or in the axillae.

ADVERSE REACTIONS: Stinging, burning, dry skin, pruritus, folliculitis, acneiform papules, irritation, hypopigmentation, skin maceration, secondary infection, skin atrophy, striae, miliaria.

PREGNANCY: Category C, (Cre, Lot) not for use in nursing; (Oint) caution in nursing.

MECHANISM OF ACTION: Corticosteroid; not established. Possesses anti-inflammatory, antipruritic, and vasoconstrictive actions.

PHARMACOKINETICS: Absorption: Percutaneous. Inflammation, use of occlusive dressings, and/or other disease states may increase absorption. **Distribution:** Systemically administered corticosteroids appear in breast milk. **Metabolism:** Liver. **Elimination:** Kidneys, bile.

DISPERMOX RX
amoxicillin (Ranbaxy)

THERAPEUTIC CLASS: Semisynthetic ampicillin derivative

INDICATIONS: Treatment of the following infections due to susceptible microorganisms: ear, nose, throat; genitourinary tract; skin and skin structure; lower respiratory tract due to susceptible (β-lactamase negative) organisms; gonorrhea (acute uncomplicated). *H. pylori* eradication to reduce the risk of duodenal ulcer recurrence.

DOSAGE: *Adults:* ENT/SSSI/GU: (Mild/Moderate): 500mg q12h or 250mg q8h. (Severe): 875mg q12h or 500mg q8h. LRTI: 875mg q12h or 500mg q8h. Gonorrhea: 3g as single oral dose. Do not chew or swallow dispersible tabs.
H. pylori Eradication: (Dual Therapy) 1g + 30mg lansoprazole, both tid for 14 days. (Triple Therapy): 1g + 30mg lansoprazole + 500mg clarithromycin, all q12h for 14 days.
Pediatrics: Neonates: ≤12 weeks: Max: 30mg/kg/day divided q12h. >3 months: ENT/SSSI/GU: (Mild/Moderate): 25mg/kg/day given q12h or 20mg/kg/day given q8h. (Severe): 45mg/kg/day given q12h or 40 mg/kg/day given q8h. LRTI: 45mg/kg/day given q12h or 40mg/kg/day given q8h. Gonorrhea: (Prepubertal) 50mg/kg with 25mg/kg probenecid as single dose (regimen not for use if <2 yrs). >40kg: Dose as adult. Do not chew or swallow dispers-ible tabs.

HOW SUPPLIED: Tab, Dispersible: 200mg, 400mg, 600mg

WARNINGS/PRECAUTIONS: Serious and fatal hypersensitivity reactions have been reported. Pseudomembranous colitis has been reported; toxin produced by *Clostridium difficile* is the primary cause. Monitor renal, hepatic, and blood with prolonged use. Dispersible tabs contain phenylalanine.

ADVERSE REACTIONS: Nausea, vomiting, diarrhea, pseudomembranous colitis, hypersensitivity reactions, blood dyscrasias, superinfection (prolonged use).

INTERACTIONS: Increased levels with probenecid. Chloramphenicol, macrolides, sulfonamides, tetracyclines may interfere with bactericidal effects. False (+) for urine glucose with Clinitest®, Benedict's or Fehling's solution. Decreased plasma concentration of total conjugated estriol, estrilglucuronide, conjugated estrone, and estradiol.

PREGNANCY: Category B, caution in nursing.

MECHANISM OF ACTION: Semi-synthetic antibiotic; has a broad spectrum bactericidal activity against susceptible organisms during active multiplication; inhibits biosynthesis of cell-wall mucopeptide.

PHARMACOKINETICS: Absorption: Rapid; administration of different doses resulted in different parameters. **Distribution:** Plasma protein binding (20%). **Elimination:** Urine (unchanged); $T_{1/2}$=61.3 min.

DITROPAN XL   RX
oxybutynin chloride (Ortho-McNeil)

OTHER BRAND NAMES: Ditropan (Ortho-McNeil)

THERAPEUTIC CLASS: Anticholinergic

INDICATIONS: (All) Overactive bladder/bladder instability with symptoms of urge urinary incontinence, urgency, and frequency. (Tab, Extended-Release) Detrusor overactivity associated with a neurological condition in pediatrics ≥6 yrs.

DOSAGE: *Adults:* (Tab, Syrup) Usual: 5mg bid-tid. Max: 5mg qid. Frail Elderly: 2.5mg bid-tid.(Tab, Extended-Release) Initial: 5 or 10mg qd. Titrate: May increase by 5mg weekly. Max: 30mg/day. Swallow XL whole with liquid; do not chew, divide or crush tab.
Pediatrics: >5 yrs: (Tab, Syrup) Usual: 5mg bid. Max: 5mg tid. ≥6 yrs: (Tab, Extended-Release) Initial: 5mg qd. Titrate: May increase by 5mg weekly. Max: 20mg/day. Swallow XL whole with liquid; do not chew, divide, or crush tab.

HOW SUPPLIED: Syrup: 5mg/5mL; Tab: 5mg*; Tab, Extended-Release: 5mg, 10mg, 15mg *scored

CONTRAINDICATIONS: Urinary retention, gastric retention and other severe decreased GI motility conditions, uncontrolled narrow-angle glaucoma, and in patients at risk for these conditions.

WARNINGS/PRECAUTIONS: Caution with hepatic or renal impairment, bladder outflow obstruction, GI obstruction/narrowing, ulcerative colitis, intestinal atony, myasthenia gravis, hyperthyroidism, CHD, CHF, arrhythmias, HTN, tachycardia, prostatic hypertrophy, and GERD. Heat prostration can occur with high environmental temperatures. Tab, Extended-Release shell may be excreted in the stool. Reduce dose or d/c if anticholinergic CNS effects occur. Caution in preexisting dementia.

ADVERSE REACTIONS: Dry mouth, constipation, somnolence, headache, diarrhea, nausea, blurred vision, dyspepsia, asthenia, pain, dizziness, dry eyes, UTI, insomnia, nervousness.

INTERACTIONS: Increased adverse effects with other anticholinergics. Increased drowsiness with alcohol or other sedatives. May alter GI absorption of other drugs due to GI motility effects. Increased levels with ketoconazole; caution with CYP3A4 inhibitors (eg, antimycotics, macrolides). Caution with bisphosphonates or other drugs that may exacerbate esophagitis.

PREGNANCY: Category B, caution in nursing.

MECHANISM OF ACTION: Antispasmodic/anticholinergic agent; inhibits muscarinic action of acetylcholine on smooth muscle exerting direct antispasmodic effect; relaxes smooth muscle of bladder.

PHARMACOKINETICS: Absorption: (Tab, Syrup) Rapid; absolute bioavailability (6%). Refer to PI for pediatric, isomer, and metabolite parameters. **Distribution**: V_d=193L. **Metabolism**: Liver via CYP3A4; desethyloxybutynin (active metabolite). **Elimination**: Urine (<0.1% unchanged); $T_{1/2}$=13.2 hrs.

DIURIL   RX
chlorothiazide (Salix)

THERAPEUTIC CLASS: Thiazide diuretic

INDICATIONS: (PO/IV) Adjunct therapy in edema associated with CHF, hepatic cirrhosis, corticosteroid and estrogen therapy, renal dysfunction. (PO) Management of hypertension.

DOSAGE: *Adults:* (PO/IV) Edema: 0.5-1g qd-bid. May give every other day or 3-5 days/week. Substitute IV for oral using same dosage. (PO) HTN: 0.5-1g qd or in divided doses. Max: 2g/day.
Pediatrics: (PO) Diuresis/HTN: Usual: 10-20mg/kg/day given qd-bid. Max: Infants up to 2 yrs: 375mg/day. 2-12 yrs: 1g/day. <6 months: Up to 15mg/kg bid may be required.

HOW SUPPLIED: Inj: 0.5g; Sus: 250mg/5mL [237mL]

CONTRAINDICATIONS: Anuria, sulfonamide hypersensitivity.

WARNINGS/PRECAUTIONS: Caution in severe renal disease, liver dysfunction, electrolyte/fluid imbalance. Monitor electrolytes. Hyperuricemia, hyperglycemia, hypokalemia, hyponatremia, hypomagnesemia, hypercalcemia may occur. Increases in cholesterol and triglyceride levels reported. May exacerbate SLE. Sensitivity reactions reported. D/C prior to parathyroid test. Enhanced effects in post-sympathectomy patient. IV use not recommended in infants or children.

ADVERSE REACTIONS: Weakness, hypotension, pancreatitis, jaundice, diarrhea, vomiting, blood dyscrasias, rash, photosensitivity, electrolyte imbalance, impotence.

INTERACTIONS: May potentiate orthostatic hypotension with alcohol, barbiturates, narcotics. Adjust antidiabetic drugs. Possible decreased response to pressor amines. Corticosteroids, ACTH increase electrolyte depletion. May potentiate nondepolarizing skeletal muscle relaxants, antihypertensives. Lithium toxicity. NSAIDs including selective cyclooxygenase-2 (COX-2) inhibitors decrease effects. Decreased PO absorption with cholestyramine, colestipol.

PREGNANCY: Category C, not for use in nursing.

MECHANISM OF ACTION: Thiazide diuretic; not established. Affects distal renal tubular mechanism of electrolyte reabsorption.

PHARMACOKINETICS: Elimination: Kidney; $T_{1/2}$=45-120 min. PO: Urine (10-15%); IV: Urine (96%).

DIVIGEL   RX
estradiol (Upsher-Smith)

> Estrogens increase the risk of endometrial cancer. Estrogens, with or without progestins, should not be used for the prevention of CVD or dementia. Increased risks of MI, stroke, invasive breast cancer, PE, and DVT in postmenopausal women (50-79 yrs of age) reported. Increased risk of developing probable dementia in postmenopausal women ≥65 yrs of age reported.

THERAPEUTIC CLASS: Estrogen

INDICATIONS: Treatment of moderate to severe vasomotor symptoms associated with menopause.

DOSAGE: *Adults:* Initial: 0.25gm qd applied on skin of right or left upper thigh. Re-evaluate periodically. Adjust dose based on individual response.

HOW SUPPLIED: Gel: 0.1% (0.25gm, 0.5gm, and 1gm single-dose foil pkts containing 0.25mg, 0.5mg, and 1mg estradiol, respectively)

CONTRAINDICATIONS: Undiagnosed abnormal genital bleeding, breast cancer, estrogen-dependent neoplasia, DVT/PE, active or recent (within past year) arterial thromboembolic disease (eg, stroke, MI), liver dysfunction or disease, pregnancy.

WARNINGS/PRECAUTIONS: May increase risk of cardiovascular events (eg, MI, stroke), venous thrombosis, and PE; d/c immediately if any occur or suspected. May increase risk of breast/endometrial cancer, dementia and gallbladder disease. May lead to severe hypercalcemia with breast cancer and bone metastases; monitor and d/c if hypercalcemia occurs. Retinal vascular thrombosis reported; monitor and d/c if papilledema or retinal vascular lesions occur. Consider addition of a progestin if no hysterectomy. May elevate BP; monitor at regular intervals. May cause elevations of plasma triglycerides with pre-existing hypertriglyceridemia. Caution with history of cholestatic jaundice associated with past estrogen use or with pregnancy; d/c with recurrence. May lead to increased TBG levels; monitor thyroid function. May cause fluid retention; caution with cardiac/renal dysfunction. Caution with severe hypocalcemia. May increase risk of ovarian cancer. May exacerbate endometriosis, asthma, DM, epilepsy, migraine, porphyria, SLE, and hepatic hemangiomas; use with caution. Alcohol-based gels are flammable; avoid fire, flame, or smoking until gel has dried.

ADVERSE REACTIONS: Nasopharyngitis, upper respiratory tract infection, vaginal mycosis, breast tenderness, metrorrhagia, headache, nausea, pruritis, abdominal cramps.

INTERACTIONS: May increase prothombin time, partial thromboplastin time, and platelet aggregation time. May require higher doses of thyroid hormone. May elevate binding proteins and decrease free hormone concentration. May increase plasma HDL concentration, reduce LDL concentration and increased triglyceride levels. Impaired glucose tolerance. Reduced response to metyrapone test.

PREGNANCY: Contraindicated in pregnancy, caution in nursing.

MECHANISM OF ACTION: Estrogen; acts through binding to nuclear receptors in estrogen responsive tissues. Circulating estrogens modulate the pituitary secretion of gonadotropins, leuteinizing hormone and follicle stimulating hormone, through a negative feedback mechanism. Acts to reduce elevated levels of these hormones seen in postmenopausal women.

PHARMACOKINETICS: Absorption: Administration of variable doses led to altered parameters. **Distribution:** Largely bound to sex hormone binding globulin and albumin; found in breast milk. **Metabolism:** Liver to estrone (metabolite), estriol (major urinary metabolite), sulfate and glucuronide conjugation (liver), intestinal hydrolysis; CYP3A4 (partial metabolism). **Elimination:** Urine (parent compound and metabolites); $T_{1/2}$=10 hrs.

DOBUTAMINE   RX
dobutamine (Various)

THERAPEUTIC CLASS: Inotropic agent

INDICATIONS: Short-term treatment of cardiac decompensation due to depressed contractility resulting from organic heart disease or from cardiac surgical procedures.

DOSAGE: *Adults:* Initial: 0.5-1mcg/kg/min. Usual: 2-20mcg/kg/min. Max: 40mcg/kg/min (rare). Adjust rate and duration based on BP, urine flow, ectopic activity, HR, and when possible on cardiac output, central venous or pulmonary wedge pressure.

HOW SUPPLIED: Inj: 12.5mg/mL [20mL, 40mL]

CONTRAINDICATIONS: Idiopathic hypertrophic subaortic stenosis.

WARNINGS/PRECAUTIONS: May increase HR or BP, especially systolic pressure; caution with atrial fibrillation and HTN. May precipitate or exacerbate ventricular ectopic activity. Hypersensitivity reactions (eg, skin rash, fever, eosinophilia, bronchospasm) reported. Contains sulfites. Monitor EKG, BP, pulmonary wedge pressure, and cardiac output. Correct hypovolemia prior to infusion. Caution in elderly. May decrease serum K⁺ levels. Improvement may not be observed with marked mechanical obstruction (eg, severe valvular aortic stenosis). Safety following acute MI has not been established.

ADVERSE REACTIONS: Increased HR, BP and ventricular ectopic activity, hypotension, infusion site reactions, nausea, headache, anginal pain, palpitations, shortness of breath, decreased K⁺ levels.

INTERACTIONS: Recent administration of β-blockers may reduce effectiveness and increase peripheral vascular resistance. Increased cardiac output and lower pulmonary wedge pressure with nitroprusside.

PREGNANCY: Category B, not for use in nursing.

MECHANISM OF ACTION: Direct-acting inotropic agent; stimulates β-receptors of the heart while producing comparatively mild chronotropic, hypertensive, arrhythmogenic, and vasodilative effects.

PHARMACOKINETICS: Metabolism: Methylation of the catechol and conjugation. **Elimination**: Urine (the conjugates of dobutamine and 3-O-methyl dobutamine; inactive metabolite).

DOLOBID   RX
diflunisal (Merck)

> NSAIDs may cause an increased risk of serious cardiovascular thrombotic events, MI, stroke and serious GI adverse events including bleeding, ulceration, and perforation of the stomach or intestines. Contraindicated for the treatment of perioperative pain in the setting of coronary artery bypass graft (CABG) surgery.

THERAPEUTIC CLASS: NSAID

INDICATIONS: Acute or long-term symptomatic treatment of mild to moderate pain, osteoarthritis (OA), rheumatoid arthritis (RA).

DOSAGE: *Adults:* Pain: Initial: 1g, then 500mg q8-12h. OA/RA: 250-500mg bid. Max: 1500mg/day.
Pediatrics: ≥12 yrs: Pain: Initial: 1g, then 500mg q12h or 500mg q8h. OA/RA: 250-500mg bid. Max: 1500mg/day.

HOW SUPPLIED: Tab: 250mg, 500mg

CONTRAINDICATIONS: ASA or other NSAID allergy that precipitates acute asthmatic attack, urticaria, or rhinitis. Treatment of perioperative pain in the setting of CABG surgery.

WARNINGS/PRECAUTIONS: May lead to onset of new HTN or worsening of pre-existing HTN; monitor BP closely. Fluid retention and edema reported; caution with fluid retention or heart failure. Renal papillary necrosis and other renal injury reported after long-term use. Not recommended for use with advanced renal disease; if therapy must be initiated, monitor renal function. Anaphylactoid reactions may occur. May cause serious skin adverse events (eg, exfoliative dermatitis, Stevens-Johnson syndrome, and toxic epidermal necrolysis). Avoid in late pregnancy; may cause premature closure of ductus arteriosis. May cause elevations of LFTs; d/c if liver disease develops or systemic manifestations occur. Caution in elderly. Anemia may occur; with long-term use, monitor Hgb/Hct if signs or symptoms of anemia develop. May inhibit platelet aggregation and prolong bleeding time; monitor with coagulation disorders. Caution with asthma and avoid with ASA-sensitive asthma. Adverse eye findings reported. Hypersensitivity syndrome reported; d/c if hypersensitivity occurs. Reye's syndrome may develop.

ADVERSE REACTIONS: Nausea, dyspepsia, GI pain, diarrhea, rash, headache, insomnia, dizziness, tinnitus, fatigue.

INTERACTIONS: May prolong PT with oral anticoagulants. Decreases hyperuricemic effect of HCTZ, furosemide. Antacids may reduce plasma levels. Avoid other NSAIDs. May potentiate methotrexate, cyclosporine toxicities. Increased plasma levels of APAP. Decreased plasma levels with ASA. Caution with nephrotoxic or hepatotoxic drugs.

PREGNANCY: Category C, not for use in nursing.

MECHANISM OF ACTION: NSAID; suspected to inhibit prostaglandin syn-thetase; exerts anti-inflammatory, analgesic, and antipyretic actions.

PHARMACOKINETICS: Absorption: Rapid and complete, T_{max}=2-3 hrs, C_{max}=41mcg/mL (250mg), 87mcg/mL (500mg), 124mcg/mL (1000mg). **Distribution:** Found in breast milk, plasma protein binding (99%). **Elimination:** Urine=90% (glucuronide conjugates); $T_{1/2}$=8-12 hrs,

DOLOPHINE   CII
methadone HCL (Roxane)

Only approved hospitals and pharmacies can dispense oral methadone for the treatment of narcotic addiction. Methadone can be dispensed in any licensed pharmacy when used as an analgesic. Deaths, cardiac and respiratory, have been reported during initiation and conversion of pain patients to methadone treatment from treatment with other opioid agonists. Respiratory depression is the main hazard associated with methadone administration. QT interval prolonga-tion and serious arrhythmias have been observed during treatment with methadone.

OTHER BRAND NAMES: Methadone (Various)

THERAPEUTIC CLASS: Opioid analgesic

INDICATIONS: Detoxification and temporary maintenance treatment of nar-cotic addiction (heroin or other morphine-like drugs). Relief of severe pain.

DOSAGE: *Adults:* Detoxification: Initial: 15-20mg/day (up to 40mg/day may be required). Stabilize for 2-3 days, then may decrease every 1-2 days depending on patient symptoms. Max: 21 days. May not repeat earlier than 4 weeks after completing previous course. Pain: Usual: 2.5-10mg q3-4h PO/IM/SQ prn.

HOW SUPPLIED: Tab: 5mg, 10mg

CONTRAINDICATIONS: Methadone is contraindicated in any patient sus-pected or having a paralytic ileus, acute bronchial asthma or hypercarbia and respiratory depression.

WARNINGS/PRECAUTIONS: Do not inject agent. Extreme caution if use narcotic antagonists in patients physically dependent on narcotics. Can cause respiratory depression and elevate CSF pressure. Caution with head injuries, acute asthma attacks, COPD, cor pulmonale, decreased respiratory reserve, pre-existing respiratory depression, hypoxia, or hypercapnia. Reduce initial dose in elderly, debilitated, severe hepatic or renal impairment, hypothyroid-ism, Addison's disease, prostatic hypertrophy, or urethral stricture. Risk of tolerance, dependence, and abuse may occur. Impairs physical and mental abilities. Ineffective in relieving anxiety. May mask symptoms of acute ab-dominal conditions. May produce hypotension. May cause incomplete cross-tolerance and iatrogenic overdose, interactions with other CNS depressants, alcohol and other drugs of abuse. May cause cardiac conduction effects like prolonged QT interval and seroius arrhythmias.

ADVERSE REACTIONS: Lightheadedness, dizziness, sedation, sweating, nau-sea, vomiting, asthenia, cardiomyopathy, ECG abnormalities, abdominal pain, agitation, siezures, confusion, hallucinations, respiratory depression.

INTERACTIONS: May increase desipramine levels. Pentazocine may precipi-tate withdrawal. Decreased serum levels with rifampin. Caution and reduce dose with CNS depressants (eg, tranquilizers, sedative-hypnotics, phenothi-azines, TCAs, alcohol). MAOIs may cause severe reactions. Use caution with concomitant administration of inducers/inhibitors of CYP450 (eg, azole antifungals, phenytoin).

PREGNANCY: Safety in pregnancy and nursing not known.

MECHANISM OF ACTION: Opioid analgesic; µ-agonist. Produces many actions similiar to morphine. Acts prominently in the CNS and in organs composed of smooth muscle. Also acts as an antagonist at the N-methyl-D-aspartate (NMDA) receptor.

PHARMACOKINETICS: Absorption: T_{max}=1-7.5 hrs.; C_{max}=124-1255ng/mL. **Distribution:** V_d=1.0-8.0L/kg. Plasma protein binding (85-90%); found in sali-va, human breast milk, amniotic fluid, and umbilical cord plasma. **Metabolism:**

Liver (N-demethylation) via CYP450 enzymes: 3A4 (primary), 2B6 (primary), 2C19 (primary); 2C9; 2D6. **Elimination:** Kidneys, feces; $T_{1/2}$=8-59 hrs.

DONNATAL

hyoscyamine sulfate - atropine sulfate - scopolamine hydrobromide - phenobarbital (PBM Pharmaceuticals)

RX

D

OTHER BRAND NAMES: Donnatal Extentabs (PBM Pharmaceuticals)

THERAPEUTIC CLASS: Anticholinergic/barbiturate

INDICATIONS: Adjunct therapy for irritable bowel syndrome, acute entero-colitis, duodenal ulcers.

DOSAGE: *Adults:* (Elixir/Tab) 1-2 tabs or 5-10mL tid-qid. (Extentabs) 1 tab q8-12h. Hepatic Disease: Use lower doses.
Pediatrics: (Elixir) 4.5kg: 0.5mL q4h or 0.75mL q6h. 9.1kg: 1mL q4h or 1.5mL q6h. 13.6kg: 1.5mL q4h or 2mL q6h. 22.7kg: 2.5mL q4h or 3.75mL q6h. 34kg: 3.75mL q4h or 5mL q6h. 45.4kg: 5mL q4h or 7.5mL q6h. Hepatic Disease: Use lower doses.

HOW SUPPLIED: (Atropine-Hyoscyamine-Phenobarbital-Scopolamine) Elixir: 0.0194mg-0.1037mg-16.2mg-0.0065mg/5mL; Tab: 0.0194mg-0.1037mg-16.2mg-0.0065mg; Tab, Extended-Release: (Extentabs) 0.0582mg-0.3111mg-48.6mg-0.0195mg

CONTRAINDICATIONS: Glaucoma, obstructive uropathy, obstructive GI disease, paralytic ileus, intestinal atony in elderly or debilitated, unstable cardiovascular status in acute hemorrhage, severe ulcerative colitis, myasthe-nia gravis, hiatal hernia with reflux esophagitis, intermittent porphyria, and for patients in whom phenobarbital produces restlessness and/or excitement.

WARNINGS/PRECAUTIONS: Inconclusive whether anticholinergic/anti-spasmodic drugs aid in duodenal ulcer healing, decrease recurrence rate, or prevent complications. Heat prostration can occur with high environmental temperatures. Avoid with intestinal obstruction. May be habit forming; cau-tion with history of physical and/or psychological drug dependence. Caution with hepatic disease, renal disease, autonomic neuropathy, hyperthyroid-ism, coronary heart disease, CHF, arrhythmias, tachycardia, HTN. May delay gastric emptying. Diarrhea may be an early symptom of incomplete intestinal obstruction, especially with ileostomy or colostomy; treatment would be inappropriate.

ADVERSE REACTIONS: Xerostomia, urinary hesitancy/retention, blurred vision, tachycardia/palpitation, mydriasis, cycloplegia, increased ocular ten-sion, loss of taste, headache, nervousness, drowsiness, weakness, dizziness, insomnia, nausea, vomiting, impotence, suppression of lactation, constipation, bloated feeling, musculoskeletal pain, allergic reaction/drug idiosyncrasies, decreased sweating.

INTERACTIONS: Phenobarbital may decrease anticoagulant effects; adjust dose.

PREGNANCY: Category C, caution in nursing.

MECHANISM OF ACTION: Anticholinergic/Barbiturate; drug combination that provides peripheral anticholinergic, antispasmodic action and mild sedation.

DOPAMINE

dopamine HCL (Various)

RX

THERAPEUTIC CLASS: Inotropic agent

INDICATIONS: For correction of hemodynamic imbalances present in shock due to MI, trauma, endotoxic septicemia, open-heart surgery, renal failure, and chronic cardiac decompensation.

DOSAGE: *Adults:* Initial: 2-5mcg/kg/min. Use 5mcg/kg/min in seriously ill. Increase in 5-10mcg/kg/min increments, up to 20-50mcg/kg/min.

D

HOW SUPPLIED: Inj: 40mg/mL, 80mg/mL, 160mg/mL

CONTRAINDICATIONS: Pheochromocytoma, uncorrected tachyarrhythmias or ventricular fibrillation.

WARNINGS/PRECAUTIONS: Contains sulfites. Monitor BP, urine flow, cardiac output and pulmonary wedge pressure. Correct hypovolemia, hypoxia, hypercapnia, and acidosis prior to use. Reduce infusion rate with increase in diastolic BP/marked decrease in pulse pressure; increase rate if hypotension occurs. D/C if hypotension persists. Reduce dose if increased ectopic beats occurs. Caution with history of occlusive vascular disease (eg, atherosclerosis, arterial embolism, Raynaud's disease, cold injury, diabetic endarteritis, and Buerger's disease); monitor for changes in skin color or temperature. Administer phentolamine if extravasation noted. Avoid abrupt withdrawal.

ADVERSE REACTIONS: Tachycardia, palpitation, ventricular arrhythmia (high doses), dyspnea, nausea, vomiting, headache, anxiety, bradycardia, hypotension, HTN, vasoconstriction.

INTERACTIONS: If treated with MAOIs within 2-3 weeks prior to administration of dopamine, reduce initial dose of dopamine to not greater than 1/10th of usual dose. Potential additive or potentiating effects on urine flow with diuretics. TCAs may potentiate cardiovascular effects of adrenergic agents. Cardiac effects antagonized by β-blockers. Peripheral vasoconstriction antagonized by α-blockers. Butyrophenones (eg, haloperidol) and phenothiazines may suppress renal and mesenteric vasodilation. Extreme caution with cyclopropane or halogenated hydrocarbon anesthetics. Concomitant use with vasopressors, vasoconstricting agents (eg, ergonovine), and some oxytocic drugs may result in severe HTN. Hypotension and bradycardia reported with phenytoin; consider alternatives.

PREGNANCY: Category C, caution in nursing.

MECHANISM OF ACTION: Catecholamine; produces positive chronotropic and inotropic effects on the myocardium, resulting in increased heart rate and cardiac contractility. Acts directly by exerting an agonist action on β-adrenoreceptor and indirectly by causing release of norepinephrine from storage sites in sympathetic nerve endings.

PHARMACOKINETICS: Metabolism: Liver, kidneys, and plasma via MAO and catechol-O-methyltransferase. **Elimination:** Urine (80%).

DORIBAX   RX
doripenem (Ortho-McNeil)

THERAPEUTIC CLASS: Carbapenem

INDICATIONS: Treatment of complicated intra-abdominal and urinary tract infections, including pyelonephritis, caused by susceptible microorganisms.

DOSAGE: Adults: ≥18 yrs: 500mg IV q8h for 5-14 days (intra-abdominal) or 10 days (UTI). Infuse over 1 hour. Renal Impairment: CrCl: >50mL/min: No dose adjustment. CrCl 30-50mL/min: 250mg IV q8h. CrCl >10 to <30mL/min: 250mg IV q12h.

HOW SUPPLIED: Inj: 500mg

CONTRAINDICATIONS: Anaphylactic reactions to β-lactams.

WARNINGS/PRECAUTIONS: Serious hypersensitivity (anaphylactic) reactions reported. *Clostridium difficile*-associated diarrhea reported (ranging from mild diarrhea to fatal colitis); evaluate if diarrhea occurs.

ADVERSE REACTIONS: Headache, nausea, diarrhea, rash, phlebitis, anemia, pruritus.

INTERACTIONS: May reduce serum valproic acid levels, which may result in loss of seizure control; monitor serum valproic levels frequently after initiation of therapy. Probenicid may increase levels; avoid co-administration.

PREGNANCY: Category B, caution in nursing.

MECHANISM OF ACTION: Broad-spectrum carbapenem; exerts bactericidal activity by inhibiting cell wall biosynthesis, resulting in cell death.

PHARMACOKINETICS: Absorption: C_{max}=23mcg/mL, AUC=36.3mcg•hr/mL. **Distribution:** Plasma protein binding (8.1%); V_d=16.8L. **Metabolism:** Via dehydropeptidase-1. **Elimination:** Urine (unchanged); $T_{1/2}$=1 hr.

DORYX   RX
doxycycline hyclate (Warner Chilcott)

D

THERAPEUTIC CLASS: Tetracycline derivative

INDICATIONS: Treatment of the following infections: respiratory, urinary, lymphogranuloma, psittacosis, trachoma, uncomplicated urethral/endocervical/ rectal, nongonococcal urethritis, Rocky Mountain spotted fever, typhus fever and the typhus group, Q fever, rickettsialpox, tick fevers, inclusion conjunctivitis, tularemia, campylobacter fetus infections, bartonellosis, granuloma chancroid, plague, cholera, brucellosis, anthrax (including inhalational anthrax, post-exposure). When penicillin is contraindicated, treatment of uncomplicated gonorrhea, syphilis, yaws, listeriosis, Vincent's infection, actinomycosis, and infections caused by *Clostridium* species. Adjunct therapy for intestinal amebiasis and severe acne. Prophylaxis of malaria in short-term travelers (<4 months) to areas with chloroquine and/or pyrimethamine-sulfadoxine resistant strains.

DOSAGE: *Adults:* Usual: 100mg q12h on 1st day, followed by 100mg/day (single dose or as 50mg q12h). Severe Infections/Chronic UTI: 100mg q12h. Uncomplicated Gonococcal Infections (Men, except anorectal infections): 100mg bid for 7 days, or 300mg followed 300mg 1 hr later. Acute Epididymo-Orchitis: 100mg bid for at least 10 days. Early Syphilis: 100mg bid for 14 days. Syphilis >1 yr: 100mg bid for 28 days. Nongonococcal Urethritis, Uncomplicated Urethral/Endocervical/Rectal Infection: 100mg bid for at least 7 days. Inhalational Anthrax (post-exposure): 100mg bid for 60 days. Treat Strep infections for 10 days. Malaria Prophylaxis: 100mg qd, begin 1-2 days before travel and continue daily during travel and for 28 days after travel to malarious area.
Pediatrics: >8 yrs: >100 lbs: 100mg q12h on 1st day, followed by 100mg/day (single dose or as 50mg q12h). Severe Infections/Chronic UTI: 100mg q12h. ≤100lbs: 2mg/lb in divided doses bid on Day 1, followed by 1mg/lb/day (single dose or divided bid) thereafter. Severe Infections: Up to 2mg/lb. Inhalational Anthrax (post-exposure): <100 lbs: 1mg/lb bid for 60 days. ≥100 lbs: 100mg bid for 60 days. Malaria Prophylaxis: 2mg/kg (up to adult dose) qd, begin 1-2 days before travel and continue daily during travel and for 28 days after travel to malarious area.

HOW SUPPLIED: Tab, Delayed-Release: 75mg, 100mg

WARNINGS/PRECAUTIONS: *Clostrium difficile*-associated diarrhea has been reported. May decrease bone growth in premature infants, and cause fetal harm during pregnancy. May cause permanent discoloration of the teeth or enamel hypoplasia if used in last half of pregnancy, infancy, or <8 yrs. Photosensitivity, increased BUN, superinfection may occur. Monitor hematopoietic, renal and hepatic values periodically with long term therapy. Bulging fontanels in infants and benign intracranial HTN in adults reported. May increase incidence of vaginal candidiasis.

ADVERSE REACTIONS: Anorexia, nausea, vomiting, diarrhea, dysphagia, enterocolitis, rash, inflammatory lesions, exfoliative dermatitis, renal toxicity, hypersensitivity reactions, blood dyscrasias, tooth discloration (<8 Yrs).

INTERACTIONS: Depress plasma PT, adjust anticoagulant dosage. May interfere with bactericidal action of penicillin; avoid concurrent use when possible. Avoid antacids containing aluminum, calcium, or magnesium, sodium bicarbonate, and iron-containing preparations. Reduced absorption with bismuth subsalicylate. Barbiturates, carbamazepine, and phenytoin decrease half-life. Fatal renal toxicity with Penthrane® (methoxyflurane). May render oral contraceptives less effective.

PREGNANCY: Category D, not for use in nursing.

MECHANISM OF ACTION: Tetracycline derivative; thought to inhibit protein synthesis.

PHARMACOKINETICS: Absorption: Complete; C_{max}=2.6 mcg/mL; T_{max}=2 hrs.
Distribution: Crosses placenta. **Metabolism:** Liver. **Elimination:** Urine, feces.

DOSTINEX   RX
cabergoline (Pharmacia & Upjohn)

THERAPEUTIC CLASS: Pituitary hormone

INDICATIONS: Treatment of hyperprolactinemic disorders, either idiopathic or due to pituitary adenomas.

DOSAGE: *Adults:* Initial: 0.25mg twice weekly. Titrate: May increase by 0.25mg twice weekly at 4 week intervals. Max: 1mg twice weekly. Discontinue after maintaining a normal serum prolactin level for 6 months. Efficacy >24 months not established.

HOW SUPPLIED: Tab: 0.5mg* *scored

CONTRAINDICATIONS: Uncontrolled HTN, hypersensitivity to ergot derivatives.

WARNINGS/PRECAUTIONS: Initial doses >1mg may produce orthostatic hypotension. Caution with hepatic impairment. Avoid with pregnancy-induced HTN (eg, preeclampsia, eclampsia). Not for inhibition/suppression of post-partum lactation. Use caution with respiratory or cardiac disorders linked to fibrotic tissue as risk of valvulopathy/fibrosis is possible; patient should be informed to notify physician if he/she develops cough.

ADVERSE REACTIONS: Nausea, constipation, abdominal pain, headache, dizziness, postural hypotension, fatigue, somnolence, depression, asthenia.

INTERACTIONS: Avoid with D_2-antagonists (eg, phenothiazines, butyrophenones, thioxanthines, metoclopramide). Caution with other drugs that lower BP.

PREGNANCY: Category B, not for use in nursing.

MECHANISM OF ACTION: Dopamine receptor agonist: Exerts a direct inhibitory effect on secretion of prolactin, decreasing serum prolactin levels (animals).

PHARMACOKINETICS: Absorption: C_{max}=30-70pg/mL, T_{max}=2-3 hrs.
Distribution: Plasma protein binding (40-42%). **Metabolism:** Liver via hydrolysis. **Elimination:** $T_{1/2}$=63-69 hrs. Urine (<4%).

DOVONEX   RX
calcipotriene (Warner Chilcott/Bristol-Myers Squibb)

THERAPEUTIC CLASS: Vitamin D_3 derivative

INDICATIONS: Treatment of plaque psoriasis.

DOSAGE: *Adults:* (Cream) Apply bid up to 8 weeks. (Oint) Apply qd-bid. Rub in gently. Wash hands after application.

HOW SUPPLIED: Cre, Oint: 0.005% [60g, 120g]

CONTRAINDICATIONS: Hypercalcemia or vitamin D toxicity. Do not use on the face.

WARNINGS/PRECAUTIONS: Avoid face and eyes. D/C if irritation or hypercalcemia occur; may continue once calcium levels are normal. Avoid excessive exposure to either natural or artificial sunlight.

ADVERSE REACTIONS: Local irritation, rash, pruritus, dermatitis, erythema, itching, worsening of psoriasis.

PREGNANCY: Category C, caution in nursing.

MECHANISM OF ACTION: Calcipotriene monohydrate; synthetic vitamin D_3 derivative.

PHARMACOKINETICS: Metabolism: Liver. **Elimination:** Bile.

DOVONEX SCALP   RX
calcipotriene (Warner Chilcott/Bristol-Myers Squibb)

THERAPEUTIC CLASS: Vitamin D$_3$ derivative

INDICATIONS: Topical treatment of chronic, moderately severe psoriasis of the scalp.

DOSAGE: *Adults:* Comb hair to remove debris. Part hair and apply bid up to 8 weeks. Rub in gently. Avoid uninvolved skin. Wash hands after application.

HOW SUPPLIED: Sol: 0.005% [60mL]

CONTRAINDICATIONS: Acute psoriatic eruptions, hypercalcemia, vitamin D toxicity.

WARNINGS/PRECAUTIONS: Avoid mucous membranes and eyes. D/C if irritation, sensitivity reaction, or hypercalcemia occur; may continue once calcium levels are normal. Avoid excessive exposure to either natural or artificial sunlight.

ADVERSE REACTIONS: Transient burning, stinging, tingling, rash, dry skin, irritation and worsening of psoriasis.

PREGNANCY: Category C, caution in nursing.

MECHANISM OF ACTION: Calcipotriene; is not fully understood. It is roughly equipotent to the natural vitamin in its effects on proliferation and differentiation of a variety of cell types.

PHARMACOKINETICS: Metabolism: Liver. **Ellimination:** Bile.

DOXEPIN   RX
doxepin HCL (Various)

> Antidepressants increased the risk of suicidal thinking and behavior (suicidality) in short-term studies in children, adolescents, and young adults with Major Depressive Disorder (MDD) and other psychiatric disorders. Doxepin is not approved for use in pediatric patients.

OTHER BRAND NAMES: Sinequan (Pfizer)

THERAPEUTIC CLASS: Tricyclic antidepressant

INDICATIONS: Depression and/or anxiety.

DOSAGE: *Adults:* Very Mild Illness: Usual: 25-50mg/day. Mild to Moderate Severity: Initial: 75mg/day. Usual: 75-150mg/day. Severely Ill: May increase up to 300mg/day. Dilute solution with 120mL of water, milk or juice. Give once daily or in divided doses. Divide dose if >150mg. Elderly: Use lower doses and monitor closely.

HOW SUPPLIED: Cap: 10mg, 25mg, 50mg, 75mg, 100mg, 150mg; Sol, Concentrate: 10mg/mL [120mL]

CONTRAINDICATIONS: Glaucoma, urinary retention.

WARNINGS/PRECAUTIONS: Monitor for suicidal tendencies and increased symptoms of psychosis. Avoid abrupt discontinuation.

ADVERSE REACTIONS: Drowsiness, dry mouth, blurred vision, constipation, urinary retention, hypotension, tachycardia, rash, edema, photosensitization, pruritus, eosinophilia, nausea, dizziness.

INTERACTIONS: Caution with drugs metabolized by CYP2D6. Potentiated by inhibitors (eg, cimetidine, quinidine, SSRIs) and substrates (other antidepressants, phenothiazines, propafenone, flecainide) of CYP2D6. Increased danger of overdose with alcohol. Hypoglycemia reported with tolazamide. Avoid within 2 weeks of MAOI therapy. Increased side effects with anticholinergics. Caution when switching from TCAs to SSRIs (≥5 weeks may be needed before initiating TCA treatment after withdrawal from fluoxetine).

PREGNANCY: Safety in pregnancy and nursing not known.

MECHANISM OF ACTION: Dibenzoxepin tricyclic; not been established, suspected to influence adrenergic activity at synapse, preventing deactivation of norepinephrine by reuptake into nerve terminals.

PHARMACOKINETICS: Metabolism: CYP2D6 (major); CYP1A2, 3A4 (minor).

DOXIL   RX
doxorubicin HCL liposome (Ortho Biotech)

D

> Myocardial damage may lead to CHF when cumulative dose approaches 550mg/m². May lead to cardiac toxicity, consider prior use of anthracyclines or anthracenediones in cumulative dose calculations. Cardiac toxicity may occur at lower cumulative doses with prior mediastinal irradiation or concurrent cardiotoxic agents, such as cyclophosphamide. Acute infusion-associated reactions reported. Severe myelosuppression, myocardial toxicity may occur. Reduce dose with impaired hepatic function. Severe side effects reported with accidental substitution for doxorubicin HCl, do not substitute on mg per mg basis.

THERAPEUTIC CLASS: Anthracycline

INDICATIONS: Treatment of ovarian cancer which has progressed or recurred after platinum-based chemotherapy. Treatment of AIDS-related Kaposi's sarcoma (KS) in patients with disease that has progressed on prior combination chemotherapy or in patients intolerant to such therapy. In combination with bortezomib for the treatment of multiple myeloma (MM) in patients who have not previously received bortezomib and have received at least one prior therapy.

DOSAGE: *Adults:* Administer as IV infusion at initial rate of 1mg/min to minimize risk of infusion-related reactions; if no reactions, may increase rate to complete infusion over 1 hr. Ovarian Cancer: 50mg/m² IV every 4 weeks for minimum of 4 courses. KS: 20mg/m² IV once every 3 weeks. MM: Give bortezomib 1.3mg/m² IV bolus on Days 1, 4, 8 and 11, every 3 weeks. Give doxorubicin 30mg/m² IV on Day 4 following bortezomib. May treat for up to 8 cycles depending on disease progression or unaccepable toxicity. Hepatic Dysfunction: If serum bilirubin 1.2-3mg/dL, give 50% of normal dose. If serum bilirubin >3mg/dL, give 25% of normal dose. Adjust dose based on toxicities (see PI).

HOW SUPPLIED: Inj: 2mg/mL

CONTRAINDICATIONS: Nursing mothers.

WARNINGS/PRECAUTIONS: Monitor cardiac function. Cardiac toxicity may occur after discontinuation. Recall of skin reaction due to radiotherapy reported. Myelosuppression may occur; obtain CBCs, including platelets frequently and at a minimum before each dose. Secondary AML reported with anthracyclines. Evaluate hepatic function before therapy. Avoid extravasation. Can cause fetal harm. Hand-foot syndrome and acute infusion-related reactions reported.

ADVERSE REACTIONS: Neutropenia, leukopenia, anemia, thromobocytopenia, stomatitis, fever, anorexia, fatigue, nausea, asthenia, vomiting, rash, alopecia, diarrhea, constipation, hand-foot syndrome.

INTERACTIONS: See Black Box Warning. May potentiate toxicity of other anticancer therapies. May exacerbate cyclophosphamide-induced hemorrhagic cystitis. May enhance hepatotoxicity of 6-mercaptopurine. May increase radiation-induced toxicity of the myocardium, mucosae, skin, and liver. Hematological toxicity may be more severe with agents that cause bone marrow suppression.

PREGNANCY: Category D, not for use in nursing.

MECHANISM OF ACTION: Anthracycline topoisomerase inhibitor; suspected to bind DNA and inhibit nucleic acid synthesis.

PHARMACOKINETICS: Absorption: (10mg/m²) C_{max}=4.12µg/mL, AUC=277µg/mL•h. (20mg/m²) C_{max}=8.34µg/mL, AUC=590µg/mL•h. **Distribution**: (10mg/m²) V_d=2.83L/m²; (20mg/m²) V_d=2.72L/m². **Metabolism:** Doxorubicinol (metabolite).

DOXORUBICIN HCL

RX

doxorubicin HCL (Various)

> Severe local tissue necrosis will occur if extravasation occurs. Do not give IM/SC route. Myocardial toxicity may occur during or after therapy. Increased risk of CHF with high cumulative doses, previous anthracycline/anthracenedione therapy, pre-existing heart disease, radiotherapy to mediastinal/pericardial area, concomitant cardiotoxic drugs. Increased risk of delayed cardiotoxicity in pediatrics. Secondary acute myelogenous leukemia reported. Reduce dose in hepatic impairment. Severe myelosuppression may occur.

THERAPEUTIC CLASS: Anthracycline

INDICATIONS: To produce regression in disseminated neoplastic conditions such as acute lymphoblastic and myeloblastic leukemias, Wilms' tumor, neuroblastoma, soft tissue/bone sarcomas, breast carcinoma, ovary, bladder and thyroid, gastric and bronchogenic carcinomas, Hodgkin's disease, malignant lymphoma in which the small-cell histologic type is the most responsive compared with other cell types. Adjuvant therapy in women with evidence of axillary lymph node involvement following resection of primary breast cancer.

DOSAGE: *Adults:* Monotherapy: 60-75mg/m^2 IV every 21 days. Use the lower dose with inadequate bone marrow reserves due to old age, prior therapy, or neoplastic marrow infiltration. Concomitant Chemotherapy: 40-60mg/m^2 IV every 21-28 days. Hyperbilirubinemia: Reduce dose by 50% if 1.2-3mg/dL; reduce dose by 75% if 3.1-5mg/dL.
Pediatrics: Monotherapy: 60-75mg/m^2 IV every 21 days. Use the lower dose with inadequate bone marrow reserves due to old age, prior therapy, or neoplastic marrow infiltration. Concomitant Chemotherapy: 40-60mg/m^2 IV every 21-28 days. Hyperbilirubinemia: Reduce dose by 50% if 1.2-3mg/dL; reduce dose by 75% if 3.1-5mg/dL.

HOW SUPPLIED: Inj: (2mg/mL) 10mg, 20mg, 50mg

CONTRAINDICATIONS: Marked myelosuppression induced by previous treatment with other antitumor agents or radiotherapy. Previous therapy with complete cumulative doses of doxorubicin, daunorubicin, idarubicin, or other anthracyclines and anthracenes.

WARNINGS/PRECAUTIONS: Irreversible myocardial toxicity may occur. Bone marrow depression and arrhythmias reported. Enhanced toxicity with hepatic impairment; evaluate hepatic function before dosing. Imparts a red coloration to urine for 1-2 days after administration. May induce tumor lysis syndrome and hyperuricemia with rapidly growing tumors. Periodically monitor CBC, hepatic function, and radionuclide left ventricular ejection fraction. May cause prepubertal growth failure and gonadal impairment.

ADVERSE REACTIONS: Myelosuppression, cardiotoxicity, alopecia, nausea, vomiting, mucositis, ulceration and necrosis of colon, fever, chills, urticaria, phlebosclerosis, facial flushing.

INTERACTIONS: May potentiate toxicity of other anticancer therapies. May exacerbate cyclophosphamide-induced hemorrhagic cystitis. May enhance hepatotoxicity of 6-mercaptopurine. May increase radiation induced toxicity of the myocardium, mucosae, skin, and liver. Acute "recall" pneumonitis in pediatrics with actinomycin-D. Paclitaxel infused before doxorubicin may decrease clearance of doxorubicin and increase neutropenia and stomatitis episodes, than the reverse sequence of administration. Enhanced neutropenia and thrombocytopenia reported with IV progesterone. Cyclosporine may prolong and exacerbate hematologic toxicity. Phenobarbital increases elimination. May decrease phenytoin levels. Streptozocin may inhibit hepatic metabolism. Live vaccines may be hazardous in those undergoing cytotoxic chemotherapy. Necrotizing colitis reported with cytarabine. Seizures and coma reported with cyclosporine, cisplatin or vincristine. Possible increased risk of cardiotoxicity with CCBs. Increased risk of CHF with radiotherapy to mediastinal/pericardial area or cardiotoxic drugs.

PREGNANCY: Category D, not for use in nursing.

MECHANISM OF ACTION: Anthracycline antineoplastic agent; inhibits nucleotide replication and action of DNA and RNA polymerases.

PHARMACOKINETICS: Distribution: V_d=809-1214L/m^2. Plasma protein binding (74-76%), excreted in breast milk. **Metabolism:** Enzymatic reduction; doxorubicinol (major metabolite). **Elimination:** Bile (40%), urine (5-12%); $T_{1/2}$=20-48 hrs.

DOXYCYCLINE IV   RX
doxycycline hyclate (Bedford)

THERAPEUTIC CLASS: Tetracycline derivative

INDICATIONS: Treatment of rickettsiae, *Mycoplasma pneumoniae*, psittacosis, ornithosis, lymphogranuloma venereum, granuloma inguinale, relapsing fever, chancroid, *Pasteurella pestis*, *Pasturella tularensis*, *Bartonella bacilliformis*, *Bacteroides* species, *Vibrio comma*, *Vibrio fetus*, *Brucella* species, *E.coli*, *Enterobacter aerogenes*, *Shigella* species, *Mima* species, *Herellea* species, *Haemophilus influenzae*, *Klebsiella* species, *Streptococcus* species, *Diplococcus pneumoniae*, *Staphylococcus aureus*, anthrax, and trachoma. When PCN is contraindicated; treatment of *Neisseria gonorrhoeae*, *N.meningitis*, syphilis, yaws, *Listeria monocytogenes*, *Clostridium* species, *Fusobacterium fusiforme*, and *Actinomyces* species. Adjunct therapy for amebiasis.

DOSAGE: *Adults:* Usual: 200mg IV divided qd-bid on Day 1 then 100-200mg/day IV depending on severity, with 200mg administered in 1 or 2 infusions. Primary/Secondary Syphilis: 300mg/day IV for at least 10 days. Inhalational Anthrax (post-exposure): 100mg IV bid. Institute oral therapy as soon as possible and continue therapy for a total of 60 days.
Pediatrics: >8 yrs: >100 lbs: Usual: 200mg IV divided qd-bid on Day 1 then 100-200mg/day IV depending on severity, with 200mg administered in 1 or 2 infusions. ≤100 lbs: 2mg/lb IV divided qd-bid on Day 1 then 1-2mg/lb/day IV divided qd-bid depending on severity. Inhalational Anthrax (post-exposure): <100 lbs: 1 mg/lb IV bid. Institute oral therapy as soon as possible and continue therapy for total of 60 days.

HOW SUPPLIED: Inj: 100mg

WARNINGS/PRECAUTIONS: May cause fetal harm during pregnancy. Permanent tooth discoloration during tooth development (last half of pregnancy and children <8 yrs) reported; avoid use in this age group except for anthrax treatment. Decreased bone growth in premature infants reported. May increase BUN. Photosensitivity, enamel hypoplasia reported. Superinfection with prolonged use. Monitor hematopoietic, renal and hepatic values periodically with long term therapy. Bulging fontanels in infants and benign intracranial HTN in adults reported.

ADVERSE REACTIONS: GI effects, increased BUN, rash, hypersensitivity reactions, hemolytic anemia, thrombocytopenia.

INTERACTIONS: May decrease PT; adjust anticoagulants. Avoid use with bactericidal agents (eg, penicillin).

PREGNANCY: Safety in pregnancy not known; not for use in nursing.

MECHANISM OF ACTION: Tetracycline derivative; thought to inhibit protein synthesis.

PHARMACOKINETICS: Absorption: Readily absorbed; C_{max}=2.5 mcg/mL. **Elimination:** $T_{1/2}$=18-22 hrs.

DRISDOL   RX
ergocalciferol (Sanofi-Aventis)

THERAPEUTIC CLASS: Vitamin D analog

INDICATIONS: Treatment of hypoparathyroidism, refractory rickets (vitamin D resistant rickets), and familial hypophosphatemia.

DOSAGE: *Adults:* Vitamin D Resistant Rickets: 12,000-500,000 IU qd. Hypoparathyroidism: 50,000-200,000 IU qd given concomitantly with calcium lactate 4g six times/day. Individualize dosage.

HOW SUPPLIED: Cap: 1.25mg (50,000 IU vitamin D)

CONTRAINDICATIONS: Hypercalcemia, malabsorption syndrome, abnormal sensitivity to the toxic effects of vitamin D, hypervitaminosis D.

WARNINGS/PRECAUTIONS: Avoid in infants with idiopathic hypercalcemia. Monitor serum calcium and phosphorous levels every 2 weeks or more frequently if necessary. X-rays of bones should be taken every month until condition is corrected and stabilized. IV calcium, parathyroid hormone, and/ or dihydrotachysterol may be needed when treating hypoparathyroidism. Maintain normal serum phosphorous levels when treating hyperphosphatemia to prevent metastatic calcification. Maintain adequate dietary calcium. Contains FD&C Yellow No. 5 (tartrazine). Protect from light.

ADVERSE REACTIONS: Anemia, anorexia, constipation, nausea, bone demineralization, stiffness, weakness, calcification of soft tissues, impaired renal function, polyuria, nocturia, polydipsia, hypercalciuria, azotemia, HTN, nephrocalcinosis.

INTERACTIONS: Impaired absorption with mineral oil. Thiazide diuretics may cause hypercalcemia.

PREGNANCY: Category C, caution in nursing.

MECHANISM OF ACTION: Calcium regulator. Antirachitic activity. After extensive metabolism, vitamin D metabolites promote the active absorption of calcium and phosphorus in the small intestine, which then elevates serum calcium and phosphate levels and promotes bone mineralization. Also mobilizes calcium and phosphate from bone and increases the reabsorption of calcium and perhaps also phosphate from renal tubules.

PHARMACOKINETICS: Metabolism: Liver via hydroxylation, 25-hydroxyvitamin D and 1,25-dihydroxyvitamin D (active major metabolites), and kidneys.

DROXIA RX
hydroxyurea (Bristol-Myers Squibb)

> Mutagenic, carcinogenic, clastogenic, and causes cellular transformation to tumorigenic phenotypes. May develop secondary leukemia with long-term therapy for myeloproliferative disorders. Administer only under supervision of a physician experienced in the use of antineoplastic agents.

THERAPEUTIC CLASS: Ribonucleotide reductase inhibitor

INDICATIONS: To reduce the frequency of painful crises and the need for blood transfusions in sickle cell anemia with recurrent moderate to severe painful crises.

DOSAGE: *Adults:* Initial: 15mg/kg/day as single dose. If blood counts are in acceptable range, increase by 5mg/kg/day every 12 weeks until maximum tolerated dose or 35mg/kg/day. If blood counts are toxic, discontinue until hematologic recovery. May resume treatment after dose reduction by 2.5mg/kg/day from dose associated with hematologic toxicity. May increase every 12 weeks by 2.5mg/kg/day until reaching a stable dose that does not result in toxicity for 24 weeks. CrCl <60mL/min or ESRD: 7.5mg/kg/day; administer in ESRD following hemodialysis.

HOW SUPPLIED: Cap: 200mg, 300mg, 400mg

WARNINGS/PRECAUTIONS: Avoid in marked bone marrow depression. Caution with renal dysfunction. Severe, life-threatening myelosuppression reported. Monitor hematologic, liver, kidney function before therapy and repeatedly thereafter. Interrupt therapy if neutrophils <2000/mm³ or platelets <80,000/mm³, Hgb <4.5g/dL or reticulocytes <80,000/mm² with Hgb <9g/dL. Monitor blood counts every 2 weeks. Cutaneous vasculitic toxicities, including vasculitic ulcerations and gangrene, reported; d/c if cutaneous vasculitic ulcerations develop. Causes macrocytosis, which mask the incidental development of folic acid deficiency.

ADVERSE REACTIONS: Neutropenia, low reticulocyte and platelet levels, hair loss, fever, GI disturbances, weight gain, bleeding, melanonychia, dermatological reactions, cutaneous vasculitic toxicities.

INTERACTIONS: Monitor for hepatoxicity and pancreatitis with didanosine, stavudine.

PREGNANCY: Category D, not for use in nursing.

MECHANISM OF ACTION: Ribonucleotide reductase inhibitor; not established, suspected to inhibit DNA synthesis by inhibiting ribonucleotide reductase without interfering with synthesis of RNA or protein.

PHARMACOKINETICS: Absorption: T_{max}=1-4 hrs. **Metabolism:** Liver; intestinal bacteria via urease (minor). **Elimination:** Urine (40%).

DRYSOL RX
aluminum chloride (Person & Covey)

THERAPEUTIC CLASS: Antiperspirant

INDICATIONS: Aid in the management of hyperhidrosis.

DOSAGE: *Adults:* Apply qhs to dry area. Wash area the following morning. Maint: After excessive sweating stops, apply once or twice weekly or as needed.

HOW SUPPLIED: Sol: 20% [35mL, 37.5mL, 60mL]

WARNINGS/PRECAUTIONS: Avoid broken, irritated or recently shaved skin. Avoid eye contact. D/C if irritation or sensitization occurs. May be harmful to certain metals and fabrics. Keep away from open flame.

ADVERSE REACTIONS: Transient stinging or itching.

PREGNANCY: Safety in pregnancy and nursing not known.

MECHANISM OF ACTION: Dermatologic agent. Unknown. Suspected to have dermatologic effects.

DTIC-DOME RX
dacarbazine (Bayer Healthcare)

> Hemopoietic toxicity and hepatotoxicity reported.

THERAPEUTIC CLASS: Purine precursor analog

INDICATIONS: Treatment of metastatic malignant melanoma and 2nd line combination therapy for Hodgkin's disease.

DOSAGE: *Adults:* Malignant Melanoma: 2-4.5mg/kg/day for 10 days. May repeat every 4 weeks. Alternate Dosage: 250mg/m²/day IV for 5 days. May repeat every 3 weeks. Hodgkin's Disease: 150mg/m²/day for 5 days. May repeat every 4 weeks. Alternate Dosage: 375mg/m²/day on day 1. May repeat every 15 days.

HOW SUPPLIED: Inj: 200mg

WARNINGS/PRECAUTIONS: Hematopoietic depression, anemia, anaphylactic reactions reported. Hepatotoxicity with hepatic vein thrombosis and hepatocellular necrosis may result in death. Extravasation may result in tissue damage and severe pain.

ADVERSE REACTIONS: Nausea, vomiting, anorexia, diarrhea, flu-like syndromes, alopecia, renal or hepatic dysfunction, rash.

PREGNANCY: Category C, safety in nursing not known.

DUAC RX
clindamycin - benzoyl peroxide (Stiefel)

THERAPEUTIC CLASS: Antibacterial/keratolytic

INDICATIONS: Topical treatment of inflammatory acne vulgaris.

DOSAGE: *Adults:* Wash face and pat dry. Apply qd in evening.
Pediatrics: ≥12 yrs: Wash face and pat dry. Apply qd in evening.

HOW SUPPLIED: Gel: (Clindamycin-Benzoyl Peroxide) 1%-5% [45g]

CONTRAINDICATIONS: Hypersensitivity to lincomycin. History of regional enteritis, ulcerative colitis, pseudomembranous colitis, or antibiotic-associated colitis.

WARNINGS/PRECAUTIONS: Severe colitis reported with oral and parenteral clindamycin. D/C if severe diarrhea occurs. Avoid contact with eyes and mucous membranes. May bleach hair or colored fabric. Limit sunlight exposure.

ADVERSE REACTIONS: Dry skin, erythema, peeling, burning.

INTERACTIONS: Cumulative irritancy possible with other topical acne agents. Avoid erythromycin agents.

PREGNANCY: Category C, not for use in nursing.

MECHANISM OF ACTION: Clindamycin: Antibacterial; binds to 50S ribosomal subunits of susceptible bacteria and prevents elongation of peptide chains by interfering with peptidyl transfer, thereby suppressing protein synthesis. Benzoyl peroxide: Keratolytic; potent oxidizing agent.

PHARMACOKINETICS: Distribution: Orally and parenterally administered clindamycin found in breast milk.

DUET STUARTNATAL   RX
folic acid - multiple vitamin - minerals (Xanodyne)

THERAPEUTIC CLASS: Prenatal vitamin

INDICATIONS: Vitamin and mineral supplementation for before, during, and after pregnancy.

DOSAGE: *Adults:* 1 tab qd.

HOW SUPPLIED: Tab: Calcium 200mg-Copper 2mg-Folic Acid 1mg-Iron 29mg-Magnesium 25mg-Niacinamide 20mg-Vitamin A 3000IU-Vitamin B_1 1.8mg-Vitamin B_2 4mg-Vitamin B_6 25mg-Vitamin B_{12} 0.012mg-Vitamin C 120mg-Vitamin D 400IU-Vitamin E 30mg-Zinc 25mg; Tab, Chewable: Calcium 100mg-Copper 2mg-Folic Acid 1mg-Iron 29mg-Magnesium 25mg-Niacinamide 20mg-Vitamin A 3000IU-Vitamin B_1 1.8mg-Vitamin B_2 4mg-Vitamin B_6 25mg-Vitamin B_{12} 0.012mg-Vitamin C 120mg-Vitamin D 400IU-Vitamin E 30mg-Zinc 25mg

WARNINGS/PRECAUTIONS: Accidental overdose of iron-containing products is a leading cause of fatal poisoning in children <6 yrs. Not for the treatment of pernicious anemia and other megaloblastic anemias where vitamin B_{12} is deficient. Folic acid >0.1mg/day may obscure pernicious anemia. Chewable tabs contain phenylalanine.

INTERACTIONS: Avoid pyridoxine in patients receiving levadopa; may antagonize effects.

MECHANISM OF ACTION: Multivitamin and mineral supplement.

DUETACT   RX
pioglitazone HCL - glimepiride (Takeda)

> Thiazolidinediones may cause or exacerbate CHF in some patients. Duetact is not recommended in patients with symptomatic heart failure.

THERAPEUTIC CLASS: Thiazolidinedione/sulfonylurea

INDICATIONS: Adjunct to diet and exercise to improve glycemic control in type 2 diabetes already being treated with combination of pioglitazone and sulfonylurea, with inadequate control on sulfonylurea alone, or with initial response to pioglitazone alone requiring additional glycemic control.

DOSAGE: *Adults:* Base recommended starting dose on current regimen of pioglitazone and/or sulfonylurea. Give with 1st meal of day. Current Glimepiride Monotherapy or Prior Therapy of Pioglitazone plus Glimepiride Separately: Initial: 30mg-2mg or 30mg-4mg qd. Current Pioglitazone or Different Sulfonylurea Monotherapy or Combination of Both: Initial: 30mg-2mg qd. Adjust dose based on response. Max: Once daily at any strength. Elderly/Debilitated/Malnourished/Renal or Hepatic Insufficiency (ALT ≤2.5x ULN): Initial: 1mg glimepiride prior to prescribing Duetact. Systolic Dysfunction: Initial: 15-30mg of pioglitazone; titrate carefully to lowest Duetact dose.

HOW SUPPLIED: Tab: (Pioglitazone-Glimepiride) 30mg-2mg, 30mg-4mg

CONTRAINDICATIONS: Established NYHA Class III or IV heart failure, diabetic ketoacidosis.

WARNINGS/PRECAUTIONS: (Glimepiride): Increased CV mortality. Hypoglycemia risk if debilitated, malnourished, or with adrenal, pituitary, renal or hepatic insufficiency. Hypoglycemia may be masked in elderly. May lose blood glucose control with stress. Secondary failure may occur. D/C if skin reactions persist or worsen. (Pioglitazone): May cause fluid retention and exacerbation/initiation of heart failure; d/c if cardiac status deteriorates. Avoid if NYHA Class III or IV cardiac status. Not for use in type 1 DM or diabetic ketoacidosis treatment. Caution with edema. Dose-related weight gain reported. Ovulation in premenopausal anovulatory patient may occur; risk of pregnancy with inadequate contraception. May decrease Hgb and Hct. Avoid with active liver disease, if ALT levels >2.5x ULN, or if jaundice occurred. Check LFTs before therapy, every 2 months for 1 yr, and periodically thereafter, or if hepatic dysfunction symptoms occur. D/C if ALT >3x ULN on therapy. Macular edema and fractures reported.

ADVERSE REACTIONS: Hypoglycemia, upper respiratory tract infection, increased weight, lower limb edema/pain, headache, UTI, diarrhea, nausea, new onset or worsening diabetic macular edema with decreased visualacuity.

INTERACTIONS: (Pioglitazone): CYP3A4 inducer. May decrease levels of ethinyl estradiol and midazolam. CYP2C8 inhibitor. May significantly increase the AUC levels of pioglitazone. CYP2C8 inducer. May significantly decrease the AUC levels of pioglitazone.(Glimepiride): Risk of hyperglycemia with thiazides, corticosteroids, phenothiazines, thyroid products, estrogens, oral contraceptives, phenytoin, nicotinic acid, sympathomimetics, or isoniazid. Hypoglycemia may be potentiated with β-blockers, MAOIs, salicylates, sulfonamides, and coumarins. Risk of severe hypoglycemia with oral miconazole.

PREGNANCY: Category C, not for use in nursing.

MECHANISM OF ACTION: Pioglitazone: Thiazolidinedione; insulin-sensitizing agent acts by enhancing peripheral glucose utilization. Glimepiride: Sulfonylurea; stimulates release of insulin from functional pancreatic β-cells.

PHARMACOKINETICS: Absorption: Administration of variable doses resulted in different parameters. Glimepiride: T_{max}=2-3 hrs. **Distribution:** Pioglitazone: V_d=0.63 L/kg, plasma protein binding (>99%); Glimepiride: (IV) V_d=8.8L, plasma protein binding (>99.5%). **Metabolism:** Pioglitazone: Extensive (hydroxylation & oxidation), CYP2C8, 3A4. Glimepiride: CYP2C9. **Elimination:** Pioglitazone: $T_{1/2}$=3-7 or 16-24 hrs, urine (15-30%), feces. Glimepiride: Urine (60%).

Dulcolax OTC
bisacodyl (Boehringer Ingelheim)

THERAPEUTIC CLASS: Stimulant laxative

INDICATIONS: Relief of occasional constipation and irregularity. For bowel cleansing regimen for surgery or endoscopic exam.

DOSAGE: *Adults:* (Tab) Take 2-3 tabs qd. Do not crush/chew. (Sup) Insert 1 sup rectally; retain for 15-20 min. May coat tip with petroleum jelly with anal fissures or hemorrhoids. X-Ray Endoscopy For Barium Enema: Avoid food after tab administration. Insert 1 sup rectally 1-2 hrs before exam.
Pediatrics ≥12 yrs: (Tab) 2-3 tabs qd. 6-12 yrs: 1 tab qd. Do not crush/chew.

(Sup) ≥12 yrs: Insert 1 sup rectally; retain for 15-20 min. 6-12 yrs: Insert 1/2 sup rectally qd. May coat tip with petroleum jelly with anal fissures or hemorrhoids. X-Ray Endoscopy for Barium Enema: ≥6 yrs: Avoid food after tab administration. Insert 1 sup 1-2 hrs before exam. <6 yrs: Avoid tab. Insert 1/2 sup rectally 1-2 hrs before exam.

HOW SUPPLIED: Sup: 10mg; Tab, Delayed-Release: 5mg

CONTRAINDICATIONS: Acute abdominal surgery, appendicitis, rectal bleeding, gastroenteritis, intestinal obstruction.

WARNINGS/PRECAUTIONS: Avoid with abdominal pain, nausea, or vomiting. Not for long-term use (>7 days). D/C with rectal bleeding or fail to have bowel movement.

ADVERSE REACTIONS: Abdominal discomfort.

INTERACTIONS: Avoid tabs within 1 hr after antacids or milk.

PREGNANCY: Safety in pregnancy and nursing not known.

DUONEB   RX
ipratropium bromide - albuterol sulfate (Dey)

THERAPEUTIC CLASS: Beta$_2$-agonist/anticholinergic

INDICATIONS: Treatment of bronchospasm in COPD in patients requiring more than one bronchodilator.

DOSAGE: *Adults:* 3mL qid via nebulizer. May give 2 additional doses/day.

HOW SUPPLIED: Sol, Inhalation: (Albuterol-Ipratropium) 3mg-0.5mg/3mL [3mL, 30^s 60^s]

CONTRAINDICATIONS: Hypersensitivity to atropine and its derivatives.

WARNINGS/PRECAUTIONS: Paradoxical bronchospasm and hypersensitivity reactions reported. Caution with cardiovascular disorders, convulsive disorders, hyperthyroidism, DM, narrow angle glaucoma, prostatic hypertrophy, and bladder-neck obstruction.

ADVERSE REACTIONS: Pain, chest pain, diarrhea, dyspepsia, nausea, leg cramps, bronchitis, lung disease, pharyngitis, pneumonia, UTI.

INTERACTIONS: Additive interactions with anticholinergic agents. Increased risk of cardiovascular side effects with sympathomimetics. Use β$_1$-selective blockers with hyper-reactive airways. Caution within 2 weeks of discontinuation of MAOIs or TCAs.

PREGNANCY: Category C (albuterol) and B (ipratropium), not for use in nursing.

MECHANISM OF ACTION: Albuterol: β$_2$-adrenergic bronchodilator; stimulates adenyl cylase, enzyme that catalyzes formation of cAMP from ATP. Increased cAMP levels are associated with relaxation of bronchial smooth muscle and inhibition of release of mediators of immediate hypersensitivity. Ipratropium: Anticholinergic bronchodilator; blocks muscarinic receptors of acetylcholine. Prevents the increase in intracellular concentration of cGMP, resulting from interaction of acetylcholine with the muscarinic receptors of bronchial smooth muscle.

PHARMACOKINETICS: Absorption: Albuterol: T$_{max}$=0.8 hrs; C$_{max}$=4.65mg/mL; AUC=24.2ng•h/mL. **Distribution:** Ipratropium: Plasma protein binding (0-9%). **Metabolism:** Albuterol: Conjugation. Ipratropium: Ester hydrolysis. **Elimination:** Albuterol: Urine (8.4% unchanged). Ipratropium: Urine (3.9% unchanged); T$_{1/2}$=6.7 hrs.

DURAGESIC

CII

fentanyl (Janssen)

> Life-threatening hypoventilation can occur. Contraindicated for acute or post-op pain and mild/intermittent pain. Avoid in patients <2 yrs. Only for use in opioid tolerant patients. Concomitant use with potent CYP450 3A4 inhibitors may result in an increase in fentanyl plasma concentrations which may cause potentially fatal respiratory depression. Monitor patients receiving potent CYP450 3A4 inhibitors.

THERAPEUTIC CLASS: Opioid analgesic

INDICATIONS: Management of persistent, moderate to severe chronic pain when continuous, around-the-clock opioid administration for an extended period of time is required and cannot be managed by other means such as nonsteroidal analgesics, opioid combination products, or immediate-release opioids.

DOSAGE: *Adults:* Individualize dose. Determine dose based on opioid tolerance. Initial: 25mcg/hr for 72 hr.
Pediatrics: ≥2 yrs: Individualize dose. Determine dose based on opioid tolerance. Initial: 25mcg/hr for 72 hr.

HOW SUPPLIED: Patch: 12.5mcg/hr, 25mcg/hr, 50mcg/hr, 75mcg/hr, 100mcg/hr [5^s]

CONTRAINDICATIONS: Non opioid-tolerant patients, management of acute/post-op pain, mild/intermittent pain. Diagnosis or suspicion of paralytic ileus. Patients who have acute or severe broncial asthma, significant respiratory depression especially in settings where there is lack of resuscitative equipment.

WARNINGS/PRECAUTIONS: Monitor patients with serious adverse events for at least 24 hrs after removal. Avoid exposing application site to direct external heat. Hypoventilation may occur; caution with chronic pulmonary diseases. Caution with brain tumors, bradyarrhythmias, renal/hepatic impairment, pancreatic/biliary tract disease. Avoid with increased ICP, impaired consciousness, or coma. May obscure clinical course of head injury. Tolerance and physical dependence can occur. May impair mental/physical abilities.

ADVERSE REACTIONS: Hypoventilation, HTN, fever, nausea, vomiting, constipation, dry mouth, somnolence, confusion, asthenia, sweating, nervousness, application site reaction, apnea, dyspnea.

INTERACTIONS: See Black Box Warning. Concomitant use with CNS depressants (opioids, sedatives, hypnotics, tranquilizers, general anesthetics, phenothiazines, skeletal muscle relaxants, alcohol) may cause respiratory depression, hypotension, profound sedation, or potentially coma or death. May increase clearance with CYP3A4 inducers (eg, rifampin, carbamazepine, phenytoin). Avoid use within 14 days of MAOI.

PREGNANCY: Category C, not for use in nursing.

MECHANISM OF ACTION: Opioid analgesic; interacts predominantly with the opioid μ-receptor. Exerts principle pharmacological actions on CNS.

PHARMACOKINETICS: Absorption: T_{max}=24-72 hrs. Transdermal administration of variable doses resulted in different parameters. **Distribution**: V_d=6 L/kg; found in breast milk. Accumulates in skeletal muscle and fat; released slowly into the blood; readily crosses placenta. **Metabolism**: Liver via CYP3A4; oxidative N-dealkylation to norfentanyl and other metabolites. **Elimination**: Urine (75%), feces (9%); $T_{1/2}$=3-12 hrs.

DURAMORPH

CII

morphine sulfate (Baxter)

THERAPEUTIC CLASS: Opioid analgesic

INDICATIONS: Management of pain unresponsive to non-narcotic analgesics.

DOSAGE: *Adults:* IV: Initial: 2-10mg/70kg. Epidural Injection: Initial: 5mg in lumbar region. Titrate: If inadequate pain relief within 1 hr, increase by 1-2mg. Max: 10mg/24hrs. Continuous Epidural: Initial: 2-4mg/24hrs. Give additional

1-2mg if needed. Intrathecal: 0.2-1mg single dose, do not repeat; may follow with 0.6mg/hr naloxone infusion to reduce incidence of side effects.

HOW SUPPLIED: Inj: 0.5mg/mL, 1mg/mL, 5mg/mL

CONTRAINDICATIONS: Allergy to opiates, acute bronchial asthma, upper airway obstruction. Severe hypotension may occur in volume depleted patients or with concurrent administration of phenothiazines or general anesthetics.

WARNINGS/PRECAUTIONS: Have resuscitation equipment, oxygen, and antidote (eg, naloxone) available; severe respiratory depression may occur. Avoid rapid administration. May be habit-forming. Caution with head injury, increased intracranial/intraocular pressure, decreased respiratory reserve, hepatic/renal dysfunction, elderly, debilitated. High doses may cause seizures. Smooth muscle hypertonicity may cause biliary colic, urinary difficulty or retention. Orthostatic hypotension may occur with hypovolemia or myocardial dysfunction. Acute respiratory failure reported with COPD or acute asthmatic attack. Limit epidural/intrathecal route to lumbar area.

ADVERSE REACTIONS: Respiratory depression, convulsions, dysphoric reactions, pruritis, urinary retention, constipation, lumbar puncture-type headache, toxic psychoses.

INTERACTIONS: CNS depressants (eg, alcohol, sedatives, antihistamines) and psychotropics potentiate CNS depression. Neuroleptics may increase respiratory depression.

PREGNANCY: Category C, safety in nursing not known.

MECHANISM OF ACTION: Opioid analgesic; analgesic effects are produced via at least 3 areas of the CNS: the periaqueductal-periventricular gray matter, the ventromedial medulla, and the spinal cord. Interacts predominantly with μ-receptor which are found distributed in the brain, spinal cord, and in the trigeminal nerve.

PHARMACOKINETICS: Absorption: (Epidural): rapid absorption; C_{max}=33-40ng/mL; T_{max}=10-15 min; (Intrathecal): C_{max}<1-7.8ng/mL; T_{max}=5-10 min. **Distribution:** Plasma protein binding (36%); Muscle tissue binding (54%). Readily passes into fetal circulation, found in breast milk. (IV): V_d=1.0-4.7L/kg. **Metabolism:** Hepatic glucuronidation. **Elimination:** Kidneys (major), urine (2-12% unchanged), feces (10%); (IV, IM) $T_{1/2}$=1.5-4.5 hrs; (epidural) $T_{1/2}$=39-249 min.

DURATUSS   RX
pseudoephedrine HCL - guaifenesin (Victory)

THERAPEUTIC CLASS: Expectorant/decongestant

INDICATIONS: Relief of nasal congestion due to the common cold, hay fever, sinusitis, or other upper respiratory allergies. Relief of eustachian tube congestion and cough. Adjunct therapy in serious otitis media.

DOSAGE: *Adults:* 1 tab q12h.
Pediatrics: ≥12 yrs: 1 tab q12h. 6-12 yrs: 1/2 tab q12h.

HOW SUPPLIED: Tab, Extended-Release: (Guaifenesin-Pseudoephedrine) 600mg-120mg* *scored

CONTRAINDICATIONS: Hypersensitivity to sympathomimetics, severe HTN, with MAOIs.

WARNINGS/PRECAUTIONS: Do not crush or chew tabs. Caution with HTN, hyperthyroidism, DM, heart disease, peripheral vascular disease, glaucoma, prostatic hypertrophy.

ADVERSE REACTIONS: Nervousness, insomnia, restlessness, headache.

INTERACTIONS: Avoid MAOIs. May reduce effects of antihypertensive drugs which interfere with sympathetic activity (eg, methyldopa, mecamylamine, reserpine). Increased ectopic pacemaker activity with digitalis. Caution with concomitant sympathomimetic amines.

PREGNANCY: Category C, not for use in nursing.

DURATUSS DM

RX

dextromethorphan hydrobromide - guaifenesin (Victory)

THERAPEUTIC CLASS: Cough suppressant/expectorant

INDICATIONS: Relief of cough due to minor throat and bronchial irritation complicated by viscous mucus.

DOSAGE: *Adults:* 5mL q4h. Max: 30mL/24 hrs.
Pediatrics: >12 yrs: 5mL q4h. Max: 30mL/24 hrs. 6-12 yrs: 2.5mL q4h. Max: 15mL/24 hrs. 2-6 yrs: 1.25mL q4h. Max: 7.5mL/24 hrs.

HOW SUPPLIED: Elixir: (Dextromethorphan-Guaifenesin) 25mg-225mg/5mL

CONTRAINDICATIONS: Within 14 days of MAOI therapy.

WARNINGS/PRECAUTIONS: Re-evaluate if cough persists >1 week or recurs.

ADVERSE REACTIONS: Nausea, GI disturbances, dizziness, drowsiness, vomiting, headache, rash.

INTERACTIONS: Avoid use within 14 days of MAOI therapy; may cause serotonin syndrome. Additive CNS depressant effects with alcohol, antihistamines, psychotropics, other CNS depressants.

PREGNANCY: Category C, caution in nursing.

DURATUSS G

RX

guaifenesin (Victory)

OTHER BRAND NAMES: Guaifenesin ER (Amide)

THERAPEUTIC CLASS: Expectorant

INDICATIONS: Temporary relief of symptoms associated with respiratory tract infections and related conditions. Loosens phlegm and thins bronchial secretions

DOSAGE: *Adults:* 1 tab q12h. Max: 2 tabs/24 hrs. May break tabs in half; do not crush or chew.
Pediatrics: >12 yrs: 1 tab q12h. Max: 2 tabs/24 hrs. 6-12 yrs: 1/2 tab q12h. Max: 1 tab/24 hrs. May break tabs in half; do not crush or chew.

HOW SUPPLIED: Tab, Extended-Release: 1200mg* *scored

ADVERSE REACTIONS: Nausea, vomiting.

PREGNANCY: Category C, caution in nursing.

DYAZIDE

RX

triamterene - hydrochlorothiazide (GlaxoSmithKline)

THERAPEUTIC CLASS: K⁺-sparing diuretic/thiazide diuretic

INDICATIONS: For hypertension or edema if hypokalemia occurs on HCTZ alone, or when a thiazide diuretic is required and cannot risk hypokalemia.

DOSAGE: *Adults:* 1-2 caps qd.

HOW SUPPLIED: Cap: (Triamterene-HCTZ) 37.5mg-25mg

CONTRAINDICATIONS: Hyperkalemia, anuria, acute or chronic renal insufficiency, sulfonamide hypersensitivity, diabetic neuropathy, K⁺-sparing agents (eg, diuretics), K⁺ supplements (except with severe hypokalemia), K⁺ salt substitutes, K⁺-rich diet.

WARNINGS/PRECAUTIONS: Risk of hyperkalemia (≥5.5mEq/L) especially with renal impairment, elderly, DM or severely ill; monitor levels frequently. Caution in severely ill in whom respiratory or metabolic acidosis may occur; monitor acid-base balance frequently. May manifest DM. Caution with hepatic dysfunction, history of renal stones. Increases uric acid levels, BUN, creatinine. May decrease PBI levels. D/C before parathyroid function tests. May potentiate electrolyte imbalance with heart failure, renal disease, cirrhosis.

ADVERSE REACTIONS: Muscle cramps, GI effects, weakness, blood dyscrasias, arrhythmia, impotence, dry mouth, jaundice, paresthesia, renal stones, hypersensitivity reactions.

INTERACTIONS: Hyperkalemia risk with ACE inhibitors, blood from blood bank, low-salt milk, K⁺-containing agents (eg, parenteral penicillin G potassium), salt substitutes. Increased risk of hyponatremia with chlorpropamide. Possible renal dysfunction with NSAIDs. Risk of lithium toxicity. Decreases arterial responsiveness to norepinephrine. ACTH, amphotericin B, and corticosteroids intensify electrolyte depletion. Adjust oral anticoagulants, antigout, and antidiabetic drugs. Increases effects of nondepolarizing muscle relaxants, antihypertensives. Overuse of laxatives or sodium polystyrene sulfonate reduces K⁺ levels. Reduces methenamine effects.

PREGNANCY: Category C, not for use in nursing.

MECHANISM OF ACTION: HCTZ: Diuretic; blocks reabsorption of Na⁺ and Cl⁻ ions. Triamterene: Antikaliuretic agent; exerts effect on distal renal tubules to inhibit reabsorption of Na⁺ in exchange for K⁺ and H⁺ ions.

PHARMACOKINETICS: Absorption: Triamterene: $AUC=148.7ng \cdot hrs/mL$; $C_{max}=46.4ng/mL$; $T_{max}=1.1$ hrs. HCTZ: $AUC=834ng \cdot hrs/mL$; $C_{max}=135.1ng/mL$; $T_{max}=2$ hrs.

DYNACIN RX
minocycline HCL (Medicis)

THERAPEUTIC CLASS: Tetracycline derivative

INDICATIONS: Treatment of inclusion conjunctivitis, nongonococcal urethritis, and other infections (eg, respiratory tract, endocervical, rectal, urinary tract, skin and skin structure) caused by susceptible strains of microorganisms. Alternative treatment in certain other infections (eg, urethritis, gonococcal, syphilis, anthrax). Adjunctive therapy in acute intestinal amebiasis and severe acne. Treatment of *Mycobacterium marinum* and asymptomatic carriers of *Neisseria meningitidis*.

DOSAGE: *Adults:* Usual: 200mg initially, then 100mg q12h; alternative is 100-200mg initially, then 50mg qid. Uncomplicated Gonococcal Infection (Men, other than urethritis and anorectal infections): 200mg initially, then 100mg q12h for minimum 4 days. Uncomplicated Gonococcal Urethritis (Men): 100mg q12h for 5 days. Syphilis: Administer usual dose for 10-15 days. Meningococcal Carrier State: 100mg q12h for 5 days. *Mycobacterium marinum:* 100mg q12h for 6-8 weeks. Uncomplicated urethral, endocervical, or rectal infection: 100mg q12h for at least 7 days. Renal Dysfunction: Reduce dose and/or extend dose intervals.
Pediatrics: >8 yrs: 4mg/kg initially followed by 2mg/kg q12h. Take with plenty of fluids.

HOW SUPPLIED: Tab: 50mg, 75mg, 100mg

WARNINGS/PRECAUTIONS: May cause fetal harm during pregnancy. Use during tooth development (last half of pregnancy, infancy, <8 yrs) may cause permanent discoloration of the teeth or enamel hypoplasia; avoid use during this period. Renal toxicity, hepatotoxicity, photosensitivity, increased BUN, superinfection, pseudotumor cerebri may occur; perform hematopoietic, renal, and hepatic monitoring. May impair mental/physical abilities. Use alternate form of contraception other than oral contraceptives. May decrease bone growth in premature infants.

ADVERSE REACTIONS: Anorexia, nausea, vomiting, diarrhea, dysphagia, enterocolitis, pancreatitis, increased LFTs, hepatitis, liver failure, renal toxicity, rash, exfoliative dermatitis, Stevens-Johnson syndrome, skin and mucous membrane pigmentation, blood dyscrasias, headache, tooth discoloration.

INTERACTIONS: May require downward adjustments of anticoagulant dosage. May interfere with bactericidal action of penicillin; avoid concurrent use when possible. May decrease efficacy of oral contraceptives. Impaired absorption with antacids containing aluminum, calcium, or magnesium and

D

iron-containing products. Fatal renal toxicity with methoxyflurane has been reported.

PREGNANCY: Category D, not for use in nursing.

MECHANISM OF ACTION: Tetracycline derivative; thought to inhibit protein synthesis.

PHARMACOKINETICS: Absorption: Rapid. **Distribution:** Crosses placenta, excreted in breast milk. **Elimination:** Urine, feces.

DynaCirc CR RX
isradipine (Reliant)

THERAPEUTIC CLASS: Calcium channel blocker (dihydropyridine)

INDICATIONS: Management of hypertension.

DOSAGE: *Adults:* Initial: 5mg qd alone or with a thiazide diuretic. Titrate: May adjust by 5mg/day at 2-4 week intervals. Max: 20mg/day. Swallow whole.

HOW SUPPLIED: Tab: Controlled-Release: 5mg, 10mg.

WARNINGS/PRECAUTIONS: May produce symptomatic hypotension. Caution in CHF, especially with concomitant β-blockers. Caution with pre-existing severe GI narrowing. Peripheral edema reported. Increased bioavailability in elderly.

ADVERSE REACTIONS: Headache, edema, dizziness, constipation, fatigue, flushing, abdominal discomfort.

INTERACTIONS: Additive effects with HCTZ. Severe hypotension possible with fentanyl and β-blockers. Increases AUC and Cmax of propranolol. Decreased levels with rifampicin.

PREGNANCY: Category C, not for use in nursing.

MECHANISM OF ACTION: Dihydropyridine calcium channel blocker; binds to calcium channels and inhibits calcium flux into cardiac and smooth muscle.

PHARMACOKINETICS: Absorption: Bioavailability (15-24%); C_{max}=3-4ng/mL; AUC=62-73ng•h/mL. **Distribution:** Plasma protein binding (95%). **Metabolism:** Oxidation, ester cleavage; CYP3A4. **Elimination:** Urine, feces.

Dyrenium RX
triamterene (WellSpring)

> Abnormal elevation of serum K+ levels (≥5.5mEq/L) can occur with all K+-sparing agents, including triamterene. Hyperkalemia is more likely to occur with renal impairment and diabetes (even without evidence of renal impairment), and in the elderly, or severely ill. Monitor serum K+ at frequent intervals.

THERAPEUTIC CLASS: K+-sparing diuretic

INDICATIONS: Treatment of edema associated with congestive heart failure, liver cirrhosis, and nephrotic syndrome. Treatment of steroid induced edema, idiopathic edema and edema due to secondary hyperaldosteronism.

DOSAGE: *Adults:* Initial: 100mg bid pc. Max: 300mg/day.

HOW SUPPLIED: Cap: 50mg, 100mg

CONTRAINDICATIONS: Anuria, severe or progressive kidney disease or dysfunction (except with nephrosis), severe hepatic disease, hyperkalemia, K+ supplements, K+ salt substitutes, K+-sparing agents (eg, diuretics).

WARNINGS/PRECAUTIONS: Check ECG if hyperkalemia occurs. May cause decreased alkali reserve with possibility of metabolic acidosis, mild nitrogen retention. Monitor BUN periodically. May contribute to megaloblastosis in folic acid deficiency. Caution with gouty arthritis; may elevate uric acid levels. May aggravate or cause electrolyte imbalances in CHF, renal disease, or cirrhosis. Caution with history of renal stones.

ADVERSE REACTIONS: Hypersensitivity reactions, hyper- or hypokalemia, azotemia, renal stones, jaundice, nausea, vomiting, diarrhea, weakness, dizziness.

INTERACTIONS: Increased risk of hyperkalemia with ACE inhibitors. Indomethacin may cause renal failure; caution with NSAIDs. Risk of lithium toxicity. Avoid K^+-sparing diuretics, K^+ supplements, K^+-containing agents or salt substitutes, low-salt milk, and blood from blood bank; may potentiate serum K^+ levels. May cause hyperglycemia; adjust antidiabetic agents. Chlorpropamide may increase risk of severe hyponatremia. May potentiate nondepolarizing muscle relaxants, antihypertensives, other diuretics, preanesthetics, and anesthetics.

PREGNANCY: Category C, not for use in nursing.

MECHANISM OF ACTION: K^+ sparing diuretic; inhibits reabsorption of sodium ions in exchange for potassium and hydrogen ions at segment of distal tubule under control of adrenal mineralocorticoids.

PHARMACOKINETICS: Absorption: Rapid; C_{max}=30ng/mL, T_{max}=3 hrs. **Distribution:** Crosses placental barrier. **Metabolism:** Hydroxytriamterene (metabolite). **Elimination:** Urine (21%).

E.E.S. RX
erythromycin ethylsuccinate (Abbott)

THERAPEUTIC CLASS: Macrolide

INDICATIONS: Treatment of mild to moderate upper/lower respiratory tract and skin and skin structure infections, listeriosis, pertussis, diphtheria, erythrasma, intestinal amebiasis, acute pelvic inflammatory disease (PID) (*N.gonorrhoeae*), primary syphilis (if PCN allergy), Legionnaires' disease, chlamydial infections (eg, newborn conjunctivitis, pneumonia of infancy, urogenital infections during pregnancy, or urethral, endocervical, or rectal infections when tetracyclines are contraindicated or not tolerated), and nongonococcal urethritis caused by susceptible strains of microorganisms. Prophylaxis of initial and recurrent attacks of rheumatic fever if PCN allergy.

DOSAGE: *Adults:* Usual: 1600mg/day in divided doses given q6h, q8h, or q12h. Max: 4g/day. Treat strep infections for at least 10 days. Streptococcal Infection Prophylaxis with Rheumatic Heart Disease: 400mg bid. Urethritis (*C.trachomatis* or *U.urealyticum*): 800mg tid for 7 days. Primary Syphilis: 48-64g in divided doses over 10-15 days. Intestinal Amebiasis: 400mg qid for 10-14 days. Pertussis: 40-50mg/kg/day in divided doses for 5-14 days. Legionnaires' Disease: 1.6-4g/day in divided doses.
Pediatrics: Usual: 30-50mg/kg/day in divided doses q6h, q8h, or q12h. Severe Infections: May double dose. Treat strep infections for at least 10 days. Streptococcal Infection Prophylaxis with Rheumatic Heart Disease: 400mg bid. Intestinal Amebiasis: 30-50mg/kg/day in divided doses for 10-14 days.

HOW SUPPLIED: Sus: 200mg/5mL, 400mg/5mL; Tab: 400mg

CONTRAINDICATIONS: Concomitant terfenadine, astemizole, cisapride, or pimozide.

WARNINGS/PRECAUTIONS: *Clostridium difficile*-associated diarrhea, hepatic dysfunction reported. Caution with impaired hepatic function. May aggravate weakness of patients with myasthenia gravis.

ADVERSE REACTIONS: Nausea, vomiting, abdominal pain, diarrhea, anorexia, hepatic dysfunction, abnormal LFTs, allergic reactions, superinfection (prolonged use).

INTERACTIONS: See Contraindications. Rhabdomyolysis reported with lovastatin. May increase levels of theophylline, digoxin, drugs metabolized by CYP450 (eg, carbamazepine, cyclosporine, tacrolimus, phenytoin, alfentanil, disopyramide, lovastatin, bromocriptine, valproate, etc). Increases effects of oral anticoagulants, triazolam, midazolam. Risk of acute ergot toxicity with ergotamine or dihydroergotamine. May increase AUC of sildenafil; consider dose reduction of sildenafil.

PREGNANCY: Category B, caution in nursing.

MECHANISM OF ACTION: Macrolide; inhibits protein synthesis by binding 50S ribosomal subunits of susceptible organisms.

PHARMACOKINETICS: Absorption: Readily absorbed. **Distribution:** Diffuses into most body fluids, crosses placental barrier. **Metabolism:** Liver. **Elimination:** Biliary excretion, urine (≤5%).

ECONAZOLE NITRATE RX
econazole nitrate (Various)

THERAPEUTIC CLASS: Azole antifungal

INDICATIONS: Treatment of tinea pedis, tinea cruris, and tinea corporis caused by *Trichophyton rubrum, Trichophyton mentagrophytes, Trichophyton tonsurans, Microsporum canis, Microsporum audouinii, Microsporum gypseum,* and *Epidermophyton floccosum.* Treatment of cutaneous candidiasis and tinea versicolor.

DOSAGE: *Adults:* T.cruris/T.corporis/T.versicolor: Apply qd for 2 weeks. T.pedis: Apply qd for 4 weeks. Cutaneous Candidiasis: Apply bid for 2 weeks.

HOW SUPPLIED: Cre: 1% [15g, 30g, 85g]

WARNINGS/PRECAUTIONS: Avoid eyes.

ADVERSE REACTIONS: Burning, itching, stinging, erythema.

PREGNANCY: Category C, caution with nursing.

MECHANISM OF ACTION: Azole antifungal; exhibits broad-spectrum antifungal activity against susceptible organisms.

PHARMACOKINETICS: Excretion: Urine and feces, (<1%).

ECOTRIN OTC
aspirin (GlaxoSmithKline Consumer)

THERAPEUTIC CLASS: Salicylate

INDICATIONS: To reduce the risk of death and nonfatal stroke with previous ischemic stroke or transient ischemia of the brain. To reduce risk of vascular mortality with suspected acute MI. To reduce risk of death and nonfatal MI with previous MI or unstable angina. To reduce risk of MI and sudden death in chronic stable angina. Indicated for patients who have undergone revascularization procedures with a pre-existing condition for which ASA is indicated. Relief of signs of rheumatoid arthritis (RA), juvenile rheumatoid arthritis (JRA), osteoarthritis (OA), spondyloarthropathies, arthritis, and pleurisy associated with systemic lupus erythematosus (SLE).

DOSAGE: *Adults:* Ischemic Stroke/TIA: 50-325mg qd. Suspected Acute MI: Initial: 160-162.5mg qd as soon as suspect MI. Maint: 160-162.5mg for 30 days post-infarction, consider further therapy for prevention/recurrent MI. Prevention or Recurrent MI/Unstable Angina/Chronic Stable Angina: 75-325mg qd. CABG: 325mg qd, start 6 hrs post-surgery. Continue for 1 yr. PTCA: Initial: 325mg, 2 hrs pre-surgery. Maint: 160-325mg qd. Carotid Endarterectomy: 80mg qd to 650mg bid, start pre-surgery. RA/Arthritis/SLE Pleurisy: Initial: 3g qd in divided doses. Increase for anti-inflammatory efficacy to 150-300mcg/mL plasma salicylate level. Spondyloarthropathies: Up to 4g/day in divided doses. OA: Up to 3g/day in divided doses.
Pediatrics: JRA: Initial: 90-130mg/kg/day in divided doses. Increase for anti-inflammatory efficacy to 150-300mcg/mL plasma salicylate level.

HOW SUPPLIED: Tab, Delayed-Release: 81mg, 325mg, 500mg

CONTRAINDICATIONS: NSAID allergy, children or teenagers for viral infections with or without fever, syndrome of asthma, rhinitis, and nasal polyps.

WARNINGS/PRECAUTIONS: Increased risk of bleeding with heavy alcohol use (≥3 drinks/day). May inhibit platelet function; can adversely affect inherited (hemophilia) or acquired (hepatic disease, vitamin K deficiency) bleeding disorders. Monitor for bleeding and ulceration. Avoid in history of active peptic ulcer, severe renal failure, severe hepatic insufficiency, and sodium restricted diets. Associated with elevated LFTs, BUN, and serum creatinine; hyperkalemia; proteinuria; and prolonged bleeding time. Avoid 1 week before and during labor.

ADVERSE REACTIONS: Fever, hypothermia, dysrhythmias, hypotension, agitation, cerebral edema, dehydration, hyperkalemia, dyspepsia, GI bleed, hearing loss, tinnitus, problems in pregnancy.

INTERACTIONS: Diminished hypotensive and hyponatremic effects of ACE inhibitors. May increase levels of acetazolamide, valproic acid. Increased risk of bleeds with heparin, warfarin. Decreased levels of phenytoin. Decreased hypotensive effects of β-blockers. Decreased diuretic effects with renal or cardiovascular disease. Decreased methotrexate clearance; increased risk of bone marrow toxicity. Avoid NSAIDs. Increased effects of hypoglycemic agents. Antagonizes uricosuric agents.

PREGNANCY: Avoid in 3rd trimester of pregnancy and nursing.

EDECRIN   RX
ethacrynic acid (Aton)

THERAPEUTIC CLASS: Aryloxyacetic acid derivative

INDICATIONS: Treatment of edema when agent of greater diuretic potential is required. Treatment of edema in CHF, hepatic cirrhosis, and renal disease. Short-term management of ascites due to malignancy, idiopathic edema, lymphedema; congenital heart disease and nephrotic syndrome in hospital-ized pediatrics.

DOSAGE: *Adults:* Initial: 50-100mg qd. Titrate: 25-50mg increments. Usual: 50-200mg/day. After diuresis achieved, give smallest effective dose continu-ously or intermittently.
Pediatrics: Initial: 25mg. Titrate: Increase by 25mg increments. Maint: Reduce dose and frequency once dry weight achieved; may give intermittently.

HOW SUPPLIED: Tab: 25mg* *scored

CONTRAINDICATIONS: Anuria, infants. D/C if increasing electrolyte imbal-ance, azotemia, or oliguria develops during treatment of severe, progressive renal disease. D/C if severe, watery diarrhea occurs.

WARNINGS/PRECAUTIONS: Caution in advanced liver cirrhosis. Monitor se-rum electrolytes, CO2, BUN early in therapy and periodically during active di-uresis. Vigorous diuresis may induce acute hypotensive episode and in elderly cardiac patients, hemoconcentration resulting in thromboembolic disorders. Ototoxicity reported with severe renal dysfunction. Hypomagnesemia and transient increase in serum urea nitrogen may occur. Reduce dose or withdraw if excessive electrolyte loss occurs. Initiate therapy in the hospital for cirrhotic patients with ascites. Liberalize salt intake and supplement with K+ if needed. Reduced responsiveness in renal edema with hypoproteinemia; use salt poor albumin.

ADVERSE REACTIONS: Anorexia, malaise, abdominal discomfort, gout, deaf-ness, tinnitus, vertigo, headache, fatigue, rash, chills.

INTERACTIONS: Risk of lithium toxicity. May increase ototoxic potential of aminoglycosides and some cephalosporins. Displaces warfarin from plasma protein; may need dose reduction. NSAIDs may decrease effects. Orthostatic hypotension may occur with antihypertensives. Increased risk of gastric hemorrhage with corticosteroids. Excessive K+ loss may precipitate digitalis toxicity. Caution with K+-depleting steroids.

PREGNANCY: Category B, not for use in nursing.

MECHANISM OF ACTION: Aryloxyacetic acid derivative; inhibits reabsorption of filtered sodium.

EDECRIN SODIUM RX
ethacrynate sodium (Aton)

THERAPEUTIC CLASS: Aryloxyacetic acid derivative

INDICATIONS: For rapid onset of diuresis (eg, acute pulmonary edema, impaired GI absorption, oral medication not practicable).

DOSAGE: *Adults:* 50mg or 0.5-1mg/kg IV single dose. May give 2nd dose if necessary.

HOW SUPPLIED: Inj: 50mg

CONTRAINDICATIONS: Anuria, infants. Discontinue if increasing electrolyte imbalance, azotemia, or oliguria develops during treatment of severe, progressive renal disease. Discontinue if severe, watery diarrhea occurs.

WARNINGS/PRECAUTIONS: Caution in advanced liver cirrhosis. Monitor serum electrolytes, CO2, BUN early in therapy and periodically during active diuresis. Vigorous diuresis may induce acute hypotensive episode and in elderly cardiac patients, hemoconcentration resulting in thromboembolic disorders. Ototoxicity reported with severe renal dysfunction. Hypomagnesemia and transient increase in serum urea nitrogen may occur. Reduce dose or withdraw if excessive electrolyte loss occurs. Initiate therapy in the hospital for cirrhotic patients with ascites. Liberalize salt intake and supplement with K$^+$ if needed. Reduced responsiveness in renal edema with hypoproteinemia; use salt poor albumin.

ADVERSE REACTIONS: Anorexia, malaise, abdominal discomfort, gout, deafness, tinnitus, vertigo, headache, fatigue, rash, chills.

INTERACTIONS: Risk of lithium toxicity. May increase ototoxic potential of aminoglycosides and some cephalosporins. Displaces warfarin from plasma protein; may need dose reduction. NSAIDs may decrease effects. Orthostatic hypotension may occur with antihypertensives. Increased risk of gastric hemorrhage with corticosteroids. Excessive K$^+$ loss may precipitate digitalis toxicity. Caution with K$^+$-depleting steroids.

PREGNANCY: Category B, not for use in nursing.

MECHANISM OF ACTION: Aryloxyacetic acid derivative; inhibits reabsorption of filtered sodium.

EFFEXOR RX
venlafaxine HCL (Wyeth)

> Antidepressants increased the risk of suicidal thinking and behavior (suicidality) in short-term studies in children, adolescents, and young adults with Major Depressive Disorder (MDD) and other psychiatric disorders. Venlafaxine is not approved for use in pediatric patients.

THERAPEUTIC CLASS: Serotonin and norepinephrine reuptake inhibitor

INDICATIONS: Treatment of MDD.

DOSAGE: *Adults:* ≥18 yrs: Initial: 75mg/day given bid-tid with food. Titrate: Increase by 75mg/day at no less than 4 day intervals. Max: 375mg/day. Hepatic Impairment (moderate): Reduce dose by 50%. Renal Impairment (mild to moderate): Reduce dose by 25%. Hemodialysis: Reduce dose by 50%. Withhold dose until after hemodialysis treatment completed. If drug used 6 weeks or longer, taper gradually (over 2 weeks or more) when discontinuing treatment.

HOW SUPPLIED: Tab: 25mg*, 37.5mg*, 50mg*, 75mg*, 100mg* *scored

CONTRAINDICATIONS: Concomitant MAOIs.

WARNINGS/PRECAUTIONS: May cause sustained increases in BP. Treatment-emergent anxiety, nervousness, insomnia, and anorexia reported. Caution with history of mania or seizures and conditions affecting hemodynamic responses. Monitor with increased IOP or if at risk of acute narrow angle glaucoma. Activation of mania/hypomania reported. Risk of hyponatremia, SIADH, skin and mucous membrane bleeding. Caution with hyperthyroidism, heart failure, recent MI, renal or hepatic impairment. Serotonin syndrome may occur. Caution with concomitant serotonergic drugs. Patients who present with progressive dyspnea, cough or chest discomfort should consider the possibility of interstitial lung disease and eosinophilic pneumonia.

ADVERSE REACTIONS: Asthenia, sweating, nausea, constipation, anorexia, vomiting, insomnia, somnolence, dry mouth, dizziness, nervousness, anxiety, tremor, blurred vision, abnormal ejaculation/orgasm, impotence in men.

INTERACTIONS: See Contraindications. Avoid within 14 days of MAOI therapy. Upon discontinuation, wait at least 7 days before starting MAOI therapy. Caution with cimetidine in elderly, HTN, hepatic dysfunction. Caution with diuretics. Decreases clearance of haloperidol. Increases risperidone and desipramine plasma levels. Decreases indinavir plasma levels. Caution with potent inhibitors of CYP3A4 and CYP2D6, CNS-active drugs (eg, triptans, SSRIs, lithium), and serotonergic drugs (eg, tramadol, tryptophans, SNRIs). Avoid alcohol.

PREGNANCY: Category C, not for use in nursing.

MECHANISM OF ACTION: 5-HT and NE reuptake inhibitor; potentiates neurotransmitter activity of CNS activity by inhibiting neuronal serotonin and norephinephrine reuptake.

PHARMACOKINETICS: Absorption: Relative bioavailability (100%). **Distribution:** Venlafaxine: Plasma protein binding (27%), V_d=7.5L/kg. ODV: Plasma protein binding (30%), V_d=5.7L/kg. **Metabolism:** Hepatic; metabolite: O-desmethylvenlafaxine (ODV). **Elimination:** Venlafaxine: $T_{1/2}$=5 hrs; urine (5%). ODV: $T_{1/2}$=11 hrs; urine.

EFFEXOR XR

RX

venlafaxine HCL (Wyeth)

> Antidepressants increased the risk of suicidal thinking and behavior (suicidality) in short-term studies in children, adolescents, and young adults with Major Depressive Disorder (MDD) and other psychiatric disorders. Venlafaxine is not approved for use in pediatric patients.

THERAPEUTIC CLASS: Serotonin and norepinephrine reuptake inhibitor

INDICATIONS: Treatment of major depressive disorder (MDD), generalized anxiety disorder (GAD), social anxiety disorder (SAD), panic disorder (PD).

DOSAGE: *Adults:* MDD/GAD/SAD: Initial: 75mg qd, or 37.5mg qd increase to 75mg qd after 4-7 days. Titrate: May increase by 75mg/day at no less than 4 day intervals. Max: 225mg/day. PD: Initial: 37.5mg qd for 7 days. Titrate: May increase 75mg/day, as needed at no less than 7 day intervals. Max: 225mg/day. Moderate Hepatic Impairment: Reduce initial dose by 50%. Renal Impairment: Reduce total daily dose by 25-50%. Hemodialysis: Reduce total daily dose by 50%. Withhold dose until after hemodialysis treatment completed. If drug used 6 weeks or longer, taper gradually (over 2 weeks or more) when discontinuing treatment. Periodically reassess need for maintenance therapy. Take with food in the am or pm, the same time each day. May sprinkle on spoonful of applesauce. Do not divide, crush, chew or place in water.

HOW SUPPLIED: Cap, Extended-Release: 37.5mg, 75mg, 150mg

CONTRAINDICATIONS: Concomitant MAOI therapy.

WARNINGS/PRECAUTIONS: May cause sustained increases in BP; monitor BP regularly. Treatment-emergent nervousness, insomnia and anorexia reported. Caution with seizures, conditions affecting hemodynamic responses or metabolism, volume-depletion, the elderly. Risk of mydriasis; monitor those with raised IOP or risk of acute narrow angle glaucoma. Abnormal bleeding (eg, ecchymosis) and activation of mania/hypomania reported. Risk of hyponatremia, SIADH. Caution with recent MI, hyperthyroidism, heart failure, renal or hepatic impairment. Serotonin syndrome may occur; caution with concomitant use of serotonergic drugs. Patients who present with progressive dyspnea, cough or chest discomfort should consider the possibility of interstitial lung disease and eosinophilic pneumonia. D/C if impaired balance occured. Cases of clinically significant hyponatremia in elderly patients.

ADVERSE REACTIONS: Asthenia, sweating, headache, nausea, constipation, anorexia, dry mouth, dizziness, insomnia, nervousness, somnolence, abnormal ejaculation, abnormal dreams.

INTERACTIONS: See Contraindications. Avoid within 14 days of MAOI therapy. Upon discontinuation, wait at least 7 days before starting MAOI therapy. Caution with cimetidine in elderly, hepatic dysfunction or pre-existing HTN. Caution with diuretics. Decreases clearance of haloperidol. Increases risperidone and desipramine plasma levels. Decreases indinavir plasma levels. Caution with potent inhibitors of CYP3A4 and CYP2D6, CNS-active drugs (eg, triptans, SSRIs, lithium), and with serotonergic drugs. Avoid alcohol.

PREGNANCY: Category C, not for use in nursing.

MECHANISM OF ACTION: 5-HT and NE reuptake inhibitor; potentiates neurotransmitter activity of CNS by inhibiting neuronal serotonin and norepinephrine reuptake.

PHARMACOKINETICS: Absorption: Venlafaxine: Absolute bioavailability (45%), C_{max}=150ng/mL, T_{max}=5.5 hrs. ODV (metabolite): C_{max}=260ng/mL, T_{max}=9 hrs. **Distribution:** Venlafaxine: Plasma protein binding (27%), V_d=7.5L/kg. ODV: Plasma protein binding (30%), V_d=5.7L/kg. **Metabolism:** Hepatic via CYP2D6; Active metabolite: O-desmethylvenlafaxine (ODV). **Elimination:** Urine (5% unchanged). Venlafaxine: $T_{1/2}$=5 hrs. ODV: $T_{1/2}$=11 hrs.

EFUDEX   RX
fluorouracil (Valeant)

OTHER BRAND NAMES: Efudex-40 (Valeant)

THERAPEUTIC CLASS: Antimetabolite

INDICATIONS: (2%, 5%) Topical treatment of actinic or solar keratoses. (5%) Treatment of superficial basal cell carcinomas when conventional methods are impractical.

DOSAGE: *Adults:* Actinic or Solar Keratosis: Apply bid until erosion occurs, usually for 2-4 weeks. Superficial Basal Cell Carcinoma: Apply 5% bid for 3-6 weeks; may use up to 10-12 weeks to obliterate lesion.

HOW SUPPLIED: Cre: 5% [25g, 40g]; Sol: 2%, 5% [10mL]

CONTRAINDICATIONS: Pregnancy.

WARNINGS/PRECAUTIONS: Avoid mucous membranes, UV light. Caution with occlusive dressings; may increase absorption. Use a porous gauze dressing for treatment of basal cell carcinoma if necessary. Ulcerations, miscarriage, and birth defects reported when applied to mucous membranes. Increased absorption with ulcerated or inflamed skin. Confirm diagnosis with biopsy.

ADVERSE REACTIONS: Burning, crusting, allergic contact dermatitis, erosions, erythema, hyperpigmentation, irritation, pain, photosensitivity, pruritus, scarring, rash, soreness, ulceration, leukocytosis.

PREGNANCY: Category X, not for use in nursing.

MECHANISM OF ACTION: Fluorinated pyrimidine; interferes with the synthesis of DNA and to a lesser extent inhibits the formation of RNA, to create a thymine deficiency that provokes unbalanced growth and cell death.

PHARMACOKINETICS: Absorption: T_{max}=2-3 weeks. **Metabolism**: via dihydropyrimidine dehydrogenase(DPD). **Elimination:** Urine (0.76%).

ELDEPRYL   RX
selegiline HCL (Somerset)

THERAPEUTIC CLASS: Monoamine oxidase inhibitor (Type B)

INDICATIONS: Adjunct to levodopa/carbidopa for management of Parkinson's disease.

DOSAGE: *Adults:* 5mg bid, at breakfast and lunch. Max: 10mg/day. May reduce levodopa/carbidopa by 10-30% after 2-3 days of therapy. May reduce further with continued therapy.

HOW SUPPLIED: Cap: 5mg

CONTRAINDICATIONS: Concomitant meperidine, other opioids.

WARNINGS/PRECAUTIONS: Do not exceed 10mg/day due to non-selective MAO inhibition. Decrease levodopa/carbidopa by 10-30% to prevent exacerbation of levodopa side effects.

ADVERSE REACTIONS: Nausea, dizziness, lightheadedness, fainting, abdominal pain, confusion, hallucinations, dry mouth.

INTERACTIONS: See Contraindications. Stupor, muscular rigidity, severe agitation, and elevated temperature reported with meperidine; avoid concomitant use. Avoid SSRIs and TCAs; severe toxicity reported. Allow 2 weeks between discontinuation of selegiline and initiation of TCAs or SSRIs. Allow 5 weeks for fluoxetine due to a longer half-life. Caution with sympathomimetics, tyramine-containing food.

PREGNANCY: Category C, not for use in nursing.

MECHANISM OF ACTION: MAO type inhibitor; increases dopaminergic activity by blocking the catabolism of dopamine.

PHARMACOKINETICS: Absorption: C_{max}=1ng/mL. **Metabolism:** Gut and liver (extensive). Metabolites: N-desmethylselegiline, L-amphetamine, L-methamphetamine. **Elimination:** $T_{1/2}$=2 hrs.

ELDOPAQUE FORTE RX
hydroquinone (Valeant)

OTHER BRAND NAMES: Eldoquin Forte (Valeant)

THERAPEUTIC CLASS: Depigmenting agent

INDICATIONS: For the gradual bleaching of hyperpigmented skin conditions (eg, chloasma, melasma, freckles, senile lentigines).

DOSAGE: *Adults:* Apply bid. Do not rub in Eldopaque Forte. Use sunscreen with Eldoquin Forte.
Pediatrics: ≥12 yrs: Apply bid. Do not rub in Eldopaque Forte. Use sunscreen with Eldoquin Forte.

HOW SUPPLIED: Cre: 4% [28.4g]

WARNINGS/PRECAUTIONS: Avoid sun exposure on bleached skin. Eldopaque Forte contains sunblock; use sunscreen. May produce unwanted cosmetic effects if not used as directed. Test for skin sensitivity. D/C if no lightening effect after 2 months. Contains sodium metabisulfite; may cause serious allergic type reactions. Limit treatment to small areas of body at one time. Avoid contact with eyes.

ADVERSE REACTIONS: Cutaneous hypersensitivity (contact dermatitis).

PREGNANCY: Category C, caution in nursing.

MECHANISM OF ACTION: Produces a reversible depigmentation of the skin by inhibiting the enzymatic oxidation of tyrosine to 3,4-dihydroxyphenylalanine and suppressing the melanocyte metabolic processes.

ELESTAT RX
epinastine HCL (Allergan)

THERAPEUTIC CLASS: H_1-antagonist

INDICATIONS: For the prevention of itching associated with allergic conjunctivitis.

DOSAGE: *Adults:* 1 drop in each eye bid.
Pediatrics: ≥3 yrs: 1 drop in each eye bid.

HOW SUPPLIED: Sol: 0.05% [5mL]

WARNINGS/PRECAUTIONS: Not for contact lens related irritation. May reinsert contact lens 10 minutes after dosing if eye is not red.

ADVERSE REACTIONS: Burning sensation in the eye, folliculosis, hyperemia, pruritus.

PREGNANCY: Category C, caution in nursing.

MECHANISM OF ACTION: Antihistaminic; topically active; direct H_1-receptor antagonist and an inhibitor of histamine release from the mast cell; selective for the histamine H_1-receptor and has affinity for the histamine H_2-receptor and possesses affinity for the $α_1$-$α_2$-and 5-HT_2-receptors.

PHARMACOKINETICS: Absorption: C_{max}=0.04ng/ml. T_{max}=2 hrs. **Distribution:** Plasma protein binding (64%). **Elimination:** Urine, feces; $T_{1/2}$=12 hrs.

ELESTRIN   RX
estradiol (Kenwood Therapeutics)

> Estrogens increase the risk of endometrial cancer. Estrogens, with or without progestins, should not be used for the prevention of cardiovascular disease or dementia. Increased risks of MI, stroke, invasive breast cancer, PE, and DVT in postmenopausal women reported.

THERAPEUTIC CLASS: Estrogen

INDICATIONS: Treatment of moderate to severe vasomotor symptoms associated with menopause.

DOSAGE: *Adults:* Individualize dose. Apply 1 pump (0.87g) qd to upper arm. Use lowest effective dose consistent with treatment goals and risks. Re-evaluate periodically.

HOW SUPPLIED: Gel: 0.06% (0.87g [0.52g estradiol] per pump actuation) [144g]

CONTRAINDICATIONS: Undiagnosed abnormal genital bleeding, breast cancer, estrogen-dependent neoplasia, DVT or PE, active or recent (within 1 year) arterial thromboembolic disease (eg, stroke, MI), liver dysfunction or disease, pregnancy.

WARNINGS/PRECAUTIONS: May increase risk of cardiovascular events (eg, MI, stroke, venous thrombosis, and PE); d/c immediately if any of these events occur or are suspected. May increase risk of breast/endometrial cancer, and gallbladder disease. May lead to severe hypercalcemia with breast cancer and bone metastases; monitor and d/c if hypercalcemia occurs. Retinal vascular thrombosis reported; monitor and d/c if papilledema or retinal vascular lesions occur. Consider addition of a progestin if no hysterectomy. May elevate BP; monitor at regular intervals. May cause elevations of plasma triglycerides with pre-existing hypertriglyceridemia. Caution with history of cholestatic jaundice associated with past estrogen use or with pregnancy; d/c with recurrence. May lead to increased thyroid-binding globulin levels; monitor thyroid function. May cause fluid retention; monitor closely with cardiac/renal dysfunction. Caution with severe hypocalcemia. May increase risk of ovarian cancer. May exacerbate endometriosis, asthma, DM, epilepsy, migraine, porphyria, SLE, and hepatic hemangiomas; use with caution. Sunscreen may increase absorption; avoid applying sunscreen to application site for ≥25 minutes or for extended period of ≥7 days. Alcohol-based gels are flammable; avoid fire, flame, or smoking until the gel dried.

ADVERSE REACTIONS: Nausea, breast tenderness, metorrhagia, vaginal discharge, nasopharyngitis, upper respiratory infection, headache.

INTERACTIONS: CYP3A4 inducers (eg, St. John's wort, phenobarbital, carbamazepine, rifampin) may decrease levels which may decrease therapeutic effects and/or change uterine bleeding profile. CYP3A4 inhibitors (eg, erythromycin, clarithromycin, ketoconazole, itraconazole, ritonavir, grapefruit juice) may increase levels and result in unwanted side effects.

PREGNANCY: Contraindicated in pregnancy, caution in nursing.

MECHANISM OF ACTION: Estrogen; acts through binding to nuclear receptors in estrogen responsive tissues. Circulating estrogens modulate the pituitary secretion of gonadropins, leutinizing hormone and follicle stimulating hormone through a negative feedback mechanism. Acts to reduce elevated levels of these hormones seen in post menopausal women.

PHARMACOKINETICS: Absorption: (0.87g): AUC= 335.2 pg•hr/mL; C_{max}=21.6pg/mL; T_{max}=18 hrs. **Distribution:** Largely bound to sex hormone binding globulin and albumin; found in breast milk. **Metabolism:** Liver to estrone (metabolite), estriol (major urinary metabolite); sulfate and glucuronide conjugation (liver) ; intestinal hydroylysis; CYP 3A4 (partial metabolism). **Elimination:** Urine (parent compound and metabolites). $T_{1/2}$=1-2 hr (parent), 4-18 hr (estrone).

ELIDEL   RX
pimecrolimus (Novartis)

THERAPEUTIC CLASS: Macrolactam ascomycin derivative

INDICATIONS: Short-term and intermittent long-term therapy of moderate to severe atopic dermatitis in nonimmunocompromised patients intolerant to or unresponsive to conventional therapy.

DOSAGE: *Adults:* Apply bid. Re-evaluate if symptoms persist after 6 weeks. *Pediatrics:* ≥2 yrs: Apply bid. Re-evaluate if symptoms persist after 6 weeks.

HOW SUPPLIED: Cre: 1% [30g, 60g, 100g]

WARNINGS/PRECAUTIONS: Increased risk of varicella zoster infection, herpes simplex virus infection or eczema herpeticum. Lymphadenopathy reported; d/c if unknown etiology of lymphadenopathy or acute mononucleosis presents. Skin papilloma or warts reported; consider discontinuation if worsening or unresponsive skin papilloma. Minimize or avoid natural or artificial sunlight exposure. Avoid with Netherton's syndrome, areas of active cutaneous viral infections, or occlusive dressings. Long-term safety has not been established. Rare cases of malignancy (eg, skin and lymphoma) reported with topical calcineurin inhibitors; therefore, continuous long-term use should be avoided and application limited to areas of involvement. Not indicated for use in children <2 yrs.

ADVERSE REACTIONS: Application site burning, headache, nasopharyngitis, influenza, pharyngitis, viral infection, pyrexia, cough, skin discoloration.

INTERACTIONS: Caution with CYP3A4 inhibitors (eg, erythromycin, itraconazole, ketoconazole, fluconazole, CCBs, cimetidine) in widespread and/or erythrodermic disease.

PREGNANCY: Category C, not for use in nursing.

MECHANISM OF ACTION: Macrolactam ascomycin derivative; not fully established. Suspected to bind with high affinity to macrophilin-12 (FKBP-12) and inhibit the calcium-dependent phosphatase, calcineurin. Consequently, this inhibits T cell activation by blocking the transcription of early cytokines.

PHARMACOKINETICS: Absorption: C_{max}=1.4ng/mL. **Distribution:** Plasma protein binding (99.5%). **Metabolism:** Liver by CYP3A. **Elimination:** Feces (78.4% metabolites) and (≤1% unchanged).

ELIGARD   RX
leuprolide acetate (Sanofi-Aventis)

THERAPEUTIC CLASS: Synthetic gonadotropin releasing hormone analog

INDICATIONS: Palliative treatment of advanced prostate cancer.

DOSAGE: *Adults:* 7.5mg SQ monthly, 22.5mg SQ every 3 months, 30mg SQ every 4 months, or 45mg SQ every 6 months. Rotate injection sites.

HOW SUPPLIED: Inj: 7.5mg, 22.5mg, 30mg, 45mg

CONTRAINDICATIONS: Women, pregnancy, pediatric patients.

WARNINGS/PRECAUTIONS: Transient worsening of symptoms or onset of new signs/symptoms may occur during 1st few weeks of therapy. Closely monitor patients with metastatic vertebral lesions and/or urinary tract obstruction during first few weeks of therapy. Ureteral obstruction and spinal cord compression reported. Monitor serum testosterone, PSA.

ADVERSE REACTIONS: Hot flashes, pain/burning/stinging/erythema/bruising at injection site, malaise/fatigue, atrophy of testes, weakness, gynecomastia, myalgia, dizziness, decreased libido, rigors, lethargy, dyspepsia, scanty urination, limb pain, insomnia, breast soreness, hypertension, clamminess, pituitary aplopexy.

PREGNANCY: Category X, safety in nursing not known.

MECHANISM OF ACTION: LH-RH agonist; acts as a potent inhibitor of gonadotropin secretion and suppresses testicular and ovarian steroidogenesis.

PHARMACOKINETICS: Absorption: (7.5mg, 1st inj) C_{max}=25.3ng/mL, T_{max}=5 hrs. (22.5mg; 1st inj, 2nd inj) C_{max}=127ng/mL, 107ng/mL, T_{max}=5 hrs. (30mg; 1st inj) C_{max}=150ng/mL, T_{max}=3.3 hrs. (45mg; 1st inj, 2nd inj): C_{max}=82ng/mL, 102ng/mL, T_{max}=4.5 hrs. **Distribution**: V_d=27L; plasma protein binding (43%-49%). **Metabolism**: Pentapeptide (major metabolite).

ELIMITE
permethrin (Allergan)
RX

THERAPEUTIC CLASS: Pyrethroid scabicidal agent

INDICATIONS: Treatment of scabies.

DOSAGE: *Adults:* Massage into skin from head to soles of feet. Wash off after 8-14 hrs. One treatment should be adequate. Retreat if living mites present after 14 days.
Pediatrics: ≥2 months: Massage into skin from head (scalp, temples and forehead) to soles of feet. Wash off after 8-14 hrs. One treatment should be adequate. Retreat if living mites present after 14 days.

HOW SUPPLIED: Cre: 5% [60g]

CONTRAINDICATIONS: Allergy to synthetic pyrethroid or pyrethrin.

WARNINGS/PRECAUTIONS: May temporarily exacerbate infection (eg, pruritus, edema, erythema). Avoid eyes. D/C if hypersensitivity occurs.

ADVERSE REACTIONS: Burning, stinging, pruritus, erythema, numbness, tingling, rash.

PREGNANCY: Category B, not for use in nursing.

ELITEK
rasburicase (Sanofi-Aventis)
RX

> May cause serious hypersensitivity reactions including anaphylaxis; discontinue if this occurs. Hemolysis may occur in G6PD deficiency; discontinue with hemolysis. Before initiate, screen patients at high risk for G6PD deficiency. Discontinue if develop methemoglobinemia. Causes enzymatic degradation of uric acid within blood samples left at room temperature. Collect blood in pre-chilled tubes containing heparin; immediately immerse and maintain in ice water bath and assay sample within 4 hrs of collection.

THERAPEUTIC CLASS: Recombinant urate-oxidase enzyme

INDICATIONS: Initial management of plasma uric acid levels in pediatrics with leukemia, lymphoma, and solid tumor malignancies who are receiving anti-cancer therapy expected to result in tumor lysis and subsequent elevation of plasma uric acid.

DOSAGE: *Pediatrics:* 1 month-17 yrs: 0.15 or 0.2mg/kg IV as single daily dose for 5 days. Administer over 30 min, not as bolus. Dosing >5 days or >1 course not recommended. Initiate chemotherapy 4-24 hrs after 1st dose.

HOW SUPPLIED: Inj: 1.5mg, 7.5mg

CONTRAINDICATIONS: G6PD deficiency, history of anaphylaxis or hypersensitivity reactions, hemolytic or methemoglobinemia reactions to rasburicase or any of the excipients.

WARNINGS/PRECAUTIONS: Screen patients at high risk for G6PD deficiency (eg, African or Mediterranean ancestry) prior to initiation. Administer IV hydration.

ADVERSE REACTIONS: Vomiting, fever, nausea, headache, abdominal pain, constipation, diarrhea, mucositis, rash, respiratory distress, sepsis, neutropenia with or without fever.

PREGNANCY: Category C, not for use in nursing.

MECHANISM OF ACTION: A recombinant urate-oxidase enzyme; catalyses enzymatic oxidation of uric acid into an inactive and soluble metabolite.

PHARMACOKINETICS: Distribution: V_d=110-127mL/kg. **Elimination:** $T_{1/2}$=18 hrs.

ELLENCE   RX
epirubicin HCL (Pharmacia & Upjohn)

> Severe local tissue necrosis with extravasation. Not for IM/SQ administration. Risk of myocardial toxicity, severe myelosuppression. Secondary acute myelogenous leukemia reported. Reduce dose with hepatic dysfunction.

THERAPEUTIC CLASS: Anthracycline

INDICATIONS: Adjuvant treatment of primary breast cancer with axillary node tumor involvement following resection of primary breast cancer.

DOSAGE: *Adults:* Initial: 100-120mg/m² IV infusion, repeat at 3-4 week cycles. May give total dose on Day 1 of each cycle or divide equally on Days 1 and 8. Bone Marrow Dysfunction: Initial: 75-90mg/m². Hepatic Dysfunction: Bilirubin 1.2-3mg/dL or AST 2-4X ULN: Give 1/2 of initial dose. Bilirubin >3mg/dL or AST 4X ULN: Give 1/4 of initial dose. Severe Renal Dysfunction: Serum Creatinine >5mg/dL: Lower dose. Give prophylactic therapy with SMZ-TMP or fluoroquinolone with 120mg/m² regimen. Consider pretreatment with antiemetics. Adjust dose after 1st treatment cycle based on hematologic and nonhematologic toxicities (see PI).

HOW SUPPLIED: Inj: 2mg/mL [25mL, 100mL]

CONTRAINDICATIONS: Baseline neutrophils <1500cells/mm³, severe myocardial insufficiency, recent MI, severe arrhythmias, previous anthracycline therapy with maximum cumulative dose, anthracenedione hypersensitivity, severe hepatic dysfunction.

WARNINGS/PRECAUTIONS: Increased risk of cardiotoxicity with active or dormant cardiovascular disease. Use extreme caution if exceeding cumulative dose of 900mg/m². Resolve acute toxicities from other cytotoxic agents prior to initiation. Monitor CBC, total bilirubin, AST, serum creatinine, and cardiac function before and during each cycle. May induce hyperuricemia. Potential for tumor lysis syndrome. Thrombophlebitis, thromboembolic phenomena reported.

ADVERSE REACTIONS: Hematologic abnormalities, amenorrhea, hot flashes, lethargy, fever, GI disturbances, infection, conjunctivitis/keratitis, alopecia, local toxicity, rash/itch, skin changes.

INTERACTIONS: Increased risk of cardiotoxicity with previous anthracycline or anthracenedione therapy, prior or concomitant radiotherapy to mediastinal/pericardial area, or with concomitant cardiotoxic drugs. Increased risk of refractory secondary leukemia with concurrent DNA-damaging antineoplastics, heavy pretreatment with cytotoxic drugs, or escalated doses of anthracyclines. Additive toxicity with other cytotoxic drugs. Cyclophosphamide and fluorouracil may cause severe leukopenia, neutropenia, thrombocytopenia, and anemia. Monitor closely with cardioactive compounds that could cause heart failure (eg, CCBs). Caution with agents that cause changes in hepatic function. AUC increased with cimetidine; stop cimetidine during therapy. Previous radiation therapy may induce inflammatory recall reaction at irradiation site.

PREGNANCY: Category D, not for use in nursing.

MECHANISM OF ACTION: Anthracycline; complexes with DNA by intercalating its planar rings between nucleotide base pairs, inhibiting nucleic acid (DNA and RNA) and protein synthesis, triggering DNA cleavage by topoisomerase II, inhibits DNA helicase activity, and generates free radicals.

PHARMACOKINETICS: Absorption: IV administration of variable doses resulted in different parameters. **Distribution:** Plasma protein binding (77%). **Metabolism:** Liver (extensive and rapid); reduction, conjugation. Epirubicinol (metabolite). **Elimination:** Biliary (major), urine (minor).

ELMIRON   RX
pentosan sodium (Ortho-McNeil)

THERAPEUTIC CLASS: Analgesic, urinary

INDICATIONS: Relief of bladder pain/discomfort associated with interstitial cystitis.

DOSAGE: *Adults:* Take 1 hr before or 2 hrs after meals with water. 100mg tid for 3 months. Re-evaluate after 3 months; may continue for another 3 months. *Pediatrics:* ≥16 yrs: Take 1 hr before or 2 hrs after meals with water. 100mg tid for 3 months. Re-evaluate after 3 months; may continue for another 3 months.

HOW SUPPLIED: Cap: 100mg

WARNINGS/PRECAUTIONS: Bleeding complications (eg, ecchymosis, epistaxis, gum hemorrhage), alopecia, increased PT/PTT reported. Caution with invasive procedures, coagulopathy, aneurysms, thrombocytopenia, hemophilia, GI ulcers, polyps, diverticula, history of heparin-induced thrombocytopenia, and hepatic impairment. Transient liver enzyme elevation reported.

ADVERSE REACTIONS: Nausea, diarrhea, alopecia, headache, rash, dyspepsia, abdominal pain.

INTERACTIONS: Increased risk of bleeding with anticoagulants, heparin, t-PA, streptokinase, high-dose ASA, and NSAIDs.

PREGNANCY: Category B, caution in nursing.

MECHANISM OF ACTION: Low molecular weight heparin-type compound; not fully established. Possesses anticoagulant and fibrinolytic effects.

PHARMACOKINETICS: Absorption: 3% of administered dose. **Distribution:** Mainly into uroepithelium. **Metabolism:** Liver and spleen, partial desulfation; depolymerization in kidney. **Elimination:** Urine (3% unchanged); $T_{1/2}$=4.8 hrs.

ELOCON   RX
mometasone furoate (Schering)

THERAPEUTIC CLASS: Corticosteroid

INDICATIONS: Corticosteroid-responsive dermatoses.

DOSAGE: *Adults:* (Cre, Oint) Apply qd. (Lot) Apply a few drops qd. Re-assess if no improvement within 2 weeks. *Pediatrics:* (Cre, Oint) ≥2 yrs: Apply qd for up to 3 weeks if needed. Avoid in diaper area. Re-assess if no improvement within 2 weeks.

HOW SUPPLIED: Cre, Oint: 0.1% [15g, 45g]; Lot: 0.1% [30mL, 60mL]

WARNINGS/PRECAUTIONS: May produce reversible HPA axis suppression, manifestations of Cushing's syndrome, hyperglycemia and glucosuria. D/C if irritation occurs. Use appropriate antifungal or antibacterial agent with dermatological infections. Pediatrics may be more susceptible to systemic toxicity. Caution when applied to large surface areas or with occlusive dressings.

ADVERSE REACTIONS: Burning, pruritus, skin atrophy, rosacea, acneiform reaction, tingling, stinging, furunculosis, folliculitis.

PREGNANCY: Category C, caution in nursing.

MECHANISM OF ACTION: Corticosteroid; possesses anti-inflammatory, antipruritic, and vasoconstrictive properties. Mechanism of anti-inflammatory effects not established. Suspected to induce phospholipase A_2 inhibitory proteins, lipocortins. Lipocortins control biosynthesis of potent mediators of inflammation (eg, prostaglandins and leukotrienes) by inhibiting release of their precursor, arachidonic acid.

PHARMACOKINETICS: Absorption: Extent of absorption depends on skin integrity, vehicle, and use of occlusive dressing.

ELOXATIN   RX
oxaliplatin (Sanofi-Aventis)

> Anaphylactic-like reactions may occur within minutes of administration.

THERAPEUTIC CLASS: Organoplatinum complex

INDICATIONS: In combination with infusional 5-fluorouracil (5-FU) and leuco-vorin (LV) for treatment of advanced metastatic carcinoma of colon or rectum and adjuvant treatment of Stage III colon cancer patients who have under-gone complete resection of the primary tumor.

DOSAGE: *Adults:* Advanced Colorectal Cancer: Day 1: 85mg/m^2 IV with LV 200mg/m^2; give over 120 min in separate bags using a Y-line; followed by 5-FU 400mg/m^2 bolus over 2-4 min, then 5-FU 600mg/m^2 as a 22 hr infusion. Day 2: LV 200mg/m^2 over 120 min; followed by 5-FU 400mg/m^2 bolus over 2-4 min, then 5-FU 600mg/m^2 as a 22 hr infusion. Repeat cycle every 2 weeks. Persistent Grade 2 Neurosensory Events: Reduce oxaliplatin to 65mg/m^2. Grade 3 Neurosensory Events: Consider d/c. After Recovery From Grade 3/4 GI or Grade 4 Hematologic Toxicity: Reduce oxaliplatin to 65mg/m^2 and 5-FU by 20%. Adjuvant Therapy Stage III Colon Cancer: Recommended cycle every 2 weeks for 6 months. Persistent Grade 2 Neurosensory Events: Reduce oxaliplatin to 75mg/m^2. Persistent Grade 3 Neurosensory Events: Consider d/c. After Recovery From Grade 3/4 GI or Grade 3/4 Hematologic Toxicity: Reduce oxaliplatin to 75mg/m^2 and 5-FU to 300mg/m^2 bolus and 500mg/m^2 22 hr infusion.

HOW SUPPLIED: Inj: 50mg, 100mg

CONTRAINDICATIONS: Hypersensitivity to platinum compounds.

WARNINGS/PRECAUTIONS: Acute and persistent neuropathy reported. Cold may exacerbate acute neurological symptoms; avoid ice for mucositis prophy-laxis. Potentially fatal pulmonary fibrosis reported. If unexplained respiratory symptoms develop, d/c until interstitial lung disease or pulmonary fibrosis is ruled out. Monitor WBC with differential, Hgb, platelets, and blood chemistries (including ALT, AST, bilirubin, creatinine) before each cycle. Caution with renal impairment.

ADVERSE REACTIONS: Neuropathy, fatigue, nausea, neutropenia, emesis, diarrhea.

INTERACTIONS: Increased 5-FU plasma levels with doses of 130mg/m^2 ox-aliplatin dosed every 3 weeks; clearance may be decreased with nephrotoxic agents.

PREGNANCY: Category D, not for use in nursing.

MECHANISM OF ACTION: Organoplatinum complex; inhibits DNA replication and transcription.

PHARMACOKINETICS: Absorption: C$_{max}$=0.814ug/mL. **Distribution**: V$_d$=440L; plasma protein binding (>90%). **Metabolism:** Rapid, nonenzymatic biotrans-formation. **Elimination**: Urine (54%), feces (2%).

EMADINE   RX
emedastine difumarate (Alcon)

THERAPEUTIC CLASS: H$_1$-receptor antagonist

INDICATIONS: Temporary relief of signs and symptoms of allergic conjunctivitis.

DOSAGE: *Adults:* 1 drop in affected eye up to qid.
Pediatrics: ≥3 yrs: 1 drop in affected eye up to qid.

HOW SUPPLIED: Sol: 0.05% [5mL]

WARNINGS/PRECAUTIONS: Wait at least 10 min after application to insert contact lens (if eye is not red). Not for irritation due to contact lens.

ADVERSE REACTIONS: Headache, abnormal dreams, asthenia, bad taste, blurred vision, burning, stinging, corneal infiltrates, corneal staining, dermatitis, discomfort, dry eye, foreign body sensation, hyperemia, keratitis, pruritus, rhinitis, sinusitis, tearing.

PREGNANCY: Category B, caution in nursing.

MECHANISM OF ACTION: Antihistaminic; relatively selective histamine H₁ antagonist; inhibits histamine-stimulated vascular permeability in the conjunctiva.

PHARMACOKINETICS: Metabolism: 5- and 6-hydroxymedastine (primary metabolites).

EMBELINE E   RX
clobetasol propionate (Healthpoint)

THERAPEUTIC CLASS: Corticosteroid

INDICATIONS: Corticosteroid-responsive dermatoses.

DOSAGE: *Adults:* Apply bid. Limit to 2 consecutive weeks. Max: 50g/week. Moderate-Severe Psoriasis: Apply to 5%-10% BSA up to 4 weeks. Max: 50g/week.
Pediatrics: ≥12 yrs: Apply bid. Limit to 2 consecutive weeks. Max: 50g/week. Moderate-Severe Psoriasis: ≥16 yrs: Apply to 5%-10% BSA up to 4 weeks. Max: 50g/week.

HOW SUPPLIED: Cre: 0.05% [15g, 30g, 60g]

WARNINGS/PRECAUTIONS: Not for use on the face, groin, or axillae, or for treatment of rosacea or perioral dermatitis. May produce reversible HPA axis suppression, manifestations of Cushing's syndrome, hyperglycemia, and glucosuria. Reassess if no improvement after 2 weeks. D/C if irritation occurs. Peds may be more susceptible to systemic toxicity. Avoid occlusive dressings.

ADVERSE REACTIONS: Burning/stinging, pruritus, irritation, erythema, folliculitis, cracking/fissuring of skin, numbness of fingers, tenderness in elbows, telangiectasia, skin atrophy.

PREGNANCY: Category C, caution in nursing.

MECHANISM OF ACTION: Corticosteroid; posssess anti-inflammatory, antipruritic, and vasoconstrictive properties. Mechanism not established; suspected to inhibit phospholipase A₂ inhibitory proteins, lipocortins. Lipocortins control biosynthesis of potent mediators of inflammation (eg, prostaglandins, leukotrienes) by inhibiting release of their precursor, arachidonic acid.

PHARMACOKINETICS: Absorption: Percutaneous; inflammation and other disease states may increase absorption. Use of occlusive dressings <24 hrs not shown to increase penetration. Use of occlusive dressings for up to 96 hrs significantly increases penetration. **Distribution:** Systemically administered corticosteroids found in breast milk.

EMCYT   RX
estramustine phosphate sodium (Pharmacia & Upjohn)

THERAPEUTIC CLASS: Estradiol/nornitrogen mustard

INDICATIONS: Palliative treatment of metastatic and/or progressive prostate carcinoma.

DOSAGE: *Adults:* Usual: 14mg/kg/day given tid-qid. Take with water at least 1 hr before or 2 hrs after meals.

HOW SUPPLIED: Cap: 140mg

CONTRAINDICATIONS: Active thrombophlebitis, thromboembolic disorders; except when the tumor mass is causing the thromboembolic phenomenon and therapy benefits outweigh risks.

WARNINGS/PRECAUTIONS: Increased risk of thrombosis and MI. Caution with CVD, CAD, metabolic bone disease associated with hypercalcemia, hepatic or renal dysfunction, or with history of thrombophlebitis, thrombosis, or thromboembolic disorders. May decrease glucose tolerance. HTN may occur; monitor BP periodically. May exacerbate pre-existing peripheral edema or CHF. Allergic reactions, angioedema reported. Gynecomastia, impotence may occur.

ADVERSE REACTIONS: Edema, dyspnea, leg cramps, nausea, diarrhea, GI upset, breast tenderness/enlargement, increased hepatic enzymes.

INTERACTIONS: Milk, milk products, and calcium-rich foods or drugs may impair absorption.

PREGNANCY: Safety in pregnancy and nursing not known.

MECHANISM OF ACTION: Estradiol/nornitrogen mustard.

PHARMACOKINETICS: Absorption: Dephosphorylated during absorption. **Metabolism:** Estramustine, estradiol, estrone (major metabolites).

EMEND
aprepitant (Merck)

RX

THERAPEUTIC CLASS: Substance P/neurokinin 1 receptor antagonist

INDICATIONS: In combination with other antiemetics for prevention of acute and delayed nausea and vomiting associated with initial and repeat courses of highly emetogenic cancer chemotherapy (eg, high-dose cisplatin) and for moderately emetogenic cancer chemotherapy. For the prevention of postoperative nausea and vomiting.

DOSAGE: *Adults:* Prevention of Chemo-Induced N/V: Day 1: 125mg 1 hr prior to chemotherapy. Days 2 and 3: 80mg qam. Regimen should include a corticosteroid and a 5-HT$_3$ antagonist. Concomitant Corticosteroid: Reduce dexamethasone PO or methylprednisolone PO by 50% and methylprednisolone IV by 25%. Prevention of Post-Op N/V: 40mg within 3 hrs prior to induction of anesthesia.

HOW SUPPLIED: Cap: 40mg, 80mg, 125mg; Tri-Pak: (one 125mg & two 80mg caps)

CONTRAINDICATIONS: Concurrent treatment with pimozide, terfenadine, astemizole, or cisapride.

WARNINGS/PRECAUTIONS: Chronic continuous use is not recommended. Caution with severe hepatic insufficiency.

ADVERSE REACTIONS: Asthenia/fatigue, nausea, constipation, diarrhea, hiccups, anorexia, headache, vomiting, dizziness, dehydration, heartburn, abdominal pain, epigastric discomfort, gastritis, tinnitis, neutropenia.

INTERACTIONS: See Contraindications. May increase levels of drugs metabolized by CYP3A4 including chemotherapy agents (eg, docetaxel, paclitaxel, etoposide, irinotecan, ifosfamide, imatinib, vinblastine, and vincristine), dexamethasone and methylprednisolone, certain benzodiazepines (eg, midazolam, alprazolam, triazolam). May reduce efficacy of oral contraceptives; use alternative contraception during treatment and for 1 month after last dose. May decrease levels of warfarin, tolbutamide, phenytoin or other drugs metabolized by CYP2C9. Caution with strong CYP3A4 inhibitors (eg, ketoconazole, itraconazole, nefazodone, troleandomycin, clarithromycin, ritonavir, nelfinavir and moderate CYP3A4 inhibitors (eg, diltiazem). Decreased efficacy with CYP3A4 inducers (eg, rifampin, carbamazepine, phenytoin). Concomitant paroxetine may decrease levels of both drugs.

PREGNANCY: Category B, not for use in nursing.

MECHANISM OF ACTION: Substance P/neurokinin 1 receptor antagonist; inhibits emesis induced by cytotoxic chemotherapeutic agents, such as cisplatin, via central actions.

PHARMACOKINETICS: Absorption: (40mg) AUC=7.8mcg•hr/mL, C_{max}=0.7mcg/mL, T_{max}=3 hrs. Refer to PI for detailed information. **Distribution:** Plasma protein binding (>95%); V_d=70L; crosses blood-brain barrier. **Metabolism:** Liver (extensive) via CYP3A4, 1A2, 2C19. **Elimination:** Urine (57%), feces (45%); $T_{1/2}$=9-13 hrs.

EMLA   RX
prilocaine - lidocaine (AstraZeneca)

THERAPEUTIC CLASS: Acetamide local anesthetic

INDICATIONS: Topical anesthetic for use on normal intact skin or on genital mucous membranes for minor surgery. Pretreatment for infiltration anesthesia.

DOSAGE: *Adults:* Apply thick layer of cream to intact skin and cover with occlusive dressing. Minor Dermal Procedure: Apply 2.5g (1/2 tube) over 20-25cm² of skin surface. Major Dermal Procedure: Apply 2g/10cm² of skin for 2 hrs. Adult Male Genital Skin: Apply 1g/10cm² of skin surface for 15 min. Female External Genitalia: Apply 5-10g for 5-10 min.
Pediatrics: 7-12 yrs and >20kg: Max: 20g/200cm² for up to 4 hrs.1-6 yrs and >10 kg: Max:10g/100cm² for up to 4 hrs. 3-12 months and ≥5 kg: Max: 2g/20cm² for up to 4 hrs. 3-12 months and ≥5 kg: Max: 2g/20cm² for up to 4 hrs. 0-3 months or <5kg: Max: 1g/10cm² for up to 1 hr.

HOW SUPPLIED: Cre: (Lidocaine-Prilocaine) 2.5%-2.5%

WARNINGS/PRECAUTIONS: Avoid application for longer than recommended times or on large areas. Avoid with methemoglobinemia. Risk of methemoglobinemia in very young or with G6P deficiency. Avoid eye contact, use in ear. Caution with severe hepatic disease, acutely ill, debilitated, elderly, history of drug sensitivities. Avoid in neonates with a gestational age <37 weeks and infants <12 months receiving treatment with methemoglobin-inducing agents.

ADVERSE REACTIONS: Local reactions such as: erythema, edema, abnormal sensations, paleness (pallor or blanching), altered temperature sensations, itching, rash.

INTERACTIONS: Caution with Class I (eg, tocainide, mexiletine) and Class III (eg, amiodarone, bretylium, sotalol) antiarrhythmic drugs. Avoid drugs associated with drug-induced methemoglobinemia (eg, sulfonamides, APAP, nitrates/nitrites, nitrofurantoin, phenobarbital, phenytoin, quinine). Caution with other products containing local anesthetics; consider the amount absorbed from all formulations.

PREGNANCY: Category B, caution in nursing.

MECHANISM OF ACTION: Amide-type local anesthetic; provides dermal analgesia by release of lidocaine and prilocaine into epidermal and dermal layers of skin and by accumulation in vicinity of dermal pain receptors and nerve endings. Also stabilizes neuronal membranes by inhibiting ionic fluxes required for initiation and conduction impulses, thereby effecting local anesthetic action.

PHARMACOKINETICS: Absorption: Lidocaine: (3 hrs 400cm²) C_{max}=0.12mcg/mL, T_{max}=4 hrs; (24 hrs 400cm²) C_{max}=0.28mcg/mL, T_{max}=10 hrs. Prilocaine: (3 hrs 400cm²) C_{max}=0.07mcg/mL, T_{max}=4 hrs; (24 hrs 400 cm²) C_{max}=0.14mcg/mL, T_{max}=10 hrs. **Distribution:** V_d=1.5L/kg (lidocaine), 2.6L/kg (prilocaine); plasma protein binding 70% (lidocaine), 55% (prilocaine). Crosses placental and blood-brain barrier; found in breast milk. **Metabolism:** Lidocaine: Liver (rapid); monoethylglycinexylidide and glycinexylidide (active metabolites). Prilocaine: Liver and kidneys by amidases; *ortho*-toluidine and propylalanine (metabolites). **Elimination:** Lidocaine: Urine (>98%); $T_{1/2}$=110 min. Prilocaine: $T_{1/2}$=70 min.

EMSAM   RX
selegiline (Bristol-Myers Squibb)

> Antidepressants increased the risk of suicidal thinking and behavior (suicidality) in short-term studies in children, adolescents and young adults with Major Depressive Disorder and other psychiatric disorders. Selegiline transdermal system is not approved for use in pediatric patients.

THERAPEUTIC CLASS: Monoamine oxidase inhibitor (Type B)

INDICATIONS: Treatment of major depressive disorder.

DOSAGE: *Adults:* Apply to dry, intact skin on the upper torso, upper thigh, or outer surface of upper arm once every 24 hrs. Initial/Target Dose: 6mg/24hrs. Titrate: May increase in increments of 3mg/24hrs at intervals no less than 2 weeks. Max: 12mg/24hrs. Elderly: 6mg/24hrs. Increase dose cautiously and monitor closely.

HOW SUPPLIED: Patch: 6mg/24hrs, 9mg/24hrs, 12mg/24hrs [30⁵]

CONTRAINDICATIONS: Pheochromocytoma. Concomitant SSRIs (eg, fluoxetine, sertraline, paroxetine), dual serotonin and norepinephrine reuptake inhibitors (eg, venlafaxine, duloxetine), TCAs (eg, imipramine, amitriptyline), bupropion, buspirone, meperidine, analgesic agents (eg, tramadol, methadone, and propoxyphene), dextromethorphan, St. John's wort, mirtazapine, cyclobenzaprine, carbamazepine, oxcarbazepine, sympathetic amines (including amphetamines), cold products and weight-reducing preparations that contain vasoconstrictors (eg, pseudoephedrine, phenylephrine, phenylpropanolamine, ephedrine), oral selegiline, other MAOIs (eg, isocarboxazid, phenelzine, tranylcypromine), general anesthesia agents, cocaine, or local anesthesia containing sympathomimetic vasoconstrictors. Dietary modifications required with 9mg/24hrs and 12mg/24hrs systems.

WARNINGS/PRECAUTIONS: Hypertensive crisis may occur with ingestion of foods with a high concentration of tyramine. Postural hypotension may occur; consider dosage adjustment with orthostatic symptoms. Activation of mania/hypomania may occur; caution with history of mania. Caution with disorders or conditions that can produce altered metabolism or hemodynamic responses. Avoid elective surgery requiring general anesthesia.

ADVERSE REACTIONS: Headache, diarrhea, dyspepsia, insomnia, dry mouth, pharyngitis, sinusitis, application site reaction, rash.

INTERACTIONS: Avoid alcohol. See Contraindications.

PREGNANCY: Category C, caution in nursing.

MECHANISM OF ACTION: MAOI; non-selectively inhibits monoamine oxidase.

PHARMACOKINETICS: Absorption: AUC=46.2ng•hr/mL. **Distribution:** Plasma protein binding (90%). **Metabolism:** Hepatic (N-dealkylation, N-depropargylation) via CYP2B6, 2C9, 3A4/5 (major), CYP2A6 (minor); N-desmethylselegiline, methamphetamine, amphetamine (metabolites). **Elimination:** Urine (0.1%); $T_{1/2}$=18-25 hrs.

EMTRIVA   RX
emtricitabine (Gilead)

> Lactic acidosis and severe hepatomegaly with steatosis, including fatal cases, reported with nucleoside analogs alone or with concomitant antiretrovirals. Not indicated for the treatment of chronic HBV infection; severe acute exacerbations of hepatitis B reported in patients co-infected with HBV and HIV upon discontinuation of emtricitabine.

THERAPEUTIC CLASS: Nucleoside analogue

INDICATIONS: Treatment of HIV-1 infection in combination with other antivirals.

DOSAGE: *Adults:* ≥18 yrs: Cap: 200mg qd. CrCl 30-49mL/min: 200mg q48h. CrCl 15-29mL/min: 200mg q72h. CrCl <15mL/min (including hemodialysis): 200mg q96h. Sol: 240mg (24mL) qd. CrCl 30-49mL/min: 120mg (12mL) qd. CrCl 15-29mL/min: 80mg (8mL) qd. CrCl <15mL/min (including hemodialysis):

E

60mg (6mL) qd.
Pediatrics: 0-3 months: Sol: 3mg/kg qd. 3 months-17 yrs: Cap: >33kg: 200mg qd. Sol: 6mg/kg qd. Max: 240mg (24mL).

HOW SUPPLIED: Cap: 200mg; Sol: 10mg/mL [170mL]

WARNINGS/PRECAUTIONS: Test for chronic hepatitis B prior to initiation; post-treatment exacerbations reported. Monitor hepatic function for several months in patients who d/c the drug and are co-infected with HIV and HBV. Reduce dose with renal dysfunction. Monitor changes in fasting cholesterol, serum amylase, creatinine kinase, and neutrophil count. Redistribution/accumulation of body fat reported. Immune reconstitution syndrome reported.

ADVERSE REACTIONS: Headache, diarrhea, nausea, rash, vomiting, dyspepsia, asthenia, abdominal pain, dizziness, insomnia, neuropathy, paresthesia, increased cough, rhinitis.

INTERACTIONS: Avoid co-administration with Atripla, Truvada, or lamivudine-containing products.

PREGNANCY: Category B, not for use in nursing.

MECHANISM OF ACTION: Nucleoside analog of cytidine; inhibits the activity of HIV-1 reverse transcriptase by competing with the natural substrate deoxycytidine 5'-triphosphate and incorporating into nascent viral DNA, resulting in chain termination.

PHARMACOKINETICS: Absorption: Rapid and extensive. C_{max}=1.8mcg/mL, T_{max}=1-2 hrs, AUC=10.0mcg•hr/mL. (Cap) Absolute bioavailabilty (93%). (Sol) Absolute bioavailabilty (75%). **Distribution:** Plasma protein binding (<4%). **Metabolism:** Hepatic (conjugation and oxidation). Metabolites: 3'sulfoxide diastereomers and 2'O-glucuronide. **Elimination:** Urine (86%), feces (14%); $T_{1/2}$=10 hrs.

ENABLEX

RX

darifenacin (Novartis)

THERAPEUTIC CLASS: Muscarinic antagonist

INDICATIONS: Treatment of overactive bladder with symptoms of urge urinary incontinence, urgency and frequency.

DOSAGE: *Adults:* Initial: 7.5mg qd with liquid. Max: 15mg qd. Moderate Hepatic Impairment/Concomitant Potent CYP3A4 Inhibitors: Do not exceed 7.5mg/d. Severe Hepatic Impairment: Avoid use. Tabs should be swallowed whole; do not chew, divide or crush.

HOW SUPPLIED: Tab, Extended-Release: 7.5mg, 15mg

CONTRAINDICATIONS: Urinary retention, gastric retention, uncontrolled narrow-angle glaucoma.

WARNINGS/PRECAUTIONS: Risk of urinary retention; caution with significant bladder outflow obstruction. Risk of gastric retention; caution with GI obstructive disorders. May decrease GI motility; caution with severe constipation, ulcerative colitis, and myasthenia gravis. Caution with moderate hepatic impairment and narrow-angle glaucoma. Avoid use with severe hepatic impairment. May produce blurred vision or dizziness.

ADVERSE REACTIONS: Dry mouth, constipation, dyspepsia, abdominal pain, nausea, diarrhea, UTI, dizziness, asthenia, dry eyes.

INTERACTIONS: Do not exceed 7.5mg/day with concomitant potent CYP3A4 inhibitors. Caution with medications metabolized by CYP2D6. Additive effects with other anticholinergic agents.

PREGNANCY: Category C, caution in nursing.

MECHANISM OF ACTION: Muscarinic receptor antagonist; inhibits cholinergic muscarinic receptors which mediate contractions of urinary bladder smooth muscle, and stimulation of salivary secretions.

PHARMACOKINETICS: Absorption: (7.5mg) Bioavailability (15%); extensive metabolizers (EM): C_{max}=2.01ng/mL, T_{max}=6.49 hrs, AUC=29.24ng•hr/mL. Poor metabolizers (PM): C_{max}=4.27ng/mL, T_{max}=5.2 hrs, AUC=67.56ng•hr/

mL. (15mg) Bioavailability (19%); EM: C_{max}=5.76ng/mL, T_{max}=7.61 hrs, AUC=88.9ng•hr/mL. PM: C_{max} = 9.99ng/mL, T_{max}=6.71 hrs, AUC=157.71ng.h/mL. **Distribution:** Plasma protein binding (98%), V_d=163L. **Metabolism:** CYP2D6, 3A4 (monohydroxylation, ring opening, N-dealkylation). **Elimination:** Urine (3%), $T_{1/2}$=13-19 hrs.

ENBREL   RX
etanercept (Amgen)

> Serious infections, including bacterial sepsis and TB, reported; d/c if severe infection develops. Evaluate for TB risk factors and test for latent TB infection prior to initiation.

THERAPEUTIC CLASS: TNF-receptor blocker

INDICATIONS: To reduce signs/symptoms, induce major clinical response, improve physical function, and inhibit progression of structural damage in moderate to severe rheumatoid arthritis (RA) (may be initiated in combination with methotrexate [MTX] or alone). To reduce signs/symptoms, inhibit progression of structural damage of active arthritis, and improve physical function in psoriatic arthritis (may be used with MTX in patients not responding to MTX alone). To reduce signs/symptoms of moderate to severe polyarticular-course juvenile rheumatoid arthritis (JRA) unresponsive to one or more DMARDs. To reduce signs/symptoms of active ankylosing spondylitis (AS). Chronic moderate to severe plaque psoriasis for candidates of systemic therapy or phototherapy.

DOSAGE: *Adults:* ≥18 yrs: RA/Psoriatic Arthritis/AS: 50mg SQ per week, given as one SQ injection. May continue MTX, glucocorticoids, salicylates, NSAIDs, or analgesics. Psoriasis: Initial: 50mg SQ twice weekly given 3 or 4 days apart for 3 months. May begin with 25-50mg/week. Maint: 50mg/week.
Pediatrics: 2-17 yrs: JRA: 0.8mg/kg SQ per week. Max: 50mg/week. May continue glucocorticoids, NSAIDs, or analgesics.

HOW SUPPLIED: Inj: (MDV) 25mg, (Syringe) 50mg/mL

CONTRAINDICATIONS: Sepsis.

WARNINGS/PRECAUTIONS: May cause autoimmune antibodies. Avoid with active infections. Monitor closely if new infection develops. Caution with pre-existing or recent onset CNS demyelinating disorders. Rare cases of pancytopenia including aplastic anemia reported; d/c if significant hematologic abnormalities occur. May cause reactivation of hepatitis B virus; evaluate prior to therapy initiation. Caution in patients with heart failure; monitor closely. JRA patients should be brought up to date with current immunization guidelines prior to initiating therapy. D/C temporarily with significant varicella virus exposure and consider prophylaxis. Avoid with Wegener's granulomatosis. Needle cap on prefilled syringe and autoinjector contains dry natural rubber; caution with latex allergy.

ADVERSE REACTIONS: (**Adults/Pediatrics**) Injection site reactions, infections, headache. (Pediatrics) Varicella, gastroenteritis, depression, cutaneous ulcer, esophagitis.

INTERACTIONS: Do not give live vaccines. Avoid with cyclophosphamide. May cause neutropenia with anakinra.

PREGNANCY: Category B, not for use in nursing.

MECHANISM OF ACTION: TNF-receptor blocker; binds specifically to tumor necrosis factor (TNF) and blocks its interaction with cell surface TNF-receptors.

PHARMACOKINETICS: Absorption: SQ administration of different doses resulted in different parameters.

ENDOMETRIN   RX
progesterone (Ferring)

THERAPEUTIC CLASS: Progesterone

ENGERIX-B

INDICATIONS: To support embryo implantation and early pregnancy by supplementation of corpus luteal function as part of an Assisted Reproductive Technology (ART) treatment program for infertile women.

DOSAGE: *Adults:* 100mg vaginally bid or tid starting at oocyte retrieval and continuing for up to 10 weeks.

HOW SUPPLIED: Vaginal Insert: 100mg [21^5]

CONTRAINDICATIONS: Known missed abortion or ectopic pregnancy, liver disease, known or suspected breast cancer. Active arterial or venous thromboembolism or severe thrombophlebitis, or a history of these events.

WARNINGS/PRECAUTIONS: D/C if signs of MI, cerebrovascular disorders, thromboembolism, thrombophlebitis, or retinal thrombosis develop. Caution with history of depression.

ADVERSE REACTIONS: Post-oocyte retrieval pain, abdominal pain, nausea, ovarian hyperstimulation syndrome, abdominal distention, headache, uterine spasm, vomiting, vaginal bleeding.

INTERACTIONS: CYP450 3A4 inducers (eg. rifampin, carbamazepine) may increase elimination. Avoid use with other vaginal products (eg, antifungals).

PREGNANCY: Safety in pregnancy and nursing not known.

MECHANISM OF ACTION: Progesterone; increases endometrial receptivity for implantation of an embryo and helps maintain pregnancy.

PHARMACOKINETICS: Absorption: C_{max}=17.0ng/mL; T_{max}=24 hr; AUC_{0-24}=217ng•hr/mL. **Distribution:** Serum plasma protein binding (approximately 96-99%). **Metabolism:** Liver and gut. **Excretion:** Kidney, 56-60% (metabolite), bile and feces, 10%.

ENGERIX-B   RX
hepatitis B (recombinant) (GlaxoSmithKline)

OTHER BRAND NAMES: Engerix-B Pediatric/Adolescent (GlaxoSmithKline)

THERAPEUTIC CLASS: Vaccine

INDICATIONS: Immunization against all known hepatitis B virus subtypes.

DOSAGE: *Adults:* >19 yrs: 20mcg IM in deltoid or thigh at 0, 1, 6 months. Hemodialysis: 40mcg IM at 0, 1, 2, 6 months. Booster: 20mcg IM. Hemodialysis Booster: 40mcg IM. May give SQ with risk of hemorrhage.
Pediatrics: ≤19 yrs: 10mcg/0.5mL IM at 0, 1, 6 months. Booster: ≤10 yrs: 10mcg IM. 11-19 yrs: 20mcg IM. See PI for special populations. May give SQ with risk of hemorrhage.

HOW SUPPLIED: Inj: 10mcg/0.5mL, 20mcg/mL

CONTRAINDICATIONS: Yeast hypersensitivity.

WARNINGS/PRECAUTIONS: Will not prevent hepatitis A, C, and E viruses infection. Vaccine may be ineffective with unrecognized hepatitis. Delay vaccine with moderate or severe febrile illnesses. May exacerbate MS (rare). Suboptimal immune response may occur with immunosuppressed persons. Have epinephrine injection (1:1000) available.

ADVERSE REACTIONS: Injection site induration, erythema, swelling, fever, headache, dizziness.

INTERACTIONS: Suboptimal immune response may occur with immunosuppressants; defer vaccine ≥3 months after immunosuppressive therapy.

PREGNANCY: Category C, caution in nursing.

MECHANISM OF ACTION: Stimulates the immune system to induce antibodies that may protect against infection caused by all known subtypes of Hepatitis B virus.

ENJUVIA

RX

conjugated estrogens (Duramed)

> Estrogens increase the risk of endometrial cancer. Estrogens and progestins should not be used for the prevention of cardiovascular disease or dementia. Increased risks of MI, stroke, invasive breast cancer, PE, and DVT in postmenopausal women (50 to 79 years of age) reported. Increased risk of developing probable dementia in postmenopausal women ≥65 yrs of age reported.

THERAPEUTIC CLASS: Estrogen

INDICATIONS: Treatment of moderate-severe vasomotor symptoms associated with menopause. Treatment of symptoms of vulvar and vaginal atrophy associated with menopause. Treatment of moderate-severe vaginal dryness and pain with intercourse; if used solely for this purpose, topical vaginal products should be considered.

DOSAGE: *Adults:* Individualize dosing. Initial: 0.3mg qd. Adjust dose based on response.

HOW SUPPLIED: Tab: 0.3mg, 0.45mg, 0.625mg, 0.9mg, 1.25mg

CONTRAINDICATIONS: Pregnancy, undiagonosed abnormal genital bleeding, breast cancer, estrogen-dependent neoplasia, DVT/PE, arterial thromboembolic disease (eg, stroke, MI), liver dysfunction.

WARNINGS/PRECAUTIONS: Increased risk of retinal vascular thrombosis, severe hypercalcemia in patients with breast cancer and bone metastases, gallbladder disease and breast and ovarian cancers. Elavated BP reported; monitor BP at regular intervals. May elevate plasma triglycerides resulting in pancreatitis. Caution in patients with impaired liver function or history of cholestatic jaundice. May increase TBG; monitor thyroid function of patients dependent on thyroid hormone replacement therapy and adjust dosage if needed. May cause fluid retention; caution with cardiac or renal dysfunction. Caution in individuals with severe hypocalcemia. May cause exacerbation of asthma, diabetes mellitus, epilepsy, migraine or porphyria, systemic lupus erythematosus, and hepatic hemangiomas.

ADVERSE REACTIONS: Abdominal pain, accidental injury, flu-syndrome, headache, pain, flatulence, nausea, dizziness, paresthesia, bronchitis, rhinitis, sinusitis, breast pain, dysmenorrhea, vaginitis.

INTERACTIONS: CYP3A4 inducers (eg, St. John's wort, phenobarbital, carbamazepine, rifampin) may decrease levels which may decrease therapeutic effects and/or uterine bleeding profile. CYP3A4 inhibitors (eg, erythromycin, clarithromycin, ketoconazole, itraconazole, ritonavir, grapefruit juice) may increase levels which may result in side effects.

PREGNANCY: Category X, caution in nursing.

MECHANISM OF ACTION: Estrogen; binds to nuclear receptors in estrogen-responsive tissues. Circulating estrogens modulate the pituitary secretion of the gonadotrophins, leuteinizing hormone and follicle stimulating hormone, through negative feedback mechanism. Reduces elevated levels of these hormones in postmenopusal women.

PHARMACOKINETICS: Absorption: Refer to package insert for conjugated and unconjugated estrogen parameters. **Distribution:** Largely bound to sex hormone binding globulin and albumin; found in breast milk. **Metabolism:** Liver to estrone (metabolite), estriol (major urinary metabolite); sulfate and glucuronide conjugation (liver); intestinal hydrolysis; CYP 3A4 (partial metabolism). **Elimination:** Urine (parent compound and metabolites); Conjugated estrone: $T_{1/2}$=14 hrs; Conjugated equilin: $T_{1/2}$=11 hrs.

ENTEX HC

CIII

phenylephrine HCL - hydrocodone bitartrate - guaifenesin (Andrx)

THERAPEUTIC CLASS: Opioid antitussive

INDICATIONS: Temporary relief of nonproductive cough.

DOSAGE: *Adults:* 5-10mL q4-6h. Max 40mL/24 hrs.
Pediatrics: ≥12 yrs: 5-10mL q4-6h. Max 40mL/24 hrs. 6-12 yrs: 5mL q4-6h. Max 20mL/24 hrs. 2-6 yrs: 2.5mL q4-6h. Max 10mL/24 hrs.

HOW SUPPLIED: Liq: (Guaifenesin-Hydrocodone-Phenylephrine) 100mg-5mg-7.5mg/5mL [473mL]

CONTRAINDICATIONS: Infants, newborns, severe HTN or CAD, hyperthyroidism, or MAOI therapy.

WARNINGS/PRECAUTIONS: May be habit-forming. May cause respiratory depression or increase CSF pressure in the presence of other intracranial pathology. May obscure head injuries or acute abdominal conditions. Caution in elderly, debilitated, hepatic/renal dysfunction, Addison's disease, hypothyroidism, postoperative use, prostatic hypertrophy, pulmonary disease, and urethral stricture. Suppresses cough reflex.

ADVERSE REACTIONS: CNS stimulation, constipation, drowsiness, dizziness, excitability, headache, insomnia, lightheadedness, nausea, vomiting, nervousness, respiratory depression, restlessness, tachycardia, tremors, urinary retention, weakness, arrhythmias, and cardiovascular.

INTERACTIONS: Additive CNS effects with alcohol, antianxiety agents, antihistamines, antipsychotics, narcotics, tranquilizers, or other CNS depressants. Increased sympathomimetic effects with MAOIs or β-blockers. Sympathomimetics may reduce antihypertensive effects of methyldopa, mecamylamine, reserpine, veratrum alkaloids. May enhance the effects of TCAs, barbiturates, alcohol, other CNS depressants.

PREGNANCY: Category C, not for use in nursing.

ENTEX LA   RX
phenylephrine HCL - guaifenesin (Andrx)

THERAPEUTIC CLASS: Expectorant/decongestant

INDICATIONS: Temporary relief of symptoms associated with upper respiratory tract disorders and cough associated with respiratory tract infections and related disorders when complicated by tenacious mucous or mucous plugs and congestion.

DOSAGE: *Adults:* 1 tab q12h. Max: 2 tabs/24hrs.
Pediatrics: ≥12 yrs: 1 tab q12h. Max: 2 tabs/24hrs. 6-12 yrs: 1/2 tab q12h. Max: 1 tab/24hrs.

HOW SUPPLIED: Tab, Extended-Release: (Guaifenesin-Phenylephrine) 400mg-30mg* *scored

CONTRAINDICATIONS: HTN, ventricular tachycardia, MAOI use within 14 days. Extreme caution in elderly, hyperthyroidism, bradycardia, partial heart block, myocardial disease, severe arteriosclerosis.

WARNINGS/PRECAUTIONS: Caution in HTN, DM, ischemic heart disease, increase IOP, hyperthyroidism, or prostatic hypertrophy. May produce CNS stimulation with convulsions or cardiovascular collapse with hypotension. Adverse effects occur more often in elderly.

ADVERSE REACTIONS: Palpitations, headache, dizziness, nausea, anxiety, restlessness, tremor, weakness, pallor, dysuria, respiratory difficulty.

INTERACTIONS: β-blockers and MAOIs may potentiate pressor response. Increased risk of arrhythmias with digitalis glycosides and halothane anesthesia. May reduce hypotensive effects of guanethidine, mecamylamine, methyldopa, reserpine, and veratrum alkaloids. TCAs may antagonize effects.

PREGNANCY: Category C, not for use in nursing.

ENTEX PSE   RX
pseudoephedrine HCL - guaifenesin (Andrx)

OTHER BRAND NAMES: Guaifenex PSE 120 (Ethex) - Ami-Tex PSE (Amide)

THERAPEUTIC CLASS: Expectorant/decongestant

INDICATIONS: Relief of nasal congestion due to common cold, hay fever, upper respiratory allergies, and nasal congestion associated with sinusitis. To promote nasal or sinus drainage. For symptomatic relief of respiratory conditions characterized by dry nonproductive cough and in the presence of tenacious mucous plugs in the respiratory tract.

DOSAGE: *Adults:* 1 tab q12h.
Pediatrics: ≥12 yrs: 1 tab q12h. 6 to <12 yrs: 1/2 tab q12h.

HOW SUPPLIED: Tab, Extended-Release: (Guaifenesin-Pseudoephedrine) 400mg-120mg* *scored

CONTRAINDICATIONS: Nursing, severe HTN, severe CAD, prostatic hypertrophy, concomitant MAOIs.

WARNINGS/PRECAUTIONS: Caution in HTN, DM, heart disease, peripheral vascular disease, increased IOP, hyperthyroidism, or prostatic hypertrophy.

ADVERSE REACTIONS: Nausea, vomiting, nervousness, dizziness, sleeplessness, lightheadedness, tremor, palpitations, tachycardia, weakness, respiratory difficulties.

INTERACTIONS: MAOI and β-blockers increase sympathomimetic effects. May reduce antihypertensive effects of methyldopa, guanethidine, mecamylamine, reserpine, and veratrum alkaloids.

PREGNANCY: Category C, contraindicated in nursing.

MECHANISM OF ACTION: Pseudoephedrine: Sympathomimetic, decongestant; produces vasoconstriction by stimulating α-receptors within the mucosa of the respiratory tract. Guaifenesin: Expectorant; promotes lower respiratory tract drainage.

ENTOCORT EC   RX
budesonide (Prometheus)

THERAPEUTIC CLASS: Corticosteroid

INDICATIONS: Treatment of mild to moderate active Crohn's disease involving the ileum and/or ascending colon. Maintenance of clinical remission of mild to moderate Crohn's disease involving the ileum and/or ascending colon for up to 3 months.

DOSAGE: *Adults:* Usual: 9mg qd, in the am for up to 8 weeks. Recurring Episodes: Repeat therapy for 8 weeks. Maint: 6mg qd for 3 months, then taper to complete cessation. Moderate to Severe Hepatic Insufficiency/Concomitant CYP3A4 Inhibitors: Reduce dose. Swallow whole; do not chew or break.

HOW SUPPLIED: Cap, Delayed-Release: 3mg

WARNINGS/PRECAUTIONS: May reduce response of HPA axis to stress. Supplement with systemic glucocorticosteroids if undergoing surgery or other stressful situations. Increased risk of infection avoid exposure to chickenpox and measles. Caution with TB, HTN, DM, osteoporosis, peptic ulcer, glaucoma, cirrhosis, cataracts, family history of DM or glaucoma. Replacement of systemic glucocorticosteroids may unmask allergies. Chronic use may cause hypercorticism and adrenal suppression.

ADVERSE REACTIONS: Headache, respiratory infection, nausea, back pain, dyspepsia, dizziness, abdominal pain, diarrhea, flatulence, vomiting, sinusitis, viral infection, arthralgia.

INTERACTIONS: Increased levels with CYP3A4 inhibitors (eg, ketoconazole, itraconazole, saquinavir, erythromycin, grapefruit, grapefruit juice); reduce budesonide dose.

PREGNANCY: Category C, not for use in nursing.

MECHANISM OF ACTION: Glucocorticosteroid.

PHARMACOKINETICS: Absorption: C_{max}=5nmol/L. T_{max}=30-600 min; AUC=30nmol•hr/L. **Distribution:** Plasma protein binding (85-90%); V_d=2.2-3.9L/kg. **Metabolism:** Liver; CYP3A4. **Elimination:** Urine (60%); $T_{1/2}$=2-3.6 hrs.

EPIFOAM RX
pramoxine HCL - hydrocortisone acetate (Schwarz)

THERAPEUTIC CLASS: Corticosteroid

INDICATIONS: Corticosteroid responsive dermatoses.

DOSAGE: *Adults:* Apply tid-qid. Use occlusive dressings for management of psoriasis or recalcitrant conditions.
Pediatrics: Use least amount necessary for effective regimen. Use occlusive dressings for management of psoriasis or recalcitrant conditions.

HOW SUPPLIED: Foam: (Hydrocortisone-Pramoxine) 1%-1% [10g]

WARNINGS/PRECAUTIONS: Avoid prolonged use. D/C use if irritation persists. May produce reversible HPA axis suppression, manifestations of Cushing's syndrome, hyperglycemia, glucosuria. Pediatrics more susceptible to systemic toxicity.

ADVERSE REACTIONS: Burning, itching, irritation, dryness, folliculitis, hypertrichosis, acneiform eruptions, hypopigmentation, perioral dermatitis, maceration, secondary infection, skin atrophy, striae, miliaria.

PREGNANCY: Category C, caution in nursing.

MECHANISM OF ACTION: Hydrocortisone: Corticosteroid; possesses anti-inflammatory, antipruritic, and vasoconstrictive properties. Anti-inflammatory activity not established. Pramoxine: Local anesthetic.

PHARMACOKINETICS: Absorption: Percutaneous; inflammation, other disease states, and use of occlusive dressings may increase absorption. **Distribution:** Systemically administered corticosteroids are found in breast milk. **Metabolism:** Liver. **Elimination:** Kidneys, bile.

EPIPEN RX
epinephrine (Dey)

OTHER BRAND NAMES: EpiPen Jr. (Dey)

THERAPEUTIC CLASS: Sympathomimetic catecholamine

INDICATIONS: Emergency treatment of allergic reactions (anaphylaxis) to insect stings or bites, foods, drugs, other allergens, and idiopathic or exercise-induced anaphylaxis.

DOSAGE: *Adults:* 0.3mg IM in thigh. May repeat with severe anaphylaxis.
Pediatrics: 0.15mg or 0.3mg (0.01mg/kg) IM in thigh. May repeat with severe anaphylaxis.

HOW SUPPLIED: Inj: (Epipen Jr) 0.5mg/mL, (Epipen) 1mg/mL

WARNINGS/PRECAUTIONS: Not for IV use. Contains sulfites. Extreme caution with heart disease. Anginal pain may be induced with coronary insufficiency. Increased risk of adverse reactions with hyperthyroidism, CVD, HTN, DM, elderly, pregnancy, pediatrics <30kg with Epipen and <15kg with Epipen, Jr.

ADVERSE REACTIONS: Palpitations, tachycardia, sweating, nausea, vomiting, respiratory difficulty, pallor, dizziness, weakness, tremor, headache, apprehension, anxiety.

INTERACTIONS: Potentiated by TCAs and MAOIs. Increased risk of arrhythmias with digitalis, mercurial diuretics, or quinidine. Pressor effects may be counteracted by rapidly acting vasodilators.

PREGNANCY: Category C, safety in nursing not known.

MECHANISM OF ACTION: Sympathomimetic drug; acts on both α and β receptors.

EPIQUIN MICRO

RX

hydroquinone (SkinMedica)

THERAPEUTIC CLASS: Depigmenting agent

INDICATIONS: Gradual treatment of UV-induced dyschromia and discoloration resulting from the use of oral contraceptives, pregnancy, hormone replacement therapy, or skin trauma.

DOSAGE: *Adults:* Apply bid (am and hs). Use sunscreen.
Pediatrics: ≥12yrs: Apply bid (am and hs). Use sunscreen.

HOW SUPPLIED: Cre: 4% [30g]

WARNINGS/PRECAUTIONS: Avoid sun exposure on bleached skin. Use sunscreen. May produce unwanted cosmetic effects if not used as directed. Test for skin sensitivity. D/C if no lightening effect after 2 months of therapy, if blue-black darkening of the skin occurs, or if itching, vesicle formation, or excessive inflammatory reactions occur. Contains sodium metabisulfite; may cause serious allergic type reactions. Avoid contact with eyes.

ADVERSE REACTIONS: Cutaneous hypersensitivity (contact dermatitis).

PREGNANCY: Category C, caution in nursing.

MECHANISM OF ACTION: Produces a reversible depigmentation of the skin by inhibition of the enzymatic oxidation of tyrosine to 3-(3,4-dihydroxyphenyl) alanine (dopa)[2] and suppresses the melanocyte metabolic processes.

EPIVIR

RX

lamivudine (GlaxoSmithKline)

> Lactic acidosis and severe hepatomegaly with steatosis, including fatal cases, reported. Epivir tablets and solution, used to treat HIV, contain higher dose of lamivudine than Epivir-HBV, used to treat hepatitis B; only use appropriate dosing forms for HIV treatment. Severe acute exacerbations of hepatitis B reported in patients coinfected with hepatitis B virus and HIV who discontinued therapy; monitor hepatic function closely.

THERAPEUTIC CLASS: Nucleoside analogue

INDICATIONS: Treatment of HIV infection in combination with other antiretrovirals.

DOSAGE: *Adults:* >16 yrs: 150mg bid or 300mg qd, concomitantly with other antiretrovirals. CrCl 30-49mL/min: 150mg qd. CrCl 15-29mL/min: 150mg first dose, then 100mg qd. CrCl 5-14mL/min: 150mg first dose, then 50mg qd. CrCl <5mL/min: 50mg first dose, then 25mg qd.
Pediatrics: Sol: 3 months-16 yrs: 4mg/kg bid, concomitantly with other antiretrovirals. Max: 150mg bid. Scored Tab: 14-21kg: 1/2 tab (75mg) in am and 1/2 tab (75mg) in pm. 21-30kg: 1/2 tab (75mg) in am and 1 tab (150mg) in pm. ≥30kg: 1 tab (150mg) in am and 1 tab (150mg) in pm. Adolescents: CrCl 30-49mL/min: 150mg qd. CrCl 15-29mL/min: 150mg first dose, then 100mg qd. CrCl 5-14mL/min: 150mg 1st dose, then 50mg qd. CrCl <5mL/min: 50mg 1st dose, then 25mg qd.

HOW SUPPLIED: Sol: 10mg/mL [240mL]; Tab: 150mg, 300mg

WARNINGS/PRECAUTIONS: Caution in pediatrics with history of prior antiretroviral nucleoside exposure, history of pancreatitis, or other significant risk factors for developing pancreatitis. D/C if pancreatitis develops. Post-treatment exacerbations of hepatitis reported. Hepatic decompensation occured when used with interferon-α w/ or w/o ribavirin. Suspend therapy if lactic acidosis or pronounced hepatotoxicity occurs. Reduce dose in renal dysfunction. Possible redistribution or accumulation of body fat. Immune reconstitution syndrome reported.

ADVERSE REACTIONS: Headache, malaise, fatigue, fever, chills, nausea, diarrhea, vomiting, anorexia, abdominal pain, neuropathy, dizziness, skin rash, musculoskeletal pain, cough.

INTERACTIONS: TMP/SMX increases levels of lamivudine. Avoid with zalcitabine, zidovudine, and fixed-dose combinations of abacavir, lamivudine, and zidovudine. Also avoid emtricitabine and fixed-dose combinations of emtricitabine, efavirenz, and tenofovir.

PREGNANCY: Category C, not for use in nursing.

MECHANISM OF ACTION: Nucleoside analogue; inhibits HIV-1 reverse transcriptase via DNA chain termination after incorporation into viral DNA.

PHARMACOKINETICS: Absorption: Rapid; (Tab) Absolute bioavailability (86%). (Sol) Absolute bioavailability (87%); C_{max}=1.5mcg/mL (HIV); T_{max}=0.9 hrs. **Distribution:** V_d=1.3L/kg; plasma protein binding (<36%). **Metabolism:** Hepatic (minor); trans-sulfoxide (metabolite). **Elimination:** Urine (unchanged); $T_{1/2}$=5-7 hrs.

EPIVIR-HBV   RX
lamivudine (GlaxoSmithKline)

> Lactic acidosis and severe, possibly fatal, hepatomegaly reported. If prescribed for patients with unrecognized or untreated HIV infection, rapid emergence of HIV resistance is likely; Epivir-HBV contains a lower dose of lamivudine than Epivir which is used to treat HIV. Severe acute exacerbations of hepatitis B reported upon discontinuation of therapy; follow-up liver function monitoring required.

THERAPEUTIC CLASS: Nucleoside analogue

INDICATIONS: Treatment of chronic hepatitis B associated with viral replication and active liver inflammation.

DOSAGE: *Adults:* 100mg qd. CrCl 30-49mL/min: 100mg Day 1, then 50mg qd. CrCl: 15-29mL/min: 100mg Day 1, then 25mg qd. CrCl 5-14mL/min: 35mg Day 1, then 15mg qd. CrCl <5mL/min: 35mg Day 1, then 10mg qd. *Pediatrics:* 2-17 yrs: 3mg/kg qd. Max: 100mg/day.

HOW SUPPLIED: Sol: 5mg/mL [240mL]; Tab: 100mg

WARNINGS/PRECAUTIONS: Reduce dose in renal dysfunction. Caution in elderly. This formulation is not appropriate in both HBV and HIV infections. Post-treatment exacerbations of hepatitis reported. Pancreatitis reported, especially in HIV-infected pediatrics with prior nucleoside exposure. Monitor patient regularly during treatment. Safety and efficacy of treatment after 1 yr is not known. Suspend therapy if lactic acidosis or pronounced hepatotoxicity develops. Emergence of resistance-associated HBV mutations.

ADVERSE REACTIONS: Pancreatitis, lactic acidosis, severe hepatomegaly, GI complaints, sore throat, infections, elevated LFTs, arthralgia.

INTERACTIONS: TMP/SMX may increase lamivudine levels. Avoid with zalcitabine.

PREGNANCY: Category C, not for use in nursing.

MECHANISM OF ACTION: Nucleoside analogue; phosphorylated to active 5'-triphosphate metabolite intracellularly; incorporation of monophosphate form into viral DNA by HBV reverse transcriptase results in DNA termination.

PHARMACOKINETICS: Absorption: Rapid; C_{max}=1.28mcg/mL (HBV), C_{max}=1.05mcg/mL (healthy); T_{max}=0.5-2.0 hrs; AUC=4.3mcg•h/mL (HBV), AUC=4.7mcg•h/mL (healthy). Tab: Absolute bioavailability (86%). Sol: Absolute bioavailability (87%). **Distribution:** Plasma protein binding (<36%); V_d=1.3L/kg. **Metabolism:** Hepatic (minor); trans-sulfoxide (metabolite). **Elimination:** Urine (unchanged); $T_{1/2}$=5-7 hrs.

EPOGEN

RX

epoetin alfa (Amgen)

> Increased mortality, serious cardiovascular/thromboembolic events, and tumor progession. (Renal Failure) Patients experienced greater risks for death and serious cardiovascular events when administered erythropoiesis-stimulating agents (ESAs) to target higher vs lower Hgb levels (13.5 vs 11.3 g/dL; 14 vs 10 g/dL) in 2 clinical studies. Individualize dosing to achieve and maintain Hgb levels within range of 10-12g/dL. (Cancer) ESAs shortened overall survival and/or time-to-tumor progression in clinical studies in patients with breast, head and neck, lymphoid, and non-small cell lung, and cervical cancers when dosed to target Hgb ≥12g/dL. The risks of shortened survival and tumor progression have not been excluded when ESAs are dosed to target Hgb <12g/dL. To minimize these risks, as well as the risk of serious cario- and thrombovascular events, use lowest dose needed to avoid RBC transfusions. Use only for treatment of anemia due to concomitant myelosuppressive chemotherapy. D/C following completion of a chemotherapy course. (Perisurgery) Epoetin alfa increased the rate of DVT in patients not receiving prophylactic anticoagulation. Consider DVT prophylaxis.

THERAPEUTIC CLASS: Erythropoiesis stimulator

INDICATIONS: Treatment of anemia of chronic renal failure (CRF), anemia related to zidovudine in HIV (serum erythropoietin ≤500 mU/mL and zidovudine ≤4200mg/week), chemotherapy-induced anemia in patients with non-myeloid malignancies, and reduction of allogeneic blood transfusions in anemic (≤13 to >10 g/dL) patients scheduled for elective, noncardiac, nonvascular surgery.

DOSAGE: *Adults:* CRF: Initial: 50-100 U/kg IV/SQ 3x/week. IV is preferred route in dialysis patients. Maint: Individually titrate. Reduce dose by 25% when Hgb approaches 12g/dL or increases >1g/dL in any 2 week period. Increase dose by 25% if Hgb is <10g/dL and has not increased by 1g/dL after 4 weeks of therapy. Zidovudine-Treated HIV Patients: If serum erythropoietin ≤500 mU/mL and zidovudine ≤4200mg/week give100 U/kg IV/SQ 3x/week for 8 weeks. Titrate: Increase by 50-100 U/kg 3x/week after 8 weeks if necessary. Max: 300 U/kg 3x/week Maint: if Hgb >13g/dL, d/c until Hgb <12g/dL, then reduce dose by 25% when resume therapy. Chemotherapy-Induced Anemia: Initial: 150 U/kg SQ 3x/week. Titrate: Reduce by 25% when Hgb approaches 12g/dL or Hgb increases >1g/dL in any 2-week period. If Hgb >13g/dL, withhold until Hgb <12g/dL then restart at 25% below previous dose. May increase to 300 U/kg 3x/week if no response after 8 weeks of therapy. Max: 300 U/kg 3x/week. Weekly Dosing: 40,000 U SQ weekly. Titrate: If Hgb not increased by ≥1g/dL after 4 weeks, increase to 60,000 U weekly. If Hgb >13g/dL, withhold until Hgb <12g/dL then restart with 25% dose reduction. Reduce dose by 25% if very rapid Hgb response (eg, increase >1g/dL in any 2-week period. Max: 60,000 U weekly. Surgery: 300 U/kg/day SQ for 10 days before, on day of, and 4 days after surgery; or 600 U/kg SQ once weekly on 21, 14, and 7 days before surgery, and a 4th dose on day of surgery.
Pediatrics: CRF: Initial: 50 U/kg 3x/week IV/SQ. Maint: Individually titrate. Reduce dose by 25% when Hgb approaches 12g/dL or increases >1g/dL in any 2 week period. Increase dose by 25% if Hgb is <10g/dL and has not increased by 1g/dL after 4 weeks of therapy. Chemotherapy Induced Anemia: Initial: 600 U/kg IV weekly. Titrate: If Hgb not increased by ≥1g/dL after 4 weeks, increase to 900 U/kg IV weekly. If Hgb >13g/dL, withhold until Hgb <12g/dL then restart with 25% dose reduction. Reduce dose by 25% if very rapid Hgb response (eg, increase >1g/dL in any 2-week period. Max: 60,000 U weekly.

HOW SUPPLIED: Inj: 2000 U/mL, 3000 U/mL, 4000 U/mL, 10,000 U/mL, 20,000 U/mL, 40,000 U/mL

CONTRAINDICATIONS: Uncontrolled HTN. Hypersensitivity to mammalian cell-derived products and Albumin (human).

WARNINGS/PRECAUTIONS: Pure red cell aplasia and severe anemia (with or without other cytopenias) may occur. Caution with porphyria, HTN or a history of seizures. Evaluate iron stores prior to and during therapy. Most patients need iron supplementation. Monitor Hct, BP, iron levels, serum chemistry, and CBC. Menses may resume. Multidose formulation contains benzyl alcohol. Increased mortality, cardiovascular, and thromboembolic events in patients with CRF reported. ESAs shortened the time to tumor progression in patients with advanced head and neck cancer receiving radiation therapy. Dose should be carefully adjusted in patients with CRF or CHF.

ADVERSE REACTIONS: HTN, headache, fatigue, arthralgias, nausea, vomiting, diarrhea, edema, rash, pyrexia, clotted vascular access, respiratory congestion, dyspnea, asthenia, dizziness, seizures, thrombotic events.

INTERACTIONS: Adjust anticoagulant dose in dialysis patients.

PREGNANCY: Category C, caution in nursing.

MECHANISM OF ACTION: Erythropoiesis stimulator.

PHARMACOKINETICS: Absorption: (SC) T_{max}=5-24 hrs. **Elimination:** (IV) $T_{1/2}$=4-13 hrs.

EPZICOM   RX
abacavir sulfate - lamivudine (GlaxoSmithKline)

> Fatal hypersensitivity reactions reported with abacavir sulfate; discontinue if hypersensitivity reaction suspected and do not restart. Lactic acidosis and severe hepatomegaly with steatosis, including fatal cases, have been reported with nucleoside analogs alone or in combination with other antivirals. Severe acute exacerbations of hepatitis B reported in patients co-infected with HBV and HIV and who have discontinued lamivudine.

THERAPEUTIC CLASS: Nucleoside analog combination

INDICATIONS: Treatment of HIV infection in combination with other antiretrovirals.

DOSAGE: *Adults:* ≥18 yrs: CrCl >50mL/min: 1 tab qd.

HOW SUPPLIED: Tab: (Abacavir Sulfate-Lamivudine) 600mg-300mg

CONTRAINDICATIONS: Hepatic impairment.

WARNINGS/PRECAUTIONS: Serious hypersensitivity reactions reported. Register abacavir hypersensitive patients at 1-800-270-0425. Suspend therapy if lactic acidosis or pronounced hepatotoxicity develops. Avoid with CrCl <50mL/min. Redistribution/accumulation of body fat reported. Hepatic decompensation has occurred in HIV/HCV co-infected patients receiving combination antiretroviral therapy for HIV and interferon alfa with or without ribavir. Immune reconstitution syndrome has been reported.

ADVERSE REACTIONS: Hypersensitivity, insomnia, depression, headache, fatigue, dizziness, nausea, diarrhea, rash, pyrexia, abdominal pain, abnormal dreams, anxiety.

INTERACTIONS: May increase methadone clearance. Decreased elimination with ethanol. TMP/SMX and/or nelfinavir may increase lamivudine exposure. Avoid with zalcitabine.

PREGNANCY: Category C, not for use in nursing.

MECHANISM OF ACTION: Abacavir: Carbocyclic nucleoside analogue. Inhibits HIV-1 reverse transcriptase (RT) by competing with natural substrate dGTP and incorporating into viral DNA. Lamivudine: Nucleoside analogue. Inhibits RT via DNA chain termination.

PHARMACOKINETICS: Absorption: Abacavir: Rapid, C_{max}=4.26mcg/mL, AUC=11.95mcg•hr/mL, bioavailability (86%); Lamivudine: Rapid, C_{max}=2.04mcg/mL, AUC=8.87mcg•hr/mL, bioavailability (86%). **Distribution:** Abacavir: V_d=0.86L/kg, plasma protein binding (50%); Lamivudine: V_d=1.3L/kg, plasma protein binding (70%). **Metabolism:** Abacavir: Via alcohol dehydrogenase. Lamivudine: Metabolite (trans-sulfoxide). **Elimination:** Abacavir: $T_{1/2}$=1.45 hrs. Lamivudine: (IV) $T_{1/2}$=5-7 hrs. Urine (70%).

EQUAGESIC   CIV
meprobamate - aspirin (Wyeth/Women First)

THERAPEUTIC CLASS: Carbamate derivative/salicylate

INDICATIONS: Adjunct in short-term treatment of pain accompanied by tension and/or anxiety in patients with musculoskeletal disease.

DOSAGE: *Adults:* 1-2 tabs tid-qid prn. Elderly/Debilitated: Use lowest effective dose.
Pediatrics: ≥12 yrs: 1-2 tabs tid-qid prn.

HOW SUPPLIED: Tab: (Meprobamate-ASA) 200mg-325mg* *scored

CONTRAINDICATIONS: Acute intermittent porphyria.

WARNINGS/PRECAUTIONS: Extreme caution with peptic ulcer, asthma, coagulation abnormalities, hypoprothrombinemia, or vitamin K deficiency. Abuse, physical and psychological dependence reported. Abrupt withdrawal after prolonged and excessive use may precipitate recurrence of pre-existing symptoms. May impair mental and physical abilities. Caution with hepatic or kidney dysfunction. May precipitate seizures in epileptic patients. Prescribe cautiously and in small amounts to suicidal patients.

ADVERSE REACTIONS: Epigastric discomfort, nausea, vomiting, drowsiness, ataxia, dizziness, slurred speech, headache, vertigo, weakness.

INTERACTIONS: Additive CNS suppression with alcohol or other psychotropic drugs. May antagonize uricosuric activity of probenecid and sulfinpyrazone. Extreme caution with anticoagulants. May enhance hypoglycemic effects of sulfonylureas.

PREGNANCY: Safety in pregnancy or nursing not known.

MECHANISM OF ACTION: Meprobamate: Carbamate derivative; affects multiple sites in CNS. ASA: Salicylate (non-narcotic analgesic); antipyretic and anti-inflammatory effects.

EQUETRO   RX
carbamazepine (Validus)

> Serious and fatal dermatologic reactions, including toxic epidermal necrolysis (TEN), Stevens-Johnsons syndrome (SJS), and presence of HLA-B*1502 allele reported. Aplastic anemia and agranulocytosis reported. Obtain complete pretreatment hematological testing as baseline. D/C if evidence of bone marrow depression develops.

THERAPEUTIC CLASS: Carboxamide

INDICATIONS: Treatment of acute manic and mixed episodes associated with bipolar I disorder.

DOSAGE: *Adults:* Initial: 400mg/day, given in divided doses, bid. Titrate: 200mg qd. Max: 1600mg/day. Do not crush or chew.

HOW SUPPLIED: Cap, Extended-Release: 100mg, 200mg, 300mg

CONTRAINDICATIONS: Avoid in patients with a history of previous bone marrow depression, hypersensitivity to the drug, or known sensitivity to any of the tricyclic compounds. Use of MAOIs is not recommended and MAOIs should be discontinued for a minimum of 14 days prior to use.

WARNINGS/PRECAUTIONS: Monitor blood levels. Avoid use with any other medication containing carbamazepine. May cause fetal harm during pregnancy. Severe dermatologic reactions, including toxic epidermal necrolysis (Lyell's syndrome), Stevens-Johnson syndrome, and presence of HLA-B*1502 allele reported with carbamazepine. Avoid abrupt discontinuation with seizure disorder. Carbamazepine has mild anticholinergic activity; observe closely with increased IOP. Caution in patients with a history of cardiac, hepatic, or renal damage; adverse hematologic reaction to other drugs may be at risk of bone marrow depression; or interrupted courses of therapy with carbamazepine. Closely monitor patients at high-risk for suicide attempts. May cause activate latent psychosis. May cause confusion/agitation in elderly. Perform eye exam and monitor LFTs and renal function at baseline and periodically.

ADVERSE REACTIONS: Dizziness, somnolence, nausea, vomiting, ataxia, headache, infection, pain, rash, diarrhea, dyspepsia, asthenia, amnesia, toxic epidermal necrolysis, Stevens-Johnson syndrome.

INTERACTIONS: See Contraindications. CYP3A4 inhibitors may increase plasma levels. CYP3A4 inducers may decrease plasma levels. May induce CYP1A2 and CYP3A4; may interact with any agent metabolized by these enzymes. May increase plasma levels of clomipramine, phenytoin, and primidone. May increase risk of neurotoxic side effects of lithium. Decreases levels of trazodone with concomitant administration. Anti-malarial drugs may antagonize the activity of carbamazepine. Caution with other centrally acting drugs and/or alcohol. Co-administration with delavirdine may lead to loss of virologic response and possible resistance to non-nucleoside reverse transcriptase inhibitors.

PREGNANCY: Category D, not for use in nursing.

MECHANISM OF ACTION: Not established. Suspected to modulate sodium and calcium ion channels, receptor-mediated neurotransmitters and intracel-lular signaling pathways.

PHARMACOKINETICS: Absorption: C_{max}=1.9mcg/mL (single dose), 11.0mcg/mL (multiple doses); T_{max}=19 hrs (single dose), 5.9 hrs (multiple doses). **Distribution:** Plasma protein binding (76%); found in breast milk. **Metabolism:** Liver, via CYP3A4; carbamazepine-10,11-epoxide (metabolite). **Elimination:** Urine 72% (3% unchanged), feces (28%); $T_{1/2}$=35-40 hrs (single dose), 12-17 hrs (multiple doses).

ERAXIS
anidulafungin (Pfizer)

RX

THERAPEUTIC CLASS: Echinocandin

INDICATIONS: Treatment of candidemia and other forms of *Candida* infec-tions (intra-abdominal abscess and peritonitis); esophageal candidiasis.

DOSAGE: *Adults:* Candidemia/*Candida* Infections: LD: 200mg on Day 1. Follow with 100mg qd thereafter. Continue therapy for at least 14 days after last positive culture. Esophageal Candidiasis: LD: 100mg on Day 1. Follow with 50mg qd thereafter. Treat for minimum of 14 days and for at least 7 days after symptoms resolve.

HOW SUPPLIED: Inj: 50mg, 100mg

WARNINGS/PRECAUTIONS: Hepatic abnormalities may occur; monitor he-patic function if abnormal LFTs develop during therapy.

ADVERSE REACTIONS: Diarrhea, nausea, rash, hypokalemia, headache, increased LFTs, neutropenia.

INTERACTIONS: Slightly increased levels with cyclosporine.

PREGNANCY: Category C, caution in nursing.

MECHANISM OF ACTION: Antifungal; inhibits synthesis of 1, 3-β-D-glucan, an essential component of fungal cell walls.

PHARMACOKINETICS: Absorption: IV infusion of variable doses resulted in different parameters. **Distribution:** V_d=30-50L; Plasma protein binding (>99%). **Elimination:** Urine, feces; $T_{1/2}$=40-50 hrs.

ERBITUX
cetuximab (Bristol-Myers Squibb)

RX

Severe infusion reactions have occurred; immediately interrupt and permanently d/c infusion if these reactions occur. Cardiopulmonary arrest and/or sudden death have occurred with squamous cell carcinoma of the head and neck treated with radiation therapy and cetuximab; closely monitor serum electrolytes during and after therapy.

THERAPEUTIC CLASS: Epidermal growth factor receptor (EGFR) antagonist

INDICATIONS: In combination with irinotecan for the treatment of epidermal growth factor receptor (EGFR)-expressing, metastatic colorectal carcinoma in patients who are refractory to irinotecan-based chemotherapy. As monother-apy, for the treatment of EGFR-expressing, metastatic colorectal carcinoma in patients after failure of both irinotecan- and oxaliplatin-based regimens. In combination with radiation therapy for the treatment of locally or regionally advanced squamous cell carcinoma of the head and neck. As monotherapy, for the treatment of patients with recurrent or metastatic squamous cell carcinoma of the head and neck for whom prior platinum-based therapy has failed.

DOSAGE: *Adults:* Premedication with H_1 antagonist (eg, diphenhydramine 50mg) IV 30-60 min prior to 1st dose is recommended. Colorectal Cancer: LD: 400mg/m² IV infusion over 120 min. Maint: 250mg/m² IV infusion over 60 min once weekly. Max Infusion Rate: 10mg/min. Squamous Cell Carcinoma of Head and Neck: Combination Therapy: Initial: 400mg/m² IV over 120 min 1 week prior to initiation of a course of radiation treatment. Maint: 250mg/m² over 60 min weekly for duration of radiation therapy. Max Infusion Rate: 10mg/min. Recurrent/Metastatic Squamous Cell Carcinoma of Head and Neck: Monotherapy: Initial: 400mg/m². Maint: 250mg/m² until disease progression or unacceptable toxicity. Mild-Moderate (Grade 1 or 2) Infusion Reactions: Reduce rate by 50%. Severe (Grade 3 or 4) Infusion Reactions: D/C. Development of Severe Acneform Rash: Delay infusion 1-2 weeks for 1st three occurrences. 1st Occurrence: If improvement, continue at 250mg/m². 2nd Occurrence: If improvement, reduce dose to 200mg/m². 3rd Occurrence: If improvement, reduce dose to 150mg/m². 4th Occurrence/No Improvement After Delaying Therapy: D/C therapy.

HOW SUPPLIED: Inj: 2mg/mL

WARNINGS/PRECAUTIONS: Infusion reactions reported; observe closely for 1 hr following infusion. Permanently d/c therapy if serious infusion reactions develop. Dermatologic (eg, acneform rash, skin drying/fissuring, paronychial inflammation, and infectious sequelae) or pulmonary toxicities may occur. D/C if interstitial lung disease confirmed. Adjust dose in cases of severe acneform rash. Apply sunscreen and limit sun exposure. Caution with hypersensitivity to murine proteins. Potential for immunogenicity. Caution with radiation therapy and cisplatin therapy. Monitor for hypomagnesemia, hypocalcemia, and hypokalemia, during and for at least 8 weeks following completion of therapy.

ADVERSE REACTIONS: Acneform rash, mucositis, asthenia/malaise, diarrhea, nausea, abdominal pain, vomiting, fatigue, fever, constipation, infusion reactions, dermatologic toxicities, infection, headache, anorexia, dyspnea, insomnia.

PREGNANCY: Category C, not for use in nursing.

MECHANISM OF ACTION: Epidermal growth factor receptor antagonist; binds specifically to EGFR on normal and tumor cells, and inhibits binding of epidermal growth factor and other ligands, such as transforming growth factor-alpha.

PHARMACOKINETICS: Absorption: C_{max}=168-235µg/mL. **Distribution:** V_d=2-3L/m². **Elimination:** $T_{1/2}$=112 hrs.

ERGOLOID MESYLATES   RX
ergoloid mesylates (Various)

THERAPEUTIC CLASS: Ergot derivative dopamine agonist

INDICATIONS: Treatment of symptomatic decline in mental capacity of unknown etiology (eg, Alzheimer's dementia, multi-infarct dementia).

DOSAGE: *Adults:* Usual: 1mg tid.

HOW SUPPLIED: Tab: 1mg

CONTRAINDICATIONS: Acute or chronic psychosis.

WARNINGS/PRECAUTIONS: Since symptoms are of unknown etiology, careful diagnosis should be attempted before prescribing.

ADVERSE REACTIONS: Transient nausea, gastric disturbances.

PREGNANCY: Safety in pregnancy and nursing is not known.

MECHANISM OF ACTION: Ergot alkaloid; not established. Suspected to enhance mental capacity.

PHARMACOKINETICS: Absorption: Rapid (via GI tract). C_{max}=0.5ng Eq/mL/mg. T_{max}=1.5-3 hrs. **Metabolism**: Hepatic (1st pass). **Elimination**: $T_{1/2}$= 2.6-5.1 hrs.

ERTACZO   RX
sertaconazole nitrate (Ortho Neutrogena)

E

THERAPEUTIC CLASS: Azole antifungal

INDICATIONS: Treatment of interdigital tinea pedis in immunocompetent patients caused by *Trichophyton rubrum*, *Trichophyton mentagrophytes*, and *Epidermophyton floccosum*.

DOSAGE: *Adults:* Apply bid to affected areas between toes and adjacent areas for 4 weeks. Re-evaluate if no clinical improvement after 2 weeks. *Pediatrics:* ≥12 yrs: Apply bid to affected areas between toes and adjacent areas for 4 weeks. Re-evaluate if no clinical improvement after 2 weeks.

HOW SUPPLIED: Cre: 2% [30g, 60g]

WARNINGS/PRECAUTIONS: Not for ophthalmic, oral, or intravaginal use. D/C if irritation or sensitivity occurs.

ADVERSE REACTIONS: Contact dermatitis, dry skin, burning skin, application site reaction, skin tenderness, hyperpigmentation.

PREGNANCY: Category C, caution in nursing.

MECHANISM OF ACTION: Azole antifungal agent; not established. Believed to act primarily by inhibiting CYP450-dependent synthesis of ergosterol, a key component of fungi cell membranes. Lack of egosterol leads to fungal cell injury through leakage of key constituents in cytoplasm from cell.

ERYC   RX
erythromycin (Warner Chilcott)

THERAPEUTIC CLASS: Macrolide

INDICATIONS: Treatment of mild to moderate upper/lower respiratory tract and skin and soft tissue infections, pertussis, diphtheria, erythrasma, intestinal amebiasis, acute pelvic inflammatory disease (PID) (*N. gonorrhea*), listeriosis, primary syphilis (if PCN allergy), Legionnaires' disease, chlamydial infections (eg, newborn conjunctivitis, pneumonia of infancy, urogenital infections during pregnancy, or urethral, endocervical, or rectal, infections in adults when tetracyclines are contraindicated or not tolerated), and nongonococcal urethritis caused by susceptible strains of microorganisms. Prophylaxis of initial or recurrent attacks of rheumatic fever if PCN allergy.

DOSAGE: *Adults:* Usual: 250mg q6h or 500mg q12h. Max: 4g/day. Do not take bid when dose is >1g/day. Treat strep infections for at least 10 days. Streptococcal Infection Prophylaxis with Rheumatic Heart Disease: 250mg bid. Chlamydial Urogenital Infection During Pregnancy: 500mg qid for at least 7 days or 250mg qid for 14 days. Urethral/Endocervical/Rectal Chlamydial Infections: 500mg qid for at least 7 days. Primary Syphilis: 30-40g in divided doses for 10-15 days. Acute PID: 500mg (erythromycin lactobionate) IV q6h for 3 days, then 250mg PO q6h for 7 days. Intestinal Amebiasis: 250mg qid for 10-14 days. Pertussis: 40-50mg/kg/day in divided doses for 5-14 days. Legionnaires' Disease: 1-4g/day in divided doses. Nongonococcal Urethritis: 500mg PO qid for at least 7 days.
Pediatrics: Usual: 30-50mg/kg/day in divided doses. Severe Infections: 60-100mg/kg/day in divided doses. Treat strep infections for at least 10 days. Streptococcal Infection Prophylaxis with Rheumatic Heart Disease: 250mg bid. Intestinal Amebiasis: 30-50mg/kg/day in divided doses for 10-14 days.

HOW SUPPLIED: Cap, Delayed-Release: 250mg

CONTRAINDICATIONS: Concomitant terfenadine or astemizole.

WARNINGS/PRECAUTIONS: *Clostridium difficile*-associated diarrhea, hepatic dysfunction, and prolonged QT syndrome reported. Caution with impaired hepatic function. May aggravate weakness of patients with myasthenia gravis.

ADVERSE REACTIONS: Nausea, vomiting, abdominal pain, diarrhea, anorexia, abnormal LFTs, allergic reaction, superinfection (prolonged use).

INTERACTIONS: See Contraindications. May increase levels of theophylline, digoxin, drugs metabolized by CYP450 (eg, carbamazepine, cyclosporine, phenytoin, tacrolimus, hexobarbital). May increase effects of oral anticoagulants and triazolam. Risk of acute ergot toxicity with ergotamine or dihydroergotamine.

PREGNANCY: Category B, caution in nursing.

MECHANISM OF ACTION: Macrolide; inhibits protein synthesis by binding 50S ribosomal subunits of susceptible organisms.

PHARMACOKINETICS: Absorption: Readily absorbed. C_{max}=1.13-1.68mcg/mL; T_{max}=3 hrs. **Distribution:** Largely bound to plasma proteins. Crosses blood-brain barrier, placenta, breast milk. Diffuses into most body fluids. **Elimination:** Bile, urine (≤5%).

ERYGEL
erythromycin (Merz)

RX

THERAPEUTIC CLASS: Macrolide

INDICATIONS: Acne vulgaris.

DOSAGE: *Adults:* Apply a thin film qd-bid after skin is cleansed and patted dry. D/C if no improvement occurs after 6-8 weeks or if condition worsens.

HOW SUPPLIED: Gel: 2% [30g, 60g]

WARNINGS/PRECAUTIONS: Avoid contact with eyes and all mucous membranes. D/C if overgrowth of antibiotic-resistant organisms occurs. Pseudomembranous colitis reported.

ADVERSE REACTIONS: Burning, peeling, dryness, itching, erythema, oiliness.

INTERACTIONS: Caution with other topical acne therapy; cumulative irritancy effect may occur with peeling, desquamating or abrasive agents.

PREGNANCY: Category B, caution in nursing.

MECHANISM OF ACTION: Macrolide; inhibits protein synthesis by binding 50 S ribosomal subunits of susceptible organisms.

PHARMACOKINETICS: Distribution: Crosses placental barrier, fetal plasma levels generally low. Following oral/parenteral administration, found in human milk.

ERYPED
erythromycin ethylsuccinate (Abbott)

RX

THERAPEUTIC CLASS: Macrolide

INDICATIONS: Treatment of mild to moderate upper and lower respiratory tract and skin and skin structure infections, listeriosis, pertussis, diphtheria, erythrasma, intestinal amebiasis, acute pelvic inflammatory disease (PID) (*N.gonorrhea*), primary syphilis in PCN allergy, Legionnaires' disease, chlamydial infections (eg, newborn conjunctivitis, urethral, endocervical, or rectal, etc.), and nongonococcal urethritis. Prophylaxis of endocarditis or rheumatic fever.

DOSAGE: *Adults:* Usual: 1600mg/day given q6h, q8h or q12h. Max: 4g/day. Treat strep infections for 10 days. Streptococcal Infection Prophylaxis with Rheumatic Heart Disease: 400mg bid. Urethritis (*C.trachomatis* or *U.urealyticum*): 800mg tid for 7 days. Primary Syphilis: 48-64g in divided doses over 10-15 days. Intestinal Amebiasis: 400mg qid for 10-14 days. Pertussis: 40-50mg/kg/day in divided doses for 5-14 days. Legionnaires' Disease: 1.6-4g/day in divided doses.

Pediatrics: Usual: 30-50mg/kg/day in divided doses q6h, q8h or q12h. Double dose for more severe infections. Treat strep infections for 10 days. Intestinal Amebiasis: 30-50mg/kg/day in divided doses for 10-14 days. Pertussis: 40-50mg/kg/day in divided doses for 5-14 days.

HOW SUPPLIED: Sus: 100mg/2.5mL [50mL], 200mg/5mL, 400mg/5mL [5mL, 100mL, 200mL]; Tab, Chewable: 200mg* *scored

CONTRAINDICATIONS: Concomitant terfenadine, astemizole, cisapride, pimozide.

WARNINGS/PRECAUTIONS: *Clostridium difficile*-associated diarrhea, hepatic dysfunction, infantile hypertrophic pyloric stenosis reported. May aggravate myasthenia gravis.

ADVERSE REACTIONS: Nausea, vomiting, abdominal pain, diarrhea, anorexia, hepatic dysfunction, abnormal LFTs, allergic reactions, superinfection (prolonged use).

INTERACTIONS: Rhabdomyolysis reported with lovastatin. May increase levels of theophylline, digoxin, drugs metabolized by CYP450 (eg, carbamazepine, cyclosporine, tacrolimus, phenytoin, alfentanil, disopyramide, lovastatin, bromocriptine, valproate, etc). Increases effects of oral anticoagulants, triazolam, midazolam. Risk of acute ergot toxicity with ergotamine or dihydroergotamine. May potentiate sildenafil. Avoid terfenadine, astemizole, cisapride, pimozide.

PREGNANCY: Category B, caution in nursing.

MECHANISM OF ACTION: Macrolide; inhibits protein synthesis by binding 50S ribosomal subunits of susceptible organisms.

PHARMACOKINETICS: Absorption: Readily and reliably absorbed (both fasting and nonfasting conditions). **Distribution:** Diffuses into most body fluids, crosses placenta and excreted in breast milk. **Elimination:** Bile, feces, urine (<5%, active form).

ERY-TAB   RX
erythromycin (Abbott)

THERAPEUTIC CLASS: Macrolide

INDICATIONS: Treatment of mild to moderate upper/lower respiratory tract and skin and skin structure infections, listeriosis, pertussis, diphtheria, erythrasma, intestinal amebiasis, acute pelvic inflammatory disease (PID) (*N.gonorrhea*), primary syphilis (if PCN allergy), Legionnaires' disease, chlamydial infections (eg, newborn conjunctivitis, pneumonia of infancy, urogenital infections during pregnancy, or urethral, endocervical, or rectal infections when tetracyclines are contraindicated or not tolerated), and nongonococcal urethritis caused by susceptible strains of microorganisms. Prophylaxis of initial and recurrent attacks of rheumatic fever if PCN allergy.

DOSAGE: *Adults:* Usual: 250mg qid, 333mg q8h or 500mg q12h. Max: 4g/day. Do not take bid when dose is >1g/day. Treat strep infections for at least 10 days. Streptococcal Infection Long-Term Prophylaxis with Rheumatic Fever: 250mg bid. Chlamydial Urogenital Infection During Pregnancy: 500mg qid or 666mg q8h for at least 7 days, or 500mg q12h, 333mg q8h or 250mg qid for at least 14 days. Urethral/Endocervical/Rectal Chlamydial Infections and Nongonococcal Urethritis: 500mg qid or 666mg q8h for at least 7 days. Primary Syphilis: 30-40g in divided doses for 10-15 days. Acute PID: 500mg (erythromycin lactobionate) IV q6h for 3 days, then 500mg PO q12h or 333mg q8h for 7 days. Intestinal Amebiasis: 500mg q12h, 333mg q8h or 250mg q6h for 10-14 days. Pertussis: 40-50mg/kg/day in divided doses for 5-14 days. Legionnaires' Disease: 1-4g/day in divided doses.
Pediatrics: Usual: 30-50mg/kg/day in divided doses. Severe Infections: May double dose. Max: 4g/day. Treat strep infections for at least 10 days. Streptococcal Infection Long-Term Prophylaxis with Rheumatic Fever: 250mg bid. Chlamydial Conjunctivitis of Newborns/Chlamydial Pneumonia in Infancy: 12.5mg/kg qid for 2 weeks and 3 weeks, respectively. Intestinal Amebiasis: 30-50mg/kg/day in divided doses for 10-14 days.

HOW SUPPLIED: Tab, Delayed-Release: 250mg, 333mg, 500mg

CONTRAINDICATIONS: Concomitant terfenadine, astemizole, pimozide, or cisapride.

WARNINGS/PRECAUTIONS: Pseudomembranous colitis, hepatic dysfunction reported. Caution with impaired hepatic function. May aggravate weakness of patients with myasthenia gravis. Erythromycin does not reach adequate concentrations in fetus to prevent congenital syphilis.

ADVERSE REACTIONS: Nausea, vomiting, abdominal pain, diarrhea, anorexia, abnormal LFTs, allergic reactions, superinfection (prolonged use).

INTERACTIONS: See Contraindications. Rhabdomyolysis reported with lovastatin. May increase levels of theophylline, digoxin, drugs metabolized by CYP450 (eg, carbamazepine, cyclosporine, phenytoin, alfentanil, disopyramide, lovastatin, bromocriptine, valproate, etc). Increases effects of oral anticoagulants, triazolam, midazolam. Risk of acute ergot toxicity with ergotamine or dihydroergotamine. May increase AUC of sildenafil; consider dose reduction of sildenafil.

PREGNANCY: Category B, caution in nursing.

MECHANISM OF ACTION: Macrolide; inhibits protein synthesis by binding 50S ribosomal subunits of susceptible organisms.

PHARMACOKINETICS: Absorption: (PO) readily absorbed. **Distribution:** Largely bound to plasma proteins. Crosses blood-brain barrier, placenta, and breast milk. Diffuses into most bodily fluids. **Elimination:** Biliary and urinary excretion (<5%).

ERYTHROCIN RX
erythromycin stearate (Abbott)

THERAPEUTIC CLASS: Macrolide

INDICATIONS: Treatment of mild to moderate upper/lower respiratory tract, and skin and skin structure infections, listeriosis, pertussis, diphtheria, erythrasma, intestinal amebiasis, acute pelvic inflammatory disease (PID) (*N.gonorrhea*), primary syphilis (if PCN allergy), Legionnaires' disease, chlamydial infections (eg, newborn conjunctivitis, pneumonia of infancy, urogenital infections during pregnancy or urethral, endocervical, or rectal infections when tetracyclines are contraindicated or not tolerated), and nongonococcal urethritis caused by susceptible strains of microorganisms. Prophylaxis of initial and recurrent attacks of rheumatic fever if PCN allergy.

DOSAGE: *Adults:* Usual: 250mg q6h or 500mg q12h without food. Max: 4g/day. Treat strep infections for at least 10 days. Streptococcal Infection Long-Term Prophylaxis in Rheumatic Fever: 250mg bid. Chlamydial Urogenital Infection During Pregnancy: 500mg qid or 666mg q8h for at least 7 days or 500mg q12h, 333mg q8h, or 250mg qid for at least 14 days. Urethral/Endocervical/Rectal Chlamydial Infections and Nongonococcal Urethritis: 500mg qid or 666mg q8h for at least 7 days. Primary Syphilis: 30-40g in divided doses over 10-15 days. Acute PID: 500mg (erythromycin lactobionate) IV q6h for 3 days, then 500mg PO q12h or 333mg PO q8h for 7 days. Intestinal Amebiasis: 500mg q12h, 333mg q8h, or 250mg q6h for 10-14 days. Pertussis: 40-50mg/kg/day in divided doses for 5-14 days. Legionnaires' Disease: 1-4g/day in divided doses.
Pediatrics: Usual: 30-50mg/kg/day in divided doses without food. Severe Infections: May double dose. Max: 4g/day. Treat strep infections for at least 10 days. Chlamydial Conjunctivitis of Newborns/Chlamydial Pneumonia in Infancy: (Sus) 12.5mg/kg qid for 2 weeks and 3 weeks, respectively. Intestinal Amebiasis: 30-50mg/kg/day in divided doses for 10-14 days.

HOW SUPPLIED: Tab: 250mg, 500mg

CONTRAINDICATIONS: Concomitant terfenadine, astenizole, pimozide, or cisapride.

WARNINGS/PRECAUTIONS: Hepatic dysfunction, pseudomembranous colitis reported. Caution with impaired hepatic function.

ADVERSE REACTIONS: Nausea, vomiting, abdominal pain, diarrhea, anorexia, abnormal LFTs, superinfection (prolonged use).

INTERACTIONS: See Contraindications. Rhabdomyolysis reported with lovastatin. May increase levels of theophylline, digoxin, drugs metabolized by CYP450 (eg, carbamazepine, cyclosporine, phenytoin, etc). Increases effects of oral anticoagulants, triazolam. Risk of acute ergot toxicity with ergotamine or dihydroergotamine. May increase AUC of sildenafil; consider dose reduction of sildenafil.

PREGNANCY: Category B, caution in nursing.

MECHANISM OF ACTION: Macrolide; inhibits protein synthesis by binding 50S ribosomal subunits of susceptible organisms.

PHARMACOKINETICS: Absorption: (PO) Readily absorbed. **Distribution:** Largely bound to plasma proteins; crosses placenta, blood-brain barrier, and is excreted in breast milk. **Metabolism:** Liver via CYP3A. **Elimination:** Bile and urine (<5% unchanged).

ERYTHROMYCIN RX
erythromycin (Various)

THERAPEUTIC CLASS: Macrolide

INDICATIONS: Topical treatment of acne vulgaris.

DOSAGE: *Adults:* (Gel) Clean and dry area. Apply qd-bid. Do not rub in. D/C if no improvement after 6-8 weeks. (Sol) Clean and dry area. Apply bid.

HOW SUPPLIED: Gel: 2% [30g]; Sol: 2% [60mL]

WARNINGS/PRECAUTIONS: Avoid eyes, nose, mouth, and other mucous membranes. D/C if overgrowth of antibiotic-resistant organisms occurs.

ADVERSE REACTIONS: Peeling, dryness, pruritus, erythema, oiliness, eye irritation, burning, desquamation.

INTERACTIONS: Caution with concomitant topical acne therapy, possible cumulative irritant effect.

PREGNANCY: (Gel) Category B, not for use in nursing; (Sol) Category C, caution in nursing.

MECHANISM OF ACTION: Macrolide; exact mechanism by which it reduces lesions in acne vulgaris not established. Inhibits protein synthesis by binding 50 *S* ribosomal subunits of susceptible organisms.

ERYTHROMYCIN BASE RX
erythromycin (Various)

THERAPEUTIC CLASS: Macrolide

INDICATIONS: Treatment of mild to moderate upper/lower respiratory tract and skin and skin structure infections, listeriosis, pertussis, diphtheria, erythrasma, intestinal amebiasis, acute pelvic inflammatory disease (PID) (*N.gonorrhea*), primary syphilis (if PCN allergy), Legionnaires' disease, chlamydial infections (eg, newborn conjunctivitis, pneumonia of infancy, urogenital infections during pregnancy or urethral, endocervical, or rectal infections when tetracyclines are contraindicated or not tolerated), and nongonococcal urethritis caused by susceptible strains of microorganisms. Prophylaxis of initial and recurrent attacks of rheumatic fever if PCN allergy.

DOSAGE: *Adults:* Usual: 250mg qid or 500mg q12h without food. Max: 4g/day. Treat strep infections for at least 10 days. Streptococcal Infection Long-Term Prophylaxis of Rheumatic Fever: 250mg bid. Chlamydial Urogenital Infection During Pregnancy: 500mg qid for at least 7 days or 500mg q12h or 250mg qid for at least 14 days. Urethral/Endocervical/Rectal Chlamydial Infections and Nongonococcal Urethritis: 500mg qid for at least 7 days. Primary Syphilis: 30-40g in divided doses over 10-15 days. Acute PID: 500mg (erythromycin lactobionate) IV q6h for 3 days, then 500mg PO q12h for 7 days. Intestinal Amebiasis: 500mg q12h or 250mg q6h for 10-14 days.

Pertussis: 40-50mg/kg/day in divided doses for 5-14 days. Legionnaires' Disease: 1-4g/day in divided doses.
Pediatrics: Usual: 30-50mg/kg/day in divided doses without food. Severe Infections: May double dose. Max: 4g/day. Treat strep infections for at least 10 days. Streptococcal Infection Long-Term Prophylaxis of Rheumatic Fever: 250mg bid. Chlamydial Conjunctivitis of Newborns/Chlamydial Pneumonia in Infancy: (Sus) 12.5mg/kg qid for 2 weeks and 3 weeks, respectively. Intestinal Amebiasis: 30-50mg/kg/day in divided doses for 10-14 days.

HOW SUPPLIED: Tab: 250mg, 500mg

CONTRAINDICATIONS: Concomitant terfenadine, astemizole, pimozide, or cisapride.

WARNINGS/PRECAUTIONS: Pseudomembranous colitis, hepatic dysfunction reported. Caution with impaired hepatic function. May aggravate weakness of patients with myasthenia gravis.

ADVERSE REACTIONS: Nausea, vomiting, abdominal pain, diarrhea, anorexia, abnormal LFTs, allergic reactions, superinfection (prolonged use).

INTERACTIONS: See Contraindications. Rhabdomyolysis reported with lovastatin. May increase levels of theophylline, digoxin, drugs metabolized by CYP450 (eg, carbamazepine, cyclosporine, phenytoin, etc). Increases effects of oral anticoagulants, triazolam. Risk of acute ergot toxicity with ergotamine or dihydroergotamine. May increase AUC of sildenafil; consider dose reduction of sildenafil.

PREGNANCY: Category B, caution in nursing.

MECHANISM OF ACTION: Macrolide; inhibits protein synthesis by binding 50S ribosomal subunits of susceptible organisms.

PHARMACOKINETICS: Absorption: (PO) readily absorbed. **Distribution:** Largely bound to plasma proteins. Crosses blood-brain barrier, placenta, breast milk. Diffuses into most body fluids. **Elimination:** Bile, urine (<5% unchanged).

ERYTHROMYCIN DELAYED-RELEASE   RX
erythromycin (Various)

THERAPEUTIC CLASS: Macrolide

INDICATIONS: Treatment of mild to moderate upper/lower respiratory tract and skin and skin structure infections, listeriosis, pertussis, diphtheria, erythrasma, intestinal amebiasis, acute pelvic inflammatory disease (PID) (*N.gonorrhea*), primary syphilis (if PCN allergy), Legionnaires' disease, chlamydial infections (eg, newborn conjunctivitis, pneumonia of infancy, urogenital infections during pregnancy, or urethral, endocervical, or rectal infections when tetracyclines are contraindicated or not tolerated), and nongonococcal urethritis caused by susceptible strains of microorganisms. Prophylaxis of initial and recurrent attacks of rheumatic fever if PCN allergy.

DOSAGE: *Adults:* Usual: 250mg q6h or 500mg q12h without food. Max: 4g/day. Treat strep infections for 10 days. Streptococcal Infection Prophylaxis with Rheumatic Heart Disease: 250mg bid. Primary Syphilis: 30-40g in divided doses over 10-15 days. Intestinal Amebiasis: 250mg q6h for 10-14 days. Legionnaires' Disease: 1-4g/day in divided doses. Chlamydial Urogenital Infection During Pregnancy: 500mg qid for 7 days or 250mg qid for 14 days. Urethral/Endocervical/Rectal Chlamydial Infections and Nongonococcal Urethritis: 500mg qid for at least 7 days. Pertussis: 40-50mg/kg/day in divided doses for 5-14 days. Acute PID: 500mg (erythromycin lactobionate) IV q6h for 3 days, then 250mg PO q6h for 7 days.
Pediatrics: Usual: 30-50mg/kg/day in divided doses without food. Severe Infections: May double dose. Max: 4g/day. Treat strep infections for 10 days. Streptococcal Infection Prophylaxis with Rheumatic Heart Disease: 250mg bid. Intestinal Amebiasis: 30-50mg/kg/day in divided doses for 10-14 days.

HOW SUPPLIED: Cap, Delayed-Release: 250mg

CONTRAINDICATIONS: Concomitant terfenadine, astenizole, pimozide, or cisapride.

WARNINGS/PRECAUTIONS: Hepatic dysfunction and pseudomembranous colitis reported. May aggravate weakness of patients with myasthenia gravis.

ADVERSE REACTIONS: Nausea, vomiting, abdominal pain, diarrhea, anorexia, hepatic dysfunction, abnormal LFTs, superinfection (prolonged use).

INTERACTIONS: See Contraindications. Rhabdomyolysis reported with lovastatin. May increase levels of theophylline, digoxin, drugs metabolized by CYP450 (eg, carbamazepine, cyclosporine, phenytoin, etc). Increases effects of oral anticoagulants, triazolam. Risk of acute ergot toxicity with ergotamine or dihydroergotamine. Extreme caution with terfenadine.

PREGNANCY: Category B, caution in nursing.

MECHANISM OF ACTION: Macrolide; inhibits protein synthesis by binding 50S ribosomal subunits of susceptible organisms.

PHARMACOKINETICS: Absorption: (PO) readily absorbed; C_{max}=1.13-1.68mcg/mL; T_{max}=3 hrs. **Distribution:** Largely bound to plasma proteins; diffuses into most bodily fluids; crosses blood-brain barrier, placenta, and breast milk. **Elimination:** Bile, urine (<5% unchanged).

ERYTHROMYCIN OPHTHALMIC RX
erythromycin (Various)

THERAPEUTIC CLASS: Macrolide

INDICATIONS: Superficial ocular infections of the conjunctiva and/or cornea. Prophylaxis of ophthalmia neonatorum due to *N.gonorrhoeae* or *C.trachomatis*.

DOSAGE: *Adults:* Superficial Ocular Infections: Apply 1cm to eye up to 6x/day, depending on severity. Do not flush ointment from eye.
Pediatrics: Superficial Ocular Infections: Apply 1 cm to eye up to 6 times/day, depending on severity. Neonatal Gonococcal or Chlamydial Ophthalmia Prophylaxis: Apply 1 cm into lower conjunctival sac. Do not flush oint from eye.

HOW SUPPLIED: Oint: 5mg/g [1g, 3.5g]

ADVERSE REACTIONS: Minor ocular irritations, redness, hypersensitivity reactions, superinfection (prolonged use).

PREGNANCY: Category B, caution in nursing.

MECHANISM OF ACTION: Macrolide; binds to 50*S* ribosomal subunits of susceptible organisms and inhibits protein synthesis

ERYTHROMYCIN TOPICAL SWABS RX
erythromycin (Various)

THERAPEUTIC CLASS: Macrolide

INDICATIONS: Topical treatment of acne vulgaris.

DOSAGE: *Adults:* Wash and dry area. Rub over area bid.

HOW SUPPLIED: Swab: 2% [60^s]

WARNINGS/PRECAUTIONS: Topical use only. Superinfection may occur. Avoid eyes, nose, mouth, and mucous membranes.

ADVERSE REACTIONS: Peeling, dryness, itching, erythema, oiliness.

INTERACTIONS: Additive irritation with other topical acne agents, especially abrasive or desquamating agents.

PREGNANCY: Category B, caution in nursing.

MECHANISM OF ACTION: Macrolide; inhibits protein synthesis by binding 50 *S* ribosomal subunits of susceptible organisms.

PHARMACOKINETICS: Distribution: Crosses placental barrier, however fetal plasma levels generally low. Following oral/parenteral administration, found in breast milk.

ESCLIM

RX

estradiol (Women First)

> Estrogens increase risk of endometrial cancer in postmenopausal women. Avoid during pregnancy.

THERAPEUTIC CLASS: Estrogen

INDICATIONS: Treatment of moderate to severe vasomotor symptoms associated with menopause and/or vulvar/vaginal atrophy. Treatment of hypoestrogenism due to hypogonadism, castration, or primary ovarian failure.

DOSAGE: *Adults:* Initial: 0.025mg twice weekly (q3-4 days). Titrate: Increase/decrease dose depending upon clinical response. Apply to clean, dry area of skin on buttocks, femoral triangle (upper inner thigh), or upper arm; avoid breasts and waistline. Rotate sites; allow 1 week between same site. Discontinue or taper at 3-6 month intervals. Wait 1 week after withdrawal of oral therapy before initiating therapy. Give continuously without intact uterus and cyclically (3 weeks on, 1 week off) with intact uterus.

HOW SUPPLIED: Patch: 0.025mg/24 hrs, 0.0375mg/24hrs, 0.05mg/24 hrs, 0.075mg/24 hrs, 0.1mg/24 hrs [8^s]

CONTRAINDICATIONS: Pregnancy, undiagnosed abnormal genital bleeding, breast cancer except in appropriately selected patients being treated for metastatic disease, estrogen-dependent neoplasia, thrombophlebitis, thromboembolic disorders.

WARNINGS/PRECAUTIONS: Risk of gallbladder disease, breast and endometrial cancer, elevated BP. Possible risk of cardiovascular disease. Caution with liver dysfunction, asthma, epilepsy, migraine, and cardiac or renal dysfunction. Increase in HDL, triglycerides, thyroid binding globulin. Acceleration of PT, PTT. Impaired glucose tolerance. Consider adding progestin in patient with intact uterus. Risk of fetal congenital reproductive tract disorder, hypercalcemia with breast cancer and bone metastases, hypercoagulability effects. Uterine bleeding and mastodynia reported.

ADVERSE REACTIONS: Breast pain, headache, infection, anxiety, emotional lability, pruritus, abdominal pain, monilia vagina, nausea, sinusitis, asthenia, diarrhea, leukorrhea.

PREGNANCY: Category X, caution in nursing.

MECHANISM OF ACTION: Estrogen; circulating estrogens modulate the pituitary secretion of the gonadotrophins, luteinizing hormone and follicle stimulating hormone, through negative feedback mechanism. In postmenopausal women, acts to reduce elevated levels of these hormones.

PHARMACOKINETICS: Absorption: T_{max}=27 hrs; (0.05mg) C_{max}=62pg/mL; (0.1 mg) C_{max}=124pg/mL. **Distribution:** Mainly bound to sex hormone binding globulin and to a lesser extent albumin. **Metabolism:** Liver to estrone and estriol (major urinary metabolite); sulfate and glucuronide conjugation (liver), gut hydrolysis. **Elimination:** Urine (parent compound and metabolites).

ESGIC

RX

acetaminophen - caffeine - butalbital (Forest)

THERAPEUTIC CLASS: Barbiturate/analgesic

INDICATIONS: Tension or muscle contraction headaches.

DOSAGE: *Adults:* 1-2 caps/tabs q4h prn. Max: 6 caps/tabs/day.
Pediatrics: ≥12 yrs: 1-2 caps/tabs q4h prn. Max: 6 caps/tabs/day.

HOW SUPPLIED: Cap/Tab: (Butalbital-APAP-Caffeine) 50mg-325mg-40mg*
*scored

CONTRAINDICATIONS: Porphyria.

WARNINGS/PRECAUTIONS: May be habit-forming; potential for abuse. Not for long-term use. Caution in elderly, debilitated, severe renal or hepatic impairment, acute abdominal conditions, suicidal tendencies, history of drug abuse.

ADVERSE REACTIONS: Drowsiness, lightheadedness, dizziness, sedation, SOB, NV, abdominal pain, intoxicated feeling.

INTERACTIONS: Enhanced CNS effects with MAOIs. May enhance CNS depressant effects of other narcotic analgesics, alcohol, general anesthetics, tranquilizers, sedative hypnotics, or other CNS depressants.

PREGNANCY: Category C, not for use in nursing.

MECHANISM OF ACTION: Butalbital: Short to intermediate acting barbiturate. Acetaminophen: Nonopiate, nonsalicylate analgesic, antipyretic. Caffeine: CNS stimulant.

PHARMACOKINETICS: Absorption: APAP, caffeine: Rapid. **Distribution:** Butalbital: Plasma protein binding (45%); crosses placenta, found in breast milk. Caffeine: Found in breast milk. **Metabolism:** APAP: Conjugation. Caffeine: Biotransformation. **Elimination:** Butalbital: Urine (3.6%); $T_{1/2}$=35 hrs. APAP: Urine; $T_{1/2}$=1.25-3 hrs. Caffeine: Urine (3%); $T_{1/2}$=3 hrs.

ESGIC-PLUS RX
acetaminophen - caffeine - butalbital (Forest)

THERAPEUTIC CLASS: Barbiturate/analgesic

INDICATIONS: Tension or muscle contraction headaches.

DOSAGE: *Adults:* 1 cap/tab q4h prn. Max: 6 caps/tabs/day. *Pediatrics:* ≥12 yrs: 1 cap/tab q4h prn. Max: 6 caps/tabs/day.

HOW SUPPLIED: Cap/Tab: (Butalbital-APAP-Caffeine) 50mg-500mg-40mg* *scored

CONTRAINDICATIONS: Porphyria.

WARNINGS/PRECAUTIONS: May be habit-forming; potential for abuse. Not for long-term use. Caution in elderly, debilitated, severe renal or hepatic impairment, acute abdominal conditions, suicidal tendencies, history of drug abuse.

ADVERSE REACTIONS: Drowsiness, lightheadedness, dizziness, sedation, SOB, NV, abdominal pain, intoxicated feeling.

INTERACTIONS: Enhanced CNS effects with MAOIs. May enhance CNS depressant effects of other narcotic analgesics, alcohol, general anesthetics, tranquilizers, sedative hypnotics, or other CNS depressants.

PREGNANCY: Category C, not for use in nursing.

MECHANISM OF ACTION: Butalbital: Short to intermediate acting barbiturate. Acetaminophen: Nonopiate, nonsalicylate analgesic, antipyretic. Caffeine: CNS stimulant.

PHARMACOKINETICS: Absorption: APAP, caffeine: Rapid. **Distribution:** Butalbital: Plasma protein binding (45%); crosses placenta; found in breast milk. Caffeine: Found in breast milk. **Metabolism:** APAP: Conjugation. Caffeine: Biotransformation. **Elimination:** Butalbital: Urine (3.6%); $T_{1/2}$=35 hrs. APAP: Urine; $T_{1/2}$=1.25-3 hrs. Caffeine: Urine (3%); $T_{1/2}$=3 hrs.

ESKALITH RX
lithium carbonate (GlaxoSmithKline)

> Lithium toxicity is related to serum levels, and can occur at doses close to therapeutic levels.

OTHER BRAND NAMES: Eskalith CR (GlaxoSmithKline)

THERAPEUTIC CLASS: Antimanic agent

INDICATIONS: Treatment of manic episodes of manic-depressive illness.

DOSAGE: *Adults:* (Cap) 300mg tid-qid. (Tab, Extended-Release) 450mg q12h. Monitor every 1-2 weeks and adjust dose if needed. When stable, monitor every 2 months to achieve levels of 0.6-1.2mEq/L. Maint: 900-1200mg/day.

Acute Mania: 1800mg/day in divided doses. Monitor levels twice weekly to achieve 1-1.5mEq/L. When switching to extended-release tabs, give same total daily dose when possible.
Pediatrics: ≥12 yrs: (Cap) 300mg tid-qid. (Tab, Extended-Release) 450mg q12h. Monitor every 1-2 weeks and adjust dose if needed. When stable, monitor every 2 months to achieve levels of 0.6-1.2 mEq/L. Maint: 900-1200mg/day. Acute Mania: 1800mg/day in divided doses. Monitor levels twice weekly to achieve 1-1.5mEq/L. When switching to extended-release tabs, give same total daily dose when possible.

HOW SUPPLIED: Cap: (Eskalith) 300mg; Tab, Extended-Release: (Eskalith CR) 450mg* *scored

WARNINGS/PRECAUTIONS: Avoid with significant renal or cardiovascular disease, severe debilitation, dehydration, or sodium depletion. Risk of encephalopathic syndrome (eg, weakness, lethargy, fever, tremulousness, confusion, EPS); d/c therapy. Maintain normal diet, adequate salt/fluid intake. Reduce dose or d/c with sweating, diarrhea, infection with elevated temperatures. Caution with hypothyroidism; may need supplemental therapy. Chronic therapy associated with diminution of renal concentrating ability, glomerular and interstitial fibrosis, and nephron atrophy.

ADVERSE REACTIONS: Fine hand tremor, polyuria, mild thirst, nausea, general discomfort, diarrhea, vomiting, drowsiness, muscular weakness.

INTERACTIONS: Increased risk of neurotoxicity with CCBs. Increased risk of toxicity with diuretics, metronidazole. Increased plasma levels with indomethacin, piroxicam, other NSAIDs, COX-2 inhibitors, ACE inhibitors, angiotensin II receptor antagonists. Caution with SSRIs. Decreased levels with acetazolamide, urea, xanthine agents, alkalinizing agents. Interacts with methyldopa, phenytoin, carbamazepine. May prolong effects of neuromuscular blockers.

PREGNANCY: Safety in pregnancy not known, not for use in nursing.

MECHANISM OF ACTION: Not established; suspected to alter sodium transport in nerve and muscle cells and effect a shift toward intraneuronal metabolism of catecholamines.

PHARMACOKINETICS: Distribution: Found in breast milk. **Elimination:** Urine (primary), feces (insignificant); $T_{1/2}$=24 hrs.

ESTAZOLAM
estazolam (Various) **CIV**

THERAPEUTIC CLASS: Benzodiazepine

INDICATIONS: Short-term management of insomnia.

DOSAGE: *Adults:* Initial: 1mg qhs. May increase to 2mg qhs. Small/Debilitated/Elderly: Initial: 0.5mg qhs.

HOW SUPPLIED: Tab: 1mg*, 2mg* *scored

CONTRAINDICATIONS: Pregnancy.

WARNINGS/PRECAUTIONS: Avoid abrupt withdrawal after prolonged use. Caution with depression, elderly/debilitated, renal/hepatic impairment. May cause respiratory depression. May impair mental/physical abilities.

ADVERSE REACTIONS: Somnolence, hypokinesia, dizziness, abnormal coordination, headache, malaise, nervousness, cold symptoms, asthenia.

INTERACTIONS: Potentiated effects with anticonvulsants, antihistamines, alcohol, barbiturates, MAOIs, narcotics, phenothiazines, psychotropic medications, or other CNS depressants. Smoking may increase clearance.

PREGNANCY: Category X, not for use in nursing.

MECHANISM OF ACTION: Trizolobendiazepine derivative.

PHARMACOKINETICS: Absorption: T_{max}=within 2 hrs. **Distribution:** Plasma protein binding (93%), found in breast milk. **Metabolism:** Liver (extensive) via CYP3A through hyroxylation. Metabolites: 1-oxo-estazolam and 4-hydroxyestazolam. **Elimination:** T$_{1/2}$=10-24 hrs. Urine; 87%, <5% (unchanged). Feces: 4%. (Elderly) T$_{1/2}$=18.4hrs.

ESTRACE

RX

estradiol (Warner Chilcott)

> Estrogens increase risk of endometrial cancer in postmenopausal women. Avoid during pregnancy.

THERAPEUTIC CLASS: Estrogen

INDICATIONS: (Cre/Tab) Treatment of vulval and vaginal atrophy. (Tab) Treatment of moderate to severe vasomotor symptoms associated with menopause. Treatment of hypoestrogenism due to hypogonadism, castration, or primary ovarian failure. Palliative treatment of metastatic breast cancer and advanced androgen-dependent prostate carcinoma. Prevention of osteoporosis.

DOSAGE: *Adults:* (Cre) Vulval/Vaginal Atrophy: Initial: 2-4g/day for 1-2 weeks, then decrease to 1-2g/day for 1-2 weeks. Maint: 1g, 1-3x/week. Discontinue or taper at 3-6 month intervals. (Tab) Vasomotor Symptoms/Vulval/Vaginal Atrophy: Initial: 1-2mg/day (3 weeks on, 1 week off). Maint: Minimum effective dose. Discontinue or taper at 3-6 month intervals. Hypoestrogenism: 1-2mg/day. Maint: Minimum effective dose. Metastatic Breast Cancer: 10mg tid for at least 3 months. Prostate Carcinoma: 1-2mg tid. Osteoporosis Prevention: 0.5mg qd cyclically (23 days on and 5 days off).

HOW SUPPLIED: Cre, Vaginal: 0.1mg/g [12g, 42.5g]; Tab: 0.5mg*, 1mg*, 2mg* *scored

CONTRAINDICATIONS: Pregnancy, undiagnosed abnormal genital bleeding, breast cancer unless being treated for metastatic disease, estrogen-dependent neoplasia, thrombophlebitis, or thromboembolic disorders.

WARNINGS/PRECAUTIONS: Risk of gallbladder disease, cardiovascular disease, endometrial and breast carcinoma, fetal congenital reproductive tract disorder, elevated BP, and hypercalcemia with breast cancer and bone metastases. Caution in liver dysfunction, asthma, epilepsy, migraine, and cardiac or renal dysfunction. Increase in HDL, triglycerides, thyroid binding globulin. Acceleration of PT, PTT. Hypercoagulability effects. Impaired glucose tolerance. Consider adding progestin in patient with intact uterus.

ADVERSE REACTIONS: Altered vaginal bleeding, vaginal candidiasis, breast tenderness/enlargement, GI effects, melasma, CNS effects, weight changes, edema, altered libido.

PREGNANCY: Category X, caution in nursing.

MECHANISM OF ACTION: Estrogen; binds to nuclear receptors in estrogen-responsive tissue. Circulating estrogens modulate the pituitary secretion of gonadotropins, luteinizing hormone and follicle stimulating hormone through negative-feedback mechanism. In postmenopausal women, reduces elevated levels of these hormones.

PHARMACOKINETICS: Absorption: (Cre) Absorbed through skin, mucous membranes, and GI tract. **Distribution**: Largely bound to sex hormone-binding globulin and albumin; found in breast milk. **Metabolism**: Liver to estrone (metabolite), estriol (major urinary metabolite); sulfate and glucuronide conjugation (liver); gut hydrolysis; CYP3A4 (partial metabolism). **Elimination**: Urine (parent compound and metabolites).

ESTRADERM
estradiol (Novartis)

> Estrogens increase the risk of endometrial cancer. Estrogens, with or without progestins, should not be used for the prevention of cardiovascular disease or dementia. Increased risks of MI, stroke, invasive breast cancer, PE, and DVT in postmenopausal women (50-79 yrs of age) reported. Increased risk of developing probable dementia in postmenopausal women ≥65 yrs of age reported.

THERAPEUTIC CLASS: Estrogen

INDICATIONS: Treatment of moderate-to-severe vasomotor symptoms and/or vulvar/vaginal atrophy associated with menopause. Treatment of hypoestrogenism due to hypogonadism, castration, or primary ovarian failure. Prevention of postmenopausal osteoporosis.

DOSAGE: *Adults:* Apply to clean, dry area on trunk of body. Do not apply to breast or waistline. Replace twice weekly. Rotate application sites. May give continuously without intact uterus. May give cyclically (3 weeks on, 1 week off) with intact uterus. Vasomotor Symptoms/Vulvar/Vaginal Atrophy: Initial: Apply 0.05mg/day twice weekly. Discontinue/Taper at 3-6 month intervals. Start 1 week after discontinuing oral hormone therapy. Osteoporosis Prevention: Initial: 0.05mg/day.

HOW SUPPLIED: Patch: 0.05mg/24 hrs, 0.1mg/24 hrs [8ˢ, 24ˢ]

CONTRAINDICATIONS: Pregnancy, undiagnosed abnormal genital bleeding, breast cancer unless being treated for metastatic disease, estrogen-dependent neoplasia, DVT/PE, active or recent (eg, within past year) arterial thromboembolic disease (eg, stroke, MI), liver dysfunction or disease.

WARNINGS/PRECAUTIONS: May increase risk of cardiovascular events (eg, MI, stroke), venous thrombosis, and PE; d/c immediately if any of these events occur or are suspected. May increase risk of breast/endometrial cancer, and gallbladder disease. May lead to severe hypercalcemia with breast cancer and bone metastases; monitor and d/c if hypercalcemia occurs. Retinal vascular thrombosis reported; monitor and d/c if papilledema or retinal vascular lesions occur. Consider addition of a progestin if no hysterectomy. May elevate BP; monitor at regular intervals. May cause elevations of plasma triglycerides with pre-existing hypertriglyceridemia. Caution with history of cholestatic jaundice associated with past estrogen use or with pregnancy; d/c with recurrence. May lead to increased thyroid-binding globulin levels; monitor thyroid function. May cause fluid retention; caution with cardiac/renal dysfunction. Caution with severe hypocalcemia. May increase risk of ovarian cancer. May exacerbate endometriosis, asthma, DM, epilepsy, migraine, porphyria, SLE, and hepatic hemangiomas; use with caution.

ADVERSE REACTIONS: Redness/irritation at application site, altered vaginal bleeding, vaginal candidiasis, breast tenderness/enlargement, GI effects, melasma, CNS effects, retinal vascular thrombosis, weight changes, edema, altered libido.

INTERACTIONS: CYP3A4 inducers (eg, St. John's wort, phenobarbital, carbamazepine, rifampin) may decrease levels resulting in decreased therapeutic effects and/or changes in uterine bleeding profile. CYP3A4 inhibitors (eg, erythromycin, clarithromycin, ketoconazole, itraconazole, ritonavir, grapefruit juice) may increase levels and result in side effects.

PREGNANCY: Category X, caution in nursing.

MECHANISM OF ACTION: Estrogen; acts through binding to nuclear receptors in estrogen-responsive tissues; modulates pituitary secretion of the gonadotropins, luteinizing hormone and follicle stimulating hormone, through negative feedback mechanism. In postmenopausal women, reduces elevated levels of these hormones.

PHARMACOKINETICS: Distribution: Largely bound to sex hormone binding globulin and albumin; found in breast milk. **Metabolism**: Liver to estrone (metabolite) and estriol (major urinary metabolite); sulfate and glucuronide conjugation (liver), gut hydrolysis; CYP3A4 (partial metabolism). **Elimination**: Urine (parent compound and metabolites); $T_{1/2}$=1 hr.

ESTRASORB　　　　　　　　　　　　RX
estradiol (Esprit)

> Estrogens increase the risk of endometrial cancer. Estrogens, with or without progestins, should not be used for the prevention of cardiovascular disease or dementia. Increased risks of MI, stroke, invasive breast cancer, PE, and DVT in postmenopausal women (50-79 yrs of age) reported. Increased risk of developing probable dementia in postmenopausal women ≥65 yrs of age reported.

THERAPEUTIC CLASS: Estrogen

INDICATIONS: Treatment of moderate to severe vasomotor symptoms associated with menopause.

DOSAGE: *Adults:* Apply 2 pouches (0.05mg/day) qAM. Apply one pouch to each leg from the upper thigh to the calf. Rub in for 3 min.

HOW SUPPLIED: Emulsion, Topical: 2.5mg/g

CONTRAINDICATIONS: Undiagnosed abnormal genital bleeding, breast cancer (unless being treated for metastatic disease), estrogen-dependent neoplasia, DVT/PE, active or recent (eg, within 1 year) arterial thromboembolic disease (eg, stroke, MI), liver dysfunction or disease, pregnancy.

WARNINGS/PRECAUTIONS: Limit use to the shortest duration consistent with goals and risks; re-evaluate periodically. Increased risk of cardiovascular events (eg, MI, stroke, venous thromboembolism, pulmonary embolism), gallbladder disease, breast and endometrial cancer. D/C 4-6 weeks before surgery associated with an increased risk of thromboembolism or during prolonged immobilization. Possible increased risk of ovarian cancer. May lead to severe hypercalcemia in patients with breast cancer and bone metastases. Consider adding progestin in patients with intact uterus to avoid endometrial hyperplasia. Increased thyroid-binding globulin levels (may need higher doses of thyroid hormone). May cause fluid retention; caution in cardiac or renal dysfunction. Retinal vascular thrombosis and elevated BP reported. May lead to severe hypercalcemia with breast cancer and bone metastases; monitor and d/c if hypercalcemia occurs. May exacerbate endometriosis, asthma, diabetes mellitus, epilepsy, migraine, porphyria, systemic lupus erythematosus (SLE), or hepatic hemangiomas; use with caution. Avoid use in close proximity to sunscreen application; may increase absorption. Potential for estradiol transfer through physical contact; wash application site 8 hours post-application. May cause elevations of plasma triglycerides with pre-existing hypertriglyceridemia. Caution with history of cholestatic jaundice associated with past estrogen use or with pregnancy;d/c with recurrence.

ADVERSE REACTIONS: Headache, infection, sinusitis, pruritus, breast pain, endometrial disorder.

INTERACTIONS: CYP3A4 inducers (eg, St. John's wort, phenobarbital, carbamazepine, rifampin) may decrease levels which may decrease therapeutic effects and/or change uterine bleeding profile. CYP3A4 inhibitors (eg, erythromycin, clarithromycin, ketoconazole, itraconazole, ritonavir, grapefruit juice) may increase levels which may result in side effects.

PREGNANCY: Contraindicated in pregnancy, caution in nursing.

MECHANISM OF ACTION: Estrogen; acts through binding to nuclear receptors in estrogen-responsive tissues. Circulating estrogens modulate the pituitary secretion of the gonadotrophins, luteinizing hormone, and follicle stimulating hormone through negative feedback mechanism. In postmenopausal women, reduces elevated levels of these hormones.

PHARMACOKINETICS: Distribution: Largely bound to sex hormone binding globulin and albumin; found in breast milk. **Metabolism:** Liver to estrone (metabolite), estriol (major urinary metabolite); sulfate and glucuronide conjugation (liver), gut hydrolysis; CYP 3A4 (partial metabolism). **Excretion:** Urine (parent compound and metabolites).

ESTRATEST   RX
esterified estrogens - methyltestosterone (Solvay)

> Estrogens increase risk of endometrial cancer in postmenopausal women. Avoid during pregnancy. Estrogens, with or without progestins, should not be used for the prevention of cardiovascular disease. Increased risks of MI, stroke, invasive breast cancer, PE, and DVT in postmenopausal women reported.

OTHER BRAND NAMES: Estratest H.S. (Solvay)

THERAPEUTIC CLASS: Estrogen/androgen combination

INDICATIONS: Treatment of moderate-severe vasomotor symptoms associated with menopause, when not improved by estrogens alone.

DOSAGE: *Adults:* Vasomotor Symptoms: 0.625-1.25mg or 1.25-2.5mg qd cyclically (3 weeks on, 1 week off). Discontinue/taper at 3-6 month intervals.

HOW SUPPLIED: (Esterified Estrogens-Methyltestosterone) Tab: (Estratest HS) 0.625-1.25mg, (Estratest) 1.25-2.5mg

CONTRAINDICATIONS: Pregnancy, nursing, severe liver damage, undiagnosed abnormal genital bleeding, breast cancer except in selected patients treated for metastatic disease, estrogen-dependent neoplasia, and thrombophlebitis or thromboembolic disease (active disease or past history associated with estrogen use, except when used in treatment of breast malignancy).

WARNINGS/PRECAUTIONS: Risk of gallbladder disease, endometrial carcinoma, thromboembolic disease, hepatic dysfunction/adenoma/neoplasm, peliosis hepatis, elevated BP, impaired glucose tolerance, hypercalcemia with breast cancer and bone metastases. Caution with metabolic bone disease associated with hypercalcemia or renal insufficiency. May increase size of pre-existing uterine leiomyomata. Caution in liver dysfunction, family history of breast cancer, breast nodules, fibrocystic disease, abnormal mammograms, diabetes, asthma, epilepsy, migraine, depression, and cardiac or renal dysfunction. D/C if cholestatic hepatitis and/or jaundice occurs, or if LFTs are abnormal. D/C 4 weeks prior to surgery if prolonged immobilization required. Increased risk of jaundice with history of jaundice during pregnancy. May effect epiphyseal closure; caution in young patients. D/C if virilization occurs. Increase in triglycerides, thyroid binding globulin, PT.

ADVERSE REACTIONS: Breakthrough bleeding, amenorrhea, virilization, inhibition of gonadotropin secretion, breast tenderness and enlargement, nausea, hirsutism, abdominal cramps, bloating, altered libido, cholestatic jaundice, weight gain, edema.

INTERACTIONS: May decrease insulin and anticoagulant requirements. May increase levels of oxyphenbutazone.

PREGNANCY: Category X, contraindicated in nursing.

MECHANISM OF ACTION: Esterified estrogen; acts by binding to nuclear receptors in estrogen-responsive tissues. Circulating estrogens modulate pituitary secretion of gonadotrophins, luteinizing hormone, and follicle stimulating hormone through negative feedback mechanism. In postmenopausal women, reduces elevated levels of these hormones. Methyltestosterone: an androgen; responsible for the normal growth and development of male sex hormones and for maintenance of secondary sex characteristics.

PHARMACOKINETICS: Distribution: Esterified estrogen: Largely bound to sex hormone-binding globulin and albumin; found in breast milk. Methyl testosterone: Bound to testosterone estradiol binding globulin (98%). **Metabolism:** Esterified estrogen: Liver to estrone (metabolite) and estriol (major urinary metabolite); sulfate and glucuronide conjugation (liver); gut hydrolysis, CYP3A4 (partial metabolism). Methyl testosterone: Liver. **Elimination:** Esterified estrogen: Urine (parent compound and metabolites). Methyltestosterone: Urine (90%), feces (6%); $T_{1/2}$=10-100 min.

ESTRING

RX

estradiol (Pharmacia & Upjohn)

> Estrogens increase risk of endometrial cancer in postmenopausal women. Estrogens with or without progestins should not be used for prevention of cardiovascular disease or dementia. Increased risk of stroke and DVT in postmenopausal women (50-79 yrs).

THERAPEUTIC CLASS: Estrogen

INDICATIONS: Treatment of urogenital symptoms associated with postmenopausal atrophy of vagina or lower urinary tract.

DOSAGE: *Adults:* Insert ring deeply into upper 1/3 of vaginal vault. Remove and replace after 90 days. Reassess at 3 or 6 month intervals.

HOW SUPPLIED: Vaginal Ring: 0.0075mg/24 hrs

CONTRAINDICATIONS: Pregnancy, undiagnosed abnormal vaginal bleeding, breast cancer, estrogen-dependent neoplasia, DVT or pulmonary embolism, arterial thromboembolic disease (eg, stroke, MI), liver dysfunction/disease.

WARNINGS/PRECAUTIONS: Increased risk of endometrial, breast, and ovarian cancer, dementia, gallbladder disease, visual abnormalities, hypercalcemia reported. Abnormal uterine bleeding, mastodynia reported. Caution with hepatic impairment, hypertriglyceridemia, hypothyroidism, hypocalcemia, vaginal stenosis, narrow vagina, prolapse, or vaginal infections. Expulsions from vagina reported. Hypercoagulation, hyperlipidemia, and fluid retention may occur.

ADVERSE REACTIONS: Headache, leukorrhea, back pain, genital moniliasis, sinusitis, vaginitis, vaginal discomfort, vaginal hemorrhage, arthralgia, insomnia, abdominal pain.

INTERACTIONS: Remove during treatment with other vaginally administered agents. CYP3A4 inhibitors (eg, erythromycin, clarithromycin, ketoconazole, itraconazole, ritonavir, grapefruit juice) may increase concentrations. CYP3A4 inducers (eg, St. John's wort, phenobarbital, carbamazepine, rifampin) may decrease concentrations.

PREGNANCY: Not for use in pregnancy or nursing.

MECHANISM OF ACTION: Estrogen; binds to nuclear receptors in estrogen-responsive tissue. Circulating estrogens modulate the pituitary secretion of the gonadotropins, luteinizing hormone and follicle stimulating hormone, through a negative feedback mechanism. In postmenopausal women, acts to reduce elevated levels of these hormones.

PHARMACOKINETICS: Absorption: Well absorbed; T_{max}=0.5-1 hr; C_{max}=63.2pg/mL. **Distribution:** Largely bound to sex hormone binding globulin and albumin; found in breast milk. **Metabolism:** Liver to estrone (metabolite) and estriol (major urinary metabolite); sulfate and glucuronide conjugation (liver); intestinal hydrolysis; CYP3A4 (partial metabolism). **Elimination:** Urine (parent compound and metabolites).

ESTROGEL

RX

estradiol (Solvay)

> Estrogens increase the risk of endometrial cancer. Estrogens, with or without progestins, should not be used for the prevention of cardiovascular disease. Increased risks of MI, stroke, invasive breast cancer, PE, and DVT in postmenopausal women reported.

THERAPEUTIC CLASS: Estrogen

INDICATIONS: Moderate to severe vasomotor symptoms and/or vulvar/vaginal atrophy associated with menopause.

DOSAGE: *Adults:* Apply one compression (1.25g) to one arm from wrist to shoulder once daily. Re-evaluate periodically.

HOW SUPPLIED: Gel: 0.06% (1.25g (0.75mg estradiol) of gel per compression) [93g]

CONTRAINDICATIONS: Undiagnosed abnormal genital bleeding, breast cancer, estrogen-dependent neoplasia, DVT or PE, active or recent (within 1 year) arterial thromboembolic disease (eg, stroke, MI), liver dysfunction or disease, pregnancy.

WARNINGS/PRECAUTIONS: May increase risk of cardiovascular events (eg, MI, stroke), venous thrombosis, and PE; d/c immediately if any of these events occur or are suspected. May increase risk of breast/endometrial cancer, and gallbladder disease. May lead to severe hypercalcemia with breast cancer and bone metastases; monitor and d/c if hypercalcemia occurs. Retinal vascular thrombosis reported; monitor and d/c if papilledema or retinal vascular lesions occur. Consider addition of a progestin if no hysterectomy. May elevate BP; monitor at regular intervals. May cause elevations of plasma triglycerides with pre-existing hypertriglyceridemia. Caution with history of cholestatic jaundice associated with past estrogen use or with pregnancy; d/c with recurrence. May lead to increased thyroid-binding globulin levels; monitor thyroid function. May cause fluid retention; caution with cardiac/renal dysfunction. Caution with severe hypocalcemia. May increase risk of ovarian cancer. May exacerbate endometriosis, asthma, DM, epilepsy, migraine, porphyria, SLE, and hepatic hemangiomas; use with caution. Alcohol-based gels are flammable; avoid fire, flame, or smoking until the gel dried.

ADVERSE REACTIONS: Headache, infection, breast pain, vaginitis, abdominal pain, rash, nausea, pruritus, diarrhea.

INTERACTIONS: CYP3A4 inducers (eg, St. John's wort, phenobarbital, carbamazepine, rifampin) may decrease levels which may decrease therapeutic effects and/or change uterine bleeding profile. CYP3A4 inhibitors (eg, erythromycin, clarithromycin, ketoconazole, itraconazole, ritonavir, grapefruit juice) may increase levels which may result in side effects. May require higher doses of thyroid hormone.

PREGNANCY: Contraindicated in pregnancy, caution in nursing.

MECHANISM OF ACTION: Estrogen; binds to nuclear receptors in estrogen-responsive tissues. Circulating estrogens modulate the pituitary secretion of the gonadotrophins, luteinizing hormone and follicle stimulating hormone, through a negative feedback mechanism. In postmenopausal women, estrogens reduce elevated levels of these hormones.

PHARMACOKINETICS: Absorption: C_{max}=46.4pg/mL. **Distribution:** Largely bound to sex hormone binding globulin and albumin; found in breast milk. **Metabolism:** Liver to estrone (metabolite) and estriol (major urinary metabolite); sulfate and glucuronide conjugation (liver); gut hydrolysis; CYP 3A4 (partial metabolism). **Elimination:** Urine (parent compound and metabolites); $T_{1/2}$=36 hrs.

ESTROSTEP FE   RX
norethindrone acetate - ethinyl estradiol (Warner Chilcott)

THERAPEUTIC CLASS: Estrogen/progestogen combination

INDICATIONS: Prevention of pregnancy. Treatment of acne vulgaris in females ≥15 yrs who want contraception (for at least 6 months), have achieved menarche, and are unresponsive to topical acne agents.

DOSAGE: *Adults:* Contraception/Acne: 1 tab qd for 28 days, then repeat. Start 1st Sunday after menses begin or the 1st day of menses.
Pediatrics: ≥15 yrs: Contraception (Postpubertal Adolescents)/Acne: 1 tab qd for 28 days, then repeat. Start 1st Sunday after menses begins or the 1st day of menses.

HOW SUPPLIED: Tab: (Ethinyl Estradiol-Norethindrone) 0.035mg-1mg, 0.030mg-1mg, 0.020mg-1mg and 75mg ferrous fumarate

CONTRAINDICATIONS: Thrombophlebitis, history of DVT, active or history of thromboembolic disorders, pregnancy, cerebrovascular disease, CAD, undiagnosed abnormal genital bleeding, cholestatic jaundice of pregnancy, jaundice with prior pill use, hepatic adenoma or carcinoma, breast carcinoma, endometrium or other estrogen-dependent neoplasia.

WARNINGS/PRECAUTIONS: Cigarette smoking increases risk of serious cardiovascular side effects. This risk increases with age (especially >35 yrs) and heavy smoking. Increased risk of MI, vascular disease, thromboembolism, stroke, and gallbladder disease. Retinal thrombosis, hepatic neoplasia reported. May cause glucose intolerance. May increase BP, elevate LDL levels or cause other lipid changes, fluid retention, breakthrough bleeding, and spotting. May cause or exacerbate migraine. May develop visual changes with contact lenses. Increased risk of MI with HTN, hyperlipidemia, obesity, and diabetes. D/C if jaundice, significant depression, or ophthalmic irregularities develop. Perform annual physical exam. Use before menarche is not indicated. May affect certain endocrine, LFTs, and blood components.

ADVERSE REACTIONS: Nausea, vomiting, breakthrough bleeding, spotting, amenorrhea, migraine, depression, vaginal candidiasis, edema, weight changes.

INTERACTIONS: Reduced effects, increased breakthrough bleeding, and menstrual irregularities with rifampin, barbiturates, phenylbutazone, phenytoin, carbamazepine, St. John's wort, and possibly with griseofulvin, ampicillin, and tetracyclines. Increased plasma levels with atorvastatin. Ascorbic acid and APAP may increase plasma levels. Decreased plasma levels of APAP. Increased clearance of temazepam, salicylic acid, morphine, and clofibric acid. Increased plasma levels of cyclosporine, prednisolone, and theophylline.

PREGNANCY: Category X, not for use in nursing.

MECHANISM OF ACTION: Estrogen/progestogen oral contraceptive; acts by suppressing gonadotropins, inhibiting ovulation, and causing other alterations, including changes in the cervical mucus (increasing difficulty of sperm entry into the uterus) and the endometrium (reducing likelihood of implantation).

PHARMACOKINETICS: Absorption: Rapid and complete. Absolute bioavailability: Norethindrone (64%), ethinyl estradiol (43%); T_{max}=1-2 hrs. **Distribution:** V_d=2-4L/kg; plasma protein binding (>95%). **Metabolism:** Norethindrone: Extensive; reduction, sulfate/glucuronide conjugation. Ethinyl estradiol: CYP3A4; oxidation, conjugation. **Elimination:** Norethindrone: $T_{1/2}$=13 hrs. Ethinyl estradiol: Urine, feces; $T_{1/2}$=19 hrs.

ETHYOL RX
amifostine (MedImmune)

THERAPEUTIC CLASS: Thiophosphate protective agent

INDICATIONS: To reduce cumulative renal toxicity with repeated cisplatin therapy in advanced ovarian cancer. To reduce incidence of moderate to severe xerostomia in post-op radiation therapy of head and neck cancer where the radiation port includes a substantial portion of parotid glands.

DOSAGE: *Adults:* Renal Toxicity Reduction: 910mg/m² IV qd over 15 min, 30 min before chemo. Interrupt if systolic BP decreases significantly from baseline. May restart if BP returns to normal within 5 min and patient asymptomatic. If cannot give full dose, give 740mg/m² for subsequent chemo. Xerostomia: 200mg/m² IV qd over 3 min, 15-30 min before radiation.

HOW SUPPLIED: Inj: 500mg

CONTRAINDICATIONS: Hypersensitivity to aminothiol compounds.

WARNINGS/PRECAUTIONS: Avoid with chemotherapy for other malignancies in which chemotherapy can produce significant survival benefit/cure, or with definitive radiotherapy. Avoid with hypotension, dehydration, or with antihypertensives that cannot be stopped for 24 hrs before chemotherapy. Keep patients well hydrated, in a supine position during infusion, and monitor BP every 5 minutes during infusion and thereafter. For infusions <5 minutes, monitor BP before and after infusion. Possible increased side effects with infusions >15 minutes. May cause serious cutaneous reactions such as Stevens-Johnson syndrome, toxic epidermal necrolysis, toxoderma, exfoliatiave dermatitis, and erythema multiforme. Monitor calcium levels if at risk for hypocalcemia (eg, nephrotic syndrome, patients receiving multiple doses). Caution in elderly, pre-existing cardiovascular or cerebrovascular disease. Administer antiemetic before and during therapy.

ADVERSE REACTIONS: Hypotension, NV, flushing, fever, dizziness, somnolence, hiccups, hypocalcemia, dyspnea, urticaria.

INTERACTIONS: Caution with antihypertensives or drugs that potentiate hypotension.

PREGNANCY: Category C, not for use in nursing.

MECHANISM OF ACTION: Thiophosphate protective agent; reduces cumulative renal toxicity of cisplatin and for the reduction of the toxic effects of radiation on normal oral tissues.

PHARMACOKINETICS: Metabolism: Metabolized to active free thiol metabolite and disulphide metabolite. **Elimination:** Urine; $T_{1/2}$=8 min.

ETODOLAC   RX
etodolac (Various)

> NSAIDs may cause an increased risk of serious cardiovascular thrombotic events, MI, stroke and serious GI adverse events including bleeding, ulceration, and perforation of the stomach or intestines. Contraindicated for the treatment of perioperative pain in the setting of coronary artery bypass graft (CABG) surgery.

THERAPEUTIC CLASS: NSAID (pyranocarboxylic acid derivative)

INDICATIONS: Management of osteoarthritis (OA), rheumatoid arthritis (RA), and pain.

DOSAGE: *Adults:* ≥18 yrs: Acute Pain: Usual: 200-400mg q6-8h. Max: 1200mg/day. OA/RA: Usual: 300mg bid-tid, or 400-500mg bid. Max: 1200mg/day.

HOW SUPPLIED: Cap: 200mg, 300mg; Tab: 400mg, 500mg

CONTRAINDICATIONS: ASA or other NSAID allergy that precipitates asthma, urticaria or other allergic type reactions. Treatment of perioperative pain in the setting of CABG surgery.

WARNINGS/PRECAUTIONS: May lead to onset of new HTN or worsening of pre-existing HTN; monitor BP closely. Fluid retention and edema reported; caution with fluid retention or heart failure. Renal papillary necrosis and other renal injury reported after long-term use. Not recommended for use with advanced renal disease; if therapy must be initiated, monitor renal function. Anaphylactoid reactions may occur. May cause serious skin adverse events (eg, exfoliative dermatitis, Stevens-Johnson syndrome, and toxic epidermal necrolysis). Avoid in late pregnancy; may cause premature closure of ductus arteriosus. May cause elevations of LFTs; d/c if liver disease develops or systemic manifestations occur. Caution in elderly. Anemia may occur; with long-term use, monitor Hgb/Hct if signs or symptoms of anemia develop. May inhibit platelet aggregation and prolong bleeding time; monitor with coagulation disorders. Caution with asthma and avoid with ASA-sensitive asthma. Risk of GI ulceration, bleeding, and perforation.

ADVERSE REACTIONS: Dyspepsia, abdominal pain, diarrhea, flatulence, nausea, constipation, gastritis, asthenia, malaise, dizziness, increased bleeding time, GI ulcers, GI bleeding/perforation, heartburn, abnormal renal function.

INTERACTIONS: May elevate digoxin, lithium, and methotrexate serum levels. May enhance nephrotoxicity associated with cyclosporine. Avoid with phenylbutazone and ASA. Increased adverse effect potential with ASA. Caution with warfarin. Diuretics may increase risk of renal toxicity. May diminish antihypertensive effects of ACE inhibitors.

PREGNANCY: Category C, not for use in nursing.

MECHANISM OF ACTION: NSAID; suspected to inhibit prostaglandin synthetase, exerts anti-inflammatory, analgesic, and antipyretic actions.

PHARMACOKINETICS: Absorption: Well absorbed. Bioavailability (100%). Mean C_{max}=14-37mcg/mL, mean T_{max}=80 min. **Distribution:** Plasma protein binding (99%), V_d=390mL/kg. **Elimination:** $T_{1/2}$=6.4 hrs. Urine, feces.

E

ETODOLAC EXTENDED-RELEASE   RX
etodolac (Various)

NSAIDs may cause an increased risk of serious cardiovascular thrombotic events, MI, stroke and serious GI adverse events including bleeding, ulceration, and perforation of the stomach or intestines. Contraindicated for the treatment of perioperative pain in the setting of coronary artery bypass graft (CABG) surgery.

THERAPEUTIC CLASS: NSAID (pyranocarboxylic acid derivative)

INDICATIONS: Relief of signs and symptoms of osteoarthritis (OA), rheumatoid arthritis (RA), and juvenile rheumatoid arthritis (JRA).

DOSAGE: *Adults:* Usual: 400-1000mg qd. Max: 1200mg/day.
Pediatrics: 6-16 yrs: JRA: >60kg: 1000mg/day. 46-60kg: 800mg/day. 31-45kg: 600mg/day. 20-30kg: 400mg/day.

HOW SUPPLIED: Tab, Extended-Release: 400mg, 500mg, 600mg

CONTRAINDICATIONS: ASA or other NSAID allergy that precipitates asthma, urticaria, or allergic reaction. Treatment of perioperative pain in the setting of CABG surgery.

WARNINGS/PRECAUTIONS: May lead to onset of new HTN or worsening of pre-existing HTN; monitor BP closely. Fluid retention and edema reported; caution with fluid retention or heart failure. Renal papillary necrosis and other renal injury reported after long-term use. Not recommended for use with advanced renal disease; if therapy must be initiated, monitor renal function. Anaphylactoid reactions may occur. May cause serious skin adverse events (eg, exfoliative dermatitis, Stevens-Johnson syndrome, and toxic epidermal necrolysis). Avoid in late pregnancy; may cause premature closure of ductus arteriosis. May cause elevations of LFTs; d/c if liver disease develops or systemic manifestations occur. Caution in elderly. Anemia may occur; with long-term use, monitor Hgb/Hct if signs or symptoms of anemia develop. May inhibit platelet aggregation and prolong bleeding time; monitor with coagulation disorders. Caution with asthma and avoid with ASA-sensitive asthma.

ADVERSE REACTIONS: Dyspepsia, abdominal pain, diarrhea, flatulence, nausea, constipation, vomiting, GI ulcers, gross bleeding/perforation.

INTERACTIONS: May elevate digoxin, lithium, and methotrexate serum levels. May enhance nephrotoxicity associated with cyclosporine. Avoid with phenylbutazone. Increased adverse effect potential with ASA. Caution with warfarin. May decrease antihypertensive effects with ACE inhibitors. May reduce natriuretic effect of furosemide and thiazides.

PREGNANCY: Category C, not for use in nursing.

MECHANISM OF ACTION: Nonsteroidal, anti-inflammatory drug; inhibits prostaglandin synthetase; exhibits anti-inflammatory, analgesic, and antipyretic activities.

PHARMACOKINETICS: Absorption: T_{max}=6 hrs. **Distribution:** V_d=566mL/kg; plasma protein binding (99%). **Metabolism:** Hydroxylation, glucuronidation. **Elimination:** Urine and feces; $T_{1/2}$=8.4 hrs.

ETOPOPHOS   RX
etoposide phosphate (Bristol-Myers Squibb)

Administer under supervision of qualified physician experienced in use of cancer chemotherapeutic agents. Severe myelosuppression with resulting infection or bleeding may occur.

THERAPEUTIC CLASS: Podophyllotoxin derivative

INDICATIONS: Adjunct therapy for management of refractory testicular tumors. First-line combination therapy for management of small cell lung cancer (SCLC).

DOSAGE: *Adults:* Testicular Cancer: Range: 50-100mg/m²/day on Days 1-5 to 100mg/m²/day on Days 1, 3, and 5. SCLC: Range: 35mg/m²/day for 4 days to

50mg/m^2/day for 5 days. After adequate recovery from toxicity, repeat course for either therapy at 3-4 week intervals. CrCl 15-50mL/min: 75% of dose.

HOW SUPPLIED: Inj: 100mg

WARNINGS/PRECAUTIONS: Observe for myelosuppression during and after therapy. Risk of anaphylactic reaction manifested by chills, fever, tachycardia, bronchospasm, dyspnea, and hypotension. Increased risk of toxicity with a low serum albumin. Perform CBC before each dose, during, and after therapy. May cause fetal harm in pregnancy. Caution with low serum albumin.

ADVERSE REACTIONS: Myelosuppression, leukopenia, neutropenia, thrombocytopenia, anemia, nausea, vomiting, anaphylactic-like reactions, BP changes, alopecia, anorexia, asthenia/malaise, chills, fever.

INTERACTIONS: Caution with drugs known to inhibit phosphatase activities (eg, levamisole). High-dose oral cyclosporine reduces clearance.

PREGNANCY: Category D, not for use in nursing.

MECHANISM OF ACTION: Podophyllotoxin derivative; induces DNA strand breaks by interacting with DNA-topoisomerase II or formation of free radicals.

PHARMACOKINETICS: Absorption: Rapid, complete; Etopophos 150mg/m^2: AUC=168.3µg•hr/mL, C_{max}=20µg/mL. **Distribution:** VePesid®: V_d=7-17L/m^2. Plasma protein binding (97%). **Metabolism:** VePesid: Liver via CYP3A4 (O-demethylation); hydroxy acid (metabolite). **Elimination:** VePesid: Biliary excretion, feces, urine; $T_{1/2}$=4-11 hrs.

ETOPOSIDE   RX
etoposide (Various)

> Administer under supervision of qualified physician experienced in use of cancer chemotherapeutic agents. Severe myelosuppression with resulting infection or bleeding may occur.

OTHER BRAND NAMES: VePesid (Bristol-Myers Squibb)

THERAPEUTIC CLASS: Podophyllotoxin derivative

INDICATIONS: (Inj) Adjunct therapy for management of refractory testicular tumors. (Cap/Inj) 1st-line combination therapy for management of small cell lung cancer (SCLC).

DOSAGE: *Adults:* (Inj) Testicular Cancer: Range: 50-100mg/m^2/day IV on Days 1-5 to 100mg/m^2/day on Days 1, 3, and 5. SCLC: Range: 35mg/m^2/day IV for 4 days to 50mg/m^2/day for 5 days. After adequate recovery from toxicity, repeat course for either therapy at 3-4 week intervals. (PO) SCLC: 2x the IV dose and round to nearest 50mg. Renal Impairment: CrCl 15-50mL/min: Use 75% of dose.

HOW SUPPLIED: Cap: 50mg; Inj: 20mg/mL

WARNINGS/PRECAUTIONS: Observe for myelosuppression during and after therapy. Risk of anaphylactic reaction manifested by chills, fever, tachycardia, bronchospasm, dyspnea, and hypotension. Perform CBC before each dose, during, and after therapy. May cause fetal harm in pregnancy. Caution with low serum albumin.

ADVERSE REACTIONS: Myelosuppression, leukopenia, thrombocytopenia, anemia, nausea, vomiting, stomatitis, anaphylactic-like reactions, hypotension (after rapid IV use), alopecia, anorexia.

INTERACTIONS: High-dose cyclosporine may reduce clearance and increase etoposide exposure.

PREGNANCY: Category D, not for use in nursing.

MECHANISM OF ACTION: Phodophyllotoxin derivative. Induces DNA strand breaks by interacting with DNA-topoisomerase II or formation of free radicals.

PHARMACOKINETICS: Absorption: Rapid, complete. (VePesid): Bioavailability (50%). **Distribution:** V_d=7-17L/m^2. Plasma protein binding (97%). **Metabolism:** Liver (O-demethylation) via CYP3A4. (Metabolite): hydroxy acid. **Elimination:** Biliary excretion; Feces (44%), urine (45%), $T_{1/2}$=4-11 hrs.

EUFLEXXA

RX

sodium hyaluronate (Ferring)

THERAPEUTIC CLASS: Hyaluronan

INDICATIONS: Treatment of pain in osteoarthritis of the knee in patients who have failed to respond adequately to conservative non-pharmacologic therapy and simple analgesics (eg, APAP).

DOSAGE: *Adults:* Inject 2mL intra-articularly into affected knee at weekly intervals for 3 weeks, for a total of 3 injections. Use strict aseptic injection procedures.

HOW SUPPLIED: Inj: 1% [2mL]

CONTRAINDICATIONS: Avoid with knee joint infections, infections or skin diseases in area of injection site.

WARNINGS/PRECAUTIONS: Avoid mixing with quaternary ammonium salts (eg, benzalkonium chloride); may result in formation of a precipitate. Avoid injecting intravascularly. Patients having repeated exposure have the potential for an immune response. Safety and effectiveness in joints other than the knee or in conjunction with other intra-articular injectables have not been established. Remove any joint effusion before injecting. Transient pain and/or swelling of the injected joint may occur. Avoid any strenuous activities or prolonged (eg, more than 1 hour) weight-bearing activities within 48 hours following injection. Safety and effectiveness have not been demonstrated in children.

ADVERSE REACTIONS: Arthralgia, nausea, back pain, rhinitis, BP increase, joint effusion/swelling, tendonitis, knee pain, skin irritation, headache, paresthesia.

PREGNANCY: Safety in pregnancy and nursing not known.

EURAX

RX

crotamiton (Ranbaxy)

THERAPEUTIC CLASS: Scabicide/antipruritic

INDICATIONS: Treatment of scabies and pruritus.

DOSAGE: *Adults:* Shake lotion well before use. Scabies: Thoroughly massage into cleansed skin from chin down to toes. Re-apply in 24 hrs. Take cleansing bath 48 hrs after last application. Pruritus: Massage into affected area. Repeat prn.

HOW SUPPLIED: Cre: 10% [60g]; Lot: 10% [60mL, 480mL]

WARNINGS/PRECAUTIONS: Avoid eyes, mouth, acutely inflamed skin or raw or weeping surfaces. D/C if severe irritation or sensitization develops.

ADVERSE REACTIONS: Allergic sensitivity, irritation.

PREGNANCY: Category C, safety in nursing not known.

MECHANISM OF ACTION: Scabicide and antipruritic agent; MOA not established.

EVAMIST

RX

estradiol (Vivus)

Estrogens increase the risk of endometrial cancer. Estrogens, with or without progestins, should not be used for the prevention of CVD or dementia. Increased risks of MI, stroke, invasive breast cancer, PE, and DVT in postmenopausal women (50-79 yrs of age) reported. Increased risk of developing probable dementia in postmenopausal women ≥65 yrs of age reported.

THERAPEUTIC CLASS: Estrogen

INDICATIONS: Treatment of moderate to severe vasomotor symptoms due to menopause.

DOSAGE: *Adults*: 1 spray qd on inner surface of forearm. Adjust dose based on response.

HOW SUPPLIED: Spray: 1.53mg/spray [56 sprays]

CONTRAINDICATIONS: Undiagnosed abnormal genital bleeding, breast cancer, estrogen-dependent neoplasia, DVT or PE, active or recent (within past year) arterial thromboembolic disease (eg, stroke, MI), liver dysfunction or disease, pregnancy.

WARNINGS/PRECAUTIONS: May increase risk of cardiovascular disorders (eg, stroke, DVT), venous thrombosis, PE, and MI; d/c immediately if any of these events occur or are suspected. May increase risk of breast/endometrial cancer, dementia, and gallbladder disease. May lead to severe hypercalcemia with breast cancer and bone metastases. Monitor and d/c if hypercalcemia occurs. Retinal vascular thrombosis reported; monitor and d/c if papilledmea or retinal vascular lesions occur. Consider addition of progestin if no hysterectomy. May elevate BP or plasma trigycerides with pre-existing hypertriglyceridemia. Caution with history of cholestatic jaundice associated with past estrogen use or with pregnancy; d/c with recurrence. May lead to increased TBG levels; monitor thyroid function. May cause fluid retention; caution with cardiac/renal dysfunction. Caution with severe hypocalcemia. May increase risk of ovarian cancer. May exacerbate endometriosis, asthma, DM, epilepsy, migraine, porphyria, SLE and hepatic hemangiomas. Avoid fire, flame or smoking until spray has dried.

ADVERSE REACTIONS: Breast tenderness, nipple pain, nausea, nasopharyngitis, back pain, arthralgia, headache.

INTERACTIONS: May increase prothrombin time, partial thromboplastin time, and platelet aggregation time. May require higher doses of thyroid hormone. May elevate binding proteins and decrease free hormone concentration. May increase plasma HDL concentration, triglyceride levels, and reduce LDL concentration. Impaired glucose tolerance. CYP3A4 inducers (St.John's wort, phenobarbital, carbamazapine, and rifampin) may reduce levels. Inhibitors of CYP3A4 (eg, erythromycin, clarithromycin, ketoconazole) may increase levels.

PREGNANCY: Contraindicated in pregnancy, caution in nursing.

MECHANISM OF ACTION: Estrogen; acts by binding to nuclear receptors in estrogen responsive tissues. Circulating estrogens modulate the pituitary secretion of the gonadotrophins, luteinizing hormone and follicle stimulating hormone, through a negative feedback mechanism. In post menopausal women, acts to reduce elevated levels of these hormones.

PHARMACOKINETICS: Absorption: Administration of various doses resulted in different parameters. **Distribution:** Largely bound to sex hormone binding globulin and albumin; found in breast milk. **Metabolism:** Liver to estriol (metabolite) and estrone (major urinary metabolite); sulfate and glucuronide conjugation (liver); intestinal hydrolysis, CYP3A4 (partial metabolism). **Elimination:** Urine (parent compound and metabolites).

EVISTA   RX
raloxifene HCL (Lilly)

> Increased risk of DVT and PE reported. Avoid use in women with active or past history of venous thromboembolism. Increased risk of death due to stroke in postmenopausal women with documented coronary heart disease or at increased risk for major coronary events.

THERAPEUTIC CLASS: Selective estrogen receptor modulator

INDICATIONS: Treatment and prevention of osteoporosis in postmenopausal women. Reduction in risk of invasive breast cancer in postmenopausal women with osteoporosis or at high risk for invasive breast cancer.

DOSAGE: *Adults:* 60mg qd.

HOW SUPPLIED: Tab: 60mg

CONTRAINDICATIONS: Nursing, pregnancy, venous thromboembolic events (eg, DVT, PE, retinal vein thrombosis).

E

WARNINGS/PRECAUTIONS: May increase risk of DVT, PE, and retinal vein thrombosis; d/c 72 hrs prior to and during prolonged immobilization. May increase risk of death due to stroke in postmenopausal women with documented coronary heart disease or in women at increased risk for coronary events. Should not be used for primary or secondary prevention of CV disease. May increase levels of triglycerides with pre-existing hypertriglyceridemia. Not for use in premenopausal women or with systemic estrogens. Caution with hepatic impairment or with moderate or severe renal impairment. Venous thromboembolism reported.

ADVERSE REACTIONS: Hot flashes, leg cramps, abdominal pain, vaginal bleeding, arthralgia, rhinitis, headache.

INTERACTIONS: Avoid concomitant use with anion exchange resins; cholestyramine decreases absorption. Monitor PT/INR with warfarin and other anticoagulants. Caution with other highly protein-bound drugs (eg, diazepam, diazoxide, lidocaine). Avoid concomitant use with other systemic estrogens.

PREGNANCY: Category X, contraindicated in nursing.

MECHANISM OF ACTION: Selective estrogen receptor modulator; binds to estrogen receptors. Results in activation of estrogenic pathways in some tissues and blockade of estrogenic pathways in others. Actions depend on the extent of recruitment of coactivators and corepressors to estrogen receptor target gene promotors. Acts as an estrogen agonist in bone. Decreases bone resorption and bone turnover, increases bone mineral density, and decreases fracture incidence.

PHARMACOKINETICS: Absorption: Rapid; Absolute bioavailability (2%); Single dose: C_{max}=0.5(ng/mL)/(mg/kg); AUC=27.2(ng•hr/mL)/(mg/kg). Multiple doses: C_{max}=1.36(ng/mL)/(mg/kg); AUC=24.2(ng•hr/mL)/(mg/kg). **Distribution:** Single dose: V_d=2348L/kg; Multiple doses: V_d=2853L/kg. Plasma protein binding (95%). **Metabolism:** Extensive; glucuronidation. **Elimination:** Feces (primary), urine (<0.2% unchanged). Single dose: $T_{1/2}$=27.7 hrs; Multiple doses: $T_{1/2}$=32.5 hr.

EVOCLIN   RX
clindamycin phosphate (Stiefel)

THERAPEUTIC CLASS: Lincomycin derivative

INDICATIONS: Treatment of acne vulgaris.

DOSAGE: *Adults:* Apply to affected area once daily.
Pediatrics: ≥12 yrs: Apply to affected area once daily.

HOW SUPPLIED: Foam: 1% [50g, 100g]

CONTRAINDICATIONS: History of regional enteritis, ulcerative colitis, or antibiotic-associated colitis.

WARNINGS/PRECAUTIONS: Diarrhea, bloody diarrhea, and colitis (including pseudomembranous colitis) reported with use of topical and systemic clindamycin. D/C if significant diarrhea occurs. Caution in atopic individuals. Avoid eye contact.

ADVERSE REACTIONS: Headache, application site burning/pruritus/dryness, pseudomembranous colitis (rare).

INTERACTIONS: May potentiate neuromuscular blockers; caution with concomitant use.

PREGNANCY: Category B, caution in nursing.

MECHANISM OF ACTION: Lincomycin derivative; shown to have activity against *Propionibacterium acnes*, which is associated with acne vulgaris.

PHARMACOKINETICS: Distribution: Orally and parenterally administered clindamycin has been found in breast milk. **Metabolism:** Liver. **Elimination:** Urine (0.024% total dose). $T_{1/2}$=2.4-3 hr.

EVOXAC
cevimeline HCL (Daiichi Sankyo)

RX

THERAPEUTIC CLASS: Cholinergic agonist

INDICATIONS: Treatment of symptoms of dry mouth in patients with Sjogren's syndrome.

DOSAGE: *Adults:* 30mg tid.

HOW SUPPLIED: Cap: 30mg

CONTRAINDICATIONS: Uncontrolled asthma, when miosis in undesirable (eg, acute iritis, narrow-angle glaucoma).

WARNINGS/PRECAUTIONS: May alter cardiac conduction and/or HR; caution with angina or MI. Potential to increase airway resistance, bronchial smooth muscle tone, and bronchial secretions; caution with controlled asthma, chronic bronchitis, or COPD. Toxicity characterized by exaggerated parasympathomimetic effects (eg, headache, visual disturbance, lacrimation, sweating, respiratory distress, GI spasm, nausea, vomiting, cardiac abnormalities, mental confusion, tremors). Caution with history of nephrolithiasis, cholelithiasis. Ophthalmic formulations decrease visual acuity; caution while night driving or hazardous activities in reduced lighting. Risk of cholecystitis.

ADVERSE REACTIONS: Excessive sweating, nausea, rhinitis, diarrhea, cough, sinusitis, upper respiratory infection.

INTERACTIONS: CYP450 2D6 and CYP450 3A3/4 inhibitors also inhibit metabolism of cevimeline. Caution with CYP450 2D6 deficiency. Possible conduction disturbances with β-antagonists. Additive effects with parasympathomimetics. May interefere with drugs with antimuscarinic effects.

PREGNANCY: Category C, not for use in nursing.

MECHANISM OF ACTION: A cholinergic agonist; increase secretion of exocrine glands, such as salivary and sweat glands, and increase tone of the smooth muscle in the GI and urinary tracts.

PHARMACOKINETICS: Absorption: T_{max}=1.5-2 hrs. **Distribution:** V_d=6L/kg. Plasma protein binding (≤20%). **Metabolism:** Via isozymes CYP2D6 and CYP3A3/4. **Elimination:** Urine, feces. Mean $T_{1/2}$=5 hrs.

EXCEDRIN MIGRAINE
acetaminophen - caffeine - aspirin (Bristol-Myers Squibb)

OTC

THERAPEUTIC CLASS: Analgesic combination

INDICATIONS: Treatment of migraine.

DOSAGE: *Adults:* Take 2 tabs with water. Max: 2 tabs/day.

HOW SUPPLIED: Tab: (APAP-ASA-Caffeine) 250mg-250mg-65mg

WARNINGS/PRECAUTIONS: Children and teenagers should not use for viral illnesses. APAP and ASA may cause liver damage and GI bleeding.

INTERACTIONS: Limit caffeine containing medications, foods, or beverages. Caution with alcohol.

PREGNANCY: Safety in pregnancy and nursing not known.

EXELON
rivastigmine tartrate (Novartis)

RX

THERAPEUTIC CLASS: Acetylcholinesterase inhibitor

INDICATIONS: Treatment of mild to moderate dementia of the Alzheimer's type and mild to moderate dementia associated with Parkinson's disease.

DOSAGE: *Adults:* Alzheimer's Dementia: Initial: 1.5mg bid. Titrate: May increase by 1.5mg bid every 2 weeks. Max: 12mg/day. If not tolerating, suspend therapy for several doses and restart at same or next lower dose.

E

If interrupted longer than several days, reinitiate with lowest daily dose and titrate as above. Dementia Associated with Parkinson's Disease: Initial: 1.5mg bid. Titrate: May increase by 1.5mg every 4 weeks. Max: 12mg/day. Take with food in am and pm. May mix solution with water, cold fruit juice, or soda. Patch: Alzheimer's Dementia/Dementia Associated with Parkinson's Disease: Initial: Apply 4.6mg/24 hrs patch qd to clean, dry, hairless intact skin. Maint: Increase dose after 4 weeks. Max: 9.5mg/24 hrs if well tolerated. Switching from Capsules/Oral Sol: Total Oral Daily Dose <6mg: Switch to 4.6mg/24 hrs patch. Total Oral Daily Dose 6-12mg: Switch to 9.5mg/24 hrs patch. Apply 1st patch on day following last oral dose.

HOW SUPPLIED: Cap: 1.5mg, 3mg, 4.5mg, 6mg; Sol: 2mg/mL [120mL]; Patch: 4.6mg/24 hrs, 9.5mg/24 hrs [30*]

CONTRAINDICATIONS: Hypersensitivity to carbamate derivatives.

WARNINGS/PRECAUTIONS: Significant GI intolerance (eg, nausea, vomiting, anorexia, and weight loss); always follow dosing guidelines. Vagotonic effect on HR (bradycardia), especially in "sick sinus syndrome" or supraventricular conduction abnormalities. May cause urinary obstruction and seizures. Monitor for peptic ulcers/GI bleeds. Caution in asthma and COPD. May exacerbate or induce extrapyramidal symptoms. (Patch) May impair mental/physical capabilities. Titrate dose with caution in patients with body weight below 50kg.

ADVERSE REACTIONS: Nausea, vomiting, abdominal pain, dyspepsia, constipation, somnolence, anorexia, asthenia, headache, dizziness, fatigue, diarrhea, tremor, depression.

INTERACTIONS: May block effects of anticholinergics. May be synergistic with succinylcholine, similar neuromuscular blockers, or cholinergic agonists (eg, bethanechol). May exaggerate succinylcholine-type muscle relaxation during anesthesia.

PREGNANCY: Category B, not for use in nursing.

MECHANISM OF ACTION: Reversible cholinesterase inhibitor; not fully established. Suspected to enhance cholinergic function by increasing concentration of acetylcholine through reversible inhibition of its hydrolysis by cholinesterase.

PHARMACOKINETICS: Absorption: Patch: T_{max}=10-16 hrs. Cap, Sol: Rapid, complete; absolute bioavailability (36%); T_{max}=1 hr. **Distribution:** Plasma protein binding (40%); V_d=1.8-2.7L/kg. **Metabolism:** Cholinesterase-mediated hydrolysis. **Elimination:** $T_{1/2}$=1.5 hrs; urine (97%), feces (0.4%).

EXFORGE   RX
amlodipine besylate - valsartan (Novartis)

> When used in pregnancy, drugs that act directly on the renin-angiotensin system can cause injury and even death to the developing fetus. D/C therapy when pregnancy is detected.

THERAPEUTIC CLASS: ARB/Calcium channel blocker (dihydropyridine)

INDICATIONS: Treatment of hypertension. Not for initial therapy.

DOSAGE: *Adults:* Combination Therapy from Monotherapy (amlodipine or valsartan): Initial: 5mg-10mg amlodipine and 160mg-320mg valsartan qd. Titrate: If inadequate control, may increase after 3-4 weeks of therapy. Max: 10mg-320mg. If receiving amlodipine and valsartan separately, may give same component doses. Elderly: Lower initial dose may be required.

HOW SUPPLIED: Tab: (Amlodipine-Valsartan) 5mg-160mg, 10mg-160mg, 5mg-320mg, 10mg-320mg.

WARNINGS/PRECAUTIONS: May cause excessive hypotension. May increase risk of angina and MI in patients with severe obstructive CAD. Caution with CHF, severe hepatic impairment, renal dysfunction, or renal artery stenosis.

ADVERSE REACTIONS: Peripheral edema, vertigo, nasopharyngitis, upper respiratory tract infection, dizziness.

INTERACTIONS: K$^+$ supplements, K$^+$-sparing diuretics (eg. spironolactone, triamterene, amiloride), or salt substitutes containing K$^+$ may increase serum K$^+$ and SrCr in heart failure patients.

PREGNANCY: Category C (1st trimester) and D (2nd and 3rd trimester), not for use in nursing.

MECHANISM OF ACTION: Amlodipine: calcium channel blocker (dihydro-pyridine); inhibits transmembrane influx of calcium ions into vascular smooth muscle and cardiac muscle. Valsartan: angiotensin II receptor blocker; blocks vasoconstrictor and aldosterone-secreting effects of angiotensin II by selectively blocking binding of angiotensin II to AT$_1$ receptor.

PHARMACOKINETICS: Absorption: Amlodipine: T$_{max}$=6-12 hrs.; Absolute bioavailability (64-90%). Valsartan: T$_{max}$=2-4 hrs; absolute bioavailability (25%). **Distribution:** Amlodipine: V$_d$=21L. Plasma protein binding (93%). Valsartan: V$_d$=17L (IV). Plasma protein binding (95%). **Metabolism:** Amlodipine: Liver (90%). Valsartan: Valeryl 4-hydroxy valsartan (metabolite). **Elimination:** Amlodipine: Urine (10%); T$_{1/2}$=30-50 hrs. Valsartan: Feces, urine; T$_{1/2}$=6 hrs.

EXJADE RX
deferasirox (Novartis)

THERAPEUTIC CLASS: Iron-chelating agent

INDICATIONS: Treatment of chronic iron overload due to blood transfusions (transfusional hemosiderosis).

DOSAGE: *Adults:* Initial: 20mg/kg/day. Titrate: May increase 5-10mg/kg q 3-6 months. Max: 30mg/kg/day. Take on empty stomach at least 30 min before food at same time each day. Tabs should be completely dispersed in 3.5oz of liquid if dose <1g or in 7oz if dose >1g. If serum ferritin falls below 500µg/L, consider interrupting therapy.
Pediatrics: ≥2 yrs: Initial: 20mg/kg/day. Titrate: May increase 5-10mg/kg q 3-6 months. Max: 30mg/kg/day. Take on empty stomach at least 30 min before food at same time each day. Tabs should be completely dispersed in 3.5oz of liquid if dose <1g or in 7oz if dose >1g. If serum ferritin falls below 500µg/L, consider interrupting therapy.

HOW SUPPLIED: Tab: 125mg, 250mg, 500mg

WARNINGS/PRECAUTIONS: Assess SCr before therapy and monitor monthly therafter; reduce dose, interrupt or d/c therapy if necessary. Intermittent proteinuria reported; monitor closely. Acute renal failure and cytopenias reported. Use caution and monitor SCr in those at risk of complications, having preexisting renal or comorbid conditions, receiving medicinal products that depress renal function, or elderly. Caution with pre-existing hematologic disorders; monitor CBC regularly. Hepatic abnormalities, increased transaminases reported; monitor LFTs monthly; modify dose for severe or persistent elevations. Reports of auditory (high frequency hearing loss, decreased hearing) and ocular distrubances (lens opacities, cataracts, elevated IOP, retinal disorders); initial and yearly auditory and ophthalmic testing recommended. Reports of skin rashes; d/c if severe, may reinitiate with short period of oral steriod.

ADVERSE REACTIONS: Diarrhea, vomiting, nausea, headache, abdominal pain, pyrexia, cough, increased SCr, rash, b-thalassemia, rare anemias, sicke cell disease.

INTERACTIONS: Avoid with aluminum-containing antacids or other iron chelator therapies.

PREGNANCY: Category B, caution in nursing.

MECHANISM OF ACTION: Iron chelating agent.

PHARMACOKINETICS: Absorption: T$_{max}$=1.5-4 hrs. **Distribution:**V$_d$=14.37; plasma protein binding (99%). **Metabolism:** Glucoronidation, deconjugation. **Elimination:** Feces (84%), urine (8%); T$_{1/2}$=8-16 hrs.

EXTINA
ketoconazole (Stiefel)

RX

THERAPEUTIC CLASS: Azole antifungal

INDICATIONS: Topical treatment of seborrheic dermatitis in immunocompetent patients ≥12 yrs of age.

DOSAGE: *Adults:* Apply to affected area(s) bid for 4 weeks.
Pediatrics: ≥12 yrs: Apply to affected area(s) bid for 4 weeks.

HOW SUPPLIED: Foam: 2% [50g, 100g]

WARNINGS/PRECAUTIONS: Contact sensitization, including photoallergicity. Contents are flammable.

ADVERSE REACTIONS: Application site burning, dryness, erythema, irritation, paresthesia, pruritis, rash, warmth, contact sensitization.

PREGNANCY: Category C, caution in nursing.

MECHANISM OF ACTION: Antifungal agent; MOA not established. Inhibits the synthesis of ergosterol, a key sterol in the cell membrane of *Malassezia furfur.*

FACTIVE
gemifloxacin mesylate (Oscient)

RX

THERAPEUTIC CLASS: Fluoroquinolone

INDICATIONS: Treatment of community-acquired pneumonia (CAP), including multi-drug resistant *Streptococcus pneumoniae* (MDRSP), and acute bacterial exacerbation of chronic bronchitis (ABECB).

DOSAGE: *Adults:* ≥18 yrs: ABECB: 320mg qd for 5 days. CAP: 320mg qd for 5 days (*S.pneumoniae, H.influenzae, M.pneumoniae,* or *C.pneumoniae*) or 7 days (MDRSP, *K.pneumoniae,* or *M.catarrhalis*). Renal Impairment: CrCl ≤ 40mL/min or Dialysis: 160mg qd. Take with fluids.

HOW SUPPLIED: Tab: 320mg

WARNINGS/PRECAUTIONS: May prolong QT interval; avoid in patients with a history of prolonged QTc interval, uncontrolled electrolyte disorders. Caution with proarrhythmic conditions, epilepsy, or if predisposed to convulsions. D/C at 1st sign of hypersensitivity (eg, rash). CNS effects, photosensitivity reactions, hypersensitivity reactions (some fatal) reported; d/c if any of these occur. *Clostridium difficile*-associated diarrhea, achilles and other tendon rupture reported. D/C therapy if rash, pain, inflammation, or ruptured tendon occurs. Caution in elderly patients taking corticosteroids. Avoid excessive sunlight and UV light. Maintain hydration. Increases of International Normalized Ratio (INR), or prothrombin time (PT), and/or clinical episodes of bleeding have been noted with concurrent administration with warfarin or derivatives.

ADVERSE REACTIONS: Diarrhea, rash, nausea, headache, abdominal pain, vomiting, dizziness.

INTERACTIONS: Magnesium- or aluminum-containing antacids, Videx® (didanosine) chewable/buffered tablets or pediatric powder, and products containing iron, and zinc, or other metal cations decrease absorption, space doses at least 3 hrs before or 2 hrs after administration. Space dosing of sucralfate by 2 hrs. Potentiated by probenecid. Monitor PT. Avoid Class IA (eg, quinidine, procainamide) or III (eg, amiodarone, sotalol) antiarrhythmics. Caution with drugs that prolong the QTc interval (eg, erythromycin, antipsychotics, TCAs).

PREGNANCY: Category C, not for use in nursing.

MECHANISM OF ACTION: Fluoroquinolone; synthetic broad-spectrum antimicrobial agent; inhibits enzymes topoisomerase II (DNA gyrase) and topoisomerase IV, which are required for bacterial DNA replication.

PHARMACOKINETICS: Absorption: Rapid; absolute bioavailability (71%); T_{max}=0.5-2 hrs; C_{max}=1.61µg/mL, AUC=8.36µg•hr/mL (respiratory infec-

tion, UTI). **Distribution:** Plasma protein binding (55%-73%); V_d=4.18L/kg.
Metabolism: Liver. **Elimination:** Feces (61%), urine (36%).

FAMVIR
famciclovir (Novartis)

RX

THERAPEUTIC CLASS: Nucleoside analogue

INDICATIONS: Treatment of acute herpes zoster (shingles). Treatment or suppression of recurrent genital herpes; or treatment of recurrent herpes labialis (cold sores) in immunocompetent patients. Treatment of recurrent mucocutaneous herpes simplex infections in HIV-infected patients;

DOSAGE: *Adults:* ≥18 yrs: Herpes Zoster: Usual: 500mg q8h for 7 days; start within 72 hrs after rash onset. CrCl 40-59mL/min: 500mg q12h. CrCl 20-39mL/min: 500mg q24h. CrCl <20mL/min: 250mg q24h. Hemodialysis: 250mg following dialysis. Recurrent Genital Herpes: 1000mg bid for 1 day; start within 6 hrs of onset of symptom. CrCl 40-59mL/min: 500mg q12h; CrCl 20-39mL/min 500mg as single dose; CrCl <20mL/min 250mg as a single dose; Hemodialysis: 250mg following dialysis. Suppression of Recurrent Genital Herpes: 250mg bid for up to 1 yr. CrCl 20-39mL/min: 125mg q12h. CrCl <20mL/min: 125mg q24h. Hemodialysis: 125mg following dialysis. Recurrent Orolabial or Genital Herpes in HIV: 500mg bid for 7 days. CrCl <20mL/min: 250mg q24h. Hemodialysis: 250mg following dialysis. Recurrent Herpes Labialis: 1500mg as a single dose; CrCl 40-59mL/min: 750mg single dose; CrCl 20-39mL/min: 500mg single dose; CrCl <20mL/min: 20mg single dose; Hemodialysis: 250mg following dialysis

HOW SUPPLIED: Tab: 125mg, 250mg, 500mg

CONTRAINDICATIONS: Hypersensitivity to penciclovir cream.

WARNINGS/PRECAUTIONS: Prodrug of penciclovir. Dose adjustment in renal disease. Not indicated for initial episode of genital herpes infection, ophthalmic zoster, disseminated zoster or in immunocompromised patients with herpes zoster.

ADVERSE REACTIONS: Headache, migraine, nausea, diarrhea, vomiting, fatigue, urticaria, hallucinations, confusion.

INTERACTIONS: Increased plasma levels of penciclovir with probenecid and other drugs significantly eliminated by active renal tubular secretion. Potential interaction with drugs metabolized by aldehyde oxidase.

PREGNANCY: Category B, safety not known in nursing.

MECHANISM OF ACTION: Nucleoside analogue; inhibits HSV-2 DNA polymerase competitively with deoxyguanosine triphosphate, inhibiting herpes viral DNA synthesis and replication.

PHARMACOKINETICS: Absorption: Penciclovir: Absolute bioavailability (77%). **Distribution:** Penciclovir (IV) V_d=1.08L/kg; lasma protein binding (<20%) **Metabolism** Hepatic; deacetylation and oxidation; famciclovir (prodrug) converted to penciclovir. **Elimination:** Urine (73%), feces (27%). Penciclovir: Urine (94%); $T_{1/2}$=2-3 hrs.

FARESTON
toremifene citrate (GTX)

RX

THERAPEUTIC CLASS: Nonsteroidal triphenylethylene derivative

INDICATIONS: Treatment of metastatic breast cancer in postmenopausal women with estrogen-receptor positive or unknown tumors.

DOSAGE: *Adults:* Usual: 60mg qd. Treat until disease progression is evident.

HOW SUPPLIED: Tab: 60mg

WARNINGS/PRECAUTIONS: Hypercalcemia and tumor flare reported with bone metastases. Endometrial hyperplasia reported. Avoid with history of thromboembolic diseases. Do not treat long-term in pre-existing endometrial hyperplasia. Leukopenia and thrombocytopenia reported (rarely). May cause fetal harm with pregnancy.

ADVERSE REACTIONS: Hot flashes, sweating, nausea, vaginal discharge, dizziness, edema, vomiting, vaginal bleeding, cataracts, dry eyes, abnormal visual fields, elevated LFTs.

INTERACTIONS: Increased risk of hypercalcemia with drugs that decrease calcium excretion (eg, thiazide diuretics). CYP450 3A4 inducers (eg, pheno-barbital, phenytoin, carbamazepine) decrease serum levels. Increased PT with coumarin-type anticoagulants. CYP450 3A4-6 inhibitors (eg, ketoconazole, erythromycin) may inhibit metabolism.

PREGNANCY: Category D, safety in nursing not known.

MECHANISM OF ACTION: Nonsteroidal antiestrogen (triphenylethylene derivative); binds to estrogen receptors and believed to exert antiestro-genic effects, ie, ability to compete with estrogen for binding sites, blocking growth-stimulating effects of estrogen in tumor.

PHARMACOKINETICS: Absorption: T_{max}=3 hrs. **Distribution:** V_d=580L; plasma protein binding (>99.5%). **Metabolism:** Liver via CYP3A4: N-demethyltoremifene (major metabolite): **Elimination:** Feces (metabolites), urine (10%), $T_{1/2}$=5 days.

FASLODEX   RX
fulvestrant (AstraZeneca)

THERAPEUTIC CLASS: Estrogen receptor antagonist

INDICATIONS: Treatment of hormone receptor positive metastatic breast cancer in postmenopausal women with disease progression following anti-estrogen therapy.

DOSAGE: *Adults:* 250mg IM into buttock once monthly as either a single 5mL injection or two concurrent 2.5mL injections. Administer slowly.

HOW SUPPLIED: Inj: 50mg/mL [2.5mL, 5mL]

CONTRAINDICATIONS: Pregnancy.

WARNINGS/PRECAUTIONS: May cause fetal harm during pregnancy; women of childbearing age should be advised not to become pregnant and preg-nancy should be ruled out prior to initiating therapy. Avoid in patients with bleeding diatheses or thrombocytopenia. Safety and efficacy have not been studied in patients with moderate or severe hepatic impairment.

ADVERSE REACTIONS: Nausea, vomiting, constipation, diarrhea, abdominal pain, headache, back pain, vasodilatation (hot flushes), pharyngitis, injection site reactions, asthenia, pain, dyspnea, increased cough.

INTERACTIONS: Avoid with concurrent anticoagulants.

PREGNANCY: Category D, not for use in nursing.

MECHANISM OF ACTION: Estrogen receptor antagonist; binds to estrogen re-ceptor, and downregulates estrogen receptor protein in human breast cancer cells.

PHARMACOKINETICS: Absorption: C_{max}=8.5ng/mL; T_{max}=7 days; AUC=131ng•d/mL. **Distribution:** Plasma protein binding (99%); V_d=3-5L/kg. **Metabolism:** CYP3A4; oxidation, aromatic hydroxylation, conjugation. **Elimination:** Feces (90%), urine (<1%); $T_{1/2}$=40 days.

FAZACLO   RX
clozapine (Avanir)

> Risk of agranulocytosis, seizures, myocarditis, and other cardiovascular and respiratory effects. Obtain baseline WBC and ANC before initiation of therapy, regularly during treatment, and for 4 weeks after discontinuation. Increased mortality in elderly patients with dementia-related psychosis.

THERAPEUTIC CLASS: Dibenzapine derivative

INDICATIONS: Management of severe schizophrenia when response to standard schizophrenia treatment fails.

DOSAGE: *Adults:* Initial: 12.5mg qd-bid. Titrate: Increase by 25-50mg/day, up to 300-450mg/day by end of 2 weeks, then increase weekly or bi-weekly by increments up to 100mg. Usual 100-900mg/day given tid. Max: 900mg/day. To d/c, gradually reduce dose over 1-2 weeks. Monitor for psychotic symptoms if abrupt discontinuation warranted (eg, leukopenia).

HOW SUPPLIED: Tab, Disintegrating: 12.5mg, 25mg*, 50mg, 100mg* *scored

CONTRAINDICATIONS: Myeloproliferative disorders, uncontrolled epilepsy, history of clozapine-induced agranulocytosis or severe granulocytopenia, severe CNS depression, coma, or with other agents with potential to cause agranulocytosis or suppress bone marrow function.

WARNINGS/PRECAUTIONS: Reserve treatment for severely ill patients unresponsive to other schizophrenia therapies. Monitor for hyperglycemia, worsening of glucose control with DM and FBG levels with diabetes risk. Significant risk of orthostatic hypotension and tachycardia. May impair alertness with initial doses. May cause high fever or pulmonary embolism. Cardiomyopathy reported; d/c unless benefit outweighs risk. Caution with prostatic enlargement, narrow angle glaucoma and renal, hepatic, or cardiac/pulmonary disease. NMS, tardive dyskinesias, impaired intestinal peristalsis and ECG changes reported. Obtain WBC and ANC at baseline, then weekly for 1st six months of therapy, then every 2 weeks for next 6 months, and then every 4 weeks thereafter if counts are acceptable. Avoid treatment if WBCs <3500/mm^3 or ANC <2000/mm^3, history of myeloproliferative disorder, previous clozapine-induced agranulocytosis, or granulocytopenia. D/C treatment if WBCs <3000/mm^3, ANC <1500/mm^3, eosinophils >4000/mm^3, or if myocarditis develops. D/C over 1-2 weeks.

ADVERSE REACTIONS: Drowsiness, vertigo, headache, tremor, salivation, sweating, dry mouth, visual disturbances, tachycardia, hypotension, syncope, constipation, nausea, fever.

INTERACTIONS: Avoid with other bone marrow suppressants, epinephrine, and carbamazepine. Caution with CNS-active drugs, anesthesia, alcohol, paroxetine, fluoxetine, fluvoxamine, sertraline, benzodiazepines, other psychotropics, or inhibitors/inducers of CYP1A2, 2D6, 3A4. Dosage reduction may be needed with drugs metabolized by CYP2D6 (eg, antidepressants, phenothiazines, carbamazepine, Type 1C antiarrhythmics). May potentiate hypotensive effects of antihypertensives and anticholinergic effects of atropine-type drugs. Caution with general anesthesia. CYP450 inducers (eg, phenytoin, nicotine, carbamazepine, rifampin) may decrease plasma levels. CYP450 inhibitors (eg, cimetidine, caffeine, fluvoxamine, erythromycin) may increase plasma levels.

PREGNANCY: Category B, not for use in nursing.

MECHANISM OF ACTION: Atypical antipsychotic agent. Interferes with the binding of dopamine specifiacally at the D_1 and D_4 receptors. Also acts as an antagonist at the adrenergic, cholinergic, histaminergic, and serotonergic receptors.

PHARMACOKINETICS: Absorption: C_{max}=413ng/mL, T_{max}=2.3 hrs. **Metabolism:** CYP1A2, 2D6; demethylation, hydroxylation. **Distribution:** Plasma protein binding (97%). **Elimination:** Urine (50%), feces (30%); $T_{1/2}$=8 hrs (initial dose), 12 hrs (multiple doses).

FELBATOL RX
felbamate (MedPointe)

Associated with aplastic anemia and fatal hepatic failure. Monitor blood, LFTs. Avoid in history of hepatic dysfunction.

THERAPEUTIC CLASS: Dicarbamate anticonvulsant

INDICATIONS: Not for first line therapy. Monotherapy or adjunct therapy in partial seizures with and without generalization in adults. Adjunct therapy for partial and generalized seizures with Lennox-Gastaut syndrome in children.

DOSAGE: *Adults:* Initial Monotherapy: 300mg qid or 400mg tid. Titrate: Increase by 600mg every 2 weeks to 2.4g/day. Max: 3.6g/day. Initial Monotherapy Conversion/Adjunct Therapy: 300mg qid or 400mg tid while reducing present AED (see literature). Titrate: For conversion, increase at week 2 to 2.4g/day, at week 3 up to 3.6g/day. Adjunct Therapy: Increase by 1.2g/day every week up to 3.6mg/day. Renal Dysfunction: May need to reduce dose with concomitant AEDs.
Pediatrics: ≥14 yrs: Initial Monotherapy: 300mg qid or 400mg tid. Titrate: Increase by 600mg every 2 weeks to 2.4g/day. Max: 3.6g/day. Initial Monotherapy Conversion/Adjunct Therapy: 300mg qid or 400mg tid while reducing present AED (see literature). Titrate: For conversion, increase at week 2 to 2.4g/day, at week 3 up to 3.6g/day. Adjunct Therapy: Increase by 1.2g/day every week up to 3.6mg/day. 2-14 yrs: Lennox-Gastaut Adjunct Therapy: Initial: 15mg/kg/day in 3-4 divided doses. Titrate: Increase by 15mg/kg/day every week to 45mg/kg/day. Renal Dysfunction: May need to reduce dose with concomitant AEDs.

HOW SUPPLIED: Sus: 600mg/5mL [240mL, 960mL]; Tab: 400mg*, 600mg* *scored

CONTRAINDICATIONS: History of blood dyscrasias, hepatic dysfunction.

WARNINGS/PRECAUTIONS: Avoid abrupt discontinuation. Caution with renal dysfunction. Obtain written, informed consent. Obtain full hematologic evaluations and LFTs before, during, and after discontinuation. D/C if bone marrow depression or liver abnormalities occur.

ADVERSE REACTIONS: Anorexia, vomiting, insomnia, nausea, headache, anemias, hepatic failure.

INTERACTIONS: Increases plasma levels of phenytoin, valproate, active carbamazepine metabolite and phenobarbital. Decreases carbamazepine levels. Decreased felbamate levels with phenytoin, carbamazepine, and phenobarbital. Caution with OCs.

PREGNANCY: Category C, safety in nursing not known.

MECHANISM OF ACTION: Anticonvulsant; weak inhibitory effects on GABA-receptor binding and benzodiazepine receptor binding. Acts as an antagonist at the strychnine-insensitive glycine recognition site of the NMDA receptor-ionophore complex.

PHARMACOKINETICS: Absorption: Well-absorbed. **Distribution:** V_d=756mL/kg; plasma protein binding (22-25%). **Metabolism:** Parahydroxyfelbamate, 2-hydroxyfelbamate, felbamatemonocarbamate (metabolites, little activity). **Elimination:** Urine (40-50% unchanged); $T_{1/2}$=20-23 hrs.

FELDENE   RX
piroxicam (Pfizer)

NSAIDs may cause an increased risk of serious cardiovascular thrombotic events, MI, stroke and serious GI adverse events including bleeding, ulceration, and perforation of the stomach or intestines. Contraindicated for the treatment of perioperative pain in the setting of coronary artery bypass graft (CABG) surgery.

THERAPEUTIC CLASS: NSAID

INDICATIONS: Relief of signs and symptoms of osteoarthritis and rheumatoid arthritis.

DOSAGE: *Adults:* 20mg qd or 10mg bid. Elderly: Start at lower end of dosing range.

HOW SUPPLIED: Cap: 10mg, 20mg

CONTRAINDICATIONS: ASA or other NSAID allergy that precipitates asthma, urticaria, or other allergic type reactions. Treatment of perioperative pain in the setting of CABG surgery.

WARNINGS/PRECAUTIONS: May lead to onset of new HTN or worsening of pre-existing HTN; monitor BP closely. Fluid retention and edema reported; caution with fluid retention or heart failure. Renal papillary necrosis and other renal injury reported after long-term use. Not recommended for use with advanced renal disease; if therapy must be initiated, monitor renal function. Anaphylactoid reactions may occur. May cause serious skin adverse events (eg, exfoliative dermatitis, Stevens-Johnson syndrome, and toxic epidermal necrolysis). Avoid in late pregnancy; may cause premature closure of ductus arteriosis. May cause elevations of LFTs; d/c if liver disease develops or systemic manifestations occur. Caution in elderly. Anemia may occur; with long-term use, monitor Hgb/Hct if signs or symptoms of anemia develop. May inhibit platelet aggregation and prolong bleeding time; monitor with coagulation disorders. Caution with asthma and avoid with ASA-sensitive asthma. Adverse eye findings reported. Dermatological and/or allergic signs and symptoms suggestive of serum sickness have occurred. Risk of GI ulceration, bleeding, and perforation.

ADVERSE REACTIONS: Edema, dyspepsia, elevated liver enzymes, dizziness, rash, tinnitus, renal dysfunction, dry mouth, weight changes, increased bleeding time, GI bleeding/perforation, ulcers, heartburn, anorexia, abdominal pain.

INTERACTIONS: Synergistic GI bleeding effects with warfarin. Diminished effect with ASA and may increase adverse effects. May decrease antihypertensive effects of ACE inhibitors. May reduce natriuretic effect of furosemide and thiazides. May increase lithium and methotrexate levels; monitor for toxicity. May displace other protein bound drugs.

PREGNANCY: Category C, not for use in nursing.

MECHANISM OF ACTION: NSAID (piroxicam); suspected to inhibit prostaglandin synthetase, exerts anti-inflammatory, analgesic, and antipyretic actions.

PHARMACOKINETICS: Absorption: T_{max}=3-5 hrs. C_{max}=1.5-2mcg/mL. **Distribution:** V_d=0.14L/kg. Plasma protein binding (99%). **Metabolism:** Via hydroxylation, conjugation and cyclodehydration. **Elimination:** Urine (approximately 5%, unchanged), feces. $T_{1/2}$=approximately 50 hrs.

FEMARA   RX
letrozole (Novartis)

THERAPEUTIC CLASS: Nonsteroidal aromatase inhibitor

INDICATIONS: First-line treatment of hormone-receptor positive or hormone-receptor unknown locally advanced or metastatic breast cancer in postmenopausal women. Treatment of advanced breast cancer with disease progression following antiestrogen therapy in postmenopausal women. Extended adjuvant treatment of early breast cancer in postmenopausal women who have received 5 yrs of adjuvant tamoxifen therapy. Adjuvant treatment of postmenopausal women with hormone-receptor positive early breast cancer.

DOSAGE: *Adults:* 2.5mg qd. Continue until tumor progression is evident. Cirrhosis/Severe Liver Dysfunction: 2.5mg every other day.

HOW SUPPLIED: Tab: 2.5mg

CONTRAINDICATIONS: Women of premenopausal endocrine status.

WARNINGS/PRECAUTIONS: May cause fetal harm in pregnancy. May elevate LFTs and total cholesterol. May decrease bone density; monitor bone mineral density (BMD). Reduce dose in cirrhosis and severe liver dysfunction. May cause fatigue and dizziness; caution when driving or using machinery.

ADVERSE REACTIONS: Bone pain, back pain, nausea, arthralgia, dyspnea, fatigue, chest pain, decreased weight, hot flushes, peripheral edema, HTN, vomiting, constipation, diarrhea, musculoskeletal pain, insomnia, cough, alopecia.

INTERACTIONS: Coadministration with tamoxifen may reduce letrozole plasma levels; if coadministered, give letrozole immediately after tamoxifen.

PREGNANCY: Category D, caution in nursing.

MECHANISM OF ACTION: Nonsteroidal aromatase inhibitor; inhibits the conversion of androgens to estrogens and competitively binds to the heme of cytochrome P450 subunit of the enzyme, resulting in a reduction of estrogen biosynthesis in all tissues.

FEMHRT

PHARMACOKINETICS: Absorption: Rapid and complete (GI tract)
Distribution: V_d=1.9L/kg. Weakly protein bound. **Metabolism:** Liver via
CYP450 isoenzymes: 3A4, 2A6. **Elimination:** Urine 90% (6% unchanged);
$T_{1/2}$=2 days.

FEMHRT   RX
norethindrone acetate - ethinyl estradiol (Warner Chilcott)

> Estrogens and progestins should not be used for prevention of cardiovascular disease or
> dementia. Increased risks of MI, stroke, invasive breast cancer, PE, and DVT in postmeno-
> pausal women (50-79 yrs of age) reported. Increased risk of developing probable dementia in
> postmenopausal women ≥65 yrs of age reported.

THERAPEUTIC CLASS: Estrogen/progestogen combination

INDICATIONS: In women with an intact uterus, treatment of moderate to
severe vasomotor symptoms associated with menopause and prevention of
postmenopausal osteoporosis.

DOSAGE: *Adults:* Vasomotor Symptoms: 1 tab qd. Re-evaluate at 3-6 month
intervals. Osteoporosis Prevention: 1 tab qd. Assess response by measuring
bone mineral density.

HOW SUPPLIED: Tab: (Ethinyl Estradiol-Norethindrone) 2.5mcg-0.5mg,
5mcg-1mg

CONTRAINDICATIONS: Pregnancy, undiagnosed abnormal genital bleeding,
breast cancer, estrogen-dependent neoplasia, DVT/PE, thrombophlebitis,
thromboembolic disorders, active or recent (eg, within past year) arterial
thromboembolic disease (eg, stroke, MI).

WARNINGS/PRECAUTIONS: Risk of gallbladder disease, endometrial and
breast carcinoma, elevated BP, visual disturbances, thromboembolism, and
hypercalcemia with breast cancer or bone metastases. Possible risk of cardiovascular disease, ovarian cancer. Caution with liver dysfunction, asthma, epilepsy, migraine, depression, and cardiac or renal dysfunction. Increase in HDL,
triglycerides, thyroxine binding globulin. Hypercoagulability effects. Impaired
glucose tolerance. D/C if sudden onset of visual abnormalities or migraine.
May exacerbate endometriosis.

ADVERSE REACTIONS: Headache, back pain, abdominal pain, nausea, vomiting, breast pain, nervousness, depression, rhinitis, sinusitis, UTI, vaginitis.

INTERACTIONS: Increases plasma levels of cyclosporine, prednisolone, and
theophylline. May decrease plasma levels of acetaminophen. May increase
clearance of temazapam, salicylic acid, morphine, and clofibric acid. CYP3A4
inducers (eg, St. John's wort, phenobarbital, carbamazepine, rifampin) may
decrease levels which may decrease therapeutic effects and/or change uterine bleeding profile. CYP3A4 inhibitors (eg, erythromycin, clarithromycin, ketoconazole, itraconazole, ritonavir, grapefruit juice) may increase levels which
may result in side effects. Reduced response to metyrapone test.

PREGNANCY: Contraindicated in pregnancy, caution in nursing.

MECHANISM OF ACTION: Ethinyl estradiol: Estrogen; binds to nuclear receptors in estrogen-responsive tissues. Circulating estrogens modulate the
pituitary secretion of the gonadotrophins, luteinizing hormone and follicle
stimulating hormone, through a negative feedback mechanism. In postmenopausal women, reduces elevated levels of these hormones. Norethindrone:
Progestin; binds to specific progesterone receptors that interact with progesterone response elements in target genes. Responsible for enhancing cellular
differentiation and opposing the actions of estrogens by decreasing estrogen
receptor levels, increasing local metabolism of estrogens to less active metabolites, or inducing gene products that blunt cellular response to estrogen.

PHARMACOKINETICS: Absorption: Ethinyl estradiol, Norethindrone: Rapidly
absorbed; T_{max}=1-2 hrs; Norethindrone: Absolute bioavailability (64%); Ethinyl
estradiol: Absolute bioavailability (55%). **Distribution:** Plasma protein binding (>95%); V_d=2-4L/kg; found in breast milk. **Metabolism:** Norethindrone:
Extensive via reduction; sulfate and glucuronide conjugation. Ethinyl estradiol: Liver to estrone (metabolite) and estriol (major urinary metabolite);

oxidation and conjugation with sulfate and glucuronide (extensive); CYP3A4 to 2-hydroxyethinyl estradiol (primary oxidative metabolite). **Elimination:** Norethindrone: Urine, feces; $T_{1/2}$=13 hrs. Ethinyl estradiol: Urine, feces; $T_{1/2}$=24 hrs.

FEMRING   RX
estradiol acetate (Warner Chilcott)

> Estrogens increase the risk of endometrial cancer. Estrogens, with or without progestins, should not be used for the prevention of cardiovascular disease or dementia. Increased risks of MI, stroke, invasive breast cancer, PE, and DVT in postmenopausal women (50-79 yrs of age) reported. Increased risk of developing probable dementia in postmenopausal women ≥65 yrs of age reported.

THERAPEUTIC CLASS: Estrogen

INDICATIONS: Treatment of moderate to severe vasomotor symptoms and vulvar/vaginal atrophy associated with menopause. Consider other vaginal products if treating solely vulvar/vaginal symptoms.

DOSAGE: *Adults:* Initial: Use lowest effective dose. Insert ring vaginally. Replace every 3 months. Re-evaluate periodically.

HOW SUPPLIED: Vaginal Ring: 0.05mg/day, 0.1mg/day

CONTRAINDICATIONS: Undiagnosed abnormal genital bleeding, known/suspected/history of breast cancer (except in appropriately selected patients being treated for metastatic disease), estrogen-dependent neoplasia, active or history of DVT or pulmonary embolism, active or recent (within 1 yr) arterial thromboembolic disease (eg, stroke, MI), pregnancy.

WARNINGS/PRECAUTIONS: May increase risk of cardiovascular events (eg, MI, stroke), venous thrombosis, and PE; d/c immediately if any of these events occur or are suspected. May increase risk of breast/endometrial cancer, and gallbladder disease. Retinal vascular thrombosis reported; monitor and d/c if papilledema or retinal vascular lesions occur. Consider addition of a progestin if no hysterectomy. May elevate BP; monitor at regular intervals. May cause elevations of plasma triglycerides with pre-existing hypertriglyceridemia. Caution with history of cholestatic jaundice associated with past estrogen use or with pregnancy; d/c with recurrence. May lead to increased thyroid-binding globulin levels; monitor thyroid function. May cause fluid retention; caution with cardiac/renal dysfunction. Caution with severe hypocalcemia. May increase risk of ovarian cancer. May exacerbate endometriosis, asthma, DM, epilepsy, migraine, porphyria; use with caution. Few cases of toxic shock syndrome reported.

ADVERSE REACTIONS: Headache, intermenstrual bleeding, vaginal candidiasis, breast tenderness, back pain, abdominal distension, nausea, vulvovaginitis, uterine pain.

INTERACTIONS: CYP3A4 inducers (eg, St. John's wort, phenobarbital, carbamazepine, rifampin) may decrease levels which may decrease therapeutic effects and/or change uterine bleeding profile. CYP3A4 inhibitors (eg, erythromycin, clarithromycin, ketoconazole, itraconazole, ritonavir, grapefruit juice) may increase levels which may result in side effects. May require higher doses of thyroid hormone.

PREGNANCY: Contraindicated in pregnancy, caution in nursing.

MECHANISM OF ACTION: Estrogen; acts by binding to nuclear receptors in estrogen responsive tissues. Circulating estrogens modulate the pituitary secretion of the gonadotropins, luteinizing hormone and follicle stimulating hormone, through a negative feedback mechanism. In postmenopausal women, acts to reduce elevated levels of these hormones.

PHARMACOKINETICS: Absorption: Rapid. 0.05mg/day: C_{max}=1129pg/ml, T_{max}=1 hr. **Distribution:** Largely bound to sex hormone binding globulin and albumin; found in breast milk. **Metabolism:** Liver to estrone (metabolite) and estriol (major urinary metablite); sulfate and glucuronide conjugation (liver); gut hydrolysis; CYP3A4 (partial metabolism). **Elimination:** Urine (parent compound and metabolites). $T_{1/2}$=1-2 hr (parent), 4-18 hr (estrone).

FEMTRACE RX
estradiol acetate (Warner Chilcott)

> Estrogens increase risk of endometrial cancer. Estrogens, with or without progestins, should not be used for the prevention of cardiovascular disease. Increased risks of MI, stroke, invasive breast cancer, PE, and DVT in postmenopausal women (50-79 yrs of age) reported.

THERAPEUTIC CLASS: Estrogen

INDICATIONS: Treatment of moderate to severe vasomotor symptoms associated with menopause.

DOSAGE: *Adults:* 1 tab qd. Use lowest effective dose for shortest duration. Re-evaluate menopausal symptoms at 3-6 month intervals.

HOW SUPPLIED: Tab: 0.45mg, 0.9mg, 1.8mg

CONTRAINDICATIONS: Pregnancy, undiagnosed abnormal genital bleeding, breast cancer, estrogen-dependent neoplasia, DVT/PE, active or recent (eg, within past year) arterial thromboembolic disease (eg, stroke, MI), liver dysfunction or disease.

WARNINGS/PRECAUTIONS: May increase risk of cardiovascular events (eg, MI, stroke), venous thrombosis, and PE; d/c immediately if any of these events occur or are suspected. May increase risk of breast/endometrial cancer, and gallbladder disease. Retinal vascular thrombosis reported; monitor and d/c if papilledema or retinal vascular lesions occur. Consider addition of a progestin if no hysterectomy. May elevate BP; monitor at regular intervals. May cause elevations of plasma triglycerides with pre-existing hypertriglyceridemia. Caution with history of cholestatic jaundice associated with past estrogen use or with pregnancy; d/c with recurrence. May lead to increased thyroid-binding globulin levels; monitor thyroid function. May cause fluid retention; caution with cardiac/renal dysfunction. Caution with severe hypocalcemia. May increase risk of ovarian cancer. May exacerbate endometriosis, asthma, DM, epilepsy, migraine, porphyria; use with caution.

ADVERSE REACTIONS: Vaginal and intermenstrual bleeding, breast tenderness, influenza, vaginal discharge, fungal infection, abdominal and back pain, headache.

INTERACTIONS: CYP3A4 inducers (eg, St. John's wort, phenobarbital, carbamazepine, rifampin) may decrease levels which may decrease therapeutic effects and/or change uterine bleeding profile. CYP3A4 inhibitors (eg, erythromycin, clarithromycin, ketoconazole, itraconazole, ritonavir, grapefruit juice) may increase levels which may result in side effects.

PREGNANCY: Contraindicated in pregnancy, caution in nursing

MECHANISM OF ACTION: Estrogens; act by binding to nuclear receptors in estrogen responsive tissues. Circulating estrogens modulate the pituitary secretion of the gonadotrophins, luteinizing hormone and follicle stimulating hormone through a negative feedback mechanism. In postmenopausal women, acts to reduce elevated levels of these hormones.

PHARMACOKINETICS: Absorption: Rapidly absorbed. Oral administration of variable doses resulted in different parameters. **Distribution:** Largely bound to sex hormone binding globulin and to albumin; found in breast milk. **Metabolism:** Liver to estrone (metabolite) and estriol (major urinary metablite); sulfate and glucuronide conjugation (liver); gut hydrolysis; CYP3A4 (partial metabolism). **Elimination:** Urine (parent compound and metabolites); $T_{1/2}$=21-26 hrs.

FENOPROFEN RX
fenoprofen calcium (Various)

> NSAIDs may cause an increased risk of serious cardiovascular thrombotic events, MI, stroke and serious GI adverse events including bleeding, ulceration, and perforation of the stomach or intestines. Contraindicated for the treatment of perioperative pain in the setting of coronary artery bypass graft (CABG) surgery.

OTHER BRAND NAMES: Nalfon (Pedinol)

THERAPEUTIC CLASS: NSAID

INDICATIONS: Management of rheumatoid arthritis (RA) and osteoarthritis (OA). Relief of mild to moderate pain.

DOSAGE: *Adults:* RA/OA: 300-600mg tid-qid. Max: 3200mg/day. Pain: 200mg q4-6h prn. Take with food or milk with GI upset.

HOW SUPPLIED: Cap: 200mg, 300mg; Tab: 600mg

CONTRAINDICATIONS: Significantly impaired renal function. ASA or other NSAID allergy that precipitates asthma, rhinitis, or urticaria. Treatment of peri-operative pain in the setting of CABG surgery.

WARNINGS/PRECAUTIONS: May lead to onset of new HTN or worsening of pre-existing HTN; monitor BP closely. Fluid retention and edema reported; caution with fluid retention, compromised cardia function, or heart failure. Renal papillary necrosis and other renal injury reported after long-term use. Not recommended for use with advanced renal disease. Anaphylactoid reactions may occur. May cause serious skin adverse events (eg, exfoliative dermatitis, Stevens-Johnson syndrome, and toxic epidermal necrolysis). Avoid in late stregnancy; may cause premature closure of ductus arteriosus. May cause elevations of LFTs; d/c if liver disease develops or systemic manifestations occur. Caution in elderly. Anemia may occur; with long-term use, monitor Hgb/Hct if signs or symptoms of anemia develop. May inhibit platelet aggregation and prolong bleeding time; monitor with coagulation disorders. Caution with asthma and avoid with ASA-sensitive asthma. Perform eye exams if visual disturbances occur. Caution with activities requiring mental alertness. With long-term use, monitor auditory function in hearing impaired patients.

ADVERSE REACTIONS: Dyspepsia, constipation, nausea, somnolence, dizziness, vomiting, abdominal pain, headache, diarrhea.

INTERACTIONS: ASA or chronic phenobarbital may decrease effects. Avoid salicylates. May potentiate hydantoins, sulfonamides, and sulfonylureas. May prolong PT with coumarin-type anticoagulants. May cause resistance to the effects of loop diuretics. May diminish antihypertensive effect of ACE inhibitors. Increases lithium levels. May enhance methotrexate toxicity; caution with concomitant use.

PREGNANCY: Category C, not for use in nursing.

MECHANISM OF ACTION: NSAID. Suspected to inhibit prostaglandin synthetase. Exerts anti-inflammatory and antiarthritic actions.

PHARMACOKINETICS: Absorption: Rapidly absorbed. C_{max}=50μ/mL, T_{max}=2 hrs. **Distribution:** Plasma protein binding (99%). **Elimination:** Urine (90%), fenoprofen glucuronide and 4'-hydroxy-fenoprofen glucuronide (major metabolites).$T_{1/2}$=3 hrs.

FENTORA CII
fentanyl citrate (Cephalon)

> Abuse liability. May cause life-threatening respiratory depression in opioid non-tolerant patients. Contraindicated in the management of acute or postoperative pain. Do not use in opioid non-tolerant patients. Adjust dose appropriately when converting from other oral fentanyl products. See Indications.

THERAPEUTIC CLASS: Opioid analgesic

INDICATIONS: Management of breakthrough pain in patients with cancer who are already receiving and who are tolerant to opioid therapy for their underlying persistent cancer pain.

DOSAGE: *Adults:* Initial: Breakthrough Pain: 100mcg. Repeat once (30 min after starting dose) during a single pain episode. Titration Above 100mcg: Use two 100mcg tabs (one on each side of buccal cavity), if not controlled use two 100mcg tabs on each side (total four 100mcg tabs). Titration Above 400mcg: Use 200mcg tab increments. Max: Not more than 4 tabs simultaneously. Re-evaluate maintenance (around-the-clock) opioid dose if >4 episodes of breakthrough pain per day occured. Do not chew, crush, swallow, or dissolve;

consume over 14-25 min. Please see the PI for more information on conversion of dosage.

HOW SUPPLIED: Tab, Buccal: 100mcg, 200mcg, 400mcg, 600mcg, 800mcg

CONTRAINDICATIONS: Opioid non-tolerant patients and management of acute or postoperative pain.

WARNINGS/PRECAUTIONS: Caution with concomitant use of other CNS depressants may cause hypoventilation, hypotension, and profound sedation. Caution wtih COPD, bradyarrhythmias, and hepatic or renal impairment. May cause physical dependence, respiratory depression. Extreme caution with evidence of increased intracranial pressure or impaired consciousness. May cause paresthesia, ulceration, or bleeding at application site.

ADVERSE REACTIONS: Respiratory depression, circulatory depression, headache, hypotension, shock, nausea, vomiting, constipation, dizziness, dyspnea, anxiety, somnolence.

INTERACTIONS: Dangerous increases in plasma concentration with potent inhibitors of CYP3A4 (eg, ketoconazole, itraconazole, clarithromycin, nelfinavir, nefazodone, ritonavir), moderate inhibitors of CYP3A4 (eg, amprenavir, diltiazem, fluconazole). CYP3A4 inducers may reduce efficacy. Increased depressant effects with other CNS depressants, including opioids, sedatives, hypnotics, general anesthetics, phenothiazines, tranquilizers, skeletal muscle relaxants, sedating antihistamines. Avoid within 14 days of MAOIs.

PREGNANCY: Category C, not for use in nursing.

MECHANISM OF ACTION: Pure opioid agonist; produces analgesia. Precise mechanism of analgesic action is not established; known to be a μ opioid receptor agonist. Specific CNS opioid receptors for endogenous compounds with opioid-like activity are found throughout the brain and spinal cord and are involved in producing analgesic effects.

PHARMACOKINETICS: Absorption: Absolute bioavailability (65%). **Distribution:** Plasma protein binding (80-85%); V_d=25.4 L/kg; found in breast milk. **Metabolism:** Liver and intestinal mucosa via CYP3A4; norfentanyl (metabolite). **Elimination:** Urine (<7% unchanged), feces.

FEOSOL   OTC
ferrous sulfate - iron carbonyl (GlaxoSmithKline Consumer)

THERAPEUTIC CLASS: Iron supplement

INDICATIONS: Treatment of iron deficiency and iron deficiency anemia.

DOSAGE: *Adults:* 1 tab qd with food.
Pediatrics: ≥12 yrs: 1 tab qd with food.

HOW SUPPLIED: Tab: Feosol Caplet (Iron Carbonyl) 50mg (45mg elemental iron), Feosol Tablet (Ferrous Sulfate) 200mg (65mg elemental iron)

WARNINGS/PRECAUTIONS: Keep product out of reach of children. Accidental overdose of iron-containing products is a leading cause of fatal poisoning in children <6 yrs.

ADVERSE REACTIONS: Nausea, GI disturbance, constipation, diarrhea.

INTERACTIONS: Decreases absorption of tetracycline; space dose by 2 hrs.

PREGNANCY: Safety in pregnancy and nursing not known.

FERRLECIT   RX
sodium ferric gluconate complex (Watson)

THERAPEUTIC CLASS: Hematinic

INDICATIONS: Treatment of iron deficiency anemia in patients ≥6 yrs old undergoing chronic hemodialysis and receiving supplemental epoetin therapy.

DOSAGE: *Adults:* 10mL (125mg) as IV infusion (diluted) over 1 hr or as slow IV injection (undiluted) at a rate of up to 12.5mg/min. Minimum Cumulative Dose: 1g elemental iron over 8 sequential dialysis sessions.

Pediatrics: ≥6 yrs: 0.12mL/kg (1.5mg/kg) as IV infusion over 1 hr at 8 sequential dialysis sessions. Max: 125mg/dose.

HOW SUPPLIED: Inj: 62.5mg elemental iron/5mL

CONTRAINDICATIONS: Anemia not associated with iron deficiency. Iron overload.

WARNINGS/PRECAUTIONS: Hypersensitivity reactions and hypotension reported. Iron overload is more common in patients with hemoglobinopathies and other refractory anemia. Should not be administered to patients with iron overload. Contains benzyl alcohol; avoid in neonates.

ADVERSE REACTIONS: Injection site reactions, nausea, vomiting, diarrhea, hypotension, cramps, HTN, dizziness, dyspnea, abnormal erythrocytes, leg cramps, pain, chest pain.

PREGNANCY: Category B, caution in nursing.

MECHANISM OF ACTION: Hematinic; used to replete the total body content of iron, which is critical for normal Hgb synthesis to maintain oxygen transport.

PHARMACOKINETICS: Absorption: Adults: Parameters varied by different dosage. (62.5mg) AUC=17.5mg-h/L; (125mg) C_{max}=19mg/L; T_{max}=7 min; AUC=35.6mg-h/L. **Pediatrics:** (1.5mg/kg) C_{max}=12.9mg/L; T_{max}=2 hrs; AUC=95mg•h/L. (3mg/kg) C_{max}=22.8mg/L; T_{max}=2.5 hrs; AUC=170.9mg•h/L. **Distribution:** V_d=6L. **Elimination:** $T_{1/2}$=1 hr.

FINACEA   RX
azelaic acid (Intendis)

THERAPEUTIC CLASS: Dicarboxylic acid antimicrobial

INDICATIONS: Topical treatment of inflammatory papules and pustules of mild to moderate rosacea.

DOSAGE: *Adults:* Wash and dry skin. Massage gently into affected area bid (am and pm) for up to 12 weeks.

HOW SUPPLIED: Gel: 15% [30g]

CONTRAINDICATIONS: Hypersensitivity to propylene glycol.

WARNINGS/PRECAUTIONS: Avoid mouth, eyes, mucous membranes, occlusive dressings, or wrappings. Hypopigmentation reported. D/C if sensitivity or severe irritation occurs. Use only very mild soap or soapless cleansing lotion for facial cleansing. Avoid foods and beverages (eg, spicy foods, alcohol, thermally hot drinks) that may provoke erythema, flushing, and/or blushing.

ADVERSE REACTIONS: Burning, stinging, tingling, pruritus, scaling, dry skin.

INTERACTIONS: Avoid alcoholic cleansers, tinctures, astringents, abrasives and peeling agents.

PREGNANCY: Category B, caution in nursing.

MECHANISM OF ACTION: Dicarboxylic acid antimicrobial; not established.

PHARMACOKINETICS: Absorption: C_{max}=24.0-90.5ng/mL. **Elimination:** Urine (mainly unchanged).

FINEVIN   RX
azelaic acid (Bayer Healthcare)

THERAPEUTIC CLASS: Dicarboxylic acid antimicrobial

INDICATIONS: Mild-to-moderate inflammatory acne vulgaris.

DOSAGE: *Adults:* Wash and dry skin. Massage gently into affected area bid (am and pm).
Pediatrics: ≥12 yrs: Wash and dry skin. Massage gently into affected area bid (am and pm).

HOW SUPPLIED: Cre: 20% [30g, 50g]

WARNINGS/PRECAUTIONS: Hypopigmentation reported after use. Avoid the mouth, eyes, mucous membranes, occlusive dressings, or wrappings.

ADVERSE REACTIONS: Pruritus, burning, stinging, tingling.

PREGNANCY: Category B, caution in nursing.

FIORICET RX
acetaminophen - caffeine - butalbital (Watson)

THERAPEUTIC CLASS: Barbiturate/analgesic

INDICATIONS: Tension or muscle contraction headaches.

DOSAGE: *Adults:* 1-2 tabs q4h prn. Max: 6 tabs/day. Not for extended use. *Pediatrics:* ≥12 yrs: 1-2 tabs q4h prn. Max: 6 tabs/day. Not for extended use.

HOW SUPPLIED: Tab: (Butalbital-APAP-Caffeine) 50mg-325mg-40mg

CONTRAINDICATIONS: Porphyria.

WARNINGS/PRECAUTIONS: May be habit forming. Not for extended use. Caution in elderly, debilitated, severe renal or hepatic impairment, acute abdominal conditions. Caution in mentally depressed and suicidal tendencies, history of drug abuse.

ADVERSE REACTIONS: Drowsiness, lightheadedness, dizziness, sedation, SOB, NV, abdominal pain, intoxicated feeling.

INTERACTIONS: Enhanced CNS effects with MAOIs. May enhance CNS depressant effects of other narcotic analgesics, alcohol, general anesthetics, tranquilizers, sedative hypnotics, or other CNS depressants.

PREGNANCY: Category C, not for use in nursing.

MECHANISM OF ACTION: Butalbital: Short to intermediate acting barbiturate. APAP: Nonopiate, nonsalicylate analgesic, antipyretic. Caffeine: CNS stimulant.

PHARMACOKINETICS: Absorption: Well absorbed (butalbital), rapid (APAP, caffeine). **Distribution:** Butalbital: Plasma protein binding (45%); found in breast milk; crosses placenta. Caffeine: Found in CNS, placenta, and breast milk. **Metabolism:** APAP: Liver (conjugation). Caffeine: Hepatic; 1-methylxanthine, 1-methyluric acid. **Elimination:** Butalbital: Urine (59-88% unchanged or metabolite); $T_{1/2}$=35 hrs. APAP: Urine (85% metabolite, unchanged); $T_{1/2}$=1.25-3 hrs. Caffeine: Urine 70% (3% unchanged); $T_{1/2}$=3 hrs.

FIORICET WITH CODEINE CIII
codeine phosphate - acetaminophen - caffeine - butalbital (Watson)

THERAPEUTIC CLASS: Barbiturate/analgesic

INDICATIONS: Tension or muscle contraction headaches.

DOSAGE: *Adults:* 1-2 caps q4h prn. Max: 6 caps/day. Not for extended use.

HOW SUPPLIED: Cap: (Butalbital-APAP-Caffeine-Codeine) 50mg-325mg-40mg-30mg

CONTRAINDICATIONS: Porphyria.

WARNINGS/PRECAUTIONS: May be habit forming. Not for extended use. Respiratory depression and CSF pressure enhanced with head injury or intracranial lesions. Caution in elderly, debilitated, severe renal or hepatic impairment, hypothyroidism, urethral stricture, Addison's disease, BPH, and history of drug abuse. May mask signs of acute abdominal conditions.

ADVERSE REACTIONS: Drowsiness, lightheadedness, dizziness, sedation, SOB, NV, abdominal pain, intoxicated feeling.

INTERACTIONS: Enhanced CNS effects with MAOIs. May enhance CNS depressant effects of other narcotic analgesics, alcohol, general anesthetics, tranquilizers, sedative hypnotics, or other CNS depressants.

PREGNANCY: Category C, not for use in nursing.

MECHANISM OF ACTION: Codeine: Narcotic analgesic and antitussive. Butalbital: Short to intermediate acting barbiturate. Caffeine: CNS stimulant. APAP: Nonopiate, nonsalicylate analgesic and antipyretic. The role each component plays in relief of complex of symptoms known as tension headache is incompletely understood.

PHARMACOKINETICS: Absorption: Butalbital: Well absorbed. Codeine, caffeine, acetaminophen: Rapid. **Distribution:** Codeine: Crosses blood-brain barrier, found in fetal tissue, breast milk. Butalbital: Plasma protein binding (45%); found in breast milk; crosses placental barrier. Caffeine: Found in fetal tissue, CNS, breast milk. **Metabolism:** Caffeine: Hepatic biotransformation to 1-methylxanthine, 1-methyluric acid. APAP: Liver (conjugation). **Elimination:** Codeine: Urine (90%), feces; $T_{1/2}$=2.9 hrs. Butalbital: Urine (59-88% unchanged or metabolites); $T_{1/2}$=35 hrs. Caffeine: Urine (70%, only 3% unchanged); $T_{1/2}$=3 hrs. APAP: Urine (85% unchanged, conjugates); $T_{1/2}$=1.25-3 hrs.

FIORINAL
caffeine - aspirin - butalbital (Watson)

CIII

THERAPEUTIC CLASS: Barbiturate/analgesic

INDICATIONS: Tension or muscle contraction headache.

DOSAGE: *Adults:* 1-2 caps q4h prn. Max: 6 caps/day. Not for extended use.

HOW SUPPLIED: Cap: (Butalbital-ASA-Caffeine) 50mg-325mg-40mg

CONTRAINDICATIONS: Porphyria, peptic ulcer disease, serious GI lesions, hemorrhagic diathesis. Syndrome of nasal polyps, angioedema, and bronchospastic reactivity to ASA or NSAIDs.

WARNINGS/PRECAUTIONS: May be habit-forming. Not for extended use. Caution in elderly, debilitated, severe renal or hepatic impairment, hypothyroidism, urethral stricture, head injuries, elevated ICP, acute abdominal conditions, Addison's disease, prostatic hypertrophy, peptic ulcer, coagulation disorders. Avoid with ASA allergy. Risk of ASA hypersensitivity with nasal polyps and asthma. Caution in children with chickenpox or flu. Preoperative ASA may prolong bleeding time.

ADVERSE REACTIONS: Drowsiness, lightheadedness, dizziness, sedation, nausea, vomiting, flatulence.

INTERACTIONS: CNS effects enhanced by MAOIs. Additive CNS depression with alcohol, other narcotic analgesics, general anesthetics, tranquilizers (eg, chloral hydrate), sedatives/hypnotics, other CNS depressants. May enhance effects of anticoagulants. May cause hypoglycemia with oral antidiabetic agents and insulin. May cause bone marrow toxicity and blood dyscrasias with 6-MP and methotrexate. Increased risk of peptic ulceration and bleeding with NSAIDs. Decreased effects of uricosuric agents (eg, probenecid, sulfinpyrazone). Withdrawal of corticosteroids may cause salicylism with chronic ASA use.

PREGNANCY: Category C, not for use in nursing.

MECHANISM OF ACTION: Combines analgesic properties of ASA with anxiolytic and muscle relaxant properties of butalbital.

PHARMACOKINETICS: Absorption: ASA: T_{max}=40 min, C_{max}=8.8mcg/mL. Butalbital: Well-absorbed; C_{max}=202ng/mL, T_{max}=1.5 hrs. Caffeine: Rapid; C_{max}=1660ng/mL, T_{max}≤1 hr. **Distribution:** ASA: Found in fetal tissue, breast milk, CNS; Plasma protein binding (50-80%). Butalbital: Crosses placenta, found in breast milk; Plasma protein binding (45%). Caffeine: Found in placenta, breast milk, CNS. **Metabolism:** ASA: Liver; salicyluric acid, phenolic/acyl glucuronides of salicylate, and gentisic and gentisuric acid (major metabolites). Caffeine: Liver; 1-methylxanthine and 1-methyluric acid (metabolites). **Elimination:** ASA: Urine; $T_{1/2}$=12 min (ASA), 3 hrs (salicylic acid/total salicylates). Butalbital: Urine (59-88%); $T_{1/2}$=35 hrs. Caffeine: Urine 70% (3% unchanged); $T_{1/2}$=3 hrs.

FIORINAL WITH CODEINE

CIII

codeine phosphate - caffeine - aspirin - butalbital (Watson)

THERAPEUTIC CLASS: Barbiturate/analgesic

INDICATIONS: Tension or muscle contraction headache.

DOSAGE: *Adults:* 1-2 caps q4h prn. Max: 6 caps/day. Not for extended use.

HOW SUPPLIED: Cap: (Butalbital-ASA-Caffeine-Codeine) 50mg-325mg-40mg-30mg

CONTRAINDICATIONS: Porphyria, peptic ulcer disease, serious GI lesions, hemorrhagic diathesis. Syndrome of nasal polyps, angioedema and bronchospastic reactivity to ASA or NSAIDs.

WARNINGS/PRECAUTIONS: May be habit-forming. Not for extended use. Respiratory depression and CSF pressure may be enhanced with head injury or intracranial lesions. Caution in elderly, debilitated, severe renal or hepatic impairment, hypothyroidism, urethral stricture, head injuries, elevated ICP, acute abdominal conditions, Addison's disease, prostatic hypertrophy, peptic ulcer, coagulation disorders. Caution in children with chickenpox or flu. May obscure acute abdominal conditions. Preoperative ASA may prolong bleeding time. Avoid with ASA allergy. Risk of ASA hypersensitivity with nasal polyps and asthma.

ADVERSE REACTIONS: Drowsiness, lightheadedness, dizziness, sedation, shortness of breath, nausea, vomiting, abdominal pain, intoxicated feeling.

INTERACTIONS: CNS effects enhanced by MAOIs. Additive CNS depression with alcohol, other narcotic analgesics, general anesthetics, tranquilizers (eg, chloral hydrate), sedatives/hypnotics, other CNS depressants. May enhance effects of anticoagulants. May cause hypoglycemia with oral antidiabetic agents, insulin. May cause bone marrow toxicity, blood dyscrasias with 6-MP and methotrexate. Increased risk of peptic ulceration, bleeding with NSAIDs. Decreased effects of uricosuric agents (eg, probenecid, sulfinpyrazone). Withdrawal of corticosteroids may cause salicylism with chronic ASA use.

PREGNANCY: Category C, not for use in nursing.

MECHANISM OF ACTION: Butalbital: short- to intermediate-acting barbiturate. ASA: analgesic, antipyretic, and anti-inflammatory. Caffeine: stimulates CNS. Codeine: narcotic analgesic and antitussive. Role each component plays in relief of complex of symptoms known as tension headache is incompletely understood.

PHARMACOKINETICS: Absorption: Codeine: Rapid; C_{max}=198ng/mL, T_{max}=1 hr. Butalbital: Well-absorbed. C_{max}=2020ng/mL, T_{max}=1.5 hrs. Caffeine: Rapid; C_{max}=1660ng/mL, T_{max}≤1 hr. **Distribution:** ASA: Found in fetal tissue, breast milk, CNS; Plasma protein binding (50-80%). Codeine: crosses BBB, placenta and breast milk. Butalbital: crosses placenta and breast milk; Plasma protein binding (45%). Caffeine: fetal tissue, breast milk and CNS. **Metabolism:** ASA: Liver; salicyluric acid, phenolic/acyl glucuronides of salicylate, and gentisic and gentisuric acid (major metabolites). Codeine: Glucuronidation. Caffeine: Liver; 1-methylxanthine and 1-methyluric acid. **Elimination:** ASA: Urine $T_{1/2}$= 12 min (ASA), 3 hrs (salicylic acid/total salicylate). Codeine: Urine (90%), feces; $T_{1/2}$=2.9 hrs. Butalbital: Urine (59-88%); $T_{1/2}$=35 hrs. Caffeine: Urine 70% (3% unchanged); $T_{1/2}$=3 hrs.

FLAGYL

RX

metronidazole (G.D. Searle)

> Metronidazole has been shown to be carcinogenic in mice and rats. Unnecessary use of the drug should be avoided.

THERAPEUTIC CLASS: Nitroimidazole

INDICATIONS: Treatment of symptomatic/asymptomatic trichomoniasis, asymptomatic consorts, acute intestinal amebiasis, amebic liver abscess, and anaerobic bacterial infections (following IV metronidazole therapy for serious infections) caused by susceptible strains of microorganisms. Treatment of intra-abdominal, skin and skin structure, bone/joint, CNS, lower respiratory tract, and gynecologic infections, septicemia, and endocarditis caused by susceptible strains of microorganisms.

DOSAGE: *Adults:* Trichomoniasis (Female/Male Sex Partner): Seven-Day Treatment: (Cap/Tab) 375mg bid or 250mg tid for 7 days. One-Day Therapy: (Tab) 2g as single dose or in two divided doses of 1g each given in the same day. If repeat course needed, reconfirm diagnosis and allow 4-6 weeks between courses. Acute Intestinal Amebiasis: 750mg PO tid for 5-10 days. Amebic Liver Abscess: 500mg or 750mg PO tid for 5-10 days. Anaerobic Bacterial Infection: Usually IV therapy initially if serious. 7.5mg/kg PO q6h for 7-10 days or longer. Max: 4g/24 hrs. Elderly: Adjust dose based on serum levels. Hepatic Disease: Give lower dose cautiously; monitor levels. *Pediatrics:* Amebiasis: 35-50mg/kg/24 hrs given tid for 10 days.

HOW SUPPLIED: Cap: 375mg; Tab: 250mg, 500mg

CONTRAINDICATIONS: Treatment during 1st trimester of pregnancy.

WARNINGS/PRECAUTIONS: Seizures and peripheral neuropathy reported. D/C if abnormal neurological signs occur. Caution with severe hepatic impairment, blood dyscrasias, or CNS diseases. Monitor leukocytes before and after therapy.

ADVERSE REACTIONS: Seizures, peripheral neuropathy, nausea, vomiting, headache, anorexia, urticaria, rash, metallic taste, dysuria, vaginal candidiasis, dizziness, leukopenia.

INTERACTIONS: Avoid alcohol during and for 3 days after use. Avoid within 2 weeks of disulfiram use; increased possibility of psychotic reactions. May potentiate anticoagulant effects of warfarin; monitor PT. Increased elimination with phenytoin, phenobarbital and other hepatic enzyme inducers. May impair phenytoin clearance. Potentiated by cimetidine and other hepatic enzyme inhibitors. May increase lithium levels.

PREGNANCY: Category B, not for use in nursing.

MECHANISM OF ACTION: Nitroimidazole antibacterial; exerts effect in anaerobic environment. Possesses bactericidal, amebicidal, and trichomonacidal activity.

PHARMACOKINETICS: Absorption: (PO) Well absorbed. PO administration of variable doses resulted in different parameters. **Distribution:** Plasma protein binding (<20%); excreted in breast milk. **Metabolism:** Side-chain oxidation and glucuronide conjugation. **Elimination:** Urine (60-80%), feces (6-15%); T$_{1/2}$=8 hrs.

FLAGYL ER   RX
metronidazole (Pharmacia & Upjohn)

> Metronidazole has been shown to be carcinogenic in mice and rats. Unnecessary use of the drug should be avoided.

THERAPEUTIC CLASS: Nitroimidazole

INDICATIONS: Treatment of bacterial vaginosis.

DOSAGE: *Adults:* 750mg qd for 7 days. Take 1 hr before or 2 hrs after meals. Elderly: Adjust dose based on serum levels. Hepatic Disease: Give lower dose cautiously; monitor levels.

HOW SUPPLIED: Tab, Extended-Release: 750mg

CONTRAINDICATIONS: Treatment during 1st trimester of pregnancy.

WARNINGS/PRECAUTIONS: Seizures and peripheral neuropathy reported. D/C if abnormal neurological signs occur. Caution with severe hepatic impairment, blood dyscrasias, or CNS diseases. Monitor leukocytes before and after therapy.

ADVERSE REACTIONS: Headache, vaginitis, nausea, metallic taste, dizziness, seizures, peripheral neuropathy, vomiting, leukopenia, urticaria, rash, dysuria, vaginal candidiasis.

INTERACTIONS: Avoid alcohol during and for 3 days after use. Avoid within 2 weeks of disulfiram; increased possibility of psychotic reactions. Potentiates anticoagulant effects of warfarin; monitor PT. Increased elimination with phenytoin, phenobarbital. May impair phenytoin clearance. Potentiated by cimetidine. Increased lithium levels.

PREGNANCY: Category B, not for use in nursing.

MECHANISM OF ACTION: Nitroimidazole antibacterial; exerts effect in anaerobic environment. Possesses bactericidal, amebicidal, and trichomonacidal activity.

PHARMACOKINETICS: Absorption: AUC=211μg/mL (fed), 198μg/mL (fasting); C_{max}=19.4μg/mL (fed), 12.5μg/mL (fasting); T_{max}=4 hrs (fed), 6.8 hrs (fasting). **Distribution:** Plasma protein binding (<20%). **Metabolism:** Side-chain oxidation and glucuronide conjugation. **Elimination:** $T_{1/2}$=8 hrs. Urine (60-80%), feces (6-15%).

FLAGYL IV   RX
metronidazole HCL (Various)

> Metronidazole has been shown to be carcinogenic in mice and rats. Unnecessary use of the drug should be avoided.

THERAPEUTIC CLASS: Nitroimidazole

INDICATIONS: Treatment of serious infections caused by susceptible anaerobic bacteria. Treatment of intra-abdominal, skin and skin structure, gynecologic, bone and joint, CNS, and lower respiratory tract infections; bacterial septicemia; and endocarditis caused by susceptible microorganisms. Prophylaxis of infection in contaminated or potentially contaminated colorectal surgery.

DOSAGE: *Adults:* Anaerobic Infections: LD: 15mg/kg IV. Maint: 7.5mg/kg IV q6h, starting 6 hrs after LD. Usual duration is 7-10 days or longer. Max: 4g/24 hrs. Surgical Prophylaxis: 15mg/kg given 1 hr before surgery, then 7.5mg/kg given 6 hrs and 12 hrs after initial dose.

HOW SUPPLIED: Inj: 500mg/100mL

WARNINGS/PRECAUTIONS: Seizures and peripheral neuropathy reported. D/C if abnormal neurological signs occur. Caution with severe hepatic impairment, blood dyscrasias, or CNS disease. Monitor leukocytes before and after therapy. Metronidazole IV is effective in *B.fragilis* infections resistant to clindamycin, chloramphenicol, or PCN.

ADVERSE REACTIONS: Convulsive seizures, peripheral neuropathy, nausea, vomiting, headache, leukopenia, rash, vaginal candidiasis, thrombophlebitis.

INTERACTIONS: Avoid alcohol during and for 3 days after use. Avoid within 2 weeks of disulfiram; increased possibility of psychotic reactions. Potentiates warfarin. Increased elimination with phenytoin, phenobarbital. May impair phenytoin clearance. Potentiated by cimetidine. Increased lithium levels.

PREGNANCY: Category B, not for use in nursing.

MECHANISM OF ACTION: Nitroimidazole antibacterial; exerts effect in anaerobic environment. Possesses bactericidal, amebicidal, and trichomonacidal activity.

PHARMACOKINETICS: Distribution: Plasma protein binding (<20%); found in breast milk. **Metabolism:** Liver via side-chain oxidation and glucuronide conjugation. **Elimination:** Urine (60-80%), feces (6-15%); $T_{1/2}$=8 hrs.

FLECTOR
diclofenac epolamine (IBSA)

RX

> NSAIDs may cause an increased risk of serious cardiovascular thrombotic events, MI, stroke and serious GI adverse events including bleeding, ulceration, and perforation of the stomach or intestines. Contraindicated for the treatment of perioperative pain in the setting of coronary artery bypass graft (CABG) surgery.

THERAPEUTIC CLASS: NSAID (benzeneacetic acid derivative)

INDICATIONS: Topical treatment of acute pain due to minor strains, sprains, and contusions.

DOSAGE: *Adults:* Apply 1 patch to most painful area bid.

HOW SUPPLIED: Patch: 180mg [5*]

CONTRAINDICATIONS: ASA or other NASID allergy that precipitates asthma, urticaria, or allergic-type reactions. Treatment of perioperative pain in the setting of CABG surgery. Application to non-intact or damaged skin (eg, exudative dermatitis, eczema, infected lesion, burns or wounds).

WARNINGS/PRECAUTIONS: May lead to onset of new HTN or worsening of pre-existing HTN; monitor BP closely. Fluid retention and edema reported; caution with fluid retention or heart failure. Renal papillary necrosis and other renal injury reported after long-term use. Not recommended for use with advanced renal disease; if therapy must be initiated, monitor renal function. Anaphylactoid reactions may occur. May cause serious skin adverse events (eg, exfoliative dermatitis, Stevens-Johnson syndrome, and toxic epidermal necrolysis). Avoid in late pregnancy; may cause premature closure of ductus arteriosus. May cause elevations of LFTs; d/c if liver disease develops or systemic manifestations occur. Rare cases of severe hepatic reactions (eg, jaundice, fatal fulminant hepatitis, liver necrosis, hepatic failure) reported. Anemia may occur; with long-term use, monitor Hgb/Hct if signs or symptoms of anemia develop. May inhibit platelet aggregation and prolong bleeding time; monitor with coagulation disorders. Caution with asthma and avoid with ASA-sensitive asthma. Wash hands after applying, handling, or removing patch. Avoid contact with eye and mucosa.

ADVERSE REACTIONS: Pruritus, dermatitis, burning, nausea, dysgeusia, dyspepsia, headache, paresthesia, somnolence.

INTERACTIONS: May diminish the antihypertensive effect of ACE inhibitors. Increased adverse effects with ASA; avoid use. May reduce natriuretic effect of furosemide and thiazides; monitor for renal failure. May enhance lithium and methotrexate toxicity; caution when co-administering. Synergistic effects on GI bleeding with warfarin.

PREGNANCY: Category C, not for use in nursing.

MECHANISM OF ACTION: NSAID; not established. Suspected to inhibit prostaglandin synthetase.

PHARMACOKINETICS: Absorption: C_{max}=0.7-6ng/mL, T_{max}=10-20 hrs. **Ditribution:** Plasma protein binding (>99%). **Elimination:** Urine, bile; $T_{1/2}$=12 hrs.

FLEET BISACODYL
bisacodyl (Fleet)

OTC

THERAPEUTIC CLASS: Stimulant laxative

INDICATIONS: Relief of occasional constipation. For bowel cleansing for X-ray and endoscopic exam. Laxative in postoperative, antepartum, or postpartum care.

DOSAGE: *Adults:* (Enema) Use 1 rectally single dose qd. (Sup) Insert 1 rectally qd. Retain for 15-20 min. (Tab) 2-3 tabs single dose qd. Swallow tabs whole; do not chew or crush.
Pediatrics: ≥12 yrs: (Enema) Use 1 rectally single dose qd. (Sup) Insert 1 rectally qd. Retain for 15-20 min. (Tab) 2-3 tabs single dose qd. 6-11 yrs: (Sup) Insert

1/2 sup rectally qd. Retain for 15-20 min. (Tab) 1 tab qd. Swallow tabs whole; do not chew or crush.

HOW SUPPLIED: Enema: 10mg; Sup: 10mg; Tab, Delayed-Release: 5mg

WARNINGS/PRECAUTIONS: Do not use with nausea, vomiting, or abdominal pain. Rectal bleeding or failure to have a bowel movement after use may indicate a serious condition. Should not be used longer than 1 week.

ADVERSE REACTIONS: Abdominal discomfort, faintness, cramps.

INTERACTIONS: Do not administer tabs within 1 hr after taking an antacid, milk, or milk products.

PREGNANCY: Safety in pregnancy and nursing is not known.

FLEET GLYCERIN LAXATIVES OTC
glycerin (Fleet)

THERAPEUTIC CLASS: Laxative

INDICATIONS: Relief of constipation.

DOSAGE: *Adults:* 1 enema (5.6g) or 1 suppository (2g or 3g) rectally. *Pediatrics:* 2-5 yrs: 1 enema (2.3g) or 1 suppository (1g) rectally. ≥ 6 yrs: 1 enema (5.6g) or 1 suppository (2g or 3g) rectally.

HOW SUPPLIED: Enema: (Babylax) 2.3g, (Liquid Glycerin) 5.6g; Sup: 1g, 2g, 3g

WARNINGS/PRECAUTIONS: Rectal irritation may occur. Do not use with nausea, vomiting, or abdominal pain. Rectal bleeding or failure to have a bowel movement after use may indicate a serious condition. Do not use longer than 1 week.

ADVERSE REACTIONS: Rectal discomfort, burning sensation.

PREGNANCY: Safety in pregnancy and nursing in not known.

FLEXERIL RX
cyclobenzaprine HCL (McNeil Consumer)

THERAPEUTIC CLASS: Skeletal muscle relaxant (central-acting)

INDICATIONS: Relief of muscle spasm associated with acute, painful musculoskeletal conditions.

DOSAGE: *Adults:* Usual: 5mg tid. Titrate: May increase to 10mg tid. Mild Hepatic Dysfunction/Elderly: Initial: 5mg qd, then slowly increase. Moderate/Severe Hepatic Dysfunction: Avoid use. Treatment should not exceed 2-3 weeks.
Pediatrics: ≥15 yrs: Usual: 5mg tid. Titrate: May increase to 10mg tid. Mild Hepatic Dysfunction/Elderly: Initial: 5mg qd, then slowly increase. Moderate/Severe Hepatic Dysfunction: Avoid use. Treatment should not exceed 2-3 weeks.

HOW SUPPLIED: Tab: 5mg, 10mg

CONTRAINDICATIONS: Acute recovery phase of MI, arrhythmias, heart block or conduction disturbances, CHF, hyperthyroidism, MAOI use during or within 14 days.

WARNINGS/PRECAUTIONS: Caution with history of urinary retention, angle-closure glaucoma, increased IOP, hepatic dysfunction. Caution in elderly due to increased risk of CNS effects. May produce arrhythmias, sinus tachycardia and conduction time prolongation. May impair mental/physical abilities.

ADVERSE REACTIONS: Drowsiness, dry mouth, headache, fatigue.

INTERACTIONS: Enhances effects of alcohol, barbiturates, and other CNS depressants. May block antihypertensive action of guanethidine and similar compounds. May enhance seizure risk with tramadol. Contraindicated with MAOIs. Caution with anticholinergic medication.

PREGNANCY: Category B, caution in nursing.

MECHANISM OF ACTION: Centrally acting skeletal muscle relaxant; relieves skeletal muscle spasm of local origin without interfering with muscle function; reduces tonic somatic motor activity by influencing both gamma and α motor systems.

PHARMACOKINETICS: Absorption: Oral bioavailability (33-55%). C_{max}=25.9ng/mL, AUC=177ng•hr/mL. **Metabolism:** Extensive; through N-demethylation pathway. Via CYP3A4, 1A2, and 2D6. **Elimination:** Urine (glucuronides); $T_{1/2}$=18 hrs.

FLOLAN   RX
epoprostenol sodium (GlaxoSmithKline)

THERAPEUTIC CLASS: Pulmonary and systemic vasodilator

INDICATIONS: Long-term treatment of primary pulmonary hypertension and pulmonary hypertension associated with the scleroderma spectrum of disease in NYHA Class III and IV patients inadequately responding to conventional therapy.

DOSAGE: *Adults:* Initial: 2ng/kg/min IV chronic infusion. Titrate: Increase by 2ng/kg/min every 15 min until no further increases are clinically warranted. May use a lower initial infusion rate if not tolerated.

HOW SUPPLIED: Inj: 0.5mg, 1.5mg

CONTRAINDICATIONS: Chronic use in CHF due to left ventricular systolic dysfunction, chronic therapy in patients who develop pulmonary edema during dose initiation.

WARNINGS/PRECAUTIONS: Abrupt withdrawal or large dose reductions may result in symptoms associated with rebound pulmonary HTN (eg, dyspnea, dizziness, and asthenia); avoid abrupt withdrawal. Unless contraindicated, administer anticoagulant therapy to reduce risk of pulmonary thromboembolism or systemic embolism through a patent foramen ovale. Monitor standing and supine BP and HR for several hours after dose adjustments.

ADVERSE REACTIONS: Flushing, headache, nausea, vomiting, hypotension, anxiety, nervousness, agitation, chest pain, dizziness, bradycardia, abdominal pain.

INTERACTIONS: Potentiates BP reduction with diuretics, antihypertensives, vasodilators. Increased risk of bleeding with antiplatelets or anticoagulants.

PREGNANCY: Category B, caution in nursing.

MECHANISM OF ACTION: Prostaglandin: Causes direct vasodilation of pulmonary and systemic arterial vascular beds; inhibits platelet aggregation.

PHARMACOKINETICS: No available chemical assay sufficient to assess in vivo human pharmacokinetics. **Metabolism:** Spontaneous degradation (6-keto-$PGF_1\alpha$); enzymatic conversion (6,15-diketo-13,14-dihydro-$PGF_1\alpha$).

FLOMAX   RX
tamsulosin HCL (Astellas/Boehringer Ingelheim)

THERAPEUTIC CLASS: $Alpha_{1a}$-antagonist

INDICATIONS: Treatment of signs and symptoms of benign prostatic hyperplasia.

DOSAGE: *Adults:* Initial: 0.4mg qd, 1/2 hr after same meal each day. Titrate: May increase to 0.8mg qd after 2-4 weeks. If therapy is interrupted, restart with 0.4mg qd.

HOW SUPPLIED: Cap: 0.4mg

WARNINGS/PRECAUTIONS: Rule out prostate cancer. Orthostasis/syncope may occur. May cause priapism (rare). Intraoperative Floppy Iris Syndrome (IFIS) has been observed during cataract surgery. Do not crush, chew or open capsules. Use with caution if has sulfa allergy.

ADVERSE REACTIONS: Headache, dizziness, somnolence, diarrhea, asthenia, back pain, pharyngitis, rhinitis, abnormal ejaculation.

INTERACTIONS: Avoid use with other α-blockers. Decreased clearance with cimetidine; caution with concomitant use especially with doses higher than 0.4mg. Caution with warfarin. Concomitant administration of flomax and an inhibitor of CYP2D6 or CYP3A4 may lead to increased flomax plasma exposure.

PREGNANCY: Category B, not for use in women.

MECHANISM OF ACTION: α_{1A} adrenoreceptor antagonist.

PHARMACOKINETICS: Absorption: Complete, (0.4mg) C_{max}=10ng/mL, T_{max}=6 hrs, AUC=151ng•hr/mL. (0.8 mg) C_{max}=29.8ng/mL, T_{max}=7 hrs, AUC=440ng•hr/mL. Refer to PI for parameters in high-fat breakfast/fasted states.
Distribution: V_d=16L, plasma protein binding (94-99%). **Metabolism:** CYP450.
Elimination: Urine (<10%), feces, $T_{1/2}$=14-15 hrs.

FLONASE   RX
fluticasone propionate (GlaxoSmithKline)

THERAPEUTIC CLASS: Corticosteroid

INDICATIONS: Management of the nasal symptoms of seasonal and perennial allergic rhinitis, and nonallergic rhinitis.

DOSAGE: *Adults:* Initial: 2 sprays per nostril qd or 1 spray per nostril bid. Maint: 1 spray per nostril qd. May dose as 2 sprays per nostril qd as needed for seasonal allergic rhinitis.
Pediatrics: ≥4 yrs: Initial: 1 sprays per nostril qd. If inadequate response, may increase to 2 sprays per nostril. Maint: 1 spray per nostril qd. Max: 2 sprays per nostril/day. ≥12 yrs: May dose as 2 sprays per nostril qd as needed for seasonal allergic rhinitis.

HOW SUPPLIED: Spray: 50mcg/spray [16g]

WARNINGS/PRECAUTIONS: Risk of adrenal insufficiency and withdrawal symptoms when replacing systemic corticosteroids with a topical corticosteroids. Caution with active or quiescent TB, ocular herpes simplex, or untreated bacterial, fungal and systemic viral infections. Avoid with recent nasal trauma, surgery or septum ulcers. Risk for more severe/fatal course of infections (eg, chickenpox, measles); avoid exposure in patients who have not had disease or been properly immunized. Candida infection of nose and pharynx reported (rare). Potential for growth velocity reduction in pediatrics. Excessive use may cause signs of hypercorticism or HPA suppression.

ADVERSE REACTIONS: Headache, pharyngitis, epistaxis, nasal burning/irritation, asthma symptoms, nausea/vomiting, cough.

INTERACTIONS: Caution with ketoconazole or other potent CYP3A4 inhibitors, may increase serum fluticasone levels. Concomitant inhaled corticosteroids increases risk of hypercorticism and/or HPA axis suppression. Increased levels with ritonavir; avoid use.

PREGNANCY: Category C, caution in nursing.

MECHANISM OF ACTION: Glucocorticosteroid; not established. Acts as anti-inflammatory agent with wide range of effects on multiple cell types (eg, mast cells, eosinophils, macrophages, and lymphocytes) and mediators (eg, histamine, eicosanoids, leukotrienes, and cytokines) involved in inflammation.

PHARMACOKINETICS: Absorption: Absolute bioavailability (<2%), C_{max}=50pg/mL.

FLOVENT HFA   RX
fluticasone propionate (GlaxoSmithKline)

THERAPEUTIC CLASS: Corticosteroid

INDICATIONS: Maintenance treatment of asthma as prophylactic therapy in patients ≥4 years; to reduce or eliminate the need for oral corticosteroidal therapy.

DOSAGE: *Adults:* Previous Bronchodilator Only: Initial: 88mcg bid. Max: 440mcg bid. Previous Inhaled Corticosteroids: Initial: 88-220mcg bid. Max: 440mcg bid. Previous Oral Corticosteroids: Initial: 440mcg bid. Max: 880mcg bid. Reduce PO prednisone no faster than 2.5 to 5mg/day weekly, beginning at least 1 week after starting fluticasone. Rinse mouth after use.
Pediatrics: ≥12 yrs: Previous Bronchodilator Only: Initial: 88mcg bid. Max: 440mcg bid. Previous Inhaled Corticosteroids: Initial: 88-220mcg bid. Max: 440mcg bid. Previous Oral Corticosteroids: Initial: 440mcg bid. Max: 880mcg bid. 4-11 yrs: Initial/Max: 88mcg bid. Reduce PO prednisone no faster than 2.5 to 5mg/day weekly, beginning at least 1 week after starting fluticasone. Rinse mouth after use.

HOW SUPPLIED: MDI: 44mcg/inh [10.6g], 110mcg/inh [12g], 220mcg/inh [12g]

CONTRAINDICATIONS: Primary treatment of status asthmaticus or other acute asthma attacks.

WARNINGS/PRECAUTIONS: Deaths due to adrenal insufficiency have occurred with transfer from systemic corticosteroids to inhaled corticosteroids. Resume oral corticosteroids during stress or severe asthma attack. Wean slowly from systemic corticosteroid therapy. Observe for adrenal insufficiency, systemic corticosteroid withdrawal effects, hypercorticism, adrenal suppression (including adrenal crisis), reduction in growth velocity (children and adolescents). May increase susceptibility to infections. Not for acute bronchospasm. D/C if bronchospasm occurs after dosing. Caution with TB of respiratory tract; untreated systemic fungal, bacterial, viral or parasitic infections; or ocular herpes simplex. *Candida* infection of mouth and pharynx reported. Glaucoma, increased IOP and cataracts reported. Rare cases of eosinophilic conditions.

ADVERSE REACTIONS: Pharyngitis, cough, bronchitis, nasal congestion, sinusitis, dysphonia, oral candidiasis, upper respiratory infection, influenza, headache, nasal discharge, allergic rhinitis, fever, paradoxical bronchospasm.

INTERACTIONS: Increased levels with ritonavir; avoid use. Caution with ketoconazole and other potent CYP3A4 inhibitors; may increase serum fluticasone levels.

PREGNANCY: Category C, caution in nursing.

MECHANISM OF ACTION: Synthetic trifluorinated corticosteroid; possesses potent anti-inflammatory activity and inhibits multiple cell types involved in asthmatic response.

PHARMACOKINETICS: Absorption: Acts locally in lung. **Distribution:** V_d=4.2 L/kg; plasma protein binding (99%). **Metabolism:** Liver via CYP3A4. **Elimination:** Feces (primary), urine (<5%); $T_{1/2}$=7.8 hrs.

Floxin RX
ofloxacin (Ortho-McNeil)

THERAPEUTIC CLASS: Fluoroquinolone

INDICATIONS: Treatment of complicated urinary tract infections (UTI), uncomplicated skin and skin structure infection (SSSI), acute bacterial exacerbation of chronic bronchitis (ABECB), community-acquired pneumonia (CAP), acute uncomplicated urethral and cervical gonorrhea, nongonococcal urethritis and cervicitis, mixed infections of urethra and cervix, acute pelvic inflammatory disease (PID), uncomplicated cystitis, and prostatitis caused by susceptible strains of microorganisms.

DOSAGE: *Adults:* ≥18 yrs: ABECB/CAP/SSSI: 400mg q12h for 10 days. Cervicitis/Urethritis: 300mg q12h for 7 days. Gonorrhea: 400mg single dose. PID: 400mg q12h for 10-14 days. Uncomplicated Cystitis: 200mg q12h for 3 days (*E.coli* or *K.pneumoniae*) or 7 days (other pathogens). Complicated UTI: 200mg q12h for 10 days. Prostatitis: (*E.coli*) 300mg q12h for 6 weeks. CrCl 20-

50mL/min: Dose q24h. CrCl <20mL/min: After regular initial dose, give 50% of normal dose q24h. Severe Hepatic Impairment: Max: 400mg/day.

HOW SUPPLIED: Tab: 200mg, 300mg, 400mg

WARNINGS/PRECAUTIONS: Convulsions, increased ICP, toxic psychosis, CNS stimulation, and serious, sometimes fatal, hypersensitivity reactions reported; d/c if any occur. *Clostridium difficile*-associated diarrhea and ruptures of shoulder, hand, and Achilles tendon reported. Not shown to be effective for syphilis. Safety and efficacy unknown in patients <18 yrs old, pregnancy, and nursing. Maintain adequate hydration. Caution with renal or hepatic dysfunction, risk for seizures, CNS disorder with predisposition to seizures. Avoid excessive sunlight. Monitor blood, renal and hepatic function with prolonged therapy. Tendon ruptures reported.

ADVERSE REACTIONS: Nausea, insomnia, headache, dizziness, diarrhea, vomiting, external genital pruritus in women, vaginitis.

INTERACTIONS: Decreased absorption with antacids, sucralfate, multivitamins, zinc, didanosine; separate dosing by 2 hrs. NSAIDs may increase risk of seizures. May potentiate theophylline, warfarin. May potentiate insulin, oral hypoglycemics; d/c if hypoglycemia occurs. May increase half-life of drugs metabolized by CYP450. Severe tendon disorder risks are increased with concomitant corticosteroid therapy.

PREGNANCY: Category C, not for use in nursing.

MECHANISM OF ACTION: Fluoroquinolone: Synthetic broad-spectrum antimicrobial agent; inhibits topoisomearase II (DNA gyrase) and topoisomerase IV, which are required for bacterial DNA replication, transcription, repair, and recombination.

PHARMACOKINETICS: Absorption: Oral administration of variable doses resulted in different parameters; T_{max}=1-2 hrs; bioavailability (98%). **Elimination:** Biphasic ($T_{1/2}$=4-5 hrs, 20-25 hrs), renal.

FLOXIN OTIC RX

ofloxacin (Daiichi Sankyo)

OTHER BRAND NAMES: Floxin Otic Singles (Daiichi Sankyo)

THERAPEUTIC CLASS: Fluoroquinolone

INDICATIONS: Otitis externa in patients ≥6 mos. Chronic suppurative otitis media in patients ≥12 yrs with perforated tympanic membranes. Acute otitis media in patients ≥1 yr with tympanostomy tubes.

DOSAGE: *Adults:* Otitis Externa: 10 drops or 2 single-dispensing containers (SDCs) once daily for 7 days. Chronic Suppurative Otitis Media with Perforated Tympanic Membrane: 10 drops or 2 SDCs bid for 14 days. *Pediatrics:* Otitis Externa: 6 mos-13 yrs: 5 drops or 1 single-dispensing container (SDC) once daily for 7 days. ≥13 yrs: 10 drops or 2 SDCs once daily for 7 days. Chronic Suppurative Otitis Media with Perforated Tympanic Membrane: ≥12 yrs: 10 drops or 2 SDCs bid for 14 days. Acute Otitis Media with Tympanostomy Tubes: 1-12 yrs: 5 drops or 1 SDC bid for 10 days.

HOW SUPPLIED: Sol: 0.3% [5mL, 10mL], (Singles) 0.3% [20s]

WARNINGS/PRECAUTIONS: D/C if hypersensitivity reaction occurs. Re-evaluate if no improvement after one week.

ADVERSE REACTIONS: Pruritus, application site reaction, taste perversion.

PREGNANCY: Category C, not for use in nursing.

MECHANISM OF ACTION: Fluoroquinilone; exerts antibacterial activity; inhibits DNA gyrase (a bacterial topoisomerase), an essential enzyme which controls DNA topology and assists in DNA replication, repair, deactivation, and transcription.

PHARMACOKINETICS: Absorption: Perforated tympanic membrane; C_{max}=10ng/ml.

FLOXURIDINE   RX
floxuridine (Various)

Hospitalize for 1st course of therapy due to possible severe toxic reactions.

OTHER BRAND NAMES: FUDR (Sterile) (Hospira)

THERAPEUTIC CLASS: Antimetabolite

INDICATIONS: Palliative management of GI adenocarcinoma metastatic to the liver.

DOSAGE: *Adults:* 0.1-0.6mg/kg/day continuous arterial infusion. Use higher dose (0.4-0.6mg) for hepatic artery infusion. Continue therapy until adverse reactions appear and resume when reactions subside. Maintain on therapy as long as response continues.

HOW SUPPLIED: Inj: 0.5g

CONTRAINDICATIONS: Poor nutritional state, depressed bone marrow function, potentially serious infections.

WARNINGS/PRECAUTIONS: Highly toxic drug with narrow margin of safety. Extreme caution in poor risk patients with renal or hepatic dysfunction, history of high-dose pelvic irradiation, or previous use of alkylating agents. Not intended as an adjuvant to surgery. D/C promptly if myocardial ischemia, stomatitis or esophagopharyngitis, leukopenia, intractable vomiting, diarrhea, GI ulceration and bleeding, thrombocytopenia, or if hemorrhage from any site occur. May cause fetal harm during pregnancy. Carefully monitor WBCs and platelets.

ADVERSE REACTIONS: Nausea, vomiting, diarrhea, enteritis, stomatitis, localized erythema, anemia, leukopenia, thrombocytopenia, LFT elevation, alopecia.

INTERACTIONS: Increased toxicity with therapies that add stress to patients, interfere with nutrition, or depress bone marrow function.

PREGNANCY: Category D, not for use in nursing.

MECHANISM OF ACTION: Antineoplastic antimetabolite; interferes with the synthesis of DNA and to lesser extent inhibits formation of RNA.

PHARMACOKINETICS: Metabolism: Liver; 5-flurorouracil (active metabolite). **Elimination:** Urine (parent compound and metabolites).

FLUDARA   RX
fludarabine phosphate (Bayer Healthcare)

Can severely suppress bone marrow function. High doses associated with severe neurologic effects, including blindness, coma, and death. Autoimmune hemolytic anemia reported. Monitor closely for hemolysis. High incidence of fatal pulmonary toxicity with pentostatin.

THERAPEUTIC CLASS: Antimetabolite

INDICATIONS: Treatment of B-cell chronic lymphocytic leukemia (CLL) unresponsive to or with disease progression during treatment with at least on standard alkylating-agent containing regimen.

DOSAGE: *Adults:* 25mg/m^2 over 30 min qd for 5 days. Repeat course every 28 days. Administer 3 additional courses after achievement of maximum response. May decrease or delay dose based on hematologic or nonhematologic toxicity. Consider delaying or discontinuing if neurotoxicity occurs. CrCl 30-70mL/min: Reduce dose by 20%. CrCl <30mL/min: Not recommended.

HOW SUPPLIED: Inj: 50mg

WARNINGS/PRECAUTIONS: Severe bone marrow suppression reported. Predisposition to increased toxicity with advanced age, renal insufficiency, and bone marrow impairment; monitor for toxicity. Caution with renal insufficiency. Tumor lysis syndrome associated with large tumor burdens. Monitor hematologic profile regularly. Can cause fetal harm during pregnancy. Use irradiated blood products if transfusion required.

ADVERSE REACTIONS: Myelosuppression, fever, chills, infection, nausea, vomiting, malaise, fatigue, anorexia, weakness, serious opportunistic infections.

INTERACTIONS: Avoid pentostatin due to the risk of severe pulmonary toxicity.

PREGNANCY: Category D, not for use in nursing.

MECHANISM OF ACTION: Antimetabolite; suspected to inhibit DNA polymerase-α, ribonucleotide reductase and DNA primase, thus inhibiting DNA synthesis.

PHARMACOKINETICS: Distribution: Plasma protein binding (19-29%). **Metabolism:** Intracellular; dephosphorylation, phosphorylation by deoxycytidine kinase. 2-fluoro-ara-A (metabolite). **Elimination:** $T_{1/2}$=20 hrs (metabolite).

FLUDROCORTISONE   RX
fludrocortisone acetate (Various)

THERAPEUTIC CLASS: Corticosteroid

INDICATIONS: Partial replacement therapy for adrenocortical insufficiency in Addison's disease. Treatment of salt-losing adrenogenital syndrome.

DOSAGE: *Adults:* Addison's Disease: Usual: 0.1mg/day with concomitant cortisone 10-37.5mg/day or hydrocortisone 10-30mg/day in divided doses. Dose Range: 0.1mg three times weekly to 0.2mg/day. If HTN develops, reduce to 0.05mg/day. Salt-Losing Adrenogenital Syndrome: 0.1-0.2mg/day.

HOW SUPPLIED: Tab: 0.1mg* *scored

CONTRAINDICATIONS: Systemic fungal infections.

WARNINGS/PRECAUTIONS: May to increase dose before, during, and after stressful situations. Caution with hypothyroidism, cirrhosis, ocular herpes simplex, HTN, ulcerative colitis, diverticulitis, peptic ulcer, osteoporosis, myasthenia gravis, renal impairment, and elderly. May mask signs of infection or cause new infection. Avoid exposure to chickenpox or measles. Marked effect on sodium retention; monitor electrolytes. May need salt restriction and potassium supplements. Monitor for psychic disturbances. Risk of glaucoma, cataracts, and eye infections. Avoid abrupt withdrawal.

ADVERSE REACTIONS: HTN, CHF, edema, convulsions, hypokalemia, hypokalemic alkalosis, muscle weakness, impaired wound healing, menstrual irregularities, cataracts, suppression of growth, hyperglycemia, HPA-suppression, acne, rash.

INTERACTIONS: Decreases serum salicylate levels. Enhanced hypokalemia with amphotericin B and potassium-depleting diuretics (eg, furosemide, ethacrynic acid). Increased risk of digitalis toxicity and arrhythmias with hypokalemia. Decreased effects with rifampin, barbiturates, and hydantoins. Monitor PT with oral anticoagulants. Decreases effects of oral hypoglycemics, insulin. Enhanced edema with other anabolic steroids (eg, oxymethalone, norethandrolone). Adjust dose with initiation or termination of estrogen. Avoid live virus vaccines (including small pox) and other immunizations. Caution with ASA.

PREGNANCY: Category C, caution in nursing.

MECHANISM OF ACTION: Synthetic adrenocortical steroid; acts on electrolyte balance and carbohydrate metabolism and on distal tubules of kidney to enhance reabsorption of sodium ions from tubular fluid into the plasma. Increases urinary excretion of both K^+ and hydrogen ions.

PHARMACOKINETICS: Distribution: Found in breast milk. **Metabolism:** Liver. **Elimination:** $T_{1/2}$=3.5 hrs (Plasama), 18-36 hr (Biological).

FLULAVAL   RX
influenza virus vaccine (GlaxoSmithKline)

THERAPEUTIC CLASS: Vaccine

INDICATIONS: Active immunization against influenza disease caused by influenza virus subtypes A and B contained in the vaccine.

DOSAGE: *Adults:* ≥18 yrs: 0.5mL IM in deltoid.

HOW SUPPLIED: Inj: 15mcg/0.5mL [5mL]

CONTRAINDICATIONS: Delay immunization with acute evolving, neurologic disorder.

WARNINGS/PRECAUTIONS: Guillain-Barre syndrome reported within 6 weeks of administration. Avoid with bleeding disorders or concomitant anticoagulants. May reduce immune response in the immunocompromised.

ADVERSE REACTIONS: Pain, redness, and/or swelling at injection site, headache, fatigue, myalgia, low grade fever, malaise.

INTERACTIONS: Do not mix with any other vaccine in same syringe or vial; administer other vaccines at different injection sites. May increase blood levels of warfarin, theophylline, phenytion. Immunosuppressive therapies (eg, irradiation, antimetabolites, alkylating agents, cytotoxic drugs, corticosteroids) may reduce effectiveness.

PREGNANCY: Category C, caution in nursing.

MECHANISM OF ACTION: Vaccine; elicits the formation of antibodies that may protect against influenza virus subtypes A and B.

FLUMADINE   RX
rimantadine HCL (Forest)

THERAPEUTIC CLASS: Adamantane class antiviral

INDICATIONS: Prophylaxis and treatment of influenza A virus.

DOSAGE: *Adults:* Prophylaxis/Treatment: 100mg bid. Elderly/Severe Hepatic Dysfunction/CrCl ≤10mL/min: 100mg qd. Initiate treatment within 48 hrs of onset of symptoms. Treat for 7 days from initial onset of symptoms.
Pediatrics: Prophylaxis: 1-9 yrs: 5mg/kg qd. Max: 150mg qd. ≥10 yrs: 100mg bid.

HOW SUPPLIED: Syrup: 50mg/5mL [240mL]; Tab: 100mg

WARNINGS/PRECAUTIONS: Caution with a history of epilepsy. D/C if seizures develop. Caution with renal or hepatic dysfunction.

ADVERSE REACTIONS: Insomnia, dizziness, nervousness, nausea, vomiting, anorexia, dry mouth, abdominal pain, asthenia.

INTERACTIONS: May be potentiated by cimetidine. APAP and ASA may decrease levels of rimantadine. Avoid use of Live Influenza Virus Vaccine within 2 weeks before or 48 hrs after use.

PREGNANCY: Category C, not for use in nursing.

MECHANISM OF ACTION: Antiviral; unknown, suspected to exert its inhibitory effect early in the viral replicative cycle, possibly inhibiting the uncoating of virus.

PHARMACOKINETICS: Absorption: C_{max}=74ng/mL; T_{max}=6 hrs. **Distribution:** Plasma protein binding (40%). **Metabolism:** Hepatic (extensive). **Elimination:** Urine (<25%); $T_{1/2}$=25.4 hrs.

FLUMIST   RX
influenza virus vaccine live (MedImmune)

THERAPEUTIC CLASS: Vaccine

INDICATIONS: Active immunization of individuals 2-49 years of age against influenza disease caused by influenza virus subtypes A and type B contained in the vaccine.

DOSAGE: *Adults:* ≤49 yrs: One 0.2mL (0.1mL per nostril) dose.
Pediatrics: ≥9 yrs: One 0.2mL (0.1mL per nostril) dose. 2-8 yrs: Not Previously Vaccinated With Influenza Vaccine: 0.2mL (0.1mL per nostril) for 2 doses at

least 1 month apart. Previously Vaccinated With Influenza Vacine: One 0.2mL (0.1mL per nostril) dose.

HOW SUPPLIED: Nasal Spray: 0.2mL [10s]

CONTRAINDICATIONS: Parenteral use. Hypersensitivity to eggs or egg products. Children and adolescents 5-17 years of age receiving ASA or ASA-containing therapy. History of Guillain-Barre syndrome. Immune deficiency diseases such as combined immuno immunodeficiency, agammaglobulinemia, and thymic abnormalities, and conditions such as HIV infection, malignancy, leukemia, or lymphoma. Immunosuppressed or altered/compromised immune status due to treatment with systemic corticosteroids, alkylating drugs, anti-metabolites, radiation, or other immunosuppressive therapies.

WARNINGS/PRECAUTIONS: Avoid with history of asthma or reactive airways disease, chronic disorders of the cardiovascular and pulmonary systems, second or third trimester of pregnancy, chronic metabolic diseases (including diabetes), renal dysfunction, hemoglobinopathies, congenital or acquired im-munosuppression. Avoid close contact with immunocompromised individuals for at least 21 days. Have epinephrine available. Delay administration until after the acute phase (at least 72 hrs) of febrile and/or respiratory illnesses.

ADVERSE REACTIONS: Runny nose, congestion, cough, irritability, headache, sore throat, fever, chills, muscle aches, vomiting, tiredness/weakness.

INTERACTIONS: See Contraindications. Avoid concurrent use with other vaccines and within 48 hrs after cessation of antiviral therapy; antiviral agents until 2 weeks after vaccination unless medically indicated; ASA or ASA-containing products in children and adolescents 5-17 yrs.

PREGNANCY: Category C, caution in nursing.

MECHANISM OF ACTION: Stimulates the immune system to produce anti-bodies (influenza-specific T cells) that may protect against influenza virus infection.

FLUNISOLIDE NASAL SPRAY RX
flunisolide (Various)

THERAPEUTIC CLASS: Corticosteroid

INDICATIONS: Relief of seasonal or perennial rhinitis.

DOSAGE: *Adults:* Initial: 2 sprays per nostril bid. Titrate: May increase to 2 sprays per nostril tid. Max: 8 sprays per nostril/day.
Pediatrics: 6-14 yrs: Initial: 1 spray per nostril tid or 2 sprays per nostril bid. Max: 4 sprays per nostril/day.

HOW SUPPLIED: Spray: 25mcg/spray [25mL]

CONTRAINDICATIONS: Untreated localized infection of the nasal mucosa.

WARNINGS/PRECAUTIONS: Risk of adrenal insufficiency and withdrawal symptoms when replacing systemic corticosteroids with a topical corticoste-roids. Caution with active or quiescent TB, ocular herpes simplex, or untreated bacterial, fungal and systemic viral infections. Avoid with recent nasal trauma, surgery or septum ulcers. Risk for more severe/fatal course of infections (eg, chickenpox, measles) and for *Candida* infections of the nose and pharynx.

ADVERSE REACTIONS: Nasal congestion, sneezing, epistaxis, bloody mu-cous, nasal irritation, watery eyes, sore throat, nausea, vomiting, headache.

INTERACTIONS: Concomitant systemic corticosteroids increases risk of hy-percorticism and/or HPA axis suppression.

PREGNANCY: Category C, caution in nursing.

MECHANISM OF ACTION: Glucocorticosteroid; not established, acts as anti-inflammatory agent with potent glucocorticoid and weak mineralocorticoid activity.

PHARMACOKINETICS: Absorption: Well absorbed. **Metabolism:** Liver. **Elimination:** Urine (65-70%, metabolites), feces, $T_{1/2}$=1-2 hrs.

FLUOCINONIDE RX
fluocinonide (Various)

OTHER BRAND NAMES: Lidex-E (Medicis) - Lidex (Medicis) - Fluocinonide-E (Various)

THERAPEUTIC CLASS: Corticosteroid

INDICATIONS: Corticosteroid-responsive dermatoses.

DOSAGE: *Adults:* Apply bid-qid. May use occlusive dressing for psoriasis or recalcitrant conditions; d/c dressings if infection develops.
Pediatrics: Apply bid-qid. May use occlusive dressing for psoriasis or recalcitrant conditions; d/c dressings if infection develops.

HOW SUPPLIED: (Fluocinonide) Cre, Gel, Oint: 0.05% [15g, 30g, 60g]; Sol: 0.05% [60mL]; (Fluocinonide-E) Cre: 0.05% [15g, 30g, 60g]

WARNINGS/PRECAUTIONS: May produce reversible HPA axis suppression, manifestations of Cushing's syndrome, hyperglycemia, and glucosuria. Caution when applied to large surface areas or under occlusive dressings. Use appropriate antifungal or antibacterial agent with dermatological infections; d/c if infection does not clear. Pediatrics may be more susceptible to systemic toxicity. Avoid eyes. D/C if irritation occurs.

ADVERSE REACTIONS: Burning, itching, irritation, dryness, folliculitis, hypertrichosis, acneiform eruptions, hypopigmentation, perioral dermatitis, allergic contact dermatitis, skin maceration, secondary infection, skin atrophy, striae, miliaria.

PREGNANCY: Category C, caution in nursing.

MECHANISM OF ACTION: Corticosteroid; possesses anti-inflammatory, anti-pruritic, and vasoconstrictive actions.

PHARMACOKINETICS: Absorption: Extent of percutaneous absorption is determined by vehicle, integrity of skin, and use of occlusive dressings. **Metabolism:** Liver. **Elimination:** Urine, bile.

FLUORESCITE RX
fluorescein sodium (Alcon)

THERAPEUTIC CLASS: Diagnostic dye

INDICATIONS: Indicated in diagnostic fluorescein angiography or angioscopy of the fundus and iris vasculature.

DOSAGE: *Adults:* Perform intradermal skin test before IV use if suspect potential allergy. Inject contents of ampule rapidly into antecubital vein. A syringe with fluorescein is attached to transparent tubing and a 25 gauge scalp vein needle for injection. Insert needle and draw patient's blood to hub of syringe so small air bubble separates patient's blood in tubing from fluorescein. With room lights on, inject blood back into vein while watching skin over needle tip. If needle extravasated, patient's blood will bulge skin; stop injection before injecting fluorescein. When certain there is no extravasation, turn room light off and complete fluorescein injection. Luminescence appears in retina and choroidal vessels in 9-14 seconds.
Pediatrics: Perform intradermal skin test before IV use if suspect potential allergy. Dose is 35mg/10lbs. Inject contents of ampule/vial rapidly into antecubital vein. A syringe with fluorescein is attached to transparent tubing and a 25 gauge scalp vein needle for injection. Insert needle and draw patient's blood to hub of syringe so small air bubble separates patient's blood in tubing from fluorescein. With room lights on, inject blood back into vein while watching skin over needle tip. If needle extravasated, patient's blood will bulge skin; stop injection before injecting fluorescein. When certain there is no extravasation, turn room light off and complete fluorescein injection. Luminescence appears in retina and choroidal vessels in 9-14 seconds.

HOW SUPPLIED: Inj: 10% [5mL], 25% [2mL]

WARNINGS/PRECAUTIONS: Not for intrathecal use. Avoid extravasation; severe local tissue damage can occur. Caution with history of allergy or bronchial asthma. Have emergency tray (eg, 0.1% epinephrine IV/IM, antihistamine, soluble steroid, IV aminophylline) and oxygen available. Avoid angiography in pregnancy, especially 1st trimester. Skin attains temporary yellowish discoloration and urine attains bright yellow color.

ADVERSE REACTIONS: Nausea, vomiting, headache, GI distress, syncope, hypotension, cardiac arrest, basilar artery ischemia, severe shock, convulsions, thrombophlebitis.

PREGNANCY: Safety in pregnancy not known, caution in nursing.

MECHANISM OF ACTION: Diagnostic dye; responds to electromagnetic radiation and light between wavelengths 465-490nm and fluoresces at wavelenghts of 520-530nm.

PHARMACOKINETICS: Distribution: V_d=0.5L/kg. **Metabolism:** Rapid via conjugation. **Elimination:** Renal.

FLUOROPLEX   RX
fluorouracil (Allergan)

THERAPEUTIC CLASS: Antimetabolite

INDICATIONS: Topical treatment of multiple actinic (solar) keratoses.

DOSAGE: *Adults:* Apply bid for 2-6 weeks. Increased frequency and longer treatment periods may be required for areas other than the head and neck. Wash hands immediately after application.

HOW SUPPLIED: Cre: 1% [30g]; Sol: 1% [30mL]

CONTRAINDICATIONS: Pregnancy.

WARNINGS/PRECAUTIONS: Avoid mucous membranes. Caution with occlusive dressings. Avoid prolonged sun/UV light exposure. Increased absorption with ulcerated or inflamed skin. Confirm diagnosis with biopsy. Skin reactions such as erosion, ulceration, and necrosis occur before re-epithelization; d/c therapy at this point. Delayed hypersensitivity reported.

ADVERSE REACTIONS: Pain, pruritus, burning, irritations, inflammation, allergic contact dermatitis, telangiectasia, hyperpigmentation, scarring.

PREGNANCY: Category X, not for use in nursing.

MECHANISM OF ACTION: Antineoplastic/antimetabolite agent; blocks the methylation reaction of deoxyuridylic acid to thymidic acid. Fluoracil interferes with the synthesis of DNA and to a lesser extent inhibits the formation of RNA.

FLUOROURACIL   RX
fluorouracil (Various)

> Hospitalize patient during initial therapy due to possible severe toxic reactions.

THERAPEUTIC CLASS: Antimetabolite

INDICATIONS: Palliative management of colon, rectum, breast, stomach, and pancreatic carcinomas.

DOSAGE: *Adults:* 12mg/kg IV qd for 4 days. Max: 800mg/day. If no toxicity, give 6mg/kg IV on 6th, 8th, 10th, and 12th days. Skip Days 5, 7, 9, and 11. Inadequate Nutritional State: 6mg/kg IV for 3 days. If no toxicity, give 3mg/kg IV on 5th, 7th, and 9th days. Max: 400mg/day. Skip Days 4, 6, and 8. Maint (Use Schedule 1 or Schedule 2): Schedule 1: If no toxicity, repeat 1st course every 30 days after last day of previous course. Schedule 2: When toxic signs from initial course subside, give 10-15mg/kg/week IV single dose; do not exceed 1g/week.

HOW SUPPLIED: Inj: 50mg/mL [10mL, 50mL, 100mL]

CONTRAINDICATIONS: Poor nutritional state, depressed bone marrow function, potentially serious infection.

WARNINGS/PRECAUTIONS: Extreme caution in poor risk patients with history of high-dose irradiation, previous use of alkylating agents, hepatic/renal dysfunction, widespread bone marrow involvement by metastatic tumors. Dipyrimidine dehydrogenase deficiency prolongs 5-FU clearance; can cause severe toxicity. May cause fetal harm in pregnancy. Other therapy interfering with nutrition or depressing bone marrow function increases toxicity. D/C with stomatitis, esophagopharyngitis, leukopenia, intractable vomiting, diarrhea, GI ulceration or bleeding, thrombocytopenia, or hemorrhage from any site. Palmar-plantar erythrodysesthesia syndrome (hand-foot syndrome) reported. Perform WBC with differential before each dose. Narrow margin of safety; monitor patients very closely.

ADVERSE REACTIONS: Stomatitis, esophagopharyngitis, diarrhea, anorexia, nausea, emesis, leukopenia, alopecia, dermatitis.

INTERACTIONS: Leucovorin calcium may enhance toxicity.

PREGNANCY: Category D, not for use in nursing.

MECHANISM OF ACTION: Antineoplastic antimetabolite; interferes with the synthesis of DNA and to a lesser extent inhibits the formation of RNA, which are essential for cell division and growth.

PHARMACOKINETICS: Distribution: Found in tumors, intestinal mucosa, bone marrow, liver; crosses the blood-brain barrier and found in brain tissue and cerebrospinal fluid. **Metabolism:** Liver. **Elimination:** Urine (7-20% unchanged); $T_{1/2}$=16 min.

FLUPHENAZINE HCL   RX
fluphenazine HCL (Various)

THERAPEUTIC CLASS: Piperazine phenothiazine

INDICATIONS: Management of psychotic disorders.

DOSAGE: *Adults:* (PO) Initial: 2.5-10mg/day in divided doses q6-8h. Titrate: May increase up to 40mg/day. Maint: 1-5mg qd. Elderly: Initial: 1-2.5mg/day. (Inj) Initial: 1.25mg IM q6-8h. Max: 10mg/day.

HOW SUPPLIED: Inj: 2.5mg/mL; Elixir: 2.5mg/5mL; Sol, Concentrate: 5mg/mL; Tab: 1mg, 2.5mg, 5mg, 10mg

CONTRAINDICATIONS: Comatose state, severe depression, concomitant large dose hypnotics, blood dyscrasia, hepatic impairment, subcortical brain damage, cross-sensitivity to phenothiazine derivatives.

WARNINGS/PRECAUTIONS: May develop tardive dyskinesia, NMS. Caution with history of cholestatic jaundice, dermatoses or allergic reactions to phenothiazine derivatives. Elevated prolactin levels reported. Avoid abrupt withdrawal. Caution if exposed to extreme heat or phosphorous insecticides, seizure disorder, cardiovascular disease, pheochromocytoma. May develop liver damage, pigmentary retinopathy, lenticular and corneal dyskinesias with prolonged therapy. Monitor for hypotension in patients on large doses undergoing surgery. May impair mental/physical abilities.

ADVERSE REACTIONS: Extrapyramidal symptoms, tardive dyskinesia, HTN, hypotension, allergic reactions, nausea, loss of appetite, dry mouth, headache, constipation, perspiration, salivation, polyuria, hepatic dysfunction.

INTERACTIONS: May potentiate alcohol effects and anticholinergics. Reduce dose of anesthetics or CNS depressants prior to surgery.

PREGNANCY: Safety in pregnancy or nursing not known.

MECHANISM OF ACTION: Trifluoromethyl phenothiazine derivative; not established. Suspected to have activity at all levels of the CNS, as well as on multiple organ systems.

FLUTAMIDE   RX
flutamide (Various)

> Hepatic injury reported; d/c if jaundice occurs or if ALT >2x ULN. Monitor LFTs monthly for first 4 months and periodically thereafter.

THERAPEUTIC CLASS: Nonsteroidal antiandrogen

INDICATIONS: In combination with lutenizing hormone releasing hormone (LHRH) agonist for treatment of locally confined Stage B_2-C and Stage D_2 metastatic prostate carcinoma.

DOSAGE: *Adults:* 250mg q8h. Max: 750mg/day.

HOW SUPPLIED: Cap: 125mg

CONTRAINDICATIONS: Severe hepatic impairment.

WARNINGS/PRECAUTIONS: Monitor PSA regularly. Not for use in women. If disease progression is evident, d/c therapy and continue LHRH agonist. Monitor methemoglobin levels in G6PD deficiency, hemoglobin M disease, or smokers.

ADVERSE REACTIONS: Hot flashes, loss of libido, impotence, diarrhea, nausea, vomiting, gynecomastia, other GI disturbances, anemia, edema, hepatitis, jaundice, skin rash.

INTERACTIONS: May increase PT; monitor warfarin.

PREGNANCY: Category D, safety in nursing is not known.

MECHANISM OF ACTION: Nonsteroidal antiandrogen; inhibits androgen uptake and/or inhibits nuclear binding of androgen target tissue.

PHARMACOKINETICS: Absorption: Rapid, complete; C_{max}=25.2ng/mL; T_{max}=2 hrs. **Distribution:** Plasma protein binding =94-96% (drug), 92-94% (metabolite). **Metabolism:** Rapid, extensive via hydroxylation. Hydroxyflutamide (active metabolite). **Elimination:** Urine, feces (4.2%); $T_{1/2}$ (Hydroxyflutamide)=6 hrs.

FLUVIRIN   RX
influenza virus vaccine (Chiron)

THERAPEUTIC CLASS: Vaccine

INDICATIONS: Immunization against influenza viruses containing antigens related to those in the vaccine.

DOSAGE: *Adults:* 0.5mL IM in deltoid or thigh single dose. Shake well. *Pediatrics:* ≥4 yrs: 0.5mL IM. <9 yrs (Not Previously Vaccinated): Repeat dose minimum 1 month apart. Administer in deltoid muscle to older children and thigh muscle in infants and young children.

HOW SUPPLIED: Inj: 45mcg/0.5mL

CONTRAINDICATIONS: Allergy to chicken eggs, chicken, chicken feathers, chicken dander, or thimerosal (a mercury derivative). Delay administration to patients with an active neurological disorder or an acute febrile illness until disease stabilizes or symptoms subside. History of any neurological signs or symptoms following administration of any vaccine is contraindicated to further use.

WARNINGS/PRECAUTIONS: Do not administer in children younger than 6 months. Caution in children between the ages of 6 months through 4 years. Caution with thrombocytopenia, coagulation disorders, and impaired immune responses.

ADVERSE REACTIONS: Soreness at the injection site, fever, malaise, myalgia.

INTERACTIONS: Immunosuppressive therapies (eg, irradiation, corticosteroids, antimetabolites, alkylating and cytotoxic agents) may reduce effectiveness. May inhibit clearance of warfarin and theophylline.

PREGNANCY: Category C, safe for use in nursing.

MECHANISM OF ACTION: Stimulates the immune response to produce antibodies that may protect against influenza.

FLUVOXAMINE   RX
fluvoxamine maleate (Various)

> Antidepressants increased the risk of suicidal thinking and behavior (suicidality) in short-term studies in children, adolescents, and young adults with major depressive disorder (MDD) and other psychiatric disorders. Fluvoxamine is not approved for use in pediatric patients except for pateints with obsessive compulsive disorder (OCD).

THERAPEUTIC CLASS: Selective serotonin reuptake inhibitor

INDICATIONS: Treatment of OCD.

DOSAGE: *Adults:* Initial: 50mg qhs. Titrate: Increase by 50mg every 4-7 days. Maint: 100-300mg/day. Give bid if total dose >100mg daily. Max: 300mg/day. Elderly/Hepatic Impairment: Modify initial dose and titration.
Pediatrics: 8-17 yrs: Initial: 25mg qhs. Titrate: Increase by 25mg every 4-7 days. Maint: 50-200mg/day. Max: 8-11 yrs: 200mg/day. Adolescents: 300mg/day. Give bid if total dose >50mg daily.

HOW SUPPLIED: Tab: 25mg, 50mg*, 100mg* *scored

CONTRAINDICATIONS: Co-administration of thioridazine, terfenadine, astemizole, cisapride, pimozide, alosetron, tizanidine.

WARNINGS/PRECAUTIONS: Activation of mania/hypomania, SIADH, and hyponatremia reported. Close supervision with high risk suicide patients. Caution with history of seizures, hepatic dysfunction, with conditions altering metabolism or hemodynamic responses. Smoking increases metabolism.

ADVERSE REACTIONS: Headache, asthenia, nausea, diarrhea, vomiting, anorexia, dyspepsia, insomnia, somnolence, nervousness, agitation, dizziness, anxiety, dry mouth, sweating, tremor, abnormal ejaculation.

INTERACTIONS: See Contraindications. May potentiate metoprolol, propranolol. Avoid alcohol, diazepam, terfenadine, astemizole, cisapride, primozide. Increases serum levels of theophylline, warfarin, clozapine, carbamazepine, methadone. Bradycardia with diltiazem. Potential for serious, fatal interactions with MAOIs. Lithium may increase serotonergic effects. Reduces clearance of mexiletine and benzodiazepines metabolized by hepatic oxidation (eg, alprazolam, midazolam, triazolam). Caution with sumatriptan, TCAs, tryptophan. Avoid thioridazine; produces dose-related QTc interval prolongation. Increases tacrine serum levels.

PREGNANCY: Category C, not for use in nursing.

MECHANISM OF ACTION: SSRI; inhibits neuronal uptake of serotonin.

PHARMACOKINETICS: Absorption: Absolute bioavailability (53%). Administration of variable doses resulted in different parameters; T_{max}=3-8 hrs. **Distribution:** V_d=25L/kg; plasma protein binding (80%). **Metabolism:** Hepatic (oxidative demethylation and deamination). **Elimination:** Urine; $T_{1/2}$=15.6 hrs.

FLUZONE   RX
influenza virus vaccine (Sanofi Pasteur)

THERAPEUTIC CLASS: Vaccine

INDICATIONS: Active immunization against influenza disease caused by influenza virus types A and B contained in vaccine in subjects from 6 months of age and older.

DOSAGE: *Adults:* 0.5mL IM in the deltoid muscle.
Pediatrics: ≥9 yrs: 0.5mL IM. 3-8 yrs: 0.5mL IM. 6-35 months: 0.25mL IM. Children <9 yrs who have not previously been vaccinated should receive two doses of vaccine ≥1 month apart. Older children should be given the IM injection in deltoid muscle, infants and young children should receive the IM injection in the anterolateral aspect of the thigh.

HOW SUPPLIED: Inj: 0.25mL, 0.5mL

CONTRAINDICATIONS: Hypersensitivity reactions to egg proteins or to chicken proteins. Vaccination may be postponed in case of febrile or acute disease. Immunization should be delayed in patients with an active neurologic disorder.

WARNINGS/PRECAUTIONS: Avoid in individuals who have a prior history of Guillain-Barre syndrome and in patients with bleeding disorders, such as hemophilia or thrombocytopenia or if patients is on anticoagulant therapy. Immunosuppressed patients may not obtain expected antibody response. Have epinephrine injection (1:1000) available.

ADVERSE REACTIONS: Local: soreness, pain, swelling. Systemic: fever, malaise, myalgia.

PREGNANCY: Category C, safety in nursing not known.

MECHANISM OF ACTION: Stimulates the immune system to produce antibodies that may protect against influenza virus.

FML RX
fluorometholone (Allergan)

OTHER BRAND NAMES: FML Forte (Allergan)

THERAPEUTIC CLASS: Corticosteroid

INDICATIONS: Treatment of inflammation of the palpebral and bulbar conjunctiva, cornea, and anterior segment of the globe.

DOSAGE: *Adults:* (Sus) 1 drop bid-qid or (Oint) apply 1/2 inch qd-tid. May give 0.1% q4h during initial 24-48 hrs. Re-evaluate after 2 days if no improvement. *Pediatrics:* ≥2 yrs: (Sus) 1 drop bid-qid or (Oint) apply 1/2 inch qd-tid. May give 0.1% q4h during initial 24-48 hrs. Re-evaluate after 2 days if no improvement.

HOW SUPPLIED: Oint: (S.O.P.) 0.1% [3.5g]; Sus: 0.1% [5mL, 10mL, 15mL]; (Forte) 0.25% [2mL, 5mL, 10mL, 15mL]

CONTRAINDICATIONS: Viral diseases of the cornea and conjunctiva including epithelial herpes simplex keratitis, vaccinia, and varicella. Mycobacterial infection and fungal diseases of the eye.

WARNINGS/PRECAUTIONS: Caution with glaucoma, herpes simplex, diseases causing thinning of cornea/sclera and other ocular viral infections. Prolonged use can cause glaucoma or secondary ocular infections (eg, fungal). Monitor IOP after 10 days of therapy. Re-evaluate if no response after 2 days. Ointment may retard corneal healing. May delay healing and increase incidence of bleb formation after cataract surgery. Avoid abrupt withdrawal with chronic use.

ADVERSE REACTIONS: Elevation of IOP, glaucoma, infrequent optic nerve damage, posterior subcapsular cataract formation, delayed wound healing, burning/stinging upon instillation, ocular irritation, taste perversion, visual disturbance.

PREGNANCY: Category C, not for use in nursing.

MECHANISM OF ACTION: Corticosteroid; suspected to act by induction of phospholipase A_2 inhibitory proteins called lipocortins which control the biosynthesis of potent inflammation mediators (eg, prostaglandins, leukotrienes) by inhibiting release of their precursor, arachidonic acid.

FML-S RX
sulfacetamide sodium - fluorometholone (Allergan)

THERAPEUTIC CLASS: Sulfonamide/corticosteroid

INDICATIONS: Ocular inflammation associated with infection or risk of infection.

DOSAGE: *Adults:* 1 drop qid. Max: 20mL for initial prescription. Re-evaluate before refill.

420   PDR® Concise Drug Guide

HOW SUPPLIED: Sus: (Sulfacetamide-Fluorometholone) 10%-0.1% [5mL, 10mL]

CONTRAINDICATIONS: Viral diseases of the cornea and conjunctiva including epithelial herpes simplex keratitis, vaccinia, and varicella. Mycobacterial infection and fungal diseases of the eye.

WARNINGS/PRECAUTIONS: Caution with glaucoma, herpes simplex, diseases causing thinning of cornea/sclera and other ocular viral infections. Prolonged use can cause glaucoma or secondary ocular infections (eg, fungal). Monitor IOP after 10 days of therapy. Fatalities reported due to severe reactions to sulfonamides. Re-evaluate before renew prescription.

ADVERSE REACTIONS: Secondary infection, elevated IOP, delayed wound healing, allergic sensitization.

INTERACTIONS: Sulfacetamide preparations are incompatible with silver preparations.

PREGNANCY: Category C, not for use in nursing.

MECHANISM OF ACTION: Sulfonamide/corticosteroid. Fluorometholone: Corticosteroid; inhibits edema, fibrin deposition, capillary dilation, leukocyte migration, capillary proliferation, fibroblast proliferation, deposition of collagen, and scar formation associated with inflammation. May also inhibit the body's defense mechanism against infection. Sulfacetamide: Anti-infective; provides activity against susceptible microorganisms.

FOCALIN `CII`
dexmethylphenidate HCL (Novartis)

THERAPEUTIC CLASS: Sympathomimetic amine

INDICATIONS: Treatment of attention deficit hyperactivity disorder (ADHD).

DOSAGE: *Adults:* Take bid at least 4 hrs apart. Methylphenidate Naive: Initial: 2.5mg bid. Titrate: Increase weekly by 2.5-5mg/day. Max: 20mg/day. Currently on Methylphenidate: Initial: Take 1/2 of methylphenidate dose. Max: 20mg/day. Reduce or d/c if paradoxical aggravation of symptoms. D/C if no improvement after appropriate dosage adjustments over 1 month.
Pediatrics: ≥6 yrs: Take bid at least 4 hrs apart. Methylphenidate Naive: Initial: 2.5mg bid. Titrate: Increase weekly by 2.5-5mg/day. Max: 20mg/day. Currently on Methylphenidate: Initial: Take 1/2 of methylphenidate dose. Max: 20mg/day. Reduce or d/c if paradoxical aggravation of symptoms. D/C if no improvement after appropriate dosage adjustments over 1 month.

HOW SUPPLIED: Tab: 2.5mg, 5mg, 10mg

CONTRAINDICATIONS: Marked anxiety, tension, and agitation; glaucoma; motor tics or family history or diagnosis of Tourette's syndrome; during or within 14 days of MAOI use.

WARNINGS/PRECAUTIONS: Caution in drug dependence or alcoholism. Avoid with known serious structural cardiac abnormalities, cardiomyopathy, serious heart rhythm abnormalities, CAD, or other serious cardiac problems. May cause modest increase in BP; caution with HTN, heart failure, recent MI, or ventricular arrhythmia. May exacerbate symptoms of behavior disturbance and thought disorder with pre-existing psychotic disorder. Caution when using stimulants to treat patients with comorbid bipolar disorder because of concern for possible induction of mixed/manic episodes in such patients. Stimulants at usual doses may cause treatment-emergent psychotic or manic symptoms (eg, hallucinations, delusional thinking, mania) in children and adolescents without prior history of psychotic illness or mania. Aggressive behavior or hostility reported in clinical trials and the postmarketing experience of some medications indicated for the treatment of ADHD. Suppression of growth reported with long-term use; monitor growth. May lower convulsive threshold; d/c in the presence of seizures. Visual disturbances reported. Monitor CBC, differential, and platelets with prolonged therapy.

ADVERSE REACTIONS: Abdominal pain, fever, anorexia, nausea, nervousness, insomnia. (Pediatrics) Loss of appetite, weight loss, tachycardia.

INTERACTIONS: See Contraindications. May decrease the effectiveness of antihypertensives. Caution with pressor agents. May inhibit metabolism of coumarin anticoagulants, anticonvulsants, and some antidepressants; adjust dose. Adverse events reported with clonidine.

PREGNANCY: Category C, caution in nursing.

MECHANISM OF ACTION: Sympathomimetic amine; blocks the reuptake of norepinephrine and dopamine into the presynaptic neuron and increases the release of these monoamines into the extraneuronal space.

PHARMACOKINETICS: Absorption: Readily absorbed; T_{max}=2.9 hrs (fed), 1.5 hrs (fasting). **Metabolism:** Via de-esterification (d-ritalinic acid; primary metabolite). **Elimination:** Urine (approximately 90%); $T_{1/2}$=2.2 hrs.

FOCALIN **XR** `CII`
dexmethylphenidate HCL (Novartis)

THERAPEUTIC CLASS: Sympathomimetic amine

INDICATIONS: Treatment of attention deficit hyperactivity disorder (ADHD) in patients aged ≥6 yrs.

DOSAGE: *Adults:* Methylphenidate Naive: Initial: 10mg/day. Titrate: May adjust weekly by 10mg/day. Max: 20mg/day. Currently on Methylphenidate: Initial: Take 1/2 of methylphenidate dose. Max: 20mg/day. Reduce or d/c if paradoxical aggravation of symptoms. Swallow capsule whole or sprinkle contents on applesauce. Contents should not be crushed, chewed or divided. D/C if no improvement after appropriate dosage adjustments over 1 month.
Pediatrics: ≥6 yrs: Methylphenidate Naive: Initial: 5mg/day. Titrate: May adjust weekly by 5mg/day. Max: 20mg/day. Currently on Methylphenidate: Initial: Take 1/2 of methylphenidate dose. Max: 20mg/day. Reduce or d/c if paradoxical aggravation of symptoms. Swallow capsule whole or sprinkle contents on applesauce: contents should not be crushed, chewed or divided. D/C if no improvement after appropriate dosage adjustments over 1 month.

HOW SUPPLIED: Cap, Extended-Release: 5mg, 10mg, 15mg, 20mg

CONTRAINDICATIONS: Marked anxiety, tension, and agitation; glaucoma; motor tics or family history or diagnosis of Tourette's syndrome; during or within 14 days of MAOI use.

WARNINGS/PRECAUTIONS: Caution in drug dependence or alcoholism. Avoid with known serious structural cardiac abnormalities, cardiomyopathy, serious heart rhythm abnormalities, CAD, or other serious cardiac problems. May cause modest increase in BP; caution with HTN, heart failure, recent MI, or ventricular arrhythmia. May exacerbate symptoms of behavior disturbance and thought disorder with pre-existing psychotic disorder. Caution when using stimulants to treat patients with comorbid bipolar disorder because of concern for possible induction of mixed/manic episodes in such patients. Stimulants at usual doses may cause treatment-emergent psychotic or manic symptoms (eg, hallucinations, delusional thinking, mania) in children and adolescents without prior history of psychotic illness or mania. Aggressive behavior or hostility reported in clinical trials and the postmarketing experience of some medications indicated for the treatment of ADHD. Suppression of growth reported with long-term use; monitor growth. May lower convulsive threshold; d/c in the presence of seizures. Visual disturbances reported. Monitor CBC, differential, and platelets with prolonged therapy.

ADVERSE REACTIONS: Dyspepsia, headache, anxiety. (Adults) dry mouth, pharyngolaryngeal pain, feeling jittery, dizziness. (Pediatrics) decreased appetite, nausea.

INTERACTIONS: See Contraindications. May decrease the effectiveness of antihypertensives. Caution with pressor agents. May inhibit metabolism of coumarin anticoagulants, anticonvulsants, and tricyclic drugs; adjust dose. Adverse events reported with clonidine. Antacids or acid supressants could alter the release of dexmethylphenidate.

PREGNANCY: Category C, caution in nursing.

MECHANISM OF ACTION: Sympathomimetic amine; CNS stimulant. Blocks reuptake of norepinephrine and dopamine into presynaptic neuron and increases release of these monoamines into extraneuronal space.

PHARMACOKINETICS: Absorption: Bimodal plasma concentration. T_{max}=1-4 hrs (first peak), 4-5.7 hrs (second peak). **Distribution:** V_d=2.65L/kg. **Metabolism:** Metabolized via de-esterification; d-ritalinic acid (metabolite). **Elimination:** Urine (90%); $T_{1/2}$=2-4.5 hrs.

FOLGARD RX 2.2 RX

vitamin B12 - vitamin B6 - folic acid (Upsher-Smith)

THERAPEUTIC CLASS: Folic acid/vitamin combination

INDICATIONS: For nutritional support and folic acid supplementation.

DOSAGE: *Adults:* 1 tab qd.

HOW SUPPLIED: Tab: Folic Acid 2.2mg-Vitamin B_6 25mg-Vitamin B_{12} 0.5mg* *scored

WARNINGS/PRECAUTIONS: Folic acid >0.1mg/day may obscure pernicious anemia.

ADVERSE REACTIONS: Allergic sensitization.

PREGNANCY: Safety in pregnancy and nursing is not known.

MECHANISM OF ACTION: Folic acid/vitamin combination.

FOLIC ACID RX

folic acid (Various)

THERAPEUTIC CLASS: Erythropoiesis agent

INDICATIONS: Treatment of megaloblastic anemia due to folic acid deficiency and in anemias of nutritional origin, pregnancy, infancy or childhood.

DOSAGE: *Adults:* Usual: Up to 1mg/day. Maint: 0.4mg qd. Pregnancy/Nursing: Maint: 0.8mg qd. Max: 1mg/day. Increase maintenance dose with alcoholism, hemolytic anemia, anticonvulsant therapy, chronic infection. *Pediatrics:* Usual: Up to 1mg/day. Maint: Infants: 0.1mg qd. <4 yrs: 0.3mg qd. ≥4 yrs: 0.4mg qd.

HOW SUPPLIED: Inj: 5mg/mL; Tab: (OTC) 0.4mg, 0.8mg, (RX) 1mg

WARNINGS/PRECAUTIONS: Not for monotherapy in pernicious anemia and other megaloblastic anemias with B_{12} deficiency. May obscure pernicious anemia in dosage >0.1 mg/day. Decreased B_{12} serum levels with prolonged therapy.

ADVERSE REACTIONS: Allergic sensitization.

INTERACTIONS: Antagonizes phenytoin effects. Methotrexate, phenytoin, primidone, barbiturates, alcohol, alcoholic cirrhosis, nitrofurantoin, and pyrimethamine increase loss of folate. Increased seizures with phenytoin, primidone and phenobarbital reported. Tetracycline may cause false low serum and red cell folate due to suppression of *Lactobacillus casei*.

PREGNANCY: Category A, requirement increases during nursing.

MECHANISM OF ACTION: Acts as cofactor for transformylation reactions in biosynthesis of purines and thymidylates of nucleic acids; acts on megaloblastic bone marrow to produce normo-blastic marrow; required for nucleo-protein synthesis and maintenance of normal erythropoiesis.

PHARMACOKINETICS: Absorption: Rapid (small intestine); T_{max}=1 hr. **Distribution:** Excreted in breast milk. **Metabolism:** Liver via reduced diphospho-pyridine nucleotide and folate reductase. **Elimination:** Urine, feces.

FOLLISTIM AQ

RX

follitropin beta (Organon)

OTHER BRAND NAMES: Follistim AQ Cartridge (Organon)

THERAPEUTIC CLASS: Follicle stimulating hormone

INDICATIONS: For the development of multiple follicles in ovulatory patients participating in Assisted Reproductive Technology (ART). For the induction of ovulation and pregnancy in anovulatory infertile patients in whom the cause of infertility is functional and not due to primary ovarian failure.

DOSAGE: *Adults:* Ovulation Induction: Cartridge: 75 IU for 7 days. Titrate: Increase by 25-50 IU at weekly intervals. Max: 175 IU daily. Inj: 75 IU for 14 days. Titrate: increase by 37.5 IU weekly. Administer hCG 5000-10,000 U when pre-ovulatory conditions are equivalent to or greater than a normal in-dividual. ART: Initial 150 to 225 IU for 5 days (cartridge) or 4 days (inj). Titrate: Adjust based upon ovarian response. Administer hCG 5000-10,000 U when a sufficient number of follicles of adequate size are present.

HOW SUPPLIED: Cartridge: 150 IU, 300 IU, 600 IU, 900 IU. Inj: 75 IU, 150 IU

CONTRAINDICATIONS: High FSH level indicating primary ovarian failure, uncontrolled thyroid or adrenal dysfunction, pregnancy, heavy or irregular vaginal bleeding of undetermined origin, ovarian cysts or enlargement not due to polycystic ovary syndrome; or tumor of the ovary, breast, uterus, hypo-thalamus or pituitary gland. Hypersensitivity to streptomycin or neomycin and to recombinant hFSH products.

WARNINGS/PRECAUTIONS: Exclude primary ovarian failure. Ovarian enlargement may occur; use the lowest effective dose and monitor ovarian response. Ovarian hyperstimulation syndrome (OHSS), multiple births, serious pulmonary and vascular complications reported. Avoid hCG if ovaries abnor-mally enlarged last day of therapy. Monitor follicular maturation by measuring estradiol levels and through sonographic visualization.

ADVERSE REACTIONS: Abdominal pain, flatulence, nausea, breast pain, injection site reaction, enlarged abdomen, back pain, constipation, headache, ovarian pain, OHSS, sinusitis, upper respiratory tract infection.

PREGNANCY: Category X, not for use in nursing.

MECHANISM OF ACTION: Follicle stimulating hormone; stimulates ovarian follicular growth in women who do not have primary ovarian failure.

PHARMACOKINETICS: Absorption: Administration of variable doses resulted in different parameters. **Distribution:** V_d=8L. **Elimination:** $T_{1/2}$=43.9 (IM).

FOLTX

RX

vitamin B12 - vitamin B6 - folic acid (PamLab)

THERAPEUTIC CLASS: Folic acid/vitamin combination

INDICATIONS: To supply nutritional requirements for those with end stage renal failure, dialysis, hyperhomocystenimia, homocystinuria, nutrient malabsorption.

DOSAGE: *Adults:* 1-2 tabs qd.

HOW SUPPLIED: Tab: Folic Acid 2.5mg-Vitamin B_6 25mg-Vitamin B_{12} 2mg

WARNINGS/PRECAUTIONS: Folic acid >0.1mg/day may obscure pernicious anemia (may be alleviated by B_{12} component).

ADVERSE REACTIONS: Allergic sensitization, paresthesia, somnolence, mild diarrhea, polycythemia vera, peripheral vascular thrombosis, itching, transi-tory exanthema, feeling of body swelling.

INTERACTIONS: Pyridoxine may antagonize levodopa; avoid concomitant use. May be used with carbidopa/levodopa. Decreases effect of phenytoin.

MECHANISM OF ACTION: Folic acid/vitamin combination.

FORADIL   RX
formoterol fumarate (Schering)

Long-acting β_2-agonists may increase the risk of asthma-related death.

THERAPEUTIC CLASS: Beta$_2$-agonist

INDICATIONS: Long-term maintenance treatment of asthma and prevention of bronchospasm with reversible obstructive airway disease (including nocturnal asthma) in patients who require regular treatment with inhaled short acting β_2-agonists. Maintenance treatment of bronchoconstriction in chronic obstructive pulmonary disease (COPD). Acute prevention of excercise-induced bronchospasm (EIB).

DOSAGE: *Adults:* Do not swallow cap; give only by inhalation with Aerolizer Inhaler. Asthma/COPD: 12mcg q12h. Max: 24mcg/day. EIB: 12mcg 15 min before exercise (do not give added dose if already on q12h dose).
Pediatrics: ≥5 yrs: Do not swallow cap; give only by inhalation with Aerolizer™ Inhaler. Asthma/COPD: 12mcg q12h. Max: 24mcg/day. ≥12 yrs: EIB: 12mcg 15 min before exercise (do not give added dose if already on q12h dose).

HOW SUPPLIED: Cap (Inhalation): 12mcg [12^s, 60^s]

WARNINGS/PRECAUTIONS: Do not d/c inhaled corticosteroids. Only use short-acting β_2-agonist inhaler for acute symptoms. D/C if paradoxical bronchospasm occurs. D/C if ECG changes, QT interval increases, or ST depression occurs. Caution with cardiovascular disorders (eg, HTN, arrhythmias), thyrotoxicosis and convulsive disorders. Anaphylactic and other allergic reactions reported. Not for use in acute asthmatic conditions. Should not be used with other long-acting β_2-agonist medications. May cause hypokalemia.

ADVERSE REACTIONS: Viral infection, dyspnea, chest pain, tremor, HTN, hypotension, tachycardia, arrhythmias, headache, nausea, vomiting, fatigue, hypokalemia, hyperglycemia, exacerbation of asthma.

INTERACTIONS: Potentiates other sympathomimetics. Hypokalemia potentiated by xanthine derivatives (eg, theophylline), steroids and non-potassium sparing diuretics. Extreme caution with MAOIs, TCAs, and drugs known to prolong QT interval. Antagonized effect with β-blockers.

PREGNANCY: Category C, caution in nursing.

MECHANISM OF ACTION: Long-acting selective β_2-adrenergic receptor agonist; acts as a bronchodilator, activates adenyl cyclase on airway smooth muscles and increases the intracellular concentration of cyclic AMP. Increased cAMP levels are associated with relaxation of bronchial smooth muscle and inhibition of release of mediators of immediate hypersensitivity.

PHARMACOKINETICS: **Absorption:** Healthy: C_{max}=92pg/mL, T_{max}=5 min. COPD patient: (12mcg) C_{max}=4.0-8.8, 8, 17.3pg/mL at 10 min, 2 hrs, 6 hrs, respectively. **Distribution:** Plasma protein binding (61-64%), serum albumin binding (31-38%). **Metabolism:** Glucuronidation, O-methylation via CYP450 enzymes 2D6, 2C19, 2CP, 2A6. **Elimination:** Healthy: Urine (59-62%), feces (32-34%). With asthma: Urine (10% unchanged). COPD: Urine (7%). $T_{1/2}$=10 hrs.

FORTAMET   RX
metformin HCL (Sciele)

THERAPEUTIC CLASS: Biguanide

INDICATIONS: Adjunct to diet or with a sulfonylurea or insulin, to improve glycemic control in type 2 diabetes mellitus.

DOSAGE: *Adults:* ≥17 yrs: Take with evening meal. Initial: 500-1000mg qd. With Insulin: Initial: 500mg qd. Titrate: May increase by 500mg/week. Max: 2500mg/day. Decrease insulin dose by 10-25% if FPG <120mg/dL. Elderly/Debilitated/Malnourished: Conservative dosing; do not titrate to max.

HOW SUPPLIED: Tab, Extended-Release: 500mg, 1000mg

CONTRAINDICATIONS: Renal disease/dysfunction (SrCr ≥1.5mg/dL [males], ≥1.4mg/dL [females], or abnormal CrCl), CHF, metabolic acidosis, diabetic ketoacidosis. D/C temporarily (48 hrs) for radiologic studies with intravascular iodinated contrast materials.

WARNINGS/PRECAUTIONS: Lactic acidosis reported (rare); increased risk with renal dysfunction, increased age, DM, CHF, and other conditions with risk of hypoperfusion and hypoxemia. Avoid use in patients ≥80 yrs unless renal function is normal. Monitor renal function and for ketoacidosis and metabolic acidosis. Avoid in renal/hepatic impairment. D/C in hypoxic states (eg, CHF, shock, acute MI), loss of blood glucose control due to stress (give insulin), acidosis, dehydration, sepsis. Temporarily d/c prior to surgery (due to restricted food intake) and procedures requiring intravascular iodinated contrast materials. May decrease serum vitamin B_{12} levels. Increased risk of hypoglycemia in elderly, debilitated/malnourished, adrenal or pituitary insufficiency, or alcohol intoxication.

ADVERSE REACTIONS: Diarrhea, nausea, dyspepsia, flatulence, abdominal pain, headache.

INTERACTIONS: Furosemide, nifedipine, cimetidine, cationic drugs (eg, digoxin, amiloride, procainamide, quinidine, quinine, ranitidine, trimethoprim, vancomycin, triamterene, morphine) may increase metformin levels. Thiazides, other diuretics, corticosteroids, phenothiazines, thyroid products, estrogens, oral contraceptives, phenytoin, nicotinic acid, sympathomimetics, CCBs, isoniazid may cause hyperglycemia. Risk of hypoglycemia with alcohol. Excess alcohol may increase potential for lactic acidosis. May decrease furosemide levels.

PREGNANCY: Category B, not for use in nursing.

MECHANISM OF ACTION: Biguanide; decreases hepatic glucose production, decreases intestinal absorption of glucose, and improves insulin selectivity by increasing peripheral glucose uptake and utilization.

PHARMACOKINETICS: Absorption: AUC=26811ng/mL, C_{max}=2849ng/mL, T_{max}=6 hrs. **Elimination:** Urine (90%); $T_{1/2}$=6.2 hrs (plasma), 17.6 hrs (blood).

FORTAZ   RX
ceftazidime (GlaxoSmithKline)

THERAPEUTIC CLASS: Cephalosporin (3rd generation)

INDICATIONS: Treatment of lower respiratory tract (eg, pneumonia), skin and skin structure (SSSI), bone/joint, gynecologic, CNS (eg, meningitis), intra-abdominal, and urinary tract infections (UTI); and septicemia caused by susceptible strains of microorganisms. Treatment of sepsis.

DOSAGE: *Adults:* Usual: 1g IM/IV q8-12h. Uncomplicated UTI: 250mg IM/IV q12h. Complicated UTI: 500mg IM/IV q8-12h. Bone and Joint Infection: 2g IV q12h. Uncomplicated Pneumonia/SSSI: 500mg-1g IM/IV q8h. Gynecological/ Intra-Abdominal/Meningitis/Severe Life-Threatening Infection: 2g IV q8h. Lung Infection Caused by *Pseudomonas* spp. in Cystic Fibrosis (Normal Renal Function): 30-50mg/kg IV q8h. Max: 6g/day. CrCl 31-50mL/min: 1g q12h. CrCl 16-30mL/min: 1g q24h. CrCl 6-15mL/min: 500mg q24h. CrCl <5mL/min: 500mg q48h. For severe infections (6g/day), increase renal impairment dose by 50% or increase dosing interval. Apply reduced dosage recommendations after initial 1g LD is given. Hemodialysis: Give 1g before, then 1g after each hemodialysis. Intra-Peritoneal Dialysis/Continuous Ambulatory Peritoneal Dialysis: Give 1g followed by 500mg q24h, or add to fluid at 250mg/2L. *Pediatrics:* 1 month-12 yrs: 30-50mg/kg IV q8h. Max: 6g/day. Neonates (0-4 weeks): 30mg/kg IV q12h. Higher doses for cystic fibrosis or meningitis. CrCl 31-50mL/min: 1g q12h. CrCl 16-30mL/min: 1g q24h. CrCl 6-15mL/min: 500mg q24h. CrCl <5mL/min: 500mg q48h. For severe infections (6g/day), increase renal impairment dose by 50% or increase dosing interval. Apply reduced dosage recommendations after initial 1g LD is given. Hemodialysis: Give 1g before, then 1g after each hemodialysis. Intra-Peritoneal Dialysis/ Continuous Ambulatory Peritoneal Dialysis: Give 1g followed by 500mg q24h, or add to fluid at 250mg/2L.

HOW SUPPLIED: Inj: 500mg, 1g, 1g/50mL, 2g, 2g/50mL, 6g

WARNINGS/PRECAUTIONS: Monitor renal function; potential for nephrotoxicity. Prolonged use may result in overgrowth of nonsusceptible organisms. Possible cross-sensitivity between PCNs, cephalosporins, and other β-lactam antibiotics. *Clostridium difficile*-associated diarrhea reported and may range in severity from mild diarrhea to fatal colitis. Elevated levels with renal insufficiency can lead to seizures, encephalopathy, coma, asterixis and neuromuscular excitability. Possible decrease in PT; caution with renal/hepatic impairment, poor nutritional state; monitor PT and give vitamin K if needed. Caution with colitis, other GI diseases, and elderly. Distal necrosis may occur after inadvertent intra-arterial administration. Continue therapy for 2 days after the signs and symptoms of infection have disappeared, but in complicated infections longer therapy may be required. False (+) for urine glucose with Benedict's solution, Fehling's solution, and Clinitest® tablets.

ADVERSE REACTIONS: Phlebitis and inflammation at injection site, pruritus, rash, fever, diarrhea.

INTERACTIONS: Nephrotoxicity reported with aminoglycosides or potent diuretics (eg, furosemide). Avoid with chloramphenicol; may decrease effect of β-lactam antibiotics. Possible decrease in PT; caution with a protracted course of antimicrobial therapy; monitor PT and give vitamin K if needed. May reduce efficacy of oral contraceptives.

PREGNANCY: Category B, caution in nursing.

MECHANISM OF ACTION: 3rd-generation cephalosporin; bactericidal, inhibits cell wall synthesis.

PHARMACOKINETICS: Absorption: (IV) Administration of variable doses resulted in different parameters. **Distribution:** Plasma protein binding (≤10%). **Elimination:** Urine (unchanged, 80-90%).

FORTEO RX
teriparatide (Lilly)

> Increased incidence of osteosarcoma seen in rats. Only prescribe when benefits outweigh risks. Not for those at increased baseline risk for osteosarcoma, including Paget's disease or unexplained alkaline phosphatase elevations, open epiphyses, or prior radiation therapy involving the skeleton.

THERAPEUTIC CLASS: Recombinant human parathyroid hormone

INDICATIONS: Treatment of postmenopausal women with osteoporosis who are at high risk for fracture. To increase bone mass in men with primary or hypogonadal osteoporosis who are at high risk for fracture.

DOSAGE: *Adults:* 20mcg qd SQ into thigh or abdominal wall. Administer initially under circumstances where patient can sit or lie down if symptoms of orthostatic hypotension occur. Discard pen after 28 days. Use for >2 yrs is not recommended.

HOW SUPPLIED: Inj: 250mcg/mL [3mL pen]

WARNINGS/PRECAUTIONS: Avoid in paget's disease of the bone, pediatrics, prior external beam or implant radiation therapy, or with bone metastases, or history of skeletal malignancies, metabolic bone diseases other than osteoporosis, or pre-existing hypercalcemia (eg, primary hyperparathyroidism). Potential exacerbation of active or recent urolithiasis. Transient episodes of symptomatic orthostatic hypotension observed infrequently. Increases serum uric acid levels. Transient calcium increases.

ADVERSE REACTIONS: Pain, arthralgia, asthenia, nausea, rhinitis, dizziness, headache, HTN, increased cough, pharyngitis, constipation, diarrhea, dyspepsia.

INTERACTIONS: Hypercalcemia may predispose to digitalis toxicity; caution with concomitant use.

PREGNANCY: Category C; not for use in nursing.

MECHANISM OF ACTION: Recombinant human parathyroid hormone; binds to specific high-affinity cell-surface receptors. Stimulates new bone

F

formation on trabecular and cortical bone surfaces by preferential stimulation of osteoblastic activity over osteoclastic activity. Produces an increase in skeletal mass, an increase in markers of bone formation and resorption, and an increase in bone strength.

PHARMACOKINETICS: Absorption: Extensive; absolute bioavailability (95%); T_{max}=30 minutes. **Distribution:** (IV) V_d= 0.12L/kg. **Metabolism:** Liver (non-specific enzymatic mechanism). **Elimination:** Kidney; (IV) $T_{1/2}$=5 min; (SC) $T_{1/2}$=1 hr.

FORTICAL   RX
calcitonin-salmon (rdna origin) (Upsher-Smith)

THERAPEUTIC CLASS: Hormonal bone resorption inhibitor

INDICATIONS: Treatment of postmenopausal osteoporosis in females >5 yrs postmenopause in conjunction with an adequate calcium and vitamin D intake.

DOSAGE: *Adults:* 200 IU qd intranasally. Alternate nostrils daily.

HOW SUPPLIED: Nasal Spray: 200 IU/inh

CONTRAINDICATIONS: Clinical allergy to calcitonin-salmon.

WARNINGS/PRECAUTIONS: Possibility of systemic allergic reactions. Consider skin testing if sensitivity suspected. If nasal mucosa ulceration occurs, d/c until healed. D/C if severe ulceration of nasal mucosa occurs. Perform periodic nasal exams. Incidence of rhinitis, irritation, erythema, and excoriation higher in geriatric patients.

ADVERSE REACTIONS: Rhinitis, nasal symptoms, back pain, arthralgia, epistaxis, headache

PREGNANCY: Category C, not for use in nursing.

MECHANISM OF ACTION: Hormonal bone resorption inhibitor; mechanism not fully established. Calcitonin receptors are found in osteoclasts and osteoblasts. Single use produces transient inhibition of bone resorptive process; persistent use causes smaller decreases in rate of bone resorption. Inhibits osteoclast function with loss of ruffled osteoclast border.

PHARMACOKINETICS: Absorption: Rapid.

FOSAMAX   RX
alendronate sodium (Merck)

THERAPEUTIC CLASS: Bisphosphonate

INDICATIONS: Treatment and prevention of osteoporosis in postmenopausal women. Treatment to increase bone mass in men with osteoporosis. Treatment of glucocorticoid-induced osteoporosis. Treatment of Paget's disease.

DOSAGE: *Adults:* Osteoporosis: Treatment: 70mg once weekly or 10mg qd. Prevention: 35mg once weekly or 5mg qd. Glucocorticoid-Induced: 5mg qd; 10mg qd for postmenopausal women not on estrogen. Paget's Disease: 40mg qd for 6 months. Take at least 30 min before the first food, beverage (other than water), or medication (Take tabs with 6-8oz plain water or 2oz with oral sol). Do not lie down for at least 30 min and until after 1st food of the day.

HOW SUPPLIED: Sol: 70mg [75mL]; Tab: 5mg, 10mg, 35mg, 40mg, 70mg

CONTRAINDICATIONS: Esophagus abnormalities which delay esophageal emptying such as stricture or achalasia; inability to stand or sit upright for at least 30 min; hypocalcemia.

WARNINGS/PRECAUTIONS: Caution with active upper GI problems. May cause local irritation of the upper GI mucosa. Correct hypocalcemia or other mineral metabolism disturbances before initiating therapy. Supplement calcium and vitamin D if needed. Not recommended with renal insufficiency (CrCl <35mL/min). D/C if symptoms of esophageal disease develop. When combined with glucocorticoids, perform BMD test at initiation and

6-12 months later. Reports of severe, incapacitating bone, joint, and/or muscle pain.

ADVERSE REACTIONS: Abdominal pain, nausea, dyspepsia, constipation, diarrhea, flatulence, acid regurgitation, musculoskeletal pain, gastric ulcers, joint swelling, asthenia, dizziness/vertigo, and rarely peripheral edema.

INTERACTIONS: Calcium supplements, antacids, other oral medications may interfere with absorption; dose at least one-half hour after alendronate. Increased GI irritation with ASA and alendronate >10mg. Caution with NSAIDs, other GI irritants.

PREGNANCY: Category C, caution in nursing.

MECHANISM OF ACTION: Biphosphonate; binds to hydroxyapatite, a component of bone. Acts as a specific inhibitor of osteoclast-mediated bone resorption.

PHARMACOKINETICS: Distribution: V_d=28L; plasma protein binding (78%). **Excretion:** Urine (50%), feces (little or none); $T_{1/2}$ >10 yrs.

FOSAMAX PLUS D
RX
alendronate sodium - cholecalciferol (Merck)

THERAPEUTIC CLASS: Bisphosphonate/vitamin D analog

INDICATIONS: Treatment of osteoporosis in postmenapausal women. Treatment to increase bone mass in men with osteoporosis.

DOSAGE: *Adults:* 1 tab (70mg/5600 IU or 70mg/2800 IU) once weekly. Take at least 30 min before 1st food, beverage (other than water), or medication. Do not lie down for at least 30 min and until after 1st food of day.

HOW SUPPLIED: Tab: (Alendronate Sodium-Cholecalciferol) 70mg-2800 IU, 70mg-5600 IU

CONTRAINDICATIONS: Esophagus abnormalities which delay esophageal emptying such as stricture or achalasia; inability to stand or sit upright for at least 30 min; hypocalcemia.

WARNINGS/PRECAUTIONS: Caution with active upper GI problems. May cause local irritation of the upper GI mucosa. Correct hypocalcemia or other mineral metabolism disturbances before initiating therapy. Do not use to treat vitamin D deficiency. May worsen hypercalcemia and/or hypercalciuria. Supplement calcium if needed. Not recommended with renal insufficiency (CrCl <35mL/min). D/C if symptoms of esophageal disease develop. Reports of severe, incapacitating bone, joint, and/or muscle pain.

ADVERSE REACTIONS: Abdominal pain, nausea, dyspepsia, constipation, diarrhea, flatulence, acid regurgitation, musculoskeletal pain, gastric ulcers, joint swelling, asthenia, dizziness/vertigo, and rarely peripheral edema.

INTERACTIONS: Calcium supplements, antacids, other oral medications may interfere with absorption; dose at least one-half hour after alendronate. Caution with NSAIDs, other GI irritants. Olestra, mineral oils, orlistat, bile acid sequestrants may impair absorption. Anticonvulsants, cimetidine, thiazides may increase catabolism.

PREGNANCY: Category C, caution in nursing.

MECHANISM OF ACTION: Alendronate: Biphosphonate; binds to hydroxyapatite found in bone. Specific inhibitor of osteoclast-mediated bone resorption. Cholecalciferol: Vitamin D analog; increases intestinal absorption of calcium and phosphate; regulates excretion of serum calcium, renal calcium and phosphate, bone formation, and bone resorption.

PHARMACOKINETICS: Absorption: Cholecalciferol: AUC=120.7ng•hr/mL; C_{max}=4.0ng/mL; T_{max}=10.6 hrs. **Distribution:** Alendronate: V_d=28L; plasma protein binding (78%). Cholecalciferol: Found in breast milk. **Metabolism:** Cholecalciferol: Liver (rapid) (hydroxylation) to 25-hydroxyvitamin D_3 (major storage form metabolite); kidney to 1,25-dihydroxyvitamin D_3 (active metabolite). **Elimination:** Alendronate: Urine (50%), feces (little or none); $T_{1/2}$ >10 years. Cholecalceferol: Urine (2.4%), feces (4.9%); $T_{1/2}$=14 hrs.

FOSRENOL
RX

lanthanum carbonate (Shire)

THERAPEUTIC CLASS: Phosphate binder

INDICATIONS: Reduction of serum phosphate in patients with end-stage renal disease.

DOSAGE: *Adults:* Initial: 750-1500mg/day in divided doses. Titrate: Every 2-3 weeks in increments of 750mg/day until acceptable serum phosphate level is reached. Take with meals and chew tablets completely before swallowing. Usual range: 1500-3000mg/day. Usual max: 3750mg/day.

HOW SUPPLIED: Tab, Chewable: 250mg, 500mg, 750mg, 1000mg

WARNINGS/PRECAUTIONS: Caution with acute peptic ulcer, ulcerative colitis, Crohn's disease or bowel obstruction.

ADVERSE REACTIONS: Nausea, vomiting, dialysis graft occulsion, abdominal pain.

INTERACTIONS: Should not be taken within 2 hrs of antacids.

PREGNANCY: Category C, caution in nursing.

MECHANISM OF ACTION: Inhibits absorption of phosphate by forming highly insoluble lanthanum phosphate complexes, consequently reducing both serum phosphate and calcium product.

PHARMACOKINETICS: Absorption: C_{max}=1.0ng/mL. **Distribution:** Plasma protein binding (>99%). **Metabolism:** Not metabolized. **Elimination:** $T_{1/2}$=53 hrs, ($T_{1/2}$=2-3.6 yrs. (from bone).

FRAGMIN
RX

dalteparin sodium (Eisai/Pfizer)

> Risk of paralysis by spinal/epidural hematoma with neuraxial anesthesia or spinal puncture. Increased risk with indwelling epidural catheters for analgesia, drugs affecting hemostasis (eg, NSAIDs, platelet inhibitors, anticoagulants), and traumatic or repeated epidural or spinal puncture. Frequently monitor for signs and symptoms of neurological impairment.

THERAPEUTIC CLASS: Low molecular weight heparin

INDICATIONS: Prevention of ischemic complications in unstable angina and non-Q-wave MI with concurrent ASA therapy. Prophylaxis of DVT in hip replacement surgery, abdominal surgery in patients who are at high risk for thromboembolic complications, and for those at risk for thromboembolic complications due to severely restricted mobility during acute illness. Extended treatment of symptomatic VTE (proximal DVT and/or PE), to reduce the recurrence of VTE in patients with cancer.

DOSAGE: *Adults:* Administer SQ. Unstable Angina/Non-Q-Wave MI: 120 IU/kg up to 10,000 IU q12h with ASA (75-165mg/day) for 5-8 days. Hip Surgery: Pre-Op Start: Initial (if start 2 hrs pre-op): 2500 IU within 2 hrs pre-op, then 2500 IU 4-8 hrs post-op. Initial (if start 10-14 hrs pre-op): 5000 IU 10-14 hrs pre-op, then 5000 IU 4-8 hrs post-op. Maint (for either initial dose): 5000 IU SQ qd for 5-10 days post-op (up to 14 days). Post-Op Start: 2500 IU 4-8 hrs post-op. Maint: 5000 IU qd. Abdominal Surgery: 2500 IU 1-2 hrs pre-op. Maint: 2500 IU qd for 5-10 days post-op. Abdominal Surgery with High Risk: 5000 IU evening before surgery. Maint: 5000 IU qd for 5-10 days post-op. Abdominal Surgery with Malignancy: Initial: 2500 IU 1-2 hrs pre-op, then 2500 IU 12 hrs later. Maint: 5000 IU qd for 5-10 days post-op. Severely Restricted Mobility During Acute Illness: 5000 IU qd for 12-14 days. Symptomatic VTE in Cancer Patients: 200 IU/kg qd for first 30 days, then 150 IU/kg qd for months 2-6. Max: 18,000 IU/day. Platelet Count 50,000-100,000/mm³: Reduce dose by 2500 IU until platelet count ≥100,000/mm³. Platelet Count <50,000/mm³: D/C therapy until platelet count >50,000/mm³. Renal Impairment (CrCl <30mL/min): Monitor anti-Xa levels to determine appropriate dose.

HOW SUPPLIED: Inj: (Syringe) 2500 IU/0.2mL, 5000 IU/0.2mL, 7500 IU/0.3mL, 10,000 IU/0.4mL, 10,000 IU/1mL, 12,500 IU/0.5mL, 15,000

IU/0.6mL, 18,000 IU/0.72mL; (MDV) 95,000 IU/mL [3.8mL], 95,000 IU/mL [9.5mL]

CONTRAINDICATIONS: Heparin or pork allergy, regional anesthesia with unstable angina, non-Q-wave MI or patients with cancer, active major bleeding, thrombocytopenia with a positive in vitro test for antiplatelet antibody.

WARNINGS/PRECAUTIONS: Not for IM injection. Cannot use interchangeably unit for unit with heparin or other low molecular weight heparins. Extreme caution with HIT, conditions with increased risk of hemorrhage (eg, bacterial endocarditis, hemorrhagic stroke, etc). Hemorrhage, thrombocytopenia, HIT may occur. May increase risk of thrombocytopenia with cancer or acute venous thromboembolism. Caution with bleeding diathesis, platelet defects, severe hepatic/kidney dysfunction, hypertensive or diabetic retinopathy, recent GI bleeding or in elderly with low body weight (<45kg) and predisposed to decreased renal function. D/C if thromboembolic event occurs. Perform periodic CBC, platelets, stool occult blood test. May increase LFTs. Multiple dose vial contains benzyl alcohol. Do not mix with other injections or infusions unless compatibilty data available.

ADVERSE REACTIONS: Hemorrhage, injection-site pain, allergic reactions, thrombocytopenia.

INTERACTIONS: Caution with oral anticoagulants, platelet inhibitors, thrombolytic agents due to increased risk of bleeding.

PREGNANCY: Category B, caution in nursing.

MECHANISM OF ACTION: Low molecular weight heparin: antithrombotic properties. Enhances inhibition of Factor Xa and thrombin by antithrombin.

PHARMACOKINETICS: Absorption: Absolute bioavailability (87%); (2500 IU) C_{max}=0.19 IU/mL; (5000 IU) C_{max}= 0.41 IU/mL; (10,000 IU) C_{max}=0.82 IU/mL; T_{max}=4 hrs. **Distribution:** V_d=40-60mL/kg. **Elimination:** (40 IU/kg) (IV): $T_{1/2}$=2.1 hrs; (60 IU/kg) (IV): $T_{1/2}$=2.3 hrs; (SQ) $T_{1/2}$=3-5 hrs.

FROVA   RX
frovatriptan succinate (Endo)

THERAPEUTIC CLASS: $5\text{-HT}_{1D\,1B}$-agonist

INDICATIONS: Acute treatment of migraine with or without aura.

DOSAGE: *Adults:* ≥18 yrs: 2.5mg with fluids. If headache recurs after initial relief, may repeat after 2 hrs. Max: 7.5mg/day. Safety of treating >4 headaches/30 days not known.

HOW SUPPLIED: Tab: 2.5mg

CONTRAINDICATIONS: Ischemic heart disease, coronary artery vasospasm (eg, Prinzmetal's angina), significant cardiovascular disease, cerebrovascular syndromes, peripheral vascular disease, uncontrolled HTN, hemiplegic or basilar migraine, use within 24 hrs of treatment with another 5-HT_1 agonist or ergot-type agent.

WARNINGS/PRECAUTIONS: Confirm diagnosis. Supervise 1st dose and monitor cardiac function in those at risk of CAD (eg, HTN, hypercholesterolemia, smoker, obesity, diabetes, CAD family history, postmenopausal women, males >40 yrs). Serious adverse cardiac events, cerebrovascular events, vasospastic reactions reported with 5-HT_1 agonists. May bind to melanin in the eye; possibility of long-term effects.

ADVERSE REACTIONS: Dizziness, headache, paresthesia, dry mouth, dyspepsia, fatigue, hot or cold sensation, chest pain, skeletal pain, flushing.

INTERACTIONS: Prolonged vasospastic reactions reported with ergot-containing drugs; avoid use within 24 hours. Avoid within 24 hours of other $5\text{-HT}_{1B/1D}$ agonists. Weakness, hyperreflexia, and incoordination reported with SSRIs (rare).

PREGNANCY: Category C, caution in nursing.

MECHANISM OF ACTION: Selective 5-HT_1-receptor agonist; binds with high affinity to $5\text{-HT}_{1B/1D}$ receptors. Believed to act on extracerebral, intracranial blood vessels, and to inhibit excessive dilation of these vessels in migraine.

PHARMACOKINETICS: Absorption: Absolute bioavailability: (20%) male, (30%) female; T_{max}=2-4 hrs. **Distribution:** V_d=4.2L/kg (male), 3L/kg (female); plasma protein binding (15%). **Metabolism:** CYP1A2. **Elimination:** Feces (62%), urine (32%); $T_{1/2}$=26 hrs.

FURADANTIN   RX
nitrofurantoin (Sciele)

THERAPEUTIC CLASS: Imidazolidinedione antibacterial

INDICATIONS: Treatment of urinary tract infection (UTI).

DOSAGE: *Adults:* Usual: 50-100mg qid with food for 1 week or at least 3 days after sterility of urine. Use lower doses for uncomplicated UTI. Long-Term Suppressive Therapy: 50-100mg qhs.
Pediatrics: >1 month: Usual: 5-7mg/kg/day given qid with food for 1 week or at least 3 days after sterility of urine. Long-Term Suppressive Therapy: 1mg/kg/day qd or bid.

HOW SUPPLIED: Sus: 25mg/5mL

CONTRAINDICATIONS: Anuria, oliguria, CrCl <60 mL/min, pregnancy at term (38-42 weeks gestation), during labor and delivery, neonates <1 month of age.

WARNINGS/PRECAUTIONS: Acute, subacute or chronic pulmonary reactions have occurred. Enhanced occurrence of peripheral neuropathy with anemia, DM, renal dysfunction, electrolyte imbalance, vitamin B deficiency, and debilitating disease. D/C therapy with acute and chronic pulmonary reactions, hepatic disorders, hemolysis, or peripheral neuropathy. Monitor renal function, LFTs and pulmonary function periodically during long-term therapy. Pseudomembranous colitis reported.

ADVERSE REACTIONS: Pulmonary disorders, hepatic damage, peripheral neuropathy, nausea, emesis, anorexia, dizziness, exfoliative dermatitis, Stevens-Johnson syndrome, anaphylaxis, blood dyscrasias.

INTERACTIONS: Antacids, especially magnesium trisilicate, decrease rate and extent of absorption. Probenecid and sulfinpyrazone increase nitrofurantoin levels.

PREGNANCY: Category B, not for use in nursing.

MECHANISM OF ACTION: Imidazolidinedione antibacterial; inhibits protein synthesis, aerobic energy metabolism, DNA, RNA, and cell wall synthesis.

PHARMACOKINETICS: Absorption: Readily absorbed (with food).
Elimination: Urine.

FUROSEMIDE   RX
furosemide (Various)

> Can lead to profound water and electrolyte depletion with excessive use.

OTHER BRAND NAMES: Lasix (Sanofi-Aventis)

THERAPEUTIC CLASS: Loop diuretic

INDICATIONS: (Inj, PO) Treatment of edema associated with CHF, liver cirrhosis, and renal disease including nephrotic syndrome. (PO) Treatment of hypertension. (Inj) Adjunct therapy for acute pulmonary edema.

DOSAGE: *Adults:* (PO) HTN: Initial: 40mg bid. Edema: Initial: 20-80mg PO. May repeat or increase by 20-40mg after 6-8 hrs. Max: 600mg/day. Alternative Regimen: Dose on 2-4 consecutive days each week. Closely monitor if on >80mg/day. (Inj) Edema: Initial: 20-40mg IV/IM. May repeat or increase by 20mg after 2 hrs. Acute Pulmonary Edema: Initial: 40mg IV. May increase to 80mg IV after 1 hr.
Pediatrics: Edema: (PO) Initial: 2mg/kg single dose. May increase by 1-2mg/kg after 6-8 hrs. Max: 6mg/kg. (Inj) Initial: 1mg/kg IV/IM single dose. May increase by 1mg/kg IV/IM after 2 hrs. Max: 6mg/kg.

HOW SUPPLIED: Inj: 10mg/mL; Sol: 10mg/mL, 40mg/5mL; Tab: 20mg, 40mg*, 80mg *scored

CONTRAINDICATIONS: Anuria.

WARNINGS/PRECAUTIONS: Monitor for fluid/electrolyte imbalance (eg, hypokalemia), renal or hepatic dysfunction. Initiate in hospital with hepatic cirrhosis and ascites. Tinnitus, hearing impairment, hyperglycemia, hyperuricemia reported. May activate SLE. Cross-sensitivity with sulfonamide allergy. Avoid excessive diuresis, especially in elderly.

ADVERSE REACTIONS: Pancreatitis, jaundice, anorexia, paresthesias, ototoxicity, blood dyscrasias, dizziness, rash, urticaria, photosensitivity, fever, thrombophlebitis, restlessness.

INTERACTIONS: Ototoxicity with aminoglycosides, ethacrynic acid. Caution with high dose salicylates. Lithium toxicity. Antagonizes tubocurarine. Potentiates antihypertensives, succinylcholine, ganglionic or peripheral adrenergic blockers. Decreases arterial response to norepinephrine. Separate sucralfate dose by 2 hrs. Indomethacin may decrease effects. Hypokalemia with ACTH, corticosteroids. Renal changes with NSAIDs. Orthostatic hypotension may be aggravated by alcohol, barbiturates, or narcotics.

PREGNANCY: Category C, caution in nursing.

MECHANISM OF ACTION: Anthranilic acid derivative (diuretic); primarily inhibits reabsorption of Na^+ and Cl^- in proximal and distal tubules and in loop of Henle.

PHARMACOKINETICS: Distribution: Plasma protein binding (91-99%). **Metabolism:** Biotransformation. Furosemide glucuronide (major metabolite). **Elimination:** Urine; $T_{1/2}$=2 hrs.

FUZEON   RX
enfuvirtide (Roche Labs)

THERAPEUTIC CLASS: Fusion inhibitor

INDICATIONS: Treatment of HIV-1 infection in combination with other antiretroviral agents in treatment-experienced patients with evidence of HIV-1 replication despite ongoing antiretroviral therapy.

DOSAGE: *Adults:* 90mg SQ bid. Inject SQ into upper arm, anterior thigh, or abdomen. Do not inject into moles, scar tissue, bruises, the navel, or near any blood vessels. Rotate sites; do not give if injection site reaction occurred from an earlier dose.
Pediatrics: 6-16 yrs: 2mg/kg SQ bid. Max: 90mg bid. 11-15.5kg: 27mg bid. 15.6-20.0kg: 36mg bid. 20.1-24.5kg: 45mg bid. 24.6-29.0kg: 54mg bid. 29.1-33.5kg: 63mg bid. 33.6-38.0kg: 72mg bid. 38.1-42.5kg: 81mg bid. ≥ 42.6kg: 90mg bid. Inject SQ into upper arm, anterior thigh, or abdomen. Do not inject into moles, scar tissue, bruises, or the navel. Rotate sites; do not give if injection site reaction occurred from an earlier dose.

HOW SUPPLIED: Inj: 90mg [60⁵]

WARNINGS/PRECAUTIONS: Monitor for signs and symptoms of pneumonia, cellulitis, or local infection. D/C if hypersensitivity reactions occur. Theoretically may lead to production of anti-enfuvirtide antibodies; may result in false positive HIV test with an ELISA assay. Immune reconstitution syndrome reported. Increased risk of bleeding or bruising in patients with coagulation disorders.

ADVERSE REACTIONS: Diarrhea, nausea, fatigue, local injection site reactions, peripheral neuropathy, insomnia, depression, anxiety, cough, sinusitis, herpes simplex, decreased weight/appetite, pancreatitis, asthenia, pruritus, myalgia, nerve pain, bruising, hematomas.

PREGNANCY: Category B, not for use in nursing.

MECHANISM OF ACTION: Fusion inhibitor; inhibits the fusion of HIV-1 with CD4+ cells by interfering with entry of HIV-1 into cells.

PHARMACOKINETICS: Absorption: (SQ) C_{max}=4.59µg/mL; T_{max}=8 hrs; AUC=55.8µg•hr/mL. (IV) Absolute bioavailabilty (84.3%). Values obtained from different parameters are different when combined with other antiretro-viral agents. **Distribution:** V_d=5.5L; plasma protein binding (92%). **Metabolism:** Hepatic (hydrolysis); metabolite (M_3). **Elimination:** (SQ) $T_{1/2}$=3.8 hrs.

GABITRIL
RX

tiagabine HCL (Cephalon)

THERAPEUTIC CLASS: Nipecotic acid derivative

INDICATIONS: Adjunctive therapy in the treatment of partial seizures.

DOSAGE: *Adults:* Initial: 4mg qd. Titrate: May increase weekly by 4-8mg until clinical response. Max: 56mg/day given bid-qid. Take with food.
Pediatrics: ≥12 yo: Initial: 4mg qd. Titrate: May increase to 8mg qd at beginning of Week 2, then increase weekly by 4-8mg until clinical response. Max: 32mg/day. Take with food.

HOW SUPPLIED: Tab: 2mg, 4mg, 12mg, 16mg

WARNINGS/PRECAUTIONS: Reports of new-onset seizure or status epilepticus in patients without epilepsy. D/C and evaluate for underlying seizure disorder. Avoid abrupt withdrawal. Monitor during initial titration for impaired concentration, speech problem, somnolence, fatigue; may require hospitalization if reaction is severe. May exacerbate EEG abnormalities; adjust dose. Status epilepticus and sudden death reported. Reduce dose or d/c if generalized weakness occurs. Reduce dose with hepatic impairment. Serious skin rash reported.

ADVERSE REACTIONS: Dizziness, asthenia, somnolence, nausea, vomiting, nervousness, tremor, abdominal pain, abnormal thinking, depression, confusion, pharyngitis, rash.

INTERACTIONS: May reduce valproate levels. Diminished effects with carbamazepine, phenytoin. Additive CNS depression with alcohol, triazolam, CNS depressants.

PREGNANCY: Category C, caution in nursing.

MECHANISM OF ACTION: Antiepileptic; not fully established. May enhance the activity of gamma aminobutytic acid (GABA), the major inhibitory neurotransmitter in the CNS. Binds to recognition sites associated with the GABA uptake carrier, thereby blocking GABA uptake into presynaptic neurons, permitting more GABA to be available for receptor binding on the surface of post-synaptic cells.

PHARMACOKINETICS: Absorption: Absolute bioavailability (90%). T_{max}=2.5 hrs. (with meals), T_{max}=45 min (fasting). **Distribution:** Plasma protein binding (96%). **Metabolism:** Hepatic via oxidation and glucoronidation, CYP3A. **Elimination:** Urine (25%), feces (63%); $T_{1/2}$=7-9 hrs. For pediatric parameters refer to full PI.

GAMMAR-P
RX

immune globulin (CSL Behring)

THERAPEUTIC CLASS: Immunoglobulin

INDICATIONS: Patients with primary defective antibody synthesis (eg, agammaglobulinemia or hypogammaglobulinemia), who are at increased risk of infection.

DOSAGE: *Adults:* 200-400mg/kg IV every 3-4 weeks. Adjust dose to maintain desired IgG levels and clinical response.
Pediatrics/Adolescents: 200mg/kg IV every 3-4 weeks. Adjust dose to maintain desired IgG levels and clinical response.

HOW SUPPLIED: Inj: 5g, 10g

CONTRAINDICATIONS: History of allergic reactions to human albumin, anaphylactic or severe systemic response to IM/IV immune globulin, isolated IgA deficiency.

WARNINGS/PRECAUTIONS: Assure patient is not volume depleted before administration. Caution if predisposed to acute renal failure (eg, any degree of pre-existing renal insufficiency, DM, >65 yrs, volume depletion, sepsis, paraproteinemia, with nephrotoxic drugs). Monitor renal function and infusion rate. Aseptic meningitis syndrome reported. Made from human blood; risk of transmitting infection.

ADVERSE REACTIONS: Acute renal failure, acute tubular necrosis, proximal tubular nephropathy, osmotic nephrosis, chills, headache, backache, neck pain.

INTERACTIONS: May interfere with response to live viral vaccines (eg, measles, mumps, rubella).

PREGNANCY: Category C, safety in nursing not known.

MECHANISM OF ACTION: Immunoglobulin (IgG); provides broad range of antibodies capable of opsonization and neutralization of microbes and toxins against bacterial and viral antigens for prevention or attenuation of infectious disease.

PHARMACOKINETICS: Elimination: $T_{1/2}$=40 days.

GAMUNEX RX
immune globulin intravenous (human) (Bayer Healthcare)

THERAPEUTIC CLASS: Immune Globulin

INDICATIONS: Primary humoral immunodeficiency (PI) states. Idiopathic thrombocytopenic purpura (ITP).

DOSAGE: *Adults:* PI: 300-600mg/kg IV every 3-4 weeks. ITP: 2g/kg IV, given as 2 doses of 1g/kg IV on 2 consecutive days (not if fluid volume is a concern) or 5 doses of 0.4g/kg IV on 5 consecutive days. May withhold 2nd dose if platelet count is adequate 24 hrs after the first 1g/kg daily dose. Infusion Rates: PI/ITP: Initial: 0.01mL/kg/min for first 30 min. Max: 0.08mL/kg/min. Risk of Renal Dysfunction/Acute Renal Failure: Reduce dose, concentration, and/or rate (<0.08mL/kg/min).

HOW SUPPLIED: Inj: 10% [10mL, 25mL, 50mL, 100mL, 200mL]

CONTRAINDICATIONS: Extreme caution in severe, selective IgA deficiences.

WARNINGS/PRECAUTIONS: Caution with pre-existing renal insufficiency, DM, elderly (≥65 yrs), volume depletion, sepsis, paraproteinemia; use minimum concentration/rate. Assess renal function prior to initial infusion and at appropriate intervals thereafter; d/c if renal fuction worsens. Risk of transmitting infectious agents. Aseptic meningitis syndrome reported with high doses and/or rapid infusion.

ADVERSE REACTIONS: Increased cough, rhinitis, pharyngitis, headache, fever, diarrhea, nausea, asthma, asthenia, ear pain, injection site reaction, ecchymosis (purpura), hemorrhage, epistaxis, petechiae, thrombocytopenia.

INTERACTIONS: Caution with concomitant nephrotoxic agents. Decreases effect of live, viral vaccines (eg, measles, mumps, rubella); separate use by 6 months.

PREGNANCY: Category C, safety in nursing not known.

MECHANISM OF ACTION: Immune globulin protein: Not established; suggested causes Fc-receptor blockade of phagocytosis and down regulation of auto-reactive β-cells by anti-idiotypic antibodies.

PHARMACOKINETICS: Absorption: 19.04mg/mL, AUC=6746.48mg•hr/mL. **Elimination:** $T_{1/2}$=35.74 days.

GANIRELIX ACETATE RX
ganirelix acetate (Organon)

THERAPEUTIC CLASS: GnRH antagonist

INDICATIONS: For inhibition of premature LH surges in women undergoing controlled ovarian stimulation.

DOSAGE: *Adults:* 250mcg SQ qd during the mid to late follicular phase. Continue until HCG administration.

HOW SUPPLIED: Inj: 250mcg/0.5mL

CONTRAINDICATIONS: Pregnancy.

WARNINGS/PRECAUTIONS: Exclude pregnancy before initiate therapy. Contains natural rubber latex.

ADVERSE REACTIONS: Abdominal pain (gynecological), fetal death, headache, ovarian hyperstimulation syndrome.

PREGNANCY: Category X, not for use in nursing.

MECHANISM OF ACTION: GnRH antagonist; stimulates the synthesis and secretion of LH and FSH.

PHARMACOKINETICS: Absorption: Rapid, T_{max}=1 hr; absolute bioavailability (91%). **Distribution:** V_d=43.7L; plasma protein binding (81.9%). **Elimination:** Feces (75.1%), urine (22.1%) $T_{1/2}$= 12.8 hrs.

GANITE   RX
gallium nitrate (Genta)

> Increased risk of severe renal insufficiency with concurrent use of other potentially nephrotoxic drugs (eg, aminoglycosides, amphotericin B). D/C if use of potentially nephrotoxic drug is indicated; hydrate for several days after administration. D/C if SCr >2.5mg/dL.

THERAPEUTIC CLASS: Calcium regulator

INDICATIONS: Treatment of symptomatic cancer-related hypercalcemia unresponsive to adequate hydration.

DOSAGE: *Adults:* 200mg/m² IV infusion over 24 hours for 5 days. May consider 100mg/m²/day with mild cases. May stop early if serum calcium levels are WNL in <5 days.

HOW SUPPLIED: Inj: 500mg [20mL]

CONTRAINDICATIONS: Severe renal impairment (SCr >2.5mg/dL).

WARNINGS/PRECAUTIONS: Monitor renal function (SCr, BUN), serum calcium (daily) and phosphorous (twice weekly). Establish and maintain adequate hydration before and after initiation. Avoid overhydration with compromised cardiovascular status. Avoid diuretics prior to correction of hypovolemia. D/C if SCr >2.5mg/dL or hypocalcemia occurs.

ADVERSE REACTIONS: Elevated BUN/SCr, hypocalcemia, transient hypophosphatemia, decreased serum bicarbonate, anemia (with high doses), decrease in BP, nausea, vomiting, tachycardia, lethargy, confusion, diarrhea, constipation.

INTERACTIONS: Avoid use with nephrotoxic drugs (eg, aminoglycosides, amphotericin B). Caution with cyclophosphamide, prednisone.

PREGNANCY: Category C, not for use in nursing.

MECHANISM OF ACTION: Calcium regulator, inhibits calcium resorption from bone, possibly by reducing increased bone turnover.

PHARMACOKINETICS: Elimination: Kidney.

GANTRISIN PEDIATRIC   RX
sulfisoxazole (Roche Labs)

THERAPEUTIC CLASS: Sulfonamide

INDICATIONS: Treatment of acute, recurrent or chronic urinary tract infection. Treatment and prophylaxis in meningococcal meningitis. Adjunct treatment of Haemophilus influenzae meningitis, acute otitis media, malaria, and toxoplasmosis. Treatment of trachoma, inclusion conjunctivitis, nocardiosis, chancroid.

DOSAGE: Pediatrics: >2 months: Initial: 1/2 of 24hr dose. Maint: 150mg/kg/24hr or 4g/m²/24hr given q4-6h. Max: 6g/24hr.

HOW SUPPLIED: Sus: 500mg/5mL

CONTRAINDICATIONS: Infants <2 months (except in congenital toxoplasmosis treatment), pregnancy at term, mothers nursing infants <2 months old.

WARNINGS/PRECAUTIONS: Fatalities reported due to Stevens-Johnson syndrome, toxic epidermal necrolysis, fulminant hepatic necrosis, agranulocytosis, aplastic anemia and other blood dyscrasias. D/C if skin rash or sign of an adverse reaction develops. Hypersensitivity reactions of the respiratory tract reported. Do not use in group A β-hemolytic streptococcal infections. Pseudomembranous colitis reported. Caution with renal/hepatic impairment, severe allergy or bronchial asthma. Hemolysis may occur in G6PD-deficient patients.

ADVERSE REACTIONS: Anaphylaxis, erythema multiforme, toxic epidermal necrolysis, tachycardia, hepatitis, nausea, anorexia, hematuria, crystalluria, BUN and creatinine elevations, blood dyscrasias, dizziness, psychosis, cough.

INTERACTIONS: May prolong PT with anticoagulants. May require less thiopental for anesthesia. May potentiate hypoglycemia effects of sulfonylureas. May displace methotrexate from plasma proteins.

PREGNANCY: Category C, not for use in nursing.

MECHANISM OF ACTION: Sulfonamide; bacteriostatic agent. Inhibits bacterial synthesis of dihydrofolic acid by preventing condensation of pteridine with aminobenzoic acid through competitive inhibition of enzyme dihydropteroate synthetase.

PHARMACOKINETICS: Absorption: Rapid, complete; C_{max}(N^1 acetyl sulfisoxazole, sulfisoxazole)=181, 169mcg/mL; T_{max}(N^1 acetyl sulfisoxazole, sulfisoxazole)=2-6 hrs, 2.5 hrs. **Distribution:** Plasma protein binding (85%); crosses placenta, blood brain barrier; excreted in breast milk. **Metabolism:** Metabolized to sulfisoxazole by digestive enzymes. **Elimination:** Urine; $T_{1/2}$(N^1 acetyl sulfisoxazole, sulfisoxazole)= 5.4-7.4, 4.6-7.8 hrs.

GARDASIL   RX
human papillomavirus recombinant vaccine, quadrivalent (Merck)

THERAPEUTIC CLASS: Vaccine

INDICATIONS: Vaccination of girls and women ages 9-26 yrs for the prevention of cervical cancer, genital warts, cervical adenocarcinoma *in situ*, cervical intraepithelial neoplasia Grades 2 and 3, vulvar intraepithelial neoplasia Grades 2 and 3, vaginal intraepithelial neoplasia Grades 2 and 3, and cervical intraepithelial neoplasia Grade 1 caused by Human Papillomavirus types 6, 11, 16, and 18.

DOSAGE: *Adults:* Give 3 separate 0.5mL IM doses in the deltoid region of upper arm or higher anterolateral area of the thigh. First dose: At elected date; Second dose: 2 months after first dose; Third dose: 6 months after first dose. *Pediatrics:* ≥9 yrs: Give 3 separate 0.5mL IM doses in the deltoid region of upper arm or higher anterolateral area of the thigh. First dose: At elected date; Second dose: 2 months after first dose; Third dose: 6 months after first dose.

HOW SUPPLIED: Inj: Vial/Syringe: 0.5mL

WARNINGS/PRECAUTIONS: Should not be administered with bleeding disorders or anticoagulant therapy unless the potential benefits outweight the risk. Patients with impaired immune responsiveness may have reduced antibody response to active immunization. Medical treatment should be readily available in case of rare anaphylactic reactions.

ADVERSE REACTIONS: Local site reactions, fever, pyrexia, nausea, nasopharyngitis, dizziness, diarrhea.

INTERACTIONS: Immunosuppressive therapies, including irradiation, anti-metabolites, alkylating agents, cytotoxic drugs, and corticosteroids (used in greater than physiologic doses) may reduce the immune responses to vaccines.

PREGNANCY: Category B, caution in nursing.

MECHANISM OF ACTION: Develops humoral immune response that may protect against human papilloma virus types 6,11,16, and 18 (animal study).

GELCLAIR RX
glycyrrhetinic acid - polyvinylpyrrolidone - sodium hyaluronate (OSI/Helsinn Healthcare)

THERAPEUTIC CLASS: Oral analgesic

INDICATIONS: Relief of oral pain from various etiologies, including oral mucositis/stomatitis, irritation from oral surgery, traumatic ulcers from braces/ill-fitting dentures, diffuse aphthous ulcers.

DOSAGE: *Adults:* Mix 1 pkt with 1-3 tbsp of water. Gargle for 1 min, then spit out. Use tid or prn. Do not eat or drink for 1 hr after treatment. May be used undiluted.

HOW SUPPLIED: Gel: 15mL/pkt [21^s]

PREGNANCY: Safety not known in pregnancy or nursing.

MECHANISM OF ACTION: Oral analgesic; forms a protective coat over the oral mucosa that soothes irritated tissues and reduces pain.

GEMZAR RX
gemcitabine HCL (Lilly)

THERAPEUTIC CLASS: Nucleoside analogue antimetabolite

INDICATIONS: Adjunct with cisplatin for 1st-line treatment of inoperable, locally advanced (Stage IIIA or IIIB) or metastatic (Stage IV) non-small cell lung cancer. If previously treated with 5-FU, 1st-line treatment of locally advanced (nonresectable Stage II or Stage III) or metastatic (Stage IV) pancreatic adenocarcinoma. Adjunct with paclitaxel for 1st-line treatment of metastatic breast cancer after failure of prior anthracycline-containing adjuvant chemotherapy, unless anthracyclines were clinically contraindicated. Combination with carboplatin for the treatment of advanced ovarian cancer that has relapsed at least 6 months after completion of platinum-based therapy.

DOSAGE: *Adults:* Pancreatic Cancer: 1000mg/m^2 IV weekly up to 7 weeks, then 1 week off. Give subsequent cycles as weekly infusions for 3 out of every 4 weeks. Lung Cancer: 4-Week Cycle: 1000mg/m^2 IV on Days 1, 8, and 15 of each 28-day cycle. Give cisplatin 100mg/m^2 IV on Day 1 after gemcitabine infusion. 3-Week Cycle: 1250mg/m^2 on Days 1 and 8 of each 21-day cycle. Give cisplatin 100mg/m^2 IV on Day 1 after gemcitabine infusion. Breast Cancer: 1250mg/m^2 IV on Days 1 and 8 of each 21-day cycle. Give paclitaxel 175mg/m^2 IV on Day 1 before gemcitabine. Ovarian Cancer: 1000mg/m^2 IV on Days 1 and 8 of each 21-day cycle. Give carboplatin AUC 4 on Day 1 after gemcitabine. Adjust dose based on hematologic toxicity.

HOW SUPPLIED: Inj: 200mg, 1g

WARNINGS/PRECAUTIONS: Increased toxicity with infusion time >60 min and more than once weekly dosing. Hemolytic-uremic syndrome, hepatotoxicity, pulmonary toxicity, renal failure, leukopenia, thrombocytopenia, and anemia reported. Myelosuppression is dose-limiting toxicity. D/C if severe lung toxicity occurs. Caution with significant renal or hepatic impairment. Pattern of tissue injury typically associated with radiation toxicity reported with concurrent and nonconcurrent use. Greater tendency for older women not to proceed to next cycle and to experience Grade 3/4 neutropenia and thrombocytopenia. Perform CBC, differential, and platelets before each dose. Decreased clearance in women and elderly.

ADVERSE REACTIONS: Myelosuppression, nausea, vomiting, diarrhea, stomatitis, elevated serum transaminases, proteinuria, hematuria, fever, rash, dyspnea, edema, flu syndrome, infection, alopecia, paresthesia.

INTERACTIONS: Monitor serum creatinine, K+, calcium, and magnesium with cisplatin. Serious hepatotoxicity reported with hepatotoxic drugs.

PREGNANCY: Category D, not for use in nursing.

MECHANISM OF ACTION: Nucleoside analogue antimetabolite; exhibits cell cycle specificity, primarily killing cells undergoing DNA synthesis (S-phase); also blocking progression of cells through the G1/S phase boundary.

PHARMACOKINETICS: Absorption: IV administration of variable doses resulted in different parameters. **Distribution:** Plasma protein binding (negligible). V_d=50L/m² (short-infusion), V_d=370L/m² (long-infusion). **Metabolism:** Intracellular by nucleoside kinases to the active diphosphate (dFdCDP) and triphosphate (dFdCTP). **Elimination:** $T_{1/2}$(short infusion, long infusion)=(42-94 minutes, 245-638 minutes). Urine.

GENOPTIC   RX
gentamicin sulfate (Allergan)

OTHER BRAND NAMES: Genoptic S.O.P. (Allergan)

THERAPEUTIC CLASS: Aminoglycoside

INDICATIONS: Treatment of ocular bacterial infections including conjunctivitis, keratitis, keratoconjunctivitis, corneal ulcers, blepharitis, blepharoconjunctivitis, acute meibomianitis and dacryocystitis.

DOSAGE: *Adults:* Usual: 1-2 drops q4h or apply 1/2 inch of ointment bid-tid. Severe Infection: 2 drops every hour.

HOW SUPPLIED: Oint: (S.O.P.) 0.3% [3.5g]; Sol: 0.3% [1mL, 5mL]

WARNINGS/PRECAUTIONS: D/C if irritation, hypersensitivity, purulent discharge, inflammation, or pain develops. Prolonged use may result in superinfection. Ointment may retard corneal healing.

ADVERSE REACTIONS: Bacterial and fungal corneal ulcers, burning, irritation, conjunctivitis, conjunctival epithelial defects, conjunctival hyperemia.

PREGNANCY: Category C, unknown use in nursing.

MECHANISM OF ACTION: Aminoglycloside; produces antimicrobial activity against susceptible strains of microorganisms.

GENOTROPIN   RX
somatropin (Pharmacia & Upjohn)

OTHER BRAND NAMES: Genotropin MiniQuick (Pharmacia & Upjohn)

THERAPEUTIC CLASS: Human growth hormone

INDICATIONS: Long-term treatment of pediatrics with growth failure due to growth hormone deficiency (GHD) or Prader-Willi syndrome (PWS) or who are born small for gestational age (SGA) and fail to catch-up by age 2. Long-term replacement therapy in adults with GHD of either childhood- or adult-onset etiology. Long-term treatment of growth failure associated with Turner Syndrome (TS) in patients who have open epiphyses.

DOSAGE: *Adults:* Individualize dose: GHD: Initial: Up to 0.04mg/kg/week. May increase at 4-8 week intervals. Max: 0.08mg/kg/week. Divide dose into 6-7 SQ injections. Elderly patients should receive a lower starting dose. *Pediatrics:* Individualize dose. GHD: 0.16-0.24mg/kg/week. PWS: 0.24mg/kg/week. SGA: 0.48mg/kg/week. TS: 0.33mg/kg/week. Divide doses into 6-7 SQ injections.

HOW SUPPLIED: Inj: 1.5mg, 5.8mg, 13.8mg; Inj, MiniQuick: 0.2mg, 0.4mg, 0.6mg, 0.8mg, 1mg, 1.2mg, 1.4mg, 1.6mg, 1.8mg, 2mg

CONTRAINDICATIONS: Evidence of neoplastic activity. Pediatrics with closed epiphyses. Patients with diabetic retinopathy or active malignancy. Acute critical illness due to complications after open heart or abdominal surgery, multiple accidental trauma, or with acute respiratory failure. Patients with PWS who are severely obese or have severe respiratory impairment.

WARNINGS/PRECAUTIONS: In PWS, evaluate for upper airway obstruction prior to initiation; monitor weight, for sleep apnea, signs of upper airway obstruction (eg, suspend therapy with onset of or increased snoring), respiratory infections (treat early and aggressively if occur). Monitor GHD secondary to intracranial lesion for progression/recurrence. Monitor gait, glucose intolerance because insulin sensitivity is decreased, for malignant transformation of skin lesions, scoliosis progression, intracranial HTN (perform fundoscopic exam at start and periodically). Caution with DM, endocrine disorders, hypopituitarism, and Turner syndrome. Tissue atrophy may occur (rotate injection site).

ADVERSE REACTIONS: Peripheral swelling/edema, arthralgia, pain/stiffness in extremities, myalgia, upper respiratory infection, paresthesia.

INTERACTIONS: Antagonized by glucocorticoids. May alter clearance of CYP450 substrates (eg, corticosteroids, sex steroids, anticonvulsants, cyclosporine). May need dose adjustment if taking oral estrogen replacement. May need insulin dose adjustment.

PREGNANCY: Category B, caution in nursing.

MECHANISM OF ACTION: Human growth hormone; stimulates linear growth synthesis, metabolizes lipids, reduces body fat stores by increasing cellular protein, and increases plasma fatty acids.

PHARMACOKINETICS: Absorption: SQ administration of variable doses resulted in different parameters. **Distribution:** V_d=1.3L/kg. **Metabolism:** Liver and kidneys (protein catabolism). **Elimination:** (IV): $T_{1/2}$=0.4 hrs. (SC): $T_{1/2}$=3 hrs.

GENTAMICIN OPHTHALMIC   RX
gentamicin sulfate (Various)

THERAPEUTIC CLASS: Aminoglycoside

INDICATIONS: Treatment of ocular bacterial infections including conjunctivitis, keratitis, keratoconjunctivitis, corneal ulcers, blepharitis, blepharoconjunctivitis, acute meibomianitis and dacryocystitis.

DOSAGE: *Adults:* Usual: 1-2 drops q4h or apply 1/2 inch of oint bid-tid. Severe Infection: 2 drops every hour.
Pediatrics: Usual: 1-2 drops q4h or apply half-inch of oint bid-tid. Severe Infection: 2 drops every hour.

HOW SUPPLIED: Oint: 0.3% [3.5g]; Sol: 0.3% [5mL]

WARNINGS/PRECAUTIONS: D/C if develop irritation, hypersensitivity, purulent discharge, inflammation or pain. Prolonged use may result in superinfection. Oint may retard corneal healing.

ADVERSE REACTIONS: Bacterial and fungal corneal ulcers, burning, irritation, conjunctivitis, conjunctival epithelial defects, conjunctival hyperemia.

PREGNANCY: Category C. Safety in nursing is not known.

MECHANISM OF ACTION: Aminoglycoside antibiotic; iInhibits normal protein synthesis in susceptible microorganisms.

GENTAMICIN SULFATE INJECTION RX
gentamicin sulfate (Various)

> Potential nephrotoxicity, neurotoxicity, ototoxicity. Risk of toxicity is greater with impaired renal function, high dosage, or prolonged therapy. Monitor serum concentrations closely. Avoid prolonged peak levels >12mcg/mL and trough levels >2mcg/mL. Monitor renal and eight cranial nerve function, urine, BUN, serum creatinine, and CrCl. Obtain serial audiograms. Advanced age and dehydration increase risk of toxicity. Adjust dose or D/C use with evidence of ototoxicity or nephrotoxicity. May cause fetal harm during pregnancy. Avoid concurrent and/or sequential systemic or topical use of other potentially neurotoxic and/or nephrotoxic drugs, such as cisplatin, cephaloridine, kanamycin, amikacin, neomycin, polymyxin B, colistin, paromomycin, streptomycin, tobramycin, vancomycin, and viomycin. Avoid concurrent use with potent diuretics, such as ethacrynic acid or furosemide.

THERAPEUTIC CLASS: Aminoglycoside

INDICATIONS: Treatment of bacterial neonatal sepsis, bacterial septicemia, and serious bacterial infections of the CNS (meningitis), urinary tract, respiratory tract, gastrointestinal tract (including peritonitis), skin, bone and soft tissue (including burns) caused by susceptible strains of microorganisms.

DOSAGE: *Adults:* IM/IV: Serious Infections: 3mg/kg/day given q8h. Life-Threatening Infections: 5mg/kg/day tid-qid; reduce to 3mg/kg/day as soon as clinically indicated. Treat for 7-10 days; may need longer course in difficult and complicated infections. Renal Impairment: Reduced dose given q8h or usual dose given at prolonged intervals based on either CrCl or serum creatinine. Dialysis: 1-1.7mg/kg, depending on severity of infection, at end of each dialysis period. Obese Patients: Calculate dose based on estimated lean body mass. *Pediatrics:* 6-7.5mg/kg/day (2-2.5mg/kg given q8h). Infants and Neonates: 7.5mg/kg/day (2.5mg/kg given q8h). Premature and Full-Term Neonates ≤1 Week: 5mg/kg/day (2.5mg/kg given q12h). Treat for 7-10 days; may need longer course in difficult and complicated infections. Renal Impairment: Reduced dose given q8h or usual dose given at prolonged intervals based on either CrCl or serum creatinine. Dialysis: 2mg/kg at end of each dialysis period. Obese Patients: Calculate dose based on estimated lean body mass.

HOW SUPPLIED: Inj: 10mg/mL, 40mg/mL

WARNINGS/PRECAUTIONS: Contains metabisulfite. Neuromuscular blockade, respiratory paralysis, ototoxicity, and nephrotoxicity may occur after local irrigation or topical application during surgical procedures. Caution with neuromuscular disorders (eg, myasthenia gravis, parkinsonism). Caution in elderly; monitor renal function. Keep patients well-hydrated during treatment. May cause fetal harm when administered to pregnant women.

ADVERSE REACTIONS: Nephrotoxicity, neurotoxicity, rash, fever, urticaria, nausea, vomiting, headache, lethargy, confusion, depression, decreased appetite, weight loss, BP changes, blood dyscrasias, elevated LFTs.

INTERACTIONS: Increased nephrotoxicity with cephalosporins. Do not premix with other drugs; administer separately. Neuromuscular blockade and respiratory paralysis may occur in anesthetized patients or those receiving neuromuscular blockers (eg, succinylcholine, tubocurarine, decamethonium). See Black Box Warning.

PREGNANCY: Category D, safety not known in nursing.

MECHANISM OF ACTION: Aminoglycoside antibiotic; inhibits synthesis of proteins in bacterial cell.

PHARMACOKINETICS: Absorption: T_{max}=30-90 mins. Administration of different doses resulted in different parameters. **Distribution:** Crosses placenta, distributed in body fluids. **Elimination:** Urine, bile.

GENTAMICIN TOPICAL RX
gentamicin sulfate (Various)

THERAPEUTIC CLASS: Aminoglycoside

INDICATIONS: Treatment of primary skin infections such as impetigo contagiosa, folliculitis, ecthyma, furunculosis, sycosis barbae, and pyoderma gangrenosum; and secondary skin infections such as infectious eczematoid dermatitis, pustular acne, pustular psoriasis, infected seborrheic dermatitis, infected contact dermatitis, infected excoriations, and bacterial superinfections.

DOSAGE: *Adults:* Apply gently tid-qid. May apply gauze dressing. *Pediatrics:* >1 yr: Apply gently tid-qid. May apply gauze dressing.

HOW SUPPLIED: Cre, Oint: 0.1% [15g, 30g]

WARNINGS/PRECAUTIONS: D/C if irritation, sensitization, or superinfection develops.

ADVERSE REACTIONS: Irritation (erythema and pruritus).

PREGNANCY: Unknown use in pregnancy and nursing.

MECHANISM OF ACTION: Aminoglycoside; wide-spectrum antibiotic that acts against primary and secondary bacterial infections of the skin.

GENTEAL   OTC
hydroxypropyl methylcellulose (Novartis Ophthalmics)

OTHER BRAND NAMES: GenTeal Mild (Novartis Ophthalmics)

THERAPEUTIC CLASS: Lubricant

INDICATIONS: Relief of dry eye (Sol 0.2% for mild, Sol 0.3% for moderate, Gel 0.3% for severe). Temporary relief of discomfort due to minor irritations of eye from exposure to wind, sun, or other irritants and to protect against further irritation.

DOSAGE: *Adults:* 1-2 drops in affected eye prn.

HOW SUPPLIED: Gel: 0.3% [10mL]; Sol: (Mild) 0.2% [15mL, 25mL]; Sol: 0.3% [15mL, 25mL]

WARNINGS/PRECAUTIONS: Do not touch container tip to any surface. D/C if eye pain, vision changes, redness, or irritation continue >72 hrs; or if condition worsens.

PREGNANCY: Safety in pregnancy or nursing not known.

GEODON   RX
ziprasidone HCL (Pfizer)

> Elderly patients with dementia-related psychosis treated with atypical antipsychotic drugs are at an increased risk of death; most appeared to be cardiovascular (eg, heart failure, sudden death) or infectious (eg, pneumonia) in nature. Ziprasidone is not approved for the treatment of patients with dementia-related psychosis.

OTHER BRAND NAMES: Geodon for Injection (Pfizer)

THERAPEUTIC CLASS: Benzisoxazole derivative

INDICATIONS: Treatment of schizophrenia. Treatment of acute manic or mixed episodes associated with bipolar disorder, with or without psychotic features. (Inj) Treatment of acute agitation in schizophrenic patients who need IM medication for rapid control of agitation.

DOSAGE: *Adults:* Schizophrenia: (Cap) Initial: 20mg bid with food. Titrate: May increase up to 80mg bid; adjust dose at intervals of not less than 2 days. Maint: 20-80mg bid for up to 52 weeks. (Inj) 10-20mg IM up to max 40mg/day. May give 10mg q2h or 20mg q4h up to 40mg/day for 3 days. Bipolar Mania: (Cap) Initial: 40mg bid with food. Titrate: Increase to 60-80mg bid on 2nd day of treatment. Maint: 40-80mg bid.

HOW SUPPLIED: Cap: (HCl) 20mg, 40mg, 60mg, 80mg; Inj: (Mesylate) 20mg/mL

CONTRAINDICATIONS: Concomitant dofetilide, sotalol, quinidine, Class Ia/III antiarrhythmics, mesoridazine, thioridazine, chlorpromazine, droperidol, pimozide, sparfloxacin, gatifloxacin, moxifloxacin, halofantrine, mefloquine, pentamidine, arsenic trioxide, levomethadyl acetate, dolasetron, probucol, tacrolimus, and drugs that prolong QT interval. History of QT prolongation, recent acute MI, uncompensated heart failure.

WARNINGS/PRECAUTIONS: D/C if persistent QTc measurements >500 msec, NMS, tardive dyskinesia occurs. Monitor for hyperglycemia in patients with DM or at risk for DM. Avoid with congenital long QT syndrome, history of arrhythmia. Caution in history of seizures. Esophageal dysmotility and aspiration reported. May elevate prolactin levels. Orthostatic hypotension reported; caution with cardiovascular or cerebrovascular disease, conditions predisposed to hypotension (eg, dehydration, hypovolemia). Caution with IM use in renal dysfunction.

ADVERSE REACTIONS: Asthenia, nausea, constipation, dyspepsia, diarrhea, dry mouth, rash, somnolence, akathisia, dizziness, EPS, dystonia, hypertonia, respiratory disorder, upper respiratory infection, vomiting, headache, injection site pain, swollen tongue, facial droop, tardive dyskinesia, enuresis, urinary incontinence.

INTERACTIONS: See Contraindications. Avoid drugs that prolong QTc intervals. Caution with centrally acting drugs. May enhance effects of antihypertensives. May antagonize effects of levodopa and dopamine agonists. Carbamazepine may decrease levels. CYP3A4 inhibitors may increase levels.

PREGNANCY: Category C, not for use in nursing.

MECHANISM OF ACTION: Psychotropic agent; not established. Actions are mediated through a combination of dopamine type 2 (D_2) and serotonin type 2 (5HT2) antagonism.

PHARMACOKINETICS: Absorption: Well absorbed orally. Absolute bioavailability: 60%; (PO) T_{max}=6-8 hrs, (IM) T_{max}=60 min. **Distribution:** Plasma protein binding (99%); V_d=1.5L/Kg. **Metabolism:** Liver (extensive) via methylation and oxidation; CYP3A4 (major), 1A2 (minor). **Elimination:** Urine: 20% (<1% unchanged), feces: 66% (<4% unchanged); (PO) $T_{1/2}$=7 hrs; (IM) $T_{1/2}$= 2 to 5 hrs.

GLEEVEC RX
imatinib mesylate (Novartis)

THERAPEUTIC CLASS: Protein-tyrosine kinase inhibitor

INDICATIONS: (Adults) Treatment of newly diagnosed adult patients with Philadelphia chromosome positive (Ph+) chronic myeloid leukemia (CML) in chronic phase. Treatment of Ph+ CML in blast crisis, accelerated phase, or in chronic phase after failure of interferon-alpha therapy. Treatment of relapsed or refractory Ph+ acute lympoblastic leukemia (ALL). Treatment of myelodysplastic/myeloproliferative diseases (MDS/MPD) associated with platelet-derived growth factor receptor (PDGFR) gene re-arrangements. Treatment of aggressive systemic mastocytosis (ASM) patients without the D816V c-Kit mutation or with unknown cKit mutational status. Treatment of hypereosinophilic syndrome (HES) and/or chronic eosinophilic leukemia (CEL) patients who have the FIP1L1-PDGFRα fusion kinase (mutational analysis or FISH demonstration of CHIC2 allele deletion) and for patients with HES and/or CEL who are FIP1L1-PDGFRα fusion kinase negative or unknown. Treatment of patients with unresectable, recurrent, and/or metastatic dermatofibrosarcoma protuberans (DFSP). Treatment of patients with Kit (CD117) positive unresectable and/or metastatic malignant gastrointestinal stromal tumors (GIST). (Pediatrics) Treatment of patients with Ph+ chronic phase CML in chronic phase who are newly diagnosed or whose disease has recurred after stem cell transplant or who are resistant to interferon-alpha therapy.

DOSAGE: *Adults:* ≥18 yrs: CML: Chronic Phase: 400mg/d, may increase to 600mg qd. Accelerated Phase/Blast Crisis: 600mg/d, may increase to 400mg bid. Relapsed/Refractory Ph+ ALL: 600mg/d. MDS or MPD/ASM/HES and/or CEL: 400mg/d. DFSP: 800mg/d. GIST: 400mg/d or 600mg/d. Severe Hepatic Impairment: Reduce dose by 25%. Co-administration with Strong CYP3A4 Inducers: Increase dose by at least 50% and monitor carefully. Hepatotoxicity/Non-Hematologic Adverse Reaction: If bilirubin >3x ULN or transaminases

>5x ULN, hold drug until bilirubin <1.5x ULN and transaminases <2.5x ULN. Continue at reduced dose. Neutropenia/Thrombocytopenia: See PI for dose adjustment. Take with food and plenty of water.
Pediatrics: ≥3 yrs: CML: Newly Diagnosed: 340mg/m2/d. Chronic Phase: 260mg/m2/day given qd or split into 2 doses (morning and evening). Severe Hepatic Impairment: Reduce dose by 25%. Co-administration with Strong CYP3A4 Inducers: Increase dose by at least 50% and monitor carefully. Hepatotoxicity/Non-Hematologic Adverse Reaction: If bilirubin >3x ULN or transaminases >5x ULN, hold drug until bilirubin <1.5x ULN and transaminases <2.5x ULN. Continue at reduced dose. Neutropenia/Thrombocytopenia: See PI for dose adjustments. Take with food and plenty of water.

HOW SUPPLIED: Tab: 100mg, 400mg

WARNINGS/PRECAUTIONS: Fluid retention/edema (pleural effusion, pericardial effusion, pulmonary edema and ascites) reported; monitor weight. Anemia/neutropenia/thrombocytopenia reported; monitor CBC weekly during 1st month, biweekly during 2nd month, and periodically thereafter. In pediatric patients, the most frequent toxicities observed were grade 3 and 4 cytopenias. May be hepatotoxic; monitor LFTs at baseline, then monthly or as needed. Avoid becoming pregnant. Interrupt treatment if severe non-hematologic adverse reaction develops (eg, severe hepatotoxicity, severe fluid retention); resume if appropriate. GI bleeds reported. Severe CHF and left ventricular dysfunction. Hypereosinophilic cardiac toxicity. Stevens-Johnson syndrome reported.

ADVERSE REACTIONS: Nausea, vomiting, fluid retention, neutropenia, thrombocytopenia, diarrhea, hemorrhage, pyrexia, rash, headache, fatigue, abdominal pain, elevated transaminases or bilirubin, edema, muscle cramps, musculoskeletal pain, flatulence, nasopharyngitis, insomnia, anemia, anorexia, rhinitis.

INTERACTIONS: Increased levels with CYP3A4 inhibitors (eg, ketoconazole, atazanavir, indinavir, nefazodone, nelfinavir, ritonavir, saquinavir, telithromycin, voriconazole, clarithromycin, itraconazole). Grapefruit juice may increase levels. Decreased levels with CYP3A4 inducers (eg, dexamethasone, phenytoin, carbamazepine, rifampin, phenobarbital, St. John's Wort). Caution with CYP3A4 substrates with narrow therapeutic windows (eg, alfentanil, cyclosporine, diergotamine, ergotamine, fentanyl, quinidine, sirolimus, tacrolimus, cyclosporine, pimozide). Increases levels of drugs metabolized by CYP3A4 (eg, dihydropyridines, triazolo-benzodiazepines, HMG-CoA reductase inhibitors). Switch patients on warfarin to low molecular weight or standard heparin.

PREGNANCY: Category D, not for nursing.

MECHANISM OF ACTION: Protein-tyrosine kinase inhibitor; inhibits the bcr-abl tyrosine kinase.

PHARMACOKINETICS: Absorption: Absolute bioavailability (98%). T_{max}=2-4 hrs. **Distribution:** Plasma protein binding (95%). **Metabolism:** Liver. N-demethyl derivative (major active metabolite). CYP3A4. **Elimination:** Urine and feces (predominant).

GLIADEL WAFER   RX
polifeprosan 20 with carmustine implant (MGI Pharma)

THERAPEUTIC CLASS: Nitrosourea oncolytic agent

INDICATIONS: Adjunct to surgery in patients with recurrent glioblastoma multiforme. Adjunct to surgery and radiation in patients with newly-diagnosed high grade malignant glioma.

DOSAGE: *Adults:* Place 8 wafers in resection cavity if size and shape allows; if not, place maximum number of wafers allowed. Max: 8 wafers per surgical procedure.

HOW SUPPLIED: Implant Wafers: (Carmustine) 7.7mg [8s]

WARNINGS/PRECAUTIONS: Avoid communication between the surgical resection cavity and ventricular system. May cause CT and MRI enhancement due to edema and inflammation. Monitor closely for known complications of craniotomy. May cause fetal harm. Risk of possible cyst formation.

ADVERSE REACTIONS: Fever, pain, abnormal healing, nausea, vomiting, brain edema, confusion, somnolence, UTI, seizures, headache, intracranial infection.

PREGNANCY: Category D, not for use in nursing.

MECHANISM OF ACTION: Nitrosourea oncolytic agent; diffuses into the surrounding brain tissue and produces an antineoplastic effect by alkylating DNA or RNA.

PHARMACOKINETICS: Distribution: Carmustine (IV): V_d=3.25L/kg. **Elimination:** Urine (60%); $T_{1/2}$=22 min.

GLIPIZIDE RX
glipizide (Various)

G

OTHER BRAND NAMES: Glucotrol (Pfizer)

THERAPEUTIC CLASS: Sulfonylurea (2nd generation)

INDICATIONS: Adjunct to diet and exercise, to improve glycemic control in type 2 diabetes mellitus.

DOSAGE: *Adults*: Take 30 min before meals. Initial: 5mg qd before breakfast. Geriatric/Hepatic Impairment: 2.5mg qd. Titrate: Increase by 2.5-5mg after several days. Max: 40mg/day. Doses >15mg should be divided. Switch From Insulin: If ≤20 U/day: Stop insulin and start Glucotrol 5mg qd. If >20 U/day, decrease dose by 50% with 5mg qd. Further insulin reductions depend on response. Elderly/Debilitated/Malnourished/Renal or Hepatic Impairment: Dose conservatively.

HOW SUPPLIED: Tab: (Glipizide) 2.5mg, 5mg, 10mg; (Glucotrol) 5mg*, 10mg* *scored

CONTRAINDICATIONS: Diabetic ketoacidosis.

WARNINGS/PRECAUTIONS: Increased risk of hypoglycemia with the elderly, debilitated, malnourished, renal and hepatic disease, adrenal or pituitary insufficiency. Increased risk of cardiovascular mortality reported. Loss of blood glucose control when exposed to stress (fever, trauma, infection or surgery); d/c therapy and start insulin. Secondary failure can occur over period of time.

ADVERSE REACTIONS: Hypoglycemia, GI disturbances, allergic skin reactions, hematologic disturbances, disulfiram-like reactions, hyponatremia, SIADH, dizziness, drowsiness, headache.

INTERACTIONS: Potentiated hypoglycemia with alcohol, NSAIDs, some azoles (eg, miconazole, fluconazole), highly protein bound drugs, salicylates, sulfonamides, chloramphenicol, probenecid, coumarins, MAOIs and β-blockers. Risk of hyperglycemia with diuretics, corticosteroids, phenothiazines, thyroid products, estrogens, oral contraceptives, phenytoin, nicotinic acid, sympathomimetics, CCBs and isoniazid. β-blockers may mask signs of hypoglycemia.

PREGNANCY: Category C, not for use in nursing.

MECHANISM OF ACTION: Sulfonylurea; lowers blood glucose acutely by stimulating the release of insulin from the pancreas.

PHARMACOKINETICS: Absorption: Rapid and complete; T_{max}=1-3 hrs. **Distribution:** V_d=11L; Plasma protein binding (98-99%). **Metabolism**: Liver. **Elimination**: $T_{1/2}$=2-4 hrs; urine.

GLUCAGON RX
glucagon (Lilly)

THERAPEUTIC CLASS: Glucagon

INDICATIONS: Treatment for severe hypoglycemia. Diagnostic aid for radiologic examination of the stomach, duodenum, small bowel, and colon.

DOSAGE: *Adults:* Severe Hypoglycemia: 1mg (1 U) SQ/IM/IV. May give another dose after 15 min if patient does not respond, but IV glucose would be a better

alternative. Use immediately after reconstitution; discard unused portion. After patient responds give supplemental carbohydrate. Diagnostic Aid: Duodenum/Small Bowel: 0.25-0.5mg (0.25-0.5 U) IV, or 1mg (1 U) IM, or 2mg (2 U) IV/IM before procedure. Stomach: 0.5mg (0.5 U) IV or 2mg (2 U) IM before procedure. Colon: 2mg (2 U) IM 10 min before procedure.
Pediatrics: Severe Hypoglycemia: ≥20kg: 1mg (1 U) SQ/IM/IV. <20kg: 0.5mg (0.5 U) or 20-30mcg/kg. May give another dose after 15 min if patient does not respond, but IV glucose would be a better alternative. Use immediately after reconstitution; discard unused portion. After patient responds give supplemental carbohydrate.

HOW SUPPLIED: Inj: 1mg

CONTRAINDICATIONS: Pheochromocytoma.

WARNINGS/PRECAUTIONS: Caution with history suggestive of insulinoma and/or pheochromocytoma. Glucagon can cause pheochromocytoma tumor to release catecholamines, which may result in a sudden and marked increase in BP. Effective in treating hypoglycemia only if sufficient liver glycogen is present. Glucagon is not effective in states of starvation, adrenal insufficiency, or chronic hypoglycemia; use glucose to treat instead.

ADVERSE REACTIONS: Nausea, vomiting, allergic reactions, urticaria, respiratory distress, hypotension.

PREGNANCY: Category B, caution in nursing.

MECHANISM OF ACTION: Anti-hypoglycemic agent; polypeptide hormone that increases blood glucose levels. Acts on liver glycogen, converting it to glucose. Relaxes smooth muscle of GI tract.

PHARMACOKINETICS: Absorption: C_{max}=7.9mg/mL (SC), 6.9ng/mL (IM); T_{max}=20 min (SC), 13 min (IM). **Distribution:** V_d=0.25L/kg; found in breast milk. **Metabolism:** Extensively degraded in liver, kidneys, plasma. **Elimination:** Urine; $T_{1/2}$=8-18 min.

GLUCOPHAGE **XR**   RX
metformin HCL (Bristol-Myers Squibb)

OTHER BRAND NAMES: Riomet (Ranbaxy) - Glucophage (Bristol-Myers Squibb)

THERAPEUTIC CLASS: Biguanide

INDICATIONS: Adjunct to diet or with a sulfonylurea or insulin, to improve glycemic control in type 2 diabetes mellitus.

DOSAGE: *Adults:* (Sol, Tab) Initial: 500mg bid or 850mg qd with meals. Titrate: Increase by 500mg/week, or 850mg every 2 weeks, or may increase from 500mg bid to 850mg bid after 2 weeks. Max: 2550mg/day. Give in 3 divided doses with meals if dose is >2g/day. (Tab, Extended-Release) Initial: ≥17 yrs: 500mg qd with evening meal. Titrate: Increase by 500mg/week. Max: 2000mg/day. With Insulin: Initial: 500mg qd. Titrate: Increase by 500mg/week. Max: 2500mg/day and 2000mg/day (XR). Decrease insulin dose by 10-25% when FPG <120mg/dL. Swallow whole; do not crush or chew. Elderly/Debilitated/Malnourished: Conservative dosing; do not titrate to Max.
Pediatrics: 10-16 yrs: (Sol, Tab) Initial: 500mg bid with meals. Titrate: Increase by 500mg/week. Max: 2000mg/day.

HOW SUPPLIED: Sol: (Riomet) 500mg/5mL; Tab: 500mg, 850mg, 1000mg*; Tab, Extended-Release: 500mg, 750mg *scored

CONTRAINDICATIONS: Renal disease/dysfunction (SrCr ≥1.5mg/dL [males], ≥1.4mg/dL [females], or abnormal CrCl), CHF, metabolic acidosis, diabetic ketoacidosis. D/C temporarily (48 hrs) for radiologic studies with intravascular iodinated contrast materials.

WARNINGS/PRECAUTIONS: Lactic acidosis reported (rare); increased risk with renal dysfunction, increased age, DM, CHF, and other conditions with risk of hypoperfusion and hypoxemia. Avoid use in patients ≥80 yrs unless renal function is normal. Monitor renal function and for ketoacidosis and metabolic acidosis. Avoid in renal/hepatic impairment. D/C in hypoxic states (eg, CHF, shock, acute MI), loss of blood glucose control due to stress (give insulin), acidosis, dehydration, sepsis. Temporarily d/c prior to surgery (due to restricted food intake) and procedures requiring intravascular iodinated contrast materials. May decrease serum vitamin B_{12} levels. Increased risk of hypoglycemia in elderly, debilitated/malnourished, adrenal or pituitary insufficiency, or alcohol intoxication. Monitor renal function.

ADVERSE REACTIONS: Lactic acidosis, diarrhea, nausea, vomiting, flatulence, abdominal discomfort, abnormal stools, hypoglycemia, myalgia, dizziness, dyspnea, nail disorder, rash, sweating, taste disorder, chest discomfort, chills, flu syndrome, palpitations, asthenia, indigestion, headache.

INTERACTIONS: Furosemide, nifedipine, cimetidine, cationic drugs (eg, digoxin, amiloride, procainamide, quinidine, quinine, ranitidine, trimethoprim, vancomycin, triamterene, morphine) may increase metformin levels. Thiazides, other diuretics, corticosteroids, phenothiazines, thyroid products, estrogens, oral contraceptives, phenytoin, nicotinic acid, sympathomimetics, CCBs, isoniazid may cause hyperglycemia. Risk of hypoglycemia with alcohol. Excess alcohol may increase potential for lactic acidosis. May decrease furosemide levels.

PREGNANCY: Category B, not for use in nursing.

MECHANISM OF ACTION: Biguanide; decreases hepatic glucose production, decreases intestinal absorption of glucose, and improves insulin selectivity by increasing peripheral glucose uptake and utilization.

PHARMACOKINETICS: Absorption: Absolute bioavailability (50-60%). T_{max}=7 hrs. **Distribution:** V_d=654L. **Elimination:** Urine (90%); $T_{1/2}$=6.2 hrs (plasma). $T_{1/2}$=17.6 hrs (blood).

GLUCOTROL XL   RX
glipizide (Pfizer)

OTHER BRAND NAMES: Glipizide ER (Watson) - Glucotrol (Pfizer)

THERAPEUTIC CLASS: Sulfonylurea (2nd generation)

INDICATIONS: Adjunct to diet and exercise, to improve glycemic control in type 2 diabetes mellitus.

DOSAGE: *Adults:* (Glucotrol XL) Do not chew, divide, or crush. Initial: 5mg qd with breakfast. Use lower doses if sensitive to hypoglycemics. Usual: 5-10mg qd. Max: 20mg/day. Combination Therapy: Initial: 5mg qd. (Glucotrol): Initial: 5mg qd 30 min before breakfast. Geriatric/Hepatic Impairment: Initial 2.5mg qd. Titrate: Increase by 2.5-5mg after several days. Max: 40mg/day. Divide doses >15mg and give 30 min before a meal. (Glucotrol XL, Glucotrol) Switch From Insulin: If on ≤20 U/day: Stop insulin; start Glucotrol XL or Glucotrol 5mg qd. If on >20 U/day: Reduce insulin dose by 50% and add Glucotrol XL or Glucotrol 5mg qd. Further insulin reductions depend on response.

HOW SUPPLIED: Tab: (Glucotrol) 5mg*, 10mg*; Tab, Extended-Release: (XL) 2.5mg, 5mg, 10mg *scored

CONTRAINDICATIONS: Diabetic ketoacidosis.

WARNINGS/PRECAUTIONS: Increased risk of hypoglycemia with the elderly, debilitated, malnourished, renal and hepatic disease, adrenal or pituitary insufficiency. Increased risk of cardiovascular mortality. Loss of blood glucose control when exposed to stress (fever, trauma, infection, or surgery); d/c therapy and start insulin. Secondary failure can occur over a period of time. (XL) GI disease will reduce retention time of the drug. Caution with pre-existing severe GI narrowing.

ADVERSE REACTIONS: Hypoglycemia, nausea, diarrhea, allergic skin reactions, disulfiram-like reactions, dizziness, drowsiness, asthenia, headache.

INTERACTIONS: Potentiated hypoglycemia with alcohol, NSAIDs, some azoles (eg, miconazole, fluconazole), highly protein bound drugs, salicylates, sulfonamides, chloramphenicol, probenecid, coumarins, MAOIs and β-blockers. Risk of hyperglycemia with diuretics, corticosteroids, phenothiazines, thyroid products, estrogens, oral contraceptives, phenytoin, nicotinic acid, sympathomimetics, CCBs and isoniazid. β-blockers may mask signs of hypoglycemia.

PREGNANCY: Category C, not for use in nursing.

MECHANISM OF ACTION: Sulfonylurea; lowers blood glucose acutely by stimulating the release of insulin from the pancreas.

PHARMACOKINETICS: Absorption: Rapid and complete; bioavailability (100%); T_{max} =6-12 hrs. **Distribution:** V_d=10L; plasma protein binding (98-99%). **Metabolism:** Liver; aromatic hydroxylation. **Elimination**: $T_{1/2}$=2-5 hrs; urine (80%), feces (10%).

GLUCOVANCE   RX
metformin HCL - glyburide (Bristol-Myers Squibb)

THERAPEUTIC CLASS: Sulfonylurea/biguanide

INDICATIONS: Adjunct to diet and exercise, to improve glycemic control in type 2 diabetes mellitus. As second-line therapy when treatment with a sulfonylurea or metformin alone is inadequate. May add a thiazolidinedione (TZD) for additional glycemic control.

DOSAGE: *Adults:* Take with meals. Initial: 1.25mg-250mg qd. If HbA_{1c} >9% or FPG >200mg/dL, give 1.25mg-250mg bid. Titrate: Increase by 1.25mg-250mg/day every 2 weeks. Do not use 50mg-500mg tab for initial therapy. Second-Line Therapy: Initial: 2.5mg-500mg or 5mg-500mg bid. Starting dose should not exceed daily doses of glyburide (or sulfonylurea equivalent) or metformin already being taken. Titrate: Increase by no more than 5mg-500mg/day. Max: 20mg-2000mg/day. With Concomitant TZD: Initiate and titrate TZD as recommended. If hypoglycemia occurs, reduce glyburide component. Elderly/Debilitated/Malnourished: Conservative dosing; do not titrate to max.

HOW SUPPLIED: Tab: (Glyburide-Metformin) 1.25mg-250mg, 2.5mg-500mg, 5mg-500mg

CONTRAINDICATIONS: Renal disease or dysfunction (SrCr ≥1.5mg/dL [males], ≥1.4mg/dL [females], or abnormal CrCl), CHF, metabolic acidosis, including diabetic ketoacidosis. D/C temporarily (48 hrs) for radiologic studies with intravascular iodinated contrast materials.

WARNINGS/PRECAUTIONS: Lactic acidosis reported (rare); increased risk with renal dysfunction, increased age, DM, CHF, and other conditions with risk of hypoperfusion and hypoxemia. Avoid use in patients ≥80 yrs unless renal function is normal. Increased risk of cardiovascular mortality. Increased risk of hypoglycemia in elderly, debilitated/malnourished, adrenal or pituitary insufficiency, or alcohol intoxication. D/C in hypoxic states (eg, CHF, shock, acute MI), loss of blood glucose control due to stress (give insulin), acidosis and prior to surgical procedures (due to restricted food intake). Monitor renal function and for ketoacidosis and metabolic acidosis. Avoid in renal/hepatic impairment. May decrease serum vitamin B_{12} levels. When used with a TZD, monitor LFTs and for weight gain. Withhold treatment with any condition associated with hypoxemia, dehydration, or sepsis.

ADVERSE REACTIONS: Hypoglycemia, nausea, vomiting, abdominal pain, upper respiratory infection, headache, dizziness, diarrhea.

INTERACTIONS: Furosemide, nifedipine, cimetidine and cationic drugs (eg, digoxin, amiloride, procainamide, quinidine, quinine, ranitidine, trimethoprim, vancomycin, triamterene, morphine) may increase metformin levels. Potentiated hypoglycemia with alcohol, ciprofloxacin, miconazole, NSAIDs, salicylates, sulfonamides, chloramphenicol, probenecid, coumarins, MAOIs, TZDs (eg, rosiglitazone), and β-blockers. Thiazides and other diuretics, corticosteroids, phenothiazines, thyroid products, estrogens, oral contraceptives, phenytoin, nicotinic acid, sympathomimetics, CCBs, and isoniazid may cause hyperglycemia. Excess alcohol may increase potential for lactic acidosis. May decrease furosemide levels.

PREGNANCY: Category B, not for use in nursing.

MECHANISM OF ACTION: Glyburide: Sulfonylurea; lowers blood glucose acutely by stimulating release of insulin from the pancreas. Metformin: Biguanide; decreases hepatic glucose production and intestinal absorption of glucose and improves insulin sensitivity by increasing peripheral glucose uptake.

PHARMACOKINETICS: Absorption: Glyburide: T_{max}=4 hrs. Metformin: Absolute bioavailability (50-60%). **Distribution:** Glyburide: Plasma protein binding (extensive). Metformin: V_d=654L. **Metabolism:** Glyburide: metabolites: 4-trans-hydroxy (major) and 3-cis hydroxyl derivatives. **Elimination:** Glyburide: $T_{1/2}$=10 hrs. Bile, urine (approx. 50% each route). Metformin: $T_{1/2}$=6.2 hrs (plasma). $T_{1/2}$=17.6 hrs (blood). Renal excretion (approx. 90%).

GLUMETZA   RX
metformin HCL (Depomed)

THERAPEUTIC CLASS: Biguanide

INDICATIONS: Adjunct to diet and exercise or with a sulfonylurea or insulin, to improve glycemic control in type 2 diabetes mellitus.

DOSAGE: *Adults:* ≥18 yrs: Take with evening meal. Initial: 1000mg qd. With Insulin: Initial: 500mg qd. Titrate: May increase by 500mg/week. Max: 2000mg/day. Decrease insulin dose by 10-25% if FPG <120mg/dL. Elderly/Debilitated/Malnourished: Conservative dosing; do not titrate to max. Swallow whole; do not crush or chew.

HOW SUPPLIED: Tab, Extended-Release: 500mg, 1000mg

CONTRAINDICATIONS: Renal disease or dysfunction (SrCr ≥1.5mg/dL [males], ≥1.4mg/dL [females], or abnormal CrCl), CHF, metabolic acidosis, including diabetic ketoacidosis. D/C temporarily (48 hrs) for radiologic studies with intravascular iodinated contrast materials.

WARNINGS/PRECAUTIONS: Lactic acidosis reported (rare); increased risk with renal dysfunction, increased age, DM, CHF, and other conditions with risk of hypoperfusion and hypoxemia. Avoid use in patients ≥80 yrs unless renal function is normal. Monitor renal function and for ketoacidosis and metabolic acidosis. Avoid in renal/hepatic impairment. D/C in hypoxic states (eg, CHF, shock, acute MI), loss of blood glucose control due to stress (give insulin), acidosis, dehydration, sepsis. Temporarily d/c prior to surgery (due to restricted food/fluid intake) or procedures requiring intravascular iodinated contrast materials. May decrease serum vitamin B12 levels. Increased risk of hypoglycemia in elderly, debilitated/malnourished, adrenal or pituitary insufficiency, or alcohol intoxication.

ADVERSE REACTIONS: Hypoglycemia, diarrhea, nausea.

INTERACTIONS: Furosemide, nifedipine, cimetidine, cationic drugs (eg, digoxin, amiloride, procainamide, quinidine, quinine, ranitidine, trimethoprim, vancomycin, triamterene, morphine) may increase metformin levels. Thiazides, other diuretics, corticosteroids, phenothiazines, thyroid products, estrogens, oral contraceptives, phenytoin, nicotinic acid, sympathomimetics, CCBs, isoniazid may cause hyperglycemia. Risk of hypoglycemia with alcohol. Excess alcohol may increase potential for lactic acidosis. May decrease furosemide levels.

PREGNANCY: Category B, not for use in nursing.

MECHANISM OF ACTION: Biguanide; decreases hepatic glucose production, decreases intestinal absorption of glucose, and improves insulin selectivity by increasing peripheral glucose uptake and utilization.

PHARMACOKINETICS: Absorption: Administration of variable doses resulted in different absorption parameters. T_{max}=7-8 hrs. **Distribution:** V_d=654L. **Elimination:** Urine (90%); $T_{1/2}$=6.2 hrs (plasma), 17.6 hrs (blood).

GLYNASE PRESTAB   RX
glyburide (Pharmacia & Upjohn)

THERAPEUTIC CLASS: Sulfonylurea (2nd generation)

INDICATIONS: Adjunct to diet and exercise, to improve glycemic control in type 2 diabetes mellitus. May use in combination with metformin.

DOSAGE: *Adults:* Initial: 1.5-3mg qd with breakfast or 1st main meal. Renal/Hepatic Disease/Elderly/Debilitated/Malnourished/Adrenal or Pituitary Insufficiency: Initial: 0.75mg qd. Titrate: Increase by no more than 1.5mg/day at weekly intervals. Maint: 0.75-12mg qd or in divided doses. Max: 12mg/day given qd or bid. Transfer from Other Sulfonylureas: Starting dose should not exceed 3mg/day. Switch from Insulin: If <20 U/day, substitute with 1.5-3mg qd. If 20-40 U/day, give 3mg qd. If >40 U/day, decrease insulin dose by 50% and give 3mg qd. Titrate: Progressive withdrawal of insulin and increase by 0.75-1.5mg every 2-10 days.

HOW SUPPLIED: Tab: 1.5mg*, 3mg*, 6mg* *scored

CONTRAINDICATIONS: Diabetic ketoacidosis, and as sole therapy of type 1 DM.

WARNINGS/PRECAUTIONS: Increased risk of cardiovascular mortality. Risk of hypoglycemia, especially with renal and hepatic disease, elderly, debilitated, malnourished, and adrenal or pituitary insufficiency. Loss of blood glucose control when exposed to stress (eg, fever, trauma, infection or surgery); d/c therapy and start insulin. Secondary failure can occur over a period of time. D/C if cholestatic jaundice or hepatitis occur. Retitrate when transferring from other glyburide products.

ADVERSE REACTIONS: Hypoglycemia, nausea, epigastric fullness, heartburn, allergic skin reactions, disulfiram-like reactions (rarely), hyponatremia, blood dyscrasias, LFT abnormalities, photosensitivity reactions.

INTERACTIONS: Hypoglycemia potentiated by alcohol, NSAIDs, miconazole, ciprofloxacin, highly protein bound drugs, salicylates, sulfonamides, chloramphenicol, probenecid, coumarins, MAOIs, and β-blockers. Risk of hyperglycemia with diuretics, corticosteroids, phenothiazines, thyroid products, estrogens, oral contraceptives, phenytoin, nicotinic acid, sympathomimetics, CCBs, and isoniazid. β-Blockers may mask hypoglycemia.

PREGNANCY: Category B, not for use in nursing.

MECHANISM OF ACTION: Sulfonylurea; lowers blood glucose acutely by stimulating the release of insulin from the pancreas.

PHARMACOKINETICS: Absorption: C_{max}=106ng/mL; T_{max}=2-3 hrs. **Distribution:** Plasma protein binding (extensive). **Metabolism:** 4-trans-hydroxy derivative (major metabolite). **Elimination:** Bile (50%), urine (50%); $T_{1/2}$=4hrs.

GLYSET   RX
miglitol (Pharmacia & Upjohn)

THERAPEUTIC CLASS: Alpha-glucosidase inhibitor

INDICATIONS: Adjunct to diet and exercise, to improve glycemic control in type 2 diabetes mellitus. May use in combination with a sulfonylurea.

DOSAGE: *Adults:* Initial: 25mg tid. May give 25mg qd (to minimize GI side effects) and gradually increase to tid. Titrate: After 4-8 weeks, increase to 50mg tid. Maint: 50mg tid. After 3 months may increase to 100mg tid if needed. Max: 100mg tid. Take with first bite of each main meal.

HOW SUPPLIED: Tab: 25mg, 50mg, 100mg

CONTRAINDICATIONS: Ketoacidosis, inflammatory bowel disease, colonic ulceration, partial intestinal obstruction or if predisposed to intestinal obstruction. Chronic intestinal diseases with digestion or absorption disorders/conditions may deteriorate with increased gas formation in the intestine.

WARNINGS/PRECAUTIONS: Use glucose (dextrose) not sucrose (cane sugar) to treat mild-moderate hypoglycemia. Temporary insulin therapy may be necessary at times of stress such as fever, trauma, infection, or surgery. Not recommended with renal impairment (SrCr >2mg/dL).

ADVERSE REACTIONS: Flatulence, diarrhea, abdominal pain, skin rash, decreased serum iron.

INTERACTIONS: Intestinal absorbents (eg, charcoal) and digestive enzyme preparations (eg, amylase, pancreatin) may reduce effects. May reduce bioavailability of ranitidine and propranolol. May interact with glyburide, metformin, and digoxin.

PREGNANCY: Category B, not for use in nursing.

MECHANISM OF ACTION: Alpha-glucosidase inhibitor; inhibits membrane-bound intestinal alpha-glucosidase hydrolase enzymes.

PHARMACOKINETICS: Absorption: Complete, T_{max}= 2.3 hrs. **Distribution:** Plasma protein binding (≤4.0%); V_d=0.18 L/Kg. **Elimination**: Urine (unchanged); $T_{1/2}$=2 hrs.

GoLYTELY

RX

polyethylene glycol 3350 - sodium bicarbonate - potassium chloride - sodium chloride - sodium sulfate (Braintree)

THERAPEUTIC CLASS: Bowel cleanser

INDICATIONS: Bowel cleansing prior to colonoscopy or barium enema X-ray.

DOSAGE: *Adults:* Oral: 240mL every 10 min until fecal discharge is clear or 4L is consumed. NG-Tube: 20-30mL/min (1.2-1.8L/hr). Patient should fast at least 3-4 hrs before administration.

HOW SUPPLIED: Sol: (Polyethylene Glycol-Potassium Chloride-Sodium Bicarbonate-Sodium Chloride-Sodium Sulfate) 236g-2.97g-6.74g-5.86g-22.74g [4000mL]

CONTRAINDICATIONS: GI obstruction, gastric retention, bowel perforation, toxic colitis, toxic megacolon, ileus.

WARNINGS/PRECAUTIONS: Do not add additional ingredients (eg, flavorings). Caution with severe ulcerative colitis. Monitor therapy with impaired gag reflex, unconsciousness/semiconsciousness and patients prone to regurgitation or aspiration. Slow administration or temporarily d/c if severe bloating, distention, or abdominal pain develops.

ADVERSE REACTIONS: Nausea, abdominal fullness, cramping, bloating, vomiting, anal irritation.

INTERACTIONS: Oral medications taken within 1 hr of start of administration may not be absorbed from GI tract.

PREGNANCY: Category C, caution in nursing.

MECHANISM OF ACTION: Stimulant laxative; induces diarrhea.

GONAL-F

RX

follitropin alfa (EMD Serono)

THERAPEUTIC CLASS: Follicle stimulating hormone

INDICATIONS: For development of multiple follicles in ovulatory patients participating in Assisted Reproductive Technology (ART). (Men) For induction of spermatogenesis in primary and secondary hypogonadotropic hypogonadism not due to primary testicular failure.

DOSAGE: *Adults:* Individualize dose. Oligo-Anovulation: Initial: 75 IU/day SQ. Titrate: Increase up to 37.5 IU/day after 14 days and further increase after 7 days if needed. Give hCG 5000 U 1 day after last dose. Do not exceed 35 days of therapy unless an E2 rise indicates imminent follicular development. Max: 300 IU/day. ART: Initial: 150 IU/day SQ on cycle Day 2 or 3 (early follicular phase). If gonadotropins suppressed, initiate at 225 IU/day. Titrate: Adjust after 5 days if needed, then at intervals no less than 3-5 days and not exceeding 75-150 IU/adjustment. Max: 450 IU/day. Once follicular development is evident, give hCG 5000-10,000 U. Hypogonadotropic Hypogonadism: Pretreat with hCG 1000-2250 U 2-3x/week to achieve normal serum testosterone levels. When normal, give 150 IU SQ and hCG 1000 U 3x/week. Max: 300 IU 3x/week.

HOW SUPPLIED: Inj: 75 IU, 450 IU, 300 IU/0.5mL, 450 IU/0.75mL, 900 IU/1.5mL

CONTRAINDICATIONS: (Men, Women) High FSH levels indicating gonadal failure, uncontrolled thyroid or adrenal dysfunction, sex hormone dependent tumors of the reproductive tract and accessory organs, organic intracranial lesions (eg, pituitary tumor). (Women) Aabnormal uterine bleeding of undetermined origin, ovarian cyst or enlargement, pregnancy.

WARNINGS/PRECAUTIONS: Ovarian enlargement may occur; monitor ovarian response. Ovarian hyperstimulation syndrome, multiple births, serious pulmonary and vascular complications reported. Avoid hCG if ovaries abnormally enlarged last day of therapy. Monitor follicular maturation by measuring estradiol levels and through ultrasonography.

ADVERSE REACTIONS: (Women) Intermenstrual bleeding, breast pain, ovarian hyperstimulation, abdominal pain, nausea, diarrhea, flatulence, headache, ovarian cysts, pain, upper respiratory tract infection. (Men) Breast pain, acne, gynecomastia, injection site pain, fatigue.

PREGNANCY: Category X, not for use in nursing.

MECHANISM OF ACTION: Follicle stimulating hormone; stimulates ovarian follicular growth in women who do not have primary ovarian failure.

PHARMACOKINETICS: Absorption: Slow (after IM, SQ). Administration of different doses resulted in different parameters. **Elimination:** (IM, SQ) $T_{1/2}$=50, 24 hrs., respectively.

GRANULEX   RX
peruvian balsam - trypsin - castor oil (Mylan Bertek)

THERAPEUTIC CLASS: Debriding agent

INDICATIONS: Treatment of decubitus ulcers, varicose ulcers, debridement of eschar, dehiscent wounds and sunburn.

DOSAGE: *Adults:* Spray wound at least bid or more often prn.
Pediatrics: Spray wound at least bid or more often prn.

HOW SUPPLIED: Spray: (Castor Oil-Peruvian Balsam-Trypsin) 650mg-72.5mg-0.1mg/0.82mL [60mL, 120mL]

WARNINGS/PRECAUTIONS: Do not spray on fresh arterial clots. Avoid spraying in eyes. Wound may be left open or a wet bandage may be applied.

PREGNANCY: Safety in pregnancy and nursing is not known.

MECHANISM OF ACTION: Assists healing of external wounds by facilitating the removal of necrotic tissue, exudate, and organic debris.

GRIFULVIN V   RX
griseofulvin (Ortho Neutrogena)

THERAPEUTIC CLASS: *Penicillium*-derived antifungal

INDICATIONS: Management of tinea capitis, tinea corporis, tinea pedis, tinea unguium, tinea barbae, and tinea cruris. Inhibits the growth of fungi that commonly cause ringworm infections of hair, skin, and nails.

DOSAGE: *Adults:* Tinea Capitis: 500mg qd for 4-6 weeks. Tinea Corporis: 500mg qd for 2-4 weeks. Tinea Pedis: 1g qd for 4-8 weeks. Tinea Cruris: 500mg qd. Tinea Unguium: 1g qd for at least 4 months (fingernail) or at least 6 months (toenails).

Pediatrics: Usual: 5mg/lb/day. 30-50lb: 125-250mg qd. >50lb: 250-500mg qd. Tinea Capitis: Treat for 4-6 weeks. Tinea Corporis: Treat for 2-4 weeks. Tinea Pedis: Treat for 4-8 weeks. Tinea Unguium: Treat for at least 4 months (fingernail) or at least 6 months (toenails).

HOW SUPPLIED: Sus: 125mg/5mL [120mL]; Tab: 250mg, 500mg

CONTRAINDICATIONS: Porphyria, hepatocellular failure, pregnancy.

WARNINGS/PRECAUTIONS: Confirm diagnosis. Not for prophylactic use. Monitor renal, hepatic, and hematopoietic functions periodically with prolonged therapy. Cross-sensitivity with PCN may exist. Photosensitivity reported. D/C if granulocytopenia occurs.

ADVERSE REACTIONS: Rash, urticaria, oral thrush, nausea, vomiting, epigastric distress, diarrhea, headache, dizziness, insomnia, mental confusion.

INTERACTIONS: Oral anticoagulants may need adjustment. Barbiturates decrease effects. Decreases effects of oral contraceptives; may increase incidence of breakthrough bleeding.

PREGNANCY: Not for use in pregnancy and in nursing.

MECHANISM OF ACTION: Acts systemically to inhibit the growth *Trichophyton, Micosporum*, and *Epidermophyton* genera of fungi. Fungistatic amounts deposit in keratin, which is gradually exfoliated and replaced by noninfected tissue.

PHARMACOKINETICS: Absorption: C_{max}=0.5gm; T_{max}=4 hrs.

GRIS-PEG   RX
griseofulvin (Pedinol)

THERAPEUTIC CLASS: *Penicillium*-derived antifungal

INDICATIONS: Treatment of t.capitis, t.corporis, t.pedis, t.unguium, t.barbae, and t.cruris.

DOSAGE: *Adults:* T.capitis: 375mg qd in single or divided doses for 4-6 weeks. T.corporis: 375mg qd in single or divided doses for 2-4 weeks. T.pedis: 375mg bid for 4-8 weeks. T.cruris: 375mg qd in single or divided doses. T.unguium: 375mg bid for at least 4 months (fingernail) or at least 6 months (toenails). *Pediatrics:* Usual: 3.3mg/lb/day. 35-60lb: 125-187.5mg qd. >60lb: 187.5-375mg qd. T.capitis: Treat for 4-6 weeks. T.corporis: Treat for 2-4 weeks. T.pedis: Treat for 4-8 weeks. T.unguium: Treat for at least 4 months (fingernail) or at least 6 months (toenails).

HOW SUPPLIED: Tab: 125mg*, 250mg* *scored

CONTRAINDICATIONS: Porphyria, hepatocellular failure, pregnancy.

WARNINGS/PRECAUTIONS: Not for prophylactic use. Periodically monitor renal, hepatic, and hematopoietic functions in prolonged therapy. Cross-sensitivity with PCN may exist. Photosensitivity reported. D/C if granulocytopenia occurs.

ADVERSE REACTIONS: Rash, urticaria, oral thrush, nausea, vomiting, epigastric distress, diarrhea, headache, dizziness, insomnia, mental confusion.

INTERACTIONS: Oral anticoagulants may need dose adjustments. Decreased effects with barbiturates. Decreased effects of oral contraceptives. Increased alcohol effects.

PREGNANCY: Not for use in pregnancy and in nursing.

MECHANISM OF ACTION: Fungistatic agent. Active against various species of *Microsporum, Epidermophyton* and *Trichophyton*. Has greater affinity for depositing in keratin precursor cells of diseased tissue. Tightly binds to new keratin, which then becomes highly resistant to fungal invasions.

PHARMACOKINETICS: Absorption: C_{max}=600ng/mL; T_{max}=4 hrs; AUC=8618ng•hr/mL.

GYNAZOLE-1 RX
butoconazole nitrate (Ther-Rx)

THERAPEUTIC CLASS: Azole antifungal

INDICATIONS: Local treatment of vulvovaginal infections caused by *Candida albicans*.

DOSAGE: *Adults:* 1 applicatorful intravaginally once.

HOW SUPPLIED: Cre: 2% [5g]

WARNINGS/PRECAUTIONS: Do not rely on condoms or diaphragm within 72 hrs after last use. Confirm diagnosis by KOH smears and/or cultures; reconfirm if no response.

ADVERSE REACTIONS: Vulvar/vaginal burning, itching, soreness, swelling, pelvic or abdominal pain, cramping.

PREGNANCY: Category C, caution in nursing.

GYNE-LOTRIMIN OTC
clotrimazole (Schering)

OTHER BRAND NAMES: Gyne-Lotrimin 3 Combination Pack (Schering) - Gyne-Lotrimin Combination Pack (Schering) - Gyne-Lotrimin 3 (Schering)

THERAPEUTIC CLASS: Azole antifungal

INDICATIONS: Treatment of vaginal candidiasis.

DOSAGE: *Adults:* 200mg sup or 2% cream intravaginally qhs for 3 days, or 100mg sup or 1% cream intravaginally qhs for 7 days. Apply 1% cream externally qd-bid prn.
Pediatrics: ≥12 yrs: 200mg sup or 2% cream intravaginally qhs for 3 days, or 100mg sup or 1% cream intravaginally qhs for 7 days. Apply 1% cream externally qd-bid prn.

HOW SUPPLIED: (Gyne-Lotrimin) Cre: 1% [5g, 45g]; Sup: 100mg [7ˢ]; (Combination Pack) Cre: 1% [7g]; Sup: 100mg [7ˢ]; (Gyne-Lotrimin 3) Sup: 200mg [3ˢ]; (3 Combination Pack) Cre: 1% [7g]; Sup: 200mg [3ˢ]

WARNINGS/PRECAUTIONS: Do not use if fever (>100°F), foul smelling vaginal discharge or abdominal, back or shoulder pain. Do not use with douches, spermicide or tampons. Do not rely on condoms or diaphragm to prevent STDs or pregnancy while using these products.

GYNODIOL RX
estradiol (Novavax)

> Estrogens increase risk of endometrial cancer in postmenopausal women. Avoid during pregnancy.

THERAPEUTIC CLASS: Estrogen

INDICATIONS: Treatment of moderate to severe vasomotor symptoms associated with menopause. Treatment of vulval/vaginal atrophy. Treatment of hypoestrogenism due to hypogonadism, castration, or primary ovarian failure. Palliative treatment of breast cancer in patients with metastatic disease and/or advanced androgen-dependent carcinoma of the prostate. Prevention of osteoporosis.

DOSAGE: *Adults:* Vasomotor Symptoms/Vulval/Vaginal Atrophy: Initial: 1-2mg/day (3 weeks on, 1 week off). Maint: Minimum effective dose. Discontinue or taper at 3-6 month intervals. Hypoestrogenism: 1-2mg/day. Maint: Minimum effective dose. Metastatic Breast Cancer: 10mg tid for at least 3 months. Prostate Carcinoma: 1-2mg tid. Osteoporosis Prevention: 0.5mg qd (23 days on and 5 days off).

HOW SUPPLIED: Tab: 0.5mg*, 1mg*, 1.5mg*, 2mg* *scored

CONTRAINDICATIONS: Pregnancy, undiagnosed abnormal genital bleeding, breast cancer unless being treated for metastatic disease, estrogen-dependent neoplasia, thrombophlebitis, thromboembolic disorders.

WARNINGS/PRECAUTIONS: Risk of endometrial and breast cancer, fetal congenital reproductive tract disorder gallbladder disease, cardiovascular disease, elevated BP, and hypercalcemia with breast cancer and bone metastases. Caution in liver dysfunction, asthma, epilepsy, migraine, and cardiac or renal dysfunction. May develop uterine bleeding and mastodynia. Accelerated PT, PTT, and platelet aggregation time. Hypercoagulability effects. Impaired glucose tolerance. Consider addition of a progestin in patient with intact uterus. Increase in HDL, triglycerides, thyroid-binding globulin.

ADVERSE REACTIONS: Altered vaginal bleeding, vaginal candidiasis, breast tenderness/enlargement, GI effects, CNS effects, chloasma, melasma, weight changes, edema, altered libido.

PREGNANCY: Category X, not for use in nursing.

HALCION

CIV

triazolam (Pharmacia & Upjohn)

THERAPEUTIC CLASS: Benzodiazepine

INDICATIONS: Short-term treatment of insomnia.

DOSAGE: *Adults:* 0.25mg qhs. Max: 0.5mg. Elderly/Debilitated: Initial: 0.125mg. Max: 0.25mg.

HOW SUPPLIED: Tab: 0.125mg, 0.25mg* *scored

CONTRAINDICATIONS: Pregnancy. With ketoconazole, itraconazole, nefazodone, medications that impair CYP3A.

WARNINGS/PRECAUTIONS: Worsening or failure of response after 7-10 days may indicate other medical conditions. Increased daytime anxiety, abnormal thinking, and behavioral changes have occurred. May impair mental/physical abilities. Anterograde amnesia reported with therapeutic doses. Caution with baseline depression, suicidal tendencies, history of drug dependence, elderly/debilitated, renal/hepatic impairment, chronic pulmonary insufficiency, and sleep apnea. Withdrawal symptoms after discontinuation; avoid abrupt withdrawal.

ADVERSE REACTIONS: Drowsiness, dizziness, lightheadedness, headache, nausea, vomiting, coordination disorders, ataxia.

INTERACTIONS: See Contraindications. Avoid the concomitant use with inhibitors of the CYP3A (eg, ketoconazole, itraconazole, all azole-type antifungals, nefazodone). Potentiated by the coadministration of isoniazid, OCs, grapefruit juice, ranitidine. Caution with fluvoxamine, diltiazem, verapamil, cimetidine, ergotamine, cyclosporine, amiodarone, nicardipine, nifedipine, sertraline, paroxetine, macrolides. Additive CNS depression with psychotropics, anticonvulsants, antihistamines, and alcohol.

PREGNANCY: Category X, not for use in nursing.

MECHANISM OF ACTION: Triazolobenzodiazepine hypnotic agent.

PHARMACOKINETICS: Absorption: C_{max}=1-6ng/mL, T_{max}=2 hrs. **Metabolism:** Hydroxylation via CYP450 3A. **Elimination:** Urine (79.9%), $T_{1/2}$=1.5-5.5 hrs.

HALFLYTELY

RX

polyethylene glycol 3350 - sodium bicarbonate - potassium chloride - sodium chloride - bisacodyl (Braintree)

THERAPEUTIC CLASS: Bowel cleanser/stimulant laxative

INDICATIONS: Bowel cleansing prior to colonoscopy.

DOSAGE: *Adults:* Consume only clear liquids on day of preparation. Swallow all 4 bisacodyl tabs at noon (do not chew or crush). After 1st bowel movement (or max of 6 hrs) begin drinking sol, 240mL every 10 min (approx. 8 glasses). Drink all sol.

HOW SUPPLIED: Kit: Tab, Delayed-Release: (Bisacodyl) 5mg [4ˢ]. Sol: (Polyethylene Glycol 3350-Potassium Chloride-Sodium Bicarbonate-Sodium Chloride) 210g-0.74g-2.86g-5.60g [2000mL].

CONTRAINDICATIONS: Ileus, GI obstruction, gastric retention, bowel perforation, toxic colitis, toxic megacolon.

WARNINGS/PRECAUTIONS: Do not add additional ingredients (eg, flavorings). Caution with severe ulcerative colitis, ileus or gastric retention. Monitor with impaired gag reflex, prone to regurgitation or aspiration. Slow administration or temporarily d/c if severe bloating, distention, or abdominal pain develops. Avoid large quantities of water during or after preparation or colonoscopy. Monitor closely with impaired water handling. Generalized tonic-clonic seizures, hives and skin rashes reported.

ADVERSE REACTIONS: Nausea, abdominal fullness, cramping, vomiting, overall discomfort.

INTERACTIONS: Oral medications taken within 1 hr of start of administration start may not be absorbed from GI tract. Avoid bisacodyl delayed release tablets within 1 hr of taking an antacid.

PREGNANCY: Category C, caution in nursing.

MECHANISM OF ACTION: Stimulant laxative that induces diarrhea.

PHARMACOKINETICS: Metabolism: Hydrolysis by intestinal brush border enzymes and colonic bacteria to form bis-(hydroxyphenyl) pyridyl-2 methane (active metabolite).

HALFPRIN   OTC
aspirin (Kramer)

THERAPEUTIC CLASS: Salicylate

INDICATIONS: To reduce the risk of vascular mortality and fatal and nonfatal cardiovascular and cerebrovascular events in patients with a suspected acute MI.

DOSAGE: *Adults:* 162mg as soon as MI suspected; continue qd for 30 days. May need to continue as prophylaxis for recurrent MI. Crush, chew, or suck the 1st dose.

HOW SUPPLIED: Tab, Delayed-Release: 81mg, 162mg

WARNINGS/PRECAUTIONS: Caution with marked HTN or renal dysfunction; monitor renal function with long-term therapy.

ADVERSE REACTIONS: Stomach pain, heartburn, nausea, vomiting, GI bleeding, small increases in BP.

PREGNANCY: Safety in pregnancy and nursing is not known.

HALOG   RX
halcinonide (Ranbaxy)

THERAPEUTIC CLASS: Corticosteroid

INDICATIONS: Corticosteroid-responsive dermatoses.

DOSAGE: *Adults:* (Cre, Oint, Sol) Apply bid-tid. May use occlusive dressings for psoriasis and recalcitrant conditions.
Pediatrics: Limit to least amount compatible with an effective therapeutic regimen.

HOW SUPPLIED: Cre, Oint: 0.1% [15g, 30g, 60g]; Sol: 0.1% [20mL, 60mL]

WARNINGS/PRECAUTIONS: May produce reversible HPA axis suppression, manifestations of Cushing's syndrome, hyperglycemia and glucosuria. Occlusive dressings and application to large surface areas may augment systemic absorption. Pediatrics may be more susceptible to systemic toxicity. D/C if irritation occurs.

ADVERSE REACTIONS: Burning, itching, irritation, dryness, folliculitis, hyper-trichosis, acneiform eruptions, hypopigmentation, perioral dermatitis, contact dermatitis, skin maceration, secondary infection.

PREGNANCY: Category C, caution in nursing.

MECHANISM OF ACTION: Corticosteroid; possesses anti-inflammatory, antipruritic, and vasoconstrictive actions. Anti-inflammatory effects not established.

PHARMACOKINETICS: Absorption: Percutaneous; inflammation, other disease states, and occlusive dressings may increase percutaneous absorption. **Distribution:** Bound to plasma proteins to varying degrees. Systemically administered corticosteroids are found in breast milk. **Metabolism:** Liver. **Elimination:** Kidneys (major), bile.

HALOPERIDOL RX
haloperidol (Various)

OTHER BRAND NAMES: Haldol (Ortho-McNeil) - Haldol Decanoate (Ortho-McNeil)

THERAPEUTIC CLASS: Butyrophenone

INDICATIONS: (Immediate-Release) Treatment of psychosis, Tourette's disorder, severe childhood behavioral problems. Short-term treatment of hyperactivity in children. (Decanoate) Prolonged management of psychosis.

DOSAGE: *Adults:* (Immediate-Release) PO: Moderate Symptoms/Elderly/Debilitated: 0.5-2mg bid-tid. Severe Symptoms/Resistant Patients: 3-5mg bid-tid. Max: 100mg/day. IM: Acute Agitation: 2-5mg every 4-8 hrs or hourly as needed for moderately severe or very severe symptoms. Max: 100mg/day. (Decanoate) For IM inj only. Give every 4 weeks or monthly. Initial:10-20 times daily oral dose up to 100mg. Give remainder of dose 3-7 days later if initial dose >100mg. Usual: 10-15 times daily oral dose. Max: 450mg/month. Elderly/Debilitated: Initial: 10-15 times daily oral dose.
Pediatrics: 3-12 yrs: (15-40kg): PO: Psychosis: Initial: 0.05-0.15mg/kg/day given bid-tid. Nonpsychotic Disorder/Tourette's: 0.05-0.075mg/kg/day given bid-tid. Max: 6mg/day.

HOW SUPPLIED: Inj: 5mg/mL; Inj: (Decanoate) 50mg/mL, 100mg/mL; Sol: 2mg/mL; Tab: 0.5mg*, 1mg*, 2mg*, 5mg*, 10mg*, 20mg** scored

CONTRAINDICATIONS: Comatose states, severe toxic CNS depression, Parkinson's disease.

WARNINGS/PRECAUTIONS: Risk of tardive dyskinesia, especially in elderly. NMS, hyperpyrexia, heat stroke, bronchopneumonia reported. Decreased cholesterol, cutaneous and/or ocular changes may occur. Neurotoxicity may occur with thyrotoxicosis. Caution with CV disease, seizures, EEG abnormalities, QT-prolonging conditions, elderly. Do not administer IV. Cases of sudden death and Torsades de Pointes reported.

ADVERSE REACTIONS: Extrapyramidal symptoms, tardive dyskinesia, tardive dystonia, ECG changes, QT prolongation, ventricular arrhythmias, tachycardia, hypotension, HTN, nausea, vomiting, constipation, diarrhea, dry mouth, blurred vision, urinary retention.

INTERACTIONS: Caution with rifampin, anticonvulsants, anticoagulants, anticholinergics, antiparkinson agents. May potentiate CNS depression with alcohol, opiates, anesthetics, and other CNS depressants. Antagonizes epinephrine. Monitor for neurological toxicity with lithium. Avoid concomitant alcohol use.

PREGNANCY: Category C, not for use in nursing.

MECHANISM OF ACTION: Butyrophenone; not established, suspected to block effects of dopamine and increase turnover rate.

PHARMACOKINETICS: Absorption: T_{max}=6 days (IM). **Elimination:** $T_{1/2}$=3 weeks (IM).

HALOTESTIN

CIII

fluoxymesterone (Pharmacia & Upjohn)

THERAPEUTIC CLASS: Androgen

INDICATIONS: Testosterone replacement therapy in males with primary hypogonadism or hypogonadotrophic hypogonadism. To stimulate puberty in males with delayed puberty. Palliation of androgen-responsive recurrent mammary cancer in females who are >1 to <5 yrs postmenopausal or who have a hormone-dependent tumor as shown by previous beneficial response to castration.

DOSAGE: *Adults:* Male Replacement Therapy: 5-20mg/day, qd or in divided doses tid-qid. Breast Cancer: 10-40mg/day in divided doses tid-qid. Continue therapy for at least 1 month for satisfactory subjective response, and for 2-3 months for objective response.
Pediatrics: Male Replacement Therapy: 5-20mg/day, qd or in divided doses tid-qid. Delayed Puberty: Initial: Use low dose, titrate carefully; use for 4-6 months. Caution in children.

HOW SUPPLIED: Tab: 2mg*, 5mg*, 10mg* *scored

CONTRAINDICATIONS: Males with breast or prostate cancer, pregnancy, serious cardiac, hepatic or renal disease.

WARNINGS/PRECAUTIONS: D/C if hypercalcemia occurs in breast cancer or immobilized patients; monitor calcium levels. Risk of hepatic adenomas, hepatocellular carcinoma, and peliosis hepatitis with prolonged high doses. D/C if jaundice, cholestatic hepatitis occurs. Caution in the elderly; increased risk of prostatic hypertrophy and prostatic carcinoma. Risk of edema; caution with pre-existing cardiac, renal, or hepatic disease. Risk of compromised stature in children; monitor bone growth every 6 months. Should not be used for enhancement of athletic performance. Monitor for virilization in females. Patients with BPH may develop acute urethral obstruction. If priapism occurs, d/c and if restarted use lower dose. Contains tartrazine; may cause allergic type reactions especially in those with ASA hypersensitivity. Monitor LFTs, Hct, Hgb periodically.

ADVERSE REACTIONS: Amenorrhea, virilization, menstrual irregularities, gynecomastia, excessive frequency/duration of penile erections, male pattern baldness, increased/decreased libido, oligospermia, hirsutism, acne, fluid and electrolyte disturbances, nausea, hypercholesterolemia, clotting factor suppression, polycythemia, altered LFTs, oligospermia, priapism, anxiety, depression.

INTERACTIONS: May potentiate oral anticoagulants and oxyphenbutazone. May decrease blood glucose and insulin requirements.

PREGNANCY: Category X, not for use in nursing.

MECHANISM OF ACTION: Endogenous androgen; responsible for normal growth and development of male sex organs and for maintenance of secondary sex characteristics.

PHARMACOKINETICS: Elimination: $T_{1/2}$=9.2 hrs.

HAVRIX

RX

hepatitis A vaccine (inactivated) (GlaxoSmithKline)

THERAPEUTIC CLASS: Vaccine

INDICATIONS: Active immunization in persons ≥12 months against hepatitis A virus.

DOSAGE: *Adults:* ≥18 yrs: 1440 EL U IM (deltoid), then booster after 6-12 months.
Pediatrics: 1-18 yrs: 720 EL U IM (deltoid), then booster after 6-12 months.

HOW SUPPLIED: Inj: 720 EL U/0.5mL, 1440 EL U/mL

CONTRAINDICATIONS: Hypersensitivity to any component, including neomycin.

WARNINGS/PRECAUTIONS: Epinephrine should be available for anaphylaxis. Delay with febrile illness. Caution with thrombocytopenia or bleeding disorders. Immunosuppressed may show suboptimal response. May not prevent hepatitis A in patients already infected.

ADVERSE REACTIONS: Injection site soreness, induration, redness, swelling, fever, fatigue, malaise, anorexia, nausea, headache.

INTERACTIONS: Caution with anticoagulant therapy and IM injection. Give immunoglobulins and other vaccines in different syringe and injection site.

PREGNANCY: Category C, caution in nursing.

MECHANISM OF ACTION: May produce immune response for protection against hepatitis A virus infection.

HECTOROL
RX

doxercalciferol (Bone Care)

THERAPEUTIC CLASS: Vitamin D analog

INDICATIONS: (Cap) Secondary hyperparathyroidism in patients with chronic kidney disease on dialysis or with Stage 3 or 4 chronic kidney disease. (Inj) Secondary hyperparathyroidism in patients with chronic kidney disease on dialysis.

DOSAGE: *Adults:* (Cap) Dialysis: Initial: 10mcg 3x/week (TTW) approximately qod at dialysis. Titrate: Adjust to obtain iPTH of 150-300 pg/mL. May increase by 2.5mcg at 8-week intervals if iPTH is not lowered by 50% and fails to reach target range. Max: 20mcg TIW (60mcg/week). Suspend therapy if iPTH <100pg/mL; restart after 1 week with dose at least 2.5mcg lower than last dose. Hypercalcemia/Hyperphosphatemia/Ca x P product >55mg^2/dL^2: Decrease or suspend therapy and/or adjust dose of phosphate binders; if suspended, restart at a dose at least 2.5mcg lower. Pre-dialysis: Initial: 1mcg qd. Titrate: May increase by 0.5mcg at 2-week intervals to achieve target iPTH range. Max: 3.5mcg qd. Hypercalcemia/Hyperphosphatemia/Ca x P product >55mg^2/dL^2: Decrease or suspend therapy and/or adjust dose of phosphate binders; if suspended, restart at a dose at least 0.5mcg lower. (Inj) Initial: 4mcg bolus TIW at the end of dialysis. Titrate: Adjust to obtain iPTH of 150-300pg/mL. May increase at 8-week intervals by 1-2mcg if iPTH is not lowered by 50% and fails to reach target range. Max: 18mcg/week. Suspend therapy if iPTH <100pg/mL; restart after 1 week with a dose at least 1mcg lower than last dose. Hypercalcemia/Hyperphosphatemia/Ca x P product >55mg^2/dL^2: Decrease or suspend therapy and/or adjust dose of phosphate binders; if suspended, restart at a dose at least 1mcg lower.

HOW SUPPLIED: Cap: 0.5mcg, 2.5mcg; Inj: 2mcg/mL [2mL]

CONTRAINDICATIONS: Tendency to develop hypercalcemia or vitamin D toxicity.

WARNINGS/PRECAUTIONS: Acute hypercalcemia may exacerbate arrythmias, seizures. Use oral Ca-based or non-aluminum containing antacids to control serum phosphate. Chronic hypercalcemia can cause calcification of soft tissues. Risk of hypercalcemia and hyperphospatemia. Maintain serum calcium times serum phosphorus at <55mg^2/dL^2 in patients with chronic kidney disease. Avoid with recent history of hypercalcemia, hyperphosphatemia, or vitamin D toxicity. Caution with hepatic dysfunction. Monitor iPTH, serum calcium, and serum phosphorus initially then weekly during dose titration. Oversuppression of iPTH can cause adynamic bone syndrome.

ADVERSE REACTIONS: Headache, malaise, bradycardia, nausea, vomiting, edema, dizziness, dyspnea, pruritus, abscess, anorexia, constipation, dyspepsia, arthralgia, weight increase, sleep disorder.

INTERACTIONS: (Cap, Inj) Magnesium-containing antacids may cause hypermagnesemia especially with chronic renal dialysis. Enzyme inducers may affect metabolism; consider adjusting dose. CYP450 inhibitors (eg, ketoconazole, erythromycin) may prevent active moiety formation. Avoid vitamin D products and derivatives during treatment. Acute hypercalcemia may affect digitalis activity. (Cap) Colestyramine, mineral oil may impair absorption.

PREGNANCY: Category B, not for use in nursing.

MECHANISM OF ACTION: Synthetic vitamin D_2 analog; regulates, along with calcitriol, blood calcium at levels required for essential body functions. Biologically active vitamin D metabolites control intestinal absorption of dietary calcium, tubular reabsorption of calcium by kidneys and, with parathyroid hormone (PTH), mobilization of calcium from the skeleton. Acts directly on bone cells to stimulate skeletal growth and on the parathyroid glands to supress PTH synthesis and secretion.

PHARMACOKINETICS: Absorptiom: (IV) $T_{max(mean)}$=8 hrs (major metabolite); (PO) $T_{max\ (mean)}$=11-12 hrs (major metabolite). **Metabolism:** Liver via CYP27 to $1a25$-$(OH)_2D_2$ (major), $1a,24$-dihydroxyvitamin D_2 (minor). **Elimination:** (PO) $T_{1/2(mean)}$=32-37 hrs.

HELIDAC   RX
tetracycline HCL - bismuth subsalicylate - metronidazole (Prometheus)

THERAPEUTIC CLASS: Antimicrobial

INDICATIONS: In combination with an H_2 antagonist for eradication of *H.pylori* and for treatment of *H.pylori* infection and duodenal ulcer disease.

DOSAGE: *Adults:* (Bismuth) 2 tabs (525mg) qid + (Metronidazole) 250mg qid + (Tetracycline) 500mg qid, all for 14 days with an H_2 antagonist. Take with meals and hs. Take metronidazole and tetracycline with a full glass of water; swallow whole.

HOW SUPPLIED: Cap: (Tetracycline) 500mg; Tab: (Metronidazole) 250mg; Tab, Chewable: (Bismuth Subsalicylate) 262.4mg

CONTRAINDICATIONS: Pregnancy, nursing, pediatrics, nitroimidazole hypersensitivity, ASA or salicylate hypersensitivity, renal/hepatic impairment.

WARNINGS/PRECAUTIONS: Do not use to treat nausea and vomiting in children or teenagers who have or are recovering from chickenpox or flu. Rare reports of neurotoxicity with excessive bismuth doses. Seizures and peripheral neuropathy reported with metronidazole; caution with CNS disease; d/c with abnormal neurological signs. Caution with blood dyscrasias. Unrecognized candidiasis may be unmasked. Avoid exposure to sunlight/UV light. Caution in elderly.

ADVERSE REACTIONS: Nausea, diarrhea, abdominal pain, melena, constipation, anorexia, asthenia, vomiting, discolored tongue, headache, dyspepsia, dizziness. Temporary, harmless darkening of tongue and black stool with bismuth. Tetracycline may cause permanent discoloration of teeth during tooth development, enamel hypoplasia, photosensitivity reactions, BUN increase, breakthrough bleeding, pseudotumor cerebri.

INTERACTIONS: Monitor anticoagulants; possible risk of bleeding and/or decreased prothrombin activity. Bismuth subsalicylate: Caution with antidiabetic agents, ASA, probenecid, and sulfinpyrazone. Tetracycline: Impaired absorption with antacids containing aluminum, calcium, magnesium; agents containing iron, zinc, sodium bicarbonate. Possible reduced absorption with dairy products, bismuth, or calcium carbonate. May interfere with bactericidal action of penicillin; avoid concomitant use. May antagonize oral contraceptive effects. Fatal renal toxicity with methoxyflurane reported. Metronidazole (MET): Decreased plasma clearance with drugs that decrease metabolism (eg, cimetidine). Increased elimination with drugs that induce metabolism (eg, phenytoin, phenobarbital). May impair phenytoin clearance. May increase lithium levels. Avoid alcohol during and at least 1 day after MET. Psychotic reactions reported in alcoholics with concomitant disulfiram and MET; space MET and disulfiram dosing by 2 weeks.

PREGNANCY: Category D, not for use in nursing.

MECHANISM OF ACTION: Combination therapy with activity against *H.pylori*. Refer to individual PI for specific mechanism of action of each component.

PHARMACOKINETICS: Absorption: Salicylic acid: C_{max}=13.1mcg/mL; metronidazole: well-absorbed. T_{max}=1-2 hrs; C_{max}=6mcg/mL; tetracycline: readily absorbed. **Distribution:** Bismuth: plasma protein binding (>90%); salicylic acid:

plasma protein binding (90%); V_d=170mL/kg; metronidazole: plasma protein binding (<20%), appears in the CSF, saliva, breast milk; tetracycline: crosses placenta, found in fetal tissues, secreted in human breast milk. **Metabolism**: Salicyclic acid: extensive; metronidazole: oxidation, glucuronide conjugation; 2-hydroxymethyl metabolite. **Elimination**: Bismuth: $T_{1/2}$=21-72 days; urine, bile; salicylic: urine (10%, unchanged). $T_{1/2}$=2-5 hrs; metronidazole: $T_{1/2}$=8 hrs, urine (60-80%), feces (6-15%); tetracycline: urine, feces.

HEMABATE   RX
carboprost tromethamine (Pharmacia & Upjohn)

THERAPEUTIC CLASS: Prostaglandin analog

INDICATIONS: Termination of pregnancy between 13th to 20th week of gestation. Termination of pregnancy in 2nd trimester if expulsion of fetus fails with other methods; premature, inadvertent, or spontaneous rupture of membranes occurs in previable fetus; or expulsion requires repeat intrauterine instillation. Treatment of postpartum hemorrhage due to uterine atony unresponsive to conventional methods.

DOSAGE: *Adults:* Consider pretreatment or concurrent use of antidiarrheals and antiemetics. Abortion/Fetal Expulsion Failure/Ruptured Membranes: May give initial optional test dose of 100mcg. Initial: 250mcg IM. Repeat 250mcg dose at 1.5-3.5 hr intervals, depending on uterine response. May increase to 500mcg if inadequate response after several doses of 250mcg. Max: 12mg total dose or continuous use for >2 days. Refractory Postpartum Uterine Bleeding: Initial: 250mcg IM. Determine additional doses and intervals based on clinical events. Max: 2mg total dose.

HOW SUPPLIED: Inj: 250mcg/mL

CONTRAINDICATIONS: Active pelvic inflammatory disease; active cardiac, pulmonary, renal or hepatic disease.

WARNINGS/PRECAUTIONS: Use in facility able to provide immediate intensive care and acute surgery. Adhere strictly to recommended dosages. Not indicated if fetus in utero is viable. If abortion fails, complete by other means. Contains benzyl alcohol. Caution with history of asthma, hypotension, HTN, cardiovascular, renal, or hepatic disease, anemia, jaundice, diabetes, epilepsy, or with compromised uteri. Transient pyrexia reported. Increased BP in postpartum hemorrhage. Use with chorioamnionitis may inhibit uterine response.

ADVERSE REACTIONS: Vomiting, diarrhea, nausea, increased temperature, flushing.

INTERACTIONS: May augment activity of other oxytocic agents; avoid concurrent use.

PREGNANCY: Category C, safety in nursing not known.

MECHANISM OF ACTION: Prostaglandin analogue; stimulates myometrial concentrations in gravid uterus, similar to labor contractions at end of full-term pregnancy.

PHARMACOKINETICS: Absorption: C_{max}=2060pg/mL; T_{max}=$^1/_2$ hr.

HEMATINIC PLUS   RX
ferrous fumarate - folic acid - multiple vitamin - minerals (Cypress)

THERAPEUTIC CLASS: Iron/vitamin

INDICATIONS: Iron and folate deficiency anemia. Iron and Vitamin C deficiencies with increased need for B-complex vitamins.

DOSAGE: *Adults:* 1 tab qd between meals.

HOW SUPPLIED: Ferrous Fumarate 324mg-Vit C 200mg, Vit B_1 10mg-Vit B_2 6mg-Vit B_6 5mg-Vit B_{12} 15mcg-Folic Acid 1mg- Niacinamide 30mg-Calcium 10mg-Zinc 18.2mg-Magnesium 6.9mg-Manganese 1.3mg-Copper 0.8mg.

CONTRAINDICATIONS: Hemochromatosis, hemosiderosis, hemolytic anemia, pernicious anemia.

WARNINGS/PRECAUTIONS: May mask pernicious anemia. May aggravate existing GI diseases. Ineffective in patients with steatorrhea and partial gastrectomy.

ADVERSE REACTIONS: Anorexia, nausea, diarrhea, constipation.

Hemocyte   OTC
ferrous fumarate (US Pharmaceutical)

INDICATIONS: Iron deficiency anemia.

DOSAGE: *Adults:* 1 tab up to bid, between meals.

HOW SUPPLIED: Tab: 324mg (106mg elemental iron)

CONTRAINDICATIONS: Hemochromatosis, hemosiderosis, hemolytic anemia.

WARNINGS/PRECAUTIONS: May aggravate existing GI disorders. Ineffective with steatorrhea, partial gastrectomy.

ADVERSE REACTIONS: Anorexia, nausea, diarrhea, constipation.

MECHANISM OF ACTION: Hematinic; used in iron deficiency anemia.

PHARMACOKINETICS: Absorption: Poor.

Hemocyte F   RX
ferrous fumarate - folic acid (US Pharmaceutical)

THERAPEUTIC CLASS: Iron/vitamin

INDICATIONS: Treatment and prevention of iron and/or folate deficiency in pregnancy, and treatment of iron and/or folate deficiency anemia.

DOSAGE: *Adults:* 1 tab qd. Elderly: Start at low end of dosing range.

HOW SUPPLIED: Tab: (Ferrous Fumarate-Folic Acid) 324mg-1mg

CONTRAINDICATIONS: Hemochromatosis, hemosiderosis, hemolytic anemia, pernicious anemia.

WARNINGS/PRECAUTIONS: Toxic when overdoses are ingested by children. Not for the treatment of pernicious anemia and other megaloblastic anemias where vitamin B_{12} is deficient. Folic acid >0.1mg-0.4mg/day may obscure pernicious anemia. Caution with peptic ulcer, regional enteritis, ulcerative colitis.

ADVERSE REACTIONS: GI disturbances, abdominal cramps, diarrhea, constipation, heartburn, nausea, vomiting, black stools, allergic sensitization.

MECHANISM OF ACTION: Iron-vitamin complex.

Hemocyte Plus   RX
ferrous fumarate - folic acid - multiple vitamin - minerals (US Pharmaceutical)

THERAPEUTIC CLASS: Vitamin/mineral

INDICATIONS: Iron and folate deficiency anemia. Iron and Vitamin C deficiencies with increased need for B-complex vitamins.

DOSAGE: *Adults:* 1 tab qd between meals.

HOW SUPPLIED: Tab: Ferrous Fumarate 324mg-Vit C 200mg-Vit B_1 10mg-Vit B_2 6mg-Vit B_6 5mg -Vit B_{12} 15mcg - Folic acid 1mg - Niacinamide 30mg - Pantothenic acid 10mg- Zinc 18.2mg - Magnesium 6.9mg - Manganese 1.3mg - Copper 0.8mg

CONTRAINDICATIONS: Hemochromatosis, hemosiderosis, hemolytic anemia, pernicious anemia.

WARNINGS/PRECAUTIONS: Folic acid doses above 0.1-0.4mg/day may mask pernicious anemia. Accidental iron overdose may lead to fatal poisoning in children <6 yrs.

ADVERSE REACTIONS: Allergic sensitization, anorexia, nausea, diarrhea, constipation.

MECHANISM OF ACTION: Iron-vitamin-mineral complex.

HEPARIN SODIUM
heparin sodium (Various)

RX

THERAPEUTIC CLASS: Glycosaminoglycan

INDICATIONS: Prophylaxis and treatment of venous thrombosis and its extension, PE in atrial fibrillation, and peripheral arterial embolism. Prevention of postoperative DVT and PE. Diagnosis and treatment of acute and chronic consumptive coagulopathies, for prevention of clotting in arterial and cardiac surgery.

DOSAGE: *Adults:* Based on 68kg: Initial: 5000 U IV, then 10,000-20,000 U SQ. Maint: 8000-10,000 U q8h or 15,000-20,000 U q12h. Intermittent IV Injection: Initial: 10,000 U. Maint: 5000-10,000 U q4-6h. Continuous IV Infusion: Initial: 5000U. Maint: 20,000-40,000 U/24 hrs. Adjust to coagulation test results. See PI for details in specific disease states.
Pediatrics: Initial: 50 U/kg IV drip. Maint: 100 U/kg IV drip q4h or 20,000 U/m²/24 hrs continuously.

HOW SUPPLIED: Inj: 1000 U/mL, 2500 U/mL, 5000 U/mL, 7500 U/mL, 10,000 U/mL

CONTRAINDICATIONS: Severe thrombocytopenia, if cannot perform appropriate blood-coagulation tests (with full-dose heparin), uncontrollable active bleeding state (except in DIC).

WARNINGS/PRECAUTIONS: Not for IM use. Hemorrhage can occur at any site; caution with increased danger of hemorrhage (severe HTN, bacterial endocarditis, surgery, etc.). Monitor blood coagulation tests frequently. Thrombocytopenia reported; d/c if platelets <100,000mm³ or if recurrent thrombosis develops. Contains benzyl alcohol. "White-clot syndrome" reported. Monitor platelets, Hct, and occult blood in the stool. Increased heparin resistance with fever, thrombosis, thrombophlebitis, infections with thrombosing tendencies, MI, cancer, and post-op. Higher bleeding incidence in women >60 yrs.

ADVERSE REACTIONS: Hemorrhage, local irritation, erythema, mild pain, hematoma, chills, fever, urticaria.

INTERACTIONS: Wait ≥5 hrs after last IV dose or 24 hrs after last SQ dose before measure PT for dicumarol or warfarin. Platelet inhibitors (eg, acetylsalicylic acid, dextran, phenylbutazone, ibuprofen, indomethacin, dipyridamole, hydroxychloroquine) may induce bleeding. Digitalis, tetracyclines, nicotine, or antihistamines may counteract anticoagulant action.

PREGNANCY: Category C, safe in nursing.

MECHANISM OF ACTION: Glycosaminoglycan; inhibits reactions that lead to blood clotting and the formation of fibrin clots. Acts at multiple sites in the normal coagulation system.

PHARMACOKINETICS: Absorption: (SC) T_{max}=2-4 hrs. **Metabolism:** Liver and reticulo-endothelial system. **Elimination:** $T_{1/2}$=10 min.

HEPSERA
adefovir dipivoxil (Gilead Sciences)

RX

> Discontinuation may result in severe acute exacerbations of hepatitis. Chronic use may result in nephrotoxicity in patients at risk of or having underlying renal dysfunction. HIV resistance may occur with unrecognized or untreated HIV infection. May cause lactic acidosis and severe hepatomegaly with steatosis.

THERAPEUTIC CLASS: Acyclic nucleotide analog

INDICATIONS: Treatment of chronic hepatitis B in patients ≥12 yrs of age with evidence of active viral replication and either evidence of persistent elevations in serum aminotransferases (ALT or AST) or histologically active disease.

DOSAGE: *Adults:* 10mg qd. Renal Impairment: CrCl 20-49mL/min: 10mg q48h. CrCl 10-19mL/min: 10mg q72h. Hemodialysis Patients: 10mg every 7 days following dialysis.
Pediatrics: ≥12 yrs: 10mg qd.

HOW SUPPLIED: Tab: 10mg

WARNINGS/PRECAUTIONS: Monitor hepatic function at repeated intervals upon discontinuation. Monitor renal function in patients with pre-existing or risk factors for renal dysfunction; adjust dosage appropriately. May require HIV antibody testing prior to treatment. Suspend treatment if lactic acidosis and severe hepatomegaly are suspected.

ADVERSE REACTIONS: Asthenia, headache, abdominal pain, nausea, flatulence, diarrhea, dyspepsia, increased creatinine, hypophosphatemia.

INTERACTIONS: Coadministration with drugs that reduce renal function or compete for active tubular secretion may increase concentrations of adefovir or the coadministered drugs.

PREGNANCY: Category C, caution in nursing.

MECHANISM OF ACTION: Acyclic nucleotide analog; inhibits HBV DNA polymerase by competing with natural substrate deoxyadenosine triphosphate and by causing DNA chain termination after incorporation into viral DNA.

PHARMACOKINETICS: Absorption: Absolute bioavailability (59%); C_{max}=18.4ng/mL; T_{max}=1.75 hrs; AUC=220ng•h/mL. **Pediatrics:** C_{max}=23.3ng/mL; AUC=248.8ng•h/mL. **Distribution:** V_d=392mL/kg (1mg/kg/day), 352mL/kg (3mg/kg/day); plasma protein binding (≤4%). **Elimination:** Urine (45%); $T_{1/2}$=7.48 hrs.

HERCEPTIN   RX
trastuzumab (Genentech)

May result in cardiac failure manifesting as CHF and decreased left ventricular ejection fraction (LVEF). Increased incidence/severity of left ventricular cardiac dysfunction in combination with anthracycline-containing regimens. Evaluate LVEF prior to and during therapy; d/c with significant decrease in left ventricular function or cardiomyopathy. Serious infusion reactions and pulmonary toxicity may result. Interrupt infusion if dyspnea or clinically significant hypotension develops. D/C with anaphylaxis, angioedema, interstitial pneumonitis, or acute respiratory distress syndrome.

THERAPEUTIC CLASS: Monoclonal antibody/HER2-blocker

INDICATIONS: Part of treatment regimen containing doxorubicin, cyclophosphamide, and either paclitaxel or docetaxel and with docetaxel and carboplatin for adjuvant treatment of HER2-overexpressing breast cancer. Single agent for adjuvant treatment of HER2-overexpressing node-negative or node-positive breast cancer, following multi-modality anthracycline based therapy. In combination with paclitaxel for treatment of HER2-overexpressing metastatic breast cancer. Single agent for treatment of HER2-overexpressing breast cancer in patients who received 1 or more chemotherapy regimens for metastatic disease.

DOSAGE: *Adults:* Adjuvant Treatment: Following Anthracycline/Concurrently With Paclitaxel for First 12 Weeks: IV infusion: Initial: 4mg/kg over 90 min. Maint: 2mg/kg/week over 30 min for total 52 doses. Following Completion of All Chemotherapy: IV Infusion: Initial: 8mg/kg. Maint: 6mg/kg every 3 weeks for total of 17 doses; give doses ≥4mg/kg over 90 min. Metastatic Breast Cancer: IV Infusion: Alone or With Paclitaxel: Initial: 4mg/kg over 90 min. Maint: 2mg/kg/week over 30 min until disease progression.

HOW SUPPLIED: Inj: 440mg

WARNINGS/PRECAUTIONS: Left ventricular cardiac dysfunction, arrhythmias, HTN, disabling cardiac failure, cardiomyopathy, and cardiac death may occur. Obtain baseline cardiac assessment (eg, history, physical, LVEF). Monitor LVEF prior to initiation, every 3 months during, and every 6 months following completion for at least 2 yrs. Fatal pulmonary toxicity may result. May exacerbate chemotherapy-induced neutropenia. HER2 testing is necessary to detect HER2 protein overexpression, which is needed to select patients for trastuzumab therapy. May increase risk of neutropenia. May cause severe infusion reactions; interrupt infusion and d/c permanently.

ADVERSE REACTIONS: Pain, asthenia, fever, nausea, chills, headache, increased cough, diarrhea, vomiting, abdominal pain, back pain, dyspnea, infection, rash, tachycardia, anemia, peripheral edema.

INTERACTIONS: Paclitaxel may increase serum levels. Concomitant anthracyclines and cyclophosphamide may increase incidence/severity of cardiac dysfunction.

PREGNANCY: Category D, caution in nursing.

MECHANISM OF ACTION: Monoclonal antibody/HER-2 blocker; inhibits the proliferation of human tumor cells that overexpress HER2.

PHARMACOKINETICS: Absorption: (500mg) C_{max}=337mcg/mL. **Distribution:** V_d=44mL/kg. **Elimination:** $T_{1/2}$=2 days (10mg), $T_{1/2}$=12 days (500mg). Mean half life increased and decreased with increasing dose level. Refer to PI for detailed information.

HEXALEN   RX
altretamine (MGI Pharma)

> Monitor peripheral blood counts at least monthly, before each course of therapy, and as clinically indicated. Possible neurotoxicity; perform neurologic exam regularly. Administer only under supervision of a physician experienced in the use of antineoplastic agents.

THERAPEUTIC CLASS: S-triazine derivative

INDICATIONS: Monotherapy for palliative treatment of persistent or recurrent ovarian cancer following 1st-line therapy with cisplatin and/or alkylating agent-based combination.

DOSAGE: *Adults:* 260 mg/m²/day in 4 divided doses for 14 or 21 consecutive days in 28 day cycle. Take after meals and qhs. Temporarily d/c for ≥14 days and restart at 200 mg/m²/day if any of the following occur: GI intolerance unresponsive to symptomatic measures; WBC <2000/mm³ or granulocytes <1000/mm³; platelets <75,000/mm³; progressive neurotoxicity. Permanently d/c if neurological symptoms do not stabilize.

HOW SUPPLIED: Cap: 50mg

CONTRAINDICATIONS: Pre-existing severe bone marrow depression or severe neurologic toxicity.

WARNINGS/PRECAUTIONS: Can cause mild to moderate myelosuppression and neurotoxicity. Perform blood counts and neurologic exam before each course of therapy and adjust dose as indicated.

ADVERSE REACTIONS: Nausea, vomiting, peripheral neuropathy, CNS symptoms (mood disorders, consciousness disorders, ataxia, dizziness, vertigo), leukopenia, thrombocytopenia, anemia, increased alkaline phosphatase.

INTERACTIONS: Severe orthostatic hypotension may occur with MAOIs. Avoid pyridoxine; possible adverse response duration effects. Cimetidine may increase levels.

PREGNANCY: Category D, not for use in nursing.

MECHANISM OF ACTION: S-triazine derivative; suspected to form covalent adducts with tissue macromolecules including DNA.

PHARMACOKINETICS: Absorption: Well-absorbed. C_{max}=0.2-20.8mg/L, T_{max}=0.5-3 hrs. **Metabolism:** Liver (extensive) via demethylation. Pentamethylmelamine and Tetramethylmelamine (active metabolites). **Elimination:** $T_{1/2}$=4.7-10.2 hrs. Urine.

HIPREX   RX
methenamine hippurate (Sanofi-Aventis)

THERAPEUTIC CLASS: Hippuric acid salt

INDICATIONS: Prophylaxis or suppression of recurrent urinary tract infections when long-term therapy is necessary. For use only after infection is eradicated by other appropriate antimicrobials.

DOSAGE: *Adults:* 1g bid.
Pediatrics: >12 yrs: 1g bid. 6 to 12 yrs: 0.5g-1g bid.

HOW SUPPLIED: Tab: 1g* *scored

CONTRAINDICATIONS: Renal insufficiency, severe hepatic insufficiency, severe dehydration, concomitant sulfonamides.

WARNINGS/PRECAUTIONS: Maintain acid urine. Doses of 8g/day may cause bladder irritation, painful and frequent micturition, albuminuria, gross hematuria. Monitor LFTs and repeated urine cultures. Contains tartrazine (FD&C Yellow No. 5), which may cause allergic-type reactions; caution with ASA hypersensitivity.

ADVERSE REACTIONS: Nausea, upset stomach, dysuria, rash.

INTERACTIONS: Avoid alkalinizing agents or foods. Sulfonamides may precipitate in the urine; avoid concomitant use.

PREGNANCY: Safety in pregnancy and nursing unknown.

MECHANISM OF ACTION: Hippuric acid salt; produces anti-bacterial effect through conversion of its methenamine component to formaldehyde in acid urine.

PHARMACOKINETICS: Absorption: Rapid. **Elimination:** Urine.

HIVID   RX
zalcitabine (Roche Labs)

> Severe peripheral neuropathy, pancreatitis (rare), hepatic failure (rare), lactic acidosis, and severe hepatomegaly with steatosis, reported. Extreme caution with pre-existing neuropathy.

THERAPEUTIC CLASS: Nucleoside analogue

INDICATIONS: Treatment of HIV infection in combination with other antiretrovirals.

DOSAGE: *Adults:* 0.75mg q8h. CrCl 10-40mL/min: 0.75mg q12h. CrCl <10mL/min: 0.75mg q24h.
Pediatrics: ≥13 yrs: 0.75mg q8h.

HOW SUPPLIED: Tab: 0.375mg, 0.75mg

WARNINGS/PRECAUTIONS: Decreased CD4 counts increase risk of adverse effects including peripheral neuropathy, pancreatitis, lactic acidosis, severe hepatomegaly with steatosis, hepatic toxicity, oral/esophageal ulcers, cardiomyopathy and CHF. Caution in elderly. Reduce dose in renal impairment. Increased risk of lymphoma with high doses. D/C if moderate peripheral neuropathy develops; may reintroduce at 50% of dose if improve to mild symptoms. Interrupt or reduce dose if serious toxicities occur (eg, peripheral neuropathy, severe oral ulcers, pancreatitis, elevated LFTs). Monitor CBC and clinical chemistry tests before therapy and at appropriate intervals thereafter. Monitor hematologic indices frequently with poor bone marrow reserve. Interrupt therapy if severe anemia or granulocytopenia occurs; reduce dose if less severe. Possible redistribution or accumulation of body fat.

ADVERSE REACTIONS: Peripheral neuropathy, oral lesions/stomatitis, headache, elevated amylase, fatigue, abdominal pain, nausea, vomiting, hepatic dysfunction, blood dyscrasias, rash, urticaria, redistribution/accumulation of body fat.

INTERACTIONS: Avoid drugs associated with peripheral neuropathy. Monitor renal function and neuropathy development with amphotericin, foscarnet, aminoglycosides. Cimetidine and probenecid decrease clearance. Metoclopramide, aluminum- and magnesium-containing antacids reduce absorption. Interrupt therapy with pancreatitis causing agents (eg, intravenous pentamidine).

PREGNANCY: Category C, not for use in nursing.

MECHANISM OF ACTION: Pyrimidine nucleoside analog; inhibits activity of HIV-reverse transcriptase both by competing for utilization of deoxycytidine 5'-triphosphate (dCTP) and by its incorporation into viral DNA.

PHARMACOKINETICS: Absorption: Pediatrics: Absolute bioavailability (54%). **Adults:** Absolute bioavailability (>80%); T_{max}=0.8 hrs, C_{max}=25.2ng/mL, AUC=72ng•h/mL (fasting); T_{max}=1.6 hrs, C_{max}=15.5ng/mL, AUC=62ng•h/mL (fed). **Distribution:** V_d=0.534L/kg. **Metabolism:** Phosphorylation (zalcitabine triphospate). Dideoxyuridine (metabolite). **Elimination:** Renal excretion: IV (80%), oral (60%). $T_{1/2}$=2 hrs.

HUMALOG   RX
insulin lispro (Lilly)

THERAPEUTIC CLASS: Insulin

INDICATIONS: To control hyperglycemia in diabetes.

DOSAGE: *Adults:* Individualize dose. Inject SQ within 15 min before or immediately after a meal. May use with external insulin pump; do not dilute or mix with other insulin when used with pump.
Pediatrics: ≥3 yrs: Individualize dose. Inject SQ within 15 min before or immediately after a meal. May use with external insulin pump; do not dilute or mix with other insulin when used with pump.

HOW SUPPLIED: Cartridge: 100 U/mL; Inj: 100 U/mL; Pen: 100 U/mL

CONTRAINDICATIONS: Hypoglycemia.

WARNINGS/PRECAUTIONS: Any change of insulin should be made cautiously. Changes in strength, manufacturer, type or method of manufacture may result in the need for a change in dosage. Hypoglycemia may occur with taking too much insulin, missing or delaying meals, exercising or working more than usual. An infection or illness (especially with diarrhea or vomiting) may change insulin requirements. With type 1 DM a longer-acting insulin is usually required to maintain glucose control; not required with type 2 DM if regimen includes sulfonylureas. May be diluted with sterile diluent. Caution with potassium-lowering drugs or drugs sensitive to serum potassium levels.

ADVERSE REACTIONS: Hypoglycemia, hypokalemia, allergic reaction, injection site reaction, lipodystrophy, pruritus, rash.

INTERACTIONS: Increased insulin requirements with corticosteroids, isoniazid, niacin, estrogens, oral contraceptives, phenothiazines, thyroid replacement therapy. Decreased insulin requirements with oral hypoglycemics, salicylates, sulfa antibiotics, MAOIs, ACEIs, ARBs, β-blockers, octreotide and alcohol. β-blockers may mask symptoms of hypoglycemia.

PREGNANCY: Category B, caution in nursing.

MECHANISM OF ACTION: Insulin lispro (rDNA origin); regulates glucose metabolism.

PHARMACOKINETICS: Absorption: Absolute bioavailability (55-77%); T_{max}=30-90 min. **Distribution:** V_d=0.26-0.36L/kg. **Elimination:** $T_{1/2}$=1 hr.

HUMALOG MIX 75/25   RX
insulin lispro protamine - insulin lispro (Lilly)

THERAPEUTIC CLASS: Insulin

INDICATIONS: To control hyperglycemia in diabetes.

DOSAGE: *Adults:* Individualize dose. Inject SQ within 15 min before a meal. May need to reduce/adjust dose with renal/hepatic impairment.

HOW SUPPLIED: (Insulin Lispro Protamine, Human-Insulin Lispro, Human) Inj: 75 U-25 U/mL; Pen: 75 U-25 U/mL

CONTRAINDICATIONS: Hypoglycemia.

WARNINGS/PRECAUTIONS: Any change of insulin should be made cautiously. Changes in strength, manufacturer, type or method of manufacture may result in the need for a change in dosage. Hypoglycemia may occur with taking too much insulin, missing or delaying meals, exercising or working more than usual. An infection or illness (especially with diarrhea or vomiting) may change insulin requirements.

ADVERSE REACTIONS: Hypoglycemia, hypokalemia, allergic reaction, injection site reaction, lipodystrophy, pruritus, rash.

INTERACTIONS: Increased insulin requirements with corticosteroids, isoniazid, niacin, estrogens, oral contraceptives, phenothiazines, thyroid replacement therapy. Decreased insulin requirements with oral hypoglycemics, salicylates, sulfa antibiotics, MAOIs, ACEIs, ARBs, β-blockers, octreotide and alcohol. β-blockers may mask symptoms of hypoglycemia.

PREGNANCY: Category B, caution in nursing.

MECHANISM OF ACTION: Insulin; 75% lispro protamine (intermediate-acting), 25% insulin lispro (rapid-acting); helps in the maintenance of blood glucose at near normal levels.

PHARMACOKINETICS: Absorption: T_{max}=60 min.

HUMATROPE   RX
somatropin (Lilly)

THERAPEUTIC CLASS: Human growth hormone

INDICATIONS: Long-term treatment of pediatrics with growth failure due to growth hormone deficiency (GHD). For short stature associated with Turner syndrome if epiphyses are not closed. Long-term treatment of idiopathic short stature in pediatrics. Treatment of short stature or growth failure in children with SHOX (short stature homeobox-containing gene) deficiency whose epiphyses are not closed. Replacement therapy in adults.

DOSAGE: *Adults:* GHD: Up to 0.006mg/kg SQ qd. Titrate: Increase by individual requirements. Max: 0.0125mg/kg/day. Alternative Dose: Initial: 0.2mg/day (range, 0.15-0.30mg/day). Titrate: Increase gradually every 1-2 months to individual requirement. Max: 0.1-0.2mg/day
Pediatrics: GHD: 0.18mg/kg weekly SQ/IM. Max: 0.3mg/kg weekly in equally divided doses given either on 3 alternate days, 6 times per week, or daily. Turner Syndrome: Up to 0.375mg/kg SQ weekly equally divided, given either daily or on 3 alternate days. Idiopathic Short Stature: Up to 0.37mg/kg SQ weekly given 6 to 7 times per week equally divided. SHOX Deficiency: 0.35mg/kg SQ weekly given daily in equally divided doses.

HOW SUPPLIED: Inj: 5mg, 6mg, 12mg, 24mg

CONTRAINDICATIONS: Pediatrics with closed epiphyses. Proliferative or preproliferative diabetic retinopathy. Active malignancy. Hypersensitivity to Metacresol or glycerin. Acute critical illness due to complications after open heart or abdominal surgery, multiple accidental trauma or acute respiratory failure. Prader-Willi syndrome who are severely obese or have severe respiratory impairment.

WARNINGS/PRECAUTIONS: If sensitivity to diluent occurs reconstitute with bacteriostatic (contains benzyl alcohol; avoid in newborns) or sterile water for injection. Monitor GHD secondary to intracranial lesion for progression/recurrence. Monitor gait, glucose intolerance, for malignant transformation of skin lesions, scoliosis progression, intracranial HTN (perform fundoscopic exam at start and periodically). Caution with DM, endocrine disorders, hypopituitarism. With Turner syndrome monitor for otic or cardiovascular disorders, autoimmune thyroid disease. Caution with endocrine disorders, monitor for otic and cardiovascular disorder.

ADVERSE REACTIONS: Injection site pain, headache, edema, myalgia, pain, rhinitis. (Adults) Arthralgia, paresthesia, HTN, back pain. (Pediatrics) Flu-syndrome, AST/ALT increases, pharyngitis, gastritis, respiratory disorder.

INTERACTIONS: Antagonized by glucocorticoids. May alter clearance of CYP450 substrates (eg, corticosteroids, sex steroids, anticonvulsants, antipyrine, cyclosporine). May require larger dose with oral estrogen replacement. Adjust dose of insulin and/or oral agent in diabetic patients.

PREGNANCY: Category C, caution in nursing.

MECHANISM OF ACTION: Human growth hormone; stimulates linear growth synthesis, metabolizes lipids, reduces body fat stores by increasing cellular protein, and increases plasma fatty acids.

PHARMACOKINETICS: Absorption: (SQ) Absolute bioavailabilty (75%). (IM) Absolute bioavailabilty (63%). **Distribution:** (IV) V_d=0.07L/kg. **Metabolism:** Liver and kidney (protein catabolism). **Elimination:** Urine: (IV) $T_{1/2}$=0.36 hrs. (SQ) $T_{1/2}$=3.8 hrs. (IM) $T_{1/2}$=4.9 hrs.

HUMIRA   RX
adalimumab (Abbott)

> Reports of TB, invasive fungal infections, and other opportunistic infections. Evaluate for latent TB and treat if necessary prior to initiation of therapy.

THERAPEUTIC CLASS: Monoclonal antibody/TNF-blocker

INDICATIONS: For reducing signs and symptoms, inducing major clinical response, inhibiting structural damage progression, and improving physical function in moderately to severely active rheumatoid arthritis (RA). For reducing signs and symptoms of moderately to severely active polyarticular juvenile idiopathic arthritis in patients ≥4 yrs. For reducing signs and symptoms of active arthritis, inhibiting the progression of structural damage, and improving physical function in patients with psoriatic arthritis (PA). For reducing signs and symptoms of active ankylosing spondylitis (AS). For reducing signs and symptoms and inducing and maintaining clinical remission of moderately to severely active Crohn's disease in patients who have had an inadequate response to conventional therapy. For reducing signs and symptoms and inducing clinical remission in patients who have lost response to or are intolerant to infliximab. For treating moderate to severe chronic plaque psoriasis in patients who are candidates for systemic therapy or phototherapy.

DOSAGE: *Adults:* (RA/PA/AS): 40mg SQ every other week. Some patients with RA not taking concomitant MTX may derive additional benefit from increasing the dosing frequency to 40mg every week. Crohn's Disease: Initial: 160mg (may be given as 4 injections on Day 1, or 2 injections/day for 2 consecutive days); then 80mg after 2 weeks (Day 15). Maint: 40mg every other week beginning at Week 4 (Day 29). Plaque Psoriasis: Initial: 80mg. Maint: 40mg every other week starting 1 week after initial dose.
Pediatrics: (4-17 yrs) 15kg-<30kg: 20mg every other week; ≥30kg: 40mg every other week.

HOW SUPPLIED: Inj: 20mg/0.4mL, 40mg/0.8mL

WARNINGS/PRECAUTIONS: Serious infections including sepsis and TB reported. Monitor for signs of infection during and after therapy; d/c if serious infection develops. Avoid with active infection. Monitor HBV carriers as reactivation may occur; if reactivation occurs, stop adalimumab and start antiviral therapy. Caution with history of recurrent infections or underlying conditions predisposing to infections or in areas where TB and histoplasmosis are endemic. Caution with pre-existing or recent-onset CNS demyelinating disorders. Lymphomas, allergic reactions observed. May affect host defenses against infections and malignancies. May result in autoantibody formation; d/c if lupus-like syndrome develops. Rare possibility of anaphylaxis and pancytopenia including aplastic anemia. May cause CHF or worsen pre-existing disease.

ADVERSE REACTIONS: URI, injection site pain/reactions, headache, rash, sinusitis, nausea, UTI, flu syndrome, abdominal pain, hyperlipidemia, hypercholesterolemia, back pain, hematuria, HTN, immunogenicity.

INTERACTIONS: Do not give concurrently with live vaccines. Reduced clearance with MTX. Do not use concurrently with anakinra due to increased risk of serious infections.

PREGNANCY: Category B, not for use in nursing.

MECHANISM OF ACTION: Monoclonal antibody/TNF-blocker; binds specifically to TNF-α and blocks its interaction with p55 and p75 cell surface TNF receptors. Lyses surface TNF-expressing cells in the presence of complement. Modulates biological responses that are induced or regulated by TNF. In plaque psoriasis, reduces the epidermal thickness and infiltration of inflammatory cells.

PHARMACOKINETICS: Absorption: Absolute bioavailability (64%); C_{max}=4.7mcg/mL; T_{max}=131 hrs. **Distribution:** V_d=4.7-6.0L. **Elimination:** $T_{1/2}$=2 weeks.

HUMULIN
OTC

insulin human, rdna origin - insulin, human isophane - insulin, human regular (Lilly)

OTHER BRAND NAMES: Humulin N (Lilly) - Humulin R (Lilly)

THERAPEUTIC CLASS: Insulin

INDICATIONS: To control hyperglycemia in diabetes.

DOSAGE: *Adults:* Individualize dose.
Pediatrics: Individualize dose.

HOW SUPPLIED: Inj: 100 U/mL (Humulin N, Humulin R), 500 U/mL (Humulin R U-500); Pen: 100 U/mL (Humulin N).

CONTRAINDICATIONS: Hypoglycemia.

WARNINGS/PRECAUTIONS: Human insulin differs from animal source insulin. Any change of insulin should be made cautiously. Changes in strength, manufacturer, type or method of manufacture may result in the need for a change in dosage. Hypoglycemia may occur with taking too much insulin, missing or delaying meals, exercising or working more than usual. An infection or illness (especially with diarrhea or vomiting) may change insulin requirements. Administration of insulin SQ can result in lipoatrophy.

ADVERSE REACTIONS: Hypoglycemia, sweating, dizziness, palpitation, tremor, hunger, restlessness, lightheadedness, inability to concentrate, headache, injection site reaction, allergic reaction.

INTERACTIONS: Increased insulin requirements with oral contraceptives, corticosteroids, or thyroid replacement therapy. Reduced insulin requirements with oral hypoglycemics, salicylates, sulfa antibiotics, and certain antidepressants. Alcoholic beverages may change insulin requirements. β-blockers may mask symptoms of hypoglycemia.

PREGNANCY: Pregnancy category is not known.

MECHANISM OF ACTION: Insulin; regular insulin human injection of rDNA origin that helps in maintenance of blood glucose at near normal level.

HUMULIN 70/30
OTC

insulin human, rdna origin - insulin, human (isophane/regular) (Lilly)

OTHER BRAND NAMES: Humulin 50/50 (Lilly)

THERAPEUTIC CLASS: Insulin

INDICATIONS: To control hyperglycemia in diabetes.

DOSAGE: *Adults:* Individualize dose. Administer SQ.
Pediatrics: Individualize dose. Administer SQ.

HOW SUPPLIED: (Isophane-Regular) Inj: (Humulin 70/30) 70 U-30 U/mL, (Humulin 50/50) 50 U-50 U/mL

WARNINGS/PRECAUTIONS: Human insulin differs from animal source insulin. Make any change of insulin cautiously. Changes in strength, manufacturer, type, or method of manufacture may result in the need for a change in dosage. Hypoglycemia may occur with too much insulin, missing or delaying meals, exercising, or working more than usual. Infection or illness (especially with diarrhea or vomiting) may change insulin requirements. Administration of insulin SQ can result in lipoatrophy.

ADVERSE REACTIONS: Hypoglycemia, sweating, dizziness, palpitation, tremor, hunger, restlessness, lightheadedness, inability to concentrate, headache, injection site reaction, allergic reaction.

INTERACTIONS: Increased insulin requirements with oral contraceptives, corticosteroids, or thyroid replacement therapy. Reduced insulin requirements with oral hypoglycemics, salicylates, sulfa antibiotics, and certain antidepressants. Alcoholic beverages may change insulin requirements. β-blockers may mask symptoms of hypoglycemia.

PREGNANCY: Pregnancy category is not known.

MECHANISM OF ACTION: Insulin; lowers blood glucose levels by stimulating peripheral glucose uptake, especially by skeletal muscle and fat, and by inhibiting hepatic glucose production. Inhibits lipolysis and proteolysis, and enhances protein synthesis.

HYALGAN RX
sodium hyaluronate (Sanofi-Synthelabo)

THERAPEUTIC CLASS: Hyaluronan

INDICATIONS: Treatment of pain in osteoarthritis of the knee in patients who have failed to respond adequately to conservative nonpharmacologic therapy, and to simple analgesics (eg, APAP).

DOSAGE: *Adults:* Administer 2mL by intra-articular injection once a week for a total of 5 injections. Some patients may experience benefit with 3 injections given at weekly intervals. Use strict aseptic technique.

HOW SUPPLIED: Inj: 2mL

CONTRAINDICATIONS: Intra-articular injections are contraindicated in cases of infections or skin disease in the area of the injection site.

WARNINGS/PRECAUTIONS: Avoid disinfectants containing quaternary ammonium salts for skin preparation; hyaluronic acid can precipitate in their presence. Anaphylactoid and allergic reactions reported. Transient increases in inflammation in the injected knee in some patients with inflammatory arthritis such as rheumatoid arthritis or gouty arthritis have been reported. Safety and effectiveness in joints other than the knee or concomitantly with other intra-articular injectables have not been established. Caution in patients who are allergic to avian proteins, feathers, and egg products. Avoid any strenuous activities or prolonged (eg, more than 1 hour) weight-bearing activities within 48 hours following the intra-articular injection. Remove any joint effusion before injecting. Safety and effectiveness have not been demonstrated in children.

ADVERSE REACTIONS: GI complaints, injection site pain, headache, local skin reactions (rash, ecchymosis), local joint pain, pruritus (local), knee swelling/effusion.

PREGNANCY: Safety in pregnancy and nursing not known.

HYCAMTIN CAPSULES RX
topotecan (GlaxoSmithKline)

> Administer only to patients with baseline neutrophil counts of ≥1,500cells/mm³ and platelet count ≥100,000cells/mm³. Monitor blood cell counts.

THERAPEUTIC CLASS: Topoisomerase I inhibitor

INDICATIONS: Treatment of relapsed small cell lung cancer in patients with a prior complete or partial response and who are at least 45 days from the end of first-line chemotherapy.

DOSAGE: *Adults:* 2.3mg/m²/day PO qd for 5 consecutive days repeated every 21 days. Round calculated dose to nearest 0.25mg and give minimum number of 1mg and 0.25mg caps. Do not treat with subsequent courses until neutrophils recover to >1000cells/m³, platelets recover to >100,000cells/mm³, and

Hgb levels recover to ≥9g/dL. If severe neutropenia (neutrophils <500cells/mm³ associated with fever or infection or lasting for ≥7 days), neutropenia (neutrophils 500-1,000cells/mm³ lasting beyond Day 21 of treatment course), or if platelet count falls below 25,000cells/mm³, reduce dose by 0.4mg/m²/day for subsequent courses. Moderate Renal Impairment (CrCl 30-49mL/min): 1.8mg/m²/day. Severe Renal Impairment (CrCl <30mL/min): Insufficient data. Swallow caps whole; do not chew, crush, or divide. If patient vomits after taking dose, do not give replacement dose.

HOW SUPPLIED: Cap: 0.25mg, 1mg

CONTRAINDICATIONS: Pregnancy, breastfeeding, severe bone marrow depression.

WARNINGS/PRECAUTIONS: Neutropenia, pancytopenia, thrombocytopenia, and/or anemia may occur. Bone marrow suppression is dose-limiting toxicity; administer only to patients with adequate bone marrow reserves and monitor peripheral blood counts. Neutropenia may lead to neutropenic colitis. Diarrhea, including severe diarrhea requiring hospitalization, reported.

ADVERSE REACTIONS: Anemia, leukopenia, neutropenia, thrombocytopenia, nausea, diarrhea, vomiting, alopecia, fatigue, anorexia, asthenia, pyrexia.

INTERACTIONS: P-glycoprotein inhibitors (eg, cyclosporine A, elacridar, ketoconazole, ritonavir, saquinavir) may cause significant increases in topotecan exposure; avoid concomitant use.

PREGNANCY: Category D, contraindicated in nursing.

MECHANISM OF ACTION: Topoisomerase 1 inhibitor; binds to topoisomerase I-DNA complex and prevents religation of DNA single strand breaks.

PHARMACOKINETICS: Absorption: (PO) Rapid. T_{max}=1-2 hrs. Absolute bioavailability (40%). **Distribution:** Plasma protein binding (35%). **Metabolism:** Reversible pH dependent hydrolysis. N-desmethyl topotecan (metabolite). **Elimination:** Urine=20% (parent), 2% (metabolite) and feces=33% (parent), 1.5% (metabolite). $T_{1/2}$=3-6 hrs.

HYCAMTIN INJECTION   RX
topotecan HCL (GlaxoSmithKline)

> Do not give if baseline neutrophils <1500cells/mm³. Monitor peripheral blood cell counts frequently due to risk of bone marrow suppression, primarily neutropenia. Administer only under supervision of a physician experienced in the use of antineoplastic agents.

THERAPEUTIC CLASS: Topoisomerase I inhibitor

INDICATIONS: Treatment of refractory metastatic ovarian carcinoma after failure of initial or subsequent chemotherapy and small cell lung cancer sensitive disease after 1st-line chemotherapy failure. Treatment of Stage IV-B, recurrent, or persistent carcinoma of the cervix which is not amenable to curative treatment with surgery and/or radiation therapy, in combination with cisplatin.

DOSAGE: *Adults:* Ovarian and Small Cell Lung Cancer: 1.5mg/m² IV qd over 30 min for 5 days, starting on Day 1 of 21-day course. Minimum of 4 courses recommended in absence of tumor progression. Severe Neutropenia During Therapy: Reduce dose by 0.25mg/m², or give G-CSF following subsequent course (before dose reduction) starting from Day 6 of the course (24 hrs after completion of topotecan administration). Renal Impairment: CrCl 39-20mL/min: 0.75mg/m². CrCl <20mL/min: Insufficient data. Cervical Cancer: 0.75mg/m² IV qd over 30 min on Days 1, 2 , and 3; followed by cisplatin 50mg/m² IV on Day 1 of every 21-day course. Severe Febrile Neutropenia (<1000cells/mm³ & temperature of 38°C): Reduce dose by 20% to 0.60mg/m² for subsequent courses (doses should be similarly reduced if platelet count falls below 10,000cells/mm³) or give G-CSF following subsequent course (before dose reduction) starting from Day 4 of course (24 hrs after completion of topotecan administration); if febrile neutropenia occurs despite use of G-CSF, reduce dose by another 20% to 0.45mg/m² for subsequent courses. Renal Impairment: CrCl 39-20mL/min: 0.75mg/m². CrCl <20mL/min: Insufficient data.

HOW SUPPLIED: Inj: 4mg

CONTRAINDICATIONS: Pregnancy, nursing, severe bone marrow depression

WARNINGS/PRECAUTIONS: Bone marrow suppression (thrombocytopenia, anemia and primarily neutropenia) is dose-limiting toxicity. Baseline neutrophils >1500 cells/mm³ and platelets >100,000cells/mm³ required. Neutrophils >1000 cells/mm³, platelets >100,000cells/mm³, and HgB ≥9g/dL required before subsequent courses. May cause fetal harm during pregnancy. Neutropenia can lead to neutropenic colitis.

ADVERSE REACTIONS: Neutropenia, leukopenia, thrombocytopenia, anemia, sepsis/fever/infection, nausea, vomiting, diarrhea, constipation, abdominal pain, anorexia, fatigue, pain, asthenia, alopecia.

INTERACTIONS: Concomitant G-CSF can prolong duration of neutropenia; should not initiate until day 6 of therapy course, 24 hrs after treatment completion with topotecan. Increased severity of myelosuppression with other cytotoxic agents, cisplatin or carboplatin.

PREGNANCY: Category D, contraindicated in nursing.

MECHANISM OF ACTION: Topoisomerase 1 inhibitor; binds to topoisomerase I-DNA complex and prevents religation of DNA single strand breaks.

PHARMACOKINETICS: Distribution: Plasma protein binding (35%). **Metabolism:** Reversible pH dependent hydrolysis. N-desmethyl topotecan (metabolite). **Elimination:** Feces, urine. $T_{1/2}$=2-3 hrs.

HYCODAN `CIII`
hydrocodone bitartrate - homatropine methylbromide (Endo)

OTHER BRAND NAMES: Hydromet (Alpharma)

THERAPEUTIC CLASS: Opioid antitussive

INDICATIONS: Symptomatic relief of cough.

DOSAGE: *Adults:* 1 tab or 5mL q4-6h prn. Max: 6 tabs/24hrs or 30mL/24hrs. *Pediatrics:* >12 yrs: 1 tab or 5mL q4-6h prn. Max: 6 tabs/24hrs or 30mL/24hrs. 6-12 yrs: 1/2 tab or 2.5mL q4-6h prn. Max: 3 tabs/24hrs or 15mL/24 hrs.

HOW SUPPLIED: (Hydrocodone-Homatropine) Syrup: 5mg-1.5mg/5mL; Tab: 5mg-1.5mg* *scored

WARNINGS/PRECAUTIONS: May be habit-forming. May cause respiratory depression. May obscure diagnosis or clinical course of acute abdominal conditions. Caution in elderly, debilitated, severe hepatic or renal impairment, hypothyroidism, Addison's disease, prostatic hypertrophy, urethral stricture, asthma, head injury, increased ICP, and narrow-angle glaucoma.

ADVERSE REACTIONS: Sedation, drowsiness, lethargy, mental/physical impairment, dizziness, psychic dependence, constipation, ureteral spasm, respiratory depression, rash.

INTERACTIONS: Narcotics, antihistamines, antipsychotics, antianxiety agents, MAOI's, TCAs, alcohol or other CNS depressants may potentiate CNS depression. Increased effect of antidepressant or hydrocodone with MAOIs or TCAs.

PREGNANCY: Category C, not for use in nursing.

MECHANISM OF ACTION: Hydrocodone: Semisynthetic opioid antitussive and analgesic; not established, believed to act directly on the cough center.

PHARMACOKINETICS: Absorption: Hydrocodone; C_{max}=23.6ng/mL, T_{max}=1.3 hrs. **Metabolism:** Hydrocodone: O-demethylation, N-demethylation and 6-keto reduction. **Elimination:** $T_{1/2}$=3.8 hrs.

HYCOTUSS `CIII`
hydrocodone bitartrate - guaifenesin (Endo)

OTHER BRAND NAMES: Vi-Q-Tuss (Vintage)

THERAPEUTIC CLASS: Cough suppressant/expectorant

INDICATIONS: Symptomatic relief of irritating nonproductive cough associated with upper and lower respiratory tract congestion.

DOSAGE: *Adults:* Initial: 5mL after meals and hs, not less than 4 hrs apart. Titrate: May increase up to 15mL after meals and hs. Max: 30mL/24 hrs. *Pediatrics:* >12 yrs: Initial: 5mL after meals and hs, not less than 4 hrs apart. Max Single Dose: 10mL. 6-12 yrs: Initial: 2.5mL after meals and hs, not less than 4 hrs apart. Max Single Dose: 5mL.

HOW SUPPLIED: Syrup: (Hydrocodone-Guaifenesin) 5mg-100mg/5mL

CONTRAINDICATIONS: Cross sensitivity to other opioids. Intracranial lesion associated with increased ICP and whenever ventilatory function is depressed.

WARNINGS/PRECAUTIONS: May be habit forming. Risk of psychic dependence, physical dependence, tolerance, and potential for abuse. Dose-related respiratory depression. Caution with head injury, other intracranial lesions or a pre-existing increase in ICP. May obscure the clinical course head injuries, acute abdominal conditions.

ADVERSE REACTIONS: Respiratory depression, HTN, postural hypotension, palpitations, urinary retention, sedation, drowsiness, mental clouding, lethargy.

INTERACTIONS: Additive CNS depression with other narcotics, analgesics, general anesthetics, phenothiazines, other tranquilizers, sedative hypnotics or other CNS depressants (including alcohol).

PREGNANCY: Category C, not for use in nursing.

MECHANISM OF ACTION: Hydrocodone: Not established; believed to act directly by depressing the cough center. Guaifenesin: Not established; believed to act by stimulating receptors in gastric mucosa that initiate a reflex secretion of respiratory tract fluid, thereby increasing the volume and decreasing the viscosity of bronchial secretions.

PHARMACOKINETICS: Absorption: Hydrocodone: C_{max}=23.6ng/mL, T_{max}=1.3 hrs. Guaifenesin: GI tract (rapid). **Metabolism:** Hydrocodone: O-demethylation, N-demethylation and 6-keto reduction. **Elimination:** Hydrocodone: $T_{1/2}$=3.8 hrs. Guaifenesin: $T_{1/2}$=1 hr.

HYDRALAZINE RX
hydralazine HCL (Various)

THERAPEUTIC CLASS: Vasodilator

INDICATIONS: Management of hypertension.

DOSAGE: *Adults:* Initial: 10mg qid for 2-4 days. Titrate: Increase to 25mg qid for the rest of the week, then increase to 50mg qid. Maint: Use lowest effective dose. Resistant Patients: 300mg/day or titrate to lower dose combined with thiazide diuretic and/or reserpine, or β-blocker.
Pediatrics: Initial: 0.75mg/kg/day given qid. Titrate: Increase gradually over 3-4 weeks to a max of 7.5mg/kg/day or 200mg/day.

HOW SUPPLIED: Inj: 20mg/mL; Tab: 10mg, 25mg, 50mg, 100mg

CONTRAINDICATIONS: CAD and mitral valvular rheumatic heart disease.

WARNINGS/PRECAUTIONS: D/C if SLE symptoms occur. May cause angina and ECG changes of MI. Caution with suspected CAD, CVA, advanced renal impairment. May increase pulmonary artery pressure in mitral valvular disease. Postural hypotension reported. Add pyridoxine if peripheral neuritis develops. Monitor CBC and ANA titer before and periodically during therapy.

ADVERSE REACTIONS: Headache, anorexia, nausea, vomiting, diarrhea, tachycardia, angina.

INTERACTIONS: Caution with MAOIs. Profound hypotension with potent parenteral antihypertensives (eg, diazoxide). May reduce pressor response to epinephrine.

PREGNANCY: Category C, safety in nursing not known.

MECHANISM OF ACTION: Vasodilator; not established. Apparently lowers BP by direct relaxation of vascular smooth muscle; interferes with calcium movement within vascular smooth muscle responsible for initiating or maintaining contraction.

PHARMACOKINETICS: Absorption: Rapid; T_{max}=1-2 hrs. **Distribution:** Plasma protein binding (87%). **Metabolism:** Acetylation. **Elimination:** Urine; $T_{1/2}$=3-7 hrs.

HYDREA   RX
hydroxyurea (Bristol-Myers Squibb)

THERAPEUTIC CLASS: Ribonucleotide reductase inhibitor

INDICATIONS: Significant tumor response demonstrated in melanoma, resistant chronic myelocytic leukemia (CML), and recurrent, metastatic, or inoperable carcinoma of the ovary. Adjunct therapy with irradiation therapy for local control of primary squamous cell carcinomas of the head and neck, excluding the lip.

DOSAGE: *Adults:* Solid Tumors: Intermittent: 80mg/kg single dose every 3rd day. Continuous: 20-30mg/kg qd. Head and Neck Carcinoma: 80mg/kg single dose every 3rd day. Start at least 7 days before irradiation. Resistant CML: 20-30mg/kg qd. Elderly/Renal Impairment: May need dose reduction.

HOW SUPPLIED: Cap: 500mg

CONTRAINDICATIONS: Marked bone marrow depression (leukopenia, thrombocytopenia, or severe anemia).

WARNINGS/PRECAUTIONS: Patients with previous irradiation therapy may have exacerbation of postirradiation erythema. Bone marrow suppression, erythrocytic abnormalities may occur. Correct severe anemia before initiating therapy. Caution with marked renal dysfunction. May develop secondary leukemia with long-term therapy for myeloproliferative disorders. Monitor CBC, bone marrow, hepatic and kidney function before therapy and repeatedly thereafter. Interrupt therapy if WBC <2500/mm^3 or platelets <100,000/mm^3. Cutaneous vasculitic toxicities reported, including vasculitic ulcerations and gangrene; d/c if cutaneous vasculitic ulcerations develop.

ADVERSE REACTIONS: Bone marrow depression (leukopenia, anemia, thrombocytopenia), GI effects (stomatitis, anorexia, nausea, vomiting, diarrhea, constipation), and dermatological reactions (maculopapular rash, skin ulceration, dermatomyositis-like skin changes, peripheral and facial erythema), cutaneous vasculitic toxicities.

INTERACTIONS: Increased risk of bone marrow depression with other myelosuppressants or radiation therapy. Uricosurics may require dose adjustment. Pancreatitis and peripheral neuropathy reported in HIV patients with concomitant didanosine. Hepatotoxicity and hepatic failure reported in HIV patients with antiretrovirals (eg, stavudine, didanosine).

PREGNANCY: Category D, not for use in nursing.

MECHANISM OF ACTION: Ribonucleotide reductase inhibitor; not established; hypothesized that it inhibits DNA synthesis, without interfering with the synthesis of ribonucleic acid or protein.

PHARMACOKINETICS: Absorption: T_{max}=1-4 hrs. **Distribution:** V_d=total body water. **Metabolism:** Hepatic (saturable); degradation by urease (minor). **Elimination:** 1st-order renal.

HYDROCHLOROTHIAZIDE   RX
hydrochlorothiazide (Various)

THERAPEUTIC CLASS: Thiazide diuretic

INDICATIONS: Adjunct therapy in edema associated with CHF, hepatic cirrhosis, corticosteroid and estrogen therapy, renal dysfunction. Management of hypertension.

DOSAGE: *Adults:* Edema: 25-100mg qd or in divided doses. May give every other day or 3-5 days/week. HTN: Initial: 25mg qd. Titrate: May increase to

50mg/day.
Pediatrics: Diuresis/HTN: 1-2mg/kg/day given qd-bid. Max: Infants up to 2 yrs: 37.5mg/day. 2-12 yrs: 100mg/day. <6 months: Up to 1.5mg/kg bid may be required.

HOW SUPPLIED: Tab: 12.5mg, 25mg*, 50mg* *scored

CONTRAINDICATIONS: Anuria, sulfonamide hypersensitivity.

WARNINGS/PRECAUTIONS: Caution in severe renal disease, liver dysfunction, electrolyte/fluid imbalance. Monitor electrolytes. Hyperuricemia, hyperglycemia, hypokalemia, hyponatremia, hypomagnesemia, hypercalcemia may occur. Increases in cholesterol and triglyceride levels reported. May exacerbate SLE. Sensitivity reactions reported. D/C prior to parathyroid test. Enhanced effects in post-sympathectomy patients.

ADVERSE REACTIONS: Weakness, hypotension, pancreatitis, jaundice, diarrhea, vomiting, blood dyscrasias, rash, photosensitivity, electrolyte imbalance, impotence.

INTERACTIONS: May potentiate orthostatic hypotension with alcohol, barbiturates, narcotics. Adjust antidiabetic drugs. Possible decreased response to pressor amines. Corticosteroids, ACTH increase electrolyte depletion. May potentiate nondepolarizing skeletal muscle relaxants, antihypertensives. Lithium toxicity. NSAIDs decrease effects. Decreased PO absorption with cholestyramine, colestipol.

PREGNANCY: Category B, not for use in nursing.

MECHANISM OF ACTION: Thiazide diuretic; affects renal tubular mechanism of electrolyte reabsorption, increasing excretion of Na$^+$ and Cl$^-$.

PHARMACOKINETICS: Distribution: Crosses placenta and found in breast milk. **Elimination:** Kidneys (61%); T$_{1/2}$=5.6-14.8 hrs.

HYDROCORTISONE ACETATE   RX
hydrocortisone acetate (Truxton)

THERAPEUTIC CLASS: Corticosteroid

INDICATIONS: By intra-articular or soft tissue injection as adjunctive therapy for short-term administration in: synovitis of osteoarthritis, rheumatoid arthritis, bursitis, gouty arthritis, epicondylitis, nonspecific tenosynovitis, and post-traumatic osteoarthritis. By intralesional injection in: keloids, localized inflammatory lesions, discoid lupus erythematosus, necrobiosis lipoidica diabeticorum, alopecia areata, and cystic tumors of an aponeurosis or tendon.

DOSAGE: *Adults:* Usual: Large joints: 25-37.5mg. Max: 50mg. Small joints: 10-25mg. Bursae: 25-37.5mg. Tendon Sheaths: 5-12.5mg. Soft Tissue Infiltration: 25-50mg, occasionally 75mg. Ganglia: 12.5-25mg. For intra-articular, intralesional, and soft tissue injection only. Injection given once every 2-3 weeks; once a week for more severe conditions.
Pediatrics: Usual: Large joints: 25-37.5mg. Max: 50mg. Small joints: 10-25mg. Bursae: 25-37.5mg. Tendon Sheaths: 5-12.5mg. Soft Tissue Infiltration: 25-50mg, occasionally 75mg. Ganglia: 12.5-25mg. For intra-articular, intralesional, and soft tissue injection only. Injection given once every 2-3 weeks; once a week for more severe conditions.

HOW SUPPLIED: Inj: 25mg/mL.

CONTRAINDICATIONS: Systemic fungal infections.

WARNINGS/PRECAUTIONS: May need to increase dose before, during, and after stressful situations. May mask signs of infection or cause new infections. Avoid with cerebral malaria. May activate latent amebiasis. Prolonged use may produce glaucoma, optic nerve damage, secondary ocular infections. Increases BP, salt/water retention, potassium excretion. More severe/fatal course of infections reported with chickenpox, measles. Caution with Strongyloides, latent TB, recent MI, hypothyroidism, cirrhosis, ocular herpes simplex, HTN, diverticulitis, fresh intestinal anastomosis, ulcerative colitis, osteoporosis, myasthenia gravis, renal insufficiency, peptic ulcer disease. May increase or decrease sperm count. Growth and development of children on prolonged therapy should be monitored. Monitor for psychic disturbances. Avoid abrupt withdrawal. Avoid injection into an infected site or unstable joint. Frequent intra-articular injections may cause joint tissue damage.

ADVERSE REACTIONS: Fluid and electrolyte disturbances, HTN, osteoporosis, muscle weakness, cushingoid state, menstrual irregularities, nervousness, insomnia, impaired wound healing, DM, ulcerative esophagitis, excessive sweating, increases intracranial pressure, carbohydrate intolerance, glaucoma, cataracts, weight gain, nausea, malaise.

INTERACTIONS: Reduced efficacy and increased clearance with hepatic enzyme inducers (eg, phenobarbital, phenytoin, ephedrine, and rifampin). Caution with ASA in hypoprothrombinemia. Effects on oral anticoagulants are variable; monitor PT. Increased insulin and oral hypoglycemic requirements in DM. Avoid live vaccines with immunosuppressive doses. Possible decreased vaccine response with killed or inactivated vaccines with immunosuppressive doses. Monitor for hypokalemia with potassium-depleting diuretics.

PREGNANCY: Safety in pregnancy not known, not for use in nursing.

H

HYDROXYZINE HCL   RX
hydroxyzine HCL (Various)

THERAPEUTIC CLASS: Piperazine antihistamine

INDICATIONS: (PO) Relief of anxiety associated with psychoneurosis and as adjunct in organic disease states with anxiety. As a sedative when used as premedication and following general anesthesia. Management of allergic pruritus. (Inj) Management of anxiety, tension, and psychomotor agitation in conditions of emotional stress. As pre-/postoperative and pre-/postpartum adjunctive medication to permit reduction in narcotic dosage, allay anxiety, and control emesis. To control nausea and vomiting, excluding pregnancy.

DOSAGE: *Adults:* PO: Anxiety: 50-100mg qid. Pruritus: 25mg tid-qid. Sedation: 50-100mg. IM: Nausea/Vomiting: 25-100mg. Pre-/Postoperative and Pre-/Postpartum Adjunct: 25-100mg. Psychiatric/Emotional Emergencies: 50-100mg q4-6h prn.
Pediatrics: PO: Anxiety/Pruritus: <6 yrs: 50mg/day in divided doses. ≥6 yrs: 50-100mg in divided doses. Sedation: 0.6mg/kg. IM: Nausea/Vomiting: 0.5mg/lb. Pre-/Postoperative Adjunct: 0.5mg/lb.

HOW SUPPLIED: Inj: 25mg/mL, 50mg/mL; Syrup: 10mg/5mL; Tab: 10mg, 25mg, 50mg, 100mg

CONTRAINDICATIONS: Early pregnancy. Injection is intended only for IM administration and should not, under any circumstances, be injected subcutaneously, intra-arterially, or IV.

WARNINGS/PRECAUTIONS: Caution in elderly. May impair mental/physical abilities. Effectiveness as an antianxiety agent for long term use (>4 months) has not been established.

ADVERSE REACTIONS: Dry mouth, drowsiness, involuntary motor activity.

INTERACTIONS: Potentiates CNS depression with other CNS depressants (eg, narcotics, non-narcotic analgesics, barbiturates, alcohol). May increase alcohol effects.

PREGNANCY: Not for use in pregnancy or nursing.

MECHANISM OF ACTION: Believed to suppress activity in key regions of subcortical area of CNS; shown to have primary skeletal muscle relaxation, bronchodilator, antihistaminic, and analgesic effects.

PHARMACOKINETICS: Absorption: Rapid (GIT).

HYDROXYZINE PAMOATE   RX
hydroxyzine pamoate (Various)

OTHER BRAND NAMES: Vistaril (Pfizer)
THERAPEUTIC CLASS: Piperazine antihistamine

477

INDICATIONS: Relief of anxiety. Allergic pruritus. For sedation as premedication and following anesthesia.

DOSAGE: *Adults:* Anxiety: 50-100mg qid. Pruritus: 25mg tid-qid. Sedation: 50-100mg.
Pediatrics: Anxiety/Pruritus: >6 yrs: 50-100mg/day in divided doses. <6 yrs: 50mg/day in divided doses. Sedation: 0.6mg/kg.

HOW SUPPLIED: Cap: 25mg, 50mg, 100mg

CONTRAINDICATIONS: Early pregnancy.

WARNINGS/PRECAUTIONS: Caution in elderly. May impair mental/physical abilities. Effectiveness as an antianxiety agent for long term use (>4 months) has not been established.

ADVERSE REACTIONS: Dry mouth, drowsiness, involuntary motor activity.

INTERACTIONS: Potentiated by CNS depressants (eg, narcotics, non-narcotic analgesics, barbiturates); reduce dose.

PREGNANCY: Safety unknown in pregnancy and is contraindicated in early pregnancy, not for use in nursing.

MECHANISM OF ACTION: Believed to suppress activity in key regions of subcortical area of CNS; shown to have primary skeletal muscle relaxation, bronchodilator, antihistaminic, and analgesic effects.

PHARMACOKINETICS: Absorption: Rapid.

HYOSCYAMINE SULFATE RX
hyoscyamine sulfate (Various)

THERAPEUTIC CLASS: Anticholinergic

INDICATIONS: Adjunct treatment of peptic ulcer, irritable bowel syndrome, neurogenic bladder, and neurogenic bowel disturbances. To reduce symptoms of functional intestinal disorders (eg, mild dysenteries, diverticulitis). To control gastric secretion, visceral spasm, and hypermotility in spastic colitis, spastic bladder, cystitis, pylorospasm, and associated abdominal cramps. Symptomatic relief of biliary and renal colic with concomitant morphine or other narcotics. "Drying agent" for symptomatic relief of acute rhinitis. To reduce rigidity and tremors of Parkinson's disease and control associated sialorrhea and hyperhidrosis. For anticholinesterase poisoning.

DOSAGE: *Adults:* 0.125-0.25mg q4h or prn. Max: 1.5mg/24hrs. Take with or without water.
Pediatrics: ≥12 yrs: 0.125-0.25mg q4h or prn. Max: 1.5mg/24hrs. 2 to <12 yrs: 0.0625-0.125mg q4h or prn. Max: 0.75mg/24hrs. Take with or without water.

HOW SUPPLIED: Tab, Disintegrating: 0.125mg

CONTRAINDICATIONS: Glaucoma, obstructive uropathy, GI tract obstruction, paralytic ileus; intestinal atony of elderly/debilitated, unstable cardiovascular status in acute hemorrhage, toxic megacolon complicating ulcerative colitis, myasthenia gravis.

WARNINGS/PRECAUTIONS: Risk of heat prostration with high environmental temperature. Avoid activities requiring mental alertness. Psychosis has been reported in sensitive patients. Caution with diarrhea, autonomic neuropathy, hyperthyroidism, coronary heart disease, CHF, arrhythmias/tachycardia, HTN, renal disease, and hiatal hernia associated with reflux esophagitis. Contains phenylalanine.

ADVERSE REACTIONS: Anticholinergic effects, drowsiness, headache, nervousness.

INTERACTIONS: Additive effects with other antimuscarinics, amantadine, haloperidol, phenothiazines, MAOIs, TCAs, and some antihistamines. Antacids interfere with absorption; take ac and antacids pc.

PREGNANCY: Category C, caution in nursing.

MECHANISM OF ACTION: Belladonna alkaloid; inhibits action of acetylcholine on structures innervated by postganglionic cholinergic nerves and on smooth muscle that respond to acetylcholine but lack cholinergic innervation, inhibiting GI propulsive motility, decreasing gastric acid secretion, and controlling excess pharyngeal, tracheal, and bronchial secretions.

PHARMACOKINETICS: Absorption: Complete. **Distribution:** Crosses placenta and BBB. **Metabolism:** Partial hydrolysis; tropic acid, tropine (metabolites). **Elimination:** Urine (primarily unchanged); $T_{1/2}$=2-3.5 hrs.

HYTONE   RX
hydrocortisone (Dermik)

THERAPEUTIC CLASS: Corticosteroid

INDICATIONS: Corticosteroid-responsive dermatoses.

DOSAGE: *Adults:* Apply bid-qid depending on the severity. May use occlusive dressings for psoriasis or recalcitrant conditions. D/C dressings if infection develops.
Pediatrics: Apply bid-qid depending on the severity. May use occlusive dressings for psoriasis or recalcitrant conditions. D/C dressings if infection develops.

HOW SUPPLIED: Cre: 2.5% [30g, 60g]; Lot: 2.5% [60mL]; Oint: 2.5% [30g]

WARNINGS/PRECAUTIONS: May produce reversible HPA axis suppression, manifestations of Cushing's syndrome, hyperglycemia, and glucosuria. Caution when applied to large surface areas or under occlusive dressings. Use appropriate antifungal or antibacterial agent with dermatological infections; d/c if infection does not clear. Pediatrics may be more susceptible to systemic toxicity. Avoid eyes. D/C if irritation occurs.

ADVERSE REACTIONS: Burning, itching, irritation, dryness, folliculitis, hypertrichosis, acneiform eruptions, hypopigmentation, perioral dermatitis, allergic contact dermatitis, skin maceration, secondary infection, skin atrophy, striae, miliaria.

PREGNANCY: Category C, caution in nursing.

MECHANISM OF ACTION: Corticosteroid; possesses anti-inflammatory, antipruritic, and vasoconstrictive actions. Anti-inflammatory effects not established.

PHARMACOKINETICS: Absorption: Percutaneous; inflammation, other skin diseases, and use of occlusive dressings may increase absorption. **Distribution:** Bound to plasma protein to varying degrees. Systemically administered corticosteroids are found in breast milk. **Metabolism:** Liver. **Elimination:** Kidneys (major), bile.

HYTONE 1%   OTC
hydrocortisone (Dermik)

THERAPEUTIC CLASS: Corticosteroid

INDICATIONS: Relief of itching associated with minor skin irritation, inflammation and rashes due to eczema, insect bites, poison ivy/oak/sumac, soaps/detergents, cosmetics, jewelry, seborrheic dermatitis, psoriasis, and/or external feminine and external anal itching.

DOSAGE: *Adults:* Apply up to tid-qid. External Anal Itching: Clean and dry area before applying.
Pediatrics: ≥2 yrs: Apply up to tid-qid. External Anal Itching: ≥12 yrs: Clean and dry area before applying.

HOW SUPPLIED: Lot: 1% [30mL, 120mL]

WARNINGS/PRECAUTIONS: Avoid eyes. D/C use if condition worsens, if symptoms persist for more than 7 days, or if symptoms recur after clearing up. Not for diaper rash. For external feminine itching, avoid use with vaginal discharge. For external anal itching, do not insert into rectum with fingers or applicator.

PREGNANCY: Safety in pregnancy and nursing is not known.

MECHANISM OF ACTION: Corticosteroid; possesses anti-inflammatory, anti-pruritic, and vasoconstrictive properties. Anti-inflammatory actions not established.

PHARMACOKINETICS: Absorption: Percutaneous; inflammation, other disease states, and the use of occlusive dressings may increase percutaneous absorption. **Distribution:** Bound to plasma proteins to varying degrees. Systemically administered corticosteroids are found in breast milk. **Metabolism:** Liver. **Excretion:** Kidneys (major), bile.

HYTRIN   RX
terazosin HCL (Abbott)

THERAPEUTIC CLASS: Alpha₁-blocker (quinazoline)

INDICATIONS: Treatment of hypertension. Treatment of symptomatic benign prostatic hyperplasia.

DOSAGE: *Adults:* HTN: Initial: 1mg hs, then slowly increase dose. Usual: 1-5mg/day. Max: 20mg/day. If response is substantially diminished at 24 hrs, may increase dose or give in 2 divided doses. BPH: Initial: 1mg qhs. Titrate: Increase stepwise as needed. Usual: 10mg/day. May increase to 20mg/day after 4-6 weeks. Max: 20mg/day. If discontinue for several days, restart at initial dose.

HOW SUPPLIED: Cap: 1mg, 2mg, 5mg, 10mg

WARNINGS/PRECAUTIONS: Monitor for orthostatic hypotension and syncope initially and with dose increase. Rule out prostate cancer. Priapism (rare) reported. Possibility of hemodilution.

ADVERSE REACTIONS: Asthenia, postural hypotension, headache, dizziness, dyspnea, nasal congestion/rhinitis, somnolence, impotence, blurred vision, palpitations, nausea, peripheral edema, priapism, thrombocytopenia, atrial fibrillation.

INTERACTIONS: Increased levels with verapamil. Possibility of significant hypotension with other antihypertensives; may need dose reduction or retitration of either agent.

PREGNANCY: Category C, caution with nursing.

MECHANISM OF ACTION: α-1 adrenoceptor blocker; (BPH) blocks receptors in bladder neck and prostate, relaxing smooth muscle; (HTN) blocks receptors decreasing total peripheral vascular resistance, causing decreased BP.

PHARMACOKINETICS: Absorption: Complete; Tₘₐₓ =1 hr. **Elimination:** Feces (20%), urine (10%); T₁/₂=12 hrs.

HYZAAR   RX
losartan potassium - hydrochlorothiazide (Merck)

> Can cause death/injury to developing fetus during 2nd and 3rd trimesters. D/C if pregnancy detected.

THERAPEUTIC CLASS: Angiotensin II receptor antagonist/thiazide diuretic

INDICATIONS: Treatment of hypertension. Initial treatment of severe hypertension only when the value of acheiving prompt BP control exceeds the risk. To reduce risk of stroke in patients with hypertension and left ventricular hypertrophy (may not apply to African-American patients).

DOSAGE: *Adults:* HTN: If BP uncontrolled on losartan monotherapy, HCTZ alone or controlled with HCTZ 25mg/day but hypokalemic: 50mg-12.5mg tab qd. Titrate/Max: If uncontrolled after 3 weeks, increase to 2 tabs of 50mg-12.5mg qd or 1 tab of 100mg-25mg qd. If uncontrolled on losartan 100mg monotherapy, may switch to 100mg-12.5mg qd. Severe HTN: Initial: 50mg-12.5mg qd. Titrate/Max: If inadequate response after 2-4 weeks, increase to 1 tab of 100mg-25mg qd. HTN With Left Ventricular Hypertrophy: Initial: Losartan 50mg qd. If BP reduction inadequate, add HCTZ 12.5mg or substitute losartan/HCTZ 50-12.5. If additional BP reduction is needed, losartan 100mg and HCTZ 12.5mg or losartan/HCTZ 100-12.5 may be substituted, followed by losartan 100mg and HCTZ 25mg or losartan/HCTZ 100-25.

HOW SUPPLIED: Tab: (Losartan-HCTZ) 50mg-12.5mg, 100mg-12.5mg, 100mg-25mg

CONTRAINDICATIONS: Anuria, sulfonamide hypersensitivity.

WARNINGS/PRECAUTIONS: Can cause fetal injury/death. Correct volume or salt depletion before therapy. Caution with hepatic or renal dysfunction, renal artery stenosis, severe CHF, history of allergies, asthma. May exacerbate or activate SLE. Monitor serum electrolytes. Avoid if CrCl ≤30mL/min. Observe for signs of fluid or electrolyte imbalance. May precipitate hyperuricemia or gout. Enhanced effects in post-sympathectomy patient. May increase cholesterol, TG levels. Angioedema reported. Not recommended with hepatic dysfunction requiring losartan titration.

ADVERSE REACTIONS: Dizziness, upper respiratory infection, back pain, cough.

INTERACTIONS: Decreased levels with rifampin. Increased levels with fluconazole. Avoid K^+-sparing diuretics (eg, spironolactone, triamterene, amiloride), K^+ supplements, K^+-containing salt substitutes. Potentiates orthostatic hypotension with alcohol, barbiturates, narcotics. Adjust insulin, antidiabetic drugs. Cholestyramine, colestipol impair absorption. Corticosteroids, ACTH deplete electrolytes. May decrease response to pressor amines (eg, norepinephrine). Potentiates other antihypertensives, skeletal muscle relaxants (eg, tubocurarine). Risk of lithium toxicity. NSAIDs, including COX-2 inhibitors, may decrease effects and may result in a further deterioration of renal function in the renally impaired.

PREGNANCY: Category C (1st trimester) and D (2nd and 3rd trimesters), not for use in nursing.

MECHANISM OF ACTION: Losartan: Angiotensin II receptor antagonist; blocks vasoconstrictor and aldosterone-secreting effects of angiotensin II by selectively blocking binding of angiotensin II to AT_1 receptor. HCTZ: Thiazide diuretic; affects renal tubular mechanism of electrolyte reabsorption, directly increasing excretion of Na^+ and Cl^- and indirectly reducing plasma volume.

PHARMACOKINETICS: Absorption: Losartan: Well absorbed, bioavailability (33%); T_{max}=1 hr, 3-4 hrs(active metabolite). **Distribution:** Losartan: V_d=34L,12L (active metabolite). HCTZ: Crosses placenta and found in breast milk. **Metabolism:** Losartan: CYP2C9, 3A4 (biotransformation), Carboxylic acid (active metabolite). **Elimination:** Losartan, Metabolite: Urine (4%, 6%), $T_{1/2}$=2 hrs, 6-9 hrs. HCTZ: Kidney (61%), $T_{1/2}$=5.6-14.8 hrs.

IBERET-FOLIC-500 RX
ferrous sulfate - folic acid - multiple vitamin (Abbott)

THERAPEUTIC CLASS: Iron/vitamin

INDICATIONS: Prevention and treatment of iron and folic acid deficiencies.

DOSAGE: *Adults:* 1 tab qd on empty stomach.

HOW SUPPLIED: Tab, Extended-Release: Ferrous Sulfate 105mg-Folic Acid 0.8mg-Vitamin B_1 6mg-Vitamin B_2 6mg-Vitamin B_3 30mg-Vitamin B_5 10mg-Vitamin B_6 5mg-Vitamin B_{12} 25mcg-Vitamin C 500mg

CONTRAINDICATIONS: Pernicious anemia.

WARNINGS/PRECAUTIONS: May mask pernicious anemia.

ADVERSE REACTIONS: Allergic sensitization.

INTERACTIONS: Iron absorption is inhibited by magnesium trisilicate, eggs, milk, carbonate-containing antacids. May interfere with absorption of tetracyclines. Pyridoxine may reverse antiparkinsonism effects of levodopa.

PREGNANCY: Category A, caution in nursing.

IC-Green
RX
indocyanine green (Akorn)

THERAPEUTIC CLASS: Diagnostic dye

INDICATIONS: To determine cardiac output, hepatic function and liver blood flow, and for ophthalmic angiography.

DOSAGE: *Adults:* For Dilution Curves: 5mg. Max: 2 mg/kg. Refer to prescribing information for further instructions for dilution curves and administration depending on study being conducted.
Pediatrics: For Dilution Curves: 2.5mg. Infants: 1.25mg. Max: 2 mg/kg. Refer to prescribing information for further instructions for dilution curves and administration depending on study being conducted.

HOW SUPPLIED: Inj: 25mg

CONTRAINDICATIONS: Caution with allergy to iodides.

WARNINGS/PRECAUTIONS: Use solvent provided for dissolution. Use aqueous solution within 6 hrs.

ADVERSE REACTIONS: Anaphylactic or urticarial reactions.

INTERACTIONS: Do not use with heparin preparations containing sodium bisulfate; may reduce absorption. Do not perform radioactive iodine uptake studies for at least 1 week following use.

PREGNANCY: Category C, caution in nursing.

MECHANISM OF ACTION: Diagnostic dye; helpful index of hepatic function.

PHARMACOKINETICS: Distribution: Plasma protein binding (95%).

Idamycin PFS
RX
idarubicin HCL (Pharmacia & Upjohn)

> Administer as freely flowing IV infusion. Severe local tissue necrosis with extravasation. Can cause myocardial toxicity and severe myelosuppression. Reduce dose with hepatic or renal dysfunction. Administer only under supervision of a physician experienced in leukemia chemotherapy and in a facility able to monitor drug tolerance and toxicity, and respond to severe hemorrhagic conditions and/or overwhelming infection.

THERAPEUTIC CLASS: Anthracycline

INDICATIONS: Treatment of acute myeloid leukemia in combination with other approved antileukemic drugs.

DOSAGE: *Adults:* Induction: 12mg/m^2 qd over 10-15 min IV qd for 3 days. Administer cytarabine 100mg/m^2 qd IV infusion for 7 days, or cytarabine 25mg/m^2 IV bolus followed by 200mg/m^2 IV infusion for 5 days. May give 2nd course if unequivocal evidence of leukemia after 1st course. If severe mucositis, delay 2nd course until recovery, then administer at 25% dose reduction. Hepatic/Renal Dysfunction: Reduce dose. Avoid if bilirubin >5mg%.

HOW SUPPLIED: Inj: 1mg/mL

WARNINGS/PRECAUTIONS: Avoid use with pre-existing bone marrow suppression induced by drug therapy or radiotherapy unless benefit warrants the risk. Monitor CBC, LFTs, and renal function tests frequently. Caution with pre-existing heart disease. Monitor cardiac function during therapy; cardiomyopathy associated with decreased left ventricular ejection fraction. Increased risk of myocardial toxicity with anemia, bone marrow depression, infections, leukemic pericarditis and/or myocarditis. May induce hyperuricemia secondary to rapid lysis of leukemic cells. Should prevent hyperuricemia and control systemic infection before starting therapy. D/C if extravasation occurs; can cause local tissue necrosis.

ADVERSE REACTIONS: Severe myelosuppression, infection, nausea, vomiting, alopecia, abdominal pain/diarrhea, hemorrhage, mucositis, rash, urticaria, bullous erythrodermatous rash of palms/soles of feet, fever, headache, cardiac toxicity (CHF, arrhythmia), pulmonary effects, mental status effects.

INTERACTIONS: Increased risk of idarubicin-induced cardiac toxicity with pre-existing heart disease, and previous therapy with high cumulative dose anthracycline therapy, other potentially cardiotoxic agents, or radiation to the mediastinal-pericardial area.

PREGNANCY: Category D, not for use in nursing.

MECHANISM OF ACTION: Anthracycline; inhibits nucleic acid synthesis by DNA intercalation and interacts with the enzyme topoisomerase II.

PHARMACOKINETICS: Distribution: (Idarubicin, idarubicinol): Plasma protein binding (97%, 94%). **Metabolism:** Liver (extensive). Metabolite: idarubicinol. **Elimination:** Biliary (major); renal (minor). (Idarubicin, idarubicinol): $T_{1/2}$=22, >45 hrs.

IFEX RX
ifosfamide (Bristol-Myers Squibb)

> Risk of urotoxic side effects, especially hemorrhagic cystitis, and CNS toxicities (eg, confusion, coma); may require discontinuation of therapy. Severe myelosuppression reported. Administer only under supervision of a physician experienced in the use of antineoplastic agents.

OTHER BRAND NAMES: Ifex/Mesnex (Bristol-Myers Squibb)

THERAPEUTIC CLASS: Cyclophosphamide analog

INDICATIONS: Third line chemotherapy of germ cell testicular cancer. Use in combination with prophylactic agent for hemorrhagic cystitis (eg, mesna).

DOSAGE: *Adults:* 1.2g/m²/day slow IV infusion over a minimum of 30 min for 5 consecutive days. Repeat treatment every 3 weeks or after recovery from hematologic toxicity (platelets ≥100,000/µL, WBC ≥4000/µL). Give with extensive hydration (eg, 2L fluid/day) and protector (eg, mesna) to prevent bladder toxicity/hemorrhagic cystitis.

HOW SUPPLIED: Inj (Ifosfamide): 1g, 3g; (Ifosfamide-Mesna) 1g-1g; 3g-1g

CONTRAINDICATIONS: Severely depressed bone marrow function.

WARNINGS/PRECAUTIONS: Hemorrhagic cystitis reported; obtain urinalysis before each dose. Withhold dose until complete resolution of microscopic hematuria. Monitor WBCs, platelets, Hgb before each dose and at appropriate intervals. Avoid with WBC <2000/µL and/or platelets <50,000/µL. D/C if somnolence, confusion, hallucinations, and/or coma occur. Caution with impaired renal function, compromised bone marrow reserve, prior radiation therapy. May interfere with normal wound healing.

ADVERSE REACTIONS: Myelosuppression, alopecia, nausea, vomiting, hematuria, CNS toxicity, infection, renal impairment, liver dysfunction, increased liver enzymes/bilirubin.

INTERACTIONS: Severe myelosuppression with other chemotherapeutic agents. Caution with other cytotoxic agents.

PREGNANCY: Category D, not for use in nursing.

MECHANISM OF ACTION: Chemotherapeutic agent; requires metabolic activation by microsomal liver enzymes and it produces active metabolites that interact with DNA.

PHARMACOKINETICS: Metabolism: Extensive; 4-carboxyifosfamide, thiodiacetic acid, cysteine conjugates of chloroacetic acid (major metabolites). **Elimination:** (3.8-5g/m²): Urine (61%), $T_{1/2}$=15 hrs. (1.6-2.4g/m²/day): Urine (12-18%), $T_{1/2}$=7 hrs.

IMDUR RX
isosorbide mononitrate (Schering)

THERAPEUTIC CLASS: Nitrate vasodilator

INDICATIONS: Prevention of angina pectoris. Not for acute attack.

DOSAGE: *Adults:* Initial: 30-60mg qd in am. Titrate: May increase after several days to 120mg/day. Swallow whole with fluids. Elderly: Start at lower end of dosing range.

HOW SUPPLIED: Tab, Extended-Release: 30mg*, 60mg*, 120mg *scored

WARNINGS/PRECAUTIONS: Not for use with acute MI or CHF. Severe hypotension may occur; caution with volume depletion and hypotension. Hypotension may increase angina pectoris. May aggravate angina caused by hypertrophic cardiomyopathy. Monitor for tolerance. May interfere with cholesterol test.

ADVERSE REACTIONS: Headache, dizziness, hypotension.

INTERACTIONS: Severe hypotension with sildenafil. Orthostatic hypotension with CCBs. Additive vasodilation with other vasodilators (eg, alcohol).

PREGNANCY: Category B, caution with nursing.

MECHANISM OF ACTION: Nitrate vasodilator; relaxes vascular smooth muscle, and consequent dilatation of peripheral arteries and veins, especially the latter. Dilatation of the veins leads to reducing the left ventricular end diastolic pressure and pulmonary capillary wedge pressure (preload). Arteriolar relaxation reduces systemic vascular resistance, systolic arterial pressure, and mean arterial pressure (afterload). It also dilates the coronary artery.

PHARMACOKINETICS: Absorption: Imdur: (60mg); C_{max} =557-572ng/mL, T_{max} =2.9-4.2 hrs., AUC=6625-7555ng•hr/mL. (120mg); C_{max} =1151-1180ng/mL, T_{max} =3.1-3.2 hrs., AUC=14241-16800ng•hr/mL. Absolute bioavailability =100%. **Distribution:** Plasma protein binding (5%). V_d =0.6-0.7L/kg. **Metabolism:** Liver. Cleared through denitration and glucuronidation pathways. **Elimination:** Urine (96%), feces (1%). (60mg); $T_{1/2}$ =6.2-6.3 hrs. (120mg); $T_{1/2}$ =6.2-6.4 hrs.

IMITREX   RX
sumatriptan (GlaxoSmithKline)

THERAPEUTIC CLASS: 5-HT₁-agonist

INDICATIONS: (Inj, Spray, Tab) Acute treatment of migraine with or without aura. (Inj) Acute treatment of cluster headaches.

DOSAGE: *Adults:* ≥18 yrs: (Inj) Initial: 6mg SQ; may repeat after 1 hr. Max: 12mg/24 hrs. (Spray) 5mg, 10mg, or 20mg single dose; may repeat after 2 hrs. Max: 40mg/24 hrs. (Tab) Initial: 25-100mg; may repeat after 2 hrs. Max: 200mg/24 hrs. May give up to 100mg/day of tabs after initial inj dose. Hepatic Disease: Max: 50mg/single dose. Safety of treating >4 headaches/30 days not known.

HOW SUPPLIED: Inj: 6mg/0.5mL; Nasal Spray: 5mg, 20mg [0.1mL 6*]; Tab: 25mg, 50mg, 100mg [9*]

CONTRAINDICATIONS: History, symptoms, or signs of ischemic cardiac, cerebrovascular, or peripheral vascular syndromes. Other significant CVD, uncontrolled HTN, hemiplegic or basilar migraine, severe hepatic impairment, MAOIs during or within 2 weeks of use, within 24 hrs of ergotamine-containing agents, ergot-type agents, or other 5-HT₁ agonists.

WARNINGS/PRECAUTIONS: Confirm diagnosis. Supervise first dose and monitor cardiac function in those at risk of CAD (eg, HTN, hypercholesterolemia, smoker, obesity, diabetes, CAD family history, postmenopausal women, males >40 yrs). Monitor cardiac function in intermittent long-term users with CAD risk factors. Serious adverse cardiac events, cerebrovascular events, vasospastic reactions reported. Avoid in elderly. Caution with hepatic or renal impairment, history of seizures or brain lesions. Possible long-term ophthalmic effects. Reconsider diagnosis before 2nd dose.

ADVERSE REACTIONS: Tingling, burning sensation, flushing, chest/mouth/tongue discomfort, injection site reaction, numbness, weakness, neck pain/stiffness.

INTERACTIONS: Prolonged vasospastic reactions with ergot-containing drugs; avoid use within 24 hrs. Weakness, hyperreflexia, and incoordination reported with SSRIs (rare). Avoid MAOIs and other 5-HT₁ agonists.

PREGNANCY: Category C, caution in nursing.

MECHANISM OF ACTION: Selective 5-hydroxytryptamine₁ receptor subtype agonist; activates vascular 5-HT₁ receptors which are located on cranial arteries, on the basilar artery, and in the vasculature of human dura mater. Responsible for mediating vasoconstriction.

PHARMACOKINETICS: Absorption: (Intranasal, 5 mg) C_{max}=5ng/mL; (Intranasal, 20 mg) C_{max}= 16ng/mL; (SQ, 6mg) C_{max}=74ng/mL, T_{max}=12 min; (PO, 25mg) C_{max}=18 ng/mL; (PO, 100 mg) C_{max}=51ng/mL. **Distribution:** (PO) V_d=2.4 L/kg, (SQ) V_d=2.7L/kg; plasma protein binding (14-21%); found in breast milk following SQ administration. **Metabolism:** Via monoamine oxidase. **Elimination:** (SQ) Urine (22% unchanged and 38% as metabolites), $T_{1/2}$=115 min; (Nasal Spray) Urine (3% unchanged and 42% as metabolites), $T_{1/2}$=2 hrs. (Oral) Urine (60%), feces (40%), $T_{1/2}$=2.5 hrs.

IMODIUM A-D   OTC
loperamide HCL (McNeil Consumer)

THERAPEUTIC CLASS: Anti-peristalsis agent

INDICATIONS: Management of diarrhea and traveler's diarrhea.

DOSAGE: *Adults:* ≥12 yrs: (Tab) Initial: 4mg after the first loose stool then 2mg after each additional loose stool, take with plenty of liquid. Max: 8mg/day for no more than 2 days. (Sol) 30mL after first loose stool then 15mL after each additional loose stool. Max: 60mL/day for no more than 2 days.
Pediatrics: 9-11 yrs (60-95 lbs): (Tab) 2mg after the first loose stool then 1mg after each additional loose stool, take with plenty of liquid. Max: 6mg/day for no more than 2 days. (Sol) 15mL after first loose stool then 7.5mL after each additional loose stool. Max: 45mL/day for no more than 2 days. 6-8 yrs (48-59 lbs): (Tab) 2mg after the first loose stool then 1mg after each additional loose stool. Max: 4mg/day for no more than 2 days. (Sol) 15mL after first loose stool then 7.5mL after each additional loose stool. Max: 30mL/day for no more than 2 days.

HOW SUPPLIED: Sol: 1mg/7.5mL [120mL]; Tab: 2mg

WARNINGS/PRECAUTIONS: Do not use if diarrhea is accompanied with high fever, blood, or mucus in stool. Caution with history of liver disease. D/C if diarrhea worsens, lasts more than 2 days, or abdominal swelling or bulging occurs.

PREGNANCY: Safety in pregnancy and nursing is not known.

IMURAN   RX
azathioprine (Prometheus)

> Increased risk of neoplasia with chronic therapy. Mutagenic potential and possible hematologic toxicities.

THERAPEUTIC CLASS: Purine antagonist antimetabolite

INDICATIONS: Adjunct therapy for prevention of rejection in renal homotransplantation. Management of severe, active rheumatoid arthritis (RA) unresponsive to rest, ASA, NSAIDs, or gold.

DOSAGE: *Adults:* Renal Homotransplantation: Initial: 3-5mg/kg/day, start at time of transplant. Maint: 1-3mg/kg/day. Rheumatoid Arthritis: Initial: 1mg/kg/day given qd-bid. Titrate: Increase by 0.5mg/kg/day after 6-8 weeks, then at 4-week intervals. Max: 2.5mg/kg/day. Maint: Lowest effective dose. Decrease by 0.5mg/kg/day or 25mg/day every 4 weeks. If no response by Week 12, then considered refractory. Renal Dysfunction: Lower dose.

HOW SUPPLIED: Tab: 50mg* *scored

CONTRAINDICATIONS: Pregnancy in RA treatment. Previous treatment of RA with alkylating agents (eg, cyclophosphamide, chlorambucil, melphalan) may increase risk of neoplasia.

WARNINGS/PRECAUTIONS: Dose-related leukopenia, thrombocytopenia, macrocytic anemia, pancytopenia, and severe bone marrow suppression may occur. Monitor CBCs, including platelets, weekly during the 1st month, twice monthly for the 2nd and 3rd months, then monthly or more frequently if dose/ therapy changes. Monitor for infections.

ADVERSE REACTIONS: Leukopenia, thrombocytopenia, infections, nausea, vomiting, hepatotoxicity.

INTERACTIONS: Caution with concomitant aminosalicylates (eg, sulphasala-zine, mesalazine, olsalazine); may inhibit TPMT. Reduce dose by 1/3-1/4 with allopurinol. Drugs affecting leukocyte production (eg, co-trimoxazole) may exaggerate leukopenia. ACE inhibitors may induce anemia, leukopenia. Inhibits anticoagulant effects of warfarin.

PREGNANCY: Category D, not for use in nursing.

MECHANISM OF ACTION: Immunosuppressive antimetabolite; an imidazolyl derivative of 6-mercaptopurine (6-MP). In homograft survival, it suppresses hypersensitivities of the cell-mediated type and causes variable alterations in antibody production. Immunoinflammatory response mechanisms have not been established; suppresses disease manifestation and underlying pathology in autoimmune disease.

PHARMACOKINETICS: Absorption: (PO) Well absorbed; T_{max}=1-2 hrs. **Distribution:** Plasma protein binding (30%); crosses placenta and found in breast milk. **Metabolism:** Liver and erythrocytes (extensive); 6-MP activated to 6-thioguanine nucleotides (major metabolites); inactivated via thiol methy-lation by thiopurine S-methyltransferase (TPMT) and oxidation by xanthine oxidase. **Elimination:** Urine; $T_{1/2}$=5 hrs.

INAPSINE   RX
droperidol (Akorn)

> QT prolongation, torsade de pointes, arrhythmias reported. Use in patients resistant or intoler-
> ant to other therapies. Monitor ECG before and 2-3 hrs after treatment. Extreme caution if at risk
> for developing prolonged QT syndrome.

THERAPEUTIC CLASS: Neuroleptic butyrophenone

INDICATIONS: To reduce incidence of nausea and vomiting associated with surgical and diagnostic procedures.

DOSAGE: *Adults:* Initial (Max): 2.5mg IM/IV. May give additional 1.25mg cau-tiously to achieve desired effect. Lower initial doses in elderly, debilitated, poor-risk patients.
Pediatrics: 2-12 yrs: Initial (Max): 0.1 mg/kg IM/IV. May give additional dose cautiously. Lower initial doses in debilitated, poor-risk patients.

HOW SUPPLIED: Inj: 2.5mg/mL

CONTRAINDICATIONS: Known or suspected QT prolongation, including con-genital long QT syndrome.

WARNINGS/PRECAUTIONS: Caution with renal/hepatic impairment. HTN, tachycardia reported with pheochromocytoma. Risk of prolonged QT syn-drome with CHF, cardiac disease, bradycardia, cardiac hypertrophy, electro-lyte imbalances (eg, hypokalemia, hypomagnesemia), >65 yrs, alcohol abuse. NMS reported; give dantrolene with increased temperature, HR, or carbon dioxide production. May decrease pulmonary arterial pressure.

ADVERSE REACTIONS: QT interval prolongation, torsade de pointes, cardiac arrest, hypotension, tachycardia, dysphoria, post-op drowsiness, restlessness, hyperactivity, anxiety, depression, syncope, irregular cardiac rhythm.

INTERACTIONS: Avoid drugs that prolong the QT interval (eg, antimalarials, CCBs, antidepressants, Class I and III antiarrhythmics, certain antihistamines, neuroleptics). Caution with MAOIs, alcohol, diuretics and drugs that induce hypokalemia, hypomagnesemia. May potentiate and be potentiated by CNS depressants (eg, barbiturates, benzodiazepines, tranquilizers, opioids, general anesthetics); use lower doses. Caution with conduction anesthesia (eg, spinal, peridural). Increased BP with fentanyl citrate or other parenteral analgesics. Epinephrine may paradoxically decrease BP.

PREGNANCY: Category C, caution in nursing.

MECHANISM OF ACTION: Neuroleptic; produces marked tranquilization and sedation, allays apprehension and provides mental detachment and indifference while maintaining reflex alertness, produces mild α-adrenergic blockade, peripheral vascular dilation, reduction of pressor effect, and produces antiemetic effects.

INDERAL RX
propranolol HCL (Wyeth)

THERAPEUTIC CLASS: Nonselective beta-blocker

INDICATIONS: (Tab) Management of hypertension, angina pectoris, hypertrophic subaortic stenosis. Migraine prophylaxis. (Inj/Tab) For cardiac arrhythmias (supraventricular, ventricular tachycardia, tachyarrhythmia of digitalis intoxication, resistant tachyarrhythmia), reduction of cardiovascular mortality post-MI, essential tremor, and pheochromocytoma.

DOSAGE: *Adults:* HTN: (Tab) Initial: 40mg bid. Titrate: Increase gradually. Maint: 120-240mg/day. Angina: (Tab) 80-320mg/day, given bid-qid. Arrhythmia: (Inj) 1-3mg IV at 1 mg/min. (Tab) 10-30mg tid-qid ac and qhs. MI: (Tab) 180-240mg/day, given bid-tid. Migraine: (Tab) Initial: 80mg/day in divided doses. Usual: 160-240mg/day in divided doses. Tremor: (Tab) Initial: 40mg bid. Maint: 120mg/day. Max: 320mg/day. Hypertrophic Subaortic Stenosis: (Tab) 20-40mg tid-qid, ac and qhs. Pheochromocytoma: (Tab) 60mg/day in divided doses for 3 days before surgery with α-blocker. Inoperable Tumor: (Tab) 30mg/day in divided doses.
Pediatrics: HTN (Tab): Initial: 1mg/kg/day PO. Usual: 1-2mg/kg bid. Max: 16mg/kg/day.

HOW SUPPLIED: Inj: 1mg/mL; Tab: 10mg*, 20mg*, 40mg*, 60mg*, 80mg*
*scored

CONTRAINDICATIONS: Cardiogenic shock, sinus bradycardia and >1st-degree block, bronchial asthma, CHF (unless failure is secondary to tachyarrhythmia treatable with propranolol).

WARNINGS/PRECAUTIONS: Caution with well-compensated cardiac failure, nonallergic bronchospasm, Wolff-Parkinson-White (WPW) syndrome, hepatic or renal dysfunction. Withdrawal before surgery is controversial. May mask hypoglycemia or hyperthyroidism symptoms. Avoid abrupt discontinuation. May reduce IOP. Can cause cardiac failure. Both digitalis glycosides and β-blockers slow atrioventricular conduction and decrease HR. Concomitant use can increase risk of bradycardia.

ADVERSE REACTIONS: Bradycardia, CHF, hypotension, lightheadedness, mental depression, nausea, vomiting, allergic reactions, agranulocytosis.

INTERACTIONS: Increased propranolol levels/toxicity with CYP2D6 inhibitors (eg, amiodarone, cimetidine, fluoxetine, paroxetine, quinidine, ritonavir), CYP1A2 inhibitors (eg, imipramine, cimetidine, ciprofloxacin, fluvoxamine, isoniazid, ritonavir, theophylline, zileuton, zolmitriptan, rizatriptan), and CYP2C19 inhibitors (eg, fluconazole, cimetidine, fluoxetine, fluvoxamine, tenioposide, tolbutamide). Decreased blood levels with hepatic enzyme inducers (eg, rifampin, ethanol, phenytoin, phenobarbital, cigarette smoking). Propafenone levels increased with concurrent administration. Lidocaine metabolism is inhibited with coadministration. Increased levels with concurrent nisoldipine and nicardipine. Zolmitriptan and rizatriptan concentrations increased with concurrent administration. Decreased theophylline clearance with concrrent administration. Increased concentrations of diazepam and its metabolites with coadministration. Increased thioridazine plasma concentrations with concurrent administration of doses ≥160mg/day. Increased plasma concentrations with chlorpromazine. Aluminum hydroxide gel may decrease plasma concentrations. Decreased plasma concentrations with coadministration of cholestyramine or colestipol. Concurrent administration increases warfarin levels and PT. Increased risk of bradycardia with concomitant digitalis glycosides.

PREGNANCY: Category C, caution in nursing. Intrauterine growth retardation, small placenta, and congenital abnormalities have been reported in neonates whose mothers received propranolol during pregnancy. Neonates whose mothers received propranolol at parturition have exhibited bradycardia, hypoglycemia, and/or respiratory depression.

MECHANISM OF ACTION: Nonselective β-adrenergic receptor blocker; not established, proposed to decrease cardiac output, inhibit renin, and diminute tonic sympathetic nerve outflow.

PHARMACOKINETICS: Absorption: T_{max}=1-4 hrs. **Distribution:** V_d=4 L/kg; plasma protein binding (90%). Crosses placenta; found in breast milk. **Metabolism:** CYP2D6 (hydroxylation), CYP1A2, 2D6 (oxidation), N-dealkylation, glucuronidation. Propranolol glucuronide, naphthyloxylactic acid, glucuronic acid, sulfate conjugates (major metabolites). **Elimination:** $T_{1/2}$=3-6 hrs.

INDERAL LA   RX
propranolol HCL (Wyeth)

THERAPEUTIC CLASS: Nonselective beta-blocker

INDICATIONS: Management of hypertension, angina pectoris, hypertrophic subaortic stenosis. Migraine prophylaxis.

DOSAGE: *Adults:* HTN: Initial: 80mg qd. Maint: 120-160mg qd. Angina: Initial: 80mg qd. Titrate: Increase gradually every 3-7 days. Maint: 160mg qd. Max: 320mg/day. Migraine: Initial: 80mg qd. Maint: 160-240mg qd. Discontinue gradually if no response within 4-6 weeks. Hypertrophic Subaortic Stenosis: 80-160mg qd.

HOW SUPPLIED: Cap, Extended-Release: 60mg, 80mg, 120mg, 160mg

CONTRAINDICATIONS: Cardiogenic shock, sinus bradycardia and >1st-degree block, bronchial asthma, CHF (unless failure is secondary to tachyarrhythmia treatable with propranolol).

WARNINGS/PRECAUTIONS: Caution with well-compensated cardiac failure, nonallergic bronchospasm, Wolff-Parkinson-White (WPW) syndrome, hepatic or renal dysfunction. Withdrawal before surgery is controversial. May mask hypoglycemia or hyperthyroidism symptoms. Avoid abrupt discontinuation. May reduce IOP. Can cause cardiac failure. Exacerbation of angina, in some cases myocardial reported. D/C if these occured. Stevens-Johnson syndrome, toxic epidermal necrolysis, exfoliative dermatitis, erythema multiforme, and urticaria reported. Hypoglycemia and postural hypotension reported.

ADVERSE REACTIONS: Bradycardia, CHF, hypotension, lightheadedness, mental depression, nausea, vomiting, allergic reactions, agranulocytosis, dry eyes, alopecia, SLE-like reactions, male impotence, Peyronie's disease

INTERACTIONS: Increased propranolol levels/toxicity with CYP2D6 inhibitors (eg, amiodarone, cimetidine, fluoxetine, paroxetine, quinidine, ritonavir), CYP1A2 inhibitors (eg, imipramine, cimetidine, ciprofloxacin, fluvoxamine, isoniazid, ritonavir, theophylline, zileuton, zolmitriptan, rizatriptan), and CYP2C19 inhibitors (eg, fluconazole, cimetidine, fluoxetine, fluvoxamine, tenioposide, tolbutamide). Decreased blood levels with hepatic enzyme inducers (eg, rifampin, ethanol, phenytoin, phenobarbital, cigarette smoking). Propafenone levels increased with concurrent administration. Lidocaine metabolism is inhibited with coadministration. Increased levels with concurrent nisoldipine and nicardipine. Zolmitriptan and rizatriptan concentrations increased with concurrent administration. Decreased theophylline clearance with concrrent administration. Increased concentrations of diazepam and its metabolites with coadministration. Increased thioridazine plasma concentrations with concurrent administration of doses ≥160mg/day. Increased plasma concentrations with chlorpromazine. Aluminum hydroxide gel may decrease plasma concentrations. Decreased plasma concentrations with coadministration of cholestyramine or colestipol. Concurrent administration increases warfarin levels and PT.

PREGNANCY: Category C, caution in nursing.

MECHANISM OF ACTION: Nonselective β-adrenergic receptor blocker; not established, proposed to decrease cardiac output, inhibit renin release, and lessen tonic sympathetic nerve outflow.

PHARMACOKINETICS: Absorption: T_{max}=6 hrs. **Distribution:** Plasma protein binding (90%); V_d=4L/kg. Crosses placenta, and found in breast milk. **Metabolism:** CYP2D6 (hydroxylation), CYP1A2, 2D6 (oxidation), N-dealkylation, glucuronidation. Propanolol glucuronide, naphthyloxylactic acid, glucuronic acid, sulfate conjugates (major metabolites). **Elimination:** $T_{1/2}$=10 hrs.

INDERIDE   RX
propranolol HCL - hydrochlorothiazide (Wyeth)

THERAPEUTIC CLASS: Nonselective beta-blocker/thiazide diuretic

INDICATIONS: Management of hypertension. Not for initial therapy.

DOSAGE: *Adults:* Initial: 80-160mg propranolol/day; 25mg-50mg HCTZ/day. Max: (propranolol-HCTZ) 160mg-50mg/day. Elderly: Start at low end of dosing range. Do not substitute mg-for-mg of extended-release cap for immediate-release tab plus HCTZ. Dose tab bid and extended-release cap qd.

HOW SUPPLIED: (Propranolol-HCTZ) Tab: (Inderide) 40mg-25mg*, 80mg-25mg* Scored

CONTRAINDICATIONS: Cardiogenic shock, sinus bradycardia and >1st-degree block, bronchial asthma, CHF (unless failure is secondary to tachyarrhythmia treatable with propranolol), anuria, sulfonamide hypersensitivity.

WARNINGS/PRECAUTIONS: Caution with well-compensated cardiac failure, nonallergic bronchospasm, Wolff-Parkinson-White syndrome, hepatic or renal dysfunction. Withdrawal before surgery is controversial. May mask hypoglycemia or hyperthyroidism symptoms. Avoid abrupt discontinuation. May reduce IOP. Can cause cardiac failure, hypokalemia, hyperuricemia, hypercalcemia, hypophosphatemia. May exacerbate or activate SLE. Monitor for fluid/electrolyte imbalance. May manifest latent DM. Enhanced effect in postsympathectomy patient. Concomitant use with alcohol may increase plasma levels of propranolol

ADVERSE REACTIONS: Bradycardia, CHF, hypotension, lightheadedness, mental depression, nausea, vomiting, allergic reactions, blood dyscrasias, pancreatitis.

INTERACTIONS: Bradycardia/hypotension with catecholamine-depleting drugs. Potentiated by chlorpromazine, cimetidine. Antagonized by NSAIDs, phenytoin, phenobarbital, rifampin. May increase cardiac effects of CCBs. Reduces clearance of antipyrine, lidocaine, and theophylline. Aluminum hydroxide gel reduces intestinal absorption. Alcohol decreases absorption rate. May block epinephrine, thyroxine effects. Hypotension and cardiac arrest reported with haloperidol. May increase response to tubocurarine. May decrease arterial response to norepinephrine. Insulin dose may need adjustment. Risk of hypokalemia with corticosteroids, ACTH. Alcohol, barbiturates, or narcotics may aggravate orthostatic hypotension. Monitor digoxin. Potentiation with ganglionic or peripheral adrenergic-blockers. Concomitant use with alcohol may increase plasma levels of propranolol

PREGNANCY: Category C, not for use in nursing. Intrauterine growth retardation, small placenta, and congenital abnormalities have been reported in neonates whose mothers received propranolol during pregnancy. Neonates whose mothers received propranolol at parturition have exhibited bradycardia, hypoglycemia, and/or respiratory depression.

MECHANISM OF ACTION: Propranolol: Nonselective β-adrenergic receptor blocker; not established, proposed to decrease cardiac output, inhibit renin, and diminute tonic sympathetic nerve outflow. HCTZ: Thiazide diuretic; not established, affects renal tubular mechanism of electrolyte reabsorption.

PHARMACOKINETICS: Absorption: Propranolol: T_{max}=1-1.5 hrs. **Metabolism:** Propranolol: Liver. **Elimination:** Propranolol: $T_{1/2}$=4 hrs. HCTZ: Kidney.

INDOCIN I.V.
indomethacin sodium trihydrate (Merck)

RX

THERAPEUTIC CLASS: NSAID (indole derivative)

INDICATIONS: To close hemodynamically significant patent ductus arteriosus in premature infants weighing between 500-1750g after 48 hrs of ineffective medical management.

DOSAGE: *Pediatrics:* Neonates 500-1750g: Therapy includes 3 doses at 12-24 hr intervals. <48 hrs old: 0.2mg/kg IV followed by 0.1mg/kg IV then 0.1mg/kg IV. 2-7 days old: 0.2mg/kg IV for 3 doses. >7 days old: 0.2mg/kg IV followed by 0.25mg/kg IV then 0.25mg/kg IV. If anuria or marked oliguria (urinary output <0.6mL/kg/hr) occurs at scheduled time of second or third dose, hold doses until renal function normalizes. May repeat course if ductus arteriosus reopens. Surgery may be needed if unresponsive after 2 courses.

HOW SUPPLIED: Inj: 1mg

CONTRAINDICATIONS: Untreated infection, bleeding, thrombocytopenia, coagulation defects, necrotizing enterocolitis, significant renal impairment, congenital heart disease when patency of ductus arteriosus is necessary for pulmonary or systemic blood flow.

WARNINGS/PRECAUTIONS: Risk of minor GI bleeding, intraventricular bleeding. May reduce urine output, CrCl, glomerular filtration rate and may increase serum creatinine, BUN. May cause renal insufficiency, including acute renal failure; caution with extracellular volume depletion, CHF, sepsis, hepatic dysfunction. Monitor renal function and serum electrolytes. May mask signs of infection. D/C if liver disease develops. Avoid extravascular injection or leakage.

ADVERSE REACTIONS: Intracranial bleeding, GI bleeding, hyponatremia, elevated serum potassium, retrolental fibroplasia.

INTERACTIONS: May prolong half-life of digitalis; monitor ECG and serum digitalis levels. May elevate gentamicin and amikacin levels. May decrease natriuretic effect of furosemide. May reduce renal function; consider reducing dosage of medications that rely on adequate renal function for elimination. Increased risk of renal insufficiency with nephrotoxic drugs. Increased risk of bleeding with anticoagulants.

PREGNANCY: Safety in pregnancy or nursing not known.

MECHANISM OF ACTION: NSAID; not fully established, believed to inhibit prostaglandin synthesis.

PHARMACOKINETICS: Elimination: Renal, biliary; half-life varies with age and weight.

INDOMETHACIN
indomethacin (Various)

RX

NSAIDs may cause an increased risk of serious cardiovascular thrombotic events, MI, stroke and serious GI adverse events including bleeding, ulceration, and perforation of the stomach or intestines. Contraindicated for the treatment of perioperative pain in the setting of coronary artery bypass graft (CABG) surgery.

OTHER BRAND NAMES: Indocin (Merck)

THERAPEUTIC CLASS: NSAID (indole derivative)

INDICATIONS: Management of moderate to severe rheumatoid arthritis (RA), ankylosing spondylitis, osteoarthritis (OA), acute painful shoulder (bursitis and/or tendinitis) and/or acute gouty arthritis.

DOSAGE: *Adults:* RA/Ankylosing Spondylitis/OA: Initial: 25mg PO bid-tid. Titrate: May increase by 25-50mg/day at weekly intervals. Max: 200mg/day.

Bursitis/Tendinitis: 75-150mg/day given tid-qid for 7-14 days. Acute Gouty Arthritis: 50mg PO tid until pain is tolerable, then d/c. Take with food. *Pediatrics:* ≥14 yrs: RA/Ankylosing Spondylitis/OA: Initial: 25mg PO bid-tid. Titrate: May increase by 25-50mg/day at weekly intervals. Max: 200mg/day. Bursitis/Tendinitis: 75-150mg/day given tid-qid for 7-14 days. Acute Gouty Arthritis: 50mg PO tid until pain is tolerable, then d/c. 2-14 yrs (safety and effectiveness not established): Initial: 1-2mg/kg/day in divided doses. Max: 3mg/kg/day or 150-200mg/day. Take with food.

HOW SUPPLIED: Cap: 25mg, 50mg; Sus: 25mg/5mL [237mL]

CONTRAINDICATIONS: ASA or other NSAID allergy that precipitates acute asthmatic attack, urticaria, or rhinitis. Do not give suppositories with history of proctitis or recent rectal bleeding. Treatment of perioperative pain in the setting of CABG surgery.

WARNINGS/PRECAUTIONS: May lead to onset of new HTN or worsening of pre-existing HTN; monitor BP closely. Fluid retention and edema reported; caution with fluid retention or heart failure. Renal papillary necrosis and other renal injury reported after long-term use. Not recommended for use with advanced renal disease; if therapy must be initiated, monitor renal function. Anaphylactoid reactions may occur. May cause serious skin adverse events (eg, exfoliative dermatitis, Stevens-Johnson syndrome, and toxic epidermal necrolysis). Avoid in late pregnancy; may cause premature closure of ductus arteriosis. May cause elevations of LFTs; d/c if liver disease develops or systemic manifestations occur. Caution in elderly. Anemia may occur; with long-term use, monitor Hgb/Hct if signs or symptoms of anemia develop. May inhibit platelet aggregation and prolong bleeding time; monitor with coagulation disorders. Caution with asthma and avoid with ASA-sensitive asthma. Corneal deposits and retinal disturbances reported with prolonged therapy; perform eye exams at periodic intervals during prolonged therapy. May aggravate depression or other psychiatric disturbances, epilepsy, and parkinsonism; use with caution. D/C if severe CNS adverse reactions develop. May impair mental/physical abilities.

ADVERSE REACTIONS: Headache, dizziness, nausea, vomiting, dyspepsia, diarrhea, abdominal pain, constipation, vertigo, somnolence, depression, fatigue.

INTERACTIONS: Avoid salicylates, diflunisal, other NSAIDs, and triamterene. Potassium-sparing diuretics may cause hyperkalemia. Increase toxicity of methotrexate, cyclosporine, lithium, and digoxin. Probenecid increases levels. Caution with antihypertensives and anticoagulants. May decrease effects of diuretics, β-blockers, captopril.

PREGNANCY: Category C, not for use in nursing.

MECHANISM OF ACTION: NSAID; not established; exhibits antipyretic, analgesic, and anti-inflammatory properties. Potent inhibitor of prostaglandin synthesis; decreases prostaglandins in peripheral tissues, suppresses inflammation in RA, and diminishes basal and CO_2-stimulated cerebral blood flow.

PHARMACOKINETICS: Absorption: Readily absorbed. Bioavailability (100%); C_{max}=1-2mcg/mL; T_{max}=2 hrs. **Distribution:** Plasma protein binding (99%); crosses blood-brain barrier and placenta; found in breast milk. **Metabolism:** Desmethyl, desbenzoyl, desmethyldesbenzoyl (metabolites). **Elimination:** Urine (60% as drug/metabolites), feces (33% as drug); $T_{1/2}$=4.5 hrs.

INFANRIX RX
pertussis vaccine, acellular - diphtheria toxoid - tetanus toxoid
(GlaxoSmithKline)

THERAPEUTIC CLASS: Vaccine/toxoid combination

INDICATIONS: Active immunization against diphtheria, tetanus, and pertussis as a 5-dose series in infants and children 6 weeks-7yrs old.

DOSAGE: *Pediatrics:* ≥6 weeks up to 7 yrs: 3 doses of 0.5mL IM at 4-8 week intervals. Start at 2 months or as early as 6 weeks if necessary. 2 Booster doses: Give at 15-20 months and at 4 to 6 years. Do not start series over again, regardless of time elapsed between doses. May use to complete primary series in infants who received 1-2 doses of whole-cell DTP vaccine.

HOW SUPPLIED: Inj: (Diphtheria-Tetanus-Pertussis) 25Lf-10Lf-25mcg/0.5mL

CONTRAINDICATIONS: Hypersensitivity to any component; serious allergic (eg, anaphylaxis) associated with previous dose. Encephalopathy not due to an identifiable cause within 7 days prior to pertussis immunization and progressive neurologic disorder, uncontrolled epilepsy, or progressive encephalopathy. Not contraindicated in individuals with HIV infection.

WARNINGS/PRECAUTIONS: Caution if within 48 hrs of previous whole-cell DTP or acellular DTP vaccine, fever ≥105°F not due to another identifiable cause, collapse or shock-like state, or inconsolable crying lasting ≥3 hrs occurs, or if convulsions occur within 3 days. For high seizure risk, give APAP at time of vaccination and q4-6h for 24 hrs. Caution with neurologic or CNS disorders. Avoid with coagulation disorders. Have epinephrine available. Suboptimal response may occur in immunocompromised patients.

ADVERSE REACTIONS: Local reactions, fever, irritability, drowsiness, anorexia, vomiting, diarrhea, crying.

INTERACTIONS: Avoid with anticoagulants. Immunosuppressive therapy (eg, irradiation, antimetabolites, alkylating agents, cytotoxic drugs, corticosteroids) may decrease response. Administer tetanus immune globulin, diphtheria antitoxin, hepatitis B vaccine, and *Haemophilus influenzae* type b vaccine at separate site.

PREGNANCY: Category C, safety in nursing not known.

MECHANISM OF ACTION: Active immunization by producing antibodies against diphtheria, tetanus, and pertussis.

INFₑD   RX
iron dextran (Watson)

> Anaphylactic-type reactions and death possible. Only use when indication clearly established and lab investigations confirm iron deficient state not amenable to oral therapy.

THERAPEUTIC CLASS: Iron supplement

INDICATIONS: Treatment of iron deficiency when oral administration is not possible.

DOSAGE: *Adults:* Iron Deficiency Anemia: Dose (mL)=0.0442 (desired Hgb-observed Hgb) x LBW + (0.26 x LBW); LBW=lean body wt (kg). See PI for details. Blood Loss: Replace equivalent amount of iron in blood loss. *Pediatrics:* ≥4 months: >15kg: Iron Deficiency Anemia: Dose (mL)=0.0442 (desired Hgb-observed Hgb) x LBW + (0.26 x LBW); LBW=lean body wt (kg). 5-15kg: Dose (mL)=0.0442 (desired Hgb-observed Hgb) x wt + (0.26 x weight). See PI for details. Blood Loss: Replace equivalent amount of iron in blood loss.

HOW SUPPLIED: Inj: 50mg/mL

CONTRAINDICATIONS: Anemia not associated with iron deficiency.

WARNINGS/PRECAUTIONS: Large IV doses associated with increased incidence of adverse effects. Caution with serious hepatic impairment, significant allergies, asthma. Avoid during acute phase of infectious kidney disease. May exacerbate cardiovascular complications in pre-existing cardiovascular disease and joint pain or swelling in rheumatoid arthritis. Hypersensitivity reactions reported after uneventful test doses. Unwarranted therapy can cause exogenous hemosiderosis. Have epinephrine (1:1000) available. Risk of carcinogenesis with IM use. Give 0.5mL test dose before IM/IV administration.

ADVERSE REACTIONS: Anaphylactic reactions, chest pain/tightness, urticaria, pruritus, abdominal pain, nausea, arthralgia, convulsions, respiratory arrest, hematuria, febrile episodes.

INTERACTIONS: Discontinue oral iron before use.

PREGNANCY: Category C, caution in nursing.

PHARMACOKINETICS: Absorption: Capillaries; lymphatic system. **Elimination:** $T_{1/2}$=5-20 hrs.

INFERGEN   RX
interferon alfacon-1 (Valeant)

> May cause or aggravate fatal or life-threatening neuropsychiatric, autoimmune, ischemic, and infectious disorders. Monitor closely with periodic clinical and laboratory evaluations.

THERAPEUTIC CLASS: Biological response modifier

INDICATIONS: Treatment of chronic hepatitis C virus (HCV) with compensated liver disease in patients with anti-HCV antibodies and/or presence of HCV RNA.

DOSAGE: *Adults:* ≥18 yrs: 9mcg 3x/week (TIW) SQ for 24 weeks, wait 48 hrs between doses. If No Response or Relapse: 15mcg TIW for up to 48 weeks. Hold dose temporarily in severe adverse effects and reduce to 7.5mcg.

HOW SUPPLIED: Inj: 9mcg/0.3mL, 15mcg/0.5mL

CONTRAINDICATIONS: Decompensated hepatic disease, autoimmune hepatitis.

WARNINGS/PRECAUTIONS: Severe psychiatric adverse events (eg, depression, suicidal ideation, suicide attempt) may occur. Avoid in decompensated hepatic disease. Monitor CBC, platelets, and clinical chemistry tests before therapy and periodically thereafter. D/C if severe decrease in neutrophils or platelets, or serious hypersensitivity reaction occurs. Caution with cardiac disease, history of endocrine disorders, or low peripheral blood cell counts. Decrease/loss of vision and retinopathy reported; perform eye examination at baseline, if any ocular symptoms develop, and periodically with pre-existing disorder. May exacerbate autoimmune disorders. Neutropenia, thrombocytopenia, hypertriglyceridemia, and thyroid disorders reported. Caution in elderly. Pancreatitis, pneumonia, interstitial pneumonitis, colitis reported; d/c when signs and symptoms develop.

ADVERSE REACTIONS: Flu-like symptoms, depression, leukopenia, granulocytopenia, hot flushes, malaise, insomnia, dizziness, headache, myalgia, abdominal pain, nausea, diarrhea, anorexia, vomiting, thrombocytopenia, nervousness.

INTERACTIONS: Caution with agents that cause myelosuppression or are metabolized by CYP450.

PREGNANCY: Category C, caution in nursing.

MECHANISM OF ACTION: Type-I interferon. Binds interferon to the cell-surface receptor, leading to the production of several interferon-stimulated gene products.

INFLAMASE   RX
prednisolone sodium phosphate (Novartis Ophthalmics)

OTHER BRAND NAMES: Inflamase Forte (Novartis Ophthalmics) - AK-Pred (Akorn)

THERAPEUTIC CLASS: Corticosteroid

INDICATIONS: Treatment of inflammation of the palpebral and bulbar conjunctiva, cornea, and anterior segment of the globe.

DOSAGE: *Adults:* Initial: 1-2 drops every hr (day) and q2h (night). Maint: 1 drop q4h, reduce to 1 drop tid-qid to control symptoms.

HOW SUPPLIED: Sol: (Inflamase) 0.125% [5mL, 10mL], (Forte) 1% [10mL, 15mL], (AK-Pred) 1% [5mL, 15mL]

CONTRAINDICATIONS: Viral diseases of the cornea and conjunctiva including superficial herpes simplex keratitis, vaccinia, and varicella. TB and fungal diseases of the eye. After uncomplicated removal of corneal foreign body.

WARNINGS/PRECAUTIONS: Prolonged use can cause optic nerve damage, visual defects, cataracts, glaucoma or secondary ocular infections (eg, fungal). Check IOP frequently. Caution with diseases causing thinning of cornea/sclera. May mask or enhance infection with acute purulent conditions. D/C if irritation develops.

ADVERSE REACTIONS: Secondary infection, visual defects, glaucoma, cataract formation.

PREGNANCY: Category C, caution in nursing.

INFUMORPH CII
morphine sulfate (Baxter)

THERAPEUTIC CLASS: Opioid analgesic

INDICATIONS: Treatment of intractable chronic pain in microinfusion devices.

DOSAGE: *Adults:* Lumbar Intrathecal: Opioid Intolerant: 0.2-1mg/day. Opioid Tolerant: 1-10mg/day. Max: Must be individualized. Caution with >20mg/day. Epidural: Opioid Intolerant: 3.5-7.5mg/day. Opioid tolerant: 4.5-10mg/day. May increase to 20-30mg/day. Max: Must be individualized. Starting dose must be based on in-hospital evaluation of response to serial single-dose intrathecal/epidural bolus injections of regular morphine sulfate.

HOW SUPPLIED: Inj: 10mg/mL (200mg), 25mg/mL (500mg)

CONTRAINDICATIONS: For neuraxial analgesia: Infection at injection site, anticoagulants, uncontrolled bleeding diathesis, any therapy or condition that may render intrathecal or epidural administration hazardous.

WARNINGS/PRECAUTIONS: Have resuscitation equipment, oxygen, and antidote (eg, naloxone) available; severe respiratory depression may occur. Use only if less invasive means of controlling pain fail. Not for single-dose IV, IM, or SQ administration. May be habit-forming. Observe patient for 24 hours following test dose, and for 1st several days after catheter implantation. Caution with determining refill frequency. Make sure needle is properly placed in the filling port of device. Myoclonic-like spasm of the lower extremities reported if dose >20mg/day; may need detoxification. Caution with head injury, increased ICP, decreased respiratory reserve, hepatic/renal dysfunction (epidural injection), elderly. Avoid with chronic asthma, upper airway obstruction, other chronic pulmonary disorders. Biliary colic reported. May cause micturition disturbances especially with BPH. Increased risk of orthostatic hypotension with reduced circulating blood volume and impaired myocardial function. Avoid abrupt withdrawal. Risk of withdrawal in patients maintained on parenteral/oral narcotics. Not for routine use in obstetric labor/delivery.

ADVERSE REACTIONS: Respiratory depression, myoclonus convulsions, dysphoric reactions, pruritus, urinary retention, constipation, lumbar puncture-type headache, peripheral edema, orthostatic hypotension.

INTERACTIONS: Depressant effect may be potentiated by CNS depressants (eg, alcohol, sedatives, antihistamines, psychotropics). Increased risk of respiratory depression with neuroleptics. Contraindicated with anticoagulants. Risk of withdrawal with narcotic antagonists. Increased risk of orthostatic hypotension with sympatholytic drugs.

PREGNANCY: Category C, safety in nursing not known.

MECHANISM OF ACTION: Opioid analgesic. Analgesic effects are produced via at least 3 areas of the CNS: the periaqueductal-periventricular gray matter, the ventromedulla, and the spinal cord. Interacts predominantly with μ-receptor. μ-binding sites are found distributed in the brain, spinal cord, and in the trigeminal nerve.

PHARMACOKINETICS: Absorption: (Epidural): rapid absorption; C_{max}=33-40ng/mL, T_{max}=10-15 min; (Intrathecal): C_{max}≤1-7.8ng/mL, T_{max}=5-10 mins. **Distribution:** Plasma protein binding (36%), Muscle tissue binding (54%). Readily passes into fetal circulation, found in breast milk. (IV):V_d=1.0-4.7L/kg. **Metabolism:** Hepatic glucuronidation. **Elimination:** Kidneys (major), urine (2-12% unchanged), feces (10%); $T_{1/2}$=1.5-4.5 hrs.

INNOHEP

RX

tinzaparin sodium (Pharmion)

> Risk of paralysis by spinal/epidural hematoma with neuraxial anesthesia or spinal puncture. Increased risk with indwelling epidural catheters for analgesia, drugs affecting hemostasis (eg, NSAIDs, platelet inhibitors, anticoagulants), and traumatic or repeated epidural or spinal puncture.

THERAPEUTIC CLASS: Low molecular weight heparin

INDICATIONS: Treatment of acute symptomatic DVT with or without PE with concomitant warfarin.

DOSAGE: *Adults:* 175 anti-Xa IU/kg SQ qd for at least 6 days and until anticoagulated with warfarin (INR is at least 2 for 2 days). Begin warfarin within 1-3 days of therapy.

HOW SUPPLIED: Inj: 20,000 anti-Xa IU/mL

CONTRAINDICATIONS: Heparin, sulfite, benzoyl alcohol, or pork allergy. Active major bleeding, with or history of heparin-induced thrombocytopenia (HIT).

WARNINGS/PRECAUTIONS: Not for IM injection. Cannot use interchangeably unit for unit with heparin or other low molecular weight heparins. Extreme caution in conditions with an increased risk of hemorrhage (eg, bacterial endocarditis, hemorrhagic stroke, etc). Bleeding can occur at any site during therapy. D/C if severe hemorrhage occurs. Perform periodic CBC, platelets, and stool occult blood test. Asymptomatic increase in AST and ALT. Priapism reported (rare). Thrombocytopenia can occur; d/c if platelets <100,000/mm^3. Multiple dose vial contains benzyl alcohol. Contains sodium metabisulfite. Caution with bleeding diathesis, uncontrolled arterial HTN, recent GI ulceration, diabetic retinopathy, hemorrhage. Reduced elimination with elderly or in renal dysfunction; use with caution.

ADVERSE REACTIONS: Hemorrhage, thrombocytopenia, elevated LFTs, local reactions (ecchymosis, hematoma), hypersensitivity reactions.

INTERACTIONS: Increased risk of bleeding with anticoagulants, platelet inhibitors (eg, salicylates, dipyridamole, sulfinpyrazone, dextran, NSAIDs, ticlopidine, clopidogrel), and thrombolytics; monitor closely if co-administered.

PREGNANCY: Category B, caution use in nursing.

MECHANISM OF ACTION: Low molecular-weight heparin with antithrombotic properties; inhibits reactions that lead to clotting of blood including the formation of fibrin clots. Acts as a potent co-inhibitor of several activated coagulation factors, including Factors Xa and IIa (thrombin). Primary inhibitory activity mediated through plasma protease inhibitor, antithrombin.

PHARMACOKINETICS: Absorption: (4,500 IU, Single Dose): C_{max}=0.25 IU/ mL, T_{max}=3.7 hrs, AUC=2.0 IU•hr/mL; (175 IU/kg, Day 1): C_{max}=0.87 IU/mL, T_{max}=4.4 hrs, AUC=9.0 IU•hr/mL; (175 IU/kg, Day 5): C_{max}=0.93 IU/mL, T_{max}=4.6 hrs, AUC=9.7 IU•hr/mL; Absolute bioavailability (86.7%). **Distribution:** V_d=3.1-5.0L. **Metabolism:** Partially metabolized by desulphation and depolymerization. **Elimination:** Renal, $T_{1/2}$=3-4 hrs.

INNOPRAN XL

RX

propranolol HCL (Reliant)

THERAPEUTIC CLASS: Nonselective beta-blocker

INDICATIONS: For the management of hypertension.

DOSAGE: *Adults:* Initial: 80mg qhs (approximately 10 PM) consistently either on empty stomach or with food. Titrate: Based on response may titrate to dose of 120mg.

HOW SUPPLIED: Cap, Extended-Release: 80mg, 120mg

CONTRAINDICATIONS: Cardiogenic shock, sinus bradycardia and >1st-degree block, bronchial asthma.

WARNINGS/PRECAUTIONS: Caution with well-compensated cardiac failure, nonallergic bronchospasm (eg, chronic bronchitis, emphysema), Wolff-Parkinson-White syndrome, hepatic or renal dysfunction or with history of severe anaphylactic reactions. Withdrawal before surgery is controversial. May mask hypoglycemia or hyperthyroidism symptoms. Avoid abrupt discontinuation. May reduce IOP. Can cause cardiac failure. Caution in patients with impaired hepatic or renal function. Not for treatment of hypertensive emrgencies.

ADVERSE REACTIONS: Fatigue, dizziness (except vertigo), constipation.

INTERACTIONS: Caution with drugs that effect CYP2D6, 1A2, or 2C19 or that slow down AV conduction (eg, digitalis, lidocaine, CCBs). ACE inhibitors can cause hypotension and certain ACE inhibitors may increase bronchial hyperactivity. May antagonize clonidine effects; caution when withdrawing from clonidine. Potentiated by α-blockers (eg, prazosin, terazosin, doxazosin), antiarrhythmics (eg, propafenone, quinidine, amiodarone), CYP2D6 substrates or inhibitors (eg, cimetidine, delavudin, fluoxetine, paroxetine, quinidine, ritonavir), CYP1A2 substrates or inhibitors (eg, imipramine, cimetidine, ciprofloxacin, fluvoxamine, isoniazid, theophylline, zileuton, zolmitriptan, rizatriptan), CYP2C19 substrates or inhibitors (eg, fluconazole, fluoxetine, fluvoxamine, teniposide, tolbutamide). Severe bradycardia, asystole, and heart failure associated with concomitant disopyramide. Decreases clearance of lidocaine and theophylline. Uncontrolled HTN may develop with concurrent epinephrine. Closely monitor for excessive reduction of resting sympathetic nervous activity (eg, hypotension, bradycardia, vertigo, orthostatic hypotension, syncope) with concurrent reserpine; reserpine may also potentiate depression. Anesthetics (eg, methoxyflurane, trichloroethylene) may depress myocardial contractility. Effects may be reversed by β-agonists (eg, dobutamine, isoproterenol). May exacerbate hypotensive effects of MAOIs or TCAs. Hypotension and cardiac arrest reported with haloperidol. Antagonized by NSAIDs. May result in lower than expected T_3 level with concomitant thyroxin. Increases level of warfarin, diazepam, zolmitriptan, rizatriptan, thioridazine. Decreased levels with aluminum hydroxide gel (1200mg), cholestyramine, colestipol, rifampin, ethanol, and cigarette smoking. Co-administration with chlorpromazine may increase levels of both drugs. Decreases levels of lovastatin and pravastatin.

PREGNANCY: Category C; caution in nursing.

MECHANISM OF ACTION: β-adrenergic receptor blocker; not established, proposed to decrease cardiac output, inhibit renin, and diminute tonic sympathetic nerve outflow.

PHARMACOKINETICS: Absorption: T_{max}=12-14 hrs. **Distribution:** V_d=4L; plasma protein binding (90%) **Metabolism:** CYP2D6 (hydroxylation), CYP1A2, 2D6 (oxidation), N-dealkylation, glucuronidation. Propranolol glucuronide, napthyloxylactic acid, glucuronic acid, sulfate conjugates (major metabolites). **Elimination:** $T_{1/2}$= 8 hrs.

INSPRA   RX
eplerenone (Pfizer)

THERAPEUTIC CLASS: Aldosterone blocker

INDICATIONS: To improve survival with left ventricular systolic dysfunction and congestive heart failure (CHF) post-MI. Treatment of hypertension, alone or with other antihypertensives.

DOSAGE: *Adults:* CHF Post-MI: Initial: 25mg qd. Titrate: To 50mg qd within 4 weeks. Maint: 50mg qd. Adjust dose based on K+ level: See PI. HTN: Initial: 50mg qd. May increase to 50mg bid if inadequate effect on BP. Max: 100mg/day. With Weak CYP3A4 Inhibitors: Initial: 25mg qd.

HOW SUPPLIED: Tab: 25mg, 50mg

CONTRAINDICATIONS: All: Serum K+ >5.5mgEq/L at initiation, CrCl ≤30mL/min, with potent CYP3A4 inhibitors (eg, ketoconazole, itraconazole, nefazodone, troleandomycin, clarithromycin, ritonavir, nelfinavir). When treating HTN: Type 2 diabetes with microalbuminuria, SCr >2mg/dL (males) or

>1.8mg/dL (females), CrCl <50mg/min, with K⁺ supplements or K⁺-sparing diuretics (eg, amiloride, spironolactone, triamterene).

WARNINGS/PRECAUTIONS: Risk of hyperkalemia (>5.5mEq/L); monitor periodically. With CHF post-MI use caution with SCr >2mg/dL (males) or >1.8mg/dL (females), CrCl ≤50mL/min, and in diabetics (also with proteinuria).

ADVERSE REACTIONS: Headache, dizziness, hyperkalemia, increased SCr/triglycerides/GGT, angina/MI.

INTERACTIONS: Avoid with potent CYP3A4 inhibitors (eg, ketoconazole, itraconazole, nefazodone, troleandomycin, clarithromycin, ritonavir, nelfinavir). Increased levels with other CYP3A4 inhibitors (eg, erythromycin, verapamil, saquinavir, fluconazole). In HTN, use caution, with ACE inhibitors and angiotensin II receptor antagonists; increased risk of hyperkalemia especially with diabetics with microalbuminuria. Monitor lithium levels. Monitor antihypertensive effect with NSAIDs.

PREGNANCY: Category B, not for use in nursing.

MECHANISM OF ACTION: Aldosterone blocker; binds to mineralocorticoid receptor and blocks binding of aldosterone.

PHARMACOKINETICS: Absorption: T_{max}=1.5 hrs. **Distribution:** Plasma protein binding (50%); V_d=43-90L. **Metabolism:** CYP3A4. **Elimination:** Urine, feces; $T_{1/2}$=4-6 hrs.

INTEGRILIN RX
eptifibatide (Schering)

THERAPEUTIC CLASS: Glycoprotein IIb/IIIa inhibitor

INDICATIONS: Treatment of acute coronary syndrome (ACS) in patients being medically managed or undergoing percutaneous coronary intervention (PCI) including intracoronary stenting.

DOSAGE: *Adults:* ACS: 180mcg/kg IV bolus, then 2mcg/kg/min IV infusion until discharge, initiation of CABG, or up to 72 hrs. If undergoing PCI, continue until discharge or 18-24 hrs post-PCI. CrCl <50mL/min: 180mcg/kg IV bolus, then 1mcg/kg/min IV infusion. PCI: 180mcg/kg IV bolus immediately before PCI, then 2mcg/kg/min IV infusion. Give 2nd bolus of 180mcg/kg 10 min after 1st bolus. Continue until discharge or 18-24 hrs post-PCI. CrCl <50mL/min: 180mcg/kg IV bolus immediately before PCI, then 1mcg/kg/min IV infusion. Give 2nd bolus of 180mcg/kg 10 min after 1st bolus. See PI for concomitant ASA and heparin doses.

HOW SUPPLIED: Sol: 0.75mg/mL, 2mg/mL

CONTRAINDICATIONS: Active abnormal bleeding, history of bleeding diathesis, or stroke within past 30 days. Severe HTN uncontrolled with antihypertensives, major surgery within preceding 6 weeks, history of hemorrhagic stroke, concomitant parenteral glycoprotein IIb/IIIa inhibitor, renal dialysis dependency.

WARNINGS/PRECAUTIONS: Bleeding reported. Caution with renal dysfunction, platelets <100,000mm³, femeral access site in PCI. Minimize vascular and other trauma. D/C if thrombocytopenia occurs. Monitor Hct, Hgb, platelets, serum creatinine (SrCr), and PT/aPTT before therapy (and activated clotting time before PCI). D/C before CABG surgery.

ADVERSE REACTIONS: Bleeding, thrombocytopenia, hypotension.

INTERACTIONS: Caution with other drugs that affect hemostasis (eg, thrombolytics, anticoagulants, NSAIDs, dipyridamole). Avoid other glycoprotein IIb/IIIa inhibitors. Cerebral, pulmonary, GI hemorrhage reported with ASA and heparin.

PREGNANCY: Category B, caution in nursing.

MECHANISM OF ACTION: Glycoprotein IIb/IIIa inhibitor; reversibly inhibits platelet aggregation by preventing the binding of fibrinogen, von Willebrand factor, and other adhesive ligands to glycoprotein IIb/IIIa.

PHARMACOKINETICS: Absorption: T_{max}=4-6 hrs. **Distribution:** Plasma protein binding (25%). **Elimination:** Urine; $T_{1/2}$= 2.5 hrs.

INTELENCE   RX
etravirine (Tibotec)

THERAPEUTIC CLASS: Non-nucleoside reverse transcriptase inhibitor

INDICATIONS: In combination with other antiretrovirals for treatment of HIV-1 infection in antiretroviral treatment-experienced adult patients, who have evidence of viral replication and HIV-1 strains resistant to a non-nucleoside reverse transcriptase inhibitor (NNRTI) and other antiretrovirals.

DOSAGE: *Adults:* 200mg (two 100mg tabs) bid following a meal.

HOW SUPPLIED: Tab: 100mg

WARNINGS/PRECAUTIONS: Severe and life-threatening skin reactions (eg, Stevens-Johnson syndrome, hypersensitivity reaction, and erythema multiforme) reported; d/c use and treat accordingly if severe rash develops. May cause body fat redistribution or accumulation. Immune reconstitution syndrome reported with combination therapy.

ADVERSE REACTIONS: Rash, nausea, abdominal pain, vomiting, fatigue, diarrhea, peripheral neuropathy, HTN, headache.

INTERACTIONS: Coadministration of drugs that induce, inhibit or are substrates of CYP3A4, CYP2C9 and CYP2C19 may alter therapeutic effect and adverse reaction profile. Concomitant use with NNRTIs (eg, efavirenz, nevirapine, delavirdine) and protease inhibitors administered without low-dose ritonavir (eg, atazanavir, fosamprenavir, nelfinavir, indinavir) are not recommended. Ritonavir 600mg bid decreases plasma levels and should not be co-administered. Do not co-administer with tipranavir/ritonavir, fosamprenavir/ritonavir, atazanavir/ritonavir. Caution with saquinavir/ritonavir. May decrease levels of antiarrhythmics; monitor drug levels. May increase warfarin concentration; monitor INR. Do not use in combination with CYP450 inducers (eg, carbamazepine, phenobarbital, phenytoin, rifampin, rifapentine, rifabutin). Adjust dose with antifungals. Consider alternatives to clarithromycin for treatment of MAC. May decrease levels of lovastatin and simvastatin. May increase levels of fluvastatin. Caution with immunosuppressants (eg, cyclosporine, sirolimus, tacrolimus). Monitor for withdrawal symptoms when coadministered with methadone. May need to alter sildenafil dose.

PREGNANCY: Category B, not for use in nursing.

MECHANISM OF ACTION: Non-nucleoside reverse transcriptase inhibitor of HIV-1; binds directly to reverse transcriptase and blocks the RNA dependent and DNA dependent DNA polymerase activities by causing a disruption of the enzyme's catalytic site.

PHARMACOKINETICS: Absorption: T_{max}=2.5-4 hrs. **Distribution:** Plasm protein binding (99.9%). **Metabolism:** Liver via CYP3A4, CYP2C9 and CYP2C19; (methyl hydroxylation). **Elimination:** Feces (93.7%); Urine (1.2%); $T_{1/2}$=41 hrs.

INTRON A   RX
interferon alfa-2b (Schering)

> May cause or aggravate fatal or life-threatening neuropsychiatric, autoimmune, ischemic, and infectious disorders. Monitor closely with periodic clinical and laboratory evaluations.

THERAPEUTIC CLASS: Biological response modifier

INDICATIONS: Treatment of hairy cell leukemia, malignant melanoma, follicular lymphoma, condylomata acuminata, AIDS-related Kaposi's sarcoma, chronic hepatitis C and B.

DOSAGE: *Adults:* ≥18 yrs: Hairy Cell Leukemia: 2 MIU/m² IM/SQ 3x/week up to 6 months. Reduce dose by 50% or stop therapy with severe reactions. Malignant Melanoma: Initial: 20 MIU/m² IV for 5 consecutive days/week for 4 weeks. Maint: 10 MIU/m² SQ 3x/week for 48 weeks. Follicular Lymphoma: 5 MIU SQ 3x/week up to 18 months. Condylomata Acuminata: 1 MIU into lesion 3x/week alternating days for 3 weeks. Max: 5 lesions/course. Kaposi's Sarcoma: 30 MIU/m² 3x/week IM/SQ. Hepatitis C: 3 MIU IM/SQ 3x/week for

18-24 months. Hepatitis B: IM/SC: 5 MIU qd or 10 MIU IM/SQ 3x/week for 16 weeks. Dose adjust according to severe adverse reactions and laboratory abnormalities (See PI for more information).

Pediatrics: ≥1 yr: Hepatitis B: 3 MIU/m^2 SQ 3x/week for 1 week, then 6 MIU/m^2 3x/week for total therapy of 16-24 weeks. Max: 10 MIU/m^2 3x/week. Reduce dose by 50% or stop therapy with severe reactions. Adjust based on WBC, granulocyte, and/or platelet counts. Dose adjust according to severe adverse reactions and laboratory abnormalities (See PI for more information).

HOW SUPPLIED: Inj: 10 MIU, 18 MIU, 50 MIU, 10 MIU/mL, 3 MIU/0.2mL, 5 MIU/0.2mL, 10 MIU/0.2mL.

CONTRAINDICATIONS: Autoimmune hepatitis, decompensated liver disease.

WARNINGS/PRECAUTIONS: Do not give IM if platelet count is less than 50,000 cells/mm^3. Hepatotoxicity, retinal hemorrhages, autoimmune diseases, pulmonary infiltrates, pneumonitis, thyroid abnormalities and pneumonia reported. Avoid with immunosuppressed transplant, autoimmune disorders, decompensated liver disease. Caution with cardiac disease, coagulation disorders, severe myelosuppression, pulmonary disease, thyroid disorders, or DM prone to ketoacidosis. Avoid with pre-existing psychiatric condition; depression, suicidal behavior, and aggressive behavior; monitor during treatment and in the 6 month follow-up period. D/C if psychiatric symptoms worsen or suicidal ideation is identified. Cases of encephalopathy observed in elderly treated with higher doses. Dental and periodontal disorders have been reported with ribavirin and interferon combination therapy. May exacerbate psoriasis or sarcoidosis. Do not interchange brands.

ADVERSE REACTIONS: Fever, headache, chills, fatigue, myalgia, GI disturbances, alopecia, dyspnea, depression.

INTERACTIONS: Increases theophylline levels by 100%. Caution with myelosuppressive agents (eg, zidovudine). Antidiabetics and thyroid agents may need adjustments. Increased risk of hemolytic anemia when coadministered with ribavirin. Risk of aplastic anemia and pure red cell aplasia with Rebetol.

PREGNANCY: Category C, Category X when used with ribavirin, not for use in nursing.

MECHANISM OF ACTION: α-interferon; binds to specific membrane receptors on cell surface initiating induction of enzymes, suppression of cell proliferation, immunomodulating activities, and inhibition of virus replication.

PHARMACOKINETICS: Absorption: (IM, SQ) C_{max}=18-116 IU/mL, T_{max}=3-12 hrs; (IV) C_{max}=135-273 IU/mL, T_{max}=30 min. **Elimination:** (IM, SQ) $T_{1/2}$=2-3 hrs; (IV) $T_{1/2}$=2 hrs.

INVANZ   RX
ertapenem sodium (Merck)

THERAPEUTIC CLASS: Carbapenem

INDICATIONS: Treatment of complicated intra-abdominal infections; complicated skin and skin structure infections (cSSSI), including diabetic foot infections without osteomyelitis; community-acquired pneumonia (CAP); complicated urinary tract infections (UTI), including pyelonephritis; acute pelvic infections, including postpartum endomyometritis, septic abortion, and post-surgical gynecologic infections caused by susceptible strains of microorganisms. Prophylaxis of surgical site infection following elective colorectal surgery.

DOSAGE: *Adults:* Treatment: 1g IM/IV qd. Duration: Intra-Abdominal Infections: 5-14 days. cSSSI: 7-14 days. CAP/UTI: 10-14 days. Acute Pelvic Infections: 3-10 days. May give IV for up to 14 days and IM for up to 7 days. Prophylaxis Following Colorectal Surgery: 1g IV as single dose given 1 hr prior to surgical incision. CrCl ≤30mL/min/1.73m^2: 500mg IM/IV qd. Hemodialysis: Give 150mg IM/IV after dialysis only if 500mg dose was given within 6 hrs prior to dialysis.

Pediatrics: ≥13 yrs: 1g IM/IV qd. 3 months-12 yrs: 15mg/kg IM/IV bid (Max: 1g/day). Treatment Duration: Intra-Abdominal Infections: 5-14 days. SSSI: 7-14

INVEGA

days. CAP/UTI: 10-14 days. Pelvic Infections: 3-10 days. May administer IV for up to 14 days and IM for up to 7 days.

HOW SUPPLIED: Inj: 1g

CONTRAINDICATIONS: Anaphylactic reactions to β-lactams, hypersensitivity to local anesthetics of the amide type (due to lidocaine diluent).

WARNINGS/PRECAUTIONS: Serious, sometimes fatal, hypersensitivity reported with β-lactam therapy. *Clostridium difficile*-associated diarrhea (CDAD) reported. D/C if CDAD confirmed. Seizures and CNS adverse experiences reported. Increased risk of seizures with CNS disorders and/or compromised renal function. Use lidocaine HCl as diluent for IM use. Monitor renal, hepatic, hematopoietic functions during prolonged therapy. Do not inject into blood vessel.

ADVERSE REACTIONS: Diarrhea, infused vein complication, nausea, headache, edema/swelling, fever, abdominal pain, constipation, altered mental status, headache, insomnia, rash, pruritis, vomiting.

INTERACTIONS: Decreased clearance with probenecid. Do not mix or coinfuse with other drugs. May decrease serum levels of valproic acid when coadministered.

PREGNANCY: Category B, caution in nursing.

MECHANISM OF ACTION: Broad-spectrum carbapenem; penetrates bacterial cells and interferes with synthesis of vital cell wall components, resulting in cell death.

PHARMACOKINETICS: Absorption: Administration of different doses resulted in different parameters. (IM): T_{max}=2.3 hrs; absolute bioavailability=90%. **Distribution:** V_d=0.12L/kg (adult); 0.2L/kg (3 months-12 yrs); 0.16L/kg (13-17 yrs). Plasma protein binding (95%); found in breast milk. **Metabolism:** Liver via hydrolysis of the β-lactam ring. **Elimination:** (Adults, 13-17 yrs old) $T_{1/2}$=4 hrs. (3 months-12 years old) Urine (38% unchanged, 37% metabolite), feces (10%); $T_{1/2}$=2.5 hrs.

INVEGA   RX
paliperidone (Janssen)

> Elderly patients with dementia-related psychosis treated with atypical antipsychotic drugs are at an increased risk of death; most appeared to be cardiovascular (eg, heart failure, sudden death) or infectious (eg, pneumonia) in nature. Paliperidone is not approved for the treatment of patients with dementia-related psychosis.

THERAPEUTIC CLASS: Benzisoxazole derivative

INDICATIONS: Acute and maintenance treatment of schizophrenia.

DOSAGE: *Adults:* 6mg qd in am. Range: 3-12mg/day. Titrate: May increase by 3mg/day at intervals of >5 days. Max: 12mg/day. Swallow whole; do not chew, divide, or crush. CrCl 50 to <80mL/min: Max of 6mg/day. CrCl 10 to <50mL/min: Max of 3mg/day. Evaluate periodically for long-term use.

HOW SUPPLIED: Tab, Extended-Release: 3mg, 6mg, 9mg

WARNINGS/PRECAUTIONS: May increase QTc interval; avoid with congenital long QT syndrome and with a history of cardiac arrhythmias. Neuroleptic malignant syndrome (NMS) and tardive dyskinesia (TD) may occur. Monitor for hyperglycemia; perform fasting blood glucose testing if symptoms develop or with risk factors for DM. Avoid with pre-existing severe GI narrowing. Cerebrovascular events (eg, stroke, TIA) reported in elderly with dementia-related psychosis. Not approved for the treatment of dementia-related psychosis. May induce priapism. May induce orthostatic hypotension and syncope; monitor closely in those vulnerable to hypotension. Caution with history of seizures or other conditions that may lower seizure threshold. May elevate prolactin levels. May cause esophageal dysmotility and aspiration; caution in those at risk for aspiration pneumonia. May disrupt body's ability to reduce core body temperature; caution in those who may experience conditions that may contribute to an elevation in core body temperature. Caution with known suicidal tendencies, cardiovascular disease, elderly, and renal impairment. Re-evaluate periodically.

ADVERSE REACTIONS: Tachycardia, nausea, akathisia, dizziness, extrapyramidal disorder, headache, somnolence, anxiety, parkinsonism, dyskinesia, hyperkinesia.

INTERACTIONS: Caution with other CNS drugs, alcohol. May antagonize the effect of levodopa and other dopamine agonists. Because of its potential for inducing orthostatic hypotension, additive effect may be observed when administered with other agents that have this potential. Avoid in combination with other drugs known to prolong QTc interval including Class 1A (eg, quinidine, procainamide) or Class III (eg, amiodarone, sotalol) antiarrhythmics, antipsychotic medications (eg, chlorpromazine, thioridazine), antibiotics (eg, gatifloxacin, moxifloxacin), or any other class of drugs known to prolong the QTc interval.

PREGNANCY: Category C, not for use in nursing.

MECHANISM OF ACTION: Benzisoxazole derivative; not fully established. Action is proposed to be mediated through a combination of central dopamine type 2 (D_2) and serotonin type 2 ($5HT_{2A}$) receptor antagonism.

PHARMACOKINETICS: Absorption: Absolute bioavailability (28%); T_{max}=24 hrs. **Distribution**: V_d=487L; plasma protein binding (74%); found in breast milk. **Metabolism**: Dealkylation, hydroxylation, dehydrogenation, benzisoxazole scission; CYP2D6, 3A4. **Elimination**: Urine (59% unchanged), feces (11%); $T_{1/2}$=23 hrs.

INVERSINE   RX
mecamylamine HCL (Targacept)

THERAPEUTIC CLASS: Ganglionic blocker

INDICATIONS: Management of moderately severe to severe essential hypertension and in uncomplicated cases of malignant hypertension.

DOSAGE: *Adults:* Initial: 2.5mg bid after meals. Titrate: Increase by 2.5mg/day at intervals of not less than 2 days. Usual: 25mg/day given tid. Give larger doses at noontime and evening. Reduce dose by 50% with thiazides.

HOW SUPPLIED: Tab: 2.5mg

CONTRAINDICATIONS: Coronary insufficiency, recent MI, uremia, glaucoma, organic pyloric stenosis, uncooperative patients, mild to moderate or labile HTN, with antibiotics or sulfonamides. Administer with great discretion in renal insufficiency.

WARNINGS/PRECAUTIONS: Caution with renal, cerebral, or cardiovascular dysfunction, marked cerebral or coronary insufficiency, prostatic hypertrophy, bladder neck obstruction, urethral stricture. Large doses in cerebral or renal insufficiency may produce CNS effects. Withdraw gradually and add other antihypertensives. May be potentiated by excessive heat, fever, infection, hemorrhage, pregnancy, anesthesia, surgery, vigorous exercise, other antihypertensive drugs, alcohol, salt depletion. D/C if paralytic ileus occurs.

ADVERSE REACTIONS: Ileus, constipation, vomiting, nausea, anorexia, dryness of mouth, syncope, postural hypotension, convulsions, tremor, interstitial pulmonary edema, urinary retention, impotence, blurred vision.

INTERACTIONS: Avoid with antibiotics and sulfonamides. Anesthesia, alcohol or other antihypertensives may potentiate effect.

PREGNANCY: Category C, not for use in nursing.

MECHANISM OF ACTION: Ganglion blocker; reduces BP.

PHARMACOKINETICS: Absorption: Complete. **Distribution:** Crosses placenta. **Elimination:** Urine.

INVIRASE

RX

saquinavir mesylate (Roche Labs)

Not interchangeable with Fortovase®.

THERAPEUTIC CLASS: Protease inhibitor

INDICATIONS: Treatment of HIV infection in combination with other antiretrovirals.

DOSAGE: *Adults:* 1000mg bid with ritonavir 100mg bid. Take within 2 hrs after a full meal.
Pediatrics: >16 yrs: 1000mg bid with ritonavir 100mg bid. Take within 2 hrs after a full meal.

HOW SUPPLIED: Cap: 200mg; Tab: 500mg

CONTRAINDICATIONS: Concomitant amiodarone, bepridil, flecainide, propafenone, quinidine, rifampin, pimozide, terfenadine, cisapride, astemizole, triazolam, midazolam, ergot derivatives.

WARNINGS/PRECAUTIONS: New onset DM, exacerbation of pre-existing DM, hyperglycemia may occur. Exacerbation of chronic liver dysfunction reported with hepatitis or cirrhosis. Spontaneous bleeding may occur with hemophilia A, B. Possible redistribution or accumulation of body fat. Caution with hepatic dysfunction. Interrupt therapy if serious toxicity occurs.

ADVERSE REACTIONS: Diarrhea, abdominal discomfort, nausea, dyspepsia, mucosa damage, headache, paresthesia, extremity numbness, asthenia, myalgia, vomiting, fatigue, pneumonia, lipodystrophy

INTERACTIONS: See contraindications. Avoid lovastatin, simvastatin, St. John's wort, garlic capsules, tipranavir, trazodone, fluticasone. Decreased plasma levels with nevirapine. Consider alternatives to CYP3A4 inducers (eg, phenobarbital, phenytoin, dexamethasone, carbamazepine). Ritonavir increases adverse effects. Risk of toxicity with substrates of CYP3A4 substrates (eg, calcium CCBs, clindamycin, dapsone, quinidine, triazolam). Delavirdine increases plasma levels; monitor LFTs frequently. Saquinavir/ritonavir increases digoxin levels; monitor digoxin serum concentration and reduce dose if needed.

PREGNANCY: Category B, not for use in nursing.

MECHANISM OF ACTION: HIV protease inhibitor; binds to the protease active site and inhibits activity of the enzyme, preventing cleavage of the viral polyproteins and resulting in formation of immature, noninfectious virus particles.

PHARMACOKINETICS: Absorption: Administration of variable doses and combinations resulted in different parameters. **Distribution:** Plasma protein binding (98%). (IV): V_d=700L. **Metabolism:** Hepatic via CYP3A4. **Elimination:** (PO): Urine (1%), feces (88%). (IV): Urine (3%), feces (81%).

IONAMIN

CIV

phentermine (Celltech)

THERAPEUTIC CLASS: Anorectic sympathomimetic amine

INDICATIONS: Short term adjunct for exogenous obesity if initial BMI ≥30kg/m² or ≥27kg/m² with other risk factors (eg, HTN, diabetes, hyperlipidemia).

DOSAGE: *Adults:* 15-30mg before breakfast or 10-14 hrs before bedtime. Swallow caps whole.
Pediatrics: ≥16 yrs: 15-30mg prior to breakfast or 10-14 hrs before bedtime. Swallow caps whole.

HOW SUPPLIED: Cap: 15mg, 30mg

CONTRAINDICATIONS: Advanced arteriosclerosis, CVD, moderate to severe HTN, hyperthyroidism, glaucoma, agitated states, history of drug abuse, within 14 days of MAOI use.

WARNINGS/PRECAUTIONS: Primary pulmonary HTN and valvular heart disease reported. D/C if tolerance occurs. Abuse potential. Caution with mild HTN.

ADVERSE REACTIONS: Primary pulmonary HTN, palpitations, tachycardia, BP elevation, restlessness, dizziness, insomnia, headache, diarrhea, constipation, impotence.

INTERACTIONS: See Contraindications. May alter insulin requirements. Avoid with weight loss products including SSRIs. Valvular heart disease and primary pulmonary hypertension reported with fenfluramine and dexfenfluramine. May decrease effects of adrenergic neuron blocking agents.

PREGNANCY: Safety in pregnancy and nursing not known.

MECHANISM OF ACTION: Anorectic sympathomimetic amine; not established as appetite suppressor; causes CNS stimulation and elevation of BP.

IOPIDINE RX
apraclonidine HCL (Alcon)

THERAPEUTIC CLASS: Alpha adrenergic agonist

INDICATIONS: (0.5%) Short-term adjunct in patients on maximally tolerated medical therapy who require additional IOP reduction. (1%) To control or prevent postsurgical IOP elevations that occur after laser surgery.

DOSAGE: *Adults:* (0.5%) 1-2 drops tid. Space dosing of other ophthalmic drugs by 5 min. (1%) 1 drop 1 hr pre-op, then 1 drop immediately post-op.

HOW SUPPLIED: Sol: 0.5% [5mL, 10mL], 1% [0.1mL 24ˢ]

CONTRAINDICATIONS: Hypersensitivity to clonidine, concomitant MAOIs.

WARNINGS/PRECAUTIONS: Vasovagal attacks may occur during laser surgery. Monitor visual fields periodically. Monitor CV parameters with renal or hepatic dysfunction. Caution with severe cardiovascular disease, HTN, coronary insufficiency, recent MI, cerebrovascular disease, chronic renal failure, Raynaud's disease, depression, or thromboangitis obliterans. D/C if allergic-like symptoms occur. May cause dizziness or somnolence.

ADVERSE REACTIONS: Hyperemia, ocular pruritus, tearing, ocular discomfort, dry mouth, taste perversion, conjunctival blanching, mydriasis.

INTERACTIONS: (0.5%, 1%) Avoid MAOIs. (0.5%) May potentiate CNS depressants. TCAs may decrease effects. May have additive hypotensive effects with neuroleptics. Caution with β-blockers, antihypertensives, and cardiac glycosides. May potentiate the risk of insulin-induced hypoglycemia. Wait 5 minutes before administering other drops.

PREGNANCY: Category C, (0.5%) caution in nursing, and (1%) not for use in nursing.

MECHANISM OF ACTION: Selective α-2-adrenergic agonist; responsible for reducing aqueous flow which leads to a decrease in intraocular pressure.

PHARMACOKINETICS: Absorption: T_{max}=3 hrs. **Metabolism:** Liver (partly metabolized) (systemic dosage form). **Excretion:** $T_{1/2}$=8 hrs,(Iopidine 0.5%).

IQUIX RX
levofloxacin (Santen)

THERAPEUTIC CLASS: Fluoroquinolone

INDICATIONS: Bacterial corneal ulcer.

DOSAGE: *Adults:* Days 1-3: 1-2 drops q30min-2h while awake and 4-6 hrs after retiring. Days 4-completion: 1-2 drops q1-4h while awake.
Pediatrics: ≥6 yrs: Days 1-3: 1-2 drops q30min-2h while awake and 4-6 hrs after retiring. Days 4-completion: 1-2 drops q1-4h while awake.

HOW SUPPLIED: Sol: 1.5% [5mL]

WARNINGS/PRECAUTIONS: D/C if hypersensitivity or superinfection occurs. Avoid contact lenses with corneal ulcer.

ADVERSE REACTIONS: Headache, taste disturbance.

INTERACTIONS: Systemic quinolone therapy increases theophylline levels, interferes with caffeine metabolism, enhances warfarin effects, and may elevate SCr with cyclosporine.

PREGNANCY: Category C, caution in nursing.

MECHANISM OF ACTION: Fluoroquinolone; antibacterial active against a broad spectrum of gram-positive and gram-negative ocular pathogens. Responsible for inhibition of bacterial topoisomerase IV and DNA gyrase, enzymes required for DNA replication, transcription, repair, and recombination.

PHARMACOKINETICS: Absorption: C_{max}=3.22ng/mL (initial dose), 10.9ng/mL (multiple doses).

ISENTRESS   RX
raltegravir potassium (Merck)

THERAPEUTIC CLASS: HIV-integrase strand transfer inhibitor

INDICATIONS: For use in combination with other antiretroviral agents for treatment of HIV-1 infection in treatment-experienced adults who have evidence of viral replication and HIV-1 strains resistant to multiple antiretroviral agents.

DOSAGE: *Adults:* 400mg bid.

HOW SUPPLIED: Tab: 400mg

WARNINGS/PRECAUTIONS: Monitor for immune reconstitution syndrome.

ADVERSE REACTIONS: Diarrhea, nausea, headache, pyrexia.

INTERACTIONS: Strong inducers of uridine diphosphate glucuronosyltransferase (UGT) 1A1 (eg, rifampin) may reduce plasma levels; use with caution.

PREGNANCY: Category C, not for use in nursing.

MECHANISM OF ACTION: HIV integrase strand transfer inhibitor; inhibits the catalytic activity of HIV-1 intergrase by preventing formation of HIV-1 provirus.

PHARMACOKINETICS: Absorption: T_{max}=3 hrs (fasting); variable doses resulted in different parameters. **Distribution:** Plasma protein binding (83%). **Metabolism:** Glucuronidation via UGT1A1. **Elimination:** $T_{1/2}$=9 hrs; urine (32%), feces (51%).

ISMO   RX
isosorbide mononitrate (ESP Pharma)

THERAPEUTIC CLASS: Nitrate vasodilator

INDICATIONS: Prevention of angina pectoris. Not for acute attack.

DOSAGE: *Adults:* 20mg bid; first dose on awakening, then 7 hrs later.

HOW SUPPLIED: Tab: 20mg* *scored

WARNINGS/PRECAUTIONS: Not for use with acute MI or CHF. Severe hypotension may occur. May aggravate angina caused by hypertrophic cardiomyopathy. Caution with volume depletion, elderly. Monitor for tolerance.

ADVERSE REACTIONS: Headache, dizziness, nausea, vomiting.

INTERACTIONS: Severe hypotension with sildenafil. Marked orthostatic hypotension with CCBs. Additive vasodilation with other vasodilators (eg, alcohol).

PREGNANCY: Category C, caution in nursing.

MECHANISM OF ACTION: Nitrate vasodilator; relaxes vascular smooth muscle, and consequent dilatation of peripheral arteries and veins, especially the latter. Dilatation of the veins leads to reducing the left ventricular end-diastolic pressure and pulmonary capillary wedge pressure (preload). Arteriolar relaxation reduces systemic vascular resistance, systolic arterial pressure and mean arterial pressure (afterload). It also dilates the coronary artery.

PHARMACOKINETICS: Absorption: Absolute bioavailability (100%). T_{max}=30-60 min. **Distribution:** V_d= 0.6L/kg. Plasma protein bound (<4%). **Metabolism:** Liver. Cleared through glucuronidation to the mononitrate glucuronide; and denitration/hydration to sorbitol. **Elimination:** Urine (<1%). $T_{1/2}$=5 hrs.

ISONIAZID RX
isoniazid (Various)

> Severe, fatal hepatitis may develop. Monitor LFTs monthly.

OTHER BRAND NAMES: Nydrazid (Sandoz)

THERAPEUTIC CLASS: Isonicotinic acid hydrazide

INDICATIONS: Prevention and treatment of TB.

DOSAGE: *Adults:* Active TB: 5mg/kg as a single dose. Max: 300mg/day or 15mg/kg 2 to 3 times/week. Max: 900mg/day. Use with other antituberculosis agents. Prevention: 300mg qd single dose.
Pediatrics: Active TB: 10-15mg/kg as a single dose. Max: 300mg qd or 20-40mg/kg 2 to 3 times/week. Max: 900mg/day. Use with other antituberculosis agents. Prevention: 10mg/kg qd single dose. Max: 300mg qd.

HOW SUPPLIED: Inj: 100mg/mL; Syrup: 50mg/5mL; Tab: 100mg, 300mg

CONTRAINDICATIONS: Severe hypersensitivity reactions including drug-induced hepatitis, previous INH-associated hepatic injury, severe adverse effects to INH (eg, drug fever, chills, arthritis), acute liver disease.

WARNINGS/PRECAUTIONS: D/C if hypersensitivity occurs. Monitor closely with liver or renal disease. Take with vitamin B_6 in malnourished and those predisposed to neuropathy.

ADVERSE REACTIONS: Peripheral neuropathy, nausea, vomiting, epigastric distress, elevated serum transaminases, bilirubinemia, jaundice, hepatitis, skin eruptions, pyridoxine deficiency.

INTERACTIONS: Alcohol is associated with hepatitis. May increase phenytoin, theophylline, and valproate serum levels. Do not take with food. Severe acetaminophen toxicity reported. Decreases carbamazepine metabolism and AUC of ketoconazole. Avoid tyramine- and histamine-containing foods.

PREGNANCY: Category C, caution in nursing.

MECHANISM OF ACTION: Inhibits mycoloic acid synthesis and acts against actively growing tuberculosis bacilli.

PHARMACOKINETICS: Distribution: Passes through placental barrier and into milk. **Metabolism:** Acetylation and dehydrazination. **Elimination:** Urine (50-70%).

ISOPTO CARBACHOL RX
carbachol (Alcon)

THERAPEUTIC CLASS: Cholinergic agent

INDICATIONS: To lower IOP in glaucoma treatment.

DOSAGE: *Adults:* 2 drops in eye up to tid.

HOW SUPPLIED: Sol: 1.5% [15mL], 3% [15mL, 30mL]

CONTRAINDICATIONS: Conditions where constriction is undesirable (eg, acute iritis).

WARNINGS/PRECAUTIONS: For topical use only. Caution with corneal abrasion; excessive penetration may produce systemic toxicity. Caution with acute cardiac failure, asthma, active peptic ulcer, hyperthyroidism, GI spasm, urinary tract obstruction, Parkinson's disease, recent MI, HTN, or hypotension. Retinal detachment reported. Caution in night driving or hazardous activity in poor light. Do not touch container tip to any surface to avoid contamination.

ADVERSE REACTIONS: Burning, stinging, headache, ciliary spasm, visual acuity decrease, salivation, syncope, arrhythmia, GI cramping, vomiting, asthma, hypotension, diarrhea, frequent urge to urinate, increased sweating, eye irritation.

PREGNANCY: Category C, caution in nursing.

MECHANISM OF ACTION: Cholinergic (parasympathomimetic) agent. Acts directly to stimulate muscarinic (smooth muscle) and nicotinic (autonomic ganglia) receptors and indirectly to inhibit cholinesterase enzyme activity.

ISOSORBIDE DINITRATE   RX
isosorbide dinitrate (Various)

OTHER BRAND NAMES: Isordil Titradose (Biovail) - Isordil (Biovail)

THERAPEUTIC CLASS: Nitrate vasodilator

INDICATIONS: Prevention of angina pectoris due to coronary artery disease.

DOSAGE: *Adults:* Prevention: Initial: 5-20mg bid-tid. Maint: 10-40mg bid-tid. Allow a dose-free interval of at least 14 hrs for both formulations. Elderly: Start at low end of dosing range.

HOW SUPPLIED: Tab: 5mg*, 10mg*, 20mg*, 30mg*; Tab, Extended-Release: 40mg; Tab, Sublingual: 2.5mg *scored

WARNINGS/PRECAUTIONS: Not for use with acute MI or CHF. Severe hypotension may occur. May aggravate angina caused by hypertrophic cardiomyopathy. Caution with volume depletion, hypotension, elderly. Monitor for tolerance.

ADVERSE REACTIONS: Headache, lightheadedness, hypotension, syncope, rebound HTN.

INTERACTIONS: Severe hypotension with sildenafil. Additive vasodilation with other vasodilators (eg, alcohol).

PREGNANCY: Category C, caution in nursing.

MECHANISM OF ACTION: Nitrate vasodilator; relaxes vascular smooth muscle, dilates peripheral arteries and veins, especially the latter. Dilatation of the veins reduces left ventricular end diastolic pressure and pulmonary capillary wedge pressure (preload). Arteriolar relaxation reduces systemic vascular resistance, systolic arterial pressure, and mean arterial pressure (afterload). It also dilates the coronary artery.

PHARMACOKINETICS: Absorption: T_{max}=1 hr. **Distribution:** V_d=2-4L/kg. **Metabolism:** Liver; extensive first-pass metabolism; 2-mononitrate, 5-mononitrate (active metabolites). **Elimination:** $T_{1/2}$=5 hrs (5-mononitrate), 2 hrs (2-mononitrate).

ISRADIPINE   RX
isradipine (Amide)

THERAPEUTIC CLASS: Calcium channel blocker (dihydropyridine)

INDICATIONS: Management of hypertension.

DOSAGE: *Adults:* Initial: 2.5mg bid alone or with a thiazide diuretic. Titrate: May adjust by 5mg/day at 2-4 week intervals. Max: 20mg/day.

HOW SUPPLIED: Cap: 2.5mg, 5mg

WARNINGS/PRECAUTIONS: May produce symptomatic hypotension. Caution in CHF, especially with concomitant β-blockers. Increased bioavailability in elderly, patients with hepatic functional impairment, and mild renal impairment.

ADVERSE REACTIONS: Headache, edema, dizziness, palpitations, chest pain, constipation, fatigue, flushing, abdominal discomfort, tachycardia, rash, pollakiura, weakness, vomiting.

INTERACTIONS: Additive effects with HCTZ. Severe hypotension possible with fentanyl and β-blockers or CCBs. Increases AUC and Cmax of propranolol. Increased mean peak plasma concentration with cimetidine. Decreased levels with rifampicin.

PREGNANCY: Category C, not for use in nursing.

MECHANISM OF ACTION: Dihydropyridine calcium channel blocker; binds to calcium channels and inhibits calcium flux into cardiac and smooth muscle.

PHARMACOKINETICS: Absorption: C_{max}=1ng/mL/mg; T_{max}=1.5 hrs. **Distribution:** Plasma protein binding (95%); V_d=3L/kg. **Metabolism:** Completely metabolized to 6 metabolites. **Elimination:** Urine (60-65%), feces (25-30%); $T_{1/2}$=8 hrs.

ISTALOL RX
timolol maleate (Ista)

THERAPEUTIC CLASS: Nonselective beta-blocker

INDICATIONS: Treatment of elevated IOP in patients with open-angle glaucoma or ocular hypertension.

DOSAGE: *Adults:* 1 drop in affected eye qam.

HOW SUPPLIED: Sol: 0.5% [2.5mL, 5mL]

CONTRAINDICATIONS: Bronchial asthma, history of bronchial asthma, severe COPD, sinus bradycardia, 2nd- or 3rd-degree AV block, overt cardiac failure, cardiogenic shock.

WARNINGS/PRECAUTIONS: Caution with cardiac failure, DM and cerebrovascular insufficiency. Severe cardiac and respiratory reactions reported. May mask symptoms of hypoglycemia and hyperthyroidism. Reinsert contact lenses 15 minutes after applying drops. Avoid with COPD, bronchospastic disease. Not for use alone in angle-closure glaucoma. May potentiate muscle weakness. D/C at 1st sign of cardiac failure. Withdrawal before surgery is controversial.

ADVERSE REACTIONS: Ocular burning, ocular stinging, blurred vision, cataract, conjunctival injection, headache, HTN, infection, itching, decreased visual acuity.

INTERACTIONS: May potentiate systemic/ophthalmic β-blockers and catecholamine-depleting drugs (eg, reserpine). Oral/IV calcium antagonists can cause AV conduction disturbances, left ventricular failure, or hypotension. Digitalis can cause additive effects in prolonging AV conduction time. Quinidine may potentiate β-blockade. May antagonize epinephrine. May exacerbate rebound HTN following clonidine withdrawal.

PREGNANCY: Category C, not for use in nursing.

MECHANISM OF ACTION: Nonselective β-blocker: does not have significant intrinsic sympathomimetic, direct myocardial depressant, or local anesthetic activity. When applied topically on eye, reduces elevated as well as normal IOP.

PHARMACOKINETICS: Absorption: T_{max}=1-2 hrs; C_{max}=0.68ng/mL (single dose), 0.88ng/mL (multiple doses).

IXEMPRA RX
ixabepilone (Bristol-Myers Squibb)

> Contraindicated in combination with capecitabine in patients with AST/ALT >2.5x ULN or bilirubin >1x ULN due to increased toxicity and neutropenia-related death.

THERAPEUTIC CLASS: Antimicrotubule agent

INDICATIONS: In combination with capecitabine for treatment of patients with metastatic or locally advanced breast cancer resistant to treatment with an anthracycline and a taxane, or whose cancer is taxane resistant and for whom further anthracycline therapy is contraindicated. As monotherapy for treatment of metastatic or locally advanced breast cancer in patients whose tumors are resistant or refractory to anthracyclines, taxanes, and capecitabine.

DOSAGE: *Adults:* 40mg/m² IV infusion over 3 hrs every 3 weeks. Adjust dose based on toxicities (see PI). Premedicate with H₁-antagonist (eg, diphenhydramine 50mg PO) and H₂-antagonist (eg, ranitidine 150-300mg PO) approximately 1 hr before infusion. Also premedicate with corticosteroid (eg, dexamethasone 20mg, IV 30 min before infusion or PO 60 min before infusion) if prior hypersensitivity reaction to ixabepilone. Hepatic Impairment: Monotherapy: Mild: AST and ALT ≤2.5x ULN and Bilirubin ≤1x ULN: 40mg/m². AST or ALT ≤10x ULN and Bilirubin ≤1x ULN: 32mg/m². Moderate (AST and ALT ≤10x ULN and Bilirubin >1.5 to ≤3x ULN): 20-30mg/m². Strong CYP3A4 Inhibitors: Avoid or reduce dose to 20mg/m².

HOW SUPPLIED: Inj: 15mg, 45mg

CONTRAINDICATIONS: Baseline neutrophil count <1500cells/mm³ or platelet count <100,000cells/mm³. In combination with capecitabine, AST or ALT >2.5x ULN or bilirubin >1x ULN. History of severe (CTC Grade 3/4) hypersensitivity reaction to Cremophor® EL or derivatives (eg, polyoxyethylated castor oil).

WARNINGS/PRECAUTIONS: Peipheral neuropathy may occur; monitor for symptoms and manage by dose adjustment and delays. Myelopsuppression, primarily neutropenia, may occur and is dose-dependent; monitor with frequent peripheral blood cell counts and adjust dose as needed. Hypersensitivity reactions may occur; premedicate all patients with H₁- and H₂-antagonists 1 hr before treatment. Caution with history of cardiac disease. Consider discontinuation of therapy if cardiac ischemia or impaired cardiac function develops. Avoid monotherapy if AST or ALT >10x ULN or bilirubin >3x ULN and use caution if AST or ALT >5x ULN.

ADVERSE REACTIONS: Peripheral neuropathy, fatigue/asthenia, myalgia/arthralgia, alopecia, nausea, vomiting, stomatitis/mucositis, diarrhea, musculoskeletal pain, palmar-plantar erythrodysesthesia (hand-foot) syndrome, anorexia, abdominal pain, nail disorder, constipation, neutropenia, leukopenia, anemia, thrombocytopenia.

INTERACTIONS: CYP3A4 inhibitors may increase levels; avoid or reduce dose with strong CYP3A4 inhibitors (eg, ketoconazole, itraconazole, clarithromycin, atazanavir, nefazodone, saquinavir, telithromycin, ritonavir, amprenavir, indinavir, nelfinavir, delavirdine, voriconazole), use caution with mild/moderate CYP3A4 inhibitors (eg, erythromycin, fluconazole, verapamil), and monitor all patients closely for acute toxicities. Strong CYP3A4 inducers (eg, dexamethasone, phenytoin, carbamazepine, rifampin, rifampicin, rifabutin, phenobarbital) may decrease levels; consider alternative agents. St. John's wort may decrease levels and should be avoided.

PREGNANCY: Category D, not for use in nursing.

MECHANISM OF ACTION: Microtubule inhibitor: binds directly to β-tubulin subunits on microtubules, leading to suppression of microtubule dynamics.

PHARMACOKINETICS: Absorption: C_{max}=252ng/mL; AUC=2143ng•hr/mL; T_{max}=3 hrs. **Distribution:** V_d=1000L. **Metabolism:** Liver (oxidation) via CYP3A4. **Elimination:** $T_{1/2}$=52 hrs; urine (1.6%), feces (5.6%).

JANUMET   RX
metformin HCL - sitagliptin (Merck)

> Lactic acidosis may occur due to metformin accumulation. If acidosis suspected, d/c drug and hospitalize patient immediately.

THERAPEUTIC CLASS: Dipeptidyl peptidase-4 inhibitor/biguanide

INDICATIONS: Adjunct to diet and exercise to improve glycemic control in adult patients with type 2 diabetes mellitus who are not adequately controlled on metformin or sitagliptin alone or in patients already being treated with the combination of sitagliptin and metformin. Not for use in patients with type 1 diabetes or for treatment of diabetic ketoacidosis.

DOSAGE: *Adults:* Individualize dosing. Patient Not Controlled on Metformin Monotherapy: Initial: 100mg/day (50mg bid) of sitagliptin + metformin dose. Patient on Metformin 850mg BID: Initial: 50mg-1000mg tab bid. Patient Not

Controlled on Sitagliptin Monotherapy: Initial: 50mg-500mg tab bid. Titrate: Gradual increase to 50mg-1000mg tab bid. Max: 100mg of sitagliptin and 2000mg of metformin. Take with meals

HOW SUPPLIED: Tab: (Sitagliptin-Metformin) 50mg-500mg, 50mg-1000mg

CONTRAINDICATIONS: Renal disease (SrCR ≥1.5mg/dL [males], ≥1.4mg/dL [females], or abnormal CrCl), metabolic acidosis, including diabetic ketoacidosis. D/C for 48 hrs in patients undergoing radiologic studies with intravascular iodinated contrast materials.

WARNINGS/PRECAUTIONS: Lactic acidosis reported (rare), increased risk with renal dysfunction. Assess renal function prior to initiation and during treatment; caution in elderly. Avoid in renal/hepatic impairment. May decrease vitamin B_{12} levels; monitor hematologic parameters. May cause hypoglycemia in elderly, debilitated/malnourished, adrenal or pituitary insufficiency, or alcohol intoxication. D/C in hypoxic states (eg, CHF, shock, acute MI), prior to surgical procedures (due to restricted food and fluid intake), and procedures requiring use of intravascular iodinated contrast materials.

ADVERSE REACTIONS: (Metformin) Diarrhea, nausea/vomiting, flatulence, abdominal discomfort, indigestion, asthenia, and headache. (Sitagliptin) Nasopharyngitis.

INTERACTIONS: Furosemide, nifedipine, and cationic drugs (eg, digoxin, amiloride, procainamide, quinidine, quinine, rantidine, trimethoprim, vancomycin, triamterene, morphine) may increase metformin levels. Caution with concomitant medications affecting renal function or metformin disposition. Thiazides and other diuretics, corticosteroids, phenothiazines, thyroid products, estrogens, oral contraceptives, phenytoin, nicotinic acid, sympathomimetics, CCB, and isoniazid may cause hyperglycemia. Alcohol may potentiate effect of metformin on lactate metabolism; avoid excessive alcohol intake. May decrease furosemide levels. Monitor digoxin levels

PREGNANCY: Category B, caution in nursing.

MECHANISM OF ACTION: Sitagliptin: Dipeptidyl peptidase-4 inhibitor; acts by slowing the inactivation of incretin hormones. Metformin: Biguanide; decreases hepatic glucose production, decreases intestinal absorption of glucose, and improves insulin selectivity by increasing peripheral glucose uptake and utilization.

PHARMACOKINETICS: Absorption: Sitagliptin: Absolute bioavailability (87%). Metformin: Absolute bioavailability (50-60%). **Distribution**: Sitagliptin: V_d=198L. Metformin: V_d=654L, Plasma protein binding (38%). **Metabolism:** Sitagliptin: CYP3A4 and CYP2C8. **Elimination**: Sitagliptin: $T_{1/2}$=12.4 hrs; feces (13%), urine (87%). Metformin: $T_{1/2}$=6.2 hrs (plasma); $T_{1/2}$=17.6 hrs (blood); urine (90%).

JANUVIA   RX
sitagliptin phosphate (Merck)

THERAPEUTIC CLASS: Dipeptidyl peptidase-4 inhibitor

INDICATIONS: Monotherapy/Combination Therapy: Adjunct to diet and exercise to improve glycemic control in patients with type 2 diabetes mellitus. Avoid use in patients with type I diabetes or for treatment of diabetic ketoacidosis. Not studied in combination with insulin.

DOSAGE: *Adults:* 100mg qd. CrCl ≥30 to <50mL/min: 50mg qd. CrCl: <30mL/min: 25mg qd.

HOW SUPPLIED: Tab: 25mg, 50mg, 100mg

CONTRAINDICATIONS: Anaphylaxis or angioedema

WARNINGS/PRECAUTIONS: Assess renal function prior to initiation of treatment. Cause hypoglycemia when used in combination with a sulfonylurea. Anaphylaxis, angioedema, and exfoliative skin conditions reported.

ADVERSE REACTIONS: (Monotherapy/Combination therapy) Upper respiratory tract infection, nasopharyngitis, headache. (Combination therapy) hypoglycemia.

INTERACTIONS: May slightly increase digoxin levels; monitor appropriately. May require lower dose of sulfonylurea to reduce risk of hypoglycemia.

PREGNANCY: Category B, caution in nursing.

MECHANISM OF ACTION: Dipeptidyl peptidase-4 inhibitor; suspected to exert its action by slowing the inactivation of incretin hormones.

PHARMACOKINETICS: Absorption: Rapidly absorbed. Absolute bioavailability (87%); T_{max}=1-4 hrs; AUC= 8.52μM•hr; C_{max}=950 nM. **Distribution:** Plasma protein bound (38%). V_d=198L. **Metabolism:** Via CYP3A4 and CYP2C8 (minor). **Elimination:** $T_{1/2}$=12.4 hrs; feces (13%), urine (87%).

KADIAN
morphine sulfate (Alpharma)

> Contains morphine sulfate, an opioid agonist and Schedule II controlled substance, with an abuse liability similar to other opioid analgesics. Indicated for management of moderate-to-severe pain when a continuous, around-the-clock opioid analgesic is needed for an extended period of time. Not for use as a prn analgesic. The 100mg and 200mg capsules are for use in opioid-tolerant patients only. Swallow capsules whole or sprinkle contents on apple sauce. Do not crush, chew, or dissolve pellets in capsules.

THERAPEUTIC CLASS: Opioid analgesic

INDICATIONS: Management of moderate to severe pain.

DOSAGE: *Adults:* Individualize dose. Conversion from other Oral Morphine: Give 50% of daily oral morphine dose q12h or give 100% oral morphine dose q24h. Do not give more frequently than q12h. Conversion from Parenteral Morphine: Oral morphine 3x the daily parenteral morphine dose may be sufficient in chronic use settings. Conversion from Other Parenteral or Oral Opioids: Initial: Give 50% of estimated daily morphine demand and supplement with immediate-release morphine. May sprinkle contents on small amount of applesauce or in water for gastrostomy tube. Do not chew, crush or dissolve pellets. Avoid administration through NG-tube.

HOW SUPPLIED: Cap, Extended-Release: 10mg, 20mg, 30mg, 50mg, 60mg, 80mg, 100mg, 200mg

CONTRAINDICATIONS: Respiratory depression in the absence of resuscitative equipment, acute or severe bronchial asthma, paralytic ileus.

WARNINGS/PRECAUTIONS: Respiratory depression possible; caution in COPD, cor pulmonale, decreased respiratory reserve. May obscure neurologic signs in head injuries, intracranial lesions, or a pre-existing increase in ICP. May cause severe hypotension. Avoid with GI obstruction. Caution in biliary tract disease, elderly, debilitated, renal/hepatic insufficiency, Addison's disease, myxedema, hypothyroidism, prostatic hypertrophy, urethral stricture, CNS depression, toxic psychosis, acute alcoholism, delirium tremens, and convulsive disorders. Depresses cough reflex. Decreases gastric, biliary, and pancreatic secretions. D/C 24 hrs before procedure that interrupts pain transmission pathways (eg, cordotomy); give short-acting parenteral opioid.

ADVERSE REACTIONS: Drowsiness, dizziness, constipation, nausea, anxiety.

INTERACTIONS: Increased risk of respiratory depression, hypotension, profound sedation or coma with CNS depressants (eg, sedatives, hypnotics, general anesthetics, antiemetics, phenothiazines, tranquilizers, alcohol); reduce initial dose of one or both agents by 50%. May enhance neuromuscular blocking action of skeletal relaxants. Mixed agonist/antagonist analgesics may reduce analgesic effects or precipitate withdrawal symptoms. Avoid MAOIs during or within 14 days of use. May reduce diuretic effects.

PREGNANCY: Category C, not for use in nursing.

MECHANISM OF ACTION: Opioid analgesic; principle actions are analgesia and sedation. Precise mechanism of analgesic effects not established. Acts as a pure agonist, binding with and activating opioid receptors at sites in the peri-aqueductal and periventricular gray matter, the ventromedial medulla, and the spinal cord to produce analgesia.

PHARMACOKINETICS: Absorption: Various doses resulted in different parameters. **Distribution:** Plasma protein binding (30-35%); V_d=3-4 L/kg; distributed to skeletal muscle, kidneys, liver, intestinal tract, lungs, spleen, brain; crossess the blood brain barrier (small amount); crosses placental membranes; found in breast milk. **Metabolism:** Liver (conjugation) to glucuronide metabolites; morphine-3-glucuronide (major metabolite), morphine-6-glucuronide (active metabolite). **Elimination:** Urine (major) (metabolites, 10% unchanged); bile (small amount); feces (7-10%); $T_{1/2}$=2-4 hrs.

KALETRA   RX
ritonavir - lopinavir (Abbott)

THERAPEUTIC CLASS: Protease inhibitor

INDICATIONS: Treatment of HIV infection in combination with other antiretrovirals.

DOSAGE: *Adults:* Therapy-Naive: 400/100mg (2 tabs or 5mL) bid or 800/200mg qd (4 tabs or 10mL). Therapy-Experienced: 400/100mg (2 tabs or 5mL) bid. Once daily administration not recommended. Concomitant Efavirenz, Nevirapine, Fosamprenavir, Nelfinavir: Therapy-Naive: 400/100mg (2 tabs) bid. Concomitant Efavirenz, Nevirapine, Amprenavir or Nelfinavir: 533/133mg (6.5mL) bid. Concomitant Efavirenz, Nevirapine, Fosamprenavir without Ritonavir, or Nelfinavir: Treatment-Experienced with Decreased Susceptibility to Lopinavir: 600/150mg (3 tabs) bid. Tabs can be taken with or without food. Oral solution must be taken with food.
Pediatrics: >12 yrs: Therapy-Naive: 400/100mg (2 tabs or 5mL) bid or 800/200mg qd (4 tabs or 10mL). Therapy-Experienced: 400/100mg (2 tabs or 5mL) bid. Once daily administration not recommended. Concomitant Efavirenz, Nevirapine, Fosamprenavir, Nelfinavir: Therapy-Naive: 400/100mg (2 tabs) bid. Concomitant Efavirenz, Nevirapine, Amprenavir or Nelfinavir: 533/133mg (6.5mL) bid. Concomitant Efavirenz, Nevirapine, Fosamprenavir without Ritonavir, or Nelfinavir: Treatment-Experienced with Decreased Susceptibility to Lopinavir: 600/150mg (3 tabs) bid. 6 months-12 yrs: >40kg: 400/100mg (4 tabs 100/25 mg, 2 tabs 200/50 mg or 5 mL) bid. 15-40kg: (Tab,Sol) 10/2.5mg/kg bid. 7-<15kg: (Sol) 12/3mg/kg bid. Concomitant Efavirenz, Nevirapine, (Fos)amprenavir: >45kg: 533/133mg (4 tabs 100/25 mg, 2 tabs 200/50 mg, or 6.5mL) bid. 15-45kg: (Tab,Sol) 11/2.75mg/kg bid. 7-<15kg: (Sol) 13/3.25mg/kg bid. Tabs can be taken with or without food. Oral solution must be taken with food.

HOW SUPPLIED: Tab: (Lopinavir-Ritonavir) 200mg-50mg, 100mg-25mg; Sol: 80mg-20mg/mL [160mL]

CONTRAINDICATIONS: Concomitant drugs dependent on CYP3A or CYP2D6 for clearance (eg, rifampin, St John's wort, lovastatin, simvastatin, dihydroergotamine, ergonovine, ergotamine, methylergonovine, cisapride, pimozide, midazolam, triazolam).

WARNINGS/PRECAUTIONS: May elevate triglyceride and total cholesterol levels; monitor levels at baseline then periodically. Possible redistribution or accumulation of body fat. D/C if symptoms of pancreatitis occur. May exacerbate DM or cause hyperglycemia. Caution in hepatic impairment. Increased bleeding may occur with hemophilia A and B. Risk of further transaminase elevation or hepatic decompensation in patients with underlying hepatitis B or C or marked transaminase elevation prior to treatment; monitor ALT/AST more frequently during first several months of therapy. Hepatic dysfunction reported.

ADVERSE REACTIONS: Abdominal pain, asthenia, headache, diarrhea, nausea, vomiting, dyspepsia, flatulence, insomnia, hepatotoxicity, pancreatitis.

INTERACTIONS: See Contraindications. Avoid use with rifampin, St. John's wort; may cause loss of virologic response and resistance. Avoid use with lovastatin and simvastatin; risk of myopathy and rhabdomyolysis. May increase levels of antiarrhythmics (eg, amiodarone, bepridil, systemic lidocaine, quinidine), dihydropyridine CCBs (eg, felodipine, nifedipine, nicardipine), immunosuppressants (eg, cyclosporine, tacrolimus, rapamycin); monitoring recommended. May increase levels of trazodone; use with caution and consider lower trazodone dose. May increase levels of fluticasone; coadministration not recommended. CYP3A inducers may decrease lopinavir levels. CYP3A inhibitors may increase lopinavir levels. May increase levels of drugs primarily metabolized by CYP3A. May increase levels of amprenavir, indinavir, saquinavir. May increase levels of clarithromycin with renal impairment; reduce clarithromycin dose by 50% if CrCl 30-60mL/min and by 75% if CrCl <30mL/min. Decreased effect with dexamethasone, carbamazepine, phenobarbital, phenytoin. Monitor PT/INR with warfarin. Space dosing with didanosine; give 1 hr before or 2 hrs after lopinavir/ritonavir. Increased levels with delavirdine. Efavirenz, nevirapine, and tipranavir may decrease levels; adjust dose. May increase levels of ketoconazole or itraconazole; avoid ketoconazole or itraconazole doses >200mg/day. May increase rifabutin levels; reduce usual rifabutin dose by 75%. Decreases atovaquone levels. Oral solution contains alcohol; disulfiram reaction may occur with disulfiram or metronidazole. May increase sildenafil, tadalafil, vardenafil levels; reduce dose of sildenafil (eg, 25mg q48h); reduce dose of tadalafil (eg, 10mg q72h); reduce dose of vardenafil (eg, 2.5mg q72h). May decrease methadone levels; may need to increase methadone dose. May decrease ethinyl estradiol levels; use alternate/additional contraception. Increased atorvastatin levels; use lowest atorvastatin or rosuvastatin dose or consider alternate HMG-CoA reductase inhibitors (eg, pravastatin, fluvastatin). Increases tenofovir levels. May increase nelfinavir levels; dosage adjustments needed. Do not administer with tipranivir coadministered with ritonavir.

PREGNANCY: Category C, not for use in nursing.

MECHANISM OF ACTION: Lopinavir: HIV-1 protease inhibitor; prevents cleavage of the Gag-Pol polyprotein, resulting in the production of immature, noninfectious viral particles. Ritonavir: CYP3A inhibitor; inhibits metabolism of lopinavir, increasing its plasma levels.

PHARMACOKINETICS: Absorption: Lopinavir: T_{max}=4 hrs, C_{max}=9.8mcg/mL, AUC=92.6mcg•h/mL. **Distribution:** Lopinavir: Plasma protein binding (98-99%). **Metabolism:** Lopinavir: Hepatic via CYP3A. Ritonavir: Induces own metabolism. **Elimination:** Urine (2.2%), feces (19.8%).

KAYEXALATE   RX
sodium polystyrene sulfonate (Sanofi-Aventis)

THERAPEUTIC CLASS: Cation-exchange resin

INDICATIONS: Treatment of hyperkalemia.

DOSAGE: *Adults:* PO: 15g qd-qid. Rectal Enema: 30-50g q6h.
Pediatrics: Use 1g per 1mEq of K^+ as basis of calculation. Avoid PO administration in neonates.

HOW SUPPLIED: Sus: 15g/60mL

CONTRAINDICATIONS: Hypokalemia, obstructive bowel disease, neonates with reduced gut motility (post-op or drug-induced), oral administration in neonates.

WARNINGS/PRECAUTIONS: Hypokalemia may occur. May be insufficient for emergency correction of hyperkalemia. Monitor for electrolyte disturbances. Caution in those intolerant to sodium increases (eg, severe CHF or HTN, or marked edema).

ADVERSE REACTIONS: Anorexia, nausea, vomiting, constipation, hypokalemia, hypocalcemia, sodium retention, diarrhea, (elderly) fecal impaction.

INTERACTIONS: Avoid nonabsorbable cation-donating antacids and laxatives; systemic alkalosis may occur (eg, magnesium hydroxide, aluminum carbonate). Hypokalemia exaggerates toxic effects of digitalis. Intestinal obstruction reported with aluminum hydroxide. May decrease absorption of lithium and thyroxine. Avoid sorbitol.

PREGNANCY: Category C, caution in nursing.

MECHANISM OF ACTION: Cation exchange resin; partially releases sodium ions and replaced by K+ ions.

K-DUR   RX
potassium chloride (Schering)

THERAPEUTIC CLASS: K+ supplement

INDICATIONS: (For those unable to tolerate liquid or effervescent potassium preparations). Treatment and prevention of hypokalemia with or without metabolic alkalosis. Treatment of digitalis intoxication and hypokalemic familial periodic paralysis.

DOSAGE: *Adults:* Prevention: 20mEq/day. Hypokalemia: 40-100mEq/day. Divide dose if >20mEq. Take with meals and a full glass of water or liquid. Tab can be broken in half or dissolved in water.

HOW SUPPLIED: Tab, Extended-Release: 10mEq, 20mEq* *scored

CONTRAINDICATIONS: Hyperkalemia, esophageal ulceration, delay in GI passage (from structural, pathological, pharmacologic causes), cardiac patients with esophageal compression due to enlarged left atrium.

WARNINGS/PRECAUTIONS: Potentially fatal hyperkalemia may occur. Extreme caution with acidosis, cardiac and renal disease; monitor ECG and electrolytes. Hypokalemia with metabolic acidosis should be treated with an alkalinizing potassium salt (eg, potassium bicarbonate, potassium citrate). May produce ulcerative or stenotic GI lesions.

ADVERSE REACTIONS: Hyperkalemia, GI effects (obstruction, bleeding, ulceration), nausea, vomiting, abdominal pain, flatulence, diarrhea.

INTERACTIONS: Risk of hyperkalemia with ACE inhibitors (eg, captopril, enalapril), K+-sparing diuretics and K+ supplements. Contraindicated with anticholinergic agents due to possible delay in tablet passage through GI tract.

PREGNANCY: Category C, safe for use in nursing.

MECHANISM OF ACTION: K+ supplement (electrolyte replenisher); potassium ions participate in maintenance of intracellular tonicity, transmission of nerve impulses, contraction of cardiac, skeletal, and smooth muscle, and maintenance of normal renal function.

KEFLEX   RX
cephalexin (Middlebrook)

THERAPEUTIC CLASS: Cephalosporin (1st generation)

INDICATIONS: Treatment of otitis media and skin and skin structure (SSSI), bone, genitourinary tract, and respiratory tract infections caused by susceptible strains of microorganisms.

DOSAGE: *Adults:* Usual: 250mg q6h. Streptococcal Pharyngitis/SSSI/Uncomplicated Cystitis (>15 yrs): 500mg q12h. Treat cystitis for 7-14 days. Max: 4g/day.
Pediatrics: Usual: 25-50mg/kg/day in divided doses. Streptococcal Pharyngitis (>1 yr)/SSSI: May divide dose and give q12h. Otitis Media: 75-100mg/kg/day in divided doses. Administer for ≥10 days in β-hemolytic streptococcal infections.

HOW SUPPLIED: Cap: 250mg, 500mg, 750mg

WARNINGS/PRECAUTIONS: Caution with markedly impaired renal function, history of GI disease. Cross-sensitivity with cephalosporins and PCNs. *Clostridium difficile*-associated diarrhea reported. Positive direct Coombs' tests reported. False (+) for urine glucose with Benedict's, Fehling's solution, and Clinitest® tabs. May result in overgrowth of nonsusceptible bacteria.

ADVERSE REACTIONS: Diarrhea, allergic reactions, dyspepsia, gastritis, abdominal pain, superinfection (prolonged use).

INTERACTIONS: Probenecid inhibits excretion.

PREGNANCY: Category B, caution in nursing.

MECHANISM OF ACTION: Cephalosporin; bactericidal due to inhibition of cell wall synthesis.

PHARMACOKINETICS: Absorption: Rapid; oral administration of variable doses resulted in different parameters. T_{max}=1 hr. **Elimination:** Urine (90%, unchanged).

KENALOG   RX
triamcinolone acetonide (Apothecon)

THERAPEUTIC CLASS: Corticosteroid

INDICATIONS: Corticosteroid responsive dermatoses.

DOSAGE: *Adults:* (Cre, Lot, Oint) Apply 0.025% bid-qid. Apply 0.1% or 0.5% bid-tid. (Spray) Apply tid-qid. May use occlusive dressings for psoriasis or recalcitrant conditions. D/C dressings if infection develops.

HOW SUPPLIED: Cre: 0.1% [15g, 60g, 80g], 0.5% [20g]; Lot: 0.025%, 0.1% [60mL]; Oint: 0.1% [15g, 60g]; Spray: 0.147mg/g [63g]

WARNINGS/PRECAUTIONS: May produce reversible HPA axis suppression, manifestations of Cushing's syndrome, hyperglycemia, and glucosuria. D/C if irritation occurs. Pediatrics may be more susceptible to systemic toxicity. Monitor for HPA suppression if applied to large surface areas or under occlusive dressings. Avoid eyes.

ADVERSE REACTIONS: Burning, itching, irritation, dryness, folliculitis, hypertrichosis, acneiform eruptions, hypopigmentation, perioral dermatitis, allergic contact dermatitis.

PREGNANCY: Category C, caution in nursing.

MECHANISM OF ACTION: Corticosteroid: Possesses anti-inflammatory, antipruritic, and vasoconstrictive actions. Mechanism of anti-inflammatory action not established.

PHARMACOKINETICS: Absorption: Percutaneous; inflammation, other disease states, and use of occlusive dressings may increase absorption. **Distribution:** Systemically administered corticosteroids found in breast milk. **Metabolism:** Liver. **Excretion:** Kidneys, bile.

KEPIVANCE   RX
palifermin (Amgen)

THERAPEUTIC CLASS: Keratinocyte growth factor

INDICATIONS: Decrease the incidence and duration of severe oral mucositis in patients with hematologic malignancies receiving myelotoxic therapy requiring hematopoietic stem cell support.

DOSAGE: *Adults:* 60mcg/kg/day IV bolus 3 consecutive days before and after myelotoxic therapy for a total of 6 doses.

HOW SUPPLIED: Inj: 6.25mg

CONTRAINDICATIONS: Known hypersensitivity to *E.coli*-derived proteins, palifermin, or any other component of the product.

WARNINGS/PRECAUTIONS: Potential for stimulation of tumor growth. Safety and efficacy have not been established in patients with non-hematologic malignancies.

ADVERSE REACTIONS: Rash, erythema, edema, fever, pruritus, dysesthesia, tongue discoloration, tongue thickening, alteration of taste, pain arthralgias.

INTERACTIONS: Do not administer 24 hrs before, during infusion, or 24 hrs after administration of myelotoxic chemotherapy due to risk of increased severity and duration of oral mucositis. If heparin is used to maintain IV line, use saline to rinse prior to and after administration.

PREGNANCY: Category C, caution in nursing.

MECHANISM OF ACTION: Keratinocyte growth factor; binds to the KGF receptor which results in proliferation, differentiation, and migration of the epithelial cells.

PHARMACOKINETICS: Elimination: $T_{1/2}$=4.5 hrs.

KEPPRA

RX

levetiracetam (UCB Pharma)

THERAPEUTIC CLASS: Pyrrolidine derivative

INDICATIONS: (PO) Adjunctive therapy for partial onset seizures in adults and children ≥4 yrs of age. Adjunctive therapy in the treatment of myoclonic seizures in adults and children ≥12 yrs with juvenile myoclonic epilepsy (JME). Adjunctive therapy in the treatment of primary generalized tonic-clonic (PGTC) seizures in adults and children ≥6 yrs with idiopathic generalized epilepsy. (Inj) Adjunctive therapy for partial onset seizures in adults with epilepsy. Adjunctive therapy for myoclonic seizures in adults with JME. Alternative for adults (≥16 yrs) when oral administration is temporarily not feasible.

DOSAGE: *Adults:* Inj/PO: Initial: 500mg bid. Titrate: Increase by 1000mg/day every 2 weeks. Max: 3000mg/day. Inj: Replacement Therapy: Initial total daily dosage and frequency should equal total daily dosage and frequency of oral therapy. Dilute injection in 100mL of compatible diluent and give as 15-min IV infusion. CrCl >80mL/min: 500mg-1500mg q12h. CrCl 50-80mL/min: 500mg-1000mg q12h. CrCl 30-50mL/min: 250mg-750mg q12h. CrCl <30mL/min: 250mg-500mg q12h. ESRD with Dialysis: 500-1000mg q24h. A supplemental dose of 250mg-500mg after dialysis is recommended.
Pediatrics: PO: Partial Onset Seizures/PGTC: ≥16 yrs or JME: ≥12 yrs: Initial: 500mg bid. Titrate: Increase by 1000mg/day every 2 weeks. Max: 3000mg/day. Partial Onset Seizures: 4 to <16 yrs or PGTC: 6-16 yrs: Initial: 10mg/kg bid: Titrate: Increase by 20mg/kg/day every 2 weeks. Max: 60mg/kg/day. Inj: Partial Onset Seizures: Initial: 500mg bid. Titrate: Increase by 1000mg/day every 2 weeks. Max: 3000mg/day. Replacement Therapy: Initial total daily dosage and frequency should equal total daily dosage and frequency of oral therapy. Dilute injection in 100mL of compatible diluent and give as 15-min IV infusion. CrCl >80mL/min: 500mg-1500mg q12h. CrCl 50-80mL/min: 500mg-1000mg q12h. CrCl 30-50mL/min: 250mg-750mg q12h. CrCl <30mL/min: 250mg-500mg q12h. ESRD with Dialysis: 500mg-1000mg q24h. A supplemental dose of 250mg-500mg after dialysis is recommended.

HOW SUPPLIED: Inj: 500mg/5mL; Sol: 100mg/mL; Tab: 250mg*, 500mg*, 750mg*, 1000mg* *scored

WARNINGS/PRECAUTIONS: Associated with somnolence, fatigue, coordination difficulties, and behavioral abnormalities (eg, psychotic symptoms, suicide ideation, and other abnormalities). Avoid abrupt withdrawal. Hematologic abnormalities reported. Caution in renal dysfunction. Myoclonic seizures reported.

ADVERSE REACTIONS: Somnolence, asthenia, headache, infection, pain, anorexia, dizziness, nervousness, vertigo, ataxia, pharyngitis, rhinitis, irritability, hepatic failure.

PREGNANCY: Category C, caution in nursing.

MECHANISM OF ACTION: Antiepileptic drug; not established, proposed that it inhibits burst firing without affecting normal neuronal excitability, suggesting that it may selectively prevent hypersynchronization of epileptiform burst firing and propagation of seizure activity.

PHARMACOKINETICS: Absorption: Rapid; complete. **Distribution:** Plasma protein binding (<10%); excreted in breast milk. **Metabolism:** Enzymatic hydrolysis (not extensive). Metabolite: Ucb L057. **Elimination:** Renal; urine (66%); $T_{1/2}$=6-8 hrs. Refer to PI for pediatric parameters.

KETAMINE
ketamine HCL (Various)

THERAPEUTIC CLASS: Nonbarbiturate anesthetic

INDICATIONS: Sole anesthetic agent for diagnostic and surgical procedures that do not require skeletal muscle relaxation. Induction of anesthesia prior to the administration of other general anesthetic agents. To supplement low-potency agents (eg, nitrous oxide).

DOSAGE: *Adults:* Initial: IV: 1-4.5mg/kg. Infuse slowly over 60 seconds. May administer with 2-5mg doses of diazepam over 60 seconds. IM: 6.5-13mg/kg. Maint: Adjust according to anesthetic needs. May increase in increments of one-half to full induction dose.
Pediatrics: Initial: IV: 1-4.5mg/kg. Infuse slowly over 60 seconds. IM: 6.5-13mg/kg. Maint: Adjust according to anesthetic needs. May increase in increments of one-half to full induction dose.

HOW SUPPLIED: Inj: 50mg/mL

CONTRAINDICATIONS: Patients in whom a significant elevation in BP would constitute a serious hazard.

WARNINGS/PRECAUTIONS: Monitor cardiac function with HTN or cardiac dysfunction. Postoperative confusional states may occur during recovery. Respiratory depression may occur; maintain airway and respiration. Do not use alone in pharynx, larynx, or bronchial tree procedures. Use with caution in chronic alcoholics and acutely intoxicated patients. May increase CSF pressure; use with extreme caution in patients with preanesthetic CSF pressure. Use with agent that obtunds visceral pain when surgical procedure involving visceral pain.

ADVERSE REACTIONS: Nausea, vomiting, anorexia, elevated blood pressure and pulse, hypotension, bradycardia, arrhythmia, respiratory depression, apnea, airway obstruction, diplopia, nystagmus, slight elevation of IOP, enhanced skeletal muscle tone.

INTERACTIONS: Prolonged recovery time with barbiturates and/or narcotics.

PREGNANCY: Not recommended with pregnancy, use in nursing unknown.

MECHANISM OF ACTION: Nonbarbiturate anesthetic; produces anesthetic state characterized by profound analgesia, normal pharyngeal-laryngeal reflexes, normal or slightly enhanced skeletal muscle tone, cardiovascular and respiratory stimulation, and occasionally a transient and minimal respiratory depression.

PHARMACOKINETICS: Metabolism: Hepatic, via N-dealkylation, hydroxylation, conjugation, and dehydration.. **Elimination:** $T_{1/2}$=10-15 min (α phase), $T_{1/2}$=2.5 hrs (β phase).

KETEK
telithromycin (Sanofi-Aventis)   **RX**

> **Contraindicated with myasthenia gravis.**

THERAPEUTIC CLASS: Ketolide antibiotic

INDICATIONS: Treatment of mild to moderate community-acquired pneumonia (CAP) due to susceptible strains of microorganisms.

DOSAGE: *Adults:* 800mg qd for 7-10 days. Severe Renal Impairment (CrCl <30mL/min): 600mg qd. Hemodialysis: Give after dialysis session on dialysis days. Severe Renal Impairment (CrCl <30mL/min) with Hepatic Impairment: 400mg qd.

HOW SUPPLIED: Tab: 300mg, 400mg [Ketek Pak, 20°]

CONTRAINDICATIONS: Myasthenia gravis. History of hepatitis and/or jaundice associated with use of telithromycin or any macrolide antibiotic. Hypersensitivity to macrolide antibiotics; concomitant use with cisapride or pimozide.

WARNINGS/PRECAUTIONS: Acute hepatic failure and severe liver injury, including fulminant hepatitis and hepatic necrosis reported; monitor closely and d/c if any signs/symptoms of hepatitis occur. Visual disturbances and loss of consciousness reported; minimize hazardous activities such as driving and operating heavy machinery. May prolong QTc interval; avoid with congenital prolongation, ongoing proarrhythmic conditions (eg, uncorrected hypokalemia or hypomagnesemia), significant bradycardia. Torsades de pointes reported. *Clostridium difficile*-associated diarrhea reported. Reduce dose with severe renal impairment.

ADVERSE REACTIONS: Diarrhea, nausea, headache, dizziness, visual disturbances, vomiting.

INTERACTIONS: See Contraindications. Increases levels of drugs metabolized by the CYP450 system (eg, carbamazepine, cyclosporine, tacrolimus, sirolimus, hexobarbital, phenytoin, triazolam, metoprolol), especially CYP3A4. Avoid cisapride, pimozide, simvastatin, lovastatin, atorvastatin, rifampin, ergot alkaloid derivatives, Class IA (eg, quinidine, procainamide) or Class III (eg, dofetilide) antiarrhythmics. Increased levels with itraconazole, ketoconazole. Monitor with midazolam, digoxin. Decreased effects with CYP3A4 inducers (eg, phenytoin, carbamazepine, phenobarbital). Decreases levels of sotalol. Space dosing of theophylline by 1 hr to reduce GI effects. Concomitant administration with oral anticoagulants may potentiate effects of the oral anticoagulants.

PREGNANCY: Category C, caution in nursing.

MECHANISM OF ACTION: Ketolide: Blocks protein synthesis by binding to domains II and V of 23S rRNA of 50S ribosomal subunit. Telithromycin may also inhibit assembly of nascent ribosomal units.

PHARMACOKINETICS: Absorption: Absolute bioavailability (57%). T_{max}=1hr; C_{max}=2mcg/mL. **Distribution:** Plasma protein binding (60-70%). V_d=2.9L/kg. **Metabolism:** Metabolized via CYP450 3A4 dependent and independent pathways. **Elimination:** $T_{1/2}$=10 hrs. Feces (7% unchanged); urine (13% unchanged).

KETOCONAZOLE TOPICAL RX

ketoconazole (Various)

THERAPEUTIC CLASS: Azole antifungal

INDICATIONS: (Cre) Tinea corporis, tinea.cruris, tinea pedis, tinea versicolor, cutaneous candidiasis, seborrheic dermatitis. (Shampoo) Tinea versicolor.

DOSAGE: *Adults:* (Cre) Cutaneous candidiasis, t.corporis, t.cruris, t.versicolor: Apply qd for 2 weeks. T.pedis: Apply qd for 6 weeks. Seborrheic Dermatitis: Apply bid for up to 4 weeks. Re-evaluate if no improvement after treatment period. (Shampoo) Apply to damp skin and lather. Rinse with water after 5 min. One application should be sufficient.

HOW SUPPLIED: Cre: 2% [15g, 30g, 60g]; Shampoo: 2% [120mL]

WARNINGS/PRECAUTIONS: Cre contains sulfites. Shampoo may remove curl from permanently waved hair. Avoid eyes.

ADVERSE REACTIONS: (Cre) Irritation, pruritus, stinging. (Shampoo) Abnormal hair texture, scalp pustules, mild skin dryness, pruritus, increase in normal hair loss, oily or dry scalp and hair.

PREGNANCY: Category C, (Cre) not for use in nursing, (Shampoo) caution in nursing.

MECHANISM OF ACTION: Azole antifungal; impairs synthesis of ergosterol, vital component of fungal cell membranes. Broad spectrum antifungal.

KETOPROFEN   RX
ketoprofen (Various)

> NSAIDs may cause an increased risk of serious cardiovascular thrombotic events, MI, stroke, and serious GI adverse events including bleeding, ulceration, and perforation of the stomach or intestines. Contraindicated for the treatment of perioperative pain in the setting of coronary artery bypass graft (CABG) surgery.

THERAPEUTIC CLASS: NSAID (propionic acid derivative)

INDICATIONS: Management of osteoarthritis (OA), rheumatoid arthritis (RA), pain and primary dysmenorrhea.

DOSAGE: *Adults:* OA/RA: 75mg tid or 50mg qid. Max: 300mg/day. Pain/Dysmenorrhea: 25-50mg q6-8h. Max: 300mg. Small Patients/Debilitated/Elderly/Hepatic or Renal Dysfunction: Reduce dose.

HOW SUPPLIED: Cap: 50mg, 75mg

CONTRAINDICATIONS: ASA or other NSAID allergy that precipitates acute asthmatic attack, urticaria, or allergic reactions. Treatment of perioperative pain in the setting of CABG surgery.

WARNINGS/PRECAUTIONS: May lead to onset of new HTN or worsening of pre-existing HTN; monitor BP closely. Fluid retention and edema reported; caution with fluid retention or heart failure. Renal papillary necrosis and other renal injury reported after long-term use. Not recommended for use with advanced renal disease; if therapy must be initiated, monitor renal function. Anaphylactoid reactions may occur. May cause serious skin adverse events (eg, exfoliative dermatitis, Stevens-Johnson syndrome, and toxic epidermal necrolysis). Avoid in late pregnancy; may cause premature closure of ductus arteriosis. May cause elevations of LFTs; d/c if liver disease develops or systemic manifestations occur. Monitor with chronic liver disease and consider dose reduction. Caution in elderly. Anemia may occur; with long-term use, monitor Hgb/Hct if signs or symptoms of anemia develop. May inhibit platelet aggregation and prolong bleeding time; monitor with coagulation disorders. Caution with asthma and avoid with ASA-sensitive asthma.

ADVERSE REACTIONS: Dyspepsia, nausea, abdominal pain, diarrhea, constipation, flatulence, headache, renal dysfunction, LFT abnormalities, CNS effects.

INTERACTIONS: Avoid ASA and probenecid. Renal toxicity potentiated by diuretics. Monitor anticoagulants. May increase levels of methotrexate and lithium.

PREGNANCY: Category C, not for use in nursing.

MECHANISM OF ACTION: NSAID; suspected to inhibit prostaglandin and leukotriene synthesis; exerts anti-inflammatory, analgesic, and antipyretic actions.

PHARMACOKINETICS: Absorption: Rapid and well-absorbed; T_{max}=1.2 hrs (fasted), 2.0 hrs (fed); C_{max}=3.9mg/L (fasted), 2.4mg/L (fed); bioavailability (90%). **Distribution:** Plasma protein binding (>99%). **Metabolism:** Glucuronide conjugation. **Elimination:** $T_{1/2}$=2-4 hrs; urine (80%).

KETOPROFEN EXTENDED-RELEASE   RX
ketoprofen (Various)

> NSAIDs may cause an increased risk of serious cardiovascular thrombotic events, MI, stroke, and serious GI adverse events including bleeding, ulceration, and perforation of the stomach or intestines. Contraindicated for the treatment of perioperative pain in the setting of coronary artery bypass graft (CABG) surgery.

THERAPEUTIC CLASS: NSAID

INDICATIONS: Management of the signs and symptoms of rheumatoid arthritis and osteoarthritis.

DOSAGE: *Adults:* 200mg qd. Max: 200mg/day.

HOW SUPPLIED: Cap, Extended-Release: 100mg, 150mg, 200mg

CONTRAINDICATIONS: ASA or other NSAID allergy that precipitates acute asthmatic attack, urticaria, or allergic reactions. Treatment of perioperative pain in the setting of CABG surgery.

WARNINGS/PRECAUTIONS: May lead to onset of new HTN or worsening of pre-existing HTN; monitor BP closely. Fluid retention and edema reported; caution with fluid retention or heart failure. Renal papillary necrosis and other renal injury reported after long-term use. Not recommended for use with advanced renal disease; if therapy must be initiated, monitor renal function. Anaphylactoid reactions may occur. May cause serious skin adverse events (eg, exfoliative dermatitis, Stevens-Johnson syndrome, and toxic epidermal necrolysis). Avoid in late pregnancy; may cause premature closure of ductus arteriosis. May cause elevations of LFTs; d/c if liver disease develops or systemic manifestations occur. Monitor with chronic liver disease and consider dose reduction. Caution in elderly. Anemia may occur; with long-term use, monitor Hgb/Hct if signs or symptoms of anemia develop. May inhibit platelet aggregation and prolong bleeding time; monitor with coagulation disorders. Caution with asthma and avoid with ASA-sensitive asthma.

ADVERSE REACTIONS: Dyspepsia, nausea, abdominal pain, diarrhea, constipation, flatulence, headache, renal dysfunction, LFT abnormalities.

INTERACTIONS: Avoid ASA, probenecid. Renal toxicity potentiated by diuretics. Monitor anticoagulants. May increase levels of methotrexate, lithium.

PREGNANCY: Category C, not for use in nursing.

MECHANISM OF ACTION: NSAID; suspected to inhibit prostaglandin and leukotriene synthesis; exerts anti-inflammatory, analgesic, and antipyretic actions.

PHARMACOKINETICS: Absorption: Rapid and well-absorbed; T_{max}=6.8 hrs (fasted), 9.2 hrs (fed); C_{max}=3.1mg/L (fasted), 3.4mg/L (fed). Bioavailability (90%). **Distribution:** Plasma protein binding (>99%). **Metabolism:** Glucorunide conjugation. **Elimination:** $T_{1/2}$=5.4 hrs; urine (80%).

KETOROLAC RX
ketorolac tromethamine (Various)

> For short-term use only (≤5 days). Contraindicated with peptic ulcer disease, GI bleeding/perforation, perioperative pain in coronary artery bypass graft (CABG) surgery, advanced renal impairment, risk of renal failure due to volume depletion, CV bleeding, hemorrhagic diathesis, incomplete hemostasis, high-risk of bleeding, intraoperatively when hemostasis is critical, intrathecal/epidural use, L&D, nursing, and with ASA, NSAIDs, or probenecid. Caution greater risk of GI events with elderly patients. NSAIDs may cause an increased risk of CV thrombotic events (MI, stroke). (PO) Contraindicated in pediatric patients and in minor or chronic painful conditions.

OTHER BRAND NAMES: Toradol (Roche Labs)

THERAPEUTIC CLASS: NSAID (pyrrolo-pyrrole derivative)

INDICATIONS: Short-term (≤5 days) management of moderately severe, acute pain as continuation therapy from IV/IM.

DOSAGE: Adults: >16 yrs to <65 yrs: Single-Dose: 60mg IM or 30mg IV. Multiple-Dose: 30mg IM/IV q6h. Max: 120mg/day. Transition from IM/IV to PO: 20mg PO single dose, then 10mg PO q4-6h. Max: 40mg/24 hrs. ≥65 yrs/Renal Impairment/<50kg: Single-Dose: 30mg IM or 15mg IV. Multiple-Dose: 15mg IM/IV q6h. Max: 60mg/day. Transition from IM/IV to PO: 10mg PO q4-6h. Max: 40mg/24 hrs.
Pediatrics: 2-16 yrs: Single-Dose: IM: 1mg/kg. Max: 30mg. IV: 0.5mg/kg. Max: 15mg.

HOW SUPPLIED: Inj: 15mg/mL, 30mg/mL; Tab: 10mg

CONTRAINDICATIONS: Active or history of peptic ulcer, GI bleeding, perioperative pain in CABG surgery, advanced renal impairment or risk of renal failure due to volume depletion, labor/delivery, nursing mothers, ASA or NSAID allergy, preoperatively or intraoperatively when hemostasis is critical, cerebrovascular bleeding, hemorrhagic diathesis, incomplete hemostasis, high risk of bleeding, neuraxial (epidural or intrathecal) administration, and concomitant ASA, NSAIDs, probenecid, or pentoxifylline.

WARNINGS/PRECAUTIONS: Do not exceed 5 days of therapy. Risk of GI ulcerations, bleeding, and perforation. Caution with renal/hepatic dysfunction, dehydration, HTN, CHF, coagulation disorders, debilitated and elderly, pre-existing asthma. Preoperative use prolongs bleeding. CV thrombotic events, fluid retention, edema, NaCl retention, oliguria, anaphylactic reactions, elevated BUN and serum creatinine, anemia reported. Correct hypovolemia before therapy.

ADVERSE REACTIONS: Nausea, dyspepsia, GI pain, diarrhea, edema, headache, drowsiness, dizziness.

INTERACTIONS: May increase risk of bleeding with anticoagulants. May reduce diuretic response to furosemide. Increased serum levels with salicylates. Avoid ASA, NSAIDs, and probenecid. Increased lithium and methotrexate levels. May increase risk of renal impairment with ACE-inhibitors. May increase seizures with phenytoin and carbamazepine. Hallucinations reported with fluoxetine, thiothixene, and alprazolam. Do not mix in the same syringe as morphine. May have adverse effects with nondepolarizing muscle relaxants.

PREGNANCY: Category C, not for use in nursing.

MECHANISM OF ACTION: NSAID; suspected to inhibit prostaglandin synthetase; exerts anti-inflammatory, analgesic, and antipyretic actions.

PHARMACOKINETICS: Absorption: Absolute bioavailability (100%). **Distribution:** V_d=13L; plasma protein binding (99%); enters breast milk. **Metabolism:** Liver; hydroxylation, conjugation. **Elimination:** Urine: 92% (40% metabolites, 60% unchanged), feces (6%); $T_{1/2}$=5-6 hrs.

KINERET   RX

anakinra (Amgen)

THERAPEUTIC CLASS: Interleukin-1 receptor antagonist

INDICATIONS: As sole or adjunct therapy with DMARDs (except TNF blockers) to reduce the signs/symptoms and slow the progression of moderate to severe rheumatoid arthritis unresponsive to one or more DMARDs.

DOSAGE: *Adults:*≥18 yrs: 100mg SQ qd at approximately same time every day. CrCl <30mL/min: 100mg SQ qod.

HOW SUPPLIED: Inj: 100mg/0.67mL

WARNINGS/PRECAUTIONS: Increased incidence of serious infections alone and with coadministration with etanercept. D/C if serious infection or hypersensitivity reaction occurs. Do not initiate with active infection. Obtain neutrophil count before therapy, monthly for 3 months, quarterly thereafter for up to one yr.

ADVERSE REACTIONS: Injection site reactions, headache, nausea, diarrhea, infections, abdominal pain, arthralgia, flu-like symptoms.

INTERACTIONS: Neutropenia and higher rate of infections reported with etanercept. Vaccines may be ineffective; avoid live vaccines. Concurrent therapy with etanercept is not recommended.

PREGNANCY: Category B, caution in nursing.

MECHANISM OF ACTION: Interleukin-1 receptor antagonist; blocks biologic activity of IL-1 by competitively inhibiting IL-1 binding to the interleukin-1 type I receptor (IL-1RI), which is expressed in a wide variety of tissues and organs.

PHARMACOKINETICS: Absorption: Absolute bioavailability (95%); T_{max}=3-7 hrs. **Elimination:** $T_{1/2}$=4-6 hrs.

KLARON   RX
sulfacetamide sodium (Dermik)

THERAPEUTIC CLASS: Sulfonamide

INDICATIONS: Topical treatment of acne vulgaris.

DOSAGE: *Adults:* Apply thin film bid.
Pediatrics: ≥12 yrs: Apply thin film bid.

HOW SUPPLIED: Lot: 10% [118mL]

WARNINGS/PRECAUTIONS: D/C if irritation, rash, or hypersensitivity reaction occurs. Avoid eyes. Contains sulfites. Caution with denuded or abraded skin.

ADVERSE REACTIONS: Erythema, itching, edema, stinging, burning, local irritation.

PREGNANCY: Category C, caution in nursing.

MECHANISM OF ACTION: Sulfonamide; acts as a competitive inhibitor of para-aminobenzoic acid (PABA) utilization, an essential component for bacterial growth.

PHARMACOKINETICS: Absorption: Percutaneous (about 4%). **Distribution:** Small amounts of orally administered sulfonamides reported to be eliminated in breast milk. **Elimination:** Urine; $T_{1/2}$=7-13 hrs.

KLONOPIN   CIV
clonazepam (Roche Labs)

OTHER BRAND NAMES: Klonopin Wafers (Roche Labs)

THERAPEUTIC CLASS: Benzodiazepine

INDICATIONS: Adjunct or monotherapy in Lennox-Gastaut syndrome, akinetic and myoclonic seizures. Absence seizures refractory to succinimides. Panic disorder with or without agoraphobia.

DOSAGE: *Adults:* Seizure Disorders: Initial: Not to exceed 1.5mg/day given tid. Titrate: May increase by 0.5-1mg every 3 days. Max: 20mg qd. Panic Disorder: Initial: 0.25mg bid. Titrate: Increase to 1mg/day after 3 days, then may increase by 0.125-0.25mg bid every 3 days. Max: 4mg/day. Wafer: Dissolve in mouth with or without water.
Pediatrics: <10 yrs or 30kg: Seizure Disorders: Initial: 0.01-0.03mg/kg/day up to 0.05mg/kg/day given bid-tid. Titrate: Increase by no more than 0.25-0.5mg every 3 days. Maint: 0.1-0.2mg/kg/day given tid. Wafer: Dissolve in mouth with or without water.

HOW SUPPLIED: Tab: 0.5mg*, 1mg, 2mg; Tab, Disintegrating (Wafer): 0.125mg, 0.25mg, 0.5mg, 1mg, 2mg *scored

CONTRAINDICATIONS: Significant liver disease, acute narrow-angle glaucoma, untreated open-angle glaucoma.

WARNINGS/PRECAUTIONS: May increase incidence of generalized tonic-clonic seizures. Monitor blood counts and LFTs periodically with long-term therapy. Caution with renal dysfunction, chronic respiratory depression. Increased fetal risks during pregnancy. Avoid abrupt withdrawal. Hypersalivation reported.

ADVERSE REACTIONS: Somnolence, depression, ataxia, CNS depression, upper respiratory tract infection, fatigue, dizziness, sinusitis, colpitis.

INTERACTIONS: Decreased serum levels with CYP450 inducers (eg, phenytoin, carbamazepine, phenobarbital). Caution with CYP3A inhibitors (eg, oral antifungals). Alcohol, narcotics, barbiturates, nonbarbiturate hypnotics, antianxiety agents, phenothiazines, thioxanthene and butyrophenone antipsychotics, MAOIs, TCAs and other anticonvulsant drugs potentiate CNS-depressant effects.

PREGNANCY: Category D, not for use in nursing.

MECHANISM OF ACTION: Benzodiazepine; not established, suspected to enhance activity of GABA, the major inhibitory neurotransmitter in the CNS.

PHARMACOKINETICS: Absorption: Rapid and complete. Absolute bio-availability (90%), T_{max}=1-4 hrs. **Distribution:** Plasma protein binding (85%). **Metabolism:** Hepatic via acetylation, hydroxylation, and glucuronidation, CYP450. **Elimination:** Renal. Urine (<2% unchanged); $T_{1/2}$=30-40 hrs.

K-Lor   RX
potassium chloride (Abbott)

THERAPEUTIC CLASS: K⁺ supplement

INDICATIONS: Treatment and prevention of hypokalemia with or without metabolic alkalosis. Treatment of digitalis intoxication and hypokalemic familial periodic paralysis.

DOSAGE: *Adults:* Prevention: 20mEq/day. Hypokalemia: 40-100mEq/day. Divide dose if >20mEq. Dissolve each 20mEq in 4oz of cold water or juice.

HOW SUPPLIED: Pow: 20mEq

CONTRAINDICATIONS: Hyperkalemia.

WARNINGS/PRECAUTIONS: Potentially fatal hyperkalemia may occur. Extreme caution with acidosis, cardiac and renal disease; monitor ECG and electrolytes. Hypokalemia with metabolic acidosis should be treated with an alkalinizing potassium salt (eg, potassium bicarbonate, potassium citrate).

ADVERSE REACTIONS: Hyperkalemia, nausea, vomiting, flatulence, abdominal pain, diarrhea.

INTERACTIONS: Risk of hyperkalemia with ACE inhibitors (eg, captopril, enalapril), K⁺-sparing diuretics and K⁺ supplements.

PREGNANCY: Category C, safe for use in nursing.

MECHANISM OF ACTION: K⁺ supplement (electrolyte replenisher); helps in maintenance of intracellular tonicity, transmission of nerve impulses, contraction of cardiac, skeletal and smooth muscles, and maintenance of normal renal function.

Klor-Con M   RX
potassium chloride (Upsher-Smith)

OTHER BRAND NAMES: Klor-Con (Upsher-Smith)

THERAPEUTIC CLASS: K⁺ supplement

INDICATIONS: (For those unable to tolerate liquid or effervescent potassium preparations). Treatment of hypokalemia with or without metabolic alkalosis, in digitalis intoxication and with hypokalemic familial periodic paralysis. Prevention of hypokalemia in patients at risk (eg, digitalized, cardiac arrhythmias).

DOSAGE: *Adults:* Prevention: 20mEq/day. Hypokalemia: 40-100mEq/day. Divide dose if >20mEq. Take with meals and fluids. Swallow tabs whole; may break Klor-Con M in half or mix with 4 ounces of water.

HOW SUPPLIED: (Klor-Con M) Tab, Extended Release: 10mEq, 15mEq, 20mEq; (Klor-Con) Pow: 20mEq, 25mEq; Tab, Extended Release: 8mEq, 10mEq

CONTRAINDICATIONS: Hyperkalemia, esophageal ulceration, delay in GI passage (from structural, pathological, pharmacologic causes), cardiac patients with esophageal compression due to enlarged left atrium.

WARNINGS/PRECAUTIONS: Potentially fatal hyperkalemia may occur. Extreme caution with acidosis, cardiac, and renal disease; monitor ECG and electrolytes. Hypokalemia with metabolic acidosis should be treated with an alkalinizing potassium salt (eg, potassium bicarbonate, potassium citrate). May produce ulcerative or stenotic GI lesions.

ADVERSE REACTIONS: Hyperkalemia, GI effects (obstruction, bleeding, ulceration), nausea, vomiting, abdominal pain, flatulence, diarrhea.

INTERACTIONS: Risk of hyperkalemia with ACE inhibitors (eg, captopril, enalapril), K⁺-sparing diuretics, and K⁺ supplements. Contraindicated with anticholinergics or other agents that decrease GI motility.

PREGNANCY: Category C, safe for use in nursing.

MECHANISM OF ACTION: K⁺ supplement (electrolyte replenisher). Intended to provide extended-release of K⁺ from matrix to minimize likelihood of high localized concentrations of K⁺ within GI tract.

PHARMACOKINETICS: Absorption: T_{max}=4-8 hrs, GI tract. **Elimination:** Urine and feces.

K-Lyte/CL RX
potassium chloride (Bristol-Myers Squibb)

OTHER BRAND NAMES: K-Lyte/CL 50 (Bristol-Myers Squibb)

INDICATIONS: Treatment or prophylaxis of potassium deficiency. Management of hypokalemia with metabolic alkalosis and hypochloremia. Treatment of digitalis intoxication.

DOSAGE: *Adults:* Usual: (K-Lyte/CL) Dissolve 25meq in 3-4 oz cold/ice water and drink bid-qid. (K-Lyte/CL 50) Dissolve 50meq in 6-8 oz cold/ice water and drink qd-bid. Dose according to patient's requirements. Take with food.

HOW SUPPLIED: Tab, Effervescent: (K-Lyte/CL) 25meq, (K-Lyte/CL 50) 50meq

CONTRAINDICATIONS: Hyperkalemia.

WARNINGS/PRECAUTIONS: Risk of hyperkalemia and cardiac arrest with impaired K⁺ excretion (eg, chronic renal disease). Potentially fatal hyperkalemia may occur rapidly and may be asymptomatic. Monitor serum K⁺ levels carefully with condtions that impair K⁺ excretion. Monitor acid-base balance, serum electrolytes, ECG, and clinical status when treating K⁺ depletion.

ADVERSE REACTIONS: Nausea, vomiting, diarrhea, abdominal discomfort.

INTERACTIONS: Risk of hyperkalemia with K⁺ sparing diuretics, and K⁺-containing salt substitutes.

PREGNANCY: Category C, not for use in nursing.

KOGENATE FS RX
antihemophilic factor (Bayer Healthcare)

THERAPEUTIC CLASS: Antihemophilic Factor (Recombinant)

INDICATIONS: Treatment of hemophilia A in which there is a deficiency of activity of clotting factor FVIII.

DOSAGE: *Adults:* Minor hemorrhage: 10-20 IU/kg IV; repeat if evidence of further bleeding. Moderate to major hemorrhage/surgery (minor): 15-30 IU/kg IV; repeat one dose at 12-24 hrs if needed. Major to life-threatening hemorrhage/fractures/head trauma: Initial: 40-50 IU/kg IV; repeat dose 20-25 IU/kg IV q 8-12 hrs. Surgery (major): Preoperative dose: 50 IU/kg IV (verify 100% FVIII activity prior to surgery); repeat as necessary after 6-12 hrs initially, and for 10-14 days until healing is complete.
Pediatrics: Minor hemorrhage: 10-20 IU/kg IV; repeat if evidence of further bleeding. Moderate to major hemorrhage/surgery (minor): 15-30 IU/kg IV; repeat one dose at 12-24 hrs if needed. Major to life-threatening hemorrhage/fractures/head trauma: Initial: 40-50 IU/kg IV; repeat dose 20-25 IU/kg IV q 8-12 hrs. Surgery (major): Preoperative dose: 50 IU/kg IV (verify 100% FVIII activity prior to surgery); repeat as necessary after 6-12 hrs initially, and for 10-14 days until healing is complete.

HOW SUPPLIED: Inj: 250 IU, 500 IU, 1000 IU, 2000 IU

CONTRAINDICATIONS: Known hypersensitivity to mouse or hamster protein.

WARNINGS/PRECAUTIONS: Development of circulating neutralizing antibodies to FVIII may occur; monitor by appropriate clinical observation and laboratory tests. Hypotension, urticaria, and chest tightness in association with hypersensitivity reported.

ADVERSE REACTIONS: Local injection site reactions, dizziness, rash, unusual taste, mild increase in BP, pruritus, depersonalization, nausea, rhinitis.

PREGNANCY: Category C, safety not known in nursing.

MECHANISM OF ACTION: Antihemophilic factor.

KRISTALOSE   RX
lactulose (Cumberland)

THERAPEUTIC CLASS: Osmotic laxative

INDICATIONS: Treatment of constipation.

DOSAGE: *Adults:* 10-20g/day. Max 40g/day. Dissolve pkt contents in 4oz of water.

HOW SUPPLIED: Powder (crystals for suspension): 10g/pkt, 20g/pkt [1⁵, 30⁵]

CONTRAINDICATIONS: Patients who require a low galactose diet.

WARNINGS/PRECAUTIONS: Caution in DM due to galactose and lactose content. Monitor electrolytes periodically in elderly or debilitated if used for >6 months. Potential for explosive reaction with electrocautery procedures during proctoscopy or colonoscopy.

ADVERSE REACTIONS: Flatulence, intestinal cramps, diarrhea, nausea, vomiting.

INTERACTIONS: Nonabsorbable antacids may decrease effects.

PREGNANCY: Category B, caution in nursing.

MECHANISM OF ACTION: Osmotic laxative; increases osmotic pressure and slight acidification of the colonic contents.

PHARMACOKINETICS: Absorption: Poorly absorbed from GI tract.
Elimination: Urine (≤3%).

K-TAB   RX
potassium chloride (Abbott)

OTHER BRAND NAMES: Klotrix (Apothecon)

THERAPEUTIC CLASS: K⁺ supplement

INDICATIONS: (For those unable to tolerate liquid or effervescent potassium preparations). Treatment and prevention of hypokalemia with or without metabolic alkalosis. Treatment of digitalis intoxication and hypokalemic familial periodic paralysis.

DOSAGE: *Adults:* Prevention: 20mEq/day. Hypokalemia: 40-100mEq/day. Divide dose if >20mEq. Take with meals and full glass of water or liquid. Do not cut, crush or chew tab.

HOW SUPPLIED: Tab, Extended-Release: 10mEq

CONTRAINDICATIONS: Hyperkalemia, esophageal ulceration, delay in GI passage (from structural, pathological, pharmacologic causes), cardiac patients with esophageal compression due to enlarged left atrium.

WARNINGS/PRECAUTIONS: Potentially fatal hyperkalemia may occur. Extreme caution with acidosis, cardiac and renal disease; monitor ECG and electrolytes. Hypokalemia with metabolic acidosis should be treated with an alkalinizing potassium salt (eg, potassium bicarbonate, potassium citrate). May produce ulcerative or stenotic GI lesions. Use with caution in elderly due to decreased renal function, start dose at low end of dosing range.

ADVERSE REACTIONS: Hyperkalemia, GI effects (obstruction, bleeding, ulceration), nausea, vomiting, abdominal pain, flatulence, diarrhea.

INTERACTIONS: Risk of hyperkalemia with ACE inhibitors (eg, captopril, enalapril), potassium-sparing diuretics and potassium supplements.

Contraindicated with anticholinergic agents due to possible delay in tablet passage through GI tract.

PREGNANCY: Category C, safe for use in nursing.

MECHANISM OF ACTION: K^+ supplement (electrolyte replenisher). Slows release of K^+, so likelihood of high localized concentrations of K^+ within GI is reduced.

KYTRIL   RX
granisetron HCL (Roche Labs)

THERAPEUTIC CLASS: $5\text{-}HT_3$-antagonist

INDICATIONS: (Inj, Sol, Tab) Prevention of nausea and vomiting associated with chemotherapy. (Sol, Tab) Prevention of nausea and vomiting associated with radiation. (Inj) Prevention and treatment of post-op nausea and vomiting.

DOSAGE: *Adults:* Prevention with Chemotherapy: (PO) 2mg qd up to 1 hr before chemotherapy or 1mg bid (up to 1 hr before chemotherapy and 12 hrs later). (IV) 10mcg/kg within 30 min before chemotherapy. Prevention with Radiation: (PO) 2mg within 1 hr of radiation. Post-Op Prevention: (IV) Administer 1mg over 30 sec before induction of anesthesia or immediately before anesthesia reversal. Post-Op Treatment: (IV) Administer 1mg over 30 sec. *Pediatrics:* 2-16 yrs: Prevention with Chemotherapy: 10mcg/kg IV within 30 min before chemotherapy.

HOW SUPPLIED: Inj: 0.1mg/mL, 1mg/mL; Sol: 2mg/10mL [30mL]; Tab: 1mg

WARNINGS/PRECAUTIONS: (Inj) Does not stimulate gastric or intestinal peristalsis. Do not use instead of nasogastric suction. May mask progressive ileus or gastric distension.

ADVERSE REACTIONS: Headache, asthenia, somnolence, diarrhea, constipation, abdominal pain, dizziness, insomnia, increased hepatic enzymes.

INTERACTIONS: Hepatic CYP450 enzyme inducers or inhibitors may alter clearance.

PREGNANCY: Category B, caution in nursing.

MECHANISM OF ACTION: $5\text{-}HT_3$ receptor antagonist; blocks serotonin stimulation on vagal nerve terminals and in chemoreceptor trigger zone and subsequent vomiting after emetogenic stimuli.

PHARMACOKINETICS: Absorption: (IV, 40mcg/kg) C_{max}=63.8 ng/mL. (PO,1mg) C_{max}=3.63ng/mL. **Distribution:** Plasma protein binding (65%). (IV) V_d=3.07L/kg; (PO) V_d=3.94L/kg. **Metabolism:** CYP3A4; N-demethylation, oxidation, conjugation. **Elimination:** PO: Urine (11% unchanged), feces. Inj: Urine (12% unchanged), feces; (IV, PO) $T_{1/2}$=8.95 hrs, 6.23hrs

LABETALOL   RX
labetalol HCL (Various)

THERAPEUTIC CLASS: Nonselective beta-blocker/$alpha_1$ blocker

INDICATIONS: (Tab) Management of hypertension. (Inj) Management of severe hypertension.

DOSAGE: *Adults:* (Tab) HTN: Initial: 100mg bid. Titrate: 100mg bid every 2-3 days. Maint: 200-400mg bid. Severe HTN: 1200-2400mg/day given bid-tid. Increments should not exceed 200mg bid for titration. (Inj) Severe HTN: Administer in supine position. Repeated IV Infusion: Initial: 20mg over 2 min. Titrate: Give additional 40-80mg at 10 min intervals if needed. Max: 300mg. Slow Continuous Infusion: 200mg at rate of 2mg/min. May adjust dose according to BP. Switch to tabs when BP is stable while in hospital. Initial: 200mg, then 200-400mg 6-12 hrs later on Day 1. Titrate: May increase at 1-day interval.

HOW SUPPLIED: Inj: 5mg/mL; Tab: 100mg*, 200mg*, 300mg *scored

CONTRAINDICATIONS: Bronchial asthma, obstructive airway disease, overt cardiac failure, >1st-degree heart block, cardiogenic shock, severe bradycardia, other conditions associated with severe and prolonged hypotension.

WARNINGS/PRECAUTIONS: Severe hepatocellular injury reported; caution with hepatic dysfunction. Monitor LFTs periodically; d/c at 1st sign of hepatic injury. Caution with well-compensated heart failure. Can cause heart failure. Exacerbation of ischemic heart disease with abrupt withdrawal. Caution in nonallergic bronchospasm patients refractory to or intolerant to other antihypertensives. May mask hypoglycemia symptoms. Withdrawal before surgery is controversial. Paradoxical HTN may occur with pheochromocytoma. Death reported during surgery. Avoid injection with low cardiac indices and elevated systemic vascular resistance.

ADVERSE REACTIONS: Fatigue, dizziness, dyspepsia, nausea, nasal stuffiness.

INTERACTIONS: Increased tremors with TCAs. Potentiated by cimetidine. Blunts reflex tachycardia of NTG without preventing hypotensive effect. Caution with calcium antagonists. Antagonizes bronchodilator effect of β-agonists. Antidiabetic agents may need dose adjustment. May block epinephrine effects. (Inj) Synergistic with halothane; do not use ≥3% halothane.

PREGNANCY: Category C, caution in nursing.

MECHANISM OF ACTION: α-1 and nonselective β-adrenergic receptor blocker; produces dose related falls in BP with out reflex tachycardia and significant reduction in heart rate.

PHARMACOKINETICS: Absorption: Complete; T_{max}=1-2 hrs. **Distribution:** Plasma protein binding (50%); crosses placenta. **Metabolism:** Conjugation. **Elimination:** Urine, feces. (Tab) $T_{1/2}$=6-8 hrs. (IV) $T_{1/2}$=5.5 hrs.

LAC-HYDRIN   RX
ammonium lactate (Ranbaxy)

THERAPEUTIC CLASS: Emollient

INDICATIONS: Treatment of ichthyosis vulgaris and xerosis.

DOSAGE: *Adults:* Apply bid and rub thoroughly.
Pediatrics: (Lot) Infants/Children: (Cre) ≥2 yrs: Apply bid and rub in thoroughly.

HOW SUPPLIED: Cre: 12% [140g, 385g]; Lot: 12% [225g, 400g]

WARNINGS/PRECAUTIONS: Avoid sun exposure to treated skin. Avoid eyes, lips, mucous membranes, intravaginal use and oral use. Caution if used on face; potential for irritation Stinging, burning may occur if applied to fissures, erosions, or abrasions. D/C if hypersensitivity observed.

ADVERSE REACTIONS: Burning, stinging, itching, erythema.

PREGNANCY: Category B, caution in nursing.

LACRISERT   RX
hydroxypropyl cellulose (Merck)

THERAPEUTIC CLASS: Lubricant

INDICATIONS: Treatment of moderate to severe dry eye syndromes (eg, keratoconjunctivitis sicca) and in patients not responsive to artificial tear solutions. Treatment of exposure keratitis, decreased corneal sensitivity, and recurrent corneal erosions.

DOSAGE: *Adults:* One insert in each eye qd, up to bid.

HOW SUPPLIED: Insert: 5mg [60ˢ]

WARNINGS/PRECAUTIONS: May result in corneal abrasion if improperly placed. May cause blurred vision; use caution while operating machinery.

ADVERSE REACTIONS: Transient blurred vision, ocular discomfort/irritation, matting/stickiness of eyelashes, photophobia, hypersensitivity, eyelid edema, hyperemia.

PREGNANCY: Safety in pregnancy and nursing not known.

MECHANISM OF ACTION: Lubricant; Acts to stabilize and thicken precorneal tear film and prolongs tear film breakup time. Also acts to lubricate and protect eye.

PHARMACOKINETICS: Elimination: Feces.

LACTULOSE RX
lactulose (Various)

OTHER BRAND NAMES: Constulose (Actavis) - Generlac (Morton Grove) - Enulose (Alpharma)

THERAPEUTIC CLASS: Osmotic laxative

INDICATIONS: Treatment of constipation. Prevention and treatment of portal-systemic encephalopathy, including stages of hepatic pre-coma and coma.

DOSAGE: *Adults:* Constipation: 15-30mL qd. Max 60mL/day. May mix with fruit juice, water, or milk. Portal-Systemic Encephalopathy: 30-45mL tid-qid. Adjust dose every 1 or 2 days to produce 2-3 soft stools daily. Rectal Use: Reversal of Coma: Mix 300mL with 700mL of water or saline and retain for 30-60 min. May repeat q4-6h. Oral doses should be started before completely stopping enema.
Pediatrics: Portal-Systemic Encephalopathy: Older Children/Adolescents: 40-90mL/day divided tid-qid adjusted to produce 2-3 soft stools daily. *Infants:* 2.5-10mL in divided doses to produce 2-3 soft stools daily.

HOW SUPPLIED: Sol: 10g/15mL

CONTRAINDICATIONS: Patients who require a low galactose diet.

WARNINGS/PRECAUTIONS: Caution in DM due to galactose and lactose content. Monitor electrolytes periodically in elderly or debilitated if used >6 months. Potential for explosive reaction with electrocautery procedures during proctoscopy or colonoscopy.

ADVERSE REACTIONS: Flatulence, intestinal cramps, diarrhea, nausea, vomiting.

INTERACTIONS: Decreased effect with nonabsorbable antacids.

PREGNANCY: Category B, caution in nursing.

MECHANISM OF ACTION: Synthetic disaccharide; broken down primarily to lactic acid, by the action of colonic bacteria, resulting in increased osmotic pressure and slight acidification of colonic content, causing an increase in stool water content and softens the stool. In portal-systemic encephalopathy, acidification of colonic contents results in retention of ammonia in colon as ammonium ion; ammonia then migrates from blood into colon to form ammonium ion, which traps and prevents absorption of ammonia; finally, laxative actions expels trapped ammonium ion from colon.

PHARMACOKINETICS: Absorption: Poor. **Elimination:** Urine (≤3%).

LAMICTAL RX
lamotrigine (GlaxoSmithKline)

> Serious life-threatening rash, including Stevens-Johnson syndrome and toxic epidermal necrolysis, reported. Occurs more often in pediatrics than adults. D/C at 1st sign of rash.

OTHER BRAND NAMES: Lamictal CD (GlaxoSmithKline)

THERAPEUTIC CLASS: Phenyltriazine

INDICATIONS: Adjunctive therapy in patients (≥2 yrs) with partial seizures and for generalized seizures of Lennox-Gastaut syndrome. For conversion to monotherapy in adults (≥16 yrs) with partial seizures receiving a single enzyme-inducing antiepileptic drug (EIAED) or valproate (VPA). Maintenance treatment of bipolar I disorder to delay the time to occurrence of mood episodes (depression, mania, hypomania, mixed episodes) in patients treated for acute mood episodes with standard therapy.

DOSAGE: *Adults:* Epilepsy: Concomitant AEDs with valproate (VPA): Weeks 1 and 2: 25mg every other day. Weeks 3 and 4: 25mg qd. Titrate: Increase every 1-2 weeks by 25-50mg/day. Maint: 100-400mg/day, given qd or bid; 100-200mg/day when added to VPA alone. Concomitant EIAEDs without VPA: Weeks 1 and 2: 50mg qd. Weeks 3 and 4: 50mg bid. Titrate: Increase every 1-2 weeks by 100mg/day. Maint: 150-250mg bid. Conversion to Monotherapy From Single EIAED: ≥16 yrs: Weeks 1 and 2: 50mg qd. Weeks 3 and 4: 50mg bid. Titrate: Increase every 1-2 weeks by 100mg/day. Maint: 250mg bid. Withdraw EIAED over 4 weeks. Conversion to Monotherapy From VPA: ≥16 yrs: Step 1: Follow Concomitant AEDs with VPA dosing regimen to achieve Lamictal dose of 200mg/day. Maintain previous VPA dose. Step 2: Maintain Lamictal 200mg/day. Decrease VPA to 500mg/day by decrements of ≤500mg/day per week. Maintain VPA 500mg/day for 1 week. Step 3: Increase to Lamictal 300mg/day for 1 week. Decrease VPA simultaneously to 250mg/day for 1 week. Step 4: D/C VPA. Increase Lamictal 100mg/day every week to maint dose of 500mg/day. Bipolar Disorder: Patients not taking carbamazepine, other enzyme-inducing drugs (EIDs) or VPA: Weeks 1 and 2: 25mg qd. Weeks 3 and 4: 50mg qd. Week 5: 100mg qd. Weeks 6 and 7: 200mg qd. Patients taking VPA: Weeks 1 and 2: 25mg every other day. Weeks 3 and 4: 25mg qd. Week 5: 50mg qd. Weeks 6 and 7: 100mg qd. Patients taking carbamazepine (or other EIDs) and not taking VPA: Weeks 1 and 2: 50mg qd. Weeks 3 and 4: 100mg qd (divided doses). Week 5: 200mg qd (divided doses). Week 6: 300mg qd (divided doses). Week 7: up to 400mg qd (divided doses). After d/c of psychotropic drugs excluding VPA, carbamazepine, or other EIDs: Maintain current dose. After d/c of VPA and current lamotrigine dose of 100mg qd: Week 1: 150mg qd. Week 2 and onward: 200mg qd. After d/c of carbamazepine or other EIDs and current lamotrigine dose of 400mg qd: Week 1: 400mg qd. Week 2: 300mg qd. Week 3 and Onward: 200mg qd. Concomitant or starting estrogen-containing oral contraceptives: not taking carbamazepine, phenytoin, phenobarbital, primidone, or rifampin, lamictal should be increased by as much as 2-fold over the recommended target maintenance dose; the dose increase should start at the same time as the initiation and continuation of contraceptives. Stopping estrogen-containing oral contraceptives: may decrease lamictal by as much as 50%. Hepatic Impairment: Initial/Titrate/Maint: Reduce by 50% for moderate (Child-Pugh Grade B) and 75% for severe (Child-Pugh Grade C) impairment. Significant Renal Impairment: Maint: Reduce dose. Elderly: Start at low end of dosing range. *Pediatrics:* Round dose down to nearest whole tab. 2-12 yrs: ≥6.7kg: Lennox-Gastaut/Partial Seizures: Concomitant AEDs with VPA: Weeks 1 and 2: 0.15mg/kg/day given qd-bid. Weeks 3 and 4: 0.3mg/kg/day given qd or bid. Titrate: Increase every 1-2 weeks by 0.3mg/kg/day. Maint: 1-5mg/kg/day given qd or bid; 1-3mg/kg/day when added to VPA alone. Max: 200mg/day. Concomitant EIAEDs without VPA: Weeks 1 and 2: 0.3mg/kg bid. Weeks 3 and 4: 0.6mg/kg bid. Titrate: Increase every 1-2 weeks by 1.2mg/kg/day. Maint: 2.5-7.5mg/kg bid. Max: 400mg/day. >12 yrs: Concomitant AEDs with VPA: Weeks 1 and 2: 25mg every other day. Weeks 3 and 4: 25mg qd. Titrate: Increase every 1-2 weeks by 25-50mg/day. Maint: 100-400mg/day, given qd or bid; 100-200mg/day when added to VPA alone. Concomitant EIAEDs without VPA: Weeks 1 and 2: 50mg qd. Weeks 3 and 4: 50mg bid. Titrate: Increase every 1-2 weeks by 100mg/day. Maint: 150-250mg bid. Hepatic Impairment: Initial/Titrate/Maint: Reduce by 50% for moderate (Child-Pugh Grade B) and 75% for severe (Child-Pugh Grade C) impairment. Significant Renal Impairment: Maint: Reduce dose.

HOW SUPPLIED: Tab: 25mg*, 100mg*, 150mg*, 200mg*; Tab, Chewable: (Lamictal CD) 2mg, 5mg, 25mg *scored

WARNINGS/PRECAUTIONS: Risk of serious life-threatening rash; d/c if rash occurs. Multiorgan failure, sudden unexplained death, hypersensitivity reactions, and pure red cell aplasia reported. Avoid abrupt withdrawal. Caution with renal, hepatic, or cardiac functional impairment. May cause ophthalmic toxicity. Do not exceed recommended initial dose and dose escalations.

Caution in elderly. Chewable tabs may be swallowed whole, chewed (with water/diluted fruit juice) or dispersed in water/diluted fruit juice; do administer partial quantities.

ADVERSE REACTIONS: Serious rash, dizziness, ataxia, somnolence, headache, diplopia, blurred vision, nausea, vomiting, insomnia, back/abdominal pain, fatigue, xerostomia, rhinitis.

INTERACTIONS: Decreased levels with phenytoin, carbamazepine, phenobarbital, primidone, rifampin, estrogen-containing oral contraceptives. Risk of life-threatening rash with valproic acid. Lamotrigine decreases valproic acid levels; valproic acid increases lamotrigine levels. Inhibits dihydrofolate reductase; may potentiate folate inhibitors.

PREGNANCY: Category C, not for use in nursing.

MECHANISM OF ACTION: Phenyltriazine; not established. Suspected to inhibit voltage-sensitive sodium channels, thereby stabilizing neuronal membranes and consequently modulating presynaptic transmitter release of excitatory amino acids.

PHARMACOKINETICS: Absorption: Rapid and complete. Absolute bioavailability (98%), T_{max}=1.4-4.8 hrs. **Distribution:** V_d=0.9-1.3L/kg; plasma protein binding (55%); Found in breast milk. **Metabolism:** Liver via glucuronic acid conjugation, 2-N-glucuronide conjugate (major metabolite, inactive). **Elimination:** Renal, urine (94%), feces (2%). Refer to full PI for pediatric parameters.

LAMISIL   RX
terbinafine HCL (Novartis)

L

THERAPEUTIC CLASS: Allylamine antifungal

INDICATIONS: (Granules) Treatment of tinea capitis in patients ≥4 yrs. (Tabs) Treatment of onychomycosis of toenail or fingernail due to dermatophytes (tinea unguium).

DOSAGE: *Adults:* Tabs: Fingernail: 250mg qd for 6 weeks. Toenail: 250mg qd for 12 weeks. Granules: Take qd with food for 6 weeks. <25 kg: 125mg/day. 25-35kg: 187.5mg/day. >35kg: 250mg/day.
Pediatrics: ≥4 yrs: Granules: Take qd with food for 6 weeks. <25 kg: 125mg/day. 25-35kg: 187.5mg/day. >35kg: 250mg/day.

HOW SUPPLIED: Granules: 125mg/pkt, 187.5mg/pkt; Tab: 250mg

WARNINGS/PRECAUTIONS: Liver disease and serious skin reactions reported; d/c therapy if these develop. Avoid with liver disease or renal impairment (CrCl ≤50 mL/min). Check serum transaminases before therapy. Monitor CBC if immunocompromised and taking terbinafine >6 weeks. Severe neutropenia reported; d/c therapy if neutrophil count ≤1,000 cells/mm³. Changes in ocular lens and retina reported (unknown significance).

ADVERSE REACTIONS: (Granules) Nasopharyngitis, headache, pyrexia, cough, vomiting, upper respiratory tract infection, upper abdominal pain, diarrhea, liver enzyme abnormalities, rash. (Tabs) Headache, diarrhea, dyspepsia, abdominal pain, liver enzyme abnormalities, rash.

INTERACTIONS: Increased clearance of cyclosporine. May potentiate levels of drugs metabolized by CYP2D6 (eg, TCAs, β-blockers, SSRIs, MAOIs-type B). Decreased clearance of IV caffeine. Clearance increased by rifampin and decreased by cimetidine.

PREGNANCY: Category B, not for use in nursing.

MECHANISM OF ACTION: Allylamine antifungal; acts by inhibiting squalene epoxidase, thus blocking biosynthesis of ergosterol, an essential component of fungal cell membranes.

PHARMACOKINETICS: Absorption: (Tab) Well-absorbed (>70%), absolute bioavailability (40%); (250mg) C_{max}=1mcg/mL; T_{max}=2 hrs; AUC =4.56mcg.h/mL. **Distribution:** Plasma protein binding (>99%). **Metabolism:** Extensive, CYP2D6. **Elimination:** Urine (70%), $T_{1/2}$=200-400 hrs.

LAMISIL AT
OTC

terbinafine HCL (Novartis Consumer)

THERAPEUTIC CLASS: Allylamine antifungal

INDICATIONS: Treatment of t.pedis, t.cruris, t.corporis.

DOSAGE: *Adults:* Wash and dry area. Tinea pedis: Apply bid for 1 week (interdigital) or for 2 weeks (bottom or sides of foot). Tinea cruris/corporis: Apply qd for 1 week.
Pediatrics: ≥12 yrs: Wash and dry area. Tinea pedis: Apply bid for 1 week (interdigital) or for 2 weeks (bottom or sides of foot). Tinea cruris/corporis: Apply qd for 1 week.

HOW SUPPLIED: Cre: 1% [12g, 24g]; Spray: 1% [30mL]

WARNINGS/PRECAUTIONS: Do not use on nails, scalp, in or near the mouth or eyes, or for vaginal yeast infections.

PREGNANCY: Not rated in pregnancy or nursing.

MECHANISM OF ACTION: Allylamine antifungal; acts by inhibiting squalene epoxidase, thus blocking the biosynthesis of ergosterol, an essential component of fungal cell membranes.

PHARMACOKINETICS: Distribution: Plasma protein binding (>99%).
Metabolism: Rapidly and extensively metabolized by CYP450:2C9, 1A2, 3A4,2C8, and 2C19. **Elimination:** Urine (approximately 70%).

LANOXIN
RX

digoxin (GlaxoSmithKline)

OTHER BRAND NAMES: Digitek (Mylan Bertek) - Lanoxicaps (GlaxoSmithKline)

THERAPEUTIC CLASS: Cardiac glycoside

INDICATIONS: Treatment of mild to moderate heart failure and to control ventricular response rate with chronic atrial fibrillation.

DOSAGE: *Adults:* Rapid Digitalization: LD: (Cap/Inj) 0.4-0.6mg PO/IV or (Tab) 0.5-0.75mg PO, may give additional (Cap/Inj) 0.1-0.3mg or (Tab) 0.125-0.375mg at 6-8 hr intervals until clinical effect. Maint: (Tab) 0.125-0.5mg qd. Elderly (>70 yrs)/Renal Dysfunction: Initial: 0.125mg qd. Marked Renal Dysfunction: Initial: 0.0625mg qd. Titrate: Increase every 2 weeks based on response. A-Fib: Titrate to minimum effective dose for desired response.
Pediatrics: (Ped Sol) Oral Digitalizing Dose: Premature Infants: 20-30mcg/kg. Full-Term Infants: 25-35mcg/kg. 1-24 months: 35-60mcg/kg. 2-5 yrs: 30-40mcg/kg. 5-10 yrs: 20-35mcg/kg. >10 yrs: 10-15mcg/kg. Maint: Premature Infants: 20-30% of PO digitalizing dose/day. Full-Term Infants to >10 yrs: 25-35% of PO digitalizing dose. (Ped Inj) IV Digitalizing Dose: Premature Infants: 15-25mcg/kg. Full-Term Infants: 20-30mcg/kg. 1-24 months: 30-50mcg/kg. 2-5 yrs: 25-35mcg/kg. 5-10 yrs: 15-30mcg/kg. >10 yrs: 8-12mcg/kg. Maint: Premature Infants: 20-30% of IV digitalizing dose. Full-Term Infants to >10 yrs: 25-35% of IV digitalizing dose/day. (Cap) Oral Digitalizing Dose: 2-5 yrs: 25-35mcg/kg. 5-10 yrs: 15-30mcg/kg. >10 yrs: 8-12mcg/kg. Maint: ≥2 yrs: 25-25% of PO or IV digitalizing dose. (Tab) Maint: 2-5 yrs: 10-15mcg/kg. 5-10 yrs: 7-10mcg/kg. >10 yrs: 3-5mcg/kg. A-Fib: Titrate to minimum effective dose for desired response.

HOW SUPPLIED: Cap: (Lanoxicaps) 0.1mg, 0.2mg; Inj: (Pediatric Inj) 0.1mg/mL, 0.25mg/mL; Sol: (Pediatric Sol) 0.05mg/mL [60mL]; Tab: 0.125mg*, 0.25mg* *scored

CONTRAINDICATIONS: Ventricular fibrillation, digitalis hypersensitivity.

WARNINGS/PRECAUTIONS: May cause severe sinus bradycardia or sinoatrial block with pre-existing sinus node disease. May cause advanced or complete heart block with pre-existing incomplete AV block. May cause very rapid ventricular response or ventricular fibrillation. Caution with thyroid disorders, AMI, hypermetabolic states, restrictive cardiomyopathy, constrictive pericarditis, amyloid heart disease, elderly, acute cor pulmonale, and idiopathic hypertrophic subaortic stenosis. Caution with renal dysfunction; high risk for toxicity. Caution with hypokalemia, hypomagnesemia, or hypercalcemia; toxicity may occur. Hypocalcemia can nullify effects of digoxin. Monitor electrolytes and renal function periodically. Risk of ventricular arrhythmia with electrical cardioversion. Bioavailability is different between dosage forms.

ADVERSE REACTIONS: Heart block, rhythm disturbances, anorexia, nausea, vomiting, diarrhea, visual disturbances, headache, weakness, dizziness, mental disturbances.

INTERACTIONS: Risk of toxicity with K⁺-depleting diuretics. Increased risk of arrhythmias with calcium, sympathomimetics, and succinylcholine. Increased serum levels with quinidine, verapamil, amiodarone, propafenone, indomethacin, itraconazole, alprazolam, and spironolactone; monitor for toxicity. Increased absorption with propantheline, diphenoxylate, macrolides, and tetracycline; monitor for toxicity. Decreased intestinal absorption with antacids, kaolin-pectin, sulfasalazine, neomycin, cholestyramine, certain anticancer drugs, and metoclopramide. Decreased serum levels with rifampin. Increased digoxin dose requirement with thyroid supplements. Additive effects on AV node conduction with β-blockers or CCBs. Caution with drugs that deteriorate renal function.

PREGNANCY: Category C, caution in nursing.

MECHANISM OF ACTION: Cardiac glycoside; inhibits Na⁺-K⁺ ATPase, leading to increase in intracellular concentration of Ca⁺.

PHARMACOKINETICS: Absorption: (Tab) Absolute bioavailability (60%-80%), T_{max}=1-3 hrs. (Sol) Absolute bioavailability (70-85%). (Lanoxicaps) Absolute bioavailability (90-100%). (Inj) Absolute bioavailability (100%). **Distribution:** Plasma protein binding (25%), crosses placenta. **Metabolism:** Hydrolysis, oxidation, and conjugation. **Elimination:** Urine (50%-70%); $T_{1/2}$=1.5-2 days.

LANTUS   RX
insulin glargine, human (Sanofi-Aventis)

THERAPEUTIC CLASS: Insulin

INDICATIONS: Treatment of adults and pediatrics with type 1 diabetes mellitus. Treatment of adults with type 2 diabetes mellitus who require basal (long-acting) insulin.

DOSAGE: *Adults:* Individualize dose. For SQ injection only. Administer qd at same time each day. Insulin naive patients on oral antidiabetic drugs, start with 10 U qd. Switching from once-daily NPH or Ultralente does not require initial dose change. Switching from bid NPH, reduce initial dose by 20%. Maint: 2-100 U/day.
Pediatrics: ≥6 yrs: Individualize dose. For SQ injection only. Administer qd at same time each day. Insulin naive patients on oral antidiabetic drugs, start with 10 U qd. Switching from once-daily NPH or Ultralente does not require initial dose change. Switching from bid NPH, reduce initial dose by 20%. Maint: 2-100 U/day.

HOW SUPPLIED: Inj: 100 U/mL; OptiClik: 100 U/mL

WARNINGS/PRECAUTIONS: Human insulin differs from animal source insulin. Any change of insulin should be made cautiously. Changes in strength, manufacturer, type or method of manufacture may result in the need for a change in dosage. Hypoglycemia may occur with taking too much insulin, missing or delaying meals, exercising or working more than usual. An infection or illness (especially with diarrhea or vomiting) may change insulin requirements. Administration of insulin SQ can result in lipodystrophy. Not for IV use. Do not mix with other insulins. May cause sodium retention and edema. Caution in patients with renal and hepatic dysfunction.

ADVERSE REACTIONS: Hypoglycemia, allergic reactions, injection site reactions, lipodystrophy, pruritus, rash.

INTERACTIONS: Increased glucose lowering effects with ACE inhibitors, disopyramide, fibrates, fluoxetine, MAOIs, propoxyphene, salicylates, somatostatin analog, sulfonamide antibiotics, and other antidiabetic agents. Decreased blood glucose lowering effects with corticosteroids, danazol, diuretics, sympathomimetic amines, isoniazid, phenothiazine derivatives, somatropin, thyroid hormones, estrogens, progestogens, protease inhibitors and atypical antipsychotics. Pentamidine may cause hypoglycemia, followed by hyperglycemia. β-blockers, clonidine, lithium salts, and alcohol may potentiate or weaken glucose lowering effect. β-blockers, clonidine, guanethidine, and reserpine may reduce or mask signs of hypoglycemia.

PREGNANCY: Category C, caution in nursing.

MECHANISM OF ACTION: Insulin glargine (rDNA origin); regulates glucose metabolism by stimulating peripheral glucose uptake by skeletal muscle and fat, inhibits hepatic glucose production, lipolysis in the adipocyte, proteolysis, and enhances protein synthesis.

PHARMACOKINETICS: Absorption: Slow, prolonged, and relatively constant. **Metabolism:** Partly metabolized into 2 active metabolites [M1 (21^A-Gly-insulin) and M2 (21^A-Gly-des-30^B-Thr-insulin)].

LARIAM   RX
mefloquine HCL (Roche Labs)

THERAPEUTIC CLASS: Quinolinemethanol derivative

INDICATIONS: Treatment and prophylaxis of mild to moderate acute malaria caused by *P.falciparum* or *P.vivax*.

DOSAGE: *Adults:* Treatment: 1250mg single dose. Prophylaxis: 250mg/week. Start 1 week before arrival in endemic area and continue weekly (same day of week) while in area. Continue for 4 weeks after leaving the area. Take with food and 8 oz of water.
Pediatrics: ≥6 months: Treatment: Usual: 20-25mg/kg, split in 2 doses. Take 6-8 hrs apart. If vomiting occurs <30 min after dose, give a 2nd full dose. If vomiting occurs 30-60 min after dose, give additional half-dose. Prophylaxis: ≥3 months: 3-5mg/kg/week. >45kg: 250mg/week. 31-45kg: 3/4 tab/week. 21-30kg: 125mg/week. 5-20kg: 1/4 tab/week. Take with food and water. May crush and mix with water.

HOW SUPPLIED: Tab: 250mg* *scored

CONTRAINDICATIONS: Hypersensitivity to related compounds (eg, quinine, quinidine). Use as prophylaxis with active or recent history of depression, generalized anxiety disorder, psychosis or schizophrenia, or other major psychiatric disorder, or with a history of convulsions.

WARNINGS/PRECAUTIONS: In life-threatening malaria infection due to *P.falciparum*, use IV antimalarials. High risk of relapse seen with acute *P.vivax*; after initial treatment, subsequently treat with 8-aminoquinoline (eg, primaquine). May cause psychiatric symptoms. During prophylaxis, d/c if symptoms of acute anxiety, depression, restlessness, or confusion occur. In long-term therapy, monitor LFTs and perform ophthalmic exams. May impair mental/physical abilities. Increase risk of convulsions in epileptic patients. Caution with cardiac disease, hepatic dysfunction and elderly.

ADVERSE REACTIONS: Nausea, vomiting, myalgia, fever, dizziness, headache, somnolence, sleep disorders, loss of balance, chills, diarrhea, abdominal pain, fatigue, tinnitus, pruritus, skin rash.

INTERACTIONS: Avoid halofantrine; may prolong QTc interval. Concomitant administration with other related compounds (eg, quinine, quinidine, chloroquine) may cause ECG abnormalities and increased risk of convulsions; delay mefloquine dose for 12 hrs after last dose of these drugs. Avoid propranolol; cardiopulmonary arrest reported. Drugs that may alter cardiac conduction (eg, anti-arrhythmic or β-blockers, CCBs, antihistamines, H$_1$-blockers, TCAs, and phenothiazines) may prolong QT$_c$ interval. May lower plasma levels of anticonvulsants (eg, valproic acid, carbamazepine, phenobarbital, phenytoin); monitor blood levels and adjust dosage accordingly. Complete vaccinations with live, attenuated vaccines (eg, typhoid vaccine) at least 3 days before mefloquine therapy. Caution with anticoagulants, antidiabetic agents.

PREGNANCY: Category C, not for use in nursing.

MECHANISM OF ACTION: Quinolinemethanol derivative; suspected to act as blood schizonticide.

PHARMACOKINETICS: Absorption: Mefloquine: C_{max}=1000 mcg/L, T_{max}=6-24 hrs; 2,8-bis-trifluoromethyl-4-quinoline carboxylic acid: T_{max}=2 weeks. **Distribution:** V_d=20l/kg; plasma protein binding (80%); crosses placenta; found in breast milk. **Metabolism:** Active metabolite: 2,8-bis-trifluoromethyl-4-quinoline carboxylic acid. **Elimination:** Bile, feces; $T_{1/2}$=2-4 weeks. Hepatic excretion.

LESCOL XL   RX
fluvastatin sodium (Novartis)

OTHER BRAND NAMES: Lescol (Novartis)

THERAPEUTIC CLASS: HMG-CoA reductase inhibitor

INDICATIONS: Adjunct to diet, to reduce elevated total cholesterol (Total-C), LDL-C, TG, and Apo B levels, and to increase HDL-C in primary hypercholesterolemia and mixed dyslipidemia (Types IIa and IIb) when response to nonpharmacological measures is inadequate. To slow coronary atherosclerosis progression in coronary heart disease by lowering Total-C and LDL-C. To reduce risk of undergoing coronary revascularization procedures in patients with coronary heart disease. Adjunct to diet, to reduce Total-C, LDL-C, and Apo B levels in adolescent boys and girls who are at least 1 yr post-menarche, 10-16 yrs of age, with heterozygous familial hypercholesterolemia when response to dietary restriction is inadequate and LDL-C remains ≥190mg/dL or if LDL-C remains ≥160mg/dL and there is positive family history of premature CV disease or 2 or more other CV disease risk factors are present.

DOSAGE: *Adults:* ≥18 yrs: (For LDL-C reduction of ≥25%) Initial: 40mg cap qpm or 80mg XL tab at any time of day or 40mg cap bid. (For LDL-C reduction of <25%) Initial: 20mg cap qpm. Range: 20-80mg/day. Severe Renal Impairment: Caution with dose >40mg/day. Take 2 hrs after bile-acid resins qhs.
Pediatrics: Heterozygous Familial Hypercholesterolemia: 10-16 yrs (≥1 yr post-menarche): Individualize dose: Initial: One 20mg cap. Titrate: Adjust dose at 6-week intervals. Max: 40mg cap bid or 80mg XL tab qd.

HOW SUPPLIED: Cap: (Lescol) 20mg, 40mg; Tab, Extended-Release: (Lescol XL) 80mg

CONTRAINDICATIONS: Active liver disease or unexplained, persistent elevations of serum transaminases, pregnancy, nursing mothers.

WARNINGS/PRECAUTIONS: Monitor LFTs prior to therapy, at 12 weeks, or with dose elevation. D/C if AST or ALT ≥3x ULN on 2 consecutive occasions. Risk of myopathy and/or rhabdomyolysis reported. D/C if markedly elevated CPK levels occur, if myopathy is diagnosed or suspected, or if predisposition to renal failure secondary to rhabdomyolysis. Less effective with homozygous familial hypercholesterolemia. Caution with heavy alcohol use and/or history of hepatic disease. Evaluate if endocrine dysfunction develops.

ADVERSE REACTIONS: Dyspepsia, abdominal pain, headache, nausea, diarrhea, abnormal LFTs, myalgia, flu-like symptoms.

INTERACTIONS: Rifampicin significantly decreases serum levels. Increases levels of glyburide, diclofenac, and phenytoin. Increased serum levels with glyburide, phenytoin, cimetidine, ranitidine, and omeprazole. Caution with drugs that decrease levels of endogenous steroid hormones (eg, ketoconazole, spironolactone, cimetidine). Avoid fibrates. Cyclosporine, colchicine, gemfibrozil, erythromycin, or niacin may increase risk of myopathy/rhabdomyolysis. Cholestyramine given within 4 hrs decreases serum levels but has additive effects when given 4 hrs after fluvastatin (immediate-release). Monitor digoxin, anticoagulants.

PREGNANCY: Category X, not for use in nursing.

MECHANISM OF ACTION: Competitive inhibition of HMG-CoA reductase; inhibits conversion of HMG-CoA to mevalonate (precursor of sterols, including cholesterol). Inhibition of cholesterol biosynthesis reduces cholesterol in hepatic cells, which stimulates the synthesis of LDL receptors, thereby increasing uptake of LDL particles, resulting in reduction of plasma cholesterol concentration.

PHARMACOKINETICS: Absorption: Rapid and complete, bioavailability (29%); T_{max}=3 hrs (fasting). **Distribution:** V_d=0.35L/kg, plasma protein binding (98%); found in breast milk. **Metabolism:** Liver via CYP2C9, 2C8 and 3A4 through N-dealkylation, β-oxidation pathways. **Elimination:** Feces, (90% metabolites, <2% unchanged), urine (5%); $T_{1/2}$=9 hrs.

LETAIRIS   RX
ambrisentan (Gilead)

> Potential liver injury and contraindicated in pregnancy. Available only through the Letairis Education and Access Program (LEAP), by calling 1-866-664-LEAP (5327).

THERAPEUTIC CLASS: Endothelin receptor antagonist

INDICATIONS: Treatment of pulmonary arterial hypertension (WHO Group 1) in patients with WHO class II or III symptoms to improve exercise capacity and delay clinical worsening.

DOSAGE: *Adults:* Initial: 5mg qd. May increase to 10mg qd if 5mg tolerated. Max: 10mg qd. Do not split, crush, or chew.

HOW SUPPLIED: Tab: 5mg, 10mg

CONTRAINDICATIONS: Pregnancy.

WARNINGS/PRECAUTIONS: Monitor liver chemistries before therapy and at least every month thereafter. Avoid therapy if elevated aminotransferase levels (>3x ULN) at baseline. If aminotransferase level is >3x ULN and ≤5x ULN, reduce daily dose or interrupt treatment and continue to monitor every 2 weeks until levels are <3x ULN. If aminotransferase elevations >5x ULN and ≤8x ULN, d/c and continue monitoring until levels are <3x ULN; may then re-initiate with more frequent monitoring of aminotransferase levels. If aminotransferase elevations >8x ULN, d/c and avoid re-initiation. May cause peripheral edema; if clinically significant, with or without weight gain, further evaluate to determine cause, such as heart failure and possible need for treatment. May decrease Hgb and Hct; measure Hgb prior to initiation, at 1 month, then periodically thereafter.

ADVERSE REACTIONS: Peripheral edema, headache, nasal congestion, palpitations, flushing, constipation, dyspnea, sinusitis, nasopharyngitis, abdominal pain.

INTERACTIONS: Cyclosporine-A may increase levels; caution when co-administering. Also use caution with strong CYP3A4 inhibitors (eg, ketoconazole), CYP2C19 inhibitors (eg, omeprazole), inducers of P-gp, CYPs, and UGTs.

PREGNANCY: Category X, not for use in nursing.

MECHANISM OF ACTION: Endothelin receptor antagonist; not established.

PHARMACOKINETICS: Absorption: Rapid, T_{max}=2 hrs. **Distribution:** Plasma protein binding (99%). **Elimination:** $T_{1/2}$=15 hrs.

LEUCOVORIN CALCIUM   RX
leucovorin calcium (Various)

THERAPEUTIC CLASS: Cytoprotective agent

INDICATIONS: (Inj, Tab) Rescue therapy after high-dose methotrexate (MTX) therapy in osteosarcoma. To reduce toxicity of impaired MTX elimination or overdose of folic acid antagonists. Adjunct to 5-fluorouracil (5-FU) for palliative treatment of advanced colorectal cancer. Treatment of megaloblastic anemia due to folic acid deficiency.

DOSAGE: *Adults:* Colorectal Cancer: 200mg/m² slow IV push over 3 min. followed by 5-FU 370mg/m² IV qd for 5 days, or 20mg/m² IV qd followed by

5-FU 425mg/m^2 IV qd for 5 days. May repeat at 4 week intervals for 2 courses then at 4-5 week intervals. May increase 5-FU dose by 10% if no toxicity. Reduce 5-FU dose by 20% with moderate GI/hematologic toxicity and by 30% with severe toxicity. Leucovorin Rescue: 15mg q6h for 10 doses starting 24 hrs after start of MTX until serum MTX is <5x10^{-8}M. Give IV/IM with GI toxicity. See PI for leucovorin adjustments and extended therapy. Impaired MTX Elimination/Overdose: 10mg/m^2 IV/IM/PO q6h until serum MTX is <10^{-8}M. Increase to 100mg/m^2 q3h if 24-hr serum creatinine is 50% over baseline, or if 24-hr serum MTX is >5x10^{-6}M, or the 48-hr level is >9x10^{-7}M. Give IV/IM with GI toxicity. Start ASAP after overdose and within 24 hrs of MTX with delayed excretion. Megaloblastic Anemia: Up to 1mg/day. Elderly: Caution with dose selection.

HOW SUPPLIED: Inj: 10mg/mL, 50mg, 100mg, 200mg, 350mg, 500mg; Tab: 5mg, 10mg, 15mg, 25mg

CONTRAINDICATIONS: Improper therapy for pernicious anemia and other megaloblastic anemias secondary to lack of vitamin B$_{12}$.

WARNINGS/PRECAUTIONS: Do not administer >160mg/min. Do not give intrathecally. Monitor serum MTX. Higher than recommended PO doses must be given IV. Increased risk of severe toxicity in elderly/debilitated colorectal cancer patients taking 5-FU with leucovorin. Monitor renal function in elderly.

ADVERSE REACTIONS: Allergic sensitization.

INTERACTIONS: Folic acid in large amounts may antagonize phenobarbital, phenytoin, and primidone, and increase seizure frequency in children. May enhance 5-FU toxicity. May reduce MTX efficacy. Increased treatment failure and morbidity in TMP-SMZ-treated HIV patients with PCP.

PREGNANCY: Category C, caution use in nursing.

MECHANISM OF ACTION: Folic acid derivative; antidote for folic acid antagonists.

PHARMACOKINETICS: Absorption: IV: (5-formyl-THF) C_{max}=1206ng/mL, T_{max}=10 minutes; (5-methyl-THF) C_{max}=258ng/mL, T_{max}=1.3 hrs. IM: (5-formyl-THF) C_{max}=360ng/mL, T_{max}=28 minutes; (5-methyl-THF) C_{max}=226ng/mL, T_{max}=2.8 hrs. Oral: (5-formyl-THF)C_{max}=51ng/mL, T_{max}=1.2 hrs; (5-methyl-THF) C_{max}=367ng/mL, T_{max}=2.4 hrs. **Metabolism:** 5-methyl-THF (metabolite via reduction).

LEUKERAN   RX
chlorambucil (GlaxoSmithKline)

> Risk of severe bone marrow suppression. Potentially carcinogenic, mutagenic, and teratogenic. Produces human infertility.

THERAPEUTIC CLASS: Nitrogen mustard alkylating agent

INDICATIONS: Treatment of chronic lymphatic (lymphocytic) leukemia (CLL), malignant lymphomas, and Hodgkin's disease.

DOSAGE: *Adults:* Usual: 0.1-0.2mg/kg qd for 3-6 weeks. Adjust according to response; reduce with abrupt WBC decline. Lymphocytic Infiltration of Bone Marrow/Hypoplastic Bone Marrow: Max: 0.1mg/kg/day. Caution within 4 weeks of full course of radiation or chemotherapy.

HOW SUPPLIED: Tab: 2mg

CONTRAINDICATIONS: Prior resistance to therapy.

WARNINGS/PRECAUTIONS: Convulsions, infertility, leukemia and secondary malignancies observed. Shown to cause chromatid or chromosome damage and sterility. Skin rash progressing to erythema multiforme, toxic epidermal necrolysis, or Stevens-Johnson syndrome reported. Avoid becoming pregnant. Lymphopenia reported, usually returns to normal upon completion. Monitor Hgb, leukocyte count and differential, platelet counts weekly. Avoid live vaccines in the immunocompromised.

L

ADVERSE REACTIONS: Bone marrow suppression, nausea, vomiting, diarrhea, tremors, muscular twitching, confusion, agitation, ataxia, urticaria, angioneurotic syndrome, pulmonary fibrosis, hepatotoxicity, jaundice.

INTERACTIONS: Cross-hypersensitivity may occur with other alkylating agents.

PREGNANCY: Category D, not for use in nursing.

MECHANISM OF ACTION: Nitrogen mustard alkylating agent.

PHARMACOKINETICS: Absorption: Rapid and complete. (0.6-1.2 mg/kg) T_{max}=1 hr; (0.2mg/kg) C_{max}=492ng/mL, AUC=883ng•h/mL, T_{max}=0.83 hrs; (Phenylacetic acid mustard) C_{max}=306ng/mL, AUC=1204ng•h/mL, T_{max}=1.9 hrs. **Distribution:** Plasma protein binding (99%); crosses placenta. **Metabolism:** Liver (rapid). Phenylacetic acid mustard (major metabolite). **Elimination:** Low urinary excretion; $T_{1/2}$=1.5 hrs (0.6-1.2mg/kg); $T_{1/2}$=1.3 hrs (0.2mg/kg); $T_{1/2}$=1.8 hrs (phenylacetic acid mustard).

LEUKINE RX
sargramostim (Berlex)

THERAPEUTIC CLASS: Granulocyte-macrophage colony stimulating factor

INDICATIONS: Acute myelogenous leukemia (AML) following induction chemotherapy in older adults (≥55 yrs) to shorten time to neutrophil recovery and to reduce incidence of severe and life-threatening infections and infections resulting in death. For mobilization of hematopoietic progenitor cells into peripheral blood for collection by leukopheresis. Myeloid recovery after autologous bone marrow transplantation (BMT) in non-Hodgkin's lymphoma (NHL), acute lymphoblastic leukemia (ALL), and Hodgkin's disease. Myeloid recovery after allogeneic BMT. BMT (allogeneic or autologous) failure or engraftment delay.

DOSAGE: *Adults:* ≥55 yrs: Neutrophil Recovery Post-Chemo in AML: Hypoplastic Bone Marrow with <5% Blasts: 250mcg/m²/day IV over 4 hrs starting on day 11 or 4 days after completion of induction chemo. If 2nd cycle of induction chemo needed, give 4 days after completion of chemo. Continue until ANC >1500 cells/mm³ for 3 consecutive days or max of 42 days. D/C immediately if leukemic regrowth occurs; reduce dose by 50% or temporarily d/c if severe adverse reaction occurs. Mobilization of Peripheral Blood Progenitor Cells (PBPC): 250mcg/m²/day IV over 24 hrs or SC once daily. Continue through PBPC collection period. Reduce dose by 50% if WBC >50,000 cells/mm³. Post Peripheral Blood Progenitor Cell Transplant: 250mcg/m²/day IV over 24 hrs or SC once daily. Begin immediately after infusion of progenitor cells and continue until ANC >1500 cells/mm³ for 3 consecutive days. Myeloid Reconstitution After BMT: 250mcg/m²/day IV over 2 hrs 2-4 hrs post bone marrow infusion and not less than 24 hrs after last dose of chemo- or radiotherapy. Do not give until ANC <500 cells/mm³. Continue until ANC >1500 cells/mm³ for 3 consecutive days. May reduce dose by 50% or temporarily d/c if severe adverse reaction occurs. D/C immediately if blast cells appear or disease progression occurs. BMT Failure/Engraftment Delay: 250mcg/m²/day IV over 2 hrs for 14 days. May repeat after 7 days if needed. Give 3rd course after another 7 days of 500mcg/m²/day IV for 14 days if needed. May reduce dose by 50% or temporarily d/c if severe adverse reaction occurs. D/C immediately if blast cells appear or disease progression occurs. Reduce dose by 50% or interrupt treatment if ANC >20,000 cells/mm³.

HOW SUPPLIED: Inj: 250mcg/vial, 500mcg/mL

CONTRAINDICATIONS: Excessive leukemic myeloid blasts in bone marrow or peripheral blood (≥10%), concomitant chemotherapy or radiotherapy.

WARNINGS/PRECAUTIONS: Contains benzyl alcohol; avoid use in neonates. Caution with pre-existing fluid retention, pulmonary infiltrate, CHF, hypoxia, cardiac disease, renal/hepatic dysfunction, or myeloid malignancies. Monitor CBC twice weekly and renal/hepatic function every other week with pre-existing dysfunction.

ADVERSE REACTIONS: Fever, nausea, diarrhea, vomiting, alopecia, rash, headache, stomatitis, anorexia, mucous membrane disorder, asthenia, malaise, abdominal pain, edema, HTN.

INTERACTIONS: Caution with drugs that may potentiate myeloproliferative effects (eg, lithium, corticosteroids).

PREGNANCY: Category C, caution in nursing.

MECHANISM OF ACTION: Recombinant human granulocyte-macrophage colony stimulating factor (GM-CSF); stimulates proliferation and differentiation of hematopoietic progenitor cells.

PHARMACOKINETICS: Absorption: IV: (liquid) C_{max}=5ng/mL, AUC=640ng/mL•min; (lyophilized) C_{max}=5.4ng/mL, AUC=677ng/mL•min. SC: T_{max}=1-3 hrs, C_{max}=1.5ng/mL; (liquid) AUC=549ng/mL•min; (lyophilized) AUC=501ng/mL•min. **Elimination:** $T_{1/2}$=60 min (IV); 162 min (SC).

LEUSTATIN   RX
cladribine (Ortho Biotech)

Anticipate reversible and dose dependent suppression of bone-marrow function. Serious neurological toxicity and acute nephrotoxicity reported with high doses (4-9x recommended dose). Acute nephrotoxicity observed especially with other nephrotoxic therapies.

THERAPEUTIC CLASS: Chlorinated purine nucleoside analog

INDICATIONS: Treatment of active Hairy Cell Leukemia.

DOSAGE: *Adults:* 0.09mg/kg/day continuous IV infusion for 7 days given as a single course. Delay or discontinue if neurotoxicity or renal toxicity occurs.

HOW SUPPLIED: Inj: 1mg/mL

WARNINGS/PRECAUTIONS: Periodically monitor peripheral blood counts, especially during 1st 4-8 weeks post-treatment. Fever reported in 1st month of therapy. Benzyl alcohol is in the diluent for 7-day infusion; it associated with fatal "Gasping Syndrome" in premature infants. Can cause fetal harm during pregnancy. Caution with renal or hepatic insufficiency, or with severe bone-marrow impairment. Assess renal and hepatic function periodically. Monitor for hematologic and non-hematologic toxicity.

ADVERSE REACTIONS: Bone-marrow suppression, neutropenia, fever, infection, fatigue, nausea, rash, headache, injection site reactions, decreased appetite, vomiting.

INTERACTIONS: Caution with drugs that cause immunosuppression or myelo-suppression. Acute nephrotoxicity with nephrotoxic agents.

PREGNANCY: Category D, not for use in nursing.

MECHANISM OF ACTION: Antineoplastic agent; inhibits DNA synthesis and repair.

PHARMACOKINETICS: Distribution: V_d=4.5L/kg, plasma protein binding (20%). **Elimination:** $T_{1/2}$=5.4 hrs, urine (18%).

LEVAQUIN   RX
levofloxacin (Ortho-McNeil)

THERAPEUTIC CLASS: Fluoroquinolone

INDICATIONS: Uncomplicated and complicated skin and skin structure (SSSI), and urinary tract infections (UTI), acute bacterial sinusitis, acute bacterial exacerbation of chronic bronchitis (ABECB), community-acquired pneumonia (CAP), including multi-drug resistant *Streptococcus pneumoniae*, nosocomial pneumonia, chronic bacterial prostatitis (CBP), and acute pyelonephritis caused by susceptible strains of microorganisms. To reduce the incidence or progression of disease of inhalational anthrax following exposure to *Bacillus anthracis* in adults and pediatric patients ≥ 6 months.

DOSAGE: *Adults:* ≥18 yrs: IV/PO: ABECB: 500mg qd for 7 days. CAP: 500mg qd for 7-14 days or 750mg qd for 5 days. Sinusitis: 500mg qd for 10-14 days

or 750mg qd for 5 days. CBP: 500mg qd for 28 days. Uncomplicated SSSI: 500mg qd for 7-10 days. Complicated SSSI/Nosocomial Pneumonia: 750mg qd for 7-14 days. Inhalational Anthrax: 500mg qd for 60 days. Complicated SSSI/Nosocomial Pneumonia/CAP/Sinusitis: CrCl 20-49mL/min: 750mg, then 750mg q48h. CrCl 10-19mL/min/Hemodialysis/CAPD: 750mg, then 500mg q48h. ABECB/CAP/Sinusitis/Uncomplicated SSSI/CBP/Inhalational Anthrax: CrCl 20-49mL/min: 500mg, then 250mg q24h. CrCl 10-19mL/min/Hemodialysis/CAPD: 500mg, then 250mg q48h. Complicated UTI/Acute Pyelonephritis: 250mg qd for 10 days or 750mg qd for 5 days. CrCl 10-19mL/min: 250mg, then 250mg q48h or 750mg, then 500mg q48h. Hemodialysis: 750mg, then 500mg q48h. Uncomplicated UTI: 250mg qd for 3 days. Take oral solution 1 hr before or 2 hrs after eating.
Pediatrics: ≥ 6 months: >50kg: 500mg q24h for 60 days. <50kg: 8mg/kg (not to exceed 250mg per dose) q12h for 60 days.

HOW SUPPLIED: Inj: 5mg/mL, 25mg/mL; Sol: 25mg/mL; Tab: 250mg, 500mg, 750mg [Leva-pak, 5^s]

WARNINGS/PRECAUTIONS: Only administer injection via IV infusion over a period of not less than 60 or 90 min depending on dosage. Convulsions, toxic psychoses, increased ICP, CNS stimulation reported; d/c if any occur. Caution with CNS disorders that may predispose to seizures/lower seizure threshold (eg, epilepsy, renal insufficiency, drug therapy). Moderate to severe photo-toxicity can occur. Serious/fatal hypersensitivity reactions; d/c at first sign of rash. Colitis and torsade de pointes (rare) reported. May permit overgrowth of Clostridia. *Clostridium difficile*-associated diarrhea reported. Liver, hemato-logic (including agranulocytosis, thrombocytopenia) and renal toxicities may occur after multiple doses. Caution in renal insufficiency. Tendon ruptures reported. D/C if pain, inflammation, or ruptured tendon occurs. Prolongation of AT interval and torsade de pointes reported; caution with any factors that may predispose to QTc prolongation or proarrhythmic conditions. Peripheral neuropathy, Stevens-Johnson syndrome reported. Causes musculoskeletal disorder in pediatrics and arthropathic effects in animals. More susceptible to QT interval prolongation and increased risk of tendon disorders with concomi-tant corticosteroid use in patients over 65 yrs.

ADVERSE REACTIONS: Nausea, diarrhea, headache, insomnia, constipation, pain, swelling, tendon tears.

INTERACTIONS: Decreased levels with antacids, sucralfate, didanosine, metal cations (eg, iron), and multivitamins with zinc; separate dosing by 2 hrs with PO dosing. Concomitant NSAIDs may increase seizure risk and CNS stimulation. Blood glucose changes with concomitant antidiabetic agents. May increase theophylline levels; monitor closely. Increases PT with warfarin; monitor closely. Severe tendon disorders are increased with concomitant corticosteroid therapy. Caution with concomitant drugs that may result in prolongation of the QT interval. Hyperglycemia or hypoglycemia may occur with insulin or oral hypoglycemics.

PREGNANCY: Category C, not for use in nursing.

MECHANISM OF ACTION: Fluoroquinolone: Synthetic broad-spectrum anti-microbial agent; inhibits topoisomerase II (DNA gyrase) and topoisomerase IV, which are required for bacterial DNA replication, transcription, repair, and recombination.

PHARMACOKINETICS: Absorption: Rapid and complete. T_{max}=1-2 hrs. **Distribution:** V_d=74-112L. Plasma protein binding (approx. 24-38%). **Metabolism:** Limited. **Elimination:** Urine, $T_{1/2}$=6-8 hrs.

LEVATOL   RX
penbutolol sulfate (Schwarz)

THERAPEUTIC CLASS: Nonselective beta-blocker

INDICATIONS: Treatment of mild to moderate arterial hypertension.

DOSAGE: *Adults:* 20mg qd.

HOW SUPPLIED: Tab: 20mg* *scored

CONTRAINDICATIONS: Cardiogenic shock, sinus bradycardia, 2nd- and 3rd-degree AV block, bronchial asthma.

WARNINGS/PRECAUTIONS: Caution with well-compensated heart failure, elderly, nonallergic bronchospasm, renal impairment. Can cause cardiac failure. Avoid abrupt withdrawal. Withdrawal before surgery is controversial. May mask hypoglycemia or hyperthyroidism symptoms.

ADVERSE REACTIONS: Diarrhea, nausea, dyspepsia, dizziness, fatigue, headache, insomnia, cough.

INTERACTIONS: Increases volume of distribution of lidocaine; may need larger LD. Synergistic hypotensive effects, bradycardia, and arrhythmias with oral CCBs. Avoid catecholamine-depleting drugs. Caution with alcohol, anesthetics that depress the myocardium. May antagonize epinephrine.

PREGNANCY: Category C, caution in nursing.

MECHANISM OF ACTION: β-receptor antagonist; not established, proposed to competitively antagonize catecholamines at peripheral adrenergic receptor sites and have CNS action leading to reduced sympathetic outflow to periphery and reduction of renin activity.

PHARMACOKINETICS: Absorption: Rapid and complete; T_{max}=2-3 hrs. **Distribution:** Plasma protein binding (80-98%). **Metabolism:** Conjugation and oxidation. 4-hydroxy penbutolol (metabolite). **Elimination:** Urine; $T_{1/2}$=5 hrs.

LEVBID RX
hyoscyamine sulfate (Alaven)

OTHER BRAND NAMES: Levsinex (Alaven) - Levsin (Alaven)
THERAPEUTIC CLASS: Anticholinergic
INDICATIONS: Adjunct treatment of peptic ulcer, irritable bowel syndrome, neurogenic bladder, and neurogenic bowel disturbances. Management of functional intestinal disorders (eg, mild dysenteries, diverticulitis). To control gastric secretion, visceral spasm, and hypermotility in spastic colitis, spastic bladder, cystitis, pylorospasm, and associated abdominal cramps. Symptomatic relief of biliary and renal colic with concomitant morphine or other narcotics. Drying agent for symptomatic relief of acute rhinitis. To reduce rigidity and tremors of Parkinson's disease and control associated sialorrhea and hyperhidrosis. For anticholinesterase poisoning. To reduce pain and hypersecretion in pancreatitis. For certain cases of partial heart block associated with vagal activity. (Elixir, Drops) Treatment of infant colic. (Inj) Facilitates GI diagnostic procedures. Reduces pain and hypersecretion in pancreatitis, in cases of partial heart block associated with vagal activity, and as antidote for anticholinesterase poisoning. In anesthesia as a pre-op antimuscarinic. In urology to improve radiologic visibility of kidneys.

DOSAGE: *Adults:* May also chew or swallow SL tab. (Drops, Elixir, Tab, and Tab, SL) 0.125-0.25mg q4h or prn. Max: 1.5mg/24 hrs. (Cap and Tab, Extended-Release) 0.375-0.75mg q12h; or 1 cap q8h. Max: 1.5mg/24 hrs. Do not crush or chew. (Inj) GI Disorders: 0.25-0.5mg IM/IV/SQ as single dose or up to qid at 4-hr intervals. Diagnostic Procedures: 0.25-0.5mg IV 5-10 min before procedure. Anesthesia: 5mcg/kg IM/IV/SQ 30-60 min before anesthesia or with narcotic/sedative administration. GI Disorders: 0.25-0.5mg IM/IV/SQ as single dose; may require bid-qid administration at 4-hr intervals. Diagnostic Procedures: 0.25-0.5mg IV 5-10 min prior. Drug-Induced Bradycardia (Surgery): Increments of 0.25mL IV; repeat prn. Neuromuscular Blockade Reversal: 0.2mg for every 1mg neostigmine or equal dose of physostigmine or pyridostigmine.
Pediatrics: May also chew or swallow SL tab. ≥12 yrs: (Drops, Elixir, Tab, and Tab, SL) 0.125-0.25mg q4h or prn. Max: 1.5mg/24 hrs. (Cap and Tab, Extended-Release) 0.375-0.75mg q12h; or 1 cap may be given q8h. Max: 1.5mg/24 hrs. Do not crush or chew. 2 to <12 yrs: (Tab and Tab, SL) 0.0625-0.125mg q4h or prn. Max: 0.75mg/24 hrs. (Elixir) Give q4h or prn. 10kg: 1.25mL. 20kg: 2.5mL. 40kg: 3.75mL. 50kg: 5mL. Max: 30mL/24 hrs. (Drops) 0.25-1mL q4h or prn. Max: 6mL/24 hrs. <2 yrs: (Drops) Give q4h or prn. 3.4kg: 4 drops. Max: 24 drops/24 hrs. 5kg: 5 drops. Max: 30 drops/24 hrs. 7kg: 6

drops. Max: 36 drops/24 hrs. 10kg: 8 drops. Max: 48 drops/24 hrs. >2 yrs: Anesthesia: (Inj) 5mcg/kg IM/IV/SQ 30-60 min before anesthesia or with narcotic/sedative administration.

HOW SUPPLIED: (Levbid) Tab, Extended-Release: 0.375mg. (Levsin) Drops: 0.125mg/mL [15mL]; Elixir: 0.125mg/5mL [473mL]; Inj: 0.5mg/mL; Tab: 0.125mg*; Tab, SL: 0.125mg*. (Levsinex) Cap, Extended-Release: 0.375mg *scored

CONTRAINDICATIONS: Glaucoma, obstructive uropathy, GI tract obstruction, paralytic ileus; intestinal atony of elderly/debilitated, unstable CV status in acute hemorrhage, toxic megacolon complicating ulcerative colitis, myasthenia gravis.

WARNINGS/PRECAUTIONS: Risk of heat prostration with high environmental temperature. Avoid activities requiring mental alertness. Psychosis has been reported. Caution with diarrhea, autonomic neuropathy, hyperthyroidism, coronary heart disease, CHF, arrhythmias/tachycardia, HTN, renal disease, and hiatal hernia associated with reflux esophagitis. D/C if diarrhea occurs.

ADVERSE REACTIONS: Anticholinergic effects, drowsiness, headache, nervousness.

INTERACTIONS: Additive effects with other antimuscarinics, amantadine, haloperidol, phenothiazines, MAOIs, TCAs, and some antihistamines. Antacids interfere with absorption; take ac and antacids pc.

PREGNANCY: Category C, caution in nursing.

MECHANISM OF ACTION: Anticholinergic/antipasmodic; inhibits specifically the actions of acetylcholine on structures innervated by postganglionic cholinergic nerves and on smooth muscles that respond to acetylcholine but lack cholinergic innervation.

PHARMACOKINETICS: Absorption: Complete. **Distribution:** Crosses blood-brain barrier and placental barrier. **Metabolism:** Hydrolyzed partially to tropic acid. **Elimination:** Urine (unchanged); $T_{1/2}$=2-3.5 hrs.

LEVEMIR RX
insulin detemir, rdna origin (Novo Nordisk)

THERAPEUTIC CLASS: Insulin

INDICATIONS: Treatment of adults and pediatrics with type 1 diabetes or adults with type 2 diabetes who require basal (long acting) insulin for the control of hyperglycemia.

DOSAGE: *Adults:* Individualize dose. Administer SQ qd or bid. Once-Daily Dosing: Administer with evening meal or bedtime. Twice-Daily Dosing: Administer evening dose with evening meal, at bedtime, or 12 hrs after morning dose. Type 1/Type 2 Diabetes on Basal-Bolus Treatment or Patients Only on Basal Insulin: Change on a unit-to-unit basis. Insulin-Naive with Type 2 Diabetes Inadequately Controlled on Oral Antidiabetics: Initial: 0.1-0.2 U/kg in evening or 10 U qd or bid.
Pediatrics: Individualize dose. Administer SQ qd or bid. Once-Daily Dosing: Administer with evening meal or bedtime. Twice-Daily Dosing: Administer evening dose with evening meal, at bedtime, or 12 hrs after morning dose. Type 1 Diabetes on Basal-Bolus Treatment or Patients Only on Basal Insulin: Change on a unit-to-unit basis.

HOW SUPPLIED: Inj: 100 U/mL [3mL, 10mL]

WARNINGS/PRECAUTIONS: Monitor glucose; may cause hypoglycemia. Not for use in an insulin infusion pump. Should not be diluted or mixed with any other insulin preparations. May cause lipodystrophy or hypersensitivity. Dose adjustment may be needed in renal or hepatic impairment and during intercurrent conditions such as illness, emotional disturbances, or other stresses.

ADVERSE REACTIONS: Allergic reactions, injection site reactions, lipodystrophy, pruritus, rash, hypoglycemia, weight gain.

INTERACTIONS: Avoid mixing with other insulins. Increased glucose lowering effects with ACE inhibitors, disopyramide, fibrates, fluoxetine, MAOIs, propoxyphene, salicylates, somatostatin analog, sulfonamide antibiotics, and other antidiabetic agents. Decreased blood glucose lowering effects with corticosteroids, danazol, diuretics, sympathomimetic agents, isoniazid, phenothiazine derivates, somatotropin, thyroid hormones, estrogens, progestogens. Pentamidine may cause hypoglycemia, followed by hyperglycemia. β-blockers, clonidine, lithium salts, and alcohol may potentiate or weaken glucose lowering effect. β-blockers, clonidine, guanethidine, and reserpine may reduce or mask signs of hypoglycemia.

PREGNANCY: Category C, caution in nursing.

MECHANISM OF ACTION: Insulin detemir (rDNA origin); regulates glucose metabolism and lowers blood glucose by facilitating cellular uptake and inhibiting the glucose output from the liver.

PHARMACOKINETICS: Absorption: Slow, prolonged; absolute bioavailability (60%); T_{max}=6-8 hrs. **Distribution:** V_d=0.1L/kg; plasma protein binding (≥98%). **Metabolism:** Liver. **Elimination:** $T_{1/2}$=5-7 hrs.

LEVITRA   RX
vardenafil HCL (Schering)

THERAPEUTIC CLASS: Phosphodiesterase type 5 inhibitor

INDICATIONS: Treatment of erectile dysfunction (ED).

DOSAGE: *Adults:* Initial: 10mg one hour prior to sexual activity at frequency of up to once daily. Titrate: May decrease to 5mg or increase to max of 20mg based on response. Elderly: ≥65 yrs: Initial: 5mg. Moderate Hepatic Impairment: Initial: 5mg; Max: 10mg. Concomitant Ritonavir: Max: 2.5mg/72 hrs. Concomitant Indinavir/Saquinavir/Atazanavir/Ketoconazole 400mg daily/Itraconazole 400mg daily: Max: 2.5mg/24 hrs. Concomitant Ketoconazole 200mg daily/Itraconazole 200mg daily/Erythromycin: Max: 5mg/24 hrs.

HOW SUPPLIED: Tab: 2.5mg, 5mg, 10mg, 20mg

CONTRAINDICATIONS: Concomitant nitrates or nitric oxide donors.

WARNINGS/PRECAUTIONS: Avoid when sexual activity is inadvisable due to underlying CV status. Increased sensitivity to vasodilation effects with left ventricular outflow obstruction. Decrease in supine BP reported. Avoid with unstable angina, hypotension (SBP<90 mmHg), uncontrolled HTN(>170/100 mmHg), recent history of stroke, life-threatening arrhythmia, MI (within last 6 months), severe cardiac failure, severe hepatic impairment (Child-Pugh C), end-stage renal disease requiring dialysis, hereditary degenerative retinal disorders including retinitis pigmentosa, congenital QT prolongation. Caution with bleeding disorders, peptic ulcers, anatomical deformation of the penis, or predisposition to priapism. Rare reports of non-arteritic anterior ischemic optic neuropathy (NAION) with PDE5 inhibitors. Sudden decrease or loss of hearing accompanied by tinnitus and dizziness reported.

ADVERSE REACTIONS: Headache, flushing, rhinitis, dyspepsia, sinusitis, flu syndrome, sudden decrease or loss of hearing, tinnitus.

INTERACTIONS: See Contraindications. Avoid use with α-blockers, nitrates, Class IA (eg, quinidine, procainamide) or Class III (eg, amiodarone, sotalol) antiarrhythmics, and other agents for ED. Increased levels with ritonavir, indinavir,saquinavir, atazanavir, ketoconazole, clarithromycin, erythromycin. May have additive hypotensive effect with nifedipine. Increased levels with CYP3A4 inhibitors.

PREGNANCY: Category B, not for use in nursing.

MECHANISM OF ACTION: Phosphodiesterase type 5 inhibitor; enhances the effect of nitric oxide by inhibiting phosphodiesterase type 5, which is responsible for the degradation of cGMP in the corpus cavernosum.

PHARMACOKINETICS: Absorption: Rapid, absolute bioavailability (15%); T_{max}=30 min-2 hrs. **Distribution:** V_d=208L; Plasma protein binding (95%). **Metabolism:** Via CYP3A4, CYP3A5, CYP2C. M1 (major metabolite). **Elimination:** $T_{1/2}$=4-5 hrs; feces (91-95%), urine (2-6%).

LEVLEN
ethinyl estradiol - levonorgestrel (Bayer Healthcare)

RX

THERAPEUTIC CLASS: Estrogen/progestogen combination

INDICATIONS: Prevention of pregnancy.

DOSAGE: *Adults*: Start 1st Sunday after menses begin. *21-day*: 1 tab qd for 21 days, stop for 7 days, then repeat. *28-day*: 1 tab qd for 28 days, then repeat.

HOW SUPPLIED: Tab: (Ethinyl Estradiol-Levonorgestrel) 0.03mg-0.15mg

CONTRAINDICATIONS: Thrombophlebitis, DVT or thromboembolic disorders, pregnancy, cerebrovascular or coronary artery disease, undiagnosed abnormal genital bleeding, cholestatic jaundice of pregnancy or jaundice with prior pill use, hepatic adenomas or carcinomas, breast cancer or other estrogen-dependent neoplasia.

WARNINGS/PRECAUTIONS: Cigarette smoking increases risk of serious cardiovascular side effects; risk increases with age (especially >35 yrs) and heavy smoking. Increased risk of MI, vascular disease, thromboembolism, stroke and gallbladder disease. Retinal thrombosis, hepatic neoplasia, carcinoma of breast and reproductive organs reported. May cause glucose intolerance. May increase BP, elevate LDL levels or cause other lipid changes, fluid retention, breakthrough bleeding, and spotting. May cause or exacerbate migraine. May develop visual changes with contact lens. Increased risk of MI with HTN, hyperlipidemia, obesity, and diabetes. D/C if jaundice, significant depression or ophthalmic irregularities develop. Perform annual physical exam. Use before menarche is not indicated. May affect certain endocrine, LFTs and blood components.

ADVERSE REACTIONS: Nausea, vomiting, breakthrough bleeding, spotting, amenorrhea, migraine, depression, vaginal candidiasis, edema, weight changes.

INTERACTIONS: Reduced effects, increased breakthrough bleeding, and menstrual irregularities with rifampin, barbiturates, phenylbutazone, phenytoin, and possibly with griseofulvin, ampicillin, and tetracyclines.

PREGNANCY: Category X, not for use in nursing.

LEVLITE
ethinyl estradiol - levonorgestrel (Bayer Healthcare)

RX

THERAPEUTIC CLASS: Estrogen/progestogen combination

INDICATIONS: Prevention of pregnancy.

DOSAGE: *Adults*: 1 tab qd for 28 days, then repeat. Start 1st Sunday after menses begin or 1st day of menses.

HOW SUPPLIED: Tab: (Ethinyl Estradiol-Levonorgestrel) 0.02mg-0.1mg

CONTRAINDICATIONS: Thrombophlebitis, DVT or thromboembolic disorders, pregnancy, cerebrovascular or CAD, undiagnosed abnormal genital bleeding, cholestatic jaundice of pregnancy or jaundice with prior pill use, hepatic adenomas or carcinomas, active liver disease (as long as liver function has not returned to normal), breast cancer or other estrogen-dependent neoplasia, thrombogenic valvulopathies, thrombogenic rhythm disorders, diabetes with vascular involvement, uncontrolled HTN.

WARNINGS/PRECAUTIONS: Cigarette smoking increases risk of serious cardiovascular side effects; risk increases with age (especially >35 yrs) and heavy smoking. Increased risk of MI, vascular disease, thromboembolism, stroke and gallbladder disease. Retinal thrombosis, hepatic neoplasia, carcinoma of breast and reproductive organs reported. May cause glucose intolerance. May increase BP, elevate LDL levels or cause other lipid changes, fluid retention, breakthrough bleeding, and spotting. May cause or exacerbate migraine. May develop visual changes with contact lens. Diarrhea and/or vomiting may reduce absorption. Increased risk of MI with HTN, hyperlipidemia, obesity, and diabetes. D/C if jaundice, significant depression or ophthalmic irregularities develop. Perform annual physical exam. Use before menarche is not indicated. May affect certain endocrine, LFTs and blood components.

ADVERSE REACTIONS: Nausea, vomiting, breakthrough bleeding, spotting, amenorrhea, migraine, depression, vaginal candidiasis, edema, weight changes.

INTERACTIONS: Reduced effects, increased breakthrough bleeding, and menstrual irregularities with rifampin, barbiturates, phenylbutazone, phenytoin, griseofulvin, topiramate, some protease inhibitors, modafinil, ampicillin, tetracyclines, and possibly with St. John's wort. Troleandomycin may increase risk of intrahepatic cholestasis. Ascorbic acid, APAP, CYP3A4 inhibitors (eg, indinavir, fluconazole, troleandomycin), atorvastatin may increase plasma levels. Increased plasma levels of cyclosporine, theophylline, and corticosteroids.

PREGNANCY: Category X, not for use in nursing.

MECHANISM OF ACTION: Estrogen/progestogen combination contraceptive; acts by suppression of gonadotropins. Primarily acts by inhibiting ovulation. Also responsible for causing changes in cervical mucus (increases difficulty of sperm entry into uterus) and in the endometrium (reduces likelihood of implantation).

PHARMACOKINETICS: Absorption: Oral administration on various days resulted in different parameters. Rapid and complete, Ethinyl estradiol: Absolute bioavailability (40%) **Distribution:** Levonorgestrel: Primarily bound to sex hormone binding globulin (SHBG). Ethinyl estradiol: Plasma protein binding (97%). **Metabolism:** Levonorgestrel: Via reduction, hydroxylation and conjugation. Ethinyl Estradiol: Hepatic via CYP3A4 (hydroxylation). **Elimination:** Levonorgestrel: $T_{1/2(mean)}$=25.4 hrs; Urine, feces. Ethinyl estradiol: $T_{1/2}$=15-25 hrs.

LEVOTHROID RX
levothyroxine sodium (Forest)

THERAPEUTIC CLASS: Thyroid replacement hormone

INDICATIONS: Hypothyroidism. As a pituitary TSH suppressant for nonendemic goiter and for chronic lymphocytic thyroiditis. Diagnostic agent in suppression tests to differentiate mild hyperthyroidism or thyroid gland autonomy. Adjunct therapy with antithyroid drugs to treat thyrotoxicosis. Adjunct to surgery and radioiodine therapy for TSH-dependent thyroid cancer.

DOSAGE: *Adults:* Hypothyroidism: Usual: 100-200mcg/day. Endocrine/Cardiovascular Complications: Initial: 50mcg/day. Titrate: Increase by 50mcg/day every 2-4 weeks until euthyroid. Hypothyroid with Angina: Initial: 25mcg/day. Titrate: Increase by 25-50mcg every 2-4 weeks until euthyroid. *Pediatrics:* Hypothyroidism: >12 yrs: Usual: 100-200mcg/day. 6-12 yrs: 4-5mcg/kg/day. 1-5 yrs: 5-6mcg/kg/day. 6-12 months: 6-8mcg/kg/day. 0-6 months: 10-15mcg/kg/day. May crush tab and sprinkle over food (applesauce) or mix with 5-10mL water, formula (non-soy), or breast milk.

HOW SUPPLIED: Tab: 25mcg*, 50mcg*, 75mcg*, 88mcg*, 100mcg*, 112mcg*, 125mcg*, 137mcg*, 150mcg*, 175mcg*, 200mcg*, 300mcg* *scored

CONTRAINDICATIONS: Untreated thyrotoxicosis, acute MI, and uncorrected adrenal insufficiency.

WARNINGS/PRECAUTIONS: Do not use in the treatment of obesity; larger doses in euthyroid patients can cause serious or even life threatening toxicity. Caution with cardiovascular disease, HTN. May aggravate diabetes mellitus or insipidus and adrenal cortical insufficiency. Excessive doses in infants may produce craniosynostosis. Add glucocorticoid with myxedema coma.

ADVERSE REACTIONS: Lactose hypersensitivity, transient partial hair loss in children.

INTERACTIONS: Monitor insulin and oral hypoglycemic requirements. May potentiate anticoagulant effects of warfarin; adjust warfarin dose and monitor PT/INR. Increased adrenergic effects of catecholamines; caution with CAD. Decreased absorption with cholestyramine and colestipol; space dosing by 4-5 hrs. Estrogens increase thyroxine-binding globulin; increase in thyroid dose may be needed. Large dose may cause life-threatening toxicities with sympathomimetic amines. Avoid mixing crushed tabs with foods/formula with large amounts of iron, soybean or fiber.

PREGNANCY: Category A, caution in nursing.

MECHANISM OF ACTION: Thyroid hormone; not understood, suspected to control DNA transcription and protein synthesis. Regulates multiple metabolic processes.

PHARMACOKINETICS: Distribution: Plasma protein binding (99%).
Metabolism: Deiodination (major pathway), conjugation (minor pathway) in liver (mainly), kidneys, and other tissues. **Elimination:** Urine; T_4 (feces; 20% unchanged); $T_{1/2}$= 6-7 days; $T_{1/2}$≤2 days (T_3).

LEVOXYL RX
levothyroxine sodium (King)

THERAPEUTIC CLASS: Thyroid replacement hormone

INDICATIONS: Hypothyroidism. As a pituitary TSH suppressant in the treatment and prevention of euthyroid goiters, including thyroid nodules, lymphocytic thyroiditis, and multinodular goiter. Adjunct to surgery and radioiodine therapy for thyrotropin-dependent well-differentiated thyroid cancer.

DOSAGE: *Adults:* Take in the AM at least one-half hour before food. Hypothyroid: Usual: 1.7mcg/kg/day. >200mcg/day (seldom). >50 yrs/<50 yrs with Cardiac Disease: Initial: 25-50mcg/day. Titrate: Increase by 12.5-25mcg/day every 6-8 weeks until euthyroid. Elderly with Cardiac Disease: Initial: 12.5-25mcg/day. Titrate: Increase by 12.5-25mcg/day every 4-6 weeks until euthyroid. Severe Hypothyroidism: Initial: 12.5-25mcg/day. Titrate: Increase by 25mcg/day every 2-4 weeks until euthyroid. Pregnancy: May increase dose requirements. Subclinical Hypothyroidism: Lower doses required. *Pediatrics:* Take in the AM at least one-half hour before food. Hypothyroidism: 0-3 months: 10-15mcg/kg/day. 3-6 months: 8-10mcg/kg/day. 6-12 months: 6-8mcg/kg/day. 1-5 yrs: 5-6mcg/kg/day. 6-12 yrs: 4-5mcg/kg/day. >12 yrs: 2-3mcg/kg/day. Growth/Puberty Complete: 1.7mcg/kg/day. Cardiac Risk: Initial: Use lower dose. Titrate: Increase dose every 4-6 weeks until euthyroid. Infants with Serum T_4 <5mcg/dL: Initial: 50mcg/day. Chronic/Severe Hypothyroidism: Children: Initial: 25mcg/day. Titrate: Increase by 25mcg/day every 2-4 weeks until desired effect. Minimize Hyperactivity in Older Children: Initial: Give 1/4 of full replacement dose. Titrate: Increase by same amount weekly until full dose achieved. May crush tab and mix with 5-10mL water.

HOW SUPPLIED: Tab: 25mcg*, 50mcg*, 75mcg*, 88mcg*, 100mcg*, 112mcg*, 125mcg*, 137mcg*, 150mcg*, 175mcg*, 200mcg* *scored

CONTRAINDICATIONS: Untreated thyrotoxicosis, acute MI, and uncorrected adrenal insufficiency.

WARNINGS/PRECAUTIONS: Do not use in the treatment of obesity; larger doses in euthyroid patients can cause serious or even life threatening toxicity. Caution with cardiovascular disease, CAD, adrenal insufficiency, and the elderly with risk of occult cardiac disease. Carefully titrate dose to avoid over or under treatment. Decreased bone mineral density with long term use. Caution with nontoxic diffuse goiter or nodular thyroid disease. With adrenal insufficiency supplement with glucocorticoids before therapy.

ADVERSE REACTIONS: Pseudotumor cerebri in children reported. Seizures (rare), hypersensitivity reactions, dysphagia, choking, gagging, hyperthyroidism (increased appetite, weight loss, heat intolerance, hyperactivity, tremors, palpitations, tachycardia, diarrhea, vomiting, hair loss).

INTERACTIONS: Sympathomimetics may increase risk of coronary insufficiency with CAD. Upward dose adjustments needed for insulin and oral hypoglycemic agents. Decreased absorption with soybean flour (infant formula), cottonseed meal, walnuts, and fiber. May potentiate oral anticoagulant effects; adjust dose and monitor PT/INR. May decrease levels and effects of digitalis glycosides. Cholestyramine, colestipol, ferrous sulfate, aluminum hydroxide, sodium polystyrene, soybean flour, sucralfate may decrease absorption. Reduced TSH secretion with dopamine/dopamine agonists, glucocorticoids, octreotide. Decreased thyroid hormone secretion with aminoglutethim-ide, amiodarone, iodine (including iodine-containing radiographic contrast agents), lithium, methimazole, PTU, sulfonamides, tolbutamide. Increased thyroid hormone secretion with amiodarone, iodide (including iodine-con-taining radiographic contrast agents). Decreased T_4 absorption with antacids (aluminum & magnesium hydroxides), simethicone, bile acid sequestrants (cholestyramine, colestipol), calcium carbonate, cation exchange resins (kayexalate), ferrous sulfate, sucralfate. Increased serum TBG concentration with clofibrate, estrogens, heroin/methadone, 5-FU, mitotane, tamoxifen. Decreased serum TBG concentration with androgens/anabolic steroids, asparaginase, glucocorticoids, nicotinic acid (slow-release). Protein-binding site displacement with furosemide, heparin, hydantoins, NSAIDs, salicylates. Increased hepatic metabolism with carbamazepine, hydantoins, phenobar-bital, rifampin. Decreased conversion of T_4 to T_3 levels with amiodarone, β-adrenergic antagonists (propranolol >160mg/day), glucocorticoids (dexa-methasone >4mg/day), PTU. Additive effects of both agents with antidepres-sants. Interferon-(alpha) may cause development of antithyroid microsomal antibodies causing transient hypothyroidism, hyperthyroidism, or both. Interleukin-2 has been associated with transient painless thyroiditis. Excessive use with growth hormones may accelerate epiphyseal closure. Ketamine use may produce marked HTN and tachycardia. May reduce uptake of iodine-containing radiographic contrast agents. Altered levels of thyroid hormone and/or TSH level with choral hydrate, diazepam, ethionamide, lovastatin, me-toclopramide, 6-mercaptopurine, nitroprusside, para-aminosalicylate sodium, perphenazine, resorcinol (excessive topical use), thiazide diuretics.

PREGNANCY: Category A, caution in nursing.

MECHANISM OF ACTION: Thyroid hormone; not understood, suspected to control DNA transcription and protein synthesis.

PHARMACOKINETICS: Distribution: Plasma protein binding (99%); found in breast milk. **Metabolism:** Deiodination (major pathway) and conjugation in liv-er (mainly), kidneys, other tissues. **Elimination:** Urine, feces (20% unchanged); (T_4) $T_{1/2}$=6-7days; (T_3) $T_{1/2}$≤2 days.

LEVULAN KERASTICK   RX
aminolevulinic acid (Dusa)

THERAPEUTIC CLASS: Protoporphyrin precursor

INDICATIONS: Adjunct to BLU-U blue light photodynamic therapy illuminator, for treatment of non-hyperkeratotic actinic keratoses of the face or scalp.

DOSAGE: *Adults:* Apply directly to target lesion. After 14-18 hrs, expose area to BLU-U blue light photodynamic illumination. May repeat treatment after 8 weeks if lesions not completely resolved.

HOW SUPPLIED: Sol: 20% [1 app, 6 app]

CONTRAINDICATIONS: Cutaneous photosensitivity at wavelengths of 400-450nm, porphyria, allergy to porphyrins.

WARNINGS/PRECAUTIONS: After application, avoid sunlight or bright indoor light. Application to perilesional areas of photodamaged skin may cause pho-tosensitization. Avoid eyes, periorbital area, and mucous membranes.

ADVERSE REACTIONS: Scaling/crusting, erythema, itching, edema, stinging, ulceration, bleeding, vesiculation, hypo/hyperpigmentation, pustules, erosion.

INTERACTIONS: Possible increased photosensitivity with photosensitizers (eg, griseofulvin, thiazide diuretics, sulfonylureas, phenothiazines, sulfon-amides, tetracyclines).

PREGNANCY: Category C, caution in nursing.

MECHANISM OF ACTION: Aminolevulinic acid (ALA) acts as metabolic pre-cursor of protoporphyrin IX (PpIX), which is a photosensitizer.

PHARMACOKINETICS: Absorption: C_{max}=4.65mcg/mL.

LEXAPRO   RX
escitalopram oxalate (Forest)

> Antidepressants increased the risk of suicidal thinking and behavior (suicidality) in short-term studies in children, adolescents, and young adults with Major Depressive Disorder (MDD) and other psychiatric disorders. Escitalopram is not approved for use in pediatric patients.

THERAPEUTIC CLASS: Selective serotonin reuptake inhibitor

INDICATIONS: Treatment of MDD and generalized anxiety disorder (GAD).

DOSAGE: *Adults:* Initial: 10mg qd, in am or pm. Titrate: May increase to 20mg after a minimum of 1 week. Elderly/Hepatic Impairment: 10mg qd. Re-evaluate periodically.

HOW SUPPLIED: Sol: 5mg/5mL [240mL]; Tab: 5mg, 10mg*, 20mg* *scored

CONTRAINDICATIONS: Concomitant MAOI or pimozide therapy.

WARNINGS/PRECAUTIONS: Avoid abrupt withdrawal. Activation of mania/hypomania, hyponatremia reported. SIADH reported with citalopram. Caution with history of mania or seizures, hepatic impairment, severe renal impairment, conditions that alter metabolism or hemodynamic responses, suicidal tendencies. May impair mental/physical abilities. Consider tapering dose during 3rd trimester of pregnancy.

ADVERSE REACTIONS: Nausea, insomnia, ejaculation disorder, increased sweating, somnolence, fatigue, diarrhea.

INTERACTIONS: See Contraindications. Avoid alcohol, citalopram, or within 14 days of MAOI therapy. Caution with other CNS drugs, lithium, carbamazepine, cimetidine, drugs metabolized by CYP2D6 (eg, desipramine). Increased risk of bleeding with NSAIDs, ASA, warfarin. May increase metoprolol levels which leads to decreased cardioselectivity. Rare reports of weakness, hyperreflexia, incoordination with an SSRI and sumatriptan. Serotonin syndrome reported with linezolid.

PREGNANCY: Category C, not for use in nursing.

MECHANISM OF ACTION: SSRI. Inhibits CNS neuronal reuptake of serotonin.

PHARMACOKINETICS: Absorption: T_{max}=5 hrs. **Distribution:** Plasma protein binding (56%). **Metabolism:** Hepatic (biotransformation: N-demethylation) via CYP3A4, 2C19. **Elimination:** $T_{1/2}$=27-36 hrs. Urine (8%).

LEXIVA   RX
fosamprenavir calcium (GlaxoSmithKline)

THERAPEUTIC CLASS: Protease inhibitor

INDICATIONS: Treatment of HIV infection in combination with other antiretrovirals.

DOSAGE: *Adults:* Therapy-naive: 1400mg bid OR 1400mg qd + ritonavir 200mg qd OR 700mg bid + ritonavir 100mg bid. PI-Experienced: 700mg bid + ritonavir 100mg bid. Mild/Moderate Hepatic Impairment (without ritonavir): 700mg bid. Mild Hepatic Impairment: 700mg bid + ritonavir 100mg qd. Moderate Hepatic Impairment: 450mg bid + ritonavir 100mg qd. Severe Hepatic Impairment: 350mg bid (without ritonavir).
Pediatrics: 2-5 yrs: Therapy-naive: 30mg/kg bid, do not exceed 1,400mg bid; Therapy-naive ≥6 yrs: : 30mg/kg bid, not to exceed 1,400mg bid. or 18mg/kg + ritonavir 3mg/kg bid, not to exceed 700mg + ritonavir 100mg bid. Therapy-experienced: ≥6 yrs: 18 mg/kg + ritonavir 3 mg/kg, not to exceed 700 mg + ritonavir 100 mg bid. For patients weighing >47 kg use adult Lexiva monotherapy. When administered in combination with ritonavir, Lexiva tabs may be used in patients weighing >39 kg and ritonavir caps for patients weighing >33 kg.

HOW SUPPLIED: Tab: 700mg; Sus: 50mg/mL [225mL]

CONTRAINDICATIONS: Concomitant drugs dependent on CYP3A4 for clearance (eg, flecainide, propafenone, rifampin, delavirdine, lovastatin, simvastatin, dihydroergotamine, ergonovine, ergotamine, methylergonovine, cisapride, pimozide, midazolam, triazolam). If used with ritonavir, refer to ritonavir monograph.

WARNINGS/PRECAUTIONS: Severe and life-threatening skin reactions (including Stevens-Johnson syndrome), hemolytic anemia, new onset, or exacerbation of, DM, hyperglycemia, diabetic ketoacidosis, and immune reconstitution syndrome reported. Caution with known sulfonamide allergy. Reduce dose and use caution in hepatic impairment. Caution with underlying hepatitis B or C or marked elevations in transaminases; monitor LFTs prior to and during therapy. Spontaneous bleeding reported with hemophilia A and B. Redistribution/accumulation of body fat observed. Increased triglycerides may occur.

ADVERSE REACTIONS: Diarrhea, nausea, vomiting, headache, rash, severe skin reactions, AST increased, ALT increased.

INTERACTIONS: See Contraindications. Concurrent nevirapine without ritonavir not recommended. Indinavir and nelfinavir may increase levels. Decreased levels with efavirenz (add additional 100mg/day ritonavir), nevirapine, lopinavir/ritonavir (also decreases lopinavir), saquinavir, carbamazepine, phenobarbital, phenytoin, dexamethasone, H$_2$ antagonists. May decrease levels of methadone (consider dose increase) and paroxetine. May increase levels of oral contraceptives (use alternate non-hormonal methods), amiodarone, lidocaine (systemic), quinidine, bepridil, ketoconazole/itraconazole (reduce dose with >400mg/day; avoid >200mg/day with concurrent ritonavir), rifabutin (reduce dose by at least 50% or 75% with ritonavir; monitor CBCs weekly), benzodiazepines, CCBs, atorvastatin, rosuvastatin (use lowest possible dose), cyclosporine, tacrolimus, rapamycin, fluticasone (use with caution and avoid with ritonavir), sildenafil/tadalafil/vardenafil (reduce dose), amitriptyline, imipramine, trazodone. May affect warfarin levels; monitor INR.

PREGNANCY: Category C, not for use in nursing.

MECHANISM OF ACTION: HIV protease inhibitor; hydrolyzed to prodrug (amprenavir) which binds to HIV-1 protease active site and prevents the processing of viral Gag and Gag-Pol polyprotein precursors; forms immature infectious viral particles.

PHARMACOKINETICS: Absorption: Oral administration of variable doses resulted in different parameters. **Distribution:** Amprenavir: Plasma protein binding (90%). **Metabolism:** Fosamprenavir: Hepatic (hydrolyzation). Amprenavir: Hepatic via CYP3A4. **Elimination**: Amprenavir: Urine (1%); T$_{1/2}$=7.7 hrs.

LIALDA RX
mesalamine (Shire)

INDICATIONS: Induction of remission in adult patients with active, mild to moderate ulcerative colitis.

DOSAGE: *Adults:* 2-4 tabs qd with meals for up to 8 weeks. Max: 2.4g or 4.8g per day.

HOW SUPPLIED: Tab, Delayed-Release: 1.2g

WARNINGS/PRECAUTIONS: Prolonged gastric retention with pyloric stenosis, delaying mesalamine release in the colon. Caution with sulfasalazine allergy. May cause acute intolerance syndrome, if suspected prompt withdrawal is required. Caution with cardiac hypersensitivity reactions, myocarditis and pericarditis reported. Renal impairment, including minimal change nephropathy, and acute or chronic interstitial nephritis reported; caution with known renal dysfunction. Monitor renal function prior to therapy and periodically after.

ADVERSE REACTIONS: Headache, flatulence.

INTERACTIONS: Concurrent use with nephrotoxic agents (eg, NSAIDs) may increase risk of renal reactions. Concurrent azathioprine or 6-mercaptopurine can increase potential for blood disorders.

PREGNANCY: Category B, caution in nursing.

MECHANISM OF ACTION: Not established; suspected to diminish inflammation by blocking cyclooxygenase and inhibiting prostaglandin production in colon.

PHARMACOKINETICS: Absorption: PO administration of variable doses resulted in different parameters. **Distribution:** Plasma protein binding (43%). **Metabolism:** Liver and intestinal mucosa (acetylation), N-acetyl-5-aminosalicylic acid (metabolite). **Elimination:** Urine (≤8%); (2.4g) $T_{1/2}$=7-9 hrs; (4.8g) $T_{1/2}$=8-12 hrs

LIBRAX   CIV
chlordiazepoxide HCL - clidinium bromide (Valeant)

THERAPEUTIC CLASS: Benzodiazepine/anticholinergic

INDICATIONS: Adjunct treatment of irritable bowel syndrome (IBS), acute enterocolitis, and peptic ulcer.

DOSAGE: *Adults:* Usual/Maint: 1-2 caps tid-qid ac and hs. Elderly/Debilitated: Initial: 2 caps/day and increase gradually, if needed.

HOW SUPPLIED: Cap: (Chlordiazepoxide-Clidinium) 5mg-2.5mg

CONTRAINDICATIONS: Glaucoma, prostatic hypertrophy, benign bladder neck obstruction.

WARNINGS/PRECAUTIONS: Risk of congenital malformations during first trimester of pregnancy; avoid use. Avoid abrupt withdrawal. Paradoxical reactions reported in psychiatric patients. Caution with depression, renal or hepatic dysfunction, the elderly. Inhibition of lactation may occur.

ADVERSE REACTIONS: Drowsiness, ataxia, confusion, skin eruptions, extrapyramidal symptoms, dry mouth, nausea, constipation, altered libido, blood dyscrasias, jaundice, hepatic dysfunction.

INTERACTIONS: Avoid with other psychotropics; if combination is indicated, use caution especially with MAOIs and phenothiazines. Caution with alcohol, other CNS depressants. Altered coagulation effects with oral anticoagulants.

PREGNANCY: Not for use in pregnancy; safety in nursing is not known.

MECHANISM OF ACTION: Anticholinergic/spasmolytic and antianxiety agent.

LIBRIUM   CIV
chlordiazepoxide HCL (Valeant)

THERAPEUTIC CLASS: Benzodiazepine

INDICATIONS: Management of anxiety disorders and short-term relief of anxiety symptoms, withdrawal symptoms of acute alcoholism, and preoperative apprehension and anxiety.

DOSAGE: *Adults:* Mild-Moderate Anxiety: 5-10mg tid-qid. Severe Anxiety: 20-25mg tid-qid. Alcohol Withdrawal: 50-100mg; repeat until agitation controlled. Max: 300mg/day. Preoperative Anxiety: 5-10mg PO tid-qid on days prior to surgery. Elderly/Debilitated: 5mg bid-qid.
Pediatrics: ≥6 yrs: 5mg bid-qid. May increase to 10mg bid-tid.

HOW SUPPLIED: Cap: 5mg, 10mg, 25mg

WARNINGS/PRECAUTIONS: Avoid in pregnancy. Paradoxical reactions reported in psychiatric patients and in hyperactive aggressive pediatrics. Caution with porphyria, renal or hepatic dysfunction. Reduce dose in elderly, debilitated. Avoid abrupt withdrawal after extended therapy. May impair mental/physical abilities.

ADVERSE REACTIONS: Drowsiness, ataxia, confusion, skin eruptions, edema, nausea, constipation, extrapyramidal symptoms, libido changes, EEG changes.

INTERACTIONS: Additive effects with CNS depressants and alcohol. Avoid other psychotropic agents.

PREGNANCY: Not for use in pregnancy, safety in nursing not known.

MECHANISM OF ACTION: MOA not established; has antianxiety, sedative, appetite stimulating, and weak analgesic actions; suspected to block EEG arousal from stimulation of brain stem reticular formation.

PHARMACOKINETICS: Elimination: Urine (1-2% unchaged, 3-6% as conjugates); $T_{1/2}$=24-48 hrs.

LIDOCAINE OINTMENT   RX
lidocaine (Fougera)

THERAPEUTIC CLASS: Acetamide local anesthetic

INDICATIONS: Topical anesthesia of the oropharynx. Anesthetic lubricant for intubation. Temporary relief of pain associated with minor burns, abrasions, and insect bites.

DOSAGE: *Adults:* Apply up to 5g (6 inches)/application. Max: 17-20g/day. *Pediatrics:* Determine dose by age and weight. Max: 4.5mg/kg.

HOW SUPPLIED: Oint: 5% [35g]

WARNINGS/PRECAUTIONS: Reduce dose in elderly, debilitated, acutely ill, and children. Avoid excessive dosage or too frequent administration; may result in serious adverse effects requiring resuscitative measures. Caution with heart block and severe shock. Extreme caution if mucosa is traumatized or sepsis is present in the area of application; risk of rapid systemic absorption.

ADVERSE REACTIONS: Lightheadedness, nervousness, confusion, euphoria, dizziness, drowsiness, blurred vision, tremors, convulsions, respiratory depression, bradycardia, hypotension, urticaria, edema, anaphylactoid reactions.

PREGNANCY: Category B, caution in nursing.

MECHANISM OF ACTION: Local anesthetic; stabilizes neuronal membrane by inhibiting ionic fluxes required for the initiation and conduction of impulses.

PHARMACOKINETICS: Absorption: Rapid (after intratracheal administration). **Distribution:** Plasma protein binding (60-80%). Crosses placenta. **Metabolism:** Hepatic (biotransformation). **Elimination:** Urine. (IV) $T_{1/2}$=1.5-2 hrs.

LIDODERM PATCH   RX
lidocaine (Endo)

THERAPEUTIC CLASS: Acetamide local anesthetic

INDICATIONS: Relief of pain associated with post-herpetic neuralgia.

DOSAGE: *Adults:* Apply to intact skin, cover most painful area. Apply up to 3 patches, once for up to 12 hrs within 24-hr period. May cut patches into smaller sizes before removal of the release liner. Debilitated/Impaired Elimination: Treat smaller areas. Remove if irritation or burning occurs; may reapply when irritation subsides.

HOW SUPPLIED: Patch: 5% [30s]

WARNINGS/PRECAUTIONS: Serious adverse events may occur in children or pets if ingested. Increased risk of toxicity in severe hepatic disease. Avoid broken or inflamed skin, eye contact, larger area or longer duration than recommended. Increased levels with application of >3 patches, small patients.

ADVERSE REACTIONS: Application site reactions such as: erythema, edema, bruising, papules, vesicles, discoloration, depigmentation, burning sensation, pruritus, dermatitis, petechia, blisters, exfoliation, abnormal sensation, irritation, allergic reactions (rare).

INTERACTIONS: Additive toxic effects with concomitant Class I antiarrhythmics (eg, tocainide, mexiletine). Consider total amount absorbed from all formulations with other local anesthetics.

PREGNANCY: Category B, caution in nursing.

MECHANISM OF ACTION: Local anesthetic; stabilizes neuronal membranes by inhibiting ionic fluxes required for initiation and conduction of impulses.

PHARMACOKINETICS: Absorption: C_{max}=0.13mcg/mL; T_{max}=11 hrs. **Distribution:** V_d=1.5L/kg; plasma protein binding (70%). Crosses placenta. **Metabolism:** Hepatic, monoethylglycinexylidide, glycinexylidide (metabolites). **Elimination:** Kidneys; $T_{1/2}$=81-149 min.

LIMBITROL   CIV
amitriptyline HCL - chlordiazepoxide (Valeant)

> Antidepressants increased the risk of suicidal thinking and behavior (suicidality) in short-term studies in children, adolescents, and young adults with Major Depressive Disorder (MDD) and other psychiatric disorders. Limbitrol is not approved for use in pediatric patients.

OTHER BRAND NAMES: Limbitrol DS (Valeant)

THERAPEUTIC CLASS: Benzodiazepine/tricyclic antidepressant

INDICATIONS: Moderate to severe depression associated with moderate to severe anxiety.

DOSAGE: *Adults:* Initial: 3-4 tabs/day in divided doses. Max: (Limbitrol DS) 6 tabs/day. Elderly: Start at low end of dosing range.

HOW SUPPLIED: (Chlordiazepoxide-Amitriptyline) Tab: (Limbitrol) 5mg-12.5mg, (Limbitrol DS) 10mg-25mg

CONTRAINDICATIONS: MAOI use during or within 14 days, acute recovery period following MI.

WARNINGS/PRECAUTIONS: Caution with urinary retention, angle-closure glaucoma, cardiovascular disorder, history of seizures, hyperthyroidism, renal or hepatic dysfunction. May produce arrhythmia, sinus tachycardia, and conduction time prolongation. May impair mental alertness. Caution in elderly. Avoid abrupt withdrawal. Monitor blood and LFT's periodically with long-term therapy.

ADVERSE REACTIONS: Drowsiness, dry mouth, constipation, blurred vision, dizziness, bloating, anorexia, fatigue, weakness, restlessness, lethargy.

INTERACTIONS: May antagonize antihypertensives (eg, guanethidine). Caution with thyroid agents. Additive effects may occur with psychotropics. Increased levels with CYP2D6 inhibitors (eg, quinidine, cimetidine, SSRIs) and enzyme substrates (eg, phenothiazines, propafenone, flecainide). Avoid within 5 weeks of fluoxetine use. Additive sedative effects with alcohol and CNS depressants. Severe constipation with anticholinergics.

PREGNANCY: Not for use in pregnancy or nursing.

MECHANISM OF ACTION: Benzodiazepine/Tricyclic Antidepressant; not established, two compenents suspected to exert their action in the central nervous sytem: 1) chlorodizoxide component; acts in limbic system producing taming action, 2) amitriptyline component; interferes with the reuptake of norepinephrine into adrenergic nerve endings leading to prolongation of the sympathatic activity of biogenic amines.

PHARMACOKINETICS: Metbolism: CYP450 2D6 (Liver).

LIMBREL   RX
flavocoxid (Primus)

THERAPEUTIC CLASS: Flavonoid

INDICATIONS: Clinical dietary management of the metabolic processes of osteoarthritis (OA).

DOSAGE: *Adults*: 250-500mg q12h for total daily dose of 500-1000mg/day. May increase to 2 or more caps q12h under physician supervision.

HOW SUPPLIED: Cap: 250mg, 500mg

CONTRAINDICATIONS: Hypersensitivity to flavocoxid or flavonoids (eg, colored fruits and vegetables, dark chocolate, tea, red wine, Brazil nuts).

ADVERSE REACTIONS: Varicose veins, HTN, fluid accumulation in knee, psoriasis, nausea, vomiting, rash, itching, synovitis, joint pain, fever.

PREGNANCY: Not recommended for pregnant or lactating patients..

MECHANISM OF ACTION: Flavonoid; acts on COX-1, COX-2 and 5-LOX pathways; restores and maintains the balance of fatty acids in OA and also acts as a strong antioxidant.

PHARMACOKINETICS: Metabolism: Liver via CYP450 enzymes (glucuronidation and sulfation).

LINCOCIN   RX
lincomycin HCL (Pharmacia & Upjohn)

> Diarrhea, colitis, pseudomembranous colitis reported; may begin up to several weeks after discontinuation. Reserve for serious infections where less toxic antimicrobials are inappropriate.

THERAPEUTIC CLASS: *Streptomyces lincolnensis* derivative

INDICATIONS: Treatment of serious infections due to streptococci, pneumococci, and staphylococci. Reserve for PCN allergy or if PCN is inappropriate.

DOSAGE: *Adults:* IM: Serious Infection: 600mg q24h. More Severe Infection: 600mg q12h or more often. IV: Dose depends on severity. Serious Infection: 600mg-1g q8-12h. More Severe Infection: Increase dose. Infuse over ≥1 hr. Life-Threatening Situation: Up to 8g/day has been given. Max: 8g/day. Severe Renal Dysfunction: 25-30% of normal dose.
Pediatrics: >1 month: IM: Serious Infection: 10mg/kg q24h. More Severe Infection: 10mg/kg q12h or more often. IV: 10-20mg/kg/day, depending on severity infused in divided doses as described for adults. Severe Renal Dysfunction: 25-30% of normal dose.

HOW SUPPLIED: Inj: 300mg/mL

CONTRAINDICATIONS: Clindamycin hypersensitivity.

WARNINGS/PRECAUTIONS: May be inadequate for meningitis treatment. Contains benzyl alcohol. Monitor elderly for change in bowel frequency. Caution with severe renal/hepatic dysfunction, or with history of GI disease (eg, colitis), asthma, significant allergies. Superinfections may occur. Perform periodic CBC, LFTs, and renal function tests with prolonged therapy. Do not administer undiluted as IV bolus. Cardiopulmonary arrest and hypotension with too rapid IV administration.

ADVERSE REACTIONS: Glossitis, stomatitis, nausea, vomiting, diarrhea, colitis, pruritus, blood dyscrasias, hypersensitivity reactions, rash, urticaria, vaginitis, tinnitus, vertigo.

INTERACTIONS: Caution with neuromuscular blockers; may enhance effects. Possible antagonism with erythromycin; avoid concomitant use. Kaolin-pectin inhibits oral lincomycin.

PREGNANCY: Category C, not for use in nursing.

LINDANE   RX
lindane (Alpharma)

> Only for patients who are intolerant or have failed first-line therapy with safer agents. Seizures and deaths reported with repeat or prolonged use. Caution in infants, children, elderly, those with other skin conditions, and those <50kg due to increased risk of neurotoxicity. Contraindicated in premature infants or those with uncontrolled seizure disorders. Instruct patients on proper use and inform that itching occurs after successful killing of scabies or lice.

THERAPEUTIC CLASS: Ectoparasiticide/ovicide

INDICATIONS: (Lot) Treatment of *Sarcoptes scabiei* (scabies) resistant to other therapies. (Shampoo) Treatment of head and pubic lice resistant to or if intolerant to other therapies.

DOSAGE: *Adults:* (Lot) Apply 1-2oz to dry skin; rub in thoroughly. Apply to whole body from neck down. Wash off after 8-12 hrs. Apply only once.

(Shampoo) Wash and dry hair with regular shampoo. Apply lindane to hair without water. Add water after 4 min; lather then rinse immediately. Towel briskly. Remove nits with comb or tweezers. Use 1oz for short hair, 1.5oz for medium length hair, and 2oz for long hair. Max: 2oz/application. Retreat if lice remain after 7 days.

Pediatrics: (Lot) Apply (≥6 yrs) 1-2oz or 1oz (<6 yrs) to dry skin; rub in thoroughly. Apply to whole body from neck down. Wash off after 8-12 hrs. Apply only once. (Shampoo) Wash and dry hair with regular shampoo. Apply lindane to hair without water. Add water after 4 min; lather then rinse immediately. Towel briskly. Remove nits with comb or tweezers. Use 1oz for short hair, 1.5oz for medium length hair, and 2oz for long hair. Max: 2oz/application. Retreat if lice remain after 7 days.

HOW SUPPLIED: Lot, Shampoo: 1% [60mL, 480mL]

CONTRAINDICATIONS: Premature infants, Norwegian (crusted) scabies, skin conditions (eg, atopic dermatitis, psoriasis) that increase systemic absorption of the drug, uncontrolled seizure disorders.

WARNINGS/PRECAUTIONS: Adverse events with serious outcomes reported. Caution in those at increased risk of seizure (eg, HIV, head trauma, prior seizure, CNS tumor, severe hepatic cirrhosis, excessive alcohol use, abrupt alchol or sedative withdrawal). Give Medication Guide to each patient when dispensing. Avoid eyes and mouth. Do not use with open wounds, cuts, or scores. Use rubber gloves to apply.

ADVERSE REACTIONS: CNS stimulation, dizziness, convulsions.

INTERACTIONS: Avoid creams, ointments, oils, oil-based hair dressings or conditioners; may enhance absorption. Caution with drugs that may lower seizure threshold (eg, antipsychotics, antidepressants, theophylline, cyclosporine, mycophenolate, tacrolimus, penicillins, imipenem, quinolones, chloroquine sulfate, pyrimethamine, isoniazid, meperidine, radiographic contrast agents, centrally active anticholinesterases, methocarbamol).

PREGNANCY: Category C, not for use in nursing.

MECHANISM OF ACTION: Ectoparasiticide/ovicide; exerts action by being directly absorbed into parasites and their ova.

PHARMACOKINETICS: Absorption: C_{max}=28ng/mL, T_{max}=6 hrs (infants and children). **Distribution:** Found in breast milk.

LIPITOR   RX
atorvastatin calcium (Parke-Davis/Pfizer)

THERAPEUTIC CLASS: HMG-CoA reductase inhibitor

INDICATIONS: Adjunct to diet, to reduce total cholesterol (total-C), LDL-C, TG, and Apo B levels, and to increase HDL-C in primary hypercholesterolemia (heterozygous familial and nonfamilial) and mixed dyslipidemia (Types IIa and IIb). Adjunct to diet for elevated serum TG levels (Type IV). Treatment of primary dysbetalipoproteinemia (Type III) inadequately responding to diet. Adjunct to other lipid-lowering treatments or if treatments are unavailable, to reduce total-C and LDL-C in homozygous familial hypercholesterolemia. Adjunct to diet to lower total-C, LDL-C and apolipoprotein B in postmenarchal adolescents with heterozygous familial hypercholesterolemia. To reduce the risk of MI, revascularization procedures, and angina in adults without clinically evident CHD but with multiple risk factors for CHD. To reduce the risk of MI and stroke in patients with Type II DM, and without clinically evident CHD, but with multiple risk factors for CHD. In patients with clinically evident CHD to reduce the risk of non-fatal MI, fatal and non-fatal stroke, revascularization procedures, hospitalization for CHF, and angina.

DOSAGE: *Adults:* Hypercholesterolemia/Mixed Dyslipidemia: Initial: 10-20mg qd (or 40mg qd for LDL-C reduction >45%). Titrate: Adjust dose if needed at 2-4 week intervals. Usual: 10-80mg qd. Homozygous Familial Hypercholesterolemia: 10-80mg qd.
Pediatrics: Heterozygous Familial Hypercholesterolemia: 10-17 yrs (post-

menarchal): Initial: 10mg/day. Titrate: Adjust dose if needed at intervals of ≥4 weeks. Max: 20mg/day.

HOW SUPPLIED: Tab: 10mg, 20mg, 40mg, 80mg

CONTRAINDICATIONS: Active liver disease, unexplained persistent elevations of serum transaminases, pregnancy, nursing mothers.

WARNINGS/PRECAUTIONS: Monitor LFTs prior to therapy, at 12 weeks or with dose elevation, and periodically thereafter. Reduce dose or withdraw if AST or ALT ≥3x ULN persist. Caution with heavy alcohol use and/or history of hepatic disease. D/C if markedly elevated CPK levels occur, if myopathy is diagnosed or suspected, or if predisposition to renal failure secondary to rhabdomyolysis. Caution in patients with recent stroke or TIA. Rare cases of rhabdomyolysis reported.

ADVERSE REACTIONS: Constipation, flatulence, dyspepsia, abdominal pain, transaminase and CK elevation in higher doses.

INTERACTIONS: Increases levels with erythromycin. Increases levels of oral contraceptives (norethindrone, ethinyl estradiol), digoxin. Monitor digoxin. Cyclosporine, fibric acid derivatives, niacin, erythromycin, and azole antifungals may increase risk of myopathy. Caution with drugs that decrease levels or activity of endogenous steroid hormones (eg, ketoconazole, spironolactone, cimetidine). Decreases levels with Maalox® TC, but LDL-C reduction not altered. Colestipol decreases levels when coadministered, but greater LDL-C reduction with coadministration than when each given alone. Avoid fibrates.

PREGNANCY: Category X, not for use in nursing.

MECHANISM OF ACTION: Competitive inhibitor of HMG-CoA reductase; inhibits conversion of HMG-CoA to mevalonate (precursor of sterols, including cholesterol).

PHARMACOKINETICS: Absorption: Rapid; absolute bioavailability (14%); T_{max}=1-2 hrs. **Distribution:** V_d=381L; plasma protein binding (≥98%); found in breast milk. **Metabolism:** Extensive; via CYP3A4 to ortho- and parahydroxylated derivatives, and various β-oxidation products. **Elimination:** Bile (drug, metabolites), urine (<2%); $T_{1/2}$=14 hrs.

LITHIUM CARBONATE

RX

lithium carbonate (Roxane)

> Lithium toxicity is related to serum lithium levels and can occur at doses close to therapeutic levels.

THERAPEUTIC CLASS: Antimanic agent

INDICATIONS: Treatment of manic episodes of bipolar disorder and maintenance treatment of bipolar disorder.

DOSAGE: *Adults:* Acute Mania: 600mg tid to achieve effective serum levels of 1-1.5mEq/L; monitor levels twice a week until stabilized. Maint: 300mg tid-qid to maintain serum levels of 0.6-1.2 mEq/L; monitor levels every 2 months. Elderly: Reduce dose.
Pediatrics: ≥12 yrs: Acute Mania: 600mg tid. Effective serum levels are 1-1.5mEq/L; monitor levels twice a week until stabilized. Maint: 300mg tid-qid to maintain serum levels of 0.6-1.2mEq/L; monitor levels every 2 months.

HOW SUPPLIED: Cap: 150mg, 300mg, 600mg; Tab: 300mg

CONTRAINDICATIONS: Renal or cardiovascular disease, severe debilitation or dehydration, sodium depletion, and diuretic use.

WARNINGS/PRECAUTIONS: May cause fetal harm; if possible withdraw for at least the 1st trimester of pregnancy. Caution in the elderly. Maintain normal diet, adequate salt/fluid intake. Assess kidney function prior to and during therapy. May impair mental/physical abilities. Reduce dose or d/c with sweating, diarrhea, infection with elevated temperatures. Caution with thyroid disorders; monitor thyroid function. Chronic therapy associated with diminution of renal concentrating ability (eg, diabetes insipidus), glomerular and interstitial fibrosis, and nephron atrophy.

ADVERSE REACTIONS: Fine hand tremor, polyuria, mild thirst, nausea, inco-ordination, diarrhea, vomiting, drowsiness, muscular weakness.

INTERACTIONS: Risk of encephalopathic syndrome (eg, weakness, lethargy, fever, tremulousness, confusion, EPS) with haloperidol and other antipsychot-ics; discontinue therapy if such signs occur. May prolong effects of neuro-muscular blockers. Increased levels with indomethacin, piroxicam and other NSAIDs. Increased risk of toxicity due to decreased clearance with diuretics and ACE inhibitors; contraindicated with diuretics.

PREGNANCY: Category D, not for use in nursing.

MECHANISM OF ACTION: Mood-stabilizing agent; mechanism not estab-lished. Suspected to alter sodium transport in nerve and muscle cells and effect a shift toward intraneuronal metabolism of catecholamines.

PHARMACOKINETICS: Distribution: Found in breast milk. **Elimination**: Urine (primary), feces; $T_{1/2}$=24 hrs.

LITHOBID

RX

lithium carbonate (JDS)

Lithium toxicity is related to serum levels, and can occur at doses close to therapeutic levels.

THERAPEUTIC CLASS: Antimanic agent

INDICATIONS: Treatment of manic episodes of manic-depressive illness.

DOSAGE: *Adults:* Acute Mania: Initial: 900mg bid or 600mg tid to achieve effective serum levels of 1-1.5mEq/L; monitor levels twice weekly until sta-bilized. Maint: 900-1200mg/day, given bid-tid to maintain serum levels of 0.6-1.2mEq/L; monitor levels every 2 months.
Pediatrics: ≥12 yrs: Acute Mania: Initial: 900mg bid or 600mg tid to achieve ef-fective serum levels of 1-1.5mEq/L; monitor levels twice weekly until stabilized. Maint: 900-1200mg/day, given bid-tid to maintain serum levels of 0.6-1.2 mEq/L; monitor levels every 2 months.

HOW SUPPLIED: Tab, Extended-Release: 300mg

WARNINGS/PRECAUTIONS: Avoid with significant renal or cardiovascular disease, severe debilitation, dehydration, or sodium depletion. Assess kidney function prior to and during therapy. Risk of encephalopathic syndrome (eg, weakness, lethargy, fever, tremulousness, confusion, EPS); d/c therapy. May impair mental/physical abilities. Reduce dose or d/c with sweating, diarrhea, infection with elevated temperatures. Caution with hypothyroidism; may need supplemental therapy. Chronic therapy associated with diminution of renal concentrating ability, glomerular and interstitial fibrosis, and nephron atrophy.

ADVERSE REACTIONS: Fine hand tremor, polyuria, mild thirst, nausea, gen-eral discomfort, diarrhea, vomiting, drowsiness, muscular weakness.

INTERACTIONS: Avoid diuretics and ACE inhibitors; risk of lithium toxic-ity due to reduced renal clearance. May prolong effects of neuromuscular blockers. Decreased levels with acetazolamide, urea, xanthine preparations, and alkalinizing agents. May produce hypothyroidism with iodide prepara-tions. Increased plasma levels with indomethacin, piroxicam, other NSAIDs. Increased risk of neurotoxic effects with carbamazepine and CCBs. Reduced renal clearance with metronidazole. Fluoxetine may increase and/or decrease lithium levels.

PREGNANCY: Category D, not for use in nursing.

MECHANISM OF ACTION: Not established; suspected to alter sodium transport in nerve and muscle cells and effects a shift toward intraneuronal metabolism of catecholamines.

PHARMACOKINETICS: Elimination: Urine (primary), feces (insignificant); $T_{1/2}$=24 hrs.

LO/OVRAL RX
norgestrel - ethinyl estradiol (Wyeth)

OTHER BRAND NAMES: Cryselle (Duramed) - Low-Ogestrel (Watson)

THERAPEUTIC CLASS: Estrogen/progestogen combination

INDICATIONS: Prevention of pregnancy.

DOSAGE: *Adults:* Start 1st Sunday after menses begins or the 1st day of menses. *21-day:* 1 tab qd for 21 days, stop 7 days, then repeat. *28-day:* 1 tab qd for 28 days, then repeat.

HOW SUPPLIED: Tab: (Ethinyl Estradiol-Norgestrel) 0.03mg-0.3mg

CONTRAINDICATIONS: Thrombophlebitis, DVT or thromboembolic disorders, pregnancy, cerebrovascular or coronary artery disease, undiagnosed abnormal genital bleeding, cholestatic jaundice of pregnancy or jaundice with prior pill use, hepatic adenomas or carcinomas, breast cancer or other estrogen-dependent neoplasia, thrombogenic valvulopathies, thrombogenic rhythm disorders, diabetes with vascular involvement, uncontrolled HTN, endometrium carcinoma, active liver disease if liver function has not returned to normal.

WARNINGS/PRECAUTIONS: Cigarette smoking increases risk of serious cardiovascular side effects; risk increases with age (especially >35 yrs) and heavy smoking. Increased risk of MI, vascular disease, thromboembolism, stroke and gallbladder disease. Retinal thrombosis, hepatic neoplasia reported. May cause glucose intolerance. May increase BP, elevate LDL levels or cause other lipid changes, fluid retention, breakthrough bleeding, and spotting. May cause or exacerbate migraine. May develop visual changes with contact lens. Increased risk of MI with HTN, hyperlipidemia, obesity, and diabetes. D/C if jaundice, significant depression or ophthalmic irregularities develop. Perform annual physical exam. Use before menarche is not indicated. May affect certain endocrine, LFTs and blood components.

ADVERSE REACTIONS: Nausea, vomiting, breakthrough bleeding, spotting, amenorrhea, migraine, depression, vaginal candidiasis, edema, weight changes.

INTERACTIONS: Reduced effects, increased breakthrough bleeding, and menstrual irregularities with rifampin, rifabutin, barbiturates, phenylbutazone, phenytoin, griseofulvin, topiramate, some protease inhibitors, modafinil and possibly with St. John's wort, some penicillins, ampicillin and tetracylines. Increased levels with ascorbic acid and acetaminophen, indinavir, fluconazole, troleandomycin, and atorvastatin. May affect cyclosporine, theophylline and corticosteroid levels.

PREGNANCY: Category X, not for use in nursing.

MECHANISM OF ACTION: Estrogen/progestogen combination oral contraceptive: acts by suppressing gonadotropins. Primarily acts by inhibiting ovulation. Also responsible for causing changes in cervical mucus (which increases difficulty of sperm entry into uterus) and in endometrium (which may reduce likelihood of implantation).

LOCOID RX
hydrocortisone butyrate (Ferndale)

THERAPEUTIC CLASS: Corticosteroid

INDICATIONS: (Cre, Oint) Corticosteroid responsive dermatoses. (Sol) Seborrheic dermatitis.

DOSAGE: *Adults:* (Cre, Oint) Apply bid-tid. May use occlusive dressings for psoriasis or recalcitrant conditions. D/C dressings if infection develops. (Sol) Apply bid-tid.
Pediatrics: (Cre, Oint) Apply bid-tid. May use occlusive dressings for psoriasis or recalcitrant conditions. D/C dressings if infection develops. (Sol) Apply bid-tid.

HOW SUPPLIED: Cre, Oint: 0.1% [15g, 45g]; Sol: 0.1% [20mL, 60mL]

L

WARNINGS/PRECAUTIONS: May produce reversible HPA axis suppression, manifestations of Cushing's syndrome, hyperglycemia, and glucosuria. D/C if irritation occurs. Use appropriate antifungal or antibacterial agent with dermatological infections. Peds may be more susceptible to systemic toxicity. Caution when applied to large surface areas. Avoid contact with eyes. Limit to least amount compatible with an effective therapeutic regimen. Chronic corticosteroid therapy may interfere with the growth and development of children.

ADVERSE REACTIONS: Burning, itching, irritation, dryness, folliculitis, hypertrichosis, acneiform eruptions, hypopigmentation, perioral dermatitis, allergic dermatitis, skin maceration, secondary infection, skin atrophy, striae, miliaria.

PREGNANCY: Category C, caution in nursing.

MECHANISM OF ACTION: Corticosteroid; possesses anti-inflammatory, anti-pruritic, and vasoconstrictive properties. Anti-inflammatory actions not established.

PHARMACOKINETICS: Absorption: Percutaneous; inflammation, other disease states, and occlusive dressings may increase absorption. **Distribution:** Bound to plasma proteins to varying degrees. Systemically administered corticosteroids found in breast milk. **Metabolism:** Liver. **Elimination:** Renal (major), bile.

LOESTRIN   RX

norethindrone acetate - ethinyl estradiol - ferrous fumarate (Duramed/Warner Chilcott)

OTHER BRAND NAMES: Junel 1.5/30 (Barr) - Junel 1/20 (Barr) - Junel Fe 1/20 (Barr) - Junel Fe 1.5/30 (Barr) - Microgestin Fe 1/20 (Watson) - Microgestin Fe 1.5/30 (Watson) - Loestrin Fe 1.5/30 (Duramed/Warner Chilcott) - Loestrin Fe 1/20 (Duramed/Warner Chilcott) - Loestrin 1.5/30 (Duramed/Warner Chilcott) - Loestrin 1/20 (Duramed/Warner Chilcott)

THERAPEUTIC CLASS: Estrogen/progestogen combination

INDICATIONS: Prevention of pregnancy.

DOSAGE: *Adults:* Start 1st Sunday after menses begin or the 1st day of menses. *21-day:* 1 tab qd for 21 days, stop 7 days, then repeat. *28-day:* 1 tab qd for 28 days, then repeat.

HOW SUPPLIED: (Ethinyl Estradiol-Norethindrone) Tab: (1/20) 20mcg-1mg, (1.5/30) 30mcg-1.5mg; (Fe 1/20) 20mcg-1mg and 75mg ferrous fumarate, (Fe 1.5/30) 30mcg-1.5mg and 75mg ferrous fumarate

CONTRAINDICATIONS: Thrombophlebitis, DVT or thromboembolic disorders, pregnancy, cerebrovascular or coronary artery disease, undiagnosed abnormal genital bleeding, cholestatic jaundice of pregnancy or jaundice with prior pill use, hepatic adenomas or carcinomas, breast cancer or other estrogen-dependent neoplasia.

WARNINGS/PRECAUTIONS: Cigarette smoking increases risk of serious cardiovascular side effects. This risk increases with age (especially >35 yrs) and heavy smoking. Increased risk of MI, vascular disease, thromboembolism, stroke, and gallbladder disease. Retinal thrombosis, hepatic neoplasia, carcinoma of breast and reproductive organs reported. May cause glucose intolerance. May increase BP, elevate LDL levels or cause other lipid changes, fluid retention, breakthrough bleeding, and spotting. May cause or exacerbate migraine. May develop visual changes with contact lens. Increased risk of MI with HTN, hyperlipidemia, obesity, and diabetes. D/C if jaundice, significant depression or ophthalmic irregularities develop. Perform annual physical exam. Use before menarche is not indicated. May affect certain endocrine, LFTs, and blood components.

ADVERSE REACTIONS: Nausea, vomiting, breakthrough bleeding, spotting, amenorrhea, migraine, depression, vaginal candidiasis, edema, weight changes.

INTERACTIONS: Reduced effects, increased breakthrough bleeding, and menstrual irregularities with rifampin, barbiturates, phenylbutazone, phenytoin, carbamazepine, and possibly with griseofulvin, ampicillin, and tetracyclines. Increased levels with atorvastatin, ascorbic acid, and APAP. Increased plasma levels of cyclosporine, prednisolone, and theophylline. Decreased levels of APAP. Increased clearance of temazepam, salicylic acid, morphine, and clofibric acid. Troglitazone reduces plasma levels of hormones.

PREGNANCY: Category X, not for use in nursing.

MECHANISM OF ACTION: Estrogen/progestogen combination oral contraceptive: acts by suppression of gonadotrophins. Primarily inhibits ovulation. Causes changes in cervical mucus (increasing difficulty of sperm entry into uterus) and endometrium (reducing likelihood of implantation) .

PHARMACOKINETICS: Absorption: Rapid and complete. Norethindrone Acetate: Absolute bioavailability (64%); Single dose: C_{max}=8420pg/mL, T_{max}=1.0 hr, AUC=33390pg/mL·hr; Multiple dose: C_{max}=16400pg/mL, T_{max}=1.3 hrs, AUC=88160pg/mL·hr. Ethinyl Estradiol: Absolute bioavailability (43%); Single dose: C_{max}=64.5pg/mL, T_{max}=1.3 hrs, AUC=465.4pg/mL·hr. Multiple doses: C_{max}= 81.9pg/mL, T_{max}=1.7 hrs, AUC= 701.3pg/mL·hr. **Distribution:** V_d=2-4L/kg; Plasma protein binding (≥95%). **Metabolism:** Norethindrone: Reduction, (sulfate-glucuronide conjugation). Ethinyl Estradiol: 1st-pass metabolism, CYP3A4 (oxidation). **Elimination:** Urine, feces. Norethindrone: $T_{1/2}$=8 hrs. Ethinyl Estradiol: $T_{1/2}$=14 hrs.

LOFIBRA RX
fenofibrate (Gate)

THERAPEUTIC CLASS: Fibric acid derivative

INDICATIONS: Adjunct to diet, for treatment of hypertriglyceridemia (Types IV and V). Adjunct to diet, for reduction of total-C, LDL-C, Apo B, and TG in primary hypercholesterolemia or mixed dyslipidemia (Types IIa and IIb).

DOSAGE: *Adults:* Hypercholesterolemia/Mixed Dyslipidemia: Initial: Cap: 200mg qd. Hypercholeserolemia/Mixed Hyperlipidemia: Tab: 160mg qd. Hypertriglyceridemia: Initial: Cap: 67-200mg/day. Tab: 54-160mg qd. Titrate: Adjust if needed after repeat lipid levels at 4-8 week intervals. Max: Cap: 200mg/day. Tab: 160mg/day. Renal Dysfunction/Elderly: Initial: Cap: 67mg/day. Tab: 54mg/day. Take with meals.

HOW SUPPLIED: Cap: 67mg, 134mg, 200mg; Tab: 54mg, 160mg

CONTRAINDICATIONS: Pre-existing gallbladder disease, unexplained persistent hepatic function abnormality, hepatic or severe renal dysfunction (including primary biliary cirrhosis).

WARNINGS/PRECAUTIONS: Monitor LFTs regularly; d/c if >3x ULN. May cause cholelithiasis; d/c if gallstones found. D/C if myopathy or marked CPK elevation occurs. Decreased Hgb, Hct, WBCs, thrombocytopenia, and agranulocytosis reported; monitor CBCs during first 12 months of therapy. Acute hypersensitivity reactions (rare) and pancreatitis reported. Monitor lipids periodically initially, d/c if inadequate response after 2 months on 200mg/day. Minimize dose in severe renal impairment. Caution in elderly.

ADVERSE REACTIONS: Abdominal pain, back pain, headache, abnormal LFTs, increased creatine phosphokinase, respiratory disorder.

INTERACTIONS: May potentiate coumarin anticoagulants; reduce anticoagulant dose and monitor PT/INR. Avoid HMG-CoA reductase inhibitors unless benefits outweigh risks. Bile acid sequestrants may impede absorption; take at least 1 hr before or 4-6 hrs after the resin. Evaluate benefits/risks with immunosuppressants (eg, cyclosporine) and other nephrotoxic agents.

PREGNANCY: Category C, not for use in nursing.

MECHANISM OF ACTION: Fenobric acid derivative; activates peroxiosome proliferator receptor alpha (PPRα); increases lipolysis and elimination of triglyceride-rich particles from plasma by activating lipoprotein lipase and reducing production of apoprotein C-III. It reduces serum uric acid levels by increasing urinary excretion of uric acid.

PHARMACOKINETICS: Absorption: Well absorbed. T_{max}=6-8 hrs. **Distribution:** Plasma protein binding (99%). **Metabolism:** Via esterases through hydrolysis and glucuronidation. **Elimination:** Urine (60%), feces (25%). $T_{1/2}$=20 hrs.

LOMOTIL
diphenoxylate HCL - atropine sulfate (Pharmacia & Upjohn)   `CV`

OTHER BRAND NAMES: Lonox (Sandoz)

THERAPEUTIC CLASS: Opioid/anticholinergic

INDICATIONS: Adjunctive therapy for management of diarrhea.

DOSAGE: *Adults:* Initial: 2 tabs or 10mL qid. Titrate: Reduce dose after symptoms are controlled. Maint: 2 tabs or 10mL qd. Max: 20mg/day diphenoxylate. D/C if symptoms not controlled after 10 days at max dose of 20mg/day (diphenoxylate).
Pediatrics: 2-12 yrs: Initial: 0.3-0.4mg/kg/day of solution given qid. 13-16 yrs: Initial: 2 tabs or 10mL tid. Titrate: Reduce dose after symptoms are controlled. Maint: 25% of initial dose. D/C if no improvement within 48 hrs.

HOW SUPPLIED: (Diphenoxylate-Atropine) Sol: 2.5mg-0.025/5mL [60mL]; Tab: 2.5mg-0.025mg

CONTRAINDICATIONS: Obstructive jaundice, diarrhea associated with pseudomembranous enterocolitis or enterotoxin-producing bacteria.

WARNINGS/PRECAUTIONS: May induce toxic megacolon in ulcerative colitis; d/c if abdominal distention occurs. May cause intestinal fluid retention. Avoid with diarrhea associated with organisms that penetrate the intestinal mucosa, and with pseudomembranous enterocolitis. Caution in pediatrics, especially with Down's syndrome. Extreme caution advanced hepatorenal disease and liver dysfunction. Do not use with severe dehydration or electrolyte imbalance until corrective therapy is initiated.

ADVERSE REACTIONS: Numbness of extremities, dizziness, anaphylaxis, hyperthermia, tachycardia, urinary retention, flushing, drowsiness, toxic megacolon, nausea, vomiting.

INTERACTIONS: May potentiate barbiturates, tranquilizers and alcohol. MAOIs may precipitate hypertensive crisis.

PREGNANCY: Category C, caution in nursing.

MECHANISM OF ACTION: Diphenoxylate: Antidiarrheal. Atropine: Anticholinergic.

PHARMACOKINETICS: Absorption: (4 tabs): C_{max}=163ng/mL. T_{max}=2 hrs. **Metabolism:** Rapid and extensive metabolism through ester hydrolysis to diphenoxylic acid (major metabolite). **Elimination:** $T_{1/2}$=12-14 hrs (diphenoxylic acid). Urine (14%, 6% conjugate), feces (49%).

LOPID
gemfibrozil (Parke-Davis)   `RX`

THERAPEUTIC CLASS: Fibric acid derivative

INDICATIONS: Types IV and V hyperlipidemia with risk of pancreatitis not responding to dietary management (usually TG >2000mg/dL). May consider therapy if TG 1000-2000mg/dL with history of pancreatitis or recurrent abdominal pain typical of pancreatitis. Risk reduction of CAD in Type IIb patients without history or symptoms of existing coronary heart disease inadequately responding to weight loss, dietary therapy, exercise, other pharmacologic agents; with triad of low HDL, and elevated LDL and TG levels.

DOSAGE: *Adults:* 600mg bid. Give 30 min before morning and evening meals.

HOW SUPPLIED: Tab: 600mg* *scored

CONTRAINDICATIONS: Hepatic or severe renal dysfunction, including primary biliary cirrhosis; pre-existing gallbladder disease, concomitant cerivastatin.

WARNINGS/PRECAUTIONS: Abnormal LFTs reported; monitor periodically. Only use if indicated and d/c if significant lipid response not obtained. Associated with myositis. D/C if suspect or diagnose myositis, if abnormal LFTs persist, or gallstones develop. Cholelithiasis reported. Monitor blood counts periodically during first 12 months. May worsen renal insufficiency.

ADVERSE REACTIONS: Dyspepsia, abdominal pain, diarrhea, fatigue, bacterial and viral infections, musculoskeletal symptoms, abnormal LFTs, hematologic changes, hypesthesia, paresthesia, taste perversion.

INTERACTIONS: Caution with anticoagulants; reduce dose and monitor PT. Increased risk of myopathy and rhabdomyolysis with HMG-CoA reductase inhibitors. Benefit with concomitant HMG-CoA reductase inhibitors does not outweigh risks. Avoid initiating therapy with repaglinide. If already on repaglinide therapy, monitor levels and adjust repaglinide dose. Avoid itraconazole in patients taking gemfibrozil and repaglinide.

PREGNANCY: Category C, not for use in nursing.

MECHANISM OF ACTION: Lipid regulating agent; decreases serum TG and VLDL cholesterol and increases HDL cholesterol. Has not been definitely established; shown to inhibit peripheral lipolysis, decrease hepatic extraction of free fatty acids, thus reducing hepatic TG production and inhibiting synthesis and increasing clearance of VLDL carrier apolipoprotein B, leading to decreased VLDL production.

PHARMACOKINETICS: Absorption: Complete. T_{max}=1-2 hr. **Metabolism:** Oxidation to hydroxymethyl and carboxyl metabolites. **Eliminition:** Urine; 70% (glucoronide conjugate), 2% (unchanged) and feces (6%).

LOPRESSOR   RX
metoprolol tartrate (Novartis)

THERAPEUTIC CLASS: Selective beta₁-blocker

INDICATIONS: Treatment of hypertension. Long-term treatment of angina pectoris. To reduce cardiovascular mortality in hemodynamically stable patients with definite or suspected AMI.

DOSAGE: *Adults:* HTN: Initial: 100mg/day in single or divided doses. Titrate: May increase at weekly (or longer) intervals. Usual: 100-450mg/day. Max: 450mg/day. Angina: Initial: 50mg bid. Titrate: May increase weekly. Usual: 100-400mg/day. Max: 400mg/day. MI (Early Phase): 5mg IV every 2 min for 3 doses (monitor BP, HR, and ECG). If tolerated, give 50mg PO q6h for 48 hrs. If not tolerated, give 25-50mg PO q6h. Initiate PO dose 15 min after last IV dose. MI (Late Phase): 100mg bid for at least 3 months. Take PO with or immediately following meals.

HOW SUPPLIED: Inj: 1mg/mL; Tab: 50mg*, 100mg* *scored

CONTRAINDICATIONS: (HTN, Angina) Sinus bradycardia, >1st-degree heart block, cardiogenic shock, overt cardiac failure, sick-sinus syndrome, severe peripheral arterial circulatory disorders, pheochromocytoma. (MI) HR <45 beats/min, 2nd- and 3rd-degree heart block, significant 1st-degree heart block, SBP <100mmHg, moderate to severe cardiac failure.

WARNINGS/PRECAUTIONS: Caution with ischemic heart disease, avoid abrupt withdrawal; taper over 1-2 weeks. Withdrawal before surgery is controversial. May mask hyperthyroidism and hypoglycemia symptoms. May exacerbate cardiac failure. Caution with hepatic dysfunction, CHF controlled by digitalis. Avoid in bronchospastic disease. May decrease sinus HR and/or slow AV conduction. D/C if heart block or hypotension occurs.

ADVERSE REACTIONS: Bradycardia, shortness of breath, fatigue, dizziness, depression, diarrhea, pruritus, rash, heart block, hypotension.

INTERACTIONS: Additive effects with catecholamine-depleting drugs (eg, reserpine). May block epinephrine effects. Caution with digitalis; both agents slow AV conduction. Potent CYP2D6 inhibitors may increase levels. Stop metoprolol several days before clonidine discontinuation when both agents given concurrently.

PREGNANCY: Category C, caution in nursing.

MECHANISM OF ACTION: β-adrenergic receptor blocker; not established, proposed to competitively antagonize catecholamines at peripheral adrenergic-neuronal sites; have central effect leading to reduced sympathetic outflow to periphery and suppression of renin activity.

PHARMACOKINETICS: Absorption: Rapid and complete. **Distribution:** Serum albumin binding (12%). **Metabolism:** CYP2D6 (oxidation). **Elimination:** Urine (<5%); $T_{1/2}$=2.8 hrs (extensive metabolizers); $T_{1/2}$=7.5 hrs (poor metabolizers). IV: Urine (10%).

LOPRESSOR HCT   RX
metoprolol tartrate - hydrochlorothiazide (Novartis)

THERAPEUTIC CLASS: Selective beta$_1$-blocker/thiazide diuretic

INDICATIONS: Management of hypertension. Not for initial therapy.

DOSAGE: *Adults:* Usual: 100-450mg metoprolol/day and 12.5-50mg HCTZ/day. Max: 50mg HCTZ/day.

HOW SUPPLIED: Tab: (Metoprolol-HCTZ) 50mg-25mg*, 100-25mg*, 100mg-50mg* *scored

CONTRAINDICATIONS: Sinus bradycardia, >1st-degree heart block, cardiogenic shock, overt cardiac failure, sick-sinus syndrome, severe peripheral arterial circulatory disorders, pheochromocytoma, anuria, sulfonamide hypersensitivity.

WARNINGS/PRECAUTIONS: Avoid abrupt withdrawal; taper over 1-2 weeks. Withdrawal before surgery is controversial. May mask hyperthyroidism and hypoglycemia symptoms. May cause cardiac failure. Caution with hepatic dysfunction, CHF controlled by digitalis, severe renal disease, allergy or asthma history. Avoid in bronchospastic disease. Monitor for fluid/electrolyte imbalance. May manifest latent DM. Hypokalemia, hyperuricemia, hypercalcemia, hypophosphatemia, and hypomagnesemia may occur. May exacerbate SLE. Enhanced effects in post-sympathectomy patient.

ADVERSE REACTIONS: Fatigue, dizziness, flu syndrome, drowsiness, hypokalemia, headache, bradycardia.

INTERACTIONS: Additive effects with catecholamine-depleting drugs (eg, reserpine). May block epinephrine effects. Caution with digitalis; both agents slow AV conduction. Potent CYP2D6 inhibitors may increase levels. Stop metoprolol several days before clonidine discontinuation when both agents given concurrently. Corticosteroids, ACTH may increase risk of hypokalemia. Risk of lithium toxicity. NSAIDs may reduce diuretic effects. Insulin may need adjustment. Impaired absorption with cholestyramine, colestipol. Additive effects with other antihypertensives. May increase responsiveness to tubocurarine. Alcohol, barbiturates, or narcotics may potentiate orthostatic hypotension. May decrease arterial responsiveness to norepinephrine.

PREGNANCY: Category C, not for use in nursing.

MECHANISM OF ACTION: Metoprolol: β-adrenergic receptor blocker; not established, proposed to competitively antagonize catecholamines at peripheral adrenergic-neuronal sites, have central effect leading to reduced sympathetic outflow to periphery and suppression of renin activity. HCTZ: Thiazide diuretic; affects renal tubular mechanism of electrolyte reabsorption.

PHARMACOKINETICS: Absorption: Metoprolol: Rapid and complete. HCTZ: Rapid; T_{max}=1-2.5 hrs. **Distribution:** Metoprolol: Plasma protein binding (12%). HCTZ: Plasma protein binding (67.9%); V_d=3.6-7.8L/kg. **Metabolism:** Metoprolol: CYP2D6 (oxidation). **Elimination:** Metoprolol: Urine (<5%); $T_{1/2}$=2.8 hrs (extensive metabolizers), 7.5 hrs (poor metabolizers). HCTZ: Urine (72-97%); $T_{1/2}$=10-17 hrs.

LOPROX

RX

ciclopirox (Medicis)

OTHER BRAND NAMES: Loprox TS (Medicis)

THERAPEUTIC CLASS: Broad-spectrum antifungal

INDICATIONS: (Cre/Sus) Treatment of dermal infections of tinea pedis, tinea cruris, tinea corporis, cutaneous candidiasis and tinea versicolor. (Gel) Treatment of interdigital tinea pedis and tinea corporis. (Gel/Shampoo) Treatment of seborrheic dermatitis of the scalp.

DOSAGE: *Adults:* (Cre/Gel/Sus) Massage affected and surrounding areas bid (am and pm) up to 4 weeks. (Shampoo) Apply about 5mL (up to 10mL for long hair) to wet scalp. Lather and rinse off after 3 min. Repeat twice weekly for 4 weeks, at least 3 days apart.
Pediatrics: ≥10 yrs: (Cre/Sus) Massage affected and surrounding areas bid (am and pm) up to 4 weeks. Gel or shampoo not recommended in pediatrics <16 yrs.

HOW SUPPLIED: Cre: 0.77% [15g, 30g, 90g]; Gel: 0.77% [30g, 45g, 100g]; Shampoo: 1% [120mL]; Sus: (Loprox TS) 0.77% [30mL, 60mL]

WARNINGS/PRECAUTIONS: Avoid eyes, mucous membranes, occlusive wrappings or dressings. D/C if sensitization or chemical irritation occurs. Hair discoloration reported in patients with lighter hair color.

ADVERSE REACTIONS: Contact dermatitis, pruritus, burning.

PREGNANCY: Pregnancy B, caution in nursing.

MECHANISM OF ACTION: Broad-spectrum antifungal; acts by chealation of polyvalent cations (Fe^{3+} or Al^{3+}) resulting in the inhibition of the metal-dependent enzymes that are responsible for degradation of peroxides in the fungal cell wall. Inhibits the growth of pathogenic dermatophytes, yeasts, and and *Malassezia furfur*.

PHARMACOKINETICS: Elimination: Renal and feces; $T_{1/2}$ = 5.5 hrs.

LORCET

CIII

hydrocodone bitartrate - acetaminophen (Forest)

OTHER BRAND NAMES: Lorcet 10/650 (Forest) - Lorcet HD (Forest) - Lorcet Plus (Forest)

THERAPEUTIC CLASS: Opioid analgesic

INDICATIONS: Relief of moderate to moderately severe pain.

DOSAGE: *Adults:* (Plus, 10/650) Usual: 1 cap/tab q4-6h prn pain. Max: 6 tabs or caps/day. (HD) 1-2 caps q4-6h prn pain. Max: 8 caps/day.

HOW SUPPLIED: (Hydrocodone-APAP) Cap: (HD) 5mg-500mg; Tab: (Plus) 7.5mg-650mg*, (10/650) 10mg-650mg* *scored

WARNINGS/PRECAUTIONS: May produce dose-related respiratory depression. May obscure acute abdominal conditions or head injuries. Caution in elderly, debilitated, severe hepatic or renal dysfunction, hypothyroidism, Addison's disease, prostatic hypertrophy, urethral stricture, pulmonary disease and postoperative use. May be habit-forming. Suppresses cough reflex.

ADVERSE REACTIONS: Dizziness, drowsiness, nausea, vomiting, dysphoria, urinary retention, urethral spasm, dyspnea, shortness of breath, rash.

INTERACTIONS: May potentiate CNS depression with narcotics, alcohol, antianxiety agents, antihistamines, antipsychotics, other CNS depressants. Increased effect of antidepressant or hydrocodone with MAOIs or TCAs.

PREGNANCY: Category C, not for use in nursing.

MECHANISM OF ACTION: Hydrocodone: Narcotic analgesic; MOA not established. Suspected to be related to existence of opiate receptors in the CNS. APAP: nonopiate, nonsalicylate analgesic and antipyretic. Mechanism of analgesic actions not established; involves peripheral influences. Antipyretic activity is mediated through hypothalamic heat regulating centers. Inhibits prostaglandin synthetase.

PHARMACOKINETICS: Absorption: Hydrocodone: C_{max}=23.6ng/mL; T_{max}=1.3 hrs. APAP: Rapidly absorbed. **Distribution:** APAP: Found in breast milk. **Metabolism**: Hydrocodone: O-demethylation, N-demethylation, and 6-keto reduction. APAP: Liver (conjugation). **Elimination**: Hydrocodone: $T_{1/2}$=3.8 hrs. APAP: Urine (85%); $T_{1/2}$=1.25-3 hrs.

LORTAB   CIII
hydrocodone bitartrate - acetaminophen (UCB Pharma)

THERAPEUTIC CLASS: Opioid analgesic

INDICATIONS: Relief of moderate to moderately severe pain.

DOSAGE: *Adults:* (2.5/500, 5/500) 1-2 tabs q4-6h prn. Max: 8 tabs/day. (7.5/500, 10/500) 1 tab q4-6h prn. Max: 6 tabs/day. (Sol) 15mL q4-6h prn. Max: 90mL/day.
Pediatrics: ≥2 yrs: (Sol) 12-15kg: 3.75mL. 16-22kg: 5mL. 23-31kg: 7.5mL. 32-45kg: 10mL. ≥46kg: 15mL. May repeat q4-6h prn.

HOW SUPPLIED: (Hydrocodone-APAP) Sol: 7.5mg-500mg/15mL; Tab: 2.5mg-500mg*, 5mg-500mg*, 7.5mg-500mg*, 10mg-500mg* *scored

WARNINGS/PRECAUTIONS: May produce dose-related respiratory depression. May obscure acute abdominal conditions or head injuries. Caution in elderly, debilitated, severe hepatic or renal dysfunction, hypothyroidism, Addison's disease, prostatic hypertrophy, urethral stricture, pulmonary disease, postoperative use. May be habit-forming. Suppresses cough reflex.

ADVERSE REACTIONS: Lightheadedness, dizziness, sedation, nausea, vomiting.

INTERACTIONS: Additive CNS depression with other narcotics, antihistamines, antipsychotics, antianxiety agents, alcohol, CNS depressants. Increased effect of antidepressant or hydrocodone with MAOIs or TCAs.

PREGNANCY: Category C, not for use in nursing.

MECHANISM OF ACTION: Hydrocodone: Narcotic analgesic and antitussive; not established. Suspected to be related to existence of opiate receptors in CNS. APAP: Nonopioid, nonsalicylate analgesic, and antipyretic. Analgesic action involves peripheral influences; specific mechanism not established. Antipyretic activity is mediated through hypothalamic heat-regulating centers. Inhibits prostaglandin synthetase.

PHARMACOKINETICS: Administration: Hydrocodone: C_{max}=23.6ng/mL; T_{max}=1.3 hrs. APAP: Rapidly absorbed. **Distribution:** Hydrocodone: Crosses placental barrier. APAP: Found in breast milk. **Metabolism:** Hydrocodone: O-demethylation, N-demethylation and 6-keto reduction. APAP: Liver (conjugation). **Elimination:** Hydrocodone: $T_{1/2}$=3.8 hrs; APAP: Urine (85%); $T_{1/2}$=1.25-3 hrs.

LOTEMAX   RX
loteprednol etabonate (Bausch & Lomb)

THERAPEUTIC CLASS: Corticosteroid

INDICATIONS: Treatment of inflammation of the palpebral and bulbar conjunctiva, cornea and anterior segment of the globe. Management of postoperative inflammation.

DOSAGE: *Adults:* Steroid-Responsive Disease: 1-2 drops qid, may increase up to 1 drop every hr within the 1st week of treatment. Re-evaluate after 2 days if no improvement. Postoperative: 1-2 drops qid starting 24 hrs post-op and continue for 2 weeks.

HOW SUPPLIED: Sus: 0.5% [2.5mL, 5mL, 10mL, 15mL]

CONTRAINDICATIONS: Viral diseases of the cornea and conjunctiva including epithelial herpes simplex keratitis, vaccinia, and varicella. Mycobacterial infection and fungal diseases of the eye.

WARNINGS/PRECAUTIONS: Caution with glaucoma, history of herpes simplex, and diseases causing thinning of cornea/sclera. Prolonged use can cause glaucoma, optic nerve damage, defects in visual acuity and fields of vision, cataracts, or secondary ocular infections (eg, fungal). Monitor IOP after 10 days of therapy. Re-evaluate if no response after 2 days. May delay healing and increase incidence of bleb formation after cataract surgery. May mask or enhance existing infection in acute, purulent conditions.

ADVERSE REACTIONS: Elevated IOP, abnormal vision, chemosis, discharge, dry eyes, burning on instillation, epiphora, itching, photophobia, foreign body sensation, optic nerve damage, visual field defects.

PREGNANCY: Category C, caution in nursing.

MECHANISM OF ACTION: Glucocorticoid; anti-inflammatory agent, no accepted explanation for mechanism of action; suspected to inhibit edema, fibrin deposition, capillary dilation and deposition of collagen and scar formation by the induction of phospholipase A_2 inhibitory proteins, lipocortins.

LOTENSIN   RX
benazepril HCL (Novartis)

> **When used in pregnancy, ACE inhibitors can cause injury and even death to the developing fetus. D/C therapy when pregnancy detected.**

THERAPEUTIC CLASS: ACE inhibitor

INDICATIONS: Treatment of hypertension. May be used alone or with thiazide diuretics.

DOSAGE: *Adults:* If possible, d/c diuretic 2-3 days prior to initiation of therapy. Initial: 10mg qd or 5mg with concomitant diuretic. Maint: 20-40mg/day given qd-bid. Resume diuretic if BP not controlled. Max: 80mg/day. CrCl <30mL/min/1.73m²: Initial: 5mg qd. Max: 40mg/day.
Pediatrics: ≥6 yrs: Initial: 0.2mg/kg qd. Max: 0.6mg/kg.

HOW SUPPLIED: Tab: 5mg, 10mg, 20mg, 40mg

WARNINGS/PRECAUTIONS: D/C if angioedema, jaundice, or if marked LFT elevation occurs. Risk of hyperkalemia with DM, renal dysfunction. Persistent nonproductive cough reported. Monitor WBCs in renal and collagen vascular disease. Anaphylactoid reactions reported. Fetal/neonatal morbidity and death reported. Monitor for hypotension in high risk patients (eg, surgery/anesthesia, prolonged diuretic therapy, heart failure, volume and/or salt depletion, etc). Caution with CHF, renal dysfunction, and renal artery stenosis. Less effective on BP in blacks and more reports of angioedema than nonblacks.

ADVERSE REACTIONS: Cough, dizziness, headache, fatigue, somnolence, postural dizziness, nausea.

INTERACTIONS: May increase lithium levels. Hypotension risk with diuretics. Increased risk of hyperkalemia with K⁺-sparing diuretics, K⁺-containing salt substitutes, or K⁺ supplements.

PREGNANCY: Category D, not for use in nursing.

MECHANISM OF ACTION: ACE inhibitor; not established, effects appear to result from suppression of renin-angiotensin-aldosterone system.

PHARMACOKINETICS: Absorption: Absolute bioavailability (≥37%); T_{max}=0.5-1 hr, 1-4 hrs (metabolite). **Distribution:** Parent, metabolite: Plasma protein binding (96.7%, 95.3%). **Metabolism:** Cleavage of ester group; benazeprilat (active metabolite). **Elimination:** Urine (7%). Benazeprilat: Urine (20%), biliary (11-12%); $T_{1/2}$=10-11 hrs (adults), 5 hrs (pediatrics).

LOTENSIN HCT   RX
benazepril HCL - hydrochlorothiazide (Novartis)

> When used in pregnancy, ACE inhibitors can cause injury and even death to the developing fetus. D/C therapy when pregnancy detected.

THERAPEUTIC CLASS: ACE inhibitor/thiazide diuretic

INDICATIONS: Treatment of hypertension. Not for initial therapy.

DOSAGE: *Adults:* Initial (if not controlled on benazepril monotherapy): 10mg-12.5mg or 20mg-12.5mg. Titrate: May increase after 2-3 weeks. Initial (if controlled on 25mg HCTZ/day with hypokalemia): 5mg-6.25mg. Replacement Therapy: Substitute combination for titrated components.

HOW SUPPLIED: Tab: (Benazepril-HCTZ) 5mg-6.25mg*, 10mg-12.5mg*, 20mg-12.5mg*, 20mg-25mg* *scored

CONTRAINDICATIONS: Anuria, sulfonamide hypersensitivity.

WARNINGS/PRECAUTIONS: Avoid if CrCl ≤30mL/min/1.73m². D/C if angioedema, jaundice, or marked LFT elevation occur. Risk of hyperkalemia with DM, renal dysfunction. May cause persistent nonproductive cough, hypokalemia, hyperuricemia, hypomagnesemia, hypercalcemia, hypophosphatemia. Monitor WBCs in renal and collagen vascular disease. Anaphylactoid reactions reported. Fetal/neonatal morbidity and death reported. Monitor for hypotension in high risk patients (eg, surgery/anesthesia, prolonged diuretic therapy, heart failure, volume and/or salt depletion, etc). Caution with CHF, renal dysfunction, and renal artery stenosis. More reports of angioedema in blacks than nonblacks. Monitor for fluid/electrolyte imbalance. May increase cholesterol and TG levels. May exacerbate/activate SLE.

ADVERSE REACTIONS: Cough, dizziness/postural dizziness, headache, fatigue.

INTERACTIONS: Increased risk of hyperkalemia with K⁺ supplements, K⁺-sparing diuretics, or K⁺-containing salt substitutes. Risk of lithium toxicity. May increase responsiveness to tubocurarine. NSAIDs reduce effects. Cholestyramine, colestipol decrease absorption. Insulin may need adjustment. May decrease arterial responsiveness to norepinephrine.

PREGNANCY: Category D, not for use in nursing.

MECHANISM OF ACTION: Benazepril: ACE inhibitor; not established, effects appear to result from suppression of renin-angiotensin-aldosterone system. HCTZ: Thiazide diuretic; affects renal tubular mechanisms of electrolyte reabsorption, directly increasing excretion of Na⁺ and Cl⁻, and indirectly reducing plasma volume.

PHARMACOKINETICS: Absorption: Benazepril: T_{max} = 0.5-1 hr, 1-4 hrs (metabolite); absolute bioavailability: (≥37%). **Distribution:** Benazepril, metabolite: plasma protein binding (96.7%, 95.3%). HCTZ: Plasma protein binding (67.9%); V_d = 3.6-7.8 L/Kg; crosses placenta. **Metabolism:** Benazepril: Cleavage of ester group; benazeprilat (active metabolite). **Elimination:** Benazepril: Urine (trace). Benazeprilat: Urine (20%), biliary (11-12%); $T_{1/2}$ = 10-11 hrs. HCTZ: Kidney; $T_{1/2}$ = 5-15 hrs.

LOTREL   RX
benazepril HCL - amlodipine besylate (Novartis)

> When used in pregnancy, ACE inhibitors can cause injury and even death to the developing fetus. D/C therapy when pregnancy detected.

THERAPEUTIC CLASS: Calcium channel blocker (dihydropyridine)/ACE inhibitor

INDICATIONS: Treatment of hypertension. Not for initial therapy.

DOSAGE: *Adults:* Usual: 2.5-10mg amlodipine and 10-80mg benazepril per day. Small/Elderly/Frail/Hepatic Impairment: Initial: 2.5mg amlodipine.

HOW SUPPLIED: Cap: (Amlodipine-Benazepril) 2.5mg-10mg, 5mg-10mg, 5mg-20mg, 5mg-40mg, 10mg-20mg, 10mg-40mg

WARNINGS/PRECAUTIONS: D/C if angioedema, jaundice, or if marked LFT elevation occurs. Risk of hyperkalemia with DM, renal dysfunction. Persistent nonproductive cough reported. Monitor WBCs in collagen vascular disease. Anaphylactoid reactions reported. Fetal/neonatal morbidity and death reported. Monitor for hypotension in high-risk patients (heart failure, surgery/anesthesia, volume and/or salt depletion, etc). Caution with CHF, severe hepatic or renal dysfunction, and renal artery stenosis. Avoid if CrCl ≤30mL/min.

ADVERSE REACTIONS: Cough, headache, dizziness, edema.

INTERACTIONS: May increase lithium levels. Hypotension risk with diuretics. Increased risk of hyperkalemia with K⁺-sparing diuretics, K⁺ supplements, or K⁺-containing salt substitutes. Caution with other peripheral vasodilators.

PREGNANCY: Category C (1st trimester) and D (2nd and 3rd trimesters), not for use in nursing.

MECHANISM OF ACTION: Benazepril: ACE inhibitor; not established, effects appear to result from suppression of renin-angiotensin-aldosterone system. Amlodipine: Ca^{2+} channel blocker (dihydropyridine); inhibits transmembrane influx of Ca^{2+} ions into vascular smooth muscle and cardiac muscle.

PHARMACOKINETICS: Absorption: Amlodipine: Absolute bioavailability (64-90%); T_{max}=6-12 hrs. Benazepril: Absolute bioavailability (≥37%); T_{max}=0.5-2 hrs, 1.5-4 hrs (metabolite). **Distribution:** Amlodipine: V_d=21 L/kg; plasma protein binding (93%). Benazepril: V_d=0.7 L/kg. **Metabolism:** Amlodipine: Liver. Benazepril: Cleavage of ester group; benazeprilat (active metabolite). **Elimination:** Amlodipine: Urine (10%); $T_{1/2}$=2 days. Benazepril: Urine (trace), biliary (11-12%). Benazeprilat: Urine (20%); $T_{1/2}$=10-11 hrs.

LOTRIMIN AF   OTC
clotrimazole (Schering)

THERAPEUTIC CLASS: Azole antifungal

INDICATIONS: Tinea pedis, t.cruris, t.corporis.

DOSAGE: *Adults:* Cleanse skin with soap and water and dry thoroughly. Apply to affected area am and pm. Athlete's Foot and Ringworm: Treat for 4 weeks. Jock Itch: Treat for 2 weeks.
Pediatrics: ≥2 yrs: Cleanse skin with soap and water and dry thoroughly. Apply to affected area am and pm. Athlete's Foot and Ringworm: Treat for 4 weeks. Jock Itch: Treat for 2 weeks.

HOW SUPPLIED: Cre: 1% [24g]; Lot: 1% [20mL]; Sol: 1% [10mL]

WARNINGS/PRECAUTIONS: D/C if irritation occurs or no improvement in 4 weeks (t.pedis or t. corporis) or 2 weeks (t. cruris). Avoid eye contact. Not effective on scalp or nails.

PREGNANCY: Safety in pregnancy and nursing not known.

LOTRIMIN AF SPRAY & POWDER   OTC
miconazole nitrate (Schering)

THERAPEUTIC CLASS: Azole antifungal

INDICATIONS: To treat and relieve the itching, cracking, burning, and scaling of athlete's foot (tinea pedis), jock itch, (tinea cruris), and ringworm (tinea corporis). Powder aids in the drying of moist areas.

DOSAGE: *Adults:* Cleanse skin with soap and water and dry thoroughly. (Powder) Sprinkle thin layer over affected area am and pm. (Spray) Spray thin layer over affected area am and pm. Athlete's Foot and Ringworm: Treat for 4 weeks. Jock Itch: Treat for 2 weeks.
Pediatrics: ≥2 yrs: Cleanse skin with soap and water and dry thoroughly. (Powder) Sprinkle thin layer over affected area am and pm. (Spray) Spray thin

L

layer over affected area am and pm. Athlete's Foot and Ringworm: Treat for 4 weeks. Jock Itch: Treat for 2 weeks.

HOW SUPPLIED: Powder: 2% [90g]; Spray, Powder: 2% [100g]; Spray: 2% [113g]

WARNINGS/PRECAUTIONS: Avoid eye contact. D/C if irritation occurs or no improvement in 4 weeks (athlete's foot or ringworm) or 2 weeks (jock itch). Avoid while smoking or near heat/flame.

PREGNANCY: Safety in pregnancy and nursing not known.

LOTRIMIN ULTRA   OTC
butenafine HCL (Schering)

THERAPEUTIC CLASS: Benzylamine antifungal

INDICATIONS: To cure and relieve itching, cracking, burning, and scaling of athlete's foot (tinea pedis), jock itch, (tinea cruris), and ringworm (tinea corporis).

DOSAGE: *Adults:* Wash and dry area. Tinea Pedis: Apply between toes bid (am and pm) for 1 week, or qd for 4 weeks. Tinea Cruris/Corporis: Apply qd for 2 weeks.
Pediatrics: ≥12 yrs: Wash and dry area. Tinea Pedis: Apply between toes bid (am and pm) for 1 week, or qd for 4 weeks. Tinea Cruris/Corporis: Apply qd for 2 weeks.

HOW SUPPLIED: Cre: 1% [12g]

WARNINGS/PRECAUTIONS: Avoid nails, scalp, mouth, and eyes. D/C if too much irritation occurs. Not for vaginal yeast infections. Effectiveness on bottom of foot unknown.

PREGNANCY: Safety in pregnancy and nursing not known.

LOTRISONE   RX
betamethasone dipropionate - clotrimazole (Schering)

THERAPEUTIC CLASS: Corticosteroid/azole antifungal

INDICATIONS: Topical treatment of tinea pedis, tinea cruris, and tinea corporis caused by *Trichophyton rubrum*, *Trichophyton mentagrophytes*, and *Epidermophyton floccosum*.

DOSAGE: *Adults:* ≥17 yrs: Massage sufficient amount bid (am and pm) to area for 2 weeks for t.cruris and t.corporis and 4 weeks for t.pedis. D/C if condition persists after 2 weeks for t.cruris and t.corporis, or after 4 weeks for t.pedis.

HOW SUPPLIED: (Betamethasone-Clotrimazole) Cre: 0.05-1% [15g, 45g]; Lot: 0.05-1% [30mL]

WARNINGS/PRECAUTIONS: May produce reversible HPA axis suppression, Cushing's syndrome, hyperglycemia, and glucosuria. D/C if irritation develops. Pediatrics may be more susceptible to systemic toxicity. Not for use with occlusive dressing.

ADVERSE REACTIONS: Paresthesia, rash, edema, secondary infection.

PREGNANCY: Category C, caution in nursing.

MECHANISM OF ACTION: Corticosteroid/azole antifungal agent.
Clotrimazole: antifungal. Inhibits 14-α-demethylation of lanosterol in fungi by binding to 1 of the cytochrome P-450 enzymes. Leads to accumulation of 14-alpha-methylsterols and reduced concentrations of ergosterol, a sterol essential for a normal fungal cytoplasmic membrane. The methylsterols may affect the electron transport system, thereby inhibiting growth of fungi. Betamethasone: corticosteroid. Possesses anti-inflammatory, antipruritic, and vasoconstrictive properties.

PHARMACOKINETICS: Absorption: Percutaneous. Inflammation, other disease states, or occlusive dressings may increase absorption. **Metabolism:** Liver. **Elimination:** Renal, biliary.

LOTRONEX
RX

alosetron HCL (GlaxoSmithKline)

> Serious GI adverse events, some fatal, reported (eg, ischemic colitis, serious constipation complications). Physicians must enroll in the Prescribing Program for Lotronex and patients must sign the Patient-Physician Agreement. Discontinue immediately if constipation or symptoms of ischemic colitis develop (rectal bleeding, bloody diarrhea, abdominal pain); do not resume therapy.

THERAPEUTIC CLASS: 5-HT$_3$-antagonist

INDICATIONS: Treatment for women with severe diarrhea-predominant IBS who have chronic symptoms (>6 months), exclusion of anatomic or biochemical abnormalities of GI tract, failure to respond to conventional therapy, frequent and severe abdominal pain/discomfort, frequent bowel urgency/fecal incontinence, and disability/restriction of daily activities due to IBS.

DOSAGE: *Adults:* Initial: 1mg qd for 4 weeks. Titrate: If tolerated and IBS symptoms not controlled, may increase to 1mg bid. Discontinue after 4 weeks if symptoms not controlled on 1mg bid.

HOW SUPPLIED: Tab: 0.5mg, 1mg

CONTRAINDICATIONS: Current constipation. History of chronic/severe constipation or sequelae of constipation, intestinal obstruction/stricture, toxic megacolon, GI perforation/adhesions, ischemic colitis, impaired intestinal circulation, thrombophlebitis, hypercoagulable state, Crohn's disease, ulcerative colitis, diverticulitis, severe hepatic impairment. Inability to understand/comply with Patient-Physician Agreement.

WARNINGS/PRECAUTIONS: Increased risk of constipation and ischemic colitis. Caution with mild or moderate hepatic impairment.

ADVERSE REACTIONS: Constipation, abdominal discomfort/pain, nausea, GI discomfort/pain.

INTERACTIONS: Increased risk of constipation with medications that decrease GI motility. Inducers and inhibitors of hepatic CYP drug-metabolizing enzymes may change the clearance of alosetron. Fluvoxamine increases AUC, concomitant administration is contraindicated. Avoid with quinolone antibiotics and cimetidine. Caution with ketoconazole, clarithromycin, telithromycin, protease inhibitors, voriconazole, itraconazole.

PREGNANCY: Category B, caution in nursing.

MECHANISM OF ACTION: 5-HT$_3$ receptor antagonist.

PHARMACOKINETICS: Absorption: Rapidly absorbed, absolute bioavailability (50-60%), C_{max}=5ng/mL (male), 9ng/mL (female); T_{max}=1 hr. **Distribution:** V_d=65-95L, plasma protein binding (82%). **Metabolism:** Extensively metabolized. **Elimination:** $T_{1/2}$=1.5 hrs, urine (73%) and feces (24%).

LOVAZA
RX

omega-3-acid ethyl esters (Reliant)

THERAPEUTIC CLASS: Lipid-regulating agent

INDICATIONS: Adjunct to diet to reduce very high (≥ 500mg/dL) triglyceride levels in adult patients.

DOSAGE: *Adults:* 4g qd. Given as single 4-g dose (4 caps) or as two 2-g doses (2 caps bid).

HOW SUPPLIED: Cap: 1g

WARNINGS/PRECAUTIONS: Caution in patients with diabetes, hypothyroidism, hepatic and pancreas problem, known sensitivity or allergy to fish. Lower alcohol use. Lose weight if you are overweight. Possible increases in alanine aminotransferase levels without a concurrent increase in aspartate aminotransferase levels. Possible increased low-density lipoprotein cholesterol levels.

ADVERSE REACTIONS: Eructation, infection, flu-syndrome, dyspepsia.

INTERACTIONS: Possible prolongation of bleeding time with concomitant anticoagulants (aspirin, warfarin, coumarin, clopidogrel).

PREGNANCY: Category C, caution in nursing.

MECHANISM OF ACTION: Lipid-regulating agent; not completely understood; inhibits acyl CoA:1,2-diacylglycerol acyltransferase, increases mitochondrial, peroxisomal β-oxidation in the liver and decreases lipogenisis in the liver, and increases plasma lipoprotein lipase activity.

LOVENOX RX
enoxaparin sodium (Sanofi-Aventis)

> Risk of paralysis by spinal/epidural hematoma with neuraxial anesthesia or spinal puncture. Increased risk with indwelling epidural catheters for analgesia, drugs affecting hemostasis (eg, NSAIDs, platelet inhibitors, anticoagulants), and traumatic or repeated epidural or spinal puncture.

THERAPEUTIC CLASS: Low molecular weight heparin

INDICATIONS: Prevention of DVT in hip or knee replacement surgery, abdominal surgery, or with severely restricted mobility during acute illness. With concomitant warfarin, inpatient treatment of acute DVT with or without PE and outpatient treatment of DVT without PE. Prevention of ischemic complications in unstable angina and non-Q-wave MI with concurrent ASA therapy. Treatment of acute ST-segment elevation MI (STEMI) in patients receiving thrombolysis and being managed medically or with percutaneous coronary intervention (PCI).

DOSAGE: *Adults:* Hip/Knee Surgery: 30mg SQ q12h, starting 12-24 hrs post-op, for 7-10 days (up to 12 days) or 40mg SQ qd for hip surgery for 3 weeks. Abdominal Surgery: 40mg SQ qd, starting 2 hrs pre-op, for 7-10 days (up to 14 days). DVT with or without PE treatment: (inpatient/outpatient) 1mg/kg SQ q12h or (inpatient) 1.5mg/kg qd with warfarin (start within 72 hrs) for 7 days (up to 17 days). Acute Illness: 40mg SQ qd for 6-11 days (up to 14 days). Unstable Angina/Non-Q-Wave MI: 1mg/kg SQ q12h with 100-325mg/day of ASA for 2-8 days (up to 12.5 days). Acute STEMI (<75 yrs): 30mg single IV bolus plus a 1mg/kg SQ dose followed by 1mg/kg SQ q12h with ASA. Max: 100mg for 1st 2 doses only. Acute STEMI (≥75 yrs): 0.75mg/kg SQ q12h (no initial bolus) with ASA. Max: 75mg for 1st 2 doses only. When given with thrombolytic, give enoxaparin dose between 15 min before and 30 min after start of fibrinolytic therapy. With PCI, if last enoxaparin SQ dose was given >8 hrs before balloon inflation, an IV bolus of 0.3mg/kg of enoxaparin should be given. CrCl <30mL/min: Surgery/Acute Illness: 30mg SQ qd. DVT with or without PE treatment (inpatient/outpatient)/Unstable Angina/Non-Q-Wave MI: 1mg/kg SQ qd. Acute STEMI: <75 yrs: 30mg single IV bolus plus a 1mg/kg SQ dose followed by 1mg/kg SQ qd. ≥75 yrs: 1mg/kg SQ qd (no initial bolus).

HOW SUPPLIED: Inj: (MDV) 300mg/3mL; (Syringe) 30mg/0.3mL, 40mg/0.4mL, 60mg/0.6mL, 80mg/0.8mL, 100mg/mL, 120mg/0.8mL, 150mg/mL

CONTRAINDICATIONS: Heparin or pork allergy, active major bleeding, thrombocytopenia with a positive in vitro test for anti-platelet antibody. Hypersensitivity to benzyl alcohol (multi-dose formulation).

WARNINGS/PRECAUTIONS: Not for IM injection. Cannot use interchangeably unit for unit with heparin or other low molecular weight heparins. Extreme caution with HIT, conditions with an increased risk of hemorrhage (eg, bacterial endocarditis, hemorrhagic stroke, etc). Major hemorrhages (eg, retroperitoneal, intracranial), thrombocytopenia reported. D/C if platelets <100,000/mm³. Perform periodic CBC, platelets, and stool occult blood test. Caution with bleeding diathesis, uncontrolled arterial HTN, recent GI ulceration, diabetic retinopathy, hemorrhage. Delayed elimination with elderly or in renal dysfunction. Monitor elderly with low body weight (<45 kg) and predisposition to decreased renal function. Higher risk of thromboembolism in pregnant women with prosthetic heart valves. Not for thromboprophylaxis in prosthetic

568 PDR® Concise Drug Guide

heart valve patients. Achieve homeostasis at puncture site before sheath removal after PCI. Caution in hepatic impairment.

ADVERSE REACTIONS: Hemorrhage, thrombocytopenia, local reactions (ecchymosis, erythema), anemia, elevation of aminotransferases.

INTERACTIONS: D/C agents that increase risk of hemorrhage (eg, anticoagulants, acetylsalicylic acid, salicylates, NSAIDs, ketorolac, dipyridamole, sulfinpyrazone), unless really needed; monitor closely if co-administered.

PREGNANCY: Category B, caution in nursing.

MECHANISM OF ACTION: Low molecular-weight heparin with antithrombotic properties.

PHARMACOKINETICS: Absorption: (1mg/kg bid) C_{max}=1.2 IU/mL. **Distribution:** V_d=4.3L. **Metabolism:** Liver. **Elimination:** Urine; (single dose) $T_{1/2}$=4.5 hrs; (multiple doses) $T_{1/2}$= 7 hrs.

LOXITANE   RX
loxapine succinate (Watson)

THERAPEUTIC CLASS: Dibenzapine derivative

INDICATIONS: Treatment of schizophrenia.

DOSAGE: *Adults:* (PO) Initial: 10mg bid, up to 50mg/day for severely disturbed. Titrate: Increase rapidly over 7-10 days. Maint: 60-100mg/day. Max: 250mg/day.

HOW SUPPLIED: Cap: 5mg, 10mg, 25mg, 50mg

CONTRAINDICATIONS: Comatose states, severe drug-induced depressed states (eg, alcohol, barbiturates, narcotics).

WARNINGS/PRECAUTIONS: Extrapyramidal symptoms, tardive dyskinesia, NMS can occur. May lower seizure threshold. May mask symptoms of overdose of other drugs. May obscure diagnosis of intestinal obstruction, brain tumor. Ocular toxicity reported. Caution in cardiovascular disease, glaucoma, urinary retention. Elevates prolactin levels. Caution with activities requiring alertness.

ADVERSE REACTIONS: Drowsiness, weakness, NMS, tachycardia, hypotension, HTN, syncope, edema, dry mouth, constipation, blurred vision.

INTERACTIONS: Significant respiratory depression and hypotension reported with lorazepam (rare). Caution with CNS-active drugs, including alcohol. Antagonizes epinephrine.

PREGNANCY: Safety in pregnancy not known. Not for use in nursing.

MECHANISM OF ACTION: Tricyclic antipsychotic. Not established. Suspected to reduce excitability of subcortical areas.

PHARMACOKINETICS: Absorption: Complete. **Distribution:** Distributed in lungs, brain, spleen, heart and kidneys. **Metabolism:** Extensive. **Elimination:** Urine (metabolites and conjugates), feces (unconjugated).

LOZOL   RX
indapamide (Sanofi-Aventis)

THERAPEUTIC CLASS: Indoline diuretic

INDICATIONS: Treatment of hypertension and salt/fluid retention associated with congestive heart failure.

DOSAGE: *Adults:* HTN: 1.25mg qam. Titrate: May increase to 2.5mg qd after 4 weeks, then to 5mg qd after another 4 weeks. Max: 5mg/day. CHF: 2.5mg qam. Titrate: May increase to 5mg qd after 1 week. Max: 5mg/day.

HOW SUPPLIED: Tab: 1.25mg, 2.5mg

CONTRAINDICATIONS: Anuria, sulfonamide hypersensitivity.

WARNINGS/PRECAUTIONS: Caution in severe renal disease, liver dysfunction. May exacerbate or activate SLE. Monitor for fluid/electrolyte imbalance. Hyperuricemia, hypercalcemia, hypokalemia, hypophosphatemia, and hyperglycemia may occur. Monitor renal function, serum uric acid levels periodically. May precipitate gout. May manifest latent DM. Enhanced effects in post-sympathectomy patient.

ADVERSE REACTIONS: Headache, infection, pain, back pain, dizziness, rhinitis, fatigue, muscle cramps, nervousness, numbness of extremities, electrolyte imbalance, anxiety, agitation.

INTERACTIONS: May decrease arterial responsiveness to norepinephrine. May potentiate other antihypertensives. Risk of lithium toxicity. Increases risk of hypokalemia with ACTH, corticosteroids. Antidiabetic agents may need adjustment.

PREGNANCY: Category B, not for use in nursing.

MECHANISM OF ACTION: Indoline diuretic.

PHARMACOKINETICS: Absorption: (2.5mg) C_{max}=115ng/mL, T_{max}=2 hrs; (5mg) C_{max}=260ng/mL, T_{max}=2 hrs. **Distribution:** Plasma protein bound (71-79%). **Metabolism:** Extensive. **Elimination:** Urine (7%), $T_{1/2}$=14 hrs.

LUCENTIS   RX
ranibizumab (Genentech)

THERAPEUTIC CLASS: Monoclonal antibody/VEGF-A blocker

INDICATIONS: Treatment of patients with neovascular (wet) age-related macular degeneration.

DOSAGE: *Adults:* Administer 0.5mg (0.05mL) by intravitreal injection once a month. May reduce to 1 injection every 3 months after the first 4 injections if monthly injections not feasible.

HOW SUPPLIED: Inj: 10mg/mL

CONTRAINDICATIONS: Ocular or periocular infections.

WARNINGS/PRECAUTIONS: Intravitreal injections have been associated with endophthalmitis and retinal detachments. Increased IOP noted within 60 min of intravitreal injection. Arterial thromboembolic events were observed.

ADVERSE REACTIONS: Conjunctival hemorrhage, eye pain, vitreous floaters, increase IOP, intraocular inflammation.

INTERACTIONS: May develop serious intraocular inflammation when used adjunctively with Verteporfin photodynamic therapy.

PREGNANCY: Category C, caution in nursing.

MECHANISM OF ACTION: Monoclonal antibody/VEGF-A blocker; responsible for binding to VEGF-A which prevents the interaction of VEGF-A with its receptors (VEGFR1 and VEGFR2) on the surface of endothelial cells. This reduces endothelial cell proliferation, vascular leakage, and new blood vessel formation.

PHARMACOKINETICS: Absorption: C_{max}=1.5ng/mL. T_{max}=1 day. **Elimination:** $T_{1/2}$= 9 days.

LUMIGAN   RX
bimatoprost (Allergan)

THERAPEUTIC CLASS: Prostaglandin analog

INDICATIONS: Reduction of elevated IOP in open-angle glaucoma. Ocular hypertension if intolerant or unresponsive to other IOP therapies.

DOSAGE: *Adults:* 1 drop qd in pm. Max: Once daily dosing. Space dosing other ophthalmic drugs by 5 min.

HOW SUPPLIED: Sol: 0.03% [2.5mL, 5mL]

WARNINGS/PRECAUTIONS: Changes to pigmented tissues, growth of eyelashes, and macular edema reported. May change eye color and eyelashes. Do not administer with contact lenses. Caution with intraocular inflammation, renal or hepatic impairment. Caution with active intraocular inflammation, aphakic patients, pseudophakic patients with a torn posterior lens capsule, patients at risk of macular edema, and renal or hepatic impairment. Not for the treatment of angle closure, inflammatory, or neovascular glaucoma.

ADVERSE REACTIONS: Conjunctival hyperemia, ocular pruritus, growth of eyelashes, ocular dryness, visual disturbances, eye burning, foreign body sensation, eye pain, periocular skin pigmentation, blepharitis, cataract, eyelid erythema, eyelash darkening, superficial punctate keratitis.

INTERACTIONS: Space dosing of other eye drops by 5 minutes.

PREGNANCY: Category C, caution in nursing.

MECHANISM OF ACTION: Prostaglandin analog: Selectively mimics the effects of naturally occuring substances, prostamides. Believed to lower intraocular pressure (IOP) by increasing outflow of aqueous humor through both the trabecular meshwork and uveoscleral routes.

PHARMACOKINETICS: Absorption: C_{max}=0.08ng/mL, AUC=0.09ng•hr/mL, T_{max}=10 min. **Distribution:** V_d=0.67L/kg. **Metabolism:** Via oxidation, N-deethylation and glucuronidation. **Elimination:** $T_{1/2}$=45 min. Urine (67%), feces (25%).

LUNESTA
eszopiclone (Sepracor)　　CIV

THERAPEUTIC CLASS: Nonbenzodiazepine hypnotic agent

INDICATIONS: Treatment of insomnia.

DOSAGE: *Adults:* Initial: 2mg qhs. Max: 3mg qhs. Elderly: Difficulty Falling Asleep: Initial: 1mg qhs. Max: 2mg qhs. Difficulty Staying Asleep: Initial/Max: 2mg qhs. Avoid high-fat meal.

HOW SUPPLIED: Tab: 1mg, 2mg, 3mg

WARNINGS/PRECAUTIONS: Abnormal thinking and behavioral changes reported. Amnesia and other neuropsychiatric symptoms may occur. Worsening of depression including suicidal thinking reported in primarily depressed patients. Avoid rapid dose decrease or abrupt discontinuation. Should only be taken immediately prior to bed or after going to bed and experiencing difficulty falling asleep. Avoid hazardous occupations. Caution in elderly, debilitated, or conditions affecting metabolism or hemodynamic responses. Reduce dose with severe hepatic impairment or concurrent use of potent CYP3A4 inhibitors. Caution with signs and symptoms of depression or suicidal tendencies.

ADVERSE REACTIONS: Headache, unpleasant taste, somnolence, dry mouth, dizziness, infection, rash, chest pain, peripheral edema, migraine.

INTERACTIONS: Possible additive effect on psychomotor performance with ethanol. Coadministration with olanzapine produced a decrease in DSST score. Strong inhibitors of CYP3A4 may significantly increase the AUC of eszopiclone.

PREGNANCY: Category C, caution in nursing.

MECHANISM OF ACTION: Not established. Pyrrolopyrazine derivative; suspected to interact with GABA-receptor complexes at binding domains located close to or allosterically coupled to benzodiazepine receptor.

PHARMACOKINETICS: Absorption: Rapidly absorbed. T_{max}=1 hr. **Distribution:** Plasma protein binding (52-59%). **Metabolism:** Liver (extensive); oxidation and demethylation pathways via CYP3A4 and CYP2E1. Primary metabolites: (S)-zopiclone-N-oxide and (S)-N-desmethyl zopiclone. **Elimination:** $T_{1/2}$=6 hrs, 9 hrs (elderly); urine (75% metabolite), (<10% parent drug).

LUPRON
leuprolide acetate (TAP)　　RX

THERAPEUTIC CLASS: Synthetic gonadotropin releasing hormone analog

Lupron Depot (GYN)

INDICATIONS: Palliative treatment of advanced prostate cancer.

DOSAGE: *Adults:* 1mg SQ qd. Rotate injection sites.

HOW SUPPLIED: Inj: 5mg/mL

CONTRAINDICATIONS: Pregnancy.

WARNINGS/PRECAUTIONS: Transient worsening of symptoms may occur during 1st few weeks of therapy. Closely monitor patients with metastatic vertebral lesions and/or urinary tract obstruction during 1st few weeks of therapy; may cause neurological problems or increase obstruction. Monitor serum testosterone, acid phosphatase levels. Contains benzyl alcohol.

ADVERSE REACTIONS: General pain, headache, hot flashes, urinary disorders, dizziness/vertigo, ECG changes/ischemia, peripheral edema, HTN, asthenia, constipation, anorexia, insomnia, myocardial infarction, diabetes, respiratory problems.

PREGNANCY: Category X, not for use in nursing.

MECHANISM OF ACTION: LH-RH agonist: Acts as a potent inhibitor of gonadotropin secretion resulting in suppression of ovarian and testicular steroidogenesis.

PHARMACOKINETICS: Absorption: (M-1): T_{max}=2-6 hrs. **Distribution:** V_d=27L, plasma protein binding (43-49%). **Metabolism:** M-I (major metabolite). **Elimination:** $T_{1/2}$=3 hrs, urine (<5%).

Lupron Depot (GYN)   RX
leuprolide acetate (TAP)

OTHER BRAND NAMES: Lupron Depot 3.75 mg (TAP) - Lupron Depot-3 Month 11.25mg (TAP)

THERAPEUTIC CLASS: Synthetic gonadotropin releasing hormone analog

INDICATIONS: Management of endometriosis alone or with norethindrone acetate 5mg, including pain relief and reduction of endometriotic lesions. Retreatment of endometriosis with norethindrone acetate 5mg daily. Adjunct with iron for preoperative hematologic improvement of anemia caused by uterine leiomyomata.

DOSAGE: *Adults:* Endometriosis: 11.25mg IM every 3 months or 3.75mg IM monthly, alone or with norethindrone acetate 5mg/day. Max: 6 months of therapy. If symptoms recur after course of therapy, may retreat with the combination (leuprolide + norethindrone) up to 6 months. Uterine Leiomyomata: 11.25mg IM single dose or 3.75mg IM monthly up to 3 months. Assess bone density before retreatment.

HOW SUPPLIED: Inj: (1 month) 3.75mg, (3 month) 11.25mg

CONTRAINDICATIONS: Undiagnosed abnormal vaginal bleeding, pregnancy, nursing.

WARNINGS/PRECAUTIONS: Exclude pregnancy before therapy. Use nonhormonal methods of contraception. D/C if pregnancy occurs. Retreatment is not recommended with endometriosis. Limit to 6 months of therapy. Use if require hormonal suppression for at least 3 months. Transient worsening of symptoms may occur during initial days of therapy. Breakthrough bleeding with skipped doses. May develop or worsen depression and cause memory disorders.

ADVERSE REACTIONS: Hot flashes, sweating, dizziness, headache, vaginitis, depression, emotional lability, general pain, asthenia, decreased libido, joint disorder, breast tenderness/pain, GI upset, edema, bone density loss.

PREGNANCY: Category X, not for use in nursing.

MECHANISM OF ACTION: GnRH analog; suppresses pituitary gonadotropins.

PHARMACOKINETICS: Absorption: (3.5mg): C_{max}=4.6-10.2 ng/mL, T_{max}=4 hrs. **Distribution:** Plasma protein binding (43-49%), V_d=27L (IV). **Elimination:** $T_{1/2}$=3 hrs.

LUPRON DEPOT (ONCOLOGY) RX
leuprolide acetate (TAP)

OTHER BRAND NAMES: Lupron Depot 7.5mg (TAP) - Lupron Depot 3-Month 22.5 mg (TAP) - Lupron Depot 4-Month (TAP)

THERAPEUTIC CLASS: Synthetic gonadotropin releasing hormone analog

INDICATIONS: Palliative treatment of advanced prostate cancer.

DOSAGE: *Adults:* 7.5mg IM as single dose monthly, 22.5mg IM single dose every 3 months, or 30mg IM single dose every 4 months. Rotate injection site.

HOW SUPPLIED: Inj: (1-month) 7.5mg, (3-month) 22.5mg, (4-month) 30mg

CONTRAINDICATIONS: Pregnancy.

WARNINGS/PRECAUTIONS: Transient worsening of symptoms may occur during 1st few weeks of therapy. Closely monitor patients with metastatic vertebral lesions and/or urinary tract obstruction during 1st few weeks of therapy. Monitor serum testosterone, PSA. (7.5mg, 30mg) Temporary increase in bone pain. Ureteral obstruction and spinal cord compression reported; may initiate with SQ formulation for 1st 2 weeks to facilitate withdrawal if needed.

ADVERSE REACTIONS: Injection site reactions, general pain, headache, hot flashes, sweating, edema, urinary disorders, dizziness/vertigo, asthenia, GI disorders, impotence.

PREGNANCY: Category X, safety in nursing not known.

MECHANISM OF ACTION: LH-RH agonist: Acts as a potent inhibitor of gonadotropin secretion resulting in suppression of ovarian and testicular steroidogenesis.

PHARMACOKINETICS: Absorption: (7.5mg, 22.5mg, 30mg): C_{max}=20ng/mL, 48.9ng/mL, 59.3ng/mL T_{max}=4 hrs; (M-1): T_{max}=2-6hrs. **Distribution:** V_d=27L, plasma protein binding (43-49%). **Metabolism:** M-I (Major metabolite). **Elimination:** $T_{1/2}$=3 hrs, urine (<5%).

LUPRON PEDIATRIC RX
leuprolide acetate (TAP)

OTHER BRAND NAMES: Lupron Depot-Ped (TAP)

THERAPEUTIC CLASS: Synthetic gonadotropin releasing hormone analog

INDICATIONS: Treatment of central precocious puberty.

DOSAGE: *Pediatrics:* Initial: 50mcg/kg/d as single SQ dose or (depot) 0.3mg/kg every 4 weeks (minimum 7.5mg) as single IM dose. Depot Start Dose: ≤25kg: 7.5mg; >25-37.5kg: 11.25mg; >37.5kg: 15mg. Titrate: Increase by 10 mcg/kg/day SQ or (depot) 3.75mg IM every 4 weeks if downregulation not achieved. Maint: Dose that produces adequate downregulation. Verify adequate downregulation with significant weight increase.

HOW SUPPLIED: Inj: 5mg/mL, (Depot) 7.5mg, 11.25mg, 15mg

CONTRAINDICATIONS: Pregnancy.

WARNINGS/PRECAUTIONS: Monitor hormonal effects after 1-2 months of therapy. Measure bone age every 6-12 months. Increase in clinical signs and symptoms may occur in early phase of therapy due to rise in gonadotropins and sex steroids. D/C before age 11 in females and age 12 in males.

ADVERSE REACTIONS: Initial exacerbation of signs and symptoms, injection site reactions, pain, acne/seborrhea, rash, urogenital bleeding/discharge, vaginitis.

PREGNANCY: Category X, not for use in nursing.

MECHANISM OF ACTION: A GnRH agonist; initially stimulates gonadotropins. Chronic stimulation results in reversible suppression of ovarian and testicular steroidogenesis.

PHARMACOKINETICS: Absorption: C_{max}=20ng/mL, T_{max}=4 hrs. **Distribution:** V_d=27L, plasma protein binding (43-49%). **Metabolism:** M-I (major metabolite). **Elimination:** Urine (<5% parent and metabolite). $T_{1/2}$=3 hrs.

Luride   RX
sodium fluoride (Colgate Oral)

THERAPEUTIC CLASS: Fluoride supplement

INDICATIONS: To prevent dental caries in areas where drinking water fluoride content is <0.6ppm.

DOSAGE: *Pediatrics:* (Drops) <0.3ppm: 6 months-3 yrs: 0.5mL qd. 3-6 yrs: 1mL qd. 6-16 yrs: 2mL qd. 0.3-0.6ppm: 3-6 yrs: 0.5mL qd. 6-16 yrs: 1mL qd. (Tab) <0.3ppm: 6 months-<3 yrs: 0.25mg qd. 3-6 yrs: 0.5mg qd. 6-16 yrs: 1mg qd. 0.3-0.6ppm: 3-6 yrs: 0.25mg qd. 6-16 yrs: 0.5mg qd. Dissolve tab in mouth or chew tab before swallowing. Take at bedtime after brushing teeth.

HOW SUPPLIED: Drops: 0.5mg/mL [50mL]; Tab, Chewable: 0.25mg, 0.5mg, 1mg

CONTRAINDICATIONS: (Drips) Areas where drinking water fluoride is >0.6 ppm, pediatrics <6 months. (Tab) 1mg: Water fluoride is >0.3ppm, pediatrics <6 yrs. 0.5mg: Water fluoride is >0.6ppm, pediatrics <6 yrs. 0.25mg: Water fluoride is >0.6ppm.

WARNINGS/PRECAUTIONS: Dental fluorosis may result from daily ingestion of excessive fluoride in pediatrics <6 yrs especially if water fluoride is >0.6ppm.

ADVERSE REACTIONS: Allergic rash.

INTERACTIONS: Do not eat or drink dairy products within 1 hour of administration.

PREGNANCY: Safety in pregnancy not known. Caution in nursing.

MECHANISM OF ACTION: Fluoride supplement; increases tooth resistance to acid dissolution by promoting remineralization and inhibiting cariogenic microbial process.

Lustra   RX
hydroquinone (Taro)

OTHER BRAND NAMES: Lustra-AF (Taro)

THERAPEUTIC CLASS: Depigmenting agent

INDICATIONS: Gradual treatment of UV-induced dyschromia and discoloration resulting from use of oral contraceptives, pregnancy, hormone replacement therapy, or skin trauma.

DOSAGE: *Adults:* Apply bid (am and hs). Use with sunscreen.
Pediatrics: ≥12 yrs: Apply bid (am and hs). Use with sunscreen.

HOW SUPPLIED: Cre: 4% [56.8g]

WARNINGS/PRECAUTIONS: Avoid sun exposure on bleached skin. Lustra-AF contains sunscreen; use sunscreen with Lustra. May produce unwanted cosmetic effects if not used as directed. Test for skin sensitivity. D/C if no lightening effect after 2 months of therapy, if blue-black darkening of the skin occurs, or if itching, vesicle formation, or excessive inflammatory reactions occur. Contains sodium metabisulfite, may cause serious allergic type reactions. Avoid contact wtih eyes.

ADVERSE REACTIONS: Cutaneous hypersensitivity (contact dermatitis).

PREGNANCY: Category C, caution in nursing.

MECHANISM OF ACTION: Produces reversible depigmentation of skin; inhibits enzymatic oxidation of tyrosine to 3-(3,4-dihydroxyphenyl) alanine (dopa) and suppresses other melanocyte metabolic processes.

LUVERIS   RX
lutropin alfa (EMD Serono)

THERAPEUTIC CLASS: Recombinant Human Luteinizing Hormore

INDICATIONS: Used in combination with Gonal-f (follitropin alfa) for stimulation of follicular development in infertile hypogonadotropic hypogonadal women with profound luteinizing hormone deficiency (LH<1.2 IU/L).

DOSAGE: *Adults:* Initial: 75 IU with 75-150 IU of Gonal-f qd SQ as two separate injections. Give hCG 1 day after last dose. Do not exceed 14 days of therapy unless signs of imminent follicular development. Do not exceed 225 IU/day of Gonal-f.

HOW SUPPLIED: Inj: 75 IU.

CONTRAINDICATIONS: Primary ovarian failure, uncontrolled thyroid or adrenal dysfunction, uncontrolled organic intracranial lesion (eg, pituitary tumor), abnormal uterine bleeding of undetermined origin, ovarian cyst or enlargement of undetermined origin, sex hormone dependent tumors of the reproductive tract and accessory organs, and pregnancy.

WARNINGS/PRECAUTIONS: Ovarian enlargement may occur; monitor ovarian response. Ovarian hyperstimulation syndrome (OHSS), multiple births, serious pulmonary and vascular complications reported. Do not administer hCG dose if evidence of OHSS. Monitor follicular maturation through ultrasonography and serum estradiol levels.

ADVERSE REACTIONS: Headache, nausea, ovarian hyperstimulation, breast pain (female), abdominal pain, ovarian cyst, flatulence, injection site reaction, dysmenorrhea, ovarian disorder, diarrhea, constipation, pain, fatigue, upper respiratory tract infection.

PREGNANCY: Category X, caution in nursing.

MECHANISM OF ACTION: Follicle stimulating hormone/lutenizing hormone; produces ovarian follicular growth in women who do not have primary ovarian failure.

PHARMACOKINETICS: **Absorption:** C_{max}=1.1IU/L, T_{max}=6 hrs. AUC=44h•IU/L. **Distribution:** V_d=approx. 10L. **Elimination:** $T_{1/2}$=14 hrs; renal (unchanged).

LUXIQ   RX
betamethasone valerate (Stiefel)

THERAPEUTIC CLASS: Corticosteroid

INDICATIONS: Corticosteroid responsive dermatoses of the scalp.

DOSAGE: *Adults:* Place foam onto saucer or other cool surface first, then apply in small amounts to scalp. Gently massage into affected area bid (am and pm) until foam disappears. Reassess if no improvement after 2 weeks.

HOW SUPPLIED: Foam: 0.12% [50g, 100g]

WARNINGS/PRECAUTIONS: May produce reversible HPA axis suppression, manifestations of Cushing's syndrome, hyperglycemia, and glucosuria. Caution when applied to large surface areas, for prolonged use, or under occlusive dressings. Use appropriate antifungal or antibacterial agent with dermatological infections; d/c if infection does not clear. Pediatrics may be more susceptible to systemic toxicity. Avoid eyes. D/C if irritation occurs.

ADVERSE REACTIONS: Burning, stinging, pruritus, paresthesia, acne, alopecia, conjunctivitis.

PREGNANCY: Category C, caution in nursing.

MECHANISM OF ACTION: Corticosteroid; possesses anti-inflammatory, antipruritic, and vasoconstrictive properties. Anti-inflammatory mechanism not established. Suspected to induce phospholipase A_2 inhibitory proteins, lipocortins. Lipocortins control biosynthesis of potent mediators of inflammation (eg, prostaglandins, leukotrienes) by inhibiting release of their precursor, arachidonic acid.

L

PHARMACOKINETICS: Absorption: Percutaneous. Occlusion, inflammation, and other disease states may increase absorption. **Distribution:** Systemically administered corticosteroids are found in human breast milk. **Metabolism:** Liver. **Elimination:** Renal (major), bile.

LYBREL   RX
ethinyl estradiol - levonorgestrel (Wyeth)

THERAPEUTIC CLASS: Estrogen/progestogen combination

INDICATIONS: Prevention of pregnancy.

DOSAGE: *Adults:* 1 tab qd. Start Day: No Current Contraceptive Therapy: Day 1 of menstrual cycle. 21- or 28-day Regimen: Day 1 of withdrawal bleed (at the latest 7 days after last active tablet). Progestin-Only Pill: Day after taking progestin-only pill. Implant: Day of implant removal. Inj: Day next inj due. Use nonhormonal back-up method of birth control for 1st 7 days of Lybrel therapy when initiating after progestin-only pill, implant, or inj.

HOW SUPPLIED: Tab: (Ethinyl Estradiol-Levonorgestrel) 0.02mg-0.09mg

CONTRAINDICATIONS: Thrombophlebitis, DVT or thromboembolic disorders, cerebrovascular or CAD, valvular heart disease with thrombogenic complications, thrombogenic rhythm disorders, hereditary or acquired thrombophilias, major surgery with prolonged immobilization, DM with vascular involvement, headaches with focal neurological symptoms, uncontrolled HTN, breast cancer, endometrial carcinoma or other estrogen-dependent neoplasia, undiagnosed abnormal genital bleeding, cholestatic jaundice of pregnancy or jaundice with prior pill use, hepatic adenomas or carcinomas, active liver disease, pregnancy.

WARNINGS/PRECAUTIONS: Cigarette smoking increases risk of serious CV side effects; risk increases with age (especially >35 yrs) and extent of smoking. Increased risk of venous and arterial thrombotic and thromboembolic events (eg, MI, thromboembolism, stroke, TIA), hepatic neoplasia, gallbladder disease, and HTN. May increase risk of breast and cervical cancer. Retinal thrombosis reported; d/c if unexplained loss of vision. May worsen existing gallbladder disease. May cause glucose tolerance; monitor prediabetic and diabetic women. May cause fluid retention and increase BP; monitor closely with HTN and d/c if significant elevation of BP occurs. May cause onset or development of migraine or development of headache. Weigh benefit of fewer planned menses against inconvenience of unscheduled breakthrough bleeding and spotting. Ectopic or intrauterine pregnancy may occur. Monitor closely with hyperlipidemias. D/C if jaundice develops. Monitor closely with depression and d/c if depression recurs to serious degree. Perform annual physical exam. Use before menarche is not indicated.

ADVERSE REACTIONS: Nausea, vomiting, spotting, amenorrhea, edema, weight or appetite (increase or decrease), spotting, dizziness, GI symptoms (eg, abdominal pain, cramps, bloating), nervousness, vaginitis, including candidiasis.

INTERACTIONS: Reduced effects, increased breakthrough bleeding with rifampin, rifabutin, barbiturates, phenylbutazone, primidone, dexamethasone, phenytoin, carbamazepine, felbamate, oxcarbazepine, griseofulvin, topiramate, St. Johns wort, modafinil, and possibly with ampicillin and tetracyclines. Atorvastatin, ascorbic acid, acetaminophen, CYP3A4 inhibitors (eg, itraconazole, ketoconazole) may increase hormones levels. Protease inhibitors may increase or decrease levels. May increase levels of cyclosporine, prednisolone, theophylline. May decrease levels of acetaminophen and lamotrigine. Increases clearance of temazepam, salicylic acid, morphine, clofibric acid.

PREGNANCY: Category X, not for use in nursing

MECHANISM OF ACTION: Estrogen/progesterone combination oral contraceptive. Acts by suppression of gonadotropins. Primarily inhibits ovulation. Also responsible for changes in cervical mucus (increasing difficulty of sperm entry into uterus) and in endometrium (reducing likelihood of implantation).

PHARMACOKINETICS: Absorption: Oral administration of variable days resulted in different parameters. Levonorgestrel: Rapid and completely absorbed, absolute bioavailability (100%); Ethinyl estradiol: Rapid and completely absorbed, absolute bioavailability (38-48%). **Distribution:** Levonorgestrel: Plasma protein binding (97%). **Metabolism:** Levonorgestrel: Reduction, hydroxylation and conjugation; Ethinyl Estradiol: Hepatic via CYP3A4 (hydroxylation). **Elimination:** Levonorgestrel: Urine (40-68%), feces (16-48%); $T_{1/2}$=36 hrs. Ethinyl Estradiol: Urine, feces; $T_{1/2}$=21 hrs.

LYRICA
pregabalin (Pfizer)

CV

THERAPEUTIC CLASS: GABA analog

INDICATIONS: Adjunct therapy for adult patients with partial onset seizures. Management of neuropathic pain associated with diabetic peripheral neuropathy. Management of post-herpetic neuralgia and fibromyalgia.

DOSAGE: *Adults:* Neuropathic Pain: Initial: 50mg tid (150mg/day). Titrate: May increase to 300mg/day within 1 week. Max: 100mg tid (300mg/day). Post-Herpetic Neuralgia: Initial: 150mg/day divided bid or tid. Max: 600mg/day divided bid or tid. Epilepsy: Initial: 150mg/day divided bid-tid. Max: 600mg/day. Fibromyalgia: Initial: 75mg bid (150mg/day). Titrate: May increase to 150mg bid (300mg/day) within 1 week based on efficacy and tolerability. May further increase to 225mg bid (450mg/day) if needed. Max: 450mg/day. Renal Impairment: CrCl 30-60 mL/min: 75-300mg/day divided bid or tid. CrCl 15-30 mL/min: 25-150mg/day divided qd or bid. CrCl <15mL/min: 25-75mg/day given qd. Give supplemental dose (25-150mg) immediately after every 4-hr hemodialysis treatment. Refer to prescribing information for further details. D/C: Taper over minimum of 1 week.

HOW SUPPLIED: Cap: 25mg, 50mg, 75mg, 100mg, 150mg, 200mg, 225mg, 300mg

WARNINGS/PRECAUTIONS: Avoid abrupt withdrawal. Gradually taper over 1 week. Possible tumorigenic potential. May impair physical/mental abilities. May cause weight gain; blurred vision, monitor for ophthalmic changes; peripheral edema, caution in heart failure; elevated creatine kinase, d/c if myopathy or markedly elevated creatine kinase levels occur; decreased platelet count; and mild PR-interval prolongation. Angioedema reported in initial and chronic treatment.

ADVERSE REACTIONS: Somnolence, dizziness, dry mouth, edema, blurred vision, weight gain, abnormal thinking (difficulty with concentration/attention), headache, nausea, diarrhea.

INTERACTIONS: Additive CNS side effects with CNS depressants (eg, opiates, benzodiazepines). May potentiate the impairment of motor skills and sedation of alcohol; avoid consumption of alcohol during therapy.

PREGNANCY: Category C, not for use in nursing.

MECHANISM OF ACTION: Gamma-aminobutyric acid derivative; not fully established. Suspected to bind to α-2-delta receptors in CNS tissues. In vitro, shown to reduce calcium-dependent release of several neurotransmitters, possibly by modulation of calcium channel function. Produces antinociceptive and antiseizure effects.

PHARMACOKINETICS: Absorption: T_{max}=1.5 hrs; bioavailability (≥90%). **Distribution:** V_d=0.5L/kg; crosses placenta and blood-brain barrier, found in milk. **Metabolism:** N-methylated derivative (major metabolite). **Elimination:** $T_{1/2}$=6.3 hrs; urine (90%, unchanged).

LYSODREN   RX
mitotane (Bristol-Myers Squibb)

> **Temporarily discontinue immediately following shock or severe trauma and administer exogenous steroids.**

THERAPEUTIC CLASS: Adrenal cytotoxic agent

INDICATIONS: Treatment of inoperable adrenal cortical carcinoma of both functional and nonfunctional types.

DOSAGE: *Adults:* Initial: 2-6g/day given tid-qid. Titrate: Increase up to 9-10g/day. If severe side effects occur, reduce to max tolerated dose (MTD). MTD varies from 2-16g/day.

HOW SUPPLIED: Tabs: 500mg* *scored

WARNINGS/PRECAUTIONS: Caution with liver disease other than metastatic lesions from the adrenal cortex. Surgically remove all possible tumor tissues from large metastatic masses before administration. Perform behavioral and neurological assessments at regular intervals when continuous treatment >2 yrs. Monitor for signs of adrenal insufficiency and institute steroid replacement where appropriate. May impair mental/physical abilities. Prolonged use may lead to brain damage and impairment of function.

ADVERSE REACTIONS: GI disturbances, depression, lethargy, somnolence, dizziness, vertigo, skin toxicity.

INTERACTIONS: May increase dosage requirements with warfarin; monitor with coumarin-type anticoagulants. Caution with drugs susceptible to hepatic enzyme induction.

PREGNANCY: Category C, not for use in nursing.

MECHANISM OF ACTION: Adrenal cytotoxic agent; not established. Can cause adrenal inhibition without cellular destruction.

PHARMACOKINETICS: Elimination: $T_{1/2}$=18-159 days.

MACROBID   RX
nitrofurantoin monohydrate (Procter & Gamble)

THERAPEUTIC CLASS: Imidazolidinedione antibacterial

INDICATIONS: Treatment of acute uncomplicated urinary tract infections (acute cystitis).

DOSAGE: *Adults:* 100mg q12h for 7 days. Take with food.
Pediatrics: >12 yrs: 100mg q12h for 7 days. Take with food.

HOW SUPPLIED: Cap: 100mg

CONTRAINDICATIONS: Anuria, oliguria, CrCl <60mL/min, pregnancy at term (38-42 weeks gestation), labor and delivery, and neonates <1 month of age.

WARNINGS/PRECAUTIONS: Acute, subacute, or chronic pulmonary reactions have occurred. Anemia, diabetes mellitus, renal dysfunction, electrolyte imbalance, vitamin B deficiency, and debilitating disease enhance occurrence of peripheral neuropathy. Stop therapy with acute and chronic pulmonary reactions, hepatic disorders, hemolysis, or peripheral neuropathy. Monitor renal function, LFTs and pulmonary function periodically during long-term therapy. Optic neuritis and hepatic reactions reported. *Clostridium difficile*- associated diarrhea has been reported.

ADVERSE REACTIONS: Pulmonary disorders, hepatic damage, peripheral neuropathy, nausea, headache, flatulence, anorexia, diarrhea, dizziness, alopecia, exfoliative dermatitis, Stevens-Johnson syndrome, anaphylaxis, blood dyscrasias, aplastic anemia.

INTERACTIONS: Antacids, especially magnesium trisilicate, decrease rate and extent of absorption. Uricosuric drugs (eg, probenecid and sulfinpyrazone) increase nitrofurantoin levels.

PREGNANCY: Category B, not for use in nursing.

MECHANISM OF ACTION: Imidazolidinedione antibacterial; inhibits protein synthesis, aerobic energy metabolism, DNA, RNA, and cell wall synthesis.

PHARMACOKINETICS: Absorption: C_{max} ≤1mcg/mL. **Elimination:** Urine (20-25%, unchanged).

MACRODANTIN   RX
nitrofurantoin macrocrystals (Procter & Gamble)

THERAPEUTIC CLASS: Imidazolidinedione antibacterial

INDICATIONS: Treatment of urinary tract infection.

DOSAGE: *Adults:* 50-100mg qid for at least 7 days. Take with food. Long-term Suppressive Use: 50-100mg at bedtime.
Pediatrics: ≥1 month: 5-7mg/kg/day given qid for at least 7 days. Take with food. Long-term Suppressive Use: 1mg/kg/day given qd-bid.

HOW SUPPLIED: Cap: 25mg, 50mg, 100mg

CONTRAINDICATIONS: Anuria, oliguria, CrCl <60mL/min, pregnancy at term (38-42 weeks gestation), labor and delivery, neonates <1 month of age.

WARNINGS/PRECAUTIONS: Acute, subacute or chronic pulmonary reactions have occurred. Anemia, diabetes mellitus, renal dysfunction, electrolyte imbalance, vitamin B deficiency, and debilitating disease enhance occurrence of peripheral neuropathy. Stop therapy with acute and chronic pulmonary reactions, hepatic disorders, hemolysis, or peripheral neuropathy. Monitor renal function, LFTs and pulmonary function periodically during long-term therapy. Optic neuritis and hepatic reactions reported. False (+) reaction for glucose in urine may occur with Benedict's and Fehling's solution.

ADVERSE REACTIONS: Pulmonary disorders, hepatic damage, peripheral neuropathy, nausea, emesis, anorexia, dizziness, alopecia, exfoliative dermatitis, Stevens-Johnson syndrome, anaphylaxis, headache, drowsiness, asthenia, vertigo.

INTERACTIONS: Antacids, especially magnesium trisilicate, decrease rate and extent of absorption. Uricosuric drugs (eg, probenecid and sulfinpyrazone) increase nitrofurantoin levels.

PREGNANCY: Category B, not for use in nursing

MECHANISM OF ACTION: Imidazolidinedione antibacterial; inhibits protein synthesis, aerobic energy metabolism, DNA, RNA, and cell wall synthesis.

MACUGEN   RX
pegaptanib sodium (Eyetech/Pfizer)

THERAPEUTIC CLASS: Vascular endothelial growth factor (VEGF) inhibitor

INDICATIONS: Treatment of neovascular (wet) age-related macular degeneration.

DOSAGE: *Adults:* 0.3mg by intravitreous injection once every 6 weeks.

HOW SUPPLIED: Inj: 0.3mg

CONTRAINDICATIONS: Ocular or periocular infections.

WARNINGS/PRECAUTIONS: Rare post-marketing cases of anaphylaxis/anaphylactoid reactions, including angioedema, reported. Endophthalmitis associated with intravitreous injections. Use proper aseptic injection technique. Monitor for increased IOP. For ophthalmic intravitreal injection only.

ADVERSE REACTIONS: Anterior chamber inflammation, blurred vision, cataract, conjunctival hemorrhage, corneal edema, eye discharge, eye irritation, eye pain, HTN, increased IOP, ocular discomfort, punctate keratitis, reduced visual acuity, visual disturbance, vitreous floaters, and vitreous opacities.

PREGNANCY: Category B, caution in nursing.

MECHANISM OF ACTION: Selective vascular endothelial growth factor (VEGF) antagonist; inhibits VEGF, which is responsible for inducing angiogenesis, increasing vascular permeability and inflammation. VEGF has also been implicated in blood retinal barrier breakdown and pathological ocular neovascularization.

PHARMACOKINETICS: Absorption: Slowly into circulation from eye. **Distribution:** Vitreous fluid, retina, aqueous fluid. **Metabolism:** Via endo- and exonucleases. **Elimination**: Urine; $T_{1/2}$=10 days.

MAG-OX   OTC
magnesium oxide (Blaine)

THERAPEUTIC CLASS: Magnesium supplement

INDICATIONS: To increase magnesium intake. For relief of acid indigestion and upset stomach.

DOSAGE: *Adults:* Supplement: 1-2 tabs qd. Antacid: 1 tab bid. Max: 2 tabs/day or 2 weeks of therapy.

HOW SUPPLIED: Tab: 400mg

WARNINGS/PRECAUTIONS: Not for use in amounts over the Recommended Daily Intake (RDI). May have a laxative effect.

INTERACTIONS: May interact with certain prescription drugs.

PREGNANCY: Safety in pregnancy and nursing not known.

MALARONE   RX
proguanil HCL - atovaquone (GlaxoSmithKline)

OTHER BRAND NAMES: Malarone Pediatric (GlaxoSmithKline)

THERAPEUTIC CLASS: Pyrimidine synthesis inhibitor

INDICATIONS: Prophylaxis or treatment of malaria caused by *P.falciparum*.

DOSAGE: *Adults:* Prevention: Begin 1-2 days before entering endemic area, continue during stay and for 7 days after return. 1 tab qd. Treatment: 4 tabs qd for 3 days. Repeat dose if vomiting occurs within 1 hr after dosing. Take as single dose with food or milky drink.
Pediatrics: Prevention: Begin 1-2 days before entering endemic area, continue during stay and for 7 days after return. 11-20kg: 1 pediatric tab qd. 21-30kg: 2 pediatric tabs qd. 31-40kg: 3 pediatric tabs qd. >40kg: Dose as adult. Treatment: Treat for 2 consecutive days. 5-8kg: 2 pediatric tabs qd. 9-10kg: 3 pediatric tabs. 11-20kg: 1 tab qd. 21-30kg: 2 tabs qd. 31-40kg: 3 tabs. >40kg: Dose as adult. Repeat dose if vomiting occurs within 1 hr after dosing. Take as single dose with food or milky drink.

HOW SUPPLIED: (Atovaquone-Proguanil) Tab: 250mg-100mg; Tab, Pediatric: 62.5mg-25mg

CONTRAINDICATIONS: For prophylaxis in severe renal impairment (CrCl <30mL/min).

WARNINGS/PRECAUTIONS: Not for cerebral malaria. Patients with severe malaria are not candidates for PO therapy. Rare cases of anaphylaxis reported.

ADVERSE REACTIONS: Vomiting, pruritus, elevation of LFTs.

INTERACTIONS: Rifampin, rifabutin may decrease levels; concomitant use is not recommended. Reduced bioavailability with metoclopramide and tetracycline.

PREGNANCY: Category C, caution in nursing.

MECHANISM OF ACTION: Pyramidine synthesis inhibitor. Atovaquone: Antiparasitic agent that acts as a selective inhibitor of parasite mitochondrial electron transport. Proguanil: Antiparasitic agent that acts on the metabolite cycloguanil, which inhibits dihydrofolate reductase in the malaria parasite, resulting in disruption of deoxythymidylate synthesis.

PHARMACOKINETICS: Absorption: Atovaquone: Absolute bioavailability (23%). Proguanil: Extensively absorbed. **Distribution:** Atovaquone: V_d=8.8L/kg; plasma protein binding (≥99%). Proguanil: V_d=1617-2502L (adult and pediatric patients ≥15 yrs with body weight 31-110kg), V_d=462-966L (pediatric patients ≤15 yrs with body weight 11-56kg). Plasma protein binding (75%). **Metabolism:** Proguanil: CYP2C19. **Elimination:** Atovaquone: Feces (unchanged), urine (≤0.6%). $T_{1/2}$=2-3 days (adult). Proguanil: Via hepatic biotransformation and renal excretion; urine (40-60%); $T_{1/2}$=12-21 hrs (adult and pediatric patients).

MARCAINE

RX

bupivacaine HCL (Hospira)

THERAPEUTIC CLASS: Local anesthetic

INDICATIONS: Production of local or regional anesthesia for surgery, dental or oral surgery procedures, diagnostic and therapeutic procedures, and for obstetrical procedures. Only 0.25% and 0.5% are indicated for obstetrical anesthesia.

DOSAGE: *Adults:* Individualize dose. Dosage varies depending on procedure, area to be anesthetized, vascularity of tissues, number of neural segments to be blocked, depth and duration of anesthesia, degree of muscle relaxation required, and patient tolerance and physical condition. Single Dose Max: 175mg. May repeat once every 3 hrs. Total Daily Dose Max: 400mg. Epidural Anesthesia: 0.5% or 0.75% in 3-5mL increments. In obstetrics, use only 0.25% or 0.5%. Use 3-5mL increments of 0.5% solution not to exceed 50-100mg at any dosing interval. Test dose using 0.5% with 1:200,000 epinephrine recommended prior to caudal and lumbar epidural blocks. Elderly/Debilitated/Cardiac or Liver Disease: Reduce dose.

Pediatrics: ≥12 yrs: Individualize dose. Dosage varies depending on procedure, area to be anesthetized, vascularity of tissues, number of neural segments to be blocked, depth and duration of anesthesia, degree of muscle relaxation required, and patient tolerance and physical condition. Single Dose Max: 175mg. May repeat once every 3 hrs. Total Daily Dose Max: 400mg. Epidural Anesthesia: 0.5% or 0.75% in 3-5mL increments. In obstetrics, use only 0.25% or 0.5%. Use 3-5mL increments of 0.5% solution not to exceed 50-100mg at any dosing interval. Test dose using 0.5% with 1:200,000 epinephrine recommended prior to caudal and lumbar epidural blocks.

HOW SUPPLIED: Inj: 0.25%, 0.5%, 0.75%

CONTRAINDICATIONS: Obstetrical paracervical block anesthesia.

WARNINGS/PRECAUTIONS: The 0.75% strength is not recommended for obstetrical anesthesia. Acidosis, cardiac arrest, death reported from delay in toxicity management. Local anesthetic solutions containing antimicrobial preservatives should not be used for epidural or caudal anesthesia. Not recommended for IV regional anesthesia. Monitor cardiovascular and respiratory vital signs and state of consciousness after each injection. Caution with hepatic disease and impaired cardiovascular function. Monitor circulation and respiration with injections into head and neck area. Respiratory arrest following local anesthetic injection during retrobulbar blocks has been reported.

ADVERSE REACTIONS: Restlessness, anxiety, dizziness, tinnitus, blurred vision, tremors, convulsions, nausea, vomiting, chills, hypotension, bradycardia, ventricular arrhythmias, urticaria, pruritus, erythema, edema.

INTERACTIONS: Avoid use with any other local anesthetics.

PREGNANCY: Category C, not for use in nursing.

MECHANISM OF ACTION: Aminoacyl local anesthetic; blocks the generation and conduction of nerve impulses, presumably by increasing the threshold for electrical excitation in the nerve by slowing the propagation of nerve impulse and by reducing rate of rise of the action potential.

PHARMACOKINETICS: Distribution: Crosses placenta, found in breast milk. Plasma protein binding (95%). **Excretion:** Urine 6% (unchanged).

MARCAINE WITH EPINEPHRINE RX
bupivacaine HCL - epinephrine (Hospira)

THERAPEUTIC CLASS: Local anesthetic

INDICATIONS: Production of local or regional anesthesia for surgery, dental, or oral surgery procedures, diagnostic and therapeutic procedures, and for obstetrical procedures. Only 0.25% and 0.5% are indicated for obstetrical anesthesia.

DOSAGE: *Adults:* Individualize dose. Dosage varies depending on procedure, area to be anesthetized, vascularity of tissues, number of neural segments to be blocked, depth and duration of anesthesia, degree of muscle relaxation required, and patient tolerance and physical condition. Single Dose Max: 225mg. May repeat once every 3 hrs. Total Daily Dose Max: 400mg. Epidural Anesthesia: 0.5% or 0.75% in 3-5mL increments. In obstetrics, use only 0.25% or 0.5%. Use 3-5mL increments of 0.5% solution not to exceed 50-100mg at any dosing interval. Test dose using 0.5% with 1:200,000 epinephrine recommended prior to caudal and lumbar epidural blocks. Dentistry: 0.5% with epinephrine. Average Dose: 1.8mL (9mg) per inj site. May repeat after 2-10 min if necessary. Max: 90mg total dose for all sites. Elderly/Debilitated/Cardiac or Liver Disease: Reduce dose.
Pediatrics: ≥12 yrs: Individualize dose. Dosage varies depending on procedure, area to be anesthetized, vascularity of tissues, number of neural segments to be blocked, depth and duration of anesthesia, degree of muscle relaxation required, and patient tolerance and physical condition. Single Dose Max: 225mg. May repeat once every 3 hrs. Total Daily Dose Max: 400mg. Epidural Anesthesia: 0.5% or 0.75% in 3-5mL increments. In obstetrics, use only 0.25% or 0.5%. Use 3-5mL increments of 0.5% solution not to exceed 50-100mg at any dosing interval. Test dose using 0.5% with 1:200,000 epinephrine recommended prior to caudal and lumbar epidural blocks. Dentistry: 0.5% with epinephrine. Average Dose: 1.8mL (9mg) per inj site. May repeat after 2-10 min if necessary. Max: 90mg total dose for all sites.

HOW SUPPLIED: Inj: (Bupivacaine-Epinephrine) 0.25%/1:200,000, 0.5%/1:200,000

CONTRAINDICATIONS: Obstetrical paracervical block anesthesia.

WARNINGS/PRECAUTIONS: The 0.75% strength is not recommended for obstetrical anesthesia. Acidosis, cardiac arrest, death reported from delay in toxicity management. Local anesthetic solutions containing antimicrobial preservatives should not be used for epidural or caudal anesthesia. Not recommended for IV regional anesthesia. Bupivacaine with epinephrine solutions contain sodium metabisulfite which may cause allergic-type reactions in susceptible people. Monitor cardiovascular and respiratory vital signs and state of consciousness after each injection. Caution when local anesthetic solutions containing a vasoconstrictor are used in areas of the body supplied by end arteries or having otherwise compromised blood supply; ischemic injury or necrosis may result with hypertensive vascular disease. Caution with hepatic disease and impaired cardiovascular function. Monitor circulation and respiration with injections into head and neck area. Respiratory arrest following local anesthetic injection during retrobulbar blocks has been reported.

ADVERSE REACTIONS: Restlessness, anxiety, dizziness, tinnitus, blurred vision, tremors, convulsions, nausea, vomiting, chills, hypotension, bradycardia, ventricular arrhythmias, urticaria, pruritus, erythema, edema.

INTERACTIONS: Avoid use with any other local anesthetics. Anesthetic solutions containing epinephrine or norepinephrine with MAOIs or TCAs may produce severe, prolonged HTN; avoid concurrent use or monitor closely if concurrent use is necessary. Concurrent administration of vasopressors and ergot-type oxytocic drugs may cause severe, persistent HTN or CVA. Phenothiazines and butyrophenones may reduce or reverse the pressor effect of epinephrine. Serious dose-related cardiac arrhythmias may occur with use during or following administration of potent inhalation anesthetics.

PREGNANCY: Category C, not for use in nursing.

MECHANISM OF ACTION: Aminoacyl local anesthetic; blocks generation and conduction of nerve impulses, presumably by increasing threshold for electrical excitation in the nerve by slowing propagation of nerve impulse and by reducing rate of rise of action potential.

PHARMACOKINETICS: Distribution: Crosses placenta; found in breast milk. Plasma protein binding (95%). **Excretion:** Urine 6% (unchanged).

MARINOL
dronabinol (Unimed)

THERAPEUTIC CLASS: Cannabinoid

INDICATIONS: Treatment of anorexia associated with weight loss in AIDS patients and nausea and vomiting associated with chemotherapy when conventional treatment has failed.

DOSAGE: *Adults:* Appetite Stimulation: Initial: 2.5mg bid before lunch and supper or 2.5mg qpm or qhs if 5mg/day is intolerable. Max: 20mg/day in divided doses. Antiemetic: Initial: 5mg/m² given 1-3 hrs before chemotherapy, then q2-4h after chemotherapy, up to 4-6 doses/day. Titrate: May increase by 2.5mg/m² increments. Max: 15mg/m²/dose.

HOW SUPPLIED: Cap: 2.5mg, 5mg, 10mg

CONTRAINDICATIONS: Hypersensitivity to sesame oil and cannabinoids.

WARNINGS/PRECAUTIONS: Do not engage in any hazardous activity until ability to tolerate drug is established. Caution with cardiac disorders due to possible HTN/hypotension, syncope, tachycardia. Caution with history of substance abuse. Monitor with mania, depression, schizophrenia; may exacerbate illness. Caution in elderly due to increased sensitivity to the psychoactive, neurological, and postural hypotensive effects. Initial dose and adjustments should be supervised by responsible adult. Caution with history of seizure disorders, may lower seizure threshold.

ADVERSE REACTIONS: Euphoria, dizziness, paranoid reaction, somnolence, abnormal thinking, abdominal pain, nausea, vomiting, diarrhea, conjunctivitis, hypotension, flushing.

INTERACTIONS: Highly protein-bound drugs may require dosage changes. Additive effects with alcohol, sedatives, hypnotics, or other psychoactive drugs. Additive HTN, tachycardia, and possible cardiotoxicity with amphetamines, cocaine, and sympathomimetics. Increased tachycardia, and drowsiness with anticholinergic agents. Potentiates effects of TCAs and CNS depressants. Decreases clearance of antipyrine and barbiturates.

PREGNANCY: Category C, not for use in nursing.

MECHANISM OF ACTION: Cannabinoid; has complex effects on the CNS, including central sympathomimetic activity.

PHARMACOKINETICS: Absorption: Complete (90-95%); (2.5mg bid) C_{max}=1.32ng/mL, T_{max}=1 hr, AUC=2.88ng•hr/mL; (5mg bid) C_{max}=2.96ng/mL, T_{max}=2.5 hr, AUC=6.16ng•hr/mL; (10mg bid) C_{max}=7.88ng/mL, T_{max}=1.5 hr, AUC=15.2ng•hr/mL. **Distribution:** V_d=10L/kg; plasma protein binding (97%). Found in breast milk. **Metabolism:** Liver via microsomal hydroxylation; 11-OH-delta-9-THC (active metabolite). **Elimination:** Urine (10-15%), and feces (<5%, unchanged); $T_{1/2}$=25-36 hrs.

MATULANE
procarbazine HCL (Sigma-Tau)

RX

To be given only by or under supervision of experienced physician in use of potent antineoplastics. Proper monitoring with adequate clinical and laboratory facilities should be conducted.

THERAPEUTIC CLASS: Hydrazine derivative

INDICATIONS: In combination with other antineoplastics for the treatment of Stage III/IV Hodgkin's disease. Used part of MOPP regimen.

DOSAGE: *Adults:* 2-4mg/kg/day as single or divided doses for first week then increase to 4-6mg/kg/day until maximum response or WBC <4000/mm³ or platelets <100,000/mm³. Maint: 1-2mg/kg/day. In MOPP: 100mg/m² qd for 14 days. Adjust dose for combination regimens.
Pediatrics: 50mg/m²/day for first week then increase to 100mg/m²/day until response is obtained or leukopenia or thrombocytopenia occurs. Maint: 50mg/m²/day. Adjust dose for combination regimens.

HOW SUPPLIED: Cap: 50mg

CONTRAINDICATIONS: Inadequate marrow reserve.

WARNINGS/PRECAUTIONS: Toxicity may occur in renal or hepatic impairment. Wait one month or longer with prior use of bone marrow suppressing radiation or chemotherapy. D/C if CNS symptoms (paresthesias, neuropathies, confusion), leukopenia, thrombocytopenia, hypersensitivity, stomatitis, diarrhea, hemorrhage or bleeding tendencies occur. Bone marrow depression often occurs 2-8 weeks after initiation. Monitor urinalysis, transaminases, LFTs weekly, hematologic status every 3-4 days.

ADVERSE REACTIONS: Leukopenia, anemia, thrombopenia, nausea, vomiting.

INTERACTIONS: Avoid sympathomimetics, TCAs, tyramine-containing drugs/foods, alcohol (may cause disulfiram-type reaction), tobacco. Caution with barbiturates, antihistamines, narcotics, hypotensives, phenothiazines.

PREGNANCY: Category D, not for use in nursing.

MECHANISM OF ACTION: Hydrazine derivative; inhibits protein, RNA, and DNA synthesis.

PHARMACOKINETICS: Absorption: Rapid and complete; T_{max}=60 min.
Metabolism: Liver and kidney. **Elimination:** Urine (70%); $T_{1/2}$=10 min (IV).

Mavik RX
trandolapril (Abbott)

> ACE inhibitors can cause death/injury to developing fetus during 2nd and 3rd trimesters. Stop therapy if pregnancy detected.

THERAPEUTIC CLASS: ACE inhibitor

INDICATIONS: Treatment of hypertension. To decrease risk of hospitalization and mortality in stable patients with signs of left-ventricular systolic dysfunction or CHF post-MI.

DOSAGE: *Adults:* HTN: If possible, d/c diuretic 2-3 days before therapy. Initial: 1mg qd in nonblack patients; 2mg qd in black patients; 0.5mg with concomitant diuretic. Titrate: Adjust at 1-week intervals. Usual: 2-4mg qd. Resume diuretic if not controlled. Max: 8mg/day. Post-MI: Initial: 1mg qd. Titrate: Increase to target dose of 4mg qd as tolerated. CrCl <30mL/min/Hepatic Cirrhosis for HTN or Post-MI: Initial: 0.5mg qd.

HOW SUPPLIED: Tab: 1mg*, 2mg, 4mg *scored

CONTRAINDICATIONS: History of ACE inhibitor-associated angioedema.

WARNINGS/PRECAUTIONS: D/C if angioedema or jaundice occurs. Risk of hyperkalemia with DM, renal dysfunction. Persistent nonproductive cough reported. Monitor WBCs in renal impairment and/or collagen vascular disease. Anaphylactoid reactions reported. Fetal/neonatal morbidity and death reported. Monitor for hypotension in high-risk patients (heart failure, surgery/anesthesia, prolonged diuretic therapy, volume and/or salt depletion, etc). Caution with CHF, renal dysfunction, and renal artery stenosis. More reports of angioedema in blacks than nonblacks.

ADVERSE REACTIONS: Cough, dizziness, hypotension, elevated serum uric acid, elevated BUN, elevated creatinine, asthenia, syncope, myalgia, gastritis, hypocalcemia, hyperkalemia, dyspepsia.

INTERACTIONS: May increase lithium levels. Hypotension risk with diuretics. Increase risk of hyperkalemia with K⁺-sparing diuretics, K⁺-containing salt substitutes or K⁺ supplements.

PREGNANCY: Category C (1st trimester) and D (2nd and 3rd trimesters), not for use in nursing.

MECHANISM OF ACTION: ACE inhibitor; inhibits ACE activity, reducing angiotensin II formation, decreasing vasoconstriction, decreasing aldosterone secretion, and increasing plasma renin.

PHARMACOKINETICS: Absorption: Parent, metabolite: Absolute bioavailability (10%, 70%); T_{max}=1 hr, 4-10 hrs. **Distribution:** V_d=18L; Plasma protein binding (80%). **Metabolism:** Cleavage of ester group; trandolaprilat (metabolite). **Elimination:** Urine, feces; $T_{1/2}$=6 hrs, 10 hrs (metabolite).

MAXAIR   RX
pirbuterol acetate (Graceway)

OTHER BRAND NAMES: Maxair Autohaler (Graceway)

THERAPEUTIC CLASS: Beta$_2$-agonist

INDICATIONS: Prevention and reversal of bronchospasm in reversible bronchospasm (eg, asthma).

DOSAGE: *Adults:* 1-2 inh q4-6h. Max: 12 inh/day.
Pediatrics: ≥12 yrs: 1-2 inh q4-6h. Max: 12 inh/day.

HOW SUPPLIED: Autohaler: 0.2mg/inh [14g, 25.6g]; MDI: 0.2mg/inh [14g]

WARNINGS/PRECAUTIONS: Caution with cardiovascular disorders, (eg, ischemic heart disease, HTN, arrhythmias), hyperthyroidism, diabetes, convulsive disorders. Fatalities reported with excessive use. Can produce paradoxical bronchospasm. Monitor BP.

ADVERSE REACTIONS: Nervousness, tremor, headache, dizziness, palpitations, tachycardia, cough, nausea.

INTERACTIONS: Avoid other aerosol β$_2$ agonists. Vascular effects may be potentiated by MAOIs, TCAs, and sympathomimetics. ECG changes and/or hypokalemia may occur with non-potassium sparing diuretics. Decreased effect with β-blockers.

PREGNANCY: Category C, caution in nursing.

MECHANISM OF ACTION: β$_2$-adrenergic bronchodilator; activates adenyl cyclase on airway smooth muscles and increases intracellular concentration of cyclic AMP. Increased cAMP levels are associated with relaxation of bronchial smooth muscle and inhibition of release of mediators of immediate hypersensitivity.

PHARMACOKINETICS: Elimination: Urine, $T_{1/2}$=2 hrs.

MAXALT   RX
rizatriptan benzoate (Merck)

OTHER BRAND NAMES: Maxalt-MLT (Merck)

THERAPEUTIC CLASS: 5-HT$_{1D,1B}$-agonist

INDICATIONS: Acute treatment of migraine attacks with or without aura.

DOSAGE: *Adults:* ≥18 yrs: 5-10mg, may repeat q2h. Max: 30mg/24 hrs. Safety of treating >4 headaches/30 days not known. MLT: Dissolve on tongue without water. Concomitant Propranolol: 5mg, up to 3 doses/24 hrs.

HOW SUPPLIED: Tab: 5mg, 10mg; Tab, Disintegrating: (MLT) 5mg, 10mg

CONTRAINDICATIONS: Ischemic heart disease, coronary artery vasospasm (eg, Prinzmetal's angina), uncontrolled HTN, significant cardiovascular disease, hemiplegic or basilar migraine, MAOI use within 14 days, other 5-HT$_1$ agonist or ergot-type agent use within 24 hrs.

WARNINGS/PRECAUTIONS: Confirm diagnosis. Supervise 1st dose and monitor cardiac function in those at risk of CAD (eg, HTN, hypercholesterolemia, smoker, obesity, diabetes, CAD family history, postmenopausal women, males >40 yrs). Serious adverse cardiac events, cerebrovascular events, vasospastic reactions, hypertensive crisis, and fatalities reported with 5-HT$_1$ agonists.

M

Disintegrating tabs contain phenylalanine. Caution with renal dialysis and hepatic dysfunction.

ADVERSE REACTIONS: Paresthesia, dry mouth, nausea, dizziness, somnolence, asthenia/fatigue.

INTERACTIONS: Increased plasma levels with propranolol. Prolonged vasospastic reactions with ergot-type agents and other 5-HT$_1$ agonists. SSRIs may cause weakness, hyperreflexia, and incoordination (rare). Avoid MAOIs during or within 14 days.

PREGNANCY: Category C, caution in nursing.

MECHANISM OF ACTION: 5-HT$_{1B/1D}$ receptor agonist; binds with high affinity to 5-HT$_{1B/1D}$ receptors on the extracerebral, intracranial blood vessels that become dilated during migraine attack; activation of these receptors results in cranial vessel constriction, inhibition of neuropeptide release, and reduced transmission in trigeminal pain pathways.

PHARMACOKINETICS: Absorption: Complete; absolute bioavailability (45%); T_{max}=1-1.5 hrs. **Distribution:** V_d=140L (male), 110L (female); plasma protein binding (14%). **Metabolism:** Oxidative deamination via MAO-A. N-monodesmethyl-rizatriptan (active metabolite). **Elimination:** Urine (82%), (14% unchanged, 51% indole acetic acid metabolite), feces (12%); $T_{1/2}$=2-3 hrs.

MAXAQUIN RX
lomefloxacin HCL (G.D. Searle)

THERAPEUTIC CLASS: Fluoroquinolone

INDICATIONS: Treatment of acute bacterial exacerbation of chronic bronchitis (ABECB) and uncomplicated/complicated urinary tract infections (UTI). Preoperatively for the prevention of infections from transrectal prostate biopsy (TRPB) and in transurethral surgical procedures (TUSP).

DOSAGE: *Adults:* ≥18 yrs: ABECB: 400mg qd for 10 days. Uncomplicated Cystitis: 400mg qd for 3 days (*E.coli*) or 10 days (*K.pneumoniae, P.mirabilis,* or *S.saprophyticus*). Complicated UTI: 400mg qd for 14 days. Hemodialysis/CrCl >10 to <40mL/min: LD: 400mg. Maint: 200mg qd. Preoperative Prevention: TRPB: 400mg single dose 1-6 hrs before procedure. TUSP: 400mg single dose 2-6 hrs before procedure.

HOW SUPPLIED: Tab: 400mg* *scored

WARNINGS/PRECAUTIONS: Rare cases of torsades de pointes have been reported; avoid with known prolongation of the QT interval, uncorrected hypokalemia, concomitant treatment with Class IA (quinidine, procainamide) or class III (amiodarone, sotalol) antiarrhythmic agents. Moderate to severe phototoxicity, convulsions, pseudomembranous colitis, serious fatal hypersensitivity reactions reported. Avoid in pregnancy and nursing. Not for empiric treatment of *Pseudomonas* bacteremia or ABECB caused by *S.pneumoniae*. Caution with CNS disorder or those predisposed to seizures. Adjust dose in renal impairment. D/C if pain, inflammation, or tendon rupture occurs. Increased risk of tendon rupture in patients receiving concomitant corticosteriods. Maintain adequate hydration. Rare cases of sensory or sensorimotor axonal polyneuropathy reported; d/c if symptoms of neuropathy occur.

ADVERSE REACTIONS: Headache, nausea, photosensitivity, dizziness, diarrhea, abdominal pain.

INTERACTIONS: Decreased bioavailability with sucralfate, divalent or trivalent cations (didanosine), and magnesium- or aluminum-containing antacids; take 4 hrs before or 2 hrs after lomefloxacin. Cimetidine may increase effects. Probenecid slows the renal elimination. May enhance cyclosporine, warfarin effects.

PREGNANCY: Category C, not for use in nursing.

MECHANISM OF ACTION: Fluoroquinolone: Synthetic broad-spectrum antimicrobial agent; inhibits topoisomerase II (DNA gyrase) and topoisomerase IV, which are required for bacterial DNA replication, transcription, repair, and recombination.

PHARMACOKINETICS: Absorption: Rapid, bioavailability (95%-98%), C_{max}(400mg)=2.8mcg/mL, AUC=25.9mcg•h/mL, T_{max}=1.5 hrs. **Elimination:** $T_{1/2}$(400mg)=7.75 hrs, urine (65% unchanged).

MAXIPIME   RX
cefepime HCL (Elan)

THERAPEUTIC CLASS: Cephalosporin (4th generation)

INDICATIONS: Treatment of uncomplicated/complicated urinary tract (UTI), uncomplicated skin and skin structure (SSSI), and complicated intra-abdominal infections, and pneumonia caused by susceptible strains of microorganisms. Emperic therapy for febrile neutropenia.

DOSAGE: *Adults:* Moderate-Severe Pneumonia: 1-2g IV q12h for 10 days. Febrile Neutropenia Emperic Therapy: 2g IV q8h for 7 days or until neutropenia resolved. Mild-Moderate UTI: 0.5-1g IM/IV q12h for 7-10 days. Severe UTI/Moderate-Severe SSSI: 2g IV q12h for 10 days. Complicated Intra-Abdominal Infections: 2g IV q12h for 7-10 days. Renal Impairment: Initial: Normal dose. Maint: CrCl >60mL/min: Normal dose. CrCl 30-60mL/min: 500mg-2g q24h or 2g q12h. CrCl 11-29mL/min: 500mg-2g q24h. CrCl <11mL/min: 250mg-1g q24h. CAPD: 500mg-2g q48h. Hemodialysis: 1g on Day 1, then 500mg q24h. *Pediatrics:* 2 months-16 yrs: ≤40kg: UTI/SSSI/Pneumonia: 50mg/kg IV q12h. Febrile Neutropenia: 50mg/kg IV q8h. Max: Do not exceed adult dose.

HOW SUPPLIED: Inj: 500mg, 1g, 2g

WARNINGS/PRECAUTIONS: Caution with PCN sensitivity; cross hypersensitivity may occur. *Clostridium difficile*-associated diarrhea reported. Treatment may result in overgrowth of nonsusceptible organisms. Caution with renal impairment or history of GI disease especially colitis. Encephalopathy, myoclonus, seizures, and/or renal failure reported. D/C if seizure occurs. Associated with a fall in PT; monitor PT with renal or hepatic impairment, poor nutritional state, and protracted course of antimicrobials; give vitamin K as indicated. Associated with (+) direct Coombs' test.

ADVERSE REACTIONS: Local reactions (eg, phlebitis) rash, diarrhea.

INTERACTIONS: Increased risk of nephrotoxicity and ototoxicity with aminoglycosides. Risk of nephrotoxicity with potent diuretics (eg, furosemide).

PREGNANCY: Category B, caution in nursing.

MECHANISM OF ACTION: Cephalosporin; bactericidal due to inhibition of cell wall synthesis.

PHARMACOKINETICS: Absorption: IV administration of variable doses resulted in different parameters. **Distribution:** V_d=18L; plasma protein binding (20%). **Metabolism:** Metabolized to N-methylpyrrolidine, which is rapidly converted to N-oxide. **Elimination:** Urine; $T_{1/2}$=2hrs.

MAXZIDE   RX
triamterene - hydrochlorothiazide (Mylan Bertek)

OTHER BRAND NAMES: Maxzide-25 (Mylan Bertek)

THERAPEUTIC CLASS: K^+-sparing diuretic/thiazide diuretic

INDICATIONS: For hypertension or edema if hypokalemia occurs on HCTZ alone, or when a thiazide diuretic is required and cannot risk hypokalemia.

DOSAGE: *Adults:* (37.5mg-25mg tab) 1-2 tabs qd. (75mg-50mg tab) 1 tab qd.

HOW SUPPLIED: (Triamterene-HCTZ) Tab: (Maxzide) 75mg-50mg*, (Maxzide-25) 37.5mg-25mg* *scored

CONTRAINDICATIONS: Hyperkalemia, anuria, acute or chronic renal insufficiency, sulfonamide hypersensitivity, diabetic neuropathy, K^+-sparing agents (eg, diuretics), K^+ supplements, K^+ salt substitutes, K^+-rich diet.

WARNINGS/PRECAUTIONS: Risk of hyperkalemia (≥5.5mEq/L) especially with renal impairment, elderly, DM or severely ill; monitor levels frequently.

Check ECG if hyperkalemia occurs. Caution with history of renal lithiasis, hepatic dysfunction. Monitor BUN and creatinine periodically. D/C if azotemia increases. May contribute to megaloblastosis in folic acid deficiency. Hyperuricemia, hypercalcemia, hypophosphatemia, hypokalemia may occur. May manifest latent DM. May decrease serum PBI levels. Monitor for fluid/electrolyte imbalance.

ADVERSE REACTIONS: Jaundice, pancreatitis, nausea, vomiting, taste alteration, drowsiness, dry mouth, depression, anxiety, tachycardia, blood dyscrasias, electrolyte disturbances.

INTERACTIONS: May potentiate other antihypertensives. Risk of lithium toxicity. Indomethacin may cause renal failure; caution with NSAIDs. Increased risk of hyperkalemia with ACE inhibitors. May increase responsiveness to tubocurarine. May decrease arterial responsiveness to norepinephrine. May alter insulin requirements. Alcohol, barbiturates, or narcotics may potentiate orthostatic hypotension.

PREGNANCY: Category C, not for use in nursing.

MECHANISM OF ACTION: HCTZ: Thiazide diuretic; block renal tubular absorption of Na^+ and Cl^+ ions. This natriuresis and diuresis is accompanied by a secondary loss of K^+ and bicarbonate. Triamterene: Potassium-sparing diuretic; acts on the distal renal tubule to inhibit the reabsorption of Na^+ in exchange for K^+ and H^+, thus increases Na^+ excretion and reduces excessive loss of K^+ and H^+ associated with HCTZ.

PHARMACOKINETICS: Absorption: HCTZ: T_{max}=2 hrs. Triamterene: Rapid, T_{max}=1 hr. **Metabolism:** Triamterene: Liver; sulfate conjugation; hydroxytriamterene (metabolite). **Elimination**: HCTZ: Urine (unchanged).

MEBARAL   `CIV`
mephobarbital (Ovation)

THERAPEUTIC CLASS: Barbiturate

INDICATIONS: As a sedative for relief of anxiety, tension, and apprehension. Treatment of grand mal and petit mal epilepsy.

DOSAGE: *Adults:* Epilepsy: 400-600mg/day. Start with small dose, gradually increase over 4-5 days until optimum dose. Elderly/Debilitated/Renal or Hepatic Dysfunction: Reduce dose. Concomitant Phenobarbital: Give 50% of each drug. Concomitant Phenytoin: Reduce phenytoin dose. Sedation: 32-100mg tid-qid. Optimum Dose: 50mg tid-qid.
Pediatrics: Epilepsy: >5 yrs: 32-64mg tid-qid. <5 yrs: 16-32mg tid-qid. Start with small dose, gradually increase over 4-5 days until optimum dose. Sedation: 16-32mg tid-qid.

HOW SUPPLIED: Tab: 32mg*, 50mg*, 100mg *scored

CONTRAINDICATIONS: Manifest or latent porphyria.

WARNINGS/PRECAUTIONS: May be habit forming; tolerance and dependence may occur with continued use. Avoid abrupt withdrawal. Caution in acute/chronic pain; paradoxical excitement may occur or symptoms masked. Can cause fetal damage. May cause marked excitement, depression, and confusion in elderly or debilitated. Reduce initial dose with hepatic damage. Careful adjustment in impaired renal, cardiac, or respiratory function, myasthenia gravis, and myxedema. May increase vitamin D requirements. Caution with depression, suicidal tendencies, and history of drug abuse.

ADVERSE REACTIONS: Somnolence, agitation, confusion, hyperkinesia, ataxia, CNS depression, hypoventilation, apnea, bradycardia, hypotension, syncope, nausea, vomiting, headache.

INTERACTIONS: MAOIs may prolong effects. Additive CNS depression with alcohol and other CNS depressants. Decreases effects of oral anticoagulants, oral contraceptives. Increases corticosteroid metabolism. Interferes with griseofulvin absorption. Decreases half-life of doxycycline. May alter phenytoin metabolism. Sodium valproate and valproic acid decrease metabolism.

PREGNANCY: Category D, caution with nursing.

MECHANISM OF ACTION: Barbiturate; depresses the sensory cortex, decreases motor activity, alters cerebellar function, and produces drowsiness, sedation, and hypnosis. Produces significant anticonvulsant activity.

PHARMACOKINETICS: Absorption: Rapid. **Distribution**: Crosses placenta, excreted in breast milk. **Metabolism**: Hepatic via N-demethylation. Phenobarbital (major metabolite). **Elimination**: Urine.

MEBENDAZOLE   RX
mebendazole (Various)

THERAPEUTIC CLASS: Broad-spectrum anthelmintic

INDICATIONS: Treatment of Enterobiasis (pinworm), Trichuriasis (whipworm), Ascariasis (common roundworm), *Ancylostoma duodenale* (common hookworm), *Necator americanus* (American hookworm).

DOSAGE: *Adults:* Pinworm: 100mg single dose. Other Parasites: 100mg bid for 3 days. May repeat in 3 weeks if needed. Chew, swallow, crush or mix tab with food.
Pediatrics: ≥2 yrs: Pinworm: 100mg single dose. Other Parasites: 100mg bid for 3 days. May repeat in 3 weeks if needed. Chew, swallow, crush or mix tab with food.

HOW SUPPLIED: Tab, Chewable: 100mg

WARNINGS/PRECAUTIONS: Neutropenia, agranulocytosis reported with prolonged use. Periodically assess organ system functions with prolonged use. Not effective for hydatid disease.

ADVERSE REACTIONS: Abdominal pain, diarrhea.

INTERACTIONS: Cimetidine may increase plasma levels.

PREGNANCY: Category C, caution in nursing.

MECHANISM OF ACTION: Broad-spectrum anthelmintic; inhibits formation of worms' microtubules and causes worms' glucose depletion.

PHARMACOKINETICS: Metabolism: 2-amine (primary metabolite). **Elimination**: Urine (approximately 2%), feces (unchanged drug or primary metabolite).

MECLOFENAMATE   RX
meclofenamate sodium (Various)

THERAPEUTIC CLASS: NSAID

INDICATIONS: Relief of mild to moderate pain, primary dysmenorrhea, and idiopathic heavy menstrual blood loss. Symptomatic treatment of acute and chronic rheumatoid arthritis (RA) and osteoarthritis (OA).

DOSAGE: *Adults:* Mild to Moderate Pain: 50mg q4-6h. Max: 400mg/day. Excessive Menstrual Blood Loss/Primary Dysmenorrhea: 100mg tid for up to 6 days starting at onset of menstrual flow. RA/OA: 200-400mg/day in 3-4 divided doses. Max: 400mg/day.
Pediatrics: ≥14 yrs: Mild to Moderate Pain: 50mg q4-6h. Max: 400mg/day. Excessive Menstrual Blood Loss/Primary Dysmenorrhea: 100mg tid for up to 6 days starting at onset of menstrual flow. RA/OA: 200-400mg/day in 3-4 divided doses. Max: 400mg/day.

HOW SUPPLIED: Cap: 50mg, 100mg

CONTRAINDICATIONS: ASA or other NSAID allergy that precipitates bronchospasm, allergic rhinitis or urticaria.

WARNINGS/PRECAUTIONS: Risk of GI ulcerations, bleeding, and perforation. Borderline LFT elevations may occur. Renal and hepatic toxicity. Extreme caution in the elderly. D/C if visual symptoms occur.

ADVERSE REACTIONS: Diarrhea, nausea, vomiting, abdominal pain, edema, urticaria, pruritus, headache, dizziness, tinnitus, pyrosis, flatulence, anorexia, constipation, peptic ulcer.

PDR Concise Drug Guide

INTERACTIONS: Enhanced effects of warfarin. ASA may lower levels.

PREGNANCY: Safety in pregnancy is not known. Not for use in nursing.

MECHANISM OF ACTION: NSAID; not established; suspected to inhibit prostaglandin synthesis and compete for binding at prostaglandin receptor site (animal studies); inhibits human leukocyte 5-lipoxygenase activity (in vitro).

PHARMACOKINETICS: Absorption: Rapid; C_{max}=4.8mcg/mL; T_{max}=0.9 hrs. Metabolite: C_{max}=1mcg/mL; T_{max}=2.4 hrs. **Distribution**: V_d=23.3L; plasma protein binding (>99%). Found in breast milk. **Metabolism**: 3-Hydroxymethyl metabolite (major metabolite). **Elimination**: Urine, feces; $T_{1/2}$=1.3 hrs. Metabolite: Urine (0.5%), feces; $T_{1/2}$=15.3 hrs.

MEDROL   RX
methylprednisolone (Pharmacia & Upjohn)

OTHER BRAND NAMES: Medrol Dose Pack (Pharmacia & Upjohn)

THERAPEUTIC CLASS: Glucocorticoid

INDICATIONS: Steroid-responsive disorders.

DOSAGE: *Adults:* Initial: 4-48mg/day depending on disease and response. Maint: Decrease dose by small amounts to lowest effective dose. MS: Initial: 160mg/day for 1 week. Maint: 64mg every other day for 1 month. Alternate Day Therapy: Twice the usual dose every other day for long-term therapy. *Pediatrics:* Initial: 4-48mg/day depending on disease and response. Maint: Decrease dose by small amounts to lowest effective dose. MS: Initial: 160mg/day for 1 week. Maint: 64mg every other day for 1 month. Alternate Day Therapy: Twice the usual dose every other day for long-term therapy.

HOW SUPPLIED: Tab: 2mg*, 4mg*, 8mg*, 16mg*, 32mg*; (Dose-Pak) 4mg* [21ˢ] *scored

CONTRAINDICATIONS: Systemic fungal infections.

WARNINGS/PRECAUTIONS: May need to increase dose before, during, and after stressful situations. May mask signs of infection or cause new infections. Prolonged use may produce glaucoma, optic nerve damage, secondary ocular infections. Increases BP, salt/water retention, potassium excretion. More severe/fatal course of infections reported with chickenpox, measles. Caution with Strongyloides, latent TB, hypothyroidism, cirrhosis, ocular herpes simplex, HTN, diverticulitis, fresh intestinal anastomoses, ulcerative colitis, osteoporosis, myasthenia gravis, renal insufficiency, peptic ulcer disease. Kaposi's sarcoma reported. Growth and development of children on prolonged therapy should be monitored. Monitor for psychic disturbances. Avoid abrupt withdrawal. The 24mg tabs contain tartrazine; caution with tartrazine sensitivity.

ADVERSE REACTIONS: Fluid and electrolyte disturbances, HTN, osteoporosis, muscle weakness, cushingoid state, menstrual irregularities, nervousness, insomnia, impaired wound healing, DM, ulcerative esophagitis, excessive sweating, increases intracranial pressure, carbohydrate intolerance, glaucoma, cataracts, weight gain, nausea, malaise.

INTERACTIONS: Reduced efficacy with hepatic enzyme inducers (eg, phenobarbital, phenytoin, and rifampin). Increases clearance of chronic high dose ASA. Caution with ASA in hypoprothrombinemia. Effects on oral anticoagulants are variable; monitor PT. Increased insulin and oral hypoglycemic requirements in DM. Avoid live vaccines with immunosuppressive doses. Possible decreased vaccine response with killed or inactivated vaccines with immunosuppressive doses. Mutual inhibition of metabolism with cyclosporine; convulsions reported. Potentiated by ketoconazole and troleandomycin.

PREGNANCY: Safety in pregnancy and nursing not known.

MECHANISM OF ACTION: Anti-inflammatory glucocorticoid; causes profound and varied metabolic effects and modifies the body's immune responses to diverse stimuli.

PHARMACOKINETICS: Absorption: Readily absorbed from GI tract.

MEGACE ES
megestrol acetate (Par)
RX

OTHER BRAND NAMES: Megace Suspension (Bristol-Myers Squibb)

THERAPEUTIC CLASS: Progesterone

INDICATIONS: Management of anorexia, cachexia, or unexplained significant weight loss in AIDS patients.

DOSAGE: *Adults:* (Megace) Initial: 800mg/day (20mL/day). Usual: 400-800mg/day. Shake well before use. Elderly: Start at lower end of dosing range. (Megace ES) Initial/Usual: 625mg/day (5mL/day).

HOW SUPPLIED: Sus: 40mg/mL [240mL], (ES) 125mg/mL [150mL]

CONTRAINDICATIONS: Pregnancy.

WARNINGS/PRECAUTIONS: May cause fetal harm; avoid in pregnancy. New onset or exacerbation of diabetes or Cushing's syndrome reported. Risk of adrenal suppression if taking or withdrawing from chronic therapy; monitor for hypotension, nausea, vomiting, dizziness, or weakness. Caution with history of thromboembolic diseases. Use in HIV-infected women has been limited. Do not use as prophylactic to avoid weight loss.

ADVERSE REACTIONS: Diarrhea, impotence, rash, flatulence, HTN, asthenia, insomnia, nausea, anemia, fever, decreased libido, dispepsia, headache, hyperglycemia, vomiting, pneumonia.

INTERACTIONS: May increase insulin requirements. Decrease in pharmacokinetic parameters of indinavir; higher dose should be considered.

PREGNANCY: Category X, not for use in nursing.

MECHANISM OF ACTION: Progesterone; has not been established; has appetite-enhancing property.

PHARMACOKINETICS: Absorption: PO administration of variable doses resulted in different parameters. **Elimination:** Urine (major), feces.

MEGESTROL
megestrol acetate (Various)
RX

THERAPEUTIC CLASS: Progesterone

INDICATIONS: (Tabs) Palliative treatment of advanced breast carcinoma or endometrial carcinoma (eg, recurrent, inoperable or metastatic disease). (Sus) Treatment of anorexia, cachexia, unexplained, significant weight loss with AIDS.

DOSAGE: *Adults:* (Tab) Breast Carcinoma: 40mg qid for a minimum of 2 months. Endometrial Carcinoma: 40-320mg/day in divided doses for a minimum of 2 months. Elderly: Start at lower end of dosing range. (Sus) 400-800mg/day (10-20mL/day); shake well.

HOW SUPPLIED: Sus: 40mg/mL [240mL]; Tab: 20mg*, 40mg* *scored

CONTRAINDICATIONS: Known or suspected pregnancy.

WARNINGS/PRECAUTIONS: May cause fetal harm; avoid in pregnancy. May cause adrenal suppression; monitor for Cushing's syndrome or new onset/exacerbation of DM. Risk of adrenal suppression if taking or withdrawing from chronic therapy; monitor for hypotension, nausea, vomiting, dizziness, weakness. Caution with history of thromboembolic diseases.

ADVERSE REACTIONS: Heart failure, nausea, vomiting, edema, breakthrough menstrual bleeding, dyspnea, glucose intolerance, alopecia, HTN, carpal tunnel syndrome, mood changes, hot flashes, malaise, weight gain.

INTERACTIONS: May increase insulin requirements.

PREGNANCY: Category D, not for use in nursing.

MECHANISM OF ACTION: Antineoplastic; unknown, suspected to inhibit pituitary gonadotropin production with resultant decrease in estrogen secretion.

PHARMACOKINETICS: Absorption: (40mg) C_{max}=27.6ng/mL, T_{max}=2.2 hrs. **Elimination:** $T_{1/2}$=34.2 hrs.

MENACTRA RX
meningococcal polysaccharide diptheria toxoid conjugate vaccine (Sanofi Pasteur)

THERAPEUTIC CLASS: Vaccine

INDICATIONS: Active immunization of adolescents and adults 2-55 yrs of age for the prevention of invasive meningococcal disease caused by *N.meningitidis* serogroups A, C, Y and W-135. Not indicated for prevention of meningitis caused by other microorganisms; prevention of invasive meningo-coccal disease caused by *N.meningitidis* serogroups B; treatment of meningo-coccal infections; or immunization against diphtheria.

DOSAGE: *Adults:* ≤55 yo: 0.5 mL IM into deltoid region.
Pediatrics: ≥2 yo: 0.5mL IM into deltoid region.

HOW SUPPLIED: Inj: 0.5mL

CONTRAINDICATIONS: Life-threatening reaction after previous administra-tion of vaccine with similar contents. Known hypersensitivity to dry natural rubber latex.

WARNINGS/PRECAUTIONS: Guillain-Barre syndrome (GBS) has been reported. Avoid with bleeding disorders (eg. hemophilia, thrombocytopenia, anticoagulant therapy). Do not administer IV, SC, or intradermally. Have epi-nephrine injection (1:1000) available, in case of anaphylatic reaction.

ADVERSE REACTIONS: Redness, swelling, induration, pain, headache, fatigue, malaise, arthralgia, anorexia, chills, fever.

INTERACTIONS: Caution with anticoagulants. Immunosuppressive therapies may reduce immune response to vaccines.

PREGNANCY: Category C, caution in nursing.

MECHANISM OF ACTION: Stimulates immune system to produce bactericidal anticapsular meningococcal antibodies (specific to capsular polysaccharides of serogroups A, C, Y and W-135) that may protect against invasive meningo-coccal disease.

MENEST RX
esterified estrogens (King)

> Estrogens increase the risk of endometrial cancer. Estrogens, with or without progestins, should not be used for the prevention of CVD. Increased risks of MI, stroke, invasive breast cancer, PE, and DVT in postmenopausal women (50-79 yrs of age) reported. Increased risk of developing probable dementia in postmenopausal women ≥65 yrs of age reported.

THERAPEUTIC CLASS: Estrogen

INDICATIONS: Treatment of moderate to severe vasomotor symptoms associ-ated with menopause, atrophic vaginitis, kraurosis vulvae, female hypogonad-ism, female castration, primary ovarian failure. Palliative therapy for meta-static breast cancer in selected men and women, and of advanced prostatic carcinoma.

DOSAGE: *Adults:* Vasomotor Symptoms: 1.25mg qd cyclically (3 weeks on, 1 week off). Start arbitrarily if not menstruating, or on Day 5 of bleeding. Atrophic Vaginitis/Kraurosis Vulvae: 0.3-1.25mg qd cyclically (3 weeks on, 1 week off). Discontinue/Taper at 3-6 month intervals. Female Hypogonadism: 2.5-7.5mg/day in divided doses for 20 days, then 10 days off therapy; repeat until menses occurs. If bleeding occurs before the end of the 10 day period, begin a 20 day estrogen-progestin cyclic regimen with Menest 2.5-7.5mg/day in divided doses, for 20 days. During the last 5 days of estrogen therapy, give an oral progestin. If bleeding occurs before this regimen is concluded, therapy is discontinued and may be resumed on the fifth day of bleeding. Female

Castration/Primary Ovarian Failure: 1.25mg qd cyclically (3 weeks on, 1 week off). Maint: Lowest effective dose. Prostate Cancer: 1.25-2.5mg tid. Breast Cancer: 10mg tid for at least 3 months.

HOW SUPPLIED: Tab: 0.3mg, 0.625mg, 1.25mg, 2.5mg

CONTRAINDICATIONS: Pregnancy, undiagnosed abnormal genital bleeding, breast cancer unless being treated for metastatic disease, estrogen-dependent neoplasia, DVT/PE, active or recent (eg, within past year) arterial thromboembolic disease (eg, stroke, MI), liver dysfunction or disease.

WARNINGS/PRECAUTIONS: May increase risk of cardiovascular events (eg, MI, stroke), venous thrombosis, and PE; d/c immediately if any of these events occur or are suspected. May increase risk of breast/endometrial cancer, and gallbladder disease. May lead to severe hypercalcemia with breast cancer and bone metastases; monitor and d/c if hypercalcemia occurs. Retinal vascular thrombosis reported; monitor and d/c if papilledema or retinal vascular lesions occur. Consider addition of a progestin if no hysterectomy. May elevate BP; monitor at regular intervals. May cause elevations of plasma triglycerides with pre-existing hypertriglyceridemia. Caution with history of cholestatic jaundice associated with past estrogen use or with pregnancy; d/c with recurrence. May lead to increased thyroid-binding globulin levels; monitor thyroid function. May cause fluid retention; caution with cardiac/renal dysfunction. Caution with severe hypocalcemia. May increase risk of ovarian cancer. May exacerbate endometriosis, asthma, DM, epilepsy, migraine, porphyria, SLE, and hepatic hemangiomas; use with caution.

ADVERSE REACTIONS: Altered vaginal bleeding, vaginal candidiasis, breast tenderness/enlargement, GI effects, melasma, CNS effects, weight changes, edema, altered libido.

INTERACTIONS: CYP3A4 inducers (eg, St. John's wort, phenobarbital, carbamazepine, rifampin) may decrease levels which may decrease therapeutic effects and/or change uterine bleeding profile. CYP3A4 inhibitors (eg, erythromycin, clarithromycin, ketoconazole, itraconazole, ritonavir, grapefruit juice) may increase levels which may result in side effects.

PREGNANCY: Contraindicated in pregnancy, caution in nursing.

MECHANISM OF ACTION: Estrogen; acts by binding to nuclear receptors in estrogen responsive tissues. Circulating estrogens modulate the pituitary secretion of the gonadotrophins, luteinizing hormone and follicle stimulating hormone, through a negative feedback mechanism. In postmenopausal women, acts to reduce elevated levels of these hormones.

PHARMACOKINETICS: Distribution: Largely bound to sex hormone binding globulin and albumin; found in breast milk. **Metabolism:** Liver to estrone (metabolite), estriol (major urinary metabolite); sulfate and glucuronide conjugation (liver); gut hydrolysis; CYP3A4 (partial metabolism). **Elimination:** Urine (parent drug and metabolites).

MENOPUR RX
menotropins (Ferring)

THERAPEUTIC CLASS: Follicle stimulating hormone/luteinizing hormone

INDICATIONS: Development of multiple follicles and pregnancy in the ovulatory patients participating in an ART program.

DOSAGE: *Adults:* Initial: 225 IU SQ. Titrate: Adjust subsequent dosing to individual response at intervals no less than every 2 days and not exceeding 150 IU/adjustment. Max: 450 IU/day. Dosing >20 days not recommended. If adequate response, administer hCG. Withhold hCG if ovaries abnormally enlarged last day of therapy.

HOW SUPPLIED: Inj: (FSH-LH) 75 IU-75 IU

CONTRAINDICATIONS: High FSH level indicating primary ovarian failure; uncontrolled thyroid and adrenal dysfunction; organic intracranial lesion (pituitary tumor); sex hormone dependent tumor of the reproductive tract and accessory organs; abnormal uterine bleeding of undetermined origin; ovarian cysts or enlargement not due to polycystic ovary syndrome; pregnant women.

WARNINGS/PRECAUTIONS: Ovarian hyperstimulation syndrome (OHSS) with or without pulmonary or vascular complications. Mild to moderate uncomplicated ovarian enlargement with abdominal distention and/or abdominal pain may occur. Reports of serious pulmonary conditions (eg, atelectasis, acute respiratory distress syndrome) and thromboembolic events (intravascular thrombosis, embolism, venous thrombophlebitis, pulmonary embolism, pulmonary infarction, cerebral vascular occlusion, arterial occlusion) which may lead to death. Potential risk of multiple births.

ADVERSE REACTIONS: Headache, abdominal pain, injection site reaction, nausea, abdominal cramps, abdominal fullness, OHSS, respiratory disorder, vomiting.

PREGNANCY: Category X, caution in nursing.

MECHANISM OF ACTION: Follicle stimulating hormone/lutenizing hormone; produces ovarian follicular growth in women who do not have primary ovarian failure.

PHARMACOKINETICS: Absorption: C_{max}=8.5(2.5)mIU/mL, T_{max}=17.9(5.8) hrs, AUC=726.2(243.0)hr•mIU/mL; (SC) C_{max}=7.8(2.4)mIU/mL, T_{max}=27.5(25.4) hrs, AUC=656.1(233.7)hr•mIU/mL. **Elimination:** $T_{1/2}$=11-13 hrs.

MENOSTAR   RX
estradiol (Bayer Healthcare)

> Estrogens increase the risk of endometrial cancer. Estrogens, with or without progestins, should not be used for the prevention of cardiovascular disease. Increased risks of MI, stroke, invasive breast cancer, PE, and DVT in postmenopausal women (50-79 yrs of age) reported. Increased risk of developing probable dementia in postmenopausal women ≥65 yrs of age reported.

THERAPEUTIC CLASS: Estrogen

INDICATIONS: Prevention of postmenopausal osteoporosis.

DOSAGE: *Adults:* Apply 1 patch weekly to lower abdomen (avoid breasts, waistline, and areas where sitting would dislodge the patch). Rotate application sites.

HOW SUPPLIED: Patch: 14mcg/day [4's]

CONTRAINDICATIONS: Pregnancy, undiagnosed abnormal genital bleeding, breast cancer, estrogen-dependent neoplasia, DVT/PE, active or recent (eg, within past year) arterial thromboembolic disease (eg, stroke, MI), liver dysfunction or disease.

WARNINGS/PRECAUTIONS: May increase risk of cardiovascular events (eg, MI, stroke), venous thrombosis, and PE; d/c immediately if any of these events occur or are suspected. May increase risk of breast/endometrial cancer, and gallbladder disease. May lead to severe hypercalcemia with breast cancer and bone metastases; monitor and d/c if hypercalcemia occurs. Retinal vascular thrombosis reported; monitor and d/c if papilledema or retinal vascular lesions occur. Consider addition of a progestin if no hysterectomy. May elevate BP; monitor at regular intervals. May cause elevations of plasma triglycerides with pre-existing hypertriglyceridemia. Caution with history of cholestatic jaundice associated with past estrogen use or with pregnancy; d/c with recurrence. May lead to increased TBG levels; monitor thyroid function. May cause fluid retention; caution with cardiac/renal dysfunction. Caution with severe hypocalcemia. May increase risk of ovarian cancer. May exacerbate endometriosis, asthma, DM, epilepsy, migraine, porphyria, SLE, and hepatic hemangiomas; use with caution.

ADVERSE REACTIONS: Pain, leukorrhea, arthralgia, application site reaction, bronchitis, cervical polyps, constipation, dyspepsia, myalgia, dizziness, breast pain.

INTERACTIONS: CYP3A4 inducers (eg, St. John's wort, phenobarbital, carbamazepine, rifampin) may reduce effects. CYP3A4 inhibitors (eg, erythromycin, clarithromycin, ketoconazole, itraconazole, ritonavir, grapefruit juice) may increase levels. May require higher doses of thyroid hormone.

PREGNANCY: Contraindicated in pregnancy, caution in nursing.

MENTAX   RX
butenafine HCL (Mylan Bertek)

THERAPEUTIC CLASS: Benzylamine antifungal

INDICATIONS: Interdigital tinea pedis, tinea corporis, tinea cruris, and tinea versicolor.

DOSAGE: *Adults:* T.pedis: Apply bid for 7 days or qd for 4 weeks. T.corporis/T.cruris/T.versicolor: Apply qd for 2 weeks.
Pediatrics: ≥12 yrs: T.pedis: Apply bid for 7 days or qd for 4 weeks. T.corporis/T.cruris/T.versicolor: Apply qd for 2 weeks.

HOW SUPPLIED: Cre: 1% [15g, 30g]

WARNINGS/PRECAUTIONS: Avoid eyes, nose, mouth, and other mucous membranes. D/C if irritation or sensitivity develops. Confirm diagnosis. Caution if sensitive to other allylamine antifungals.

ADVERSE REACTIONS: Burning, stinging, itching, contact dermatitis, irritation, erythema, worsening of condition.

PREGNANCY: Category B, caution in nursing.

MECHANISM OF ACTION: Benzylamine antifungal; inhibits epoxidation of squalene, thus blocking the biosynthesis of ergosterol, which is an essential component of fungal cell membranes.

PHARMACOKINETICS: Absorption: Topical administration of variable doses result in different parameters.

MEPERIDINE/PROMETHAZINE   CII
meperidine HCL - promethazine HCL (Ethex)

OTHER BRAND NAMES: Meprozine (Vintage)

THERAPEUTIC CLASS: Opioid analgesic/phenothiazine

INDICATIONS: Management of moderate pain and sedation for postoperative and postpartum use, and pain associated with malignancies.

DOSAGE: *Adults:* 1 cap q4-6h prn.

HOW SUPPLIED: Cap: (Meperidine-Promethazine) 50mg-25mg

CONTRAINDICATIONS: During or within 14 days of MAOIs.

WARNINGS/PRECAUTIONS: May cause tolerance and dependence; potential for abuse. Extreme caution with head injury, increased ICP, intracranial lesions, acute asthma, COPD, cor pulmonale, decreased respiratory reserve, respiratory depression, hypoxia, hypercapnia. Severe hypotension may occur with depleted blood volume. Orthostatic hypotension may occur. Caution with atrial flutter and other supraventricular tachycardias. May obscure diagnosis or clinical course of acute abdominal conditions. Reduce initial dose in elderly, debilitated, severe hepatic or renal dysfunction, hypothyroidism, Addison's disease, prostatic hypertrophy, urethral stricture. May aggravate seizure disorders. Not for use in pregnant women prior to labor.

ADVERSE REACTIONS: Lightheadedness, dizziness, sedation, nausea, vomiting, sweating.

INTERACTIONS: See Contraindications. Additive sedative effects with CNS depressants (eg, narcotics, anesthetics, phenothiazines, tranquilizers, sedative-hypnotics, TCAs, alcohol). Reduce analgesic depressant dose by 25-50% and dose of barbiturates by 50%. Severe hypotension possible with concurrent phenothiazines, certain anesthetics.

PREGNANCY: Safety in pregnancy and nursing not known.

MECHANISM OF ACTION: Meperidine: Narcotic analgesic. Promethazine: Phenothiazine derivative; has antiemetic, sedative, antihistaminic actions.

MEPHYTON
phytonadione (Aton)

RX

THERAPEUTIC CLASS: Vitamin K derivative

INDICATIONS: For coagulation disorders caused by vitamin K deficiency or interference with vitamin K activity, including anticoagulant-induced prothrombin deficiency caused by coumarin or indanedione derivatives; and hypoprothrombinemia secondary to antibacterials, salicylates, obstructive jaundice, or biliary fistulas.

DOSAGE: *Adults:* Anticoagulant-Induced Prothrombin Deficiency: Initial: 2.5-10mg up to 25mg (rarely 50mg). May repeat if PT is still elevated 12-48 hrs after initial dose. Hypoprothrombinemia Due to Other Causes: 2.5-25mg or more (rarely up to 50mg). Give bile salts when endogenous bile supply to GIT is deficient.

HOW SUPPLIED: Tab: 5mg* *scored

WARNINGS/PRECAUTIONS: Does not produce an immediate coagulant effect. Maintain lowest possible dose to prevent original thromboembolic events. Avoid repeated large doses with hepatic disease. Failure to respond may indicate a congenital coagulation defect or a condition unresponsive to vitamin K. Avoid large doses in liver disease. Monitor PT regularly.

ADVERSE REACTIONS: Severe hypersensitivity reactions (anaphylactoid reactions, death), flushing, peculiar taste sensations, dizziness, rapid and weak pulse, profuse sweating, hypotension, dyspnea, cyanosis.

INTERACTIONS: Does not counteract anticoagulant effects of heparin. Temporary resistance to prothrombin-depressing anticoagulants, especially with large doses.

PREGNANCY: Category C, caution in nursing.

MECHANISM OF ACTION: Vitamin K derivative; promotes the hepatic biosynthesis of vitamin K-dependent clotting factors.

PHARMACOKINETICS: Absorption: Adequately absorbed if bile salts are present. **Metabolism:** Liver.

MEPROBAMATE
meprobamate (Various)

CIV

THERAPEUTIC CLASS: Carbamate derivative

INDICATIONS: Management of anxiety disorders or short-term relief of symptoms of anxiety.

DOSAGE: *Adults:* Usual: 1200-1600mg/day given tid-qid. Max: 2400mg/day. Elderly: >65 yrs: Start at low end of dosing range.
Pediatrics: 6-12 yrs: 200-600mg/day given bid-tid.

HOW SUPPLIED: Tab: 200mg, 400mg

CONTRAINDICATIONS: Porphyria, allergic or idiosyncratic reactions to carisoprodol, mebutamate, tybamate, carbromal.

WARNINGS/PRECAUTIONS: Physical and psychological dependence reported. Avoid abrupt withdrawal after prolonged or excessive use. Increased risk of congenital malformations with use during 1st trimester of pregnancy. Caution with liver or renal dysfunction, and in elderly. May precipitate seizures in epileptic patients. Prescribe small quantities in suicidal patients.

ADVERSE REACTIONS: Drowsiness, ataxia, slurred speech, vertigo, weakness, nausea, vomiting, diarrhea, tachycardia, transient ECG changes, rash, leukopenia, petechiae.

INTERACTIONS: Administration with other CNS depressants, alcohol, psychotropics have additive effects.

PREGNANCY: Safety in pregnancy and nursing not known.

MECHANISM OF ACTION: Anxiolytic agent; acts on the thalamus and limbic system.

PHARMACOKINETICS: Distribution: Passes placental barrier; found in umbilical cord blood and breast milk. **Metabolism:** Liver. **Elimination:** Renal excretion.

MEPRON RX
atovaquone (GlaxoSmithKline)

THERAPEUTIC CLASS: Napthoquinone antiprotozoal

INDICATIONS: Prevention and treatment of mild to moderate *Pneumocystis carinii* pneumonia (PCP) in those intolerant to trimethoprim-sulfamethoxazole.

DOSAGE: *Adults:* Take with food. Prevention: 1500mg qd. Treatment: 750mg bid for 21 days.
Pediatrics: 13-16 yrs: Take with food. Prevention: 1500mg qd. Treatment: 750mg bid for 21 days.

HOW SUPPLIED: Sus: 750mg/5mL [5mL, 42^s; 210mL]

WARNINGS/PRECAUTIONS: Monitor with severe hepatic impairment. Absorption significantly increased with food.

ADVERSE REACTIONS: Rash, nausea, GI effects, cough increased, rhinitis, asthenia, infection, dyspnea, insomnia, asthenia, pruritus.

INTERACTIONS: Significantly decreased plasma levels with rifampin. Caution with other highly protein-bound drugs.

PREGNANCY: Category C, caution in nursing.

MECHANISM OF ACTION: Naphthoquinone antiprotozoal; site of action appears to be cytochrome bc$_1$ complex which is linked to mitochondrial electron transport. Inhibition of electron transport by atovaquone will result in indirect inhibition of these enzymes, resulting in nucleic acid and ATP synthesis inhibition.

PHARMACOKINETICS: Absorption: Absolute bioavailability (47%); PO administration of variable doses resulted in different parameters. **Distribution:** V_d=0.6L/kg; plasma protein binding (99.9%). **Elimination:** Feces (≥94%, unchanged), urine (≤0.6%).

MERIDIA CIV
sibutramine HCL monohydrate (Abbott)

THERAPEUTIC CLASS: Dopamine/norepinephrine/serotonin reuptake inhibitor

INDICATIONS: To induce and maintain weight loss in obese patients with an initial BMI ≥30kg/m^2 or ≥27kg/m^2 with risk factors (eg, HTN, diabetes, dyslipidemia).

DOSAGE: *Adults:* Initial: 10mg qd. Titrate: May increase after 4 weeks to 15mg qd. Max: 15mg/day. Use 5mg/day in patients unable to tolerate 10mg/day. May continue for up to 2 yrs.
Pediatrics: ≥16 yrs: Initial: 10mg qd. Titrate: May increase after 4 weeks to 15mg qd. Use 5mg/day in patients unable to tolerate 10mg/day. Max: 15mg/day. May continue for up to 2 yrs.

HOW SUPPLIED: Cap: 5mg, 10mg, 15mg

CONTRAINDICATIONS: Concomitant MAOIs or centrally acting appetite suppressants, eating disorders (eg, anorexia/bulimia nervosa).

WARNINGS/PRECAUTIONS: May increase BP and/or pulse. Avoid with uncontrolled or poorly controlled HTN, CAD, CHF, arrhythmias, stroke, severe hepatic or renal dysfunction. Monitor BP and pulse before therapy and regularly thereafter. Caution with narrow angle glaucoma, mild to moderate renal impairment, seizures and if predisposed to bleeding. Exclude organic causes of obesity. Gallstones precipitated with weight loss.

ADVERSE REACTIONS: Anorexia, constipation, increased appetite, nausea, dyspepsia, dry mouth, insomnia, dizziness, nervousness, HTN, tachycardia, dysmenorrhea, headache.

INTERACTIONS: Avoid excess alcohol, CNS-active drugs, other serotonergic agents (eg, SSRIs, migraine therapy agents, certain opioids), within 14 days of MAOI use. Caution with drugs affecting hemostasis or platelet function; ephedrine, pseudoephedrine; and other agents that increase BP, heart rate. Possible decreased metabolism with ketoconazole and erythromycin.

PREGNANCY: Category C, not for use in nursing.

MECHANISM OF ACTION: Inhibits norepinephrine, serotonin, and dopamine reuptake.

PHARMACOKINETICS: Absorption: Rapid; T_{max}=1.2 hrs; (15mg Dose, M_1, M_2) C_{max}=4ng/mL, 6.4ng/mL; T_{max}=3.6 hrs, 3.5 hrs; AUC=25.5ng•h/mL, 92.1ng•h/mL. **Distribution:** Plasma protein binding (97%); M_1, M_2 (94%). **Metabolism:** Liver via CYP3A4; M_1 and M_2 (active metabolites). **Elimination:** Urine (77%), feces; $T_{1/2}$=1.1 hrs, 14 hrs (M_1), 16 hrs (M_2).

MERREM   RX
meropenem (AstraZeneca)

THERAPEUTIC CLASS: Carbapenem

INDICATIONS: Treatment of intra-abdominal infections, bacterial meningitis, and complicated skin and skin structure infections (cSSSI) caused by susceptible strains of microorganisms.

DOSAGE: *Adults:* IV: Intra-Abdominal: 1g q8h. CrCl 26-50mL/min: 1g q12h. CrCl 10-25mL/min: 500mg q12h. CrCl <10mL/min: 500mg q24h. cSSSI: 500mg q8h. CrCl 26-50mL/min: 500mg q12h. CrCl 10-25mL/min: 250mg q12h. CrCl <10mL/min: 250mg q24h.
Pediatrics: IV: ≥3 months: >50kg: Intra-Abdominal: 1g q8h. Meningitis: 2g q8h. cSSSI: 500mg q8h. ≤50kg: Intra-Abdominal: 20mg/kg q8h. Max: 1g q8h. Meningitis: 40mg/kg q8h. Max: 2g q8h. cSSSI: 10mg/kg q8h. Max: 500mg q8h.

HOW SUPPLIED: Inj: 500mg, 1g

CONTRAINDICATIONS: Hypersensitivity to β-lactams.

WARNINGS/PRECAUTIONS: Severe and fatal hypersensitivity reactions reported; increased risk with allergens and/or PCN sensitivity. *Clostridium difficile*-associated diarrhea reported. Seizures and other CNS effects reported particularly with pre-existing CNS disorders, bacterial meningitis, and renal dysfunction. Thrombocytopenia reported with severe renal impairment. Prolonged use may result in superinfection. Use as monotherapy for meningitis caused by penicillin nonsusceptible strains of *Streptococcus pneumoniae* has not been established.

ADVERSE REACTIONS: Headache, rash, local reactions, diarrhea, nausea, vomiting, constipation.

INTERACTIONS: Probenecid inhibits renal excretion; avoid concomitant use. May reduce valproic acid levels.

PREGNANCY: Category B, caution in nursing.

MECHANISM OF ACTION: Broad-spectrum carbapenem; penetrates bacterial cells and interferes with synthesis of vital cell wall components, resulting in cell death.

PHARMACOKINETICS: Absorption: 30 min infusion: C_{max}=23μg/mL (500mg); 49μg/mL (1g). 5-min bolus injection: C_{max}=45μg/mL (500mg); 112μg/mL (1g). **Distribution:** Plasma protein binding (2%). **Elimination:** Urine (70%); $T_{1/2}$=1 hr, 1.5 hrs (3mo-2yrs).

MERUVAX II
rubella vaccine live (Merck) RX

THERAPEUTIC CLASS: Vaccine

INDICATIONS: Vaccination against rubella.

DOSAGE: *Adults:* 0.5mL SQ in outer aspect of upper arm.
Pediatrics: Primary Vaccination at 12-15 months: 0.5mL SQ in outer aspect of upper arm. Revaccinate with MMR II prior to elementary school entry.

HOW SUPPLIED: Inj: 1000 $TCID_{50}$

CONTRAINDICATIONS: Avoid pregnancy for 3 months after vaccine, anaphylactic reaction to neomycin, febrile/active respiratory illness, immunosuppressive therapy (except corticosteroids as replacement therapy), blood dyscrasias, leukemia, lymphoma, malignant neoplasms affecting bone marrow or lymphatic system, immunodeficiency states.

WARNINGS/PRECAUTIONS: May worsen thrombocytopenia. Defer vaccination for at least 3 months after blood or plasma transfusions, immune globulin (except susceptible postpartum patients with follow-up HI titer after 6-8 weeks). Do not vaccinate with active untreated TB. Temperature elevation may occur after vaccination. Contains albumin, remote risk of viral infection transmission. Have epinephrine (1:1000) available.

ADVERSE REACTIONS: Fever, syncope, headache, dizziness, malaise, irritability, thrombocytopenia, arthritis, vasculitis, diarrhea, local reactions.

INTERACTIONS: Do not give with immune globulin. May depress TB skin sensitivity, administer test either simultaneously or before. Do not give <1 month before or after other live viral vaccines. Do not give simultaneously with DTP or oral poliovirus vaccine.

PREGNANCY: Category C, contraindicated in pregnancy and caution in nursing.

MECHANISM OF ACTION: Induces a broader profile of circulating antibodies, including anti-theta and anti-iota antibodies against RA 27/3 rubella virus.

MESNEX
mesna (Baxter/Bristol-Myers Squibb) RX

THERAPEUTIC CLASS: Sodium 2-mercaptoethane sulfonate

INDICATIONS: Prophylactic agent to reduce incidence of ifosfamide-induced hemorrhagic cystitis.

DOSAGE: *Adults:* (IV) IV bolus as 20% of ifosfamide dose given concurrently, and 4 and 8 hrs after each ifosfamide dose. Max: 60% of ifosfamide dose/day. (IV/PO) IV bolus as 20% of ifosfamide dose given concurrently, then give tabs as 40% of ifosfamide dose 2 and 6 hrs after each ifosfamide dose. Max: 100% of ifosfamide dose/day.

HOW SUPPLIED: Inj: 100mg/mL; Tab: 400mg

CONTRAINDICATIONS: Hypersensitivity to thiol compounds.

WARNINGS/PRECAUTIONS: Allergic reaction reported; higher incidence with autoimmune disorders. Does not prevent hemorrhagic cystitis in all patients. Hematuria reported; examine morning urine specimen daily prior to therapy. Multi-dose vial contains benzyl alcohol. False positive test for urinary ketones may occur.

ADVERSE REACTIONS: Nausea, vomiting, constipation, leukopenia, fatigue, fever, anorexia, thrombocytopenia, anemia, granulocytopenia, asthenia, abdominal pain, alopecia.

PREGNANCY: Category B, not for use in nursing.

MECHANISM OF ACTION: Sodium 2-mercaptoethane sulfonate; detoxifying agent which inhibits the hemorrhagic cystitis induced by ifosfamide.

PHARMACOKINETICS: Absorption: Administration of variable doses resulted in different pharmacokinetic parameters. **Distribution:** Plasma protein binding

(69-75%). **Metabolism:** Liver via oxidation. Mesna disulfide (major metabolite). **Elimination:** Urine (32-33%, unchanged). T$_{1/2}$=0.5 hr (Mesna IV), 1.2-8.3 hr (Mesna IV&PO).

MESTINON   RX
pyridostigmine bromide (Valeant)

THERAPEUTIC CLASS: Cholinesterase inhibitor

INDICATIONS: Treatment of myasthenia gravis.

DOSAGE: *Adults:* Adjust dose and frequency based on the needs of the individual patient. (Syrup, Tab) 600mg qd in divided doses. (Tab, Extended-Release) 180-540mg given qd-bid. Dosing interval should be at least 6 hrs apart.

HOW SUPPLIED: Syrup: 60mg/5mL; Tab: 60mg*; Tab, Extended-Release: 180mg* *scored

CONTRAINDICATIONS: Mechanical intestinal or urinary obstruction.

WARNINGS/PRECAUTIONS: Caution with bronchial asthma. Cholinergic crisis or myasthenic crisis may occur; it is important to differentiate. May need dose adjustment with renal disease.

ADVERSE REACTIONS: Nausea, vomiting, diarrhea, abdominal cramps, increased peristalsis, increased salivation, increased bronchial secretions, miosis, diaphoresis.

INTERACTIONS: Effects may be antagonized by atropine; caution when counteracting side effects.

PREGNANCY: Safety in pregnancy and nursing not known.

MECHANISM OF ACTION: Inhibits the destruction of ACh by cholinesterase and thereby permits free transmission of nerve impulses across the neuromuscular junction.

PHARMACOKINETICS: Excertion: Urine.

METADATE CD   CII
methylphenidate HCL (UCB)

THERAPEUTIC CLASS: Sympathomimetic amine

INDICATIONS: Treatment of attention deficit hyperactivity disorder (ADHD).

DOSAGE: *Pediatrics:* ≥6 yrs: Usual: 20mg qam before breakfast. Titrate: Increase weekly by 20mg depending on tolerability/efficacy. Max: 60mg/day. Reduce dose or discontinue if paradoxical aggravation of symptoms occur. D/C if no improvement after appropriate dose adjustments over 1 month. Swallow whole with liquids or open and sprinkle on 1 tbs applesauce followed by water. Do not crush, chew, or divide.

HOW SUPPLIED: Cap, Extended-Release: 10mg, 20mg, 30mg, 40mg, 50mg, 60mg

CONTRAINDICATIONS: Marked anxiety, tension, and agitation; glaucoma; motor tics, family history or diagnosis of Tourette's syndrome, severe HTN, angina pectoris, cardiac arrhythmias, heart failure, recent MI, hyperthyroidism or thyrotoxicosis; during or within 14 days of MAOI use.

WARNINGS/PRECAUTIONS: Monitor growth in children. Not for severe depression or fatigue. May exacerbate symptoms of behavior disturbance and thought disorder in psychotic patients. Caution when using stimulants to treat patients with comorbid bipolar disorder because of concern for possible induction of mixed/manic episode in such patients. Stimulants at usual doses can cause treatment emergent psychotic or manic symptoms (eg, hallucinations, delusional thinking, mania) in children and adolescents without prior history of psychotic illness. Aggressive behavior or hostility reported in clinical trials and postmarketing experience of some medications indicated for the treatment of ADHD. May lower seizure threshold, especially in known EEG abnormalities. Caution with HTN, conditions affected by BP or HR elevation, history of drug abuse or alcoholism. Monitor during withdrawal from abusive use. Visual disturbances may occur (rare). Monitor CBC, differential, and platelets with prolonged use. Avoid with serious structural cardiac abnormalities, cardiomyopathy, serious heart rhythm abnormalities, CAD, or other serious cardiac problems.

ADVERSE REACTIONS: Headache, abdominal pain, anorexia, insomnia.

INTERACTIONS: See Contraindications. Potentiates anticoagulants, anticonvulsants (eg, phenobarbital, phenytoin, primidone), TCAs, and SSRIs. Caution with α₂-agonist (eg, clonidine) and pressor agents.

PREGNANCY: Category C, caution in nursing.

MECHANISM OF ACTION: CNS stimulant; not established, thought to block reuptake of norepinephrine and dopamine into presynaptic neuron and increase release of these monoamines into extraneuronal space.

PHARMACOKINETICS: Absorption: (PO) Readily absorbed. Administration of variable doses resulted in different parameters. **Metabolism:** Via de-esterification. Metabolite: Alpha-phenyl-piperidine acetic acid (ritalinic acid). **Elimination:** $T_{1/2}$=6.8 hrs.

METADATE ER
methylphenidate HCL (UCB) `CII`

THERAPEUTIC CLASS: Sympathomimetic amine

INDICATIONS: Treatment of attention deficit disorder and narcolepsy.

DOSAGE: *Adults:* (Immediate-Release Methylphenidate) 10-60mg/day given bid-tid 30-45 min ac. Take last dose before 6 pm if insomnia occurs. (Tab, Extended-Release) May use in place of immediate release tabs when the 8 hr dose corresponds to the titrated 8 hr immediate release dose. Swallow whole; do not chew or crush.
Pediatrics: ≥6 yrs: (Immediate-Release Methylphenidate) Initial: 5mg bid before breakfast and lunch. Titrate: Increase gradually by 5-10mg weekly. Max: 60mg/day. (Tab, Extended-Release) May use in place of immediate release tabs when the 8 hr dose corresponds to the titrated 8hr immediate release dose. Swallow whole; do not chew or crush. Reduce dose or discontinue if paradoxical aggravation of symptoms occur. Discontinue if no improvement after appropriate dose adjustment over 1 month.

HOW SUPPLIED: Tab, Extended-Release: 10mg, 20mg

CONTRAINDICATIONS: Marked anxiety, tension, and agitation; glaucoma; motor tics or family history or diagnosis of Tourette's syndrome; during or within 14 days of MAOI use.

WARNINGS/PRECAUTIONS: Caution with comorbid bipolar disorder. Monitor growth in children. Not for severe depression or fatigue. May exacerbate symptoms of behavior disturbance and thought disorder in psychotic children. Treatment emergent psychotic/manic symptoms in children and adolescents may occur. Aggressive behavior or hostility observed. May lower seizure threshold, especially in known EEG abnormalities. Caution with HTN, emotionally-unstable patients. Monitor during withdrawal. Visual disturbances may occur (rare). Monitor CBC, differential, and platelets with prolonged use. Periodically d/c to assess condition.

ADVERSE REACTIONS: Nervousness, insomnia, hypersensitivity reactions, anorexia, nausea, dizziness, palpitations, headache, dyskinesia, drowsiness, BP and pulse changes, tachycardia, angina, arrhythmia, abdominal pain.

INTERACTIONS: See Contraindications. May decrease hypotensive effect of guanethidine. Caution with pressor agents. Potentiates anticoagulants, anticonvulsants (eg, phenobarbital, phenytoin, primidone), phenylbutazone, TCAs (eg, imipramine, clomipramine, desipramine).

PREGNANCY: Safety in pregnancy and nursing not known.

MECHANISM OF ACTION: Not established, suspected to have sympathomimetic activity in the brain stem arousal system and cortex.

PHARMACOKINETICS: Absorption: Slowly absorbed. T_{max} =1.3-8.2 hrs (sustained-release tab), 0.3-4.4 hrs (immediate release tab).

METAGLIP   RX
metformin HCL - glipizide (Bristol-Myers Squibb)

THERAPEUTIC CLASS: Sulfonylurea/biguanide

INDICATIONS: Adjunct to diet and exercise, as initial therapy to improve glycemic control in type 2 diabetes, and as 2nd-line therapy when treatment with a sulfonylurea or metformin is inadequate.

DOSAGE: *Adults:* Initial: 2.5mg-250mg qd. If FBG 280-320mg/dL, give 2.5mg-500mg bid. Titrate: Increase by 1 tab/day every 2 weeks. Max: 10mg-1g/day or 10mg-2g/day given in divided doses. Second-Line Therapy: Initial: 2.5mg-500mg or 5mg-500mg bid (with morning and evening meals). Starting dose should not exceed daily dose of metformin or glipizide already being taken. Titrate: Increase by no more than 5mg-500mg/day. Max: 20mg-2g/day. Elderly/Debilitated/Malnourished: Do not titrate to max dose. Take with meals.

HOW SUPPLIED: Tab: (Glipizide-Metformin) 2.5mg-250mg, 2.5mg-500mg, 5mg-500mg

CONTRAINDICATIONS: Renal disease/dysfunction (SrCr ≥1.5mg/dL [males], ≥1.4mg/dL [females], abnormal CrCl), metabolic acidosis, diabetic ketoacidosis. D/C temporarily (48 hrs) for radiologic studies with intravascular iodinated contrast materials.

WARNINGS/PRECAUTIONS: Lactic acidosis reported (rare); increased risk with renal dysfunction, increased age, DM, CHF, and other conditions with risk of hypoperfusion and hypoxemia. Avoid use in patients≥80 yrs unless renal function is normal. Increased risk of cardiovascular mortality. Increased risk of hypoglycemia in elderly, debilitated/malnourished, adrenal or pituitary insufficiency, or alcohol intoxication. D/C in hypoxic states (eg, CHF, shock, acute MI) and prior to surgical procedures (due to restricted food intake). Avoid in renal/hepatic impairment. May decrease serum vitamin B_{12} levels. Impaired renal and/or hepatic function may slow glipizide excretion. Withhold treatment with any condition associated with dehydration or sepsis. Monitor renal function.

ADVERSE REACTIONS: Upper respiratory tract infection, HTN, headache, diarrhea, dizziness, musculoskeletal pain, nausea, vomiting, abdominal pain.

INTERACTIONS: Furosemide, nifedipine, cimetidine and cationic drugs (eg, digoxin, amiloride, procainamide, quinidine, quinine, ranitidine, trimethoprim, vancomycin, triamterene, morphine) may increase metformin levels. Potentiated hypoglycemia with alcohol, NSAIDs, some azoles, and other highly protein bound drugs, salicylates, sulfonamides, chloramphenicol, probenecid, coumarins, MAOIs, and β-blockers. Severe hypoglycemia reported with concomitant oral miconazole. Thiazides and other diuretics, corticosteroids, phenothiazines, thyroid products, estrogens, oral contraceptives, phenytoin, nicotinic acid, sympathomimetics, CCBs, and isoniazid may cause hyperglycemia. Alcohol potentiates effect of metformin on lactate metabolism. May decrease furosemide levels.

PREGNANCY: Category C, not for use in nursing.

MECHANISM OF ACTION: Sulfonylurea; lowers blood glucose acutely by stimulating release of insulin from the pancreas. Biguanide; decreases hepatic glucose production and intestinal absorption of glucose and improves insulin sensitivity by increasing peripheral glucose uptake.

PHARMACOKINETICS: Absorption: Glipizide: Rapid, complete, T_{max}=1-3 hrs; Metformin: Absolute bioavailability (50-60%). **Distribution:** Glipizide: Plasma protein binding (98%); V_d=11L (IV). Metformin: V_d=654L. **Metabolism:** Glipizide: Liver (extensive) **Elimination:** Glipizide: $T_{1/2}$=2-4 hrs, urine; Metformin: $T_{1/2}$(plasma, blood)=(6.2,17.6 hrs); renal excretion (approx. 90%).

METANX   RX
vitamin B12 - vitamin B6 - L-methylfolate (PamLab)

THERAPEUTIC CLASS: Folate/vitamin combination

INDICATIONS: Dietary management of endothelial dysfunction or hyperhomocysteinemia with particular emphasis for individuals with or at risk for atherosclerotic vascular disease in the coronary, peripheral, or cerebral vessels; C677T mutation of the MTHFR gene; or Vitamin B_{12} deficiency.

DOSAGE: *Adults:* 1-2 tabs qd.

HOW SUPPLIED: Tab: L-methylfolate 2.8mg-Vitamin B_6 25mg-Vitamin B_{12} 2mg

WARNINGS/PRECAUTIONS: Folates >0.1mg/day may obscure pernicious anemia (may be alleviated by B_{12} component).

ADVERSE REACTIONS: Paresthesia, somnolence, nausea, headache, diarrhea, polycythemia vera, itching, transitory exanthema, feeling of body swelling.

INTERACTIONS: Pyridoxal 5'-phosphate may antagonize levodopa; avoid concomitant use. May be used with carbidopa/levodopa.

MECHANISM OF ACTION: Folate/vitamin combination: Containing L-methylfolate, Pyridoxal 5'-phosphate, Methylcobalamin.

PHARMACOKINETICS: Absorption: Pyridoxal 5'-phosphate: Readily absorbed in GI. Methylcobalamin: GI. **Distribution:** L-methylfolate: Crosses blood-brain barrier.

METAPROTERENOL   RX
metaproterenol sulfate (Various)

OTHER BRAND NAMES: Alupent (Boehringer Ingelheim)

THERAPEUTIC CLASS: Beta$_2$-agonist

INDICATIONS: For bronchial asthma and reversible bronchospasm.

DOSAGE: *Adults:* (MDI) 2-3 inh q3-4h. Max: 12 inh/day. (Sol 0.4%, 0.6%) 2.5mL by IPPB tid-qid, up to q4h. (Syr, Tab) 20mg tid-qid.
Pediatrics: (MDI) ≥12 yrs: 2-3 inh q3-4h. Max: 12 inh/day. (Sol 0.4%, 0.6%) ≥12 yrs: 2.5mL by IPPB tid-qid, up to q4h. (Syr, Tab) >9 yrs or >60 lbs: 20mg tid-qid. 6-9 yrs or <60 lbs: 10mg tid-qid.

HOW SUPPLIED: MDI: 0.65mg/inh [14g]; Sol, Inhalation: 0.4% [2.5mL], 0.6% [2.5mL]; Syrup: 10mg/5mL [480mL]; Tab: 10mg, 20mg

CONTRAINDICATIONS: Cardiac arrhythmias associated with tachycardia.

WARNINGS/PRECAUTIONS: Caution with cardiovascular disorders, (eg, ischemic heart disease, HTN, arrhythmias), hyperthyroidism, diabetes, convulsive disorders. Fatalities reported with excessive use. Can produce paradoxical bronchospasm. Monitor BP. Nebulized solution single dose may not abort an asthma attack.

ADVERSE REACTIONS: Headache, dizziness, HTN, GI distress, throat irritation, cough, asthma exacerbation, nervousness, tremor, nausea, vomiting.

INTERACTIONS: Avoid other aerosol β$_2$ agonists. Vascular effects may be potentiated by MAOIs, TCAs, and sympathomimetics.

PREGNANCY: Category C, caution in nursing.

MECHANISM OF ACTION: β-adrenergic stimulator (bronchodilator); activates adenyl cylase, the enzyme that catalyzes the formation of cAMP from ATP. Increased cAMP levels are associated with relaxation of bronchial smooth muscle and inhibition of release of mediators of immediate hypersensitivity.

PHARMACOKINETICS: Absorption: 40% absorbed after oral dosing.

M

METHADOSE
methadone HCL (Mallinckrodt)

> Deaths, cardiac and respiratory, reported during initiation and conversion from other other opioid agonists. Respiratory depression and QT prolongation observed. Only certified/approved opioid treatment programs can dispense oral methadone for treatment of narcotic addiction. Use as analgesic should be initiated only if benefits outweigh risks.

THERAPEUTIC CLASS: Opioid analgesic

INDICATIONS: Detoxification and maintenance treatment of narcotic addiction (heroin or other morphine-like drugs) in conjunction with appropriate social and medical services.

DOSAGE: *Adults:* Detoxification: Initial/Induction: 20-30mg/day. Give 5-10mg 2-4 hrs later if needed. Max: 40mg on first day. Adjust dose to control withdrawl symptoms over 1st week. Stabilize for 2-3 days, then may decrease every 1-2 days depending on symptoms. Maintenance: Titrate to a dose at which symptoms prevented for 24 hrs. Usual: 80-120mg/day. Pain in Opioid Non-Tolerant: Usual: 2.5-10mg q8-12h, slowly titrated to effect. Conversion From Parenteral: Initial: Use a 1:2 dose ratio parenteral to oral. Switching From Other Chronic Opioids: Use caution; see PI for dosing details.

HOW SUPPLIED: Oral Concentrate: 10mg/mL; Tab: 5mg, 10mg, 40mg; Tab, Dispersible: 40mg

CONTRAINDICATIONS: Respiratory depression. Acute bronchial asthma or hypercarbia. Paralytic ileus.

WARNINGS/PRECAUTIONS: Do not inject agent. Extreme caution if use narcotic antagonists in patients physically dependent on narcotics. Can cause respiratory depression and elevate CSF pressure. Caution with head injuries, acute asthma attacks, COPD, cor pulmonale, decreased respiratory reserve, pre-existing respiratory depression, hypoxia, or hypercapnia. Reduce initial dose in elderly, debilitated, severe hepatic or renal impairment, hypothyroidism, Addison's disease, prostatic hypertrophy, or urethral stricture. Risk of tolerance, dependence, and abuse may occur. Impairs physical and mental abilities. Ineffective in relieving anxiety. May mask symptoms of acute abdominal conditions. May produce hypotension.

ADVERSE REACTIONS: Lightheadedness, dizziness, sedation, sweating, nausea, vomiting.

INTERACTIONS: Concurrent μ-agonists (eg, pentazocine, nalaxone, buprenorphine), or St. John's wort may precipitate withdrawal. Decreased levels with CYP3A4 inducers (eg, rifampin). Increased levels with CYP3A4 inhibitors (eg, ketoconazole). Caution and reduce dose with CNS depressants (eg, tranquilizers, sedative-hypnotics, phenothiazines, TCAs, alcohol). MAOIs may cause severe reactions.

PREGNANCY: Category C, not for use in nursing.

MECHANISM OF ACTION: Synthetic opioid analgesic; μ-agonist. Produces actions similiar to morphine; acts on CNS and organs composed of smooth muscle. May also act as N-methyl-D-aspartate (NMDA) receptor antagonist.

PHARMACOKINETICS: Absorption: Bioavailability (36-100%); T_{max}=1-7.5 hrs; C_{max}=124-1255ng/mL. **Distribution:**V_d=1-8 L/kg; bound to $α_1$-acid glycoprotein (85-90%); secreted in saliva, breast milk, amniotic fluid, and umbilical cord plasma. **Metabolism:** Hepatic N-demethylation; CYP3A4, 2B6, 2C19 (major); 2C9, 2D6 (minor). **Elimination**: Urine, feces; $T_{1/2}$=7-59 hrs.

METHERGINE RX
methylergonovine maleate (Novartis)

THERAPEUTIC CLASS: Ergot alkaloid

INDICATIONS: Management after delivery of the placenta. To treat postpartum atony and hemorrhage. For subinvolution.

DOSAGE: *Adults:* (Inj) 0.2mg IM/IV after delivery of the anterior shoulder, placenta, or during puerperium. May be repeated q2-4h. (Tab) 0.2mg PO tid-qid in the puerperium. Max: 1 week.

HOW SUPPLIED: Inj: 0.2mg/mL; Tab: 0.2mg

CONTRAINDICATIONS: HTN, toxemia, pregnancy.

WARNINGS/PRECAUTIONS: Risk of hypertensive or cerebrovascular accidents with IV administration. Caution in sepsis, obliterative vascular disease, hepatic/renal involvement, and during second stage of labor.

ADVERSE REACTIONS: Seizures, headache, hypotension, nausea, vomiting, acute MI, dyspnea, hematuria, thrombophlebitis, water intoxication, hallucinations, leg cramps, dizziness, nasal congestion, diarrhea.

INTERACTIONS: Caution with vasoconstrictors or ergot alkaloids.

PREGNANCY: Category C, caution in nursing.

MECHANISM OF ACTION: Ergot alkaloid; acts directly on smooth muscle of uterus, increasing tone, rate and amplitude of rhythmic contractions; inducing rapid and sustained tetanic uterotonic effect, which shortens third stage of labor and reduces blood loss.

PHARMACOKINETICS: Absorption: (PO): Bioavailability (60%), C_{max}=3243pg/mL, T_{max}=1.12 hrs. (IM): Bioavailability (78%), C_{max}=5918pg/mL, T_{max}=0.41 hrs. **Distribution:** Rapid. V_d=56.1L. **Elimination:** $T_{1/2}$=3.39 hrs.

METHOTREXATE RX
methotrexate (Various)

> Should only be used by physicians whose knowledge and experience includes the use of antimetabolite therapy. Only for life-threatening neoplastic diseases, or with severe, recalcitrant, disabling disease not adequately responsive to other forms of therapy. Fetal death/congenital anomalies reported. Elimination reduced with impaired renal function, ascites, or pleural effusions; monitor carefully. Severe, sometimes fatal, bone marrow suppression and GI toxicity reported with concomitant NSAIDs. May cause hepatotoxicity, fibrosis, and cirrhosis (usually after prolonged use). Lung disease, malignant melanomas, and potentially fatal opportunistic infections may occur. Interrupt therapy if diarrhea or ulcerative colitis occur. May induce tumor lysis syndrome. Severe, occasionally fatal, skin reactions reported. Concomitant radiotherapy may increase risk of soft tissue necrosis and osteonecrosis.

OTHER BRAND NAMES: Rheumatrex (Stada)

THERAPEUTIC CLASS: Dihydrofolic acid reductase inhibitor

INDICATIONS: (Inj/PO) Treatment of neoplastic diseases (eg, acute lymphocytic leukemia, gestational choriocarcinoma, chorioadenoma destruens, hydatidiform mole, breast cancer, epidermoid cancer of the head and neck, advanced mycosis fungoides, lung cancer, advanced stage non-Hodgkin's lymphomas). Prophylaxis and treatment of meningeal leukemia, and maintenance with other chemotherapeutics. For prolonging relapse-free survival in non-metastatic osteosarcoma followed by leucovorin. Symptomatic control of severe, recalcitrant, disabling psoriasis. (PO) Management of rheumatoid arthritis (RA) or polyarticular-course juvenile rheumatoid arthritis (JRA) unresponsive to other therapies.

DOSAGE: *Adults:* Choriocarcinoma/Trophoblastic Disease: 15-30mg qd PO/IM for 5 days. May repeat 3-5 times as required with rest period of ≥1 week. Leukemia: Induction: 3.3mg/m² with prednisone 60mg/m² qd. Remission Maintenance: 15mg/m² PO/IM twice weekly or 2.5mg/kg IV every 14 days. Burkitt's Tumor: Stages I-II: 10-25mg/day PO for 4-8 days. Administer several courses with rest periods of 7-10 days in between. Lymphosarcoma: Stage III: 0.625-2.5mg/kg/day with other antitumor agents. Mycosis Fungoides: 5-50mg once weekly. If poor response, give 15-37.5mg twice weekly. Adjust dose based on response and hematologic monitoring. Osteosarcoma: Initial: 12g/m² IV, increase to 15g/m² if peak serum levels of 1000 micromolar not reached at end of infusion. Meningeal Leukemia: Dilute preservative free MTX to 1mg/mL. Give 12mg intrathecally at 2-5 day intervals. Psoriasis: Initial: 10-25mg PO/IM/IV weekly until response or use divided oral dose schedule, 2.5mg at 12 hr intervals for 3 doses. Titrate: Increase gradually until

M

optimal response. Maint: Reduce to lowest effective dose. Max: 30mg/week. Rheumatoid Arthritis: Initial: 7.5mg PO once weekly, or 2.5mg q12h for 3 doses given as a course once weekly. Titrate: Gradual increase. Max: 20mg weekly. After response, reduce dose to lowest effective amount of drug.
Pediatrics: Meningeal Leukemia: Dilute preservative free MTX to 1mg/mL. <1 yr: 6mg. 1 yr: 8mg. 2 yrs: 10mg. ≥3yrs: 12mg. Give intrathecally at 2-5 day intervals. JRA: 2-16 yrs: Initial: 10mg/m² once weekly. Adjust dose gradually to achieve optimal response.

HOW SUPPLIED: Inj: (Generic) (Methotrexate Sodium) 25mg/mL, 1g; Tab: (Generic) (Methotrexate) 2.5mg*; Tab: (Rheumatrex) (Methotrexate) 2.5mg* [Dose Pack 15mg, 4 x 6 tabs; 12.5mg, 4 x 5 tabs; 10mg, 4 x 4 tabs; 7.5mg, 4 x 3 tabs; 5mg, 4 x 2 tabs] *scored

CONTRAINDICATIONS: Pregnant women with psoriasis or RA (should be used in treatment of pregnant women with neoplastic diseases only when potential benefit outweighs risk), nursing mothers. Psoriasis or RA patients with alcoholism, alcoholic liver disease, chronic liver disease, immunodeficiency syndromes, and pre-existing blood dyscrasias (eg, bone marrow hypoplasia, leukopenia, thrombocytopenia, significant anemia).

WARNINGS/PRECAUTIONS: Monitor closely; toxicity may be related to dose and frequency of administration. When reactions do occur, doses should be reduced or discontinued and corrective measures should be taken. Avoid pregnancy if either partner is receiving therapy. Avoid intrathecal administration or high-dose therapy. Injection contains benzyl alcohol; avoid use in neonates (<1 month), may cause gasping syndrome.

ADVERSE REACTIONS: Ulcerative stomatitis, leukopenia, nausea, abdominal distress, malaise, fatigue, chills, fever, dizziness, decreased resistance to infection, anemia, photosensitivity, rash, pruritus, hepatotoxicity.

INTERACTIONS: See Black Box Warning. Avoid NSAIDs with high doses. Caution with nephrotoxic agents (eg, cisplatin), NSAIDs, probenecid, and highly protein bound drugs (eg, sulfonamides, phenytoin, phenylbutazone, salicylates). Oral antibiotics (eg, tetracycline, chloramphenicol) may decrease absorption or interfere with enterohepatic circulation. Penicillins may decrease clearance. Closely monitor with hepatotoxins (eg, azathioprine, retinoids, sulfasalazine). Folic acid may decrease response to MTX. TMP/SMZ may increase bone marrow suppression. May decrease theophylline clearance.

PREGNANCY: Category X, contraindicated in nursing.

MECHANISM OF ACTION: Dihydrofolic acid reductase inhibitor; interferes with DNA synthesis, repair, and cellular replication. MOA in rheumatoid arthritis not established; may affect immune function.

PHARMACOKINETICS: Absorption: (PO, Healthy) T_{max}=1-2 hrs. (IM) T_{max}=30-60 min. Oral administration resulted in different parameters according to disease state and dosing; refer to PI for further information. **Distribution:** (IV, Initial) V_d=0.18L/kg; (Steady state) V_d=0.4-0.8L/kg; plasma protein binding (50%); found in breast milk. **Metabolism:** Hepatic and intracellular; 7-hydroxymethotrexate (metabolite). **Elimination:** Renal (primary route), bile (≤10%). (Psoriasis, rheumatoid arthritis, low-dose chemotherapy at <30mg/m²) $T_{1/2}$=3-10 hrs; (High dose) $T_{1/2}$=8-15 hrs.

METHYCLOTHIAZIDE   RX
methyclothiazide (Various)

OTHER BRAND NAMES: Enduron (Abbott)

THERAPEUTIC CLASS: Thiazide diuretic

INDICATIONS: Adjunct therapy in edema associated with CHF, hepatic cirrhosis, renal dysfunction, corticosteroid and estrogen therapy. Management of hypertension.

DOSAGE: *Adults:* Edema: 2.5-10mg qd. Max: 10mg/dose. HTN: 2.5-5mg qd.

HOW SUPPLIED: Tab: 5mg* *scored

CONTRAINDICATIONS: Anuria, sulfonamide hypersensitivity.

WARNINGS/PRECAUTIONS: Caution in severe renal disease, liver dysfunction, electrolyte/fluid imbalance. Monitor electrolytes. Hyperuricemia, hyperglycemia, hypokalemia, hyponatremia, hypomagnesemia, hypercalcemia may occur. Increases in cholesterol and triglyceride levels reported. May exacerbate SLE. Sensitivity reactions reported. D/C prior to parathyroid test. Enhanced effects in post-sympathectomy patient.

ADVERSE REACTIONS: Headache, cramping, weakness, orthostatic hypotension, pancreatitis, hyperglycemia, hyperuricemia, electrolyte imbalance, blood dyscrasias, hypersensitivity reactions.

INTERACTIONS: Hypokalemia may develop with steroids or ACTH. May: 1) affect insulin requirements 2) decrease arterial responsiveness to norepinephrine 3) increase responsiveness to tubocurarine 4) potentiate other antihypertensives. Lithium toxicity

PREGNANCY: Category B, not for use in nursing.

MECHANISM OF ACTION: Thiazide diuretic; inhibits renal tubular reabsorption of electrolytes.

PHARMACOKINETICS: Absorption: Rapid. **Elimination:** Kidneys.

METHYLDOPA   RX
methyldopa (Various)

THERAPEUTIC CLASS: Central alpha-adrenergic agonist

INDICATIONS: Treatment of hypertension.

DOSAGE: *Adults:* Initial: 250mg bid-tid for 48 hrs. Adjust dose at intervals of not less than 2 days. Maint: 500mg-2g/day given bid-qid. Max: 3g/day. Concomitant Antihypertensives (other than thiazides): Initial: Limit to 500mg/day. Renal Impairment: May respond to lower doses.
Pediatrics: Initial: 10mg/kg/day given bid-qid. Max: 65mg/kg/day or 3g/day, whichever is less.

HOW SUPPLIED: Tab: 125mg, 250mg, 500mg

CONTRAINDICATIONS: Active hepatic disease, history of methyldopa associated liver disorder, concomitant MAOIs.

WARNINGS/PRECAUTIONS: Positive Coombs test, hemolytic anemia, and liver disorders may occur. Fever reported within the first 3 weeks of therapy. HTN has recurred after dialysis. Caution with liver disease or dysfunction. D/C if signs of heart failure, or involuntary choreoathetotic movements develop. Edema and weight gain reported. Blood count, Coombs test and LFTs prior to therapy and periodically thereafter.

ADVERSE REACTIONS: Sedation, headache, asthenia, edema/weight gain, hepatic disorders, vomiting, diarrhea, nausea, sore or "black" tongue, blood dyscrasias, BUN increase, gynecomastia, impotence.

INTERACTIONS: See Contraindications. May potentiate other antihypertensives. Anesthetics may need dose reduction. Monitor for lithium toxicity. Ferrous sulfate and ferrous gluconate may decrease bioavailability; avoid coadministration.

PREGNANCY: Category B, caution in nursing.

MECHANISM OF ACTION: Aromatic-aminoacid decarboxylase inhibitor; not established, antihypertensive effect probably due to metabolism to α-methylnorepinephrine, which lowers arterial pressure by stimulation of central inhibitory α-adrenergic receptors, false neurotransmission, and reduction of plasma renin activity.

PHARMACOKINETICS: Distribution: Crosses placenta, found in breast milk. **Metabolism:** Extensive. **Elimination:** Urine; $T_{1/2}$=105 min.

M

METHYLDOPA/HCTZ
methyldopa - hydrochlorothiazide (Various)

RX

> Not for initial therapy of HTN.

THERAPEUTIC CLASS: Central alpha-adrenergic agonist/thiazide diuretic

INDICATIONS: Treatment of HTN. Not for initial treatment.

DOSAGE: *Adults:* Initial: 250mg-15mg tab bid-tid, 250mg-25mg tab bid, or 500mg-30mg qd. Max: 50mg HCTZ/day or 3g methyldopa/day.

HOW SUPPLIED: Tab: (HCTZ-Methyldopa) 15mg-250mg, 25mg-250mg

CONTRAINDICATIONS: Active hepatic disease, anuria, sulfonamide allergy, concomitant MAOIs, history of methyldopa associated liver disorder.

WARNINGS/PRECAUTIONS: Positive Coombs test, hemolytic anemia, liver disorders, sensitivity reactions, hypokalemia, hyperuricemia, hyperglycemia, hypomagnesemia, hypercalcemia may occur. Fever reported within the first 3 weeks of therapy. HTN has recurred after dialysis. Caution with liver disease or dysfunction, severe renal disease. D/C if signs of heart failure, progressive renal dysfunction, or involuntary choreoathetotic movements develop. Edema and weight gain reported. Blood count, Coombs test and LFTs before therapy and periodically thereafter. Monitor electrolytes. May exacerbate or activate SLE. May increase cholesterol and TG levels. Enhanced effects in postsympathectomy patient.

ADVERSE REACTIONS: Weakness, asthenia, headache, pancreatitis, diarrhea, vomiting, constipation, nausea, blood dyscrasias, rash, electrolyte imbalance, renal failure, impotence, vertigo.

INTERACTIONS: See Contraindications. Potentiates orthostatic hypotension with alcohol, barbiturates, narcotics. Lithium toxicity. Adjust antidiabetic drugs. NSAIDs decrease diuretic effects. Reduce dose of anesthetics. Ferrous sulfate and ferrous gluconate may decrease bioavailability; avoid coadministration. May potentiate nondepolarizing skeletal muscle relaxants, antihypertensives. May decrease response to pressor amines. Corticosteroids, ACTH intensify electrolyte depletion. Impaired absorption with cholestyramine, colestipol.

PREGNANCY: Category C, not for use in nursing.

MECHANISM OF ACTION: Methyldopa; central α-adrenergic agonist. Aromatic-amino-acid decarboxylase inhibitor; lowers arterial pressure by stimulating central inhibitory α-adrenergic receptor, false neurotransmission, and/or reduction of plasma renin activity. HCTZ: thiazide diuretic. Affects renal tubular mechanism of electrolyte reabsorption, directly increasing excretion of sodium salt and chloride.

PHARMACOKINETICS: Distribution: Methyldopa: Crosses placental barrier, appears in breast milk and cord blood. HCTZ: Crosses placenta, excreted in breast milk. **Metabolism:** Methyldopa: extensive. **Elimination:** Methyldopa: Urine (70%); $T_{1/2}$=105 min; HCTZ: Urine (61% unchanged); $T_{1/2}$=5.6-14.8 hrs.

METHYLDOPATE HCL
methyldopate HCL (American Regent)

RX

THERAPEUTIC CLASS: Central alpha-adrenergic agonist

INDICATIONS: Treatment of hypertension and hypertensive crises.

DOSAGE: *Adults:* 250-500mg IV q6h as needed. Max: 1gm q6h. Elderly/Renal Dysfunction: May reduce dose. Switch to oral therapy once BP is controlled. *Pediatrics:* 20-40mg/kg/day IV given q6h. Max: 65mg/kg/day or 3 g/day, whichever is less. Switch to oral therapy once BP is controlled.

HOW SUPPLIED: Inj: 50mg/mL

CONTRAINDICATIONS: Hypersensitivity to sulfites, active hepatic disease, liver disorders previously associated with methyldopa therapy, concomitant MAOIs.

WARNINGS/PRECAUTIONS: Positive Coombs test, hemolytic anemia, and liver disorders may occur. Fever reported within the first 3 weeks of therapy. HTN has recurred after dialysis. Caution with liver disease or dysfunction. D/C if signs of heart failure develop. Edema and weight gain reported. Blood count, Coombs test and LFTs prior to therapy and periodically thereafter. Caution with cerebrovascular disease.

ADVERSE REACTIONS: Sedation, headache, asthenia, weakness, edema, weight gain, liver disorders, vomiting, diarrhea, nausea, sore or "black" tongue, blood dyscrasias, BUN increase, gynecomastia, impotence.

INTERACTIONS: See Contraindications. May potentiate other antihypertensives. Anesthetics may need dose reduction. May increase lithium levels. Ferrous sulfate and ferrous gluconate may decrease bioavailability; avoid coadministration.

PREGNANCY: Category C, caution in nursing.

MECHANISM OF ACTION: Aromatic-amino-acid decarboxylase inhibitor; not established, antihypertensive effect probably due to metabolism to α-methyl-norepinephrine, which lowers arterial pressure by stimulating central inhibitory α-adrenergic receptors, false neurotransmission, and/or reduction of plasma renin activity.

PHARMACOKINETICS: Distribution: Crosses placental barrier; appears in breast milk and cord blood. **Metabolism:** Extensive. **Elimination:** Urine (49%); $T_{1/2}$=90-127 min.

METHYLIN
methylphenidate HCL (Mallinckrodt) CII

OTHER BRAND NAMES: Methylin ER (Mallinckrodt)
THERAPEUTIC CLASS: Sympathomimetic amine
INDICATIONS: Treatment of attention deficit disorder and narcolepsy.
DOSAGE: *Adults:* (Sol/Tab/Tab, Chewable) 10-60mg/day given bid-tid 30-45 min ac. Take last dose before 6 pm if insomnia occurs. (Tab, Extended-Release) May use in place of immediate release tabs when 8 hr dose corresponds to titrated 8 hr immediate release dose. Swallow whole; do not chew or crush.
Pediatrics: ≥ 6 yrs: (Sol/Tab/Tab, Chewable) Initial: 5mg bid before breakfast and lunch. Titrate: Increase gradually by 5-10mg weekly. Max: 60mg/day. (Tab, Extended-Release) May be use in place of immediate release tabs when 8 hr dose corresponds to titrated 8 hr immediate release dose. Swallow whole; do not chew or crush. Reduce dose or d/c if paradoxical aggravation of symptoms occur. D/C if no improvement after appropriate dose adjustment over 1 month.
HOW SUPPLIED: Sol: 5mg/5mL [500mL], 10mg/5mL [500mL]; Tab: 5mg, 10mg, 20mg; Tab, Chewable: 2.5mg, 5mg, 10mg; Tab, Extended-Release: 10mg, 20mg
CONTRAINDICATIONS: Marked anxiety, tension, and agitation; glaucoma; motor tics or family history or diagnosis of Tourette's syndrome; during or within 14 days of MAOI use.
WARNINGS/PRECAUTIONS: Monitor growth in children. Not for severe depression or fatigue. May exacerbate symptoms of behavior disturbance or thought disorder in psychotic children. Caution when using stimulants to treat patients with comorbid bipolar disorder because of concern for possible induction of mixed/manic episode in such patients. Stimulants at usual doses can cause treatment emergent psychotic or manic symptoms (hallucinations, delusional thinking, mania) in children and adolescents without prior history of psychotic illness. Aggressive behavior or hostility has been reported in clinical trials and the postmarketing experience of some medications indicated for the treatment of ADHD. May lower seizure threshold, especially in known EEG abnormalities. Caution with HTN, heart failure, recent MI, ventricular arrhythmia, or emotionally-unstable patients. Monitor during withdrawal. Visual disturbances may occur (rare). Monitor CBC, differential, and platelets with

prolonged use. Periodically d/c to assess condition. Avoid with serious structural cardiac abnormalities, cardiomyopathy, serious heart rhythm abnormalities, CAD, or other serious cardiac problems. Caution in emotionally unstable patients with history of drug dependence or alcoholism.

ADVERSE REACTIONS: Nervousness, insomnia, hypersensitivity reactions, anorexia, nausea, dizziness, palpitations, headache, dyskinesia, drowsiness, BP and pulse changes, tachycardia, angina, arrhythmia, abdominal pain.

INTERACTIONS: May decrease hypotensive effect of guanethidine. Caution with pressor agents. Avoid during or within 14 days of MAOI use. Potentiates anticoagulants, anticonvulsants (phenobarbital, diphenylhydantoin, primidone), phenylbutazone, TCAs (imipramine, clomipramine, desipramine). Caution with α_2 agonists (eg, clonidine); serious adverse reactions reported with concurrent use.

PREGNANCY: Category C, caution in nursing.

MECHANISM OF ACTION: CNS stimulant; activates the brain-stem arousal system and cortex to produce its stimulant effect. Blocks the reuptake of norepinephrine and dopamine into the presynaptic neuron and increases the release of monoamines into the extraneuronal space.

PHARMACOKINETICS: Absorption: (20mg, Sol) C_{max}=9ng/mL, T_{max}=1-2 hrs. **Metabolism:** Deesterification to α-phenyl-piperidine acetic acid. **Elimination:** Urine (90%), $T_{1/2}$=2.7 hrs (sol), 3 hrs (chewable).

METOCLOPRAMIDE RX
metoclopramide HCL (Various)

OTHER BRAND NAMES: Reglan Injection (Baxter) - Reglan (Schwarz)

THERAPEUTIC CLASS: Dopamine antagonist/prokinetic

INDICATIONS: (PO) Symptomatic treatment of gastroesophageal reflux in patients who fail to respond to conventional therapy. (Inj, PO) Symptomatic relief of diabetic gastroparesis. (Inj) Prevention of post-op or chemo-induced nausea/vomiting. Diagnostic aid during radiological examination and facilitates intubation of small intestine.

DOSAGE: *Adults:* GERD: PO: 10-15mg qid 30 min ac and hs. Elderly: 5 mg qid. Max: 12 weeks of therapy. Intermittent Symptoms: Up to 20mg as single dose prior to provoking situation. Gastroparesis: 10mg PO 30 min ac and hs for 2-8 weeks. Severe Gastroparesis: May give same doses IV/IM for up to 10 days if needed. Antiemetic: (Post-op) 10-20mg IM near end of surgery. (Chemotherapy-Induced) 1-2mg/kg 30 min before chemotherapy then q2h for 2 doses, then q3h for 3 doses. Give 2mg/kg for highly emetogenic drugs for initial 2 doses. Small Bowel Intubation/Radiological Exam: 10mg IV as single dose. CrCl <40mL/min: 50% of normal dose.
Pediatrics: Small Bowel Intubation: 6-14 yrs: 2.5-5mg IV single dose. <6 yrs: 0.1mg/kg IV single dose. CrCl <40mL/min: 50% of normal dose.

HOW SUPPLIED: Inj: 5mg/mL; Syr: 5mg/5mL; Tab: 5mg, 10mg* *scored

CONTRAINDICATIONS: Where GI mobility stimulation is dangerous (eg, perforation, obstruction, hemorrhage), pheochromocytoma, seizure disorder, concomitant drugs that cause EPS effects.

WARNINGS/PRECAUTIONS: Caution with HTN, Parkinson's disease, depression. EPS, tardive dyskinesia, Parkinsonian-like symptoms, neuroleptic malignant syndrome reported. Administer IV injection slowly. Risk of developing fluid retention and volume overload especially with cirrhosis or CHF; d/c if these occur. May increase pressure of suture lines.

ADVERSE REACTIONS: Restlessness, drowsiness, fatigue, EPS effects (acute dystonic reactions), galactorrhea, hyperprolactinemia, hypotension, arrhythmia, diarrhea, dizziness, urinary frequency.

INTERACTIONS: See Contraindications. May decrease gastric absorption of drugs (eg, digoxin) and increase intestinal absorption of drugs (eg, APAP, tetracycline, levodopa, ethanol, and cyclosporine). Additive sedation with alcohol, hypnotics, narcotics, or tranquilizers. Caution with MAOIs. Antagonized by anticholinergics, narcotics. Insulin dose or timing of dose may need adjustment to prevent hypoglycemia.

PREGNANCY: Category B, caution with nursing.

MECHANISM OF ACTION: Dopamine antagonist/promotility agent; not established, stimulates motility of upper GI tract, increases tone of gastric contractions, relaxes pyloric sphincter and duodenal bulb, increases peristalsis of duodenum and jejunum resulting in increased gastric emptying and intestinal transit, increases resting tone of LES, antagonizes central and peripheral dopamine receptors blocking stimulation of CTZ.

PHARMACOKINETICS: Absorption: Rapid; absolute bioavailability (80%). (Peds) C_{max} at tenth dose =56.8mcg/L, T_{max} =2.5 hrs. (Adults) T_{max}=1-2 hrs. **Distribution:** Plasma protein binding (30%); (adults)V_d=3.5L/kg; (peds) V_d =4.4L/kg. **Elimination:** Urine; (adults) $T_{1/2}$=5-6 hrs, (peds) $T_{1/2}$=4.1 hrs.

METROGEL RX
metronidazole (Galderma)

OTHER BRAND NAMES: MetroLotion (Galderma) - MetroCream (Galderma)

THERAPEUTIC CLASS: Imidazole antibiotic

INDICATIONS: Treatment of inflammatory papules and pustules of rosacea.

DOSAGE: *Adults:* (Cre, Gel 0.75%, Lot) Wash affected area(s) then apply bid, am and pm. (Gel 1%) Wash affected area(s) then apply qd.

HOW SUPPLIED: Cre: 0.75% [45g]; Gel: 0.75%, 1% [45g]; Lot: 0.75% [59mL]

WARNINGS/PRECAUTIONS: Avoid eye contact. Decrease frequency or d/c if skin irritation occurs. Caution with blood dyscrasias.

ADVERSE REACTIONS: Burning, skin irritation, dryness, redness, metallic taste, tingling/numbness of extremities, nausea.

INTERACTIONS: Oral metronidazole may potentiate warfarin; unknown effect with topical formulation.

PREGNANCY: Category B, not for use in nursing.

MECHANISM OF ACTION: Imidazole antibiotic; not established. Suspected to have an anti-inflammatory effect.

PHARMACOKINETICS: Absorption: (1g of 1% Gel) C_{max}=32ng/mL, AUC_{0-24}=595ng•hr/mL, T_{max}=6-10 hrs. (1g of 0.75% Lot) C_{max}=96ng/mL, AUC_{0-24}=962ng•hr/mL.

METROGEL-VAGINAL RX
metronidazole (Graceway)

THERAPEUTIC CLASS: Imidazole antibacterial

INDICATIONS: Treatment of bacterial vaginosis.

DOSAGE: *Adults:* One applicatorful intravaginally qd-bid for 5 days. For once daily dosing, administer at bedtime .

HOW SUPPLIED: Gel: 0.75% [70g]

CONTRAINDICATIONS: Hypersensitivity to other nitroimidazole derivatives.

WARNINGS/PRECAUTIONS: Caution with CNS or severe hepatic disease. D/C if abnormal neurologic signs appear. Avoid vaginal intercourse during therapy. May develop *Candida* vaginitis. May interfere with lab tests (ALT, SGPT, AST, SGOT, LDH, triglycerides, and glucose hexokinase).

ADVERSE REACTIONS: *Candida* cervicitis/vaginitis, vaginal discharge, pelvic discomfort, nausea, vomiting, headache, vulva/vaginal irritation, GI discomfort, change in WBC count.

INTERACTIONS: May potentiate warfarin, other anticoagulants, and lithium. Cimetidine may potentiate metronidazole. Avoid alcohol; possible disulfiram-like reaction may occur. Do not administer gel within 2 weeks of discontinuing disulfiram therapy.

PREGNANCY: Category B, not for use in nursing.

MECHANISM OF ACTION: Antibacterial/antiprotozoal agent: mechanism not been established. Suspected that 5-nitro group of metronidazole is reduced by metabolically active anaerobes and the reduced form of the drug interacts with bacterial DNA.

PHARMACOKINETICS: Absorption: C_{max}=237ng/mL; T_{max}=6-12 hrs.
Distribution: Found in breast milk and crosses placental barrier.

MEVACOR   RX
lovastatin (Merck)

THERAPEUTIC CLASS: HMG-CoA reductase inhibitor

INDICATIONS: To reduce risk of MI, unstable angina, and coronary revascularization procedures in patients without symptomatic coronary disease, average to moderately elevated total-C and LDL-C, and below average HDL-C. To slow coronary atherosclerosis progression in patients with coronary heart disease to reduce total-C and LDL-C. Adjunct to diet to lower total-C and LDL-C in primary hypercholesterolemia (Types IIa and IIb). Adjunct to diet to lower total-C, LDL-C and apolipoprotein B in adolescents at least 1-yr postmenarchal with heterozygous familial hypercholesterolemia.

DOSAGE: *Adults:* Initial: 20mg qd at dinner (10mg/day if need LDL-C reduction <20%). Usual: 10-80mg/day given qd or bid. May adjust every 4 weeks. Max: 80mg/day. Concomitant Cyclosporine: Initial: 10mg/day. Max: 20mg/day. Fibrates/Niacin (≥1g/day): Max: 20mg/day. Concomitant Amiodarone/ Verapamil: Max: 40mg/day. CrCl <30mL/min: Consider dose increase of >20mg/day carefully and implement cautiously.
Pediatrics: Heterozygous Familial Hypercholesterolemia: 10-17 yrs (at least 1-yr postmenarchal): Initial: If <20% LDL-C Reduction Needed: 10mg qd. If ≥20% LDL-C Reduction Needed: 20mg qd. May adjust every 4 weeks. Max: 40mg/day. Concomitant Cyclosporine: Initial: 10mg/day. Max: 20mg/day. Fibrates/Niacin (≥1g/day): Max: 20mg/day. Concomitant Amiodarone/ Verapamil: Max: 40mg/day. CrCl <30mL/min: Consider dose increase of >20mg/day carefully and implement cautiously.

HOW SUPPLIED: Tab: 20mg, 40mg

CONTRAINDICATIONS: Active liver disease, unexplained persistent elevations of serum transaminases, pregnancy, nursing mothers.

WARNINGS/PRECAUTIONS: May increase serum transaminases and CPK levels; consider in differential diagnosis of chest pain. D/C if AST or ALT ≥3x ULN persist, or if myopathy diagnosed or suspected. Monitor LFTs prior to therapy, at 6 weeks, 12 weeks, then periodically or with dose elevation. Caution with heavy alcohol use and/or history of hepatic disease. Caution with dose escalation in renal insufficiency. Less effective with homozygous familial hypercholesterolemia. Rhabdomyolysis (rare), myopathy reported. D/C a few days before elective major surgery and when any major acute medical or surgical condition supervenes.

ADVERSE REACTIONS: Headache, constipation, flatulence, dizziness, rash, elevated transaminases or CK levels, GI upset, blurred vision.

INTERACTIONS: Increased risk of myopathy with CYP3A4 inhibitors (eg, cyclosporine, itraconazole, ketoconazole, erythromycin, clarithromycin, telithromycin, protease inhibitors, nefazodone, >1 quart/day of grapefruit juice), verapamil, amiodarone, fibrates (eg, gemfibrozil), danazol, and ≥1g/day of niacin. Monitor anticoagulants. Caution with drugs that diminish levels or activity of steroid hormones (eg, ketoconazole, spironolactone, cimetidine).

PREGNANCY: Category X, not for use in nursing.

MECHANISM OF ACTION: HMG-CoA reductase inhibitor; causes reduction of VLDL-C concentration and induction of LDL-receptor, leading to reduced production and/or increased catabolism of LDL-C. Also causes lowering of apolipoprotein B, component of LDL particles, consequently leading to reduction in concentration of circulating LDL.

PHARMACOKINETICS: Absorption: T_{max}=2-4 hrs. **Distribution:** Plasma protein binding (>95%). **Metabolism:** Liver (first pass); CYP450 3A4. β-hydroxyacid, 6´-hydroxy derivative (major active metabolites). **Elimination:** Urine (10%), feces (83%).

MEXILETINE   RX
mexiletine HCL (Various)

THERAPEUTIC CLASS: Class IB antiarrhythmic

INDICATIONS: Treatment of life-threatening ventricular arrhythmias.

DOSAGE: *Adults:* Initial: 200mg q8h when rapid control is not essential. Titrate: Adjust by 50-100mg, not less than every 2-3 days. Usual: 200-300mg q8h. Max: 1200mg/day. If control with ≤300mg q8h, then may divide daily dose and give q12h. Max: 450mg q12h. For Rapid Control: LD: 400mg, then 200mg in 8 hrs. Transfer from Class I Oral Agents: Initial: 200mg and titrate as above, 6-12 hrs after last quinidine sulfate or disopyramide dose, 3-6 hrs after last procainamide dose, or 8-12 hrs after last tocainide dose. Severe Hepatic Disease: May need lower dose. Take with food or antacid.

HOW SUPPLIED: Cap: 150mg, 200mg, 250mg

CONTRAINDICATIONS: Cardiogenic shock, pre-existing 2nd- or 3rd-degree AV block (without a pacemaker).

WARNINGS/PRECAUTIONS: Reserve for life-threatening arrhythmias. May treat patients with 2nd- or 3rd-degree AV block with a pacemaker; monitor continuously. Can worsen arrhythmias. Caution with hypotension, severe CHF, seizure disorder, hepatic impairment, sinus node dysfunction, or intraventricular conduction abnormalities. Leukopenia, agranulocytosis, and abnormal LFTs reported. Monitor ECG.

ADVERSE REACTIONS: Coordination difficulties, tremor, GI distress, lightheadedness.

INTERACTIONS: Avoid drugs or diet regimens that may alter urinary pH. Enzyme inducers (eg, rifampin, phenobarbital, phenytoin) lower plasma levels. May increase theophylline levels. Decreases caffeine clearance. Cimetidine may alter levels.

PREGNANCY: Category C, not for use in nursing.

MECHANISM OF ACTION: Class IB antiarrhythmic; local anesthetic; inhibits inward Na^+ current, thus reducing the action potential rise rate, and decreases the effective refractory period in Purkinje fibers.

PHARMACOKINETICS: Absorption: Well absorbed; T_{max}=2-3 hrs. **Distribution:** Plasma protein binding (50-60%), V_d=5-7L/kg. Found in breast milk. **Metabolism:** Liver, through CYP2D6 and CYP1A2 metabolism, aromatic/aliphatic hydroxylation, dealkylation, deamination, N-oxidation, and glucuronidation pathways. P-hydroxymexiletine, hydroxy-methylmexiletine, and N-hydroxy-mexiletine (major metabolites). **Elimination:** Urine, (10% unchanged); $T_{1/2}$=10-12hrs.

MIACALCIN   RX
calcitonin-salmon (Novartis)

THERAPEUTIC CLASS: Hormonal bone resorption inhibitor

INDICATIONS: (Inj) Treatment of Paget's disease, hypercalcemia, and postmenopausal osteoporosis. (Spray) Treatment of postmenopausal osteoporosis in females >5yrs postmenopause.

DOSAGE: *Adults:* (Inj) Paget's Disease: Usual: 100 IU IM/SQ qd. Hypercalcemia: Initial: 4 IU/kg IM/SQ q12h. Titrate: May increase to 8 IU/kg q12h after 1-2 days, then to 8 IU/kg q6h after 2 days if unsatisfactory response. Osteoporosis: (Inj) 100 IU IM/SQ every other day. If >2mL, use IM injection. (Spray) 200 IU qd intranasally. Alternate nostrils daily. Take with supplemental calcium and vitamin D for postmenopausal osteoporosis.

M

HOW SUPPLIED: Inj: 200 IU/mL; Nasal Spray: 200 IU/inh [2mL 2^s]

WARNINGS/PRECAUTIONS: Possibility of systemic allergic reactions. Monitor urine sediment periodically with chronic use. If nasal mucosa ulceration occurs, d/c until healed. D/C if severe ulceration of the nasal mucosa occurs. Perform periodic nasal exams. Monitor drug effects.

ADVERSE REACTIONS: (Inj) Nausea, vomiting, injection site inflammation, flushing of face or hands, nocturia, ear lobe pruritus, poor appetite, abdominal pain. (Spray) Nasal symptoms, back pain, headache, arthralgia, epistaxis.

INTERACTIONS: Prior diphosphonate use with Paget's disease may reduce anti-resorptive response.

PREGNANCY: Category C, not for use in nursing.

MECHANISM OF ACTION: Hormonal bone resorption inhibitor; actions on bone not fully established. Calcitonin receptors have been found in osteoclasts and osteoblasts. Initially causes a marked transient inhibition of the ongoing bone resorptive process. Prolonged use causes a smaller decrease in the rate of bone resorption. Thought to be associated with decrease in number of osteoclasts as well as decrease in resorptive activity.

PHARMACOKINETICS: Absorption: (Intranasal): Rapid, T_{max}=31-39 min; (Inj): T_{max}=16-25 min. **Elimination:** Urine; (Intranasal): $T_{1/2}$=43 min.

MICARDIS   RX
telmisartan (Boehringer Ingelheim)

Can cause death/injury to developing fetus during 2nd and 3rd trimesters. Stop therapy if pregancy detected.

THERAPEUTIC CLASS: Angiotensin II receptor antagonist

INDICATIONS: Treatment of hypertension, alone or with other antihypertensives.

DOSAGE: *Adults:* Initial: 40mg qd. Usual: 20-80mg/day. May add diuretic if need additional BP reduction after 80mg/day.

HOW SUPPLIED: Tab: 20mg, 40mg*, 80mg* *scored

WARNINGS/PRECAUTIONS: Can cause fetal injury/death. Correct volume or salt depletion before therapy. Changes in renal function may occur; caution with renal artery stenosis, severe CHF. Closely monitor with biliary obstructive disorders or hepatic dysfunction.

ADVERSE REACTIONS: Upper respiratory infection, back pain, sinusitis, diarrhea, bradycardia, eosinophilia, thrombocytopenia, increased uric acid, increased CPK, increased sweating, abnormal hepatic function/liver disorder, renal impairment including acute renal failure, anemia, edema and cough.

INTERACTIONS: Increases digoxin levels. May alter warfarin levels.

PREGNANCY: Category C (1st trimester) and D (2nd and 3rd trimesters), not for use in nursing

MECHANISM OF ACTION: Angiotensin II receptor antagonist; blocks the vasoconstrictor and aldosterone-secreting effects of angiotensin II by selectively blocking the binding of angiotensin II to the AT_1 receptor.

PHARMACOKINETICS: Absorption: Absolute bioavailability (40mg,160mg), =42%, 58%; T_{max}=0.5-1 hr. **Distribution:** Plasma protein binding (>99.5%); V_d=500L. **Metabolism:** Conjugation. **Elimination**: Feces (>97%), urine; $T_{1/2}$=24 hrs.

MICARDIS HCT   RX
telmisartan - hydrochlorothiazide (Boehringer Ingelheim)

Can cause death/injury to developing fetus during 2nd and 3rd trimesters. Stop therapy if pregnancy detected.

THERAPEUTIC CLASS: Angiotensin II receptor antagonist/thiazide diuretic

INDICATIONS: Treatment of hypertension. Not for initial therapy.

DOSAGE: *Adults:* If BP not controlled on 80mg telmisartan, or 25mg HCTZ/day, or controlled on 25mg HCTZ/day but serum K+ decreased, 80mg-12.5mg tab qd. Titrate/Max: If uncontrolled after 2-4 weeks, increase to 160mg-25mg. Biliary Obstruction/Hepatic Dysfunction: Initial: 40mg-12.5mg tab qd; monitor closely.

HOW SUPPLIED: Tab: (HCTZ-Telmisartan) 12.5mg-40mg, 12.5mg-80mg, 25mg-80mg

CONTRAINDICATIONS: Anuria, sulfonamide hypersensitivity.

WARNINGS/PRECAUTIONS: Can cause fetal injury/death. Correct volume or salt depletion before therapy. Caution with hepatic or renal dysfunction, biliary obstructive disorders, renal artery stenosis, severe CHF, history of allergies, and asthma. May exacerbate or activate SLE. Monitor serum electrolytes. Avoid if CrCl ≤30mL/min. Hyperuricemia, hyperglycemia, hypokalemia, hypomagnesemia, hypercalcemia may occur. Enhanced effects in post-sympathectomy patient. May increase cholesterol and triglyceride levels.

ADVERSE REACTIONS: Dizziness, fatigue, sinusitis, upper respiratory infection, diarrhea, bradycardia, eosinophilia, thrombocytopenia, uric acid increased, abnormal hepatic function/liver disorder, renal impairment including acute renal failure, anemia, and increased CPK.

INTERACTIONS: Potentiates orthostatic hypotension with alcohol, barbiturates, and narcotics. Adjust insulin and antidiabetic drugs. Impaired absorption with cholestyramine, colestipol. Corticosteroids and ACTH deplete electrolytes. May decrease response to pressor amines. Potentiates other antihypertensives. May increase responsiveness to skeletal muscle relaxants. Risk of lithium toxicity. NSAIDs decrease diuretic effects. Increases digoxin levels. May alter warfarin levels.

PREGNANCY: Category C (1st trimester) and D (2nd and 3rd trimesters), not for use in nursing.

MECHANISM OF ACTION: Telmisartan: Angiotensin II receptor antagonist; blocks the vasoconstrictor and aldosterone-secreting effects of angiotensin II by selectively blocking the binding of angiotensin II to the AT_1 receptor in vascular smooth muscle and adrenal gland. HCTZ: Thiazide diuretic; affects renal tubular mechanism of electrolyte reabsorption, directly increasing excretion of sodium salt and chloride.

PHARMACOKINETICS: Absorption: Telmisartan: T_{max}=0.5-1 hr; Absolute bioavailability =42% (40mg), 58% (160mg). **Distribution:** Telmisartan: Plasma protein binding (≥99.5%); V_d= 500L. HCTZ: Crosses the placenta and excreted in breast milk. **Metabolism:** Telmisartan: Conjugation. **Elimination:** Telmisartan: $T_{1/2}$=24 hrs; feces (≥97%), urine. HCTZ: Urine (61%, unchanged); $T_{1/2}$=5.6-14.8 hrs.

Micro-K

RX

potassium chloride (Ther-Rx)

THERAPEUTIC CLASS: K+ supplement

INDICATIONS: (For those unable to tolerate liquid or effervescent potassium preparations). Treatment and prevention of hypokalemia with or without metabolic alkalosis. Treatment of digitalis intoxication and hypokalemic familial periodic paralysis.

DOSAGE: *Adults:* Prevention: 20mEq/day. Hypokalemia: 40-100mEq/day. Divide dose if >20mEq. Take with meal and full glass of water or liquid. May sprinkle on soft food; swallow without chewing.

HOW SUPPLIED: Cap, Extended-Release: 8mEq, 10mEq

CONTRAINDICATIONS: Hyperkalemia, esophageal ulceration, delay in GI passage (from structural, pathological, pharmacologic causes), cardiac patients with esophageal compression due to enlarged left atrium.

WARNINGS/PRECAUTIONS: Potentially fatal hyperkalemia may occur. Extreme caution with acidosis, cardiac and renal disease; monitor ECG and electrolytes. Hypokalemia with metabolic acidosis should be treated with an alkalinizing potassium salt (eg, potassium bicarbonate, potassium citrate). May produce ulcerative or stenotic GI lesions.

ADVERSE REACTIONS: Hyperkalemia, GI effects (obstruction, bleeding, ulceration), nausea, vomiting, abdominal pain, diarrhea.

INTERACTIONS: Risk of hyperkalemia with ACE inhibitors (eg, captopril, enalapril), K⁺-sparing diuretics, and K⁺ supplements. Contraindicated with anticholinergic agents due to possible delay in tablet passage through GI tract.

PREGNANCY: Category C, safe for use in nursing.

MECHANISM OF ACTION: K⁺ supplement; helps in maintenance of intracellular tonicity, transmission of nerve impulses, contraction of cardiac, skeletal, and smooth muscle, and maintenance of normal renal function.

MICRONASE   RX
glyburide (Pharmacia & Upjohn)

THERAPEUTIC CLASS: Sulfonylurea (2nd generation)

INDICATIONS: Adjunct to diet and exercise, to improve glycemic control in type 2 diabetes mellitus. May use in combination with metformin.

DOSAGE: *Adults:* Initial: 2.5-5mg qd with breakfast or 1st main meal; give 1.25mg if sensitive to hypoglycemia. Titrate: Increase by no more than 2.5mg/day at weekly intervals. Maint: 1.25-20mg given qd or in divided doses. Max: 20mg/day. May give bid with >10mg/day. Renal or Hepatic Disease/Elderly/Debilitated/Malnourished/Adrenal or Pituitary Insufficiency: Initial: 1.25mg qd. Transfer From Other Oral Antidiabetic Agents: Initial: 2.5-5mg/day. Switch From Insulin: If <20 U/day: 2.5-5mg qd. If 20-40 U/day: 5mg qd. If >40 U/day, decrease dose by 50% and give 5mg qd. Titrate: Progressive withdrawal of insulin, and increase by 1.25-2.5mg/day every 2-10 days. Concomitant Metformin: Add glyburide gradually to max dose of metformin monotherapy after 4 weeks if needed.

HOW SUPPLIED: Tab: 1.25mg*, 2.5mg*, 5mg* *scored

CONTRAINDICATIONS: Diabetic ketoacidosis, and as sole therapy for type 1 DM.

WARNINGS/PRECAUTIONS: Increased risk of cardiovascular mortality. Risk of hypoglycemia, especially with renal and hepatic disease, elderly, debilitated or malnourished patients, and those with adrenal or pituitary insufficiency. May need to d/c and give insulin with stress (eg, fever, trauma). Secondary failure may occur. D/C if jaundice, hepatitis, or persistent skin reaction occur. Hematologic reactions and hyponatremia reported.

ADVERSE REACTIONS: Hypoglycemia, nausea, epigastric fullness, heartburn, allergic skin reactions, disulfiram-like reactions (rarely), hyponatremia, liver function abnormalities, photosensitivity reactions.

INTERACTIONS: Hypoglycemia potentiated by alcohol, NSAIDs, miconazole, fluoroquinolones, highly protein-bound drugs, salicylates, sulfonamides, chloramphenicol, probenecid, coumarins, MAOIs, and β-blockers. Risk of hyperglycemia with diuretics, corticosteroids, phenothiazines, thyroid products, estrogens, oral contraceptives, phenytoin, nicotinic acid, sympathomimetics, CCBs, and INH. β-blockers may mask hypoglycemia. Disulfiram-like reactions (rarely) with alcohol.

PREGNANCY: Category B, not for use in nursing.

MECHANISM OF ACTION: Sulfonylurea; lowers blood glucose acutely by stimulating the release of insulin from the pancreas.

PHARMACOKINETICS: Absorption: T_{max}=4 hrs. **Distribution:** Serum protein binding (extensive). **Metabolism:** 4-trans-hydroxy derivative (major metabolite). **Elimination:** $T_{1/2}$=10 hrs; bile (50%), urine (50%).

MICRONOR
RX

norethindrone (Ortho-McNeil)

OTHER BRAND NAMES: Camila (Barr) - Errin (Barr)

THERAPEUTIC CLASS: Progestogen

INDICATIONS: Prevention of pregnancy.

DOSAGE: *Adults:* 1 tab qd without interruption (continuous regimen) on 1st day of menstrual period. If fully nursing, start 6 weeks postpartum. If partially nursing, start 3 weeks postpartum.

HOW SUPPLIED: Tab: 0.35mg

CONTRAINDICATIONS: Pregnancy, breast carcinoma, undiagnosed abnormal genital bleeding, benign or malignant liver tumors, acute liver disease.

WARNINGS/PRECAUTIONS: Avoid smoking. Perform annual physical exam. Not for use before menarche. May affect certain endocrine tests (eg, sex hormone binding globulin, thyroxine binding globulin). Monitor glucose tolerance in prediabetics and diabetics. May alter lipid metabolism. May increase risk of breast cancer and hepatic adenomas. May cause irregular menstrual patterns. Delayed follicular atresia/ovarian cysts and ectopic pregnancy may occur. D/C with recurrent migraines or severe headaches.

ADVERSE REACTIONS: Menstrual irregularities, frequent or irregular bleeding, headache, breast tenderness, nausea, dizziness, androgenic effects (rare).

INTERACTIONS: Reduced efficacy with hepatic enzyme inducers (eg, rifampin, phenytoin, carbamazepine, barbiturates).

PREGNANCY: Not for use in pregnancy, caution in nursing.

MECHANISM OF ACTION: Progestogen oral contraceptive: suppresses ovulation. Thickens cervical mucus to inhibit sperm penetration, lowers midcycle LH and FSH peaks, slows movement of ovum through fallopian tubes, and alters endometrium.

PHARMACOKINETICS: Absorption: T$_{max}$=2 hrs. **Distribution:** Rapid.

MICROZIDE
RX

hydrochlorothiazide (Watson)

THERAPEUTIC CLASS: Thiazide diuretic

INDICATIONS: Management of hypertension.

DOSAGE: *Adults:* Initial: 12.5mg qd. Max: 50mg/day.

HOW SUPPLIED: Cap: 12.5mg

CONTRAINDICATIONS: Anuria, sulfonamide hypersensitivity.

WARNINGS/PRECAUTIONS: Caution in severe renal disease, liver dysfunction, electrolyte/fluid imbalance. Monitor electrolytes. Hyperuricemia, hyperglycemia, hypokalemia, hyponatremia, hypomagnesemia, hypercalcemia may occur. Increases in cholesterol and triglyceride levels reported. May exacerbate SLE. Sensitivity reactions reported. D/C prior to parathyroid test. Enhanced effects in post-sympathectomy patient.

ADVERSE REACTIONS: Weakness, hypotension, pancreatitis, jaundice, diarrhea, vomiting, blood dyscrasias, rash, photosensitivity, electrolyte imbalance, impotence.

INTERACTIONS: May potentiate orthostatic hypotension with alcohol, barbiturates, narcotics. Adjust antidiabetic drugs. Possible decreased response to pressor amines. Corticosteroids, ACTH increase electrolyte depletion. May potentiate nondepolarizing skeletal muscle relaxants, antihypertensives. Lithium toxicity. NSAIDs decrease effects. Decreased PO absorption with cholestyramine, colestipol.

PREGNANCY: Category B, not for use in nursing.

MECHANISM OF ACTION: Thiazide diuretic; affects renal tubular mechanism of electrolyte reabsorption directly increasing excretion of sodium salt and chloride.

PHARMACOKINETICS: Absorption: Well absorbed (65-75%). T_{max}=1-5 hrs. C_{max}=70-490ng/mL. **Distribution:** Plasma protein binding (40-68%). **Elimination:** Urine (unchanged), $T_{1/2}$ =6-15 hrs.

MIDAZOLAM INJECTION   CIV
midazolam HCL (Various)

> Associated with respiratory depression and respiratory arrest especially when used for sedation in noncritical care settings. Do not administer by rapid injection to neonates. Continuous monitoring required.

THERAPEUTIC CLASS: Benzodiazepine

INDICATIONS: For sedation, anxiolysis, and amnesia induction pre-op, prior to or during diagnostic, therapeutic, or endoscopic procedures, either alone or in combination with other CNS depressants. For induction of general anesthesia. For sedation of intubated and ventilated patients.

DOSAGE: *Adults:* IV: Sedation/Anxiolysis/Amnesia Induction: <60 yrs: Initial: 1-2.5mg IV over 2 min. Max: 5mg. Titrate: In small increments at 2 min intervals if needed. Concomitant Narcotics/Other CNS Depressants: Reduce by 30%. ≥60 yrs/Debilitated/Chronically Ill: Initial: 1-1.5mg IV over 2 min. Max: 3.5mg. Titrate: In small increments at 2 min intervals if needed. Concomitant Narcotics/Other CNS Depressants. Reduce by 50%. Maint: 25% of sedation dose by slow titration. IM: Preoperative Sedation/Anxiolysis/Amnesia: <60 yrs: 0.07-0.08mg/kg IM up to 1 hr before surgery. ≥60 yrs/Debilitated: 1-3mg IM. Anesthesia Induction: Unpremedicated: <55 yrs: Initially: 0.3-0.35mg/kg IV over 20-30 seconds. May give additional doses of 25% of initial dose to complete induction. ≥55 yrs: Initial: 0.3mg/kg IV. Debilitated: Initial: 0.15-0.25mg/kg IV. Premedicated: <55 yrs: Initial: 0.25mg/kg IV over 20-30 seconds. ≥55 yrs: Initial: 0.2mg/kg IV. Debilitated: 0.15mg/kg IV. Maintenance Sedation: LD: 0.01-0.05mg/kg IV. May repeat dose at 10-15 min intervals until adequate sedation. Maint: 0.02-0.1mg/kg/hr. Titrate to desired level of sedation using 25-50% adjustments. Infusion rate should be decreased 10-25% every few hrs to find minimum effective infusion rate.
Pediatrics: Sedation/Anxiolysis/Amnesia Induction: IV: <6 months: Limited information; titrate with small increments and monitor. 6 months-5 yrs: Initial: 0.05-0.1mg/kg IV over 2-3 min, up to 0.6mg/kg if needed. Max: 6mg. 6-12 yrs: Initial: 0.025-0.05mg/kg IV over 2-3 min, up to 0.4mg/kg if needed. Max: 10mg. 12-16 yrs: 1-2.5mg IV over 2 min. Titrate: In small increments at 2 min intervals if needed. Max: 10mg. IM: 0.1-0.15mg/kg IM, up to 0.5mg/kg if needed. Max: 10mg. Sedation: LD: 0.05-0.2mg/kg IV infusion over 2-3 min. Maint: 0.06-0.12mg/kg/hr IV infusion. May adjust dose by 25%. Sedation in Critical Care: Neonatal Dose: <32 weeks: Initial: 0.03mg/kg/hr IV infusion. >32 weeks: Initial: 0.06mg/kg/hr IV infusion. Adjust to lowest effective dose.

HOW SUPPLIED: Inj: 1mg/mL, 5mg/mL

CONTRAINDICATIONS: Acute narrow-angle glaucoma, untreated open-angle glaucoma, intrathecal or epidural use.

WARNINGS/PRECAUTIONS: Agitation, involuntary movements, hyperactivity, and combativeness reported. Caution with CHF, chronic renal failure, pulmonary disease, uncompensated acute illnesses (eg, severe fluid or electrolyte disturbances), elderly or debilitated. Avoid use with shock or coma, or in acute alcohol intoxication with depression of vital signs. Contains benzyl alcohol. Administer IM or IV only.

ADVERSE REACTIONS: Decreased tidal volume and/or respiratory rate, BP/HR variations, apnea, hypotension, pain and local reactions at injection site, hiccoughs, nausea, vomiting.

INTERACTIONS: Prolonged sedation with CYP450 3A4 inhibitors (eg, erythromycin, diltiazem, verapamil, ketoconazole, itraconazole, saquinavir, cimetidine). Increased sedative effects with morphine, meperidine, fentanyl, secobarbital, droperidol or other CNS depressants. Avoid use with acute alcohol intoxication. May decrease concentration of halothane and thiopental required for anesthesia. May cause severe hypotension with concomitant use of fentanyl in neonates.

PREGNANCY: Category D, caution in nursing.

MECHANISM OF ACTION: Benzodiazepine; short-acting CNS depressant.

PHARMACOKINETICS: Absorption: (IM) Absolute bioavailability (>90%), C_{max}=90ng/mL, T_{max}=0.5 hr; (1-hydroxy-midazolam) C_{max}=8 ng/ml, T_{max}=1 hr. **Distribution:** Crosses placenta, found in breast milk and CSF. V_d=1.0-3.1L/kg; plasma protein binding (97%). **Metabolism:** Liver via CYP450-3A4;1-hydroxy-midazolam (major metabolite). **Elimination:** Urine; (0.5% unchanged, 45%-57% as 4-hydroxy-midazolam); $T_{1/2}$= approximately 3 hrs.

MIDAZOLAM SYRUP   CIV
midazolam HCL (Various)

> Associated with respiratory depression and respiratory arrest especially when used for sedation in noncritical care settings. Reports of airway obstruction, desaturation, hypoxia, and apnea especially with other CNS depressants. Continuous monitoring required.

THERAPEUTIC CLASS: Benzodiazepine

INDICATIONS: Use in pediatric patients for sedation, anxiolysis and amnesia prior to diagnostic procedures or before induction of anesthesia.

DOSAGE: *Pediatrics:* single dose of 0.25-1mg/kg. 6 months-5 yrs or less cooperative patients: 1mg/kg. Max: 20mg. 6-15 yrs or cooperative patients: 0.25mg/kg. Max: 20mg. Cardiac/respiratory compromised, higher risk surgical patients, or patients who have received concomitant narcotics or other CNS depressants: 0.25mg/kg. Max: 20mg.

HOW SUPPLIED: Syrup: 2mg/mL [118mL]

CONTRAINDICATIONS: Acute narrow-angle glaucoma.

WARNINGS/PRECAUTIONS: Monitor for respiratory adverse events and paradoxical reactions. Agitation, involuntary movements, hyperactivity, and combativeness reported. Caution with CHF, chronic renal failure, chronic hepatic disease, pulmonary disease, cardiac or respiratory compromised patients. Avoid use with shock or coma, or in acute alcohol intoxication with depression of vital signs.

ADVERSE REACTIONS: Emesis, nausea, agitation, hypoxia, laryngospasm, agitation.

INTERACTIONS: Decreased levels with CYP3A4 inducers (eg, rifampin, carbamazepine, phenytoin). Increased levels with CYP3A4 inhibitors (eg, azole antimycotics, protease inhibitors, CCBs, macrolide antibiotics, cimetidine). Increased sedative and respiratory effects with narcotics, propofol, ketamine, nitrous oxide, droperidol, barbiturates, alcohol and other CNS depressants. Caution with anesthetics.

PREGNANCY: Category D, caution in nursing.

MECHANISM OF ACTION: Benzodiazepine; short-acting CNS depressant.

PHARMACOKINETICS: Absorption: Rapidly absorbed; T_{max}=0.17-2.65 hrs (0.25, 0.5, 1 mg/kg). **Distribution:** V_d=1.24-2.02L/kg; plasma protein binding (97% midazolam), (89% α-hydroxymidazolam). **Metabolism:** Liver and gut via CYP3A4 and glucuronidation; α-hydroxymidazolam (major metabolite), 4-hydroxy metabolite and 1,4-dihydroxy metabolite (minor metabolites). **Elimination:** Urine (63%-80% as α-hydroxymidazolam glucuronide); $T_{1/2}$=2.2-6.8 hrs.

M

MIDRIN
isometheptene mucate - dichloralphenazone - acetaminophen (Women First)

CIV

OTHER BRAND NAMES: Migrazone (Various) - Migquin (Qualitest) - Duradrin (Duramed) - Amidrine (Amide)

THERAPEUTIC CLASS: Analgesic/sedative/sympathomimetic

INDICATIONS: Relief of tension and vascular headaches. FDA has classified this agent as "possibly" effective in the treatment of migraine headache.

DOSAGE: *Adults:* Migraine: 2 caps, then 1 cap every hr until relieved. Max: 5 caps/12hrs. Tension Headache: 1-2 caps q4h. Max: 8 caps/day.

HOW SUPPLIED: Cap: (APAP-Dichloralphenazone-Isometheptene) 325mg-100mg-65mg

CONTRAINDICATIONS: Glaucoma, severe renal disease, HTN, organic heart disease, hepatic disease, concomitant MAOI therapy.

WARNINGS/PRECAUTIONS: Caution with HTN, peripheral vascular disease, or recent cardiovascular attacks.

ADVERSE REACTIONS: Transient dizziness, skin rash.

PREGNANCY: Safety in pregnancy and nursing are not known.

MECHANISM OF ACTION: Isometheptene: Sympathomimetic amine; acts by constricting dilated cranial and cerebral arterioles, reducing stimuli. Dichloralphenazone: Mild sedative; reduces emotional reaction to pain. Acetaminophen: Non-salicylate; raises threshold to painful stimuli exerting analgesic effect.

MIFEPREX
mifepristone (Danco Laboratories)

RX

> Serious and sometimes fatal infections and bleeding occur very rarely following spontaneous, surgical, and medical abortions, including following Mifeprex use. Before prescribing Mifeprex, inform the patient about the risk of these serious events and discuss Medication Guide and Patient Agreement. Ensure that patient knows whom to call and what to do, including going to the ER if none of provided contacts are reachable, if she experiences sustained fever, severe abdominal pain, prolonged heavy bleeding, or syncope.

THERAPEUTIC CLASS: Abortifacient

INDICATIONS: Medical termination of intrauterine pregnancy through 49 days of pregnancy.

DOSAGE: *Adults:* Day 1: 600mg single dose. Day 3: Unless abortion is confirmed, give 400mcg PO of misoprostol. Day 14: Assess if complete termination of pregnancy has occurred. Perform surgical termination if mifeprex and misoprostol fail.

HOW SUPPLIED: Tab: 200mg

CONTRAINDICATIONS: Ectopic pregnancy, undiagnosed adnexal mass, IUD in place, chronic adrenal failure, concurrent long-term corticosteroid therapy, hemorrhagic disorders, concurrent anticoagulant therapy, inherited porphyrias, prostaglandin hypersensitivity. Patients who do not have access to medical facilities or who are unable to understand the treatment or comply with regimen.

WARNINGS/PRECAUTIONS: Vaginal bleeding lasts for average 9-16 days. Infection and sepsis, including rare cases of fatal septic shock. Conduct follow-up visit 14 days after initial dose to confirm pregnancy termination. Preventive measures required to prevent rhesus immunization. Patients should review medication guide and patient agreement prior to procedure. Caution with women >35 yrs who smoke ≥10 cigarettes daily. Risk of fetal malformation if treatment fails. May cause decreases in Hgb, Hct and RBCs. Very rare cases of fatal septic shock reported.

ADVERSE REACTIONS: Abdominal pain, uterine cramping, nausea, headache, vomiting, diarrhea, dizziness, fatigue, back pain, uterine hemorrhage, fever, viral infections, vaginitis.

INTERACTIONS: Ketoconazole, itraconazole, erythromycin, and grapefruit juice may inhibit metabolism. Rifampin, dexamethasone, St. John's wort and certain anticonvulsants may induce metabolism.

PREGNANCY: Not for use in pregnancy or nursing.

MECHANISM OF ACTION: Abortifacient; has anti-progestational activity, it inhibits the activity of endogenous and exogenous progesterone which results from competitive interaction with progesterone at progesterone-receptor sites.

PHARMACOKINETICS: Absorption: Rapid. C_{max}=1.98mg/L; T_{max}=approximately 90 min; absolute bioavailability (20mg)=69%. **Distribution**: Plasma protein binding (98%). **Metabolism**: N-demethylation, terminal hydroxylation via CYP3A4, (major metabolites: RU 42 633, RU 42 848, RU 42 698). **Elimination**: $T_{1/2}$=18 hrs. Feces (83%), urine (9%).

MIGRANAL   RX
dihydroergotamine mesylate (Valeant)

> Serious and life-threatening peripheral ischemia reported with potent CYP3A4 inhibitors (eg, protease inhibitors, macrolides). Elevated levels of dihydroergotamine increases risk of vasospasm leading to cerebral ischemia or ischemia of the extremities. Concomitant use with CYP3A4 inhibitors is contraindicated.

THERAPEUTIC CLASS: Ergot alkaloid

INDICATIONS: Acute treatment of migraine headache with or without aura.

DOSAGE: *Adults:* 1 spray per nostril, repeat in 15 min. Max: 6 sprays/24 hrs or 8 sprays/week.

HOW SUPPLIED: Nasal Spray: 0.5mg/spray [3.5mL]

CONTRAINDICATIONS: Ischemic heart disease (angina, history of MI, documented silent ischemia), coronary artery vasospasm (Prinzmetal's variant angina), uncontrolled HTN, known peripheral artery disease, sepsis, following vascular surgery, severe renal or hepatic dysfunction, hemiplegic or basilar migraine, pregnancy, or nursing, with potent CYP3A4 inhibitors (eg, ritonavir, nelfinavir, indinavir, erythromycin, clarithromycin, troleandomycin, ketoconazole, itraconazole). Do not use with peripheral and central vasoconstrictors or within 24 hrs of 5-HT₁ agonists, ergot-type drugs, or methysergide.

WARNINGS/PRECAUTIONS: Confirm diagnosis. Monitor and consider ECG with 1st dose in patients with CAD risk factors (eg, HTN, hypercholesterolemia, smoker, obesity, DM, strong family history, postmenopausal women, men >40 yrs). Risk of elevated BP, MI, and other adverse cardiac or vasospastic effects. Monitor cardiovascular function with intermittent long-term use. Fibrotic complications (eg, pleural and retroperitoneal fibrosis) reported.

ADVERSE REACTIONS: Rhinitis, altered taste, application site reactions, dizziness, nausea, vomiting, pharyngitis, somnolence.

INTERACTIONS: Potentiated BP elevation with peripheral and central vasoconstrictors. Additive coronary vasospastic effect with sumatriptan; avoid within 24 hrs of each other. Propranolol and nicotine may potentiate the vasoconstrictive action. Increased plasma levels and peripheral vasoconstriction with macrolides. Contraindicated with CYP3A4 inhibitors (eg, macrolides, protease inhibitors). Caution with less potent CYP3A4 inhibitors (eg, saquinavir, nefazodone, fluconazole, grapefruit juice, fluoxetine, fluvoxamine, zileuton, clotrimazole).

PREGNANCY: Category X, not for use in nursing.

MECHANISM OF ACTION: Ergot alkaloid; activates 5-HT$_{1D}$ receptors located on intracranial blood vessels causing vasoconstriction or activates 5-HT$_{1D}$ receptors located on sensory nerve endings of trigeminal system, inhibiting pro-inflammatory neuropeptide release.

M

PHARMACOKINETICS: Absorption: Bioavailability (32%).
Distribution: Plasma protein binding (93%); V_d=800L. **Metabolism:**
8-β-hydroxydihydroergotamine (major metabolite). **Elimination:** Bile (major),
urine (2%).

MINIPRESS   RX
prazosin HCL (Pfizer)

THERAPEUTIC CLASS: Alpha$_1$-blocker (quinazoline)

INDICATIONS: Treatment of hypertension.

DOSAGE: *Adults:* Initial: 1mg bid-tid. Maint: 6-15mg/day in divided doses. Max:
40mg/day. Concomitant Diuretic/Antihypertensive: Reduce to 1-2mg tid, then
retitrate.

HOW SUPPLIED: Cap: 1mg, 2mg, 5mg

WARNINGS/PRECAUTIONS: Syncope may occur, usually after initial dose
or dose increase. Excessive postural hypotensive effects. Avoid driving for
24 hrs after 1st dose or dose increase. Always start on 1mg cap. False (+) for
pheochromocytoma.

ADVERSE REACTIONS: Dizziness, headache, drowsiness, lack of energy,
weakness, palpitations, nausea.

INTERACTIONS: Additive hypotensive effects with diuretics, β-blockers, or
other antihypertensives. Dizziness or syncope may occur with alcohol.

PREGNANCY: Category C, caution in nursing.

MECHANISM OF ACTION: α$_1$ blocker; blockade of postsynaptic
α-adrenoreceptors causes a reduction in total peripheral resistance.

PHARMACOKINETICS: Absorption: T_{max}=3 hrs. **Distribution:** Plasma protein binding (highly bound). **Metabolism:** Demethylation and conjugation.
Elimination: Bile and feces; $T_{1/2}$=2-3 hrs.

MINIZIDE   RX
prazosin HCL - polythiazide (Pfizer)

> Not for initial therapy of HTN.

THERAPEUTIC CLASS: Diuretic/alpha$_1$-blocker

INDICATIONS: Treatment of HTN.

DOSAGE: *Adults:* 1 cap bid-tid. Determine strength by individual component
titration.

HOW SUPPLIED: Cap: (Polythiazide-Prazosin) 0.5mg-1mg, 0.5mg-2mg,
0.5mg-5mg

CONTRAINDICATIONS: Anuria, thiazide or sulfonamide sensitivity.

WARNINGS/PRECAUTIONS: Syncope may occur, usually after initial dose
or dose increase. Excessive postural hypotensive effects. Avoid driving for
24 hrs after 1st dose or dose increase. Always start on 1mg prazosin. Caution
with severe renal disease, hepatic dysfunction, or progressive liver disease.
Sensitivity reactions may occur with history of allergy or bronchial asthma.
May exacerbate or activate SLE. Hyperuricemia, hypokalemia or frank gout
may occur. Monitor electrolytes. May manifest latent DM. Enhanced effects in
the post-sympathectomy patient. May decrease serum protein-bound iodine
levels. False (+) for pheochromocytoma.

ADVERSE REACTIONS: Dizziness, headache, drowsiness, lack of energy,
weakness, palpitations, nausea, blood dyscrasias, rash.

INTERACTIONS: Additive effects with other antihypertensives. Potentiation
with ganglionic or peripheral adrenergic blockers. Increased risk of hypokalemia with ACTH, corticosteroids. May increase responsiveness to
tubocurarine. May alter insulin requirements. May decrease arterial respon-

siveness to norepinephrine. Orthostatic hypotension aggravated by alcohol, barbiturates, or narcotics.

PREGNANCY: Category C, not for use in nursing.

MECHANISM OF ACTION: Prazosin: Suspected to cause blockade of post-synaptic alpha-adrenoreceptors, causing a reduction in total peripheral resistance. Polythiazide: Interferes with renal tubular mechanism of electrolyte reabsorption.

PHARMACOKINETICS: Absorption: Prazosin: T_{max}=3 hrs. Polythiazide: well absorbed; T_{max}=5 hrs. **Distribution:** Prazosin: Plasma protein binding (highly bound). **Metabolism:** Prazosin: Demethylation and conjugation. **Elimination:** Prazosin: Bile and feces; $T_{1/2}$=2-3 hrs. Polythiazide: Urine, feces. $T_{1/2}$=27 hrs.

MINOCIN RX
minocycline HCL (Triax)

THERAPEUTIC CLASS: Tetracycline derivative

INDICATIONS: Treatment of inclusion conjunctivitis, nongonococcal urethritis, and other infections (eg, respiratory tract, endocervical, rectal, urinary tract, skin and skin structure) caused by susceptible strains of microorganisms. Alternative treatment, when penicillin is contraindicated, in certain other infections (eg, urethritis, gonococcal, syphilis, anthrax). Adjunctive therapy in acute intestinal amebiasis and severe acne. Treatment of *Mycobacterium marinum* and asymptomatic carriers of *Neisseria meningitidis*.

DOSAGE: *Adults:* Usual: 200mg initially, then 100mg q12h; alternative is 100-200mg initially, then 50mg qid. Uncomplicated Gonococcal Infection (Men, other than urethritis and anorectal infections): 200mg initially, then 100mg q12h for minimum 4 days. Uncomplicated Gonococcal Urethritis (Men): 100mg q12h for 5 days. Syphilis: Administer usual dose for 10-15 days. Meningococcal Carrier State: 100mg q12h for 5 days. *Mycobacterium marinum:* 100mg q12h for 6-8 weeks. Uncomplicated Urethral, Endocervical, or Rectal Infection Caused by *Chlamydia trachomatis* or *Ureaplasma urealyticum*: 100mg q12h for at least 7 days. Gonorrhea in Patients Sensitive to PCN: 200mg initially, then 100mg q12h for at least 4 days, with post-therapy cultures within 2-3 days. Take with plenty of fluids. Renal Dysfunction: Max: 200mg/24 hrs. *Pediatrics:* >8 yrs: 4mg/kg initially followed by 2mg/kg q12h, not to exceed adult dose. Take with plenty of fluids. Renal Dysfunction: Max: 200mg/24 hrs.

HOW SUPPLIED: Cap: 50mg, 100mg; Inj: 100mg; Sus: 50mg/5mL [60mL]

WARNINGS/PRECAUTIONS: May cause fetal harm during pregnancy. Use during tooth development (last half of pregnancy, infancy, <8 yrs) may cause permanent discoloration of the teeth or enamel hypoplasia; avoid use during this period. Renal toxicity, hepatotoxicity, photosensitivity, increased BUN, superinfection, pseudotumor cerebri may occur; perform hematopoietic, renal, and hepatic monitoring. Caution with hepatic dysfunction. Caution in renal impairment; may lead to azotemia, hyperphosphatemia, and acidosis. Use alternate form of contraception other than oral contraceptives. May decrease bone growth in premature infants. If *Clostridium difficile*-associated diarrhea (CDAD) develops, appropriate therapy should be initiated.

ADVERSE REACTIONS: Anorexia, nausea, vomiting, diarrhea, dysphagia, enterocolitis, pancreatitis, increased LFTs, renal toxicity, rash, exfoliative dermatitis, Stevens-Johnson syndrome, skin and mucous membrane pigmentation, blood dyscrasias, headache, tooth discoloration.

INTERACTIONS: May require downward adjustments of anticoagulant dosage. May interfere with bactericidal action of penicillin; avoid concurrent use when possible. May decrease efficacy of oral contraceptives. Impaired absorption with antacids containing aluminum, calcium, or magnesium- and iron-containing products. Fatal renal toxicity with methoxyflurane has been reported. Avoid isotretinoin shortly before, during and after therapy. Caution with other hepatotoxic drugs. Risk of ergotism with ergot alkaloids.

PREGNANCY: Category D, not for use in nursing.

MECHANISM OF ACTION: Tetracycline; bacteriostatic, thought to inhibit protein synthesis.

PHARMACOKINETICS: Absorption: Rapid; C_{max}=3.5mcg/mL; T_{max}=2.1 hrs. **Elimination:** Urine, feces; $T_{1/2}$=15.5 hrs.

MINOXIDIL   RX
minoxidil (Par)

> May cause pericardial effusion, occasionally progressing to tamponade, and angina pectoris may be exacerbated. Only for nonresponders to maximum therapeutic doses of two other antihypertensives and a diuretic. Administer under supervision with a β-blocker and diuretic. Monitor in hospital for a decrease in BP in those receiving guanethidine with malignant hypertension.

THERAPEUTIC CLASS: Peripheral vasodilator

INDICATIONS: Treatment of hypertension that is symptomatic or associated with target organ damage and is not manageable with maximum therapeutic doses of diuretic plus 2 other antihypertensive drugs.

DOSAGE: *Adults:* Initial: 5mg qd. Titrate: Increase by no less than 3 days; may increase every 6 hrs if closely monitored. Usual: 10-40mg/day. Max: 100mg/day. Frequency: Give qd if diastolic BP is reduced to <30mmHg and if reduced to >30mmHg give bid. Give with a diuretic (eg, HCTZ 50mg bid, furosemide 40mg bid) and a β-blocker (equivalent to propranolol 80-160mg/day) or methyldopa (250-750mg bid starting 24 hrs before therapy). Renal Failure/Dialysis: Reduce dose.
Pediatrics: >12 yrs: Initial: 5mg qd. Titrate: Increase by no less than 3 days; may increase every 6 hrs if closely monitored. Usual: 10-40mg/day. Max: 100mg/day. Frequency: Give qd if diastolic BP is reduced to <30mmHg and if reduced to >30mmHg give bid. Give with a diuretic (eg, HCTZ 50mg bid, furosemide 40mg bid) and a β-blocker (equivalent to propranolol 80-160mg/day) or methyldopa (250-750mg bid starting 24 hrs before therapy). <12 yrs: 0.2mg/kg qd. Titrate: May increase by 50-100% increments. Usual: 0.25-1mg/kg/day. Max: 50mg/day. Renal Failure/Dialysis: Reduce dose.

HOW SUPPLIED: Tab: 2.5mg*, 10mg* *scored

CONTRAINDICATIONS: Pheochromocytoma.

WARNINGS/PRECAUTIONS: Administer with a diuretic and β-blocker. Pericarditis, pericardial effusion and tamponade reported. With renal failure or dialysis, reduce dose to prevent renal failure exacerbation and precipitation of cardiac failure. Avoid rapid control with severe HTN. Monitor body weight, fluid and electrolyte balance. Extreme caution with post-MI. Hypersensitivity reactions reported.

ADVERSE REACTIONS: Salt and water retention, pericarditis, pericardial effusion, tamponade, hypertrichosis, nausea, vomiting, rash, ECG changes, hemodilution effects.

INTERACTIONS: Severe orthostatic hypotension with guanethidine.

PREGNANCY: Category C, not for use in nursing.

MECHANISM OF ACTION: Antihypertensive peripheral vasodilator; reduces systolic and diastolic blood pressure by decreasing peripheral vascular resistance.

PHARMACOKINETICS: Absorption: Almost complete (90%); T_{max}=1 hr. **Metabolism:** Glucuronide conjugation. **Elimination:** Urine; $T_{1/2}$=4.2 hrs.

MINTEZOL   RX
thiabendazole (Merck)

THERAPEUTIC CLASS: Vermicidal and/or vermifugal agent

INDICATIONS: Treatment of strongyloidiasis (threadworm), cutaneous larva migrans (creeping eruption), visceral larva migrans, and trichinosis. Second line or adjunct treatment for uncinariasis, trichuriasis, ascariasis (intestinal roundworms).

DOSAGE: *Adults:* 100 lbs: 1g or 10mL bid. 125 lbs: 1.25g or 12.5mL bid. ≥150 lbs: 1.5g or 15mL bid. Max: 3g/day. Take with meals. Treatment Duration: Strongyloidiasis/Cutaneous Larva Migrans/Intestinal Roundworms: 2 days. Trichinosis: 2-4 days. Visceral Larva Migrans: 7 days.
Pediatrics: 30 lbs: 250mg or 2.5mL bid. 50 lbs: 500mg or 5mL bid. 75 lbs: 750mg or 7.5mL bid. Max: 3g/day. Take with meals. Treatment Duration: Strongyloidiasis/Cutaneous Larva Migrans/Intestinal Roundworms: 2 days. Trichinosis: 2-4 days. Visceral Larva Migrans: 7 days.

HOW SUPPLIED: Sus: 500mg/5mL [120mL]; Tab, Chewable: 500mg* *scored

CONTRAINDICATIONS: Prophylactic treatment for pinworm infestation.

WARNINGS/PRECAUTIONS: D/C if hypersensitivity reactions occurs. Erythema multiforme and Stevens-Johnson syndrome, jaundice, cholestasis, and parenchymal hepatic damage reported. Prolonged use may cause abnormal sensation in eyes, xanthopsia, and blurred vision. Not for mixed infections with ascaris, prophylaxis, or first line treatment of enterobiasis. Monitor with hepatic or renal dysfunction. CNS side effects may occur; avoid activities requiring mental alertness.

ADVERSE REACTIONS: Anorexia, nausea, vomiting, diarrhea, weariness, drowsiness, dizziness, abnormal sensation in eyes, xanthopsia, hypotension, hyperglycemia, leukopenia, hematuria, pruritus, fever.

INTERACTIONS: Decreases metabolism of xanthine derivatives; monitor blood levels and/or reduce dose.

PREGNANCY: Category C, not for use in nursing.

MECHANISM OF ACTION: Vermicidal agent; suspected to inhibit helminth-specific enzyme fumarate reductase.

PHARMACOKINETICS: Absorption: Rapidly absorbed. T_{max}=1-2 hrs.
Metabolism: Almost completely metabolized in liver to 5-hydroxy form.
Elimination: Urine (90%), feces (5%).

MIRALAX
OTC
polyethylene glycol 3350 (Schering-Plough)

THERAPEUTIC CLASS: Osmotic laxative

INDICATIONS: Treatment of occasional constipation.

DOSAGE: *Adults:* Stir and dissolve 17g in 4-8 oz of beverage and drink qd. Use no more than 7 days.
Pediatrics: ≥17 yrs: Stir and dissolve 17g in 4-8 oz of beverage and drink qd. Use no more than 7 days.

HOW SUPPLIED: Powder: 17g/dose [119g, 238g]

WARNINGS/PRECAUTIONS: Avoid in kidney disease.

MIRAPEX
RX
pramipexole dihydrochloride (Boehringer Ingelheim)

THERAPEUTIC CLASS: Non-ergot dopamine agonist

INDICATIONS: Treatment of signs and symptoms of idiopathic Parkinson's disease. Treatment of moderate-to-severe primary Restless Legs Syndrome (RLS).

DOSAGE: *Adults:* Parkinson's: Initial: 0.125mg tid. Titrate: May increase every 5-7 days (eg, Week 2: 0.25mg tid; Week 3: 0.5mg tid; Week 4: 0.75mg tid; Week 5: 1mg tid; Week 6: 1.25mg tid; Week 7: 1.5mg tid). Maint: 0.5-1.5mg tid. Max: 1.5mg tid. CrCl >60mL/min: Initial: 0.125mg tid. CrCl 35-59mL/min: Initial: 0.125mg bid. Max: 1.5mg bid. CrCl 15-34mL/min: Initial: 0.125mg qd. Max: 1.5mg qd. RLS: Initial: 0.125mg once daily, 2-3 hours before bedtime. Titrate: May double dose every 4-7 days up to 0.5mg/day.

HOW SUPPLIED: Tab: 0.125mg, 0.25mg*, 0.5mg*, 0.75mg, 1mg*, 1.5mg* *scored

WARNINGS/PRECAUTIONS: Somnolence, symptomatic hypotension, hallu-cinations and rhabdomyolysis reported. Caution with renal insufficiency. May potentiate dyskinesia. May cause retinal pathology, fibrotic complications, withdrawal-emergent hyperpyrexia and confusion. Consider discontinuation if significant daytime sleepiness or sudden onset of sleep occurs during daily activities. Cases of pathological gambling, hypersexuality, and compulsive eating reported. Rebound and augmentation in RLS reported. Falling asleep during activities of daily living.

ADVERSE REACTIONS: Nausea, dizziness, somnolence, insomnia, constipa-tion, asthenia, hallucination, vision abnormalities, peripheral edema, arthritis, dry mouth, postural hypotension, chest pain, malaise

INTERACTIONS: Cimetidine, ranitidine, diltiazem, triamterene, verapamil, quinidine, and quinine may decrease clearance. Dopamine antagonists (eg, phenothiazines, butyrophenones, thioxanthenes, metoclopramide) may de-crease effects.

PREGNANCY: Category C, not for use in nursing.

MECHANISM OF ACTION: Non-ergot dopamine agonist; suspected to stimu-late dopamine receptors on the striatum.

PHARMACOKINETICS: Absorption: Rapid, absolute bioavailability (>90%), T_{max}=2 hrs. **Distribution:** Plasma protein binding (15%), V_d=500L. **Elimination:** $T_{1/2}$=12hrs (elderly), urine (90%, unchanged).

MIRCETTE   RX
desogestrel - ethinyl estradiol (Organon)

OTHER BRAND NAMES: Kariva (Barr)

THERAPEUTIC CLASS: Estrogen/progestogen combination

INDICATIONS: Prevention of pregnancy.

DOSAGE: *Adults:* Start 1st Sunday after menses begins or 1st day of menses. 28-day: 1 tab qd for 28 days, then repeat.

HOW SUPPLIED: Tab: (Ethinyl Estradiol-Desogestrel) 0.02mg-0.15mg and 0.01mg-NA

CONTRAINDICATIONS: Thrombophlebitis, DVT or thromboembolic disorders, pregnancy, cerebrovascular or coronary artery disease, undiagnosed abnor-mal genital bleeding, cholestatic jaundice of pregnancy or jaundice with prior pill use, hepatic adenomas or carcinomas, breast cancer or other estrogen-dependent neoplasia.

WARNINGS/PRECAUTIONS: Cigarette smoking increases risk of serious cardiovascular side effects. This risk increases with age (especially >35 yrs) and heavy smoking. Increased risk of MI, vascular disease, thromboembo-lism, stroke and gallbladder disease. Retinal thrombosis, hepatic neoplasia, carcinoma of breast and reproductive organs reported. May cause glucose intolerance. May increase BP, elevate LDL levels or cause other lipid changes, fluid retention, breakthrough bleeding, and spotting. May cause or exacerbate migraine. May develop visual changes with contact lens. Increased risk of MI with HTN, hyperlipidemia, obesity, and diabetes. D/C if jaundice, significant depression, or ophthalmic irregularities develop. Perform annual physical exam. Use before menarche is not indicated. May affect certain endocrine, LFTs and blood components.

ADVERSE REACTIONS: Nausea, vomiting, breakthrough bleeding, spot-ting, amenorrhea, migraine, depression, vaginal candidiasis, edema, weight changes.

INTERACTIONS: Reduced effects, increased breakthrough bleeding, and menstrual irregularities with rifampin, barbiturates, phenylbutazone, phenytoin, carbamazepine, and possibly with griseofulvin, ampicillin, and tetracyclines.

PREGNANCY: Category X, not for use in nursing.

MECHANISM OF ACTION: Oral contraceptive combination; supresses gonad-otropins, inhibits ovulation, increases difficulty of sperm entry into uterus, and reduces likelihood of implantation by producing changes in cervical mucus and endometrium, respectively.

PHARMACOKINETICS: Absorption: Desogestrel: Rapid, complete; relative bioavailability (100%). Ethinyl estradiol: Rapid, complete; absolute bioavailability (93-99%). **Distribution:** Desogestrel: Sex hormone-binding globulin (99%, metabolite). Ethinyl estradiol: Plasma protein binding (98.3%). **Metabolism:** Desogestrel: Hydroxylation in intestinal mucosa; etonogestrel (metabolite). Ethinyl estradiol: Conjugation. **Elimination:** Urine, bile, feces; Desogestrel: $T_{1/2}$=27.8 hrs (metabolite). Ethinyl estradiol: $T_{1/2}$=23.9 hrs.

Mirena   RX
levonorgestrel (Bayer Healthcare)

THERAPEUTIC CLASS: Progestogen

INDICATIONS: For intrauterine contraception.

DOSAGE: *Adults:* Insert intravaginally for contraception. Initial insertion is recommended within 7 days of the onset of menses. Replacement may be done at any time in the cycle. May insert 6 weeks postpartum or until involution of uterus is complete, and immediately after 1st trimester abortion. Reexamine within 3 months after insertion. Replace every 5 yrs.

HOW SUPPLIED: Intrauterine Insert: 52mg

CONTRAINDICATIONS: Pregnancy, congenital or acquired uterine anomaly, acute or history of PID, postpartum endometriosis, infected abortion in the past 3 months, uterine or cervical neoplasia, abnormal Pap smear, genital bleeding of unknown etiology, untreated acute cervicitis or vaginitis, acute liver disease, liver tumor, women or partner with multiple sexual partners, conditions associated with increased susceptibility to microorganisms, genital actinomycosis, previously inserted IUD that is not removed, breast carcinoma, and predisposition to ectopic pregnancy.

WARNINGS/PRECAUTIONS: Risk of ectopic pregnancy, glucose intolerance. Pregnancy with IUD in place, increases risk of septic abortion, congenital anomalies, premature labor, miscarriage. Increased risk of PID, sepsis, ovarian cysts. Can alter bleeding patterns. Partial penetration or embedment in myometrium may decrease effectiveness. May perforate the uterus or cervix during insertion. Displacement may occur.

ADVERSE REACTIONS: Abdominal pain, leukorrhea, headache, vaginitis, back pain, breast pain, acne, depression, HTN, upper respiratory infection, nausea, dysmenorrhea, weight increase, skin disorder, decreased libido, abnormal pap smear.

INTERACTIONS: Enzyme inducers may decrease effectiveness.

PREGNANCY: Category X, not for use in nursing.

MECHANISM OF ACTION: Progestrone; mechanism not conclusively demonstrated. Thickening of cervical mucus preventing passage of sperm into uterus, inhibition of sperm capacitation or survival, and alteration of endometrium.

PHARMACOKINETICS: Absorption: C_{max}(20mcg/day)=150-200pg/mL. **Distribution:** Found in breast milk.

M-M-R II   RX
rubella vaccine live - measles vaccine live - mumps vaccine live (Merck)

THERAPEUTIC CLASS: Vaccine

INDICATIONS: Vaccination against measles, mumps, and rubella.

DOSAGE: *Adults:* 0.5mL SQ into outer aspect of upper arm.
Pediatrics: 12-15 months: 0.5mL SQ into outer aspect of upper arm. Repeat before elementary school entry. If vaccinated at 6-12 months due to measles outbreak, give another dose between 12-15 months and then before elementary school entry.

HOW SUPPLIED: Inj: 0.5mL

CONTRAINDICATIONS: Avoid pregnancy for 3 months after vaccine, anaphylactic reaction to neomycin, febrile/active respiratory illness, immunosuppressive therapy (except corticosteroids as replacement therapy), blood dyscrasias, leukemia, lymphoma, malignant neoplasms affecting bone marrow or lymphatic system, immunodeficiency states.

WARNINGS/PRECAUTIONS: Caution with egg allergy, cerebral injury, and individual/family history of convulsions. Defer vaccination for 3 months after blood or plasma transfusions or administration of human immune globulin. Avoid pregnancy for 3 months after vaccination. May worsen thrombocytopenia. Contains albumin, remote risk of viral infection transmission. Have epinephrine (1:1000) available.

ADVERSE REACTIONS: Atypical measles, fever, syncope, headache, dizziness, malaise, diarrhea, local reactions, vomiting, nausea, arthralgia, pneumonitis, sore throat, Stevens-Johnson Syndrome.

INTERACTIONS: Do not give with immune globulin. May depress TB skin sensitivity, administer test either simultaneously or before. Do not give <1 month before or after other live viral vaccines. Do not give simultaneously with DTP or oral poliovirus vaccine.

PREGNANCY: Category C, caution in nursing.

MECHANISM OF ACTION: May induce antibodies that may protect against measles, mumps, and rubella.

MOBAN   RX
molindone HCL (Endo)

THERAPEUTIC CLASS: Dihydroindolone

INDICATIONS: Management of schizophrenia.

DOSAGE: *Adults:* Initial: 50-75mg/day. Titrate: Increase to 100mg/day in 3-4 days; adjust to patient response. Maint: Mild: 5-15mg tid-qid. Moderate: 10-25mg tid-qid. Severe: 225mg/day.
Pediatrics: ≥12 yrs: Initial: 50-75mg/day. Titrate: Increase to 100mg/day in 3-4 days; adjust to patient response. Maint: Mild: 5-15mg tid-qid. Moderate: 10-25mg tid-qid. Severe: 225mg/day.

HOW SUPPLIED: Tab: 5mg, 10mg, 25mg*, 50mg* *scored

CONTRAINDICATIONS: Severe CNS depression (alcohol, barbiturates, narcotics), comatose states.

WARNINGS/PRECAUTIONS: Tardive dyskinesia, NMS may occur. Concentrate contains sulfites. Caution with activities requiring alertness. Convulsions, increased activity reported. May obscure signs of intestinal obstruction or brain tumor. May elevate prolactin levels.

ADVERSE REACTIONS: Drowsiness, depression, hyperactivity, euphoria, extrapyramidal reactions, akathisia, Parkinson's syndrome, blurred vision, nausea, dry mouth.

INTERACTIONS: Tabs contain calcium sulfate; may interfere with phenytoin sodium and tetracycline absorption.

PREGNANCY: Safety in pregnancy and nursing not known.

MECHANISM OF ACTION: Dihydroindolone compound; exerts effect on the ascending reticular activating system. Causes reduction of spontaneous locomotion and aggressiveness, suppression of a conditioned response, and antagonism of hyperactivity induced by amphetamines in lab animals.

PHARMACOKINETICS: Absorption: Rapidly absorbed, T_{max}=1.5 hrs.
Elimination: Urine; feces (unchanged).

MOBIC
RX

meloxicam (Boehringer Ingelheim)

> NSAIDs may cause an increased risk of serious cardiovascular thrombotic events, MI, stroke and serious GI adverse events including bleeding, ulceration, and perforation of the stomach or intestines. Contraindicated for the treatment of perioperative pain in the setting of coronary artery bypass graft (CABG) surgery.

THERAPEUTIC CLASS: NSAID

INDICATIONS: Relief of signs and symptoms of osteoarthritis (OA) and rheumatoid arthritis (RA). Relief of the signs and symptoms of pauciarticular or polyarticular course juvenile rheumatoid arthritis (JRA) in patients ≥2 yrs.

DOSAGE: *Adults:* ≥18 yrs: OA/RA: Initial/Maint: 7.5mg qd. Max: 15mg/day. *Pediatrics:* >2 yrs: JRA: 0.125mg/kg qd. Max: 7.5mg/day.

HOW SUPPLIED: Sus: 7.5mg/5mL; Tab: 7.5mg, 15mg

CONTRAINDICATIONS: ASA or other NSAID allergy that precipitates asthma, urticaria, or allergic-type reactions. Treatment of perioperative pain in the setting of CABG surgery.

WARNINGS/PRECAUTIONS: May lead to onset of new HTN or worsening of pre-existing HTN; monitor BP closely. Fluid retention and edema reported; caution with fluid retention, HTN, or heart failure. Renal papillary necrosis, renal insufficiency, acute renal failure, and other renal injury reported after long-term use. Not recommended for use with advanced renal disease; if therapy must be initiated, monitor renal function. Anaphylactoid reactions may occur. May cause serious skin adverse events (eg, exfoliative dermatitis, Stevens-Johnson syndrome, and toxic epidermal necrolysis). Avoid in late pregnancy; may cause premature closure of ductus arteriosis. May cause elevations of LFTs; d/c if liver disease develops or systemic manifestations occur. Caution with considerable dehydration and in elderly. Anemia may occur; with long-term use, monitor Hgb/Hct if signs or symptoms of anemia develop. May inhibit platelet aggregation and prolong bleeding time; monitor with coagulation disorders. Caution with asthma and avoid with ASA-sensitive asthma.

ADVERSE REACTIONS: Abdominal pain, constipation, diarrhea, dyspepsia, nausea, vomiting, headache, anemia, arthralgia, insomnia, upper respiratory tract infection, UTI.

INTERACTIONS: May decrease antihypertensive effects of ACE inhibitors. Potentiates GI bleeds with ASA; avoid concomitant use. Increased clearance with cholestyramine. May decrease natriuretic effects of furosemide, thiazides. Decreased lithium clearance/increased serum levels. Monitor PT/INR with warfarin. Caution with methotrexate.

PREGNANCY: Category C, not for use in nursing.

MECHANISM OF ACTION: NSAIDs; unknown, may inhibit prostaglandin synthetase.

PHARMACOKINETICS: Absorption: Absolute bioavailability (89%), C_{max}=1.05mcg/mL, T_{max}=4.9 hrs. **Distribution:** V_d=10 L/kg, plasma protein binding (99.4%). **Metabolism:** Hepatic (oxidation) via CYP2C9 (major), CYP3A4 (minor). **Elimination:** Urine (0.2%), feces (1.6%); $T_{1/2}$=20.1 hrs. Significant biliary and/or enteral secretion.

MODICON
RX

ethinyl estradiol - norethindrone (Ortho-McNeil)

OTHER BRAND NAMES: Necon 0.5/35 (Watson) - Nortrel 0.5/35 (Barr) - Brevicon (Watson)

THERAPEUTIC CLASS: Estrogen/progestogen combination

INDICATIONS: Prevention of pregnancy.

DOSAGE: *Adults:* 21-day: 1 tab qd for 21 days, stop 7 days, then repeat. 28-day: 1 tab qd for 28 days continuously, then repeat. Start 1st Sunday after onset of menstruation or the 1st day of menstruation.

HOW SUPPLIED: Tab: (Ethinyl Estradiol-Norethindrone) 0.035mg-0.5mg

CONTRAINDICATIONS: Thrombophlebitis, DVT or thromboembolic disorders, pregnancy, cerebrovascular or coronary artery disease, undiagnosed abnormal genital bleeding, cholestatic jaundice of pregnancy or jaundice with prior pill use, hepatic adenomas or carcinomas, breast cancer or other estrogen-dependent neoplasia.

WARNINGS/PRECAUTIONS: Cigarette smoking increases risk of serious cardiovascular side effects; risk increases with age (especially >35 yrs) and heavy smoking. Increased risk of MI, vascular disease, thromboembolism, stroke, and gallbladder disease. Retinal thrombosis, hepatic neoplasia, carcinoma of breast and reproductive organs reported. May cause glucose intolerance. May increase BP, elevate LDL levels or cause other lipid changes, fluid retention, breakthrough bleeding, and spotting. May cause or exacerbate migraine. May develop visual changes with contact lens. Increased risk of MI with HTN, hyperlipidemia, obesity, and diabetes. D/C if jaundice, significant depression or ophthalmic irregularities develop. Perform annual physical exam. Use before menarche is not indicated. May affect certain endocrine, LFTs, and blood components.

ADVERSE REACTIONS: Nausea, vomiting, breakthrough bleeding, spotting, amenorrhea, migraine, depression, vaginal candidiasis, edema, weight changes.

INTERACTIONS: Reduced effects, increased breakthrough bleeding, and menstrual irregularities with rifampin, barbiturates, phenylbutazone, phenytoin, carbamazepine, griseofulvin, topiramate, St. John's wort, and possibly with ampicillin and tetracyclines.

PREGNANCY: Category X, not for use in nursing.

MECHANISM OF ACTION: Oral contraceptive. Inhibits ovulation, other alterations include changes in the cervical mucus (which increases difficulty of sperm entry into the uterus) and the endometrium (which may reduce likelihood of implantation).

MONISTAT OTC
miconazole nitrate (Personal Products Company)

OTHER BRAND NAMES: Monistat 3 (Personal Products Company) - Monistat 7 (Personal Products Company)

THERAPEUTIC CLASS: Azole antifungal

INDICATIONS: Treatment of vaginal yeast infections.

DOSAGE: *Adults:* 100mg sup or 2% cream intravaginally qhs for 7 days or 200mg sup or 4% cream intravaginally qhs for 3 days.
Pediatrics: ≥12 yrs: 100mg sup or 2% cream intravaginally qhs for 7 days or 200mg sup or 4% cream intravaginally qhs for 3 days.

HOW SUPPLIED: (Monistat 3) Cre: 4% [15g, 25g]; Sup: 200mg [3s]; (Monistat 7) Cre: 2% [35g, 45g]; Sup: 100mg [7s]

WARNINGS/PRECAUTIONS: Avoid or d/c if abdominal pain, fever (>100°F), shoulder pain, back pain, or foul smelling discharge occurs. Do not use with tampons. Do not rely on condoms or diaphragm to prevent STDs or pregnancy.

ADVERSE REACTIONS: Vulvovaginal burning.

PREGNANCY: Safety in pregnancy and nursing not known.

MONISTAT-DERM RX
miconazole nitrate (Ortho-McNeil)

THERAPEUTIC CLASS: Azole antifungal

INDICATIONS: Treatment of tinea pedis, tinea cruris, tinea corporis, tinea versicolor, cutaneous candidiasis.

DOSAGE: *Adults:* T.pedis/T.cruris/T.corporis/Candidiasis: Apply bid (am and pm). T.versicolor: Apply qd. Treat t. pedis for 1 month and other infections for 2 weeks.

HOW SUPPLIED: Cre: 2% [15g, 30g, 85g]

WARNINGS/PRECAUTIONS: D/C if irritation occurs. If no improvement after a month, reassess diagnosis. Avoid eyes.

ADVERSE REACTIONS: Irritation, burning, skin maceration, allergic contact dermatitis.

PREGNANCY: Safety in pregnancy and nursing not known.

MONODOX   RX
doxycycline monohydrate (Watson)

THERAPEUTIC CLASS: Tetracycline derivative

INDICATIONS: Treatment of rocky mountain spotted fever, typhus fever and the typhus group, Q fever, rickettsialpox, and ticks fever, respiratory tract, urinary tract, skin and skin structure, inclusion conjunctivitis, uncomplicated urethral/endocervical/rectal infection caused by *C.trachomatis*, nongonococcal urethritis caused by *C.trachomatis* and *U.urealyticum*, lymphogranuloma, psittacosis, trachoma, tularemia, campylobacter fetus, yaws, vincent's infection, actinomycosis, chancroid, plague, cholera, brucellosis. Treatment of uncomplicated gonorrhea, syphilis, listeriosis, anthrax, *Clostridium* species when PCN is contraindicated. Adjunct therapy for amebicides and severe acne.

DOSAGE: *Adults:* Usual: 100mg q12h or 50mg q6h for 1 day, then 100mg/day. Severe Infection: 100mg q12h. Uncomplicated Gonococcal Infections (except anorectal infections in men): 100mg bid for 7 days or 300mg stat, then repeat in 1 hr. Acute Epididymo-Orchitis caused by *N.gonorrhea* or *C.trachomatis:* 100mg bid for at least 10 days. Primary/Secondary Syphilis: 300mg/day in divided dose for at least 10 days. Uncomplicated Urethral/Endocervical/Rectal Infection caused by *C.trachomatis:* 100mg bid for at least 7 days. Nongonococcal Urethritis caused by *C.trachomatis* and *U.urealyticum:* 100mg bid for at least 7 days. Take with full glass of water. Take with food if GI upset occurs. Inhalational Anthrax (post-exposure): 100mg bid for 60 days. *Pediatrics:* >8 yrs: ≤100 lbs: 2mg/lb divided in 2 doses for 1 day, then 1mg/lb daily in single or 2 divided doses. Severe Infection: May use up to 2mg/lb/day. >100 lbs: 100mg q12h or 50mg q6h for 1 day, then 100mg/day. Severe Infection: 100mg q12h. Take with full glass of water. Take with food if GI upset occurs.

HOW SUPPLIED: Cap: 50mg, 75mg, 100mg

WARNINGS/PRECAUTIONS: Avoid direct sunlight or UV light. May cause permanent tooth discoloration during tooth development (last half of pregnancy and children <8 years). Enamel hypoplasia reported. Monitor renal/hepatic function, and blood with long-term therapy. May increase BUN. Photosensitivity, pseudotumor cerebri reported. D/C if superinfection occurs. Bulging fontanels in infants and intracranial HTN in adults reported. *Clostridium difficile*-associated diarrhea reported.

ADVERSE REACTIONS: GI effects, photosensitivity, rash, blood dyscrasias, hypersensitivity reactions.

INTERACTIONS: Carbamazepine, barbiturates, phenytoin decrease half-life of doxycycline. May decrease PT; adjust anticoagulants. May decrease bactericidal agents (eg, penicillin). May decrease effects of oral contraceptives. Take 1 hr before or 2 hrs after dairy products. Aluminum-, calcium-, iron-, and magnesium-containing products and bismuth subsalicylate impair absorption. Fatal renal toxicity may occur with methoxyflurane.

PREGNANCY: Category D, not for use in nursing.

MECHANISM OF ACTION: Tetracycline; bacteriostatic, thought to inhibit protein synthesis.

PHARMACOKINETICS: Absorption: C_{max}=3.61mcg/mL; T_{max}=2.6 hrs.
Elimination: Urine, feces; $T_{1/2}$=16.33 hrs.

MONOKET   RX
isosorbide mononitrate (Schwarz)

THERAPEUTIC CLASS: Nitrate vasodilator

INDICATIONS: Prevention and treatment of angina pectoris. Not for acute attack.

DOSAGE: *Adults:* 20mg bid (space doses 7 hours apart). Small Patients: Initial: 5mg per dose for 1 day, then increase to 10mg by 2nd or 3rd day.

HOW SUPPLIED: Tab: 10mg*, 20mg* *scored

WARNINGS/PRECAUTIONS: Not for use with acute MI or CHF. Severe hypotension may occur; caution with volume depletion or hypotension. May aggravate angina caused by hypertrophic cardiomyopathy. Monitor for tolerance.

ADVERSE REACTIONS: Headache, dizziness, fatigue, GI upset.

INTERACTIONS: Severe hypotension with sildenafil. Marked orthostatic hypotension with CCBs. Additive vasodilation with other vasodilators (eg, alcohol).

PREGNANCY: Category B, caution with nursing.

MECHANISM OF ACTION: Nitrate vasodilator; relaxes vascular smooth muscle, and consequent dilatation of peripheral arteries and veins, especially the latter. Dilatation of the veins leads to reducing the left ventricular end-diastolic pressure and pulmonary capillary wedge pressure (preload). Arteriolar relaxation reduces systemic vascular resistance, systolic arterial pressure, and mean arterial pressure (afterload). It also dilates the coronary artery.

PHARMACOKINETICS: Absorption: (Tab, 60mg) C_{max}=557-572ng/mL, T_{max}=2.9-4.2 hrs, AUC=6625-7555ng•hr/mL; (120mg); C_{max}=1151-1180ng/mL, T_{max}=3.1-3.2 hrs, AUC=14241-16800ng•hr/mL. **Distribution:** Plasma protein binding (5%), V_d=0.6-0.7L/kg. **Metabolism:** Liver. Cleared through glucuronidation pathways. **Elimination:** Urine (96%), feces (1%); (60mg): $T_{1/2}$=6.2-6.3 hrs; (120mg): $T_{1/2}$=6.2-6.4 hrs.

MONOPRIL   RX
fosinopril sodium (Bristol-Myers Squibb)

> ACE inhibitors can cause death/injury to developing fetus during 2nd and 3rd trimesters. Stop therapy if pregnancy detected.

THERAPEUTIC CLASS: ACE inhibitor

INDICATIONS: Treatment of hypertension. Adjunct therapy for heart failure.

DOSAGE: *Adults:* If possible, d/c diuretic 2-3 days before therapy. Initial: 10mg qd, monitor carefully if cannot d/c diuretic. Maint: 20-40mg/day. Resume diuretic if BP not controlled. Max: 80mg/day. Heart Failure: Initial: 10mg qd, 5mg with moderate to severe renal failure or vigorous diuresis. Titrate: Increase over several weeks. Maint: 20-40mg qd. Max: 40mg qd. Elderly: Start at low end of dosing range.

HOW SUPPLIED: Tab: 10mg*, 20mg, 40mg *scored

CONTRAINDICATIONS: History of ACE inhibitor associated angioedema.

WARNINGS/PRECAUTIONS: D/C if angioedema, jaundice, or if marked LFT elevation occur. Risk of hyperkalemia with DM, renal dysfunction. Persistent non-productive cough reported. Monitor WBCs in renal and collagen vascular disease. Anaphylactoid reactions reported. Fetal/neonatal morbidity and death reported. Monitor for hypotension in high-risk patients (heart failure, volume and/or salt depletion, surgery/anesthesia, etc.). Less effective on BP in blacks and more reports of angioedema than nonblacks. Caution with

CHF, renal or hepatic dysfunction, renal artery stenosis. May cause false low measurement of serum digoxin level.

ADVERSE REACTIONS: Dizziness, cough, hypotension, musculoskeletal pain.

INTERACTIONS: May increase lithium levels. Hypotension risk with diuretics. Increase risk of hyperkalemia with K^+-sparing diuretics, K^+-containing salt substitutes or K^+ supplements. Decreased absorption with antacids; space dosing by 2 hrs.

PREGNANCY: Category C (1st trimester) and D (2nd and 3rd trimesters), not for use in nursing.

MECHANISM OF ACTION: ACE inhibitor; inhibition results in decreased plasma angiotensin II, which leads to decreased vasopressor activity and decreased aldosterone secretion.

PHARMACOKINETICS: Absorption: Slow; T_{max}=3 hrs. **Distribution**: Plasma protein binding (99.4%). **Metabolism:** Hepatic, glucoronidation. **Elimination:** Renal, $T_{1/2}$=11.5 hrs.

MONOPRIL HCT RX
fosinopril sodium - hydrochlorothiazide (Bristol-Myers Squibb)

> ACE inhibitors can cause death/injury to developing fetus during 2nd and 3rd trimesters. Stop therapy if pregnancy detected.

THERAPEUTIC CLASS: ACE inhibitor/thiazide diuretic

INDICATIONS: Hypertension. Not for initial therapy.

DOSAGE: *Adults:* Initial (if not controlled with fosinopril/HCTZ monotherapy): 12.5mg-10mg tab or 12.5mg-20mg tab qd.

HOW SUPPLIED: Tab: (Fosinopril-HCTZ) 10mg-12.5mg, 20mg-12.5mg

CONTRAINDICATIONS: Anuria, sulfonamide hypersensitivity.

WARNINGS/PRECAUTIONS: D/C if angioedema, jaundice, or marked LFT elevation occurs. Risk of hyperkalemia with DM, renal dysfunction. Persistent nonproductive cough reported. Monitor WBCs in renal and collagen vascular disease. Anaphylactoid reactions reported. Fetal/neonatal morbidity and death reported. Monitor for hypotension in high-risk patients (eg, surgery/anesthesia, volume/salt depletion). Caution with CHF, renal or hepatic dysfunction. More reports of angioedema in blacks than nonblacks. May exacerbate or activate SLE. Monitor electrolytes. Avoid if CrCl ≤30mL/min/1.7m². May increase cholesterol, TG. Hypercalcemia, hypomagnesemia, hyperuricemia may occur.

ADVERSE REACTIONS: Headache, cough, fatigue, dizziness, upper respiratory infection, musculoskeletal pain.

INTERACTIONS: Increase risk of hyperkalemia with K^+-sparing diuretics, K^+ supplements, or K^+-containing salt substitutes. Risk of lithium toxicity. Antacids may impair absorption; separate dose by 2 hrs. May alter insulin requirements. May increase responsiveness to tubocurarine. NSAIDs reduce effects. May decrease effects of methenamine. Reduced absorption with cholestyramine, colestipol. Caution with other antihypertensives. May decrease response to norepinephrine.

PREGNANCY: Category C (1st trimester) and D (2nd and 3rd trimesters), not for use in nursing.

MECHANISM OF ACTION: ACE inhibitor; inhibition results in decreased plasma angiotensin II, which leads to decreased vasopressor activity and decreased aldosterone secretion. Thiazide diuretic; affects renal tubular mechanism of electrolyte reabsorption directly increasing excretion of sodium salt and chloride.

PHARMACOKINETICS: Absorption: Fosinopril: Slow, T_{max}=3 hrs; HCTZ: T_{max}=1-2.5 hrs. **Distribution**: Fosinopril: plasma protein binding (95%); HCTZ: Vd =3.6-7.8L; plasma protein binding (67.9%).**Metabolism:** Hepatic, glucoronidation. **Elimination:** Fosinopril: Renal, $T_{1/2}$=11.5 hrs; HCTZ: Renal; $T_{1/2}$=5-15 hrs.

MONUROL RX
fosfomycin tromethamine (Forest)

THERAPEUTIC CLASS: Phosphonic acid derivative

INDICATIONS: Uncomplicated urinary tract infection (acute cystitis) in women.

DOSAGE: *Adults:* ≥18 yrs: 1 single-dose sachet. Mix with 3-4oz of water before ingesting.

HOW SUPPLIED: Powder: 3g/sachet

WARNINGS/PRECAUTIONS: Maximum of 1 dose per episode. *Clostridium difficile* associated diarrhea reported.

ADVERSE REACTIONS: Diarrhea, headache, vaginitis, nausea.

INTERACTIONS: Metoclopramide and other drugs that increase GI motility may decrease serum levels and urinary excretion.

PREGNANCY: Category B, not for use in nursing.

MECHANISM OF ACTION: Phosphonic acid derivative; inactivates enolpyruvyl transferase, irreversibly blocking condensation of uridine diphosphate-N-acetylglucosamine with p-enolpyruvate; reduces adherence of bacteria to uroepithelial cells.

PHARMACOKINETICS: Absorption: Rapid; absolute bioavailability (37%); C_{max}=26.1µg/mL, 17.6µg/mL (fed); T_{max}=2 hrs, 4 hrs (fed). **Distribution:** V_d=136.1L; crosses placenta. **Elimination:** Urine (38%), feces (18%); $T_{1/2}$=5.7 hrs.

MORPHINE SULFATE IMMEDIATE RELEASE CII
morphine sulfate (Various)

THERAPEUTIC CLASS: Opioid analgesic

INDICATIONS: Relief of severe pain.

DOSAGE: *Adults:* (Sol) 10-20mg q4h. (Tab) 15-30mg q4h.

HOW SUPPLIED: Sol: 10mg/5mL, 20mg/5mL [100mL, 500mL]; Tab: 15mg*, 30mg* *scored

CONTRAINDICATIONS: Respiratory insufficiency or depression; severe CNS depression; attack of bronchial asthma; heart failure secondary to chronic lung disease; cardiac arrhythmias; increased ICP or CSF pressure; head injuries; brain tumor; acute alcoholism; delirium tremens; convulsive disorders; after biliary tract surgery; suspected surgical abdomen; surgical anastomosis; concomitantly with MAOIs or within 14 days of such treatment.

WARNINGS/PRECAUTIONS: May cause tolerance, psychological/physical dependence; avoid abrupt withdrawal. Caution with head injury, increased ICP, acute asthma attack, chronic COPD or cor pulmonale, decreased respiratory reserve, pre-existing respiratory depression, hypoxia, hypercapnia, elderly, debilitated, severe hepatic/renal impairment, hypothyroidism, Addison's disease, prostatic hypertrophy, or urethral stricture. May cause severe hypotension. May obscure diagnosis or clinical course with abdominal conditions. May impair mental/physical abilities.

ADVERSE REACTIONS: Respiratory depression, lightheadedness, dizziness, sedation, nausea, vomiting, sweating.

INTERACTIONS: See Contraindications. Effects may be potentiated by alkalinizing agents and antagonized by acidifying agents. Analgesic effect may be potentiated by chlorpromazine and methocarbamol. Depressant effects may be enhanced by other CNS depressants (eg, anesthetics, sedatives, hypnotics, TCAs, barbiturates, phenothiazines, chloral hydrate, glutethimide, antihistamines, β-blockers (propranolol), alcohol, furazolidone, and other narcotic analgesics). May increase anticoagulant activity of coumarin and other anticoagulants.

PREGNANCY: Category C, caution in nursing.

MECHANISM OF ACTION: Opioid analgesic; binds to CNS opiate receptors, producing analgesic effects. Also produces respiratory depression by direct action on brain stem respiratory centers, and depresses cough reflex by direct action on cough center in the medulla.

PHARMACOKINETICS: Absorption: Bioavailability (40%). **Distribution:** Skeletal muscle, kidneys, liver, intestinal tract, lungs, spleen, and brain; crosses placenta and found in breast milk; V_d=4L/kg. **Metabolism:** Gut wall and liver; morphine-3-glucuronide (inactive metabolite). **Elimination:** Urine, bile; $T_{1/2}$=2-4 hrs.

MOTRIN   RX
ibuprofen (Pharmacia & Upjohn)

NSAIDs may cause an increased risk of serious cardiovascular thrombotic events, MI, stroke and serious GI adverse events including bleeding, ulceration, and perforation of the stomach or intestines. Contraindicated for the treatment of perioperative pain in the setting of coronary artery bypass graft (CABG) surgery.

THERAPEUTIC CLASS: NSAID

INDICATIONS: Adults: Relief of mild-to-moderate pain. Dysmenorrhea. Rheumatoid arthritis (RA) Osteoarthritis (OA). **Pediatrics:** Fever. Relief of mild to moderate pain. Juvenile arthritis (JA).

DOSAGE: *Adults:* Pain: 400mg q4-6h prn. Max: 2400mg/day. Dysmenorrhea: 400mg q4-6h prn. Max: 2400mg/day. RA/OA: 300mg qid or 400mg, 600mg or 800mg tid-qid. Max: 3200mg/day. Fever: 200-400mg q4-6h. Max: 1200mg/day. Take with meals/milk. Renal Impairment: Reduce dose. *Pediatrics:* Fever: 6 months-12 yrs: 5mg/kg for temp <102.5°F; 10mg/kg if temp ≥102.5°F q6-8h. Max: 40mg/kg/day. Pain: 6 months-12 yrs: 10mg/kg q6-8h. Max: 40mg/kg/day. JA: 30-40mg/kg/day divided into 3 or 4 doses. Milder disease may use 20mg/kg/day.

HOW SUPPLIED: Sus: 100mg/5mL; Tab: 400mg, 600mg, 800mg

CONTRAINDICATIONS: Syndrome of nasal polyps, angioedema, and bronchospastic reactions to ASA or other NSAIDs. Treatment of perioperative pain in the setting of CABG surgery.

WARNINGS/PRECAUTIONS: May lead to onset of new HTN or worsening of pre-existing HTN; monitor BP closely. Fluid retention and edema reported; caution with fluid retention or heart failure. Renal papillary necrosis and other renal injury reported after long-term use. Not recommended for use with advanced renal disease; if therapy must be initiated, monitor renal function. Anaphylactoid reactions may occur. May cause serious skin adverse events (eg, exfoliative dermatitis, Stevens-Johnson syndrome, and toxic epidermal necrolysis). Avoid in late pregnancy; may cause premature closure of ductus arteriosis. May cause elevations of LFTs; d/c if liver disease develops or systemic manifestations occur. Caution in elderly. Anemia may occur; with long-term use, monitor Hgb/Hct if signs or symptoms of anemia develop. May inhibit platelet aggregation and prolong bleeding time; monitor with coagulation disorders. Caution with asthma and avoid with ASA-sensitive asthma. D/C if visual disturbances occur. Aseptic meningitis with fever and coma reported.

ADVERSE REACTIONS: Nausea, epigastric pain, heartburn, dizziness, rash.

INTERACTIONS: Use caution with anticoagulants. May enhance methotrexate toxicity. May decrease natriuretic effects of furosemide or thiazides. Avoid use with ASA. May decrease lithium clearance; monitor for toxicity. May diminish antihypertensive effect of ACE inhibitors. Caution with concomitant warfarin use.

PREGNANCY: Category C, not for use in nursing.

MECHANISM OF ACTION: NSAIDs; unknown, suspected to inhibit prostaglandin synthetase.

PHARMACOKINETICS: Absorption: (Tab) Rapid. (Susp) **Adults:** C_{max}=19µg/mL; T_{max}=0.79 hrs; AUC=64µg•h/mL. Febrile children: C_{max}=55µg/mL; T_{max}=0.97 hrs; AUC=155µg•h/mL. **Distribution:** (Susp): Plasma

protein binding (>99%). **Adults:** V_d=0.12L/kg; febrile children: V_d=0.2L/kg.
Metabolism: Hepatic. **Elimination:** (Tab): $T_{1/2}$=1.8-2 hrs. (Sus): Urine (1%); $T_{1/2}$=2 hrs.

MOTRIN IB   OTC
ibuprofen (McNeil Consumer)

THERAPEUTIC CLASS: NSAID

INDICATIONS: Temporarily relieves minor aches and pains due to headache, muscular aches, arthritis, toothache, backache, the common cold, menstrual cramps. Temporarily reduces fever.

DOSAGE: *Adults:* 200mg q4-6h. 400mg if symptoms do not respond. Max: 1200mg/24 hrs.
Pediatrics: ≥12 yrs: 200mg q4-6h. 400mg if symptoms do not respond. Max: 1200mg/24 hrs.

HOW SUPPLIED: Tab: 200mg

WARNINGS/PRECAUTIONS: Do not take for >10 days for pain or >3 days for fever. May cause severe allergic reaction, especially in people allergic to ASA. Do not use if history of allergic reaction to other pain relievers/fever reducers or right before or after heart surgery. May cause stomach bleeding; increased risk ≥60 yrs; stomach ulcers or bleeding problems; concomitant blood thinning or steroid drug, and other NSAIDs; ≥3 alcoholic drinks every day; longer course of therapy. Caution if taking ASA for heart attack or stroke, it may decrease this benefit of ASA.

INTERACTIONS: Avoid other ibuprofen-containing products.

PREGNANCY: Safety in pregnancy and nursing not known.

MOVIPREP   RX
ascorbic acid - sodium ascorbate - polyethylene glycol 3350 - potassium chloride - sodium chloride - sodium sulfate (Salix)

THERAPEUTIC CLASS: Bowel cleanser

INDICATIONS: Colon cleansing as a preparation for colonoscopy in adults ≥18 yrs of age.

DOSAGE: *Adults:* ≥18 yrs: Split-Dose Regimen: 8oz every 15 min (first liter) followed by 0.5 liters of clear liquid the evening prior, then another liter over 1 hr followed by 0.5 liters of clear liquid in the morning at least 1 hr prior to colonoscopy. Evening-Only Regimen: Around 6 pm take 8oz every 15 min (first liter), then 1.5 hrs later take second liter over one hour, additionally take 1 liter of clear liquid.

HOW SUPPLIED: Pow: (PEG 3350-Sodium Sulfate-Sodium Chloride-Potassium Chloride-Ascorbic Acid-Sodium Ascorbate) 100g-7.5g-2.69g-1.015g-4.7g-5.9g

WARNINGS/PRECAUTIONS: Rare reports of generalized tonic-clonic seizures with use of PEG colon preparations. Caution with concomitant medications that increase risk of electrolyte abnormalities (eg, diuretics, ACEIs) or in patients with hyponatremia; consider baseline and post-colonoscopy lab tests (eg, sodium, potassium, calcium, creatinine, BUN).

ADVERSE REACTIONS: Abdominal distension, anal discomfort, thirst, nausea, abdominal pain, sleep disorder, rigors, hunger, malaise, vomiting, dizziness.

INTERACTIONS: Oral medications given within 1 hour of administration may be flushed from GI and may not be absorbed.

PREGNANCY: Category C, caution in nursing.

MECHANISM OF ACTION: Laxative/evacuant: produces watery stool leading to cleansing of colon.

MS CONTIN
morphine sulfate (Purdue Pharma)

> Contains morphine sulfate with an abuse liability similar to other opioid analgesics. Not intended for use as a prn analgesic. MS Contin 100mg and 200mg tablets are for use in opioid-tolerant patients only. Tablets are to be swallowed whole, do not break, crush, chew, or dissolve.

THERAPEUTIC CLASS: Opioid analgesic

INDICATIONS: Management of moderate to severe pain when a continuous, around-the-clock opioid analgesic is needed for an extended period of time.

DOSAGE: *Adults:* Conversion from MSIR: Give 1/2 of total daily MSIR dose as MS Contin q12h or give 1/3 of total daily MSIR dose as MS Contin q8h. Conversion from Parenteral Morphine: Initial: If daily morphine dose ≤120mg/day, give MS Contin 30mg. Titrate: Switch to 60mg or 100mg MS Contin. Swallow whole; do not crush, chew, or break. Taper dose; do not d/c abruptly.

HOW SUPPLIED: Tab, Extended-Release: 15mg, 30mg, 60mg, 100mg, 200mg

CONTRAINDICATIONS: Paralytic ileus, respiratory depression in the absence of resuscitative equipment, acute or severe bronchial asthma.

WARNINGS/PRECAUTIONS: Extreme caution with COPD, cor pulmonale, decreased respiratory reserve, hypoxia, hypercapnia, respiratory depression. Caution with elderly, debilitated, head injury, increased ICP, circulatory shock, severe hepatic/renal/pulmonary dysfunction, myxedema, hypothyroidism, adrenocortical insufficiency, CNS depression, coma, toxic psychosis, prostatic hypertrophy, urethral stricture, alcoholism, delirium tremens, kyphoscoliosis, inability to swallow, convulsive disorder, acute abdominal problems, biliary tract surgery, acute pancreatitis secondary to biliary tract disease. May cause hypotension and drug dependence. Reserve 200mg tabs for opioid-tolerant patients requiring ≥400mg/day of morphine. May cause neonatal withdrawal syndrome.

ADVERSE REACTIONS: Constipation, lightheadedness, dizziness, sedation, nausea, vomiting, sweating, dysphoria, euphoria, respiratory depression.

INTERACTIONS: Additive depressant effects with other CNS depressants (eg, sedatives, hypnotics, general anesthetics, phenothiazines, tranquilizers, alcohol). Enhances neuromuscular blocking effects and increases respiratory depression with skeletal muscle relaxants. Avoid agonist/antagonist analgesics (eg, pentazocine, nalbuphine, butorphanol, buprenorphine); may reduce analgesic effect or cause withdrawal symptoms. Risk of hypotension with phenothiazines or general anesthetics.

PREGNANCY: Category C, not for use in nursing.

MECHANISM OF ACTION: Opioid analgesic; pure opioid agonist whose principal therapeutic action is analgesia. Precise mechanism of analgesic action not established. Specific CNS opiate receptors for endogenous compounds with opioid like activity are found throughout the brain and spinal cord and are likely to play a role in analgesic effects.

PHARMACOKINETICS: Distribution: V_d = 4L/kg; found in skeletal muscle, kidneys, liver, intestinal tract, lungs, spleen, and brain; crosses placental membranes and found in breast milk. **Metabolism:** Liver to glucuronide metabolites, M3G (major metabolite), M6G (active metabolite). **Elimination:** Renal (primary), bile; (IV): $T_{1/2}$=2-4 hrs.

MUCINEX
guaifenesin (Adams)

OTC

THERAPEUTIC CLASS: Expectorant

INDICATIONS: To help loosen phlegm, thin bronchial secretions and make coughs more productive.

DOSAGE: *Adults:* 1-2 tabs every 12hrs. Max: 4 tabs/24hrs. Take with full glass of water. Do not crush, chew or break.

Pediatrics: ≥12 yrs: 1-2 tabs every 12hrs. Max: 4 tabs/24hrs. Take with full glass of water. Do not crush, chew or break.

HOW SUPPLIED: Tab, Extended-Release: 600mg

WARNINGS/PRECAUTIONS: D/C if cough lasts >7 days, recurs, or occurs with fever, rash, or persistent headache.

PREGNANCY: Safety in pregnancy or nursing not known.

MUCINEX D   OTC
pseudoephedrine HCL - guaifenesin (Adams)

THERAPEUTIC CLASS: Expectorant/decongestant

INDICATIONS: Help loosen phlegm and thin bronchial secretions. Temporarily relieves nasal congestion due to common cold, hay fever, or upper respiratory allergies. Temporarily restores freer breathing through the nose. Promotes nasal and sinus drainage. Temporarily relieves sinus congestion and pressure.

DOSAGE: *Adults:* 2 tabs every 12hrs. Max: 4 tabs/24hrs. Take with full glass of water. Do not crush, chew or break.
Pediatrics: ≥12 yrs: 2 tabs every 12hrs. Max: 4 tabs/24hrs. Take with full glass of water. Do not crush, chew or break.

HOW SUPPLIED: Tab, Extended-Release: (Guaifenesin-Pseudoephedrine HCl) 600mg-60mg

WARNINGS/PRECAUTIONS: Avoid use during or for 2 weeks after stopping MAOI therapy. Caution with heart disease, high BP, thyroid disease, diabetes, difficulty urinating due to enlarged prostate, persistent or chronic cough. D/C if cough lasts >7 days, or occurs with fever, rash or persistent headache.

INTERACTIONS: See Warnings and Precautions.

PREGNANCY: Safety in pregnancy and nursing not known.

MUCINEX DM   OTC
dextromethorphan hydrobromide - guaifenesin (Adams)

THERAPEUTIC CLASS: Cough suppressant/expectorant

INDICATIONS: To help loosen phlegm, thin bronchial secretions and make coughs more productive. Temporarily relieves cough due to minor throat and bronchial irritations, intensity of coughing, and impulse to cough.

DOSAGE: *Adults:* 1-2 tabs q12hrs. Max: 4 tabs/24hrs. Take with full glass of water. Do not crush, chew or break.
Pediatrics: ≥12 yrs: 1-2 tabs q12hrs. Max: 4 tabs/24hrs. Take with full glass of water. Do not crush, chew or break.

HOW SUPPLIED: Tab: (Dextromethorphan-Guaifenesin) 30mg-600mg

WARNINGS/PRECAUTIONS: D/C if cough lasts >7 days, recurs, or occurs with fever, rash, or persistent headache. Avoid during or within 14 days of MAOIs.

INTERACTIONS: See Warnings and Precautions.

PREGNANCY: Safety in pregnancy or nursing not known.

MUMPSVAX   RX
mumps virus vaccine live (Merck)

THERAPEUTIC CLASS: Vaccine

INDICATIONS: Vaccination against mumps.

DOSAGE: *Adults:* 0.5mL SQ into outer aspect of upper arm.
Pediatrics: ≥12 mos: 0.5mL SQ in outer aspect of upper arm. Give primary vaccine at 12-15 months. Revaccinate prior to elementary school.

HOW SUPPLIED: Inj: 20,000 TCID$_{50}$

CONTRAINDICATIONS: Avoid pregnancy for 3 months after vaccine, anaphylactic reaction to neomycin, febrile/active respiratory illness, immunosuppressive therapy (except corticosteroids as replacement therapy), blood dyscrasias, leukemia, lymphoma, malignant neoplasms affecting bone marrow or lymphatic system, immunodeficiency states.

WARNINGS/PRECAUTIONS: Caution with hypersensitivity to eggs and neomycin. May worsen thrombocytopenia. Defer vaccine for at least 3 months after blood or plasma transfusion and immune globulin. Do not revaccinate with active untreated TB. Monitor for temperature elevation after administration. Contains albumin, remote risk of viral infection transmission. Have epinephrine (1:1000) available.

ADVERSE REACTIONS: Fever, syncope, irritability, diarrhea, diabetes, purpura, cough, febrile seizures, local site reactions.

INTERACTIONS: Do not give with immune globulin. May depress TB skin sensitivity, administer test either simultaneously or before. Do not give <1 month before or after other live viral vaccines. Do not give simultaneously with DTP or oral poliovirus vaccine.

PREGNANCY: Category C, caution in nursing.

MECHANISM OF ACTION: Induces the immune system to produce antibodies that may protect against mumps.

MURINE TEARS PLUS   OTC
tetrahydrozoline HCL - polyvinyl alcohol - povidone (Ross)

THERAPEUTIC CLASS: Decongestant/lubricant

INDICATIONS: Temporary relief or prevention of further discomfort due to minor irritations and symptoms related to dry eyes plus removal of redness.

DOSAGE: *Adults:* 1-2 drops in affected eye up to qid.

HOW SUPPLIED: Sol: (Tetrahydrozoline-Polyvinyl alcohol-Povidone) 0.05%-0.5%-0.6% [15mL, 30mL]

WARNINGS/PRECAUTIONS: May temporarily enlarge pupils. Overuse may cause increased eye redness. Do not touch container tip to any surface to avoid contamination. D/C if eye pain or vision changes occur, if redness or irritation continues, or if condition worsens or persists >72 hrs. Supervision required in patients with narrow angle glaucoma.

PREGNANCY: Safety in pregnancy and nursing not known.

MURO 128   OTC
sodium chloride (Bausch & Lomb)

THERAPEUTIC CLASS: Hypertonic agent

INDICATIONS: Temporary relief of corneal edema.

DOSAGE: *Adults:* (Sol) 1-2 drops q3-4h. (Oint) Apply 1/4 inch q3-4h.

HOW SUPPLIED: Oint: 5% [3.5g]; Sol: 2% [15mL], 5% [15mL, 30mL]

WARNINGS/PRECAUTIONS: Temporary burning and irritation may occur. Do not use if solution becomes cloudy or changes color. D/C if eye pain, vision changes, continued eye redness or irritation occur, or if condition worsens or persists for ≥72 hrs.

ADVERSE REACTIONS: Burning, irritation.

PREGNANCY: Safety in pregnancy and nursing not known.

M

MUTAMYCIN   RX
mitomycin (Bristol-Myers Squibb)

> Bone marrow suppression (eg, thrombocytopenia, leukopenia) may occur. Hemolytic Uremic Syndrome (HUS) reported, mostly with high doses (≥60mg). Blood product transfusion may exacerbate HUS. Administer only under supervision of a physician experienced in the use of antineoplastic agents.

THERAPEUTIC CLASS: DNA synthesis inhibitor

INDICATIONS: Disseminated adenocarcinoma of the stomach or pancreas as an adjunct to other chemotherapeutic agents or as palliative treatment when other modalities have failed. Not recommended as single-agent.

DOSAGE: *Adults:* Usual: (after full hematological recovery): 20mg/m^2 IV single dose q6-8 weeks. Dosage Adjustments: Leukocytes 2000-2999/mm^3, Platelets 25,000-74,999/mm^3: Give 70% of prior dose. Leukocytes <2000/mm^3, Platelets <25,000/mm^3: Give 50% of prior dose. No repeat dosage should be given until leukocyte count has returned to 4000/mm^3 and platelet count to 100,000/mm^3.

HOW SUPPLIED: Inj: 5mg, 20mg, 40mg

CONTRAINDICATIONS: Thrombocytopenia, coagulation disorder, increased bleeding tendency due to other causes.

WARNINGS/PRECAUTIONS: See Black Box Warning, Drug Interactions. Monitor platelets, WBCs, differential and Hgb repeatedly during therapy and for at least 8 weeks after. May cause renal toxicity, avoid if serum creatinine is >1.7mg %. Bladder fibrosis/contraction reported with intravesical administration.

ADVERSE REACTIONS: Bone marrow toxicity, integument and mucous membrane toxicity (eg, cellulitis, stomatitis, alopecia, skin necrosis), renal/pulmonary/cardiac toxicity, fever, anorexia, nausea, vomiting.

INTERACTIONS: Acute shortness of breath and bronchospasm reported following concomitant vinca alkaloids use. Adult respiratory distress syndrome reported with concomitant chemotherapy; monitor oxygen and fluid balance.

PREGNANCY: Safety in pregnancy unknown, not for use in nursing.

MECHANISM OF ACTION: DNA synthesis inhibitor; selectively inhibits synthesis of DNA and suppresses cellular RNA and protein synthesis at high concentrations.

PHARMACOKINETICS: Absorption: (IV) C_{max}=2.4mcg/mL, 1.7mcg/mL, 0.52mcg/mL (30mg, 20mg, 10mg). **Metabolism**: Liver. **Elimination**: Urine (approximately 10% unchanged). $T_{1/2}$(30mg)=17 min.

MYAMBUTOL   RX
ethambutol HCL (X-Gen)

THERAPEUTIC CLASS: Cell metabolism inhibitor

INDICATIONS: Adjunct treatment of pulmonary TB with at least 1 other anti-TB drug.

DOSAGE: *Adults:* Initial: 15mg/kg q24h. Retreatment: 25mg/kg q24h. After 60 days, decrease to 15mg/kg q24h. Renal Dysfunction: Reduce dose.
Pediatric: ≥13 yrs: Initial: 15mg/kg q24h. Retreatment: 25mg/kg q24h. After 60 days, decrease to 15mg/kg q24h. Renal Dysfunction: Reduce dose.

HOW SUPPLIED: Tab: 100mg, 400mg* *scored

CONTRAINDICATIONS: Optic neuritis. Patients unable to appreciate and report visual side effects or changes in vision.

WARNINGS/PRECAUTIONS: Test visual acuity before and periodically during therapy; monthly with dose >15mg/kg/day. Liver toxicity reported; monitor hepatic function at baseline and periodically. Evaluate renal and hematopoietic functions periodically.

ADVERSE REACTIONS: Decreased visual acuity, optic neuropathy, anaphylactic reactions, dermatitis, pruritus, joint pain, GI effects, malaise, dizziness, elevated uric acid levels, pulmonary infiltrates, abnormal LFTs, eosinophilia.

INTERACTIONS: Avoid concurrent administration with aluminum hydroxide containing antacids.

PREGNANCY: Category C, safety in nursing not known.

MECHANISM OF ACTION: Antitubercular agent; inhibits synthesis of one or more metabolites, thus causing impairment of cell metabolism, arrest of multiplication, and cell death.

PHARMACOKINETICS: Absorption: C_{max} =2-5mcg/mL; T_{max} =2-4 hrs. **Distribution:** Excreted in breast milk. **Metabolism:** Initial oxidation of alcohol to aldehydic metabolite, followed by conversion to dicarboxylic acid. **Elimination:** Urine (50% unchanged), (8-15%, metabolites), feces (20-22%, unchanged).

MYCAMINE RX
micafungin sodium (Astellas)

THERAPEUTIC CLASS: Glucan synthesis inhibitor

INDICATIONS: Treatment of candidemia, acute disseminated candiadiasis, *Candida* peritonitis, abscesses, and esophageal candidiasis. Prophylaxis of *Candida* infections in patients undergoing hematopoietic stem cell transplantation (HSCT).

DOSAGE: *Adults:* Candidemia/Acute Disseminated Candiadiasis/*Candida* Peritonitis/Abscesses: 100mg IV qd (usual range 10-47 days). Esophageal Candidiasis: 150mg IV qd (usual range 10-30 days). *Candida* Infection Prophylaxis in HSCT: 50mg IV qd (usual range 6-51 days). Do not mix or co-infuse with other drugs.

HOW SUPPLIED: Inj: 50mg, 100mg

WARNINGS/PRECAUTIONS: Reports of serious hypersensitivity reactions (eg, anaphylaxis, anaphylactoid, shock). LFT abnormalities, monitor for evidence of worsening. Reports of significant renal dysfunction, acute renal failure, and elevations in BUN and creatinine. Reports of acute intravascular hemolysis and hemoglobinuria. May precipitate when mixed or co-infused with other drugs. Hepatic carcinomas and adenomas observed.

ADVERSE REACTIONS: Hyperbilirubinemia, neutropenia, headache, rash, phlebitis, nausea, diarrhea, vomiting, pyrexia, hypokalemia, thrombocytopenia.

INTERACTIONS: Monitor for sirolimus, nifedipine, or itraconazole toxicity; reduce their dose if toxicity occurs.

PREGNANCY: Category C, caution in nursing.

MECHANISM OF ACTION: Antifungal agent. Inhibits the synthesis of 1,3-β-F-glucan, a component of fungal cell walls.

PHARMACOKINETICS: Absorption: IV infusion of variable doses resulted in different parameters. **Distribution:** V_d=0.39±0.11L/kg (terminal phase). Plasma protein binding (≥99%). **Metabolism:** Metabolized to M-1 (catechol form) by arylsulfatase and further metabolized to M-2 (methoxy form) by catechol-O-methyltransferase. Catalyzed by CYP450 isoenzymes. **Elimination:** Urine and feces (major route).

MYCELEX TROCHE RX
clotrimazole (Ortho-McNeil)

THERAPEUTIC CLASS: Azole antifungal

INDICATIONS: Local treatment of oropharyngeal candidiasis. Prophylactically to reduce the incidence of oropharyngeal candidiasis in immunocompromised conditions (eg, chemotherapy, radiotherapy, steroid therapy).

DOSAGE: *Adults:* Treatment: Slowly dissolve 1 troche in mouth 5 times/day for 14 days. Prophylaxis: Slowly dissolve 1 troche in mouth tid for duration of chemotherapy or until steroids reduced to maint levels.
Pediatrics: ≥3 yrs: Treatment: Slowly dissolve 1 troche in mouth 5 times/day for 14 days. Prophylaxis: Slowly dissolve 1 troche in mouth tid for duration of chemotherapy or until steroids reduced to maint levels.

HOW SUPPLIED: Tab: 10mg

WARNINGS/PRECAUTIONS: Not for systemic mycoses. May cause abnormal LFTs; monitor hepatic function. Only use in patients mentally and physically able to dissolve the troche. Confirm diagnosis by KOH smear and/or culture.

ADVERSE REACTIONS: Abnormal LFTs, nausea, vomiting, unpleasant mouth sensations, pruritus.

PREGNANCY: Category C, safety in nursing is not known.

MECHANISM OF ACTION: Broad-spectrum antifungal agent; inhibits growth of pathogenic yeasts by altering cell membrane permeability.

PHARMACOKINETICS: Absorption: C_{max} = 4.98ng/mL (30 min), 3.23ng/mL (60 min).

MYCELEX-3   OTC
butoconazole nitrate (Bayer Healthcare)

THERAPEUTIC CLASS: Azole antifungal

INDICATIONS: Treatment of vaginal yeast infection.

DOSAGE: *Adults:* Insert 1 applicatorful vaginally qhs for 3 days.
Pediatrics: ≥12 yrs: Insert 1 applicatorful vaginally qhs for 3 days.

HOW SUPPLIED: Cre: 2% [5g, 20g]

WARNINGS/PRECAUTIONS: Do not use if abdominal pain, fever, foul smelling discharge, pregnancy, diabetes, HIV positive and AIDS patients. Avoid tampons. Do not rely on condoms or diaphragms to prevent STDs or pregnancy while on therapy; use alternate birth control method.

PREGNANCY: Safety in pregnancy or nursing not known.

MYCELEX-7   OTC
clotrimazole (Bayer Healthcare)

THERAPEUTIC CLASS: Azole antifungal

INDICATIONS: (Cre, Combination Pack) Treatment of vaginal yeast infection. (Combination Pack) For relief of external vulvar itching and irritation associated with vaginal yeast infections.

DOSAGE: *Adults:* (Cre) Insert 1 applicatorful vaginally qhs for 7 days. (Combination Pack) 1 insert vaginally qhs for 7 days. Apply small amount of cream onto irritated area of vulva qd-bid for up to 7 days.
Pediatrics: ≥12 yrs: (Cre) Insert 1 applicatorful vaginally qhs for 7 days. (Combination Pack) 1 insert vaginally qhs for 7 days. Apply small amount of cream onto irritated area of vulva qd-bid for up to 7 days.

HOW SUPPLIED: Cre: 1% [45g]; (Combination Pack) Cre: 1% [7g], Vaginal Insert: 100 mg [7's]

WARNINGS/PRECAUTIONS: Do not use if abdominal pain, fever, foul smelling discharge, during pregnancy. Avoid tampons. May reduce effectiveness of condoms, diaphragm or vaginal spermicides.

PREGNANCY: Safety in pregnancy or nursing not known.

MYCOBUTIN   RX
rifabutin (Pharmacia & Upjohn)

THERAPEUTIC CLASS: Semisynthetic ansamycin (RNA polymerase inhibitor)

INDICATIONS: Prevention of disseminated *Mycobacterium avium* complex (MAC) in advanced HIV infection.

DOSAGE: *Adults:* 300mg qd; give 150mg bid with food if intolerant to GI side effects. Concomitant Nelfinavir/Indinavir or CrCl <30mL/min: Reduce dose by 50%.

HOW SUPPLIED: Cap: 150mg

WARNINGS/PRECAUTIONS: Avoid with active TB. *Clostridium difficile*-associated diarrhea reported. Neutropenia and thrombocytopenia may occur; obtain hematologic studies periodically. May permanently stain soft contact lenses. May cause discoloration of body fluids and skin. Caution in elderly.

ADVERSE REACTIONS: Rash, abdominal pain, nausea, vomiting, neutropenia, leukopenia, headache, rash, urine discoloration, taste perversion, increased SGOT/SGPT.

INTERACTIONS: May reduce levels of drugs metabolized by CYP3A enzymes (eg, itraconazole, clarithromycin, saquinavir). Increased levels with CYP3A inhibitors (eg, fluconazole, clarithromycin). Avoid delavirdine; rifabutin levels increase and delavirdine levels decrease. Avoid ritonavir; increased risk of adverse effects. Increased levels with nelfinavir, indinavir. May decrease efficacy of oral contraceptives.

PREGNANCY: Category B, not for use in nursing.

MECHANISM OF ACTION: Ansamycin antibiotic; inhibits DNA-dependent RNA polymerase in susceptible strains but not mammalian cells.

PHARMACOKINETICS: Absorption: C_{max}=375ng/mL; T_{max}=3.3 hrs; absolute bioavalability (20%). **Distribution:** V_d=9.3L/kg; plasma protein binding (85%). **Metabolism:** CYP3A; 25-O-desacetyl, 31-hydroxy (metabolites). **Elimination:** Urine, feces; $T_{1/2}$=45 hrs.

M

MYFORTIC   RX
mycophenolic acid (Novartis)

> Increased susceptibility to infection. Possible development of lymphoma and other neoplasms. Female users of childbearing potential must use contraception. Increased risk of pregnancy loss and congenital malformations.

THERAPEUTIC CLASS: Inosine monophosphate dehydrogenase inhibitor

INDICATIONS: Prophylaxis of organ rejection in patients receiving allogeneic renal transplants, administered in combination with cyclosporine and corticosteroids.

DOSAGE: *Adults:* 720mg bid on empty stomach, 1 hr before or 2 hrs after food intake.
Pediatrics: 400mg/m² bid. Max: 720mg bid. BSA 1.19-1.58m²: 540mg bid. BSA >1.58m²: 720mg bid. BSA <1.19m² cannot be accurately adminsitered with current formulations.

HOW SUPPLIED: Tab, Delayed-Release: 180mg, 360mg

WARNINGS/PRECAUTIONS: Risk of lymphomas and other malignancies, especially of the skin. Avoid sunlight to decrease risk of skin cancer. May cause fetal harm during pregnancy. Must have negative serum/urine pregnancy test within 1 week before therapy. Two reliable forms of contraception required before and during therapy, and 6 weeks following discontinuation. Monitor for bone marrow suppression. Risk of GI ulceration, hemorrhage, and perforation; caution with active digestive system disease. Caution with delayed renal graft function post-transplant. Oral suspension contains phenylalanine; caution with phenylketonurics. Monitor CBC weekly during the 1st month, twice monthly for the 2nd and 3rd months, and then monthly through 1st year. Avoid with rare hereditary deficiency of hypoxanthine-guanine phosphoribosyl-transferase (eg, Lesch-Nyhan and Kelley-Seegmiller syndrome). Female users of childbearing potential must use contraception. Increased risk of pregnancy loss and congenital malformations.

ADVERSE REACTIONS: Infections, diarrhea, leukopenia, sepsis, vomiting, GI bleeding, pain, abdominal pain, fever, headache, asthenia, chest pain, back pain, anemia, leukopenia, thrombocytopenia.

INTERACTIONS: Additive bone marrow suppression with azathioprine; avoid use. Reduced efficacy with drugs that interfere with enterohepatic recirculation (eg, cholestyramine). Efficacy/safety with other immunosuppressive agents not determined. Avoid live attenuated vaccines. Increased levels of both drugs with acyclovir, ganciclovir. Decreased levels with magnesium- and aluminum-containing antacids; space dosing. Decreased effects of oral contraceptives. Increased levels with probenecid. Other drugs that compete for renal tubular secretion may raise levels of both drugs.

PREGNANCY: Category D, not for use in nursing.

MECHANISM OF ACTION: Inosine monophosphate dehydrogenase inhibitor; inhibits the de novo pathway of guanosine nucleotide synthesis without incorporation to DNA.

PHARMACOKINETICS: Absorption: Absolute bioavailability (72%); T_{max}=1.5-2.75 hrs. **Distribution:** V_d=54L (steady state). Plasma protein binding: ≥98% (mycophenolic acid (MPA), 82% (mycophenolic acid glucuronide (MPAG). **Metabolism:** (MPA) metabolized by glucuronyl transferase to MPAG (major metabolite). **Elimination:** Urine: >60% (MPAG), 3% (unchanged), and bile; $T_{1/2}$=8-16 hrs (MPA), 13-17 hrs (MPAG).

MYLANTA GAS MAXIMUM STRENGTH OTC
simethicone (J&J -- Merck)

OTHER BRAND NAMES: Mylanta Gas Maximum Strength Softgels (J&J -- Merck) - Mylanta Gas Maximum Strength Chewable Tablets (J&J -- Merck)

THERAPEUTIC CLASS: Antigas

INDICATIONS: For the relief of bloating, pressure, and discomfort of gas caused by food or air swallowing.

DOSAGE: *Adults:* Softgels/Chewable Tabs: 1-2 prn. Max: 4 per day. Take after meals and at bedtime.

HOW SUPPLIED: Softgels, Maximum Strength: 125mg; Tab, Maximum Strength Chewable: 125mg

MYLANTA MAXIMUM STRENGTH LIQUID OTC
aluminum hydroxide - magnesium hydroxide - simethicone (J&J -- Merck)

OTHER BRAND NAMES: Mylanta Regular Strength Liquid (J&J -- Merck)

THERAPEUTIC CLASS: Antacid/antigas

INDICATIONS: For the relief of heartburn, acid indigestion, sour stomach, upset stomach, pressure and bloating.

DOSAGE: *Adults:* ≥12 yrs: 2-4 tsp between meals or at bedtime. Max: 24 tsp/day for 2 weeks. Shake well.
Pediatrics: ≥12 yrs: 2-4 tsp between meals or at bedtime. Max: 24 tsp/day for 2 weeks. Shake well.

HOW SUPPLIED: Liq: (Aluminum Hydroxide-Magnesium Hydroxide-Simethicone) Maximum Strength: 400mg/5mL-400mg/5mL-40mg/5mL. Regular Strength: 200mg/5mL-200mg/5mL-20mg/5mL

MYLANTA SUPREME
calcium carbonate - magnesium hydroxide (J&J -- Merck)

OTC

OTHER BRAND NAMES: Mylanta Ultra Tabs (J&J -- Merck) - Mylanta Gelcaps Antacid (J&J -- Merck)

THERAPEUTIC CLASS: Antacid

INDICATIONS: For the relief of acid indigestion, heartburn, sour and upset stomach associated with these symptoms.

DOSAGE: *Adults:* (Gelcaps) 2-4 caps prn. Max: 12 caps/24hrs. (Ultra Tabs) Chew 2-4 tabs between meals or at bedtime. Max: 10 tabs/24hrs. (Supreme Liquid) 2-4 tsp between meals or at bedtime. Max: 18 tsp/24hrs. Shake well.

HOW SUPPLIED: Cap: (Calcium Carbonate-Magnesium Hydroxide) 550mg-125mg. Tab: 700mg-300mg. Liq: 400mg/5mL-135mg/5mL

WARNINGS/PRECAUTIONS: Caution with kidney disease.

INTERACTIONS: Antacids may interact with other prescription drugs.

MYLERAN
busulfan (GlaxoSmithKline)

RX

> **Do not use unless CML diagnosis is established. May induce severe bone marrow hypoplasia; reduce dose or d/c if unusual depression of bone marrow function occurs.**

THERAPEUTIC CLASS: Alkylating agent

INDICATIONS: Palliative treatment of chronic myelogenous leukemia (CML).

DOSAGE: *Adults:* 60mcg/kg/day or 1.8mg/m²/day. Range: 4-8mg/day. Reserve dose >4mg/day for the most compelling symptoms.
Pediatrics: 60mcg/kg/day or 1.8mg/m²/day. Range: 4-8mg/day. Reserve dose >4mg/day for the most compelling symptoms.

HOW SUPPLIED: Tab: 2mg* *scored

CONTRAINDICATIONS: Lack of definitive diagnosis of CML.

WARNINGS/PRECAUTIONS: Induction of bone marrow failure resulting in severe pancytopenia reported. Bronchopulmonary dysplasia with pulmonary fibrosis, cellular dysplasia, malignant tumors, acute leukemias, hepatic veno-occlusive disease reported. Ovarian suppression and amenorrhea with menopausal symptoms have occurred. Cardiac tamponade in patients with thalassemia and seizures reported. Caution with compromised bone marrow reserve from prior irradiation/chemotherapy. Seizures reported.

ADVERSE REACTIONS: Myelosuppression, pulmonary fibrosis, cardiac tamponade, hyperpigmentation, weakness, fatigue, weight loss, nausea, vomiting, melanoderma, hyperuricemia, myasthenia gravis, hepatic veno-occlusive disease.

INTERACTIONS: Additive myelosuppression with myelosuppressive drugs. Additive pulmonary toxicity with myelotoxic drugs. Increased clearance of cyclophosphamide and busulfan with phenytoin pretreatment. Decreased clearance with concomitant cyclophosphamide alone. Reduced clearance with itraconazole; monitor for signs of toxicity. Concurrent thioguanine was associated with portal HTN and esophageal varices with abnormal LFTs; caution with long-term therapy.

PREGNANCY: Category D, not for use in nursing.

MECHANISM OF ACTION: Bifunctional alkylating agent.

PHARMACOKINETICS: Absorption: (IV, PO) Absolute bioavailability (adults 80%, children 68%); C$_{max}$(2mg, 4mg)=30ng/mL, 68ng/mL; T$_{max}$=0.9 hrs; AUC (4mg) =269ng•hr/mL **Distribution**: Crosses blood-brain barrier; plasma protein binding (32%). **Metabolism**: Liver (extensive); 3-hydroxytetrahydrothiopene-1, 1-dioxide (major metabolite). **Elimination**: Urine (>2%, unchanged); T$_{1/2}$=2.69 hrs.

M

MYLOTARG RX
gemtuzumab ozogamicin (Wyeth)

> Only use as monotherapy. Severe myelosuppression, severe hypersensitivity reactions (eg, anaphylaxis, pulmonary events, infusion related-reactions) can occur. Hepatotoxicity, including severe hepatic veno-occlusive disease (VOD) reported.

THERAPEUTIC CLASS: IgG_4 kappa antibody/calicheamicin conjugate

INDICATIONS: Treatment of patients with CD33 positive acute myeloid leukemia (AML) in 1st relapse patients ≥60 yrs who are not candidates for chemotherapy.

DOSAGE: *Adults:* ≥60 yrs: $9mg/m^2$ as 2 hr IV infusion, for 2 doses with 14 days between doses. Premedicate 1 hr prior with diphenhydramine 50mg and APAP 650-1000mg (may give additional APAP dose q4h for 2 doses as needed). Monitor vital signs during infusion and for 4 hrs after.

HOW SUPPLIED: Inj: 5mg

CONTRAINDICATIONS: Lactating mothers.

WARNINGS/PRECAUTIONS: Monitor CBC, LFTs, and electrolytes. Monitor vital signs during infusion and 4 hrs after. Interrupt infusion if dyspnea or significant hypotension develops. Consider discontinuing if develop anaphylaxis, pulmonary edema, or ARDS. Increased risk of severe VOD if used before or after hematopoietic stem-cell transplant, underlying hepatic disease or abnormal liver function, or with combination chemotherapy. Extra caution with hepatic impairment. Administer in appropriate facility. Tumor lysis syndrome may occur. Not for IV push or bolus use.

ADVERSE REACTIONS: Chills, fever, nausea, vomiting, headache, hypotension, HTN, hypoxia, dyspnea, hyperglycemia, antibody formation, myelosuppression, anemia, thrombocytopenia, sepsis, pneumonia, epistaxis, mucositis, hepatotoxicity, neutropenia.

PREGNANCY: Category D, not for use in nursing.

MECHANISM OF ACTION: IgG4 kappa antibody/calicheamicin conjugate; binds to CD33 antigen, resulting in formation of a complex that is internalized. Upon internalization, the calicheamicin derivative is released inside lysosomes of myeloid cell, which then binds to DNA in the minor groove, resulting in DNA double strand breaks and cell death.

PHARMACOKINETICS: Elimination: $T_{1/2}$ =41 hrs(total), 143hrs (congugated).

MYOZYME RX
alglucosidase alfa (Genzyme)

> Risk of hypersensitivity reactions. Life-threatening anaphylactic reactions, including anaphylactic shock observed during infusion. Appropriate medical support should be readily available when administered.

THERAPEUTIC CLASS: Enzyme

INDICATIONS: Treatment of Pompe Disease.

DOSAGE: *Adults:* 20 mg/kg IV every 2 weeks. Administer over 4 hrs. *Pediatrics:* 20 mg/kg IV every 2 weeks. Administer over 4 hrs.

HOW SUPPLIED: Inj: 50 mg

WARNINGS/PRECAUTIONS: See Black Box Warning. Risk of cardiac arrhythmia, sudden cardiac death during general anesthesia for central venous catheter placement, and acute cardiorespiratory failure. Infusion reactions observed. Caution with acutely ill patients.

ADVERSE REACTIONS: Pyrexia, cough, respiratory distress/failure, pneumonia, otitis media, upper respiratory tract infection, gastroenteritis, pharyngitis, diarrhea, vomiting, rash, decreased oxygen saturation, anemia, oral candidiasis.

PREGNANCY: Category B, caution in nursing.

MECHANISM OF ACTION: Enzyme; provides exogenous source of human enzyme α-glucosidase (GAA). Binds to mannose-6-phosphate receptors on cell surface via carbohydrate groups on GAA molecule. It is then internalized and transported into lysosomes where it undergoes proteolytic cleavage, producing an increase in enzymatic activity (cleaving glycogen).

PHARMACOKINETICS: Absorption: (20mg/kg single dose) C_{max}=162mcg/mL, AUC=811mcg-hr/mL; (40mg/kg single Dose) C_{max}=276mcg/mL, AUC=1781mcg-hr/mL. **Distribution:** (20mg/kg single dose) V_d=69ml/kg; (40mg/kg single dose) V_d=119mL/kg. **Elimination:** (20mg/kg Single Dose) $T_{1/2}$=2.6 hrs; (40mg/kg Single Dose) $T_{1/2}$=2.9 hrs.

MYSOLINE RX
primidone (Valeant)

THERAPEUTIC CLASS: Pyrimidinedione derivative

INDICATIONS: For control of grand mal, psychomotor, and focal epileptic seizures.

DOSAGE: *Adults:* Initial: Day 1-3: 100-125mg qhs. Day 4-6: 100-125mg bid. Day 7-9: 100-125mg tid. Day 10-Maint: 250mg tid. Max: 500mg qid. Effective serum level is 5-12mcg/mL. Prior Anticonvulsant Therapy: Initial: 100-125mg qhs. Titrate: Increase gradually to maintenance dose as other drug is discontinued over 2 weeks.
Pediatrics: ≥8 yrs: Initial: Day 1-3: 100-125mg qhs. Day 4-6: 100-125mg bid. Day 7-9: 100-125mg tid. Day 10-Maint: 250mg tid. Max: 500mg qid. <8 yrs: Day 1-3: 50mg qhs. Day 4-6: 50mg bid. Day 7-9: 100mg bid. Day 10-Maint: 125-250mg tid or 10-25mg/kg/day in divided doses. Effective serum level is 5-12mcg/mL. Prior Anticonvulsant Therapy: Initial: 100-125mg qhs. Titrate: Increase gradually to maintenance dose as other drug is discontinued over 2 weeks.

HOW SUPPLIED: Tab: 50mg*, 250mg* *scored

CONTRAINDICATIONS: Porphyria, phenobarbital hypersensitivity.

WARNINGS/PRECAUTIONS: Avoid abrupt withdrawal. May take several weeks to assess therapeutic efficacy. Pregnant women should receive prophylactic vitamin K_1 therapy for one month prior to, and during, delivery. Perform CBC and a SMA-12 test every 6 months. Phenobarbital is a metabolite of primidone.

ADVERSE REACTIONS: Ataxia, vertigo, nausea, anorexia, vomiting, fatigue, hyperirritability, emotional disturbances, sexual impotency, diplopia, nystagmus, drowsiness, morbilliform skin eruptions.

PREGNANCY: Safety in pregnancy not known, caution in nursing.

MECHANISM OF ACTION: Pyrimidinedione. Not established; suspected to raise electro- or chemoshock seizure thresholds or alter seizure patterns. Has anticonvulsant activity.

PHARMACOKINETICS: Distribution: Found in breast milk. **Metabolism:** Metabolites: Phenobarbital and phenylethylmalonamide (PEMA) (Both active).

NABUMETONE RX
nabumetone (Various)

> NSAIDs may cause an increased risk of serious cardiovascular thrombotic events, MI, stroke and serious GI adverse events including bleeding, ulceration, and perforation of the stomach or intestines. Contraindicated for the treatment of perioperative pain in the setting of coronary artery bypass graft (CABG) surgery.

THERAPEUTIC CLASS: NSAID (naphthylalkanone derivative)

INDICATIONS: Relief of signs and symptoms of osteoarthritis and rheumatoid arthritis.

DOSAGE: *Adults:* Initial: 1000mg qd. Max: 2000mg/day.

HOW SUPPLIED: Tab: 500mg, 750mg

CONTRAINDICATIONS: Allergy to ASA or other NSAID that precipitates asthma, urticaria, or other allergic-type reaction. Treatment of perioperative pain in the setting of CABG surgery.

WARNINGS/PRECAUTIONS: May lead to onset of new HTN or worsening of pre-existing HTN; monitor BP closely. Fluid retention and edema reported; caution with fluid retention or heart failure. Renal papillary necrosis and other renal injury reported after long-term use. Not recommended for use with advanced renal disease; if therapy must be initiated, monitor renal function. Anaphylactoid reactions may occur. May cause serious skin adverse events (eg, exfoliative dermatitis, Stevens-Johnson syndrome, and toxic epidermal necrolysis). Avoid in late pregnancy; may cause premature closure of ductus arteriosis. May cause elevations of LFTs; d/c if liver disease develops or systemic manifestations occur. Caution in elderly. Anemia may occur; with long-term use, monitor Hgb/Hct if signs or symptoms of anemia develop. May inhibit platelet aggregation and prolong bleeding time; monitor with coagulation disorders. Caution with asthma and avoid with ASA-sensitive asthma. May induce photosensitivity. Risk of GI ulceration, bleeding, and perforation.

ADVERSE REACTIONS: Diarrhea, dyspepsia, abdominal pain, constipation, flatulence, nausea, positive stool guaiac, dizziness, headache, pruritus, rash, tinnitus, edema.

INTERACTIONS: Caution with warfarin, other protein bound drugs. Nephrotoxicity risk with diuretics. May elevate lithium and methotrexate levels. May diminish antihypertensive effect of ACE inhibitors. Avoid concomitant ASA.

PREGNANCY: Category C, not for use in nursing.

MECHANISM OF ACTION: NSAID (napthylalkanone derivative); suspected to inhibit prostaglandin synthetase, exerts anti-inflammatory, analgesic, and antipyretic actions.

PHARMACOKINETICS: Absorption: Well-absorbed (GIT). PO administration of variable doses resulted in different parameters. **Distribution:** Plasma protein binding (≥99%). **Metabolism:** Liver (extensive biotransformation), 6-methoxy-2-naphthylacetic acid (active metabolite). **Elimination:** Urine (approximately 75%), feces; $T_{1/2}$=24 hrs.

NAFTIN   RX
naftifine HCL (Merz)

THERAPEUTIC CLASS: Allylamine antifungal

INDICATIONS: Topical treatment of tinea pedis, tinea cruris, and tinea corporis caused by *Trichophyton rubrum, Trichophyton mentagrophytes,* and *Epidermophyton floccosum.*

DOSAGE: *Adults:* Massage into affected and surrounding area(s) (Cre) qd or (Gel) bid (am and pm). Wash hands after use. Re-evaluate if no improvement after 4 weeks.

HOW SUPPLIED: Cre: 1% [15g, 30g, 60g]; Gel: 1% [20g, 40g, 60g]

WARNINGS/PRECAUTIONS: Stop therapy if irritation develops. Avoid eyes, nose, and mucous membranes.

ADVERSE REACTIONS: Burning/stinging, rash, erythema, itching, dryness, skin tenderness.

PREGNANCY: Category B, caution in nursing.

MECHANISM OF ACTION: Allylamine antifungal; mechanism not established. Suspected to interfere with sterol biosynthesis by inhibiting the enzyme squalene 2,3-epoxidase. Results in decreased amounts of sterols, especially ergosterol, and corresponding accumulation of squalene in cells.

PHARMACOKINETICS: Absorption: Penetrates stratum corneum. Systemic absorption: Cre: (6% of applied dose); Gel: (up to 4.2% of applied dose). **Elimination:** Urine, feces (metabolites). $T_{1/2}$=2-3 days.

NALOXONE RX
naloxone HCL (Various)

OTHER BRAND NAMES: Narcan (Endo)

THERAPEUTIC CLASS: Opioid antagonist

INDICATIONS: For complete or partial opioid depression reversal induced by natural and synthetic opioids. Diagnosis of suspected opioid tolerance or acute opioid overdose. Adjunct in management of septic shock to increase blood pressure.

DOSAGE: *Adults:* Opioid Overdose: Initial: 0.4-2mg IV every 2-3 minutes up to 10mg. IM/SQ if IV route not available. Post-op Opioid Depression: 0.1-0.2mg IV every 2-3 minutes to desired response. May repeat in 1-2 hr intervals. Supplemental IM doses last longer. Narcan Challenge Test: IV: 0.1-0.2mg, observe 30 secs for signs of withdrawal, then 0.6mg, observe for 20 min. SQ: 0.8mg, observe for 20 min.
Pediatrics: Opioid Overdose: Initial: 0.01mg/kg IV. Inadequate Response: repeat 0.1mg/kg once. IM/SQ in divided doses if IV route not available. Post-op Opioid Depression: 0.005-0.01mg IV every 2-3 min to desired response. May repeat in 1-2 hr intervals. Supplemental IM doses last longer. Neonates: Opioid-induced Depression: 0.01mg/kg IV/IM/SQ, may repeat every 2-3 min until desired response.

HOW SUPPLIED: Inj: 0.4mg/mL, 1mg/mL

WARNINGS/PRECAUTIONS: Caution in patients including newborns of mothers known or suspected of opioid physical dependence. May precipitate acute withdrawal syndrome. Have other resuscitative measures available. Caution with cardiac, renal, or hepatic disease. Monitor patients satisfactorily responding due to extended opioid duration of action. Abrupt postoperative opioid depression reversal may result in serious adverse effects leading to death.

ADVERSE REACTIONS: HTN, hypotension, ventricular tachycardia and fibrillation, dyspnea, pulmonary edema, cardiac arrest, nausea, vomiting, sweating, seizures, body aches, fever, nervousness.

INTERACTIONS: Caution using drugs with potential adverse cardiac effects. Reversal of buprenorphine-induced respiratory depression may be incomplete.

PREGNANCY: Category B, caution in nursing.

MECHANISM OF ACTION: Narcotic antagonist; prevents or reverses effects of opioids, including respiratory depression, sedation, and hypotension, by competing for same receptor sites. Also reverses psychotomimetic and dysphoric effects of agonist-antagonists (eg, pentazocine).

PHARMACOKINETICS: Distribution: Rapid; plasma protein binding (weak). **Metabolism:** Liver; via glucuronide conjugation; naloxone-3-glucuronide (major metabolite). **Elimination:** Urine (25-40%); $T_{1/2}$=30-80 min (adults), 3.1 hrs (neonates).

NAMENDA RX
memantine HCL (Forest)

THERAPEUTIC CLASS: NMDA receptor antagonist

INDICATIONS: Treatment of moderate to severe dementia of the Alzheimer's type.

DOSAGE: *Adults:* Initial: 5mg qd. Titrate: Increase at intervals of at least one week to 5mg bid, then 5mg and 10mg as separate doses, then to 10mg bid. Severe Renal Impairment: Reduce dose.

HOW SUPPLIED: Sol: 2mg/mL; Tab: 5mg, 10mg; Titration-Pak: 5mg [28s], 10mg [21s].

WARNINGS/PRECAUTIONS: Use not evaluated with seizure disorders. Alkalinized urine (eg, renal tubular acidosis, severe urinary tract infections) may increase levels. Reduce dose with severe renal impairment. Should be administered with caution to patients with severe hepatic impairment.

ADVERSE REACTIONS: Dizziness, confusion, headache, constipation, coughing, HTN, pain, vomiting, somnolence, hallucinations.

INTERACTIONS: Caution with other NMDA antagonists (eg, amantadine, ketamine, dextromethorphan), urinary alkalinizers (eg, carbonic anhydrase inhibitors, sodium bicarbonate). Other renally-excreted drugs (eg, HCTZ, triamterene, metformin, cimetidine, ranitidine, quinidine, nicotine) may alter levels of both agents.

PREGNANCY: Category B, caution in nursing.

MECHANISM OF ACTION: NMDA receptor antagonist; postulated to exert effect by binding to NMDA receptor-operated cation channels.

PHARMACOKINETICS: Absorption: T_{max}=3-7 hrs. **Distribution:** V_d=9-11L/kg. Plasma protein binding (45%) **Metabolism:** Hepatic (partial). **Elimination:** Urine (48%). $T_{1/2}$=60-80 hrs.

NAPHCON-A   OTC
naphazoline HCL - pheniramine maleate (Alcon)

THERAPEUTIC CLASS: H_1-antagonist/alpha-agonist (imidazoline)

INDICATIONS: Temporary relief of ocular itching and redness caused by ragweed, pollen, grass, animal hair and dander.

DOSAGE: *Adults:* 1-2 drops up to 4 times daily.
Pediatrics: ≥6 yrs: 1-2 drops up to 4 times daily.

HOW SUPPLIED: Sol: (Pheniramine-Naphazoline) 0.3%-0.025% [15mL]

CONTRAINDICATIONS: Heart disease, high BP, enlargement of the prostate, narrow-angle glaucoma.

WARNINGS/PRECAUTIONS: Do not use if solution changes color or becomes cloudy. D/C with eye pain, changes in vision, continued redness or irritation, and if the condition worsens or persists for more than 72 hrs. Remove contact lenses before use. Supervision required with heart disease, high BP, difficulty in urination due to prostate enlargement or narrow angle glaucoma.

PREGNANCY: Safety in pregnancy and nursing not known.

NAPRELAN   RX
naproxen sodium (Elan)

> NSAIDs may cause an increased risk of serious cardiovascular thrombotic events, MI, stroke and serious GI adverse events including bleeding, ulceration, and perforation of the stomach or intestines. Contraindicated for the treatment of perioperative pain in the setting of coronary artery bypass graft (CABG) surgery.

THERAPEUTIC CLASS: NSAID (arylacetic acid derivative)

INDICATIONS: Treatment of rheumatoid arthritis (RA), osteoarthritis (OA), ankylosing spondylitis (AS), tendinitis, bursitis, primary dysmenorrhea and acute gout. Relief of mild to moderate pain.

DOSAGE: *Adults:* RA/OA/AS: Usual: 750mg-1g qd. Max: 1.5g/day. Pain/Primary Dysmenorrhea/Tendinitis/Bursitis: 1g/day or 1.5g for a limited period. Max: 1g/day thereafter. Acute Gout: 1-1.5g qd for 1 day, then 1g qd until attack subsides.

HOW SUPPLIED: Tab, Extended-Release: 375mg, 500mg

CONTRAINDICATIONS: History of angioedema, urticaria, bronchospastic reactivity, nasal polyps. NSAID allergy that precipitates asthma, nasal polyps, urticaria, and hypotension. Treatment of perioperative pain in the setting of CABG surgery.

WARNINGS/PRECAUTIONS: May lead to onset of new HTN or worsening of pre-existing HTN; monitor BP closely. Fluid retention and edema reported; caution with fluid retention or heart failure. Renal papillary necrosis and other renal injury reported after long-term use. Not recommended for use with advanced renal disease; if therapy must be initiated, monitor renal function. Anaphylactoid reactions may occur. May cause serious skin adverse events (eg, exfoliative dermatitis, Stevens-Johnson syndrome, and toxic epidermal necrolysis). Avoid in late pregnancy; may cause premature closure of ductus arteriosis. May cause elevations of LFTs; d/c if liver disease develops or systemic manifestations occur. Caution in elderly. Anemia may occur; with long-term use, monitor Hgb/Hct if signs or symptoms of anemia develop. May inhibit platelet aggregation and prolong bleeding time; monitor with coagulation disorders. Caution with asthma and avoid with ASA-sensitive asthma.

ADVERSE REACTIONS: Headache, dyspepsia, flu syndrome, pain, infection, nausea, diarrhea, constipation, abdominal pain, heartburn, drowsiness, edema, skin rash, ecchymoses.

INTERACTIONS: Avoid with other products containing naproxen. May inhibit natriuretic effect of furosemide. Probenecid increases plasma levels and extends its plasma half-life. May increase methotrexate toxicity. Avoid ASA. Caution with coumarin-type anticoagulants, hydantoins, sulfonamides or sulfonylureas; monitor for toxicity. ACE inhibitors may potentiate renal disease states. May displace albumin-bound drugs. May reduce antihypertensive effect of β-blockers. May increase lithium levels.

PREGNANCY: Category C, not for use in nursing.

MECHANISM OF ACTION: NSAID; not fully established, suspected to inhibit prostaglandin synthetase.

PHARMACOKINETICS: Absorption: Rapid, complete; bioavailability (95%); T_{max}=5 hrs; C_{max}=94mcg/mL; AUC=1448mcg•hr/mL. **Distribution:** Plasma protein binding (>99%); V_d=0.16L/kg. **Metabolism:** Hepatic; 6-O-desmethyl naproxen (metabolite). **Elimination:** Urine, feces (≤5%); $T_{1/2}$=15 hrs.

NAPROSYN   RX
naproxen (Roche Labs)

N

> NSAIDs may cause an increased risk of serious cardiovascular thrombotic events, MI, stroke and serious GI adverse events including bleeding, ulceration, and perforation of the stomach or intestines. Contraindicated for the treatment of perioperative pain in the setting of coronary artery bypass graft (CABG) surgery.

OTHER BRAND NAMES: EC-Naprosyn (Roche Labs)

THERAPEUTIC CLASS: NSAID

INDICATIONS: (Naprosyn, EC-Naprosyn) Relief of signs and symptoms of rheumatoid arthritis (RA), osteoarthritis (OA), ankylosing spondylitis, and juvenile arthritis (JA). (Naprosyn) Relief of signs and symtoms of tendinitis, bursitis, and acute gout. Management of pain and primary dysmenorrhea. EC-Naprosyn not recommended for initial treatment of acute pain.

DOSAGE: *Adults:* RA/OA/Ankylosing Spondylitis: Naprosyn: 250, 375, or 500mg bid; EC-Naprosyn: 375 or 500mg bid. Max: 1500mg/day. Acute Gout: Naprosyn: 750mg followed by 250mg q8h until attack subsides. Pain/Dysmenorrhea/Tendinitis/Bursitis: Naprosyn: 500mg followed by 500mg q12h or 250mg q6-8h prn. Max: 1250mg on Day 1, then 1000mg/day. EC-Naprosyn should not be chewed, crushed, or broken.
Pediatrics: ≥2 yrs: JA: (Sus) 5mg/kg bid. Max: 15mg/kg/day.

HOW SUPPLIED: (Naproxen) Sus: 25mg/mL; Tab: 250mg*, 375mg, 500mg*; Tab, Delayed-Release: (EC-Naprosyn) 375mg, 500mg *scored

CONTRAINDICATIONS: History of ASA or NSAID allergy that cause symptoms of asthma, rhinitis, nasal polyps, and hypotension. Treatment of perioperative pain in the setting of CABG surgery.

WARNINGS/PRECAUTIONS: May lead to onset of new HTN or worsening of pre-existing HTN; monitor BP closely. Fluid retention, edema, and peripheral edema reported; caution with fluid retention, HTN, or heart failure. Renal papillary necrosis and other renal injury reported after long-term use. Not recommended for use with advanced renal disease; if therapy must be initiated, monitor renal function. Anaphylactoid reactions may occur. May cause serious skin adverse events (eg, exfoliative dermatitis, Stevens-Johnson syndrome, and toxic epidermal necrolysis). Avoid in late pregnancy; may cause premature closure of ductus arteriosis. Monitor Hgb levels with long-term therapy if initial Hgb ≤10g. Monitor for visual changes or disturbances. May cause elevations of LFTs; d/c if liver disease develops or systemic manifestations occur. Caution with high doses in chronic alcoholic liver disease and elderly. Anemia may occur; with long-term use, monitor Hgb/Hct if signs or symptoms of anemia develop. May inhibit platelet aggregation and prolong bleeding time; monitor with coagulation disorders. Caution with asthma and avoid with ASA-sensitive asthma.

ADVERSE REACTIONS: Edema, drowsiness, dizziness, constipation, heartburn, abdominal pain, nausea, headache, tinnitus, dyspnea, pruritus, skin eruptions, ecchymoses.

INTERACTIONS: (Naprosyn, EC-Naprosyn) Avoid with other products containing naproxen. Decreased plasma levels with ASA. May reduce tubular secretion of methotrexate; monitor for toxicity. May increase nephrotoxicity of cyclosporine; caution when coadministering. May diminish antihypertensive effect and potentiate renal disease with ACE inhibitors. May reduce natriuretic effect of furosemide and thiazides; monitor for renal failure. May increase lithium levels; monitor for toxicity. Synergistic effects on GI bleeding with warfarin. Observe for dose adjustment with hydantoins, sulfonamides, or sulfonylureas. May reduce antihypertensive effects of propranolol and other β-blockers. Probenecid may increase half-life. (EC-Naprosyn) Avoid with H_2-blockers, sucralfate, or intensive antacid therapy.

PREGNANCY: Category C, not for use in nursing.

MECHANISM OF ACTION: NSAIDs; unknown, suspected to inhibit prostaglandin synthetase.

PHARMACOKINETICS: Absorption: Rapid and complete. Bioavailability (95%), T_{max}=1.9 hrs; C_{max}=97.4mcg/mL; AUC_{0-12h}=767mcg•hr/mL. (Tab, Delayed-Release) T_{max}=4 hrs; C_{max}=94.9mcg/mL; AUC_{0-12h}=845mcg•hr/mL. (Sus) T_{max}=1-4 hrs. **Distribution:** V_d=0.16L/kg; plasma protein binding (>99%), excreted in breast milk. **Metabolism:** Hepatic. Metabolite (6-O-desmethyl naproxen). **Elimination:** Urine (95%), feces (≤3%), $T_{1/2}$=12-17 hrs.

NARDIL   RX
phenelzine sulfate (Parke-Davis)

> Antidepressants increased the risk of suicidal thinking and behavior (suicidality) in short-term studies in children, adolescents, and young adults with Major Depressive Disorder (MDD) and other psychiatric disorders. Phenelzine is not approved for use in pediatric patients.

THERAPEUTIC CLASS: Monoamine oxidase inhibitor

INDICATIONS: Treatment of atypical, nonendogenous or neurotic depression not responsive to other antidepressants.

DOSAGE: *Adults:* Initial: 15mg tid. Titrate: Increase to 60-90mg/day at a fairly rapid pace until maximum benefit. Maint: Reduce slowly over several weeks to 15mg qd or 15mg every other day.

HOW SUPPLIED: Tab: 15mg

CONTRAINDICATIONS: Pheochromocytoma, CHF, history of liver disease, abnormal LFT's, severe renal impairment or renal disease, meperidine, MAOIs, dextromethorphan, CNS depressants, alcohol, certain narcotics, sympathomimetic drugs (eg, amphetamines, cocaine, methylphenidate, dopamine, epinephrine, norepinephrine), or related compounds (eg, methyldopa, L-dopa, L-tryptophan, L-tyrosine, phenylalanine), high tyramine-containing food (eg, cheese, pickled herring, beer, wine, yeast extract, salami, yogurt), excessive caffeine and chocolate, dextromethorphan, CNS depressants, buspirone, serotoninergic agents (eg, dexfenfluramine, fluoxetine, fluvoxamine, paroxetine, sertraline, venlafaxine), bupropion, guanethidine.

WARNINGS/PRECAUTIONS: Hypertensive crisis, postural hypotension reported; monitor BP frequently. Caution with epilepsy, asthma, DM, or psychosis.

D/C if palpitations or headache occur. Excessive stimulation in schizophrenics. D/C 10 days prior to elective surgery. Avoid abrupt withdrawal.

ADVERSE REACTIONS: Dizziness, headache, drowsiness, sleep disturbances, constipation, dry mouth, GI disturbances, elevated serum transaminases, weight gain, edema, sexual disturbances.

INTERACTIONS: See Contraindications. Hypertensive crisis with other MAOIs, sympathomimetics, high tyramine-containing foods. Allow 10 days between starting another MAOI, or antidepressant or buspirone. Serious reactions reported with serotoninergic agents. Allow 5 weeks after discontinuing fluoxetine before starting therapy. Allow 2 weeks after discontinuing therapy before starting bupropion. Avoid cocaine, local, general, and spinal anesthesia. Reduce dose of barbiturates. Caution with rauwolfia alkaloids. Exaggerated hypotensive effects with antihypertensives. Excitation, seizures, delirium, hyperpyrexia, circulatory collapse, coma, and death have been reported with meperidine.

PREGNANCY: Safety in pregnancy and nursing not known.

MECHANISM OF ACTION: MAOI; inhibits MAO activity.

PHARMACOKINETICS: Absorption: (30mg): C_{max}=19.8ng/mL, T_{max}=43 mins. **Metabolism:** Oxidation via MAO. Acetylation (minor). **Elimination:** (30mg): $T_{1/2}$=11.6 hrs.

NAROPIN   RX
ropivacaine HCL (Abraxis)

THERAPEUTIC CLASS: Local anesthetic

INDICATIONS: Production of local or regional anesthesia in surgery. Management of acute pain.

DOSAGE: *Adults:* Dose may vary by procedure, area to be anesthetized, tissue vascularity, duration and depth of anesthesia needed. Administer test dose of 3-5mL before induction of complete block. Surgical: Lumbar Epidural: Usual: 75-200mg in 15-30mL. Thoracic Epidural for Surgery: 25-113mg in 5-15mL. Lumbar Epidural in Cesarean: 100-150mg in 15-30mL. Major Nerve Block: 75-300mg in 10-50mL. Field Block: 5-200mg in 1-40mL Labor: Lumbar Epidural: Initial: 20-40mg. Maint: 12-28mg/h. Postoperative: Lumbar/Thoracic Epidural: 12-28mg/hr. Infiltration: 2-200mg in 1-100mL.

HOW SUPPLIED: Inj: 2mg/mL, 5mg/mL, 7.5mg/mL, 10mg/mL

WARNINGS/PRECAUTIONS: Administer in incremental doses. High risk of arrhythmias, circulatory arrest, and death reported in pregnant patients. Not for production of obstetrical paracervical block, retrobulbar block, or spinal anesthesia. Use lowest effective dose. Perform syringe aspiration to avoid extravasation and subarachnoid injection. Administer test dose with epidural anesthesia. Anxiety, dizziness, blurred vision, tremors, depression, and tinnitus are early signs of CNS toxicity. Caution in hepatic impairment, cardiovascular disorders, hypotension, hypovolemia, heart block. Should cardiac arrest occur, prolonged resuscitative efforts may be required to improve the probability of a successful outcome.

ADVERSE REACTIONS: Hypotension, bradycardia, nausea, vomiting, paresthesia, back pain, fever, chills, headache, pain, urinary retention, dizziness, pruritus, HTN, anemia.

INTERACTIONS: Caution with other local anesthetics, amide-type anesthetics; additive toxic effects may occur. Caution with class III antiarrhythmics. Increased levels with inhibitors of CYP450 1A2 (eg, fluvoxamine) and CYP450 3A4 (eg, ketoconazole).

PREGNANCY: Category B, caution in nursing.

MECHANISM OF ACTION: Mono amide class of local anesthetic agent; blocks the generation and the conduction of nerve impulses, presumably by increasing the threshold for electrical excitation in the nerve, by slowing the propagation of the nerve impulse, and by reducing the rate of rise of the action potential.

PHARMACOKINETICS: Absorption: Complete and biphasic absorption (epidural space). Sytemic concentration of drug is dependent on total dose, concentration, and route of administration; refer to PI for more information. **Distribution:** Plasma protein binding (94%), V_d=41L (IV). Crosses placenta and excreted in breast milk. **Metabolism:** Liver (extensive); aromatic hydroxylation, CYP4501A; 3-hydroxyropivacaine. **Elimination:** Urine: IV (86%), (1% unchanged); $T_{1/2}$=1.8 hrs and 4.2 hrs (epidural).

NASACORT AQ   RX
triamcinolone acetonide (Sanofi-Aventis)

THERAPEUTIC CLASS: Corticosteroid

INDICATIONS: Nasal treatment of seasonal and perennial allergic rhinitis symptoms.

DOSAGE: *Adults:* Initial/Max: 2 sprays per nostril qd. With improvement, may reduce dose to 1 spray per nostril qd.
Pediatrics: ≥12 yrs: Initial/Max: 2 sprays per nostril qd. With improvement, may reduce dose to 1 spray per nostril qd. 6-12 yrs: Initial: 1 spray per nostril qd. Max: 2 sprays per nostril qd.

HOW SUPPLIED: AQ Spray: 55mcg/spray [16.5g]

WARNINGS/PRECAUTIONS: Risk of adrenal insufficiency and withdrawal symptoms when replacing systemic corticosteroid with a topical corticosteroids. Caution with active or quiescent TB, ocular herpes simplex, or untreated bacterial, fungal and systemic viral infections. Avoid with recent nasal trauma, surgery or septum ulcers. Risk for more severe/fatal course of infections (eg, chickenpox, measles) and for *Candida* infections of the nose and pharynx. Potential for growth velocity reduction in pediatrics.

ADVERSE REACTIONS: Pharyngitis, epistaxis, infection, otitis media, headache, sneezing, rhinitis, nasal irritation, cough, sinusitis, vomiting.

PREGNANCY: Category C, caution in nursing.

MECHANISM OF ACTION: Corticosteroid; not established; anti-inflammatory action.

PHARMACOKINETICS: Absorption: C_{max}=0.5ng/mL; T_{max}=1.5 hrs; AUC (110mcg, 400mcg)=1.4ng•hr/mL, 4.7ng•hr/mL. **Elimination:** $T_{1/2}$=3.1 hrs.

NASAREL   RX
flunisolide (Ivax)

THERAPEUTIC CLASS: Corticosteroid

INDICATIONS: Relief of seasonal or perennial rhinitis.

DOSAGE: *Adults:* Initial: 2 sprays per nostril bid. Titrate: May increase to 2 sprays per nostril tid. Max: 8 sprays per nostril/day.
Pediatrics: 6-14 yrs: Initial: 1 spray per nostril tid or 2 sprays per nostril bid. Max: 4 sprays per nostril/day.

HOW SUPPLIED: Spray: 29mcg/spray [25mL]

CONTRAINDICATIONS: Untreated localized infection of the nasal mucosa.

WARNINGS/PRECAUTIONS: Risk of adrenal insufficiency and withdrawal symptoms when replacing systemic corticosteroids with a topical corticosteroids. Caution with active or quiescent TB, ocular herpes simplex, or untreated bacterial, fungal and systemic viral infections. Avoid with recent nasal trauma, surgery or septum ulcers. Risk for more severe/fatal course of infections (eg, chickenpox, measles) and for *Candida* infections of the nose and pharynx. Potential for growth velocity reduction in pediatrics.

ADVERSE REACTIONS: Aftertaste, nasal burning/stinging, cough, epistaxis, nasal dryness, pharyngitis, sinusitis.

INTERACTIONS: Concomitant systemic corticosteroids increases risk of hypercorticism and/or HPA axis suppression.

PREGNANCY: Category C, caution in nursing.

MECHANISM OF ACTION: Glucocorticosteroid; anti-inflammatory agent with potent glucucorticoid and weak mineralocorticoid activity.

PHARMACOKINETICS: Absorption: Well absorbed. **Metabolism:** Liver (rapidly). **Elimination:** Urine (65-70%) primary metabolite, feces.

NASCOBAL   RX
cyanocobalamin (Questcor)

THERAPEUTIC CLASS: Synthetic Vitamin B_{12}

INDICATIONS: Maintenance of hematologic status of patients in remission following IM vitamin B_{12} therapy for the following conditions: pernicious anemia; dietary deficiency in vegetarians; malabsorption resulting from structural/functional damage to the stomach (eg, HIV, AIDS, Crohn's disease); lesions that destroy gastric mucosa and conditions associated with gastric atrophy (eg, MS, HIV, AIDS); intestinal parasites; and inadequate utilization of vitamin B_{12} (antimetabolites used to treat neoplasia).

DOSAGE: *Adults:* 500mcg (1 spray) intranasally once weekly. Patients should be in hematologic remission before treatment.

HOW SUPPLIED: Gel, Spray: 500mcg/0.1mL (per actuation) [2.3mL]

CONTRAINDICATIONS: Sensitivity to cobalt.

WARNINGS/PRECAUTIONS: Severe and swift optic atrophy reported with Leber's disease. Hypokalemia and sudden death may occur in severe megaloblastic anemia treated intensely. Folic acid is not a substitute for vitamin B_{12}-deficient anemia. Perform intradermal test dose if sensitivity suspected. Vitamin B_{12} deficiency may suppress signs of polycythemia vera. Hypokalemia and thrombocytosis may occur upon conversion of severe megaloblastic to normal erythropoiesis. Avoid use with nasal congestion, allergic rhinitis, upper respiratory infection. Monitor vitamin B_{12} levels and peripheral blood counts prior to and periodically during therapy.

ADVERSE REACTIONS: Nausea, headache, rhinitis.

INTERACTIONS: Antibiotics, MTX, pyrimethamine invalidate folic acid and vitamin B_{12} blood assays. Colchicine, para-aminosalicylic acid and heavy alcohol intake for >2 weeks may produce vitamin B_{12} malabsorption.

PREGNANCY: Category C, consume recommended amount by the Food and Nutrition Board during nursing.

MECHANISM OF ACTION: Synthetic vitamin B_{12}. Essential to growth, cell reproduction, hematopoiesis, and nucleoprotein and myelin synthesis.

PHARMACOKINETICS: Absorption: C_{max}=757.96pg/mL, T_{max}=1.25 hrs, Bioavailability (6.1%). **Distribution:** Bound to plasma proteins. **Elimination:** Urine.

NASONEX   RX
mometasone furoate monohydrate (Schering)

THERAPEUTIC CLASS: Corticosteroid

INDICATIONS: Treatment of the nasal symptoms of seasonal and perennial allergic rhinitis. Prophylaxis of the nasal symptoms of seasonal allergic rhinitis. Treatment of nasal polyps in patients 18 years of age and older.

DOSAGE: *Adults:* Allergic Rhinitis: Treatment/Prophylaxis: 2 sprays per nostril qd. For prophylaxis, start 2-4 weeks before allergy season. Nasal Polyps: 2 sprays per nostril bid.
Pediatrics: ≥12 yrs: Treatment/Prophylaxis: 2 sprays per nostril qd. For prophylaxis, start 2-4 weeks before allergy season. 2-11 yrs: Treatment: 1 spray per nostril qd.

HOW SUPPLIED: Spray: 50mcg/spray [17g]

WARNINGS/PRECAUTIONS: Risk of adrenal insufficiency and withdrawal symptoms when replacing systemic corticosteroids with a topical corticosteroids. Caution with active or quiescent TB, ocular herpes simplex, or untreated bacterial, fungal and systemic viral infections. Avoid with recent nasal trauma, surgery or septum ulcers. Risk for more severe/fatal course of infections (eg, chickenpox, measles) and for *Candida* infections of the nose and pharynx. Potential for growth velocity reduction in pediatrics.

ADVERSE REACTIONS: Headache, viral infection, pharyngitis, epistaxis, cough, upper respiratory tract infection, dysmenorrhea, myalgia, sinusitis.

PREGNANCY: Category C, caution with nursing.

MECHANISM OF ACTION: Corticosteroid; not established; demonstrates anti-inflammatory properties, shown to have a wide range of effects on multiple cell types (eg, mast cells, eosinophils, neutrophils, macrophages, lymphocytes) and mediators (eg, histamine, eicosanoids, leukotrienes, cytokines) involved in inflammation.

PHARMACOKINETICS: Distribution: Plasma protein binding (98-99%). **Metabolism**: Liver (extensive) via CYP3A4. **Elimination**: Bile (as metabolites), $T_{1/2}$=5.8 hrs.

NATACHEW   RX
folic acid - multiple vitamin - minerals (Warner Chilcott)

THERAPEUTIC CLASS: Prenatal vitamin

INDICATIONS: Vitamin and mineral supplementation for before, during, and after pregnancy.

DOSAGE: *Adults:* 1 tab qd.

HOW SUPPLIED: Tab, Chewable: Folic Acid 1mg-Iron 29mg-Niacinamide 20mg-Vitamin A 1000 IU-Vitamin B_1 2mg-Vitamin B_2 3mg-Vitamin B_6 10mg-Vitamin B_{12} 0.012mg-Vitamin C 120mg-Vitamin D 400 IU-Vitamin E 11 IU

WARNINGS/PRECAUTIONS: Accidental overdose of iron-containing products is a leading cause of fatal poisoning in children <6 yrs. Folic acid may partially correct hematological damage due to vitamin B_{12} deficiency of pernicious anemia, while neurological damage progresses.

MECHANISM OF ACTION: Vitamin and mineral supplement.

NATACYN   RX
natamycin (Alcon)

THERAPEUTIC CLASS: Tetraene polyene antifungal

INDICATIONS: Treatment of fungal blepharitis, conjunctivitis, and keratitis. Not recommended as monotherapy for fungal endophthalmitis.

DOSAGE: *Adults:* Keratitis: 1 drop q1-2h for 3-4 days, then 1 drop 6-8 times daily for 14-21 days or until the resolution of infection. Reduce dose at 4-7 day intervals. Blepharitis/Conjunctivitis: 1 drop 4-6 times daily.

HOW SUPPLIED: Sus: 5% [15mL]

WARNINGS/PRECAUTIONS: Re-evaluate if no improvement after 7-10 days. Monitor twice weekly for toxicity.

ADVERSE REACTIONS: Conjunctival chemosis, hyperemia.

PREGNANCY: Category C, caution in nursing.

MECHANISM OF ACTION: Tetraene polyene antifungal: Binds to sterol moiety of fungal cell membrane. The polyenesterol complex alters permeability of membrane to produce depletion of essential cellular constituents.

PHARMACOKINETICS: Absorption: GI (poor).

NATAFORT RX
folic acid - multiple vitamin - iron (Warner Chilcott)

THERAPEUTIC CLASS: Prenatal vitamin

INDICATIONS: Vitamin and mineral supplementation for before, during, and after pregnancy.

DOSAGE: *Adults:* 1 tab qd.

HOW SUPPLIED: Tab: Folic Acid 1mg-Iron 60mg-Niacinamide 20mg-Vitamin A 1000 IU-Vitamin B$_1$ 2mg-Vitamin B$_2$ 3mg-Vitamin B$_6$ 10mg-Vitamin B$_{12}$ 12mcg-Vitamin C 120mg-Vitamin D3 400 IU-Vitamin E 11 IU

WARNINGS/PRECAUTIONS: Accidental overdose of iron-containing products is leading cause of fatal poisoning in children <6 yrs. Folic acid may partially correct hematological damage due to vitamin B$_{12}$ deficiency of pernicious anemia, while neurological damage progresses.

NATALCARE CFE 60 RX
folic acid - multiple vitamin - minerals (Ethex)

THERAPEUTIC CLASS: Prenatal vitamin

INDICATIONS: Vitamin and mineral supplementation for before, during, and after pregnancy.

DOSAGE: *Adults:* 1 tab qd.

HOW SUPPLIED: Tab: Folic Acid 1mg-Iron 60mg-Niacinamide 20mg-Vitamin A 1000 IU-Vitamin B$_1$ 2mg-Vitamin B$_2$ 3mg-Vitamin B$_6$ 10mg-Vitamin B$_{12}$ 0.012mg-Vitamin C 120mg-Vitamin D 400 IU-Vitamin E 11 IU

WARNINGS/PRECAUTIONS: Accidental overdose of iron-containing products is a leading cause of fatal poisoning in children <6 yrs. Folic acid may partially correct hematological damage due to vitamin B$_{12}$ deficiency of pernicious anemia, while neurological damage progresses.

ADVERSE REACTIONS: Allergic hypersensitivity.

MECHANISM OF ACTION: Vitamin and mineral supplement.

NATRECOR RX
nesiritide (Scios Inc.)

THERAPEUTIC CLASS: Human B-type natriuretic peptide

INDICATIONS: Treatment of acutely decompensated congestive heart failure with dyspnea at rest or with minimal activity.

DOSAGE: *Adults:* 2mcg/kg IV bolus over 60 seconds, then 0.01mcg/kg/min IV infusion. Reduce dose or d/c if hypotension occurs.

HOW SUPPLIED: Inj: 1.5mg

CONTRAINDICATIONS: Primary therapy with cardiogenic shock or systolic BP <90mmHg.

WARNINGS/PRECAUTIONS: Avoid with low cardiac filling pressures. Use precautions for parenteral administration of protein pharmaceuticals or *E.coli*-derived products; may cause allergic reaction. Avoid when vasodilators are inappropriate (eg, significant valvular stenosis, restrictive/obstructive cardio-myopathy, constrictive pericarditis, pericardial tamponade, conditions where cardiac output is dependent on venous return). May affect renal function; azotemia reported. Monitor BP closely; hypotension reported. Caution with BP <100 mmHg at baseline. Reduce dose or d/c if hypotension occurs.

ADVERSE REACTIONS: Hypotension, ventricular tachycardia, ventricular extrasystoles, headache, back pain, dizziness, anxiety, nausea, abdominal pain, insomnia

INTERACTIONS: Increased risk of hypotension with drugs that cause hypotension such as oral ACE inhibitors. Do not co-administer through the same IV catheter with heparin, insulin, ethacrynate sodium, bumetamide, enalaprilat, hydralazine, furosemide, or injectable drugs containing sodium metabisulfite. Flush catheter between uses with incompatible drugs.

PREGNANCY: Category C, caution in nursing.

MECHANISM OF ACTION: Human B-type natriuretic peptide; binds to the particulate guanylate cyclase receptor of vascular smooth muscle and endothelial cells, leading to increased intracellular concentrations of cGMP and smooth muscle relaxation.

PHARMACOKINETICS: Distribution: V_{ss}=0.19L/kg. **Elimination:** Renal; $T_{1/2}$=18 min.

NAVANE   RX
thiothixene (Pfizer)

THERAPEUTIC CLASS: Thioxanthene

INDICATIONS: Management of schizophrenia.

DOSAGE: *Adults:* Mild Condition: Initial: 2mg tid. Titrate: May increase to 15mg/day. Severe Condition: Initial: 5mg bid. Usual: 20-30mg/day. Max: 60mg/day.
Pediatrics: ≥12 yrs: Mild Condition: Initial: 2mg tid. Titrate: May increase to 15mg/day. Severe Condition: Initial: 5mg bid. Usual: 20-30mg/day. Max: 60mg/day.

HOW SUPPLIED: Cap: 1mg, 2mg, 5mg, 10mg, 20mg

CONTRAINDICATIONS: Circulatory collapse, comatose states, CNS depression, blood dyscrasias.

WARNINGS/PRECAUTIONS: May develop tardive dyskinesia, NMS. May mask symptoms of overdose of toxic drugs. May obscure conditions such as intestinal obstruction and brain tumor. May lower seizure threshold. Monitor for pigmentary retinopathy and lenticular pigmentation. Caution with cardiovascular disease, extreme heat exposure, activities requiring alertness. May elevate prolactin levels.

ADVERSE REACTIONS: Tachycardia, hypotension, lightheadedness, syncope, drowsiness, agitation, insomnia, hyperreflexia, cerebral edema, pseudoparkinsonism, LFT elevation, blood dyscrasias, rash, photosensitivity, dry mouth, blurred vision.

INTERACTIONS: Possible additive effects including hypotension with CNS depressants, alcohol. Caution with atropine or related drugs. Paradoxical effects with pressor agents.

PREGNANCY: Safety in pregnancy and nursing not known.

MECHANISM OF ACTION: Thioxanthene derivative.

NAVELBINE   RX
vinorelbine tartrate (GlaxoSmithKline)

For IV use only; fatal if given intrathecally. Severe granulocytopenia may occur; granulocyte counts should be ≥1000cells/mm³ prior to administration. Use extreme caution to prevent extravasation (can cause local tissue necrosis); if this occurs, d/c and restart in another vein. Administer only under supervision of a physician experienced in the use of antineoplastic agents.

THERAPEUTIC CLASS: Vinca alkaloid

INDICATIONS: Single agent or in combination with cisplatin for 1st-line treatment of unresectable, advanced nonsmall cell lung cancer (NSCLC), including Stage IV NSCLC. For use in combination with cisplatin for Stage III NSCLC .

DOSAGE: *Adults:* Single-Agent: 30mg/m² IV weekly over 6-10 min. With Cisplatin: 25mg/m² weekly with cisplatin 100mg/m² every 4 weeks, or 30mg/m² weekly with cisplatin 120mg/m² on Days 1 and 29, then every

6 weeks. Adjustments Based on Granulocytes: If 1000-1499cells/mm³ give 50% starting dose. If <1000cells/mm³, hold dose and repeat count in 1 week. D/C if hold 3 consecutive weekly doses because granulocyte <1000cells/mm³. If fever and/or sepsis occurs while granulocytopenic or if hold 2 consecutive weekly doses due to granulocytopenia; give 75% of the starting dose if granulocytes ≥1500cells/mm³, and 37.5% of the starting dose if granulocytes 1000-1499cells/mm³. Hepatic Insufficiency: (bilirubin 2.1-3mg/dL) 50% of starting dose or (bilirubin >3mg/dL) 25% of starting dose. If both hematologic toxicity and hepatic insufficiency, use lowest dose. Neurotoxicity: D/C if Grade ≥2 develops.

HOW SUPPLIED: Inj: 10mg/mL

CONTRAINDICATIONS: Pretreatment granulocytes <1000cells/mm³.

WARNINGS/PRECAUTIONS: Monitor for myelosuppression during and after therapy, and for infection and/or fever with developing severe granulocytopenia. Interstitial pulmonary changes, ARDS, acute shortness of breath and severe bronchospasm reported. Extreme caution with compromised bone marrow reserve due to prior irradiation or chemotherapy. Radiation recall reactions may occur. Monitor for new or worsening signs/symptoms of neuropathy. D/C if moderate or severe neurotoxicity develops. Avoid contact with skin, mucosa, and eyes. Avoid pregnancy. May cause severe constipation, paralytic ileus, intestinal obstruction, necrosis, and/or perforation.

ADVERSE REACTIONS: Granulocytopenia, leukopenia, thrombocytopenia, anemia, asthenia, injection site reactions/pain, phlebitis, peripheral neuropathy, nausea, vomiting, diarrhea, severe constipation, paralytic ileus, intestinal obstruction, necrosis, and/or perforation, dyspnea, alopecia, chest pain, fatigue.

INTERACTIONS: Risk of acute pulmonary reactions with mitomycin. Increased incidence of granulocytopenia with cisplatin. Monitor for signs/symptoms of neuropathy with paclitaxel, either concomitantly or sequentially. Radiosensitizing effects may occur with prior or concomitant radiation therapy. Caution with CYP450 3A inhibitors, or with hepatic dysfunction; earlier onset and/or increased severity of side effects may occur.

PREGNANCY: Category D, not for use in nursing.

MECHANISM OF ACTION: Vinca alkaloid; its antitumor activity is thought to be due primarily to inhibition of mitosis at metaphase through its interaction with tubulin. It also interferes with amino acid, cyclic AMP, and glutathione metabolism; calmodulin-dependent Ca⁺⁺-transport ATPase activity; cellular respiration; and nucleic acid and lipid biosynthesis.

PHARMACOKINETICS: Distribution: V_d=25.4-40.1L/kg, plasma protein binding (79.6%-91.2%). **Metabolism**: CYP450, 3A4: deacetylvinorelbine (major metabolite), vinorelbine N-oxide. **Elimination**: $T_{1/2}$=27.7-43.6 hrs. Feces (46%), urine (18%).

NEFAZODONE RX
nefazodone HCL (Various)

Antidepressants increased the risk of suicidal thinking and behavior (suicidality) in short-term studies in children, adolescents, and young adults with Major Depressive Disorder (MDD) and other psychiatric disorders. Nefazodone is not approved for use in pediatric patients. Life-threatening hepatic failure reported. Avoid with active liver disease or elevated serum transaminases. D/C and do not retreat if symptoms of hepatic disease develop or if ALT/AST ≥3x ULN.

THERAPEUTIC CLASS: Serotonin and norepinephrine reuptake inhibitor

INDICATIONS: Treatment of depression.

DOSAGE: *Adults:* Initial: 100mg bid. Usual: 300-600mg/day. Titrate: May increase by 100-200mg/day at intervals of no less than 1 week. Elderly/Debilitated: Initial: 50mg bid.

HOW SUPPLIED: Tab: 50mg, 100mg*, 150mg*, 200mg, 250mg *scored

CONTRAINDICATIONS: Coadministration of terfenadine, astemizole, cisapride, pimozide, carbamazepine, triazolam. Liver injury from previous treatment.

WARNINGS/PRECAUTIONS: May cause postural hypotension. Caution with cardiovascular or cerebrovascular disease that could be exacerbated by hypotension and conditions with predisposition to hypotension (eg, dehydration, hypotension). May activate mania/hypomania. Priapism reported. Caution with history of MI, unstable heart disease, seizures, liver cirrhosis. Avoid with active liver disease.

ADVERSE REACTIONS: Hepatic failure, somnolence, dry mouth, nausea, dizziness, insomnia, agitation, constipation, asthenia, lightheadedness, blurred vision, confusion, abnormal vision.

INTERACTIONS: Avoid MAOIs within 14 days of use. Avoid alcohol, terfenadine, astemizole, cisapride, pimozide. Reduce triazolam dose by 75% and avoid in elderly. Reduce alprazolam dose by 50%. Effects antagonized by carbamazepine. Caution with highly protein bound drugs, drugs metabolized by CYP3A4, CNS-active drugs. Discontinue prior to general anesthesia. Haloperidol may need dose adjustment. Increases plasma levels of cyclosporine, tacrolimus. Rhabdomyolysis (rare) reported with simvastatin and lovastatin. Monitor digoxin. Institute a wash-out period and lower doses if used after fluoxetine therapy. May increase buspirone levels; decrease buspirone dose to 2.5mg qd.

PREGNANCY: Category C, caution in nursing.

MECHANISM OF ACTION: 5-HT and NE reuptake inhibitor (phenylpiperazine); potentiates neurotransmitter activity of CNS activity by inhibiting neuronal serotonin and norephinephrine reuptake.

PHARMACOKINETICS: Absorption: Rapid. Absolute bioavailability (20%), T_{max}=1 hr. **Distribution:** Plasma protein binding (>99%), V_d=0.22-0.87L/kg. **Metabolism:** N-dealkylation and aliphatic and aromatic hydroxylation. **Elimination:** $T_{1/2}$=2-4 hrs, urine (<1%).

NEMBUTAL SODIUM SOLUTION   CII

pentobarbital sodium (Ovation)

THERAPEUTIC CLASS: Barbiturate

INDICATIONS: Short-term treatment of insomnia; sedation; preoperative anesthesia; anticonvulsant in the emergency control of certain acute convulsive episodes.

DOSAGE: *Adults:* Usual: 150-200mg as a single IM injection. IV: 100mg (commonly used initial dose for 70kg adult); if needed additional small increments may be given up to 200-500mg total dose. Rate of IV injection should not exceed 50mg/min. Elderly/Debilitated/Renal or Hepatic Impairment: Reduce dose.
Pediatrics: 2-6mg/kg as a single IM injection. Max: 100mg. IV: Proportional reduction in dosage. Slow IV injection is essential.

HOW SUPPLIED: Inj: 50mg/mL

CONTRAINDICATIONS: History of manifest or latent porphyria.

WARNINGS/PRECAUTIONS: May be habit forming; avoid abrupt cessation after prolonged use. Avoid rapid administration. Tolerance to hypnotic effect can occur. Prehepatic coma use not recommended. Use with caution in patients with chronic or acute pain, mental depression, suicidal tendencies, history of drug abuse or hepatic impairment. Monitor blood, liver and renal function. May impair mental/physical abilities. Avoid alcohol.

ADVERSE REACTIONS: Agitation, confusion, hyperkinesia, ataxia, CNS depression, somnolence, bradycardia, hypotension, nausea, vomiting, constipation, headache, hypersensitivity reactions, liver damage.

INTERACTIONS: May produce additive CNS depression with other CNS depressants (eg, other sedatives/hypnotics, antihistamines, tranquilizers, alcohol). May decrease levels of oral anticoagulants, corticosteroids, griseofulvin, and doxycycline. Dosage adjustments may be required for anticoagulants and corticosteroids. Variable effects on phenytoin and increased levels with valproic acid, sodium valproate; monitor blood levels and adjust dose appropriately. May decrease effects of estradiol; alternative contraceptive method should be suggested. Prolonged effect with MAOIs.

PREGNANCY: Category D, caution with nursing.

MECHANISM OF ACTION: Not established; barbiturates are nonslective CNS depressants; depress the sensory cortex, decrease motor activity, alter cerebellar function, and produce drowsiness, sedation, and hypnosis.

PHARMACOKINETICS: Distribution: Found in breast milk, crosses placental barrier. **Metabolism:** Liver. **Elimination:** Urine (25-50%, unchanged), feces; $T_{1/2}$=15-50 hrs.

NEORAL   RX
cyclosporine (Novartis)

> Increased susceptibility to infection, and development of neoplasia, HTN, nephrotoxicity.
> Monitor blood levels to avoid toxicity. Neoral is not bioequivalent to Sandimmune. Risk of skin
> malignancies if previously treated with PUVA, UVB, coal tar, radiation, MTX, or other immuno-
> suppressives.

THERAPEUTIC CLASS: Cyclic polypeptide immunosuppressant

INDICATIONS: Organ rejection prophylaxis in kidney, liver, and heart allogeneic transplants. Treatment of severe active, rheumatoid arthritis (RA) unresponsive to methotrexate (MTX). Treatment of nonimmunocompromised adults with severe, recalcitrant, plaque psoriasis unresponsive to at least 1 systemic therapy (eg, PUVA, retinoids, MTX) or when other systemic therapies are contraindicated/not tolerated.

DOSAGE: *Adults:* Transplant: Give initial oral dose 4-12 hrs before transplant or post-op. Dose bid. Initial: Renal Transplant: 9 ± 3mg/kg/day. Liver Transplant: 8±4mg/kg/day. Heart Transplant: 7 ± 3mg/kg/day. Give with corticosteroids initially. Conversion from Sandimmune: 1:1 dose conversion. Adjust to trough levels. Monitor every 4-7 days. RA: Initial: 1.25mg/kg bid. Titrate: May increase by 0.5-0.75mg/kg/day after 8 weeks, again after 12 weeks. Max: 4mg/kg/day. Discontinue if no benefit by week 16. Psoriasis: Initial: 1.25mg/kg bid for 4 weeks. Titrate: May increase by 0.5mg/kg/day every 2 weeks. Max: 4mg/kg/day. Decrease dose by 25-50% to control adverse events. Take at the same time every day. Dilute sol in orange or apple juice that is room temp.

HOW SUPPLIED: Cap: 25mg, 100mg; Sol: 100mg/mL [50mL]

CONTRAINDICATIONS: Abnormal renal function, uncontrolled HTN, malignancies. PUVA or UVB therapy, MTX, other immunosuppressants, coal tar, or radiation in psoriasis patients.

WARNINGS/PRECAUTIONS: Risk of hepatotoxicity and nephrotoxicity. Caution in elderly. Hyperkalemia, hyperuricemia, thrombocytopenia, microangiopathic hemolytic anemia, and encephalopathy reported in transplant patients. Monitor CBC and LFTs monthly with MTX. Monitor BP and renal function before therapy, every 2 weeks during 1st 3 months, then monthly if stable with RA or psoriasis. Monitor SCr after initiate or increase NSAID dose in RA. Monitor CBC, uric acid, K⁺, lipids, and magnesium every 2 weeks during 1st 3 months, then monthly if stable in RA. Monitor LFTs repeatedly. Monitor CBC, SCr with transplants.

ADVERSE REACTIONS: Renal dysfunction, HTN, hirsutism, muscle cramps, acne, tremor, headache, gingival hyperplasia, diarrhea, nausea, vomiting, paresthesia, flushing, dyspepsia, hypertrichosis, stomatitis, hypomagnesemia.

INTERACTIONS: Phenytoin, phenobarbital, rifampin, nafcillin, carbamazepine, orlistat, ticlopidine, octreotide, St. John's wort, oxcarbazepine, and bosentan decrease cyclosporine levels. Increases MTX levels. Potentiated by clarithromycin, diltiazem, fluconazole, erythromycin, itraconazole, ketoconazole, voriconazole, verapamil, nicardipine, quinupristin/dalfopristin, allopurinol, bromocriptine, danazol, metoclopramide, colchicine, amiodarone, grapefruit juice. Aminoglycosides, ciprofloxacin, vancomycin, SMZ/TMP, melphalan, ketoconazole, NSAIDs, colchicine, cimetidine, ranitidine, tacrolimus, amphotericin B, bezafibrate, fenofibrate, and methotrexate may potentiate renal dysfunction. Digitalis toxicity reported. Myotoxicity with statins, frequent gingival hyperplasia with nifedipine, and convulsions with high dose methylprednisolone reported. Avoid potassium-sparing diuretics, grapefruit juice. Decreased clearance of prednisolone, digoxin, and lovastatin. Caution with HIV protease inhibitors, ACEIs, angiotensin II blockers. Decreased effects of vaccinations; avoid live attenuated vaccines.

PREGNANCY: Category C, not for use in nursing.

MECHANISM OF ACTION: Cyclosporine; immunosuppressive agent. Inhibits immunocompetent lymphocytes in the G_0-and G_1 phase of cell cycle, T-lymphocytes, T-helper and T-suppressor cells. Also inhibits lymphokine production and release, including interleukin-2.

PHARMACOKINETICS: Absorption: Incomplete; T_{max}=1.5-2 hrs. Pharmacokinetic parameters varied with different indications (renal, liver, rheumatoid arthritis and/or psoriasis). **Distribution:** V_d=3.5L/kg (IV); Plasma protein binding (90%); Found in human breast milk. **Metabolism:** (extensive) Via CYP3A, in liver, GI tract, kidneys. Major metabolites (M1, M9, and M4N); oxidation and demethylation pathways. **Elimination:** Bile (primary), urine (6% unchanged and metabolites); $T_{1/2}$=8.4 hrs.

NEOSPORIN OINTMENT OTC
bacitracin zinc - polymyxin B sulfate - neomycin (McNeil)

THERAPEUTIC CLASS: Antibacterial combination

INDICATIONS: To help prevent infection in minor cuts, scrapes, and burns.

DOSAGE: *Adults:* Clean area and apply a small amount qd-tid. May cover with sterile bandage.
Pediatrics: Clean area and apply a small amount qd-tid. May cover with sterile bandage.

HOW SUPPLIED: Oint: (Neomycin-Polymyxin-Bacitracin) 3.5mg-5000 U-400 U/g [15g, 30g], [Neo To Go, 10 x 0.9g pkts]

WARNINGS/PRECAUTIONS: Avoid eyes. Do not use over large areas. D/C if condition persists, worsens, or if a rash or other allergic reaction develops, or if needed longer than 1 week.

PREGNANCY: Safety in pregnancy and nursing not known.

NEOSPORIN OPHTHALMIC RX
bacitracin zinc - polymyxin B sulfate - neomycin sulfate (King)

THERAPEUTIC CLASS: Antibacterial combination

INDICATIONS: Superficial ocular infections including conjunctivitis, keratitis and keratoconjunctivitis, blepharitis and blepharoconjunctivitis.

DOSAGE: *Adults:* (Oint) Apply q3-4h for 7-10 days. (Sol) Instill 1-2 drops q4h for 7-10 days. Severe Infection: 2 drops q1h.

HOW SUPPLIED: Oint: (Bacitracin-Neomycin-Polymyxin B) 400U-3.5mg-10,000U/g [3.5g]; Sol: (Gramicidin-Neomycin-Polymixin B) 0.025mg-1.75mg-10,000U/mL [10mL]

WARNINGS/PRECAUTIONS: May cause cutaneous sensitization. Ointment may retard corneal wound healing.

ADVERSE REACTIONS: Itching, swelling, conjunctival erythema, local irritation, superinfection.

PREGNANCY: Category C, caution in nursing.

MECHANISM OF ACTION: Antibacterial combination. Neomycin: Aminoglycoside antibiotic. Inhibits protein synthesis by binding with ribosomal RNA and causing misreading of the bacterial genetic code. Polymyxin B: Increases permeability of the bacterial cell membrane by interacting with the phospholipid components of the membrane. Gramicidin: Increases permeability of the bacterial cell membrane to inorganic cations by forming a network of channels through the normal lipid bilayer of the membrane.

NEPHROCAPS RX
multiple vitamin (Fleming)

THERAPEUTIC CLASS: Vitamin supplement

INDICATIONS: Vitamin supplement for wasting syndrome in chronic renal failure, uremia, impaired metabolic functions of the kidney to maintain or replace depleted vitamins. Effective as a stress vitamin.

DOSAGE: *Adults:* 1 cap qd. Take after treatment if on dialysis.

HOW SUPPLIED: Cap: Biotin 0.15mg-Calcium Pantothenate 5mg-Folate 1mg-Niacin 20mg-Vitamin B$_1$ 1.5mg-Vitamin B$_2$ 1.7mg-Vitamin B$_6$ 10mg-Vitamin B$_{12}$ 0.006mg-Vitamin C 100mg

WARNINGS/PRECAUTIONS: Folic acid may mask symptoms of pernicious anemia.

PREGNANCY: Safety in pregnancy and nursing not known.

MECHANISM OF ACTION: Vitamin supplement.

NEPHRO-VITE RX RX
multiple vitamin (R&D)

THERAPEUTIC CLASS: Vitamin supplement

INDICATIONS: Vitamin supplement for dialysis patients and azotemic patients not on dialysis who eat poorly.

DOSAGE: *Adults:* 1 tab qd.

HOW SUPPLIED: Tab: Biotin 0.3mg-Calcium Pantothenic Acid 10mg-Folic Acid 1mg-Niacinamide 20mg-Vitamin B$_1$ 1.5mg-Vitamin B$_2$ 1.7mg-Vitamin B$_6$ 10mg-Vitamin B$_{12}$ 0.006mg-Vitamin C 60mg

WARNINGS/PRECAUTIONS: Folic acid may partially correct the hematological damage due to vitamin B$_{12}$ deficiency of pernicious anemia, while neurological damage progresses.

PREGNANCY: Safety in pregnancy and nursing not known.

MECHANISM OF ACTION: Vitamin B complex and vitamin C supplement

NESACAINE RX
chloroprocaine HCL (Abraxis)

OTHER BRAND NAMES: Nesacaine-MPF (Abraxis)

THERAPEUTIC CLASS: Local anesthetic

INDICATIONS: (Nesacaine) Production of local anesthesia by infiltration and peripheral nerve block. (Nesacaine-MPF) Production of local anesthesia by infiltration, peripheral and central nerve block, including lumbar and caudal epidural blocks.

DOSAGE: *Adults:* Dosage varies depending on procedure, vascularity of tissues, depth and duration of anesthesia, degree of muscle relaxation required, and patient physical condition. Max: 11mg/kg (800mg total dose) without epinephrine or 14mg/kg (1000mg total dose) with epinephrine. MPF: Caudal/Lumbar Epidural Block: Test dose: 3mL of 3% or 5mL of 2% prior to complete block. Caudal Epidural: 15-25mL of 2% or 3% solution. Repeat dose may be given at 40-60 min intervals. Lumbar Epidural: 2-2.5mL/segment of 2% or 3% solution. Usual: 15-25mL. Repeat doses of 2-6mL less than original dose at 40-50 min intervals. Elderly/Debilitated/Acutely Ill/Cardiac or Liver Disease: Reduce dose.

Pediatrics: >3 yrs: Max: 11mg/kg. Use 0.5-1% for infiltration and 1-1.5% for nerve block.

HOW SUPPLIED: Inj: 1%, 2%; (MPF) 2%, 3%

CONTRAINDICATIONS: Extreme caution with lumbar and caudal epidural anesthesia in existing neurological disease, spinal deformities, septicemia, severe HTN.

WARNINGS/PRECAUTIONS: Acidosis, cardiac arrest, death reported from delay in toxicity management. Nesacaine contains methylparaben and should not be used for lumbar or caudal epidural anesthesia. MPF formulation contains no preservative; discard any unused injection after initial use. Use lowest effective dose. Perform syringe aspiration to avoid intravascular injection. Caution with hepatic disease or impaired cardiovascular function. Monitor cardiovascular and respiratory vital signs and state of consciousness after each injection. Caution when local anesthetic injections containing a vasoconstrictor are used in areas of the body supplied by end arteries or having otherwise compromised blood supply; ischemic injury or necrosis may result with peripheral or hypertensive vascular disease due to exaggerated vasoconstrictor response. Do not rely on lack of corneal sensation after retrobulbar block to determine if patient is ready for surgery.

ADVERSE REACTIONS: Restlessness, anxiety, dizziness, tinnitus, blurred vision, tremors, convulsions, drowsiness, hypotension, bradycardia, ventricular arrhythmias, urticaria, pruritus, nausea, vomiting, loss of bladder/bowel control, loss of sexual function.

INTERACTIONS: Caution regarding toxic equivalence when using local anesthetic mixtures. Vasopressors, ergot-type oxytocic drugs may cause severe, persistent HTN or CVA. Anesthetic solutions containing epinephrine or norepinephrine with MAOIs, TCAs, or phenothiazines may produce severe, prolonged hypotension or HTN. Avoid sulfonamides.

PREGNANCY: Category C, caution in nursing.

MECHANISM OF ACTION: Local anesthetic agent; blocks the generation and conduction of nerve impulses, presumably by increasing the threshold for electrical excitation in the nerve by slowing the propagation of the nerve impulse and by reducing the rate of rise of the action potential.

PHARMACOKINETICS: Absorption: Rapid absorption. **Distribution:** Crosses placenta. **Metabolism:** (Rapid) by hydrolysis of the ester linkage by pseudocholinesterase. **Elimination:** Urine.

NEULASTA RX
pegfilgrastim (Amgen)

THERAPEUTIC CLASS: Pegylated granulocyte colony stimulating factor

INDICATIONS: To decrease the incidence of infection, as manifested by febrile neutropenia, in patients with nonmyeloid malignancies receiving myelosuppressive anticancer drugs.

DOSAGE: *Adults:* 6mg SQ once per chemotherapy cycle. Do not administer in the period between 14 days before and 24 hrs after chemotherapy.

HOW SUPPLIED: Inj: 6mg/0.6mL

CONTRAINDICATIONS: Hypersensitivity to *E.coli*-derived proteins.

WARNINGS/PRECAUTIONS: Rare cases of splenic rupture reported, some fatal. Evaluate for enlarged spleen or splenic rupture if complaints of upper abdominal and/or shoulder tip pain. Acute respiratory distress syndrome (ARDS), allergic reactions (eg, anaphylaxis, rash) reported with filgrastim. Caution with sickle cell disease; monitor for sickle cell crises. Obtain CBC, platelets before chemotherapy. Monitor Hct, platelets regularly. Do not use in infants, children, and smaller adolescents <45kg.

ADVERSE REACTIONS: Bone pain, myalgia, arthralgia, peripheral edema, nausea, fatigue, alopecia, diarrhea, vomiting, constipation, fever, anorexia, headache.

INTERACTIONS: Lithium may potentiate release of neutrophils; monitor neutrophil counts. Increased hematopoetic activity of the bone marrow in response to growth factor therapy has been associated with transient positive bone-imaging changes. This should be considered when interpreting bone-imaging results.

PREGNANCY: Category C, caution in nursing.

MECHANISM OF ACTION: Pegylated granulocyte colony stimulating factor; acts on hematopoietic cells by binding to specific cell surface receptors, thereby stimulating proliferation, differentiation, commitment, and end cell functional activation.

PHARMACOKINETICS: Elimination: (SQ) $T_{1/2}$=80 hrs.

NEUMEGA RX
oprelvekin (Wyeth)

Allergic or hypersensitivity reactions, including anaphylaxis, reported; permanently d/c if an allergic or hypersensitivity reaction develops.

THERAPEUTIC CLASS: Thrombopoietic agent

INDICATIONS: Prevention of severe thrombocytopenia and reduction of the need for platelet transfusions following myelosuppressive chemotherapy in nonmyeloid malignancy patients at high risk.

DOSAGE: *Adults:* 50mcg/kg qd SQ. Severe renal impairment (CrCl<30mL/min) 25mcg/kg qd SQ.Initiate 6-24 hrs after chemotherapy completion. Monitor platelets to assess optimal duration of therapy. Continue therapy until post-nadir platelets ≥50,000 cells/mcL. D/C at least 2 days before next chemotherapy cycle. Max: 21 days of therapy.

HOW SUPPLIED: Inj: 5mg

WARNINGS/PRECAUTIONS: Fluid retention reported; caution in CHF and patients receiving aggressive hydration. Capillary leak syndrome, pleural/pericardial effusion, renal failure, visual disturbances, papilledema, stroke, and rash reported. Monitor fluid and electrolyte balance with chronic diuretic therapy. Permanently d/c if significant allergic reactions occur. Moderate decreases in Hgb, Hct, and RBCs reported. Caution with history of atrial arrhythmias. May develop antibodies to therapy. Obtain CBC before therapy, then regularly. Monitor platelets during expected nadir time and until adequate recovery.

ADVERSE REACTIONS: Edema, dyspnea, tachycardia, conjunctival injection, palpitations, atrial arrhythmias, pleural effusions, syncope, pneumonia, neutropenic fever, headache, nausea/vomiting, fever, mucositis, diarrhea.

PREGNANCY: Category C, not for use in nursing.

MECHANISM OF ACTION: Thrombopoietic agent; stimulates megakaryocytopoiesis and thrombopoiesis.

PHARMACOKINETICS: Absorption: C_{max}=17.4ng/mL; T_{max}=3.2 hrs; absolute bioavailability (>80%). **Elimination:** Kidneys (animal studies); $T_{1/2}$=6.9 hrs.

NEUPOGEN RX
filgrastim (Amgen)

THERAPEUTIC CLASS: Granulocyte colony stimulating factor

INDICATIONS: To decrease incidence of infection, as manifested by febrile neutropenia, in nonmyeloid malignancies with myelosuppressive anti-cancer drugs (eg, bone marrow transplants). To reduce duration of neutropenia and fever in adults after induction or consolidation chemotherapy with acute myeloid leukemia. For peripheral blood progenitor cell collection (PBPC) and therapy. For severe chronic neutropenia.

DOSAGE: *Adults:* Myelosuppressive Chemotherapy: Initial: 5mcg/kg qd SQ bolus, short IV infusion, or continuous SQ/IV infusion. Monitor CBCs and platelets before therapy, twice weekly during therapy. Titrate: Increase 5mcg/kg for each chemotherapy cycle according to duration and severity of ANC nadir. Avoid 24 hours before through 24 hours after cytotoxic chemotherapy. Perform CBC twice weekly during therapy. Continue therapy after chemotherapy until the post nadir ANC =10,000/mm³. BMT: Following BMT, 10mcg/kg/day by IV infusion of 4 or 24 hrs, or by continuous 24-hr SQ infusion. First dose at least 24 hrs after chemotherapy and at least 24 hrs after bone marrow infusion. Dose Adjustment: If ANC >1000/mm³ for 3 days, 5mcg/kg/day; increase to 10mcg/kg/day if ANC <1000/mm³. If ANC >1000/mm³ for 3 more days, stop therapy. If ANC drops to <1000/mm³, resume 5mcg/kg/day. PBPC: 10mcg/kg/day bolus or continuous SQ 4 days before and for 6-7 days with leukapheresis on days 5, 6 and 7. Monitor neutrophils after 4 days and adjust if WBC >100,000/mm³. Chronic Neutropenia: Congenital Neutropenia: Initial: 6mcg/kg SQ bid. Idiopathic or Cyclic Neutropenia: Initial: 5mcg/kg SQ qd. Adjust dose based on clinical course and ANC.

HOW SUPPLIED: Inj: 300mcg/0.5mL, 300mcg/mL, 480mcg/0.8mL, 480mcg/1.6mL [10⁵]

CONTRAINDICATIONS: Hypersensitivity to *E coli*-derived proteins.

WARNINGS/PRECAUTIONS: Allergic-type reactions may occur. Rare cases of splenic rupture reported, some fatal. Evaluate for enlarged spleen or splenic rupture if complaints of left upper abdominal and/or shoulder tip pain. Acute respiratory distress syndrome reported with sepsis; d/c until resolved. Sickle cell crisis reported with sickle cell disease; keep patient well hydrated. Potential for immunogenicity. The patient may be at greater risk of thrombocytopenia, anemia, and nonhematologic consequences due to the potential of receiving higher doses of chemotherapy. Regular monitoring of Hct and platelet count recommended. Alveolar hemorrhage manifesting as pulmonary infiltrates and hemoptysis requiring hospitalization reported.

ADVERSE REACTIONS: Bone pain, nausea, vomiting, rash, alopecia, diarrhea, neutropenic fever, mucositis, fatigue, anorexia, dyspnea.

INTERACTIONS: Caution with drugs that may potentiate the release of neutrophils (eg, lithium). Transient positive bone imaging changes has been associated with increased hematopoetic activity of the bone marrow in response to growth factor therapy. This should be considered when interpreting bone-imaging results.

PREGNANCY: Category C, caution in nursing.

MECHANISM OF ACTION: Granulocyte colony-stimulating factor (G-CSF); acts on hematopoietic cells by binding to specific cell surface receptors. Stimulates proliferation, differentiation commitment, and some end-cell functional activation.

PHARMACOKINETICS: Absorption: (IV, 20mcg/kg over 24 hrs): C_{max}=48ng/mL; (SQ, 3.45mcg/kg, 11.5mcg/kg): C_{max}=4ng/mL, 49ng/mL. **Distribution**: V_d=150mL/kg. **Elimination**: (IV) $T_{1/2}$=231 min (34.5mcg/kg). (SQ) $T_{1/2}$=210 min (3.45mcg/kg).

NEURONTIN   RX
gabapentin (Parke-Davis)

THERAPEUTIC CLASS: GABA analog

INDICATIONS: Adjunct therapy for partial seizures with or without secondary generalization in patients ≥12 yrs. Adjunct therapy for partial seizures in pediatrics 3-12 yrs. Management of postherpetic neuralgia (PHN).

DOSAGE: *Adults:* Epilepsy: Initial: 300mg tid. Titrate: Increase up to 1800mg/day. Max: 3600mg/day. PHN: 300mg single dose on Day 1, then 300mg bid on Day 2, and 300mg tid on Day 3. Increase further prn for pain. Max: 600mg tid. Renal Impairment: CrCl 30-59mL/min: 400-1400 mg/day. CrCl 15-29mL/min: 200-700 mg/day. CrCl 15mL/min: 100-300mg/day. CrCl <15 mL/min: Reduce dose in proportion to CrCl. Hemodialysis: Maint: Base on CrCl. Give supplemental dose (125-350mg) after 4 hrs of hemodialysis. Refer to prescribing information for dose-adjustment.

Pediatrics: Epilepsy: >12 yrs: Initial: 300mg tid. Titrate: Increase up to 1800mg/day. Max: 3600mg/day. 3-12 yrs: Initial: 10-15mg/kg/day given tid. Titrate: Increase over 3 days. Usual: 3-4 yrs: 40mg/kg/day given tid. ≥5 yrs: 25-35mg/kg/day given tid. Max: 50mg/kg/day. Renal Impairment: ≥12 yrs: CrCl 30-59mL/min: 400-1400 mg/day. CrCl 15-29mL/min: 200-700 mg/day. CrCl 15mL/min: 100-300mg/day. CrCl <15 mL/min: Reduce dose in proportion to CrCl. Hemodialysis: Maint: Base on CrCl. Give supplemental dose (125-350 mg) after 4 hrs of hemodialysis. Refer to prescribing information for dose-adjustment.

HOW SUPPLIED: Cap: 100mg, 300mg, 400mg; Sol: 250mg/5mL; Tab: 600mg*, 800mg* *scored

WARNINGS/PRECAUTIONS: Avoid abrupt withdrawal. Possible tumorigenic potential. Sudden and unexplained deaths reported. Neuropsychiatric adverse events in pediatrics (3-12 yrs).

ADVERSE REACTIONS: Somnolence, dizziness, ataxia, nystagmus, fatigue, tremor, rhinitis, weight gain, nausea, vomiting, viral infection, fever, dysarthria, diplopia.

INTERACTIONS: Take 2 hrs after antacids. Increased levels with controlled-release morphine.

PREGNANCY: Category C, caution in nursing.

MECHANISM OF ACTION: Anticonvulsant; not established. Anticonvulsant activity: Suspected to bind to different areas of the brain including neocortex and hippocampus. Analgesic effects: Prevents allodynia and hyperalgesia.

PHARMACOKINETICS: Absorption: PO administration of variable doses resulted in different parameters. **Distribution:** V_d =58L; plasma protein binding (<3%); found in breast milk. **Metabolism:** Not appreciably metabolized. **Elimination:** Renal excretion (unchanged); $T_{1/2}$=5-7 hrs. Refer to PI for pediatric parameters.

NEVANAC   RX
nepafenac (Alcon)

THERAPEUTIC CLASS: NSAID

INDICATIONS: Treatment of pain and inflammation associated with cataract surgery.

DOSAGE: *Adults:* 1 drop tid, start 24 hrs prior to surgery, continue to 2 weeks post-op.

HOW SUPPLIED: Sus: 0.1% [3mL]

WARNINGS/PRECAUTIONS: Possible cross-sensitivity to acetylsalicylic acid, phenylacetic acid derivatives, and other NSAIDs. May cause increased bleeding of ocular tissue; slowed or delayed healing; keratitis. With continued use, may cause epithelial breakdown, corneal thinning, erosion, ulceration, perforation. Caution with bleeding tendencies and in complicated ocular surgeries, corneal denervation, corneal epithelial defects, diabetes mellitus, ocular surface diseases, rheumatoid arthritis, or repeat ocular surgeries.

ADVERSE REACTIONS: Capsular opacity, decreased visual acuity, foreign body sensation, increased IOP, and sticky sensation.

PREGNANCY: Category C, caution in nursing.

MECHANISM OF ACTION: NSAID; inhibits the cyclo-oxygenase that is essential for the biosynthesis of prostaglandins.

NEXAVAR   RX
sorafenib (Bayer/Onyx)

THERAPEUTIC CLASS: Multikinase inhibitor

INDICATIONS: Treatment of advanced renal cell carcinoma or unresectable hepatocellular carcinoma.

DOSAGE: *Adults:* 400mg bid without food (1 hr before or 2 hrs after eating). Continue until no clinical benefit or unacceptable toxicity. Temporary interruption or dose reduction to 400mg qd or qod may be necessary if serious adverse events suspected.

HOW SUPPLIED: Tab: 200mg

WARNINGS/PRECAUTIONS: Risk of ischemia and/or infarction occured; temporary or permenent discontinuation may be necessary. Increased risk of bleeding may occur; consider discontinuation if bleeding necessitates medical intervention. HTN reported; monitor BP weekly during first 6 weeks and periodically thereafter. Hand-foot skin reaction and rash may occur; may require topical treatment, temporary treatment interruption, dose modification, or permanent discontinuation. D/C if GI perforation occurs. Temporary interruption of therapy recommended when undergoing surgical procedures. May cause fetal harm; women of childbearing potential should avoid becoming pregnant during therapy. Hepatic impairment may reduce plasma levels. Caution when co-administered with docetaxel and doxorubicin.

ADVERSE REACTIONS: HTN, fatigue, weight loss, rash/desquamation, hand-foot skin reaction, alopecia, pruritus, diarrhea, nausea, anorexia, vomiting, constipation, hemorrhage, dyspnea, abdominal pain, liver dysfunction, cardiac ischemia.

INTERACTIONS: Caution with compounds metabolized/eliminated predominantly by the UGT1A1 pathway (eg, irinotecan); systemic exposure to substrates of UGT1A1 and UGT1A9 may increase with co-administration. May increase AUC of docetaxel and doxorubicin; co-administer with caution. May alter AUC of fluorouracil; co-administer with caution. Systemic exposure to substrates of CYP2B6 and CYP2C8 may increase with co-administration. CYP3A4 inducers may increase metabolism and decrease levels of sorafenib. May increase INR; monitor with concomitant warfarin.

PREGNANCY: Category D, not for use in nursing.

MECHANISM OF ACTION: Multikinase inhibitor; inhibits multiple intracellular and cell surface kinases which are thought to be involved in tumor cell signaling, angiogenesis, and apoptosis.

PHARMACOKINETICS: Absorption: Relative bioavailability (38-49%), T_{max}=3 hrs. **Distribution:** Plasma protein binding (99.5%). **Metabolism:** Liver via oxidation and glucuronidation; CYP3A4, UGT1A9: Pyridine N-oxide. **Elimination:** $T_{1/2}$=25-48 hrs, Feces (77%, 51% unchanged), urine (19% as glucuronidated metabolites).

NEXIUM   RX
esomeprazole magnesium (AstraZeneca)

THERAPEUTIC CLASS: Proton pump inhibitor

INDICATIONS: Symptomatic treatment of GERD; healing and maintenance treatment of erosive esophagitis. Reduction in occurrence of gastric ulcers associated with continuous NSAID therapy in patients at risk for developing gastric ulcers. Adjunct therapy (with amoxicillin and clarithromycin) for *H.pylori* eradication to reduce the risk of duodenal ulcer recurrence. Long-term treatment of pathological hypersecretory conditions including Zollinger-Ellison syndrome.

DOSAGE: *Adults:* Erosive Esophagitis: Healing: 20mg or 40mg qd for 4-8 weeks; may extend treatment for 4-8 weeks if not healed. Maint: 20mg qd for up to 6 months. Risk Reduction of NSAID-Associated Gastric Ulcer: 20mg or 40mg qd for up to 6 months. Symptomatic GERD: 20mg qd for 4 weeks; may extend treatment for 4 weeks if symptoms do not resolve. *H.pylori:* Triple Therapy: 40mg qd + amoxicillin 1000mg bid + clarithromycin 500mg bid, all for 10 days. Zollinger-Ellison Syndrome: 40mg bid. Severe Hepatic Dysfunction: Max: 20mg/day. Take 1 hr before meals. Swallow capsule whole. Contents may be mixed with soft food (eg, applesauce, yogurt) that does not require chewing.
Pediatrics: GERD: 12-17 yrs: 20mg or 40mg qd for up to 8 weeks. 1-11 yrs: 10mg qd for up to 8 weeks. Erosive Esophagitis: 1-11 yrs: ≥20kg: 10mg or 20mg qd

for 8 weeks. <20kg: 10mg qd for 8 weeks. Severe Hepatic Dysfunction: Max: 20mg/day. Take 1 hr before meals. Swallow capsule whole. Contents may be mixed with soft food (eg, applesauce, yogurt) that does not require chewing.

HOW SUPPLIED: Cap, Delayed-Release: 20mg, 40mg; Sus, Delayed-Release: 20mg, 40mg (granules/pkt).

CONTRAINDICATIONS: Hypersensitivity to substituted benzimidazoles. Clarithromycin is contraindicated with pimozide.

WARNINGS/PRECAUTIONS: Atrophic gastritis may occur. Symptomatic response does not preclude gastric malignancy.

ADVERSE REACTIONS: Headache, diarrhea, abdominal pain, constipation, nausea, flatulence, dry mouth.

INTERACTIONS: Potentiates diazepam. May alter absorption of pH-dependent drugs (eg, ketoconazole, digoxin, iron salts). May reduce levels of atazanavir when used concomitantly. Increased levels with amoxicillin and clarithromycin. Clarithromycin is contraindicated with pimozide. Concomitant use with warfarin may increase INR and PT.

PREGNANCY: Category B, not for use in nursing.

MECHANISM OF ACTION: Proton pump inhibitor; suppresses gastric acid secretion by specific inhibition of the H^+/K^+-ATPase in the gastric parietal cell.

PHARMACOKINETICS: Absorption: (40 mg) C_{max}=4.7μmol/L; T_{max}=1.6 hrs; AUC=12.6μmol•hr/L. (20mg) C_{max}=2.1μmol/L; T_{max}=1.6 hrs; AUC=4.2μmol•hr/L. **Distribution:** V_d=16L; plasma protein binding (97%). **Metabolism:** Liver (extensive) via CYP2C19, CYP3A4. **Elimination:** Urine (80%), feces; $T_{1/2}$=1-1.5 hrs. For pediatric parameters, refer to full PI.

NEXIUM IV   RX
esomeprazole sodium (AstraZeneca)

THERAPEUTIC CLASS: Proton pump inhibitor

INDICATIONS: Short-term treatment (up to 10 days) of GERD with history of erosive esophagitis when oral therapy not possible or appropriate.

DOSAGE: *Adults:* 20mg or 40mg qd IV injection (no less than 3 min) or infusion (10-30 min). D/C as soon as patient able to resume oral therapy. Severe Hepatic Dysfunction: Max: 20mg/day.

HOW SUPPLIED: Inj: 20mg, 40mg

CONTRAINDICATIONS: Hypersensitivity to substituted benzimidazoles.

WARNINGS/PRECAUTIONS: Atrophic gastritis may occur. Symptomatic response does not preclude gastric malignancy. D/C and convert to oral therapy as soon as possible.

ADVERSE REACTIONS: Headache, flatulence, dyspepsia, nausea, abdominal pain, diarrhea, dry mouth,

INTERACTIONS: Potentiates diazepam. May alter absorption of gastric pH-dependent drugs (eg, ketoconazole, iron salts, digoxin).

PREGNANCY: Category B, not for use in nursing.

MECHANISM OF ACTION: Proton pump inhibitor. Suppresses gastric acid secretion by specific inhibition of the H^+/K^+-ATPase in the gastric parietal cell.

PHARMACOKINETICS: Absorption: (20mg): AUC=5.11μmol•hr/L; C_{max}=3.86μmol/L; (40mg): AUC=16.21μmol•hr/L. **Distribution:** Plasma protein binding (97%); V_d= 16L. **Metabolism:** Liver (extensive) via CYP2C19, 3A4. **Elimination:** Urine (primary), (<1%, unchanged), feces. $T_{1/2}$=1.1-1.4 hrs.

NIASPAN   RX
niacin (Abbott)

THERAPEUTIC CLASS: Nicotinic acid

INDICATIONS: Adjunct to diet, to reduce total cholesterol (total-C), LDL-C, TG, and Apo B levels, and to increase HDL-C in primary hypercholesterolemia (heterozygous familial and nonfamilial) and mixed dyslipidemia (Types IIa and IIb). With concomitant lovastatin, to further reduce LDL-C and TG, or increase HDL-C in primary hypercholesterolemia (heterozygous familial and nonfamilial) and mixed dyslipidemia (Types IIa and IIb). To reduce risk of recurrent nonfatal MI with history of MI and hypercholesterolemia. With concomitant bile acid binding resin, to slow progression/promote regression of atherosclerotic disease with history of CAD and hypercholesterolemia. Adjunct to diet with concomitant bile acid binding resin to reduce total-C and LDL-C in primary hypercholesterolemia (Type IIa) inadequately responding to diet or diet plus monotherapy. Adjunct for very high TG levels (Type IV and Type V hyperlipidemia) with risk of pancreatitis, inadequately responding to diet.

DOSAGE: *Adults:* Take qhs after low-fat snack. Initial: 500mg qhs. Titrate: Increase by 500mg every 4 weeks. Maint: 1-2g qhs. Max: 2g/day. Take ASA or NSAIDs 30 min before to reduce flushing. Do not chew, crush, or break; swallow whole. Women may respond to lower doses than men.

HOW SUPPLIED: Tab, Extended-Release: 500mg, 750mg, 1000mg

CONTRAINDICATIONS: Unexplained or significant hepatic dysfunction, active peptic ulcer disease, arterial bleeding.

WARNINGS/PRECAUTIONS: Do not substitute with equivalent doses of immediate-release niacin (severe hepatic toxicity may occur). Associated with abnormal LFTs; monitor LFTs before therapy, every 6-12 weeks during 1st yr, then periodically thereafter. D/C if LFTs ≥3x ULN persists or develop signs of hepatotoxicity. Monitor for rhabdomyolysis. Observe closely with history of jaundice, hepatobiliary disease, and peptic ulcer; monitor LFTs and blood glucose frequently. Dose-related rise in glucose tolerance in diabetics. Caution with history of hepatic disease, heavy alcohol use, renal dysfunction, unstable angina, and acute phase of MI. Elevated uric acid levels reported. May reduce platelet and phosphorous levels.

ADVERSE REACTIONS: Flushing episodes (eg, warmth, redness, itching, tingling), dizziness, tachycardia, shortness of breath, sweating, chills, edema, headache, diarrhea.

INTERACTIONS: Rhabdomyolysis may occur with HMG-CoA reductase inhibitors. May potentiate antihypertensives (eg, ganglionic blockers, vasoactive drugs). Separate dosing from bile acid resins by at least 4-6 hrs. Avoid concomitant alcohol or hot drinks; may increase flushing and pruritus. High dose niacin or nicotinamide may potentiate adverse effects. Caution with anticoagulants. Antidiabetic agents may need adjustment.

PREGNANCY: Category C, not for use in nursing.

MECHANISM OF ACTION: Nicotinic acid; not well established. May partially inhibit release of free fatty acids from adipose tissue, and increases lipoprotein lipase activity, which increases rate of chylomicron triglyceride removal from plasma. Decreases rate of hepatic synthesis of VLDL and LDL.

PHARMACOKINETICS: Absorption: Rapid and extensive. **Distribution:** Liver, kidney, adipose tissue; found in breast milk. **Metabolism:** Liver (extensive) to nicotinamide and other metabolites. **Elimination:** Urine; Parent and metabolites (60-76%), unchanged (12%).

NICARDIPINE RX
nicardipine HCL (Various)

THERAPEUTIC CLASS: Calcium channel blocker (dihydropyridine)

INDICATIONS: Treatment of hypertension. Management of chronic stable angina.

DOSAGE: *Adults:* ≥18 yrs: Initial: 20mg tid. Titrate: Increase dose every 3 days if needed. Usual: 20-40mg tid. Hepatic Dysfunction: Initial: 20mg bid.

HOW SUPPLIED: Cap: 20mg, 30mg

CONTRAINDICATIONS: Advanced aortic stenosis.

WARNINGS/PRECAUTIONS: Increased angina reported in patients with angina. Caution with CHF when titrating dose. Caution in hepatic/renal impairment, or reduced hepatic blood flow. May cause symptomatic hypotension. Measure BP 1-2 hrs and 8 hrs after dosing.

ADVERSE REACTIONS: Headache, pedal edema, vasodilation, palpitations, nausea, dizziness, asthenia, flushing, increased angina.

INTERACTIONS: Increased levels with cimetidine. Elevates cyclosporine levels. With β-blocker withdrawal, gradually reduce over 8-10 days. Monitor digoxin levels. Caution with fentanyl anesthesia.

PREGNANCY: Category C, not for use in nursing.

MECHANISM OF ACTION: Ca^{2+} channel blocker; inhibits transmembrane influx of Ca^{2+} ions into cardiac and smooth muscle without changing serum Ca^{2+} concentrations.

PHARMACOKINETICS: Absorption: Complete; Absolute bioavailability (35%). T_{max}=1 hr, C_{max}=36ng/mL (20mg), 88ng/mL (30mg), 133ng/mL (40mg). **Distribution**: Plasma protein binding (>95%). **Metabolism**. Liver. **Elimination:** Urine (<1%), feces; $T_{1/2}$=8.6 hrs (steady state), 2-4 hrs (inital).

NICODERM CQ   OTC
nicotine (GlaxoSmithKline Consumer)

THERAPEUTIC CLASS: Nicotine

INDICATIONS: To reduce withdrawal symptoms associated with smoking cessation.

DOSAGE: *Adults:* Stop smoking completely. >10 cigarettes/day: 21mg qd for 6 weeks, then 14mg qd for 2 weeks, then 7mg qd for 2 weeks, then discontinue. ≤10 cigarettes/day: 14mg qd for 6 weeks, then 7mg qd for 2 weeks, then discontinue. Apply to clean, dry, hairless area; hold for 10 seconds; wash hands. Rotate application sites. Remove after 16 or 24 hours; if crave cigarettes when wake up, wear patch for 24 hrs. If vivid dreams occur, remove before sleep. Do not wear >1 patch at a time. Do not cut patch in half. Do not use same patch >24 hrs.

HOW SUPPLIED: Patch: 7mg/24hrs [14ˢ], 14mg/24hrs [14ˢ], 21mg/24hrs [7ˢ 14ˢ]

WARNINGS/PRECAUTIONS: Avoid with serious arrhythmias, severe or worsening angina, accelerated HTN, and immediately post-MI. Tachycardia, palpitations reported. D/C with irregular heartbeat, palpitations, symptoms of nicotine overdose (eg, nausea, vomiting, dizziness, weakness, rapid heartbeat), skin redness or swelling, or rash >4 days. Avoid creams or lotions at application site.

ADVERSE REACTIONS: Skin irritation, tobacco withdrawal symptoms, tachycardia.

INTERACTIONS: Antidepressants and antiasthmatic drugs may need adjustment. Avoid smoking, chewing tobacco, snuff, nicotine gum, or other nicotine products.

PREGNANCY: Safety in pregnancy and nursing not known.

NICOMIDE   RX
cupric oxide - zinc oxide - folic acid - nicotinamide (Sirus Laboratories)

THERAPEUTIC CLASS: Vitamin and mineral combinations

INDICATIONS: Treatment of acne vulgaris, acne rosacea, or other inflammatory skin disorders in nonpregnant patients.

DOSAGE: *Adults:* 1 tab qd-bid.

HOW SUPPLIED: Tab: (Cupric Oxide-Folic Acid-Nicotinamide-Zinc Oxide) 1.5mg-500mcg-750mg-25mg

CONTRAINDICATIONS: Wilson's disease (hepatolenticular degeneration).

N

WARNINGS/PRECAUTIONS: Folic acid is improper treatment of pernicious anemia and other megaloblastic anemias with vitamin B$_{12}$-deficiency. Folic acid >0.1mg/day may obscure pernicious anemia. Caution with history of jaundice, liver disease, DM, or in elderly.

ADVERSE REACTIONS: Nausea, vomiting, transient LFT elevations, allergic sensitization.

INTERACTIONS: Reduced clearance of primidone and carbamazepine. Decreased absorption of quinolones and tetracyclines. Concomitant use of penicillamine and copper can decrease absorption of both.

PREGNANCY: Avoid in pregnancy, caution in nursing.

MECHANISM OF ACTION: Nicotinamide: water soluble component of vitamin B complex. Incorporated into nicotinamide adenine dinucleotide and nicotinamide adenine dinucleotide phosphate. Produces anti-inflammatory actions including suppression of antigen-induced lymphocytic transformation and inhibition of 3'-5' cyclic AMP phosphodiesterase. Also blocks inflammatory actions of iodides. Zinc: inhibits inflammatory polymorphonuclear leukocyte chemotaxis. Also produces inhibitory effect on lipase of Propionibacterium species found in pilosebaceous follicles. Copper: essential trace mineral in nutrition. Folic acid: essential cofactor for biosynthesis of thymidine and purine nucleotides required for normal cellular DNA synthesis.

NICORETTE OTC
nicotine polacrilex (GlaxoSmithKline Consumer)

THERAPEUTIC CLASS: Nicotine

INDICATIONS: To reduce withdrawal symptoms associated with smoking cessation.

DOSAGE: *Adults:* Stop smoking completely before use. <25 Cigarettes/Day: Use 2mg. >25 Cigarettes/Day: Use 4mg. Chew 1 piece for 30 min q1-2h for 6 weeks, then 1 piece q2-4h for 3 weeks, then 1 piece q4-8h for 3 weeks. Max 24 pieces/day and 12 weeks of therapy. Chew at least 9 pieces/day. Do not eat/drink for 15 min before or while chewing gum.

HOW SUPPLIED: Gum: 2mg, 4mg

WARNINGS/PRECAUTIONS: Do not use if continue to smoke, chew tobacco, use snuff, use a nicotine patch, or other nicotine products. Caution with heart disease, recent MI, irregular heartbeat, HTN, stomach ulcers. May increase BP and HR. D/C with mouth, teeth, or jaw problems, or with symptoms of nicotine overdose (nausea, vomiting, dizziness, weakness, palpitations). Use under medical supervision if <18 yrs of age.

ADVERSE REACTIONS: Headache, nausea, upset stomach, dizziness.

INTERACTIONS: Insulin, antidepressants, and asthma agents may need adjustment. Reduced effect with coffee, juices, wine, or soft drinks.

PREGNANCY: Safety in pregnancy and nursing is not known.

NICOTROL INHALER RX
nicotine (Pharmacia & Upjohn)

THERAPEUTIC CLASS: Nicotine

INDICATIONS: To reduce withdrawal symptoms associated with smoking cessation.

DOSAGE: *Adults:* Initial: At least 6 cartridges/day for 3-6 weeks. Usual: 6-16 cartridges/day. Max: 16 cartridges/day for 12 weeks. Best effect achieved by frequent continuous puffing (20 min). Continue for 3 months. Wean by gradual reduction of daily dose over the following 6-12 weeks. Do not treat >6 months.

HOW SUPPLIED: Inh: 4mg/inh

CONTRAINDICATIONS: Hypersensitivity or allergy to menthol.

WARNINGS/PRECAUTIONS: Can be toxic and addictive. Keep away from children and pets. Stop smoking completely before start therapy. May cause bronchospasm; caution with bronchospastic disease. Caution with coronary heart disease, arrhythmias, vasospastic diseases, renal/hepatic insufficiency, hyperthyroidism, pheochromocytoma, insulin-dependent diabetes, active peptic ulcers and in elderly. Tachycardia and palpitations reported; avoid in post-MI, severe arrhythmias, severe or worsening angina. Increased risk for malignant HTN with accelerated HTN.

ADVERSE REACTIONS: Mouth and throat local irritation, coughing, rhinitis, dizziness, anxiety, sleep disorder, depression, withdrawal syndrome, drug dependence, fatigue, dyspepsia, nausea, diarrhea.

INTERACTIONS: TCAs and theophylline may need dose adjustment.

PREGNANCY: Category D, not for use in nursing.

MECHANISM OF ACTION: Binds stereo-selectively to nicotinic-cholinergic receptors at autoimmune ganglia, in adrenal medulla, at neuromuscular junctions, and in brain.

PHARMACOKINETICS: Absorption: Cmax=23ng/mL. **Distribution:** Vd=2-3L/kg; Plasma protein binding (<5%). **Metabolism:** Metabolites: Cotinine and trans-3-hydroxycotinine; $T_{/2}$=15-20 hrs. **Elimination**: Urine=10% (unchanged); $T_{1/2}$=1-2 hrs.

NICOTROL NASAL SPRAY   RX
nicotine (Pharmacia & Upjohn)

THERAPEUTIC CLASS: Nicotine

INDICATIONS: To reduce withdrawal symptoms associated with smoking cessation.

DOSAGE: *Adults:* Initial: 2-4 sprays/hr, up to 10 sprays/hr, for up to 8 weeks. Minimum: 16 sprays/day. Max: 80 sprays/day. Elderly: Start at low end of the dosing range. May d/c abruptly or over 4-6 weeks. Do not treat >3 months. Do not sniff, swallow, or inhale through nose as spray is being administered. Tilt head back slightly to administer.

HOW SUPPLIED: Nasal Spray: 0.5mg/inh [10mL]

WARNINGS/PRECAUTIONS: Avoid with known chronic nasal disorders. Can be toxic and addictive. Keep away from children and pets. Stop smoking completely before start therapy. May cause bronchospasm; caution with bronchospastic disease. Caution with coronary heart disease, arrhythmias, vasospastic diseases, renal or hepatic insufficiency, hyperthyroidism, pheochromocytoma, insulin-dependent diabetes, active peptic ulcers, and elderly. Tachycardia and palpitations reported. Increased risk for malignant HTN with accelerated HTN.

ADVERSE REACTIONS: Local irritation, chest tightness, dyspepsia, numbness, constipation, stomatitis, anxiety, irritability, restlessness, cravings, dizziness, impaired concentration, weight increase, increased sweating, insomnia.

INTERACTIONS: May need dose reduction of APAP, caffeine, imipramine, oxazepam, pentazocine, theophylline, insulin, adrenergic antagonists, propranolol or other β-blockers after smoking cessation.

PREGNANCY: Category D, not for use in nursing.

NIFEDIPINE   RX
nifedipine (Various)

OTHER BRAND NAMES: Procardia (Pfizer)

THERAPEUTIC CLASS: Calcium channel blocker (dihydropyridine)

INDICATIONS: Management of vasospastic angina and chronic stable angina.

DOSAGE: *Adults:* Initial: 10mg tid. Titrate over 7-14 days. Usual: 10-20mg tid. Max: 180mg/day. Elderly: Start at low end of dosing range.

HOW SUPPLIED: Cap: 10mg, 20mg

WARNINGS/PRECAUTIONS: May cause hypotension; monitor BP initially or with titration. May exacerbate angina from β-blocker withdrawal. CHF risk, especially with aortic stenosis or β-blockers. Peripheral edema reported. Not for acute reduction of BP or essential HTN. May increase angina or MI with severe obstructive CAD. Avoid with acute coronary syndrome or within 1-2 weeks of MI. Caution in elderly.

ADVERSE REACTIONS: Dizziness, lightheadedness, giddiness, flushing, muscle cramps, headache, weakness, nausea, peripheral edema, nervousness/mood changes.

INTERACTIONS: β-Blockers may increase risk of CHF, severe hypotension, or angina exacerbation. Possible hypotension with fentanyl. Potentiates digoxin. Monitor quinidine, coumarin. Potentiated by cimetidine and grapefruit juice. Avoid grapefruit juice.

PREGNANCY: Category C, unknown use in nursing.

MECHANISM OF ACTION: Calcium channel blocker; inhibits the transmembrane influx of calcium ions into cardiac muscle and smooth muscle. Angina: MOA has not been fully determined; believed to act by relaxation and prevention of coronary artery spasm, and reduction of oxygen utilization.

PHARMACOKINETICS: Absorption: Rapid and full; T_{max}=30 min. **Distribution:** Plasma protein binding (92-98%). **Metabolism:** Liver, via biotransformation. **Elimination:** Urine (80%).

NIFEREX   OTC
iron (Ther-Rx)

THERAPEUTIC CLASS: Iron supplement

INDICATIONS: Treatment of uncomplicated iron deficiency anemias.

DOSAGE: *Adults:* 1-2 tabs bid or 5-10mL qd.
Pediatrics: ≥6 yrs: 1-2 tabs qd or 5mL qd. <6 yrs: (Sol): Individualize dose.

HOW SUPPLIED: Cap: 60mg; Sol: 100mg/5mL

WARNINGS/PRECAUTIONS: Fatal poisoning reported in children <6 yrs with accidental overdose of iron-containing products.

PREGNANCY: Safety in pregnancy and nursing not known.

NIFEREX-150   OTC
iron - vitamin C (Ther-Rx)

OTHER BRAND NAMES: Fe-Tinic 150 (Ethex)

THERAPEUTIC CLASS: Iron supplement

INDICATIONS: Treatment of uncomplicated iron deficiency anemias.

DOSAGE: *Adults:* 1-2 caps qd.

HOW SUPPLIED: Cap: (Iron-Vitamin C) 150mg-50mg

WARNINGS/PRECAUTIONS: Fatal poisoning reported in children <6 yrs with accidental overdose of iron-containing products.

PREGNANCY: Safety in pregnancy and nursing not known.

NIFEREX-150 FORTE   RX
vitamin B12 - folic acid - iron - vitamin C (Ther-Rx)

OTHER BRAND NAMES: Fe-Tinic 150 Forte (Ethex)

THERAPEUTIC CLASS: Iron/vitamin

INDICATIONS: Prevention and treatment of iron deficiency anemia and/or nutritional megaloblastic anemias.

DOSAGE: *Adults:* 1 cap qd.

HOW SUPPLIED: Cap: (Folic Acid-Iron-Vitamin B₁₂-Vitamin C) 1mg-150mg-25mcg-60mg

CONTRAINDICATIONS: Hemochromatosis, hemosiderosis.

WARNINGS/PRECAUTIONS: Fatal poisoning reported in children <6 yrs with accidental overdose of iron-containing products. Determination of type, cause of anemia is recommended before starting therapy. Folic acid >0.1mg/day may obscure pernicious anemia.

ADVERSE REACTIONS: Constipation, diarrhea, nausea, vomiting, dark stools, abdominal pain.

PREGNANCY: Safety in pregnancy and nursing not known.

NIFEREX-PN   RX
folic acid - multiple vitamin - iron (Ther-Rx)

THERAPEUTIC CLASS: Iron/vitamin/mineral

INDICATIONS: Prevention and treatment of dietary vitamin and mineral deficiencies associated with pregnancy and lactation.

DOSAGE: *Adults:* 1 tab qd.

HOW SUPPLIED: Tab: Calcium 125mg-Folic Acid 1mg-Iron 60mg-Niacinamide 10mg-Vitamin A 4000IU-Vitamin B₁ 2.43mg-Vitamin B₂ 3mg-Vitamin B₆ 1.64mg-Vitamin B₁₂ 0.003mg-Vitamin C 50mg-Vitamin D 400IU-Zinc 18mg

CONTRAINDICATIONS: Hemochromatosis, hemosiderosis.

WARNINGS/PRECAUTIONS: Fatal poisoning reported in children <6 yrs with accidental overdose of iron-containing products. Folic acid >0.1mg/day may obscure pernicious anemia. High doses of vitamin A may be associated with birth defects.

ADVERSE REACTIONS: Constipation, diarrhea, nausea, vomiting, dark stools, abdominal pain.

PREGNANCY: Safety in pregnancy and nursing not known.

NIFEREX-PN FORTE   RX
folic acid - multiple vitamin - minerals - iron (Ther-Rx)

THERAPEUTIC CLASS: Iron/vitamin/mineral

INDICATIONS: Prevention and treatment of dietary vitamin and mineral deficiencies associated with pregnancy and lactation.

DOSAGE: *Adults:* 1 tab qd.

HOW SUPPLIED: Tab: Calcium 250mg-Copper 2mg-Folic Acid 1mg-Iodine 0.2mg-Iron 60mg-Magnesium 10mg-Niacinamide 20mg-Vitamin A 5000IU-Vitamin B₁ 3mg-Vitamin B₂ 3.4mg-Vitamin B₆ 4mg-Vitamin B₁₂ 0.012mg-Vitamin C 80mg-Vitamin D 400IU-Vitamin E 30IU-Zinc 25mg

CONTRAINDICATIONS: Hemochromatosis, hemosiderosis.

WARNINGS/PRECAUTIONS: Fatal poisoning reported in children <6 yrs with accidental overdose of iron-containing products. Folic acid >0.1mg/day may obscure pernicious anemia. High doses of vitamin A may be associated with birth defects.

ADVERSE REACTIONS: Constipation, diarrhea, nausea, vomiting, dark stools, abdominal pain.

PREGNANCY: Safety in pregnancy and nursing not known.

NILANDRON RX
nilutamide (Sanofi-Aventis)

> Interstitial pneumonitis reported. Perform routine chest X-ray and baseline pulmonary function test before therapy. D/C if symptoms occur.

THERAPEUTIC CLASS: Nonsteroidal antiandrogen

INDICATIONS: Treatment of metastatic prostatic cancer (Stage D_2) in combination with surgical castration.

DOSAGE: *Adults:* Initial: 300mg/day for 30 days. Maint: 150mg qd. Begin on the same day or the day after surgical castration.

HOW SUPPLIED: Tab: 150mg

CONTRAINDICATIONS: Severe hepatic impairment, respiratory insufficiency.

WARNINGS/PRECAUTIONS: Hepatotoxicity, aplastic anemia reported. D/C if develop jaundice or ALT >2x ULN. Delay in adaptation to dark; caution with driving at night or in tunnels; wear tinted glasses to alleviate effect. Evaluate baseline hepatic enzymes before therapy, at regular intervals for 1st 4 months, and periodically thereafter.

ADVERSE REACTIONS: Hot flushes, decreased libido, abnormal vision, increased LFTs, dyspnea, GI effects, dry skin, sweating, dizziness, HTN, anemia, testicular atrophy, gynecomastia.

INTERACTIONS: May potentiate vitamin K antagonists, phenytoin, and theophylline. Intolerance to alcohol (eg, hypotension, malaise).

PREGNANCY: Category C, safety in nursing not known.

MECHANISM OF ACTION: Nonsteroidal antiandrogen; acts by blocking effects of testosterone at the androgen receptor sites.

PHARMACOKINETICS: Absorption: Rapid and complete. **Elimination:** Urine (62%), feces (1.4%-7%); $T_{1/2}$=38-59.1 hrs (100-300mg single dose).

NIMBEX RX
cisatracurium besylate (Abbott)

THERAPEUTIC CLASS: Skeletal muscle relaxant (nondepolarizing)

INDICATIONS: Adjunct to general anesthesia, to facilitate tracheal intubation, and to provide skeletal muscle relaxation during surgery/mechanical ventilation.

DOSAGE: *Adults:* Initial: 0.15mg/kg (3 x ED_{95}) or 0.20mg/kg (4 x ED_{95}) IV. Serious Cardiovascular Disease: Up to 8 x ED_{95}. Maint/Prolonged Surgical Procedures: 0.03mg/kg IV (for 20 min blockade) 40-50 min after initial 0.15mg/kg, and 50-60 min after initial 0.20mg/kg. Operating Room Infusion: After initial bolus dose, give 3mcg/kg/min to counteract recovery from bolus, then 1-2mcg/kg/min. ICU: 3mcg/kg/min IV; dose requirements may increase/decrease with time.
Pediatrics: >12 yrs: Initial: 0.15mg/kg (3 x ED_{95}) or 0.20mg/kg (4 x ED_{95}) IV. Serious Cardiovascular Disease: Up to 8 x ED_{95}. Maint/Prolonged Surgical Procedures: 0.03mg/kg IV (for 20 min blockade) 40-50 min after initial 0.15mg/kg, and 50-60 min after initial 0.20mg/kg. 2-12 yrs: Initial: 0.10-0.15mg/kg over 5-10 seconds during halothane or opioid anesthesia. (1-23 months): Initial: 0.15mg/kg over 5-10 sec during halothane or opioid anesthesia. (≥ 2 yrs): Operating Room Infusion: After initial bolus dose, give 3mcg/kg/min to counteract recovery from bolus, then 1-2mcg/kg/min.

HOW SUPPLIED: Inj: 2mg/mL, 10mg/mL

CONTRAINDICATIONS: Hypersensitivity to bisbenzylisoquinolinium agents and benzyl alcohol.

WARNINGS/PRECAUTIONS: Avoid administration before unconsciousness has been induced. Use in facility with resuscitation and life support, and have antagonist available. Monitor neuromuscular function with peripheral nerve stimulator during administration. Multi-dose vials contain benzyl alcohol. Not for rapid sequence endotracheal intubation. May have profound effect with neuromuscular diseases (eg, myasthenia gravis, carcinomatosis); monitor neuromuscular function with peripheral nerve stimulator. Resistance may develop in burn victims; consider increasing dose. Resistance with hemiparesis or paraparesis. Acid-base and/or serum electrolyte abnormalities may potentiate or antagonize effect. Monitor for malignant hyperthermia.

ADVERSE REACTIONS: Bradycardia, hypotension, flushing, bronchospasm, rash, muscle weakness, myopathy, prolonged/inadequate neuromuscular blockade.

INTERACTIONS: Prolonged duration of action and required infusion rate decreased with isoflurane or enflurane with nitrous oxide/oxygen. Enhanced neuromuscular blocking action with certain antibiotics (eg, aminoglycosides, tetracyclines, bacitracin, polymyxins, lincomycin, clindamycin, colistin, sodium colistimethate), magnesium salts, lithium, local anesthetics, procainamide, and quinidine. Antagonized effect with phenytoin and carbamazepine. May not be compatible with pH >8.5 alkaline solutions (eg, barbiturate solutions).

PREGNANCY: Category B, caution in nursing.

MECHANISM OF ACTION: Non depolarizing skeletal muscle relaxant; binds competitively to cholinergic receptors on the motor end-plate to antagonize the action of acetylcholine, resulting in block of neuromuscular transmission.

PHARMACOKINETICS: Distribution: V_d=145mL/kg. **Metabolism:** Laudanosine (major active metabolite). **Elimination:** Hoffmann elimination (80%); hepatic/renal elemination (20%). Urine (95% metabolites), (<10% unchanged), feces (4%); $T_{1/2}$=22-29 min.

NIMOTOP   RX
nimodipine (Bayer Healthcare)

> Do not administer IV or by other parenteral routes. Deaths and serious, life-threatening adverse events have occurred when contents of capsules injected parenterally.

THERAPEUTIC CLASS: Calcium channel blocker

INDICATIONS: Improvement of neurological outcome in patients with subarachnoid hemorrhage (SAH) from ruptured intracranial berry aneurysms regardless of their post-ictus neurological condition.

DOSAGE: *Adults:* 60mg q 4 hrs for 21 days, 1 hr before or 2 hrs after meals. Hepatic Cirrhosis: 30mg q 4 hrs for 21 days. Start therapy within 96 hrs of SAH. If cannot swallow cap, extract contents into syringe and empty into NG tube, then flush with 30mL of 0.9% NaCl.

HOW SUPPLIED: Cap: 30mg

WARNINGS/PRECAUTIONS: Carefully monitor BP. Monitor BP and HR closely with hepatic dysfunction. Do not administer IV or by other parenteral routes.

ADVERSE REACTIONS: Decreased BP, headache, rash, diarrhea, bradycardia, nausea, abnormal LFTs.

INTERACTIONS: May enhance cardiovascular effects of other CCBs. Increased serum levels with cimetidine. May intensify effects of antihypertensives.

PREGNANCY: Category C, not for use in nursing.

MECHANISM OF ACTION: Calcium channel blocker; not established; suspected to inhibit calcium ion transfer into smooth muscle cells, thereby inhibiting contractions of vascular smooth muscle.

PHARMACOKINETICS: Absorption: Rapid. T_{max}=1 hr. **Distribution:** Plasma protein binding (≥95%). Crosses blood-brain barrier. **Elimination:** Urine (≤1%, unchanged). $T_{1/2}$=8-9 hrs.

NIRAVAM   CIV
alprazolam (Schwarz)

THERAPEUTIC CLASS: Benzodiazepine

INDICATIONS: Management of anxiety disorders and short-term relief of anxiety symptoms. Treatment of panic disorder with or without agoraphobia.

DOSAGE: *Adults:* Anxiety: Initial: 0.25-0.5mg tid. Titrate: May increase every 3-4 days. Max: 4mg/day. Panic Disorder: Initial: 0.5mg tid. Titrate: Increase by no more than 1mg/day every 3-4 days; slower titration if ≥4mg/day. Usual: 1-10mg/day. Decrease dose slowly (no more than 0.5mg every 3 days). Elderly/Advanced Liver Disease/Debilitated: Initial: 0.25mg bid-tid. Titrate: Increase gradually as tolerated.

HOW SUPPLIED: Tab, Orally Disintegrating: 0.25mg*, 0.5mg*, 1mg*, 2mg*
*scored

CONTRAINDICATIONS: Acute narrow angle glaucoma, untreated open angle glaucoma, concomitant ketoconazole or itraconazole.

WARNINGS/PRECAUTIONS: Risk of dependence. Withdrawal symptoms, including seizure, reported with dose reduction or abrupt discontinuation; avoid abrupt withdrawal. Risk of CNS depression and impaired performance. May cause fetal harm. Caution with impaired renal, hepatic, or pulmonary function, severe depression, obesity, elderly and debilitated. Hypomania/mania reported with depression. Weak uricosuric effect.

ADVERSE REACTIONS: Drowsiness, fatigue/tiredness, impaired coordination, irritability, memory impairment, cognitive disorder, dysarthria, decreased libido, confusional state, light-headedness, dry mouth, hypotension, increased salivation.

INTERACTIONS: Avoid with potent CYP3A inhibitors (eg, azole antifungals). Potentiated by nefazodone, fluvoxamine, cimetidine, fluoxetine, oral contraceptives. Decreased plasma levels with propoxyphene and carbamazepine. Caution with diltiazem, isoniazid, macrolides, grapefruit juice, sertraline, paroxetine, ergotamine, cyclosporine, amiodarone, nicardipine, nifedipine and other CYP3A inhibitors. Increases levels of imipramine and desipramine. Additive CNS depressant effects with psychotropic agents, anticonvulsants, antihistamines, ethanol.

PREGNANCY: Category D, not for use in nursing.

MECHANISM OF ACTION: Benzodiazepine; not established, CNS depressant, believed to exert its effects by binding at stereo specific receptor at several sites within the CNS.

PHARMACOKINETICS: Absorption: Readily absorbed, T_{max}=1.5-2 hrs, C_{max}=8-37ng/mL. **Distribution:** Plasma protein binding (80%). **Metabolism:** Metabolized (extensively), hydroxylation, 4-hydroxyalprazolam and α-hydroxyalprazolam (major metabolites). **Elimination:** $T_{1/2}$=12.5 hrs; urine.

NITRO-BID   RX
nitroglycerin (Fougera)

THERAPEUTIC CLASS: Nitrate vasodilator

INDICATIONS: Prevention of angina pectoris. Not for acute attacks.

DOSAGE: *Adults:* Initial: Apply 0.5 inch bid (once in the am and 6 hrs later). Titrate: May increase to 1 inch bid, then to 2 inches bid. Should have 10-12 hr nitrate-free period.

HOW SUPPLIED: Oint: 2% (15mg/inch) [1g (48ˢ), 30g, 60g]

WARNINGS/PRECAUTIONS: Monitor with acute MI or CHF. Severe hypotension may occur; caution with volume depletion and hypotension. May aggravate angina caused by hypertrophic cardiomyopathy. Tolerance to other nitrates may decrese effects. Topical use only. See Drug Interactions.

ADVERSE REACTIONS: Headache, lightheadedness, hypotension, flushing, syncope, rebound HTN.

INTERACTIONS: Additive vasodilating effects with other vasodilators (eg, alcohol). Severe hypotension with sildenafil. Marked orthostatic hypotension reported with CCBs.

PREGNANCY: Category C, caution in nursing.

MECHANISM OF ACTION: Nitrate vasodilator; relaxes vascular smooth muscle, and consequent dilatation of peripheral arteries and veins, especially the latter. Dilatation of the veins leads to reduced left ventricular end-diastolic pressure and pulmonary capillary wedge pressure (preload). Arteriolar relaxation reduces systemic vascular resistance, systolic arterial pressure and mean arterial pressure (afterload). It also dilates the coronary artery.

PHARMACOKINETICS: Distribution: V_d=3L/kg. **Metabolism:** Extrahepatic metabolism (RBC and vascular walls), inorganic nitrate and 1,2-and 1,3-dinitrogylcerin (metabolites). Dinitrates are metabolized to mononitrates, gycerol and CO_2. **Elimination:** $T_{1/2}$ =3 min.

NITRO-DUR   RX
nitroglycerin (Schering)

OTHER BRAND NAMES: Nitrek (Mylan Bertek) - Minitran (Graceway)

THERAPEUTIC CLASS: Nitrate vasodilator

INDICATIONS: Prevention of angina pectoris. Not for acute attack.

DOSAGE: *Adults:* Initial: 0.2-0.4mg/hr for 12-14 hrs. Remove for 10-12 hrs.

HOW SUPPLIED: Patch: (Minitran) 0.1mg/hr, 0.2mg/hr, 0.4mg/hr, 0.6mg/hr [30^s]; (Nitrek) 0.2mg/hr, 0.4mg/hr, 0.6mg/hr [30^s]; (Nitro-Dur) 0.1mg/hr, 0.2mg/hr, 0.3mg/hr, 0.4mg/hr, 0.6mg/hr, 0.8mg/hr [30^s]

CONTRAINDICATIONS: Allergy to adhesives in NTG patches.

WARNINGS/PRECAUTIONS: Severe hypotension may occur; caution with volume depletion or hypotension. Vasodilatory effects with phosphodiesterase inhibitors (eg, sildenafil) can result in severe hypotension. May aggravate angina caused by hypertrophic cardiomyopathy. Tolerance to other nitrate forms may decrease effects. Monitor with acute MI or CHF. Do not discharge defibrillator/cardioverter through the patch.

ADVERSE REACTIONS: Headache, lightheadedness, hypotension, syncope.

INTERACTIONS: Additive vasodilating effects with other vasodilators (eg, alcohol). Marked orthostatic hypotension reported with CCBs. Severe hypotension with sildenafil.

PREGNANCY: Category C, caution in nursing.

N

NITROLINGUAL SPRAY   RX
nitroglycerin (Sciele)

OTHER BRAND NAMES: NitroMist (NovaDel Pharma)

THERAPEUTIC CLASS: Nitrate vasodilator

INDICATIONS: For acute relief of angina attack. Prophylaxis of angina pectoris.

DOSAGE: *Adults:* Acute: 1-2 sprays at onset of attack onto or under tongue. Max: 3 sprays/15 min. Prophylaxis: 1-2 sprays onto or under tongue 5-10 min before activity that may cause acute attack. Do not expectorate medication or rinse mouth for 5-10 min after administration.

HOW SUPPLIED: Spray: 400mcg/spray

CONTRAINDICATIONS: Concomitant use with phosphodiesterase type 5 (PDE5) inhibitors such as sildenafil, vardenafil, and tadalafil.

WARNINGS/PRECAUTIONS: Severe hypotension may occur; caution with volume depletion or hypotension. May aggravate angina caused by hypertrophic cardiomyopathy. Tolerance and cross-tolerance to other nitrates/nitrites may occur. Monitor during early days of AMI.

ADVERSE REACTIONS: Headache, hypotension, flushing, dizziness, weakness, rash, exfoliative dermatitis.

INTERACTIONS: See Contraindications. Avoid PDE5 inhibitors (eg, sildenafil, vardenafil, tadalafil); severe hypotension may occur. Concomitant use with CCBs may cause orthostatic hypotension. Alcohol may cause hypotension.

(NitroMist) Increased hypotensive effects with β-adrenergic blockers (eg, labetolol). ASA may increase levels. May decrease anticoagulant effect of heparin. Avoid ergotamine. Caution with tissue-type plasminogen activator.

PREGNANCY: Category C, caution in nursing.

MECHANISM OF ACTION: Nitrate vasodilator; activates guanylate cyclase, resulting in an increase cyclic GMP in smooth muscle and other tissues; leads to dephosphorylation of myosin light chains, which regulates the contractile state in smooth muscle and results in vasodilation.

PHARMACOKINETICS: Absorption: Rapid, C_{max}=0.8ng/mL, T_{max}=8 min. **Distribution:** V_d=3.3L/kg. **Metabolism:** Extrahepatic metabolism (red cells and vascular walls); 1,2-dinitroglycerin and 1,3-dinitroglycerin (major metabolites). **Elimination:** $T_{1/2}$=3 min (nitroglycerin), 10 min (1,2-dinitroglycerin), 11 min (1,3-dinitroglycerin).

NITROSTAT RX
nitroglycerin (Parke-Davis)

OTHER BRAND NAMES: Nitroquick (Ethex)

THERAPEUTIC CLASS: Nitrate vasodilator

INDICATIONS: For acute relief of angina attack. Prophylaxis of angina pectoris.

DOSAGE: *Adults:* Treatment: 1 tab SL or in buccal pouch at onset of attack. May repeat in 5 min. Max: 3 tabs in 15 min. Prophylaxis: Take 5-10 min before activity that may cause acute attack. Administer in sitting position.

HOW SUPPLIED: Tab, Sublingual: 0.3mg, 0.4mg, 0.6mg

CONTRAINDICATIONS: Early MI, severe anemia, increased ICP, concomitant sildenafil.

WARNINGS/PRECAUTIONS: Do not swallow tabs. Severe hypotension may occur; caution with volume depletion or hypotension. May aggravate angina caused by hypertrophic cardiomyopathy. D/C if develop blurred vision or dry mouth. May interfere with cholesterol test. Monitor with acute MI or CHF. Tolerance to other nitrate forms may decrease effects. Caution in elderly.

ADVERSE REACTIONS: Headache, vertigo, dizziness, weakness, palpitation, syncope, flushing, postural hypotension, drug rash, exfoliative dermatitis.

INTERACTIONS: Additive hypotension with alcohol, β-blockers, phenothiazines, CCBs, other antihypertensives. Avoid ergotamine (related drugs), sildenafil. Vasodilatory and hemodynamic effects potentiated by ASA. Caution with alteplase. TCAs, anticholinergics may make sublingual dissolution difficult. Long-acting nitrates may decrease effects.

PREGNANCY: Category C, caution in nursing.

MECHANISM OF ACTION: Nitrate vasodilator; relaxes the vascular smooth muscle; activates guanylate cyclase, resulting in an increase of guanosine 3'5' monophosphate in smooth muscle and other tissues, resulting in vasodilatation.

PHARMACOKINETICS: Absorption: (SL) rapid, absolute bioavailability (40%); (0.3mg) T_{max}=6.4 min, C_{max}=2.3ng/mL, AUC=14.9ng•mL/min; (0.6mg) T_{max}=7.2 min, C_{max}=2.1ng/mL, AUC=14.9ng•mL/min. **Distribution:** V_d=3.3 L/kg, plasma protein binding (60%). **Metabolism:** Liver via reductase, extrahepatic (red cells and vascular wall). 1,2- and 1,3-dinitroglycerin (major metabolites). **Elimination:** (0.3mg) $T_{1/2}$=2.8 min, (0.6mg) 2.6 min.

NIX OTC
permethrin (Insight Pharmaceuticals)

THERAPEUTIC CLASS: Pyrethroid pediculicide

INDICATIONS: (Liquid) Treatment of head lice and prophylactic use during epidemics (at least 20% of population are infested). (Spray) To kill lice on bedding and furniture. Not for use in humans.

DOSAGE: *Adults:* (Liquid) Treatment: Wash then towel dry hair. Apply liquid and saturate hair and scalp. Rinse with water after 10 min. Remove nits with comb provided. Repeat after 7 days if live lice is observed. Prophylaxis: Same as treatment. Repeat therapy after 2 weeks in epidemic setting. (Spray) Use from an 8-10 inch distance. Treat only garments, bedding, and furniture that cannot be washed or dry cleaned. Allow area to dry completely.
Pediatrics: ≥2 months: (Liquid) Treatment: Wash and dry hair, then saturate hair and scalp. Rinse with water after 10 min. Remove nits with comb provided. Repeat after 7 days if observe lice. Prophylaxis: Same as treatment. Do not use nit comb.

HOW SUPPLIED: Liq: (Creme Rinse) 1% [60mL]; Spray: 0.25% [148mL]

WARNINGS/PRECAUTIONS: (Liquid) Protect from getting into eyes, inside nose, mouth, or vagina. May cause breathing difficulty or asthmatic episodes in susceptible persons. D/C if skin irritation persists or infection develops. (Spray) Do not use in food serving areas or while food is exposed. Do not apply in classrooms while in use.

ADVERSE REACTIONS: Itching, redness, swelling of the scalp.

PREGNANCY: Safety in pregnancy and nursing not known.

NIZORAL   RX
ketoconazole (Janssen)

> Risk of fatal hepatotoxicity. Concomitant terfenadine, astemizole and cisapride are contraindicated due to serious cardiovascular adverse events.

THERAPEUTIC CLASS: Azole antifungal

INDICATIONS: Treatment of the following systemic fungal infections: candidiasis, chronic mucocutaneous candidiasis, oral thrush, candiduria, blastomycosis, coccidioidomycosis, histoplasmosis, chromomycosis, and paracoccidioidomycosis. Treatment of severe recalcitrant cutaneous dermatophyte infections not responsive to topical therapy or oral griseofulvin. Not for treatment of fungal meningitis.

DOSAGE: *Adults:* Initial: 200mg qd. Max: 400mg qd.
Pediatrics: >2 yrs: 3.3-6.6mg/kg/day.

HOW SUPPLIED: Tab: 200mg* *scored

CONTRAINDICATIONS: Concomitant terfenadine, astemizole, cisapride or oral triazolam.

WARNINGS/PRECAUTIONS: Hepatotoxicity reported. Monitor LFTs prior to therapy and periodically thereafter. Serum testosterone levels may be lowered. Hypersensitivity reactions reported. Tablets require acidity for dissolution. Not for use in children unless benefit outweighs risk.

ADVERSE REACTIONS: Nausea, vomiting, abdominal pain, pruritus.

INTERACTIONS: See Contraindications. Give antacids, anticholinergics, and H_2 blockers 2 hrs after ketoconazole. May potentiate midazolam, triazolam, oral hypoglycemics. May enhance anticoagulant effect of coumarin-like drugs. Avoid rifampin, isoniazid. Monitor digoxin, phenytoin. May alter metabolism of cyclosporine, tacrolimus, methylprednisolone and drugs metabolized by CYP3A4.

PREGNANCY: Category C, not for use in nursing.

MECHANISM OF ACTION: Azole antifungal: Impairs synthesis of ergosterol, a vital component of fungal cell membranes.

PHARMACOKINETICS: Absorption: C_{max}=3.5µg/mL; T_{max}=1-2 hrs. **Distribution**: Plasma protein binding (99%). **Metabolism**: Via oxidation, degradation of imidazole and piperazine rings, oxidative dealkylation and aromatic hydroxylation. CYP3A4 inhibitor. **Elimination:** Biphasic. $T_{1/2}$=2 hrs (during first 10 hrs); $T_{1/2}$=8 hrs (thereafter); bile (major), urine (13%).

NIZORAL A-D   OTC
ketoconazole (McNeil Consumer)

THERAPEUTIC CLASS: Azole antifungal

INDICATIONS: Controls flaking, scaling and itching associated with dandruff.

DOSAGE: *Adults:* Wet hair. Apply and lather. Rinse thoroughly and repeat. Apply every 3-4 days up to 8 weeks if needed.
Pediatrics: >12 yrs: Wet hair. Apply and lather. Rinse thoroughly and repeat. Apply every 3-4 days up to 8 weeks if needed.

HOW SUPPLIED: Shampoo: 1% [4oz, 7oz]

CONTRAINDICATIONS: Scalp that is broken or inflamed.

WARNINGS/PRECAUTIONS: Avoid eyes. D/C if rash appears, or if condition worsens or does not improve in 2-4 weeks.

PREGNANCY: Use in pregnancy and nursing not known.

NIZORAL SHAMPOO   RX
ketoconazole (McNeil Consumer)

THERAPEUTIC CLASS: Azole antifungal

INDICATIONS: Tinea versicolor.

DOSAGE: *Adults:* Apply to damp skin and lather. Rinse with water after 5 min. One application should be sufficient.

HOW SUPPLIED: Shampoo: 2% [4oz]

WARNINGS/PRECAUTIONS: Shampoo may remove curl from permanently waved hair. Avoid eyes. D/C if chemical irritation occurs. Do not use on broken or inflamed scalp.

ADVERSE REACTIONS: Abnormal hair texture, scalp pustules, mild skin dryness, pruritus, increase in normal hair loss, oily or dry scalp and hair.

PREGNANCY: Category C, caution in nursing.

MECHANISM OF ACTION: Azole antifungal; impairs synthesis of ergosterol, a vital component of fungal membranes.

NORCO   CIII
hydrocodone bitartrate - acetaminophen (Watson)

THERAPEUTIC CLASS: Opioid analgesic

INDICATIONS: Relief of moderate to moderately severe pain.

DOSAGE: *Adults:* Usual: (5/325) 1-2 tabs q4-6h prn pain. Usual: (7.5/325, 10/325) 1 tab q4-6h prn pain. Max: 6 tabs/day.

HOW SUPPLIED: Tab: (Hydrocodone-APAP) 5mg-325mg*, 7.5mg-325mg*, 10mg-325mg* *scored

WARNINGS/PRECAUTIONS: May produce dose-related respiratory depression. May obscure diagnosis of acute abdominal conditions or head injuries. Caution in elderly, debilitated, severe hepatic or renal dysfunction, hypothyroidism, Addison's disease, prostatic hypertrophy, urethral stricture, pulmonary disease and postoperative use. May be habit-forming. Suppresses cough reflex.

ADVERSE REACTIONS: Lightheadedness, dizziness, sedation, nausea, vomiting.

INTERACTIONS: Additive CNS depression with narcotics, antipsychotics, antihistamines, antianxiety agents, alcohol, or other CNS depressants. Increased effect of antidepressant or hydrocodone with MAOIs or TCAs.

PREGNANCY: Category C, not for use in nursing.

MECHANISM OF ACTION: Hydrocodone: opioid analgesic; most effects involve the CNS and smooth muscles. Precise MOA not established; suspected to relate to existence of opiate receptors in the CNS. APAP: nonopiate, nonsalicylate analgesic and antipyretic. Analgesic activity involves peripheral influences; specific mechanism has not been established. Antipyretic activity is mediated through hypothalmic heat regulating centers; inhibits prostaglandin synthetase.

PHARMACOKINETICS: Absorption: Hydrocodone: C_{max}=23.6ng/mL; T_{max}=1.3 hrs. APAP: rapidly absorbed. **Distribution:** APAP: excreted in breast milk. **Metabolism:** Hydrocodone: O-demethylation, N-demethylation and 6-ketoreduction; APAP: Liver via conjugation. **Elimination:** Hydrocodone: $T_{1/2}$=3.8 hrs; APAP: Urine (85%). $T_{1/2}$=1.25-3 hrs.

NORDETTE-28   RX
ethinyl estradiol - levonorgestrel (Duramed)

OTHER BRAND NAMES: Portia (Barr) - Levora (Watson)

THERAPEUTIC CLASS: Estrogen/progestogen combination

INDICATIONS: Prevention of pregnancy.

DOSAGE: *Adults:* 1 tab qd for 28 days, then repeat. Start 1st Sunday after menses begins.

HOW SUPPLIED: Tab: (Ethinyl Estradiol-Levonorgestrel) 0.03mg-0.15mg

CONTRAINDICATIONS: Thrombophlebitis, DVT or thromboembolic disorders, pregnancy, cerebrovascular or coronary artery disease, undiagnosed abnormal genital bleeding, cholestatic jaundice of pregnancy or jaundice with prior pill use, hepatic adenomas or carcinomas, breast cancer or other estrogen-dependent neoplasia.

WARNINGS/PRECAUTIONS: Cigarette smoking increases risk of serious cardiovascular side effects; risk increases with age (especially >35 yrs) and heavy smoking. Increased risk of MI, vascular disease, thromboembolism, stroke and gallbladder disease. Retinal thrombosis, hepatic neoplasia, carcinoma of breast and reproductive organs reported. May cause glucose intolerance. May increase BP, elevate LDL levels or cause other lipid changes, fluid retention, breakthrough bleeding, and spotting. May cause or exacerbate migraine. May develop visual changes with contact lens. Increased risk of MI with HTN, hyperlipidemia, obesity, and diabetes. D/C if jaundice, significant depression or ophthalmic irregularities develop. Perform annual physical exam. Use before menarche is not indicated. May affect certain endocrine, LFTs and blood components.

ADVERSE REACTIONS: Nausea, vomiting, breakthrough bleeding, spotting, amenorrhea, migraine, depression, vaginal candidiasis, edema, weight changes.

INTERACTIONS: Reduced effects, increased breakthrough bleeding, and menstrual irregularities with rifampin, barbiturates, phenylbutazone, phenytoin, griseofulvin, topiramate, some protease inhibitors, modafinil, and possibly St. John's wort, penicillins, and tetracyclines. Increased plasma levels with ascorbic acid, APAP, indinavir, fluconazole, troleandomycin, and atorvastatin. May affect cyclosporine, theophylline, and corticosteroid levels.

PREGNANCY: Category X, not for use in nursing.

MECHANISM OF ACTION: Estrogen/progestogen oral contraceptive: acts by suppressing gonadotropins. Primarily responsible for inhibiting ovulation. Also causes changes in the cervical mucus (increases difficulty of sperm entry into the uterus) and in the endometrium (reduces the likelihood of implantation).

PHARMACOKINETICS: Distribution: Found in breast milk.

NORDITROPIN RX
somatropin (Novo Nordisk)

OTHER BRAND NAMES: Norditropin Nordiflex (Novo Nordisk)

THERAPEUTIC CLASS: Human growth hormone

INDICATIONS: (Adults) Replacement of endogenous growth hormone deficiency who meet either of the following criteria: (1) adult onset-patients with growth hormone deficiency, either alone or associated with multiple hormone deficiencies (hypopituitarism), as a result of pituitary disease, hypothalamic disease, surgery, radiation therapy, or trauma: or (2) childhood onset-patients who were growth hormone deficient during childhood should have growth hormone deficiency confirmed as an adult before replacement therapy is started. (Pediatrics) Long-term treatment of children with growth failure due to inadequate growth hormone secretion. Treatment of children with short stature associated with Noonan syndrome.

DOSAGE: *Adults:* Initial: No more than 0.004mg/kg/day. Increase to no more than 0.016mg/kg/day after 6 weeks.
Pediatrics: Growth Hormone Deficiency: 0.024-0.034mg/kg SQ 6-7x/week.
Noonan Syndrome: Dose up to 0.066mg/kg/day.

HOW SUPPLIED: Inj: (Norditropin (cartridge) and Norditropin Nordiflex (prefilled pen)) 5mg/1.5mL, 10mg/1.5ml,15mg/1.5mL

CONTRAINDICATIONS: Presence of active neoplasia; acute critical illness due to complications following open heart or abdominal surgery, multiple accidental trauma or acute respiratory failure; proliferative or preproliferative diabetic retinopathy; closed epiphyses; and Prader-Willi syndrome with severe obesity or severe respiratory impairment.

WARNINGS/PRECAUTIONS: Monitor for recurrence or progression of underlying disease in growth hormone deficiency secondary to intracranial lesions. Hypothyroidism reported. May develop slipped capital epiphyses. Intracranial HTN with papilledema, visual changes, headache, nausea, and vomiting reported. Progression of scoliosis may occur in rapid growth. Monitor for any form of malignant skin lesion prior to and during therapy. May decrease insulin sensitivity; monitor blood sugar. Dose dependent/transient fluid retention may occur. Increased occurrence of otitis media in patients with Turner syndrome.Monitor closely for cardiovascular disorders (e.g., stroke, aortic aneurysm/dissection, hypertension).

ADVERSE REACTIONS: (Pediatrics) Headache, injection site reaction, localized muscle pain, rash, weakness, mild hyperglycemia, glucosuria, arthralgia, leukemia. (Adults) Edema, arthralgia, myalgia, infection, parasthesia, skeletal pain, headache, bronchitis.

INTERACTIONS: Diminished effects with glucocorticoid therapy. Insulin resistance reported. May reduce plasma levels of oral estrogens.

PREGNANCY: Category C, caution in nursing.

MECHANISM OF ACTION: Human growth hormone; binds to dimeric GH receptor in cell membrane of target cells resulting in intracellular signal transduction.

PHARMACOKINETICS: Absorption: T_{max}=4-5 hrs; (4mg) C_{max}=13.8ng/mL; (8mg) C_{max}=17.1ng/mL. **Elimination**: $T_{1/2}$=7-10 hrs.

NORITATE RX
metronidazole (Dermik)

THERAPEUTIC CLASS: Imidazole antibiotic

INDICATIONS: Inflammatory lesions and erythema of rosacea.

DOSAGE: *Adults:* Apply thin film to clean area qd.

HOW SUPPLIED: Cre: 1% [30g, 60g]

WARNINGS/PRECAUTIONS: Conjunctivitis reported with use on face. Avoid eye contact. Caution with blood dyscrasias.

ADVERSE REACTIONS: Local irritation, condition aggravated.

INTERACTIONS: May potentiate anticoagulant effects of warfarin.

PREGNANCY: Category B, not for use in nursing.

MECHANISM OF ACTION: Imidazole antibiotic; not established. Suspected to reduce inflammatory lesions of rosacea.

PHARMACOKINETICS: Absorption: C_{max}=27.6ng/mL; T_{max}=8-12 hrs.
Distribution: Crosses placental barrier and secreted in human breast milk.

NOROXIN RX
norfloxacin (Merck)

THERAPEUTIC CLASS: Fluoroquinolone

INDICATIONS: Treatment of complicated and uncomplicated urinary tract infection (UTI), uncomplicated urethral and cervical gonorrhea, and prostatitis due to *E.coli.*

DOSAGE: *Adults:* ≥18 yrs: Uncomplicated UTI Due To *E.coli, K.pneumonia, P.mirabilis*: 400mg q12h for 3 days. Uncomplicated UTI Due To Other Organisms: 400mg q12h for 7-10 days. Complicated UTI: 400mg q12h for 10-21 days. CrCl ≤30mL/min: 400mg qd. Uncomplicated Gonorrhea: 800mg single dose. Acute/Chronic Prostatitis: 400mg q12h for 28 days. Take 1 hr before or 2 hrs after meals or milk/dairy products.

HOW SUPPLIED: Tab: 400mg

CONTRAINDICATIONS: History of tendinitis or tendon rupture associated with use of quinolones.

WARNINGS/PRECAUTIONS: Pseudomembranous colitis, convulsions, phototoxicity, peripheral neuropathy and ruptures of the shoulder, hand, and Achilles tendons reported. Avoid in pregnancy and nursing mothers. Convulsions reported. Caution with renal dysfunction. D/C if CNS stimulation, increase in ICP, or toxic psychoses occurs. Not effective for treatment of syphilis. May exacerbate myasthenia gravis. Hemolytic reactions reported with G6P deficiency. *Clostridium difficile*-associated diarrhea reported.

ADVERSE REACTIONS: Dizziness, nausea, headache, abdominal pain, asthenia.

INTERACTIONS: May increase theophylline and cyclosporine levels. May enhance effects of warfarin. Diminished urinary excretion with probenecid. Antagonized effects with nitrofurantoin. Iron- or zinc-containing products, antacids, or didanosine (chewable/buffered tabs, pediatric oral solution) may interfere with absorption; space dose by 2 hrs. May reduce clearance of caffeine. Coadministration with NSAIDs may increase risk of CNS stimulation and convulsive seizures. May cause hypoglycemia if coadministered with glyburide.

PREGNANCY: Category C, not for use in nursing.

MECHANISM OF ACTION: Fluoroquinolone; inhibits bacterial DNA synthesis, ATP-dependent DNA supercoiling reaction catalyzed by DNA gyrase, relaxation of supercoiled DNA, and promotes double-stranded DNA breakage.

PHARMACOKINETICS: Absorption: C_{max}=0.8μg/mL (200mg), 1.5μg/mL (400mg), 2.4μg/mL (800mg); T_{max}=1 hr. **Elimination:** Urine (26-32%), feces; $T_{1/2}$=3-4 hrs.

NORPACE RX
disopyramide phosphate (Pharmacia & Upjohn)

OTHER BRAND NAMES: Norpace CR (Pharmacia & Upjohn)
THERAPEUTIC CLASS: Class I antiarrhythmic

INDICATIONS: Treatment of documented life-threatening ventricular arrhythmias.

DOSAGE: *Adults:* Usual: 400-800mg/day in divided dose. Recommended: 150mg q6h immediate-release (IR) or 300mg q12h extended-release (CR). Adjust dose with anticholinergic effects. Weight <110lbs/Moderate Hepatic or Renal Insufficiency (CrCl >40mL/min): 100mg q6h IR or 200mg q12h CR. Severe Renal Insufficiency (with or without initial 150mg LD): CrCl 30-40mL/min: 100mg q8h IR. CrCl 30-15mL/min: 100mg q12h IR. CrCl <15mL/min: 100mg q24h IR. Rapid Control of Ventricular Arrhythmia: LD: 300mg IR (200mg if <110lbs). Follow with maint dose. Cardiomyopathy/Cardiac Decompensation: Initial: 100mg q6-8h IR. Adjust gradually. See PI if no response or toxicity occurs. Elderly: Start at low end of dosing range. *Pediatrics:* <1 yr: 10-30mg/kg/day. 1-4 yrs: 10-20mg/kg/day. 4-12 yrs: 10-15mg/kg/day. 12-18 yrs: 6-15mg/kg/day. Give in equally divided doses q6h. Hospitalize patient during initial therapy. Start dose titration at lower end of range.

HOW SUPPLIED: Cap: (Norpace) 100mg, 150mg; Cap, Extended-Release: (Norpace CR) 100mg, 150mg

CONTRAINDICATIONS: Cardiogenic shock, 2nd- or 3rd-degree AV block (if no pacemaker present), congenital QT prolongation.

WARNINGS/PRECAUTIONS: Proarrhythmic; reserve for life-threatening ventricular arrhythmias. May cause or worsen CHF and produce hypotension due to negative inotropic properties. Reduce dose if 1st-degree heart block occurs. Avoid with urinary retention, glaucoma, and myasthenia gravis unless adequate overriding measures taken. Atrial flutter/fibrillation; digitalize first. Monitor closely or withdraw if QT prolongation >25% occurs and ectopy continues. D/C if QRS widening >25% occurs. Avoid LD with cardiomyopathy or cardiac decompensation. Correct K$^+$ abnormalities before therapy. Reduce dose with renal/hepatic dysfunction; monitor ECG. Avoid CR formulation with CrCl ≤40mL/min. Caution with sick sinus syndrome, Wolff-Parkinson-White syndrome, bundle branch block, or elderly. May significantly lower blood glucose.

ADVERSE REACTIONS: Dry mouth, urinary retention/frequency/urgency, constipation, blurred vision, GI effects, dizziness, fatigue, headache.

INTERACTIONS: Avoid type IA and IC antiarrhythmics, and propranolol except in unresponsive, life-threatening arrhythmias. Hepatic enzyme inducers may lower levels. Avoid within 48 hrs before or 24 hrs after verapamil. Possible fatal interactions with CYP3A4 inhibitors. Monitor blood glucose with β-blockers, alcohol.

PREGNANCY: Category C, not for use in nursing.

MECHANISM OF ACTION: Type I antiarrhythmic; decreases rate of diastolic depolarization in cells with augmented automaticity, decreases upstroke velocity, and increases action potential duration of normal cardiac cells. Decreases disparity in refractoriness between infracted and adjacent normally perfused myocardium and has no effect on α- or β-adrenergic receptors.

PHARMACOKINETICS: Absorption: Rapid and complete; C_{max}=2.22mcg/mL, T_{max}=4.5 hrs. **Distribution:** Plasma protein binding (50-65%). **Metabolism:** Liver. **Elimination:** Urine (50% unchanged), (20% mono-N-dealkylated metabolite), (10% other metabolite); $T_{1/2}$=11.65 hrs.

NORPLANT II   RX
levonorgestrel (Population Council)

OTHER BRAND NAMES: Jadelle (Population Council)

THERAPEUTIC CLASS: Progestogen

INDICATIONS: Long-term (up to 5 yrs) prevention of pregnancy.

DOSAGE: *Adults:* Implant 150mg (2 implants) in midportion of upper arm during 1st 7 days of onset of menses. Place in a "V" shape 30° apart. Replace by end of 5th year.

HOW SUPPLIED: Implant: 75mg

CONTRAINDICATIONS: Active thrombophlebitis or thromboembolic disorders, undiagnosed abnormal genital bleeding, pregnancy, acute live disease or liver tumors, carcinoma of the breast, and idiopathic intracranial HTN.

WARNINGS/PRECAUTIONS: Complications related to insertion and removal of capsules reported. Bleeding irregularities have occurred. Retinal thrombosis leading to partial or complete loss of vision, hepatic neoplasia, carcinoma of breast and reproductive organs reported. Risk of thromboembolic and thrombotic diseases, MI, ectopic pregnancy, ovarian cysts, breast cancer, gall bladder and autoimmune diseases, cerebrovascular diseases. Cigarette smoking increases risk of serious cardiovascular side effects; risk increases with age (especially >35 yrs) and the extent of smoking. Idiopathic intracranial HTN and increases in BP reported. Caution with fluid retention. Vision changes reported; caution with contact lenses. Weight gain, thrombosis, and thrombophlebitis reported. May worsen depression, increase LDL levels. If jaundice develops, remove implants. Altered glucose tolerance; monitor diabetics. Rare reports of congenital anomalies with use during early pregnancy.

ADVERSE REACTIONS: Menorrhagia, amenorrhea, oligomenorrhea, irregular bleeding, pain/itching or infection at implant site, headache, nervousness, GI effects, dizziness, rash, acne, weight gain, cervicitis.

INTERACTIONS: Not recommended with chronic phenytoin, carbamazepine, phenobarbital, or oxcarbazepine use; decreased effectiveness. Back-up method of contraception with short-term therapy with CYP450 inducers. Rifampicin and St. John's wort may decreases levels and effectiveness.

PREGNANCY: Use in pregnancy not known, caution in nursing.

MECHANISM OF ACTION: Progestin; inhibits ovulation and thickens cervical mucus.

PHARMACOKINETICS: Absorption: C_{max} =722pg/mL (day 2), T_{max} =2-3 days. **Distribution:** Highly bound to sex-hormone-binding globulin. **Metabolism:** β-hydroxylation. **Excretion:** Urine (40-68%), feces (16-48%); $T_{1/2}$ =13-18 hrs

NORPRAMIN RX
desipramine HCL (Sanofi-Aventis)

> Antidepressants increased the risk of suicidal thinking and behavior (suicidality) in short-term studies in children, adolescents, and young adults with Major Depressive Disorder (MDD) and other psychiatric disorders. Desipramine is not approved for use in pediatric patients.

THERAPEUTIC CLASS: Tricyclic antidepressant

INDICATIONS: Treatment of depression.

DOSAGE: *Adults:* Usual: 100-200mg/day given qd or in divided doses. Max: 300mg/day. Elderly/Adolescents: Usual: 25-100mg/day given qd or in divided doses. Max: 150mg/day.

HOW SUPPLIED: Tab: 10mg, 25mg, 50mg, 75mg, 100mg, 150mg

CONTRAINDICATIONS: MAOI use within 14 days, acute recovery period following MI.

WARNINGS/PRECAUTIONS: Hypomania with manic-depressive disease. D/C prior to elective surgery. Do not withdraw abruptly. Extreme caution with urinary retention, glaucoma, seizure disorders, cardiovascular disease, thyroid disease, alcohol abuse. May exacerbate psychosis; caution with schizophrenia. May impair mental or physical abilities. May alter blood glucose levels.

ADVERSE REACTIONS: Arrhythmias, hypotension, HTN, tachycardia, confusion, hallucination, dizziness, anxiety, numbness, tingling, ataxia, tremors, dry mouth, urinary retention, urticaria, photosensitivity, SIADH, altered libido.

INTERACTIONS: See Contraindications. Additive sedative effects with benzodiazepines (eg, diazepam, chlordiazepoxide), other CNS depressants (eg, sedatives/hypnotics, psychotropics). Blocks antihypertensive effects of guanethidine. Exaggerates response to alcohol. Monitor with other anticholinergic or sympathomimetic drugs. Potentiated by CYP2D6 inhibitors (eg, quinidine, cimetidine, SSRIs) or substrates of CYP2D6 (eg, other antidepressants, phenothiazines, propafenone, flecainide). Caution with thyroid medications.

PREGNANCY: Safety in pregnancy and nursing not known.

MECHANISM OF ACTION: Tricyclic; unknown, suspected to restore normal levels of neurotransmitters (NE and 5-HT) by blocking their re-uptake from the CNS synapse.

PHARMACOKINETICS: Absorption: Rapid (via GI tract). **Metabolism:** Liver. **Elimination:** Urine.

Nor-QD

RX

norethindrone (Watson)

OTHER BRAND NAMES: Camila (Barr)

THERAPEUTIC CLASS: Progestogen

INDICATIONS: Prevention of pregnancy.

DOSAGE: *Adults:* 1 tab qd without interruption (continuous regimen) on 1st day of menstrual period. If fully nursing, start 6 weeks postpartum. If partially nursing, start 3 weeks postpartum.

HOW SUPPLIED: Tab: 0.35mg

CONTRAINDICATIONS: Pregnancy, breast carcinoma, undiagnosed abnormal genital bleeding, benign or malignant liver tumors, acute liver disease.

WARNINGS/PRECAUTIONS: Avoid smoking. Perform annual physical exam. Not for use before menarche. May affect certain endocrine tests (eg, sex hormone binding globulin, thyroxine binding globulin). Monitor glucose tolerance in prediabetics and diabetics. May alter lipid metabolism. May increase risk of breast cancer and hepatic adenomas. May cause irregular menstrual patterns. Delayed follicular atresia/ovarian cysts and ectopic pregnancy may occur. D/C with recurrent migraines or severe headaches.

ADVERSE REACTIONS: Menstrual irregularities, frequent or irregular bleeding, headache, breast tenderness, nausea, dizziness.

INTERACTIONS: Reduced effects with hepatic enzyme inducers (eg, rifampin, phenytoin, carbamazepine, barbiturates).

PREGNANCY: Category X, caution in nursing.

MECHANISM OF ACTION: Progestin oral contraceptive: prevents conception by suppressing ovulation in approx half of users, thickens cervical mucus to inhibit sperm penetration, lowers mid-cycle LH and FSH peaks, slows movement of ovum through fallopian tubes, and alters endometrium.

PHARMACOKINETICS: Absorption: Absolute bioavailability (65%); $T_{max(mean)}$=1.2 hrs; $C_{max(mean)}$=4816.8pg/mL; $AUC_{(mean)}$=21233pg•h/mL. **Distribution:** 36% bound to sex hormone binding globulin (SHBG), 61% bound to albumin Vd=4L/kg; Found in breastmilk. **Metabolism:** Via reduction, sulfate and glucuronide conjugation. **Elimination:** Urine (≥50%), feces (20-40%); $T_{1/2}$=8 hrs.

Nortriptyline

RX

nortriptyline HCL (Various)

> Antidepressants increased the risk of suicidal thinking and behavior (suicidality) in short-term studies in children, adolescents, and young adults with Major Depressive Disorder (MDD) and other psychiatric disorders. Patients of all ages who are started on antidepressant therapy should be monitored appropriately and observed closely for clinical worsening, suicidality, or unusual changes in behavior. Nortriptyline is not approved for use in pediatric patients.

THERAPEUTIC CLASS: Tricyclic antidepressant

INDICATIONS: Relief of symptoms of depression.

DOSAGE: *Adults:* 25mg tid-qid. Max: 150mg/day. Total daily dose may be given once a day. Monitor serum levels if dose >100mg/day. Elderly/Adolescents: 30-50mg/day in single or divided doses.

HOW SUPPLIED: Cap: 10mg, 25mg, 50mg, 75mg; Sol: 10mg/5mL

CONTRAINDICATIONS: MAOI use within 14 days, acute recovery period following MI.

WARNINGS/PRECAUTIONS: MI, arrhythmia, strokes have occurred. Caution with cardiovascular disease, glaucoma, history of urinary retention, hyperthyroidism. May lower seizure threshold. Caution with operating machinery. May exacerbate psychosis or activate schizophrenia. May cause symptoms of mania in bipolar disease. D/C several days prior to elective surgery. May alter glucose levels.

ADVERSE REACTIONS: Arrhythmias, hypotension, HTN, tachycardia, MI, heart block, stroke, confusion, hallucination, insomnia, tremors, ataxia, anxiety, dry mouth, blurred vision, skin rash, extrapyramidal symptoms, anorexia.

INTERACTIONS: May block guanethidine effects. Arrhythmia risk with thyroid agents. Alcohol may potentiate effects. "Stimulating" effect with reserpine. Monitor with anticholinergic and sympathomimetic drugs. Increased plasma levels with cimetidine. Hypoglycemia reported with chlorpropamide. Antidepressants, phenothiazines, carbamazepine, propafenone, flecainide, encainide, and CYP2D6 inhibitors (eg, quinidine) may potentiate effects. Avoid MAOIs.

PREGNANCY: Safety during pregnancy and nursing not known.

MECHANISM OF ACTION: Tricyclic; inhibits activity of histamine, 5-hydroxytryptamine, and acetylcholine; increases pressor effect of NE, blocks pressor response of phenethylamine, and interferes with transport, release and storage of catecholamine.

NORVASC RX
amlodipine besylate (Pfizer)

THERAPEUTIC CLASS: Calcium channel blocker (dihydropyridine)

INDICATIONS: Treatment of hypertension and Coronary Artery Disease (CAD) including chronic stable or vasospastic angina (Prinzmetal's or Variant Angina).

DOSAGE: *Adults:* HTN: Initial: 5mg qd. Titrate over 7-14 days. Max: 10mg qd. Small, Fragile, or Elderly/Hepatic Dysfunction/Concomitant Antihypertensive: Initial: 2.5mg qd. Angina: 5-10mg qd. Elderly/Hepatic Dysfunction: 5mg qd. CAD: 5-10mg qd.
Pediatrics: 6-17 yrs: HTN: 2.5-5mg qd.

HOW SUPPLIED: Tab: 2.5mg, 5mg, 10mg

WARNINGS/PRECAUTIONS: May increase angina or MI with severe obstructive CAD. Caution with severe aortic stenosis, CHF, severe hepatic impairment, and in elderly.

ADVERSE REACTIONS: Edema, flushing, palpitation, dizziness, headache, fatigue.

PREGNANCY: Category C, not for use in nursing.

MECHANISM OF ACTION: A dihydropyridine calcium antagonist (calcium ion antagonist or slow-channel blocker) that inhibits transmembrane influx or calcium ions into vascular smooth muscle and cardiac muscle. Binds to both dihydropyridine and nondihydropyridine binding sites which results in peripheral arterial vasodilation and reduction in BP.

PHARMACOKINETICS: Absorption: Absolute bioavailability (64-90%); T_{max}=6-12 hrs. **Distribution:** Plasma protein binding (93%). **Metabolism:** Hepatic. **Elimination:** Urine, $T_{1/2}$=30-50 hrs.

NORVIR
RX

ritonavir (Abbott)

> Use with certain non-sedating antihistamines, sedative hypnotics, antiarrhythmics, or ergot alkaloids may result in life-threatening adverse events.

THERAPEUTIC CLASS: Protease inhibitor

INDICATIONS: Treatment of HIV infection in combination with other antiretrovirals.

DOSAGE: *Adults:* Initial: 300mg bid. Titrate: Increase every 2-3 days by 100mg bid. Maint: 600mg bid. If combined with saquinavir, adjust dose to 400mg bid. Elderly: Start at low end of dosing range. Take with meals if possible. *Pediatrics:* >1 month: Initial: 250mg/m² po bid. Titrate: Increase by 50mg/m² every 2-3 days. Maint: 350-400mg/m² po bid or highest tolerated dose. Max: 600mg bid.

HOW SUPPLIED: Cap: 100mg; Sol: 80mg/mL [240mL]

CONTRAINDICATIONS: Alfuzosin, amiodarone, bepridil, flecainide, propafenone, quinidine, voriconazole, astemizole, terfenadine, ergot derivatives, midazolam, triazolam, cisapride, pimozide, dihydroergotamine, ergonovine, ergotamine, methylergonovine, midazolam, triazolam.

WARNINGS/PRECAUTIONS: Allergic reactions (eg, urticaria, mild skin eruptions, bronchospasm, and angioedema) pancreatitis, new onset/exacerbation of pre-existing diabetes mellitus, hyperglycemia, immune reconstitution syndrome, hepatic transaminase elevations and hepatic dysfunction reported. Caution with moderate to severe hepatic impairment and in elderly. Monitor LFTs, especially 1st three months. Increased bleeding may occur with hemophilia A and B. Possible redistribution or accumulation of body fat. May increase total triglyceride and cholesterol levels.

ADVERSE REACTIONS: Diarrhea, anorexia, vomiting, nausea, abdominal pain, asthenia, headache, malaise, vasodilation, constipation, dizziness, taste perversion, peripheral paresthesia.

INTERACTIONS: See Contraindications. Avoid use with rifampin, St. John's wort; may cause loss of virologic response and resistance. Avoid use with lovastatin and simvastatin; risk of myopathy and rhabdomyolysis. Neurologic and cardiac events reported with disopyramide, mexiletine, nefazodone, fluoxetine, and β-blockers. Concomitant use with tipranavir may cause hepatitis and hepatic decompensation. May increase levels of saquinavir, atazanavir, darunavir, fosamprenavir, desipramine, indinavir, rifabutin. May increase levels of clarithromycin with renal impairment; reduce clarithromycin dose by 50% if CrCl 30-60mL/min and by 75% if CrCl<30mL/min. May increase ketoconazole levels; avoid ketoconazole doses >200mg/day. May increase sildenafil levels; do not exceed sildenafil 25mg/48 hrs. May increase levels of tramadol, propoxyphene, disopyramide, lidocaine, mexiletine, carbamazepine, clonazepam, ethosuximide, bupropion, nefazodone, SSRIs, TCAs, dronabinol, itraconazole, quinine, metoprolol, timolol, diltiazem, nifedipine, verapamil, atorvastatin, rosuvastatin, cyclosporine, tacrolimus, sirolimus, perphenazine, risperidone, thioridazine, clorazepate, diazepam, estazolam, flurazepam, zolpidem, dexamethasone, fluticasone, prednisone, methamphetamine. May increase levels of trazodone; use with caution and consider lower trazodone dose. Decreases levels of theophylline, meperidine, methadone. May decrease levels of phenytoin, divalproex, lamotrigine, and atovaquone. Separate dosing with didanosine by 2.5 hrs. May increase plasma levels of drugs metabolized by CYP3A or CYP2D6. May decrease ethinyl estradiol levels; use alternative contraceptive measures. Monitor PT/INR with warfarin. Contains alcohol; may produce disulfiram-like reactions with disulfiram, metronidazole.

PREGNANCY: Category B, not for use in nursing.

MECHANISM OF ACTION: HIV protease inhibitor; renders enzyme incapable of processing *gag-pol* polyprotein precursor, which leads to production of non-infectious immature HIV particles.

PHARMACOKINETICS: Absorption: C_{max}=11.2mcg/mL; T_{max}=2 hrs (fasting), 4 hrs (fed); AUC=121.7mcg•h/mL (Cap), 129mcg•hr/mL (Sol). **Metabolism:**

CYP3A, 2D6 (oxidation); isopropylthiazole (major metabolite). **Elimination:** Urine (3.5%), feces (33.8%); T$_{1/2}$=3-5 hrs.

NOVACORT

RX

pramoxine HCL - hydrocortisone acetate (Primus)

THERAPEUTIC CLASS: Corticosteroid/anesthetic

INDICATIONS: Relief of the inflammatory and pruritic manifestations of corticosteroid-responsive dermatoses.

DOSAGE: *Adults:* Apply to affected area(s) tid-qid. May use occlusive dressings for psoriasis or recalcitrant conditions. D/C dressings if infection develops.
Pediatrics: Apply to affected area(s) tid-qid. May use occlusive dressings for psoriasis or recalcitrant conditions. D/C dressings if infection develops.

HOW SUPPLIED: Gel: (Hydrocortisone-Pramoxine) 2%-1% [29g]

WARNINGS/PRECAUTIONS: May produce reversible HPA axis suppression, manifestations of Cushing's syndrome, hyperglycemia, and glucosuria. Caution when applied to large surface areas, under occlusive dressings, or with prolonged use. Use appropriate antifungal or antibacterial agent with dermatological infections; d/c if infection does not clear. Pediatrics may be more susceptible to systemic toxicity. D/C if irritation develops. Avoid eyes.

ADVERSE REACTIONS: Burning, itching, irritation, dryness, folliculitis, hypertrichosis, acneiform eruptions, hypopigmentation, perioral dermatitis, allergic dermatitis, skin maceration, secondary infection, skin atrophy, striae, miliaria.

PREGNANCY: Category C, caution in nursing.

MECHANISM OF ACTION: Topical corticosteroid/anesthetic. Hydrocortisone: Possesses anti-inflammatory, anti-pruritic, and vasoconstrictive properties. Anti-inflammatory mechanism not established. Pramoxine: Stabilizes neuronal membrane of nerve endings with which it comes into contact.

PHARMACOKINETICS: Absorption: Percutaneous; occlusion, inflammation, other disease states may increase absorption. **Distribution:** Bound to plasma protein in varying degrees. Systemically administered corticosteroids found in breast milk. **Metabolism:** Liver. **Elimination:** Kidney (major), bile.

NOVANTRONE

RX

mitoxantrone (EMD Serono)

> Severe local tissue damage with extravasation. Administer only as slow IV infusion; not for IM, SQ, intra-arterial, or intrathecal use. Should not be given to patients with baseline neutrophil count <1,500cells/mm³. Cardiotoxicity can occur at any time and risk increases with cumulative dose; toxicity can occur during therapy or months to years after discontinuation. CHF may occur during or after termination of therapy. Secondary AML reported in MS and cancer patients treated with Novatrone.

THERAPEUTIC CLASS: Topoisomerase II inhibitor

INDICATIONS: With corticosteroids, for initial treatment of advanced hormone-refractory prostate cancer with pain. Initial therapy of acute non-lymphocytic leukemia (ANLL) in combination with other agents. To reduce neurologic disability and/or frequency of clinical relapses in secondary (chronic) progressive, progressive relapsing, or worsening relapsing-remitting multiple sclerosis (MS).

DOSAGE: *Adults:* Prostate Cancer: 12-14mg/m²/day IV every 21 days. ANLL: Induction: 12mg/m²/day IV on days 1-3 and 100mg/m²/day IV of cytarabine on days 1-7. Consolidation: 12mg/m²/day on days 1-2 and cytarabine 100mg/m²/day on days 1-5. MS: 12mg/m²/day IV every 3 months.

HOW SUPPLIED: Inj: 2mg/mL

WARNINGS/PRECAUTIONS: Can cause myelosuppression at any dose. Severe myelosuppression with high doses (leukemia); assure full hematologic recovery before consolidation therapy. Avoid with pre-existing myelosuppression. Increased risk of cardiac toxicity with prior anthracyclines or mediastinal radiotherapy, or with pre-existing cardiovascular disease. Irreversible CHF has been reported. Avoid in MS when baseline left ventricular ejection fraction <50%. Caution in hepatic impairment. Risk of hyperuricemia in leukemia; monitor serum uric acid levels. Obtain CBC, platelet count, and LFTs before each course. May cause blue-green urine and bluish sclera 24 hrs after administration. Perform pregnancy test in women with MS before each dose. Caution in elderly.

ADVERSE REACTIONS: Nausea, alopecia, menstrual disorder, upper respiratory infection, UTI, stomatitis, arrhythmia, diarrhea, constipation, back pain, abnormal ECG, asthenia, headache, cardiac toxicity.

INTERACTIONS: Development of acute leukemia associated with other concomitant antineoplastics. Possible danger of cardiac toxicity if previously treated with anthracyclines.

PREGNANCY: Category D, not for use in nursing.

MECHANISM OF ACTION: Synthetic Anthracenedione Topoisomerase II inhibitor and DNA-reactive agent; it intercalates into DNA through hydrogen bonding, causes crosslinks and strands breaks. Also interferes with RNA and inhibits topoisomerase II, responsible for uncoiling and repairing damaged DNA.

PHARMACOKINETICS: Distribution: Plasma protein binding (78%), V_d>1000L/m². **Metabolism:** Monocarboxylic and dicarboxylic acid derivatives and their glucuronide conjugates. **Elimination:** Urine (11%), feces (25%) both as unchanged and metabolites, $\alpha T_{1/2}$=6-12 min, $\beta T_{1/2}$=1.1-3.1 hrs, gamma $T_{1/2}$=23-215 hrs.

NOVAREL   RX
chorionic gonadotropin (Ferring)

THERAPEUTIC CLASS: Human chorionic gonadotropin

INDICATIONS: For prepubertal cryptorchidism not due to anatomic obstruction. For hypogonadotropic hypogonadism (secondary to a pituitary deficiency) in males. To induce ovulation (OI) and pregnancy in anovulatory, infertile women in whom anovulation is not due to primary ovarian failure and pretreated with human menotropins.

DOSAGE: *Adults:* Hypogonadism: 500-1000 U IM 3x/week (TIW) for 3 weeks, then twice weekly for 3 weeks; or 4000 U IM TIW for 6-9 months, then reduce to 2000 U TIW for 3 months. OI: 5000-10,000 U IM 1 day after last dose of menotropins.
Pediatrics: ≥4 yrs: Cryptorchidism: 4000 U IM TIW for 3 weeks; or 5000 U IM every 2nd day for 4 doses; or 15 doses of 500-1000 U over 6 weeks; or 500 U TIW for 4-6 weeks (if treatment fails, give 1000 U/injection starting 1 month later). Initiate therapy between 4-9 yrs. Hypogonadism: 500-1000 U IM TIW for 3 weeks, then twice weekly for 3 weeks; or 4000 U IM TIW for 6-9 months, then reduce to 2000 U TIW for 3 months.

HOW SUPPLIED: Inj: 10,000 U

CONTRAINDICATIONS: Precocious puberty, prostatic carcinoma or other androgen-dependent neoplasms, pregnancy.

WARNINGS/PRECAUTIONS: Potential ovarian hyperstimulation, enlargement or rupture of ovarian cysts, multiple births, and arterial thromboembolism with infertility treatment. D/C if precocious puberty occurs in cryptorchidism patients. Caution with cardiac or renal disease, epilepsy, migraine, asthma. Not effective treatment for obesity.

ADVERSE REACTIONS: Headache, irritability, restlessness, depression, fatigue, edema, precocious puberty, gynecomastia, injection site pain.

PREGNANCY: Category C, caution in nursing.

MECHANISM OF ACTION: Human chorionic gonadotropin; stimulates production of gonadal steriod hormones by stimulating the interstitial cells (leydig cells) of testis to produce androgens and the corpus luteum of the ovary to produce progesterone.

NOVOLIN   OTC
insulin human, rdna origin - insulin, human isophane - insulin, human regular (Novo Nordisk)

OTHER BRAND NAMES: Novolin R (Novo Nordisk) - Novolin N (Novo Nordisk)

THERAPEUTIC CLASS: Insulin

INDICATIONS: To control hyperglycemia in diabetes.

DOSAGE: *Adults:* Individualize dose.
Pediatrics: Individualize dose.

HOW SUPPLIED: Inj: 100 U/mL (Novolin N, Novolin R); PenFill: 100 U/mL (Novolin N, Novolin R); Prefilled: 100 U/mL (Novolin N, Novolin R)

WARNINGS/PRECAUTIONS: Human insulin differs from animal source insulin. Any change in insulin should be made cautiously. Changes in strength, manufacturer, type or method of manufacture may result in the need for a change in dosage. Hypoglycemia may occur with taking too much insulin, missing or delaying meals, exercising or working more than usual. An infection or illness (especially if accompanied by diarrhea or vomiting) may change insulin requirements. Administration of insulin SQ can result in lipoatrophy. Novolin R is not recommended for use in insulin pumps.

ADVERSE REACTIONS: Hypoglycemia, sweating, dizziness, palpitations, tremor, hunger, restlessness, lightheadedness, inability to concentrate, headache, injection-site reaction, allergic reaction.

INTERACTIONS: Increased insulin requirements with oral contraceptives, corticosteroids, or thyroid replacement therapy. Reduced insulin requirements with oral hypoglycemics, salicylates, sulfa antibiotics, and certain antidepressants. Alcoholic beverages may change insulin requirements. β-blockers may mask symptoms of hypoglycemia.

PREGNANCY: Pregnancy category is not known.

MECHANISM OF ACTION: Insulin (rDNA origin); regulates glucose metabolism, lowers blood glucose by facilitating cellular uptake of glucose and simultaneously inhibiting the glucose output from the liver.

NOVOLIN 70/30   OTC
insulin human, rdna origin - insulin, human (isophane/regular) (Novo Nordisk)

THERAPEUTIC CLASS: Insulin

INDICATIONS: To control hyperglycemia in diabetes.

DOSAGE: *Adults:* Individualize dose. Administer SQ.
Pediatrics: Individualize dose. Administer SQ.

HOW SUPPLIED: (Isophane/Regular) Inj: 70 U-30 U/mL; PenFill: 70 U-30 U/mL; Prefilled: 70 U-30 U/mL

WARNINGS/PRECAUTIONS: Human insulin differs from animal source insulin. Any change of insulin should be made cautiously. Changes in strength, manufacturer, type or method of manufacture may result in the need for a change in dosage. Hypoglycemia may occur with taking too much insulin, missing or delaying meals, exercising or working more than usual. An infection or illness (especially with diarrhea or vomiting) may change insulin requirements. Caution with diseases of adrenal, pituitary, or thyroid glands, or progression of kidney or liver disease. Administration of insulin SQ can result in lipoatrophy.

ADVERSE REACTIONS: Hypoglycemia, sweating, dizziness, palpitation, tremor, hunger, restlessness, lightheadedness, inability to concentrate, headache, injection site reaction, allergic reaction.

INTERACTIONS: Increased insulin requirements with oral contraceptives, corticosteroids, or thyroid replacement therapy. Reduced insulin requirements with oral hypoglycemics, salicylates, sulfa antibiotics, and certain antidepressants. Alcoholic beverages may change insulin requirements. β-blockers may mask symptoms of hypoglycemia.

PREGNANCY: Pregnancy category is not known.

MECHANISM OF ACTION: Insulin (rDNAorigin); has 70% NPH human insulin isophane suspension and 30% regular human insulin. Regulates glucose metabolism, lowers blood glucose by facilitating cellular uptake of glucose and simultaneously inhibiting the glucose output from the liver.

NOVOLOG RX
insulin aspart (Novo Nordisk)

THERAPEUTIC CLASS: Insulin

INDICATIONS: To control hyperglycemia in diabetes.

DOSAGE: *Adults:* Individualize dose. Inject SQ within 5-10 min before a meal. Draw first when mixing with NPH human insulin; inject immediately. Do not mix with crystalline zinc insulins, animal source insulins, or other manufacturer insulins. (External Pump) Do not use or mix with any other insulin or diluent in pump.
Pediatrics: ≥4 yrs: Individualize dose. Inject SQ within 5-10 min before a meal. Draw first when mixing with NPH human insulin; inject immediately. Do not mix with crystalline zinc insulins, animal source insulins, or other manufacturer insulins. (External Pump) Do not use or mix with any other insulin or diluent in pump.

HOW SUPPLIED: Inj: 100 U/mL; PenFill: 100 U/mL; Prefilled: 100 U/mL

CONTRAINDICATIONS: Hypoglycemia.

WARNINGS/PRECAUTIONS: Any change of insulin should be made cautiously. Changes in strength, manufacturer, type or method of manufacture may result in the need for a change in dosage. Hypoglycemia may occur with taking too much insulin, missing or delaying meals, exercising or working more than usual, diseases of adrenal, pituitary, or thyroid glands, or progression of kidney or liver disease. May cause hypokalemia. Dosage adjustments may be needed with hepatic or renal dysfunction, during any infection, illness (especially with diarrhea or vomiting) or pregnancy. A longer-acting insulin is usually required to maintain adequate glucose control. Infusion sets and the insulin in the infusion sets should be changed q48h or sooner. Do not use in quick-release infusion sets or cartridge adapters.

ADVERSE REACTIONS: Hypoglycemia, hypokalemia, lipodystrophy, hypersensitivity reaction, injection site reactions, pruritus, rash.

INTERACTIONS: Increased glucose lowering effects with ACE inhibitors, disopyramide, fibrates, fluoxetine, MAOIs, propoxyphene, salicylates, somatostatin analog, sulfonamide antibiotics and other antidiabetic agents. Decreased blood glucose lowering effects with corticosteroids, niacin, danazol, diuretics, sympathomimetic agents, isoniazid, phenothiazine derivatives, somatropin, thyroid hormones, estrogens, progesterones. Pentamidine may cause hypoglycemia followed by hyperglycemia. β-blockers, clonidine, lithium salts, and alcohol may potentiate or weaken glucose lowering effect. Masked or reduced hypoglycemic symptoms with β-blockers, clonidine, guanethidine, and reserpine.

PREGNANCY: Category B, caution in nursing.

MECHANISM OF ACTION: Insulin aspart (rDNAorigin); regulates glucose metabolism, lowers blood glucose by facilitating cellular uptake of glucose and simultaneously inhibiting glucose output from the liver.

PHARMACOKINETICS: Absorption: C_{max}=82.1 mU/L; T_{max}=40-50 min.
Distribution: Plasma protein binding (0-9%). **Elimination:** $T_{1/2}$=81 min.

NOVOLOG MIX 70/30   RX
insulin aspart protamine - insulin aspart (Novo Nordisk)

THERAPEUTIC CLASS: Insulin

INDICATIONS: To control hyperglycemia in diabetes.

DOSAGE: *Adults:* Individualize dose. For SQ inj only. Inject SQ bid within 15 min before breakfast and dinner. Do not mix with other insulins or use in insulin pumps.

HOW SUPPLIED: (Insulin Aspart Protamine-Insulin Aspart) Inj: 70 U-30 U/mL; PenFill: 70 U-30 U/mL; Prefilled: 70 U-30 U/mL

CONTRAINDICATIONS: Hypoglycemia.

WARNINGS/PRECAUTIONS: Any change of insulin should be made cautiously. Changes in strength, manufacturer, type or method of manufacture may result in the need for a change in dosage. Hypoglycemia and hypokalemia may occur; caution with fasting and autonomic neuropathy. Illness, stress, change in meals and exercise may change insulin requirements. Smoking, temperature, and exercise affect insulin absorption. Caution with liver or kidney disease. Administration of insulin SQ can result in lipoatrophy.

ADVERSE REACTIONS: Hypoglycemia, hypokalemia, lipodystrophy, hypersensitivity reaction, injection site reactions, pruritus, rash.

INTERACTIONS: Increased glucose lowering effects with ACE inhibitors, disopyramide, fibrates, fluoxetine, MAOIs, propoxyphene, salicylates, somatostatin analog, sulfonamide antibiotics and oral antidiabetics. Decreased blood glucose lowering effects with corticosteroids, niacin, danazol, diuretics, sympathomimetics, isoniazid, phenothiazine derivatives, somatropin, thyroid hormones, estrogens, progesterones. β-blockers, clonidine, lithium salts, and alcohol may potentiate or weaken glucose lowering effect. β-blockers, clonidine, guanethidine, and reserpine may reduce or mask signs of hypoglycemia. Do not mix with other insulin products. Caution with potassium-lowering drugs or drugs sensitive to serum potassium levels. Pentamidine may cause hypoglycemia, followed by hyperglycemia.

PREGNANCY: Category C, safety in nursing not known.

MECHANISM OF ACTION: Insulin; regulates glucose metabolism. Lowers blood glucose by facilitating cellular uptake of glucose, simultaneously inhibiting output of glucose from liver.

PHARMACOKINETICS: Absorption: (0.2, 0.3 U/kg): C_{max}=23.4, 61.3m U/L; T_{max}=60, 85 min. **Distribution:** Plasma protein binding (0-9%). **Elimination:** $T_{1/2}$=8-9 hrs.

NOXAFIL   RX
posaconazole (Schering)

THERAPEUTIC CLASS: Azole antifungal

INDICATIONS: Prophylaxis of invasive *Aspergillus* and *Candida* infections in patients, ≥13 yrs, who are at high risk of developing these infections due to being severely immunocompromised. Treatment of oropharyngeal candidiasis, including oropharyngeal candidiasis refractory to itraconazole and/or fluconazole.

DOSAGE: *Adults:* Prophylaxis of Invasive Fungal Infections: 200mg (5mL) tid. Base duration of therapy on recovery from neutropenia or immunosuppression. Oropharyngeal Candidiasis: LD: 100mg (2.5mL) bid on 1st day, then 100mg qd for 13 days. Oropharyngeal Candidiasis Refractory to Itraconazole and/or Fluconazole: 400mg (10mL) bid. Base duration of therapy on severity of underlying disease and clinical response. Give each dose with full meal or nutritional supplement.
Pediatrics: ≥13 yrs: Prophylaxis of Invasive Fungal Infections: 200mg (5mL) tid. Base duration of therapy on recovery from neutropenia or immunosuppression. Oropharyngeal Candidiasis: LD: 100mg (2.5mL) bid on 1st day, then

100mg qd for 13 days. Oropharyngeal Candidiasis Refractory to Itraconazole and/or Fluconazole: 400mg (10mL) bid. Base duration of therapy on severity of underlying disease and clinical response. Give each dose with full meal or nutritional supplement.

HOW SUPPLIED: Susp: 40mg/mL

CONTRAINDICATIONS: Concomitant ergot alkaloids, terfenadine, astemizole, cisapride, pimozide, halofantrine, or quinidine.

WARNINGS/PRECAUTIONS: Hepatic reactions (eg, mild to moderate elevations in ALT, AST, alkaline phosphatase, total bilirubin, and/or clinical hepatitis) reported; monitor LFTs at start of and during therapy. Caution with hepatic impairment. Monitor closely with severe renal impairment. Prolongation of QT interval reported; caution with potentially proarrhythmic conditions.

ADVERSE REACTIONS: Fever, headache, rigors, HTN, anemia, neutropenia, diarrhea, nausea, vomiting, abdominal pain, constipation, hypokalemia, thrombocytopenia, coughing, dyspnea.

INTERACTIONS: See Contraindications. May elevate cyclosporine and tacrolimus levels; consider dose reduction and more frequent clinical monitoring of cyclosporine, tacrolimus, and sirolimus when therapy is initiated. Avoid use with drugs that are known to prolong the QTc interval and are metabolized through CYP3A4. Avoid concurrent use of cimetidine, rifabutin, and phenytoin unless benefits outweigh risks. If concomitant phenytoin is required, monitor closely and consider phenytoin dose reduction. If concomitant rifabutin is required, monitor CBC and adverse events. Monitor adverse events with concomitant benzodiazepines metabolized by CYP3A4; consider dose reduction of these benzodiazepines during coadministration. May increase levels of vinca alkaloids; consider dose adjustment of vinca alkaloid. Consider dose reduction of concomitant HMG-CoA reductase inhibitors (statins). Monitor for adverse events and toxicity with concomitant CCBs; dose reduction of CCBs may be needed.

PREGNANCY: Category C, not for use in nursing.

MECHANISM OF ACTION: Antifungal agent; blocks synthesis of ergosterol, a key component of fungal cell membrane, through inhibition of the enzyme lanosterol 14α-demethylase and accumulation of methylated sterol precursors.

PHARMACOKINETICS: Administration: Oral administration of variable doses resulted in different parameters. **Distribution:** V_d=1774L, plasma protein binding (≥98%). **Metabolism:** Via UDP glucuronidation; CYP3A4 enzyme. **Elimination:** $T_{1/2}$=35 hrs. Feces (71%), urine (13%).

NUBAIN   RX
nalbuphine HCL (Endo)

THERAPEUTIC CLASS: Agonist-antagonist analgesic

INDICATIONS: Relief of moderate to severe pain. Adjunct to balanced anesthesia for pre- and postoperative analgesia, and for obstetrical analgesia during labor and delivery.

DOSAGE: *Adults:* ≥18 yrs: Pain: Initial: 10mg/70kg IV/IM/SQ q3-6h prn. Adjust according to severity, physical status and concomitant agents. Max: 20mg/dose or 160mg/day. Anesthesia Adjunct: Induction: 0.3-3mg/kg IV over 10-15 min. Maint: 0.25-0.5mg/kg IV.

HOW SUPPLIED: Inj: 10mg/mL, 20mg/mL

WARNINGS/PRECAUTIONS: Increased risk of respiratory depression with head injury, intracranial lesions, or pre-existing increased ICP. Only for use by specifically trained persons. Naloxone, resuscitative and intubation equipment, and oxygen should be readily available. Caution with emotionally unstable patients, narcotic abuse, impaired respiration, MI with nausea and vomiting, biliary tract surgery. May impair ability to drive or operate machinery. Caution with renal or hepatic dysfunction; reduce dose. Caution during labor and delivery; monitor newborns for respiratory depression, apnea, bradycardia, and arrhythmias.

ADVERSE REACTIONS: Sedation, sweating, nausea/vomiting, dizziness/vertigo, dry mouth, headache, injection site reactions.

INTERACTIONS: Possible additive effects with narcotic analgesics, general anesthetics, phenothiazines, tranquilizers, sedatives, hypnotics, or other CNS depressants. Incompatible with nafcillin and ketorolac.

PREGNANCY: Category B, caution in nursing.

MECHANISM OF ACTION: Opioid agonist-antagonist analgesic; kappa agonist/partial mu antagonist analgesic.

PHARMACOKINETICS: Metabolism: Liver. **Elimination:** Kidney; $T_{1/2}$=5 hrs.

NUCOFED `CIII`
pseudoephedrine HCL - codeine phosphate (King)

THERAPEUTIC CLASS: Antitussive/decongestant

INDICATIONS: Relief of cough and congestion associated with respiratory infections, bronchitis, influenza, and sinusitis.

DOSAGE: *Adults:* 1 cap q6h. Max: 4 caps/24 hrs.
Pediatrics: ≥12 yrs: 1 cap q6h. Max: 4 caps/24 hrs.

HOW SUPPLIED: (Codeine-Pseudoephedrine) Cap: 20mg-60mg; Syrup: 20mg-60mg/5mL

WARNINGS/PRECAUTIONS: Not for cough associated with smoking, emphysema, asthma, or excessive secretions. May cause constipation. Caution with pulmonary disease, shortness of breath, HTN, heart disease, DM, thyroid disease, prostatic hypertrophy, Addison's disease, children, ulcerative colitis, drug dependence, liver or kidney dysfunction. May impair alertness.

ADVERSE REACTIONS: Nervousness, restlessness, insomnia, drowsiness, dysuria, dizziness, headache, nausea, vomiting, constipation, trembling, dyspnea, sweating, paleness, weakness, heart rate changes.

INTERACTIONS: β-blockers, MAOIs, sympathomimetics may increase the effects of pseudoephedrine. Avoid within 14 days of MAOI use. TCAs may antagonize effects of pseudoephedrine. Caution with CNS depressants, general anesthetics, alcohol. Anticholinergics may cause paralytic ileus. Digitalis glycosides may cause cardiac arrhythmias. Decreases effects of antihypertensive agents.

PREGNANCY: Category C, caution in nursing.

MECHANISM OF ACTION: Codeine: Antitussive-decongestant; causes cough suppression by direct effect on the cough center in the medulla oblongata, exerts a drying effect on respiratory tract mucosa, increases viscosity of bronchial secretions. Pseudoephedrine: Directly stimulates α-adrenergic receptors, causing vasoconstriction. Directly stimulates β-adrenergic receptors to a lesser degree, causing bronchial smooth muscle relaxation.

PHARMACOKINETICS: Absorption: Codeine: GIT (well-absorbed). T_{max}=1-2 hrs. Pseudoephedrine: T_{max}=4-6 hrs. **Distribution:** Codeine: Found in breast milk; crosses placenta. Pseudoephedrine: Crosses placenta and enters CSF. **Metabolism:** Codeine: Liver (O-demethylation, N-demethylation, and partial conjugation with glucuronic acid). Pseudoephedrine: Liver (incomplete). N-demethylation. **Elimination:** Both in urine; pseudoephedrine (55-75% unchanged).

NUCOFED PEDIATRIC EXPECTORANT `CV`
pseudoephedrine HCL - codeine phosphate - guaifenesin (King)

OTHER BRAND NAMES: Mytussin DAC (Morton Grove)

THERAPEUTIC CLASS: Antitussive/expectorant/decongestant

INDICATIONS: Relief of cough and congestion associated with respiratory infections, bronchitis, influenza, and sinusitis.

DOSAGE: *Adults:* 10mL q6h. Max: 40mL/24 hrs.
Pediatrics: ≥12 yrs: 10mL q6h. Max: 40mL/24hrs. 6 to <12 yrs: 5mL q6h. Max: 20mL/24hrs. 2 to <6 yrs: 2.5mL q6h. Max: 10mL/24hrs.

HOW SUPPLIED: (Codeine-Guaifenesin-Pseudoephedrine) Syrup: 10mg-100mg-30mg/5mL

WARNINGS/PRECAUTIONS: Not for cough associated with smoking, emphysema, asthma, or excessive secretions. May cause constipation. Caution with pulmonary disease, shortness of breath, HTN, heart disease, DM, thyroid disease, prostatic hypertrophy, Addison's disease, children, ulcerative colitis, drug dependence, liver or kidney dysfunction. May impair alertness.

ADVERSE REACTIONS: Nervousness, restlessness, insomnia, drowsiness, dysuria, dizziness, headache, nausea, vomiting, constipation, trembling, dyspnea, sweating, paleness, weakness, heart rate changes.

INTERACTIONS: β-blockers, MAOIs, sympathomimetics may increase the effects of pseudoephedrine. Avoid within 14 days of MAOI use. TCAs may antagonize effects of pseudoephedrine. Caution with CNS depressants, general anesthetics, alcohol. Anticholinergics may cause paralytic ileus. Digitalis glycosides may cause cardiac arrhythmias. Decreases effects of antihypertensive agents.

PREGNANCY: Category C, caution in nursing.

NuLYTELY   RX
polyethylene glycol 3350 - sodium bicarbonate - potassium chloride - sodium chloride (Braintree)

OTHER BRAND NAMES: Trilyte (Schwarz Pharma)

THERAPEUTIC CLASS: Bowel cleanser

INDICATIONS: Bowel cleansing prior to colonoscopy.

DOSAGE: *Adults:* Oral: 240mL every 10 min until fecal discharge is clear or 4L is consumed. NG Tube: 20-30mL/min (1.2-1.8L/hr). Patient should fast at least 3-4 hours before administration.
Pediatrics: ≥6 months: Oral/Nasogastric Tube: 25mL/kg/hr until fecal discharge is clear. Patient should fast at least 3-4 hours before administration.

HOW SUPPLIED: Sol: (Polyethylene Glycol-Potassium Chloride-Sodium Bicarbonate-Sodium Chloride) 420g-1.48g-5.72g-11.2g [4000mL]

CONTRAINDICATIONS: GI obstruction, gastric retention, bowel perforation, toxic colitis, toxic megacolon, ileus.

WARNINGS/PRECAUTIONS: Do not add additional ingredients (eg, flavorings). Caution with severe ulcerative colitis. Monitor therapy with impaired gag reflex, unconsciousness/semiconsciousness and patients prone to regurgitation and aspiration. Temporarily d/c if develop severe bloating, distention, or abdominal pain. Monitor for hypoglycemia in pediatrics <2 yrs of age.

ADVERSE REACTIONS: Nausea, abdominal fullness/cramps, bloating, vomiting, anal irritation.

INTERACTIONS: Oral medications taken within 1 hr of start of administration may not be absorbed from GI tract.

PREGNANCY: Category C, caution in nursing.

MECHANISM OF ACTION: Omotic laxative which induces diarrhea..

NUTROPIN   RX
somatropin (Genentech)

OTHER BRAND NAMES: Nutropin AQ (Genentech)

THERAPEUTIC CLASS: Human growth hormone

INDICATIONS: (Adults) Replacement of endogenous growth hormone (GH) in GH deficiency (GHD). (Pediatrics) Long-term treatment of growth failure due to lack of adequate endogenous GH secretion, in short stature associated with Turner Syndrome, and in idiopathic short stature (ISS). Treatment of growth failure associated with chronic renal insufficiency (CRI) up to the time of renal transplantation.

DOSAGE: *Adults:* GHD: Initial: Up to 0.006mg/kg/day SQ. Max: <35 yrs: 0.025mg/kg/day. ≥35 yrs: 0.0125mg/kg/day. Alternatively may use 0.2mg/day (range: 0.15-0.30mg/day). Increase every 1-2 months by increments of 0.1-0.2mg/day.
Pediatrics: GHD: Usual: 0.3mg/kg/week divided into daily SQ doses. Pubertal Patients: Up to 0.7mg/kg/week divided into daily SQ doses. CRI: 0.35mg/kg/week divided into daily SQ doses. Continue until renal transplantation. Hemodialysis: Give qhs or 3-4 hrs post dialysis. Chronic Cycling Peritoneal Dialysis: Give in am after dialysis. Chronic Ambulatory Peritoneal Dialysis: Give qhs during overnight exchange. Turner Syndrome: Up to 0.375mg/kg/week SQ in divided doses 3-7x/week. ISS: 0.3mg/kg/week divided into daily SQ doses.

HOW SUPPLIED: Inj: 5mg, 10mg, (AQ) 5mg/mL

CONTRAINDICATIONS: Acute critical illness after serious surgeries (eg, open heart or abdominal surgery, accidental trauma, acute respiratory failure), closed epiphyses in pediatrics, active proliferative or severe non-proliferative diabetic retinopathy, active neoplasia, evidence of recurrence or progression of an intracranial tumor. Prader-Willi syndrome (unless also diagnosed with GH deficiency) with severe obesity or respiratory impairment.

WARNINGS/PRECAUTIONS: Caution with epiphyseal closure in adults treated with GH-replacement therapy in childhood. Recurrence/progression reported with intracranial lesions. Renal osteodystrophy may occur with growth failure secondary to renal impairment. Scoliosis and slipped capital femoral epiphysis may develop in rapid growth. Caution with Turner syndrome and ISS. Intracranial hypertension with papilledema, visual changes, headache, nausea, and/or vomiting has been reported. Funduscopic exam should be done before and during treatment. Monitor for malignant transformation of skin lesions. Injecting SQ in same site over long period of time may cause tissue atrophy. May decrease insulin sensitivity; monitor blood sugar.

ADVERSE REACTIONS: Antibodies to the protein, leukemia, transient peripheral edema, arthralgia, carpal tunnel syndrome, malignant transformations, gynecomastia, pancreatitis.

INTERACTIONS: Decreased effects with glucocorticoids. May reduce insulin sensitivity; may need insulin adjustment. May need to increase dose in adult women on estrogen replacement.

PREGNANCY: Category C, caution in nursing.

MECHANISM OF ACTION: Human growth hormone; increases growth rate and serum insulin-like growth factor-I levels.

PHARMACOKINETICS: Absorption: (SQ) Absolute bioavailability (81%), C_{max}=71.1mcg/L, T_{max}=3.9 hrs, AUC=677 mcg•hr/L. **Distribution:** V_d=50mL/kg. **Metabolism:** Liver and kidneys. **Elimination:** (SQ): $T_{1/2}$=2.3 hrs. (IV): $T_{1/2}$=19.5 min.

NuvaRing
etonogestrel - ethinyl estradiol (Organon)

RX

THERAPEUTIC CLASS: Estrogen/progestogen combination

INDICATIONS: Prevention of pregnancy.

DOSAGE: *Adults:* Insert ring vaginally on or before the 5th day of cycle. Remove ring after 3 consecutive weeks. Insert new ring 1 week later on same day of the week and same time of day.

HOW SUPPLIED: Vaginal ring: (Ethinyl estradiol-Etonogestrel) 0.015mg-0.120mg/day

CONTRAINDICATIONS: Thrombophlebitis, active or history of thromboembolic disorders, history of DVT, cerebrovascular or coronary artery disease, valvular heart disease with complications, severe HTN, diabetes with vascular complications, headaches with focal neurological symptoms, major surgery with prolonged immobilization, breast carcinoma, endometrial carcinoma or other estrogen-dependent neoplasia, undiagnosed abnormal genital bleeding, cholestatic jaundice of pregnancy or jaundice with prior hormonal contraceptive use, hepatic tumors, active liver disease, pregnancy, heavy smoking and >35 yrs.

WARNINGS/PRECAUTIONS: Cigarette smoking increases risk of serious cardiovascular side effects. This risk increases with age (especially >35 yrs) and heavy smoking. Increases risk of MI, thromboembolism, stroke, and gallbladder disease, and hypertension. Retinal thrombosis and benign hepatic adenomas reported. May decrease glucose tolerance. May increase BP, PT, sex hormone-binding globulins, thyroid hormone, or LDL levels. May cause other lipid changes, fluid retention, breakthrough bleeding and spotting, or exacerbate migraines. May develop visual changes with contact lens. D/C if jaundice, significant depression, severe headaches or migraines develop. Toxic shock syndrome with tampon use reported. Increased risk of morbidity and mortality in certain inherited thrombophilias, obesity, and diabetes. Older women who take hormonal contraceptive should take the lowest possible dose formulation that is effective.

ADVERSE REACTIONS: Vaginitis, headache, upper respiratory tract infection, leukorrhea, sinusitis, weight gain, nausea.

INTERACTIONS: Reduced effects with barbiturates, griseofulvin, rifampin, phenylbutazone, phenytoin, carbamazepine, felbamate, oxycarbazepine, topiramate, modafinil, St. John's wort, and possibly with ampicillin and tetracyclines. Increases levels of cyclosporine, prednisolone, and theophylline. Protease inhibitors may affect efficacy. Increased levels of ethinyl estradiol with atorvastatin, ascorbic acid, APAP, and CYP3A4 inhibitors (eg, ketoconazole, itraconazole). Increased levels of etonogestrel and ethinyl estradiol with vaginal miconazole nitrate. Decreases levels of APAP and increases clearance of temazepam, salicylic acid, morphine, and clofibric acid. Elevations of triglycerides leading to pancreatitis reported. D/C if depression observed and recurs to a serious degree.

PREGNANCY: Category X, not for use in nursing.

MECHANISM OF ACTION: Combination hormonal contraceptive; suppresses gonadotropins leading to inhibition of ovulation, and increases difficulty of sperm entry into uterus and reduces likelihood of implantation by producing changes in cervical mucus and endometrium, respectively.

PHARMACOKINETICS: Absorption: Etonorgestrel: Rapid; Bioavailability (100%); C_{max}=1716pg/mL; T_{max}=200.3 hrs. Ethinyl estradiol: Rapid; Absolute bioavailability (56%); C_{max}=34.7pg/mL; T_{max}= 59.3 hrs. **Distribution:** Etonorgestrel: Serum albumin binding (66%), sex hormone-binding globulin (32%). Ethinyl estradiol: Serum albumin binding (98.5%). **Metabolism:** Hepatic via CYP3A4. **Elimination:** Urine, bile, feces; Etonorgestrel: $T_{1/2}$=29.3 hrs; Ethinyl estradiol: $T_{1/2}$=44.7 hrs.

NUVIGIL CIV
armodafinil (Cephalon)

THERAPEUTIC CLASS: Wakefulness-promoting agent

INDICATIONS: To improve wakefulness in patients with excessive daytime sleepiness associated with narcolepsy, obstructive sleep apnea/hypopnea syndrome (OSAHS), shiftwork sleep disorder (SWSD). As adjunct to standard treatment for underlying obstruction in OSAHS.

DOSAGE: *Adults:* OSAHS/Narcolepsy: 150mg or 250mg qd in AM. SWSD: 150mg qd 1 hour prior to work shift. Hepatic Dysfunction: Reduce dose. Elderly: Consider dose reduction.

HOW SUPPLIED: Tab: 50mg, 150mg, 250mg

WARNINGS/PRECAUTIONS: May cause serious rash, including Stevens-Johnson syndrome, anaphylactoid reactions, angioedema, and multi-organ hypersensitivity. May impair mental/physical abilities. Psychiatric adverse experiences reported; consider discontinuing treatment if psychiatric symptoms develop and use caution with history of psychosis, depression, or mania. Caution with history of MI or unstable angina. Avoid with history of left ventricular hypertrophy, ischemic ECG changes, chest pain, arrhythmia, or other manifestations of mitral valve prolapse with CNS stimulants. Monitor hypertensive patients.

ADVERSE REACTIONS: Headache, nausea, dizziness, insomnia, diarrhea, dry mouth, anxiety, depression, rash.

INTERACTIONS: Potent CYP3A4/5 inducers, (eg, carbamazepine, phenobarbital, rifampin) or inhibitors, (eg, ketoconazole, erythromycin) may alter plasma levels. Effectiveness of CYP3A substrates (eg, cyclosporine, ethinyl estradiol, midazolam, triazolam) may be reduced. May cause moderate inhibition of CYP2C19 activity; dosage reduction may be required for some CYP2C19 substrates (eg, omeprazole, diazepam, phenytoin, propranolol). Methylphenidate or dextroamphetamine may delay absorption. Caution with MAOIs. Monitor PT/INR with warfarin. Effectiveness of steroidal contraceptives may be reduced during and for 1 month after discontinuation of therapy; alternate or concomitant methods of contraception are recommended.

PREGNANCY: Category C, caution in nursing.

MECHANISM OF ACTION: Not known; suspected to bind to the dopamine transporter and inhibit dopamine reuptake.

PHARMACOKINETICS: Absorption: Readily absorbed. T_{max}=2 hrs (fasted), 2-4 hrs (fed). **Distribution**: V_d=42L. Plasma protein binding (60%). **Metabolism**: Liver via amide hydrolysis with sulfone formation by CYP450, 3A4, 3A5: R-modafinil acid, modafinil sulfone. **Elimination**: Feces, urine. $T_{1/2}$=15 hrs.

NYSTATIN ORAL RX
nystatin (Various)

THERAPEUTIC CLASS: Polyene antifungal

INDICATIONS: (Sus) Treatment of oral candidiasis. (Tab) Treatment of non-esophageal mucous membrane GI candidiasis.

DOSAGE: *Adults:* Oral Candidiasis: (Sus) 4-6mL qid. Retain in mouth as long as possible before swallowing. GI Candidiasis: (Tab) 500,000-1,000,000 U tid.
Pediatrics: Oral Candidiasis: (Sus) 4-6mL qid. Infants: 2mL qid. Retain in mouth as long as possible before swallowing.

HOW SUPPLIED: Sus: 100,000 U/mL [60mL, 480mL]; Tab: 500,000 U

WARNINGS/PRECAUTIONS: Not for systemic mycoses. D/C if irritation/hypersensitivity occurs. Confirm diagnosis with KOH smear and/or cultures if symptoms persist after course of therapy. Continue at least 48 hrs after clinical response.

ADVERSE REACTIONS: Diarrhea, nausea, vomiting, GI distress, rash, urticaria, Stevens-Johnson syndrome, oral irritation.

PREGNANCY: Category C, caution in nursing.

MECHANISM OF ACTION: Fungistatic and fungicidal agent. Acts by binding to sterols in the cell membrane of susceptible *Candida* species with a resultant change in membrane permeability, allowing leakage of intracellular components.

PHARMACOKINETICS: Absorption: GI (insignificant). **Elimination:** Stool (unchanged).

NYSTATIN TOPICAL RX
nystatin (Various)

THERAPEUTIC CLASS: Polyene antifungal

INDICATIONS: Treatment of cutaneous or mucocutaneous mycotic infections caused by susceptible *Candida* species.

DOSAGE: Adults: (Cre) Apply to affected area bid until healing is complete. (Powder) Apply to lesions bid-tid until healing is complete. For fungal infections of the feet, dust powder on feet and in shoes also.
Pediatrics: Neonates and Older: (Cre) Apply to affected area bid until healing is complete. (Powder) Apply to lesions bid-tid until healing is complete. For fungal infections of the feet, dust powder on feet and in shoes also.

HOW SUPPLIED: Cre: 100,000 U/g [30g]; Powder, Topical: 100,000 U/g [15g]

WARNINGS/PRECAUTIONS: D/C if irritation or sensitization occurs. Confirm diagnosis. Not for systemic, oral, intravaginal, or ophthalmic use. For fungal infections of the feet, dust powder on feet as well as in all footwear. Moist lesions are best treated with topical dusting powder.

ADVERSE REACTIONS: Allergic reactions, burning, itching, rash, eczema, pain at application site.

PREGNANCY: Category C, caution in nursing.

MECHANISM OF ACTION: Polyene antifungal; binds sterols in the cell membrane of susceptible species, causing a change in membrane permeability and subsequent leakage of intracellular components. Fungistatic and fungicidal.

PHARMACOKINETICS: Absorption: Not absorbed from intact skin or mucous membranes.

NYSTATIN VAGINAL   RX
nystatin (Odyssey)

THERAPEUTIC CLASS: Polyene antifungal

INDICATIONS: Local treatment of vulvovaginal candidiasis.

DOSAGE: *Adults:* Insert 1 tablet vaginally qd for 2 weeks. Deposit tablets high in the vagina by means of the applicator.

HOW SUPPLIED: Tab, Vaginal: 100,000U [15s]

WARNINGS/PRECAUTIONS: D/C if sensitization or irritation occurs. Confirm diagnosis by KOH smears and/or cultures.

PREGNANCY: Category A, safety in nursing not known.

MECHANISM OF ACTION: Antimycotic polyene antibiotic; fungistatic and fungicidal against yeast and yeast-like fungi; acts by binding to sterols in the cell membrane of fungus with a resultant change in membrane permeability allowing leakage of intracellular components.

PHARMACOKINETICS: Absorption: None from intact skin or mucous membrane.

NYSTATIN/TRIAMCINOLONE   RX
triamcinolone acetonide - nystatin (Various)

THERAPEUTIC CLASS: Polyene antifungal/corticosteroid

INDICATIONS: Topical treatment of cutaneous candidiasis.

DOSAGE: *Adults:* Apply bid (am and pm). Max: 25 days of treatment.
Pediatrics: Apply bid (am and pm). Max: 25 days of treatment.

HOW SUPPLIED: Cre, Oint: (Nystatin-Triamcinolone) 100,000 U/g-0.1% [15g, 30g, 60g]

WARNINGS/PRECAUTIONS: Avoid occlusive dressing. Monitor periodically for HPA axis suppression with prolonged use or when applied over a large area. D/C if hypersensitivity or irritation develops. Systemic absorption with topical corticosteroids reported; children are more prone to systemic toxicity. May cause Cushing's syndrome, hyperglycemia, and glucosuria.

ADVERSE REACTIONS: Acneiform eruption, burning, itching, irritation, secondary infection.

PREGNANCY: Category C, caution in nursing.

MECHANISM OF ACTION: Nystatin: Polyene antifungal; binds to sterols in cell membrane, which renders cell membrane incapable of functioning as selective barrier. Triamcinolone: Synthetic corticosteroid; produces anti-inflammatory, antipruritic, and vasoconstrictive actions. Dermatological effects not established.

PHARMACOKINETICS: Absorption: Triamcinolone: Percutaneous; inflammation, other disease states, and the use of occlusive dressings may increase absorption. **Metabolism**: Triamcinolone: Liver. **Excretion**: Triamcinolone: Urine (primary); bile.

NYSTOP RX
nystatin (Paddock)

THERAPEUTIC CLASS: Polyene antifungal

INDICATIONS: Treatment of cutaneous and mucocutaneous mycotic infections caused by susceptible *Candida* species.

DOSAGE: *Adults:* Apply to lesions bid-tid until healing is complete. For fungal infections of the feet, dust powder on feet and also in shoes.
Pediatrics: Neonates and Older: Apply to lesions bid-tid until healing is complete. For fungal infections of the feet, dust powder on feet and in shoes also.

HOW SUPPLIED: Powder, Topical: 100,000 U/g [15g, 30g, 60g]

WARNINGS/PRECAUTIONS: D/C if irritation or sensitization occurs. Confirm diagnosis. Not for systemic, oral, intravaginal, or ophthalmic use.

ADVERSE REACTIONS: Allergic reactions, burning, itching, rash, eczema, pain at application site.

PREGNANCY: Category C, caution in nursing.

MECHANISM OF ACTION: Polyene antifungal; binds sterols in the cell membrane of susceptible species, causing a change in membrane permeability and subsequent leakage of intracellular components. Fungistatic and fungicidal.

PHARMACOKINETICS: Absorption: Not absorbed from intact skin or mucous membranes.

OCUFEN RX
flurbiprofen sodium (Allergan)

THERAPEUTIC CLASS: Phenylalkanoic acid NSAID

INDICATIONS: Inhibition of intraoperative miosis.

DOSAGE: *Adults:* 1 drop every 1/2 hr starting 2 hrs prior to surgery (total 4 drops).

HOW SUPPLIED: Sol: 0.03% [2.5mL]

WARNINGS/PRECAUTIONS: Increased risk of bleeding of ocular tissue with ocular surgery. Caution in surgical patients with known bleeding tendencies or with agents that may prolong bleeding time. Caution with salicylate allergy. May delay wound healing.

ADVERSE REACTIONS: Fibrosis, miosis, mydriasis, transient burning and stinging, increased bleeding of ocular tissue with ocular surgery.

INTERACTIONS: May diminish effects of acetylcholine chloride and carbachol. Potential cross-sensitivity to acetylsalicylic acid and other NSAIDS.

PREGNANCY: Category C, not for use in nursing.

MECHANISM OF ACTION: NSAID; inhibits the cyclo-oxygenase that is essential in the biosynthesis of prostaglandins; which are mediators for ceratin kind of intraocular inflammation, cause disruption of the blood-aqueous humor barrier, vasodilataion, increased vascular permeabiltiy, leukocytosis, and increased IOP, and also play a role in the miotic response during ocular surgery.

OCUFLOX

RX

ofloxacin (Allergan)

THERAPEUTIC CLASS: Fluoroquinolone

INDICATIONS: Management of bacterial infections in conjunctivitis and corneal ulcers.

DOSAGE: *Adults:* Conjunctivitis: 1-2 drops q2-4h for 2 days, then 1-2 drops qid for 5 days. Corneal Ulcer: 1-2 drops every 30 min while awake and 1-2 drops 4-6 hrs after retiring for 2 days, then 1-2 drops q1h while awake for 5-7 days, then 1-2 drops qid for 2 days or until treatment completion.
Pediatrics: ≥1 yr: Conjunctivitis: 1-2 drops q2-4h for 2 days, then 1-2 drops qid for 5 days. Corneal Ulcer: 1-2 drops every 30 min while awake and 1-2 drops 4-6 hrs after retiring for 2 days, then 1-2 drops q1h while awake for 5-7 days, then 1-2 drops qid for 2 days or until treatment completion.

HOW SUPPLIED: Sol: 0.3% [5mL, 10mL]

WARNINGS/PRECAUTIONS: Not for injection into eye. Do not inject subconjunctivally nor into the eye's anterior chamber. Superinfection may result with prolonged use. Fatal hypersensitivity reactions reported after 1st dose of systemic quinolone therapy. Avoid allowing tip of container to contact fingers, eye or surrounding structures.

ADVERSE REACTIONS: Transient ocular burning or discomfort, stinging, redness, itching, keratitis, ocular periocular/facial edema, photophobia, blurred vision, tearing, dryness, eye pain.

INTERACTIONS: Systemic quinolone therapy may increase theophylline levels, interfere with caffeine metabolism, enhance warfarin effects, and elevate serum creatinine with cyclosporine.

PREGNANCY: Category C, not for use in nursing.

MECHANISM OF ACTION: Fluoroquinolone; exerts bactericidal effect on susceptible bacteria by inhibiting DNA gyrase, an essential bacterial enzyme that is a critical catalyst in the duplication, transcription, and repair of bacterial DNA.

PHARMACOKINETICS: Absorption: C_{max}=1.1 ng/mL (Day one, qid dosing), 1.9 ng/mL (Day 11, qid dosing). **Excretion:** Urine.

OCUPRESS

RX

carteolol HCL (Novartis Ophthalmics)

THERAPEUTIC CLASS: Nonselective beta-blocker

INDICATIONS: Reduction of intraocular pressure intraocular pressure (IOP) in chronic open-angle glaucoma and intraocular hypertension.

DOSAGE: *Adults:* 1 drop bid.

HOW SUPPLIED: Sol: 1% [5mL, 10mL, 15mL]

CONTRAINDICATIONS: Bronchial asthma, severe COPD, sinus bradycardia, 2nd- and 3rd-degree AV block, overt cardiac failure, cardiogenic shock.

WARNINGS/PRECAUTIONS: May be absorbed systemically. Caution with cardiac failure, bronchospasm, diminished pulmonary function, and DM. May mask symptoms of hypoglycemia and hyperthyroidism. Not for use alone in angle-closure glaucoma. May potentiate muscle weakness. D/C if cardiac failure develops. Withdrawal before surgery is controversial.

ADVERSE REACTIONS: Eye irritation, burning, tearing, conjunctival hyperemia, conjunctival edema, photophobia, decreased night vision, ptosis, bradycardia, decreased BP, dyspnea, asthenia, headache, dizziness, taste perversion.

INTERACTIONS: May potentiate systemic effects with oral β-blockers. Possible hypotension and bradycardia with catecholamine-depleting drugs (eg, reserpine). May antagonize epinephrine.

PREGNANCY: Category C, caution in nursing.

MECHANISM OF ACTION: Nonselective β-adrenergic blocker: reduces normal and elevated levels of IOP. Exact mechanism of ocular hypotensive effect not definitely demonstrated. β-adrenergic blockers also associated with reducing cardiac output and increasing airway resistance in bronchi and bronchioles.

OCUVITE OTC
selenium - lutein - copper - zinc - vitamin E - vitamin C - vitamin A (Bausch & Lomb)

THERAPEUTIC CLASS: Vitamin/mineral combination

INDICATIONS: To provide nutritional support for the eye.

DOSAGE: *Adults:* 1 tab qd-bid.

HOW SUPPLIED: Tab: Copper 2mg-Lutein 2mg-Selenium 55mcg-Vitamin A 1000IU-Vitamin C 200mg-Vitamin E 60IU-Zinc 40mg

PREGNANCY: Safety in pregnancy or nursing not known.

OCUVITE EXTRA OTC
niacinamide - riboflavin - L-glutathione - selenium - lutein - copper - zinc - vitamin E - vitamin C - vitamin A - manganese (Bausch & Lomb)

THERAPEUTIC CLASS: Vitamin/mineral combination

INDICATIONS: To provide nutritional support for the eye.

DOSAGE: *Adults:* 1 tab qd-bid.

HOW SUPPLIED: Tab: Copper 2mg-L-Glutathione 5mg-Lutein 2mg-Manganese 5mg-Niacinamide 40mg-Riboflavin 3mg-Selenium 55mcg-Vitamin A 1000IU-Vitamin C 300mg-Vitamin E 100IU-Zinc 40mg

PREGNANCY: Safety in pregnancy or nursing not known.

OCUVITE LUTEIN OTC
lutein - copper - zinc - vitamin E - vitamin C (Bausch & Lomb)

THERAPEUTIC CLASS: Vitamin/mineral combination

INDICATIONS: To provide nutritional support for the eye.

DOSAGE: *Adults:* 1 cap qd-bid.

HOW SUPPLIED: Cap: Copper 2mg-Lutein 6mg-Vitamin C 60mg-Vitamin E 30IU-Zinc 15mg

PREGNANCY: Safety in pregnancy or nursing not known.

OCUVITE PRESERVISION OTC
copper - zinc - vitamin E - vitamin C - vitamin A (Bausch & Lomb)

THERAPEUTIC CLASS: Vitamin/mineral combination

INDICATIONS: To help preserve eye health.

DOSAGE: *Adults:* 2 tabs bid.

HOW SUPPLIED: Tab: Copper 0.4mg-Vitamin A 7160IU-Vitamin C 113mg-Vitamin E 100IU-Zinc 17.4mg

PREGNANCY: Safety in pregnancy or nursing not known.

O

OGEN

RX

estropipate (Pharmacia & Upjohn)

> Estrogens increase the risk of endometrial cancer. Estrogens, with or without progestins, should not be used for the prevention of cardiovascular disease. Increased risks of MI, stroke, invasive breast cancer, PE, and DVT in postmenopausal women (50-79 yrs of age) reported. Increased risk of developing probable dementia in postmenopausal women ≥65 yrs of age reported.

THERAPEUTIC CLASS: Estrogen

INDICATIONS: Treatment of moderate to severe vasomotor symptoms and/or vulval/vaginal atrophy associated with menopause. Treatment of hypoestrogenism due to hypogonadism, castration, or primary ovarian failure. Prevention of postmenopausal osteoporosis.

DOSAGE: *Adults:* Vasomotor Symptoms: 0.75-6mg/day (as estropipate). Start cyclic administration arbitrarily if not menstruating, or on day 5 of bleeding if menstruating. Vulval/Vaginal Atrophy: 0.75-6mg/day (as estropipate), administer cyclically. Discontinue/Taper over 3-6 month interval. Hypoestrogenism: 1.5-9mg/day (as estropipate) for 1st 3 weeks of cycle, then 8-10 days off. Maint: Lowest effective dose. For female hypogonadism, repeat dose if bleeding doesn't occur or add progestogen in 3rd week of cycle. Osteoporosis Prevention: 0.75mg (as estropipate) qd for 25 days of 31-day cycle.

HOW SUPPLIED: Tab: 0.625mg* (0.75mg estropipate), 1.25mg* (1.5mg estropipate), 2.5mg* (3mg estropipate) *scored

CONTRAINDICATIONS: Pregnancy, undiagnosed abnormal genital bleeding, breast cancer, estrogen-dependent neoplasia, DVT/PE, active or recent (eg, within past year) arterial thromboembolic disease (eg, stroke, MI), liver dysfunction or disease.

WARNINGS/PRECAUTIONS: May increase risk of cardiovascular events (eg, MI, stroke), venous thrombosis, and PE; d/c immediately if any of these events occur or are suspected. May increase risk of breast/endometrial cancer, and gallbladder disease. May lead to severe hypercalcemia with breast cancer and bone metastases; monitor and d/c if hypercalcemia occurs. Retinal vascular thrombosis reported; monitor and d/c if papilledema or retinal vascular lesions occur. Consider addition of a progestin if no hysterectomy. May elevate BP; monitor at regular intervals. May cause elevations of plasma triglycerides with pre-existing hypertriglyceridemia. Caution with history of cholestatic jaundice associated with past estrogen use or with pregnancy; d/c with recurrence. May lead to increased thyroid-binding globulin levels; monitor thyroid function. May cause fluid retention; caution with cardiac/renal dysfunction. Caution with severe hypocalcemia. May increase risk of ovarian cancer. May exacerbate endometriosis, asthma, DM, epilepsy, migraine, porphyria, SLE, and hepatic hemangiomas; use with caution.

ADVERSE REACTIONS: Altered vaginal bleeding, vaginal candidiasis, breast tenderness/enlargement, GI effects, melasma, CNS effects, weight changes, edema, altered libido.

INTERACTIONS: CYP3A4 inducers (eg, St. John's wort, phenobarbital, carbamazepine, rifampin) may decrease levels which may decrease therapeutic effects and/or change uterine bleeding profile. CYP3A4 inhibitors (eg, erythromycin, clarithromycin, ketoconazole, itraconazole, ritonavir, grapefruit juice) may increase levels which may result in side effects.

PREGNANCY: Contraindicated in pregnancy, caution in nursing

MECHANISM OF ACTION: Estrogen; binds to nuclear receptors in estrogen-responsive tissues. Circulating estrogens modulate the pituitary secretion of the gonadotrophins, luteinizing hormone and follicle stimulating hormone, through negative feedback mechanism. In postmenopausal women, reduces elevated levels of these hormones.

PHARMACOKINETICS: Absorption: Well-absorbed. **Distribution:** Largely bound to sex hormone binding globulin and albumin; found in breast milk. **Metabolism:** Liver, to estrone (metabolite) and estriol (major urinary metabolite); sulfate and glucuronide conjugation (liver). **Excretion:** Urine (parent drug and metabolites).

Olux   RX
clobetasol propionate (Stiefel)

THERAPEUTIC CLASS: Corticosteroid

INDICATIONS: Short-term treatment of inflammatory and pruritic manifestations of moderate to severe corticosteroid responsive dermatoses of the
scalp. Short-term treatment of mild to moderate plaque-type psoriasis of non-
scalp regions excluding the face and intertriginous areas.

DOSAGE: *Adults:* Apply to affected area bid (am and pm). No more than 1.5
capfuls/application. Limit to 2 consecutive weeks. Avoid with occlusive dressings. Max 50g/week.
Pediatrics: ≥12 yrs: Apply to affected area bid (am and pm). No more than 1.5
capfuls/application. Limit to 2 consecutive weeks. Avoid with occlusive dressings. Max 50g/week.

HOW SUPPLIED: Foam: 0.05% [50g, 100g]

WARNINGS/PRECAUTIONS: May produce reversible HPA axis suppression, manifestations of Cushing's syndrome, hyperglycemia, and glucosuria.
Caution when applied to large surface areas or under occlusive dressings. Use
appropriate antifungal or antibacterial agent with dermatological infections;
d/c if infection does not clear. Pediatrics may be more susceptible to systemic
toxicity. Avoid eyes. D/C if irritation occurs.

ADVERSE REACTIONS: Burning/stinging, pruritus, irritation, erythema, folliculitis, cracking/fissuring of skin, numbness of fingers, telangiectasia, skin
atrophy.

PREGNANCY: Category C, caution in nursing.

MECHANISM OF ACTION: Corticosteroid; possesses anti-inflammatory,
antipruritic, and vasoconstrictive properties. Anti-inflammatory effects not
established; suspected to act by induction of phospholipase A_2 inhibitory
proteins, lipocortins. Lipocortins control biosynthesis of inflammation mediators (prostaglandins and leukotrienes) by inhibiting release of their common
precursor, arachidonic acid.

PHARMACOKINETICS: Absorption: Percutaneous; occlusion, inflammation,
and other disease states may increase absorption. **Distribution:** Systemically
administered corticosteroids are found in breast milk. **Metabolism:** Liver.
Elimination: Kidney (major), bile.

Olux-E   RX
clobetasol propionate (Stiefel)

THERAPEUTIC CLASS: Corticosteroid

INDICATIONS: Treatment of inflammatory and pruritic manifestations of
corticosteroid-responsive dermatoses.

DOSAGE: *Adults:* Apply thin layer to affected area bid (am and pm). Limit to 2
consecutive weeks. Avoid with occlusive dressings. Max: 50g/week.
Pediatrics: ≥12 yrs: Apply thin layer to affected area bid (am and pm). Limit to
2 consecutive weeks. Avoid with occlusive dressings. Max: 50g/week.

HOW SUPPLIED: Foam: 0.05% [50g,100g]

WARNINGS/PRECAUTIONS: May produce reversible HPA axis suppression, manifestations of Cushing's syndrome, hyperglycemia, and glucosuria.
Caution when applied to large surface area or under occlusive dressings. Use
appropriate antifungal or antibacterial agent with dermatological infections;
d/c if infection does not clear. Pediatrics may be more susceptible to systemic
toxicity. D/C if irritation occurs. Should not be used to treat rosacea or perioral dermatitis. Avoid use on face, groin, axillae, or other intertriginous areas.

ADVERSE REACTIONS: Folliculitis, acneiform eruptions, hypopigmentation,
perioral dermatitis, allergic contact dermatitis, secondary infection, irritation,
striae, miliaria.

PREGNANCY: Category C, caution in nursing.

MECHANISM OF ACTION: Corticosteroid; possesses anti-inflammatory, antipruritic, and vasoconstrictive properties. Anti-inflammatory effect not established; suspected to act by induction of phospholipase A_2 inhibitory proteins called lipocortins. Lipocortins control biosynthesis of inflammation mediators (prostaglandins and leukotrienesn) by inhibiting release of their common precursor, arachidonic acid.

PHARMACOKINETICS: Absorption: Percutaneous; occlusion, inflammation, and other disease states may increase absorption; C_{max}=59pg/mL; T_{max}=5 hrs. **Distribution:** Systemically administered corticosteroids are found in breast milk. **Metabolism:** Liver. **Elimination**: Kidneys, bile.

OMNARIS   RX
ciclesonide (Nycomed)

THERAPEUTIC CLASS: Non-halogenated glucocorticoid

INDICATIONS: Treatment of nasal symptoms associated with seasonal allergic rhinitis in adults and children ≥6 yrs of age. Treatment of nasal symptoms associated with perennial allergic rhinitis in adults and adolescents ≥12 yrs of age.

DOSAGE: *Adults:* Seasonal Allergic Rhinitis/Perennial Allergic Rhinitis: 2 sprays (50mcg/spray) each nostril qd.
Pediatrics: Seasonal Allergic Rhinitis: ≥6 yrs: 2 sprays (50mcg/spray) each nostril qd. Perennial Allergic Rhinitis: ≥12 yrs: 2 sprays (50mcg/spray) each nostril qd.

HOW SUPPLIED: Spray: 50mcg/spray [12.5g]

WARNINGS/PRECAUTIONS: Risk of acute adrenal insufficiency and withdrawal symptoms when replacing systemic corticosteroids with a topical corticosteroids; monitor closely. Risk for more severe/fatal course of infections (eg, chickenpox, measles); avoid exposure in patients who have not had the disease or been properly immunized. May cause growth velocity reduction in pediatrics. Monitor routinely the growth of pediatrics. May impair wound healing; avoid in recent nasal septal ulcers, nasal surgery, or nasal trauma until healed. Candida infections of the nose or pharynx may occur; examine periodically and treat accordingly. Caution in patients with active or quiescent tuberculosis infections, untreated local or systemic fungal or bacterial infections, systemic viral or parasitic infections, or ocular herpes simplex. Taper dose if symptoms of hypercorticism occur. Caution in patients with history of glaucoma and/or cataracts; monitor IOP accordingly.

ADVERSE REACTIONS: Headache, epistaxis, nasopharyngitis, ear pain, pharyngolaryngeal pain.

INTERACTIONS: Ketoconazole may increase levels of the pharmacologically active metabolite des-ciclesonide; co-administer with caution.

PREGNANCY: Category C, caution in nursing.

MECHANISM OF ACTION: Not established; glucocorticoid has an anti-inflammatory effect and other effects on multiple cell types (eg, mast cells, eosinophils, macrophages, and lymphocytes) and mediators (eg, histamine, eicosanoids, leukotrienes, and cytokines) involved in allergic inflammation.

PHARMACOKINETICS: Absorption: (50-800mcg) C_{max}<30pg/mL (adults); (25-200mcg) C_{max}<45pg/mL (pediatrics). **Metabolism:** Nasal mucosa estrases to des-ciclesonide (active metabolite) followed by liver CYP3A4, 2D6.

OMNICEF   RX
cefdinir (Abbott)

THERAPEUTIC CLASS: Cephalosporin (3rd generation)

INDICATIONS: Community-acquired pneumonia (CAP), acute exacerbations of chronic bronchitis (AECB), acute maxillary sinusitis, pharyngitis/tonsillitis, uncomplicated skin and skin structure infections (SSSI), and acute bacterial otitis media.

DOSAGE: *Adults:* (Cap) SSSI/CAP: 300mg q12h for 10 days. AECB/ Pharyngitis/Tonsillitis: 300mg q12h for 5-10 days or 600mg q24h for 10 days. Sinusitis: 300mg q12h or 600mg q24h for 10 days. CrCl <30mL/min: 300mg qd.
Pediatrics: (Sus) 6 months-12 yrs: Otitis Media/Pharyngitis/Tonsillitis: 7mg/kg q12h for 5-10 days or 14mg/kg q24h for 10 days. Sinusitis: 7mg/kg q12h or 14mg/kg q24h for 10 days. SSSI: 7mg/kg q12h or 14mg/kg q24h for 10 days. (Cap) ≥13 yrs: CAP/SSSI: 300mg q12h for 10 days. AECB/Pharyngitis/ Tonsillitis: 300mg q12h for 5-10 days or 600mg q24h for 10 days. Sinusitis: 300mg q12h or 600mg q24h for 10 days. CrCl <30mL/min/1.73m²: 7mg/kg qd. Max: 300mg qd.

HOW SUPPLIED: Cap: 300mg; Sus: 125mg/5mL, 250mg/5mL [60mL, 100mL]

WARNINGS/PRECAUTIONS: Cross-sensitivity to PCNs and other cephalosporins may occur. *Clostridium difficile*-associated diarrhea has been reported. Positive direct Coombs' tests may occur. Caution with renal dysfunction, history of colitis. Suspension contains 2.86g/5mL of sucrose; caution in diabetes. False (+) for urine glucose with Clinitest® and Benedict's or Fehling's solution.

ADVERSE REACTIONS: Diarrhea, vaginal moniliasis, nausea, headache, abdominal pain, superinfection (prolonged use).

INTERACTIONS: Iron-fortified foods, iron supplements, and aluminum- or magnesium-containing antacids reduce absorption; separate doses by 2 hrs. Probenecid inhibits the renal excretion. Reddish stools reported with iron-containing products.

PREGNANCY: Category B, safe in nursing.

MECHANISM OF ACTION: Extended-spectrum cephalosporin; bactericidal activity from inhibition of cell wall synthesis.

PHARMACOKINETICS: Absorption: Cap: (300mg) Bioavailability (21%), C_{max}=1.6µg/mL, T_{max}=2.9 hrs, AUC=7.05µg•h/mL. (600mg) Bioavailability (16%), C_{max}=2.87µg/mL, T_{max}=3 hrs, AUC=11.1µg•h/mL. Sus: (7mg/kg) Bioavailability (25%), C_{max}=2.3µg/mL, T_{max}=2.2 hrs, AUC=8.31µg•h/mL. (14mg/kg) C_{max}=3.86µg/mL, T_{max}=1.8 hrs, AUC=13.4µg•h/mL. **Distribution:** V_d=0.35L/kg (adults), 0.67L/kg (pediatrics); plasma protein binding (60-70%). **Elimination:** (300mg) Urine (18.4%); (600mg) Urine (11.6%); $T_{1/2}$=1.7 hrs.

OMNITROPE   RX
somatropin (Sandoz)

THERAPEUTIC CLASS: Human growth hormone

INDICATIONS: Long-term treatment of pediatric patients who have growth failure due to an inadequate secretion of endogenous growth hormone. Long-term replacement therapy in adults with growth hormone deficiency (GHD) of either childhood- or adult-onset etiology.

DOSAGE: *Adults:* Individualize dose. GHD: ≤0.04mg/kg/week. May increase at 4-8 week intervals. Max: 0.08mg/kg/week. Divide dose into daily SQ injections (give preferably in the evening).
Pediatrics: Individualize dose. GHD: 0.16-0.24mg/kg/week. Divide dose into daily SQ injections (give preferably in the evening).

HOW SUPPLIED: Inj: 1.5mg, 5.8mg

CONTRAINDICATIONS: Evidence of neoplastic activity. Pediatrics with fused epiphyses. Acute critical illness due to complications after open heart or abdominal surgery, multiple accidental trauma, or with acute respiratory failure. Patients with Prader-Willi syndrome who are severely obese or have severe respiratory impairment.

WARNINGS/PRECAUTIONS: Contains benzyl alcohol; avoid use in newborns. Patients with GHD secondary to an intracranial lesion should be monitored closely for progression or recurrence of underlying disease process. Monitor closely for any malignant transformation of skin lesions, scoliosis progression, or gait abnormalities. Monitor closely with DM, glucose intolerance, hypopituitarism. Intracranial HTN reported. Funduscopic exam recomended at initiation, and periodically during course of therapy.

ADVERSE REACTIONS: Hypothyroidism, elevated HbA$_{1c}$, eosinophilia, hematoma, headache, hypertriglyceridemia, leg pain.

INTERACTIONS: Growth promoting effects may be inhibited by glucocorticoids. May alter clearance of CYP450 substrates (eg, corticosteroids, sex steroids, anticonvulsants, cyclosporine); monitor closely. May need insulin dose adjustment.

PREGNANCY: Category B, caution in nursing.

MECHANISM OF ACTION: Human growth hormone; binds to dimeric GH receptor in cell membrane of target cells resulting in intracellular signal transduction.

PHARMACOKINETICS: Absorption: C$_{max}$=72mcg/mL, T$_{max}$=4 hrs. **Elimination:** T$_{1/2}$=2.8 hrs.

ONCASPAR   RX
pegaspargase (Enzon)

THERAPEUTIC CLASS: Protein synthesis inhibitor

INDICATIONS: Acute lymphoblastic leukemia in patients who have developed hypersensitivity to the native forms of L-asparaginase. May be given as monotherapy if multi-agent therapy is inappropriate.

DOSAGE: *Adults:* Usual: 2500 IU/m^2 IM or IV every 14 days.
Pediatrics: 1-9 yrs: 2500 IU/m^2 IM on Day 3 of 4-Week induction phase and on Day 3 of each of two 8-Week delayed intensifications phases.

HOW SUPPLIED: Inj: 750 IU/mL [5mL]

CONTRAINDICATIONS: Pancreatitis. History of pancreatitis, significant hemorrhagic events, or serious thrombosis with prior L-asparaginase therapy.

WARNINGS/PRECAUTIONS: May be a contact irritant. Avoid inhalation or contact with skin or mucous membranes. Serious allergic reaction, pancreatitis, or glucose intolerance can occur. Increased prothrombin time, partial thromboplastin time, and hypofibrinogenemia can occur; monitor coagulation parameters. May predispose to infections, bleeding, thrombosis. D/C in patients with serious thrombotic event including sagittal sinus thrombosis.

ADVERSE REACTIONS: Allergic reactions (including anaphylaxis), CNS thrombosis, coagulopathy, elevated transaminases, hyperbilirubinemia, hyperglycemia, pancreatitis.

INTERACTIONS: May increase toxicity of protein bound drugs. May interfere with the action of drugs that require cell replication for their lethal effects (eg, methotrexate), and the enzymatic detoxification of other drugs, particularly in the liver. Caution with concomitant anticoagulants (eg, coumadin, heparin, dipyridamole, ASA, or NSAIDs), hepatotoxic agents.

PREGNANCY: Category C, not for use in nursing.

MECHANISM OF ACTION: Protein synthesis inhibitor; selectively kills leukemic cells due to depletion of plasma asparagine.

PHARMACOKINETICS: Elimination: T$_{1/2}$=5.8 days.

ONTAK   RX
denileukin diftitox (Eisai)

> Should only be administered under the supervision of a physician experienced in the use of antineoplastic therapy and management of cancer patients. Facility must be equipped and staffed for cardiopulmonary resuscitation.

THERAPEUTIC CLASS: Fusion protein

INDICATIONS: Treatment of persistent or recurrent cutaneous T-cell lymphoma whose malignant cells express the CD25 component of the interleukin-2 (IL-2) receptor.

DOSAGE: *Adults:* Treatment Cycle: 9 or 18mcg/kg/day IV for 5 consecutive days, every 21 days. Infuse over at least 15 min. D/C or reduce infusion rate (up to 80 min) if infusional adverse reactions occur.

HOW SUPPLIED: Inj: 150mcg/mL

CONTRAINDICATIONS: Hypersensitivity to IL-2 or diphtheria toxin.

WARNINGS/PRECAUTIONS: Hypersensitivity reactions reported. Vascular leak syndrome reported; caution with pre-existing cardiovascular disease. Pre-existing low serum albumin may increase risk of syndrome; monitor weight, edema, BP, and serum albumin levels. Monitor for infection. Test malignant cells for CD25 expression prior to therapy. Perform CBC, blood chemistry panel, liver and renal function, and serum albumin prior to and weekly during therapy. Hypoalbuminemia reported; delay therapy until serum albumin ≥3g/dL. Loss of visual acuity, usually with loss of color vision, with or without retinal pigment mottling reported.

ADVERSE REACTIONS: Chills/fever, asthenia, hypotension, nausea, vomiting, infection, pain, headache, anorexia, diarrhea, hypoalbuminemia, anemia, transaminase increase, myalgia, dizziness, dyspnea, cough increase, rash, infusion-associated reactions.

PREGNANCY: Category C, not for use in nursing.

MECHANISM OF ACTION: Fusion protein; interacts with high affinity IL-2 receptor on cell surface and inhibits cellular protein synthesis resulting in cell death.

PHARMACOKINETICS: Distribution: V_d=0.06-0.08L/kg. **Metabolism:** Proteolytic degradation. **Elimination:** $T_{1/2}$ =70-80 min.

OPANA ER CII
oxymorphone HCL (Endo)

> (Tab, Extended-Release) Abuse liability and potential. For continuous analgesia only; not intended for prn use. To be swallowed whole; not to be broken, chewed, dissolved, or crushed. Must not be taken with alcohol.

OTHER BRAND NAMES: Opana (Endo)

THERAPEUTIC CLASS: Opioid analgesic

INDICATIONS: (Tab) Relief of moderate to severe acute pain. (Tab, Extended-Release) Relief of moderate to severe pain in patients requiring continuous, around-the-clock opioid treatment for extended period of time.

DOSAGE: *Adults:* Individualize dose. Opana: Opioid-Naive: Initial: 5-20mg q4-6h. Titrate based on response. Max: 20mg/dose. Conversion from Parenteral Oxymorphone: Give 10x total daily parenteral oxymorphone dose in 4 or 6 equally divided doses. Conversion from Other Oral Opioids: Give half of calculated total daily dose in 4-6 equally divided doses, q4-6h. Opana ER: Swallow whole; do not break, chew, crush, or dissolve. Opioid-Naive: Initial: 5mg q12h. Titrate based on response. Usual: Increase dose by 5-10mg q12h every 3-7 days. Conversion from Opana: Divide 24h Opana dose in half to obtain q12h dose. Conversion from Parenteral Oxymorphone: Give 10x total daily parenteral oxymorphone dose in 2 equally divided doses. Conversion from Other Oral Opioids: Divide calculated 24h Opana dose (refer to PI for conversion ratios) in half to obtain q12h dose. Mild Hepatic Impairment or Renal Impairment (CrCl <50mL/min): Start with lowest dose and titrate slowly while carefully monitoring side effects. With CNS Depressants: Start at 1/3 to 1/2 of usual dose. Elderly: Start at lower end of dosing range.

HOW SUPPLIED: Tab: (Opana) 5mg, 10mg; Tab, Extended-Release: (Opana ER) 5mg, 7.5mg, 10mg, 15mg, 20mg, 30mg, 40mg

CONTRAINDICATIONS: Respiratory depression (except in monitored settings with resuscitative equipment), acute/severe bronchial asthma or hypercarbia, paralytic ileus, moderate/severe hepatic impairment. (Opana ER) Not indicated for pain in immediate post-operative period (12-24 hrs following surgery) for patients not previously taking opioids or, if the pain is mild or not expected to persist for extended period of time.

WARNINGS/PRECAUTIONS: Schedule II controlled substance with abuse liability. May have additive effects in conjunction with alcohol, other opioids, or illicit drugs that cause CNS depression; respiratory depression, hypotension, and profound sedation or coma may result. Extreme caution with hypoxia, hypercapnia, or decreased respiratory reserve. With head injury, intracranial lesions or a pre-existing increase in ICP, possible respiratory depressant effects and potential to elevate CSF pressure may be markedly exaggerated; effects on pupillary response and consciousness may obscure neurologic signs of further increases in ICP with head injuries. May cause severe hypotension with compromised ability to maintain BP due to depleted blood volume. Caution in elderly or debilitated patients sensitive to CNS depressants. Caution with circulatory shock, acute alcoholism, adrenocortical insufficiency (eg, Addison's disease), CNS depression or coma, delirium tremens, kyphoscoliosis associated with respiratory depression, myxedema or hypothyroidism, prostatic hypertrophy or urethral stricture, severe impairment of pulmonary or renal function, mild/moderate hepatic impairment and toxic psychosis. May aggravate convulsions with convulsive disorders; may induce or aggravate seizures in some clinical settings. Monitor for decreased bowel motility in post-op patients. May cause spasm of the sphincter of Oddi; caution with biliary tract disease (including acute pancreatitis). May produce tolerance and dependence. Should not abruptly d/c, may cause abstinence syndrome in physically-dependent patients.

ADVERSE REACTIONS: Constipation, nausea, pyrexia, somnolence, headache, dizziness, vomiting, pruritis, increased sweating, xerostomia, sedation, diarrhea, insomnia, fatigue, tachycardia, miosis, biliary colic, hypotension.

INTERACTIONS: Additive CNS depression with other CNS depressants (eg, sedatives, hypnotics, tranquilizers, general anesthetics, phenothiazines, other opioids, alcohol); reduce dose of either/both agents. Caution with concomitant use of MAOIs; reduce dose of either/both agents. Anticholinergics may increase risk of urinary retention and/or severe constipation, which may lead to paralytic ileus. CNS toxicity (eg, confusion, disorientation, respiratory depression, apnea, seizures) reported with cimetidine. Avoid use with mixed agonist/antagonist opioid analgesics, may reduce effect and/or precipitate withdrawal symptoms.

PREGNANCY: Category C, caution with nursing.

MECHANISM OF ACTION: Opioid analgesic; an opioid agonist. Prescise mechanism of analgesic action not established. However, specific CNS opioid receptors for endogenous compounds with opioid-like activity have been found throughout the brain and spinal cord and play a role in the analgesic effects. Opioid receptors have also been found in the peripheral nervous system.

PHARMACOKINETICS: Absorption: Absolute bioavailability (10%); various doses led to altered parameters. **Distribution:** Plasma protein binding (10-12%); crosses the placenta. **Metabolism:** Liver (conjugation) to form oxymorphone-3-glucuronide (major metabolite), 6-OH-oxymorphone (major active metabolite). **Elimination:** Urine (<1% unchanged), feces.

Opcon-A   OTC
naphazoline HCL - pheniramine maleate (Bausch & Lomb)

THERAPEUTIC CLASS: H₁-antagonist/alpha-agonist (imidazoline)

INDICATIONS: Temporary relief of redness and itching of the eye due to various allergens.

DOSAGE: *Adults:* 1-2 drops up to qid.
Pediatrics: ≥6 yrs: 1-2 drops up to qid.

HOW SUPPLIED: Sol: (Pheniramine-Naphazoline) 0.3%-0.027% [15mL]

CONTRAINDICATIONS: Cardiovascular disease, HTN, narrow angle glaucoma, BPH.

WARNINGS/PRECAUTIONS: D/C if pain, vision changes, no improvement, condition worsens or persists >72 hrs. Remove contact lens before use. Overuse may produce increased redness of eye. Temporary pupil enlargement may occur. Supervision required with heart disease, high BP, difficulty in urination due to prostate enlargement, or narrow angle glaucoma.

ADVERSE REACTIONS: Brief tingling sensation.

PREGNANCY: Safety in pregnancy and nursing not known.

OptiNate
folic acid - multiple vitamin - minerals - iron (Sciele)
RX

THERAPEUTIC CLASS: Prenatal vitamin

INDICATIONS: Vitamin and mineral supplementation for before, during, and after pregnancy.

DOSAGE: *Adults:* One tablet and one L-Vcaps capsule qd. Max: Do not exceed 1g/day of DHA.

HOW SUPPLIED: Cap: (L-Vcaps) Docosahexaenoic Acid (DHA) 250mg. Tab: Biotin 0.03mg-Calcium 200mg-Copper 2mg-Docusate Sodium 50mg-Folate 1mg-Iron 90mg-Magnesium 30mg-Niacinamide 20mg-Pantothenic Acid 6mg-Vitamin B_1 3mg-Vitamin B_2 3.4mg-Vitamin B_6 20mg-Vitamin B_{12} 0.012mg-Vitamin C 120mg-Vitamin D_3 400 IU-Vitamin E 10 IU-Zinc 15mg

WARNINGS/PRECAUTIONS: Accidental overdose of iron-containing products is a leading cause of fatal poisoning in children <6 yrs. Omega-3 fatty acids >3g/day may increase bleeding time and INR; avoid in patients with inherited or acquired bleeding diathesis. Folic acid alone is improper treatment of pernicious anemia and other megaloblastic anemias with vitamin B_{12}-deficiency. Folic acid >0.1mg/day may obscure pernicious anemia.

ADVERSE REACTIONS: Allergic sensitization

INTERACTIONS: Avoid with anticoagulants. DHA component has potential antithrombotic effects.

MECHANISM OF ACTION: Multivitamin/multimineral nutritional supplement.

OptiPranolol
metipranolol (Bausch & Lomb)
RX

THERAPEUTIC CLASS: Nonselective beta-blocker

INDICATIONS: Treatment of elevated intraocular pressure (IOP) in ocular hypertension or open angle glaucoma.

DOSAGE: *Adults:* 1 drop in affected eye bid.

HOW SUPPLIED: Sol: 0.3% [5mL, 10mL]

CONTRAINDICATIONS: Bronchial asthma, severe COPD, symptomatic sinus bradycardia, greater than 1st-degree AV block, cardiogenic shock, overt cardiac failure.

WARNINGS/PRECAUTIONS: May be absorbed systemically. Severe respiratory and cardiac reactions may occur. Caution with heart failure, DM, cerebrovascular insufficiency, and in those with a history of anaphylactic reactions. May mask signs of hyperthyroidism; abrupt withdrawal may precipitate a thyroid storm. May cause muscle weakness. Withdraw gradually before surgery. Avoid with COPD.

ADVERSE REACTIONS: Abnormal vision, blepharitis, photophobia, uveitis, conjunctivitis, eyelid dermatitis, allergic reactions.

INTERACTIONS: Additive systemic blockade with oral β-blockers. Additive hypotension or bradycardia with catecholamine-depleting agents (eg, reserpine). CCBs may precipitate left ventricular dysfunction and hypotension. Digoxin and CCBs may prolong AV conduction. Caution with adrenergic psychotropics. Effects can be reversed by β-agonists. Use with miotic agent in angle-closure glaucoma.

O

PREGNANCY: Category C, caution in nursing.

MECHANISM OF ACTION: Nonselective β-adrenoreceptor blocker: Reduces elevated as well as normal IOP. Responsible for reducing aqueous humor production and possibly increasing the outflow of aqueous humor. β-adrenergic blockers, when administered orally, produce a reduction in cardiac output and an increase in bronchi and bronchioles airway resistance.

PHARMACOKINETICS: Absorption: T_{max}=2 hrs.

OPTIVAR RX
azelastine HCL (MedPointe)

THERAPEUTIC CLASS: H_1-antagonist

INDICATIONS: Treatment of itching of the eye associated with allergic conjunctivitis.

DOSAGE: *Adults:* 1 drop bid.
Pediatrics: ≥3 yrs: 1 drop bid.

HOW SUPPLIED: Sol: 0.05% [6mL]

WARNINGS/PRECAUTIONS: Not for injection or oral use. Do not wear contact lens if the eye is red. Not for treatment of contact-lens irritation. Wait 10 min after instilling drops to insert contact lens.

ADVERSE REACTIONS: Transient eye burning/stinging, headaches, asthma, conjunctivitis, dyspnea, eye pain, fatigue, influenza-like symptoms, pharyngitis, pruritus, rhinitis, temporary blurring.

PREGNANCY: Category C, caution in nursing.

MECHANISM OF ACTION: Antihistaminic agent; relatively selective H_1-receptor antagonist; inhibits release of histamine and other mediators from cells (eg, mast cells) involved in the allergic response and decreases chemotaxis and activation of eosinophils.

PHARMACOKINETICS: Metabolism: N-desmethylazelastine (principle metabolite).

ORACEA RX
doxycycline (CollaGenex)

THERAPEUTIC CLASS: Tetracycline derivative

INDICATIONS: Treatment of only inflammatory lesions (papules and pustules) of rosacea.

DOSAGE: *Adults:* 40mg qd in am. Take on empty stomach.

HOW SUPPLIED: Cap: 40mg (30mg Immediate-Release and 10mg Delayed-Release beads)

WARNINGS/PRECAUTIONS: May cause fetal harm during pregnancy. Use during tooth development (last half of pregnancy, infancy, ≤8 yrs) may cause permanent discoloration of teeth or enamel hypoplasia. Pseudomembranous colitis reported. Caution in patients with renal impairment. May cause superinfection, photosensitivity, increase in BUN, bacterial resistance, autoimmune syndromes and hyperpigmentation. Bulging fontanels in infants and benign intracranial HTN in adults reported.

ADVERSE REACTIONS: Nasopharyngitis, sinusitis, fungal infection, influenza, diarrhea, HTN, pharyngolaryngeal pain, nasal congestion, abdominal pain, dry mouth, anxiety, sinus headache.

INTERACTIONS: May require downward adjustments of anticoagulant dosage. May interfere with bactericidal action of penicillin; avoid concurrent use when possible. Concomitant use with methoxyflurane may result in fatal renal toxicity. Bismuth subsalicylate, proton pump inhibitors, antacids containing aluminum, calcium or magnesium and iron-containing preparations may impair absorption. May interfere with the effectiveness of oral contraceptives.

Avoid concurrent use with oral retinoids (eg, isotetinoin). False elevations of urinary catecholamine levels may occur.

PREGNANCY: Category D, not for use in nursing.

MECHANISM OF ACTION: Tetracycline derivative. Antibacterial agent; does not produce any long-term effects on bacterial flora in the oral cavity, skin, intestinal tract, or vagina.

PHARMACOKINETICS: Absorption: Single Dose: C_{max}=510ng/mL; T_{max}=3 hrs; AUC=9227ng•hr/mL. Multiple Doses: C_{max}=600ng/mL; T_{max}=2 hrs; AUC=7543ng•hr/mL. **Distribution**: Plasma protein binding (>90%), crosses the placenta, excreted in human breast milk. **Elimination**: Urine, feces; $T_{1/2}$=21.2 hrs (single dose), 23.2 hrs (multiple doses).

ORAMORPH SR
morphine sulfate (Xanodyne)

CII

> This is a sustained-release tablet. Swallow tab whole; do not break in half, crush or chew.

THERAPEUTIC CLASS: Opioid analgesic

INDICATIONS: Relief of pain in patients who require opioid analgesics for more than a few days.

DOSAGE: *Adults:* Conversion from Parenteral or Immediate Release Oral Morphine: Daily dose determined by daily requirement of immediate-release formulation. Single dose is 1/2 of daily requirement given q12h. Initial: 30mg is recommended if daily morphine requirement is ≤120mg. Use 15mg for low daily morphine requirements. Titrate: Increase to 60mg or 100mg after stable dose reached.

HOW SUPPLIED: Tab, Extended-Release: 15mg, 30mg, 60mg, 100mg

CONTRAINDICATIONS: Respiratory depression in the absence of resuscitative equipment, acute or severe bronchial asthma, paralytic ileus.

WARNINGS/PRECAUTIONS: Not for initial treatment. Caution with hepatic and renal dysfunction, increased ICP or with head injury, decreased respiratory reserve (eg, emphysema, severe obesity, kyphoscoliosis, or paralysis of the phrenic nerve), chronic asthma, upper airway obstruction, or in other chronic pulmonary disorders. Tolerance, psychological and physical dependence may develop. Avoid abrupt discontinuation. Not for pediatrics or use in women during or immediately before labor.

ADVERSE REACTIONS: Constipation, nausea, vomiting, dizziness, sedation, dysphoria, euphoria, and sweating, respiratory depression.

INTERACTIONS: Potentiated depressant effects with CNS depressants, alcohol, sedatives, antihistaminics, or psychotropics. Increased risk of respiratory depression, hypotension, sedation and coma with neuroleptics. Mixed agonist/antagonist opioid analgesics (eg, pentazocine, nalbuphine, butorphanol, or buprenorphine) may alter effect or precipitate withdrawal symptoms.

PREGNANCY: Category C, not for use in nursing.

MECHANISM OF ACTION: Opioid analgesic; interacts predominantly with μ-receptor. μ binding sites are found distributed in the brain, spinal cord, and in trigeminal nerve. Primary actions are analgesia and sedation.

PHARMACOKINETICS: Absorption: Absolute bioavailability (40%), oral administration of variable doses resulted in different parameters. **Distribution:** V_d=4L/kg; crosses the placental membrane, found in breast milk. **Metabolism:** Liver to glucuronide metabolites; morphine-3-glucuronide (major metabolite), morphine-6-glucuronide (active metabolite). **Elimination:** Kidneys (major), feces (10%), bile (small amount); $T_{1/2}$=2-4 hrs.

ORAP
pimozide (Gate)

RX

THERAPEUTIC CLASS: Diphenylbutylperidine

INDICATIONS: Suppression of motor and phonic tics in Tourette's syndrome in patients that failed standard therapy.

DOSAGE: *Adults:* Initial: 1-2mg/day in divided doses. May increase every other day. Maint: <0.2mg/kg/day or 10mg/day, whichever is less. Max: 0.2mg/kg/day or 10mg/day.
Pediatrics: >12 yrs: Initial: 0.05mg/kg qhs. Titrate: May increase every 3 days. Max: 0.2mg/kg/day or 10mg/day.

HOW SUPPLIED: Tab: 1mg*, 2mg* *scored

CONTRAINDICATIONS: Severe CNS depression, comatose states, congenital long QT syndrome, history of cardiac arrhythmias, hypokalemia, hypomagnesemia, simple tics or tics not associated with Tourette's syndrome. CYP3A4 inhibitors (eg, nefazadone, macrolide antibiotics, azole antifungals, protease inhibitors), sertraline, and drugs that cause motor and phonic tics (eg, pemoline, methylphenidate, amphetamines) or prolong the QT interval.

WARNINGS/PRECAUTIONS: May cause tardive dyskinesia, NMS, hyperpyrexia. Caution with history of seizures, EEG abnormalities, severe hepatic/renal impairment. Perform ECG before therapy, periodically thereafter, with dose adjustment. Produces anticholinergic effects. Sudden death reported. May impair mental/physical abilities.

ADVERSE REACTIONS: Akinesia, QT prolongation, tardive dyskinesia, sedation, loss of libido, constipation, dry mouth, visual disturbances, headache, asthenia, increased salivation.

INTERACTIONS: May potentiate CNS depressants (eg, analgesics, sedatives, anxiolytics, alcohol). Bradycardia reported with fluoxetine. Avoid grapefruit juice, CYP3A4 inhibitors (eg, azole antifungal drugs, macrolides, protease inhibitors, zileuton, fluvoxamine), sertraline. May interact with CYP1A2 inhibitors. Avoid other drugs that may potentiate QT prolongation such as phenothiazines, TCAs, antiarrhythmics, sparfloxacin, gatifloxacin, moxifloxacin, halofantrine, mefloquine, pentamidine, arsenic trioxide, levomethadyl acetate, dolasetron mesylate, probucol, tacrolimus, ziprasidone.

PREGNANCY: Category C, not for use in nursing.

MECHANISM OF ACTION: Antipsychotic agent; not established. Blocks dopaminergic receptors on neurons in the CNS.

PHARMACOKINETICS: Absorption: T_{max}=6-8 hrs. **Metabolism:** Liver (extensive) through N-dealkylation mediated CYP 3A4. Metabolites: 1-(4-piperidyl)-2-benzimidazoline and 4,4-bis (4-fluorophenyl) butyric acid. **Elimination:** Urine; $T_{1/2}$=55 hrs.

ORAPRED RX
prednisolone sodium phosphate (Biomarin)

OTHER BRAND NAMES: Orapred ODT (Alliant)

THERAPEUTIC CLASS: Glucocorticoid

INDICATIONS: Steroid-responsive disorders.

DOSAGE: *Adults:* (Sol) Initial: 5-60mg/day depending on disease and response. (Tab) Initial: 10-60mg/day depending on disease and response. Maint: Decrease dose by small amounts to lowest effective dose. (Sol/Tab) MS Exacerbations: 200mg qd for 1 week, then 80mg every other day for 1 month. *Pediatrics:* (Sol/Tab) Initial: 0.14-2mg/kg/day, depending on disease and response, given tid-qid. Nephrotic Syndrome: 20mg/m² tid for 4 weeks, then 40mg/m² every other day for 4 weeks. Uncontrolled Asthma: 1-2mg/kg/day in single or divided doses until peak expiratory flow rate of 80% is achieved (usually 3-10 days).

HOW SUPPLIED: Sol: 15mg/5mL [237mL]; Tab, Orally Disintegrating: 10mg, 15mg, 30mg

CONTRAINDICATIONS: Systemic fungal infections.

WARNINGS/PRECAUTIONS: May produce reversible HPA axis suppression. Adjust dose during stress or change in thyroid status. May mask signs of infection or cause new infections. May activate latent amebiasis. Avoid with cerebral malaria. Avoid exposure to chickenpox or measles. Not for treatment of optic neuritis or active ocular herpes simplex. May cause elevation of BP or IOP, cataracts, glaucoma, optic nerve damage, Kaposi's sarcoma, psychic derangements, salt/water retention, increased excretion of potassium and/or calcium, osteoporosis, growth suppression in children, secondary ocular infections. Caution with Strongyloides, CHF, diverticulitis, HTN, renal insufficiency, fresh intestinal anastomoses, active or latent peptic ulcer, ulcerative colitis. Enhanced effect in hypothyroidism or cirrhosis. Avoid abrupt withdrawal.

ADVERSE REACTIONS: Edema, fluid/electrolyte disturbances, osteoporosis, muscle weakness, pancreatitis, peptic ulcer, impaired wound healing, increased intracranial pressure, cushingoid state, hirsutism, menstrual irregularities, growth suppression in children, glaucoma, nausea, weight gain.

INTERACTIONS: Enhanced metabolism with barbiturates, phenytoin, ephedrine, and rifampin. Use with cyclosporine may increase activity of both drugs; convulsions reported with concomitant use. Decreased metabolism with estrogens or ketoconazole. May inhibit response to warfarin. Increased risk of GI side effects with ASA or other NSAIDs. May increase clearance of salicylates. High doses or concurrent neuromuscular drugs may cause acute myopathy. Enhanced possibility of hypokalemia when given with potassium-depleting agents. May produce severe weakness in myasthenia gravis patients on anticholinesterase agents. Avoid live vaccines with immunosuppressive doses. Possible diminished response with killed or inactivated vaccines. May increase blood glucose; adjust antidiabetic agents. May suppress reactions to skin tests.

PREGNANCY: Category C, caution in nursing.

MECHANISM OF ACTION: Synthetic adrenocorticoid steroid; promotes gluconeogenesis, increases deposition of glycogen in the liver, inhibits glucose utilization, increases catabolism of protein, lipolysis, glomerular filtration that leads to increased urinary excretion of urate and calcium.

PHARMACOKINETICS: Absorption: Readily absorbed from GI tract. **Distribution:** Plasma protein binding (70-90%), found in breast milk. **Metabolism:** Liver. **Elimination:** Urine (as sulfate and glucuronide conjugates), $T_{1/2}$=2-4 hrs.

ORENCIA   RX
abatacept (Bristol-Myers Squibb)

THERAPEUTIC CLASS: Selective costimulation modulator

INDICATIONS: To reduce signs and symptoms, inducing major clinical response, inhibiting the progression of structural damage, and improving physical function in adult patients with moderately to severely active rheumatoid arthritis who have had an inadequate response to one or more disease-modifying, anti-rheumatic drugs (DMARDs) (eg, MTX, TNF antagonists). May be used as monotherapy or concomitantly with DMARDs other than TNF-antagonists. For reducing signs and symptoms in pediatric patients ≥6 yrs with moderately to severely active polyarticular juvenile idiopathic arthritis. May be used as monotherapy or concomitantly with MTX.

DOSAGE: *Adults:* Initial: <60kg: 500mg; 60-100kg: 750mg; >100kg: 1g IV over 30 min. Maint: Give at 2 and 4 weeks after initial infusion, then every 4 weeks thereafter.
Pediatrics: 6-17 yrs: >75 kg: Follow adult dosing regimen. Max: 1000mg; <75kg: Initial: 10mg/kg IV over 30 min. Maint: Give at 2 and 4 weeks after initial infusion, then every 4 weeks thereafter.

HOW SUPPLIED: Inj: 250mg

WARNINGS/PRECAUTIONS: Increased risk of infections and serious infections with concomitant TNF-antagonist therapy; concurrent use not recommended. Anaphylaxis or anaphylactoid reactions reported. Caution with history of recurrent infections; d/c if serious infections develop. Screen for latent TB prior to initiation. Avoid live vaccines. Caution with COPD. Concurrent use with anakinra is not recommended. Cases of lung cancer and lymphoma reported. Screening for viral hepatitis is recommended before initiation of therapy. Juvenile idiopathic arthritis patients should be brought up to date with all immunizations prior to therapy.

ADVERSE REACTIONS: Headache, nasopharyngitis, dizziness, cough, back pain, HTN, dyspepsia, UTI, rash, pain in extremities.

INTERACTIONS: See Warnings/Precautions.

PREGNANCY: Category C, not for use in nursing.

MECHANISM OF ACTION: Selective costimulation modulator; inhibits T cell activation by binding to CD80 and CD86, thereby blocking interaction with CD28.

PHARMACOKINETICS: Absorption: C_{max}=292mcg/mL. **Distribution:** V_d=0.09L/Kg. **Elimination:** $T_{1/2}$=16.7 days.

ORFADIN   RX
nitisinone (Rare Disease Therapeutics)

THERAPEUTIC CLASS: Nitisinone

INDICATIONS: Adjunct to dietary restriction of tyrosine and phenylalanine in the treatment of hereditary tyrosinemia type I.

DOSAGE: *Adults:* Initial: 1mg/kg/day in divided doses, qam and qpm. Titrate: Increase to 1.5mg/kg/day if biochemical parameters (except plasma succinylacetone) are not normalized within 1 month. Max: 2mg/kg/day. Take at least 1 hr before a meal. May sprinkle contents of capsule in small amount of water, formula, or applesauce immediately before use.
Pediatrics: Initial: 1mg/kg/day in divided doses, qam and qpm. Titrate: Increase to 1.5mg/kg/day if biochemical parameters (except plasma succinylacetone) are not normalized within 1 month. Max: 2mg/kg/day. Take at least 1 hr before a meal. May sprinkle contents of capsule in small amount of water, formula, or applesauce immediately before use.

HOW SUPPLIED: Cap: 2mg, 5mg, 10mg

WARNINGS/PRECAUTIONS: Inadequate restriction of tyrosine and phenylalanine can result in elevated tyrosine levels. Maintain tyrosine levels <500μmol/L to avoid toxicity. Transient thrombocytopenia and leucopenia reported; monitor platelet and WBC count. Perform slit-lamp eye examination before initiation and if patient develops photophobia, eye pain or inflammation. Do not adjust dose further to lower tyrosine levels; may deteriorate patient's condition; use diet restriction instead. Increased risk of porphyric crises, liver failure, or hepatic neoplasms; monitor liver by imaging and lab tests including serum alpha-fetoprotein. Monitor urine succinylacetone levels to guide dose adjustment. Monitor serum phosphate to screen for renal involvement.

ADVERSE REACTIONS: Hepatic neoplasm, liver failure, conjunctivitis, corneal opacity, keratitis, photophobia, thrombocytopenia, leucopenia.

PREGNANCY: Category C, caution in nursing.

MECHANISM OF ACTION: Competitevely inhibits 4-hydroxyphenyl-pyruvate dioxygenase, an enzyme upstream of FAH in the tyrosine catabolic pathways, thereby preventing accumulation of the catabolic intermediates maleylacetoacetate and fumarylacetoacetate, which is converted to the toxic metabolite succinylacetone and succinylacetoacetate.

PHARMACOKINETICS: Absoption: T_{max}=3 hrs. **Elimination:** $T_{1/2}$=54 hrs.

ORTHO EVRA   RX
ethinyl estradiol - norelgestromin (Ortho-McNeil)

THERAPEUTIC CLASS: Estrogen/progestogen combination

INDICATIONS: Prevention of pregnancy.

DOSAGE: *Adults:* Start 1st Sunday after menses begin or 1st day of menses. Apply patch every week on same day for 3 weeks. Week 4 is patch-free. Apply to clean, dry intact skin on buttock, abdomen, upper arm, or upper torso.

HOW SUPPLIED: Patch: (Ethinyl Estradiol-Norelgestromin): 0.75mg-6mg [1ˢ, 3ˢ]

CONTRAINDICATIONS: Thrombophlebitis, DVT, thromboembolic disorders, pregnancy, cerebrovascular or coronary artery disease, valvular heart disease with complications, undiagnosed abnormal genital bleeding, cholestatic jaundice of pregnancy or jaundice with prior pill use, hepatic adenomas or carcinomas, breast cancer or other estrogen-dependent neoplasia, severe HTN, diabetes with vascular involvement, headaches with focal neurological symptoms, major surgery with prolonged immobilization, acute/chronic hepatocellular disease with abnormal liver function.

WARNINGS/PRECAUTIONS: Cigarette smoking increases risk of serious cardiovascular side effects. This risk increases with age (especially >35 yrs) and heavy smoking. Increased risk of MI, vascular disease, thromboembolism, stroke, and gallbladder disease. Retinal thrombosis, hepatic neoplasia reported. May cause glucose intolerance. May increase BP, elevate LDL levels or cause other lipid changes, fluid retention, breakthrough bleeding, and spotting. May cause or exacerbate migraine. May develop visual changes with contact lens. Increased risk of MI with HTN, hyperlipidemia, and diabetes. D/C if jaundice or depression develops. Perform annual physical exam. Use before menarche is not indicated. May affect certain endocrine, LFTs, and blood components. May be less effective in women with body weight ≥198 lbs.

ADVERSE REACTIONS: Breast symptoms, headache, application site reaction, nausea, upper respiratory infection, menstrual cramps, abdominal pain.

INTERACTIONS: Reduced effects and increased breakthrough bleeding with rifampin, barbiturates, phenylbutazone, phenytoin, carbamazepine, topiramate, St. John's wort, griseofulvin, felbamate, oxycarbazepine, possibly with ampicillin. Protease inhibitors alter levels. Increased levels with atorvastatin, ascorbic acid, acetaminophen, and CYP3A4 inhibitors (eg, itraconazole, ketoconazole). May increase levels of cyclosporine, prednisolone, theophylline. May decrease levels of acetaminophen and increase clearance of temazepam, salicylic acid, morphine, and clofibric acid.

PREGNANCY: Category X, not for use in nursing.

MECHANISM OF ACTION: Contraceptive; suppresses gonadotropin, inhibits ovulation, promotes changes in cervical mucus (which increases difficulty of sperm entry into uterus) and the endometrium (which reduce likelihood of implantation).

PHARMACOKINETICS: Absorption: Norelgestromin: C_{max}=0.305-1.53ng/mL, AUC_{0-168}=107ng•h/mL. Ethinyl estradiol: C_{max}=11.2-137pg/mL, AUC_{0-168}=6796pg•h/mL. **Distribution:** Norelgestromin: Serum protein binding (>97%). Ethinyl estradiol: Serum albumin binding (extensive). **Metabolism:** GI tract and/or liver (1st pass metabolism). **Elimination:** Norelgestromin: Urine, feces; $T_{1/2}$=28 hrs. Ethinyl estradiol: Urine, feces; $T_{1/2}$=17 hrs.

ORTHO TRI-CYCLEN   RX
ethinyl estradiol - norgestimate (Ortho-McNeil)

OTHER BRAND NAMES: Tri-Previfem (Teva) - Tri-Sprintec (Barr)

THERAPEUTIC CLASS: Estrogen/progestogen combination

INDICATIONS: Prevention of pregnancy. Treatment of acne vulgaris in females ≥15 yrs who want contraception, have achieved menarche and are unresponsive to topical acne agents.

DOSAGE: *Adults:* Contraception/Acne: 28-day: 1 tab qd for 28 days, then repeat. Start 1st Sunday after menses begin or 1st day of menses.
Pediatrics: Contraception (postpubertal adolescents)/Acne: 28-day: 1 tab qd for 28 days, then repeat. Start 1st Sunday after menses begin or 1st day of menses.

HOW SUPPLIED: Tab: (Ethinyl Estradiol-Norgestimate) 0.035mg-0.18mg, 0.035mg-0.215mg, 0.035mg-0.25mg

CONTRAINDICATIONS: Thrombophlebitis, deep vein thrombophlebitis, thromboembolic disorders, pregnancy, cerbrovascular or coronary artery disease, migraine with focal aura, acute or chronic hepatocellular disease with abnormal liver function, undiagnosed abnormal genital bleeding, cholestatic jaundice of pregnancy or jaundice with prior pill use, hepatic adenomas or carcinomas, breast cancer, endometrium carcinoma, or other estrogen-dependent neoplasia.

WARNINGS/PRECAUTIONS: Cigarette smoking increases risk of serious cardiovascular side effects. This risk increases with age (especially >35 yrs) and heavy smoking. Increased risk of MI, vascular disease, thromboembolism, stroke, and gallbladder disease. Retinal thrombosis, hepatic neoplasia, carcinoma of breast and reproductive organs reported. May cause glucose intolerance, fluid retention, breakthrough bleeding, and spotting. May increase BP, elevate LDL levels, or cause other lipid changes. May cause or exacerbate migraine. May develop visual changes with contact lens. Increased risk of morbidity and mortality with HTN, hyperlipidemia, obesity, and diabetes. D/C if jaundice, significant depression, or ophthalmic irregularities develop. Perform annual physical exam. Use before menarche is not indicated. May affect certain endocrine, LFTs, and blood components.

ADVERSE REACTIONS: Nausea, vomiting, breakthrough bleeding, spotting, amenorrhea, migraine, depression, vaginal candidiasis, edema, weight changes.

INTERACTIONS: Reduced effects, increased breakthrough bleeding, and menstrual irregularities with rifampin, barbiturates, phenylbutazone, phenytoin, carbamazepine, griseofulvin, topiramate, St. John's wort, and possibly with ampicillin and tetracyclines.

PREGNANCY: Category X, not for use in nursing.

MECHANISM OF ACTION: Estrogen/progestogen oral contraceptive; acts by suppressing gonadotropin, inhibiting ovulation, and causing other alterations, including changes in cervical mucus, (which increases difficulty of sperm entry into uterus) and endometrium (which reduces likehood of implantation).

PHARMACOKINETICS: Absorption: Rapid. Oral administration on various days during dosing led to altered parameters. **Distribution:** Norgestimate: Albumin binding (>97%). Ethinyl estradiol: Albumin binding (>97%). **Metabolism:** Norgestimate: GI tract and/or liver (1st pass mechanism). Norelgestromin (primary active metabolite): Hepatic, norgestrel (active metabolite). Ethinyl estradiol: Hydroxylated, glucuronide, sulfate conjugates. **Elimination:** Norgestimate: Urine (47%), feces (37%).

ORTHO TRI-CYCLEN LO   RX
ethinyl estradiol - norgestimate (Ortho-McNeil)

THERAPEUTIC CLASS: Estrogen/progestogen combination

INDICATIONS: Prevention of pregnancy.

DOSAGE: *Adults:* 1 tab qd for 28 days, then repeat. Start 1st Sunday after menses begin or 1st day of menses.

HOW SUPPLIED: Tab: (Ethinyl Estradiol-Norgestimate) 0.025mg-0.18mg, 0.025mg-0.215mg, and 0.025mg-0.25mg

CONTRAINDICATIONS: Thrombophlebitis, deep vein thrombophlebitis, thromboembolic disorders, pregnancy, cerebrovascular or CAD, valvular heart disease with complications, severe HTN, DM with vascular involvement, headaches with focal neurological symptoms, major surgery with prolonged immobilization, undiagnosed abnormal genital bleeding, cholestatic jaundice of pregnancy or jaundice with prior pill use, hepatic adenomas or carcinomas, breast cancer, endometrial carcinoma or other estrogen-dependent neoplasia.

WARNINGS/PRECAUTIONS: Cigarette smoking increases risk of serious CV side effects; risk increases with age (especially >35 yrs) and heavy smoking.

Increased risk of MI, vascular disease, thromboembolism, stroke, and gallbladder disease. Retinal thrombosis, hepatic neoplasia, carcinoma of breast and reproductive organs reported. May cause glucose intolerance, fluid retention, breakthrough bleeding, and spotting. May increase BP, elevate LDL levels or cause other lipid changes. May cause or exacerbate migraine. May develop visual changes with contact lens. Increased risk of morbidity and mortality with HTN, hyperlipidemia, obesity, and DM. D/C if jaundice, significant depression, or ophthalmic irregularities develop. Perform annual physical exam. Use before menarche is not indicated. May affect certain endocrine, LFTs, and blood components.

ADVERSE REACTIONS: Nausea, vomiting, breakthrough bleeding, spotting, amenorrhea, migraine, depression, vaginal candidiasis, edema, weight changes.

INTERACTIONS: Reduced effects, increased breakthrough bleeding with rifampin, barbiturates, phenylbutazone, phenytoin, carbamazepine, felbamate, oxcarbazepine, griseofulvin, topiramate, St. John's wort, and possibly with ampicillin and tetracyclines. Atorvastatin, ascorbic acid, APAP, CYP3A4 inhibitors (eg, itraconazole, ketoconazole) may increase hormone levels. HIV protease inhibitors may increase or decrease levels. Increases levels of cyclosporine, prednisolone, theophylline. Decreases levels of APAP. Increases clearance of temazepam, salicylic acid, morphine, clofibric acid.

PREGNANCY: Category X, not for use in nursing.

MECHANISM OF ACTION: Estrogen/progestogen oral contraceptive: acts by suppressing gonadotropin, inhibits ovulation, changes in cervical mucus, (which increases difficulty of sperm entry into uterus) and endometrium (which reduces likelihood of implantation).

PHARMACOKINETICS: Absorption: Rapidly absorbed. Oral administration on various days during dosing schedule led to altered parameters. **Distribution:** Found in breast milk. Norgestimate: Serum protein binding (>97%). Ethinyl Estradiol: Serum albumin binding (>97%). **Metabolism:** Norgestimate: 1st pass metabolism, GI tract and/or liver. norelgestromin (active major metabolite) norgestrel (active major metabolite). Norrelgestromin: Hepatic. Ethinyl Estradiol: Hydroxylated, glucuronide and sulfate congugates. **Elimination:** Urine, feces; T$_{1/2}$=28.1 hrs (norelgestromin), 36.4 hrs (norgestrel), 17.7 hrs (ethinyl estradiol)

ORTHO-CEPT   RX
desogestrel - ethinyl estradiol (Ortho-McNeil)

THERAPEUTIC CLASS: Estrogen/progestogen combination

INDICATIONS: Prevention of pregnancy.

DOSAGE: *Adults:* 1 tab qd for 28 days, then repeat. Start 1st Sunday after menses begin or 1st day of menses.

HOW SUPPLIED: Tab: (Ethinyl Estradiol-Desogestrel) 0.03mg-0.15mg

CONTRAINDICATIONS: Thrombophlebitis, DVT or thromboembolic disorders, pregnancy, cerebrovascular or coronary artery disease, undiagnosed abnormal genital bleeding, cholestatic jaundice of pregnancy or jaundice with prior pill use, hepatic adenomas or carcinomas, breast cancer or other estrogen-dependent neoplasia.

WARNINGS/PRECAUTIONS: Cigarette smoking increases risk of serious cardiovascular side effects. This risk increases with age (especially >35 yrs) and heavy smoking. Increased risk of MI, vascular disease, thromboembolism, stroke, and gallbladder disease. Retinal thrombosis, hepatic neoplasia, carcinoma of breast and reproductive organs reported. May cause glucose intolerance. May increase BP, elevate LDL levels or cause other lipid changes, fluid retention, breakthrough bleeding, and spotting. May cause or exacerbate migraine. May develop visual changes with contact lens. Increased risk of MI with HTN, hyperlipidemia, obesity, and diabetes. D/C if jaundice, significant depression, or ophthalmic irregularities develop. Perform annual physical exam. Use before menarche is not indicated. May affect certain endocrine, LFTs, and blood components.

ADVERSE REACTIONS: Nausea, vomiting, breakthrough bleeding, spotting, amenorrhea, migraine, depression, vaginal candidiasis, edema, weight changes.

INTERACTIONS: Reduced effects, increased breakthrough bleeding, and menstrual irregularities with rifampin, barbiturates, phenylbutazone, phenytoin, carbamazepine, griseofulvin, topiramate, St. John's wort, and possibly with ampicillin and tetracyclines.

PREGNANCY: Category X, not for use in nursing.

MECHANISM OF ACTION: Estrogen/progestogen combination oral contraceptive. Responsible for suppressing gonadotropins. Primarily inhibits ovulation. Also causes changes in cervical mucus (increases difficulty of sperm entry into uterus) and changes in endometrium (which reduces likelihood of implantation).

PHARMACOKINETICS: Absorption: Desogestrel: Rapid, C_{max}=2,805pg/mL (single dose), 5840 (multiple doses), T_{max}=1.4 hrs (single dose), 1.4 hrs (after multiple doses); AUC=33,858pg/mL•hr (single dose), 52,299pg/mL•hr (after multiple doses); Ethinyl estradiol: C_{max}=95pg/mL (single dose), 141pg/mL (multiple doses), T_{max}=1.5 hrs (single dose), 1.4 hrs (multiple doses) AUC=1471pg/mL•hr. **Distribution:** Found in breast milk. **Metabolism:** Desogestrel: 3-keto-desogestrel (major active metabolite), conjugation into sulfates and glucuronides. Ethinyl estradiol: Phase I metabolism: 2-OH-ethinyl estradiol, 2-methoxy-ethinyl-estradiol (major metabolites), hepatic conjugation. **Elimination:** 3-ketodesogestrel: $T_{1/2}$=38 hrs; Ethinyl estradiol: $T_{1/2}$=26 hrs.

Ortho-Cyclen   RX
ethinyl estradiol - norgestimate (Ortho-McNeil)

OTHER BRAND NAMES: MonoNessa (Watson) - Sprintec (Barr)

THERAPEUTIC CLASS: Estrogen/progestogen combination

INDICATIONS: Prevention of pregnancy.

DOSAGE: *Adults:* 1 tab qd for 28 days, then repeat. Start 1st Sunday after menses begin or 1st day of menses.

HOW SUPPLIED: Tab: (Ethinyl Estradiol-Norgestimate) 0.035mg-0.25mg

CONTRAINDICATIONS: Thrombophlebitis, deep vein thrombophlebitis, thromboembolic disorders, pregnancy, cerebrovascular or coronary artery disease, migraine with focal aura, acute or chronic hepatocellular disease with abnormal liver function, undiagnosed abnormal genital bleeding, cholestatic jaundice of pregnancy or jaundice with prior pill use, hepatic adenomas or carcinomas, breast cancer, endometrium carcinoma, or other estrogen-dependent neoplasia.

WARNINGS/PRECAUTIONS: Cigarette smoking increases risk of serious cardiovascular side effects; risk increases with age (especially >35 yrs) and heavy smoking. Increased risk of MI, vascular disease, thromboembolism, stroke, and gallbladder disease. Retinal thrombosis, hepatic neoplasia, carcinoma of breast and reproductive organs reported. May cause glucose intolerance. May increase BP, elevate LDL levels or cause other lipid changes, fluid retention, breakthrough bleeding, and spotting. May cause or exacerbate migraine. May develop visual changes with contact lens. Increased risk of MI with HTN, hyperlipidemia, obesity, and diabetes. D/C if jaundice, significant depression, or ophthalmic irregularities develop. Perform annual physical exam. Use before menarche is not indicated. May affect certain endocrine, LFTs, and blood components.

ADVERSE REACTIONS: Nausea, vomiting, breakthrough bleeding, spotting, amenorrhea, migraine, depression, vaginal candidiasis, edema, weight changes.

INTERACTIONS: Reduced effects, increased breakthrough bleeding, and menstrual irregularities with rifampin, barbiturates, phenylbutazone,

VISUAL IDENTIFICATION GUIDE*

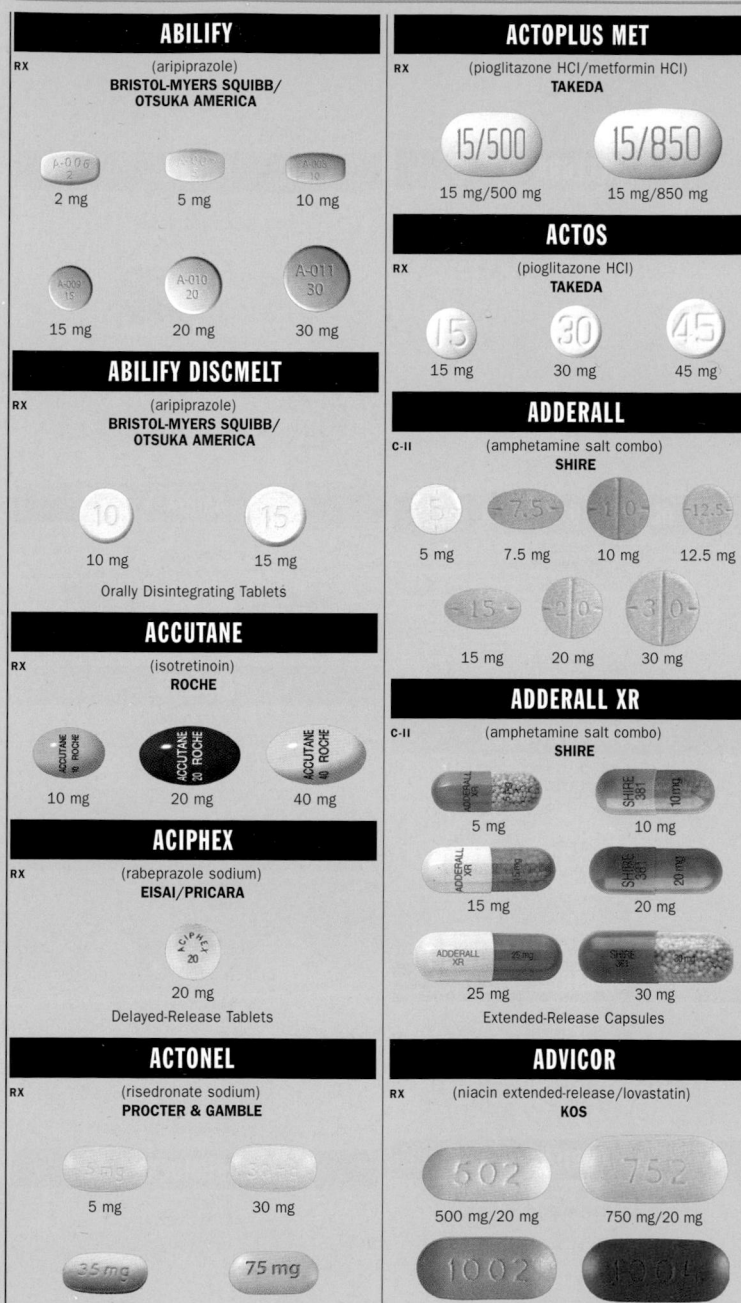

ABILIFY

RX

(aripiprazole)
**BRISTOL-MYERS SQUIBB/
OTSUKA AMERICA**

2 mg   5 mg   10 mg

15 mg   20 mg   30 mg

ABILIFY DISCMELT

RX

(aripiprazole)
**BRISTOL-MYERS SQUIBB/
OTSUKA AMERICA**

10 mg   15 mg

Orally Disintegrating Tablets

ACCUTANE

RX

(isotretinoin)
ROCHE

10 mg   20 mg   40 mg

ACIPHEX

RX

(rabeprazole sodium)
EISAI/PRICARA

20 mg

Delayed-Release Tablets

ACTONEL

RX

(risedronate sodium)
PROCTER & GAMBLE

5 mg   30 mg

35 mg   75 mg

ACTOPLUS MET

RX

(pioglitazone HCl/metformin HCl)
TAKEDA

15/500   15/850

15 mg/500 mg   15 mg/850 mg

ACTOS

RX

(pioglitazone HCl)
TAKEDA

15 mg   30 mg   45 mg

ADDERALL

C-II

(amphetamine salt combo)
SHIRE

5 mg   7.5 mg   10 mg   12.5 mg

15 mg   20 mg   30 mg

ADDERALL XR

C-II

(amphetamine salt combo)
SHIRE

5 mg   10 mg

15 mg   20 mg

25 mg   30 mg

Extended-Release Capsules

ADVICOR

RX

(niacin extended-release/lovastatin)
KOS

500 mg/20 mg   750 mg/20 mg

1000 mg/20 mg   1000 mg/40 mg

AGGRENOX

RX   (aspirin/extended-release dipyridamole)
BOEHRINGER INGELHEIM

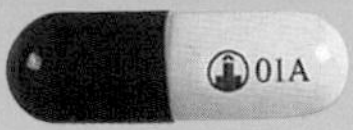

01A

25 mg/200 mg

ALLEGRA

RX   (fexofenadine HCl)
SANOFI-AVENTIS

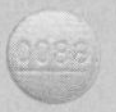

0088

30 mg

014

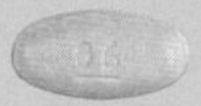

60 mg

018

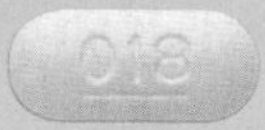

180 mg

ALLEGRA-D 12 HOUR

RX   (fexofenadine HCl/pseudoephedrine HCl)
SANOFI-AVENTIS

06/012D

60 mg/120 mg
Extended-Release Tablets

ALLEGRA-D 24 HOUR

RX   (fexofenadine HCl/pseudoephedrine HCl)
SANOFI-AVENTIS

308
AV

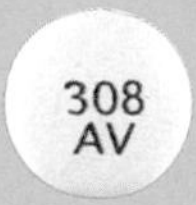

180 mg/240 mg
Extended-Release Tablets

AMARYL

RX   (glimepiride)
SANOFI-AVENTIS

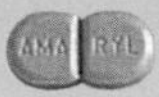

AMA RYL   AMA RYL   AMA RYL

1 mg 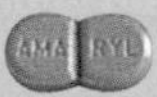   2 mg 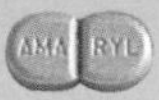   4 mg

AMBIEN

C-IV   (zolpidem tartrate)
SANOFI-AVENTIS

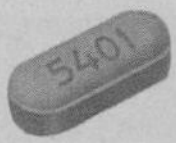

5401   5421

5 mg 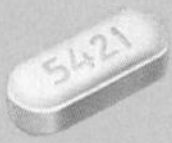   10 mg

AMERGE

RX   (naratriptan HCl)
GLAXOSMITHKLINE

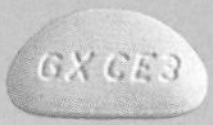

GX CE3   GX CE5

1 mg 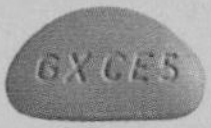   2.5 mg

AMOXIL

RX   (amoxicillin)
GLAXOSMITHKLINE

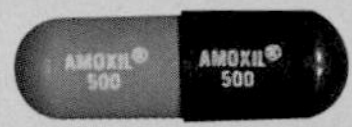

AMOXIL 500   AMOXIL 500

500 mg

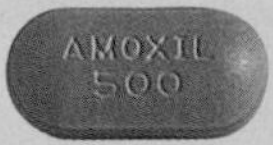

AMOXIL 500   AMOXIL 875

500 mg 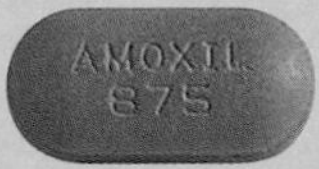   875 mg

AMRIX

RX   (cyclobenzaprine HCl)
CEPHALON

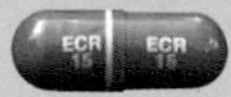

ECR 15 ECR 15   ECR 30 ECR 30

15 mg 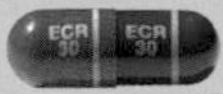   30 mg
Extended-Release Capsules

ARICEPT

RX   (donepezil HCl)
EISAI/PFIZER

5 mg 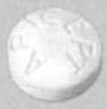   10 mg

ARICEPT ODT

RX   (donepezil HCl)
EISAI/PFIZER

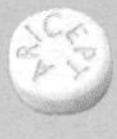

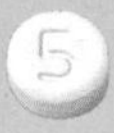

ACEPT   5

5 mg

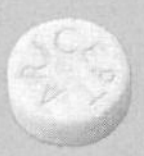

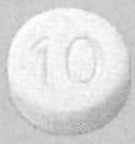

5   10

10 mg
Orally Disintegrating Tablets

ARIMIDEX

RX   (anastrozole)
ASTRAZENECA

Acix 1   A

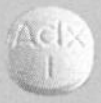

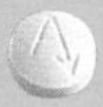

1 mg

ATACAND

RX   (candesartan cilexetil)
ASTRAZENECA LP

4 mg   8 mg

16 mg   32 mg

ATACAND HCT

RX   (candesartan cilexetil/hydrochlorothiazide)
ASTRAZENECA LP

16 mg/12.5 mg

32 mg/12.5 mg

ATRIPLA

RX   (efavirenz/emtricitabine/tenofovir
disoproxil fumarate)
**BRISTOL-MYERS SQUIBB/
GILEAD SCIENCES**

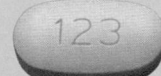

600 mg/200 mg/300 mg

AUGMENTIN

RX   (amoxicillin/clavulanate potassium)
GLAXOSMITHKLINE

   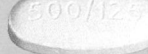

250 mg/125 mg   500 mg/125 mg

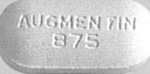

875 mg/125 mg

AUGMENTIN XR

RX   (amoxicillin/clavulanate potassium)
GLAXOSMITHKLINE

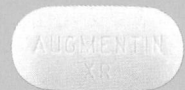

1000 mg/62.5 mg
Extended-Release Tablets

AVALIDE

RX   (irbesartan/hydrochlorothiazide)
BRISTOL-MYERS SQUIBB/SANOFI-AVENTIS

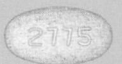

150 mg/12.5 mg   300 mg/12.5 mg

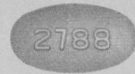

300 mg/25 mg

AVANDAMET

RX   (rosiglitazone maleate/metformin HCl)
GLAXOSMITHKLINE

2 mg/500 mg   2 mg/1000 mg

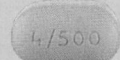

4 mg/500 mg   4 mg/1000 mg

AVANDARYL

RX   (rosiglitazone maleate/glimepiride)
GLAXOSMITHKLINE

4 mg/1 mg   4 mg/2 mg   4 mg/4 mg

8 mg/2 mg   8 mg/4 mg

AVANDIA

RX   (rosiglitazone maleate)
GLAXOSMITHKLINE

     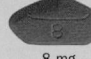

2 mg   4 mg   8 mg

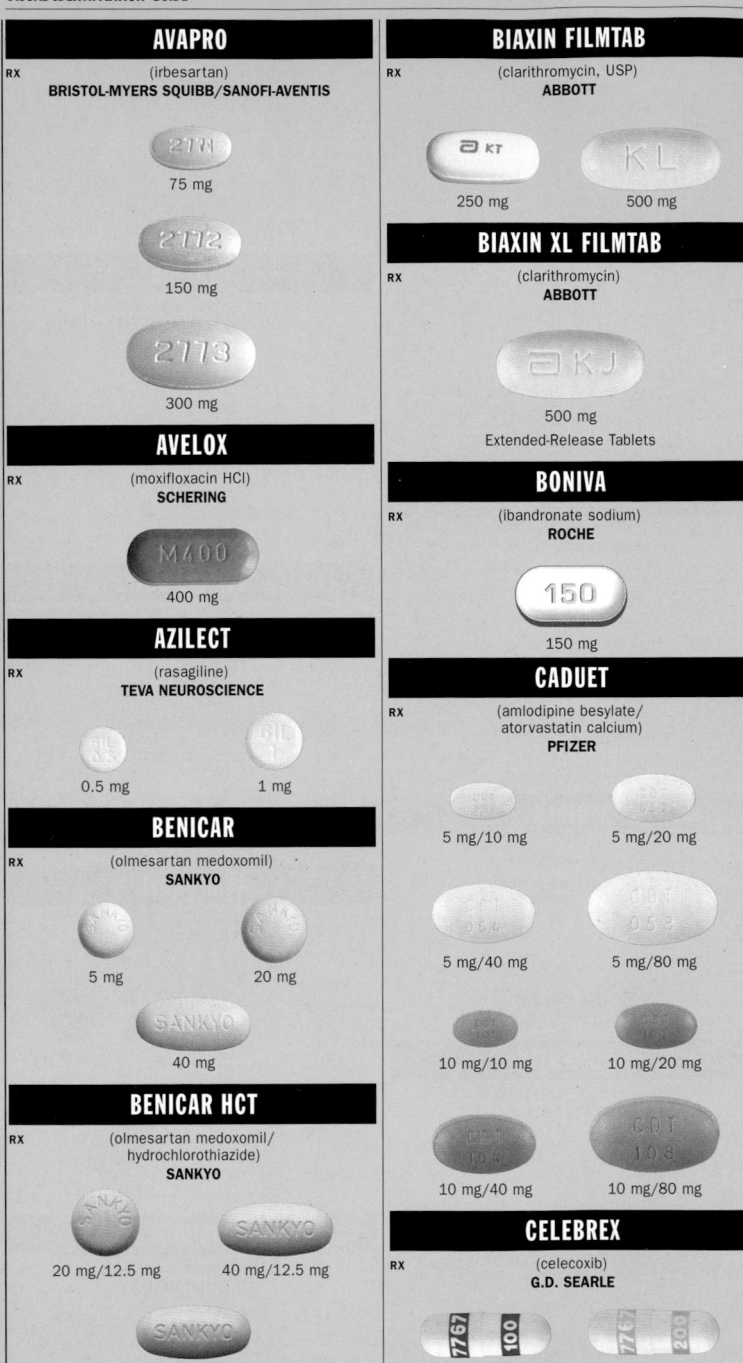

AVAPRO

RX

(irbesartan)
BRISTOL-MYERS SQUIBB/SANOFI-AVENTIS

75 mg

150 mg

300 mg

AVELOX

RX

(moxifloxacin HCl)
SCHERING

400 mg

AZILECT

RX

(rasagiline)
TEVA NEUROSCIENCE

0.5 mg   1 mg

BENICAR

RX

(olmesartan medoxomil)
SANKYO

5 mg   20 mg

40 mg

BENICAR HCT

RX

(olmesartan medoxomil/
hydrochlorothiazide)
SANKYO

20 mg/12.5 mg   40 mg/12.5 mg

40 mg/25 mg

BIAXIN FILMTAB

RX

(clarithromycin, USP)
ABBOTT

250 mg   500 mg

BIAXIN XL FILMTAB

RX

(clarithromycin)
ABBOTT

500 mg
Extended-Release Tablets

BONIVA

RX

(ibandronate sodium)
ROCHE

150 mg

CADUET

RX

(amlodipine besylate/
atorvastatin calcium)
PFIZER

5 mg/10 mg   5 mg/20 mg

5 mg/40 mg   5 mg/80 mg

10 mg/10 mg   10 mg/20 mg

10 mg/40 mg   10 mg/80 mg

CELEBREX

RX

(celecoxib)
G.D. SEARLE

100 mg   200 mg

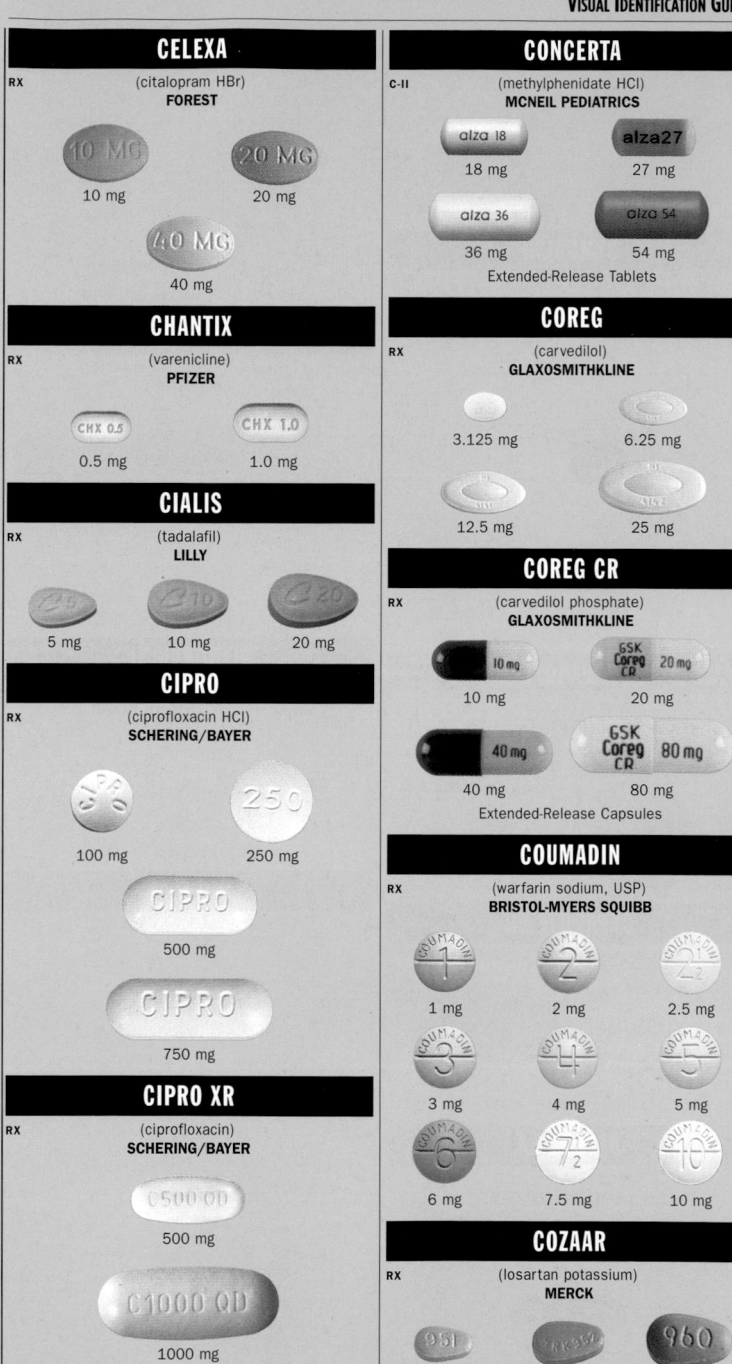

CELEXA
RX
(citalopram HBr)
FOREST

10 mg

20 mg

40 mg

CHANTIX
RX
(varenicline)
PFIZER

CHX 0.5 — 0.5 mg

CHX 1.0 — 1.0 mg

CIALIS
RX
(tadalafil)
LILLY

5 mg

10 mg

20 mg

CIPRO
RX
(ciprofloxacin HCl)
SCHERING/BAYER

100 mg

250 mg

CIPRO 500 mg

CIPRO 750 mg

CIPRO XR
RX
(ciprofloxacin)
SCHERING/BAYER

C 500 QD — 500 mg

C 1000 QD — 1000 mg

Extended-Release Tablets

CONCERTA
C-II
(methylphenidate HCl)
MCNEIL PEDIATRICS

alza 18 — 18 mg

alza 27 — 27 mg

alza 36 — 36 mg

alza 54 — 54 mg

Extended-Release Tablets

COREG
RX
(carvedilol)
GLAXOSMITHKLINE

3.125 mg

6.25 mg

12.5 mg

25 mg

COREG CR
RX
(carvedilol phosphate)
GLAXOSMITHKLINE

10 mg

GSK Coreg CR 20 mg — 20 mg

40 mg

GSK Coreg CR 80 mg — 80 mg

Extended-Release Capsules

COUMADIN
RX
(warfarin sodium, USP)
BRISTOL-MYERS SQUIBB

1 mg

2 mg

2.5 mg

3 mg

4 mg

5 mg

6 mg

7.5 mg

10 mg

COZAAR
RX
(losartan potassium)
MERCK

951 — 25 mg

50 mg

960 — 100 mg

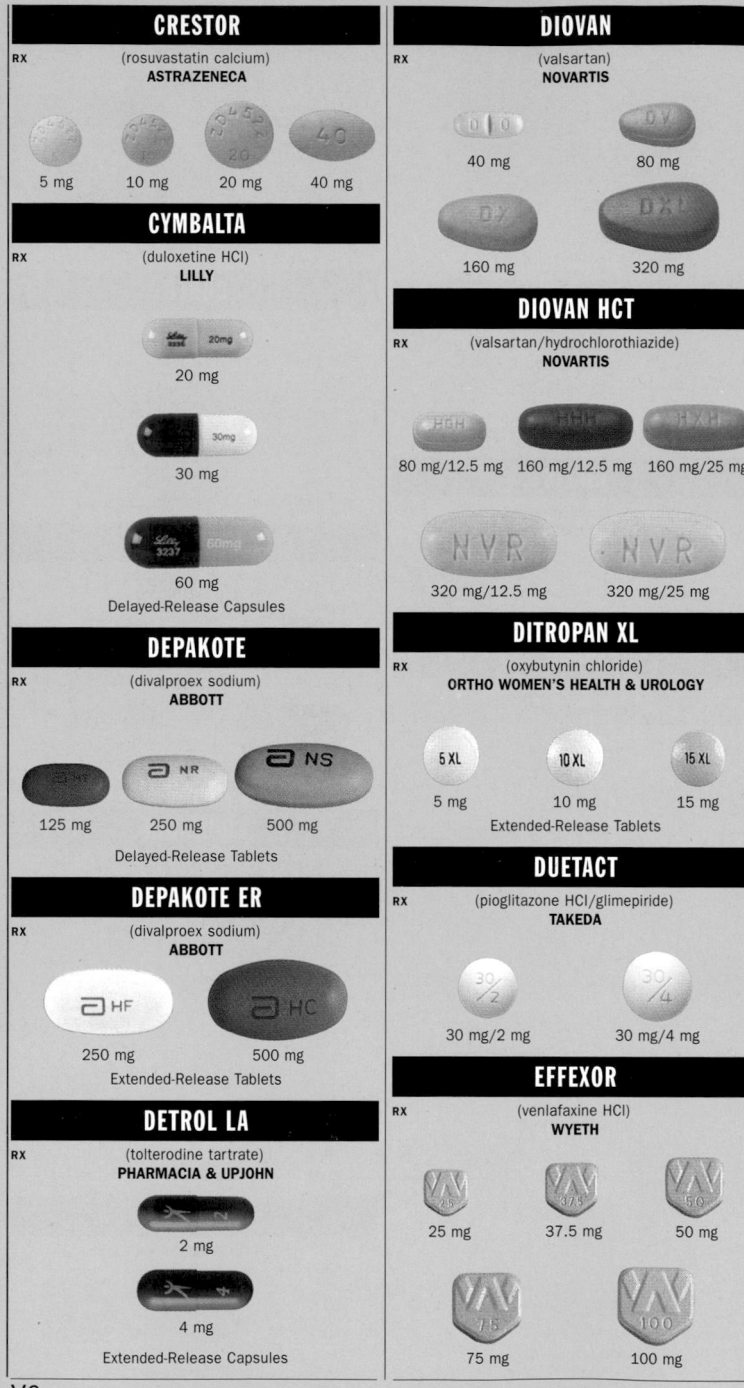

CRESTOR

RX

(rosuvastatin calcium)
ASTRAZENECA

5 mg | 10 mg | 20 mg | 40 mg

CYMBALTA

RX

(duloxetine HCl)
LILLY

20 mg

30 mg

60 mg
Delayed-Release Capsules

DEPAKOTE

RX

(divalproex sodium)
ABBOTT

125 mg | 250 mg | 500 mg

Delayed-Release Tablets

DEPAKOTE ER

RX

(divalproex sodium)
ABBOTT

250 mg | 500 mg

Extended-Release Tablets

DETROL LA

RX

(tolterodine tartrate)
PHARMACIA & UPJOHN

2 mg

4 mg

Extended-Release Capsules

DIOVAN

RX

(valsartan)
NOVARTIS

40 mg | 80 mg

160 mg | 320 mg

DIOVAN HCT

RX

(valsartan/hydrochlorothiazide)
NOVARTIS

80 mg/12.5 mg | 160 mg/12.5 mg | 160 mg/25 mg

320 mg/12.5 mg | 320 mg/25 mg

DITROPAN XL

RX

(oxybutynin chloride)
ORTHO WOMEN'S HEALTH & UROLOGY

5 mg | 10 mg | 15 mg

Extended-Release Tablets

DUETACT

RX

(pioglitazone HCl/glimepiride)
TAKEDA

30 mg/2 mg | 30 mg/4 mg

EFFEXOR

RX

(venlafaxine HCl)
WYETH

25 mg | 37.5 mg | 50 mg

75 mg | 100 mg

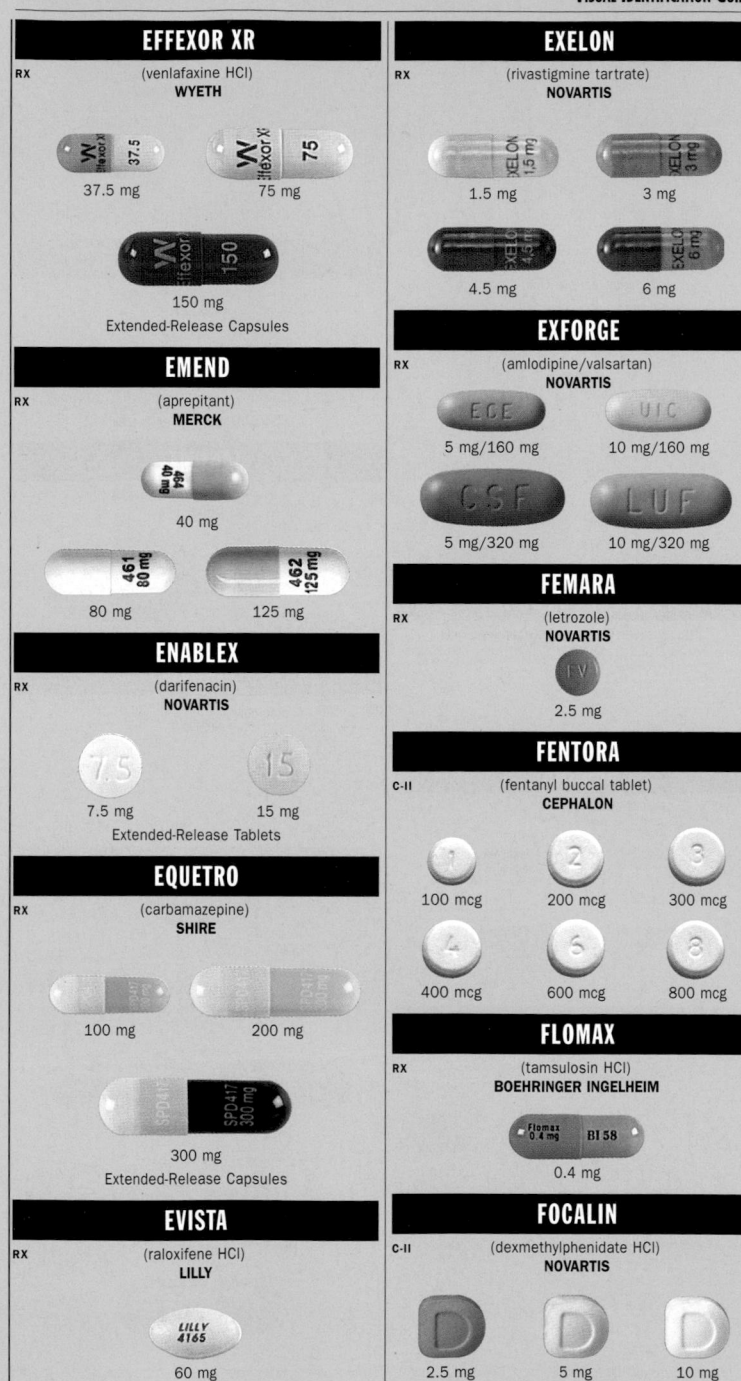

EFFEXOR XR
RX
(venlafaxine HCl)
WYETH

37.5 mg

75 mg

150 mg

Extended-Release Capsules

EMEND
RX
(aprepitant)
MERCK

40 mg

80 mg

125 mg

ENABLEX
RX
(darifenacin)
NOVARTIS

7.5 mg

15 mg

Extended-Release Tablets

EQUETRO
RX
(carbamazepine)
SHIRE

100 mg

200 mg

300 mg

Extended-Release Capsules

EVISTA
RX
(raloxifene HCl)
LILLY

LILLY
4165

60 mg

EXELON
RX
(rivastigmine tartrate)
NOVARTIS

1.5 mg

3 mg

4.5 mg

6 mg

EXFORGE
RX
(amlodipine/valsartan)
NOVARTIS

ECE
5 mg/160 mg

UIC
10 mg/160 mg

CSF
5 mg/320 mg

LUF
10 mg/320 mg

FEMARA
RX
(letrozole)
NOVARTIS

FV
2.5 mg

FENTORA
C-II
(fentanyl buccal tablet)
CEPHALON

1
100 mcg

2
200 mcg

3
300 mcg

4
400 mcg

6
600 mcg

8
800 mcg

FLOMAX
RX
(tamsulosin HCl)
BOEHRINGER INGELHEIM

Flomax
0.4 mg   BI 58

0.4 mg

FOCALIN
C-II
(dexmethylphenidate HCl)
NOVARTIS

2.5 mg

5 mg

10 mg

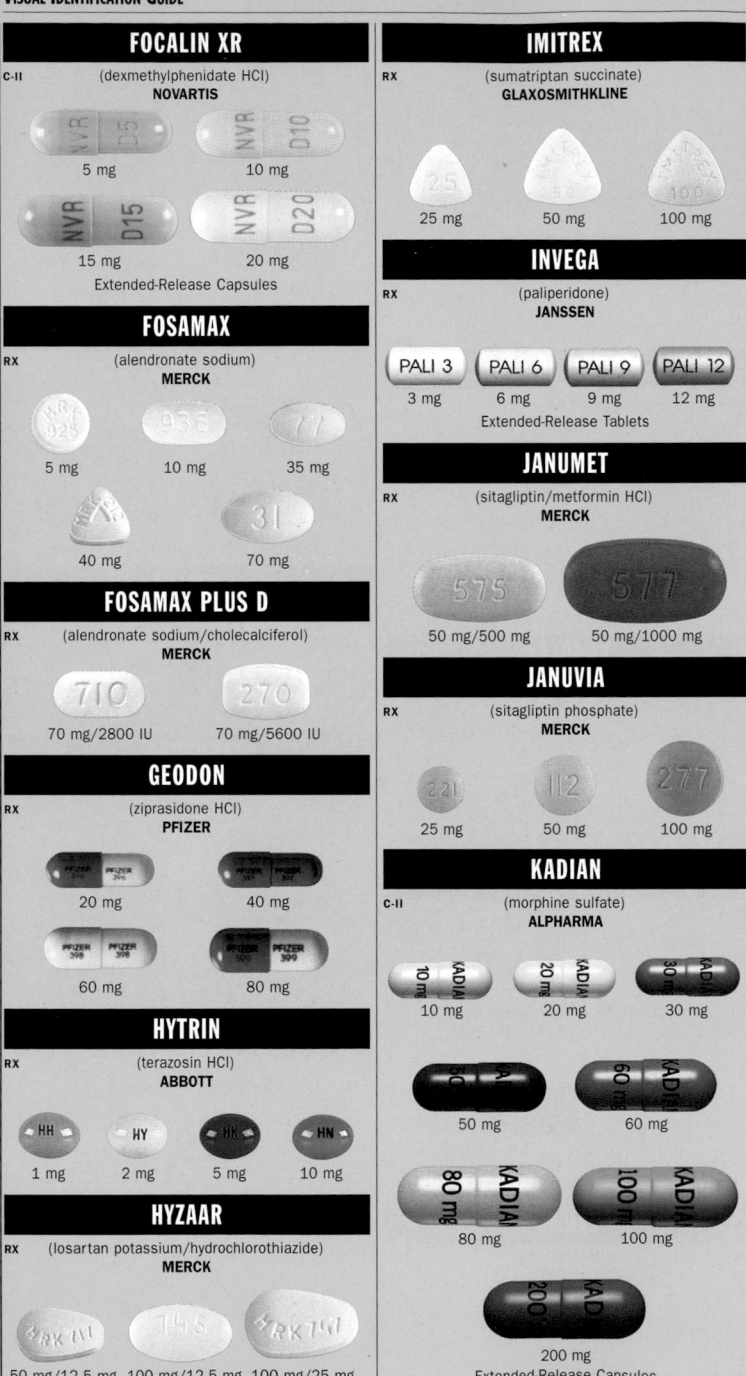

FOCALIN XR

C-II

(dexmethylphenidate HCl)
NOVARTIS

5 mg   10 mg

15 mg   20 mg

Extended-Release Capsules

FOSAMAX

RX

(alendronate sodium)
MERCK

5 mg   10 mg   35 mg

40 mg   70 mg

FOSAMAX PLUS D

RX

(alendronate sodium/cholecalciferol)
MERCK

70 mg/2800 IU   70 mg/5600 IU

GEODON

RX

(ziprasidone HCl)
PFIZER

20 mg   40 mg

60 mg   80 mg

HYTRIN

RX

(terazosin HCl)
ABBOTT

1 mg   2 mg   5 mg   10 mg

HYZAAR

RX

(losartan potassium/hydrochlorothiazide)
MERCK

50 mg/12.5 mg   100 mg/12.5 mg   100 mg/25 mg

IMITREX

RX

(sumatriptan succinate)
GLAXOSMITHKLINE

25 mg   50 mg   100 mg

INVEGA

RX

(paliperidone)
JANSSEN

PALI 3   PALI 6   PALI 9   PALI 12

3 mg   6 mg   9 mg   12 mg

Extended-Release Tablets

JANUMET

RX

(sitagliptin/metformin HCl)
MERCK

50 mg/500 mg   50 mg/1000 mg

JANUVIA

RX

(sitagliptin phosphate)
MERCK

25 mg   50 mg   100 mg

KADIAN

C-II

(morphine sulfate)
ALPHARMA

10 mg   20 mg   30 mg

50 mg   60 mg

80 mg   100 mg

200 mg

Extended-Release Capsules

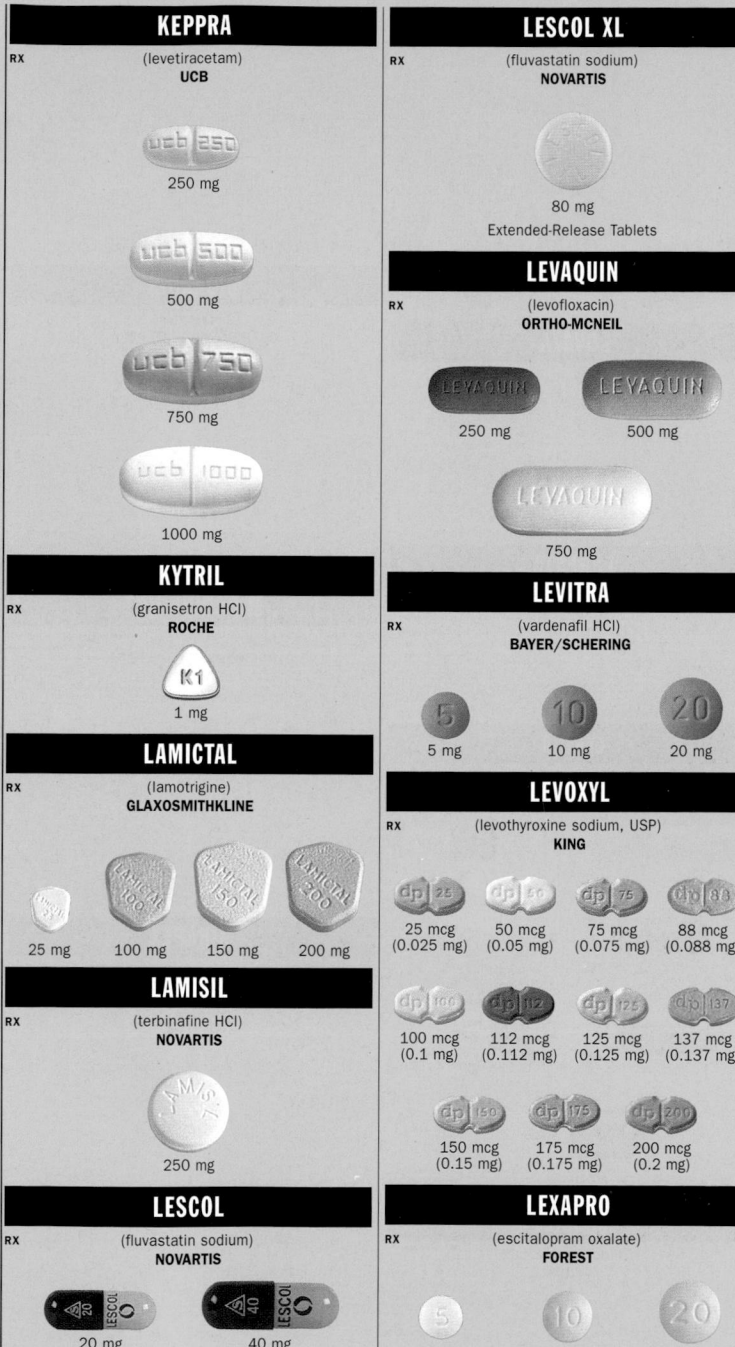

KEPPRA

RX

(levetiracetam)
UCB

250 mg

500 mg

750 mg

1000 mg

KYTRIL

RX

(granisetron HCl)
ROCHE

1 mg

LAMICTAL

RX

(lamotrigine)
GLAXOSMITHKLINE

25 mg   100 mg   150 mg   200 mg

LAMISIL

RX

(terbinafine HCl)
NOVARTIS

250 mg

LESCOL

RX

(fluvastatin sodium)
NOVARTIS

20 mg   40 mg

LESCOL XL

RX

(fluvastatin sodium)
NOVARTIS

80 mg
Extended-Release Tablets

LEVAQUIN

RX

(levofloxacin)
ORTHO-MCNEIL

250 mg   500 mg

750 mg

LEVITRA

RX

(vardenafil HCl)
BAYER/SCHERING

5 mg   10 mg   20 mg

LEVOXYL

RX

(levothyroxine sodium, USP)
KING

25 mcg (0.025 mg)	50 mcg (0.05 mg)	75 mcg (0.075 mg)	88 mcg (0.088 mg)
100 mcg (0.1 mg)	112 mcg (0.112 mg)	125 mcg (0.125 mg)	137 mcg (0.137 mg)
150 mcg (0.15 mg)	175 mcg (0.175 mg)	200 mcg (0.2 mg)	

LEXAPRO

RX

(escitalopram oxalate)
FOREST

5 mg   10 mg   20 mg

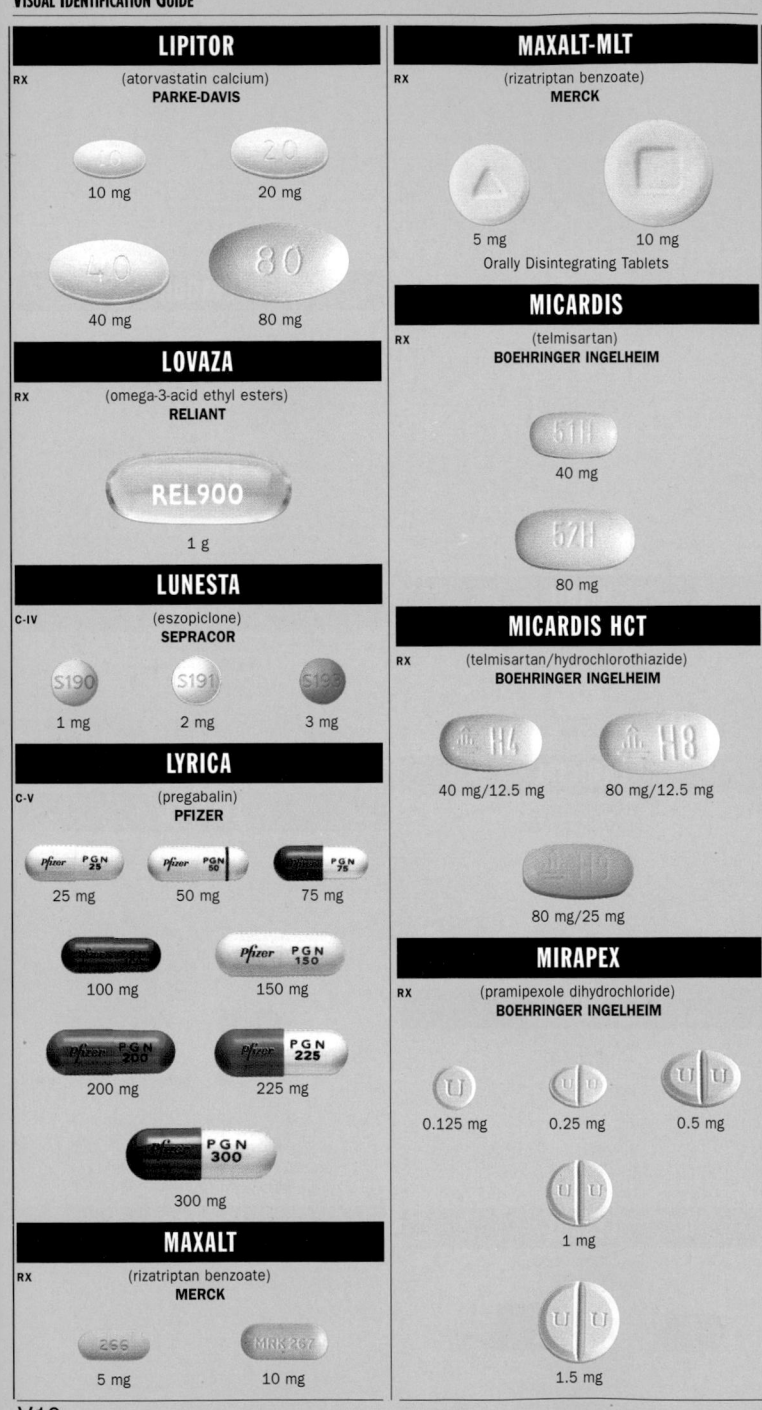

LIPITOR

RX — (atorvastatin calcium)
PARKE-DAVIS

10 mg
20 mg
40 mg
80 mg

LOVAZA

RX — (omega-3-acid ethyl esters)
RELIANT

REL900

1 g

LUNESTA

C-IV — (eszopiclone)
SEPRACOR

S190 — 1 mg
S191 — 2 mg
S193 — 3 mg

LYRICA

C-V — (pregabalin)
PFIZER

Pfizer PGN 25 — 25 mg
Pfizer PGN 50 — 50 mg
PGN 75 — 75 mg

100 mg
Pfizer PGN 150 — 150 mg
Pfizer PGN 200 — 200 mg
Pfizer PGN 225 — 225 mg
Pfizer PGN 300 — 300 mg

MAXALT

RX — (rizatriptan benzoate)
MERCK

266 — 5 mg
MRK 267 — 10 mg

MAXALT-MLT

RX — (rizatriptan benzoate)
MERCK

5 mg
10 mg
Orally Disintegrating Tablets

MICARDIS

RX — (telmisartan)
BOEHRINGER INGELHEIM

51H — 40 mg
52H — 80 mg

MICARDIS HCT

RX — (telmisartan/hydrochlorothiazide)
BOEHRINGER INGELHEIM

H4 — 40 mg/12.5 mg
H8 — 80 mg/12.5 mg
H9 — 80 mg/25 mg

MIRAPEX

RX — (pramipexole dihydrochloride)
BOEHRINGER INGELHEIM

U — 0.125 mg
U|U — 0.25 mg
U|U — 0.5 mg
U|U — 1 mg
U|U — 1.5 mg

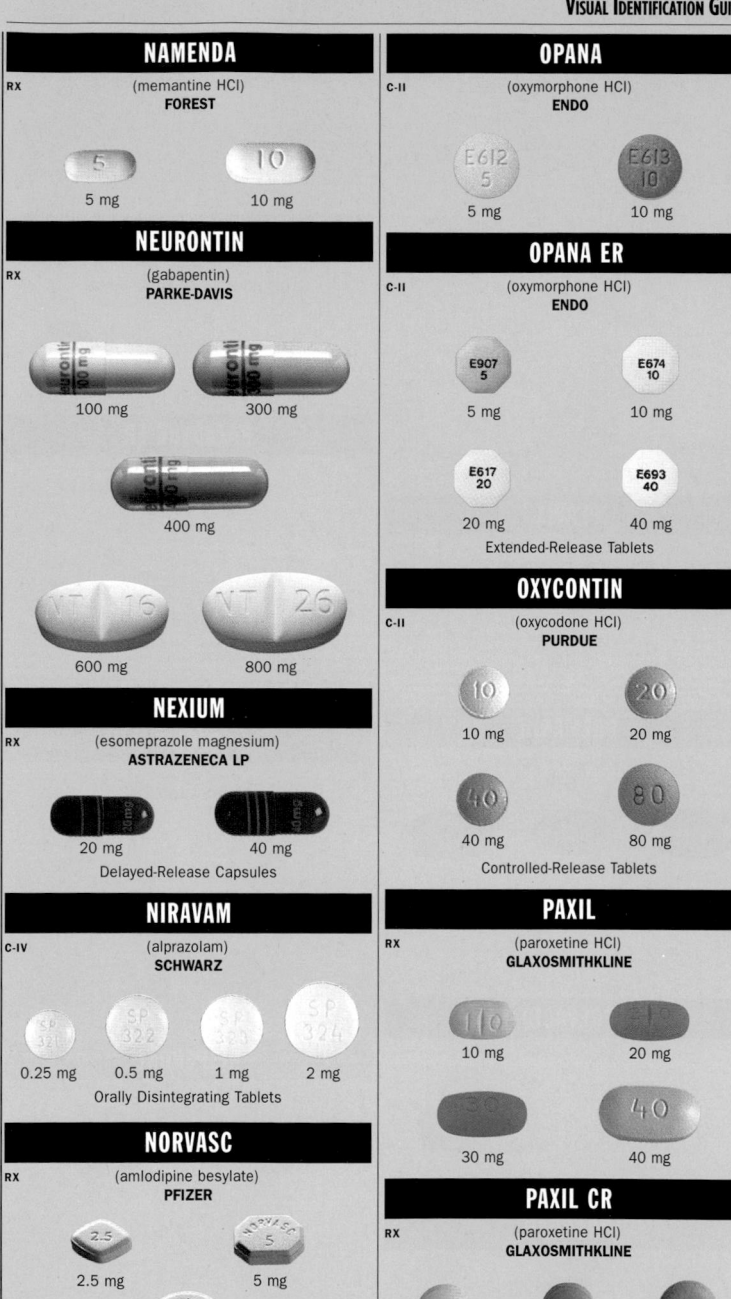

NAMENDA

RX

(memantine HCl)
FOREST

5 mg — 10 mg

NEURONTIN

RX

(gabapentin)
PARKE-DAVIS

100 mg — 300 mg

400 mg

600 mg — 800 mg

NEXIUM

RX

(esomeprazole magnesium)
ASTRAZENECA LP

20 mg — 40 mg

Delayed-Release Capsules

NIRAVAM

C-IV

(alprazolam)
SCHWARZ

0.25 mg — 0.5 mg — 1 mg — 2 mg

Orally Disintegrating Tablets

NORVASC

RX

(amlodipine besylate)
PFIZER

2.5 mg — 5 mg

10 mg

OPANA

C-II

(oxymorphone HCl)
ENDO

5 mg — 10 mg

OPANA ER

C-II

(oxymorphone HCl)
ENDO

5 mg — 10 mg

20 mg — 40 mg

Extended-Release Tablets

OXYCONTIN

C-II

(oxycodone HCl)
PURDUE

10 mg — 20 mg

40 mg — 80 mg

Controlled-Release Tablets

PAXIL

RX

(paroxetine HCl)
GLAXOSMITHKLINE

10 mg — 20 mg

30 mg — 40 mg

PAXIL CR

RX

(paroxetine HCl)
GLAXOSMITHKLINE

12.5 mg — 25 mg — 37.5 mg

Controlled-Release Tablets

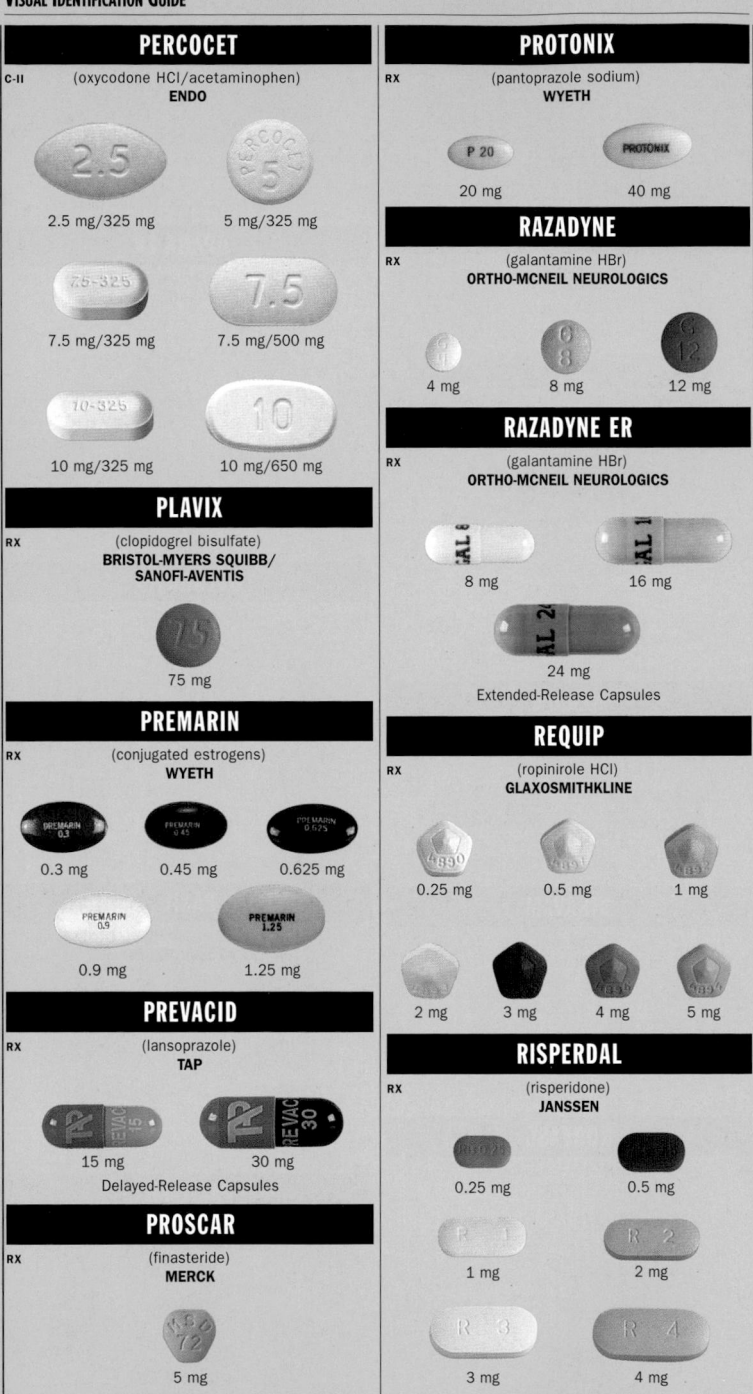

PERCOCET

C-II (oxycodone HCl/acetaminophen)
ENDO

2.5 mg/325 mg

5 mg/325 mg

7.5 mg/325 mg

7.5 mg/500 mg

10 mg/325 mg

10 mg/650 mg

PLAVIX

RX (clopidogrel bisulfate)
**BRISTOL-MYERS SQUIBB/
SANOFI-AVENTIS**

75 mg

PREMARIN

RX (conjugated estrogens)
WYETH

0.3 mg

0.45 mg

0.625 mg

0.9 mg

1.25 mg

PREVACID

RX (lansoprazole)
TAP

15 mg

30 mg

Delayed-Release Capsules

PROSCAR

RX (finasteride)
MERCK

5 mg

PROTONIX

RX (pantoprazole sodium)
WYETH

20 mg

40 mg

RAZADYNE

RX (galantamine HBr)
ORTHO-MCNEIL NEUROLOGICS

4 mg

8 mg

12 mg

RAZADYNE ER

RX (galantamine HBr)
ORTHO-MCNEIL NEUROLOGICS

8 mg

16 mg

24 mg

Extended-Release Capsules

REQUIP

RX (ropinirole HCl)
GLAXOSMITHKLINE

0.25 mg

0.5 mg

1 mg

2 mg

3 mg

4 mg

5 mg

RISPERDAL

RX (risperidone)
JANSSEN

0.25 mg

0.5 mg

1 mg

2 mg

3 mg

4 mg

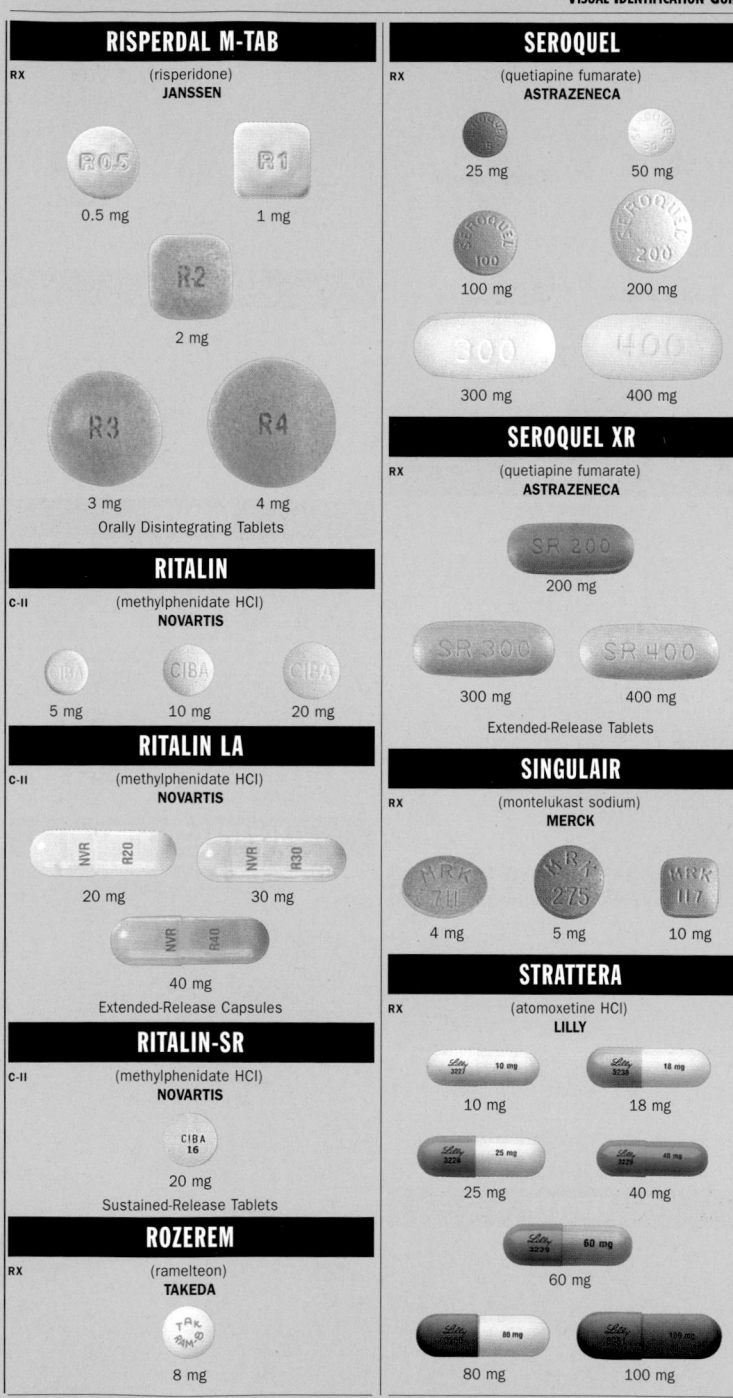

RISPERDAL M-TAB

RX

(risperidone)
JANSSEN

0.5 mg — 1 mg — 2 mg — 3 mg — 4 mg

Orally Disintegrating Tablets

RITALIN

C-II

(methylphenidate HCl)
NOVARTIS

5 mg — 10 mg — 20 mg

RITALIN LA

C-II

(methylphenidate HCl)
NOVARTIS

20 mg — 30 mg — 40 mg

Extended-Release Capsules

RITALIN-SR

C-II

(methylphenidate HCl)
NOVARTIS

20 mg

Sustained-Release Tablets

ROZEREM

RX

(ramelteon)
TAKEDA

8 mg

SEROQUEL

RX

(quetiapine fumarate)
ASTRAZENECA

25 mg — 50 mg — 100 mg — 200 mg — 300 mg — 400 mg

SEROQUEL XR

RX

(quetiapine fumarate)
ASTRAZENECA

200 mg — 300 mg — 400 mg

Extended-Release Tablets

SINGULAIR

RX

(montelukast sodium)
MERCK

4 mg — 5 mg — 10 mg

STRATTERA

RX

(atomoxetine HCl)
LILLY

10 mg — 18 mg — 25 mg — 40 mg — 60 mg — 80 mg — 100 mg

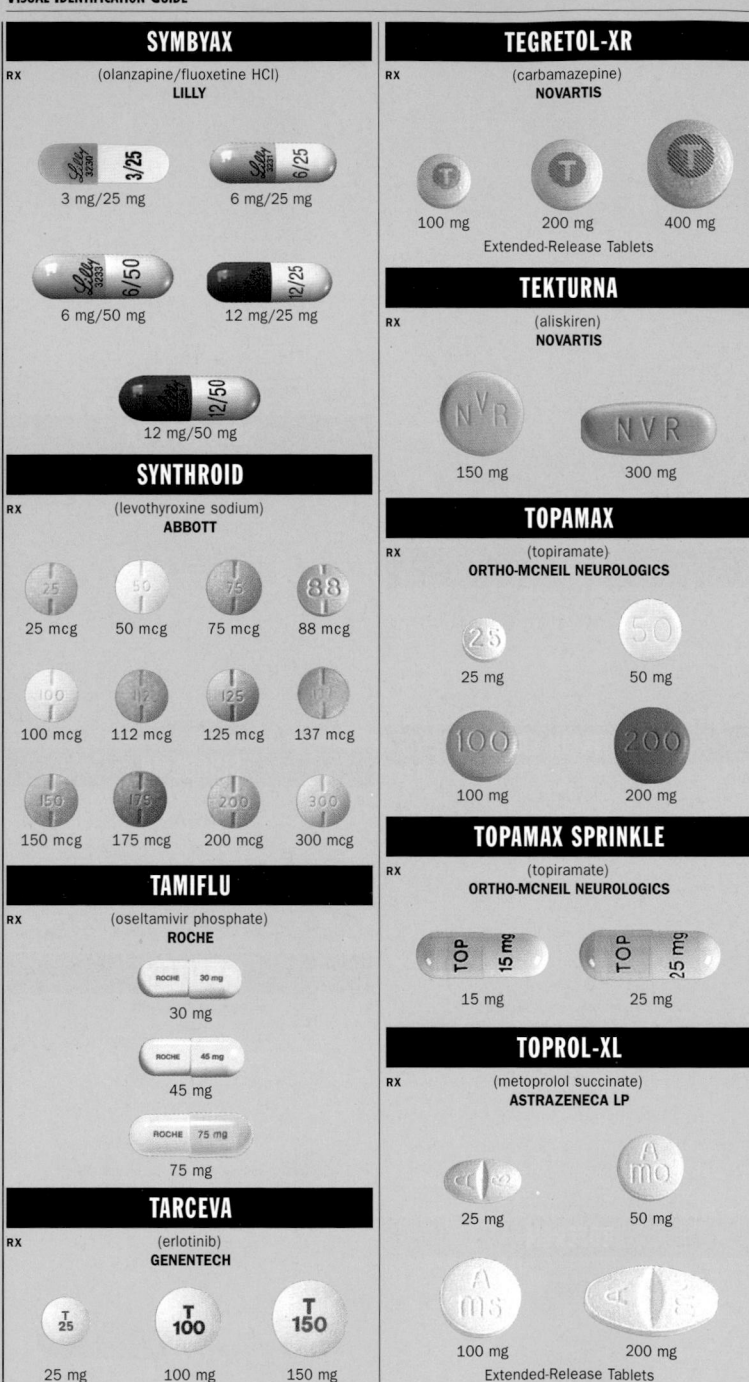

SYMBYAX

RX

(olanzapine/fluoxetine HCl)
LILLY

3 mg/25 mg   6 mg/25 mg

6 mg/50 mg   12 mg/25 mg

12 mg/50 mg

SYNTHROID

RX

(levothyroxine sodium)
ABBOTT

25 mcg   50 mcg   75 mcg   88 mcg

100 mcg   112 mcg   125 mcg   137 mcg

150 mcg   175 mcg   200 mcg   300 mcg

TAMIFLU

RX

(oseltamivir phosphate)
ROCHE

ROCHE 30 mg
30 mg

ROCHE 45 mg
45 mg

ROCHE 75 mg
75 mg

TARCEVA

RX

(erlotinib)
GENENTECH

T 25 — 25 mg

T 100 — 100 mg

T 150 — 150 mg

TEGRETOL-XR

RX

(carbamazepine)
NOVARTIS

100 mg   200 mg   400 mg

Extended-Release Tablets

TEKTURNA

RX

(aliskiren)
NOVARTIS

NVR — 150 mg

NVR — 300 mg

TOPAMAX

RX

(topiramate)
ORTHO-MCNEIL NEUROLOGICS

25 — 25 mg   50 — 50 mg

100 — 100 mg   200 — 200 mg

TOPAMAX SPRINKLE

RX

(topiramate)
ORTHO-MCNEIL NEUROLOGICS

TOP 15 mg — 15 mg

TOP 25 mg — 25 mg

TOPROL-XL

RX

(metoprolol succinate)
ASTRAZENECA LP

25 mg   A mo — 50 mg

A m5 — 100 mg   200 mg

Extended-Release Tablets

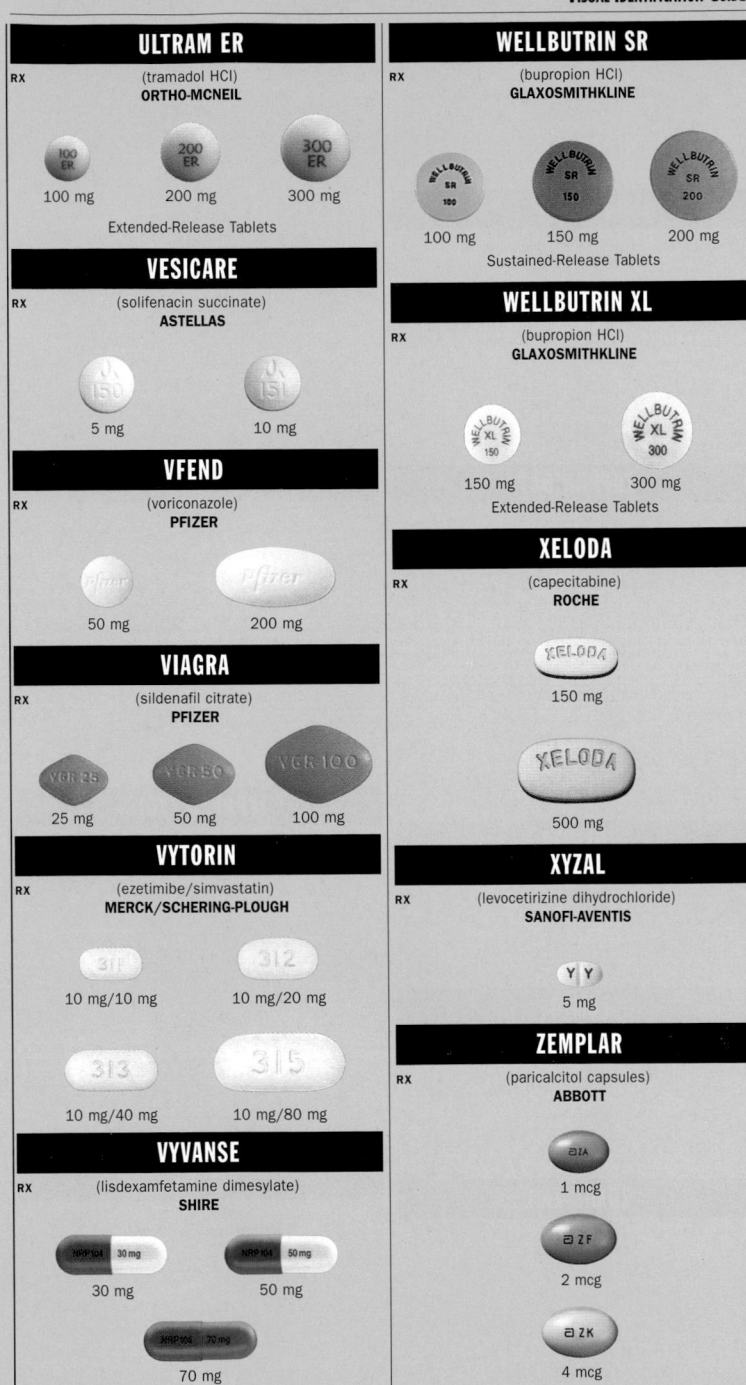

ULTRAM ER

RX

(tramadol HCI)
ORTHO-MCNEIL

100 mg   200 mg   300 mg

Extended-Release Tablets

VESICARE

RX

(solifenacin succinate)
ASTELLAS

5 mg   10 mg

VFEND

RX

(voriconazole)
PFIZER

50 mg   200 mg

VIAGRA

RX

(sildenafil citrate)
PFIZER

25 mg   50 mg   100 mg

VYTORIN

RX

(ezetimibe/simvastatin)
MERCK/SCHERING-PLOUGH

10 mg/10 mg   10 mg/20 mg

10 mg/40 mg   10 mg/80 mg

VYVANSE

RX

(lisdexamfetamine dimesylate)
SHIRE

30 mg   50 mg

70 mg

WELLBUTRIN SR

RX

(bupropion HCI)
GLAXOSMITHKLINE

100 mg   150 mg   200 mg

Sustained-Release Tablets

WELLBUTRIN XL

RX

(bupropion HCI)
GLAXOSMITHKLINE

150 mg   300 mg

Extended-Release Tablets

XELODA

RX

(capecitabine)
ROCHE

150 mg

500 mg

XYZAL

RX

(levocetirizine dihydrochloride)
SANOFI-AVENTIS

5 mg

ZEMPLAR

RX

(paricalcitol capsules)
ABBOTT

1 mcg

2 mcg

4 mcg

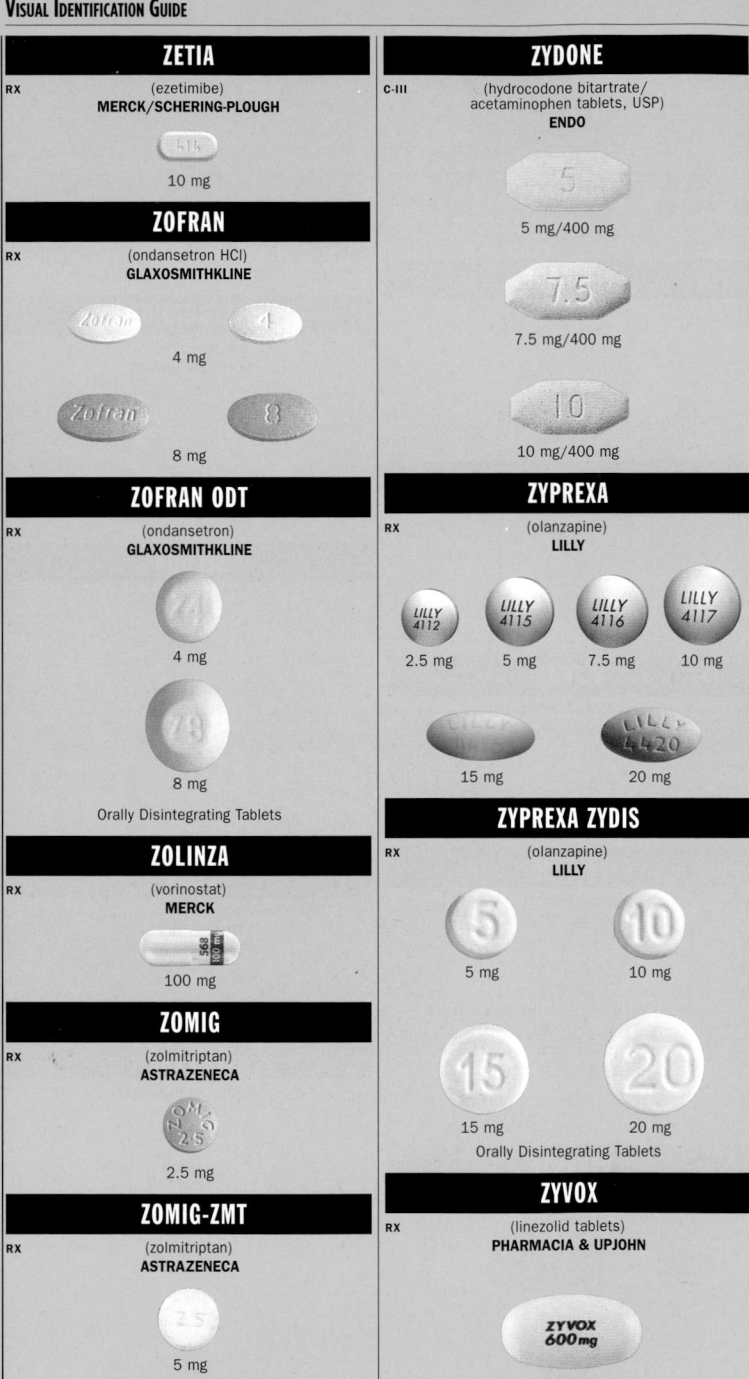

ZETIA

RX

(ezetimibe)
MERCK/SCHERING-PLOUGH

10 mg

ZOFRAN

RX

(ondansetron HCl)
GLAXOSMITHKLINE

4 mg

8 mg

ZOFRAN ODT

RX

(ondansetron)
GLAXOSMITHKLINE

4 mg

8 mg

Orally Disintegrating Tablets

ZOLINZA

RX

(vorinostat)
MERCK

100 mg

ZOMIG

RX

(zolmitriptan)
ASTRAZENECA

2.5 mg

ZOMIG-ZMT

RX

(zolmitriptan)
ASTRAZENECA

5 mg

Orally Disintegrating Tablets

ZYDONE

C-III

(hydrocodone bitartrate/
acetaminophen tablets, USP)
ENDO

5 mg/400 mg

7.5 mg/400 mg

10 mg/400 mg

ZYPREXA

RX

(olanzapine)
LILLY

2.5 mg   5 mg   7.5 mg   10 mg

15 mg   20 mg

ZYPREXA ZYDIS

RX

(olanzapine)
LILLY

5 mg   10 mg

15 mg   20 mg

Orally Disintegrating Tablets

ZYVOX

RX

(linezolid tablets)
PHARMACIA & UPJOHN

600 mg

phenytoin, carbamazepine, griseofulvin, topiramate, St. John's wort, and possibly with ampicillin and tetracyclines.

PREGNANCY: Category X, not for use in nursing.

MECHANISM OF ACTION: Estrogen/progestogen combination oral contraceptive: Acts by suppressing gonadotropins. Primarily inhibits ovulation. Also causes changes to the cervical mucus (increases the difficulty of sperm entry into the uterus), and causes changes in the endometrium (reduces the likehood of implantation).

PHARMACOKINETICS: Absorption: Rapid. Oral administration of various doses led to altered parameters. **Distribution:** Norgestimate: Albumin binding (>97%). Ethinyl estradiol: albumin binding (>97%). **Metabolism:** Norgestimate: GI tract and/or liver (1st pass mechanism), hepatic. Norelgestromin (major active metabolite), norgestrel (major active metabolite) Ethinyl estradiol: Hydroxylated, glucuronide, and sulfate conjugates. **Elimination:** Norgestimate: Urine (47%), feces (37%).

ORTHO-EST   RX
estropipate (Women First)

> Estrogens increase risk of endometrial cancer in postmenopausal women. Avoid during pregnancy.

THERAPEUTIC CLASS: Estrogen

INDICATIONS: Treatment of moderate to severe vasomotor symptoms of menopause and/or vulval/vaginal atrophy. Treatment of hypoestrogenism due to hypogonadism, castration, or primary ovarian failure. Prevention of osteoporosis.

DOSAGE: *Adults:* Vasomotor Symptoms: 0.75-6mg/day (as estropipate). Start cyclic administration arbitrarily if not menstruating, or on day 5 of bleeding if menstruating. Vulval/Vaginal Atrophy: 0.75-6mg/day (as estropipate), administer cyclically. Discontinue/Taper over a 3-6 month interval. Female Hypogonadism/Castration/Primary Ovarian Failure: 1.5-9mg/day (as estropipate) for 1st 3 weeks of cycle, then 8-10 days off. For female hypogonadism, repeat dose if bleeding does not occur, or add progestogen in 3rd week of cycle. Maint: Lowest effective dose. Osteoporosis Prevention: 0.75mg (as estropipate) qd for 25 days of a 31-day cycle.

HOW SUPPLIED: Tab: 0.625mg* (0.75mg estropipate), 1.25mg* (1.5mg estropipate) *scored

CONTRAINDICATIONS: Pregnancy, undiagnosed abnormal genital bleeding, breast cancer unless being treated for metastatic disease, estrogen-dependent neoplasia, thrombophlebitis, or thromboembolic disorders.

WARNINGS/PRECAUTIONS: Risk of gallbladder disease, endometrial and breast carcinoma, fetal congenital reproductive tract disorder, elevated BP, and hypercalcemia with breast cancer and bone metastases. Possible risk of cardiovascular disease. Caution in liver dysfunction, asthma, epilepsy, migraine, and cardiac or renal dysfunction. Increase in HDL, triglycerides, thyroid binding globulin. Acceleration of PT, PTT. Hypercoagulability effects. Impaired glucose tolerance. Consider adding progestin in patient with intact uterus.

ADVERSE REACTIONS: Altered vaginal bleeding, vaginal candidiasis, breast tenderness/enlargement, GI effects, melasma, CNS effects, weight changes, edema, altered libido.

PREGNANCY: Category X, caution in nursing.

ORTHO-NOVUM 1/35   RX
ethinyl estradiol - norethindrone (Ortho-McNeil)

OTHER BRAND NAMES: Nortrel 1/35 (Barr) - Norinyl 1/35 (Watson) - Necon 1/35 (Watson)

THERAPEUTIC CLASS: Estrogen/progestogen combination

INDICATIONS: Prevention of pregnancy.

DOSAGE: *Adults:* 1 tab qd for 28 days, then repeat. Start 1st Sunday after menses begin or 1st day of menses.

HOW SUPPLIED: (Ethinyl Estradiol-Norethindrone) Tab: 0.035mg-1mg

CONTRAINDICATIONS: Thrombophlebitis, DVT or thromboembolic disorders, pregnancy, cerebrovascular or coronary artery disease, undiagnosed abnormal genital bleeding, cholestatic jaundice of pregnancy or jaundice with prior pill use, hepatic adenomas or carcinomas, breast cancer or other estrogen-dependent neoplasia.

WARNINGS/PRECAUTIONS: Cigarette smoking increases risk of serious cardiovascular side effects. This risk increases with age (especially >35 yrs) and heavy smoking. Increased risk of MI, vascular disease, thromboembolism, stroke and gallbladder disease. Retinal thrombosis, hepatic neoplasia, carcinoma of breast and reproductive organs reported. May cause glucose intolerance. May increase BP, elevate LDL levels or cause other lipid changes, fluid retention, breakthrough bleeding, and spotting. May cause or exacerbate migraine. May develop visual changes with contact lens. Increased risk of MI with HTN, hyperlipidemia, obesity, and diabetes. D/C if jaundice, significant depression, or ophthalmic irregularities develop. Perform annual physical exam. Use before menarche is not indicated. May affect certain endocrine, LFTs and blood components.

ADVERSE REACTIONS: Nausea, vomiting, breakthrough bleeding, spotting, amenorrhea, migraine, depression, vaginal candidiasis, edema, weight changes.

INTERACTIONS: Reduced effects, increased breakthrough bleeding, and menstrual irregularities with rifampin, barbiturates, phenylbutazone, phenytoin, carbamazepine, griseofulvin, topiramate, St. John's wort, and possibly with ampicillin and tetracyclines.

PREGNANCY: Category X, not for use in nursing.

MECHANISM OF ACTION: Estrogen/progestogen combination oral contraceptive: acts by suppressing gonadotropins, primarily inhibiting ovulation, and causing changes in cervical mucus (increasing difficulty of sperm entry into uterus) and endometrium (reducing likelihood of implantation).

Ortho-Novum 1/50   RX
norethindrone - mestranol (Ortho-McNeil)

OTHER BRAND NAMES: Brevicon (Watson) - Necon 1/50 (Watson) - Norinyl 1/50 (Watson)

THERAPEUTIC CLASS: Estrogen/progestogen combination

INDICATIONS: Prevention of pregnancy.

DOSAGE: *Adults:* 1 tab qd for 28 days, then repeat. Start 1st Sunday after menses begins or 1st day of menses.

HOW SUPPLIED: Tab: (Mestranol-Norethindrone) 0.05mg-1mg

CONTRAINDICATIONS: Thrombophlebitis, DVT or thromboembolic disorders, pregnancy, cerebrovascular or coronary artery disease, undiagnosed abnormal genital bleeding, cholestatic jaundice of pregnancy or jaundice with prior pill use, hepatic adenomas or carcinomas, breast cancer or other estrogen-dependent neoplasia.

WARNINGS/PRECAUTIONS: Cigarette smoking increases risk of serious cardiovascular side effects. This risk increases with age (especially >35 yrs) and heavy smoking. Increased risk of MI, vascular disease, thromboembolism, stroke, and gallbladder disease. Retinal thrombosis, hepatic neoplasia, carcinoma of breast and reproductive organs reported. May cause glucose intolerance. May increase BP, elevate LDL levels or cause other lipid changes, fluid retention, breakthrough bleeding, and spotting. May cause or exacerbate migraine. May develop visual changes with contact lenses. Increased risk of MI with HTN, hyperlipidemia, obesity, and diabetes. D/C if jaundice, significant depression, or ophthalmic irregularities develop. Perform annual physical exam. Use before menarche is not indicated. May affect certain endocrine, LFTs, and blood components.

ADVERSE REACTIONS: Nausea, vomiting, breakthrough bleeding, spotting, amenorrhea, migraine, depression, vaginal candidiasis, edema, weight changes.

INTERACTIONS: Reduced effects, increased breakthrough bleeding, and menstrual irregularities with rifampin, barbiturates, phenylbutazone, phenytoin, carbamazepine, griseofulvin, topiramate, St. John's wort, and possibly with ampicillin and tetracyclines.

PREGNANCY: Category X, not for use in nursing.

MECHANISM OF ACTION: Estrogen/progestogen combination oral contraceptive: acts by suppressing gonadotropin, inhibiting ovulation, causing changes in cervical mucus, increasing difficulty of sperm entry into uterus and endometrium, reducing likehood of implantation.

PHARMACOKINETICS: Distribution: Found in breast milk.

ORTHO-NOVUM 10/11   RX
ethinyl estradiol - norethindrone (Ortho-McNeil)

OTHER BRAND NAMES: Necon 10/11 (Watson)

THERAPEUTIC CLASS: Estrogen/progestogen combination

INDICATIONS: Prevention of pregnancy.

DOSAGE: *Adults:* 1 tab qd for 28 days, then repeat. Start 1st Sunday after menses begin or 1st day of menses.

HOW SUPPLIED: Tab: (Ethinyl Estradiol-Norethindrone) 0.035mg-0.5mg and 0.035mg-1mg

CONTRAINDICATIONS: Thrombophlebitis, DVT or thromboembolic disorders, pregnancy, cerebrovascular or coronary artery disease, undiagnosed abnormal genital bleeding, cholestatic jaundice of pregnancy or jaundice with prior pill use, hepatic adenomas or carcinomas, breast cancer or other estrogen-dependent neoplasia.

WARNINGS/PRECAUTIONS: Cigarette smoking increases risk of serious cardiovascular side effects; risk increases with age (especially >35 yrs) and heavy smoking. Increased risk of MI, vascular disease, thromboembolism, stroke, and gallbladder disease. Retinal thrombosis, hepatic neoplasia reported. May cause glucose intolerance. May increase BP, elevate LDL levels or cause other lipid changes, fluid retention, breakthrough bleeding, and spotting. May cause or exacerbate migraine. May develop visual changes with contact lens. Morbidity and mortality risk increased with HTN, hyperlipidemia, obesity, and diabetes. D/C if jaundice, significant depression, or ophthalmic irregularities develop. Perform annual physical exam. Use before menarche is not indicated. May affect certain endocrine, LFTs, and blood components.

ADVERSE REACTIONS: Nausea, vomiting, breakthrough bleeding, spotting, amenorrhea, migraine, depression, vaginal candidiasis, edema, weight changes.

INTERACTIONS: Reduced effects, increased breakthrough bleeding, and menstrual irregularities with rifampin, barbiturates, phenylbutazone, phenytoin, carbamazepine, and possibly with griseofulvin, ampicillin, and tetracyclines.

PREGNANCY: Category X, not for use in nursing.

MECHANISM OF ACTION: Estrogen/progestogen combination oral contraceptive: acts by suppression of gonadotrophins. Primary mechanism inhibits ovulation. Also causes changes in cervical mucus (which increases difficulty of sperm entry into uterus) and in endometrium (which reduces likelihood of implantation).

PHARMACOKINETICS: Distribution: Found in breast milk.

ORTHO-NOVUM 7/7/7   RX
ethinyl estradiol - norethindrone (Ortho-McNeil)

OTHER BRAND NAMES: Nortrel 7/7/7 (Barr)

THERAPEUTIC CLASS: Estrogen/progestogen combination

INDICATIONS: Prevention of pregnancy.

DOSAGE: *Adults:* 1 tab qd for 28 days, then repeat. Start 1st Sunday after menses begin or 1st day of menses.

HOW SUPPLIED: Tab: (Ethinyl Estradiol-Norethindrone) 0.035mg-0.5mg, 0.035mg-0.75mg and 0.035mg-1mg

CONTRAINDICATIONS: Thrombophlebitis, DVT or thromboembolic disorders, pregnancy, cerebrovascular or coronary artery disease, undiagnosed abnormal genital bleeding, cholestatic jaundice of pregnancy or jaundice with prior pill use, hepatic adenomas or carcinomas, breast cancer or other estrogen-dependent neoplasia.

WARNINGS/PRECAUTIONS: Cigarette smoking increases risk of serious cardiovascular side effects; risk increases with age (especially >35 yrs) and heavy smoking. Increased risk of MI, vascular disease, thromboembolism, stroke and gallbladder disease. Retinal thrombosis, hepatic neoplasia, carcinoma of breast and reproductive organs reported. May cause glucose intolerance. May increase BP, elevate LDL levels or cause other lipid changes, fluid retention, breakthrough bleeding, and spotting. May cause or exacerbate migraine. May develop visual changes with contact lens. Increased risk of MI with HTN, hyperlipidemia, obesity, and diabetes. D/C if jaundice, significant depression or ophthalmic irregularities develop. Perform annual physical exam. Use before menarche is not indicated. May affect certain endocrine, LFTs, and blood components.

ADVERSE REACTIONS: Nausea, vomiting, breakthrough bleeding, spotting, amenorrhea, migraine, depression, vaginal candidiasis, edema, weight changes.

INTERACTIONS: Reduced effects, increased breakthrough bleeding, and menstrual irregularities with rifampin, barbiturates, phenylbutazone, phenytoin, carbamazepine, griseofulvin, topiramate, St. John's wort, and possibly with ampicillin and tetracyclines.

PREGNANCY: Category X, not for use in nursing.

MECHANISM OF ACTION: Estrogen/progestogen combination oral contraceptive: acts by suppression of gonadotropins. Primary mechanism inhibits ovulation. Also causes changes in cervical mucus (which increases difficulty of sperm entry into uterus) and in endometrium (which reduces likelihood of implantation).

PHARMACOKINETICS: Distribution: Found in breast milk.

OVACE   RX
sulfacetamide sodium (Healthpoint)

THERAPEUTIC CLASS: Sulfonamide

INDICATIONS: Topical application for seborrheic dermatitis, seborrhea sicca (dandruff). Treatment of secondary bacterial infections of the skin.

DOSAGE: *Adults:* Seborrheic Dermatitis/Dandruff: (Cre/Gel/Foam) Apply to affected area bid for 8-10 days. (Wash) Wash affected area bid for 8-10 days. To prevent recurrence, apply once or twice weekly, or every other week. Bacterial Infection: (Cre/Gel) Apply to affected area bid for 8-10 days. (Foam) Apply to affected area qd for 8-10 days. (Wash) Wash affected area qd for 8-10 days.

HOW SUPPLIED: Cre: 10% [30g, 60g]; Gel: 10% [30g, 60g]; Foam: 10% [50g, 100g]; Wash: 10% [170mL, 340mL]

CONTRAINDICATIONS: Hypersensitivity to sulfonamides.

WARNINGS/PRECAUTIONS: Stevens-Johnson syndrome in hypersensitive individuals, and systemic lupus erythematous reported with sulfonamides. May cause proliferation of nonsusceptible organisms. D/C if hypersensitivity or untoward reactions occur. Greater systemic absorption in application to large, infected, abraded, denuded or severely burned area.

ADVERSE REACTIONS: Irritation, hypersensitivity.

INTERACTIONS: Incompatible with silver preparations.

PREGNANCY: Category C, caution in nursing.

MECHANISM OF ACTION: Sulfonamide; exerts a bacteriostatic effect against susceptible gram-positive and gram-negative microorganisms. Acts by restricting the synthesis of folic acid required by bacteria for growth, through competition with paraminobenzoic acid (PABA).

Ovcon-35   RX
ethinyl estradiol - norethindrone (Warner Chilcott)

OTHER BRAND NAMES: Balziva (Barr) - Ovcon-50 (Warner Chilcott)

THERAPEUTIC CLASS: Estrogen/progestogen combination

INDICATIONS: Prevention of pregnancy.

DOSAGE: *Adults:* 1 tab qd for 28 days, then repeat. Start 1st Sunday after menses begin or the 1st day of menses.

HOW SUPPLIED: (Ethinyl Estradiol-Norethindrone) Tab: (Ovcon 35, Balziva) 0.035mg-0.4mg; (Ovcon 50) 0.05mg-1mg

CONTRAINDICATIONS: Thrombophlebitis, DVT or thromboembolic disorders, pregnancy, cerebrovascular or coronary artery disease, valvular heart disease with thrombogenic complications, uncontrolled HTN, DM with vascular involvement, HA with focal neurological symptoms, major surgery with prolonged immobilization, undiagnosed abnormal genital bleeding, cholestatic jaundice of pregnancy or jaundice with prior pill use, hepatic adenomas or carcinomas, breast cancer, endometrial cancer or other estrogen-dependent neoplasia.

WARNINGS/PRECAUTIONS: Cigarette smoking increases risk of serious cardiovascular side effects. This risk increases with age (especially >35 yrs) and heavy smoking. Increased risk of MI, vascular disease, thromboembolism, stroke and gallbladder disease. Retinal thrombosis, hepatic neoplasia, carcinoma of breast and reproductive organs reported. May cause glucose intolerance. May increase BP, elevate LDL levels or cause other lipid changes, fluid retention, breakthrough bleeding, and spotting. May cause or exacerbate migraine. May develop visual changes with contact lens. Increased risk of MI with HTN, hyperlipidemia, obesity, and diabetes. D/C if develop jaundice, significant depression or ophthalmic irregularities. Perform annual physical exam. Use before menarche is not indicated. May affect certain endocrine, LFTs and blood components.

ADVERSE REACTIONS: Nausea, vomiting, breakthrough bleeding, spotting, amenorrhea, migraine, depression, vaginal candidiasis, edema, weight changes.

INTERACTIONS: Reduced effects, increased breakthrough bleeding, and menstrual irregularities with rifampin, barbiturates, phenylbutazone, phenytoin, carbamazepine, felbamate, oxcarbazepine, topiramate, griseofulvin, ampicillin, and tetracyclines. Anti-HIV PIs may change (increase or decrease) the levels of OCs. Herbal products, such as St. John's Wort may reduce the levels of OCs and result in breakthrough bleeding. Atorvastatin, ascorbic acid, acetaminophen, CYP3A4 inhibitors (itraconazole or ketoconazole) may increase the levels of ehinyl estradiol. Increased levels of cyclosporin, prednisolone, theophylline reported. Decreased levels of actaminophen and increased clearance of temazepam, salicylic acid, morphine, clofibric acid reported.

PREGNANCY: Category X, not for use in nursing.

MECHANISM OF ACTION: Estrogen/progestogen combination oral contraceptive: acts by suppressing gonadotropins, primarily inhibiting ovulation, and causing changes in cervical mucus (increasing difficulty of sperm entry into uterus) and endometrium (reducing likelihood of implantation).

PHARMACOKINETICS: Distribution: Found in breast milk.

OVCON-35 FE   RX
ethinyl estradiol - ferrous fumarate - norethindrone (Warner Chilcott)

THERAPEUTIC CLASS: Estrogen/progestogen combination

INDICATIONS: Prevention of pregnancy.

DOSAGE: *Adults:* 1 tab qd for 28 days, then repeat. Start 1st Sunday after menses begin or the 1st day of menses.

HOW SUPPLIED: Tab, Chewable: (Ethinyl Estradiol-Norethindrone) 0.035mg-0.4mg [21^s], (Ferrous Fumarate) 75mg [7^s]

CONTRAINDICATIONS: Thrombophlebitis, DVT or thromboembolic disorders, pregnancy, cerebrovascular or coronary artery disease, valvular heart disease with thrombogenic complications, uncontrolled HTN, DM with vascular involvement, HA with focal neurological symptoms, major surgery with prolonged immobilization, undiagnosed abnormal genital bleeding, cholestatic jaundice of pregnancy or jaundice with prior pill use, hepatic adenomas or carcinomas, breast cancer, endometrial cancer or other estrogen-dependent neoplasia.

WARNINGS/PRECAUTIONS: Cigarette smoking increases risk of serious cardiovascular side effects; risk increases with age (especially >35 yrs) and heavy smoking. Increased risk of MI, vascular disease, thromboembolism, stroke and gallbladder disease. Retinal thrombosis, hepatic neoplasia, carcinoma of breast and reproductive organs reported. May cause glucose intolerance. May increase BP, elevate LDL levels or cause other lipid changes, fluid retention, breakthrough bleeding, and spotting. May cause or exacerbate migraine. May develop visual changes with contact lens. Increased risk of MI with HTN, hyperlipidemia, obesity, and diabetes. D/C if jaundice, significant depression, or ophthalmic irregularities develop. Perform annual physical exam. Use before menarche is not indicated. May affect certain endocrine, LFTs and blood components.

ADVERSE REACTIONS: Nausea, vomiting, breakthrough bleeding, spotting, amenorrhea, migraine, depression, vaginal candidiasis, edema, weight changes.

INTERACTIONS: Reduced effects, increased breakthrough bleeding, and menstrual irregularities with rifampin, barbiturates, phenylbutazone, phenytoin, carbamazepine, felbamate, oxcarbazepine, topiramate, griseofulvin, ampicillin, and tetracyclines. Anti-HIV PIs may change (increase or decrease) the levels of OCs. Herbal products, such as St. John's Wort may reduce the levels of OCs and result in breakthrough bleeding. Atorvastatin, ascorbic acid, acetaminophen, CYP3A4 inhibitors (itraconazole or ketoconazole) may increase the levels of ehinyl estradiol. Increased levels of cyclosporin, prednisolone, theophylline reported. Decreased levels of actaminophen and increased clearance of temazepam, salicylic acid, morphine, clofibric acid reported.

PREGNANCY: Category X, not for use in nursing.

MECHANISM OF ACTION: Estrogen/progestogen combination oral contraceptive: Acts by suppression of gonadotropins. Primary mechanism is through inhibition of ovulation. Also causes changes in cervical mucus (which increases difficulty of sperm entry ino uterus) and endometrium (which reduces likelihood of implantation).

PHARMACOKINETICS: Absorption: Rapid. Norethindrone: Absolute bioavailability (65%), C_{max}=4210.6pg/mL, T_{max}=1.24 hr, AUC=18034.9pg•h/mL; Ethinyl estradiol: Absolute bioavailability (43%), C_{max}=131.4pg/mL, T_{max}=1.44 hrs, AUC=1065.8pg•h/mL. **Distribution:** V_d=2-4L/kg; Norethindone: Sex hormone-binding globulin binding (36%), albumin binding (61%). Ethinyl estradiol: Albumin binding (98.5%). **Metabolism:** Norethindone: Reduction, sulfate, glucoronide conjugation. Ethinyl estradiol: CYP3A4, via oxidation (conjugation with sulfate and glucuronide), 2-hydroxy-ethinyl estradiol (primary oxidative metabolite). **Elimination:** Norethindrone: $T_{1/2}$=9 hrs; Urine (50%), feces (20-40%). Ethinyl Estradiol: $T_{1/2}$=17 hrs; Urine, feces.

OVIDE
malathion (Taro)   RX

THERAPEUTIC CLASS: Organophosphate/cholinesterase inhibitor

INDICATIONS: For infections of *Pediculus humanus capitis* (head lice and their ova) of scalp hair.

DOSAGE: *Adults:* Apply sufficient amount on dry hair to thoroughly wet hair and scalp. Allow hair to dry naturally. Shampoo after 8-12 hrs. Rinse and use a fine-toothed comb to remove dead lice and eggs. Repeat with 2nd application if lice present after 7-9 days.
Pediatrics: ≥6 yrs: Apply sufficient amount on dry hair to thoroughly wet hair and scalp. Allow hair to dry naturally. Shampoo after 8-12 hrs. Rinse and use a fine-toothed comb to remove dead lice and eggs. Repeat with 2nd application if lice present after 7-9 days.

HOW SUPPLIED: Lot: 0.5% [59mL]

CONTRAINDICATIONS: Neonates, infants.

WARNINGS/PRECAUTIONS: Lotion is flammable; do not expose lotion or wet hair to open flames or electric heat sources (eg, hair dryers, electric curlers). If contact with eyes, flush immediately with water. If skin irritation develops, d/c until irritation clears. Slight stinging sensations reported. Adult supervision is required with use in children.

ADVERSE REACTIONS: Skin and scalp irritation, mild conjunctivitis (with eye contact).

PREGNANCY: Category B, caution in nursing.

MECHANISM OF ACTION: Organophosphate/cholinesterase inhibitor; acts as a pediculocide by inhibiting cholinesterase activity.

OVIDREL
choriogonadotropin alfa (EMD Serono)   RX

THERAPEUTIC CLASS: Recombinant human chorionic gonadotropin

INDICATIONS: For induction of final follicular maturation and early luteinization in infertile women who have undergone pituitary desensitization and pretreated with follicle stimulating hormone in an Assisted Reproductive Technology program. To induce ovulation and pregnancy in anovulatory, infertile women in whom anovulation is not due to primary ovarian failure.

DOSAGE: *Adults:* 250mcg SQ 1 day following the last dose of follicle stimulating agent. Withhold if excessive ovarian response.

HOW SUPPLIED: Inj: 250mcg/0.5mL

CONTRAINDICATIONS: Primary ovarian failure, uncontrolled thyroid or adrenal function, uncontrolled organic intracranial lesion (eg, pituitary tumor), abnormal uterine bleeding of undetermined origin, ovarian cyst or enlargement of undetermined origin, sex hormone dependent tumors of reproductive tract and accessory organs, pregnancy.

WARNINGS/PRECAUTIONS: Ovarian hyperstimulation syndrome (OHSS), multiple births, and elevated ALTs reported. Potential for arterial thromboembolism. Withhold hCG if ovarian enlargement or OHSS occurs. Administer when adequate follicular development indicated by serum estradiol and vaginal ultrasonography occurs.

ADVERSE REACTIONS: Injection site pain/bruising, abdominal pain, nausea, vomiting.

PREGNANCY: Category X, caution in nursing.

O

MECHANISM OF ACTION: Recombinant human chorionic gonadotropin; stimulates late follicle maturation and resumption of oocyte meiosis and initiates rupture of pre-ovulatory ovarian follicle.

PHARMACOKINETICS: Absorption: C_{max}=121 IU/L, T_{max}=24 hrs, AUC=7701h•IU/L, absolute bioavailability (40%). **Elimination:** Urine, $T_{1/2}$=9 hrs.

OXANDRIN

oxandrolone (Savient)

THERAPEUTIC CLASS: Anabolic steroid

INDICATIONS: Adjunctive therapy to promote weight gain after weight loss following extensive surgery, chronic infections, severe trauma, and for those who fail to gain or maintain normal weight without pathophysiologic reasons, to offset protein catabolism associated with prolonged administration of corticosteroids, for the relief of osteoporotic bone pain.

DOSAGE: *Adults:* Usual: 2.5-20mg/day given bid-qid for 2-4 weeks. May repeat course intermittently as indicated. Elderly: 5mg bid.
Pediatrics: ≤0.1mg/kg/day. May repeat intermittently as indicated.

HOW SUPPLIED: Tab: 2.5mg*, 10mg *scored

CONTRAINDICATIONS: Carcinoma of the prostate or breast, carcinoma of the breast in females with hypercalcemia, pregnancy, nephrosis, hypercalcemia.

WARNINGS/PRECAUTIONS: D/C if peliosis hepatis, liver cell tumors, cholestatic hepatitis, jaundice, LFT abnormalities, hypercalcemia or signs of virilization (females) occur. Edema, with or without CHF, may occur with pre-existing cardiac, renal, or hepatic disease. Monitor bone growth in children every 6 months. Increased risk of prostatic hypertrophy/carcinoma in the elderly. May decrease levels of thyroxine-binding globulin, suppress clotting factors II, V, VII, and X and increase PT. Caution with CAD and history of MI. Lower dose recommended in elderly.

ADVERSE REACTIONS: Cholestatic jaundice, gynecomastia, edema, CNS effects, acne, phallic enlargement, increased frequency/persistence of erections, inhibition of testicular function, chronic priapism, epididymitis, impotence, testicular atrophy, oligospermia, bladder irritability, menstrual irregularities, virilization.

INTERACTIONS: Increased sensitivity to oral anticoagulants (eg, warfarin). May increase edema with adrenal cortical steroids or ACTH. May inhibit metabolism of oral hypoglycemics.

PREGNANCY: Category X, not for use in nursing.

MECHANISM OF ACTION: Anabolic steroid; inhibits endogenous testosterone release through inhibition of pituitary luteinizing hormone.

PHARMACOKINETICS: Elimination: $T_{1/2}$=13.3 hrs (elderly), 10.4 hrs (young).

OXAZEPAM

oxazepam (Various)

THERAPEUTIC CLASS: Benzodiazepine

INDICATIONS: Management of anxiety and alcohol withdrawal.

DOSAGE: *Adults:* Anxiety: Mild-Moderate: 10-15mg tid-qid. Severe: 15-30mg tid-qid. Elderly: Initial: 10mg tid. Titrate: Increase to 15mg tid-qid. Alcohol Withdrawal: 15-30mg tid-qid.

HOW SUPPLIED: Cap: 10mg, 15mg, 30mg; Tab: 15mg

CONTRAINDICATIONS: Psychoses.

WARNINGS/PRECAUTIONS: May impair mental/physical abilities. Withdrawal symptoms with abrupt discontinuation. Caution in sensitivity to hypotension, elderly. Caution with tablets in tartrazine or ASA allergy. Risk of congenital malformations; avoid in pregnancy.

ADVERSE REACTIONS: Drowsiness, dizziness, vertigo, headache, paradoxical excitement, transient amnesia, memory impairment.

INTERACTIONS: Additive effects with alcohol and other CNS depressants.

PREGNANCY: Not for use in pregnancy or nursing.

MECHANISM OF ACTION: Benzodiazepine; binds to benzodiazepine receptors and enhances GABA effects.

PHARMACOKINETICS: Absorption: C_{max}=450mg/mL. T_{max}=3 hrs. **Metabolism:** Liver via CYP450. Glucuronide (major inactive metabolite). **Elimination:** Urine. $T_{1/2}$=8.2 hrs.

OXISTAT   RX
oxiconazole nitrate (GlaxoSmithKline)

THERAPEUTIC CLASS: Azole antifungal

INDICATIONS: (Cre/Lot) Topical treatment of tinea pedis, tinea cruris and tinea corporis due to *Trichophyton rubrum*, *Trichophyton mentagrophytes* , or *Epidermophyton floccosum*. (Cre) Topical treatment of tinea versicolor due to *Malassezia furfur*.

DOSAGE: *Adults:* (Cre/Lot) T.pedis/T.corporis/T.cruris: Apply qd-bid. (Cre) T.versicolor: Apply qd. Treat t.pedis for 1 month and other infections for 2 weeks.
Pediatrics: ≥12 yrs: (Cream) T.pedis/T.corporis/T.cruris: Apply qd-bid. T.versicolor: Apply qd. Treat t.pedis for 1 month and other infections for 2 weeks.

HOW SUPPLIED: Cre: 1% [15g, 30g, 60g]; Lot: 1% [30mL]

WARNINGS/PRECAUTIONS: Not for ophthalmic or intravaginal use. D/C if irritation or sensitivity occurs.

ADVERSE REACTIONS: Pruritus, burning/stinging.

PREGNANCY: Category B, caution in nursing.

MECHANISM OF ACTION: Azole antifungal; acts by inhibition of ergosterol biosynthesis, which is critical for cellular membrane integrity.

PHARMACOKINETICS: Distribution: Excreted in breast milk. **Elimination**: Urine (<0.3%).

OXYCONTIN   CII
oxycodone HCL (Purdue Pharma)

> For continuous analgesia. Abuse potential. 80mg tabs only for opioid-tolerant patients. Swallow tabs whole.

THERAPEUTIC CLASS: Opioid analgesic

INDICATIONS: Management of moderate to severe pain when a continuous analgesic is needed for an extended period. Only for postoperative use in patients already receiving the drug before surgery or those expected to have moderate-severe postoperative pain for an extended period of time.

DOSAGE: *Adults:* ≥18 yrs: Opioid Naive: 10mg q12h. Titrate: May increase to 20mg q12h, then may increase the total daily dose by 25-50% of the current dose. Increase every 1-2 days. Conversion from Oxycodone: Divide 24 hr oxycodone dose in half to obtain q12h dose. Round down to appropriate tab strength. Opioid Tolerant Patients: May use 80mg tabs. D/C other around-the-clock opioids. With CNS Depressants: Reduce dose by 1/3 or 1/2. Swallow whole; do not break, crush, or chew.

HOW SUPPLIED: Tab, Extended-Release: 10mg, 20mg, 40mg, 80mg

CONTRAINDICATIONS: Significant respiratory depression, acute or severe bronchial asthma, hypercarbia, paralytic ileus.

WARNINGS/PRECAUTIONS: Do not break, chew, or crush tabs. Extreme caution with COPD, cor pulmonale, decreased respiratory reserve, hypoxia,

OxyIR

hypercapnia, pre-existing respiratory depression. Caution with circulatory shock, delirium tremens, acute alcoholism, adrenocortical insufficiency, CNS depression, myxedema or hypothyroidism, BPH, severe hepatic/renal/pulmonary impairment, toxic psychosis, biliary tract disease, increased ICP or head injury, elderly or debilitated. May cause severe hypotension. May produce drug dependence; caution in known drug abuse. May aggravate convulsive disorders and mask abdominal disorders.

ADVERSE REACTIONS: Respiratory depression, constipation, nausea, somnolence, dizziness, vomiting, pruritus, headache, dry mouth, sweating, asthenia.

INTERACTIONS: Respiratory depression, hypotension and profound sedation with other CNS depressants (eg, sedatives, anesthetics, phenothiazines, alcohol). Mixed agonist/antagonist analgesics may reduce the analgesic effect and/or cause withdrawal. Risk of severe hypotension with phenothiazines, or other agents that compromise vasomotor tone. May enhance skeletal muscle relaxant effects and increase respiratory depression. May interact with CYP2D6 inhibitors (eg, amiodarone, quinidine, polycyclic antidepressants). Caution with MAOIs.

PREGNANCY: Category B, not for use in nursing.

MECHANISM OF ACTION: Opioid analgesic; pure agonist opioid whose principle therapeutic action is analgesia. Precise mechanism of analgesic action has not been established. However, specific CNS opioid receptors for endogenous compounds with opioid-like activity have been found throughout the brain and spinal cord and play a role in the analgesic effects.

PHARMACOKINETICS: Absorption: Well absorbed, various doses resulted in altered parameters. **Distribution:** Plasma protein binding (45%); V_d=2.6L/kg, found in breast milk. **Metabolism:** Extensively to noroxycodone (major metabolite), CYP2D6 to oxymorphone (active metabolite). **Elimination:** Urine (major); $T_{1/2}$=4.5 hrs.

OxyIR
oxycodone HCL (Purdue Pharma)

CII

THERAPEUTIC CLASS: Opioid analgesic

INDICATIONS: Moderate to moderately severe pain.

DOSAGE: *Adults:* Usual: 5mg q6h prn for pain. May add to 30mL of juice or other liquid, applesauce, pudding, or other semi-solid foods.

HOW SUPPLIED: Cap: 5mg

CONTRAINDICATIONS: Respiratory depression, acute or severe bronchial asthma, hypercarbia, paralytic ileus, situations where opioids are contraindicated.

WARNINGS/PRECAUTIONS: Extreme caution with COPD, cor pulmonale, decreased respiratory reserve, hypoxia, hypercapnia, pre-existing respiratory depression. Caution with circulatory shock, delirium tremens, acute alcoholism, adrenocortical insufficiency, CNS depression, myxedema or hypothyroidism, BPH, severe hepatic/renal/pulmonary impairment, toxic psychosis, biliary tract disease, increased ICP, or head injury, elderly or debilitated. May cause severe hypotension. May produce drug dependence; caution in known drug abuse. May aggravate convulsive disorders and mask abdominal disorders. May impair mental/physical abilities.

ADVERSE REACTIONS: Lightheadedness, dizziness, nausea, vomiting, sedation.

INTERACTIONS: Respiratory depression, hypotension and profound sedation with other CNS depressants (eg, sedatives, anesthetics, phenothiazines, alcohol). Mixed agonist/antagonist analgesics may reduce the analgesic effect and/or cause withdrawal. Risk of severe hypotension with phenothiazines, or other agents that compromise vasomotor tone. May enhance skeletal muscle relaxant effects and increase respiratory depression. May interact with CYP2D6 inhibitors (eg, amiodarone, quinidine, polycyclic antidepressants). Caution with MAOIs.

PREGNANCY: Category B, not for use in nursing.

MECHANISM OF ACTION: Opioid analgesic; pure agonist opioid whose principle therapeutic effect is analgesia. Precise mechanism of analgesic action not established. However, specific CNS opioid receptors for endogenous compounds with opioid-like activity are found throughout the brain and spinal cord and play a role in analgesic effects.

PHARMACOKINETICS: Distribution: Found in breast milk. **Metabolism:** Via CYP2D6 to oxymorphone (metabolite).

OXYTROL   RX
oxybutynin (Watson)

THERAPEUTIC CLASS: Anticholinergic

INDICATIONS: Treatment of overactive bladder with symptoms of urge urinary incontinence, urgency, and frequency.

DOSAGE: *Adults:* Apply to dry, intact skin on the abdomen, hip, or buttock twice weekly (every 3-4 days). Rotate sites.

HOW SUPPLIED: Patch: 3.9mg/day [8^s]

CONTRAINDICATIONS: Urinary retention, gastric retention, uncontrolled narrow-angle glaucoma, and in patients at risk for these conditions.

WARNINGS/PRECAUTIONS: Caution with hepatic or renal impairment, bladder outflow obstruction, GI obstructive disorders, ulcerative colitis, intestinal atony, myasthenia gravis, and gastroesophageal reflux. Heat prostration may occur when used in a hot environment.

ADVERSE REACTIONS: Application site reactions, dry mouth, diarrhea, constipation, drowsiness, dizziness, blurred vision.

INTERACTIONS: Increased adverse events with other anticholinergics. Alcohol may enhance drowsiness effect. Caution with bisphosphonates or other drugs that may exacerbate esophagitis. May alter GI absorption of other drugs due to GI motility effects.

PREGNANCY: Category B, caution in nursing.

MECHANISM OF ACTION: Antispasmodic, anticholinergic agent; acts as competitive antagonist of acetylcholine at postganglionic muscarinic receptor, resulting in relaxation of bladder smooth muscle.

PHARMACOKINETICS: Absorption: (Single dose) C_{max}=3-3.4ng/mL, T_{max}=36-48 hrs. (Multiple dose) C_{max}=4.2-6.6ng/mL, T_{max}=10-28 hrs. **Distribution:** V_d=193L. **Metabolism:** CYP3A4, N-desethyloxybutynin (active metabolite). **Elimination:** $T_{1/2}$=7-8 hrs, urine (<0.1%).

PACERONE   RX
amiodarone HCL (Upsher-Smith)

THERAPEUTIC CLASS: Class III antiarrhythmic

INDICATIONS: Treatment of documented, life-threatening recurrent ventricular fibrillation and recurrent hemodynamically unstable ventricular tachycardia.

DOSAGE: *Adults:* Give LD in hospital. LD: 800-1600mg/day in divided doses for 1-3 weeks. After control is achieved, then 600-800mg/day for 1 month. Maint: 400mg/day; up to 600mg/day if needed. Use lowest effective dose. Take with meals. Elderly: Start at low end of dosing range.

HOW SUPPLIED: Tab: 100mg, 200mg*, 300mg*, 400mg* *scored

CONTRAINDICATIONS: Severe sinus-node dysfunction causing marked sinus bradycardia; 2nd- and 3rd-degree AV block; when episodes of bradycardia have caused syncope (except when used with a pacemaker).

WARNINGS/PRECAUTIONS: Only for life-threatening arrhythmias due to its substantial toxicity (eg, pulmonary toxicity, hepatic injury, arrhythmia exacerbation). Hospitalize when giving LD. May cause a clinical syndrome of cough and progressive dyspnea. D/C if LFTs are 3x the normal or if an elevated baseline doubles; monitor LFTs regularly. Optic neuropathy, optic neuritis reported. Fetal harm in pregnancy. May develop reversible corneal micro deposits (eg, visual halos, blurred vision), photosensitivity, peripheral neuropathy (rare). May decrease T_3 levels, increase thyroxine levels, increase inactive reverse T_3 levels and can cause hypo- or hyperthyroidism. Adult Respiratory Distress Syndrome reported with surgery. Correct K^+ or magnesium deficiency before therapy. Caution in elderly.

ADVERSE REACTIONS: Pulmonary toxicity (inflammation, fibrosis), arrhythmia exacerbation, hepatic injury, malaise, fatigue, tremor, poor coordination, paresthesis, nausea, vomiting, constipation, anorexia, ophthalmic abnormalities, photosensitivity.

INTERACTIONS: Risk of interactions after discontinuation due to long half-life. May increase sensitivity to myocardial depressant and conduction effects of halogenated inhalation anesthetics. Elevates cyclosporine plasma levels. D/C or reduce digoxin dose by 50%. D/C or decrease warfarin dose by 1/3-1/2. Caution with β-blockers, calcium blockers. May increase levels of quinidine, procainamide and phenytoin. Initiate added antiarrhythmic drug at lower than usual dose. D/C or decrease quinidine dose by 1/3-1/2. D/C or decrease procainamide dose by 1/3.

PREGNANCY: Category D, not for use in nursing.

MECHANISM OF ACTION: Class III antiarrhythmic; prolongs the myocardial cell-action potential duration and refractory period and noncompetitively inhibits α- and β-adrenergic receptors, which leads to decreased sinus rate, increased PR and QT interval, development of U-waves and changes in T-wave contour.

PHARMACOKINETICS: Absorption: Slow; bioavailability (50%). T_{max}=3-7 hrs. **Distribution:** Protein binding (96%). V_d=60L/kg. Found in breast milk. **Metabolism:** Liver via CYP3A4, 2C8; desethylamidarone (major metabolite). **Elimination:** Bile (major), urine.

PAMELOR   RX
nortriptyline HCL (Mallinckrodt)

> Antidepressants increased the risk of suicidal thinking and behavior (suicidality) in short-term studies in children, adolescents, and young adults with Major Depressive Disorder (MDD) and other psychiatric disorders. Nortriptyline is not approved for use in pediatric patients.

THERAPEUTIC CLASS: Tricyclic antidepressant

INDICATIONS: Relief of symptoms of depression.

DOSAGE: *Adults:* 25mg tid-qid. Max: 150mg/day. Total daily dose may be given once a day. Monitor serum levels if dose >100mg/day. Elderly/Adolescents: 30-50mg/day in single or divided doses.

HOW SUPPLIED: Cap: 10mg, 25mg, 50mg, 75mg; Sol: 10mg/5mL

CONTRAINDICATIONS: MAOI use within 14 days, acute recovery period following MI.

WARNINGS/PRECAUTIONS: MI, arrhythmia, strokes have occurred. Caution with cardiovascular disease, glaucoma, history of urinary retention, hyperthyroidism. May lower seizure threshold, exacerbate psychosis or activate schizophrenia, cause symptoms of mania in bipolar disease, or alter glucose levels. D/C several days prior to elective surgery.

ADVERSE REACTIONS: Arrhythmias, hypotension, HTN, tachycardia, MI, heart block, stroke, confusion, hallucination, insomnia, tremors, ataxia, anxiety, dry mouth, blurred vision, skin rash, extrapyramidal symptoms, photosensitivity, SIADH, anorexia.

INTERACTIONS: See Contraindications. May block guanethidine effects. Arrhythmia risk with thyroid agents. Alcohol may potentiate effects. "Stimulating" effect with reserpine. Monitor with anticholinergic and sympathomimetic drugs. Increased plasma levels with cimetidine. Hypoglycemia reported with chlorpropamide. SSRIs, antidepressants, phenothiazines, propafenone, flecainide and CYP2D6 inhibitors (eg, quinidine) may potentiate effects. Decreased clearance with quinidine.

PREGNANCY: Safety during pregnancy and nursing not known.

MECHANISM OF ACTION: Tricyclic; inhibits activity of histamine, 5-hydroxytryptamine, and acetylcholine; increases pressor effect of NE, blocks pressor response of phenethylamine, and interferes with transport, release and storage of catecholamine.

PAMINE RX
methscopolamine bromide (Kenwood Therapeutics)

OTHER BRAND NAMES: Pamine Forte (Kenwood Therapeutics)

THERAPEUTIC CLASS: Anticholinergic

INDICATIONS: Adjunctive therapy for the treatment of peptic ulcer.

DOSAGE: *Adults:* 2.5mg tid 30 min ac and 2.5-5mg qhs. Severe Symptoms: 5mg 30 min ac and qhs. Max: 30mg/day.

HOW SUPPLIED: Tab: 2.5mg; (Forte) 5mg

CONTRAINDICATIONS: Glaucoma, obstructive uropathy, obstructive GI disease, paralytic ileus, intestinal atony of the elderly or debilitated, unstable cardiovascular status in acute hemorrhage, severe ulcerative colitis, toxic megacolon, myasthenia gravis.

WARNINGS/PRECAUTIONS: Heat prostration may occur with high environmental temperatures. Avoid or d/c use if diarrhea develops, especially with ileostomy or colostomy. Caution in elderly, autonomic neuropathy, hepatic/renal disease, ulcerative colitis, hyperthyroidism, coronary heart disease, CHF, tachyrhythmia, tachycardia, HTN, or prostatic hypertrophy. May impair mental/physical abilities.

ADVERSE REACTIONS: Constipation, decreased sweating, headache, drowsiness, dizziness.

INTERACTIONS: Additive anticholinergic effects with antipsychotics, TCAs, and other drugs with anticholinergic effects. Antacids may interfere with absorption.

PREGNANCY: Category C, caution in nursing.

MECHANISM OF ACTION: Anticholinergic; reduces volume and total acid content of gastric secretion, inhibits gastrointestinal motility and inhibits salivary excretion.

PHARMACOKINETICS: Absorption: Poorly absorbed. **Distribution:** Crosses blood-brain barrier. **Elimination:** (Primary): Urine, bile; (Unabsorped): feces.

PANAFIL RX
chlorophyllin copper complex sodium - papain - urea (Healthpoint)

THERAPEUTIC CLASS: Proteolytic enzyme (debriding/healing agent)

INDICATIONS: Treatment of acute and chronic lesions such as varicose, diabetic and decubitus ulcers, burns, postoperative wounds, pilonidal cyst wounds, carbuncles and other traumatic or infected wounds.

DOSAGE: *Adults:* (Oint, Spray) Clean wound, then apply qd-bid. Cover with dressing.

HOW SUPPLIED: Oint: (Chlorophyllin-Papain-Urea) 0.5%-10%-10% [6g, 30g]; Spray: (Chlorophyllin-Papain-Urea) 0.5%-10%-10% [33mL]

WARNINGS/PRECAUTIONS: Not for ophthalmic use.

ADVERSE REACTIONS: Transient burning, skin irritation.

INTERACTIONS: May be inactivated by hydrogen peroxide, salts of heavy metals (eg, lead, silver, mercury).

PREGNANCY: Safety in pregnancy and nursing not known.

P

MECHANISM OF ACTION: Papain: Proteolytic enzyme; potent digestant of nonviable protein matter. Urea: Combines with papain to produce two chemical actions; 1) to expose activators of papain by solvent action, 2) denature the nonviable protein matter in lesions thereby rendering it more susceptible to enzymatic digestion. Chlorophyllin Copper Complex Sodium: Promotes healthy granulations, controls local inflammation, and reduces wound odors. Responsible for inhibiting the hemagglutinating and inflammatory properties of protein degradation products in the wound, including products of enzymatic digestion.

PANCREASE MT   RX
protease - amylase - lipase (McNeil Consumer)

THERAPEUTIC CLASS: Pancreatic enzyme supplement

INDICATIONS: Treatment of steatorrhea secondary to pancreatic insufficiency such as cystic fibrosis (CF) and chronic alcoholic pancreatitis.

DOSAGE: *Adults:* Initial: 400 U lipase/kg/meal. Max: 2500 U lipase/kg/meal. Adjust dose based on 3-day fecal fat studies. Take with plenty of water. Do not chew/crush caps. May add capsule contents to soft food (pH <7.3) and swallow immediately without chewing.
Pediatrics: ≤12 months: 2000-4000 U lipase/120mL formula or per breast feeding. 13 months-3 yrs: Initial: 1000 U lipase/kg/meal. Max: 2500 U lipase/kg/meal. ≥4 yrs: Initial: 400U lipase/kg/meal. Max: 2500 U lipase/kg/meal. Adjust dose based on 3-day fecal fat studies. Take with plenty of water. Do not chew/crush caps. May add capsule contents to soft food (pH <7.3) and swallow immediately without chewing.

HOW SUPPLIED: Cap: (Amylase-Lipase-Protease) (MT 4) 12,000 U-4000 U-12,000 U, (MT 10) 30,000 U-10,000 U-30,000 U, (MT 16) 48,000 U-16,000 U-48,000 U, (MT 20) 56,000 U-20,000 U-44,000 U

CONTRAINDICATIONS: Pork protein hypersensitivity.

WARNINGS/PRECAUTIONS: May cause fibrotic strictures in colon of primarily CF patients. Caution when changing dose or brand of medication.

ADVERSE REACTIONS: Diarrhea, abdominal pain, intestinal obstruction, vomiting, flatulence, nausea, constipation, melena, perianal irritation, weight loss, pain.

PREGNANCY: Category B, safety in nursing not known.

PANDEL   RX
hydrocortisone probutate (PharmaDerm)

THERAPEUTIC CLASS: Corticosteroid

INDICATIONS: Relief of the inflammatory and pruritic manifestations of corticosteroid-responsive dermatoses in patients ≥18 yrs.

DOSAGE: *Adults:* Apply qd-bid depending on severity of condition. May use occlusive dressing for refractory lesions of psoriasis and other deep-seated dermatoses.

HOW SUPPLIED: Cre: 0.1% [15g, 45g, 80g]

WARNINGS/PRECAUTIONS: May produce reversible HPA axis suppression, manifestations of Cushing's syndrome, hyperglycemia, glucosuria. D/C if irritation occurs. Use appropriate antifungal or antibacterial agent with dermatological infections. Pediatrics may be more susceptible to systemic toxicity. Caution when applied to large surface areas. Avoid eyes.

ADVERSE REACTIONS: Burning, stinging, moderate paresthesia, itching, dryness, folliculitis, hypertrichosis, acneiform eruptions, hypopigmentation, perioral dermatitis, skin atrophy, secondary infections, striae, millaria.

PREGNANCY: Category C, caution in nursing.

MECHANISM OF ACTION: Corticosteroid: posesses anti-inflammatory, anti-pruritic, and vasoconstrictive actions. Mechanism of anti-inflammatory activity not established. Suspected to act by the induction of phospholipase A_2 inhibitory proteins, lipocortins. Lipocortins control the biosynthesis of potent mediators of inflammation (eg, prostaglandins, leukotrienes) by inhibiting the release of their common precursor, arachidonic acid.

PHARMACOKINETICS: Absorption: Percutaneous. Inflammation, other disease states, or the use of occlusive dressings may increase absorption. Use of occlusive dressings ≤24 hrs does not increase penetration. Use of occlusive dressings ≥96 hrs markedly enhances penetration. **Distribution:** Systemically administered corticosteroids have been found in breast milk.

PANIXINE   RX
cephalexin (Ranbaxy)

THERAPEUTIC CLASS: Cephalosporin (1st generation)

INDICATIONS: Skin and skin structure (SSSI), bone, genitourinary and respiratory tract infections, otitis media, acute prostatitis.

DOSAGE: *Adults*: ≥15 yrs: Usual: 250mg q6h. Streptococcal pharyngitis/SSSI: 500mg q12h. Cystitis: 500mg q12h for minimum of 7-14 days. Max: 4g/day. Do not crush, cut, or chew tab. Treat β-hemolytic streptococcal infections for ≥10 days.
Pediatrics: Usual: 25-50mg/kg/day in divided doses. Streptococcal Pharyngitis (>1 yr)/SSSI: May divide into 2 doses, give q12h. Otitis Media: 75-100mg/kg/day given qid. Treat β-hemolytic streptococcal infections for ≥10 days.

HOW SUPPLIED: Tab, Dispersible: 125mg, 250mg

WARNINGS/PRECAUTIONS: Caution with PCN sensitivity. Caution with markedly impaired renal function, history of GI disease. Cross-sensitivity with cephalosporins and penicillins. Pseudomembranous colitis reported. False (+) direct Coombs' tests reported. False (+) for urine glucose with Benedict's, Fehling's solution, and Clinitest® tablets.

ADVERSE REACTIONS: Diarrhea, dyspepsia, gastritis, abdominal pain, allergic reactions, genital and anal pruritus, moniliasis, vaginitis, dizziness, fatigue, headache, superinfection (prolonged use).

INTERACTIONS: Probenecid inhibits excretion. Concomitant usage with metformin may require monitoring and dose adjustment.

PREGNANCY: Category B, caution in nursing.

MECHANISM OF ACTION: Cephalosporin; bactericidal due to inhibition of cell wall synthesis.

PHARMACOKINETICS: Absorption: Rapid; C_{max}=15.25 mcg/mL; T_{max}=1 hr. **Elimination:** Urine (>90%).

PANRETIN   RX
alitretinoin (Eisai)

THERAPEUTIC CLASS: Retinoid

INDICATIONS: Topical treatment of cutaneous lesions in patients with AIDS-related Kaposi's sarcoma (KS).

DOSAGE: *Adults:* Initial: Apply bid to lesions. Titrate: Gradually increase to tid-qid as tolerated. Allow to dry before covering with clothing. Reduce frequency if application site toxicity occurs. D/C temporarily if severe irritation occurs.

HOW SUPPLIED: Gel: 0.1% [60g]

WARNINGS/PRECAUTIONS: Avoid mucous membranes, normal skin. Not for use when systemic anti-KS therapy is required. Possible photosensitizing effects, minimize exposure of treated areas to sunlight and sunlamps. Treatment-limiting toxicities. Avoid occlusive dressings or in pregnancy.

ADVERSE REACTIONS: Rash, pain, pruritus, erythema, exfoliative dermatitis, skin disorder, paresthesia, edema.

P

INTERACTIONS: Avoid DEET-containing products (eg, insect repellents).

PREGNANCY: Category D, not for use in nursing.

MECHANISM OF ACTION: Binds to and activates intracellular retinoid receptor subtypes that regulate the expression of genes and control the process of cellular differentiation and proliferation in both normal and neoplastic cells.

PHARMACOKINETICS: Metabolism: Liver via CYP2C9, 3A4, 1A1, and 1A2; 4-oxo-9-*cis*-retinoic acid (major metabolite).

PARCOPA   RX
levodopa - carbidopa (Schwarz)

THERAPEUTIC CLASS: Dopa-decarboxylase inhibitor/dopamine precursor

INDICATIONS: Treatment of symptoms of idiopathic Parkinson's disease, postencephalitic parkinsonism, and symptomatic parkinsonism.

DOSAGE: *Adults:* ≥18yrs: 25mg-100mg tab: Initial: 1 tab tid. Titrate: Increase by 1 tab qd or qod until 8 tabs/day. 10mg-100mg tab: Initial: 1 tab tid-qid. Titrate: Increase 1 tab qd or qod until 2 tabs qid. 70-100mg/day carbidopa required. Max 200mg/day carbidopa. Levodopa must be discontinued 12 hrs before starting carbidopa-levodopa.

HOW SUPPLIED: Tab, Disintegrating: (Carbidopa-Levodopa) 10mg-100mg*, 25mg-100mg*, 25mg-250mg* *scored

CONTRAINDICATIONS: MAOIs during or within 14 days of use, narrow-angle glaucoma, suspicious, undiagnosed skin lesions, history of melanoma.

WARNINGS/PRECAUTIONS: Dyskinesias and mental disturbances may occur. Caution with severe cardiovascular or pulmonary disease, bronchial asthma, renal or hepatic disease, endocrine disease, chronic wide-angle glaucoma, peptic ulcer, and MI with residual arrhythmias. NMS reported during dose reduction or withdrawal. Dark color may appear in saliva, urine, or sweat. May cause false (+) ketonuria or false (-) glucosuria (glucose-oxidase method).

ADVERSE REACTIONS: Dyskinesias, choreiform, dystonic, other involuntary movements, nausea.

INTERACTIONS: See Contraindications. Risk of postural hypotension with antihypertensives, selegiline. HTN and dyskinesia may occur with TCAs. Reduced effects with dopamine D_2 antagonists (eg, phenothiazines, butyrophenones, risperidone), isoniazid. Antagonized by phenytoin, papaverine, metoclopramide. Reduced bioavailability with iron salts, high-protein diets.

PREGNANCY: Category C, caution in nursing

MECHANISM OF ACTION: Carbidopa: inhibits decarboxylation of peripheral levodopa. Levodopa: Crosses the blood-brain barrier, converting into dopamine and thereby increasing concentrations in the brain.

PHARMACOKINETICS: Absorption: Carbidopa: bioavailability (99%). **Elimination:** Urine.

PARLODEL   RX
bromocriptine mesylate (Novartis)

THERAPEUTIC CLASS: Dopamine receptor agonist

INDICATIONS: Management of hyperprolactinemia including amenorrhea with or without galactorrhea, infertility, or hypogonadism. Treatment of prolactin-secreting adenomas, acromegaly, and symptoms of Parkinson's disease.

DOSAGE: *Adults:* Take with food. Parkinson's Disease: Initial: 1.25mg bid. Titrate: if needed, increase by 2.5mg/day every 2-4 weeks. Max: 100mg/day. Hyperprolactinemia: Initial: 1.25mg-2.5mg qd. Titrate: If needed, increase by 2.5mg every 2-7 days. Usual: 2.5-15mg/day. Acromegaly: Initial: 1.25-2.5mg qhs for 3 days. Titrate: Increase by 1.25-2.5mg every 3-7 days until optimal response. Usual: 20-30mg/day. Max: 100mg/day. Withdraw for 4-8 weeks every year in patients treated with pituitary irradiation.

Pediatrics: Take with food. 11-15 yrs: Prolactin-Secreting Pituitary Adenomas: Initial: 1.25-2.5mg/day. Titrate: Increase as tolerated. Usual: 2.5-10mg/day.

HOW SUPPLIED: Cap: 5mg; Tab: 2.5mg* *scored

CONTRAINDICATIONS: Uncontrolled HTN, ergot alkaloid sensitivity, postpartum with CVD unless withdrawal is medically contraindicated, pregnancy if treating hyperprolactinemia, HTN in pregnancy.

WARNINGS/PRECAUTIONS: Caution with renal or hepatic dysfunction, psychosis, CVD, peptic ulcer, dementia. D/C with macroadenomas associated with rapid regrowth of tumor and increased prolactin levels and if severe headache or HTN develops. Risk of pulmonary infiltrates, pleural effusion, thickening of pleura, and retroperitoneal fibrosis with long-term use. Not for prevention of physiological lactation. Monitor BP for symptomatic hypotension and HTN.

ADVERSE REACTIONS: Headache, dizziness, GI effects, orthostatic hypotension, fatigue, arrhythmia, insomnia, hallucinations, abnormal involuntary movements, depression, syncope.

INTERACTIONS: Decreased effects with dopamine antagonists (eg, butyrophenones, haloperidol, phenothiazines, pimozide, metoclopramide). Levodopa may cause hallucinations. Caution with antihypertensives. Alcohol may potentiate side effects. Not for use with other ergot alkaloids.

PREGNANCY: Category B, not for use in nursing.

MECHANISM OF ACTION: Dopamine receptor agonist; activates post-synaptic dopamine receptors and modulates prolactin secretion from anterior pituitary by secreting prolactin inhibitory factor.

PHARMACOKINETICS: Absorption: GI tract (28%); C_{max}=0.4652ng/mL (5mg); T_{max}=1-3 hrs. **Distribution:** Serum albumin binding (90-96%). **Metabolism:** Liver, via CYP3A and hydroxylation. **Elimination:** Liver and kidneys (6%); $T_{1/2}$=8-20 hrs.

PARNATE   RX
tranylcypromine sulfate (GlaxoSmithKline)

Antidepressants increased the risk of suicidal thinking and behavior (suicidality) in short-term studies in children, adolescents, and young adults with Major Depressive Disorder and other psychiatric disorders. Tranylcypromine is not approved for use in pediatric patients.

THERAPEUTIC CLASS: Monoamine oxidase inhibitor

INDICATIONS: Treatment of major depressive episode without melancholia.

DOSAGE: *Adults:* Usual: 30mg/day in divided doses. Titrate: After 2 weeks, may increase by 10mg/day every 1-3 weeks depending on signs of improvement. Max: 60mg/day.

HOW SUPPLIED: Tab: 10mg

CONTRAINDICATIONS: Cardiovascular or cerebrovascular disorder, HTN, history of headache, pheochromocytoma. Concomitant MAOIs, dibenzazepine derivatives, sympathomimetics (including amphetamines), some CNS depressants (including narcotics and alcohol), antihypertensives, diuretics, antihistamines, sedatives, anesthetics, bupropion, buspirone, meperidine, SSRIs, dexfenfluramine, dextromethorphan, foods with high tyramine content (cheese) and excessive quantities of caffeine. Elective surgery requiring general anesthesia. History of liver disease or abnormal LFTs. Caution with anti-parkinsonism drugs.

WARNINGS/PRECAUTIONS: Use in patients who are resistant to other therapies. Hypotension reported. Drug dependency possible in doses excessive of the therapeutic range. May suppress anginal pain in myocardial ischemia. Caution with hyperthyroidism, renal dysfunction, diabetes, elderly. May aggravate depression symptoms. May lower seizure threshold. Inhibits MAO 10 days after discontinuation. D/C at least 10 days before elective surgery. D/C if palpitations or frequent headaches occur.

ADVERSE REACTIONS: Restlessness, insomnia, weakness, drowsiness, nausea, diarrhea, tachycardia, anorexia, edema, tinnitis, muscle spasm, overstimulation, dizziness, dry mouth, blood dyscrasias.

INTERACTIONS: See Contraindications. Caution with disulfiram. Additive hypotensive effects with phenothiazines. Tryptophan may precipitate disorientation, memory impairment and other neurological and behavioral signs. Avoid metrizamide; d/c 48 hrs before myelography and may resume 24 hrs post-procedure.

PREGNANCY: Safety in pregnancy and nursing not known.

MECHANISM OF ACTION: Non-hydrazine MAOI; inhibits monoamine oxidase, increasing concentration of epinephrine, norepinephrine, and serotonin in storage sites throughout nervous system.

PASER   RX
aminosalicylic acid (Jacobus)

THERAPEUTIC CLASS: Hydroxybenzoic acid derivative

INDICATIONS: Treatment of TB in combination with other agents.

DOSAGE: *Adults:* 4g tid. Sprinkle on apple sauce, yogurt, or mix with tomato or orange juice.
Pediatrics: Use correspondingly smaller doses to the adult dose. Sprinkle on apple sauce, yogurt, or mix with tomato or orange juice.

HOW SUPPLIED: Pkt: 4g

CONTRAINDICATIONS: Severe renal disease.

WARNINGS/PRECAUTIONS: Monitor for rash, or signs of intolerance during 1st 3 months. D/C if hypersensitivity occurs. Can desensitize by administering small, gradually increasing doses.

ADVERSE REACTIONS: Diarrhea, nausea, vomiting, abdominal pain, fever, dermatitis, lymphoma-like syndrome, agranulocytosis, thrombocytopenia, anemia, jaundice, hepatitis, hypoglycemia.

INTERACTIONS: Reduces acetylation of isoniazid, especially in rapid acetylators. Decreases vitamin B_{12} absorption; consider vitamin B_{12} maintenance treatment. Decreases digoxin levels.

PREGNANCY: Category C, safety in nursing not known.

MECHANISM OF ACTION: Bacteriostatic agent; believed to inhibit folic acid synthesis and/or inhibition of synthesis of the cell wall component, mycobactin, thus reducing iron uptake by *M.tuberculosis*.

PHARMACOKINETICS: Absorption: C_{max}=20mcg/mL; T_{max}=6 hrs. **Distribution:** Plasma protein binding (50-60%), CSF penetration occurs only if the meninges is inflamed. **Metabolism:** Via acetylation. **Excretion:** Urine (80%); aminosalicylic acid (metabolite); $T_{1/2}$=26.4 min.

PATANOL   RX
olopatadine HCL (Alcon)

THERAPEUTIC CLASS: H_1-antagonist and mast cell stabilizer

INDICATIONS: Allergic conjunctivitis.

DOSAGE: *Adults:* 1 drop bid, q6-8h.
Pediatrics: ≥3 yrs: 1 drop bid, q6-8h.

HOW SUPPLIED: Sol: 0.1% [5mL]

WARNINGS/PRECAUTIONS: May re-insert contact lens 10 min after dosing if eye is not red.

ADVERSE REACTIONS: Headache, asthenia, blurred vision, burning, stinging, cold syndrome, dry eye, foreign body sensation, hyperemia, hypersensitivity, keratitis, lid edema, nausea, pharyngitis, pruritus, rhinitis, sinusitis, taste perversion.

PREGNANCY: Category C, caution in nursing.

MECHANISM OF ACTION: Antihistaminic drug; relatively selective histamine H_1-antagonist; inhibits the type 1 immediate hypersensitivity reaction, including inhibition of histamine induced effects on human conjunctival epithelial cells.

PHARMACOKINETICS: Absorption: C_{max}=0.5-1.3ng/mL; T_{max}=2 hrs. **Metabolism:** Metabolites: Mono-desmethyl and N-oxide. **Elimination:** Urine (60-70% parent drug).

PAXIL   RX
paroxetine HCL (GlaxoSmithKline)

> Antidepressants increased the risk of suicidal thinking and behavior (suicidality) in short-term studies in children, adolescents, and young adults with Major Depressive Disorder (MDD) and other psychiatric disorders. Paroxetine is not approved for use in pediatric patients.

THERAPEUTIC CLASS: Selective serotonin reuptake inhibitor

INDICATIONS: Treatment of major depressive disorder (MDD), panic disorder with or without agoraphobia. Treatment of obsessive compulsive disorder (OCD), social anxiety disorder (SAD), generalized anxiety disorder (GAD), and posttraumatic stress disorder (PTSD).

DOSAGE: *Adults:* Give qd, usually in the AM. MDD: Initial: 20mg/day. Max: 50mg/day. OCD: Initial: 20mg qd. Usual: 40mg qd. Max: 60mg/day. Panic Disorder: Initial: 10mg qd. Usual: 40mg/day. Max: 60mg/day. GAD: Initial: 20mg/day. Usual: 20-50mg/day. SAD: Initial/Usual: 20mg/day. Max: 60mg/day. PTSD: Initial: 20mg/day. Usual: 20-50mg/day. To titrate, may increase weekly by 10mg/day. Elderly/Debilitated/Severe Renal/Hepatic Impairment: Initial: 10mg qd. Max: 40mg/day.

HOW SUPPLIED: Sus: 10mg/5mL [250mL]; Tab: 10mg*, 20mg*, 30mg, 40mg *scored

CONTRAINDICATIONS: Concomitant MAOIs, thioridazine, or pimozide.

WARNINGS/PRECAUTIONS: Caution with history of mania or seizures, conditions that affect metabolism or hemodynamic responses, narrow angle glaucoma. D/C if seizures occur. Altered platelet function, hyponatremia, mydriasis reported. Avoid abrupt withdrawal. Re-evaluate periodically. Monitor for clinical worsening and/or suicidality, especially at initiation of therapy or dose changes.

ADVERSE REACTIONS: Somnolence, insomnia, nausea, asthenia, abnormal ejaculation, dry mouth, constipation, dizziness, diarrhea, decreased libido, sweating.

INTERACTIONS: See Contraindications. Avoid alcohol, tryptophan. May shift concentrations with plasma-bound drugs. Increased risk of bleeding with NSAIDs, aspirin, oral anticoagulants. May inhibit metabolism of TCAs. Rare reports of weakness, hyperreflexia, incoordination with an SSRI and sumatriptan. Caution with other agents that may affect serotonergic systems (eg, triptans, serotonin reuptake inhibitors, linezolid, lithium, tramadol, St. John's wort); increased risk of serotonin syndrome. Monitor theophylline. Increased levels with cimetidine. Reduce procyclidine dose if anticholinergic effects occur. Caution with diuretics, digoxin, lithium, cimetidine, warfarin, phenobarbital, phenytoin, drugs metabolized by CYP2D6 (eg, antidepressants, phenothiazines, Type 1C antiarrhythmics), or drugs that inhibit CYP2D6 (eg, quinidine). May increase levels of risperidone. May increase levels of atomoxetine; dosage adjustment of atomoxetine may be necessary and initiate atomoxetine at reduced dose. Fosamprenavir/ritonavir may decrease levels.

PREGNANCY: Category D, caution in nursing.

MECHANISM OF ACTION: SSRI; inhibits CNS neuronal reuptake of serotonin.

PHARMACOKINETICS: Absorption: Complete; C_{max}=61.7ng/mL; T_{max}=5.2 hrs. **Distribution:** Plasma protein bound (95%). **Metabolism:** Oxidation and methylation via CYP2D6. **Elimination:** Urine (2%), feces (<1%); $T_{1/2}$=21 hrs.

PAXIL CR   RX
paroxetine HCL (GlaxoSmithKline)

> Antidepressants increased the risk of suicidal thinking and behavior (suicidality) in short-term studies in children, adolescents, and young adults with Major Depressive Disorder (MDD) and other psychiatric disorders. Paroxetine is not approved for use in pediatric patients.

THERAPEUTIC CLASS: Selective serotonin reuptake inhibitor

INDICATIONS: Treatment of major depressive disorder (MDD), panic disorder with or without agoraphobia, social anxiety disorder (SAD), and premenstrual dysphoric disorder (PMDD).

DOSAGE: *Adults:* Give qd, usually in the AM. Swallow whole. MDD: Initial: 25mg/day. Titrate: May increase weekly by 12.5mg/day. Max: 62.5mg/day. Panic Disorder: Initial: 12.5mg/day. May increase weekly by 12.5mg/day. Max: 75mg/day. SAD: Initial: 12.5mg/day. May increase weekly by 12.5mg/day. Max: 37.5mg/day. PMDD: Initial: 12.5mg/day continuous or limited to luteal phase of cycle. May increase weekly by 12.5mg/day. Elderly/Debilitated/Severe Renal/Hepatic Impairment: Initial: 12.5mg/day. Max: 50mg/day.

HOW SUPPLIED: Tab, Controlled-Release: 12.5mg, 25mg, 37.5mg

CONTRAINDICATIONS: Concomitant MAOIs, thioridazine, or pimozide.

WARNINGS/PRECAUTIONS: Caution with history of mania or seizures, conditions that affect metabolism or hemodynamic responses, narrow angle glaucoma. D/C if seizures occur. Hyponatremia, mydriasis reported. Avoid abrupt withdrawal. Re-evaluate periodically. Monitor for clinical worsening and/or suicidality, especially at initiation of therapy or dose changes.

ADVERSE REACTIONS: Somnolence, insomnia, nausea, asthenia, abnormal ejaculation, dry mouth, constipation, dizziness, diarrhea, decreased libido, sweating.

INTERACTIONS: See Contraindications. Avoid alcohol, tryptophan. May shift concentrations with plasma-bound drugs. May inhibit metabolism of TCAs. Rare reports of weakness, hyperreflexia, incoordination with an SSRI and sumatriptan. Caution with other drugs or agents that may affect the serotonergic neurotransmitter systems, such as tryptophan, triptans, serotonin reuptake inhibitors, linezolid, lithium, tramadol, or St. John's wort. Monitor theophylline. Increased risk of bleeding with NSAIDs, aspirin, oral anticoagulants. Reduce procyclidine dose if anticholinergic effects occur. Caution with TCAs, diuretics, digoxin, lithium, cimetidine, warfarin, phenobarbital, phenytoin, drugs metabolized by CYP2D6 (eg, antidepressants, phenothiazines, Type 1C antiarrhythmics), or drugs that inhibit CYP2D6 (eg, quinidine). May increase levels of risperidone. May increase levels of atomoxetine; dosage adjustment of atomoxetine may be necessary and initiate atomoxetine at reduced dose. Fosamprenavir/ritonavir may decrease levels.

PREGNANCY: Category C, caution in nursing.

MECHANISM OF ACTION: SSRI; inhibits CNS neuronal reuptake of serotonin.

PHARMACOKINETICS: Absorption: Complete; administration of variable doses resulted in different parameters; T_{max}=6-10 hrs. **Distribution:** Plasma protein binding (95%). **Metabolism:** Oxidation and methylation via CYP2D6. **Elimination:** Urine (2%), feces (<1%); $T_{1/2}$=15-20 hrs.

PCE   RX
erythromycin (Abbott)

THERAPEUTIC CLASS: Macrolide

INDICATIONS: Treatment of mild to moderate upper/lower respiratory tract and skin and skin structure infections, listeriosis, pertussis, diphtheria, erythrasma, intestinal amebiasis, acute pelvic inflammatory disease (PID) (*N.gonorrhea*), primary syphilis (if PCN allergy), Legionnaires' disease, chlamydial infections (eg, newborn conjunctivitis, pneumonia of infancy, urogenital infections during pregnancy or urethral, endocervical, or rectal infections when tetracyclines are contraindicated or not tolerated), and nongonococcal urethritis caused by susceptible strains of microorganisms. Prophylaxis of initial and recurrent attacks of rheumatic fever if PCN allergy.

DOSAGE: *Adults:* Usual: 333mg q8h or 500mg q12h without food. Max: 4g/day. Do not take bid when dose is ≥1g/day. Treat strep infections for at least 10 days. Streptococcal Infection Long-Term Prophylaxis of Rheumatic Fever: 250mg bid. Chlamydial Urogenital Infection During Pregnancy: 500mg qid or 666mg q8h for at least 7 days, or 500mg q12h, 333mg q8h, or 250mg qid for at least 14 days. Urethral/Endocervical/Rectal Chlamydial Infections and Nongonococcal Urethritis: 500mg qid or 666mg q8h for at least 7 days. Primary Syphilis: 30-40g in divided doses over 10-15 days. Acute PID: 500mg (erythromycin lactobionate) IV q6h for 3 days, then 500mg PO q12h or 333mg PO q8h for 7 days. Intestinal Amebiasis: 500mg q12h, 333mg q8h, or 250mg q6h for 10-14 days. Pertussis: 40-50mg/kg/day in divided doses for 5-14 days. Legionnaires' Disease: 1-4g/day in divided doses.
Pediatrics: Usual: 30-50mg/kg/day in divided doses without food. Severe Infections: May double dose. Max: 4g/day. Treat strep infections for at least 10 days. Streptococcal Infection Long-Term Prophylaxis of Rheumatic Fever: 250mg bid. Chlamydial Conjunctivitis of Newborns/Chlamydial Pneumonia in Infancy: (Sus) 12.5mg/kg qid for 2 weeks and 3 weeks, respectively. Intestinal Amebiasis: 30-50mg/kg/day in divided doses for 10-14 days.

HOW SUPPLIED: Tab, Extended-Release: 333mg, 500mg

CONTRAINDICATIONS: Concomitant terfenadine, astemizole, pimozide, or cisapride.

WARNINGS/PRECAUTIONS: *Clostridium difficile*-associated diarrhea, hepatic dysfunction reported. Caution with impaired hepatic function. May aggravate weakness of patients with myasthenia gravis. Erythromycin does not reach adequate concentrations in fetus to prevent congenital syphilis.

ADVERSE REACTIONS: Nausea, vomiting, abdominal pain, diarrhea, anorexia, hepatic dysfunction, abnormal LFTs, allergic reactions, superinfection (prolonged use).

INTERACTIONS: See Contraindications. Rhabdomyolysis reported with lovastatin. May increase levels of theophylline, digoxin, drugs metabolized by CYP450 (eg, carbamazepine, cyclosporine, phenytoin, alfentanil, disopyramide, lovastatin, bromocriptine, valproate, etc). Increases effects of oral anticoagulants, triazolam, midazolam. Risk of acute ergot toxicity with ergotamine or dihydroergotamine. May increase AUC of sildenafil; consider dose reduction of sildenafil.

PREGNANCY: Category B, caution in nursing.

MECHANISM OF ACTION: Macrolide; inhibits protein synthesis by binding 50S ribosomal subunits of susceptible organisms.

PHARMACOKINETICS: Distribution: Crosses placenta, found in breast milk. **Elimination:** Biliary excretion, urine (<5%).

PEDIAPRED   RX
prednisolone sodium phosphate (Celltech)

THERAPEUTIC CLASS: Glucocorticoid

INDICATIONS: Steroid-responsive dermatoses.

DOSAGE: *Adults:* Initial: 5-60mg/day depending on disease and response. Maint: Decrease dose by small amounts to lowest effective dose. MS Exacerbations: 200mg qd for 1 week, then 80mg every other day for 1 month. *Pediatrics:* Initial: 0.14-2mg/kg/day given tid-qid. Nephrotic Syndrome: 20mg/m² tid for 4 weeks, then 40mg/m² every other day for 4 weeks. Uncontrolled Asthma: 1-2mg/kg/day in single or divided doses peak expiratory rate of 80% is achieved (usually 3-10 days).

HOW SUPPLIED: Sol: 5mg/5mL [120mL]

CONTRAINDICATIONS: Systemic fungal infections.

WARNINGS/PRECAUTIONS: May produce reversible HPA axis suppression. Adjust dose during stress or change in thyroid status. May mask signs of infection or cause new infections. May activate latent amebiasis. Avoid with cerebral malaria. Avoid exposure to chickenpox or measles. Not for treatment of optic neuritis or active ocular herpes simplex. May cause elevation of BP or IOP, cataracts, glaucoma, optic nerve damage, Kaposi's sarcoma, psychic derangements, salt/water retention, increased excretion of potassium and/or calcium, osteoporosis, growth suppression in children, secondary ocular infections. Caution with Strongyloides, CHF, diverticulitis, HTN, renal insufficiency, fresh intestinal anastomoses, active or latent peptic ulcer, ulcerative colitis. Enhanced effect in hypothyroidism or cirrhosis. Avoid abrupt withdrawal. Use with caution in elderly, increased risk of corticosteroid-induced side effects; start at low end of dosing range; monitor bone mineral density.

ADVERSE REACTIONS: Edema, fluid/electrolyte disturbances, osteoporosis, muscle weakness, pancreatitis, peptic ulcer, impaired wound healing, increased intracranial pressure, cushingoid state, hirsutism, menstrual irregularities, growth suppression in children, glaucoma, nausea, weight gain.

INTERACTIONS: Enhanced metabolism with barbiturates, phenytoin, ephedrine, and rifampin. Use with cyclosporine may increase activity of both drugs; convulsions reported with concomitant use. Decreased metabolism with estrogens or ketoconazole. May inhibit response to warfarin. Increased risk of GI side effects with ASA or other NSAIDs. May increase clearance of salicylates. High doses or concurrent neuromuscular drugs may cause acute myopathy. Enhanced possibility of hypokalemia when given with potassium-depleting agents. May produce severe weakness in myasthenia gravis patients on anticholinesterase agents. Avoid live vaccines with immunosuppressive doses. Possible diminished response with killed or inactivated vaccines. May increase blood glucose; adjust antidiabetic agents. May suppress reactions to skin tests.

PREGNANCY: Category C, caution in nursing.

MECHANISM OF ACTION: Synthetic adrenocorticoid steroid; promotes gluconeogenesis, increases deposition of glycogen in the liver, inhibits glucose utilization, increases catabolism of protein, lipolysis, glomerular filtration that leads to increased urinary excretion of urate and calcium.

PHARMACOKINETICS: Absorption: Rapidly absorbed from GI tract. **Distribution:** Plasma protein binding (70-90%), found in breast milk. **Metabolism:** Liver. **Elimination:** Urine (as sulfate and glucuronide conjugates). $T_{1/2}$=2-4 hrs.

PEDIARIX   RX

pertussis vaccine, acellular - hepatitis B (recombinant) - poliovirus vaccine, inactivated - diphtheria toxoid - tetanus toxoid (GlaxoSmithKline)

THERAPEUTIC CLASS: Vaccine/toxoid combination

INDICATIONS: Active immunization against diphtheria, tetanus, pertussis, hepatitis B, and poliomyelitis (polioviruses Types 1, 2, and 3).

DOSAGE: *Pediatrics:* ≥6 weeks-up to 7 yrs: 3 doses of 0.5mL IM at 6-8 week intervals. Start at 2 months old or as early as 6 weeks old if necessary. May use to complete primary series in infants who have received 1 or 2 doses of Infanrix® or IPV or to complete a hepatitis B vaccine (Recombinant) series. Not recommended for completion of the first 3 doses of the DTaP vaccination series initiated with a DTaP vaccine from a different manufacturer.

HOW SUPPLIED: Inj: 0.5mL

CONTRAINDICATIONS: Hypersensitivity to yeast, neomycin, and polymyxin B. Anaphylaxis associated with previous dose or encephalopathy within 7 days of previous vaccine, progressive neurologic disorder (including infantile spasms, uncontrolled epilepsy, progressive encephalopathy).

WARNINGS/PRECAUTIONS: Higher rates of fever reported. Tip cap and plunger contains latex. Caution if within 48 hrs of previous whole-cell DTP or vaccine containing an acellular pertussis component, fever ≥105°F not due to another identifiable cause, collapse or shock-like state, or inconsolable crying lasting ≥3 hrs occurs, or if seizures occur within 3 days. Re-evaluate need if Guillain-Barre syndrome occurs within 6 weeks of receipt of tetanus toxoid-containing vaccine. Defer vaccination with moderate or severe illness, with or without fever. Administer antipyretic for initial 24 hours for those with higher risk for seizures. Caution with bleeding disorders (eg, hemophilia, thrombocytopenia). Have epinephrine available. Suboptimal response may occur in immunocompromised patients.

ADVERSE REACTIONS: Local injection-site reactions, fever, fussiness.

INTERACTIONS: Avoid with anticoagulants unless benefit outweighs risk. Immunosuppressive therapy (eg, irradiation, antimetabolites, alkylating agents, cytotoxic drugs, large doses of corticosteroids) may decrease response. Do not mix with other vaccines in same syringe/vial. Tetanus immune globulin or diphtheria antitoxin should be given at separate site with separate needle/syringe.

PREGNANCY: Category C, safety in nursing not known.

MECHANISM OF ACTION: Multivalent vaccine; stimulates immune system to elicit an immune response which produces antibodies that may protect against diphtheria, tetanus, pertussis, hepatitis B, and poliovirus infections.

PEDIOTIC   RX
polymyxin B sulfate - neomycin sulfate - hydrocortisone (King)

THERAPEUTIC CLASS: Antibacterial/corticosteroid combination

INDICATIONS: Superficial bacterial infections of the external auditory canal. Infections of mastoidectomy and fenestration cavities.

DOSAGE: *Adults:* Clean and dry ear canal. Instill 4 drops tid-qid. Max: 10 days. *Pediatrics:* Clean and dry ear canal. Instill 4 drops tid-qid. Max: 10 days.

HOW SUPPLIED: Sus: (Neomycin-Hydrocortisone-Polymyxin B) 0.35%-1%-10,000 U/mL [7.5mL]

CONTRAINDICATIONS: Herpes simplex, vaccinia, and varicella infections.

WARNINGS/PRECAUTIONS: Caution with perforated eardrum or chronic otitis media; ototoxicity may develop. Re-evaluate if no improvement after 10 days.

ADVERSE REACTIONS: Allergic sensitization, superinfection.

INTERACTIONS: Cross-reactivity with kanamycin, paromomycin, streptomycin, and gentamycin.

PREGNANCY: Category C, caution in nursing.

MECHANISM OF ACTION: Antibacterial and anti-inflammatory otic suspension.

PHARMACOKINETICS: Distribution: Found in breast milk.

PEGASYS   RX
peginterferon alfa-2a (Roche)

> May cause or aggravate fatal or life-threatening neuropsychiatric, autoimmune, ischemic, and infectious disorders. Monitor closely with periodic clinical and laboratory evaluations. D/C with persistently severe or worsening signs or symptoms of these conditions. When used with ribavirin, refer to the individual monograph.

THERAPEUTIC CLASS: Pegylated virus proliferation inhibitor

INDICATIONS: Treatment of chronic hepatitis C, alone or in combination with Copegus®, in adults with compensated liver disease not previously treated with interferon alfa. Treatment of adult patients with HBeAg positive and HBeAg negative chronic hepatitis B who have compensated liver disease and evidence of viral replication and liver inflammation.

DOSAGE: *Adults:* ≥18 yrs: HCV: Monotherapy: 180mcg SQ (in abdomen or thigh) once weekly for 48 weeks. Combination Therapy With Copegus®:

180mcg SQ once weekly for 24 weeks with genotypes 2 and 3 or 48 weeks with genotypes 1 and 4. HCV w/ HIV: Monotherapy: 180mcg SQ once weekly for 48 weeks. Combination Therapy with Copegus®: 180mcg SQ once weekly for 48 weeks, regardless of genotype. HBV: Monotherapy: 180mcg SQ once weekly for 48 weeks. Adjust dose based on hematological parameters and depression severity. (See PI for dose modifications.)

HOW SUPPLIED: Inj: Syringe: 180mcg/0.5mL; Single Dose Vial: 180mcg/mL

CONTRAINDICATIONS: Autoimmune hepatitis, hepatic decompensation; neonates and infants (contains benzyl alcohol). When used with ribavirin, refer to the individual monograph.

WARNINGS/PRECAUTIONS: Life-threatening neuropsychiatric reactions may occur; extreme caution with history of depression. Risk of bone marrow suppression; obtain CBCs prior to initiation and routinely thereafter. HTN, arrhythmias, chest pain, and MI reported; caution with pre-existing cardiac disease. Decrease/loss of vision and retinopathy reported; perform eye exam at baseline (periodically with pre-existing disorder); d/c if patient develops new or worsening of ophthalmologic disorders. Monitor for signs/symptoms of toxicity with impaired renal function and caution with CrCl <50mL/min. Development or exacerbation of autoimmune disorders reported. Caution in elderly. May induce or aggravate dyspnea, pulmonary infiltrates, pneumonia, bronchiolitis obliterans, interstitial pneumonitis, and sarcoditis; d/c if persistent or unexplained pulmonary infiltrates or pulmonary function impairment. Hypersensitivity reactions, hemorrhagic/ischemic colitis, and pancreatitis reported; d/c if any of these develop. May cause or aggravate hypothyroidism or hyperthyroidism. Hypoglycemia, hyperglycemia, and DM reported. Avoid if failed other alpha interferon treatments, liver or other organ transplant recipients, or with HIV or HBV coinfection. Monitor for severe viral, bacterial, fungal infections. Exacerbation of hepatitis B reported. Chronic hepatitis C patients with cirrhosis may be at risk for hepatic decompensation; monitor hepatic function and serum ALT's.

ADVERSE REACTIONS: Injection site reaction, fatigue/asthenia, pyrexia, rigors, nausea/vomiting, neutropenia, myalgia, headache, irritability/anxiety/nervousness, insomnia, depression, alopecia.

INTERACTIONS: May inhibit CYP1A2 and increase theophylline AUC; monitor theophylline serum levels. Hepatic decompensation can occur with concomitant use of NRTIs and peginterferon alfa-2a/ribavirin. May increase methadone levels; monitor for methadone toxicity.

PREGNANCY: Category C (monotherapy) and Category X (with ribavirin), not for use in nursing.

MECHANISM OF ACTION: α-2a interferon; binds to specific receptors on the cell surface initiating intracellular signaling leading to rapid activation of gene transcription.

PHARMACOKINETICS: Absorption: T_{max}=72-96 hrs. **Elimination:** $T_{1/2}$=160 hrs. (chronic HCV).

PEG-INTRON RX
peginterferon alfa-2b (Schering)

> May cause or aggravate fatal or life-threatening neuropsychiatric, autoimmune, ischemic, and infectious disorders. Monitor closely with periodic clinical and laboratory evaluations. D/C with severe or worsening signs or symptoms of these conditions. When used with Rebetol, refer to the individual monograph.

THERAPEUTIC CLASS: Pegylated virus proliferation inhibitor

INDICATIONS: Treatment of chronic hepatitis C alone or in combination with Rebetol®, in patients with compensated liver disease not previously treated with interferon alpha.

DOSAGE: *Adults:* ≥18 yrs: Administer SQ once weekly for 1 yr. Monotherapy: 1mcg/kg/week. Combination Therapy With Rebetol: 1.5mcg/kg/week plus Rebetol 800mg/day in 2 divided doses. CrCl <50mL/min: D/C ribavirin. Monotherapy or With Rebetol: D/C if HCV levels remain high after 6 months.

Adjust dose based on hematological parameters and depression severity. Renal Impairment: CrCl 30-50mL/min, reduce dose by 25%. CrCl 10-29mL/min, reduce dose by 50%. D/C if renal function decreases.

HOW SUPPLIED: Inj: 50mcg/0.5mL, 80mcg/0.5mL, 120mcg/0.5mL, 150mcg/0.5mL

CONTRAINDICATIONS: Autoimmune hepatitis, decompensated liver disease. When used with Rebetol, refer to the individual monograph.

WARNINGS/PRECAUTIONS: Life-threatening neuropsychiatric reactions may occur; caution with history of depression or psychiatric symptoms/disorders. Risk of bone marrow suppression; monitor CBCs and blood chemistry at initiation and periodically thereafter. Hypotension, arrhythmia, tachycardia, angina pectoris, MI reported; caution with cardiovascular disease. Conduct baseline eye exam in all patients and periodical exams with pre-existing ophthalmologic disorders; d/c if new or worsening ophthalmologic disorders occur. Caution with CrCl <50mL/min, autoimmune disorders, and the elderly. D/C if persistent or unexplained pulmonary infiltrates, or pulmonary dysfunction, or hypersensitivity reaction occurs, or if hemorrhagic/ischemic colitis or pancreatitis develops. May cause or aggravate hypothyroidism/hyperthyroidism. Hyperglycemia and DM reported. Avoid if failed other alpha interferon treatments, liver or other organ transplant recipients, or with HIV or HBV coinfection. May elevate triglyceride levels. Monitor renal impairment for toxicity.

ADVERSE REACTIONS: Headache, fatigue, rigors, dizziness, nausea, anorexia, depression, insomnia, irritability, myalgia, arthralgia, weight loss, alopecia, pruritus, decreased platelets/Hgb/neutrophils.

INTERACTIONS: Hemolytic anemia reported with ribavirin. May increase AUC of methadone, resulting in an increased narcotic effect. Caution with medications metabolized by CYP2C8/9 (eg, warfarin and phenytoin) or CYP2D6 (eg, flecainide).

PREGNANCY: Category C, safety in nursing not known.

MECHANISM OF ACTION: α-2b interferon. Binds to specific membrane receptors on cell surface, initiating induction of enzymes, suppression of cell proliferation, immunomodulating activities, and inhibition of virus replication.

PHARMACOKINETICS: Absorption: T_{max}=15-44 hrs. **Elimination:** $T_{1/2}$=approx. 40 hrs (HCV).

PENICILLIN VK   RX

penicillin V potassium (Various)

OTHER BRAND NAMES: Veetids (Sandoz)

THERAPEUTIC CLASS: Penicillin

INDICATIONS: Treatment of mild to moderately severe bacterial infections including conditions of the respiratory tract, oropharynx, skin and soft tissue caused by susceptible strains of microorganisms. Prevention of recurrence following rheumatic fever and/or chorea.

DOSAGE: *Adults:* Usual: Streptococcal Infections (Scarlet Fever/Erysipelas/Upper Respiratory Tract): 125-250mg q6-8h for 10 days. Pneumococcal Infections (Otitis Media/Respiratory Tract): 250-500mg q6h until afebrile for at least 2 days. Staphylococcus Infections (Skin/Soft Tissue): 250-500mg q6-8h. Fusospirochetosis Infections (Oropharynx): 250-500mg q6-8h. Rheumatic Fever/Chorea Prevention: 125-250mg bid.
Pediatrics: ≥12 yrs: Usual: Streptococcal Infections (Scarlet Fever/Erysipelas/Upper Respiratory Tract): 125-250mg q6-8h for 10 days. Pneumococcal Infections (Otitis Media/Respiratory Tract): 250-500mg q6h until afebrile for at least 2 days. Staphylococcus Infections (Skin/Soft Tissue): 250-500mg q6-8h. Fusospirochetosis Infections (Oropharynx): 250-500mg q6-8h. Rheumatic Fever/Chorea Prevention: 125-250mg bid.

HOW SUPPLIED: Sus: 125mg/5mL, 250mg/5mL [100mL, 200mL]; Tab: 250mg, 500mg

WARNINGS/PRECAUTIONS: Not for severe pneumonia, empyema, bacteremia, pericarditis, meningitis and arthritis during the acute stage. Serious, fatal anaphylactic reactions reported. Pseudomembranous colitis reported. Oral administration may not be effective with severe illnesses, nausea, vomiting, gastric dilation, cardiospasm, intestinal hypermotility. Cross-sensitivity with cephalosporins. Caution with asthma and allergies.

ADVERSE REACTIONS: Nausea, vomiting, epigastric distress, diarrhea, hypersensitivity reactions, black hairy tongue, anaphylaxis, superinfection (prolonged use).

PREGNANCY: Category B, caution in nursing.

MECHANISM OF ACTION: Phenoxymethyl analog of penicillin G; exerts bactericidal action during stage of active multiplication by inhibiting biosynthesis of cell wall mucopeptide.

PHARMACOKINETICS: Distribution: Plasma protein binding (80%). **Elimination:** Urine.

PENLAC   RX
ciclopirox (Dermik)

THERAPEUTIC CLASS: Broad-spectrum antifungal

INDICATIONS: Mild to moderate onychomycosis of fingernails or toenails without lunula involvement due to *Trichophyton rubrum* (in immunocompetent patients).

DOSAGE: *Adults:* Apply qhs or 8 hrs before washing to nail bed, hyponychium, and under surface when it is free of nail bed. Apply daily over previous coat and remove with alcohol every 7 days. Repeat cycle up to 48 weeks.

HOW SUPPLIED: Sol: 8% [6.6mL]

WARNINGS/PRECAUTIONS: Only for use on nails and adjacent skin. Caution with removal of infected nail in insulin-dependent DM or diabetic neuropathy.

ADVERSE REACTIONS: Periungual erythema, erythema of proximal nail fold, nail shape change, nail irritation, ingrown toenail, nail discoloration.

INTERACTIONS: Avoid nail polish or other nail cosmetics on treated nails.

PREGNANCY: Category B, caution in nursing.

MECHANISM OF ACTION: Broad spectrum antifungal: acts by chelation of polyvalent cations (Fe^{+3} or Al^{+3}), resulting in the inhibition of the metal-dependent enzymes responsible for degradation of peroxides within fungal cell.

PHARMACOKINETICS: Absorption: Serum levels range from 12-80ng/mL following topical administration. **Elimination:** Urine (<5% of applied topical dose).

PENTASA   RX
mesalamine (Shire)

THERAPEUTIC CLASS: Anti-inflammatory Agent

INDICATIONS: Induction of remission and for treatment of mild to moderate active ulcerative colitis.

DOSAGE: *Adults:* 1g qid. Can be given up to 8 weeks.

HOW SUPPLIED: Cap, Extended-Release: 250mg, 500mg

CONTRAINDICATIONS: Hypersensitivity to salicylates.

WARNINGS/PRECAUTIONS: Caution with hepatic and renal dysfunction; monitor closely. D/C if acute intolerance syndrome develops (eg, cramping, bloody diarrhea, abdominal pain, headache). If rechallenge is considered, perform under careful observation.

ADVERSE REACTIONS: Diarrhea, headache, nausea, abdominal pain.

PREGNANCY: Category B, caution in nursing.

MECHANISM OF ACTION: Unknown, suspected to act as anti-inflammatory agent for blocking cyclooxygenase and inhibiting prostaglandin in gastrointestinal use.

PHARMACOKINETICS: Absorption: C_{max}=1mcg/mL, T_{max}=3 hrs. (N-acetylmesalamine): C_{max}=1.8mcg/mL, T_{max}=3 hrs. **Metabolism:** N-acetylmesalamine (Metabolite). **Elimination:** Feces (130 mg). N-acetylmesalamine: urine (19-30%).

PENTOTHAL CIII
thiopental sodium (Hospira)

THERAPEUTIC CLASS: Thiobarbiturate

INDICATIONS: Sole anesthetic agent for brief (15 minute) procedures. For induction of anesthesia prior to administration of other anesthetic agents. To supplement regional anesthesia. To provide hypnosis during balanced anesthesia with other agents for analgesia or muscle relaxation. For the control of convulsive states during or following inhalation/local anesthesia or other causes. In neurosurgical patients with increased ICP, if adequate ventilation is provided. For narcoanalysis and narcosynthesis in psychiatric disorders.

DOSAGE: *Adults:* Individualize dose. IV: Test Dose: 25-75mg. Anesthesia: 50-75mg at 20-40 sec intervals. Once anesthesia established, additional inj of 25-50mg may be given whenever patient moves. Induction in Balanced Anesthesia: Initial: 3-4mg/kg. Convulsive States: Following anesthesia, give 75-125mg as soon as possible after convulsion begins. Convulsions following use of local anesthetic may require 125-250mg over 10 min period. Neurosurgical Patients with Increased ICP: 1.5-3.5mg/kg bolus. Psychiatric Disorders: After test dose, infuse at 100mg/min with patient counting backwards from 100; d/c shortly after counting becomes confused but before actual sleep is produced.

HOW SUPPLIED: Inj: 20mg/mL, 25mg/mL

CONTRAINDICATIONS: Absolute: Absence of suitable veins for IV administration, variegate porphyria (South Africa) or acute intermittent porphyria. Relative: Severe cardiovascular disease, hypotension, shock, conditions in which the hypnotic effect may be prolonged or potentiated (excessive premedication, Addison's disease, hepatic/renal dysfunction, myxedema, increased blood urea, severe anemia, asthma, and myasthenia gravis), and status asthmaticus.

WARNINGS/PRECAUTIONS: Avoid extravasation or intra-arterial injection. May be habit forming. Reduce dose and administer slowly with relative contraindications. Caution with advanced cardiac disease, increased ICP, ophthalmoplegia plus, asthma, myasthenia gravis, and endocrine insufficiency (pituitary, thyroid, adrenal, pancreas).

ADVERSE REACTIONS: Respiratory/myocardial depression, cardiac arrhythmias, prolonged somnolence and recovery, sneezing, coughing, bronchospasm, laryngospasm, shivering, anaphylactic and anaphylactoid reactions.

INTERACTIONS: Prolonged action with probenecid. Hypotension with diazoxide. Antagonism with zimelidine or aminophylline. Decreased antinociceptive action with opioid analgesics. Synergism with midazolam.

PREGNANCY: Category C, caution in nursing.

MECHANISM OF ACTION: Thiobarbiturate; ultrashort-acting depressant of CNS, which induces hypnosis and anesthesia, but not analgesia.

PHARMACOKINETICS: Distribution: Plasma protein binding (80%), crosses placental barrier, found in breast milk. **Metabolism:** Liver, kidneys, and brain. **Elimination:** Urine, $T_{1/2}$=3-8 hrs.

PEPCID

RX

famotidine (Merck)

OTHER BRAND NAMES: Pepcid RPD (Merck)

THERAPEUTIC CLASS: H$_2$-blocker

INDICATIONS: (PO/Inj) Short term treatment of active duodenal ulcer (DU), active benign gastric ulcer (GU), gastroesophageal reflux disease (GERD) and esophagitis due to GERD. Maintenance therapy for DU. Treatment of hypersecretory conditions (eg, Zollinger-Ellison syndrome). (Inj) For hospitalized patients with hypersecretory conditions or intractable ulcers. As an alternative in patients unable to take oral forms.

DOSAGE: *Adults:* (PO) Acute DU: 40mg qhs or 20mg bid for 4-8 weeks. Maint DU: 20mg qhs. GU: 40mg qhs. GERD: 20mg bid up to 6 weeks. GERD with Esophagitis: 20-40mg bid up to 12 weeks. Hypersecretory Conditions: Initial: 20mg q6h. Max: 160mg q6h. (Inj) 20mg IV q12h, hypersecretory conditions may require higher doses. CrCl <50mL/min: Reduce to 1/2 dose, or increase interval to q36-48h.
Pediatrics: 1-16 yrs: (PO) DU/GU: Usual: 0.5mg/kg/day qhs or divided bid. Max: 40mg/day. GERD With or Without Esophagitis: 0.5mg/kg PO bid. Max: 40mg bid. (Inj) 0.25mg/kg IV q12h up to 40mg/day. Base duration of therapy on clinical response, and/or pH, and endoscopy. (PO) GERD: 3 months-1yr: 0.5mg/kg bid for up to 8 weeks. <3 months: 0.5mg/kg qd for up to 8 weeks. CrCl <50mL/min: Reduce to 1/2 dose, or increase interval to q36-48h.

HOW SUPPLIED: Inj: 0.4mg/mL, 10mg/mL; Sus: 40mg/5mL [50mL]; Tab: 20mg, 40mg; Tab, Disintegrating: (RPD) 20mg, 40mg

CONTRAINDICATIONS: Hypersensitivity to other H$_2$ antagonists.

WARNINGS/PRECAUTIONS: CNS adverse effects reported with moderate to severe renal insufficiency; adjust dose. Disintegrating tabs contain phenylalanine; caution in phenylketonurics. Symptomatic response does not preclude the presence of gastric malignancy.

ADVERSE REACTIONS: Headache, dizziness, constipation, diarrhea, convulsions, interstitial pneumonia, Stevens-Johnson syndrome.

INTERACTIONS: May give with antacids.

PREGNANCY: Category B, not for use in nursing.

MECHANISM OF ACTION: Histamine H$_2$-receptor antagonist; inhibits both acid concentration and volume of gastric secretion.

PHARMACOKINETICS: Absorption: (Adults PO): Incompletely absorbed; T$_{max}$=1.3 hrs. (Adults, IV): T$_{max}$=20-30 min. **Distribution:** (Adult) Plasma protein binding (15-20%); excreted in breast milk. **Metabolism:** S-oxide (metabolite). **Elimination:** Renal (65-70%), (PO) 25-30% unchanged; (IV) 65-70% unchanged. Metabolic (65-70%); (Adults) T$_{1/2}$=2.5-3.5 hrs. Refer to package insert for pediatric parameters.

PEPCID AC

OTC

famotidine (J&J - Merck)

THERAPEUTIC CLASS: H$_2$-blocker

INDICATIONS: Relief and prevention of heartburn, acid indigestion, and sour stomach.

DOSAGE: *Adults:* Relief: 1 tab/cap prn. Max: 2 doses/24 hrs. Prevention: 1 tab/cap 15-60 min before food or beverages that cause heartburn. Max: 2 doses/24 hrs.
Pediatrics: ≥12yrs: 1 tab/cap prn. Max: 2 doses/24 hrs. Prevention: 1 tab/cap 15-60 min before food or beverages that cause heartburn. Max: 2 doses/24 hrs.

HOW SUPPLIED: Cap: 10mg; Tab: 10mg, 20mg; Tab, Chewable: 10mg

INTERACTIONS: Avoid with other acid reducers.

PEPCID COMPLETE OTC
calcium carbonate - magnesium hydroxide - famotidine (J&J - Merck)

THERAPEUTIC CLASS: H_2-blocker/antacid

INDICATIONS: To relieve heartburn associated with acid indigestion and sour stomach.

DOSAGE: *Adults:* Chew 1 tab to relieve symptoms. Max: 2 tabs/24hrs.
Pediatrics: ≥12 yrs: Chew 1 tab to relieve symptoms. Max: 2 tabs/24hrs.

HOW SUPPLIED: Tab, Chewable: (Famotidine-Calcium Carbonate-Magnesium Hydroxide) 10mg-800mg-165mg

WARNINGS/PRECAUTIONS: Not for use in those with trouble swallowing. Avoid use with other acid reducers.

PREGNANCY: Safety in pregnancy and nursing not known.

PEPTO-BISMOL OTC
bismuth subsalicylate (Procter & Gamble)

OTHER BRAND NAMES: Pepto-Bismol Maximum Strength (Procter & Gamble)

THERAPEUTIC CLASS: Antimicrobial

INDICATIONS: To control diarrhea within 24 hrs, relieving associated abdominal cramps; soothes heartburn, and indigestion without constipation; and relieves nausea and upset stomach.

DOSAGE: *Adults:* (Sus) 30mL every 0.5-1 hr prn. Max: 8 doses/24hrs. (Sus, Max Strength) 30mL hourly prn. Max: 4 doses/24 hrs. (Tab; Tab, Chewable) 2 tabs every 0.5-1 hr prn. Max: 8 doses/24hrs. Drink plenty of clear fluids.
Pediatrics: (Sus) 9-12 yrs: 15mL every 0.5-1 hr prn. 6-9 yrs: 10mL every 0.5-1 hr prn. 3-6 yrs: 5mL every 0.5-1 hr. Max: 8 doses/24hrs. (Sus, Max Strength) 9-12 yrs: 15mL hourly prn. 6-9 yrs: 10mL hourly prn. 3-6 yrs: 5mL hourly prn. Max: 4 doses/24hrs. (Tab; Tab, Chewable) 9-12 yrs: 1 tab every 0.5-1 hr prn. 6-9 yrs: 2/3 tab every 0.5-1 hr prn. 3-6 yrs: 1/3 tab every 0.5-1 hr prn. Max: 8 doses/24 hrs. Drink plenty of clear fluids.

HOW SUPPLIED: Sus: 262mg/15mL; Sus, Maximum Strength: 525mg/15mL; Tab: 262mg; Tab, Chewable: 262mg

WARNINGS/PRECAUTIONS: Avoid in children and teenagers with or recovering from chickenpox or flu. Do not give with ASA or non-ASA salicylate allergy. May cause temporary darkening of tongue or stool. Product may contain small amounts of naturally occurring lead.

INTERACTIONS: May cause ringing in ears with ASA; d/c if this occurs. Caution with anticoagulants, antidiabetic, and antigout agents.

PREGNANCY: Safety in pregnancy and nursing not known.

PERCOCET CII
oxycodone HCL - acetaminophen (Endo)

OTHER BRAND NAMES: Endocet (Endo)

THERAPEUTIC CLASS: Opioid analgesic

INDICATIONS: Relief of moderate to moderately severe pain.

DOSAGE: *Adults:* (2.5/325): 1-2 tabs q6h. Max: 12 tabs/day. (5/325): 1 tab q6h prn. Max: 12 tabs/day. (7.5/500): 1 tab q6h prn. Max: 8 tabs/day. (10-650) 1 tab q6h prn. Max: 6 tabs/day. (7.5/325): 1 tab q6h prn. Max: 8 tabs/day. (10/325): 1 tab q6h prn. Max: 6 tabs/day. Do not exceed APAP 4g/day.

HOW SUPPLIED: Tab: (Oxycodone-APAP) 2.5mg-325mg, 5mg-325mg, 7.5mg-325mg, 7.5mg-500mg, 10mg-325mg, 10mg-650mg

WARNINGS/PRECAUTIONS: May cause drug dependence and tolerance; potential for abuse. Risk of respiratory depression. Capacity to elevate CSF pressure may be exaggerated with head injury, other intracranial lesions or a pre-existing increase in ICP. May obscure the diagnosis or clinical course with head injuries or with acute abdominal conditions. Caution with severe hepatic impairment, renal dysfunction, hypothyroidism, Addison's disease, prostatic hypertrophy, urethral stricture, the elderly or debilitated.

ADVERSE REACTIONS: Lightheadedness, dizziness, sedation, nausea, vomiting, euphoria, dysphoria, constipation, skin rash, pruritus.

INTERACTIONS: Potentiates CNS depression with other opioid analgesics, general anesthetics, phenothiazines, tranquilizers, sedative-hypnotics, alcohol and other CNS depressants. Risk of paralytic ileus with anticholinergics.

PREGNANCY: Category C, caution in nursing.

MECHANISM OF ACTION: Oxycodone: Opioid analgesic; semisynthetic pure opioid agonist whose principal therapeutic action is analgesia. Other pharmacological effects include anxiolysis, euphoria, and feelings of relaxation. Effects mediated by CNS receptors (eg, mu and kappa) for endogenous opioid-like compounds (eg, endorphins, enkephalins). APAP: Non-opiate, non-salicyclic analgesic, and antipyretic. Site and mechanism of analgesic effect not established. Antipyretic effect produced through inhibition of endogenous pyrogen action on the hypothalmic heat-regulating centers.

PHARMACOKINETICS: Absorption: Oxycodone: Absolute bioavailability (87%). APAP: Rapid absorption. **Distribution:** Oxycodone: Plasma protein binding (45%); (IV):V_d= 211.9L; found in breast milk. APAP: Plasma protein binding (20-50%) (variable). **Metabolism:** Oxycodone: N-dealkylation to noroxycodone (metabolite); CYP2D6 (O-demethylation) to oxymorphone (metabolite). Acetaminophen: Liver via cytochrome P450 (conjugation), NAPQI (toxic metabolite). **Elimination:** Oxycodone: Urine (parent compound and metabolites); $T_{1/2}$=3.51 hrs. APAP: Urine (90-100%).

PERCODAN CII
oxycodone HCL - aspirin (Endo)

OTHER BRAND NAMES: Endodan (Endo)

THERAPEUTIC CLASS: Opioid analgesic

INDICATIONS: Relief of moderate to moderately severe pain.

DOSAGE: *Adults:* Usual: 1 tab q6h prn. Max: 12 tabs/day or ASA 4g/day.

HOW SUPPLIED: Tab: (Oxycodone HCl-ASA) 4.8355mg-325mg* *scored

WARNINGS/PRECAUTIONS: May cause drug dependence and tolerance; potential for abuse. Risk of respiratory depression. Capacity to elevate CSF pressure may be exaggerated with head injury, other intracranial lesions or a pre-existing increase in ICP. May obscure the diagnosis or clinical course with head injuries or with acute abdominal conditions. Caution with severe of hepatic impairment, renal dysfunction, hypothyroidism, Addison's disease, prostatic hypertrophy, urethral stricture, peptic ulcer, coagulation abnormalities, and the elderly or debilitated. May increase the risk of developing Reye's syndrome in children and teenagers. May impair mental/physical abilities.

ADVERSE REACTIONS: Lightheadedness, dizziness, sedation, nausea, vomiting, euphoria, dysphoria, constipation, pruritus.

INTERACTIONS: Additive CNS depression with other opioid analgesics, general anesthetics, phenothiazines, tranquilizers, sedative-hypnotics, or other CNS depressants (including alcohol). ASA may enhance effect of anticoagulants and inhibit effects of uricosuric agents.

PREGNANCY: Category B (Oxycodone) and D (ASA), not for use in nursing.

MECHANISM OF ACTION: Oxycodone: Semisynthetic pure opioid agonist. Principle therapeutic effect is analgesia. Other effects include anxiolysis, euphoria, and feelings of relaxation. Effects mediated by CNSb receptors (ex, mu, kappa) for endogenous opioid-like compounds (eg, endorphins, enkephalins). ASA: Inhibits prostaglandin production, including those involved in inflammation. (Prostaglandins cause pain sensation by stimulating muscle contractions and dilating blood vessels throughout body.) In CNS, works on hypothalmus heat-regulating center to reduce fever.

PHARMACOKINETICS: Absorption: Oxycodone: Absolute bioavailability (87%). ASA: Rapidly absorbed. **Distribution:** Oxycodone: Plasma protein binding (45%); found in breast milk; (IV) V_d=211.9L. ASA: Found in most body tissues, fluids (eg, fetal tissues, breast milk, CNS, liver, kidneys); variable serum protein binding. **Metabolism:** Oxycodone: N-dealkylation to noroxycodone (metabolite); CYP2D6 (O-demethylation) to oxymorphone (metabolite). ASA: Liver, hydrolysis to salicylate, salicyluric acid, salicyl phenolic glucuronide, salicyl acyl glucuronide, gentisic acid, gentisuric acid (major metabolites). **Elimination:** Oxycodone: Urine (parent compound and metabolites); $T_{1/2}$=3.51 hrs. ASA: Urine (parent compound and metabolites) (80-100%); $T_{1/2}$=2-3 hrs.

PERFOROMIST   RX
formoterol fumarate (Dey)

> Long-acting β_2-agonists may increase risk of asthma-related death.

THERAPEUTIC CLASS: Beta$_2$-agonist

INDICATIONS: Long-term maintenance treatment of bronchoconstriction in patients with chronic obstructive pulmonary disease (COPD), including chronic bronchitis and emphysema.

DOSAGE: *Adults:* 20mcg bid q12h. Administer by nebulizer.

HOW SUPPLIED: Sol, Inhalation: 20mcg/2mL [2.5mL, 60^s]

WARNINGS/PRECAUTIONS: Only use short-acting B$_2$-agonist inhaler for acute symptoms. Should not be used with other long acting B$_2$-agonist medications. D/C if paradoxical bronchospasm occurs. D/C if ECG changes, QT interval increases, or ST depression occurs. Caution with cardiovascular disorders (eg.coronary insufficiency, arrythmias, and HTN), convulsive disorders, thyrotoxicosis, and DM. May cause hypokalemia and hyperglycemia.

ADVERSE REACTIONS: Diarrhea, nausea, nasopharyngitis, dry mouth, angina, HTN, hypotension, tachycardia, arrythmias, nervousness, headache, tremor, muscle cramps, palpitations, dizziness.

INTERACTIONS: Adrenergic drugs may potentiate effects. Xanthine derivatives, steroids, diuretics, or non-potassium sparing diuretics may potentiate hypokalemia or ECG changes; use with caution. MAOIs, TCAs, and drugs known to prolong QTc interval may potentiate effect on cardiovascular system; use with extreme caution. β-blockers may decrease effectiveness; use with caution.

PREGNANCY: Category C, caution in nursing.

MECHANISM OF ACTION: Long acting β_2-agonist; acts as bronchodilator, stimulates intracellular adenyl cyclase, the enzyme that catalyzes the conversion of ATP to cAMP. Increased cAMP levels cause relaxation of bronchial smooth muscle and inhibition of release of mediators of immediated hypersensitivity from cells such as mast cells.

PHARMACOKINETICS: Absorption: C_{max}=72pg/mL; T_{max}=12 min. **Distribution:** Plasma protein binding (61-64%). **Metabolism:** Glucuronidation, O-demethylation; CYP2D6, 2C19, 2C19, 2A6. **Elimination:** Urine (unchanged); $T_{1/2}$=7 hrs.

PERI-COLACE   OTC
docusate sodium - senna (Purdue Products)

THERAPEUTIC CLASS: Stool softener/laxative combination

INDICATIONS: Management of constipation.

DOSAGE: *Adults:* 2-4 tabs daily.
Pediatrics: ≥12yrs: 2-4 tabs daily. 6-<12yrs: 1-2 tabs daily. 2-<6yrs: Max of 1 tab daily.

HOW SUPPLIED: (Docusate Sodium-Sennosides) Tab: 50mg-8.6mg
WARNINGS/PRECAUTIONS: Caution with use >1 week.
INTERACTIONS: Caution with mineral oil.
PREGNANCY: Safety in pregnancy and nursing not known.

PERIDEX   RX
chlorhexidine gluconate (Zila)

THERAPEUTIC CLASS: Antimicrobial

INDICATIONS: For use between dental visits for treatment of gingivitis.

DOSAGE: *Adults:* Swish for 30 seconds and expectorate 15mL bid, am and hs, after brushing. Initiate after a dental prophylaxis. Max: 6 month intervals.

HOW SUPPLIED: Liq: 0.12%

WARNINGS/PRECAUTIONS: May stain oral surfaces and alter taste perception.

ADVERSE REACTIONS: Staining of teeth and other oral surfaces, calculus formation, taste perception alteration, minor gum irritation.

PREGNANCY: Category B, caution in nursing.

MECHANISM OF ACTION: Microbial agent; suspected to reduce bacterial assay count, both aerobic and anaerobic.

PHARMACOKINETICS: Absorption: Poor. C_{max}=0.206µg/g, T_{max}=30 min. **Elimination:** Feces (90%), urine (<1%).

PERIOGARD   RX
chlorhexidine gluconate (Colgate Oral)

THERAPEUTIC CLASS: Antimicrobial

INDICATIONS: Treatment of gingivitis between dental visits, including gingival bleeding.

DOSAGE: *Adults:* Rinse with 15mL for 30 seconds bid, am and pm, after toothbrushing. Expectorate after rinsing; do not ingest. Do not rinse with water or other mouthwashes, brush teeth, or eat immediately after use.

HOW SUPPLIED: Liq: 0.12%

WARNINGS/PRECAUTIONS: Effect in periodontitis not known. May increase supragingival calculus. Hypersensitivity, allergic reactions and altered taste reported. May stain tooth, oral surfaces and dorsum of the tongue. Caution with anterior facial restoration.

ADVERSE REACTIONS: Increases staining of teeth and other oral surfaces, increases calculus formation, alteration in taste perception, oral irritation, local allergy-type symptoms, stomatitis, gingivitis, glossitis, ulcer, dry mouth, hypesthesia, glossal edema, paresthesia.

PREGNANCY: Category B, caution in nursing.

MECHANISM OF ACTION: Microbial agent; suspected to reduce bacterial assay count, both aerobic and anaerobic.

PHARMACOKINETICS: Absorption: Poorly absorbed from GI tract; C_{max}=0.206mcg/g; T_{max}=30 min. **Elimination**: Feces (90%), urine (<1%).

PERIOSTAT   RX
doxycycline hyclate (CollaGenex)

THERAPEUTIC CLASS: Tetracycline derivative

INDICATIONS: Adjunct to scaling and root planing to promote attachment level gain and reduces pocket depth in patients with adult periodontitis.

DOSAGE: *Adults:* Following scaling and root planing, 20mg bid, 1 hour prior to morning and evening meals for up to 9 months. Maintain adequate fluid intake with caps to reduce risk of esophageal irritation and ulceration.

HOW SUPPLIED: Tab: 20mg

WARNINGS/PRECAUTIONS: Do not exceed recommended dosage. May cause permanent tooth discoloration during tooth development (last half of pregnancy and up to 8 years old). Risk of fetal harm in pregnancy. May increase BUN and risk of vaginal candidiasis. Photosensitivity reported. Superinfection with nonsusceptible microorganism. Caution with history of oral candidiasis.

ADVERSE REACTIONS: Headache, common cold, flu symptoms, toothache, periodontal abscess, tooth disorder, nausea, sinusitis, dyspepsia, sore throat, joint pain, diarrhea, sinus congestion, coughing, rash.

INTERACTIONS: Decreased effects with barbiturates, phenytoin and car-bamazepine. Interferes with bactericidal effects of β-lactam (eg, penicillin) antibiotics. Depresses plasma PT activity; adjust oral anticoagulant dose. Absorption impaired by aluminum-, calcium- or magnesium-containing antacids, iron-containing products and bismuth subsalicylate. Decreases effects of oral contraceptives. Fatal renal toxicity reported with concurrent methoxyflurane.

PREGNANCY: Category D, contraindicated in nursing.

MECHANISM OF ACTION: Tetracycline; inhibits collagenase activity; reduces elevated collagenase activity of gingival crevicular fluid in periodontitis.

PHARMACOKINETICS: Absorption: Rapid; C_{max}=790mcg/mL, T_{max}=2 hrs. **Distribution:** Plasma protein binding (>90%). V_d=52.6-134L. **Elimination:** Urine, feces. (20mg) $T_{1/2}$=18 hrs.

PERMAPEN   RX
penicillin G benzathine (Pfizer)

THERAPEUTIC CLASS: Penicillin

INDICATIONS: Treatment of microorganisms susceptible to low and very prolonged serum levels in upper respiratory tract infections (streptococci group A - without bacteremia), syphilis, yaws, bejel, and pinta. Prophylaxis for rheumatic fever and/or chorea. Follow-up prophylactic therapy for rheumatic heart disease and acute glomerulonephritis.

DOSAGE: *Adults:* Streptococcal Infection: 1.2 MU IM single dose. Primary/Secondary/Latent Syphilis: 1 MU IM single dose. Late (Tertiary/Neurosyphilis) Syphilis: 3 MU IM every 7 days for total of 6-9 MU. Yaws/Bejel/Pinta: 1.2 MU IM single dose. Rheumatic Fever/Glomerulonephritis Prophylaxis: 1.2 MU IM once monthly or 600,000 U IM twice monthly. Use upper outer quadrant of buttock. Rotate injection site.
Pediatrics: ≤12 yrs: Adjust dose according to age and weight and severity of infection. Streptococcal Infection: 900,000 U IM single dose in older children. Congenital Syphilis: <2 yrs: 50,000 U/kg IM single dose. 2-12 yrs: Adjust dose based on adult schedule. Use midlateral aspect of thigh in infants and small children. May divide dose between 2 buttocks in peds <2 yrs. Rotate injection site.

HOW SUPPLIED: Inj: 600,000 U/mL

WARNINGS/PRECAUTIONS: Caution in newborns; evaluate organ system function frequently. Evaluate renal, hepatic and hematopoietic systems with prolonged therapy. Serious, fatal anaphylactic reactions reported; increased risk with hypersensitivity to PCNs, cephalosporins, and other allergens. Avoid IV, intra-arterial administration, or injection into/near major peripheral nerves or blood vessels may cause severe neurovascular damage. May result in overgrowth of nonsusceptible organisms. Avoid subcutaneous and fat-layer injections. Take culture after therapy completion to determine streptococci eradication.

ADVERSE REACTIONS: Skin eruptions, urticaria, laryngeal edema, anaphylaxis, fever, eosinophilia.

INTERACTIONS: Bacteriostatic agents (eg, tetracycline, erythromycin) may diminish effects. Prolonged levels with probenecid.

PREGNANCY: Category B, caution in nursing.

MECHANISM OF ACTION: Penicillin; exerts bactericial action during stage of multiplication by inhibiting biosynthesis of cell-wall mucopeptide.

PHARMACOKINETICS: Absorption: Slow. **Distribution:** Plasma protein binding (60%). **Metabolism:** Hydrolysis. **Elimination:** Kidneys, bile.

PERPHENAZINE RX
perphenazine (Various)

THERAPEUTIC CLASS: Phenothiazine

INDICATIONS: Treatment of schizophrenia. To control severe nausea and vomiting.

DOSAGE: *Adults:* Moderately Disturbed Non-Hospitalized With Schizophrenia: Initial: 4-8mg tid. Maint: Reduce to minimum effective dose. Hospitalized Psychotic Patients With Schizophrenia: 8-16mg bid-qid. Max: 64mg/day. Severe Nausea/Vomiting: 8-16mg/day in divided doses. Max: 24mg/day. Elderly: Lower dosages recommended.
Pediatrics: ≥12 yrs: Use lowest limits of adult dose.

HOW SUPPLIED: Tab: 2mg, 4mg, 8mg, 16mg

CONTRAINDICATIONS: Comatose or greatly obtunded patients, large doses of CNS depressants (eg, barbiturates, alcohol, narcotics, analgesics, or antihistamines), blood dyscrasias, bone marrow depression, liver damage, subcortical brain damage with or without hypothalamic involvement.

WARNINGS/PRECAUTIONS: Tardive dyskinesia may develop. NMS, photosensitivity reported. May lower convulsive threshold; caution with alcohol withdrawal. Caution with psychic depression, renal impairment, respiratory impairment. May impair mental/physical abilities. May mask signs of overdosage to other drugs. May obsure diagnosis of intestinal obstruction, brain tumor. Severe hypotension may occur in surgery. May elevate prolactin levels. Monitor hepatic/renal functions, blood counts. Increased risk of liver damage, jaundice, corneal and lenticular deposits, and irreversible dyskinesias with long-term use.

ADVERSE REACTIONS: Extrapyramidal reactions, tardive dyskinesia, cerebral edema, seizures, drowsiness, dry mouth, salivation, nausea, vomiting, diarrhea, anorexia, constipation, urticaria, erythema, eczema, postural hypotension, tachycardia.

INTERACTIONS: See Contraindications. Additive effects with CNS depressants and phenothiazine; use reduced amount of added drug. Additive anticholinergic effects with atropine/atropine-like drugs, exposure to phosphorous insecticide. Additive effects and hypotension may occur with alcohol. Cytochrome P450 2D6 inhibitors (TCAs, SSRIs) may increase levels; lower doses may be required.

PREGNANCY: Safety in pregnancy and nursing not known.

MECHANISM OF ACTION: Piperazinyl phenothiazine; mechanism not known, has actions at all levels of the CNS, particularly the hypothalamus.

PHARMACOKINETICS: Absorption: C_{max}=984(43)pg/mL; T_{max}=1-3 hrs. **Metabolism:** Liver (extensive) via sulfoxidation, hydroxylation mediated by CYP450 (2D6), dealkylation, and glucoronidation. **Elimination:** Urine (primarly), feces, bile; $T_{1/2}$=9-12 hrs.

PERSANTINE RX
dipyridamole (Boehringer Ingelheim)

THERAPEUTIC CLASS: Platelet aggregation inhibitor

INDICATIONS: Adjunct to coumarin anticoagulants for prevention of postoperative thromboembolic complications of cardiac valve replacement.

DOSAGE: *Adults:* 75-100mg qid.

HOW SUPPLIED: Tab: 25mg, 50mg, 75mg

WARNINGS/PRECAUTIONS: Caution with hypotension or severe CAD (eg, unstable angina or recent MI); may aggravate chest pain. Elevated hepatic enzymes and hepatic failure reported.

ADVERSE REACTIONS: Dizziness, abdominal distress.

INTERACTIONS: Increases levels of adenosine. May counteract effects of cholinesterase inhibitors.

PREGNANCY: Category B, caution in nursing.

MECHANISM OF ACTION: Platelet inhibitor; inhibits the uptake of adenosine into platelets, endothelial cells, and erythrocytes. Inhibition results in an increase in adenosine concentrations that act on the platelet A$_2$ receptor to stimulate platelet adenylate cyclase and increase platelet cyclic-3',5'-adenosine monophosphate (cAMP) levels. Platelet aggregation is thereby inhibited in response to various stimuli (eg, platelet activating factor (PAF), collagen, adenosine diphosphate). Also inhibits phosphodiesterase (PDE) in various tissues. Inhibits cyclic-3'5'-guanosine monophosphate-PDE (cGMP-PDE), which thereby augments the increase in cGMP produced by EDRF (endothelium-derived relaxing factor [nitric oxide]).

PHARMACOKINETICS: Absorption: T$_{max}$=75 min. **Distribution:** Highly bound to plasma proteins. Found in human breast milk. **Metabolism:** Liver (conjugation). **Elimination:** Bile; T$_{1/2}$=40 min. (initial); T$_{1/2}$=10 hrs.

PEXEVA RX
paroxetine mesylate (Synthon)

> Antidepressants increased the risk of suicidal thinking and behavior (suicidality) in short-term studies in children, adolescents, and young adults with Major Depressive Disorder (MDD) and other psychiatric disorders. Pexeva is not approved for use in pediatric patients.

THERAPEUTIC CLASS: Selective serotonin reuptake inhibitor

INDICATIONS: Treatment of major depressive disorder (MDD), obsessive compulsive disorder (OCD), panic disorder with or without agoraphobia, and generalized anxiety disorder (GAD).

DOSAGE: *Adults:* MDD: Initial: 20mg/day. Max: 50mg/day. OCD: Initial: 20mg/day. Titrate: Increase by 10mg/day. Usual: 40mg/day. Max: 60mg/day. Panic Disorder: Initial: 10mg/day. Titrate: 10mg/day increments at intervals of at least 1 week. Max: 60mg/day. GAD: Initial: 20mg/day. Titrate: Increase by 10mg/day. Max: 50mg/day. Elderly/Debilitated/Severe Renal or Hepatic Impairment: Initial: 10mg qd. Max: 40mg/day.

HOW SUPPLIED: Tab: 10mg, 20mg, 30mg, 40mg

CONTRAINDICATIONS: Concomitant MAOIs, thioridazine, and pimozide.

WARNINGS/PRECAUTIONS: Caution with history of mania, seizures, history of suicidal thoughts or attempts (adolescents have an increased risk of suicidal thoughts and/or attempts), conditions that affect metabolism or hemodynamic responses, narrow angle glaucoma. Risk of serotonin syndrome with contomitant use of triptans, tramadol, and other serotonergic agents. D/C if seizures occur. Altered platelet function, hyponatremia, mydriasis reported. Avoid abrupt withdrawal. Re-evaluate periodically. Monitor for clinical worsening and/or suicidality, especially at initiation of therapy or dose changes.

ADVERSE REACTIONS: Asthenia, sweating, nausea, decreased appetite, somnolence, dizziness, insomnia, tremor, nervousness, abnormal ejaculation, dry mouth, constipation, decreased libido, impotence, headache, tinnitus.

INTERACTIONS: Avoid alcohol, tryptophan, thioridazine, and within 14 days of MAOI therapy. May shift concentrations with plasma-bound drugs. Increased risk of bleeding with NSAIDS, aspirin, oral anticoagulants. May inhibit metabolism of TCAs. Rare reports of weakness, hyperreflexia, incoordination with an SSRI and sumatriptan; avoid triptans unless necessary-carefully monitor patient when on paroxetine and triptan with initiation and dose changes. Monitor theophylline. Reduce procyclidine dose if anticholinergic effects occur.

Increased levels with cimetidine. Caution with diuretics, digoxin, lithium, cimetidine, warfarin, phenobarbital, phenytoin, drugs metabolized by CYP2D6 (eg, antidepressants, phenothiazines, Type 1C antiarrhythmics), quinidine, avoid concomitant use with SSRIs and SNRIs. Fosamprenavir/ritonavir decreases paroxetine levels. Pimozide levels may be increased with concomitant administration of paroxetine, which could result in QT prolongation.

PREGNANCY: Category D, increased risk of cardiovascular malformations (ventrciular/atrial septal defects) in newborns; avoid unless benefit outweighs risk.

MECHANISM OF ACTION: SSRI; inhibits CNS neuronal reuptake of serotonin.

PHARMACOKINETICS: Absorption: Complete; C_{max}=81.3ng/mL; T_{max}=8.1 hr. **Distribution:** Plasma protein binding (95%). **Metabolism:** Oxidation and methylation via CYP2D6. **Elimination:** Urine (2%), feces (<1%); $T_{1/2}$=33.2 hrs.

Pfizerpen   RX
penicillin G potassium (Pfizer)

THERAPEUTIC CLASS: Penicillin

INDICATIONS: For therapy of severe infections when rapid and high blood levels of penicillin required. Management of streptococcal, pneumococcal, staphylococcal, clostridial, fusospirochetal, listeria, and gram negative bacillary, and pasteurella infections. For anthrax, actinomycosis, diphtheria, erysipeloid, meningitis, endocarditis, bacteremia, rat-bite fever, syphilis, and gonorrheal endocarditis and arthritis. With combined oral therapy, prophylaxis against endocarditis in patients with congenital heart disease, rheumatic, or other acquired valvular heart disease undergoing dental procedures or surgical procedures of upper respiratory tract.

DOSAGE: *Adults:* Anthrax/Gonorrheal Endocarditis/Severe Infections (Streptococci, Pneumococci, Staphylococci): Minimum of 5MU/day. Syphilis: Administer in hospital. Determine dose and duration based on age and weight. Meningococcic Meningitis: 1-2MU IM q2h or 20-30MU/day continuous IV. Actinomycosis: 1-6MU/day for cervicofacial cases; 10-20MU/day for thoracic and abdominal disease. Clostridial Infections: 20MU/day (adjunct to antitoxin). Fusospirochetal Severe Infections: 5-10MU/day for oropharynx, lower respiratory tract, and genital area infection. Rat-bite Fever: 12-15MU/day for 3-4 weeks. Listeria Endocarditis: 15-20MU/day for 4 weeks. Pasteurella Bacteremia/Meningitis: 4-6MU/day for 2 weeks. Erysipeloid Endocarditis: 2-20MU/day for 4-6 weeks. Gram Negative Bacillary Bacteremia: 20-80MU/day. Diphtheria (carrier state): 0.3-0.4MU/day in divided doses for 10-12 days. Endocarditis Prophylaxis: 1MU IM mixed with 0.6MU procaine penicillin G 0.5-1 hr before procedure. Renal/Cardiac/Vascular Dysfunction: Consider dose reduction. For streptococcal infection, treat for minimum 10 days.
Pediatrics: Listeria Infections: Neonates: 0.5-1MU/day. Congenital Syphilis: Administer in hospital. Determine dose and duration based on age and weight. Endocarditis Prophylaxis: 30,000U/kg IM mixed with 0.6MU procaine penicillin G 0.5-1 hr before procedure. For streptococcal infection, treat for minimum 10 days.

HOW SUPPLIED: Inj: 1MU, 5MU, 20MU

WARNINGS/PRECAUTIONS: Serious, fatal anaphylactic reactions reported; increased risk with hypersensitivity to PCNs, cephalosporins, and other allergens. Avoid IV, intra-arterial administration, or injection into/near major peripheral nerves or blood vessels; may cause severe neurovascular damage. Take culture after therapy completion to determine streptococci eradication. Caution with history of significant allergies or asthma. May result in overgrowth of nonsusceptible organisms. Evaluate renal, hepatic and hematopoietic systems with prolonged therapy. Administer slowly to avoid electrolyte imbalance from potassium or sodium content; monitor electrolytes and consider dose reductions with renal, cardiac, or vascular dysfunction. Caution in newborns; evaluate organ system function frequently.

ADVERSE REACTIONS: Skin rash (eg, maculopapular eruption, exfoliative dermatitis) urticaria, chills, fever, edema, arthralgia, prostration, anaphylaxis, arrhythmias, cardiac arrest, Jarisch-Herxheimer reaction.

INTERACTIONS: Bacteriostatic agents (eg, tetracycline, erythromycin) may diminish effects. Prolonged levels with probenecid.

PREGNANCY: Category B, caution in nursing.

MECHANISM OF ACTION: Penicillin; exerts bactericidal action during stage of active multiplication by inhibiting biosynthesis of cell-wall mucopeptide.

PHARMACOKINETICS: Absorption: Rapid. **Distribution:** Found in breast milk. **Elimination:** Urine.

PHENERGAN INJECTION RX
promethazine HCL (Baxter)

THERAPEUTIC CLASS: Phenothiazine derivative

INDICATIONS: For blood or plasma allergic reactions, allergic reactions where oral therapy is not possible, sedation, and special surgical situations (eg, repeated bronchoscopy). Adjunct for anaphylactic reactions and postoperative pain. Treatment of motion sickness. Prevention and control of nausea and vomiting in surgery.

DOSAGE: *Adults:* (IM/IV) IM is preferred. Allergy: Initial: 25mg, may repeat within 2 hrs. Sedation: 25-50mg qhs. Nausea/Vomiting: 12.5-25mg q4h. Preoperative/Postoperative: 25-50mg. Obstetrics: 50mg in early labor, 25-75mg in established labor, may repeat once or twice q4h. Max: 100mg/24 hrs of labor. Do not give IV administration >25mg/mL and at a rate >25mg/min. *Pediatrics:* ≥2 yrs: Dose should not exceed half of adult dose. Premedication: Usual: 0.5mg/lb. Do not give IV administration >25mg/mL and at a rate >25mg/min.

HOW SUPPLIED: Inj: 25mg/mL, 50mg/mL

CONTRAINDICATIONS: Comatose states, intra-arterial or subcutaneous injection. Hypersensitivity to other phenothiazines.

WARNINGS/PRECAUTIONS: Caution in patients ≥2 yrs. Not recommended for uncomplicated vomiting in pediatrics. May cause marked drowsiness; caution with operating machinery. Fatal respiratory depression reported; avoid with respiratory dysfunction (eg, COPD, sleep apnea). Avoid prolonged sun exposure. May lower seizure threshold. Caution with bone marrow depression. NMS reported. Caution in acutely ill pediatric patients. Avoid in pediatrics with Reye's syndrome or hepatic disease. Avoid perivascular extravasation or inadvertent intra-arterial injection. Caution with narrow-angle glaucoma, prostatic hypertrophy, stenosing peptic ulcer, bladder-neck or pyloroduodenal obstruction, cardiovascular disease, hepatic dysfunction. Cholestatic jaundice reported. Alters HCG pregnancy test reading. May increase blood glucose.

ADVERSE REACTIONS: Drowsiness, dizziness, tinnitus, blurred vision, dry mouth, increased or decreased blood pressure, urticaria, nausea, vomiting, blood dyscrasia.

INTERACTIONS: Added sedative effects with CNS depressants (eg, alcohol, narcotics, narcotic analgesics, sedatives, hypnotics, general anesthetics, tranquilizers, TCAs); reduce dose or eliminate these agents. Reduce barbiturate dose by one-half and analgesic depressant dose by one-quarter to one-half. Caution with drugs that alter seizure threshold (eg, narcotics, local anesthetics). Do not use epinephrine for promethazine injection overdose. Caution with anticholinergics. Possible adverse reactions with MAOIs.

PREGNANCY: Category C, caution in nursing.

MECHANISM OF ACTION: Phenothiazine derivative/H_1 receptor antagonist; possesses antihistamine (does not block release of histamine), sedative, anti-motion sickness, antiemetic, and anticholinergic effects.

PHARMACOKINETICS: Metabolism: Liver; sulfoxides, N-desmethylpromethazine (metabolites). **Elimination:** Urine; $T_{1/2}$=9-16 hrs (IV), 9.8 hrs (IM).

P

PHENOBARBITAL
phenobarbital (Various) `CIV`

THERAPEUTIC CLASS: Barbiturate

INDICATIONS: Treatment of generalized, tonic-clonic and cortical focal seizures. For relief of anxiety, tension and apprehension. Short-term treatment of insomnia.

DOSAGE: *Adults:* Sedation: 30-120mg/day given bid-tid. Max: 400mg/24h. Hypnotic: 100-200mg. Seizures: 60-200mg/day. Elderly/Debilitated/Renal or Hepatic Dysfunction: Reduce dosage.
Pediatrics: Seizures: 3-6mg/kg/day.

HOW SUPPLIED: Elixir: 20mg/5mL; Tab: 15mg, 30mg, 32.4mg, 60mg, 64.8mg, 100mg

CONTRAINDICATIONS: Respiratory disease with dyspnea or obstruction, porphyria, severe liver dysfunction. Large doses with nephritic patients.

WARNINGS/PRECAUTIONS: May be habit forming. Avoid abrupt withdrawal. Caution with acute or chronic pain; may mask symptoms or paradoxical excitement may occur. Cognitive deficits reported in children with febrile seizures. May cause excitement in children and excitement, depression or confusion in elderly, debilitated. Caution with hepatic dysfunction, borderline hypoadrenal function, depression.

ADVERSE REACTIONS: Drowsiness, residual sedation, lethargy, vertigo, somnolence, respiratory depression, hypersensitivity reactions, nausea, vomiting, headache.

INTERACTIONS: May be potentiated by MAOIs, antihistamines, alcohol, tranquilizers, sedative/hypnotics, other CNS depressants. Decreases effects of oral anticoagulants. Increases corticosteroid metabolism. Decreases effects of oral contraceptives. Decreases absorption of griseofulvin. Decreases half-life of doxycycline. May alter phenytoin metabolism. Increased levels with sodium valproate and valproic acid.

PREGNANCY: Category D, caution in nursing.

MECHANISM OF ACTION: Barbiturate; nonselective CNS depressant. Capable of producing all levels of CNS mood alteration. Responsible for depressing the sensory cortex, decreasing motor activity, altering cerebellar function, causing sedation and hypnosis.

PHARMACOKINETICS: Distribution: Distributed to all tissues and fluids. High concentrations found in the brain, liver, and kidneys. Found in breast milk. **Metabolism:** Hepatic. **Elimination:** Urine (primary), feces; $T_{1/2}$=79 hrs (adults), 110 hrs (children and newborns less than 48 hrs old).

PHENYTEK `RX`
phenytoin sodium (Mylan Bertek)

THERAPEUTIC CLASS: Hydantoin

INDICATIONS: Control of generalized tonic-clonic (grand mal) and complex partial (psychomotor, temporal lobe) seizures. Prevention and treatment of neurosurgically induced seizures.

DOSAGE: *Adults:* No Previous Treatment: Initial: 100mg extended phenytoin sodium capsule tid. Titrate: May increase at 7-10 day intervals. Usual: 100mg tid-qid. May increase up to 200mg Phenytek tid. Once Daily Dosing: 300mg Phenytek qd may replace 100mg extended phenytoin sodium capsule tid if seizures are controlled. LD (clinic/hospital): 1g in 3 divided doses (400mg, 300mg, 300mg) given 2 hrs apart. Start maintenance 24 hrs later. Avoid LD with renal and hepatic disease.
Pediatrics: Initial: 5mg/kg/day given bid-tid. Titrate: May increase at 7-10 day intervals. Maint: 4-8mg/kg/day. Max: 300mg/day. >6 yrs: May require the minimum adult dose (300mg/day).

HOW SUPPLIED: Cap, Extended-Release: 200mg, 300mg

WARNINGS/PRECAUTIONS: Avoid abrupt discontinuation. Caution with porphyria, hepatic dysfunction, elderly, diabetes, debilitated. D/C if rash occurs. Lymphadenopathy reported. Serum sickness may occur with lymph node involvement. Gingival hyperplasia reported; maintain proper dental hygiene. Hyperglycemia, birth defects, and osteomalacia reported. Monitor levels. Confusional states reported with toxic levels. Increased seizure frequency during pregnancy. Neonatal coagulation defects reported within first 24 hrs of birth; give vitamin K to mother before delivery and to neonate after birth. Avoid use with seizures due to hypoglycemia or other metabolic causes. Hemopoietic complications reported.

ADVERSE REACTIONS: Nystagmus, ataxia, slurred speech, decreased coordination, confusion, dizziness, insomnia, transient nervousness, motor twitchings, headaches, nausea, vomiting, constipation, rash, hypersensitivity reactions.

INTERACTIONS: Increased levels with acute alcohol intake, amiodarone, chloramphenicol, chlordiazepoxide, diazepam, dicumarol, disulfiram, estrogens, H_2-antagonists, halothane, isoniazid, methylphenidate, phenothiazines, phenylbutazone, salicylates, succinamides, sulfonamides, tolbutamide, trazodone. Decreased levels with chronic alcohol abuse, carbamazepine, reserpine, sucralfate. Decreases effects of corticosteroids, coumarin anticoagulants, digitoxin, doxycycline, estrogens, furosemide, oral contraceptives, quinidine, rifampin, theophylline, vitamin D. Phenobarbital, sodium valproate, valproic acid may increase or decrease levels. May increase or decrease levels of phenobarbital, sodium valproate, valproic acid. Calcium antacids decrease absorption; space dosing. Moban® contains calcium ions that interfere with absorption. TCAs may precipitate seizures. Increased risk of phenytoin hypersensitivity with barbiturates, succinamides, oxazolidinediones.

PREGNANCY: Possibly teratogenic, weigh benefits versus risk; not for use in nursing.

MECHANISM OF ACTION: Inhibits spread of seizure activity; primary site of action appears to be the motor cortex. Possibly promotes sodium efflux from neurons, stabilizing the threshold against hyperexcitability caused by excessive stimulation or environmental changes capable of reducing membrane sodium gradient. Also reduces the posttetanic potentiation at synapses, which prevents cortical seizure foci from detonating adjacent cortical areas.

PHARMACOKINETICS: Absorption: T_{max}=4-12 hrs. **Metabolism:** Hepatic via hydroxylation. **Elimination:** Renal; bile (inactive metabolite) and urine; $T_{1/2}$=22 hrs.

pHisoHex   RX
hexachlorophene (Sanofi-Aventis)

THERAPEUTIC CLASS: Detergent cleanser

INDICATIONS: As a surgical scrub and a bacteriostatic skin cleanser. Also to control outbreak of gram-positive infection, when other infection control methods failed.

DOSAGE: *Adults:* Surgical Scrub: Apply 5mL with water and lather over hands and forearms. Scrub well with a wet brush for 3 min, including nails and interdigital spaces. Rinse thoroughly then repeat. Bacteriostatic Cleansing: Apply 5mL with water and lather, apply to areas that need cleansing. Rinse thoroughly.
Pediatrics: Bacteriostatic Cleansing: Apply 5mL with water and lather, apply to areas that need cleansing. Rinse thoroughly. Do not use routinely for bathing infants.

HOW SUPPLIED: Liq: 3% [150mL, 480mL, 3840mL]

CONTRAINDICATIONS: Burned/denuded skin. Should not use as wet pack, vaginal pack, tampon, occlusive dressing, lotion, on mucous membranes, or as a routine prophylactic bath. Light sensitivity to halogenated phenol derivatives.

WARNINGS/PRECAUTIONS: D/C promptly if cerebral irritability occurs. Infants are more susceptible to CNS toxicity. Avoid skin lesions; may cause toxic blood levels. Do not apply to burns; may cause neurotoxicity and death. Avoid eye contact.

ADVERSE REACTIONS: Dermatitis, photosensitivity, redness, mild scaling, dryness.

INTERACTIONS: Skin products containing alcohol may decrease efficacy.

PREGNANCY: Category C, not for use in nursing.

MECHANISM OF ACTION: Bacteriostatic cleansing agent; cleanses the skin thoroughly and has bacteriostatic action against staphylococci and other gram-positive bacteria.

PHOSPHOLINE IODIDE   RX
echothiophate iodide (Wyeth)

THERAPEUTIC CLASS: Cholinesterase inhibitor

INDICATIONS: Treatment of glaucoma and accommodative esotropias.

DOSAGE: *Adults:* Early Chronic Simple Glaucoma: (0.3%) 1 drop bid, am and hs. Advanced Chronic Simple Glaucoma/Glaucoma Secondary to Cataract Surgery: Initial: (0.3%) 1 drop bid, am and hs. Titrate: May increase to higher strengths prn.
Pediatrics: Accommodative Esotropia: Diagnosis: (0.125%) 1 drop qhs for 2-3 weeks. Treatment: Decrease dose to 1 drop (0.125%) every other day or (0.6%) 1 drop qd. Titrate: Decrease strength gradually. Max: (0.125%) 1 drop qd.

HOW SUPPLIED: Sol: 0.03%, 0.06%, 0.125%, 0.25% [5mL]

CONTRAINDICATIONS: Active uveal inflammation, angle-closure glaucoma.

WARNINGS/PRECAUTIONS: Avoid with quiescent uveitis. Should hold nose for 1-2 min to prevent absorption. D/C with cardiac irregularities, salivation, urinary incontinence, diarrhea, profuse sweating, muscle weakness, or respiratory difficulties. Caution with vagotonia, bronchial asthma, spastic GI disturbance, peptic ulcer, bradycardia, hypotension, recent MI, epilepsy, parkinsonism, retinal detachment. Tolerance may develop.

ADVERSE REACTIONS: Stinging, burning, lacrimation, lid muscle twitching, conjunctival and ciliary redness, browache, induced myopia, visual blurring.

INTERACTIONS: Risk of respiratory or cardiovascular collapse with succinylcholine during general anesthesia. May potentiate effects of other cholinesterase inhibitors (eg, succinylcholine, organophosphate, carbamate insecticides, myasthenia gravis drugs).

PREGNANCY: Category C, not for use in nursing.

MECHANISM OF ACTION: Long-acting cholinesterase inhibitor; enhances the effect of endogenously liberated acetylcholine in the iris, ciliary muscle, and other parasympathetically innervated structures of the eye. Responsible for causing miosis, an increase in aqueous humor outflow, decrease in IOP, and potentiation of accomodation.

PHRENILIN FORTE   RX
acetaminophen - butalbital (Amarin)

OTHER BRAND NAMES: Phrenilin (Amarin)

THERAPEUTIC CLASS: Barbiturate/analgesic

INDICATIONS: Tension or muscle contraction headaches.

DOSAGE: *Adults:* (Phrenilin Forte) 1 cap q4h. (Phrenilin) 1-2 tabs q4h. Max: 6 caps/tabs/day.
Pediatrics: ≥12 yrs: (Phrenilin Forte) 1 cap q4h. (Phrenilin) 1-2 tabs q4h. Max: 6 caps/tabs/day.

HOW SUPPLIED: (Butalbital-APAP) Cap: (Phrenilin Forte) 50mg-650mg; Tab: (Phrenilin)50mg-325mg.

CONTRAINDICATIONS: Porphyria.

WARNINGS/PRECAUTIONS: Abuse potential. Caution in elderly/debilitated, severe renal/hepatic impairment, and acute abdominal conditions.

ADVERSE REACTIONS: Drowsiness, lightheadedness, dizziness, sedation, shortness of breath, nausea, vomiting, abdominal pain, intoxicated feeling.

INTERACTIONS: Enhanced CNS effects with MAOIs. May enhance CNS depression effects of narcotic analgesics, alcohol, general anesthetics, tranquilizers (eg, chlordiazepoxide, sedative hypnotics, CNS depressants).

PREGNANCY: Category C, not for use in nursing.

MECHANISM OF ACTION: Butalbital: Short-intermediate acting barbiturate; not established. Acetaminophen (APAP): Non-opiate, non-salicylate analgesic, and antipyretic; not established.

PHARMACOKINETICS: Absorption: APAP: Rapid; GIT. Butalbital: GIT. **Metabolism:** APAP: Liver (conjugation). **Distribution:** Butalbital: Crosses placental barrier, found in breast milk. **Elimination:** Butalbital: Urine (3.6%), $T_{1/2}$=35 hrs. APAP: $T_{1/2}$=1.25-3 hrs.

PHYTONADIONE RX
phytonadione (Various)

> Severe, fatal reactions reported during or immediately after IV or IM use. Only use IV or IM route when SC route is not feasible.

THERAPEUTIC CLASS: Vitamin K derivative

INDICATIONS: For coagulation disorders caused by vitamin K deficiency or interference with vitamin K activity, including prophylaxis and therapy of hemorrhagic disease of the newborn; anticoagulant-induced prothrombin deficiency caused by coumarin or indanedione derivatives; and hypoprothrombinemia caused by antibacterials, secondary factors that limit absorption or synthesis of vitamin K (obstructive jaundice, biliary fistula), or by drugs that interfere with vitamin K metabolism (eg, salicylates).

DOSAGE: *Adults:* Administer SQ when possible. Anticoagulant-Induced PT Deficiency: Initial: 2.5-10mg up to 25mg (rarely 50mg). May repeat if PT is still elevated 6-8 hrs after initial dose. Hypoprothrombinemia Due to Other Causes: 2.5-25mg or more (rarely up to 50mg); route depends on severity of condition and response.
Pediatrics: Prophylaxis of Hemorrhagic Disease in Newborn: 0.5-1mg IM within 1 hr of birth. Treatment of Hemorrhagic Disease in Newborn: 1mg SQ/IM (may need higher dose if mother has received oral anticoagulants).

HOW SUPPLIED: Inj: 1mg/0.5 mL, 10mg/mL.

WARNINGS/PRECAUTIONS: Contains benzyl alcohol; toxicity in newborns may occur. Takes 1-2 hrs to observe improvement in PT. Maintain lowest possible dose to prevent original thromboembolic events. Avoid repeated large doses with hepatic disease. Failure to respond may indicate a congenital coagulation defect or a condition unresponsive to vitamin K. Monitor PT regularly.

ADVERSE REACTIONS: Anaphylactoid reactions, flushing, peculiar taste sensations, dizziness, rapid and weak pulse, profuse sweating, hypotension, dyspnea, cyanosis, injection site tenderness or swelling, hyperbilirubinemia (in newborns).

INTERACTIONS: Does not counteract anticoagulant effects of heparin. Temporary resistance to prothrombin-depressing anticoagulants, especially with large doses.

PREGNANCY: Category C, caution in nursing.

MECHANISM OF ACTION: Vitamin K derivative; works in the liver as a necessary component in the production of active clotting factors: prothrombin (fac-

P

tor II), proconvertin (factor VII), plasma thromboplastin component (factor IX), and Stuart factor (factor X).

PHARMACOKINETICS: Absorption: (IM) Readily absorbed. **Metabolism:** Liver.

PILOCARPINE

pilocarpine HCL (Various)

RX

OTHER BRAND NAMES: Isopto Carpine (Alcon)

THERAPEUTIC CLASS: Cholinergic agent

INDICATIONS: To control IOP.

DOSAGE: *Adults:* 2 drops tid-qid or more if needed. Heavily pigmented irises may require higher strengths.

HOW SUPPLIED: Sol: 0.5%, 1%, 2%, 3%, 4%, 6% [15mL]

CONTRAINDICATIONS: Where constriction is undesirable (eg, acute iritis) or pupillary block glaucoma.

WARNINGS/PRECAUTIONS: Difficulty adapting in the dark. Caution while night driving and in poor illumination. Risk of retinal detachment.

ADVERSE REACTIONS: Local irritation, ciliary spasm, conjunctival vascular congestion, temporal or supraorbital headache, induced myopia, reduced visual acuity in poor illumination (elderly), lens opacity (prolonged use).

PREGNANCY: Category C, caution in nursing.

MECHANISM OF ACTION: Cholinergic agent; acts through direct stimulation of muscarinic neuroreceptors and smooth muscle such as iris and secretory glands. Produces miosis through contraction of iris sphincter, causing increased tension on scleral spur and opening of trabecular mesh work spaces to facilitate outflow of aqueous humor, thereby reducing outflow resistance and lowering IOP.

PINDOLOL

pindolol (Various)

RX

THERAPEUTIC CLASS: Nonselective beta-blocker

INDICATIONS: Management of hypertension.

DOSAGE: *Adults:* Initial: 5mg bid. Titrate: May increase by 10mg/day after 3-4 weeks. Max: 60mg/day.

HOW SUPPLIED: Tab: 5mg, 10mg

CONTRAINDICATIONS: Bronchial asthma, overt cardiac failure, cardiogenic shock, 2nd- and 3rd-degree heart block, severe bradycardia.

WARNINGS/PRECAUTIONS: Caution with well-compensated heart failure, nonallergic bronchospasm, renal or hepatic impairment. Can cause cardiac failure. Avoid abrupt withdrawal. Withdrawal before surgery is controversial. May mask hypoglycemia or hyperthyroidism symptoms.

ADVERSE REACTIONS: Dizziness, fatigue, insomnia, nervousness, dyspnea, edema, joint pain, muscle cramps/pain.

INTERACTIONS: Additive hypotension and/or bradycardia with catecholamine-depleting drugs. Both thioridazine and pindolol levels may increase when used concomitantly.

PREGNANCY: Category B, not for use in nursing.

MECHANISM OF ACTION: Nonselective β-blocker; inhibits β-andrenergic receptor with intrinsic sympathomimetic activity.

PHARMACOKINETICS: Absorption: Rapid; T_{max}=1 hr. **Distribution:** Plasma protein binding (40%) V_d= 2L/Kg. **Metabolism:** Metabolized to hydroxy-metabolites, which are excreted as glucoronides and ethereal sulfates. **Elimination:** Urine (35-40%), feces (6-9%); $T_{1/2}$=approximately 3-4 hrs, $T_{1/2}$=8 hrs (metabolites).

PIPERACILLIN
piperacillin sodium (Various)

RX

THERAPEUTIC CLASS: Broad-spectrum penicillin

INDICATIONS: Treatment of serious infections caused by susceptible strains of microorganisms in the following conditions: intra-abdominal, urinary tract, gynecologic, lower respiratory tract, skin and skin structure, bone/joint, and uncomplicated gonococcal urethritis, and septicemia. Perioperative surgical prophylaxis during certain procedures.

DOSAGE: *Adults:* Usual: 3-4g IM/IV q4-6h. Max: 24g/day; IM: 2g/site. Serious Infections: 200-300mg/kg/day IV divided q4-6h. Complicated UTI: 125-200mg/kg/day IV divided q6-8h. Uncomplicated UTI/CAP: 100-125mg/kg/day IM/IV divided q6-12h. Uncomplicated Gonorrhea: 2g IM single dose with 1g PO probenecid 1/2 hr before injection. Surgical Prophylaxis: 2g IV 20-30 min just prior to anesthesia (See PI for follow-up dosing). Renal Impairment: Uncomplicated/Complicated UTI: CrCl <20mL/min: 3g q12h. Complicated UTI: CrCl 20-40mL/min: 3g q8h. Serious Infection: CrCl 20-40mL/min: 4g q8h. CrCl <20mL/min: 4g q12h. Hemodialysis: Give 1g additional dose after each dialysis. Max: 2g q8h. Usual treatment is for 7-10 days; treat gynecologic infections for 3-10 days; treat *S.pyogenes* infections for at least 10 days.
Pediatrics: ≥12 yrs: Usual: 3-4g IM/IV q4-6h. Max: 24g/day; IM: 2g/site. Serious Infections: 200-300mg/kg/day IV divided q4-6h. Complicated UTI: 125-200mg/kg/day IV divided q6-8h. Uncomplicated UTI/CAP: 100-125mg/kg/day IM/IV divided q6-12h. Uncomplicated Gonorrhea: 2g IM single dose with 1g PO probenecid 1/2 hr before injection. Surgical Prophylaxis: 2g IV 20-30 min just prior to anesthesia (See PI for follow-up dosing). Renal Impairment: Uncomplicated/Complicated UTI: CrCl <20mL/min: 3g q12h. Complicated UTI: CrCl 20-40mL/min: 3g q8h. Serious Infection: CrCl 20-40mL/min: 4g q8h. CrCl <20mL/min: 4g q12h. Hemodialysis: Give 1g additional dose after each dialysis. Max: 2g q8h. Usual treatment is for 7-10 days; treat gynecologic infections for 3-10 days; treat *S.pyogenes* infections for at least 10 days.

HOW SUPPLIED: Inj: 2g, 3g, 4g

CONTRAINDICATIONS: Hypersensitivity to cephalosporins.

WARNINGS/PRECAUTIONS: Serious, sometimes fatal, hypersensitivity reactions reported with PCN therapy. *Clostridium difficile*-associated diarrhea reported. Cross-sensitivity to cephalosporins. Monitor renal, hepatic and hematopoietic functions with prolonged use. D/C if bleeding manifestations occur; increased risk with renal failure. Prolonged use may cause superinfections. May experience neuromuscular excitability or convulsions with higher than recommended doses. Contains 1.85mEq/g sodium; caution with salt restriction. Monitor electrolytes periodically with low potassium levels. Increased incidence of rash and fever in cystic fibrosis. Continue treatment for at least 48-72 hrs after patient becomes asymptomatic.

ADVERSE REACTIONS: Thrombophlebitis, erythema and pain at injection site, diarrhea, headache, dizziness, anaphylaxis, rash, superinfections.

INTERACTIONS: Do not mix with aminoglycoside in a syringe or infusion bottle; may cause inactivation of aminoglycoside. May prolong neuromuscular blockade of nondepolarizing muscle relaxants (eg, vecuronium). Increased risk of hypokalemia with cytotoxic therapy or diuretics. May reduce methotrexate clearance. Probenecid may increase levels. Monitor coagulation parameters closely with concomitant anticoagulants.

PREGNANCY: Category B, caution in nursing.

MECHANISM OF ACTION: Broad-spectrum penicillin; exerts bacterial activity by inhibiting both septum and cell wall synthesis; active against a variety of gram-positive and gram-negative aerobic and anaerobic bacteria.

PHARMACOKINETICS: Absorption: (2g) Rapid; T_{max} =30 min., C_{max} =36mcg/mL. **Distribution:** Plasma protein binding (16%). **Elimination:** Urine (60%-80%); (2g) $T_{1/2}$=54 min., (6g) 63 min.

PITOCIN RX
oxytocin (King)

THERAPEUTIC CLASS: Uterine Stimulant

INDICATIONS: For induction, stimulation or reinforcement of labor. Adjunct for management of incomplete or inevitable abortion. To control postpartum bleeding or hemorrhage.

DOSAGE: *Adults:* Labor Induction or Stimulation: Initial: 0.5-1mU/min IV infusion. Titrate: Increase by 1-2mU/min every 30-60 min until desired contraction pattern established. Once 5-6cm dilation achieved, reduce dose by similar increments. Rates >9-10mU/min rarely required. Postpartum Bleeding: IV Infusion: Add 10-40U. Max: 40 U/1000mL. Adjust infusion rate to sustain contraction and control uterine atony. IM: Give 10 U after placenta delivery. Incomplete/Inevitable/Elective Abortion: Add 10 U to 500mL physiologic saline IV sol or 5% dextrose-in-water IV sol after a suction or sharp curettage. Midtrimester Elective Abortion: 10-20mU/min IV. Max: 30U/12 hrs.

HOW SUPPLIED: Inj: 10U/mL

CONTRAINDICATIONS: Significant cephalopelvic disproportion, unfavorable fetal positions or presentations, obstetrical emergencies, fetal distress if delivery is not imminent, unsatisfactory progress with adequate uterine activity, hyperactive or hypertonic uterus, when vaginal delivery is contraindicated (eg, invasive cervical carcinoma, active herpes genitalis, total placenta previa, vasa previa, cord presentation or prolapse).

WARNINGS/PRECAUTIONS: Continuously monitor by trained personnel. Not indicated for elective induction of labor. D/C if uterine hyperactivity or fetal distress occurs. Except in unusual circumstances, avoid with fetal distress, hydramnios, partial placenta previa, prematurity, borderline cephalopelvic disproportion, and with predisposition to uterine rupture. Hypertonic contractions can occur. Has intrinsic antidiuretic effect; water intoxication may occur.

ADVERSE REACTIONS: Mother: Anaphylaxis, postpartum hemorrhage, arrhythmias, fatal fibrinogenemia, nausea, vomiting, pelvic hematoma, subarachnoid hemorrhage, hypertensive episodes, uterine rupture. Fetus: Bradycardia, arrhythmias, CNS damage, seizures, low Apgar scores, jaundice, retinal hemorrhage.

INTERACTIONS: Severe HTN reported 3-4 hrs after prophylactic administration of a vasoconstrictor with caudal block anesthesia. Hypotension, maternal sinus bradycardia with abnormal AV rhythms reported with cyclopropane anesthesia.

MECHANISM OF ACTION: Pituitary nonapeptide: Promotes contractions by increasing the intracellular Ca^{2+}.

PHARMACOKINETICS: Elimination: $T_{1/2}$=1-6 min.

PLAN B RX
levonorgestrel (Duramed)

THERAPEUTIC CLASS: Emergency contraceptive kit

INDICATIONS: To prevent pregnancy after known or suspected contraceptive failure or unprotected intercourse.

DOSAGE: *Adults:* 1 tab as soon as possible, within 72 hrs after unprotected intercourse, then 1 tab 12 hrs after 1st dose. May use during menstrual cycle.

HOW SUPPLIED: Tab: 0.75mg

CONTRAINDICATIONS: Pregnancy and undiagnosed abnormal genital bleeding.

WARNINGS/PRECAUTIONS: Not for routine use as a contraceptive. Risk of glucose intolerance; monitor women with DM. Not effective in terminating an existing pregnancy. Risk of ectopic pregnancy. Irregular menstrual bleeding may occur. Vomiting within 1 hr after doses may decrease effectiveness.

ADVERSE REACTIONS: Nausea, abdominal pain, fatigue, headache, menstrual changes, dizziness, breast tenderness, vomiting, diarrhea.

INTERACTIONS: Hepatic enzyme inducers (eg, phenytoin, carbamazepine, barbiturates, rifampin) may reduce effectiveness.

PREGNANCY: Pregnancy category unknown, caution in nursing.

PLAQUENIL   RX
hydroxychloroquine sulfate (Sanofi-Aventis)

> Be familiar with complete prescribing information before prescribing hydroxychloroquine.

THERAPEUTIC CLASS: Quinine derivative

INDICATIONS: Suppression and treatment of acute attacks of malaria in adults and children. Treatment of discoid and systemic lupus erythematosus and rheumatoid arthritis (RA) in adults.

DOSAGE: *Adults:* Malaria Suppression: 400mg weekly. Begin 2 weeks before exposure and continue for 8 weeks after leaving endemic area. Give 400mg q6h for 2 doses if therapy is not begun before exposure. Acute Attack: 800mg, then 400mg 6-8 hrs later, then 400mg for 2 more days. RA: Initial: 400-600mg qd with food or milk; increase until optimum response. Maint: After 4-12 weeks, 200-400mg qd with food or milk. Lupus Erythematosus: Initial: 400mg qd-bid for several weeks depending on response. Maint: 200-400mg/day.
Pediatrics: Malaria Suppression: 5mg/kg (base) weekly, max 400mg/dose. Begin 2 weeks before exposure and continue for 8 weeks after leaving endemic area. q6h for 2 doses if therapy is not begun before exposure. Acute Attack: 10mg base/kg, max 800mg/dose; then 5mg base/kg, max 400mg/dose at 6, 24 and 48 hrs after 1st dose.

HOW SUPPLIED: Tab: 200mg (200mg tab=155mg base)

CONTRAINDICATIONS: Long term therapy in children or if retinal/visual field changes due to 4-aminoquinoline compounds.

WARNINGS/PRECAUTIONS: Caution with hepatic disease, G6PD deficiency, alcoholism, psoriasis, and porphyria. Perform baseline and periodic (3 months) ophthalmologic exams and blood cell counts with prolonged therapy. Test periodically for muscle weakness. D/C if blood disorders occur. Avoid if possible in pregnancy. D/C after 6 months if no improvement in RA.

ADVERSE REACTIONS: Headache, dizziness, diarrhea, loss of appetite, muscle weakness, nausea, abdominal cramps, bleaching of hair, dermatitis, ocular toxicity, visual field defects.

INTERACTIONS: Caution with hepatotoxic drugs.

PREGNANCY: Safety in pregnancy and nursing not known.

MECHANISM OF ACTION: Quinine derivative; has antimalarial action. Precise mechanism not established.

PLATINOL-AQ   RX
cisplatin (Bristol-Myers Squibb)

> Cumulative renal toxicity is severe. Myelosuppression, nausea, and vomiting are also dose-related toxicities. Ototoxicity is significant. Anaphylactic-like reactions reported. Avoid inadvertent confusion with carboplatin. Doses >100mg/m²/cycle once every 3-4 weeks are rarely used.

THERAPEUTIC CLASS: Heavy-metal platinum complex

INDICATIONS: Combination therapy for metastatic testicular or ovarian tumors after surgery and/or radiotherapy. Monotherapy as secondary therapy for metastatic ovarian tumors refractory to standard treatment. Monotherapy for transitional cell bladder cancer no longer amenable to local treatments.

DOSAGE: *Adults:* Testicular Tumor: 20mg/m² IV qd for 5 days per cycle. Ovarian Tumor: Cyclophosphamide Combination Therapy: 75-100mg/m² IV per cycle once every 4 weeks. Monotherapy: 100mg/m² IV per cycle once every 4 weeks. Bladder Cancer: 50-70mg/m² IV per cycle every 3-4 weeks. Pretreatment hydration with 1-2L of fluid 8-12 hrs before therapy, and maintain adequate hydration and urinary output for the 24 hrs after infusion. Hold repeat course until SCr <1.5mg/100mL, BUN <25mg/100mL, platelets ≥100,000/mm³, WBC ≥4000/mm³. Hold subsequent doses until audiometric analysis is within normal limits.

HOW SUPPLIED: Inj: 50mg, 100mg

CONTRAINDICATIONS: Renal impairment, myelosuppression, hearing impairment, allergy to platinum-containing compounds.

WARNINGS/PRECAUTIONS: Severe neuropathies reported with higher doses or greater frequency than recommended. Loss of motor function reported. Perform audiometric testing and measure SrCr, BUN, CrCl, magnesium, sodium, potassium, and calcium before each dose. Can cause fetal harm during pregnancy. Perform peripheral blood counts weekly, LFTs periodically, and neurologic exam regularly. Avoid aluminum containing IV sets; may cause precipitate. Caution in elderly.

ADVERSE REACTIONS: Nephrotoxicity, ototoxicity, vestibular toxicity, myelosuppression, Coombs' positive hemolytic anemia, immediate or delayed nausea and vomiting, serum electrolyte disturbances, hyperuricemia, neurotoxicity, hepatotoxicity.

INTERACTIONS: Cumulative nephrotoxicity potentiated with aminoglycosides. Anticonvulsant levels may become subtherapeutic. Response duration adversely affected with pyridoxine and altretamine.

PREGNANCY: Category D, not for use in nursing.

MECHANISM OF ACTION: Heavy metal platinum complex.

PHARMACOKINETICS: Distribution: V_d=11-12L/m²; Plasma platinum protein binding (90%). **Excretion:** Urine; $T_{1/2}$=20-30 min (cisplatin), ≥5 days (albumin-platinum complex)

PLAVIX   RX
clopidogrel bisulfate (Bristol-Myers Squibb/Sanofi-Aventis)

THERAPEUTIC CLASS: Platelet aggregation inhibitor

INDICATIONS: For reduction of thrombotic events in those with recent stroke or MI, established peripheral arterial disease (PAD); or with non-ST-segment elevation acute coronary syndrome (unstable angina/non-Q-wave MI); and patients with ST-segment elevation acute myocardial infarction (STEMI).

DOSAGE: *Adults:* MI/Stroke/PAD: 75mg qd. Acute Coronary Syndrome: Take with 75-325mg ASA qd. LD: 300mg. Maint: 75mg qd. STEMI: 75mg, with 75-325mg ASA, qd with or without LD.

HOW SUPPLIED: Tab: 75mg, 300mg

CONTRAINDICATIONS: Active pathological bleeding (eg, peptic ulcer, intracranial hemorrhage).

WARNINGS/PRECAUTIONS: Caution with risk of increased bleeding, ulcers or lesions with a propensity to bleed, severe hepatic or renal impairment. D/C 5 days before surgery if antiplatelet effect is not desired. Monitor blood cell count and other appropriate tests if symptoms of bleeding or undesirable hematological effects arise. Thrombotic thrombocytopenic purpura (TTP) reported (rare).

ADVERSE REACTIONS: Chest pain, influenza-like symptoms, pain, edema, HTN, headache, dizziness, abdominal pain, dyspepsia, diarrhea, arthralgia, purpura, upper respiratory tract infection, back pain, dyspnea.

INTERACTIONS: Potentiates effect of ASA on collagen-induced platelet aggregation. Caution with warfarin. Increased occult GI loss with NSAIDs. Inhibits CYP2C9; caution with phenytoin, tamoxifen, tolbutamide, warfarin, torsemide, fluvastatin, and many NSAIDs. Caution with drugs that may induce GI lesions.

PREGNANCY: Category B, not for use in nursing.

MECHANISM OF ACTION: Platelet aggregation inhibitor; selectively inhibits the binding of adenosine diphosphate (ADP) to its platelet receptor and subsequent ADP-mediated activation of the glycoprotein GIIb/IIIa complex. Platelet aggregation is thereby inhibited.

PHARMACOKINETICS: Absorption: Rapidly; C_{max}=3mg/L; T_{max}=1 hr. **Distribution:** Plasma protein binding (98%). **Metabolism:** Liver (hydrolysis); carboxylic acid derivative (major metabolite). **Elimination:** Urine (50%), feces (46%); $T_{1/2}$=8 hrs.

PLENDIL   RX
felodipine (AstraZeneca)

THERAPEUTIC CLASS: Calcium channel blocker (dihydropyridine)

INDICATIONS: Treatment of hypertension.

DOSAGE: *Adults:* Initial: 5mg qd. Titrate: Adjust at no less than 2 week intervals. Maint: 2.5-10mg qd. Elderly/Hepatic Dysfunction: Initial: 2.5mg qd. Take without food or with a light meal. Swallow tab whole.

HOW SUPPLIED: Tab, Extended-Release: 2.5mg, 5mg, 10mg

WARNINGS/PRECAUTIONS: May cause hypotension and lead to reflex tachycardia with precipitation of angina. Caution with heart failure or ventricular dysfunction, especially with concomitant β-blockers. Monitor dose adjustment with hepatic dysfunction or elderly. Peripheral edema reported. Maintain good dental hygiene; gingival hyperplasia reported.

ADVERSE REACTIONS: Peripheral edema, headache, flushing, dizziness.

INTERACTIONS: CYP3A4 inhibitors (eg, itraconazole, ketoconazole, erythromycin, grapefruit juice, cimetidine) may increase plasma levels. Levels decreased with long-term anticonvulsant therapy. May increase metoprolol levels.

PREGNANCY: Category C, not for use in nursing.

MECHANISM OF ACTION: Calcium channel blocker; reversibly competes with nitrendipine and/or other calcium channel blockers for dihydropyridine binding sites and blocks voltage-dependent calcium ion currents in vascular smooth muscle.

PHARMACOKINETICS: Absorption: Complete, T_{max}=2.5-5 hrs. (oral). Systemic bioavailability approx (20%). **Distribution:** Plasma protein binding (99%). V_d=10 L/kg. **Elimination:** Urine (70%) and feces (10%). $T_{1/2}$(immediate release)=11-16 hrs.

PLETAL   RX
cilostazol (Otsuka America)

> Contraindicated with CHF of any severity due to possible decrease in survival.

THERAPEUTIC CLASS: Phosphodiesterase III inhibitor

INDICATIONS: Reduction of symptoms with intermittent claudication.

DOSAGE: *Adults:* 100mg bid, 1/2 hr before or 2 hrs after breakfast and dinner. Concomitant CYP3A4 and CYP2C19 Inhibitors: Consider 50mg bid.

HOW SUPPLIED: Tab: 50mg, 100mg

CONTRAINDICATIONS: CHF of any severity. Haemostatic disorders or active pathologic bleeding (eg, peptic ulcer, intracranial bleeding).

WARNINGS/PRECAUTIONS: Risks not known in patients with severe underlying heart disease, moderate or severe hepatic impairment, or with long-term use. Rare cases of thrombocytopenia or leukopenia reported.

ADVERSE REACTIONS: Headache, palpitation, tachycardia, abnormal stool, diarrhea, peripheral edema, dizziness, infection, rhinitis, blood pressure increase, aplastic anemia.

INTERACTIONS: Caution with CYP3A4 inhibitors (eg, ketoconazole, diltiazem, erythromycin) or CYP2C19 inhibitors (eg, omeprazole); may increase cilostazol levels. Avoid grapefruit juice.

PREGNANCY: Category C, not for use in nursing.

MECHANISM OF ACTION: Phosphodiesterase III inhibitor; not fully established. Inhibits phosphodiesterase activity and suppresses cyclic AMP (cAMP) degradation. Results in an increase of cAMP in platelets and blood vessels. Leads to reversible inhibition of platelet aggregation and produces vasodilation.

PHARMACOKINETICS: Distribution: Plasma protein binding (95-98%). **Metabolism:** Liver via CYP450 3A4 (primary), 2C19; 3,4-dehydro-cilostazol, 4'-trans-hydroxy-cilostazol (major active metabolites). **Elimination:** Urine (74%), feces (20%); $T_{1/2}$=11-13 hrs.

PLEXION RX
sulfacetamide sodium - sulfur (Medicis)

OTHER BRAND NAMES: Plexion SCT (Medicis) - Plexion TS (Medicis)

THERAPEUTIC CLASS: Sulfonamide/sulfur combination

INDICATIONS: Topical treatment of acne vulgaris, acne rosacea, and seborrheic dermatitis.

DOSAGE: *Adults:* (Cleanser) Wash qd-bid. Massage into skin for 10-20 sec, then rinse and dry. (TS) Apply qd-tid. (Cre) Apply to wet skin. Rinse off with water after 10 min or if dry.
Pediatrics: ≥12 yrs: (Cleanser) Wash qd-bid. Massage into skin for 10-20 sec, then rinse and dry. (TS) Apply qd-tid. (Cre) Apply to wet skin. Rinse off with water after 10 min or if dry.

HOW SUPPLIED: Cleanser: (Sulfacetamide-Sulfur) 10%-5% [170.3g, 340.2g]; Cre: (SCT) 10%-5% [120g]; Lot: (TS) 10%-5% [30g]; Pads: 10%-5% [30s]

CONTRAINDICATIONS: Kidney disease.

WARNINGS/PRECAUTIONS: D/C if irritation occurs. Avoid eye contact or mucous membranes. Caution with denuded or abraded skin, patients prone to topical sulfonamide hypersensitivity. Can cause reddening and scaling of epidermis.

ADVERSE REACTIONS: Local irritation.

PREGNANCY: Category C, caution in nursing.

MECHANISM OF ACTION: Sulfonamide/sulfur combination. Sodium sulfacetamide: Acts as a competitive antagonist to para-aminobenzoic acid (PABA). Sulfur: Not established. Responsible for inhibiting the growth of *Propionibacterium acnes* and the formation of free fatty acids.

PHARMACOKINETICS: Absorption: (PO) Readily absorbed **Excretion:** (PO) Urine (unchanged).

PNEUMOVAX 23 RX
pneumococcal vaccine (Merck)

THERAPEUTIC CLASS: Vaccine

INDICATIONS: Immunization against pneumococcal disease caused by those pneumococcal types included in the vaccine.

DOSAGE: *Adults:* Usual: 0.5mL SQ/IM in deltoid muscle or lateral mid-thigh. *Pediatrics:* ≥2 yrs: 0.5mL SQ/IM in deltoid muscle or lateral mid-thigh.

HOW SUPPLIED: Inj: 575mcg/0.5mL

WARNINGS/PRECAUTIONS: Vaccination timing is critical for chemotherapy or immunosuppressive therapy. Suboptimal response may occur in immunocompromised patients. Caution with severely compromised cardiovascular or pulmonary function where systemic reaction would be a significant risk. Delay vaccine with febrile respiratory illness or other active infection. Do not revaccinate immunocompetent patients. Continue prophylaxis pneumococ-cal antibiotics. May not prevent pneumococcal meningitis with chronic CSF leakage.

ADVERSE REACTIONS: Local injection site reactions (eg, soreness, warmth, erythema, swelling, induration), fever (≤102°F).

PREGNANCY: Category C, caution use in nursing.

MECHANISM OF ACTION: Active immunization that may protect against pneumococcal infection.

PODOCON-25 RX
podophyllin (Paddock)

THERAPEUTIC CLASS: Cytotoxic agent

INDICATIONS: Removal of soft genital warts (condylomata acuminata).

DOSAGE: *Adults:* Cleanse area. Initial: Apply to lesion; remove after 30-45 min to determine sensitivity. Usual: Apply to lesion; remove with alcohol or soap and water when achieve desired result (1-4 hrs).

HOW SUPPLIED: Liq: 25% [15mL]

CONTRAINDICATIONS: Diabetes, steroid therapy, poor blood circulation, bleeding warts, moles, birthmarks, unusual warts with hair, pregnancy, nursing.

WARNINGS/PRECAUTIONS: Powerful caustic and severe irritant; avoid healthy tissue. Avoid inflamed or irritated tissue, eyes, bleeding warts, moles, birthmarks, or unusual warts with hair.

ADVERSE REACTIONS: Paresthesia, polyneuritis, paralytic ileus, pyrexia, leukopenia, thrombocytopenia, coma, death.

PREGNANCY: Contraindicated in pregnancy and nursing.

MECHANISM OF ACTION: Cytotoxic agent; arrests mitosis in metaphase.

POLYCITRA RX
potassium citrate - citric acid (Ortho-McNeil)

THERAPEUTIC CLASS: Alkalinizing agent

INDICATIONS: Alkalinizing agent for uric acid and cystine calculi of the uri-nary tract. Adjunct to uricosuric agents for gout. Correction of renal tubular acidosis.

DOSAGE: *Adults:* 15mL or 1 pkt qid, pc and hs. Dilute in 6 oz of water or juice.

HOW SUPPLIED: Pkt: 1002mg-3300mg/pack [100s]; Sol: (Citric Acid-Potassium Citrate) 334mg-550mg/5mL [480mL]

CONTRAINDICATIONS: Severe renal impairment with oliguria or azotemia, untreated Addison's disease, adynamia episodica hereditaria, acute dehydra-tion, heat cramps, anuria, severe myocardial damage, hyperkalemia.

WARNINGS/PRECAUTIONS: Large doses can cause hyperkalemia and alka-losis. Caution with low urinary output. Dilute adequately in water to minimize GI injury.

ADVERSE REACTIONS: Diarrhea and other GI effects.

INTERACTIONS: Risk of toxicity with K⁺-containing agents, K⁺-sparing diuret-ics, ACE inhibitors, cardiac glycosides.

PREGNANCY: Safety in pregnancy and nursing not known.

MECHANISM OF ACTION: Potassium supplement.

P

POLY-PRED

RX

prednisolone acetate - polymyxin B sulfate - neomycin sulfate (Allergan)

THERAPEUTIC CLASS: Antibacterial/corticosteroid

INDICATIONS: Ocular inflammation associated with infection or risk of infection.

DOSAGE: *Adults:* Eye Treatment: 1-2 drops q3-4h prn, or more often if needed (up to every 30 min for acute infection). Lid Treatment: 1-2 drops in the eye q3-4h. Close eyes and rub excess on the lid. Max: 20mL for initial prescription.

HOW SUPPLIED: Sus: (Neomycin-Polymyxin B-Prednisolone) 0.35%-10,000 U/mL-0.5% [5mL]

CONTRAINDICATIONS: Viral diseases of the cornea and conjunctiva including epithelial herpes simplex keratitis, vaccinia, and varicella. Mycobacterial infection and fungal diseases of the eye. After uncomplicated removal of corneal foreign body.

WARNINGS/PRECAUTIONS: Not for injection into eye. Prolonged use can cause optic nerve damage, visual defects, glaucoma or secondary ocular infections (eg, fungal). Monitor IOP after 10 days of therapy. Caution with diseases causing thinning of cornea/sclera. May mask or enhance infection with acute purulent conditions. May cause cutaneous sensitization.

ADVERSE REACTIONS: Secondary infection, elevated IOP, delayed wound healing, allergic sensitization.

PREGNANCY: Category C, caution in nursing

MECHANISM OF ACTION: Antibacterial/Corticosteroid. Prednisolone: Suppresses the inflammatory response to a variety of agents. May inhibit the body's defense mechanism against infection. Neomycin and Polymixin B: Provides action against specific organisms susceptible to them (*Staphyloccus aureus, Escherida coli, Hemophilus influenzae, Klebsiella/Enterobacter* species, *Neisseria* species, and *Pseudomonas aeruginosa*).

PHARMACOKINETICS: Distribution: Found in breast milk.

POLYTRIM

RX

polymyxin B sulfate - trimethoprim sulfate (Allergan)

THERAPEUTIC CLASS: Dihydrofolate reductase inhibitor/antibiotic

INDICATIONS: Surface ocular bacterial infections, including blepharoconjunctivitis, acute bacterial conjunctivitis.

DOSAGE: *Adults:* Mild-Moderate Infections: 1 drop q3h for 7-10 days. Max: 6 doses/day.
Pediatrics: ≥2 months: Mild-Moderate Infections: 1 drop q3h for 7-10 days. Max: 6 doses/day.

HOW SUPPLIED: Sol: (Trimethoprim-Polymyxin B) 1mg-10,000U/mL [10mL]

WARNINGS/PRECAUTIONS: Not indicated for the prophylaxis or treatment of ophthalmia neonatorum.

ADVERSE REACTIONS: Local irritation, lid edema, itching, increased redness, tearing, burning, stinging, circumocular rash, superinfection (prolonged use).

PREGNANCY: Category C, caution in nursing.

MECHANISM OF ACTION: Dihydrofolate reductase inhibitor/antibiotic. Polymyxin B: Increases permeability of bacterial cell membrane by interacting with phospholipid components of membrane. Trimethoprim: Blocks production of tetrahydrofolic acid from dihydrofolic acid by binding to and reversibly inhibiting the enzyme dihydrofolate reductase. Binding is stronger for the bacterial enzyme than for corresponding mammalian enzyme, and therefore selectively interferes with bacterial biosynthesis of nucleic acids and proteins.

PHARMACOKINETICS: Absorption: C_{max}=0.03mcg/mL (trimethoprim), 1 unit/mL (polymyxin B) (following two-time dosing of 2 drops of ophthalmic solution containing 1mg of trimethoprim and 10,000 units of polymyxin B).

POLY-VI-FLOR RX
multiple vitamin - sodium fluoride (Mead Johnson)

THERAPEUTIC CLASS: Multiple vitamin/fluoride supplement

INDICATIONS: Vitamin supplement. Fluoride supplement for caries prophy-laxis in areas where water contains less than optimal fluoride levels.

DOSAGE: *Pediatrics:* (Sol) 6 months-3 yrs and <0.3 ppm Fluoride or 3-6 yrs and 0.3-0.6 ppm Fluoride: 1mL (0.25mg) qd. 3-6 yrs and <0.3 ppm Fluoride or >6 yrs and 0.3-0.6 ppm Fluoride: 1mL (0.5mg) qd. (Tab) 4-6 yrs and 0.3-0.6 ppm Fluoride: 0.25mg qd. 4-6 yrs and <0.3 ppm Fluoride or ≥6 yrs and 0.3-0.6 ppm Fluoride: 0.5mg qd. 6-16 yrs and <0.3 ppm Fluoride: 1mg qd.

HOW SUPPLIED: Sol: Vitamin A 1500 IU-Vitamin C 35mg-Vitamin D 400 IU-Vitamin E 5 IU-Thiamin 0.5mg-Riboflavin 0.6mg-Niacin 8mg-Vitamin B$_6$ 0.4mg-Vitamin B$_{12}$ 2mcg. 0.25mg drops contains 0.25mg Fluoride [50mL], 0.5mg drops contain 0.5mg Fluoride [50mL]; Tab, Chewable: Vitamin A 2500 IU-Vitamin C 60mg-Vitamin D 400 IU-Vitamin E 15 IU-Thiamin 1.05mg-Riboflavin 1.2mg-Niacin 13.5mg-Vitamin B$_6$ 1.05mg-Folate 0.3mg-Vitamin B$_{12}$ 4.5mcg. 0.25mg tabs contain 0.25mg Fluoride; 0.5mg tabs contain 0.5mg Fluoride; 1mg tabs contain 1mg Fluoride

WARNINGS/PRECAUTIONS: Must chew tab; not for pediatrics <4yrs. Risk of dental fluorosis from ingestion of large amounts of fluoride. Children up to 16 yrs, in areas where water contains less than optimal fluoride levels, should receive daily fluoride supplementation.

ADVERSE REACTIONS: Allergic rash.

PREGNANCY: Safety in pregnancy and nursing not known.

PONSTEL RX
mefenamic acid (Sciele)

NSAIDs may cause an increased risk of serious cardiovascular thrombotic events, MI, stroke, and serious GI adverse events including bleeding, ulceration, and perforation of the stomach or intestines. Contraindicated for the treatment of perioperative pain in the setting of coronary artery bypass graft (CABG) surgery.

THERAPEUTIC CLASS: NSAID (fenamate derivative)

INDICATIONS: Relief of mild to moderate pain in patients ≥14 yrs, when therapy will not exceed 7 days. Treatment of primary dysmenorrhea.

DOSAGE: *Adults:* Acute Pain: Usual: 500mg, then 250mg q6h prn up to 1 week. Primary Dysmenorrhea: Usual: 500mg, then 250mg q6h up to 3 days. Take with food.
Pediatrics: ≥14 yrs: Acute Pain: Usual: 500mg, then 250mg q6h prn up to 1 week. Primary Dysmenorrhea: Usual: 500mg, then 250mg q6h up to 3 days. Take with food.

HOW SUPPLIED: Cap: 250mg

CONTRAINDICATIONS: Pre-existing renal disease, active ulceration or chronic inflammation of the GI tract. Allergic-type reactions, including asthma and urticaria, after taking ASA or other NSAIDs. Treatment of perioperative pain in the setting of CABG surgery.

WARNINGS/PRECAUTIONS: May lead to onset of new HTN or worsening of pre-existing HTN; monitor BP closely. Fluid retention and edema reported; caution with fluid retention or heart failure. Renal papillary necrosis and other renal injury reported after long-term use. Not recommended for use with advanced renal disease. Anaphylactoid reactions may occur. May cause serious skin adverse events (eg, exfoliative dermatitis, Stevens-Johnson syn-drome, and toxic epidermal necrolysis). Avoid in late pregnancy; may cause premature closure of ductus arteriosis. May cause elevations of LFTs; d/c if liver disease develops or systemic manifestations occur. Caution in elderly. Anemia may occur; with long-term use, monitor Hgb/Hct if signs or symptoms of anemia develop. May inhibit platelet aggregation and prolong bleeding time; monitor with coagulation disorders. Caution with asthma and avoid with ASA-sensitive asthma.

ADVERSE REACTIONS: Abdominal pain, constipation, diarrhea, dyspepsia, flatulence, gross bleeding/perforation, heartburn, nausea, GI ulcers, vomiting, abnormal renal function, anemia, dizziness, edema, elevated liver enzymes, headache, increased bleeding time, pruritus, rash, tinnitus.

INTERACTIONS: Caution with CYP2C9 inhibitors. ASA may increase adverse effects; avoid use. Warfarin may increase GI bleeding. May prolong PT with oral anticoagulants. May enhance methotrexate toxicity. Decreases effects of ACE inhibitors, furosemide, and thiazides; monitor for renal toxicity. Increases lithium levels. Magnesium hydroxide may increase mefenamic acid levels. Enhances methotrexate toxicity; caution with concomitant use.

PREGNANCY: Category C, not for use in nursing.

MECHANISM OF ACTION: NSAID (fenamate derivative); suspected to inhibit prostaglandin synthetase, exerts anti-inflammatory, analgesic, and antipyretic actions.

PHARMACOKINETICS: Absorption: Rapid; C_{max}=10-20mcg/mL^3, T_{max}=2-4 hrs. **Distribution:** V_d=1.06L/kg^2; plasma protein binding (90%). **Metabolism**: Via CYP2C9. **Elimination:** Urine (52%), feces (20%); $T_{1/2}$=2 hrs.

Pramosone RX
pramoxine HCL - hydrocortisone acetate (Ferndale)

THERAPEUTIC CLASS: Corticosteroid/anesthetic

INDICATIONS: Relief of the inflammatory and pruritic manifestations of corticosteroid-responsive dermatoses.

DOSAGE: *Adults:* Apply tid-qid. May use occlusive dressings for psoriasis or recalcitrant conditions. D/C dressings if infection develops.
Pediatrics: Apply tid-qid. May use occlusive dressings for psoriasis or recalcitrant conditions. D/C dressings if infection develops.

HOW SUPPLIED: (Pramoxine-Hydrocortisone) Cre: 1%-1%, 1%-2.5% [30g, 60g]; Lot: 1%-1% [60mL, 120mL, 240mL], 1%-2.5% [60mL, 120mL]; Oint: 1%-1%, 1%-2.5% [30g]

WARNINGS/PRECAUTIONS: May produce reversible HPA axis suppression, manifestations of Cushing's syndrome, hyperglycemia, and glucosuria. Caution when applied to large surface areas or under occlusive dressings. Use appropriate antifungal or antibacterial agent with dermatological infections; d/c if infection does not clear. Peds may be more susceptible to systemic toxicity. Avoid eyes. D/C if irritation occurs.

ADVERSE REACTIONS: Burning, itching, irritation, dryness, folliculitis, hypertrichosis, acneiform eruptions, hypopigmentation, perioral dermatitis, allergic dermatitis, skin maceration, secondary infection, skin atrophy, striae, miliaria.

PREGNANCY: Category C, caution in nursing.

MECHANISM OF ACTION: Corticosteroid/anesthetic. Hydrocortisone: Possesses anti-inflammatory, anti-pruritic, and vasoconstrictive properties. Anti-inflammatory action not established. Pramoxine: Provides temporary relief from itching and pain. Stabilizes neuronal membrane of nerve endings with which it comes into contact.

PHARMACOKINETICS: Absorption: Percutaneous; occlusion, inflammation, and other disease states may increase absorption. **Distribution:** Bound to plasma proteins in varying degrees. Systemically administered corticosteroids found in breast milk. **Metabolism:** Liver. **Excretion:** Kidneys (major), bile.

Prandin RX
repaglinide (Novo Nordisk)

THERAPEUTIC CLASS: Meglitinide

INDICATIONS: Adjunct to diet and exercise, to improve glycemic control in type 2 diabetes mellitus. May use in combination with metformin or thiazolidinediones (TZDs).

DOSAGE: *Adults:* Take within 15-30 min before meals. Skip dose if skipping meal and add dose if adding meal. Initial: Treatment-Naive or HbA$_{1c}$ <8%: 0.5mg with each meal. Previous Oral Therapy/Combination Therapy and HbA$_{1c}$ ≥8%: 1-2mg with each meal. Titrate: May double preprandial dose up to 4mg (bid-qid) at no less than 1 week intervals. Maint: 0.5-4mg with meals. Max: 16mg/day. If hypoglycemia with combination metformin or TZD occurs, reduce repaglinide dose. Renal Dysfunction: CrCl 20-40mg/dL: Initial: 0.5mg with each meal; titrate carefully. Hepatic Dysfunction: Increase intervals between dose adjustments.

HOW SUPPLIED: Tab: 0.5mg, 1mg, 2mg

CONTRAINDICATIONS: Diabetic ketoacidosis and type 1 diabetes.

WARNINGS/PRECAUTIONS: Hypoglycemia risk especially with renal/hepatic insufficiency, elderly, malnourished and adrenal/pituitary insufficiency. Loss of blood glucose control when exposed to stress (fever, trauma, infection or surgery); d/c therapy and start insulin. Secondary failure can occur over a period of time. Caution with hepatic and renal dysfunction. Not indicated for use in combination with NPH insulin.

ADVERSE REACTIONS: Hypoglycemia, cardiovascular effects, respiratory infections, URI, bronchitis, sinusitis, rhinitis, paresthesia, nausea, diarrhea, constipation, vomiting, dyspepsia, arthralgia, back pain, headache, chest pain.

INTERACTIONS: Increased metabolism with CYP3A4 inducers (eg, rifampin, barbiturates, carbamazepine). Ketoconazole, miconazole, and erythromycin (CYP3A4 inhibitors) and trimethoprim, gemfibrozil, and montelukast (CYP2C8 inhibitors) may inhibit metabolism. Increased levels with gemfibrozil; caution and monitor levels if already on both drugs, avoid initiation of concurrent use. Avoid itraconazole if already on gemfibrozil and repaglinide; synergistic effect may occur. Potentiated hypoglycemia with alcohol, β-blockers, NSAIDs, and other highly protein bound drugs, salicylates, sulfonamides, chloramphenicol, coumarins, probenecid, MAOIs. Risk of hyperglycemia with diuretics, corticosteroids, phenothiazines, thyroid products, estrogens, phenytoin, nicotinic acid, sympathomimetics, CCBs, and isoniazid. β-blockers may mask hypoglycemia. Increases levonorgestrel and ethinyl estradiol levels. Increased levels with simvastatin, levonorgestrel, and ethinyl estradiol.

PREGNANCY: Category C, not for use in nursing.

MECHANISM OF ACTION: Meglitinide; lowers blood glucose levels by stimulating the release of insulin from the pancreas.

PHARMACOKINETICS: Absorption: Rapid and complete; T$_{max}$=1 hr; bioavailability (56%). **Distribution:** V$_d$=31L; plasma protein binding (98%). **Metabolism:** CYP2C8, 3A4; oxidation, glucuronidation. **Elimination:** Feces (90%), urine (8%); T$_{1/2}$=1 hr.

PRAVACHOL RX
pravastatin sodium (Bristol-Myers Squibb)

THERAPEUTIC CLASS: HMG-CoA reductase inhibitor

INDICATIONS: As adjunct to diet, to reduce elevated total-C, LDL-C, Apo B, TG levels, and to increase HDL-C in primary hypercholesterolemia and mixed dyslipidemia (Type IIa and IIb). Treatment of primary dysbetalipoproteinemia (Type III) and heterozygous familial hypercholesterolemia. To reduce elevated serum TG levels (Type IV). In hypercholesterolemic patients without coronary heart disease, to reduce risk of: MI, undergoing myocardial revascularization procedures, and cardiovascular mortality with no increase in death from non-cardiovascular causes. In patients with coronary heart disease, to reduce risk of: mortality by reducing coronary death, undergoing myocardial revascularization procedures, MI, stroke, and TIA; and to slow progression of coronary atherosclerosis.

P

DOSAGE: *Adults:* ≥18 yrs: Initial: 40mg qd. Perform lipid tests within 4 weeks and adjust according to response and guidelines. Titrate: May increase to 80mg qd if needed. Significant Renal/Hepatic Dysfunction: Initial: 10mg qd. Concomitant Immunosuppressives (eg, cyclosporine): Initial:10mg qhs. Max: 20mg/day.
Pediatrics: Heterozygous Familial Hypercholesterolemia: 14-18 yrs: Initial: 40mg qd. 8-13 yrs: 20mg qd. Concomitant Immunosuppressives (eg, cyclosporine): Initial: 10mg qhs. Max: 20mg/day.

HOW SUPPLIED: Tab: 10mg, 20mg, 40mg, 80mg

CONTRAINDICATIONS: Active liver disease, unexplained persistent elevations of LFTs, pregnancy, nursing mothers.

WARNINGS/PRECAUTIONS: Perform LFTs before therapy, before dose increases, and if clinically indicated. Risk of myopathy, myalgia, and rhabdomyolysis. D/C if AST or ALT ≥3x ULN persists, if elevated CPK levels occur, or if myopathy diagnosed or suspected. Less effective with homozygous familial hypercholesterolemia. Monitor for endocrine dysfunction. Closely monitor with heavy alcohol use, recent history or signs of hepatic disease, or renal dysfunction.

ADVERSE REACTIONS: Rash, nausea, vomiting, diarrhea, headache, chest pain, influenza, abdominal pain, dizziness, increases ALT, AST, CPK.

INTERACTIONS: Risk of myopathy with fibrates, niacin, cyclosporine, erythromycin. Increased levels with gemfibrozil, itraconazole. Avoid fibrates unless benefit outweighs drug combination risk. Decreased levels with concomitant cholestyramine/colestipol; take 1 hr before or 4 hrs after resins. Caution with drugs that diminish levels or activity of steroid hormones (eg, ketoconazole, spironolactone, cimetidine).

PREGNANCY: Category X, not for use in nursing.

MECHANISM OF ACTION: HMG-CoA reductase inhibitor; causes increased number of LDL-receptors on cell surfaces and enhanced receptor mediated catabolism and clearance of circulating LDL. Inhibits LDL production by inhibiting hepatic synthesis of VLDL, LDL precursor.

PHARMACOKINETICS: Absorption: Rapid. Absolute bioavailability (17%); T_{max}=1-1.5 hrs. **Distribution:** Plasma protein binding (50%). **Metabolism:** Liver. **Elimination:** Feces (70%), urine (20%); $T_{1/2}$=77 hrs.

PreCare RX
folic acid - multiple vitamin - minerals (Ther-Rx)

THERAPEUTIC CLASS: Prenatal vitamin

INDICATIONS: Vitamin and mineral supplementation for before, during, and after pregnancy.

DOSAGE: *Adults:* 1 tab qd.

HOW SUPPLIED: Tab, Chewable: Calcium 250mg-Copper 2mg-Folic Acid 1mg-Iron 40mg-Magnesium 50mg-Vitamin B_6 2mg-Vitamin C 50mg-Vitamin D 0.006mg-Vitamin E 3.5mg-Zinc 15mg

WARNINGS/PRECAUTIONS: Accidental overdose of iron-containing products is a leading cause of fatal poisoning in children <6 yrs. Not for the treatment of pernicious anemia and other megaloblastic anemias where vitamin B_{12} is deficient. Folic acid >0.1mg/day may obscure pernicious anemia.

ADVERSE REACTIONS: Allergic sensitization.

MECHANISM OF ACTION: Vitamin and mineral supplement.

PreCare Conceive RX
folic acid - multiple vitamin - minerals (Ther-Rx)

THERAPEUTIC CLASS: Prenatal vitamin

INDICATIONS: Vitamin and mineral supplementation for before and during pregnancy.

DOSAGE: *Adults:* 1 tab qd.

HOW SUPPLIED: Tab: Calcium 200mg-Copper 2mg-Folic Acid 1mg-Iron 30mg-Magnesium 100mg-Niacin 20mg-Vitamin B₁ 3mg-Vitamin B₂ 3.4mg-Vitamin B₆ 50mg-Vitamin B₁₂ 0.012mg-Vitamin C 60mg-Vitamin E 30IU-Zinc 15mg

WARNINGS/PRECAUTIONS: Accidental overdose of iron-containing products is a leading cause of fatal poisoning in children <6 yrs. Not for the treatment of pernicious anemia and other megaloblastic anemias where vitamin B₁₂ is deficient. Folic acid >0.1mg/day may obscure pernicious anemia.

ADVERSE REACTIONS: Allergic sensitization.

MECHANISM OF ACTION: Multivitamin/mineral nutritional supplement.

PRECARE PRENATAL

RX

docusate sodium - folic acid - multiple vitamin - minerals (Ther-Rx)

OTHER BRAND NAMES: PreCare Premier (Ther-Rx)

THERAPEUTIC CLASS: Prenatal vitamin

INDICATIONS: Vitamin and mineral supplementation for before, during, and after pregnancy.

DOSAGE: *Adults:* 1 tab qd.

HOW SUPPLIED: Tab: Calcium 250mg-Copper 2mg-Folic Acid 1mg-Iron 40mg-Magnesium 50mg-Niacin 20mg-Vitamin B₁ 3mg-Vitamin B₂ 3.4mg-Vitamin B₆ 50mg-Vitamin B₁₂ 0.012mg-Vitamin C 50mg-Vitamin D 0.006mg-Vitamin E 3.5mg-Zinc 15mg* *scored

WARNINGS/PRECAUTIONS: Accidental overdose of iron-containing products is a leading cause of fatal poisoning in children <6 yrs. Not for the treatment of pernicious anemia and other megaloblastic anemias where vitamin B₁₂ is deficient. Folic acid >0.1mg/day may obscure pernicious anemia.

ADVERSE REACTIONS: Allergic sensitization.

PRECOSE

RX

P

acarbose (Bayer Healthcare)

THERAPEUTIC CLASS: Alpha-glucosidase inhibitor

INDICATIONS: Adjunct to diet and exercise, to improve glycemic control in type 2 diabetes mellitus. May use with insulin, metformin, or a sulfonylurea.

DOSAGE: *Adults:* Initial: 25mg tid with first bite of each main meal. To minimize GI effects: 25mg qd, increase gradually to 25mg tid. Titrate: After reaching 25mg tid, may increase at 4-8 week intervals. Maint: 50-100mg tid. Max: ≤60kg: 50mg tid. >60kg: 100mg tid. If no further reduction in post prandial or HbA₁c with 100mg tid, consider reducing dose.

HOW SUPPLIED: Tab: 25mg, 50mg, 100mg

CONTRAINDICATIONS: Diabetic ketoacidosis, cirrhosis, inflammatory bowel disease, colonic ulceration, partial or predisposition to intestinal obstruction, chronic intestinal disease with marked disorders of digestion or absorption, and conditions that may deteriorate from increased intestinal gas formation.

WARNINGS/PRECAUTIONS: Avoid with significant renal dysfunction (SrCr >2mg/dL). May need to d/c and give insulin with stress (eg, fever, trauma). Dose related elevated serum transaminase levels reported. Monitor serum transaminases every 3 months for first year then periodically. Reduce dose or d/c if elevated serum transaminases persist. Use glucose (dextrose) instead of sucrose (sugar cane) to treat mild to moderate hypoglycemia.

ADVERSE REACTIONS: Transient flatulence, diarrhea, abdominal pain.

INTERACTIONS: Risk of hyperglycemia with diuretics, corticosteroids, phenothiazines, thyroid products, estrogens, oral contraceptives, phenytoin, nicotinic acid, sympathomimetics, CCBs, and isoniazid. Reduced effect with intestinal adsorbents (eg, charcoal) and digestive enzymes containing carbohydrate-splitting enzymes (eg, amylase, pancreatin); avoid concomitant use. May affect digoxin bioavailability; may require dose adjustment of digoxin. Monitor for hypoglycemia with insulin and sulfonylureas.

PREGNANCY: Category B, not for use in nursing.

MECHANISM OF ACTION: Alpha-glucosidase inhibitor; reversibly inhibits pancreatic alpha-amylase and membrane-bound intestinal alpha-glucoside hydrolase enzymes.

PHARMACOKINETICS: Absorption: Poor; T_{max}=1 hr. **Metabolism:** GI tract by intestinal bacteria or digestive enzymes; 4-methylpyrogallol derivatives (major metabolites). **Elimination:** $T_{1/2}$=2 hrs; urine (unchanged).

PRED FORTE   RX
prednisolone acetate (Allergan)

THERAPEUTIC CLASS: Corticosteroid

INDICATIONS: Treatment of inflammation of the palpebral and bulbar conjunctiva, cornea and anterior segment of the globe.

DOSAGE: *Adults:* 1-2 drops bid-qid. May dose more frequently during initial 24-48 hrs. Re-evaluate after 2 days if no improvement.

HOW SUPPLIED: Sus: 1% [1mL, 5mL, 10mL, 15mL]

CONTRAINDICATIONS: Viral diseases of the cornea and conjunctiva including epithelial herpes simplex keratitis, vaccinia, and varicella. Mycobacterial infection and fungal diseases of the eye.

WARNINGS/PRECAUTIONS: Caution with glaucoma, herpes simplex, diseases causing thinning of cornea/sclera and other ocular viral infections. Prolonged use can cause glaucoma or secondary ocular infections (eg, fungal). Monitor IOP after 10 days of therapy. Re-evaluate if no response after 2 days. May delay healing and increase incidence of bleb formation after cataract surgery. Avoid abrupt withdrawal with chronic use. Contains sodium bisulfite.

ADVERSE REACTIONS: Elevation of IOP, glaucoma, infrequent optic nerve damage, posterior subcapsular cataract formation, delayed wound healing, burning/stinging upon instillation, ocular irritation, secondary infection, visual disturbance.

PREGNANCY: Category C, not for use in nursing.

MECHANISM OF ACTION: Glucocorticoid; anti-inflammatory agent; inhibits edema, fibrin deposition, capillary dilation, deposition of collagen, and scar formation.

PRED MILD   RX
prednisolone acetate (Allergan)

THERAPEUTIC CLASS: Corticosteroid

INDICATIONS: Treatment of noninfectious ocular inflammation.

DOSAGE: *Adults:* 1-2 drops bid-qid. May dose more frequently during initial 24-48 hrs. Re-evaluate after 2 days if no improvement.

HOW SUPPLIED: Sus: 0.12% [5mL, 10mL]

CONTRAINDICATIONS: Viral diseases of the cornea and conjunctiva including epithelial herpes simplex keratitis, vaccinia, and varicella. Mycobacterial infection and fungal diseases of the eye.

WARNINGS/PRECAUTIONS: Caution with glaucoma, herpes simplex, diseases causing thinning of cornea/sclera and other ocular viral infections. Prolonged use can cause glaucoma or secondary ocular infections (eg, fungal). Monitor IOP after 10 days of therapy. Re-evaluate if no response after 2 days. May delay healing and increase incidence of bleb formation after cataract surgery. Avoid abrupt withdrawal with chronic use. Contains sodium bisulfite.

ADVERSE REACTIONS: Elevation of IOP, glaucoma, infrequent optic nerve damage, posterior subcapsular cataract formation, delayed wound healing, burning/stinging upon instillation, ocular irritation, secondary infection, visual disturbance.

PREGNANCY: Category C, not for use in nursing.

MECHANISM OF ACTION: Glucocorticoid; inhibits edema, fibrin disposition, capillary dilation, and phagocytic migration of acute inflammatory response as well as capillary proliferation, deposition of collagen and scar formation.

PRED-G   RX
prednisolone acetate - gentamicin sulfate (Allergan)

OTHER BRAND NAMES: Pred-G S.O.P. (Allergan)

THERAPEUTIC CLASS: Aminoglycoside/corticosteroid

INDICATIONS: Ocular inflammation associated with infection or risk of infection.

DOSAGE: *Adults:* (Sus) 1 drop bid-qid. May increase dose to every hour during initial 24-48 hrs. Max: 20mL for initial prescription. (Oint) Apply 1/2 inch in conjunctival sac qd-tid. Max: 8g for initial prescription.

HOW SUPPLIED: (Gentamicin-Prednisolone) Oint: (S.O.P.) 0.3%-0.6% [3.5g]; Sus: 0.3%-1% [2mL, 5mL, 10mL]

CONTRAINDICATIONS: Viral diseases of the cornea and conjunctiva including epithelial herpes simplex keratitis, vaccinia, and varicella. Mycobacterial infection and fungal diseases of the eye.

WARNINGS/PRECAUTIONS: Not for injection into eye. Caution with glaucoma, herpes simplex, diseases causing thinning of cornea/sclera and other ocular viral infections. Prolonged use can cause glaucoma or secondary ocular infections (eg, fungal). Monitor IOP after 10 days of therapy. Re-evaluate if no response after 2 days. May delay healing and increase incidence of bleb formation after cataract surgery. Ocular irritation and punctate keratitis reported. Cataract formation and optic nerve damage with prolonged use.

ADVERSE REACTIONS: Elevation of IOP, glaucoma, infrequent optic nerve damage, posterior subcapsular cataract formation, delayed wound healing, irritation upon instillation, ocular discomfort, secondary infection, allergic sensitization, burning, stinging, eye irritation.

PREGNANCY: Category C, not for use in nursing.

MECHANISM OF ACTION: Aminoglycoside/corticosteroid. Gentamicin: Anti-infective component that provides action against susceptible organisms. Prednisolone: Corticosteroid that suppresses the inflammatory response and delays or slows healing.

PREDNISONE   RX
prednisone (Roxane)

OTHER BRAND NAMES: Deltasone (Pharmacia & Upjohn)

THERAPEUTIC CLASS: Glucocorticoid

INDICATIONS: Steroid-responsive disorders.

DOSAGE: *Adults:* Initial: 5-60mg/day depending on disease and response. Maint: Decrease dose by small amounts to lowest effective dose.
Pediatrics: Initial: 5-60mg/day depending on disease and response. Maint: Decrease dose by small amounts to lowest effective dose.

HOW SUPPLIED: Sol: 5mg/mL, 5mg/5mL; Tab: 1mg, 2.5mg*, 5mg*, 10mg*, 20mg*, 50mg* *scored

CONTRAINDICATIONS: Systemic fungal infections.

WARNINGS/PRECAUTIONS: May need to increase dose before, during, and after stressful situations. May mask signs of infection or cause new infections. Prolonged use may produce glaucoma, optic nerve damage, secondary ocular

P

infections. Increases BP, salt/water retention, potassium excretion. More severe/fatal course of infections reported with chickenpox, measles. Caution with latent TB, hypothyroidism, cirrhosis, ocular herpes simplex, HTN, diverticulitis, fresh intestinal anastomosis, ulcerative colitis, osteoporosis, myasthenia gravis, renal insufficiency, peptic ulcer disease. Growth and development of children on prolonged therapy should be monitored. Monitor for psychic disturbances. Avoid abrupt withdrawal.

ADVERSE REACTIONS: Fluid and electrolyte disturbances, HTN, osteoporosis, muscle weakness, cushingoid state, menstrual irregularities, nervousness, insomnia, impaired wound healing, DM, ulcerative esophagitis, excessive sweating, increases intracranial pressure, carbohydrate intolerance, glaucoma, cataracts, weight gain, nausea, malaise.

INTERACTIONS: Increases clearance of high dose ASA; caution in hypoprothrombinemia. Increased insulin and oral hypoglycemic requirements in DM. Avoid small pox vaccine, and live vaccines with immunosuppressive doses. Possible decreased vaccine response with killed or inactivated vaccines with immunosuppressive doses. Increased clearance with hepatic enzyme inducers. Decreased metabolism with troleandomycin, ketoconazole. Variable effect on oral anticoagulants.

PREGNANCY: Safety in pregnancy and nursing not known.

MECHANISM OF ACTION: Anti-inflammatory glucocorticoid; causes profound and varied metabolic effects and modifies the body's immune responses to diverse stimuli.

PHARMACOKINETICS: Absorption: Readily absorbed (GI tract).

PREFEST RX
norgestimate - estradiol (King)

Estrogens and progestins should not be used for the prevention of cardiovascular disease. Increased risks of MI, stroke, invasive breast cancer, PE, and DVT in postmenopausal women (50-79 yrs of age) reported. Increased risk of developing probable dementia in postmenopausal women ≥65 yrs of age reported.

THERAPEUTIC CLASS: Estrogen/progestogen combination

INDICATIONS: In women with an intact uterus, treatment of moderate to severe vasomotor symptoms and/or vulvar/vaginal atrophy associated with menopause and prevention of postmenopausal osteoporosis.

DOSAGE: *Adults:* Vasomotor Symptoms/Vulvar/Vaginagil Atrophy/Osteoporosis Prevention: 1mg (estradiol) qd for 3 days followed by 1mg-0.09mg (estradiol-norgestimate) qd for 3 days. Repeat regimen continuously. Re-evaluate at 3-6 month intervals when treating menopausal symptoms.

HOW SUPPLIED: Tab: (Estradiol) 1mg and (Estradiol-Norgestimate) 1mg-0.09mg

CONTRAINDICATIONS: Pregnancy, undiagnosed abnormal genital bleeding, breast cancer, estrogen-dependent neoplasia, DVT/PE, active or recent (eg, within past year) arterial thromboembolic disease (eg, stroke, MI), liver dysfunction or disease.

WARNINGS/PRECAUTIONS: May increase risk of cardiovascular events (eg, MI, stroke), venous thrombosis, and PE; d/c immediately if any of these events occur or are suspected. May increase risk of breast/endometrial cancer, and gallbladder disease. May lead to severe hypercalcemia with breast cancer and bone metastases; monitor and d/c if hypercalcemia occurs. Retinal vascular thrombosis reported; monitor and d/c if papilledema or retinal vascular lesions occur. May elevate BP; monitor at regular intervals. May cause elevations of plasma triglycerides with pre-existing hypertriglyceridemia. Caution with history of cholestatic jaundice associated with past estrogen use or with pregnancy; d/c with recurrence. May lead to increased thyroid-binding globulin levels; monitor thyroid function. May cause fluid retention; caution with cardiac/renal dysfunction. Caution with severe hypocalcemia. May increase risk of ovarian cancer. May exacerbate endometriosis, asthma, DM, epilepsy, migraine, porphyria, SLE, and hepatic hemangiomas; use with caution.

ADVERSE REACTIONS: Altered vaginal bleeding, vaginal candidiasis, breast tenderness/enlargement, nausea, vomiting, melasma, headache, weight changes, edema, altered libido.

INTERACTIONS: CYP3A4 inducers (eg, St. John's wort, phenobarbital, carbamazepine, rifampin) may decrease levels which may decrease therapeutic effects and/or change uterine bleeding profile. CYP3A4 inhibitors (eg, erythromycin, clarithromycin, ketoconazole, itraconazole, ritonavir, grapefruit juice) may increase levels which may result in side effects.

PREGNANCY: Contraindicated in pregnancy, caution in nursing.

MECHANISM OF ACTION: Estradiol: estrogen; binds to nuclear receptors in estrogen-responsive tissues and modulates the pituitary secretion of the gonadotropins, luteinizing hormone and follicle stimulating hormone, through a negative feedback mechanism. In postmenopausal women, reduces elevated levels of these hormones. Norgestimate: Progestin; binds to androgen and progestogen receptors. Counters estrogenic effects by decreasing number of estradiol receptors and suppressing epithelial DNA synthesis in endometrial tissue.

PHARMACOKINETICS: Absorption: Oral administration of variable doses resulted in different parameters. **Distribution:** Found in breast milk. Estradiol: Largely bound to sex hormone binding globulin and albumin. Norgestimate: (17-deacetylnorgestimate) (primary active metabolite): Plasma protein binding (99%). **Metabolism:** Estradiol: Liver to estrone (metabolite) and estriol (major urinary metabolite); sulfate and glucuronide conjugation (liver); gut hydrolysis; CYP 3A4 (partial metabolism). Norgestimate: Extensively in GI tract and liver; 17-deacetylnorgestimate (primary active metabolite). **Elimination:** Estradiol: Urine (parent compound and metabolites); $T_{1/2}$=16 hrs. Norgestimate: Urine, feces; (Active metabolite): $T_{1/2}$=37 hrs.

PREGNYL   RX
chorionic gonadotropin (Organon)

THERAPEUTIC CLASS: Human chorionic gonadotropin

INDICATIONS: For prepubertal cryptorchidism not due to anatomic obstruction. For hypogonadotropic hypogonadism (secondary to a pituitary deficiency) in males. To induce ovulation (OI) and pregnancy in anovulatory, infertile women in whom anovulation is not due to primary ovarian failure and pretreated with human menotropins.

DOSAGE: *Adults:* Hypogonadism: 500-1000 U IM 3x/week (TIW) for 3 weeks, then twice weekly for 3 weeks; or 4000 U IM TIW for 6-9 months, then reduce to 2000 U TIW for 3 months. OI: 5000-10,000 U IM 1 day after last dose of menotropins.
Pediatrics: Cryptorchidism: 4000 U IM TIW for 3 weeks; or 5000 U IM every 2nd day for 4 doses; or 15 doses of 500-1000 U over 6 weeks; or 500 U TIW for 4-6 weeks (if treatment fails, give 1000 U/injection starting 1 month later). Initiate therapy between 4-9 yrs. Hypogonadism: 500-1000 U IM TIW for 3 weeks, then twice weekly for 3 weeks; or 4000 U IM TIW for 6-9 months, then reduce to 2000 U TIW for 3 months.

HOW SUPPLIED: Inj: 10,000 U

CONTRAINDICATIONS: Precocious puberty, prostatic carcinoma or other androgen-dependent neoplasms, pregnancy.

WARNINGS/PRECAUTIONS: Potential ovarian hyperstimulation, enlargement or rupture of ovarian cysts, multiple births, and arterial thromboembolism with infertility treatment. D/C if precocious puberty occurs in cryptorchidism patients. Caution with cardiac or renal disease, epilepsy, migraine, asthma. Not effective treatment for obesity.

ADVERSE REACTIONS: Headache, irritability, restlessness, depression, fatigue, edema, precocious puberty, gynecomastia, injection site pain.

PREGNANCY: Safety in pregnancy and nursing not known.

MECHANISM OF ACTION: Human chorionic gonadotropin; stimulates production of gonadal sterioid hormones by stimulating interstitial cells (leydig cells) of testis to produce androgens and the ovary's corpus luteum to produce progesterone.

PRELONE   RX
prednisolone (Muro)

THERAPEUTIC CLASS: Glucocorticoid

INDICATIONS: Treatment of steroid-responsive disorders.

DOSAGE: *Adults:* Initial: 5-60mg/day depending on disease and response. Maint: Decrease dose by small amounts to lowest effective dose. *Pediatrics:* Initial: 5-60mg/day depending on disease and response. Maint: Decrease dose by small amounts to lowest effective dose.

HOW SUPPLIED: Syrup: 5mg/5mL [120mL], 15mg/5mL [240mL, 480mL]

CONTRAINDICATIONS: Systemic fungal infections.

WARNINGS/PRECAUTIONS: Adjust dose during stress or change in thyroid status. May mask signs of infection or or cause new infections. Prolonged use may produce glaucoma, optic nerve damage, secondary ocular infections. Increases BP, salt/water retention, potassium excretion. Avoid exposure to chickenpox, measles. Caution with latent TB, hypothyroidism, cirrhosis, ocular herpes simplex, HTN, diverticulitis, fresh intestinal anastomosis, ulcerative colitis, osteoporosis, myasthenia gravis, renal insufficiency, peptic ulcer disease. Growth and development of children on prolonged therapy should be monitored. Monitor for psychic disturbances. Avoid abrupt withdrawal.

ADVERSE REACTIONS: Fluid and electrolyte disturbances, osteoporosis, muscle weakness, cushingoid state, menstrual irregularities, nervousness, insomnia, impaired wound healing, excessive sweating, carbohydrate intolerance, glaucoma, cataracts, weight gain, nausea, malaise.

INTERACTIONS: Avoid ASA with hypoprothrombinemia. May increase blood glucose; adjust antidiabetic agents. Avoid smallpox vaccination, and live vaccines with immunosuppressive doses. Possible decreased vaccine response with killed or inactivated vaccines with immunosuppressive doses.

PREGNANCY: Safety in pregnancy and nursing not known.

MECHANISM OF ACTION: Systemic corticosteroid. Unkown, suspected to cause profound and varied metabolic effects.

PREMARIN IV   RX
conjugated estrogens (Wyeth)

> Estrogens increase the risk of endometrial cancer. Estrogens, with or without progestins, should not be used for the prevention of CVD or dementia. Increased risks of MI, stroke, invasive breast cancer, PE, and DVT in postmenopausal women (50-79 yrs of age) reported. Increased risk of developing probable dementia in postmenopausal women ≥65 yrs of age reported.

THERAPEUTIC CLASS: Estrogen

INDICATIONS: Treatment of abnormal uterine bleeding due to hormonal imbalance in the absence of organic pathology.

DOSAGE: *Adults:* 25mg IV or IM. Repeat in 6-12 hrs if needed.

HOW SUPPLIED: Inj: 25mg

CONTRAINDICATIONS: Pregnancy, undiagnosed abnormal genital bleeding, breast cancer, estrogen-dependent neoplasia, DVT/PE, active or recent (eg, within past year) arterial thromboembolic disease (eg, stroke, MI), liver dysfunction or disease.

WARNINGS/PRECAUTIONS: May increase risk of cardiovascular events (eg, MI, stroke), venous thrombosis, and PE; d/c immediately if any of these events occur or are suspected. May increase risk of breast/endometrial cancer, and gallbladder disease. May lead to severe hypercalcemia with breast cancer and bone metastases; monitor and d/c if hypercalcemia occurs. Retinal vascular thrombosis reported; monitor and d/c if papilledema or retinal vascular lesions occur. Consider addition of a progestin if no hysterectomy. May elevate BP; monitor at regular intervals. May cause elevations of plasma triglycerides with pre-existing hypertriglyceridemia. Caution with history of cholestatic jaundice associated with past estrogen use or with pregnancy; d/c with recurrence. May lead to increased thyroid-binding globulin levels; monitor thyroid function. May cause fluid retention; caution with cardiac/renal dysfunction. Caution with severe hypocalcemia. May increase risk of ovarian cancer. May exacerbate endometriosis, asthma, DM, epilepsy, migraine, porphyria, SLE, and hepatic hemangiomas; use with caution.

ADVERSE REACTIONS: Abnormal vaginal bleeding, vaginal candidiasis, nausea, vomiting, abdominal cramps, bloating, breast pain/tenderness/enlargement, erythema multiforme, headache, dizziness, nervousness, weight changes, libido changes.

INTERACTIONS: CYP3A4 inducers (eg, St. John's wort, phenobarbital, carbamazepine, rifampin) may decrease levels which may decrease therapeutic effects and/or change uterine bleeding profile. CYP3A4 inhibitors (eg, erythromycin, clarithromycin, ketoconazole, itraconazole, ritonavir, grapefruit juice) may increase levels which may result in side effects.

PREGNANCY: Contraindicated in pregnancy, caution in nursing.

MECHANISM OF ACTION: Estradiol: Estrogen; responsible for development and maintenance of female reproductive system and secondary sexual characteristics by modulating pituitary secretion of gonadotropins, LH and FSH.

PHARMACOKINETICS: Absorption: Skin, mucous membranes, GI tract. **Metabolism:** Partial, via CYP3A4. Estrone (metabolite); estriol (major urinary metabolite). **Elimination:** Urine.

PREMARIN TABLETS   RX
conjugated estrogens (Wyeth)

> Estrogens increase the risk of endometrial cancer. Estrogens, with or without progestins, should not be used for the prevention of cardiovascular disease or dementia. Increased risks of MI, stroke, invasive breast cancer, PE, and DVT in postmenopausal women (50-79 yrs of age) reported. Increased risk of developing probable dementia in postmenopausal women ≥65 yrs of age reported.

THERAPEUTIC CLASS: Estrogen

INDICATIONS: Treatment of moderate to severe vasomotor symptoms and/or vulvar/vaginal atrophy associated with menopause. Treatment of hypoestrogenism due to hypogonadism, castration, or primary ovarian failure. Palliative treatment of breast cancer in patients with metastatic disease and/or advanced androgen-dependent carcinoma of the prostate. Prevention of postmenopausal osteoporosis.

DOSAGE: *Adults:* Vasomotor Symptoms/Vulvar/Vaginal Atrophy: 0.3mg qd continuously or cyclically (eg, 25 days on, 5 days off). Adjust dose based on response. Re-evaluate at 3-6 month intervals. Osteoporosis Prevention: 0.3mg qd continuously or cyclically (eg, 25 days on, 5 days off). Female Hypogonadism: 0.3-0.625mg qd cyclically (eg, 3 weeks on, 1 week off). Titrate at 6-12 month intervals. Female Castration/Ovarian Failure: 1.25mg qd cyclically. Breast Cancer (palliation): 10mg tid for minimum 3 months. Prostate Cancer (palliation): 1.25-2.5mg tid.

HOW SUPPLIED: Tab: 0.3mg, 0.45mg, 0.625mg, 0.9mg, 1.25mg

CONTRAINDICATIONS: Pregnancy, undiagnosed abnormal genital bleeding, breast cancer unless being treated for metastatic disease, estrogen-dependent neoplasia, DVT/PE, active or recent (eg, within past year) arterial thromboembolic disease (eg, stroke, MI), liver dysfunction or disease.

WARNINGS/PRECAUTIONS: May increase risk of cardiovascular events (eg, MI, stroke), venous thrombosis, and PE; d/c immediately if any of these events occur or are suspected. May increase risk of breast/endometrial cancer, and gallbladder disease. May lead to severe hypercalcemia with breast cancer and bone metastases; monitor and d/c if hypercalcemia occurs. Retinal vascular thrombosis reported; monitor and d/c if papilledema or retinal vascular lesions occur. Consider addition of a progestin if no hysterectomy. May elevate BP; monitor at regular intervals. May cause elevations of plasma triglycerides with pre-existing hypertriglyceridemia. Caution with history of cholestatic jaundice associated with past estrogen use or with pregnancy; d/c with recurrence. May lead to increased thyroid-binding globulin levels; monitor thyroid function. May cause fluid retention; caution with cardiac/renal dysfunction. Caution with severe hypocalcemia. May increase risk of ovarian cancer. May exacerbate endometriosis, asthma, DM, epilepsy, migraine, porphyria, SLE, and hepatic hemangiomas; use with caution.

ADVERSE REACTIONS: Abdominal pain, back pain, headache, infection, pain, arthralgia, leg cramps, breast pain, vaginal hemorrhage, vaginitis

INTERACTIONS: CYP3A4 inducers (eg, St. John's wort, phenobarbital, carbamazepine, rifampin) may decrease levels which may decrease therapeutic effects and/or change uterine bleeding profile. CYP3A4 inhibitors (eg, erythromycin, clarithromycin, ketoconazole, itraconazole, ritonavir, grapefruit juice) may increase levels which may result in side effects. Reduced response to metyrapone test.

PREGNANCY: Contraindicated in pregnancy, caution in nursing.

MECHANISM OF ACTION: Estrogen; binds to nuclear receptors in estrogen-responsive tissues. Circulating estrogens modulate the pituitary secretion of the gonadotrophins, luteinizing hormone and follicle stimulating hormone, through a negative feedback mechanism. In postmenopausal women, reduces elevated levels of these hormones.

PHARMACOKINETICS: Absorption: Well absorbed; oral administration of variable doses resulted in different parameters. **Distribution:** Largely bound to sex hormone binding globulin and albumin; found in breast milk. **Metabolism:** Liver, to estrone (metabolite) and estriol (major urinary metabolite); sulfate and glucuronide conjugation (liver); gut hydrolysis; CYP3A4 (partial metabolism). **Elimination:** Urine (parent drug and metabolites).

PREMARIN VAGINAL   RX
conjugated estrogens (Wyeth)

> Estrogens increase risk of endometrial cancer. Estrogens, with or without progestins, should not be used for the prevention of cardiovascular disease or dementia. Increased risks of MI, stroke, invasive breast cancer, PE, and DVT in postmenopausal women (50-79 yrs of age) reported. Increased risk of developing probable dementia in postmenopausal women ≥65 yrs of age reported. Estrogens with or without progestins should be prescribed at the lowest effective dose and for the shortest duration consistent with treatment goals and risks for the individual woman.

THERAPEUTIC CLASS: Estrogen

INDICATIONS: Treatment of atrophic vaginitis and kraurosis vulvae.

DOSAGE: *Adults:* Usual: 1/2-2g intravaginally qd cyclically (3 weeks on, 1 week off). Discontinue or taper at 3-6 month intervals.

HOW SUPPLIED: Cre: 0.625mg/g [42.5g]

CONTRAINDICATIONS: Pregnancy, undiagnosed abnormal genital bleeding, breast cancer, estrogen-dependent neoplasia, DVT/PE, active or recent (eg, within past year) arterial thromboembolic disease (eg, stroke, MI), liver dysfunction or disease.

WARNINGS/PRECAUTIONS: May increase risk of cardiovascular events (eg, MI, stroke), venous thrombosis, and PE; d/c immediately if any of these events occur or are suspected. Risk factors for arterial vascular disease and/or venous thromboembolism should be managed appropriately. May increase risk of breast/endometrial cancer, dementia and gallbladder disease. May lead to severe hypercalcemia with breast cancer and bone metastases; monitor and d/c if hypercalcemia occurs. Retinal vascular thrombosis reported; monitor and d/c if papilledema or retinal vascular lesions occur. Consider addition of a progestin if no hysterectomy. May elevate BP; monitor at regular intervals. May cause elevations of plasma triglycerides with pre-existing hypertriglyceridemia. Caution with history of cholestatic jaundice associated with past estrogen use or with pregnancy; d/c with recurrence. May lead to increased thyroid-binding globulin levels; monitor thyroid function. May cause fluid retention; caution with cardiac/renal dysfunction. Caution with severe hypocalcemia. May increase risk of ovarian cancer. May exacerbate endometriosis, asthma, DM, epilepsy, migraine, porphyria, SLE, and hepatic hemangiomas; use with caution. May weaken and contribute to the failure of condoms, diaphragms, or cervical caps made of latex or rubber.

ADVERSE REACTIONS: Breakthrough bleeding, vaginal candidiasis, change in cervical secretion, breast tenderness and enlargement, nausea, vomiting, abdominal cramps, bloating, chloasma, melasma, venous thromboembolism, pulmonary embolism, headache.

INTERACTIONS: CYP3A4 inducers (eg, St. John's wort, phenobarbital, carbamazepine, rifampin) may decrease levels which may decrease therapeutic effects and/or change uterine bleeding profile. CYP3A4 inhibitors (eg, erythromycin, clarithromycin, ketoconazole, itraconazole, ritonavir, grapefruit juice) may increase levels which may result in side effects.

PREGNANCY: Contraindicated in pregnancy, caution in nursing.

MECHANISM OF ACTION: Estrogen; binds to nuclear receptors in estrogen-responsive tissues. Circulating estrogens modulate the pituitary secretion of the gonadotrophins, luteinizing hormone and follicle stimulating hormone, through negative feedback mechanism. In postmenopausal women, reduces elevated levels of these hormones.

PHARMACOKINETICS: Absorption: Well-absorbed. **Distribution:** Largely bound to sex hormone binding globulin and albumin; found in breast milk. **Metabolism:** Liver to estrone (metabolite), estriol (major urinary metabolite); sulfate and glucuronide conjugation (liver); gut hydrolysis; CYP 3A4 (partial metabolism). **Elimination:** Urine (parent compound and metabolites).

PREMESIS RX   RX
folic acid - multiple vitamin - minerals (Ther-Rx)

THERAPEUTIC CLASS: Prenatal vitamin

INDICATIONS: Vitamin and mineral supplementation during pregnancy.

DOSAGE: *Adults:* 1 tab qd.

HOW SUPPLIED: Tab: Calcium 200mg-Folic Acid 1mg-Vitamin B$_6$ 75mg-Vitamin B$_{12}$ 0.012mg

WARNINGS/PRECAUTIONS: Not for the treatment of pernicious anemia and other megaloblastic anemias where vitamin B$_{12}$ is deficient. Folic acid >0.1mg/day may obscure pernicious anemia.

ADVERSE REACTIONS: Allergic sensitization.

MECHANISM OF ACTION: Prenatal vitamin.

PREMPHASE   RX
medroxyprogesterone acetate - conjugated estrogens (Wyeth)

> Estrogens and progestins should not be used for prevention of cardiovascular disease or dementia. Increased risks of MI, stroke, invasive breast cancer, PE, and DVT in postmenopausal women (50-79 yrs of age) reported. Increased risk of developing probable dementia in postmenopausal women ≥65 yrs of age reported.

THERAPEUTIC CLASS: Estrogen/progestogen combination

INDICATIONS: In women with intact uterus, treatment of moderate to severe vasomotor symptoms and/or vulvar/vaginal atrophy associated with menopause and prevention of postmenopausal osteoporosis.

DOSAGE: *Adults:* Vasomotor Symptoms/Vulvar/Vaginal Atrophy/Osteoporosis Prevention: 0.625mg tab qd on days 1-14 and 0.625mg-5mg tab qd on days 15-28. Re-evaluate after 3-6 months.

HOW SUPPLIED: Tab: 0.625mg (Estrogens, Conjugated) and 0.625mg-5mg (Estrogens, Conjugated-Medroxyprogesterone)

CONTRAINDICATIONS: Pregnancy, undiagnosed abnormal genital bleeding, breast cancer, estrogen dependent neoplasia, DVT/PE, active or recent (eg, within past year) arterial thromboembolic disease (eg, stroke, MI), liver dysfunction or disease.

WARNINGS/PRECAUTIONS: May increase risk of cardiovascular events (eg, MI, stroke), venous thrombosis, and PE; d/c immediately if any of these events occur or are suspected. May increase risk of breast/endometrial cancer, and gallbladder disease. May lead to severe hypercalcemia with breast cancer and bone metastases; monitor and d/c if hypercalcemia occurs. Retinal vascular thrombosis reported; monitor and d/c if papilledema or retinal vascular lesions occur. May elevate BP; monitor at regular intervals. May cause elevations of plasma triglycerides with pre-existing hypertriglyceridemia. Caution with history of cholestatic jaundice associated with past estrogen use or with pregnancy; d/c with recurrence. May lead to increased thyroid-binding globulin levels; monitor thyroid function. May cause fluid retention; caution with cardiac/renal dysfunction. Caution with severe hypocalcemia. May increase risk of ovarian cancer. May exacerbate endometriosis, asthma, DM, epilepsy, migraine, porphyria, SLE, and hepatic hemangiomas; use with caution.

ADVERSE REACTIONS: Abdominal pain, dysmenorrhea, vaginal moniliasis, breast pain, nausea, arthralgia, headache, depression, back pain, infection, pain, vaginal hemorrhage, vaginitis.

INTERACTIONS: CYP3A4 inducers (eg, St. John's wort, phenobarbital, carbamazepine, rifampin) may decrease levels which may decrease therapeutic effects and/or change uterine bleeding profile. CYP3A4 inhibitors (eg, erythromycin, clarithromycin, ketoconazole, itraconazole, ritonavir, grapefruit juice) may increase levels which may result in side effects.

PREGNANCY: Contraindicated in pregnancy, caution in nursing.

MECHANISM OF ACTION: Conjugated estrogens: Estrogen; binds to nuclear receptors in estrogen-responsive tissues. Circulating estrogens modulate the pituitary secretion of the gonadotropins, luteinizing hormone and follicle stimulating hormone. Medroxyprogesterone: Progesterone derivative; inhibits gonadotropin production which prevents follicular maturation and ovulation.

PHARMACOKINETICS: Absorption: Well-absorbed. Oral administration of various doses resulted in different parameters. **Distribution:** Found in breast milk. Conjugated Estrogen: Largely bound to sex hormone binding globulin and albumin. Medroxyprogesterone: Plasma protein binding (90%). **Metabolism:** Estrogen: Liver to estrone (metabolite) and estriol (major urinary metabolite); sulfate and glucuronide conjugation (liver); gut hydrolysis; CYP3A4 (partial metabolism). Medroxyprogesterone: Liver via hydroxylation, conjugation. **Elimination:** Estrogen: Urine (parent compound and metabolites); Medroxyprogesterone: Urine (metabolites).

PREMPRO RX

medroxyprogesterone acetate - conjugated estrogens (Wyeth)

> Estrogens and progestins should not be used for prevention of cardiovascular disease or dementia. Increased risks of MI, stroke, invasive breast cancer, PE, and DVT in postmenopausal women (50-79 yrs of age) reported. Increased risk of developing probable dementia in postmenopausal women ≥65 yrs of age reported.

THERAPEUTIC CLASS: Estrogen/progestogen combination

INDICATIONS: In women with intact uterus, treatment of moderate to severe vasomotor symptoms and/or vulvar/vaginal atrophy associated with menopause and prevention of postmenopausal osteoporosis.

DOSAGE: *Adults:* Vasomotor Symptoms/Vulvar/Vaginal Atrophy/ Osteoporosis Prevention: Initial: 0.3mg-1.5mg qd. Adjust dose based on response. Re-evaluate after 3-6 months.

HOW SUPPLIED: Tab: (Estrogens, Conjugated-Medroxyprogesterone) 0.3mg-1.5mg, 0.45mg-1.5mg, 0.625mg-2.5mg, 0.625mg-5mg

CONTRAINDICATIONS: Pregnancy, undiagnosed abnormal genital bleeding, breast cancer, estrogen dependent neoplasia, DVT/PE, active or recent (eg, within past year) arterial thromboembolic disease (eg, stroke, MI), liver dysfunction or disease.

WARNINGS/PRECAUTIONS: May increase risk of cardiovascular events (eg, MI, stroke), venous thrombosis, and PE; d/c immediately if any of these events occur or are suspected. May increase risk of breast/endometrial cancer, and gallbladder disease. May lead to severe hypercalcemia with breast cancer and bone metastases; monitor and d/c if hypercalcemia occurs. Retinal vascular thrombosis reported; monitor and d/c if papilledema or retinal vascular lesions occur. May elevate BP; monitor at regular intervals. May cause elevations of plasma triglycerides with pre-existing hypertriglyceridemia. Caution with history of cholestatic jaundice associated with past estrogen use or with pregnancy; d/c with recurrence. May lead to increased thyroid-binding globulin levels; monitor thyroid function. May cause fluid retention; caution with cardiac/renal dysfunction. Caution with severe hypocalcemia. May increase risk of ovarian cancer. May exacerbate endometriosis, asthma, DM, epilepsy, migraine, porphyria, SLE, and hepatic hemangiomas; use with caution.

ADVERSE REACTIONS: Abdominal pain, dysmenorrhea, vaginal moniliasis, breast pain, nausea, arthralgia, headache, depression, back pain, infection, pain, vaginal hemorrhage, vaginitis.

INTERACTIONS: CYP3A4 inducers (eg, St. John's wort, phenobarbital, carbamazepine, rifampin) may decrease levels which may decrease therapeutic effects and/or change uterine bleeding profile. CYP3A4 inhibitors (eg, erythromycin, clarithromycin, ketoconazole, itraconazole, ritonavir, grapefruit juice) may increase levels which may result in side effects. Reduced response to metyrapone test. Concomitant aminoglutethimide may significantly depress bioavailability of medroxyprogesterone.

PREGNANCY: Contraindicated in pregnancy, caution in nursing.

MECHANISM OF ACTION: Estrogen: Responsible for development and maintenance of female reproductive system, and secondary sexual characteristics by modulating pituitary secretion of gonadotropins, LH and FSH. Medroxyprogesterone (MPA): Progesterone derivative; decreases nuclear estrogen receptors and suppression of epithelial DNA synthesis in endometrial tissue.

PHARMACOKINETICS: Absorption: Oral administration of different doses resulted in different parameters. **Distribution**: MPA: Plasma protein binding (90%). **Metabolism**: Estrogen: Liver; Estrone (metabolite), estriol (major urinary metabolite). MPA: Hydroxylation, conjugation. **Elimination**: Estrogen: Urine. MPA: Urine.

PREPIDIL RX
dinoprostone (Pharmacia & Upjohn)

THERAPEUTIC CLASS: Prostaglandin E$_2$

INDICATIONS: For ripening of an unfavorable cervix in pregnant women at or near term with a medical or obstetrical need for labor induction.

DOSAGE: *Adults:* Bring to room temperature before administration. Choose appropriate length shielded catheter. Use 20mm endocervical catheter if no effacement present or 10mm catheter if cervix is 50% effaced. Patient should remain in supine position for 15-30 min after administration. May give repeat dose of 0.5mg with dosing interval of 6 hrs. Max: 1.5mg/24hrs.

HOW SUPPLIED: Gel: 0.5mg/3g [3g]

CONTRAINDICATIONS: Patients in whom oxytocic drugs are contraindicated or where prolonged contractions of the uterus are inappropriate (eg, history of cesarean section, major uterine surgery, history of difficult labor or traumatic delivery, cephalopelvic disproportion, grand multiparae with ≥6 previous term pregnancy cases with non-vertex presentation, hyperactive or hypertonic uterine patterns, fetal distress where delivery is not imminent, obstetric emergencies where benefit-to-risk ratio for fetus or mother favors surgical intervention). Placenta previa, unexplained vaginal bleeding during this pregnancy, vaginal delivery not indicated (eg, vasa previa, active herpes genitalia).

WARNINGS/PRECAUTIONS: Strictly adhere to recommended dosage. Monitor uterine activity, fetal status, and character of cervix. Continuously monitor uterine activity and fetal status with history of hypertonic uterine contractility or tetanic uterine contractions. Caution with asthma, glaucoma, increased IOP, renal/hepatic dysfunction, ruptured membranes. Avoid administration above level of internal os. Evaluate feto-pelvic relationship before therapy.

ADVERSE REACTIONS: (Maternal) Abnormal uterine contractility, GI effects, back pain, warm feeling in vagina, fever. (Fetal) Abnormal heart rate, brady-cardia, altered deceleration.

INTERACTIONS: May augment activity of other oxytocic agents; avoid con-comitant use. Use 6-12 hr dosing interval with sequential use of oxytocin.

PREGNANCY: Category C, safety in nursing not known.

MECHANISM OF ACTION: Prostaglandin E_2; stimulates myometrium of gravid uterus to contract similar to contractions seen in term uterus during labor.

PHARMACOKINETICS: Absorption: Rapid. T_{max}=0.5-0.75 hrs. C_{max}=433pg/mL. **Metabolism:** Lungs. (Metabolite) 13,14-dihydro-15-keto-PGE_2 (DHK-PGE_2). **Elimination:** Kidneys.

PREVACID
lansoprazole (TAP)

RX

OTHER BRAND NAMES: Prevacid IV (TAP) - Prevacid Solutab (TAP)

THERAPEUTIC CLASS: Proton pump inhibitor

INDICATIONS: (PO) Treatment of active duodenal ulcer (DU), active benign gastric ulcer (GU), erosive esophagitis, symptomatic GERD. Maintain healing of erosive esophagitis and duodenal ulcers. Treatment of pathological hyper-secretory conditions (eg, Zollinger-Ellison syndrome). Combination therapy with amoxicillin +/- clarithromycin for H.pylori eradication in duodenal ulcer disease, to reduce risk of ulcer recurrence. Treatment and risk reduction in NSAID induced gastric ulcer. (Inj) Short-term treatment of erosive esophagitis.

DOSAGE: *Adults:* >17 yrs: (PO) DU: 15mg qd for 4 weeks. Maint: 15mg qd. GU: 30mg qd up to 8 weeks. GERD: 15mg qd up to 8 weeks. Erosive Esophagitis: 30mg qd up to 8 weeks. May repeat for 8 weeks if needed. Maint: 15mg qd. NSAID-Induced GU: 30mg qd for 8 weeks. Reduce Risk of NSAID Induced GU: 15mg qd for 12 weeks. Hypersecretory Conditions: Initial: 60mg qd, then adjust. Max: 90mg bid. Divide dose if >120mg/day. H.pylori: Triple Therapy: 30mg + clarithromycin 500mg + amoxicillin 1000mg, all bid (q12h) for 10-14 days. Dual Therapy: 30mg + amoxicillin 1000mg both tid (q8h) for 14 days. Take before eating. Caps: Swallow whole or sprinkle cap contents on 1 tbsp of applesauce, ENSURE® pudding, cottage cheese, yogurt, strained pears, or in 60mL orange juice or tomato juice; swallow immediately. Sus: Do not chew or crush. Mix pkt with 30mL of water; stir well and drink immediately; not for use with NG tube. Solutab: Place on tongue with or without water. Oral Syringe: (SoluTab) Place 15mg tab in oral syringe and draw up 4mL of water, or 30mg tab in oral syringe and draw up 10mL of water. Shake contents and administer after tablet has dispersed within 15 mins. Refill syringe with 2mL (5mL for 30mg tab) of water, shake, and give any remaining contents. NG Tube: (Cap) Mix cap contents with 40mL apple juice and inject into NG tube; flush with additional juice to clear tube. (SoluTab) Place 15mg tab and draw up 4mL of water, or 30mg tab and draw up 10mL of water. Shake contents and after tab-let has dispersed, inject through NG tube into stomach within 15 mins. Refill syringe with 5mL of water, shake, and flush NG tube. (Inj) Erosive Esophagitis: 30mg IV qd over 30 mins for 7 days. May switch to PO formulation for total of 6 to 8 weeks of therapy once patient is able to take oral medications. Severe Hepatic Impairment: Adjust dose.
Pediatrics: 12-17 yrs: Short-Term Symptomatic GERD: 15mg qd for up to 8 weeks. Erosive Esophagitis: 30mg qd for up to 8 weeks. 1-11 yrs: Short-Term Symptomatic GERD/Erosive Esophagitis: ≤30kg: 15mg qd for up to 12 weeks.

>30kg: 30mg qd for up to 12 weeks. Titrate: May increase up to 30mg bid after 2 weeks if symptomatic. Severe Hepatic Impairment: Adjust dose. Take before eating. Caps: Swallow whole or sprinkle contents on 1 tbsp of applesauce, ENSURE® pudding, cottage cheese, yogurt, strained pears, or in 60mL orange juice or tomato juice; swallow immediately. Sus: Do not chew or crush. Mix pkt with 30mL water; stir well and drink immediately; not for use with NG tube. Solutab: Place on tongue with or without water. Oral Syringe: (SoluTab) Place 15mg tab in oral syringe and draw up 4mL of water, or 30mg tab in oral syringe and draw up 10mL of water. Shake contents and administer after tablet has dispersed within 15 mins. Refill syringe with 2mL (5mL for 30mg tab) of water, shake, and give any remaining contents. NG Tube: (Cap) Mix cap contents with 40mL apple juice and inject into NG tube; flush with additional juice to clear tube. (SoluTab) Place 15mg tab and draw up 4mL of water, or 30mg tab and draw up 10mL of water. Shake contents and after tablet has dispersed, inject through NG tube into stomach within 15 mins. Refill syringe with 5mL of water, shake, and flush NG tube.

HOW SUPPLIED: Cap, Delayed-Release: 15mg, 30mg; Inj: 30mg; Sus, Delayed-Release: 15mg, 30mg (granules/pkt); Tab, Disintegrating (SoluTab): 15mg, 30mg.

WARNINGS/PRECAUTIONS: Symptomatic response does not preclude the presence of gastric malignancy. Adjust dose with hepatic impairment.

ADVERSE REACTIONS: Abdominal pain, constipation, diarrhea, nausea, myositis, interstitial nephritis

INTERACTIONS: May alter absorption of pH-dependent drugs (eg, ketoconazole, ampicillin esters, digoxin, and iron salts). Give at least 30 minutes prior to sucralfate. Theophylline may need dose adjustment. Concomitant use with warfarin may increase INR and prothrombin time.

PREGNANCY: Category B, not for use in nursing.

MECHANISM OF ACTION: Proton pump inhibitor; suppresses gastric acid secretion by specific inhibition of the (H^+, K^+)-ATPase enzyme system at the secretory surface of the gastric parietal cell.

PHARMACOKINETICS: Absorption: (PO, adult) absolute bioavailability (>80%); T_{max}=1.7 hrs. (IV, adult) C_{max}=1705ng/mL; AUC=3192ng•hr/mL. **Distribution:** V_d=15.7L; plasma protein binding (97%). **Metabolism:** Liver (extensive) via CYP3A4 and CYP2C19. **Elimination:** Urine, feces; $T_{1/2}$≤2 hrs. Refer to package insert for pediatric parameters.

PREVACID NAPRAPAC   RX
lansoprazole - naproxen (TAP)

> NSAIDs may cause an increased risk of serious cardiovascular thrombotic events, MI, and stroke. Risk may increase with duration of use and in patients with cardiovascular disease or risk factors for cardiovascular disease. NSAIDs may cause an increased risk of serious GI events which may be fatal. Patients with history of gastric and/or duodenal ulcers (especially patients with history of bleeding or perforation) and geriatric patients are at greater risk for serious GI events. Contraindicated for the treatment of perioperative pain in the setting of coronary artery bypass graft (CABG) surgery.

THERAPEUTIC CLASS: NSAID/Proton Pump Inhibitor

INDICATIONS: To reduce the risk of NSAID-associated gastric ulcers in patients with a history of documented gastric ulcers who require the use of an NSAID for treatment of rheumatoid arthritis, osteoarthritis, and ankylosing spondylitis.

DOSAGE: *Adults:* Take am dose before eating. Lansoprazole 15mg qam + naproxen 500mg bid in am and pm. Max: 1000mg naproxen/day. Swallow lansoprazole whole.

HOW SUPPLIED: Cap, Delayed-Release: (Naproxen-Lansoprazole): 500mg-15mg [14 tabs naproxen + 7 caps lansoprazole/weekly blister card; 4 cards/pkg]

CONTRAINDICATIONS: Presence or history of NSAID/ASA-related asthma, urticaria, or allergic-type reactions. Perioperative pain in the setting of CABG surgery.

WARNINGS/PRECAUTIONS: Risk of GI ulceration, bleeding, and perforation. Monitor for visual disturbances, fluid retention/edema, Hgb levels (if initial ≤10g), and LFTs with chronic use. Acute interstitial nephritis, hematuria, proteinuria, nephrotic syndrome and severe hepatic reactions reported. Caution with impaired renal (CrCl <20mL/min) or hepatic function, elderly, heart failure, and high doses with chronic alcoholic liver disease. NSAIDs can lead to onset or worsening of pre-existing HTN; monitor BP closely. Naproxen can cause exfoliative dermatitis, Stevens-Johnson syndrome, toxic epidermal necrolysis.

ADVERSE REACTIONS: Nausea, abdominal pain, constipation, heartburn, headache, dizziness, drowsiness, pruritus, skin eruptions, ecchymoses, tinnitus, edema, dyspnea.

INTERACTIONS: Avoid other forms of naproxen, ASA. May potentiate renal disease with ACE inhibitors. Naproxen may displace other albumin-bound drugs. Caution with warfarin. Monitor for toxicity with hydantoin, sulfonamide, or sulfonylureas. Decreased plasma levels with ASA. May antagonize natriuretic effect of furosemide and thiazides. Decreases renal clearance of lithium and methotrexate. May decrease antihypertensive effects of propranolol and other β-blockers. Increased levels and half-life with probenecid. Take lansoprazole 30 min prior to sucralfate. Lansoprazole may alter absorption of pH-dependent drugs (eg, ketoconazole, ampicillin, iron, digoxin).

PREGNANCY: Category C, not for use in nursing.

MECHANISM OF ACTION: Naproxen: NSAID; inhibits prostaglandin synthetase. Lansoprazole: PPI; inhibits gastric acid secretion by blocking proton pumps.

PHARMACOKINETICS: Absorption: Naproxen: Rapid, complete; bioavailability (95%); T_{max}=2-4 hrs. Lansoprazole: Rapid; bioavailability (80%); T_{max}=1.7 hrs. **Distribution:** Naproxen: Plasma protein binding (≥99%); V_d=0.16 L/kg; found in breast milk. Lansoprazole: Plasma protein binding (97%). **Metabolism:** Naproxen: Hepatic; 6-O-desmethyl naproxen (metobolite). Lansoprazole: Hepatic. **Elimination:** Naproxen: Kidney; urine (95%), feces (≤3%); $T_{1/2}$=12-17 hrs. Lansoprazole: Biliary; $T_{1/2}$= <2 hrs.

PreviDent RX
sodium fluoride (Colgate Oral)

OTHER BRAND NAMES: PreviDent 5000 Plus (Colgate Oral)

THERAPEUTIC CLASS: Fluoride preparation

INDICATIONS: Prevention of dental caries.

DOSAGE: *Adults:* Apply thin ribbon to teeth with toothbrush or mouth tray qhs for at least 1 min with gel and 2 min with cream after regular brushing. Expectorate after use. Do not eat, drink, or rinse for 30 min.
Pediatrics: 6-16 yrs: Apply thin ribbon to teeth with toothbrush or mouth tray qhs for at least 1 min with gel and 2 min with cream after regular brushing. Expectorate and rinse mouth thoroughly after use.

HOW SUPPLIED: Gel: (PreviDent) 1.1%; Cre: (PreviDent 5000 Plus) 1.1%

CONTRAINDICATIONS: Not for children <6 years of age, unless recommended by dentist or physician.

WARNINGS/PRECAUTIONS: Prolonged ingestion may lead to dental fluorosis in children <6 years of age. Not for systemic treatment. Do not swallow.

ADVERSE REACTIONS: Allergic reactions.

PREGNANCY: Category B, caution in nursing.

MECHANISM OF ACTION: Fluoride preparation; increases tooth resistance to acid dissolution and enhances penetration of fluoride ion into tooth enamel.

PREVNAR

RX

pneumococcal vaccine, diphtheria conjugate (Wyeth)

THERAPEUTIC CLASS: Vaccine

INDICATIONS: Active immunization of children against invasive disease caused by *S.pneumoniae*. Active immunization of children against otitis media caused by serotypes included in the vaccine.

DOSAGE: *Pediatrics:* 6 weeks-2 months: 4 doses of 0.5mL IM. Give 3 doses at 2 month intervals and 4th dose at 12-15 months old. Unvaccinated Children: 7-11 months: 3 doses of 0.5mL IM. Give 1st 2 doses at least 4 weeks apart and 3rd dose after 1yr birthday; separate from 2nd dose by at least 2 months. 12-23 months: 2 doses of 0.5mL IM at least 2 months apart. ≥24 months-9 yrs: 0.5mL IM single dose.

HOW SUPPLIED: Inj: 16mcg/0.5mL

CONTRAINDICATIONS: Severe or moderate febrile illness.

WARNINGS/PRECAUTIONS: Avoid with thrombocytopenia or coagulation disorder. Impaired immune responses may cause reduced response to active immunization. Not a substitute for diphtheria or 23-valent pneumococcal vaccinations. Do not give IV. Have epinephrine (1:1000) available. Caution with latex sensitivity; packaging contains dry natural rubber. Fever and rarely febrile seizures reported.

ADVERSE REACTIONS: Injection site reactions, irritability, drowsiness, restless sleep, decreased appetite, vomiting, diarrhea, fever.

INTERACTIONS: Suboptimal response with immunosuppressants. Caution with anticoagulants.

PREGNANCY: Category C, not for use in nursing.

MECHANISM OF ACTION: Immunostimulant; elicits formation of antibodies that may protect against invasive pneumococcal disease and otitis media.

PREVPAC

RX

amoxicillin - clarithromycin - lansoprazole (TAP)

THERAPEUTIC CLASS: *H.pylori* treatment combination

INDICATIONS: Treatment of *H.pylori* infection associated with active duodenal ulcer and to reduce the risk of duodenal ulcer recurrence.

DOSAGE: *Adults:* 1g amoxicillin, 500mg clarithromycin and 30mg lansoprazole, all bid (am and pm) before meals for 10 or 14 days. Swallow each pill whole. Renal Impairment (with or without hepatic impairment): Decrease clarithromycin dose or prolong intervals. Avoid with CrCl <30mL/min.

HOW SUPPLIED: Cap: (Amoxicillin) 500mg, Tab: (Clarithromycin) 500mg, Cap, Delayed-Release: (Lansoprazole) 30mg

CONTRAINDICATIONS: Concomitant cisapride, pimozide, astemizole, terfenadine, ergotamine or dihydroergotamine. Hypersensitivity to prevacid, macrolide or penicillin antibiotics.

WARNINGS/PRECAUTIONS: Avoid if CrCl <30mL/min. Caution with cephalosporin/PCN allergy; anaphylactic reactions have been reported. Pseudomembranous colitis reported. Possibility of superinfections. Caution in elderly. Clarithromycin may increase colchicine; monitor for toxicity. Do not use clarithromycin during pregnancy. Symptomatic response to lansoprazole does not preclude the presence of gastric malignancy. *Clostridium difficile* associated diarrhea (CDAD) reported. D/C if confirmed.

ADVERSE REACTIONS: Diarrhea, taste perversion, headache.

INTERACTIONS: Contraindicated with cisapride, pimozide, astemizole, terfenadine, ergotamine or dihydroergotamine. May interfere with absorption of drugs dependent on gastric pH for bioavailability (eg, atazanavir, ketoconazole, ampicillin esters, iron salts, digoxin). Clarithromycin increases plasma levels of carbamazepine, digoxin. Clarithromycin potentiates oral

P

anticoagulants and may decrease triazolam clearance. Erythromycin or clarithromycin can cause acute ergot toxicity with ergotamine or dihydroer-gotamine. Clarithromycin increases levels of HMG CoA reductase inhibitors (eg, lovastatin, simvastatin). Theophylline may need dose adjustment. Take lansoprazole and other proton pump inhibitors 30 minutes before sucralfate. Caution with drugs metabolized by CYP450 (eg, cyclosporine, tacrolimus, phenytoin); monitor levels. QTc prolongation has occurred with coadminis-tration of clarithromycin and antiarrhythmics (eg, quinidine, disopyramide). Concomitant clarithromycin and colchine may lead to increased exposure to colchicine.

PREGNANCY: Category C, not for use in nursing.

MECHANISM OF ACTION: Lansoprazole: Substituted benzimidazole; inhibits gastric acid secretion. Amoxicillin: Semi-synthetic antibiotic; has broad spec-trum of bactericidal activity against many gram-positive and gram-negative organisms. Clarithromycin: Semi-synthetic macrolide antibiotic.

PHARMACOKINETICS: Absorption: Lansoprazole: Rapidly absorbed; Absolute bioavailability (80%); T_{max}=1.7 hrs. Amoxicillin: Rapidly absorbed. Clarithromycin: Rapidly absorbed; Absolute bioavailability (50%); T_{max}=2-3 hrs. **Distribution:** Lansoprazole: Plasma protein binding (97%); found in breast milk. Amoxicillin: Plasma protein binding (approx. 20%). Clarithromycin: Found in breast milk. **Metabolism:** Lansoprazole: Liver (extensive). Clarithromycin: 14-OH clarithromycin (active metabolite). **Elimination:** Lansoprazole: Urine and feces; $T_{1/2}$=1.5 hrs. Amoxicillin: Urine (60%). Clarithromycin: Urine (30%); $T_{1/2}$=5-7 hrs; (metabolite); $T_{1/2}$=7-9 hrs.

PREZISTA   RX
darunavir (Tibotec)

THERAPEUTIC CLASS: Protease inhibitor

INDICATIONS: For use with 100mg ritonavir, and other antiretroviral agents, for the treatment of HIV infection in antiretroviral treatment-experienced adult patients.

DOSAGE: *Adults:* 600mg bid with ritonavir 100mg bid. Take with food.

HOW SUPPLIED: Tab: 300mg, 600mg

CONTRAINDICATIONS: Concomitant antihistamines (eg, astemizole, ter-fenadine), ergot derivatives (eg, dihydroergotamine, ergonovine, ergotamine, methylergonovine), cisapride, pimozide, sedative hypnotics (eg, midazolam, triazolam).

WARNINGS/PRECAUTIONS: Severe skin rash, including erythema multi-forme and Stevens-Johnson syndrome, reported. Caution with sulfonamide allergy. New onset DM, exacerbation of pre-existing DM, and hyperglycemia reported. Caution with hepatic impairment. Drug-induced hepatitis (eg, acute hepatitis, cytolytic hepatitis) may occur. Increased frequency of liver function abnormalities reported with pre-existing liver dysfunction, including chronic active hepatitis. Increased bleeding, including spontaneous skin hematomas and hemarthrosis in hemophilia type A and B reported. Redistribution/ac-cumulation of body fat, including central obesity, dorsocervical fat enlarge-ment, peripheral wasting, facial wasting, breast enlargement, and cushingoid appearance observed with antiretroviral therapy. Immune reconstitution syndrome may occur.

ADVERSE REACTIONS: Diarrhea, nausea, vomiting, nasopharyngitis, abdomi-nal pain, constipation, headache.

INTERACTIONS: See Contraindications. Avoid with carbamazepine, pheno-barbital, phenytoin, rifampin, St. John's wort; significant decreases in plasma concentrations may occur. Potential for serious reactions (eg, myopathy, rhabdomyolysis) with HMG-CoA reductase inhibitors. Concomitant darunavir/ritonavir and efavirenz may decrease darunavir and increase efavirenz levels; use with caution. Concentrations of antiarrhythmics (eg, bepridil, lidocaine, quinidine, amiodarone) may be increased with concomitant use; caution is warranted and therapeutic concentration monitoring recommended. Monitor

INR with concomitant warfarin use. Trazadone concentrations may increase; use combination with caution. Therapeutic concentration monitoring recommended for concomitant immunosuppressants (eg, cyclosporine, tacrolimus, sirolimus). May decrease methadone concentrations. Alternative/additional measures of contraception should be used with concurrent use. Refer to Prescribing Information for a complete list of drug interactions.

PREGNANCY: Category B, not for use in nursing.

MECHANISM OF ACTION: Protease inhibitor; inhibits cleavage of HIV encoded Gag-Pol polyproteins in infected cells, preventing the formation of mature virus particles.

PHARMACOKINETICS: Absorption: Darunavir: Absolute bioavailability (37%). Darunavir/Ritonavir: Absolute bioavailability (82%). T_{max}=2.5-4 hrs. **Distribution:** Darunavir: Plasma protein binding (95%). **Metabolism:** Darunavir: Hepatic (oxidation) via CYP3A. **Elimination:** Darunavir: urine (7.7%), feces (41.2%). Darunavir/Ritonavir: $T_{1/2}$=15 hrs.

PRIALT RX
ziconotide acetate (Elan)

Severe psychiatric symptoms and neurological impairment may occur during treatment. Patients with a pre-existing history of psychosis should not be treated with ziconotide. Monitor patients for evidence of cognitive impairment, hallucinations, or changes in mood or consciousness. Therapy can be interrupted or discontinued abruptly without evidence of withdrawal effects in the event of serious neurological or psychiatric signs or symptoms.

THERAPEUTIC CLASS: N-type Calcium Channel Blocker

INDICATIONS: Management of severe chronic pain in patients for whom intrathecal (IT) therapy is warranted, and who are intolerant of or refractory to other treatment, such as systemic analgesics, adjunctive therapies, or IT morphine.

DOSAGE: *Adults*: Initial: No more than 2.4mcg/d IT (0.1mcg/hr). Titrate by 2.4mcg/d no more than 2-3x/week. Max: 19.2mcg/d (0.8mcg/hr) by Day 21.

HOW SUPPLIED: Sol: 25mcg/mL [20mL], 100mcg/mL [1mL, 2mL, 5mL]

CONTRAINDICATIONS: Pre-existing history of psychosis. Contraindications to the use of IT analgesia: presence of infection at the microinfusion injection site, uncontrolled bleeding diathesis, and spinal canal obstruction that impairs circulation of CSF.

WARNINGS/PRECAUTIONS: Caution against engaging in hazardous activity requiring complete mental alertness or motor coordination. Dosage adjustments may be necessary when combined with other CNS-depressants due to additive effects. Ziconotide is not an opiate and cannot prevent or relieve the symptoms associated with the withdrawal of opiates. Risk of meningitis due to inadvertent contamination of the microinfusion device. Monitor for signs and symptoms of meningitis. Reports of CNS-related adverse events: psychiatric symptoms, cognitive impairment, and decreased alertness/unresponsiveness. Discontinue if patient becomes unresponsive or stuporous. Monitor for elevations in serum creatine kinase levels.

ADVERSE REACTIONS: Dizziness, nausea, confusion, headache, somnolence, nystagmus, asthenia, pain, vertigo, blurred vision, constipation, dry mouth, anorexia.

INTERACTIONS: Coadministration with CNS depressants increases the risk of CNS adverse effects.

PREGNANCY: Category C, caution in nursing.

MECHANISM OF ACTION: Has not been established; suggested that it binds to N-type calcium channels, which leads to a blockade of excitatory neurotransmitter release from the primary afferent nerve terminals and antinociception.

PHARMACOKINETICS: Absorption: T_{max}= 1 hr, AUC=83.6-608ng•h/mL, C_{max}=16.4-132ng/mL. **Distribution**: Plasma protein binding (50%), V_d=155mL.

Metabolism: Kidneys, liver, lungs, muscle via endopeptidases, exopeptidases and proteases. **Elimination**: $T_{1/2}$=4.6 hrs.

PRIFTIN RX

rifapentine (Sanofi-Aventis)

THERAPEUTIC CLASS: Rifamycin derivative

INDICATIONS: Treatment of pulmonary TB. Do not use alone, as initial or retreatment.

DOSAGE: *Adults:* Intensive Phase: Initial: 600mg twice weekly with an interval of not <3 days (72 hrs) between doses. Continue for 2 months. Maint: 600mg once weekly for 4 months. Elderly: Start at low end of dosing range. *Pediatrics:* ≥12 yrs: Intensive Phase: Initial: 600mg twice weekly with an interval of not <3 days (72 hrs) between doses. Continue for 2 months. Maint: 600mg once weekly for 4 months.

HOW SUPPLIED: Tab: 150mg

WARNINGS/PRECAUTIONS: Give with pyridoxine in the malnourished, if predisposed to neuropathy (eg, alcoholics, diabetics), and adolescents. Caution with hepatic impairment; monitor LFTs before and every 2-4 weeks during therapy. May cause postnatal hemorrhages in mother and infant during last weeks of pregnancy; monitor clotting parameters; may need vitamin K. May produce a red-orange discoloration of body tissues, fluids. May stain/discolor contact lenses, breast milk, or dentures. Pseudomembranous colitis reported. Avoid with porphyria. Caution in elderly.

ADVERSE REACTIONS: Hyperuricemia, increased ALT/AST, neutropenia, pyuria, proteinuria, lymphopenia, urinary casts, rash, pruritus, acne, anorexia, anemia.

INTERACTIONS: Antagonizes drugs metabolized by CYP3A4, CYP2C8, and CYP2C9 due to enzyme induction (eg, anticonvulsants, antiarrhythmics, oral anticoagulants, antibiotics, antifungals, barbiturates, benzodiazepines, β-blockers, CCB, corticosteroids, cardiac glycosides, clofibrate, hormonal contraceptives, oral hypoglycemics, haloperidol, immunosuppressants, levothyroxine, narcotic analgesics, progestins, quinine, reverse transcriptase inhibitors, sildenafil, theophylline, TCAs). Increases indinavir metabolism; extreme caution with protease inhibitors. Avoid hormonal contraceptives. Consider hepatotoxic effects of other antituberculosis drug therapies (eg, isoniazid, pyrazinamide).

PREGNANCY: Category C, not for use in nursing.

MECHANISM OF ACTION: Cyclopentyl rifamycin; inhibits DNA-dependent RNA polymerase in susceptible strains of *Mycobacterium tuberculosis* (but not in mammalian cells). It also exhibits bactericidal activity against both intracellular and extracellular *M. tuberculosis* organisms.

PHARMACOKINETICS: Absorption: Relative bioavailabilty (70%); C_{max}=15.05±4.62μg/mL; AUC=319.54±91.52μg•hr/mL; T_{max}=4.83±1.8 hrs. **Distribution:** V_d=70.2±9.1L; Plasma protein binding: 97.7% (rifapentine), 93.2% (metabolite). **Metabolism:** Metabolite: 25-desacetyl rifapentine. **Elimination:** Urine (17%), feces (70%).

PRILOSEC RX

omeprazole (AstraZeneca)

THERAPEUTIC CLASS: Proton pump inhibitor

INDICATIONS: Short-term treatment of active duodenal ulcer and active benign gastric ulcer in adults. Treatment of heartburn and other symptoms associated with GERD in adults and pediatrics. Short-term treatment of erosive esophagitis and to maintain healing of erosive esophagitis in adults and pediatrics. Long-term treatment of pathological hypersecretory conditions (eg, Zollinger-Ellison syndrome, multiple endocrine adenomas, systemic mastocytosis) in adults. Combination therapy with clarithromycin +/- amoxicillin for *H.pylori* eradication in duodenal ulcer disease, and to reduce risk of ulcer recurrence, in adults.

DOSAGE: *Adults:* Duodenal Ulcer: 20mg qd for 4-8 weeks. Gastric Ulcer: 40mg qd for 4-8 weeks. GERD: 20mg qd up to 4 weeks without esophageal lesions. Treatment Erosive Esophagitis with GERD: 20mg qd for 4-8 weeks. Maint: 20mg qd. Hypersecretory Conditions: Initial: 60mg qd, then adjust if needed. Divide dose if >80mg/day. Doses up to 120mg tid have been given. *H.pylori* Triple Therapy: 20mg + clarithromycin 500mg + amoxicillin 1g, all bid for 10 days. Give additional 18 days of omeprazole 20mg every morning if ulcer present initially. Dual Therapy: 40mg qd + clarithromycin 500mg tid for 14 days. Give additional 14 days of omeprazole 20mg every morning if ulcer present initially. Do not crush or chew. Take before eating. Can add contents of caps to applesauce if difficulty swallowing; swallow immediately without chewing.
Pediatrics: 1-16 yrs: GERD/Erosive Esophagitis: ≥20kg: 20mg qd. 10 to <20kg: 10mg qd. 5 to <10kg: 5mg qd. Do not crush or chew. Take before eating. Can add contents of caps to applesauce if difficulty swallowing; swallow immediately without chewing.

HOW SUPPLIED: Cap, Delayed-Release: 10mg, 20mg, 40mg; Sus, Delayed-Release: 2.5mg, 10mg granules/packet

WARNINGS/PRECAUTIONS: Atrophic gastritis reported with long-term use. Symptomatic response does not preclude the presence of gastric malignancy.

ADVERSE REACTIONS: Headache, diarrhea, abdominal pain, asthenia, nausea, vomiting.

INTERACTIONS: May potentiate diazepam, warfarin, phenytoin and drugs metabolized by oxidation. May alter absorption of pH-dependent drugs (eg, ketoconazole, ampicillin esters, iron salts). Monitor drugs metabolized by CYP450 (eg, cyclosporine, disulfiram, benzodiazepines). Increased levels with clarithromycin. Increases levels of clarithromycin. Voriconazole may increase levels. May reduce plasma levels of atazanavir. May increase levels of tacrolimus.

PREGNANCY: Category C, not for use in nursing.

MECHANISM OF ACTION: Proton pump inhibitor; suppresses gastric acid secretion by specific inhibition of the H^+/K^+ ATPase enzyme system at the secretory surface of the gastric parietal cell.

PHARMACOKINETICS: Absorption: Rapid; Absolute bioavailability (30-40%); T_{max}=0.5-3.5 hrs. (Adult, single dose) C_{max}=668ng/mL; AUC=1220ng•hr/mL. (Children<20 kg, 2-5yrs, 10 mg single dose) C_{max}=288ng/mL; AUC=511ng•hr/mL. (Children >20kg, 6-16yrs, 20 mg single dose) C_{max}=495ng/mL; AUC=1140ng•hr/mL. **Distribution:** Plasma protein binding (95%); found in breast milk. **Metabolism:** Hydroxyomeprazole and corresponding carboxylic acid (metabolites). **Elimination:** Urine (77%), feces; $T_{1/2}$=0.5-1 hr.

PRILOSEC OTC OTC
omeprazole magnesium (Procter & Gamble)

THERAPEUTIC CLASS: Proton pump inhibitor

INDICATIONS: Treatment of frequent heartburn (≥2 days per week).

DOSAGE: *Adults:* 20mg qd for 14 days. Take with water in morning before food. May repeat q 4 months.

HOW SUPPLIED: Tab, Delayed-Release: 20mg

CONTRAINDICATIONS: Trouble or pain swallowing food, vomiting with blood, or bloody or black stools.

INTERACTIONS: Caution with warfarin, diazepam, digoxin, antifungals, tacrolimus, and atazanavir.

PREGNANCY: Safety in pregnancy and nursing not known.

PrimaCare
folic acid - multiple vitamin - minerals (Ther-Rx)

RX

THERAPEUTIC CLASS: Prenatal vitamin

INDICATIONS: Vitamin, mineral, and fatty acid supplementation for before, during, and after pregnancy.

DOSAGE: *Adults:* 1 cap qam and 1 tab qpm.

HOW SUPPLIED: Cap: (AM) Calcium 150mg-Linoleic Acid 30mg-Omega-3 Fatty Acids 330mg-Vitamin D 170 IU-Vitamin E 30 IU; Tab: (PM) Biotin 0.035mg-Calcium 250mg-Chromium 0.045mg-Copper 1.3mg-Folic Acid 1mg-Iron 30mg-Molybdenum 0.05mg-Pantothenic Acid 7mg-Selenium 0.075mg-Vitamin B_1 3mg-Vitamin B_2 3.4mg-Vitamin B_3 20mg-Vitamin B_6 50mg-Vitamin B_{12} 0.012mg-Vitamin C 100mg-Vitamin D 230 IU-Vitamin K 0.09mg-Zinc 11mg* *scored

WARNINGS/PRECAUTIONS: Accidental overdose of iron-containing products is a leading cause of fatal poisoning in children <6 yrs. Not for the treatment of pernicious anemia and other megaloblastic anemias where vitamin B_{12} is deficient. Folic acid >0.1mg/day may obscure pernicious anemia.

ADVERSE REACTIONS: Allergic sensitization.

MECHANISM OF ACTION: Prenatal vitamin.

PrimaCare One
folic acid - multiple vitamin - minerals (Ther-Rx)

RX

THERAPEUTIC CLASS: Prenatal vitamin

INDICATIONS: Vitamin, mineral, essential fatty acid supplementation throughout pregnancy, during the postnatal period for both lactating and non-lactating mothers, and throughout childbearing years. Also to improve nutritional status prior to conception.

DOSAGE: *Adults:* 1 cap qd.

HOW SUPPLIED: Cap: Omega-3 Fatty Acids 330mg-Linolenic Acid 30mg-Folic Acid 1mg-Vitamin B_6 25mg-Vitamin C 25mg-Vitamin D_3 170 IU-Vitamin E 30 IU-Calcium 150mg-Iron 27mg.

CONTRAINDICATIONS: Known hypersensitivity to any of the ingredients.

WARNINGS/PRECAUTIONS: Folic acid in doses above 1mg daily may obscure pernicious anemia (hematologic remission can occur while neurological manifestations remain progressive). Accidental overdose of iron-containing products is leading cause of fatal poisoning in children <6 yrs; keep out of reach of children. In case of overdose, call doctor or poison control center immediately.

ADVERSE REACTIONS: Allergic sensitization.

MECHANISM OF ACTION: Prenatal vitamin.

Primaxin I.M.
imipenem - cilastatin (Merck)

RX

THERAPEUTIC CLASS: Thienamycin/dehydropeptidase I inhibitor

INDICATIONS: Treatment of lower respiratory tract (LRTI), skin and skin structure (SSSI), intra-abdominal, and gynecologic infections caused by susceptible strains of microorganisms. Not for severe or life-threatening infections.

DOSAGE: *Adults:* Dose according to imipenem. Mild to Moderate LRTI/SSSI/Gynecologic Infection: 500mg or 750mg IM q12h depending on severity. Intra-Abdominal Infection: 750mg IM q12h. Continue for at least 2 days after symptoms resolve. Elderly: Start at low end of dosing range. Continue for at least 2 days after symptoms resolve; do not treat >14 days. Max: 1500mg/day. Avoid if CrCl <20mL/min.

Pediatrics: ≥12 yrs: Dose according to imipenem. Mild to Moderate LRTI/SSSI/ Gynecologic Infections: 500mg or 750mg IM q12h depending on severity. Intra-Abdominal Infection: 750mg IM q12h. Continue for at least 2 days after symptoms resolve; do not treat >14 days. Max: 1500mg/day. Avoid if CrCl <20mL/min.

HOW SUPPLIED: Inj: (Imipenem-Cilastatin) 500mg-500mg, 750mg-750mg

CONTRAINDICATIONS: Severe shock, heart block, hypersensitivity to local anesthetics of amide type (due to lidocaine diluent).

WARNINGS/PRECAUTIONS: Serious, sometimes fatal, hypersensitivity reactions reported with β-lactam therapy. *Clostridium difficile*-associated diarrhea reported. Prolonged use may result in overgrowth of nonsusceptible organisms. Avoid injection into blood vessel. Caution in elderly. CNS adverse events (eg, myoclonic activity, confusion, seizures) reported most commonly with CNS disorders and renal dysfunction; d/c if any occur. Positive Coombs test reported.

ADVERSE REACTIONS: Injection site pain, nausea, diarrhea, fever, vomiting, rash, hypotension, seizures, dizziness, pruritus, urticaria, somnolence.

INTERACTIONS: Avoid probenecid. Do not mix or physically add with other antibiotics. May give concomitantly with other antibiotics. May decrease levels of valproic acid.

PREGNANCY: Category C, caution in nursing.

MECHANISM OF ACTION: Imipenem: Thienamycin; inhibits cell-wall synthesis. Cilastatin: Dehydropeptidase I inhibitor; prevents renal metabolism of parent drug.

PHARMACOKINETICS: Absorption: Imipenem: C_{max}=10mcg/mL (500mg), 12mcg/mL (750mg); T_{max}=2 hrs. Cilastatin: C_{max}=24mcg/mL (500mg), 33mcg/mL (750mg); T_{max}=1 hr. **Distribution:** Imipenem: Plasma protein binding (20%). Cilastatin: Plasma protein binding (40%). **Metabolism:** Imipenem: Kidneys. **Elimination:** Imipenem: Urine; Cilastatin: Urine.

PRIMAXIN I.V. RX
imipenem - cilastatin (Merck)

THERAPEUTIC CLASS: Thienamycin/dehydropeptidase I inhibitor

INDICATIONS: Treatment of serious lower respiratory tract, urinary tract (UTI), intra-abdominal, gynecologic, skin and skin structure, bone and joint, septicemia, endocarditis, and polymicrobic infections caused by susceptible strains of microorganisms.

DOSAGE: *Adults:* ≥70kg and CrCl >70mL/min: Dose based on imipenem component. Uncomplicated UTI: 250mg q6h. Complicated UTI: 500mg q6h. Mild Infection: 250-500mg q6h. Moderate Infection: 500mg q6-8h or 1g q8h. Severe, Life-Threatening Infection: 500mg-1g q6h or 1g q8h. Max: 50mg/kg/day or 4g/day, whichever lower. Renal Impairment and/or <70kg: Refer to PI. CrCl 6-20mL/min: 125-250mg q12h. CrCl ≤5mL/min: Administer hemodialysis within 48 hrs of dose.
Pediatrics: ≥3 months: Dose based on imipenem component. Non-CNS Infections: 15-25mg/kg q6h. Max: 2g/day if susceptible or 4g/day if moderately susceptible. May use up to 90mg/kg/day in older cystic fibrosis children. 4 weeks-3 months and ≥1500g: 25mg/kg q6h. 1-4 weeks and ≥1500g: 25mg/kg q8h. <1 week and ≥1500g: 25mg/kg q12h. Not recommended with CNS infection, and <30kg with impaired renal function.

HOW SUPPLIED: Inj: (Imipenem-Cilastatin) 250mg-250mg, 500mg-500mg

WARNINGS/PRECAUTIONS: Serious, sometimes fatal, hypersensitivity reactions reported with β-lactam therapy. *Clostridium difficile*-associated diarrhea reported. Prolonged use may result in overgrowth of nonsusceptible organisms. CNS adverse events (eg, myoclonic activity, confusion, seizures) reported most commonly with CNS disorders and renal dysfunction.

ADVERSE REACTIONS: Phlebitis/thrombophlebitis, nausea, diarrhea, vomiting, rash, fever, hypotension, seizures, dizziness, pruritus, urticaria, somnolence, hepatitis (including fulminant hepatitis), hepatic failure.

INTERACTIONS: Seizures reported with ganciclovir; avoid concomitant use. Avoid probenecid. Do not mix or physically add to other antibiotics. May give concomitantly with other antibiotics. May decrease levels of valproic acid.

PREGNANCY: Category C, caution in nursing.

MECHANISM OF ACTION: Imipenem: Thienamycin; inhibits cell-wall synthesis. Cilastatin: Dehydropeptidase I inhibitor; prevents renal metabolism of parent drug.

PHARMACOKINETICS: Absorption: Variable doses resulted in different parameters. **Distribution:** Imipenem: Plasma protein binding (20%). Cilastatin: Plasma protein binding (40%). **Metabolism:** Imipenem: Kidneys. **Elimination:** Imipenem: Urine (70%); Cilastatin: Urine (70%).

PRIMSOL RX
trimethoprim HCL (FSC Laboratories)

THERAPEUTIC CLASS: Tetrahydrofolic acid inhibitor

INDICATIONS: Treatment of acute otitis media in pediatrics and urinary tract infection (UTI) in adults due to susceptible microorganisms.

DOSAGE: *Adults:* UTI: Usual: 100mg q12h or 200mg q24h for 10 days. CrCl: 15-30mL/min: Give 50% of usual dose.
Pediatrics: Otitis Media: ≥6 months: 5mg/kg q12h for 10 days. CrCl: 15-30mL/min: Give 50% of usual dose.

HOW SUPPLIED: Sol: 50mg/5mL

CONTRAINDICATIONS: Megaloblastic anemia due to folate deficiency.

WARNINGS/PRECAUTIONS: May interfere with hematopoiesis. Serious blood disorders; monitor for sore throat, fever, pallor, and purpura. Caution with folate deficiency and renal/hepatic impairment, diarrhea, rash.

ADVERSE REACTIONS: Epigastric distress, nausea, vomiting, anemia, methemoglobinemia, hyperkalemia, hyponatremia, fever, elevation of serum transaminases and bilirubin, increases BUN and serum creatinine.

INTERACTIONS: May inhibit phenytoin metabolism.

PREGNANCY: Category C, caution in nursing.

MECHANISM OF ACTION: Dihydrofolate reductase inhibitor; blocks production of tetrahydrofolic acid from dihydrofolic acid by binding to and reversibly inhibiting dihydrofolate reductase.

PHARMACOKINETICS: Absorption: Rapid; C_{max}=1mcg/mL; T_{max}=1-4 hrs. **Distribution:** Crosses placenta; found in breast milk. **Metabolism:** Liver. 1- and 3-oxide, 3'- and 4'-hydroxy derivative (principal metabolites). **Elimination:** Urine; $T_{1/2}$=9 hrs.

PRINIVIL RX
lisinopril (Merck)

ACE inhibitors can cause death/injury to developing fetus during 2nd and 3rd trimesters. Stop therapy if pregnancy detected.

THERAPEUTIC CLASS: ACE inhibitor

INDICATIONS: Treatment of hypertension. Adjunct therapy in heart failure if inadequately controlled by diuretics and digitalis. Adjunct therapy in stable patients within 24 hrs of AMI to improve survival.

DOSAGE: *Adults:* HTN: If possible, d/c diuretic 2-3 days prior to therapy. Initial: 10mg qd; 5mg qd with diuretic. Usual: 20-40mg qd. Resume diuretic if BP not controlled. Max: 80mg/day. CrCl 10-30mL/min: Initial: 5mg/day. Max: 40mg/day. CrCl <10mL/min: Initial: 2.5mg/day. Max: 40mg/day. Heart Failure:

Initial: 5mg qd. Usual: 5-20mg qd. Hyponatremia or CrCl ≤30mL/min: Initial: 2.5mg qd. AMI: Initial: 5mg within 24 hrs, then 5mg after 24 hrs, then 10mg after 48 hrs, then daily. Use 2.5mg during first 3 days with low systolic BP. Maint: 10mg qd for 6 weeks, 2.5-5mg with hypotension. D/C with prolonged hypotension. Elderly: Caution with dose adjustment.
Pediatrics: ≥6 yrs: HTN: Initial: 0.07mg/kg qd (up to 5mg total). Adjust dose based on BP response. Max: 0.61mg/kg qd (40mg/day).

HOW SUPPLIED: Tab: 5mg*, 10mg*, 20mg* *scored

CONTRAINDICATIONS: History of ACE inhibitor-associated angioedema and hereditary or idiopathic angioedema.

WARNINGS/PRECAUTIONS: Intestinal/head/neck angioedema reported. D/C if angioedema, jaundice, or if marked LFT elevation occurs. Risk of hyperkalemia with DM, renal dysfunction. Persistent nonproductive cough reported. Monitor WBCs in renal and collagen vascular disease. Anaphylactoid reactions reported. Fetal/neonatal morbidity and death reported. Monitor for hypotension in high-risk patients (eg, heart failure with systolic BP <100mmHg, surgery/anesthesia, hyponatremia, high dose diuretic therapy, severe volume and/or salt depletion). Caution with renal artery stenosis, CHF, renal dysfunction, or if obstruction to left ventricle outflow tract. Less effective on BP in blacks and more reports of angioedema than nonblacks. Caution in hypoglycemia and leukopenia/neutropenia. Patients should report any indication of infection which may be sign of leukopenia/neutropenia.

ADVERSE REACTIONS: Hypotension, diarrhea, headache, dizziness, cough, chest pain.

INTERACTIONS: May increase lithium levels. Hypotension risk with diuretics. May further decrease renal dysfunction with NSAIDs. Hyperkalemia with K^+-sparing diuretics, K^+-containing salt substitutes, or K^+ supplements. Nitroid reactions have been reported rarely in patients on therapy with injectable gold and concomitant ACE inhibitor therapy. NSAIDs may diminish antihypertensive effects.

PREGNANCY: Category C (1st trimester) and D (2nd and 3rd trimesters), not for use in nursing.

MECHANISM OF ACTION: ACE inhibitor; inhibition results in decreased plasma angiotensin II, which leads to decreased vasopressor activity and aldosterone secretion.

PHARMACOKINETICS: Absorption: 25%; T_{max}=7 hrs. **Elimination:** Urine (unchanged); $T_{1/2}$=12 hr.

PRINZIDE   RX
lisinopril - hydrochlorothiazide (Merck)

> ACE inhibitors can cause death/injury to developing fetus during 2nd and 3rd trimesters. Stop therapy if pregnancy detected.

THERAPEUTIC CLASS: ACE inhibitor/thiazide diuretic

INDICATIONS: Treatment of hypertension. Not for initial therapy.

DOSAGE: *Adults:* Initial (if not controlled with lisinopril/HCTZ monotherapy): 10mg-12.5mg tab or 20mg-12.5mg tab daily. Titrate: May increase after 2-3 weeks. Initial (if controlled on 25mg HCTZ/day with hypokalemia): 10mg-12.5mg tab. Replacement Therapy: Substitute combination for titrated components.

HOW SUPPLIED: Tab: (Lisinopril-HCTZ) 10mg-12.5mg, 20mg-12.5mg, 20mg-25mg

CONTRAINDICATIONS: History of ACE inhibitor associated angioedema and hereditary or idiopathic angioedema. Anuria, sulfonamide hypersensitivity.

WARNINGS/PRECAUTIONS: D/C if angioedema, jaundice, or if marked LFT elevation occurs. Risk of hyperkalemia with DM, renal dysfunction. Persistent nonproductive cough reported. Agranulocytosis and bone marrow depression in renal impairment, especially with collagen vascular disease; monitor WBCs in renal disease and collagen vascular disease. Anaphylactoid reactions reported. Fetal/neonatal morbidity and death reported. Monitor for hypotension in high-risk patients (eg, surgery/anesthesia, volume/salt depletion). Caution with CHF, renal or hepatic dysfunction, obstruction to left ventricle outflow tract, renal artery stenosis, elderly. More reports of angioedema in blacks than nonblacks. May exacerbate or activate SLE. Monitor electrolytes. Avoid if CrCl ≤30mL/min/1.73m². May increase cholesterol, TG. Hypercalcemia, hyperglycemia, hypomagnesemia, hyperuricemia may occur.

ADVERSE REACTIONS: Dizziness, cough, fatigue, orthostatic effects, diarrhea, nausea, muscle cramps, angioedema.

INTERACTIONS: Increase risk of hyperkalemia with K⁺-sparing diuretics, K⁺ supplements, or K⁺-containing salt substitutes. Potentiates orthostatic hypotension with alcohol, barbiturates, and narcotics. Adjust antidiabetic drugs. Reduced absorption with cholestyramine, colestipol. Corticosteroids, ACTH deplete electrolytes. May decrease response to pressor amines. Potentiates other antihypertensives. May increase responsiveness to skeletal muscle relaxants. Risk of lithium toxicity. NSAIDs reduce effects and worsen renal dysfunction. Nitroid reactions have been reported rarely in patients on therapy with injectable gold and concomitant ACE inhibitor therapy. Patients on diuretics may experience an excessive reduction of blood pressure.

PREGNANCY: Category C (1st trimester) and D (2nd and 3rd trimesters), not for use in nursing.

MECHANISM OF ACTION: Lisinopril: ACE inhibitor. Inhibition results in decreased plasma angiotensin II, which leads to decreased vasopressor activity and decreased aldosterone secretion. HCTZ: Thiazide diuretic. Affects renal tubular mechanism of electrolyte reabsorption, directly increasing excretion of sodium salt and chloride.

PHARMACOKINETICS: Absorption: Lisinopril: T_{max}=7 hrs. **Distribution:** Lisinopril: Crosses blood-brain barrier. HCTZ: Crosses placental barrier. **Elimination:** Lisinopril: Urine (unchanged); $T_{1/2}$=12 hrs. HCTZ: Renal (61%-unchanged); $T_{1/2}$=5.6-14.8 hrs.

PRISTIQ   RX
desvenlafaxine (Wyeth)

> Antidepressants increased the risk of suicidal thinking and behavior (suicidality) in short-term studies in children, adolescents, and young adults with Major Depressive Disorder (MDD) and other psychiatric disorders. Desvenlafaxine is not approved for use in pediatric patients.

THERAPEUTIC CLASS: Serotonin and norepinephrine reuptake inhibitor

INDICATIONS: Treatment of major depressive disorder (MDD).

DOSAGE: *Adults:* ≥18 yrs: 50mg qd. Renal Impairment (CrCl<30mL/min) or ESRD: 50mg every other day. Supplemental doses should not be given to patients after dialysis. Hepatic Impairment: Max: 100mg/day. Upon discontinuation: Gradually reduce dose (giving 50mg less frequently) rather than abrupt cessation. Do not divide, crush, chew or place in water.

HOW SUPPLIED: Tab, Extended-Release: 50mg, 100mg

CONTRAINDICATIONS: Concomitant MAOI or within 14 days of stopping.

WARNINGS/PRECAUTIONS: Worsening of depression and/or emergence of suicidal behavior may occur. Serotonin syndrome reported; caution with concomitant serotonergic drugs. May cause sustained increases in BP; monitor BP regularly. May increase the risk of bleeding events. Monitor with increased IOP or if at risk of acute narrow-angle glaucoma. Activation of mania/hypomania reported. Caution with cardiovascular or cerebrovascular disease, recent MI, renal impairment, and seizure disorder. Cholesterol and triglyceride elevation may occur; consider monitoring. Discontinuation symptoms occurred; taper dose and monitor symptoms. Hyponatremia may occur. Interstitial lung disease and eosinophilic pneumonia may occur.

ADVERSE REACTIONS: Headache, nausea, dry mouth, diarrhea, dizziness, insomnia, somnolence, hyperhidrosis, fatigue, constipation, vomiting, palpitations, anxiety, decreased appetite, specific male sexual disorders.

INTERACTIONS: See Contraindications. Avoid within 14 days of MAOI therapy. Upon discontinuation, wait at least 7 days before starting MAOI therapy. Caution with potent inhibitors of CYP3A4 and CYP2D6, CNS-active drugs (eg, triptans, SSRIs, lithium), and with serotonergic drugs (eg, tramadol, tryptophans, SNRIs). Aspirin, NSAIDs, warfarin, and other anticoagulants may increase the risk of bleeding. Avoid alcohol. Avoid products containing venlafaxine and desvenlafaxine.

PREGNANCY: Category C, not for use in nursing.

MECHANISM OF ACTION: Potent and selective serotonin and norepinephrine reuptake inhibitor; potentiates neurotransmitter activity of CNS activity by inhibiting neuronal serotonin and norepinephrine reuptake.

PHARMACOKINETICS: Absorption: Absolute oral bioavailability (80%); T_{max}=7.5 hrs. **Distribution:** Plasma protein binding (30%); V_d=3.4L/kg. **Metabolism:** Conjugation and via CYP3A4 mediated oxidation (minor). **Elimination:** Urine (45% unchanged).

ProAir HFA RX
albuterol sulfate (Ivax)

THERAPEUTIC CLASS: Beta$_2$-agonist

INDICATIONS: Prevention and treatment of bronchospasm with reversible obstructive airway disease; prevention of exercise-induced bronchospasm (EIB) in patients ≥12 yrs.

DOSAGE: *Adults:* Bronchospasm or Asthmatic Symptoms: 2 inh q4-6h or 1 inh q4h. EIB: 2 inh 15-30 min before activity.
Pediatrics: ≥12 yrs: Bronchospasm or Asthmatic Symptoms: 2 inh q4-6h or 1 inh q4h. EIB: 2 inh 15-30 min before activity.

HOW SUPPLIED: MDI: 90mcg/inh [8.5g]

WARNINGS/PRECAUTIONS: Hypersensitivity reactions reported. Monitor for worsening asthma. Fatalities reported with excessive use. Caution with cardiovascular disorders, especially coronary insufficiency, arrhythmias and HTN. May need concomitant corticosteroids. Can produce paradoxical bronschospasm. Caution with DM, hyperthyroidism, and seizures. May cause transient hypokalemia.

ADVERSE REACTIONS: Pharyngitis, headache, rhinitis, dizziness, pain, tachycardia, tremor, nervousness.

INTERACTIONS: Avoid other sympathomimetic agents. Extreme caution with MAOIs and TCAs, and β-blockers. Monitor digoxin. May worsen ECG changes and/or hypokalemia with nonpotassium-sparing diuretics.

PREGNANCY: Category C, not for use in nursing.

MECHANISM OF ACTION: β$_2$-adrenergic bronchodilator; stimulates adenyl cylase, the enzyme that catalyzes the formation of cAMP from ATP. Increased cAMP levels are associated with relaxation of bronchial smooth muscle and inhibition of release of mediators of immediate hypersensitivity.

PHARMACOKINETICS: Absorption: C_{max}=4100pg/mL; AUC=28,426pg•hr/mL. **Metabolism:** GI tract by SULTIA3. **Elimination:** Renal excretion (80-100%), urine (unchanged), feces (≤20%); $T_{1/2}$=6 hrs.

ProAmatine RX
midodrine HCL (Shire)

> Can cause marked elevation of supine BP. Clinical benefits of improving ability to carry out activities of daily living have not been verified.

THERAPEUTIC CLASS: Alpha$_1$-agonist

INDICATIONS: Treatment of symptomatic orthostatic hypotension.

DOSAGE: *Adults:* Initial: 10mg tid; at 3-4 hr intervals, while awake. Max: 30mg/day. To avoid supine HTN during sleep, do not give <4 hrs before bedtime or after evening meal. Renal Dysfunction: Initial: 2.5mg tid.

HOW SUPPLIED: Tab: 2.5mg*, 5mg*, 10mg *scored

CONTRAINDICATIONS: Severe organic heart disease, acute renal disease, urinary retention, pheochromocytoma, thyrotoxicosis, persistent and excessive HTN.

WARNINGS/PRECAUTIONS: Risk of supine HTN; monitor for symptoms (eg, pounding in ears, headache, blurred vision), supine and standing BP; d/c if supine HTN persists. Caution with urinary retention, diabetes, renal or hepatic dysfunction. Decreased HR due to vagal reflex.

ADVERSE REACTIONS: Supine and siting HTN, paresthesia, scalp pruritus, goosebumps, chills, urinary urge/retention/frequency.

INTERACTIONS: Monitor BP with vasoconstrictors (eg, phenylephrine, ephedrine, dihydroergotamine, pseudoephedrine). Fludrocortisone may potentiate supine HTN due to salt-retaining properties. OTC cold and diet products may potentiate pressor effects. Antagonized by -blockers (eg, prazosin, terazosin, doxazosin). Metformin, cimetidine, ranitidine, procainamide, triamterene, flecainide, and quinidine may increase clearance. Caution with cardiac glycosides, psychopharmacologics, and β-blockers.

PREGNANCY: Category C, caution in nursing.

MECHANISM OF ACTION: Desglymidodrine; (major metabolite); Alpha$_1$-agonist; It exerts its actions via activation of the alpha-adrenergic receptors of the arteriolar and venous vasculature, producing an increase in vascular tone and elevation of BP.

PHARMACOKINETICS: Absorption: Rapid; absolute bioavailability (93%), Midodrine; (prodrug); T_{max}=1/2 hr. Desglymidodrine; T_{max}=1-2 hrs. **Distribution:** Poorly, across blood-brain barrier. **Metabolism:** Liver; via; deglycination to desglymidodrine (major metabolite). **Elimination:** Urine; (metabolite; 80%).

PROBENECID   RX
probenecid (Various)

THERAPEUTIC CLASS: Uricosuric

INDICATIONS: Treatment of hyperuricemia associated with gout and gouty arthritis. Adjunct to penicillin, ampicillin, methicillin, oxacillin, cloxacillin, or nafcillin for elevation and prolongation of plasma levels.

DOSAGE: *Adults:* Gout: Initial: 250mg bid for 1 week. Titrate: May increase by 500mg every 4 weeks. Maint: 500mg bid. Max: 2g/day. May reduce by 500mg every 6 months if acute attack has been absent ≥6 months and serum urate levels are normal. Renal Impairment: Usual: 1g/day. Adjunct Antibiotic Therapy: 500mg qid. Elderly/Renal Impairment: Reduce dose. Decrease dose with gastric intolerance. May not be effective if CrCl ≤30mL/min.
Pediatrics: 2-14 yrs: Adjunct Antibiotic Therapy: Initial: 25mg/kg. Maint: 10mg/kg qid. ≥50kg: 500mg qid.

HOW SUPPLIED: Tab: 500mg

CONTRAINDICATIONS: Blood dyscrasias, uric acid kidney stones and children <2 yrs. Do not use in acute gout attack.

WARNINGS/PRECAUTIONS: Initiate therapy when acute gout attack subsides. Exacerbation of gout may occur; treat with colchicine. Use APAP if analgesic needed. Severe allergic reactions and anaphylaxis reported. D/C if hypersensitivity occurs. Caution with peptic ulcer. Monitor for glycosuria. Maintain liberal fluid intake and alkalization of urine.

ADVERSE REACTIONS: Headache, acute gouty arthritis, dizziness, hepatic necrosis, vomiting, nausea, anorexia, sore gums, nephrotic syndrome, uric acid stones, renal colic, costovertebral pain, urinary frequency, anaphylaxis, fever, urticaria, pruritus, blood dyscrasias, dermatitis, alopecia, flushing.

INTERACTIONS: Probenecid increases plasma levels of penicillin and other β-lactams; psychic disturbances reported. Avoid use with penicillin in the presence of renal impairment. Salicylates and pyrazinamide antagonize uricosuric effects. Increased plasma levels of methotrexate, sulfonamides, sulfonylureas, thiopental or ketamine-induced anesthesia, some NSAIDs (eg, indomethacin, naproxen), lorazepam, APAP, and rifampin. Possible false high plasma levels of theophylline.

PREGNANCY: Safety in pregnancy and nursing is not known.

MECHANISM OF ACTION: Uricosuric/renal tubular blocking agent; inhibits tubular reabsorption of urate, increasing urinary excretion of uric acid and decreasing serum urate levels.

PROCARDIA XL   RX
nifedipine (Pfizer)

THERAPEUTIC CLASS: Calcium channel blocker (dihydropyridine)

INDICATIONS: Management of vasospastic angina and chronic stable angina. Treatment of hypertension.

DOSAGE: *Adults:* Angina/HTN: Initial: 30-60mg qd. Titrate over 7-14 days. Max: 120mg/day. Caution if dose >90mg with angina.

HOW SUPPLIED: Tab, Extended-Release: 30mg, 60mg, 90mg

WARNINGS/PRECAUTIONS: May cause hypotension; monitor BP initially or with titration. May exacerbate angina from β-blocker withdrawal. CHF risk, especially with aortic stenosis or β-blockers. Peripheral edema reported. May increase angina or MI with severe obstructive CAD. Caution in pre-existing severe GI narrowing.

ADVERSE REACTIONS: Dizziness, lightheadedness, giddiness, flushing, muscle cramps, headache, weakness, nausea, peripheral edema, nervousness/mood changes.

INTERACTIONS: β-Blockers may increase risk of CHF, severe hypotension, or angina exacerbation. Possible hypotension with fentanyl. Potentiates digoxin. Monitor quinidine, coumarin. Potentiated by cimetidine and grapefruit juice. Avoid grapefruit juice.

PREGNANCY: Category C, unknown use in nursing.

MECHANISM OF ACTION: Calcium channel blocker: inhibits calcium ion influx into cardiac muscle and smooth muscle.

PHARMACOKINETICS: Absorption: Complete. **Distribution:** Plasma protein binding (92-98%). **Metabolism:** Hepatic Biotransformation. **Elimination:** Urine, feces; $T_{1/2}$=2 hrs.

PROCHLORPERAZINE   RX
prochlorperazine (Various)

THERAPEUTIC CLASS: Phenothiazine derivative

INDICATIONS: Control of severe nausea and vomiting. Management of psychotic disorders (eg, schizophrenia). Short-term treatment of generalized non-psychotic anxiety.

DOSAGE: *Adults:* Nausea/Vomiting: (Tab) Usual: 5-10mg tid-qid. Max: 40mg/day. (IM) 5-10mg IM q3-4h prn. Max: 40mg/day. (IV) 2.5-10mg IV (not bolus). Max: 10mg single dose and 40mg/day. Nausea/Vomiting with Surgery: 5-10mg IM 1-2 hrs or 5-10mg IV 15-30 min before anesthesia, or during or after surgery; repeat once if needed. Non-Psychotic Anxiety: (Tab) 5mg tid-qid; Psychosis: Mild/Outpatient: 5-10mg PO tid-qid. Moderate-Severe/Hospitalized: Initial: 10mg PO tid-qid. May increase in small increments every 2-3 days. Severe: (PO) 100-150mg/day. (IM) 10-20mg, may repeat q2-4 hrs if needed. Switch to oral after obtain control or if needed, 10-20mg IM q4-6h. Elderly: use lower dosing range and titrate more gradually.
Pediatrics: Nausea/Vomiting: >2 yrs and >20 lbs: (PO/PR) 20-29 lbs: Usual: 2.5mg qd-bid. Max: 7.5mg/day. 30-39 lbs: 2.5mg bid-tid. Max: 10mg/day. 40-85 lbs: 2.5mg tid or 5mg bid. Max: 15mg/day. (IM) 0.06mg/lb, usually single

dose for control. Psychosis: (PO/PR) 2-12 yrs: Initial: 2.5mg bid-tid, up to 10mg/day on 1st day. Max: 2-5 yrs: 20mg/day. 6-12 yrs: 25mg/day. (IM) <12 yrs: 0.06mg/lb single dose. Switch to oral after obtain control.

HOW SUPPLIED: Inj: (Edisylate) 5mg/mL; Sup: 5mg, 25mg; Tab: (Maleate) 5mg, 10mg

CONTRAINDICATIONS: Comatose states, concomitant large dose CNS depressants (alcohol, barbiturates, narcotics), pediatric surgery, pediatrics <2 yrs or <20lbs.

WARNINGS/PRECAUTIONS: Secondary extrapyramidal symptoms can occur. Tardive dyskinesia, NMS may develop. Caution with activities requiring alertness. May mask symptoms of overdose of other drugs. May obscure diagnosis of intestinal obstruction, brain tumor, and Reye's syndrome. May interfere with thermoregulation. Caution with glaucoma, cardiac disorders. Caution in children with dehydration or acute illness and the elderly. D/C 48 hrs before myelography and may resume after 24 hrs post-procedure.

ADVERSE REACTIONS: Drowsiness, dizziness, amenorrhea, blurred vision, skin reactions, hypotension, NMS, cholestatic jaundice.

INTERACTIONS: May decrease oral anticoagulant effects. May potentiate α-adrenergic blockade. Thiazide diuretics potentiate orthostatic hypotension. Increased levels of both drugs with propranolol. Anticonvulsants may need adjustment. Risk of encephalopathic syndrome with lithium. May antagonize antihypertensive effects of guanethidine and related compounds.

PREGNANCY: Safety in pregnancy is not known; caution in nursing.

MECHANISM OF ACTION: Phenothiazine derivative; anti-emetic and antipsychotic.

PROCRIT   RX
epoetin alfa (Ortho Biotech)

> Increased mortality, serious cardiovascular/thromboembolic events, and tumor progression. (Renal Failure) Patients experienced greater risks for death and serious cardiovascular events when administered erythropoiesis-stimulating agents (ESAs) to target higher vs lower Hgb levels (13.5 vs 11.3 g/dL; 14 vs 10 g/dL) in 2 clinical studies. Individualize dosing to achieve and maintain Hgb levels within range of 10-12g/dL. (Cancer) ESAs shortened overall survival and/or time-to-tumor progression in clinical studies in patients with breast, head and neck, lymphoid, non-small cell lung, and cervical cancers when dosed to target Hgb ≥12g/dL. The risks of shortened survival and tumor progression have not been excluded when ESAs are dosed to target Hgb <12g/dL. To minimize these risks, as well as the risk of serious cardio- and thrombovascular events, use lowest dose needed to avoid RBC transfusions. Use only for treatment of anemia due to concomitant myelosuppressive chemotherapy. D/C following completion of a chemotherapy course. (Perisurgery) Epoetin alfa increased the rate of DVT in patients not receiving prophylactic anticoagulation. Consider DVT prophylaxis.

THERAPEUTIC CLASS: Erythropoiesis stimulator

INDICATIONS: Treatment of anemia due to chronic renal failure (CRF), anemia related to zidovudine treatment of HIV, chemotherapy-induced anemia in non-myeloid malignancies, and reduction of allogeneic blood transfusions in anemic patients (>10 to ≤13g/dL) scheduled for elective, noncardiac, nonvascular surgery.

DOSAGE: *Adults:* CRF: Initial: 50-100 U/kg IV/SQ 3x/week. IV is preferred route in dialysis patients. Maint: Individually titrate. Reduce if Hgb approaches 12g/dL or if Hgb increases >1g/dL in any 2-week period. Increase when Hgb does not increase by 2g/dL after 8 weeks of therapy and Hgb is below target range (10-12g/dL). Zidovudine-Treated HIV Patients: If serum erythropoietin levels ≤500 mU/mL and zidovudine ≤4200mg/week, give 100 U/kg IV/SQ 3x/week for 8 weeks. Titrate: Increase by 50-100 U/kg 3x/week after 8 weeks if necessary. Max: 300 U/kg 3x/week. Maint: If Hgb >13g/dL, d/c until Hgb <12g/dL, then reduce dose by 25% when therapy resumes. Chemotherapy-Induced Anemia: Initial: 150 U/kg SQ 3x/week. Titrate: Reduce by 25% when Hgb approaches 12g/dL or Hgb increases >1g/dL in any 2-week period. If Hgb >13g/dL, withhold until Hgb <12g/dL then restart at 25% below previous dose. May increase to 300 U/kg 3x/week if no response after 8 weeks of therapy.

Max: 300 U/kg 3x/week. Weekly Dosing: 40,000 U SQ weekly. Titrate: If Hgb not increased by ≥1g/dL after 4 weeks, increase to 60,000 U weekly. If Hgb >13g/dL, withhold until Hgb <12g/dL then restart with 25% dose reduction. Reduce dose by 25% if very rapid Hgb response (eg, increase >1g/dL in any 2-week period). Max: 60,000 U weekly. Surgery: 300 U/kg/day SQ for 10 days before surgery, on surgery day, and 4 days post-op or 600 U/kg SQ once weekly on 21, 14, and 7 days before surgery and a 4th dose on surgery day, with adequate iron supplement.

Pediatrics: CRF: Initial: 50 U/kg 3x/week IV/SQ. Titrate: Reduce if Hgb approaches 12g/dL or if Hgb increases by >1g/dL in any 2-week period. Increase if Hgb does not increase by 2g/dL after 8 weeks of therapy and Hgb is below target range (10-12g/dL). Maint: Individually titrate. Chemotherapy Induced Anemia: Initial: 600 U/kg IV weekly. Titrate: If Hgb not increased by ≥1g/dL after 4 weeks, increase to 900 U/kg IV weekly. If Hgb >13g/dL, withhold until Hgb <12g/dL then restart with 25% dose reduction. Reduce dose by 25% if very rapid Hgb response (eg, increase >1g/dL in any 2-week period). Max: 60,000 U weekly.

HOW SUPPLIED: Inj: 2000 U/mL, 3000 U/mL, 4000 U/mL, 10,000 U/mL, 20,000 U/mL, 40,000 U/mL

CONTRAINDICATIONS: Uncontrolled HTN. Hypersensitivity to mammalian cell-derived products and albumin (human).

WARNINGS/PRECAUTIONS: Pure red cell aplasia and severe anemia (with or without other cytopenias) may occur. Caution with porphyria, HTN, or history of seizures. Monitor patients with pre-existing CV disease closely. Evaluate iron stores before and during therapy; most patients need iron supplementation. Monitor Hgb, BP, iron levels, serum chemistry, and CBC. Multidose formulation contains benzyl alcohol, which has been associated with an increased incidence of neurological and other complications in premature infants; these compilcations are sometimes fatal.

ADVERSE REACTIONS: HTN, headache, fatigue, arthralgias, nausea, vomiting, diarrhea, edema, rash, pyrexia, constipation, respiratory congestion, dyspnea, asthenia, skin reaction.

INTERACTIONS: Adjust anticoagulant dose in dialysis patients.

PREGNANCY: Category C, caution in nursing.

MECHANISM OF ACTION: Erythropoiesis stimulator.

PHARMACOKINETICS: Absorption: (SQ) T_{max}=5-24 hrs. **Elimination:** (IV) $T_{1/2}$=4-13 hrs.

P

PROCTOCORT CREAM   RX
hydrocortisone (Salix)

THERAPEUTIC CLASS: Corticosteroid

INDICATIONS: Corticosteroid responsive dermatoses.

DOSAGE: *Adults:* Apply bid-qid. May use occlusive dressings for psoriasis or recalcitrant conditions; d/c dressings if infection develops.
Pediatrics: Apply bid-qid. May use occlusive dressings for psoriasis or recalcitrant conditions; d/c dressings if infection develops.

HOW SUPPLIED: Cre: 1% [30g]

WARNINGS/PRECAUTIONS: May produce reversible HPA axis suppression, manifestations of Cushing's syndrome, hyperglycemia, and glucosuria. Caution when applied to large surface areas or under occlusive dressings. Use appropriate therapy with infections. Pediatrics may be more susceptible to systemic toxicity. D/C if irritation occurs. Avoid eyes.

ADVERSE REACTIONS: Burning, itching, irritation, dryness, folliculitis, hypertrichosis, acneiform eruptions, hypopigmentation, perioral dermatitis, allergic contact dermatitis, maceration skin, secondary infection, skin atrophy, striae, miliaria.

PREGNANCY: Category C, caution in nursing.

MECHANISM OF ACTION: Topical corticosteroid; not established. Suspected to have anti-inflammatory, antipruritic, and vasoconstrictive activities.

PHARMACOKINETICS: Absorption: Skin. **Metabolism:** Liver. **Elimination:** Kidneys (major); bile (minor).

PROCTOCORT SUPPOSITORY

RX

hydrocortisone acetate (Salix)

THERAPEUTIC CLASS: Corticosteroid

INDICATIONS: For use in inflamed hemorrhoids and post irradiation (factitial) proctitis. Adjunct for chronic ulcerative colitis, cryptitis, other anorectum inflammation and pruritus ani.

DOSAGE: *Adults:* Nonspecific Proctitis: 1 sup rectally bid for 2 weeks. More Severe Cases: 1 sup rectally tid or 2 sup rectally bid. Factitial Proctitis: Use up to 6-8 weeks.

HOW SUPPLIED: Sup: 30mg [12^s 24^s]

WARNINGS/PRECAUTIONS: D/C if irritation develops. D/C if infection that does not respond to appropriate therapy develops. May stain fabric. Only use after adequate proctologic exam.

ADVERSE REACTIONS: Burning, itching, irritation, dryness, folliculitis, hypo-pigmentation, allergic contact dermatitis, secondary infection.

PREGNANCY: Category C, not for use in nursing.

MECHANISM OF ACTION: Corticosteroid; has anti-inflammatory, antipruritic, and vasoconstrictive action.

PROGRAF

RX

tacrolimus (Astellas)

> Increased susceptibility to infection and development of lymphoma.

THERAPEUTIC CLASS: Macrolide immunosuppressant

INDICATIONS: Prophylaxis of organ rejection in allogenic liver, kidney, or heart transplants with concomitant adrenal corticosteroids. In heart transplant patients, azathioprine or mycophenolate mofetil co-administration is recommended.

DOSAGE: *Adults:* Initial (6h after transplantation): 0.03-0.05mg/kg/day (liver, kidney) or 0.01mg/kg/day (heart) IV infusion if cannot tolerate PO. Hepatic Transplant: 0.05-0.075mg/kg PO q12h with grapefruit juice; start 8-12 hrs after last IV dose. Kidney Transplant: 0.1mg/kg PO q12h, 24 hrs after transplant or until renal function recovered. Heart Transplant: 0.0375mg/kg PO q12h; start 8-12 hrs after last IV dose. Renal/Hepatic Impairment: Give lowest recommended dose. Severe Hepatic Impairment (Pugh ≥10): May require lower doses. Wait at least 48 hrs with post-op oliguria.
Pediatrics: Liver Transplant: Initial: 0.03-0.05mg/kg/day IV or 0.15-0.2mg/kg/day PO. Severe Hepatic Impairment (Pugh ≥10): May require lower doses.

HOW SUPPLIED: Cap: 0.5mg, 1mg, 5mg; Inj: 5mg/mL

CONTRAINDICATIONS: Hypersensitivity to HCO-60.

WARNINGS/PRECAUTIONS: Insulin-dependent post-transplant DM, HTN, myocardial hypertrophy, neurotoxicity, hyperkalemia, nephrotoxicity reported. Monitor drug levels frequently to prevent organ rejection and/or reduce potential toxicity. Monitor for anaphylaxis with infusion. Monitor levels closely with hepatic impairment.

ADVERSE REACTIONS: HTN, headache, insomnia, fever, pruritus, hyperglycemia, hyperkalemia, hypomagnesemia, diarrhea, nausea, vomiting, increased BUN, anorexia, constipation, tremor, rash, pleural effusion, gastroenteritis.

INTERACTIONS: CYP450 3A inducers (eg, carbamazepine, phenobarbital, phenytoin, rifabutin, rifampin, St. John's wort, etc.) may decrease plasma levels. Caution with other nephrotoxic drugs (eg. aminoglycosides, ampho-tericin B, cisplatin). May affect drugs metabolized by CYP450 3A. Avoid grapefruit juice. CYP450 3A inhibitors (eg, diltiazem, nicardipine, nifedipine, verapamil, azole antifungal, macrolides, cisapride, metoclopramide, etc) may increase plasma levels. Vaccination may be less effective. Avoid live vaccines, cyclosporine (when switching to tacrolimus, wait at least 24 hrs. after last cyclosporine dose), and K+ sparing diuretics.

PREGNANCY: Category C, not for use in nursing.

MECHANISM OF ACTION: Macrolide immunosuppressant; not established. Suspected to inhibit T-lymphocyte activation. Binds to intracellular protein (FKBP-12). Complex of tacrolimus-FKBP-12, calcium, calmodulin, and calcineurin is then formed and phosphatase activity of calcineurin inhibited. Effect may prevent dephosphorylation and translocation of nuclear factor of activated T cells (NF-AT), a nuclear component responsible for initiating gene transcription for the formation of lymphokines. Results in inhibition of T-lymphocyte activation.

PHARMACOKINETICS: Absorption: (PO) Incomplete and variable, absolute bioavailability (18%), C_{max}=29.7ng/mL, T_{max}=1.6 hrs, AUC=243ng•hr/mL; (IV) AUC=598ng•hr/mL. **Distribution:** Plasma protein binding (99%), appears in breast milk; (PO) V_d=1.94L/kg; (IV) V_d=1.91 L/kg. **Metabolism:** Hepatic, via CYP3A (demethylation and hydroxylation); 13-methyl tacrolimus (major metabolite); 31-demethyl (active metabolite). **Elimination:** (PO) Feces (92%), urine (2.3%); $T_{1/2}$=34.8 hrs. (IV) Feces (92.4%); $T_{1/2}$=34.2 hrs. Refer to PI for parameters in patients with renal, hepatic, and cardiac transplants.

PROLASTIN   RX
alpha1-proteinase inhibitor (human) (Talecris)

THERAPEUTIC CLASS: Alpha$_1$-Proteinase Inhibitor

INDICATIONS: Chronic replacement therapy of individuals having congenital deficiency of alpha$_1$-proteinase inhibitor (alpha$_1$-antitrypsin deficiency) with clinically demonstrable panacinar emphysema.

DOSAGE: *Adults:* 60mg/kg IV once weekly.

HOW SUPPLIED: Inj: 500mg, 1000mg

CONTRAINDICATIONS: IgA deficiencies with known antibodies against IgA.

WARNINGS/PRECAUTIONS: May contain infectious agents (eg, viruses). May cause increase in plasma volume.

ADVERSE REACTIONS: Delayed fever, lightheadedness, dizziness, flu-like symptoms, allergic-like reactions, chills, dyspnea, rash, tachycardia.

PREGNANCY: Category C, caution in nursing.

MECHANISM OF ACTION: Alpha$_1$-proteinase enzyme inhibitor.

PROLEUKIN   RX
aldesleukin (Chiron)

> Caution with history of cardiac or pulmonary disease. Associated with capillary leak syndrome and impaired neutrophil function. Increased risk of infection. Withhold treatment with moderate to severe lethargy or somnolence.

THERAPEUTIC CLASS: Biological response modifier

INDICATIONS: Treatment of metastatic renal cell carcinoma and metastatic melanoma.

DOSAGE: *Adults:* 600,000IU/kg IV q8h. Max: 14 doses. After 9-day rest period, repeat for 14 doses. Max: 28 doses/course. Retreatment: Evaluate response after 4 weeks of course completion. Give additional courses if tumor shrinks. Separate courses by at least 7 weeks. Hold dose or interrupt therapy if toxicity occurs.

HOW SUPPLIED: Inj: 22MIU

CONTRAINDICATIONS: See Black Box Warning. Abnormal thallium stress test, abnormal pulmonary function tests, or organ allografts. Do not retreat if previous treatment caused sustained ventricular tachycardia, chest pain with ECG changes showing angina or MI, unresponsive cardiac arrythymias, cardiac tamponade, intubation >72 hrs, renal failure requiring dialysis >72 hrs, coma >48 hrs, uncontrollable seizures, bowel ischemia/perforation, and GI bleeding requiring surgery.

WARNINGS/PRECAUTIONS: May exacerbate or cause autoimmune/inflammatory disorders. May exacerbate Crohn's disease, scleroderma, thyroiditis, inflammatory arthritis, DM, oculo-bulbar myasthemia gravis, crescentic IgA glomerulonephritis, cholecystitis, cerebral vasculitis, Stevens-Johnson syndrome and bullous pemphigoid reported. Confirm negative CNS metastases before treatment. Neurologic impairments reported without CNS metastases. Caution with history of seizures. May cause reduced kidney and hepatic function.

ADVERSE REACTIONS: Chills, fever, malaise, infection, hypotension, abdominal pain, tachycardia, vasodilation, arrhythmia, diarrhea, vomiting, nausea, stomatitis, anorexia, anemia, bilirubinemia, edema, weight gain, confusion, dyspnea.

INTERACTIONS: Increased CNS effects with psychotropics (eg, narcotics, analgesics, antiemetics, sedatives, and tranquilizers). Nephrotoxic, myelotoxic, cardiotoxic, or hepatotoxic drugs may increase toxicity to that organ system. Increased risk of MI, myocarditis, ventricular hypokinesia, and severe rhabdomyolysis. Hypersensitivity reactions reported with high dose antineoplastics. Glucocorticoids decrease antitumor effects; avoid concomitant use. Antihypertensives can potentiate hypotension. Iodinated contrast media may cause hypersensitivity reactions up to several months after therapy.

PREGNANCY: Category C, not for use in nursing.

MECHANISM OF ACTION: Human recombinant interleukin-2; not established; enhances lymphocyte mitogenesis and stimulates long-term growth of human interleukin-2 dependent cell lines; enhances lymphocyte cytotoxicity and inducts killer cells and interferon-gamma production.

PHARMACOKINETICS: Metabolism: Kidneys. **Elimination:** Kidneys; $T_{1/2}$=85 min.

PROMETHAZINE   RX
promethazine HCL (Various)

OTHER BRAND NAMES: Promethegan (G & W Labs) - Phenergan (Wyeth)

THERAPEUTIC CLASS: Phenothiazine derivative

INDICATIONS: Allergic and vasomotor rhinitis, allergic conjunctivitis, blood or plasma allergic reactions, dermographism, urticaria, angioedema. Pre- and postoperative sedation. Adjunct in anaphylaxis, postoperative pain. Prevention and control of nausea, vomiting, and motion sickness.

DOSAGE: *Adults:* Allergy: 25mg qhs or 12.5mg ac and hs. Motion Sickness: Initial: 25mg 30-60 min before travel, then 25mg 8-12 hrs later if needed. Maint: 25mg bid. Prevention/Control of Nausea/Vomiting: 25mg initially, then 12.5-25mg q4-6h prn. Sedation: 25-50mg qhs. Preoperative: 50mg night before surgery, then 50mg preoperatively. Postoperative: 25-50mg. *Pediatrics:* ≥2 yrs: Allergy: 25mg or 0.5mg/lb qhs or 6.25-12.5 tid. Motion Sickness: 12.5-25mg bid. Prevention/Control of Nausea/Vomiting: 25mg or 0.5mg/lb initially then 12.5-25mg or 0.5mg/lb q4-6h prn. Sedation: 12.5-25mg hs. Preoperative: 12.5-25mg night before surgery, then 0.5mg/lb preoperatively. Postoperative: 12.5-25mg.

HOW SUPPLIED: Sup: (Promethegan, Phenergan, Promethazine)12.5mg, 25mg, 50mg; Tab: (Phenergan, Promethazine)12.5mg*, 25mg*, 50mg *scored

CONTRAINDICATIONS: Treatment of lower respiratory tract symptoms (eg, asthma). Pediatric patients <2 yrs.

WARNINGS/PRECAUTIONS: Potential for fatal respiratory depression in pediatric patients <2 yrs. Caution in patients ≥2 yrs. Avoid with compromised respiratory function (eg, COPD, sleep apnea). Caution with bone marrow depression, narrow-angle glaucoma, stenosing peptic ulcer, bladder or pyloroduodenal obstruction, prostatic hypertrophy, CVD, hepatic dysfunction. Cholestatic jaundice reported. Alters HCG pregnancy tests. May lower seizure threshold, increase blood glucose, cause sun sensitivity. May impair mental/physical abilities.

ADVERSE REACTIONS: Drowsiness, sedation, blurred vision, dizziness, increased or decreased blood pressure, urticaria, dry mouth, nausea, vomiting.

INTERACTIONS: Additive sedative effects with CNS depressants (eg, alcohol, narcotic analgesics, sedatives, hypnotics, tranquilizers); reduce dose or eliminate these agents. Reduce barbiturate dose by one-half and analgesic depressant dose by one-quarter to one-half. Caution with drugs that alter seizure threshold (eg, narcotics, local anesthetics). Avoid sedatives and CNS depressants with sleep apnea.

PREGNANCY: Category C, not for use in nursing.

MECHANISM OF ACTION: Phenothiazine derivative; H_1 receptor-blocking agent. Also has sedative and antiemetic properties.

PHARMACOKINETICS: Absorption: GI tract (well absorbed). **Metabolism:** Liver. **Elimination:** Urine.

PROMETHAZINE DM   RX
dextromethorphan hbr - promethazine HCL (Various)

THERAPEUTIC CLASS: Phenothiazine derivative/antitussive

INDICATIONS: Temporary relief of coughs and upper respiratory symptoms associated with allergy or the common cold.

DOSAGE: *Adults:* 5mL q4-6h. Max: 30mL/24 hr.
Pediatrics: ≥12 yrs: 5mL q4-6h. Max: 30mL/24hr. 6-11 yrs: 2.5-5mL q4-6h. Max: 20mL/24hr. 2-5 yrs: 1.25-2.5mL q4-6h. Max: 10mL/24hr.

HOW SUPPLIED: Syrup: (Promethazine-Dextromethorphan) 6.25mg-15mg/5mL

CONTRAINDICATIONS: Concomitant MAOIs, comatose states, treatment of lower respiratory tract symptoms (eg, asthma), pediatric patients <2 yrs.

WARNINGS/PRECAUTIONS: Caution in pediatrics ≥2 yrs. Avoid in pediatric patients whose signs and symptoms may suggest Reye's syndrome or other hepatic diseases. May impair mental/physical abilities. May lower seizure threshold; caution with seizure disorders. May lead to potentially fatal respiratory depression; avoid with compromised respiratory function (eg, COPD, sleep apnea). Caution with bone marrow depression; leukopenia and agranulocytosis reported. Neuroleptic malignant syndrome reported. Caution with narrow-angle glaucoma, prostatic hypertrophy, stenosing peptic ulcer, bladder neck or pyloroduodenal obstruction, cardiovascular disease, hepatic impairment, atopic children, sedated, elderly, or debilitated patients, and patients confined to supine position. Cholestatic jaundice reported. May alter HCG pregnancy test reading. May increase blood glucose. Avoid prolonged exposure to sunlight.

ADVERSE REACTIONS: Drowsiness, dizziness, sedation, GI disturbance, blurred vision, dry mouth, increased or decreased BP, rash, nausea, vomiting.

INTERACTIONS: See Contraindications. Hyperpyrexia, hypotension and death associated with MAOIs. May increase, prolong, or intensify sedative action of other CNS depressants, such as alcohol, sedatives/hypnotics (including barbiturates), narcotics, narcotic analgesics, general anesthetics, TCAs, and tranquilizers; avoid such agents or administer in reduced dosages. Reduce barbiturate dose by at least one-half and narcotic analgesics by one-quarter to one-half. May reverse epinephrines's vasopressor effect. May lower seizure threshold; caution with concomitant medications which may also affect seizure threshold (eg, narcotics, local anesthetics). Avoid concomitant administration with other respiratory depressants in pediatrics. Caution with concomitant use of other agents with anticholinergic properties.

P

PREGNANCY: Category C, caution in nursing.

MECHANISM OF ACTION: Dextromethorphan: Antitussive agent; acts centrally and elevates the threshold for coughing. Promethazine: Phenothiazine derivative, (antihistaminic); H₁ receptor blocking agent and provides clinically useful sedative and antiemetic effects.

PHARMACOKINETICS: Absorption: Dextromethorphan (rapid); Promethazine (well-absorbed). **Metabolism:** Promethazine: Liver. Dextromethorphan: Liver via O-demethylation, N-demethylation, and partial conjugation with glucuronic acid and sulfate. **Elimination:** Promethazine: Urine (sulfoxides and N-demethylpromethazine). Dextromethorphan: Urine.

PROMETHAZINE VC   RX
phenylephrine HCL - promethazine HCL (Various)

THERAPEUTIC CLASS: Phenothiazine derivative/ sympathomimetic

INDICATIONS: Temporary relief of upper respiratory symptoms (eg, nasal congestion) associated with allergy or the common cold.

DOSAGE: *Adults:* 5mL q4-6h. Max: 30mL/24 hr.
Pediatrics: ≥12 yrs: 5mL q4-6h. Max: 30mL/24 hr. 6-11 yrs: 2.5-5mL q4-6h. Max: 30mL/24 hr. 2-5 yrs: 1.25-2.5mL q4-6h.

HOW SUPPLIED: Syrup: (Promethazine-Phenylephrine) 6.25mg-5mg/5mL

CONTRAINDICATIONS: Concomitant MAOIs, comatose states, treatment of lower respiratory tract symptoms (eg, asthma), HTN, peripheral vascular insufficiency, pediatric patients <2 yrs.

WARNINGS/PRECAUTIONS: Caution in pediatrics ≥2 yrs. Avoid in pediatric patients whose signs and symptoms may suggest Reye's syndrome or other hepatic diseases. May impair mental/physical abilities. May lower seizure threshold; caution with seizure disorders. May lead to potentially fatal respiratory depression; avoid with compromised respiratory function (eg, COPD, sleep apnea). Caution with bone marrow depression; leukopenia and agranulocytosis reported. Neuroleptic malignant syndrome reported. Caution with narrow-angle glaucoma, prostatic hypertrophy, stenosing peptic ulcer, bladder neck or pyloroduodenal obstruction, cardiovascular disease, and elderly patients. Cholestatic jaundice reported. May alter HCG pregnancy test reading. May increase blood glucose. Avoid prolonged exposure to sunlight.

ADVERSE REACTIONS: Drowsiness, dizziness, anxiety, tremor, sedation, blurred vision, dry mouth, increased or decreased blood pressure, rash, nausea, vomiting.

INTERACTIONS: See Contraindications. May increase, prolong, or intensify the sedative action of other CNS depressants, such as alcohol, sedatives/hypnotics (including barbiturates), narcotics, narcotic analgesics, general anesthetics, TCAs, and tranquilizers. avoid such agents or administer in reduced dosages. Reduce barbiturate dose by at least one-half and narcotic analgesics by one-quarter to one-half. Cardiac pressor response potentiated and possible hypertensive crisis with MAOIs. Pressor response increased with TCAs. Excessive rise in BP with ergot alkaloids. Tachycardia or other arrhythmias may occur with sympathomimetics. Reflex bradycardia blocked and pressor response enhanced with atropine. Cardiostimulating effects blocked with β-blockers. Pressor response decreased with α-adrenergic blockers. Synergistic adrenergic response with amphetamines or phenylpropanolamine. Avoid concomitant administration with other respiratory depressants in pediatrics. May lower seizure threshold; caution with concomitant medications which may also affect seizure threshold (eg, narcotics, local anesthetics). Relex bradycardia blocked; pressor response enhanced with atropine.

PREGNANCY: Category C, caution in nursing.

MECHANISM OF ACTION: Promethazine: Phenothiazine derivative; H₁-receptor blocking agent. Phenylephrine: Sympathomimetic; α-receptor agonist with little effect on β-receptors of heart; increases resistance and decreases capacitance of blood vessels; has mild central stimulant effect.

PHARMACOKINETICS: Absorption: Promethazine: Well-absorbed (GI tract). Phenylephrine: Irregularly absorbed. **Metabolism:** Promethazine: Liver, sulfoxides and N-demethylpromethazine (metabolites). Phenylephrine: Liver and intestine via monoamine oxidase. **Elimination:** Promethazine: Urine (sulfoxides and N-demethylpromethazine).

PROMETHAZINE VC/CODEINE
phenylephrine HCL - promethazine HCL - codeine phosphate (Various)

THERAPEUTIC CLASS: Phenothiazine derivative/antitussive/sympathomimetic

INDICATIONS: Temporary relief of cough and upper respiratory symptoms (eg, nasal congestion) associated with allergy or the common cold.

DOSAGE: *Adults:* 5mL q4-6h. Max: 30mL/24hr.
Pediatrics: ≥16 yrs: 5mL q4-6h. Max: 30mL/24hr.

HOW SUPPLIED: Syrup: (Promethazine-Codeine-Phenylephrine) 6.25mg-10mg-5mg/5mL

CONTRAINDICATIONS: Concomitant MAOIs, comatose states, treatment of lower respiratory tract symptoms (eg, asthma), HTN, peripheral vascular insufficiency, pediatric patients <16 yrs.

WARNINGS/PRECAUTIONS: May cause or aggravate constipation. May lead to potentially fatal respiratory depression; avoid with compromised respiratory function (eg, COPD, sleep apnea). Caution in atopic children. May elevate CSF pressure; caution with head injury, intracranial lesions, or pre-existing increase in ICP. Avoid with asthma, acute febrile illness with chronic cough, or with chronic respiratory disease where interference with ability to clear tracheobronchial tree of secretions would have a deleterious effect on patient's respiratory function. May cause orthostatic hypotension. May impair mental/physical abilities. May lower seizure threshold; caution with seizure disorders. Caution with bone marrow depression; leukopenia and agranulocytosis reported. Neuroleptic malignant syndrome reported. Hallucinations and convulsions have occurred in pediatrics. Cholestatic jaundice reported. Caution with acute abdominal conditions, convulsive disorders, significant hepatic/renal impairment, fever, hypothyroidism, Addison's disease, ulcerative colitis, prostatic hypertrophy, recent GI or urinary tract surgery, elderly, debilitated, narrow-angle glaucoma, stenosing peptic ulcer, pyloroduodenal or bladder-neck obstruction, cardiovascular disease, thyroid disease, DM, heart disease. Urinary retention may occur with BPH. May decrease cardiac output; use extreme caution with arteriosclerosis, elderly, and patients with initially poor cerebral or coronary circulation. May alter HCG pregnancy test reading. May increase blood glucose. Avoid prolonged exposure to sunlight.

ADVERSE REACTIONS: Drowsiness, dizziness, sedation, tremor, anxiety, blurred vision, dry mouth, increased or decreased blood pressure, rash, nausea, vomiting, constipation, urinary retention.

INTERACTIONS: See Contraindications. May increase, prolong, or intensify the sedative action of other CNS depressants such as alcohol, sedatives/hypnotics (including barbiturates), narcotics, narcotic analgesics, general anesthetics, TCAs, and tranquilizers. Reduce barbiturate dose by at least one-half and narcotic analgesics by one-quarter to one-half. Cardiac pressor response potentiated and acute hypertensive crisis may occur with MAOIs; consider small test dose. May reverse epinephrine's vasopressor effect. Caution with concomitant use of other agents with anticholinergic properties. Pressor response increased with TCAs. Excessive rise in BP with ergot alkaloids. Tachycardia or other arrhythmias may occur with other sympathomimetics. Cardiostimulating effects blocked with β-blockers. Reflex bradycardia blocked and pressor response enhanced with atropine. Pressor response decreased with α-adrenergic blockers. Synergistic adrenergic response with diet preparations (eg, amphetamines or phenylpropanolamine). Avoid concomitant administration with other respiratory agents in pediatrics. May lower seizure threshold; caution with concomitant medications which may also affect seizure threshold (eg, narcotics, local anesthetics).

PREGNANCY: Category C, caution in nursing.

MECHANISM OF ACTION: Promethazine: phenothiazine derivative. Blocks H_1-receptor. Phenylephrine; sympathomimetic. Potent postsynaptic-α-receptor agonist with little effect on β-receptors of heart; increases resistance and decreases capacitance of blood vessels. Codeine: narcotic analgesic/antitussive. Primary effects on central CNS and GI tract.

PHARMACOKINETICS: Absorption: Codeine: Well-absorbed. Promethazine: Well-absorbed (GI tract). Phenylephrine: Irregularly-absorbed. **Distribution:** Codeine: Found in breast milk. **Metabolism:** Promethazine: Liver. Phenylephrine: Liver and intestine, via monoamine oxidase. Codeine: Liver, via O-demethylation, N-demethylation, and partial conjugation with glucuronic acid. **Elimination:** Promethazine: Urine (sulfoxides and N-demethylpromethazine). Codeine: Urine (inactive metabolite and free/conjugated morphine), feces.

PROMETHAZINE W/CODEINE   `CV`
promethazine HCL - codeine phosphate (Various)

THERAPEUTIC CLASS: Phenothiazine derivative/antitussive

INDICATIONS: Temporary relief of coughs and upper respiratory symptoms associated with allergy or the common cold.

DOSAGE: *Adults:* 5mL q4-6h. Max: 30mL/24 hr.
Pediatrics: ≥16 yrs: 5mL q4-6h. Max: 30mL/24 hr.

HOW SUPPLIED: Syrup: (Promethazine-Codeine) 6.25mg-10mg/5mL

CONTRAINDICATIONS: Comatose states, reatment of lower respiratory tract symptoms (eg, asthma), pediatric patients <16 yrs.

WARNINGS/PRECAUTIONS: May cause or aggravate constipation. May lead to potentially fatal respiratory depression; avoid with compromised respiratory function (eg, COPD, sleep apnea). Caution in atopic children. May elevate CSF pressure; caution with head injury, intracranial lesions, or pre-existing increase in ICP. Avoid with asthma, acute febrile illness with chronic cough, or with chronic respiratory disease where interference with ability to clear tracheobronchial tree of secretions would have a deleterious effect on patient's respiratory function. May cause orthostatic hypotension. May impair mental/physical abilities. May lower seizure threshold; caution with seizure disorders. Caution with bone marrow depression; leukopenia and agranulocytosis reported. Neuroleptic malignant syndrome reported. Hallucinations and convulsions have occurred in pediatrics. Cholestatic jaundice reported. Caution with acute abdominal conditions, convulsive disorders, significant hepatic/renal impairment, fever, hypothyroidism, Addison's disease, ulcerative colitis, prostatic hypertrophy, recent GI or urinary tract surgery, elderly, debilitated, narrow-angle glaucoma, stenosing peptic ulcer, pyloroduodenal or bladder-neck obstruction, or cardiovascular disease. May alter HCG pregnancy test reading. May increase blood glucose. Avoid prolonged exposure to sunlight.

ADVERSE REACTIONS: Drowsiness, dizziness, sedation, blurred vision, dry mouth, increased or decreased blood pressure, rash, nausea, vomiting, constipation, urinary retention.

INTERACTIONS: May increase, prolong, or intensify the sedative action of other CNS depressants such as alcohol, sedative/hypnotics (including barbiturates), narcotics, narcotic analgesics, general anesthetics, TCAs, and tranquilizers; avoid such agents or administer in reduced dosages. Reduce barbiturate dose by at least one-half and narcotic analgesics by one-quarter to one-half. May reverse epinephrine's vasopressor effect. Caution with concomitant use of other agents with anticholinergic properties. May lower seizure threshold; caution with concomitant medications which may also affect seizure threshold (eg, narcotics, local anesthetics). Avoid concomitant administration with other respiratory depressants in pediatrics. Possible interaction with MAOIs; consider small test dose.

PREGNANCY: Category C, caution in nursing.

MECHANISM OF ACTION: Promethazine: phenothiazine derivative; blocks H₁ receptor (antihistaminic action) and provides sedative and antiemetic effects. Codeine: Narcotic analgesic and antitussive; primary effects are on CNS and GI tract.

PHARMACOKINETICS: Absorption: Promethazine and codeine (well absorbed). **Distribution:** Codeine: Found in breast milk. **Metabolism:** Promethazine: Liver. Codeine: Liver via O-demethylation, N-demethylation, and partial conjugation with glucuronic acid. **Elimination:** Promethazine: Urine (sulfoxides and N-demethylpromethazine). Codeine: Urine (inactive metabolites and free/conjugated morphine), feces (codeine and metabolites).

PROMETRIUM

RX

progesterone (Solvay)

> Progestins and estrogens should not be used for the prevention of cardiovascular disease.
> Increased risks of MI, stroke, invasive breast cancer, pulmonary emboli, DVT, and development
> of probable dementia in postmenopausal women.

THERAPEUTIC CLASS: Progestogen

INDICATIONS: Prevention of endometrial hyperplasia in non-hysterectomized postmenopausal women receiving conjugated estrogens. For secondary amenorrhea.

DOSAGE: *Adults:* Prevention of Endometrial Hyperplasia: 200mg qpm for 12 days sequentially per 28 day cycle. Secondary Amenorrhea: 400mg qhs for 10 days.

HOW SUPPLIED: Cap: 100mg, 200mg

CONTRAINDICATIONS: Peanut allergy, undiagnosed abnormal genital bleeding, breast cancer, DVT, PE, thromboembolic disorders (stroke, myocardial infarction), liver dysfunction or disease, pregnancy.

WARNINGS/PRECAUTIONS: D/C if thrombotic disorders, papilledema, or retinal vascular lesions develop. D/C pending exam if sudden onset of proptosis, sudden partial or complete loss of vision, diplopia, or migraine. Include pap smear in pretreatment exam. Caution with depression, DM, and conditions aggravated by fluid retention (eg, epilepsy, migraine, asthma, cardiac/renal dysfunction).

ADVERSE REACTIONS: Dizziness, headache, breast pain, nausea, diarrhea, dizziness, abdominal pain and distension, emotional lability, upper respiratory infection.

INTERACTIONS: CYP3A4 inhibitors (eg, ketoconazole) may increase bioavailability of progesterone.

PREGNANCY: Category B, caution in nursing.

MECHANISM OF ACTION: Progesterone.

PHARMACOKINETICS: Absorption: Oral administration of variable doses resulted in different parameters. **Distribution:** Plasma protein binding (96-99%). **Metabolism:** Liver; pregnanediols, pregnanolones (metabolites). **Elimination:** Bile, urine.

PROPECIA

RX

finasteride (Merck)

THERAPEUTIC CLASS: Type II 5 alpha-reductase inhibitor

INDICATIONS: Treatment of male pattern hair loss (androgenetic alopecia). For men only.

DOSAGE: *Adults:* 1mg qd. Continue use to sustain benefit.

HOW SUPPLIED: Tab: 1mg [ProPak, 3 x 30 tabs]

CONTRAINDICATIONS: Pregnancy or women who may potentially become pregnant.

WARNINGS/PRECAUTIONS: Caution with hepatic dysfunction. Consider doubling PSA level results in men >41 yrs of age, without BPH, who are undergoing PSA test. Women who are pregnant or may become pregnant should not handle crushed or broken tablets; potential risk to a male fetus. Do not use in pediatrics or women.

ADVERSE REACTIONS: Decreased libido, erectile dysfunction, decreased volume of ejaculate, breast tenderness, hypersensitivity reactions.

PREGNANCY: Category X, not for use in nursing.

MECHANISM OF ACTION: Competitive and specific inhibitor of type II 5-α reductase; blocks peripheral conversion of testosterone to DHT, resulting in significant decreases in serum and tissue DHT concentrations.

PHARMACOKINETICS: Absorption: C_{max}=9.2ng/mL; T_{max}=1-2 hrs. AUC=53ng•hr/mL. **Distribution:** Plasma protein binding (approx. 90%); V_d=76L. Crosses blood-brain barrier. **Metabolism:** Liver (extensive); via CYP3A4. **Elimination:** Urine (39%, metabolites), feces (57%).$T_{1/2}$=4.5 hrs.

PROPINE   RX
dipivefrin HCL (Allergan)

THERAPEUTIC CLASS: Epinephrine (sympathomimetic) prodrug

INDICATIONS: Control of IOP in open-angle glaucoma.

DOSAGE: *Adults:* Usual: 1 drop q12h.

HOW SUPPLIED: Sol: 0.1% [5mL, 10mL, 15mL]

CONTRAINDICATIONS: Narrow-angle glaucoma.

WARNINGS/PRECAUTIONS: Macular edema may occur in aphakic patients; d/c if develop.

ADVERSE REACTIONS: Tachycardia, arrhythmias, HTN, burning, stinging, follicular conjunctivitis, mydriasis, blurry vision, eye pruritus/pain, headache.

PREGNANCY: Category B, caution in nursing.

MECHANISM OF ACTION: Epinephrine prodrug; converted to epinephrine inside the eye by hydrolysis. Ephinephrine: An adrenergic agonist. Exerts its action by decreasing aqueous production and enhancing outflow facility.

PHARMACOKINETICS: Absorption: T_{max}=1 hr.

PROPYLTHIOURACIL   RX
propylthiouracil (Various)

THERAPEUTIC CLASS: Thiourea-derivative antithyroid agent

INDICATIONS: Treatment of hyperthyroidism.

DOSAGE: *Adults:* Initial: 300mg/day in 3 divided doses, q8h. Severe Hyperthyroidism/Very Large Goiters: Initial: 400mg/day in 3 divided doses; may give up to 600-900mg/day if needed. Maint: 100-150mg/day. *Pediatrics:* 6-10 yrs: Initial: 50-150mg/day. ≥10 yrs: Initial: 150-300mg/day. Maint: Determine by patient response.

HOW SUPPLIED: Tab: 50mg

CONTRAINDICATIONS: Nursing mothers.

WARNINGS/PRECAUTIONS: D/C with agranulocytosis, aplastic anemia, hepatitis, fever, or exfoliative dermatitis. Rare reports of severe hepatic reactions exist. D/C with significant hepatic abnormality, including transaminases >3x ULN. Caution with pregnancy, may cause fetal harm. Monitor PT and TFTs.

ADVERSE REACTIONS: Agranulocytosis, granulopenia, thrombocytopenia, aplastic anemia, drug fever, hepatitis, periarteritis, hypoprothrombinemia, skin rash, urticaria, nausea, vomiting, epigastric distress, arthralgia, paresthesias.

INTERACTIONS: May potentiate anticoagulant effects. Hyperthyroidism increases clearance of β-blockers; reduce β-blocker dose when patient becomes euthyroid. Increased digitalis glycoside levels when patient becomes euthyroid; reduce digitalis dose. Decreased theophylline clearance when patient becomes euthyroid; reduce theophylline dose. Caution with other drugs that cause agranulocytosis.

PREGNANCY: Category D, contraindicated in nursing.

MECHANISM OF ACTION: Antithyroid agent; inhibits synthesis of thyroid hormones.

PHARMACOKINETICS: Absorption: GI tract (readily absorbed). **Distribution:** Found in breast milk, crosses the placental membranes. **Elimination:** Urine (35%); $T_{1/2}$= 24 hrs.

PROQUAD   RX
varicella virus vaccine live - rubella vaccine live - measles vaccine live - mumps vaccine live (Merck)

THERAPEUTIC CLASS: Vaccine

INDICATIONS: Vaccination against measles, mumps, rubella, and varicella in children 12 months to 12 yrs of age.

DOSAGE: *Pediatrics:* 12 months-12 yrs: 0.5mL SQ. At least 1 month should elapse between dose of measles-containing vaccine and dose of ProQuad. If for any reason a 2nd dose of varicella-containing vaccine is required, at least 3 months should elapse between doses.

HOW SUPPLIED: Inj: 0.5mL

CONTRAINDICATIONS: Anaphylactic reactions to neomycin; hypsensitivity to gelatin; blood dyscrasias, leukemia, lymphomas, or other malignant neoplasms affecting the bone marrow or lymphatic system; immunosuppressive therapy; primary and acquired immunodeficiency states (e.g., AIDS/HIV); congenital or hereditary immunodeficiency; active untreated tuberculosis; active afebrile illness with fever >101.3°F; pregnant. Disseminated varicella vaccine virus infection has been reported in children with underlying immunodeficiency disorders who were inadvertently vaccinated with a varicella-containing vaccine.

WARNINGS/PRECAUTIONS: Caution with egg allergy. May cause thrombocytopenia. Contains albumin, remote risk of viral infection transmission. Have epinephrine (1:1000) available.

ADVERSE REACTIONS: Injection Site: Pain/tenderness/soreness, erythema, swelling. Systemic: Fever, irritability, measles-like rash, herpes zoster and varicella infection, anaphylactic reaction, ataxia, convulsion, febrile seizure, pruritus.

INTERACTIONS: Do not give with immune globulin. Avoid use of salicylates for 6 weeks after vaccination. Avoid use of immunosuppressive doses of corticosteriods or other immunosuppressive drugs.

PREGNANCY: Category C, not for use in nursing.

MECHANISM OF ACTION: Vaccine; stimulates immune system to elicit immune response to produce antibodies that may protect against measles, mumps, rubella, and varicella disease.

PROQUIN XR   RX
ciprofloxacin HCL (Esprit)

THERAPEUTIC CLASS: Fluoroquinolone

INDICATIONS: Treatment of uncomplicated urinary tract infections (acute cystitis) caused by *E.coli* and *K.pneumoniae.*

DOSAGE: *Adults:* 500mg qd with pm meal for 3 days. Administer at least 4 hrs before or 2 hrs after magnesium-or aluminum-containing antacids, sucralfate, Videx (didanosine) chewable/buffered tablets of pediatric powder, metal cations (eg, iron), multivitamins with zinc. Do not split, crush, or chew. Swallow tab whole.

P

HOW SUPPLIED: Tab, Extended-Release: 500mg

WARNINGS/PRECAUTIONS: Convulsions, increased ICP and toxic psychosis reported. D/C if dizziness, confusion, tremors, hallucinations, depression, or suicidal thoughts/acts. Caution with CNS disorders or if predisposed to seizures. Severe, fatal hypersensitivity reactions may occur. Pseudomembranous colitis; achilles, and other tendon ruptures reported. D/C at first sign of rash, jaundice or if pain, inflammation, or ruptured tendon occurs. Maintain hydration; avoid alkaline urine. Avoid excessive sunlight and UV light. Not interchangeable with immediate-release or other extended-release oral formulations. D/C if phototoxicity occurs.

ADVERSE REACTIONS: Fungal infection, nasopharyngitis, headache, micturition urgency.

INTERACTIONS: Increases theophylline and caffeine levels and prolongs effects. Serious/fatal reactions have occurred with theophylline. Magnesium or aluminum containing antacids, sucralfate, Videx (didanosine) chewable/buffered tablets or pediatric powder, and products containing calcium, iron, or zinc decrease serum and urine levels; administer at least 4 hrs before or 2 hrs after administration. Altered serum levels of phenytoin. Severe hypoglycemia with glyburide (rare). Potentiated by probenecid. Transient serum creatinine elevations with cyclosporine. Enhances oral anticoagulant effects. May increase risk of methotrexate toxic reactions due to inhibition of renal tubular transport. High dose quinolones shown to provoke convulsions with NSAIDs (not ASA).

PREGNANCY: Category C, not for use in nursing.

MECHANISM OF ACTION: Broad-spectrum fluoroquinolone; inhibits topoisomerase II (DNA gyrase) and topoisomerase IV (both type II topoisomerases), which are required for bacterial DNA replication, transcription, repair, and recombination.

PHARMACOKINETICS: Absorption: 500mg: AUC=7.67mcg•h/mL; C_{max}=0.82mcg/mL; T_{max}=6.1 hrs. 250mg bid: AUC=7.83mcg•h/mL; C_{max}=0.57mcg/mL (pm), 0.93mcg/mL (am); T_{max}=2.5 hrs. **Distribution:** Plasma protein binding (9.9-36.6%). **Metabolism:** Desethyleneciprofloxacin, sulfociprofloxacin, oxociprofloxacin and formylciprofloxacin (metabolites). **Elimination:** Urine (26.9%), feces; $T_{1/2}$=4.5 hrs.

PROSCAR   RX
finasteride (Merck)

THERAPEUTIC CLASS: Type II 5 alpha-reductase inhibitor

INDICATIONS: Treatment of symptomatic benign prostatic hypertrophy (BPH) to improve symptoms, reduce the risk of acute urinary retention, and reduce the risk of the need for prostate surgery. To reduce the risk of symptomatic progression of BPH in combination with doxazosin.

DOSAGE: *Adults:* 5mg qd.

HOW SUPPLIED: Tab: 5mg

CONTRAINDICATIONS: Pregnancy.

WARNINGS/PRECAUTIONS: Not for use in pediatrics or women. Risk to male fetus in pregnancy. Pregnant women should not handle crushed or broken tablets. Rule out infection, prostate cancer, stricture disease, hypotonic bladder prior to initiating therapy. Caution with liver dysfunction. Decreases serum PSA levels by ~50% in patients with BPH, even with prostate cancer; adjust (double) PSA results to compare with normal values. Monitor for obstructive uropathy with large residual urinary volume and/or severely diminished urinary flow.

ADVERSE REACTIONS: Impotence, decreased libido, decreased ejaculate volume, hypersensitivity reactions (pruritus, urticaria, swelling of lips and face), testicular pain.

PREGNANCY: Category X, not for use in nursing.

MECHANISM OF ACTION: Type II 5α-reductase inhibitor; inhibits type II 5α-reductase which metabolizes testosterone to 5α-dihydrotestosterone (DHT), a potent androgen needed for development and enlargement of prostate gland.

PHARMACOKINETICS: Absorption: Absolute bioavailability (63%). C_{max}=37ng/mL. T_{max}=1-2 hrs. **Distribution:** V_d=76L, Plasma protein binding (90%). **Metabolism:** CYP3A4. **Elimination:** $T_{1/2}$=6 hrs. Feces (major), urine.

PROSED EC   RX
hyoscyamine sulfate - atropine sulfate - benzoic acid - methenamine - phenyl salicylate - methylene blue (Esprit)

OTHER BRAND NAMES: Prosed DS (Star)

THERAPEUTIC CLASS: Urinary tract analgesic

INDICATIONS: Relief of lower urinary tract discomfort due to hypermotility. Treatment of formaldehyde-susceptible cystitis, urethritis, trigonitis.

DOSAGE: *Adults:* 1 tab qid with plenty of fluid.
Pediatrics: >12 yrs: Individualize dose. Take with plenty of fluid.

HOW SUPPLIED: Tab, Enteric Coated: Atropine 0.06mg-Benzoic Acid 9mg-Hyoscyamine 0.06mg-Methenamine 81.6mg-Methylene Blue 10.8mg-Phenyl Salicylate 36.2mg

CONTRAINDICATIONS: Risk-benefit assessment in glaucoma, urinary bladder neck obstruction, pyloric or duodenal obstruction, cardiospasm.

WARNINGS/PRECAUTIONS: D/C if tachycardia, dizziness, or blurred vision occurs. Delay in gastric emptying time may obscure gastric ulcer therapy.

ADVERSE REACTIONS: Rapid pulse, flushing, blurred vision, dizziness, shortness of breath, difficult micturition, acute urinary retention, dry mouth, nausea, vomiting.

INTERACTIONS: May decrease absorption of other oral agents (dose 2 hrs after ketoconazole). Reduced effectiveness with urinary alkaliners, thiazide diuretics, antacids/antidiarrheals (space dosing by 1 hr). Antimuscarinic effects potentiated with other antimuscarinics, MAOIs. Caution with antimyasthenics. Increased risk of constipation with opioids. Increased risk of crystalluria with sulfonamides.

PREGNANCY: Category C, caution in nursing.

MECHANISM OF ACTION: Methenamine: Degrades in an acidic urine environment, releasing formaldehyde, which provides bactericidal or bacteriostatic action. Phenyl salicylate: Releases salicylate, a mild analgesic for pain. Methylene blue: Possesses weak antiseptic properties. Benzoic acid: Has mild antibacterial and antifungal action; helps maintain an acid pH in the urine, necessary for the degradation of methenamine. Hyoscyamine sulfate: Parasympathetic drug which relaxes smooth muscles.

PHARMACOKINETICS: Absorption: Well (methenamine, methylene blue, and hyoscyamine). **Distribution:** Methenamine and hyoscyamine, crosses placenta; found in breast milk. **Metabolism:** Methenamine: Hydrolizes in acidic urine to formaldehyde. Methylene blue: Reduced to leukomethylene blue (metabolite). Hyoscyamine: Hepatic biotransformation. **Elimination:** Methenamine: Urine (70-90% unchanged). Methylene blue: Urine (75% unchanged). Hyoscyamine: Unchanged.

PROSTIN E2   RX
dinoprostone (Pharmacia & Upjohn)

THERAPEUTIC CLASS: Prostaglandin E_2

INDICATIONS: Termination of pregnancy between 12th to 20th week of gestation. Evacuation of uterine contents in the management of missed abortion or intrauterine fetal death up to 28 weeks gestation. Management of nonmetastatic gestational trophoblastic disease.

DOSAGE: *Adults:* Insert 1 sup high into vagina; remain in supine position for 10 min. Insert additional sups at 3-5 hr intervals until abortion occurs. Max: 2 days of continuous use.

HOW SUPPLIED: Sup: 20mg [1ˢ, 5ˢ]

CONTRAINDICATIONS: Active pelvic inflammatory disease; active cardiac, pulmonary, renal, or hepatic disease.

WARNINGS/PRECAUTIONS: Adhere strictly to recommended dose. Use in facility able to provide intensive care and acute surgery. Not a feticidal agent. Can induce bone proliferation. If abortion fails, complete by other means. Caution with asthma, hypotension, HTN, CVD, renal/hepatic disease, anemia, jaundice, diabetes, epilepsy, cervicitis, infected endocervical lesions, acute vaginitis, and compromised uteri. Transient pyrexia reported.

ADVERSE REACTIONS: Vomiting, diarrhea, nausea, temperature elevation, shivering, chills, transient BP decrease, headache.

INTERACTIONS: May augment activity of other oxytocic drugs; avoid concomitant use.

PREGNANCY: Category C, safety in nursing not known.

MECHANISM OF ACTION: Prostaglandin E2: stimulates myometrium of gravid uterus to contract, similar to term uterus in labor.

PROSTIN VR PEDIATRIC   RX
alprostadil (Pharmacia & Upjohn)

> Apnea occurs in about 10-12% of neonates, usually appearing during the 1st hr of drug infusion. Monitor respiratory status throughout treatment.

THERAPEUTIC CLASS: Prostaglandin E₁

INDICATIONS: Palliative therapy to maintain patency of the ductus arteriosus until corrective surgery in neonates with congenital heart defects.

DOSAGE: Pediatrics: Initial: 0.05-0.1mcg/kg/min IV. Maint: 0.025-0.01mcg/kg/min IV. Max: 0.4mcg/kg/min.

HOW SUPPLIED: Inj: 0.5mg/mL

WARNINGS/PRECAUTIONS: May cause gastric outlet obstruction secondary to antral hyperplasia, monitor closely after 120 hrs of therapy. Limit infusion to minimum effective dose and time. May inhibit platelet aggregation; caution with bleeding tendencies. Cortical proliferation of long bones, localized and aneurysmal dilatations, vessel wall edema, intimal lacerations, decrease in medial muscularity and disruption of medial and internal lamina reported. Avoid in respiratory distress syndrome. Monitor arterial pressure intermittently; decrease rate of infusion with significant fall in pressure.

ADVERSE REACTIONS: Apnea, fever, seizures, bradycardia, flushing, diarrhea, hypotension, tachycardia.

PREGNANCY: Safety in pregnancy and nursing not known.

MECHANISM OF ACTION: Prostaglandin; causes vasodilation, inhibits platelet aggregation, stimulates intestinal and uterine smooth muscles.

PHARMACOKINETICS: Metabolism: Rapid. Lungs (β- and omega oxidation). **Elimination**: Kidneys.

PROTAMINE SULFATE RX
protamine sulfate (Various)

> May cause severe hypotension, cardiovascular collapse, noncardiogenic pulmonary edema, catastrophic pulmonary vasoconstriction, and pulmonary HTN; risk factors include high dose/overdose, rapid/previous administration, repeated doses, and current/previous use of protamine-containing drugs. Risk to benefit of administration should be carefully considered with presence of any risk factors. Should not be given when bleeding occurs without prior heparin use.

THERAPEUTIC CLASS: Heparin antagonist

INDICATIONS: Management of heparin overdose.

DOSAGE: *Adults:* Administer as very slow IV infusion over 10 min in doses not to exceed 50mg. Determine dose by blood coagulation studies. Each mg neutralizes not less than 100 USP heparin units.

HOW SUPPLIED: Inj: 10mg/mL [5mL, 25mL]

WARNINGS/PRECAUTIONS: May cause allergic reactions with fish hypersensitivity. Rapid administration may cause severe hypotensive and anaphylactoid-like reactions. Caution in cardiac surgeries; hyperheparinemia or bleeding reported. Previous exposure to protamine/protamine-containing insulin may induce humoral immune response; severe hypersensitivity reaction, including life-threatening anaphylaxis reported. Increased risk of antiprotamine antibodies in infertile or vasectomized men.

ADVERSE REACTIONS: Hypotension, bradycardia, transitory flushing/feeling of warmth, lassitude, dyspnea, nausea, vomiting, back pain, anaphylaxis that causes severe respiratory distress, circulatory collapse, noncardiogenic pulmonary edema, acute pulmonary HTN.

INTERACTIONS: Incompatible with certain antibiotics, such as cephalosporins and penicillins. Concomitant or previous use of protamine-containing drugs (eg, NPH insulin, protamine zinc insulin, certain beta-blockers) is risk factor for severe adverse events; see Black Box Warning.

PREGNANCY: Category C, caution in nursing.

MECHANISM OF ACTION: Heparin antagonist; has anticoagulant effects when administered alone; however, when given in presence of heparin, a stable salt is formed and anticoagulant activity of both drugs is lost.

PROTONIX RX
pantoprazole sodium (Wyeth)

OTHER BRAND NAMES: Protonix IV (Wyeth)

THERAPEUTIC CLASS: Proton pump inhibitor

INDICATIONS: (PO) Short-term treatment (up to 8 weeks) and maintenance of healing of erosive esophagitis associated with GERD. Long-term treatment of pathological hypersecretory conditions (eg, Zollinger-Ellison syndrome). (Inj) Short-term treatment (7-10 days) of GERD with a history of erosive esophagitis. Treatment of pathological hypersecretory conditions associated with Zollinger-Ellison syndrome or other neoplastic conditions.

DOSAGE: *Adults:* (PO) Erosive Esophagitis Treatment: 40mg qd for up to 8 weeks. May repeat for 8 weeks if needed. Maint: 40mg qd. Hypersecretory Conditions: Initial: 40mg bid. Adjust to patient's needs. Max: 240mg/day. (Inj) GERD: 40mg IV qd for 7-10 days. Pathological Hypersecretory Conditions: 80mg IV q12h. May adjust up to 80mg IV q8h based on acid output. Max: 240mg/day. Duration >6 days not studied. Do not split, crush or chew tabs.

HOW SUPPLIED: Inj: 40mg; Sus, Delayed-Release: 40mg (granules/pkt); Tab, Delayed-Release: 20mg, 40mg

WARNINGS/PRECAUTIONS: Symptomatic response does not preclude the presence of gastric malignancy. Atrophic gastritis has been noted occasionally in gastric corpus biopsies from patients treated for long-term. False (+) urine screening test for THC reported. Vitamin B-12 deficiency reported with long-term use (>3 yrs). (Inj) Immediate hypersensitivity reactions reported (eg, thrombophlebitis, LFT elevation).

ADVERSE REACTIONS: (Inj) Abdominal pain, headache, constipation, dyspepsia, nausea, inj site reactions. (PO) Headache, flatulence, diarrhea, abdominal pain.

INTERACTIONS: May alter absorption of pH-dependent drugs (eg, ketoconazole, ampicillin esters, and iron salts). May substantially decrease atazanavir levels; avoid concomitant use. May increase INR and prothrombin time with concomitant warfarin therapy.

PREGNANCY: Category B, not for use in nursing.

MECHANISM OF ACTION: Proton pump inhibitor; suppresses final step in gastric acid production by covalently binding to the (H^+,K^+)-ATPase enzyme system at the secretory surface of the gastric parietal cell. Leads to inhibition of both basal and stimulated gastric acid secretion irrespective of the stimulus.

PHARMACOKINETICS: Absorption: (PO): Well absorbed; absolute bioavailability (77%); C_{max}=2.52mcg/mL;(IV): C_{max}=5.52mcg/mL; AUC=5.4mcg•hr/mL. Bioavailability 77%, C_{max}=2.5mcg/mL, T_{max}=2.5 hr, AUC=4.8mcg•hr/mL, (PO) **Distribution:** V_d=11.0-23.6L; plasma protein binding (98%); found in breast milk. **Metabolism:** Liver (extensive) via CYP2C19 (demethylation), sulfation; CYP3A4 (oxidation). **Elimination:** Urine (71%), feces (18%); $T_{1/2}$=1 hr.

Protopic   RX
tacrolimus (Astellas)

THERAPEUTIC CLASS: Macrolide immunosuppressant

INDICATIONS: Short-term and intermittent long-term therapy of moderate to severe atopic dermatitis intolerant or unresponsive to conventional therapy.

DOSAGE: *Adults:* (0.03% or 0.1%) Apply thin layer bid. Rub in gently. Stop use when signs and symptoms resolve.
Pediatrics: ≥16 yrs: (0.03% or 0.1%) Apply thin layer bid. Rub in gently. 2-15 yrs: (0.03%) Apply thin layer bid. Rub in gently. Stop use when signs and symptoms resolve.

HOW SUPPLIED: Oint: 0.03%, 0.1% [30g, 60g, 100g]

WARNINGS/PRECAUTIONS: Do not use with occlusive dressings. Increased risk of varicella zoster, herpes simplex, or eczema herpeticum. Lymphadenopathy reported; monitor closely. D/C if unknown etiology of lymphadenopathy or presence of acute infectious mononucleosis. Avoid in Netherton's syndrome. Minimize or avoid exposure to natural or artificial sunlight. Long-term safety not established. Rare cases of malignancy (eg, skin and lymphoma) reported with topical calcineurin inhibitors; therefore, continuous long-term use should be avoided and application limited to areas of involvement. Should not use in immunocompromised adults and children. Caution in patients predisposed to renal impairment. Not indicated for use in children <2 yrs. Only 0.03% oint is indicated for use in children 2-15 yrs.

ADVERSE REACTIONS: Skin burning, pruritus, flu-like symptoms, allergic reaction, skin erythema, headache, skin infection, fever, herpes simplex, rhinitis.

INTERACTIONS: Caution with CYP3A4 inhibitors (eg, erythromycin, itraconazole, ketoconazole, fluconazole, CCBs, cimetidine) in widespread and/or erythrodermic disease. Increased risk for lymphomas in transplant patients receiving other immunosuppressive therapy.

PREGNANCY: Category C, not for use in nursing.

MECHANISM OF ACTION: Macrolide immunosuppressant; not known in atopic dermatitis. Inhibits T-lymphocyte activation by first binding to an intracellular protein, FKBP-12. A complex of tacrolimus-FKBP-12, calcium, calmodulin, and calcineurin is then formed and the phosphate activity of calcineurin is inhibited. This has been shown to prevent the dephosphorylation and translocation of nuclear factor of activated T-cells.

PHARMACOKINETICS: Absorption: Absolute bioavailability (0.5%), C_{max}<2ng/mL (90% of population). **Distribution:** V_d=99%. **Metabolism:** CYP3A (extensive); demethylation and hydroxylation; 13-demethyl tacrolimus (major metabolite). **Elimination:** Feces (major).

PROVENTIL HFA RX
albuterol sulfate (Schering)

THERAPEUTIC CLASS: Beta$_2$-agonist

INDICATIONS: Prevention and treatment of bronchospasm with reversible obstructive airway disease; prevention of exercise-induced bronchospasm (EIB) in patients ≥4 yrs old.

DOSAGE: *Adults:* Bronchospasm: 2 inh q4-6h or 1 inh q4h. EIB: 2 inh 15-30 min before activity.
Pediatrics: ≥4 yrs: Bronchospasm: 2 inh q4-6h or 1 inh q4h. EIB: 2 inh 15-30 min before activity.

HOW SUPPLIED: MDI: 90mcg/inh [6.7g]

WARNINGS/PRECAUTIONS: Hypersensitivity reactions reported. Monitor for worsening asthma. Fatalities reported with excessive use. Caution with cardiovascular disorders, especially coronary insufficiency, arrhythmias and HTN. May need concomitant corticosteroids. Can produce paradoxical bronschospasm. Caution with DM, hyperthyroidism, and seizures. May cause transient hypokalemia.

ADVERSE REACTIONS: Tachycardia, tremor, dizziness, nausea/vomiting, palpitations, rihinitis, upper respiratory tract infection, fever, inhalation site and taste sensation, back pain, and nervousness.

INTERACTIONS: Avoid other sympathomimetic agents. Extreme caution wtih MAOIs and TCAs. Monitor digoxin. May worsen ECG changes and/or hypokalemia with nonpotassium-sparing diuretics. Antagonized by β-blockers.

PREGNANCY: Category C, not for use in nursing.

MECHANISM OF ACTION: β$_2$-adrenergic bronchodilator; stimulates adenyl cylase, the enzyme that catalyzes the formation of cAMP from ATP. Increased cAMP levels are associated with relaxation of bronchial smooth muscle and inhibition of release of mediators of immediate hypersensitivity.

PROVERA RX
medroxyprogesterone acetate (Pharmacia & Upjohn)

> Not for use for prevention of cardiovascular disease or dementia. Increased risk of MI, stroke, invasive breast cancer, pulmonary emboli, and DVT in postmenopausal women (50-79 yrs) reported. Increased risk of developing probable dementia in postmenopausal women (≥65 yrs) reported.

THERAPEUTIC CLASS: Progestogen

INDICATIONS: Secondary amenorrhea and for abnormal uterine bleeding due to hormonal imbalance in the absence of organic pathology, such as fibroids or uterine cancer. To reduce the incidence of endometrial hyperplasia in non-hysterectomized postmenopausal women receiving 0.625mg conjugated estrogen.

DOSAGE: *Adults:* Secondary Amenorrhea: 5-10mg qd for 5-10 days. Abnormal Uterine Bleeding: 5-10mg qd for 5-10 days beginning on day 16 or day 21 of cycle. Endometrial Hyperplasia: 5-10mg qd for 12-14 consecutive days per month beginning on day 1 or day 16 of cycle.

HOW SUPPLIED: Tab: 2.5mg*, 5mg*, 10mg* *scored

CONTRAINDICATIONS: Thrombophlebitis, thromboembolic disorders, cerebral apoplexy, liver dysfunction, malignancy of breast or genital organs, undiagnosed vaginal bleeding, missed abortion, pregnancy, as a diagnostic test for pregnancy.

WARNINGS/PRECAUTIONS: D/C if develop thrombotic disorders, papilledema, or retinal vascular lesions. D/C pending exam if sudden onset of proptosis, sudden partial or complete loss of vision, diplopia, or migraine. Include pap smear in pretreatment exam. Caution with depression, DM, and conditions aggravated by fluid retention (eg, epilepsy, migraine, asthma, cardiac, renal dysfunction). Increased risk of endometrial and ovarian cancer reported.

ADVERSE REACTIONS: Abnormal uterine bleeding, breast tenderness, galactorrhea, urticaria, pruritus, edema, rash, thromboembolic phenomena, menstrual changes, change in weight, cervical changes, cholestatic jaundice, depression, insomnia, nausea, somnolence.

PREGNANCY: Category X, not for use in nursing.

MECHANISM OF ACTION: Progesterone derivative; transforms proliferative into secretory endometrium.

PHARMACOKINETICS: Absorption: (10mg) Rapid; C_{max}=0.71ng/mL; T_{max}=2.83 hrs; AUC=6.01ng•h/mL. **Distribution:** Plasma protein binding (90%); V_d=40564L. **Metabolism:** hydroxylation, conjugation. **Elimination:** Urine.

PROVIGIL
modafinil (Cephalon)

THERAPEUTIC CLASS: Wakefulness-promoting agent

INDICATIONS: To improve wakefulness in patients with excessive daytime sleepiness associated with narcolepsy, obstructive sleep apnea/hypopnea syndrome (OSAHS), shiftwork sleep disorder (SWSD). As adjunct treatment for underlying obstruction in OSAHS.

DOSAGE: *Adults:* 200mg qd. Narcolepsy/OSAHS: Take in AM. SWSD: Take 1 hr prior to start of work shift. Hepatic Dysfunction: 100mg qd. Elderly: Consider dose reduction.

HOW SUPPLIED: Tab: 100mg, 200mg* *scored

WARNINGS/PRECAUTIONS: Avoid in history of left ventricular hypertrophy, ischemic ECG changes, chest pain, arrhythmia or other manifestations of mitral valve prolapse with CNS stimulants. Caution if recent MI, unstable angina, history of psychosis. Monitor hypertensive patients. Rare cases of severe or life-threatening rash, including Stevens-Johnson syndrome (SJS), toxic epidermal necrolysis (TEN), and drug rash with eosinophilia and systemic symptoms (DRESS) have been reported with the use of modafinil. Angioedema and anaphylactoid reactions reported.

ADVERSE REACTIONS: Headache, infection, nausea, nervousness, anxiety, insomnia, rhinitis, diarrhea, back pain, dizziness, dyspepsia, hostility.

INTERACTIONS: Methylphenidate may delay absorption. May reduce efficacy of steroidal contraceptives up to 1 month after discontinuation. Caution with MAOIs. CYP3A4 inducers (eg, carbamazepine, phenobarbital, rifampin) may decrease levels. CYP3A4 inhibitors (eg, ketoconazole, itraconazole) may increase levels. May increase levels of drugs metabolized by CYP2C19 (eg, diazepam, propranolol, phenytoin) or CYP2C9 (eg, warfarin). Monitor for toxicity with phenytoin and PT with warfarin. May increase levels of clomipramine, desipramine. May decrease levels of drugs metabolized by CYP3A4 (eg, cyclosporine, steroidal contraceptives, theophylline). Avoid alcohol.

PREGNANCY: Category C, caution in nursing.

MECHANISM OF ACTION: Wakefulness promoting agent: Psychoactive and euphoric effects, alterations in mood, perception, thinking and feelings typical of other CNS stimulants: Modafinil binds to dopamine transporter, inhibits dopamine reuptake, and results in increased extracellular dopamine levels in some brain regions.

PHARMACOKINETICS: Absorption: T_{max}=2-4 hrs. **Distribution:** Plasma protein binding (60%). V_d=0.9L/kg. **Metabolism:** Liver via hydrolytic deamination, S-oxidation, aromatic ring hydroxylation, and glucuronide conjugation through CYP3A4. **Elimination:** Urine, feces.

PROZAC   RX
fluoxetine HCL (Lilly)

> Antidepressants increased the risk of suicidal thinking and behavior (suicidality) in short-term studies of children, adolescents, and young adults with Major Depressive Disorder (MDD) and other psychiatric disorders.

THERAPEUTIC CLASS: Selective serotonin reuptake inhibitor

INDICATIONS: Treatment of MDD, OCD, bulimia nervosa, panic disorder with or without agoraphobia.

DOSAGE: *Adults:* MDD: Daily Dosing: Initial: 20mg qam; increase dose if no improvement after several weeks. Doses >20mg/day, give qam or bid (am and noon). Max: 80mg/day. OCD: Initial: 20mg qam; may increase dose if no significant improvement after several weeks. Maint: 20-60mg/day given qd-bid, am and noon. Max: 80mg/day. Bulimia Nervosa: 60mg qam. Max: 60mg/day. Panic Disorder: Initial: 10mg/day. May increase to 20mg/day after 1 week. May increase further after several weeks if no clinical improvement. Max: 60mg/day. Hepatic Impairment/Elderly: Use lower or less frequent dosage. *Pediatrics:* MDD: ≥8 yrs: Higher Weight Peds: Initial: 10 or 20mg/day. After 1 week at 10mg/day, may increase to 20mg/day. Lower Weight Peds: Initial: 10mg/day. Titrate: May increase to 20mg/day after several weeks if clinical improvement is not observed. OCD: ≥7 yrs: Adolescents and Higher Weight Peds: Initial: 10mg/day. Titrate: Increase to 20mg/day after 2 weeks. Consider additional dose increases after several more weeks if clinical improvement is not observed. Usual: 20-60mg/day. Lower Weight Peds: Initial: 10mg/day. Titrate: Consider additional dose increases after several weeks if clinical improvement is not observed. Usual: 20-30mg/day. Max: 60mg/day.

HOW SUPPLIED: Cap: 10mg, 20mg, 40mg; Sol: 20mg/5mL [120mL]

CONTRAINDICATIONS: During or within 14 days of MAOI therapy. Thioridazine during or within 5 weeks of discontinuation. Concomitant use of pimozide.

WARNINGS/PRECAUTIONS: D/C if unexplained allergic reaction occurs. Monitor for symptoms of mania/hypomania. Caution with diseases or conditions that could affect metabolism or hemodynamic responses, diabetes, history of seizures, suicidal tendencies. Altered platelet function, hyponatremia reported. Periodically monitor height and weight in pediatrics. Monitor for clinical worsening and/or suicidality, especially at initiation of therapy or dose changes. Avoid abrupt withdrawal. Monitor for discontinuation symptoms. Caution in third trimester of pregnancy due to risk of serious neonatal complications. May interfere with cognitive and motor performance.

ADVERSE REACTIONS: Nausea, diarrhea, insomnia, anxiety, nervousness, dizziness, somnolence, tremor, decreased libido, sweating, anorexia, asthenia, dry mouth, dyspepsia, headache.

INTERACTIONS: See Contraindications. Antidiabetic drugs may need adjustment. May shift concentrations with plasma-bound drugs (eg, coumadin, digitoxin). May alter warfarin effects. May increase benzodiazepine, phenytoin, carbamazepine levels. Increased adverse effects with tryptophan. Caution with CNS drugs. Lithium levels may increase/decrease; monitor lithium levels. May potentiate drugs metabolized by CYP2D6, antipsychotics (eg, haloperidol, clozapine), other antidepressants. Avoid alcohol. Caution with drugs that interfere with hemostasis (eg, non-selective NSAIDs, ASA, warfarin) due to increased risk of bleeding. Serotonin syndrome reported with use of an SSRI and a triptan; monitor closely. Altered appetite and weight loss reported.

PREGNANCY: Category C, not for use in nursing.

MECHANISM OF ACTION: SSRI; inhibits CNS neuronal reuptake of serotonin.

PHARMACOKINETICS: Absorption: C_{max}=15-55ng/mL, T_{max}=6-8 hrs. **Distribution:** Plasma protein binding (94.5%); excreted in breast milk. **Metabolism:** Liver (extensive) via demethylation, norfluoxetine (active metabolite). **Elimination:** Urine; $T_{1/2}$=1-3 days (fluoxetine), 4-16 days (norfluoxetine).

PROZAC WEEKLY   RX
fluoxetine HCL (Lilly)

> Antidepressants increased the risk of suicidal thinking and behavior (suicidality) in short-term studies in children, adolescents, and young adults with Major Depressive Disorder (MDD) and other psychiatric disorders. Fluoxetine is approved for use in pediatric patients with MDD and obsessive compulsive disorder (OCD).

THERAPEUTIC CLASS: Selective serotonin reuptake inhibitor

INDICATIONS: Treatment of MDD.

DOSAGE: *Adults:* One 90mg capsule every week starting 7 days after last daily dose of fluoxetine 20mg.

HOW SUPPLIED: Cap, Extended-Release: 90mg

CONTRAINDICATIONS: During or within 14 days of MAOI therapy. Thioridazine during or within 5 weeks of discontinuation. Concomitant use of pimozide.

WARNINGS/PRECAUTIONS: Rash with systemic involvement and urticaria reported. Anxiety, nervousness, insomnia or activation of mania/hypomania reported. Weight loss and altered appetite; monitor weight changes. Caution with diseases or conditions that could affect metabolism or hemodynamic responses, diabetes, or history of seizures. May impair judgment, thinking or motor skills. Altered platelet function and hyponatremia reported. Monitor for clinical worsening and/or suicidality, especially at initiation of therapy or dose changes. Avoid abrupt withdrawal. Monitor for discontinuation symptoms. Caution in third trimester of pregnancy due to risk of neonatal complications.

ADVERSE REACTIONS: Nausea, diarrhea, insomnia, anxiety, nervousness, dizziness, somnolence, tremor, decreased libido, sweating, anorexia, asthenia, dry mouth, dyspepsia, headache.

INTERACTIONS: See Contraindications. Antidiabetic drugs may need adjustment. May shift concentrations with plasma-bound drugs (eg, coumadin, digitoxin). May alter warfarin effects. May increase benzodiazepine, phenytoin and carbamazepine levels. Increased adverse effects with tryptophan. Caution with CNS drugs. Lithium levels may increase/decrease; monitor lithium levels. May potentiate drugs metabolized by CYP2D6, antipsychotics (eg, haloperidol, clozapine) and other antidepressants. Avoid alcohol. Caution with drugs that interfere with hemostasis (eg, non-selective NSAIDs, ASA, warfarin) due to increased risk of bleeding. Serotonin syndrome reported with use of an SSRI and a triptan; monitor closely.

PREGNANCY: Category C, not for use in nursing.

MECHANISM OF ACTION: SSRI; inhibits CNS neuronal reuptake of serotonin.

PHARMACOKINETICS: Absorption: Delayed onset by 1-2 hrs. **Distribution:** Plasma protein binding (94.5%). Excreted in breast milk. **Metabolism:** Liver (extensive) via demethylation, norfluoxetine (active metabolite). **Elimination:** Kidney. $T_{1/2}$=1-3 days (fluoxetine), 4-16 days (norfluoxetine).

PSORCON E   RX
diflorasone diacetate (Dermik)

THERAPEUTIC CLASS: Corticosteroid

INDICATIONS: Corticosteroid responsive dermatoses.

DOSAGE: *Adults:* Apply qd-tid depending on severity. May use occlusive dressings for psoriasis or recalcitrant conditions. D/C dressings if infection develops.

HOW SUPPLIED: Cre: 0.05% [30g, 60g]

WARNINGS/PRECAUTIONS: May produce reversible HPA axis suppression, manifestations of Cushing's syndrome, hyperglycemia, and glucosuria. Caution when applied to large surface areas or under occlusive dressings. Use appropriate antifungal or antibacterial agent with dermatological infections;

d/c if infection does not clear. Pediatrics may be more susceptible to systemic toxicity. Avoid eyes. D/C if irritation occurs. Cre has an increased risk of producing adrenal suppression than Oint. Cre should not be used in treatment of rosacea or perioral dermatitis; avoid face, groin, or axillae.

ADVERSE REACTIONS: Burning, itching, irritation, dryness, folliculitis, hypertrichosis, acneiform eruptions, hypopigmentation, perioral dermatitis, allergic contact dermatitis, skin maceration, secondary infection, skin atrophy, striae, miliaria.

PREGNANCY: Category C, caution in nursing.

MECHANISM OF ACTION: Corticosteroid; posesses anti-inflammatory, antipruritic, and vasoconstrictive actions. Mechanism of anti-inflammatory activity not established. Suspected to act by the induction of phospholipase A_2 inhibitory proteins, lipocortins. Lipocortins control the biosynthesis of potent mediators of inflammation (eg, prostaglandins, leukotrienes) by inhibiting release of their common precursor, arachidonic acid.

PHARMACOKINETICS: Absorption: Percutaneous. Inflammation, other disease states, and the use of occlusive dressing may increase absorption. Use of occlusive dressings for ≤24 hrs does not increase penetration. Use of occlusive dressings for ≥96 hrs markedly enhances penetration. **Distribution:** Bound to plasma proteins in varying degrees. Systemically administered corticosteroids secreted in breast milk. **Metabolism:** Liver. **Elimination:** Kidneys (major), bile.

PULMICORT RX
budesonide (AstraZeneca)

OTHER BRAND NAMES: Pulmicort Respules (AstraZeneca) - Pulmicort Flexhaler (AstraZeneca)

THERAPEUTIC CLASS: Corticosteroid

INDICATIONS: (Respules) Treatment of asthma and as prophylactic therapy in children 12 months to 8 yrs. (Flexhaler) Maintenance treatment of asthma as prophylactic therapy in patients ≥6 yrs and to reduce or eliminate the need for oral systemic corticosteroidal therapy.

DOSAGE: *Adults:* (Flexhaler) Initial: 180-360mcg bid. Max: 720mcg bid. Individualize dose.
Pediatrics: (Flexhaler) ≥6 yrs: Initial: 180-360mcg bid. Max: 360mcg bid. Individualize dose. (Respules) 1-8 yrs: Previous Bronchodilator Only: Initial: 0.5mg qd or 0.25mg bid. Administer via jet nebulizer. Max: 0.5mg/day. Previous Inhaled Corticosteroid: 0.5mg qd or 0.25mg bid. Max: 1mg/day. Previous Oral Corticosteroid: 1mg qd or 0.5mg bid. Max: 1mg/day. Gradually reduce PO corticosteroid after 1 week of budesonide.

HOW SUPPLIED: Powder, Inhalation: (Flexhaler) 90mcg/dose, 180mcg/dose; Sus, Inhalation: (Respules) 0.25mg/2mL; 0.5mg/2mL [2mL, 30*]

CONTRAINDICATIONS: Primary treatment of status asthmaticus or other acute episodes of asthma where intensive measures are required.

WARNINGS/PRECAUTIONS: Deaths due to adrenal insufficiency have occurred with transfer from systemic corticosteroids to inhaled corticosteroids. Resume oral corticosteroids during stress or severe asthma attack. Transferring from oral to inhalation therapy may unmask allergic conditions (eg, rhinitis, conjunctivitis, arthritis, eosinophilic conditions, eczema). Observe for adrenal insufficiency, systemic corticosteroid withdrawal effects, and growth suppression (children). More susceptible to infections. Not for acute bronchospasm. D/C if bronchospasm occurs after dosing. Caution with TB of respiratory tract; untreated systemic fungal, bacterial, viral or parasitic infections; or ocular herpes simplex. *Candida* infection of mouth and pharynx reported. Patients requiring oral corticosteroids should be weaned slowly from systemic corticosteroid use.

ADVERSE REACTIONS: Nasopharyngitis, pharyngitis, headache, fever, sinusitis, pain, bronchospasm, bronchitis, respiratory infection, monoliasis.

INTERACTIONS: Oral ketoconazole increases plasma levels. CYP3A4 inhibitors (eg, itraconazole, clarithromycin, erythromycin) may inhibit metabolism and increase systemic exposure. (Respules) Slight decrease in clearance and increase in oral bioavailabilty with cimetidine.

PREGNANCY: (Respules) Category B, caution in nursing; (Flexhaler) Category B, caution in nursing.

MECHANISM OF ACTION: Corticosteroid; not established. Shown to have inhibitory effects on multiple cell types (mast cells, eosinophils, neutrophils, macrophages and lymphocytes) and mediators (histamine, eicosanoids, leukotrienes and cytokines) involved in inflammatory and asthmatic response.

PHARMACOKINETICS: Absorption: Respules: (4-6 yrs) Absolute bioavailability (6%); C_{max}=2.6nmol/L, T_{max}=20 min. Turbuhaler: T_{max}=30 min. Flexhaler: (Adults) T_{max}=10 min, (180mg qd) C_{max}=0.6nmol/L. (360mg bid) C_{max}=1.6nmol/L. (Peds) T_{max}=15-30 mins, (180mg qd) C_{max}=0.4nmol/L. (360mg bid) C_{max}=1.5nmol/L. **Distribution:** V_d=3L/kg; Plasma protein binding (85-90%). **Metabolism:** Liver (biotransformation), via CYP3A4. **Elimination:** (Respules) $T_{1/2}$=2.3 hrs. (Turbuhaler, Flexhaler) $T_{1/2}$=2-3 hrs.

PULMOZYME   RX
dornase alfa (Genentech)

THERAPEUTIC CLASS: Protein

INDICATIONS: Adjunct therapy in cystic fibrosis to improve pulmonary function.

DOSAGE: *Adults:* 2.5mg qd-bid via nebulizer.
Pediatrics: ≥5 yrs: 2.5mg qd-bid via nebulizer.

HOW SUPPLIED: Sol: 2.5mg/2.5mL [2.5mL: 1^5, 30^s]

CONTRAINDICATIONS: Hypersensitivity to chinese hamster ovary cell products.

WARNINGS/PRECAUTIONS: Use with standard therapies for cystic fibrosis.

ADVERSE REACTIONS: Voice alteration, pharyngitis, rash, laryngitis, chest pain, conjunctivitis, rhinitis, fever, dyspnea.

PREGNANCY: Category B, caution in nursing.

MECHANISM OF ACTION: Protein; hydrolyzes the DNA in sputum and reduces sputum viscoelasticity.

PURINETHOL   RX
mercaptopurine (Gate)

THERAPEUTIC CLASS: Purine analog

INDICATIONS: Remission induction and maintenance therapy of acute lymphatic leukemia (ALL).

DOSAGE: *Adults:* Maint: 1.5-2.5mg/kg/day as single dose. Renal/Hepatic Impairment: Reduce dose. Concomitant Allopurinol: Reduce mercaptopurine dose by 1/3-1/4 of usual dose. TPMT Deficiency: Consider dose reduction. *Pediatrics:* Maint: 1.5-2.5mg/kg/day as single dose. Renal/Hepatic Impairment: Reduce dose. Concomitant Allopurinol: Reduce mercaptopurine dose by 1/3-1/4 of usual dose. TPMT Deficiency: Consider dose reduction.

HOW SUPPLIED: Tab: 50mg* *scored

CONTRAINDICATIONS: Lack of definitive diagnosis of ALL. Prior resistance to mercaptopurine or thioguanine.

WARNINGS/PRECAUTIONS: Risk of dose-related bone marrow suppression. Monitor weekly platelet counts, Hgb, Hct, total WBC with differential; increase frequency during induction phase. Monitor closely for life-threatening infection or bleeding. Risk of hepatotoxicity, anorexia, diarrhea, jaundice, and ascites (especially with >2.5mg/kg dose). Perform LFTs weekly initially, then monthly; monitor more frequently with hepatotoxic drugs or pre-existing liver disease. Increased sensitivity to myelosuppressive effects with thiopurine-

P

S-methyltransferase (TPMT) gene deficiency; consider TPMT testing with evidence of severe toxicity.

ADVERSE REACTIONS: Bone marrow toxicity, hepatotoxicity, hyperuricemia (reduce incidence by prehydration, urine alkalinization, prophylactic allopurinol), intestinal ulceration, rash, hyperpigmentation, alopecia, transient oligospermia.

INTERACTIONS: Reduce to 1/3-1/4 of usual dose with allopurinol to avoid toxicity. Reduce dose with myelosuppressants. Bone marrow suppression reported with trimethoprim-sulfamethoxazole. Cross-resistance with thioguanine. Increased bone marrow toxicity with concomitant TPMT inhibitors (eg, olsalazine, mesalazine, sulphasalazine). Inhibition of anticoagulant effect of warfarin with concomitant administration.

PREGNANCY: Category D, not for use in nursing.

MECHANISM OF ACTION: Purine analog; competes with hypoxanthine and guanine for hypoxanthine-guanine phosphoribosyltransferase and gets converted to thiosinic acid, which then inhibits glutamine-5-phosphoribosylpyrophosphate amidotransferase of de novo pathway for purine ribonucleotide synthesis.

PHARMACOKINETICS: Absorption: Incomplete. **Distribution:** Plasma protein binding (19%). **Elimination:** $T_{1/2}$=21 min (pediatric); 47 min (adult).

PYRAZINAMIDE   RX
pyrazinamide (Various)

THERAPEUTIC CLASS: Nicotinamide analogue

INDICATIONS: Adjunctive initial treatment of active TB. For use after treatment failure with other primary drugs.

DOSAGE: *Adults:* Usual: 15-30mg/kg qd. Max: 3g/day. (CDC recommends Max: 2g/day). Alternate Regimen: 50-75mg/kg twice weekly. Dose based on lean body weight. Take initial 2 months of 6 month or longer regimen. *Pediatrics:* Usual: 15-30mg/kg qd. Max: 3g/day. (CDC recommends Max: 2g/day). Alternate Regimen: 50-75mg/kg twice weekly. Dose based on lean body weight. Take initial 2 months of 6 month or longer regimen.

HOW SUPPLIED: Tab: 500mg* *scored

CONTRAINDICATIONS: Severe hepatic damage and active gout.

WARNINGS/PRECAUTIONS: Obtain baseline serum uric acid and LFTs before therapy. Caution with hepatic dysfunction or those at risk for drug-related hepatitis (eg, alcoholics) and DM. D/C if hyperuricemia with gouty arthritis or hepatocellular damage occurs. Inhibits renal excretion of urates.

ADVERSE REACTIONS: Gout, hepatotoxicity, nausea, vomiting, anorexia, arthralgia, myalgia, rash, urticaria, pruritus.

PREGNANCY: Category C, caution in nursing.

MECHANISM OF ACTION: Nicotinamide analogue; suspected to act as bacteriostatic and bactericidal against *Mycobacterium* tuberculosis.

PHARMACOKINETICS: Absorption: GI tract (well-absorbed); T_{max}=2hrs. **Distribution:** Plasma protein binding (10%); distributed in liver, lungs, and CSF; found in breast milk. **Metabolism:** Liver, via hydroxylation; pyrazinoic acid (major active metabolite). **Elimination:** Urine (70%); $T_{1/2}$=9-10 hrs.

PYRIDIUM   RX
phenazopyridine HCL (Warner Chilcott)

THERAPEUTIC CLASS: Urinary tract analgesic

INDICATIONS: Symptomatic relief of urinary pain, burning, frequency and urgency associated with infection, trauma, and urinary procedures.

DOSAGE: *Adults:* 200mg tid pc. Concomitant Antibiotic for UTI: Do not exceed 2 days of phenazopyridine therapy.

PDR® Nursing Drug Guide

HOW SUPPLIED: Tab: 100mg, 200mg

CONTRAINDICATIONS: Renal insufficiency.

WARNINGS/PRECAUTIONS: D/C if skin or sclera develops a yellow color; may indicate impaired renal excretion. Caution in elderly, renal impairment. May produce orange to red urine; may stain fabric and contact lenses.

ADVERSE REACTIONS: Headache, rash, pruritus, GI distress, methemoglobinemia, hemolytic anemia, anaphylactoid-like reactions.

PREGNANCY: Category B, safety in nursing not known.

MECHANISM OF ACTION: Not established; urinary tract analgesic agent excreted in urine where it exerts a topical analgesic effect on urinary tract mucosa.

PHARMACOKINETICS: Elimination: Urine (rapid); (65% unchanged).

PYRIDIUM PLUS RX
phenazopyridine HCL - hyoscyamine hydrobromide - butabarbital (Warner Chilcott)

THERAPEUTIC CLASS: Anticholinergic/barbiturate/analgesic

INDICATIONS: Symptomatic relief of urinary pain, burning, frequency and urgency associated with infection, trauma, and urinary procedures.

DOSAGE: *Adults:* 1 tab qid (pc and hs). Concomitant Antibiotic for UTI: Do not exceed 2 days of therapy.

HOW SUPPLIED: Tab: (Butabarbital-Hyoscyamine-Phenazopyridine) 15mg-0.3mg-150mg

CONTRAINDICATIONS: Renal or hepatic insufficiency, glaucoma, bladder neck obstruction, porphyria.

WARNINGS/PRECAUTIONS: D/C if skin or sclera develops yellow color; may indicate impaired renal excretion. Caution in elderly, renal impairment. Produces orange to red urine; may stain fabric and contact lenses.

ADVERSE REACTIONS: Headache, rash, pruritus, GI distress, methemoglobinemia, hemolytic anemia, anaphylactoid-like reactions, dry mouth, dizziness, drowsiness, blurred vision.

PREGNANCY: Category C, safety in nursing not known.

MECHANISM OF ACTION: Phenazopyridine: Analgesic agent excreted in urine where it exerts a topical analgesic effect on urinary tract mucosa. Hyoscyamine: Parasympatholytic; acts to relieve detrusor muscle spasm. Butabarbital: Short-to-intermediate acting sedative, helps to allay associated anxiety and apprehension.

QUESTRAN RX
cholestyramine (Par)

OTHER BRAND NAMES: Questran Light (Par)

THERAPEUTIC CLASS: Bile acid sequestrant

INDICATIONS: Adjunct to reduce elevated cholesterol in primary hypercholesterolemia not responding to diet or to reduce LDL in hypertriglyceridemia. Relief of pruritus associated with partial biliary obstruction.

DOSAGE: *Adults:* Initial: 1 pkt or scoopful qd or bid. Maint: 2-4 pkts or scoopfuls/day, given bid. Titrate: Adjust at no less than 4 week intervals. Max: 6 pkts/day or 6 scoopfuls/day. May also give as 1-6 doses/day. Mix with fluid or highly fluid food.
Pediatrics: Usual: 240mg/kg/day of anhydrous cholestyramine resin in 2-3 divided doses. Max: 8g/day.

HOW SUPPLIED: Powder: 4g/pkt [60s, 378g], (Light) 4g/scoopful [60s, 268g]

CONTRAINDICATIONS: Complete biliary obstruction.

WARNINGS/PRECAUTIONS: May produce hyperchloremic acidosis with prolonged use. Caution in renal insufficiency, volume depletion, and with concomitant spironolactone. Chronic use may produce or worsen constipation. Avoid constipation with symptomatic CAD. May increase bleeding tendency due to vitamin K deficiency. Serum or red cell folate reduced with chronic use. Constipation may aggravate hemorrhoids. Light formulation contains phenylalanine. Measure cholesterol during 1st few months; periodically thereafter. Measure TG periodically.

ADVERSE REACTIONS: Constipation, heartburn, nausea, vomiting, abdominal pain, flatulence, diarrhea, anorexia, osteoporosis, rash, hyperchloremic acidosis (children), vitamin A and D deficiency, steatorrhea, hypoprothrombinemia (vitamin K deficiency).

INTERACTIONS: May interfere with absorption of fat-soluble vitamins (A, D, E, K), drugs that undergo enterohepatic circulation, and oral phosphate supplements. Take concomitant drugs 1hr before or 4-6 hrs after. Additive effects with HMG-CoA reductase inhibitors and nicotinic acid. Caution with spironolactone. May reduce or delay absorption of phenylbutazone, warfarin, thiazide diuretics, propranolol, tetracycline, penicillin G, phenobarbital, thyroid and thyroxine agents, estrogens, progestins, digitalis.

PREGNANCY: Category C, caution in nursing.

MECHANISM OF ACTION: Bile acid sequestrant; absorbs and combines with bile acids in intestine to form insoluble complex excreted in the feces, resulting in partial removal of bile acids from enterohepatic circulation by preventing their absorption. This leads to increased oxidation of cholesterol to bile acids and decreased plasma LDL and serum cholesterol levels.

PHARMACOKINETICS: Elimination: Feces.

QUINIDINE GLUCONATE INJECTION   RX

quinidine gluconate (Various)

THERAPEUTIC CLASS: Class IA antiarrhythmic/schizonticide antimalarial

INDICATIONS: Treatment of life-threatening *Plasmodium falciparum* malaria. Conversion of atrial fibrillation/flutter (A-Fib/Flutter) to normal sinus rhythm. Treatment of ventricular arrhythmias.

DOSAGE: *Adults:* Malaria: LD: 15mg/kg base (24mg/kg gluconate) over 4 hrs. Maint: After 8 hrs, 7.5mg/kg (12mg/kg gluconate) IV q8h for 7 days. Alternate: Initial: 6.25mg/kg base (10mg/kg gluconate) IV over 1-2 hrs. Maint: 12.5mcg/kg/min base (20mcg/kg/min gluconate) for 72h. Switch to PO therapy when possible. A-Fib/Flutter and Ventricular Arrhythmia: 0.25mg/kg/min. Max: 5-10mg/kg. Consider alternate therapy if conversion to sinus rhythm not achieved. Renal/Hepatic Impairment or CHF: Reduce dose. Elderly: Start at low end of dosing range.
Pediatrics: Malaria: LD: 15mg/kg base (24mg/kg gluconate) over 4 hrs. Maint: After 8 hrs, 7.5mg/kg (12mg/kg gluconate) IV q8h for 7 days. Alternate: Initial: 6.25mg/kg base (10mg/kg gluconate) IV over 1-2 hrs. Maint: 12.5mcg/kg/min base (20mcg/kg/min gluconate) for 72h. Switch to PO therapy when possible.

HOW SUPPLIED: Inj: 80mg/mL

CONTRAINDICATIONS: Cardiac rhythm dependent upon a junctional or idio-ventricular pacemaker (absent of functioning pacemaker), thrombocytopenic purpura with previous treatment, patients adversely affected by anticholinergics (eg, myasthenia gravis).

WARNINGS/PRECAUTIONS: Rapid infusion can cause peripheral vascular collapse and hypotension. May prolong QTc interval. Paradoxical increase in ventricular rate in A-Fib/Flutter. Caution in those at risk of complete AV block without implanted pacemakers, renal/hepatic dysfunction, elderly, and CHF. Physical/pharmacologic maneuvers to terminate paroxysmal supraventricular tachycardia may be ineffective. Exacerbated bradycardia in sick sinus syndrome.

ADVERSE REACTIONS: GI distress, lightheadedness, fatigue, palpitations, weakness, visual problems, nausea, vomiting, diarrhea, sleep disturbances, rash, headache, cinchonism, hepatotoxicity, autoimmune/inflammatory syndromes.

INTERACTIONS: Urine alkalinizers (eg, carbonic anhydrase inhibitors, sodium bicarbonate, thiazide diuretics) reduce renal elimination. CYP3A4 inducers (eg, phenobarbital, phenytoin, rifampin) may accelerate elimination. Verapamil, diltiazem decrease clearance. Caution with drugs metabolized by CYP2D6 (eg, mexiletine, phenothiazines, polycyclic antidepressants, codeine, hydrocodone) or by CYP3A4 (eg, nifedipine, felodipine, nicardipine, nimodipine). β-blockers may decrease clearance. May slow metabolism of nifedipine. Increases levels of digoxin, digitoxin, procainamide and haloperidol. Increased levels with ketoconazole, amiodarone, cimetidine. Potentiates warfarin, depolarizing and nondepolarizing neuromuscular blockers. Additive effects with anticholinergics, vasodilators, and negative inotropes. Antagonistic effects with cholinergics, vasoconstrictors, and positive inotropes.

PREGNANCY: Category C, not for use in nursing.

MECHANISM OF ACTION: Antimalarial schizonticide and antiarrhythmic agent with class 1a activity. Slows phase-0 depolarization by depressing the inward depolarizing Na+ current, which slows conduction, prolongs effective refractory period, and reduces automaticity in the heart. Also has anticholinergic activity, negative ionotropic activity, and acts peripherally as an α-adrenergic antagonist.

PHARMACOKINETICS: Absorption: T_{max} ≤2 hrs. **Distribution:** V_d=2-3 L/kg; plasma protein binding (80-88%), (50-70%) in pregnant women, infants and neonates; found in breast milk. **Metabolism:** Liver, via CYP3A4 pathway. 3-hydroxy-quinidine (3HQ); major metabolite. **Elimination:** Urine, 20% (unchanged); $T_{1/2}$=6-8 hrs (adults), 3-4 hrs (pediatrics), and 12 hrs (3HQ).

QUINIDINE GLUCONATE ORAL RX
quinidine gluconate (Various)

THERAPEUTIC CLASS: Class IA antiarrhythmic

INDICATIONS: Conversion of symptomatic atrial fibrillation/flutter (A-Fib/Flutter) to normal sinus rhythm, reduction of relapse frequency into A-Fib/Flutter, and suppression of ventricular arrhythmias.

DOSAGE: *Adults:* A-Fib/Flutter Conversion: Initial: 2 tabs q8h. Titrate: Increase cautiously if no effect after 3-4 doses. Alternate Regimen: 1 tab q8h for 2 days, then 2 tabs q12h for 2 days, then 2 tabs q8h up to 4 days. A-Fib/Flutter Relapse Reduction: 1 tab q8-12h. Titrate: Increase cautiously if needed. Ventricular Arrhythmia: Dosing regimens not adequately studied. Generally similar to A-Fib/Flutter. Renal/Hepatic Impairment or CHF: Reduce dose. May break tab in half. Do not chew or crush.

HOW SUPPLIED: Tab, Extended-Release: 324mg

CONTRAINDICATIONS: Cardiac rhythm dependent upon a junctional or idioventricular pacemaker (absent of functioning pacemaker), thrombocytopenic purpura with previous treatment, myasthenia gravis.

WARNINGS/PRECAUTIONS: Increases risk of mortality, especially with structural heart disease. May prolong QTc interval. Paradoxical increase in ventricular rate in A-Fib/Flutter. Caution in those at risk of complete AV block without implanted pacemakers, renal/hepatic dysfunction, and CHF. Physical/pharmacologic maneuvers to terminate paroxysmal supraventricular tachycardia may be ineffective. Exacerbated bradycardia in sick sinus syndrome.

ADVERSE REACTIONS: Diarrhea, fever, rash, arrhythmia, abnormal ECG, nausea, vomiting, dizziness, headache.

INTERACTIONS: Urine alkalinizers (eg, carbonic anhydrase inhibitors, sodium bicarbonate, thiazide diuretics) reduce renal elimination. CYP3A4 inducers (eg, phenobarbital, phenytoin, rifampin) may accelerate elimination. Verapamil, diltiazem, β-blockers decrease clearance. Caution with drugs metabolized by CYP450 3A4 (eg, nifedipine, felodipine, nicardipine, nimodipine) and 2D6 (eg, mexiletine, phenothiazines, polycyclic antidepressants, codeine, hydrocodone). Increases levels of digoxin, digitoxin, procainamide and haloperidol. Increased levels with ketoconazole, amiodarone, cimetidine. Potentiates warfarin, depolarizing and nondepolarizing neuromuscular blockers. Additive effects with anticholinergics, vasodilators, and negative inotropics. Antagonistic effects with cholinergics, vasoconstrictors, and positive inotropes. Avoid grapefruit juice. Dietary salt may affect absorption.

PREGNANCY: Category C, not for use in nursing.

MECHANISM OF ACTION: Antimalarial schizonticide and antiarrhythmic agent with class Ia activity. Slows phase-0 depolarization by depressing the inward depolarizing Na+ current, slows conduction, prolongs effective refractory period and reduces automaticity in the heart. Also has anticholinergic activity, negative ionotropic activity, and acts peripherally as an α-adrenergic antagonist.

PHARMACOKINETICS: Absorption: Absolute bioavailability (70-80%), T_{max} =3-5 hrs. **Distribution:** V_d= 2-3L/kg; plasma protein binding (80-88% in adults), (50-70% in pregnant, pediatrics). Found in breast milk. **Metabolism:** Liver, via CYP3A4. 3-hydroxy-quinidine (3HQ); major metabolite. **Elimination:** Urine (20%, unchanged). $T_{1/2}$= 6-8 hrs (adults), 3-4 hrs (pediatrics), 12 hrs (3HQ).

QUINIDINE SULFATE   RX
quinidine sulfate (Watson)

THERAPEUTIC CLASS: Class IA antiarrhythmic/schizonticide antimalarial

INDICATIONS: Conversion of symptomatic A-fib/flutter to normal sinus rhythm, reduction of relapse frequency into A-fib/flutter, and suppression of ventricular arrhythmias. Treatment of life-threatening *Plasmodium falciparum* malaria.

DOSAGE: *Adults:* A-Fib/Flutter Conversion: Initial: 400mg q6h. Titrate: Increase cautiously if no effect after 4-5 doses. A-Fib/Flutter Relapse Reduction: 200mg q6h. Titrate: Increase cautiously if needed. Ventricular Arrhythmia: Dosing regimens not adequately studied. Malaria: After LD of quinidine gluconate, 300mg q8h for 7 days. Alternate: After LD of quinidine gluconate, 300mg q8h for 72h or until parasitemia had decreased to ≤1%. *Pediatrics:* Malaria: After LD of quinidine gluconate, 300mg q8h for 7 days. Alternate: After LD of quinidine gluconate, 300mg q8h for 72h or until parasitemia had decreased to ≤1%.

HOW SUPPLIED: Tab: 200mg, 300mg

CONTRAINDICATIONS: Cardiac rhythm dependent upon a junctional or idioventricular pacemaker (in the absence of functioning pacemaker), thrombocytopenic purpura with previous treatment, patients adversely affected by anticholinergics (eg, myasthenia gravis).

WARNINGS/PRECAUTIONS: Increases risk of mortality, especially with structural heart disease. May prolong QTc interval. Paradoxical increase in ventricular rate in A-fib/flutter. Adjust dose in renal/hepatic dysfunction and CHF. Caution if at risk of complete AV-block in those without implanted pacemakers or in elderly. Physical/pharmacologic maneuvers to terminate paroxysmal supraventricular tachycardia may be ineffective. Exacerbated bradycardia in sick sinus syndrome. Monitor blood counts, hepatic, and renal function periodically with long-term therapy. D/c if blood dyscrasia or hepatic/renal dysfunction occurs.

ADVERSE REACTIONS: Diarrhea, nausea, vomiting, headache, esophagitis, lightheadedness, fatigue, palpitations, angina-like pain, weakness, rash, visual problems, cinchonism, hepatotoxicity, autoimmune/inflammatory syndromes.

INTERACTIONS: Urine alkalinizers (eg, carbonic anhydrase inhibitors, sodium bicarbonate, thiazide diuretics) reduce renal elimination. CYP3A4 inducers (eg, phenobarbital, phenytoin, rifampin) may accelerate hepatic elimination. Verapamil, diltiazem, β-blockers decrease clearance. Caution with drugs metabolized by CYP3A4 and 2D6. Increases levels of procainamide and haloperidol. Increased levels with ketoconazole, amiodarone, cimetidine. Decreased

Q

levels with nifedipine. Potentiates warfarin, depolarizing (eg, succinylcholine, decamethonium) and nondepolarizing (eg, d-tubocurarine, pancuronium) neuromuscular blockers. Additive effects with anticholinergics, vasodilators, and negative inotropics. Avoid grapefruit juice. Dietary salt may affect absorption. Digoxin may need dose reduction.

PREGNANCY: Category C, not for use in nursing.

MECHANISM OF ACTION: An antimalarial schizonticide and an antiarrhythmic agent with class 1a activity. Quinidine depresses rapid inward depolarizing Na current, thereby slowing phase-0 depolarization and reducing the amplitude of action potentials without affecting resting potentials resulting in slowed conduction and reduced automaticity in all parts of the heart, with increase in effective refractory period relative to the duration of action potentials in the atria, ventricles, and Purkinje tissues, also raises fibrillation thresholds of the atria and ventricles, and it raises ventricular defibrillation threshold. It can interrupt or prevent reentrant arrhythemias and arrhythemias due to increased automaticity, including atrial flutter, AF, and PST. It has anticholinergic activity, negative inotropic activity, and acts peripherally as an α-adrenergic antagonist.

PHARMACOKINETICS: Absorption: Absolute bioavailability (70%), T_{max}=6 hrs. **Distribution:** Plasma protein binding (80-88%), and (50-70%) in pregnant women, infants and neonates. Vd=2-3 L/kg. Found in breast milk. **Metabolism:** Liver via CYP3A4 pathway; 3-hydroxy-quinidine (3HQ) major metabolite. **Elimination:** Urine, (70%) unchanged. $T_{1/2}$=6-8 hrs (adults), 3-4 hrs (pediatrics), and 12 hrs (3HQ).

QUININE SULFATE   RX
quinine sulfate (Various)

THERAPEUTIC CLASS: Cinchona alkaloid

INDICATIONS: For use in malaria.

DOSAGE: *Adults:* 1-3 tabs/caps tid for 6-12 days.

HOW SUPPLIED: Cap: 325mg; Tab: 260mg

CONTRAINDICATIONS: Pregnancy, glucose-6-phosphate dehydrogenase (G-6PD) deficiency, history of thrombocytopenic purpura associated with quinine sulfate, tinnitus, optic neuritis, and history of blackwater fever.

WARNINGS/PRECAUTIONS: May cause cinchonism (eg, headache, tinnitus, nausea, vision disturbance). Hemolysis reported with G-6PD deficiency; d/c if hemolysis appears. D/C if hypersensitivity occurs. Caution with atrial fibrillation.

ADVERSE REACTIONS: Headache, nausea, vomiting, epigastric pain, tinnitus, blurred vision, photophobia, hemolysis, thrombocytopenic purpura, diplopia, vertigo, restlessness, asthma symptoms, anginal symptoms.

INTERACTIONS: Decreased absorption with aluminum-containing antacids. May enhance the effect of warfarin and other oral anticoagulants. Potentiates neuromuscular blocking agents (eg, pancuronium, succinylcholine, tubocurarine). Increases digoxin and digitoxin plasma levels. Urinary alkalizers (eg, acetazolamide and sodium bicarbonate) may increase levels.

PREGNANCY: Category X, caution in nursing.

MECHANISM OF ACTION: Cinchona alkaloid; inhibits nucleic acid synthesis, protein synthesis, and glycolysis in *Plasmodium falciparum* and can bind with hemazoin in parasitized erthrocytes.

PHARMACOKINETICS: Absorption: Absolute bioavailability (76-88%); (healthy) T_{max}=2.8 hrs. C_{max}=3.2mcg/mL, AUC=28.0mcg•h/mL. (Malaria patients): T_{max}=5.9 hrs. C_{max}=8.4mcg/mL, AUC=73.0mcg•h/mL. **Distribution:** V_d=2.5-7.1L/kg; plasma protein binding (69-92%). **Metabolism:** Via hepatic oxidative CYP3A4 and CYP2D6, 3-hydroxyquinine (major metabolite). **Elimination:** Via hepatic biotransformation; urine (approximately 20% unchanged). $T_{1/2}$=9.7-12.5 hrs.

QUIXIN
levofloxacin (Vistakon)

RX

THERAPEUTIC CLASS: Fluoroquinolone

INDICATIONS: Treatment of bacterial conjunctivitis.

DOSAGE: *Adults:* Days 1-2: 1-2 drops q2h while awake, up to 8x/day. Days 3-7: 1-2 drops q4h while awake, up to qid.
Pediatrics: ≥1 yr: Days 1-2: 1-2 drops q2h while awake, up to 8x/day. Days 3-7: 1-2 drops q4h while awake, up to qid.

HOW SUPPLIED: Sol: 0.5% [5mL]

WARNINGS/PRECAUTIONS: D/C if hypersensitivity or superinfection occurs. Avoid contact lenses with conjunctivitis.

ADVERSE REACTIONS: Transient ocular burning, decreased vision, fever, foreign body sensation, headache, ocular pain, pharyngitis, photophobia.

INTERACTIONS: Systemic quinolone therapy may increase theophylline levels, interfere with caffeine metabolism, enhance warfarin effects, and elevate serum creatinine with cyclosporine.

PREGNANCY: Category C, caution in nursing.

MECHANISM OF ACTION: Fluroquinlone; antibacterial active against broad spectrum of gram-positive and gram-negative organisms. Responsible for inhibition of bacterial topoisomerase IV and DNA gyrase, enzymes required for DNA replication, transcription, repair, and recombination.

PHARMACOKINETICS: Absorption: C_{max}=0.94ng/mL (single dose), 2.15ng/mL (multiple doses).

QVAR
beclomethasone dipropionate (Ivax)

RX

THERAPEUTIC CLASS: Corticosteroid

INDICATIONS: Maintenance treatment of asthma as prophylactic therapy in patients ≥5 tears; to reduce or eliminate the need for oral corticosteroidal therapy.

DOSAGE: *Adults:* Previous Bronchodilator Only: 40-80mcg bid. Max: 320mcg bid. Previous Inhaled Corticosteroid (CS) Therapy: 40-160mcg bid. Max: 320mcg bid. Maint With Oral CS: May attempt gradual reduction of oral dose after 1 week on inhaled therapy.
Pediatrics: Adolescents: Previous Bronchodilator Only: 40-80mcg bid. Max: 320mcg bid. Previous Inhaled Corticosteroid (CS) Therapy: 40-160mcg bid. Max: 320mcg bid. 5-11 yrs: Previous Bronchodilator Only or Inhaled CS Therapy: 40mcg bid. Max: 80mcg bid. ≥5 yrs: Maint With Oral CS: May attempt gradual reduction of oral dose after 1 week on inhaled therapy.

HOW SUPPLIED: MDI: 40mcg/inh, 80mcg/inh [7.3g]

CONTRAINDICATIONS: Status asthmaticus, acute asthmatic attacks.

WARNINGS/PRECAUTIONS: Deaths due to adrenal insufficiency have occurred with transfer from systemic corticosteroids to inhaled corticosteroids. Resume oral corticosteroids during stress or severe asthma attack. Risk of adrenal insufficiency and withdrawal symptoms when replacing systemic corticosteroids. May unmask allergic conditions previously suppressed by systemic steroid therapy. Caution with TB, ocular herpes simplex, or untreated systemic bacterial, fungal, parasitic or viral infections. May suppress growth in children. Exposure to chickenpox or measles requires prophylaxis treatment. Not for rapid relief of bronchospasm.

ADVERSE REACTIONS: Headache, pharyngitis, upper respiratory tract infection, rhinitis, increased asthma symptoms, sinusitis.

PREGNANCY: Category C, not for use in nursing.

MECHANISM OF ACTION: Corticosteroid; inhibits both inflammatory cells and release of inflammatory mediators.

PHARMACOKINETICS: Absorption: C_{max}=88pg/mL; T_{max}=0.5 hr. (17-BMP) C_{max}=1419pg/mL, T_{max}=0.7hr. **Metabolism:** Biotransformation, via CYP3A. (Metabolites) beclomethasone-17-monopropionate (17-BMP), beclonethasone-21-monopropionate (21-BMP) and beclomethasone (BOH). **Elimination:** Feces (major). (17-BMP) $T_{1/2}$=2.8 hrs.

RABAVERT   RX
rabies vaccine (Chiron)

THERAPEUTIC CLASS: Vaccine

INDICATIONS: Pre-exposure immunization and post-exposure prophylaxis against rabies.

DOSAGE: *Adults:* Pre-exposure: Primary: 1mL IM on Day 0, 7, either 21 or 28. Booster: 1mL IM in high-risk patients to maintain >1:5 serum dilution by RFFIT. Post-exposure: 1mL IM on days 0, 3, 7, 14, and 28 with rabies immune globulin 20 IU/kg on Day 0. Post-exposure if Previously Immunized: 1mL IM on Day 0 and Day 3.
Pediatrics: Pre-exposure: Primary: 1mL IM on Day 0, 7, either 21 or 28. Booster: 1mL IM in high-risk patients to maintain >1:5 serum dilution by RFFIT. Post-exposure: 1mL IM on days 0, 3, 7, 14, and 28 with rabies immune globulin 20 IU/kg on Day 0. Post-exposure if Previously Immunized: 1mL IM on Day 0 and Day 3.

HOW SUPPLIED: Inj: 2.5 IU

CONTRAINDICATIONS: Caution in sensitivity to bovine gelatin, chicken protein, neomycin, chlortetracycline, and amphotericin B in preexposure vaccination. There is no contraindication to postexposure prophylaxis, including pregnancy.

WARNINGS/PRECAUTIONS: Do not use SQ, intradermally, or IV. Postpone pre-exposure vaccination in the sick, convalescent, or during the incubation period of an infectious disease. Avoid in patients with egg-sensitivity. Active immunity can be impaired in immunocompromised patients. Have epinephrine available.

ADVERSE REACTIONS: Local reactions (eg, induration, swelling, reddening), lymphadenopathy, headache, dizziness, flu-like symptoms (asthenia, fatigue, fever, myalgia, malaise), nausea, rash, arthralgia.

INTERACTIONS: Active immunity can be impaired with corticosteroids, immunosuppressants, and antimalarials. Do not give immunosuppressants during post-exposure unless essential. Do not give rabies immune globulin at greater than the recommended dose.

PREGNANCY: Category C, safety in nursing not known.

MECHANISM OF ACTION: Stimulates the immune system to produce antibodies that may protect against rabies.

RANEXA   RX
ranolazine (CV Therapeutics)

THERAPEUTIC CLASS: Miscellaneous antianginal

INDICATIONS: Treatment of chronic angina. Because it prolongs the QT interval, use should be reserved for patients who have not achieved an adequate response with other antianginal drugs. For use in combination with amlodipine, β-blockers or nitrates. The effect on angina rate or exercise tolerance appeared to be smaller in women than men.

DOSAGE: *Adults:* Initial: 500mg bid. Max: 1000mg bid. Swallow whole; do not crush, break, or chew.

HOW SUPPLIED: Tab, Extended-Release: 500mg, 1mg

CONTRAINDICATIONS: Pre-existing QT prolongation; hepatic impairment (Child-Pugh Classes A [mild], B [moderate], C [severe]); with QT prolonging drugs; with potent and moderately potent CYP3A inhibitors (including diltiazem).

WARNINGS/PRECAUTIONS: May prolong QTc interval in a dose-related manner; avoid with known QT prolongation (including congenital long QT syndrome, uncorrected hypokalemia), known history of ventricular tachycardia, hepatic dysfunction. Monitor BP with severe renal impairment.

ADVERSE REACTIONS: Dizziness, headache, constipation, nausea.

INTERACTIONS: See Contraindications. Increased levels with ketoconazole, diltiazem, verapamil, paroxetine. Avoid use with potent or moderately potent CYP3A inhibitors such as ketoconazole and other azole antifungals, diltiazem, verapamil, macrolide antibiotics, HIV protease inhibitors, grapefruit juice or grapefruit-containing products. May increase levels of digoxin, simvastatin; consider dosage reduction of digoxin, simvastatin. Avoid with drugs that may prolong the QTc interval, such as Class Ia (eg, quinidine) and Class III (eg, dofetilide, sotalol) antiarrhythmics, and antipsychotics (eg, thioridazine, ziprasidone). May increase levels of drugs metabolized by CYP2D6 such as TCAs and some antipsychotics; consider dosage reduction of these drugs.

PREGNANCY: Category C, not for use in nursing.

MECHANISM OF ACTION: Not been established; suspected to have antianginal and anti-ischemic effects that do not depend upon reductions of HR and BP.

PHARMACOKINETICS: Absorption: T_{max}=2-5hrs., C_{max}=2569ng/mL. **Distribution:** Plasma protein binding (62%). **Metabolism:** Gut and liver (extensive), via CYP3A and CYP2D6. **Elimination:** $T_{1/2}$=7 hrs. Urine (75%), feces (25%), and (<5% unchanged).

RAPAMUNE   RX
sirolimus (Wyeth)

> Increased susceptibility to infection and development of lymphoma.

THERAPEUTIC CLASS: Macrocyclic lactone immunosuppressant

INDICATIONS: Prophylaxis of organ rejection in renal transplant patients. Recommended to be used initially with cyclosporine and corticosteroids. In low-moderate risk patients, withdraw cyclosporine 2-4 months after transplantation and increase sirolimus dose to reach recommended blood levels.

DOSAGE: *Adults:* LD: 6mg. Maint: 2mg qd. Hepatic Impairment: Reduce maintenance dose by one-third.
Pediatrics: ≥13 yrs and <40kg: LD: 3mg/m² Maint: 1mg/m²/day. Hepatic Impairment: Reduce maintenance dose by one-third. Take 4 hrs after cyclosporine.

HOW SUPPLIED: Sol: 1mg/mL [60mL]; Tab: 1mg, 2mg

WARNINGS/PRECAUTIONS: Increased cholesterol and triglycerides that may require treatment. Reduction in renal function due to long-term concomitant cyclosporine. Proteinuria observed in maintenance renal transplant patients, periodic monitoring recommended. May delay recovery of renal function in patients with delayed graft function. Increased risk of lymphocele. Provide 1 year prophylaxis for *Pneumocystis carinii* pneumonia and 3 months for cytomegalovirus after transplant. Limit exposure to sunlight and UV light. Not for use in liver or lung transplants. Interstitial lung disease reported. Increased susceptability to infection and the possible development of lymphoma and malignancy, especially of the skin, may result from immnosupression. Avoid in liver or lung transplant patients. Increased risk of angioedema, caution with concomitant use of angioedema-causing drugs, such as ACEI. Impaired wound healing and fat accummulation reported.

ADVERSE REACTIONS: Hypercholesterolemia, hyperlipemia, HTN, rash, acne, anemia, leukopenia, arthralgia, diarrhea, hypokalemia, thrombocytopenia, fever, abdominal pain, headache, constipation, creatinine increase, arthralgia, insomnia, dyspnea, upper respiratory infection, anaphylactic/anaphylactoid reactions, angioedema, hypersensitivity vasculitis, incisional hernia, azoospermia, pericardial effusion, tuberculosis.

INTERACTIONS: Increased levels with diltiazem. CYP3A4 inhibitors (eg, CCBs, antifungals, macrolide antibiotics) may increase levels of sirolimus, while CYP3A4 inducers (eg, anticonvulsants, rifabutin, St. John's wort) may decrease levels. Avoid live vaccines, grapefruit juice, rifampin, ketoconazole. Caution with other nephrotoxic drugs (eg, aminoglycosides, amphotericin B). Hepatic artery thrombosis reported with cyclosporine or tacrolimus, and increased death rate and graft loss with tacrolimus in liver transplant patients. Bronchial anastomotic dehiscence reported with immunosupressives in lung transplant patients. Cyclosporine is a substrate and inhibitor of CYP3A4 and P-gp. Caution with dosing. Monitor for rhabdomyolysis with cyclosporine and HMG Co-A reductase inhibitors/fibrates. Monitor renal function with cyclosporine. Grapefruit juice reduces CYP3A4 medicated drug metabolism, should not be administered with rapamune or used for dilution. Increased risk of deterioration of renal function, serum lipid abnormalities, and urinary tract infections with calcineurin inhibitors and corticosteriods.

PREGNANCY: Category C, not for use in nursing.

MECHANISM OF ACTION: Immunosuppressant; inhibits T-lymphocyte activation and proliferation that occurs in response to antigenic and cytokine (interleukin [IL]-2, IL-4, and IL-15) stimulation by a mechanism that is distinct from that of other immunosuppressants. Also inhibits antibody production. Prolongs allograft survival and suppresses immune-mediated events (animal study).

PHARMACOKINETICS: Absorption: T_{max}=1-2 hrs. **Distribution:** V_d=12L/kg; plasma protein binding (approximately 92%). **Metabolism:** CYP3A4 and P-gp, intestinal wall, liver (extensive) via O-demethylation and hydroxylation; hydroxy, demethyl and hydroxymethyl (major metabolites). **Elimination:** Feces (91%), urine (2.2%), $T_{1/2}$=62 hrs. Different pharmacokinetic data resulted from concentration-controlled trials of pediatric renal transplants.

RAPTIVA   RX
efalizumab (Genentech)

THERAPEUTIC CLASS: Monoclonal antibody/LFA-1 blocker

INDICATIONS: Chronic moderate to severe plaque psoriasis for candidates of systemic therapy or phototherapy.

DOSAGE: *Adults:* ≥18 yrs: Initial: 0.7mg/kg SQ single dose. Maint: 1mg/kg SQ once weekly. Max: 200mg/dose.

HOW SUPPLIED: Inj: 125mg

WARNINGS/PRECAUTIONS: May increase risk of infection or reactivate latent, chronic infections. Avoid with clinically important infections. Serious infections may occur. Caution with chronic or history of recurrent infections or malignancies; d/c if serious infection or malignancy develops. Obtain baseline platelet counts and monitor periodically; d/c if thrombocytopenia develops. D/C if hemolytic anemia occurs. Infrequent or recurrent severe arthritis has been reported.

ADVERSE REACTIONS: Headache, chills, fever, nausea, myalgia, flu syndrome, pain, back pain, acne, infections (may be serious), malignancies, thrombocytopenia, psoriasis worsening.

INTERACTIONS: Avoid other immunosuppressives, acellular, live and live-attenuated vaccines.

PREGNANCY: Category C, not for use in nursing.

MECHANISM OF ACTION: Efalizumab: inhibits the binding LFA-1 to intercellular adhesion molecule-1 (ICAM-1). Inhibits the adhesion of leukocytes to other cell types.

PHARMACOKINETICS: Absorption: (Last dose); C_{max}=12mcg/mL. **Elimination:** $T_{1/2}$=25 days.

RAZADYNE ER RX
galantamine hydrobromide (Ortho-McNeil)

OTHER BRAND NAMES: Razadyne (Ortho-McNeil)

INDICATIONS: Treatment of mild to moderate dementia of the Alzheimer's type.

DOSAGE: *Adults:* (Sol, Tab) Initial: 4mg bid with am and pm meals. Titrate: Increase to 8mg bid after 4 weeks if tolerated, then increase to 12mg bid after 4 weeks if tolerated. Usual: 16-24mg/day. Max: 24mg/day. (Cap, ER) Initial: 8mg qd with am meal. Titrate: Increase to 16mg qd after 4 weeks, then increase to 24mg qd after 4 weeks if tolerated. Usual: 16-24mg/day. Max: 24mg/day. If therapy is interrupted, restart at lowest dose and increase to current dose. Moderate Renal/Hepatic Impairment (Child-Pugh: 7-9): Caution during dose titration. Max: 16mg/day. Avoid use with severe renal (CrCl <9mL/min) and severe hepatic impairment (Child-Pugh: 10-15).

HOW SUPPLIED: Sol: (Razadyne) 4mg/mL [100mL]; Tab: (Razadyne) 4mg, 8mg, 12mg. Cap, Extended-Release: (Razadyne ER) 8mg, 16mg, 24mg.

WARNINGS/PRECAUTIONS: Vagotonic effects; caution with supraventricular conduction disorder. May cause bradycardia and/or heart block. Caution with asthma or obstructive pulmonary disease. Monitor for active or occult GI bleeding and ulcers due to increased gastric acid secretion. Risk of generalized convulsions or bladder outflow obstruction. Ensure adequate fluid intake during treatment. Deaths reported with mild cognitive impairment.

ADVERSE REACTIONS: Nausea, vomiting, diarrhea, anorexia, weight loss, fatigue, dizziness, headache, depression, insomnia, abdominal pain, dyspepsia, UTI.

INTERACTIONS: Potential to interfere with anticholinergics. Synergistic effect with succinylcholine, other cholinesterase inhibitors, similar neuromuscular blockers, or cholinergic agonists (eg, bethanechol). Increased levels with cimetidine, ketoconazole, and paroxetine. Caution with drugs that slow heart rate due to vagotonic effects. Monitor for GI bleeding with NSAIDs.

PREGNANCY: Category B, not for use in nursing.

MECHANISM OF ACTION: Unknown; suspected to inhibit acetylcholinesterase-enhancing cholinergic function by increasing concentration of acetylcholine through reversible inhibition of its hydrolysis.

PHARMACOKINETICS: Absorption: Bioavailability: (90%, rapid and complete), T_{max}=1 hr. **Distribution:** V_d=175L. Plasma protein binding (18%). **Metabolism:** Liver (glucuronidation). CYP450 enzymes: 2D6, 3A4. **Elimination:** Urine (unchanged). $T_{1/2}$=7 hrs.

REBETOL RX
ribavirin (Schering)

> Not for monotherapy treatment of chronic hepatitis C. Primary toxicity is hemolytic anemia. Avoid with significant or unstable cardiac disease. Contraindicated in pregnancy and male partners of pregnant women. Use 2 forms of contraception during therapy and for 6 months after discontinuation.

THERAPEUTIC CLASS: Nucleoside analogue

INDICATIONS: In combination with Intron A® for treatment of chronic hepatitis C in patients ≥3 yrs with compensated liver disease previously untreated with alpha interferon or in patients ≥18 yrs who relapsed after alpha interferon therapy. In combination with Peg-Intron™ for treatment of chronic hepatitis C in patients ≥18 yrs with compensated liver disease previously untreated with alpha interferon.

DOSAGE: *Adults:* ≥18 yrs: With Intron A: ≤75kg: 400mg qam and 600mg qpm. >75kg: 600mg qam and 600mg qpm. Treat for 24-48 weeks interferon-naive; 24 weeks in relapse. With Peg-Intron: 400mg bid, qam and qpm with food. Reduce to 600mg qd if Hgb <10g/dL with no cardiac history, or if Hgb

R

decreases by ≥2g/dL during a 4 week-period with a cardiac history. D/C if Hgb <8.5g/dL with no cardiac history or if Hgb <12g/dL after 4 weeks of dose reduction with a cardiac history. CrCl <50mL/min: Avoid use.

Pediatrics: ≥3 yrs: 15mg/kg/day in divided doses qam and qpm. Use sol if ≤25kg or cannot swallow caps. With Intron A: 25-36kg: 200mg bid, qam and qpm. 37-49kg: 200mg qam and 400mg qpm. 50-61kg: 400mg bid, qam and qpm. >61kg: Dose as adult. Genotype 1: Treat for 48 weeks. Genotype 2/3: Treat for 24 weeks. Reduce to 7.5mg/day if Hgb <10g/dL with no cardiac history, or if Hgb decreases by ≥2g/dL during a 4 week-period with a cardiac history. D/C if Hgb <8.5g/dL with no cardiac history or if Hgb <12g/dL after 4 weeks of dose reduction with a cardiac history.

HOW SUPPLIED: Cap: 200mg; Sol: 40mg/mL [100mL]

CONTRAINDICATIONS: Pregnancy, male partners of pregnant women, hemoglobinopathies (eg, thalassemia major, sickle cell anemia). When used with Intron A or PEG-Intron, refer to individual monograph.

WARNINGS/PRECAUTIONS: Severe depression, suicidal ideation, bone marrow suppression, autoimmune and infectious disorders, pulmonary dysfunction, pancreatitis, and DM reported. Assess for underlying cardiac disease (obtain EKG); fatal and nonfatal MI reported with anemia. Hemolytic anemia reported; monitor Hgb or Hct initially then at Week 2 and 4 (or more if needed) of therapy. Suspend therapy if symptoms of pancreatitis arise. Avoid if CrCl <50mL/min. Obtain negative pregnancy test prior to initiation then monthly, and for 6 months post-therapy.

ADVERSE REACTIONS: Hemolytic anemia, headache, fatigue, rigors, fever, nausea, anorexia, myalgia, arthralgia, insomnia, irritability, depression, dyspnea, alopecia.

INTERACTIONS: Dental and periodontal disorders reported with interferon or peginterferon combination therapy. Coadminstration not recommended with didanosine. Caution with stavudine and zidovudine.

PREGNANCY: Category X, not for use in nursing.

MECHANISM OF ACTION: Nucleoside analog; not established.

PHARMACOKINETICS: Absorption: Rapid; (Sol) C_{max}=872ng/mL, T_{max}=1 hr, AUC=14098ng•h/mL. (Cap) C_{max}=782ng/mL, T_{max}=1.7 hrs, AUC=13400ng•h/mL; absolute bioavailability (64%). **Distribution:** (Cap) V_d=2825L. **Metabolism:** Nucleated cells (phosphorylation); deribosylation and amide hydrolysis. **Elimination:** Urine (61%), feces (12%). (Cap) $T_{1/2}$=43.6 hrs.

Rebif   RX
interferon beta-1a (Pfizer/Serono)

THERAPEUTIC CLASS: Biological response modifier

INDICATIONS: Treatment of patients with relapsing forms of multiple sclerosis.

DOSAGE: *Adults:* Initial: 20% of prescribed dose SQ 3x/week (TIW); 4.4mcg for prescribed dose of 22mcg, 8.8mcg for prescribed dose of 44mcg. Titrate: Increase over a 4 week period to either 22mcg or 44mcg SQ TIW. Maint: 22mcg or 44mcg SQ TIW. Leukopenia/Elevated LFTs: Reduce dose until toxicity resolves. Administer dose at the same time everyday (late afternoon, evening) on the same 3 days/week at least 48 hrs apart.

HOW SUPPLIED: Inj: 22mcg/0.5mL, 44mcg/0.5mL; Titration Pack: 8.8mcg/0.2mL [6ˢ] and 22mcg/0.5mL [6ˢ]

CONTRAINDICATIONS: Hypersensitivity to human albumin.

WARNINGS/PRECAUTIONS: Caution with depression, alcohol abuse, active hepatic disease, increased serum SGPT (>2.5x ULN), history of significant hepatic disease, seizure disorder. Consider discontinuing therapy if depression, jaundice/hepatic dysfunction develops. Reduce dose if serum SGPT >5x ULN. Contains albumin; risk of viral disease transmission. Monitor blood cell counts and LFTs at 1, 3, and 6 months after initiation, then periodically. Monitor thyroid function tests every 6 months with history of thyroid dysfunction.

ADVERSE REACTIONS: Psychiatric disorders, injection site disorders, influenza-like symptoms (eg, headache, fatigue, fever, rigors, chest pain), back pain, myalgia, abdominal pain, depression, elevation of liver enzymes, hematologic abnormalities.

INTERACTIONS: Monitor with myelosuppressive agents.

PREGNANCY: Category C, caution in nursing.

MECHANISM OF ACTION: Interferon β-1a; possesses immunomodulatory, antiviral, and antiproliferative biological activities. Its effects in MS have not been fully defined.

PHARMACOKINETICS: Absorption: C_{max}=5.1 IU/mL, T_{max}=16 hrs, AUC=294 IU•h/mL. **Elimination:** $T_{1/2}$=69 hrs.

RECLAST
zoledronic acid (Novartis)
RX

THERAPEUTIC CLASS: Bisphosphonate

INDICATIONS: Treatment of osteoporosis in postmenopausal women and to reduce incidence of new clinical fractures in patients at high risk of fractures. Treatment of Paget's disease of bone in men and women.

DOSAGE: *Adults:* Osteoporosis: 5mg IV once a year. Paget's disease: 5mg IV as single dose. Infuse for >15 mins at constant rate. Hydrate prior to administration.

HOW SUPPLIED: Sol: 5mg/100mL [100mL]

CONTRAINDICATIONS: Hypocalcemia

WARNINGS/PRECAUTIONS: Increases risk of hypocalcemia; monitor calcium and mineral levels regularly. May need calcium and vitamin D supplements. Not recommended for use in patients with severe renal impairment (CrCl <35mL/min); monitor serum creatinine before each dose. May cause osteonecrosis of the jaw; routine oral or dental exam needed prior to treatment. Avoid during pregnancy. Musculoskeletal pain may occur; D/C if severe symptoms develop.

ADVERSE REACTIONS: Influenza, hypocalcemia, headache, lethargy, dyspnea, HTN, A-fib, arthralgia, myalgia, pyrexia, rigors, peripheral edema, paresthesia, dyspnea, angioedema.

INTERACTIONS: Caution with aminoglycosides; may have an additive effect to lower serum calcium for prolonged periods. Caution when used in combination with loop diuretics; may increase risk of hypocalcemia. Caution with other nephrotoxic drugs such as NSAIDs. Avoid use in patients treated with Zometa. Caution in patients sensitive to aspirin; may cause bronchoconstriction.

PREGNANCY: Category D, not for use in nursing.

MECHANISM OF ACTION: Bisphosphonate; acts primarily on bone. Inhibits osteoclast-mediated bone resorption.

PHARMACOKINETICS: Distribution: Plasma protein binding (28-53%). **Elimination:** Urine, $T_{1/2}$=146 hrs.

R

RECOMBIVAX HB
hepatitis B (recombinant) (Merck)
RX

OTHER BRAND NAMES: Recombivax HB Adult (Merck) - Recombivax HB Dialysis (Merck) - Recombivax HB Pediatric/Adolescent (Merck)

THERAPEUTIC CLASS: Vaccine

INDICATIONS: Vaccination against hepatitis B virus.

DOSAGE: *Adults:* Give IM into deltoid muscle. Give SQ if risk of hemorrhage. ≥20 yrs: 3-Dose Regimen: 10mcg at 0,1,6 months. Predialysis/Dialysis (Dialysis Formulation): 40mcg at 0,1,6, months; consider booster if anti-HBs level <10MIU/mL.
Pediatrics: Give IM into anterolateral thigh in infants/young children. Give

SQ if risk of hemorrhage. 0-19 yrs: 3-Dose Regimen (Pediatric/Adolescent Formulation) 5mcg at 0,1,6 months. 11-15 yrs: 2-Dose Regimen (Adult Formulation): 10mcg 1st dose, 10mcg 4-6 months later. Infants Born to HBsAg Positive/Unknown Status Mothers: Give 3-dose regimen vaccine and 0.5mL HBIG in opposite anterolateral thigh.

HOW SUPPLIED: Inj: (Pediatric/Adolescent-Preservative Free) 5mcg/0.5mL, (Adult) 10mcg/mL, (Dialysis) 40mcg/mL

CONTRAINDICATIONS: Yeast hypersensitivity.

WARNINGS/PRECAUTIONS: Do not continue therapy if hypersensitivity occurs after injection. May not prevent hepatitis B with unrecognized infection. Caution with severely compromised cardiopulmonary status and those where febrile or systemic reaction is a significant risk. May delay use with serious active infection (eg, febrile illness). Have epinephrine available. Do not give intradermally or IV.

ADVERSE REACTIONS: Irritability, fever, diarrhea, fatigue/weakness, diminished appetite, rhinitis, injection site reactions.

PREGNANCY: Category C, caution in nursing.

MECHANISM OF ACTION: Stimulation of immune response to produce antibodies that may protect against all subtypes of hepatitis B virus infection.

REFLUDAN   RX
lepirudin (Bayer Healthcare)

THERAPEUTIC CLASS: Thrombin inhibitor

INDICATIONS: Anticoagulant for heparin-induced thrombocytopenia (HIT) and associated thromboembolic disease.

DOSAGE: *Adults:* LD: 0.4mg/kg (max 44mg) IV over 15-20 seconds. Initial: 0.15mg/kg/hr (max 16.5mg/hr) continuous infusion for 2-10 days. Adjust dose based on aPTT. If aPTT is above target range, stop infusion for 2 hrs and restart at 50% of previous rate. Check aPTT 4 hrs later. If aPTT is below target range, increase rate in steps of 20% and check aPTT 4 hrs later. Do not exceed 0.21mg/kg/hr. Renal Impairment: LD: 0.2mg/kg. Initial: CrCl 45-60 mL/min: 0.075mg/kg/hr. CrCl 30-44mL/min: 0.045mg/kg/hr. CrCl 15-29 mL/min: 0.0225mg/kg/hr. CrCl <15mL/min/Hemodialysis: Avoid or stop infusion. Concomitant Thrombolytic Therapy: LD: 0.2mg/kg. Initial: 0.1mg/kg/hr.

HOW SUPPLIED: Inj: 50mg

WARNINGS/PRECAUTIONS: Risk of bleeding. Weigh risks/benefits with recent puncture of large vessels or organ biopsy, anomaly of vessels or organs, recent CVA, stroke, intracerebral surgery or other neuraxial procedures, severe uncontrolled HTN, bacterial endocarditis, advanced renal impairment, hemorrhagic diathesis, recent major surgery or bleeding. Avoid with baseline aPTT ≥2.5. Monitor aPTT 4 hrs after initiate infusion and at least once daily. Liver injury may enhance anticoagulant effects. Antihirudin antibodies reported; may increase anticoagulant effects.

ADVERSE REACTIONS: Hemorrhagic events (eg, bleeding, anemia, hematoma, hematuria, epistaxis, hemothorax), fever, liver dysfunction, pneumonia, sepsis, allergic skin reactions, multiorgan failure.

INTERACTIONS: Thrombolytics increase risk of life-threatening intracranial bleeding or other bleeding complications and may enhance the effect on aPTT prolongation. Increased risk of bleeding with coumarin derivatives and other drugs that affect platelet function.

PREGNANCY: Category B, not for use in nursing.

MECHANISM OF ACTION: Thrombin inhibitor; binds to thrombin and thereby blocks its thrombogenic activity.

PHARMACOKINETICS: Absorption: C_{max}=1500ng/mL. **Distribution:** V_d=12.2L. **Metabolism:** Catabolic hydrolysis. **Elimination:** Urine(48%); $T_{1/2}$=1.3 hrs.

REGRANEX
becaplermin (Ortho-McNeil)

RX

> Increased rate of mortality secondary to malignancy in patients treated with 3 or more tubes of regranex gel reported in a post-marketing study. Should only be used when the benefits can be expected to outweigh the risks. Use with caution in patients with known malignancy.

THERAPEUTIC CLASS: Platelet-derived growth factor (recombinant human)

INDICATIONS: Treatment of lower extremity diabetic neuropathic ulcers that extend into the subcutaneous tissue or beyond and have an adequate blood supply.

DOSAGE: *Adults:* Amount applied will vary depending on ulcer size. Measure the greatest length by the greatest width of the ulcer to determine amount of gel to apply. To calculate in inches: (For 15g tube) length x width x 0.6; (For 2g tube) length x width x 1.3. To calculate in centimeters: (For 15g tube) length x width/4; (For 2g tube) length x width/2. Adjust amount weekly or biweekly depending on the change in ulcer area. Squeeze gel onto clean measuring surface (eg, wax paper), then apply to ulcer with an application aid. Apply 1/16 of an inch thickness over entire ulcer area qd, then cover with moist saline dressing for 12 hrs. Remove dressing, rinse off residual gel with saline or water and cover again with moist saline dressing for 12 hrs and repeat. Reassess if ulcer does not decrease by 30% after 10 weeks or is not completely healed in 20 weeks.
Pediatrics: ≥16 yrs: Amount applied will vary depending on ulcer size. Measure the greatest length by the greatest width of the ulcer to determine amount of gel to apply. To calculate in inches: (For 15g tube) length x width x 0.6; (For 2g tube) length x width x 1.3. To calculate in centimeters: (For 15g tube) length x width/4; (For 2g tube) length x width/2. Adjust amount weekly or biweekly depending on the change in ulcer area. Squeeze gel onto clean measuring surface (eg, wax paper), then apply to ulcer with an application aid. Apply 1/16 of an inch thickness over entire ulcer area qd, then cover with moist saline dressing for 12 hrs. Remove dressing, rinse off residual gel with saline or water and cover again with moist saline dressing for 12 hrs and repeat. Reassess if ulcer does not decrease by 30% after 10 weeks or is not completely healed in 20 weeks.

HOW SUPPLIED: Gel: 0.01% [2g, 15g]

CONTRAINDICATIONS: Known neoplasm at application site.

WARNINGS/PRECAUTIONS: Do not use in wounds that close by primary intention. For external use only. May cause application site reactions; consider the possibility of sensitization or irritation caused by parabens or m-cresol.

ADVERSE REACTIONS: Erythematous rash.

PREGNANCY: Category C, caution in nursing.

MECHANISM OF ACTION: Recombinant human platelet-derived growth factor; promotes chemotactic recruitment and proliferation of cells involved in wound repair. Enhances formation of granulation tissue.

RELENZA
zanamivir (GlaxoSmithKline)

RX

THERAPEUTIC CLASS: Neuraminidase inhibitor

INDICATIONS: Treatment of uncomplicated acute illness due to influenza A and B virus in patients symptomatic for ≤2 days. Prophylaxis of influenza.

DOSAGE: *Adults:* Treatment: Usual: 2 inh (10mg) q12h for 5 days. Take 2 doses at least 2 hrs apart on 1st day. Prophylaxis: Household Setting: 2 inh (10mg) qd for 10 days. Community Setting: 2 inh (10mg) qd for 28 days. Administer at same time every day.
Pediatrics: Treatment: ≥7 yrs: Usual: 2 inh (10mg) q12h for 5 days. Take 2 doses at least 2 hrs apart on 1st day. Prophylaxis: ≥5 yrs: Household Setting: 2 inh

(10mg) qd for 10 days. Community Setting: ≥12 yrs: 2 inh (10mg) qd for 28 days. Administer at same time every day.

HOW SUPPLIED: Inh: 5mg/inh [20 blisters]

WARNINGS/PRECAUTIONS: Not recommended for use with underlying airways disease (eg, asthma, COPD). Serious cases of bronchospasm reported during treatment; d/c if bronchospasm or decline in respiratory function develops. D/C if allergic reaction occurs. Postmarketing neuropsychiatric events (seizures, delerium, hallucinations) reported.

ADVERSE REACTIONS: Dizziness, headaches, diarrhea, nausea, sinusitis, bronchitis, cough, ear/nose/throat infections, nasal symptoms.

INTERACTIONS: Use inhaled bronchodilator before zanamivir. Avoid administration of live attenuated influenza vaccine within 2 weeks before or 48 hours after.

PREGNANCY: Category C, caution in nursing

MECHANISM OF ACTION: Neuraminidase inhibitor; inhibits influenza virus neuraminidase, affecting release of particles.

PHARMACOKINETICS: Absorption: Absolute bioavailabilty (4-17%); C_{max}=17-142ng/mL; T_{max}=1-2 hrs; AUC=111-1364ng•hr/mL. **Distribution:** Plasma protein binding (<10%). **Elimination**: Renal; $T_{1/2}$=2.5-5.1 hrs.

Relpax   RX
eletriptan hydrobromide (Pfizer)

THERAPEUTIC CLASS: 5-HT$_{1D,1B}$-agonist

INDICATIONS: Acute treatment of migraine with or without aura.

DOSAGE: *Adults:* ≥18 yrs: Initial: 20 or 40mg at onset of headache. If recurs after initial relief, may repeat after 2 hrs. Max: 40mg/dose or 80mg/day. Safety of treating >3 headaches/30 days not known. Severe Hepatic Impairment: Avoid use. Avoid within 72 hrs of potent CYP3A4 inhibitors.

HOW SUPPLIED: Tab: 20mg, 40mg

CONTRAINDICATIONS: Ischemic heart disease, coronary artery vasospasm (eg, Prinzmetal's angina) or other significant underlying cardiovascular disease, peripheral vascular disease, cerebrovascular syndromes, uncontrolled HTN, hemiplegic or basilar migraine, use within 24 hrs of other 5-HT$_1$ agonist or ergot-type agent (eg, dihydroergotamine, methysergide), severe hepatic impairment.

WARNINGS/PRECAUTIONS: Confirm diagnosis. Supervise 1st dose and monitor cardiac function in those at risk of CAD (eg, HTN, hypercholesterolemia, smoker, obesity, diabetes, CAD family history, postmenopausal women, males >40 yrs). Consider ECG during interval immediately following initial administration in patients with CAD risk factors. Monitor cardiac function in intermittent long-term users with CAD risk factors. Serious adverse cardiac events, increased BP, cerebrovascular events, vasospastic reactions reported. Caution in elderly. Possible long-term ophthalmic effects.

ADVERSE REACTIONS: Asthenia, chest tightness, dizziness, dry mouth, headache, nausea, paresthesia, somnolence, pain/pressure/heaviness in precordium/throat/jaw.

INTERACTIONS: Prolonged vasospastic reactions reported with ergot-containing drugs; avoid within 24 hours of each other. Avoid within 72 hrs of potent CYP3A4 inhibitors (eg, ketoconazole, itraconazole, nefazodone, troleandomycin, clarithromycin, ritonavir, nelfinavir). Avoid within 24 hours of other 5-HT$_1$ agonists. Propranolol, erythromycin, verapamil, fluconazole may increase levels.

PREGNANCY: Category C, caution in nursing.

MECHANISM OF ACTION: Selective 5HT$_{1D/1B}$ agonist; binds with high affinity to 5HT$_{1D/1B/1F}$ receptors. Believed to activate these receptors located on intracranial blood vessels, including those on arteriovenous ananstomoses, which leads to vasoconstriction and is correlated with relief of migraine headache.

Activation of those located on sensory nerve endings in trigeminal system results in inhibition of pro-inflammatory neuropeptide release.

PHARMACOKINETICS: Absorption: Complete; absolute bioavailability (50%); T_{max}=1.5 hrs. **Distribution:** V_d=138L; plasma protein binding (85%). **Metabolism:** N-demethylated (active metabolite). **Elimination:** $T_{1/2}$= 4 hrs (parent drug), 13 hrs (metabolite).

REMERON
mirtazapine (Organon)

RX

Antidepressants increased the risk of suicidal thinking and behavior (suicidality) in short-term studies in children, adolescents, and young adults with Major Depressive Disorder (MDD) and other psychiatric disorders. Mirtazapine is not approved for use in pediatric patients.

OTHER BRAND NAMES: Remeron SolTab (Organon)

THERAPEUTIC CLASS: Piperazino-azepine

INDICATIONS: Treatment of MDD.

DOSAGE: *Adults:* Initial: 15mg qhs. Titrate: May increase every 1-2 weeks. Max: 45mg/day. Disintegrating tabs disintegrate rapidly on tongue and can be swallowed with saliva; no water needed. Do not cut tabs in half.

HOW SUPPLIED: Tab: 15mg*, 30mg*, 45mg; Tab, Disintegrating: 15mg, 30mg, 45mg *scored

WARNINGS/PRECAUTIONS: Risk of agranulocytosis. D/C if sore throat, fever, or stomatitis, along with low WBC count, develop. May increase appetite, cholesterol, and triglycerides. Caution in history of seizures, mania/hypomania, hepatic or renal impairment, altered metabolic or hemodynamic conditions, elderly. Somnolence, dizziness reported. Close supervision with high risk suicide patients. May impair judgement, thinking, or motor skills.

ADVERSE REACTIONS: Somnolence, appetite increase, weight gain, dizziness, dry mouth, constipation, asthenia, flu syndrome, abnormal dreams.

INTERACTIONS: Alcohol and diazepam increase cognitive and motor skill impairment. Avoid MAOIs within 14 days of use.

PREGNANCY: Category C, caution in nursing.

MECHANISM OF ACTION: Antidepressant belonging to the piperazino-azepine group, suspected to enhance central noradrenergic and serotonergic activity.

PHARMACOKINETICS: Absorption: Rapidly and completely absorbed; T_{max}=2 hrs. Absolute bioavailability: 50%. **Distribution:** Plasma protein binding (85%). **Metabolism:** Demethylation and hydroxylation followed by glucuronide conjugation. **Elimination:** Urine (75%), feces (15%). $T_{1/2}$=37 hrs (female), 26 hrs (male).

R

REMICADE
infliximab (Centocor)

RX

Reports of TB, invasive fungal infections, and other opportunistic infections. Evaluate for latent TB and treat if necessary prior to initiation of therapy.

THERAPEUTIC CLASS: Monoclonal antibody/TNF-alpha receptor blocker

INDICATIONS: In combination with methotrexate (MTX), for reducing signs/symptoms, inhibiting structural damage progression and improving physical function in moderately to severely active rheumatoid arthritis (RA). For reducing signs/symptoms and inducing and maintaining clinical remission of moderately to severely active Crohn's disease, when response to conventional therapy is inadequate. For reducing the number of draining enterocutaneous and rectovaginal fistulas and maintaining fistula closure in fistulizing Crohn's disease. For reducing signs/symptoms in patients with active ankylosing spondylitis (AS). For reducing signs/symptoms of active arthritis, inhibiting structural damage progression, and improving physical function in patients with psoriatic arthritis. For reducing signs/symptoms, inducing and maintaining clinical remission and mucosal healing, and eliminating corticosteroid use in patients with moderately to severely active ulcerative colitis (UC) who have inadequate response to conventional therapy. Treatment of patients with chronic, severe plaque psoriasis who are candidates for systemic therapy and when other systemic therapies are medically less appropriate.

DOSAGE: *Adults:* RA (Combo with MTX): 3mg/kg as IV infusion; repeat at 2 and 6 weeks. Maint: 3mg/kg every 8 weeks. Incomplete Response: May increase to 10mg/kg or give every 4 weeks. Crohn's Disease/Fistulizing Crohn's Disease: Induction Regimen: 5mg/kg IV at 0, 2, and 6 weeks. Maint: 5mg/kg every 8 weeks. For patients who respond then lose their response, may increase to 10mg/kg. Consider discontinuing therapy if no response to by Week 14. Alkylosing Spondylitis: 5mg/kg as IV infusion; repeat at 2 and 6 weeks. Maint: 5mg/kg every 6 weeks. Psoriatic Arthritis: 5mg/kg as IV infusion; repeat at 2 and 6 weeks. Maint: 5mg/kg every 8 weeks. May be used with or without MTX. Ulcerative Colitis: 5mg/kg at 0, 2, and 6 weeks. Maint: 5mg/kg every 8 weeks. Plaque Psoriasis: 5mg/kg IV infusion; repeat at 2 and 6 weeks. Maint: 5mg/kg every 8 weeks.
Pediatrics: ≥6 yrs: Crohn's Disease: Induction Regimen: 5mg/kg IV at 0, 2, and 6 weeks. Maint: 5mg/kg every 8 weeks.

HOW SUPPLIED: Inj: 100mg

CONTRAINDICATIONS: Hypersensitivity to murine proteins. Moderate or severe CHF (NYHA Class III/IV) with doses >5mg/kg.

WARNINGS/PRECAUTIONS: Leukopenia, neutropenia, thrombocytopenia, and pancytopenia reported. Serious infections, including sepsis and pneumonia, reported. Avoid with active infection. Monitor for signs of infection during and after therapy; d/c if serious infection develops. Caution in patients who have resided in areas where histoplasmosis or coccidioidomycosis are endemic. Hypersensitivity reactions reported. Caution with optic neuritis, chronic and recurrent infections, CNS demyelinating disease (eg, MS) and seizure disorder. May result in autoantibody formation; d/c if lupus-like syndrome develops. Monitor closely and d/c if new or worsening symptoms of heart failure appear. Lymphoma reported; caution with malignancies. Severe hepatic reactions, including acute liver failure, jaundice, hepatitis and cholestasis reported rarely. Caution in elderly.

ADVERSE REACTIONS: Nausea, infections, infusion reactions, headache, sinusitis, pharyngitis, coughing, abdominal pain, diarrhea, bronchitis, dyspepsia, fatigue, rhinitis, pain, arthralgia, hepatotoxicity.

INTERACTIONS: Do not give concurrently with live vaccines. May increase risk of serious infections and neutropenia with anakinra.

PREGNANCY: Category B, not for use in nursing.

MECHANISM OF ACTION: Monoclonal antibody; neutralizes biological activity of TNF-a by binding with high affinity to the soluble and transmembrane forms of TNF-a and inhibiting binding of TNF-a with its receptors.

PHARMACOKINETICS: Elimination: $T_{1/2}$=7.7-9.5 days.

REMODULIN   RX
treprostinil sodium (United Therapeutics)

THERAPEUTIC CLASS: Pulmonary and systemic vasodilator

INDICATIONS: Treatment of pulmonary arterial hypertension (PAH) in patients with NYHA Class II-IV symptoms to diminish symptoms associated with exercise.

DOSAGE: *Adults:* Initial: 1.25ng/kg/min SQ continuous infusion. Reduce rate to 0.625ng/kg/min if not tolerated. Titrate: Increase by no more than 1.25ng/kg/min per week for first 4 weeks, then no more than 2.5ng/kg/min per week thereafter, depending on clinical response.

HOW SUPPLIED: Inj: 1mg/mL, 2.5mg/mL, 5mg/mL, 10mg/mL [20mL]

WARNINGS/PRECAUTIONS: For SQ use only. Initiate therapy in adequate setting for monitoring and emergency care. Abrupt withdrawal or sudden large dose reduction may worsen PAH symptoms. Caution with hepatic or renal impairment.

ADVERSE REACTIONS: Infusion site pain/reactions, headache, diarrhea, nausea, rash, jaw pain, vasodilatation, dizziness, edema, pruritus, hypotension.

INTERACTIONS: Drugs that alter BP (eg, diuretics, antihypertensives, vasodilators) may potentiate BP reduction. Increased risk of bleeding with anticoagulants.

PREGNANCY: Category B, caution in nursing.

MECHANISM OF ACTION: Pulmonary and systemic vasodilator: causes direct vasodilation of pulmonary and systemic arterial vascular beds; inhibits platelet aggregation.

PHARMACOKINETICS: Absorption: (SQ): Rapid, complete. Absolute bioavailability (100%). **Distribution:** V_d=14L/70kg, plasma protein binding (91%). **Metabolism:** Liver. **Elimination:** Urine (4%) .

RENOVA   RX
tretinoin (Ortho Neutrogena)

THERAPEUTIC CLASS: Retinoid

INDICATIONS: Adjunct to comprehensive skin care and sunlight avoidance programs, for mitigation of fine facial wrinkles.

DOSAGE: *Adults:* 18-71 yrs: Wash face with mild soap, pat skin dry, and wait 20-30 min before use. Apply once daily in evening. Max: 52 weeks of therapy. May apply cosmetics 1 hr later. Use moisturizer every morning to prevent dryness.

HOW SUPPLIED: Cre: 0.02% [40g]

WARNINGS/PRECAUTIONS: Avoid with sunburned skin, eczema, chronic skin conditions, and pregnancy. Larger amounts will not lead to better or faster results and may increase adverse effects. Avoid contact with eyes, mouth, paranasal creases, and mucous membranes. D/C if sensitivity, irritation, or systemic adverse reaction develops. Minimize sunlight exposure; avoid sunlamps. Wear protective clothing and use SPF ≥15. Causes photosensitivity. Extreme weather may increase skin irritation.

ADVERSE REACTIONS: Peeling, dry skin, burning, stinging, erythema, pruritus at the site of application.

INTERACTIONS: Caution with topical agents with strong drying effects, high concentration of alcohol, astringents, spices or lime, permanent wave solutions, electrolysis, hair depilatories, waxes or medicated or abrasive soaps, shampoos and cleansers. Increased phototoxicity with photosensitizers (eg, thiazides, tetracyclines, fluoroquinolones, phenothiazines, sulfonamides).

PREGNANCY: Category C, not for use in nursing.

MECHANISM OF ACTION: Endogenous retinoid metabolite of vitamin A; binds to intracellular receptors in the cytosol and nucleus. Activates three members of the retinoic acid (RAR) nuclear receptors (RARα, RARβ, RAR-gamma), which may act to modify gene expression, subsequent protein synthesis, and epithelial cell growth and differentiation.

RENVELA   RX
sevelamer carbonate (Genzyme)

THERAPEUTIC CLASS: Phosphate binder

INDICATIONS: Control of serum phosphorus in patients with chronic kidney disease on dialysis.

DOSAGE: *Adults:* Take with meals. Initial: Not Taking Phosphate Binder: Serum Phosphorus >5.5 and <7.5mg/dL: 800mg tid. Serum Phosphorus ≥7.5mg/dL:

R

1600mg tid. Switching from Sevelamer HCl: May prescibe on a gram per gram basis. Switching from Calcium Acetate: May switch on a tab per tab basis. Titrate: All Patients: May increase or decrease by 1 tab per meal at 2 week intervals as needed.

HOW SUPPLIED: Tab: 800mg

CONTRAINDICATIONS: Hypophosphatemia or bowel obstruction.

WARNINGS/PRECAUTIONS: Caution with dysphagia, swallowing disorders, severe GI motility disorders, or major GI tract surgery. Monitor bicarbonate and chloride levels. Monitor for reduced vitamins D, E, K (clotting factors) and folic acid.

ADVERSE REACTIONS: Nausea, vomiting, diarrhea, dyspepsia, abdominal pain, flatulence, constipation.

INTERACTIONS: May decrease ciprofoxacin levels. When giving oral medicaton where reduction in bioavailability of that medication would have a clinically significant effect on its safety or efficacy, the drug should be given at least 1 hour before or 3 hours after sevelamer carbonate or consider monitoring blood levels of drug. Caution in patients taking anti-arrhythmics and anti-seizure medications.

PREGNANCY: Category C, safety in nursing unknown.

ReoPro

RX

abciximab (Lilly)

THERAPEUTIC CLASS: Glycoprotein IIb/IIIa inhibitor

INDICATIONS: Adjunct to percutaneous coronary intervention (PCI) for prevention of cardiac ischemic complications in patients undergoing PCI or with unstable angina unresponsive to conventional therapy when PCI is planned within 24 hrs. Intended for use with aspirin and heparin.

DOSAGE: *Adults:* PCI: 0.25mg/kg IV bolus given 10-60 min before start PCI, followed by 0.125mcg/kg/min IV infusion (Max: 10mcg/min) for 12 hrs. Unstable Angina: 0.25mg/kg IV bolus followed by 10mcg/min infusion for 18-24 hrs, concluding 1 hr after PCI.

HOW SUPPLIED: Inj: 2mg/mL

CONTRAINDICATIONS: Active internal bleeding, recent (within 6 weeks) significant GI or GU bleeding, CVA within 2 yrs, CVA with significant residual neurological deficit, bleeding diathesis, oral anticoagulants within 7 days (unless PT ≤1.2x control), thrombocytopenia, recent (within 6 weeks) major surgery or trauma, intracranial neoplasm, arteriovenous malformation, aneurysm, severe uncontrolled HTN, history of vasculitis, IV dextran use before PCI or during an intervention. Hypersensitivity to murine proteins.

WARNINGS/PRECAUTIONS: Increased risk of bleeding. Monitor all potential bleeding sites (eg, catheter insertion sites, arterial and venous puncture sites, cutdown sites). Minimize vascular and other trauma. D/C if serious, uncontrollable bleeding, thrombocytopenia, or emergency surgery occurs. Anaphylaxis may occur. Antibody (HACA) formation may occur; risk of hypersensitivity, thrombocytopenia, decreased benefit with readministration. Monitor platelets, PT, APTT, ACT before infusion.

ADVERSE REACTIONS: Bleeding, thrombocytopenia, hypotension, bradycardia, nausea, vomiting, back/chest pain, headache.

INTERACTIONS: Caution with other drugs that affect hemostasis (eg, thrombolytics, heparin, oral anticoagulants, NSAIDs, dipyridamole, ticlopidine). Increased risk of bleeding with anticoagulants, thrombolytics, and antiplatelets. If have HACA titers, possible allergic reactions with monoclonal antibody agents.

PREGNANCY: Category C, caution in nursing.

MECHANISM OF ACTION: Glycoprotein IIb/IIIa inhibitor; binds to the GPIIb/IIIa receptor and inhibits platelet aggregation by preventing the binding of fibrinogen, von Willebrand factor, and other adhesive molecules to GPIIb/IIIa receptor sites on activated platelets. Also binds to vitronectin receptor, which mediates the procoagulant properties of platelets and the proliferative properties of vascular endothelial and smooth muscle cells.

PHARMACOKINETICS: Elimination: $T_{1/2}$=30 min.

REPRONEX   RX
menotropins (Ferring)

THERAPEUTIC CLASS: Follicle stimulating hormone/luteinizing hormone

INDICATIONS: With hCG, for multiple follicular development and ovulation in women who received pituitary suppression.

DOSAGE: *Adults:* Oligo-anovulation: Individualize dose. Initial: 150 IU SQ/IM qd for 5 days. Adjust subsequent dose to individual response at intervals no less than every 2 days and not exceeding 75-150 IU/adjustment. Max: 450 IU/day. Dosing >12 days is not recommended. If adequate response, give 5000-10,000 U hCG. May repeat course if inadequate response. Assisted Reproductive Technology: Initial: 225 IU SQ/IM. Adjust subsequent dose to individual response at intervals no less than every 2 days and not exceeding 75-150 IU/adjustment. Max: 450 IU/day. Dosing >12 days is not recommended. If adequate response, give 5000-10,000 U hCG.

HOW SUPPLIED: Inj: (FSH-LH) 75 IU-75 IU

CONTRAINDICATIONS: High FSH levels indicating primary ovarian failure, uncontrolled thyroid or adrenal dysfunction, organic intracranial lesions (eg, pituitary tumor), any cause of infertility other than anovulation (unless candidate for in vitro fertilization), abnormal bleeding of undetermined origin, ovarian cysts or enlargement not due to polycystic ovary syndrome, pregnancy.

WARNINGS/PRECAUTIONS: Exclude primary ovarian failure. Ovarian enlargement may occur; monitor ovarian response. Ovarian hyperstimulation syndrome (OHSS), hypersensitivity/anaphylactic reactions, multiple pregnancies, serious pulmonary and vascular complications reported. Avoid hCG if ovaries abnormally enlarged last day of therapy. Monitor follicular maturation by measuring estradiol levels and through ultrasonography.

ADVERSE REACTIONS: Pulmonary and vascular complications, OHSS, hemoperitoneum, adnexal torsion, ovarian enlargement, ovarian cysts, abdominal pain, GI symptoms, injection site reactions, rash.

PREGNANCY: Category X, caution in nursing.

MECHANISM OF ACTION: Follicle stimulating hormone/lutenizing hormone; produces ovarian follicular growth in women who do not have primary ovarian failure.

PHARMACOKINETICS: Absorption: (SQ) C_{max}=5.62mIU/mL , AUC=385.2mIU-h/mL, T_{max}=12 hrs; (IM) C_{max}=4.15mIU/mL, AUC=320.1mIU-h/mL, T_{max}=18 hrs. **Elimination:** $T_{1/2}$(SQ, IM)=53.7 hrs, 59.2 hrs.

REQUIP   RX
ropinirole HCL (GlaxoSmithKline)

OTHER BRAND NAMES: Requip XL (GlaxoSmithKline)

THERAPEUTIC CLASS: Non-ergoline dopamine agonist

INDICATIONS: (Tab/Tab, Extended-Release) Treatment of signs and symptoms of idiopathic Parkinson's disease. (Tab) Treatment of moderate-to-severe primary Restless Legs Syndrome (RLS).

DOSAGE: *Adults:* Parkinson's: Tab: Initial: 0.25mg tid. Titrate: May increase weekly by 0.25mg tid (0.75mg/day) for 4 weeks. After week 4, may increase weekly by 1.5mg/day up to 9mg/day, then by 3mg/day weekly to 24mg/day. Max: 24mg/day. Withdrawal: Decrease dose to bid for 4 days, then qd for 3 days. Tab, Extended-Release: Initial: 2mg qd for 1-2 weeks. Titrate: May increase by 2mg/day at ≥1 week intervals, depending on therapeutic response and tolerability. Max: 24mg/day. Swallow whole; do not chew, crush, or divide. Switching from Immediate-Release (IR) to XL: Initial dose should match total

PDR® Concise Drug Guide

daily dose of IR formulation. See PI for more info. **RLS: Tab:** Initial: 0.25mg qd, 1-3 hours before bedtime. Titrate: 0.5mg qd days 3-7, 1mg qd week 2, then increase by 0.5mg weekly. Max: 4mg.

HOW SUPPLIED: Tab: 0.25mg, 0.5mg, 1mg, 2mg, 3mg, 4mg, 5mg; Tab, Extended-Release: (XL) 2mg, 4mg, 8mg

WARNINGS/PRECAUTIONS: (Tab/Tab, Extended-Release) Falling asleep during activities of daily living reported; if significant, d/c or warn patient to refrain from dangerous activities. Syncope, symptomatic hypotension, and hallucinations reported. Caution with severe renal or hepatic dysfunction. May cause or exacerbate pre-existing dyskinesia. Neuroleptic malignant syndrome, fibrotic complications, and melanoma reported. Augmentation and rebound in RLS reported. Avoid rapid dose reduction or abrupt withdrawal. Compulsive behaviors reported. (Tab, Extended-Release) May cause elevation of BP and changes in HR.

ADVERSE REACTIONS: (Tab) Neuralgia, increased BUN, hallucinations, somnolence, vomiting, headache, sweating, asthenia, edema, fatigue, syncope, orthostatic symptoms. (Tab, Extended-Release) Nausea, somnolence, dizziness, constipation, abdominal pain/discomfort.

INTERACTIONS: Adjust dose if CYP1A2 inhibitor or estrogen is stopped or started during treatment. Potentiated by ciprofloxacin. Decreased effects with dopamine antagonists (eg, phenothiazines, butyrophenones, thioxanthenes, metoclopramide). Drowsiness increased with sedatives. Caution with dopamine antagonists or alcohol.

PREGNANCY: Category C, not for use in nursing.

MECHANISM OF ACTION: Nonergoline dopamine agonist; believed to stimulate the post synaptic D_2-type receptors within the caudate-putamen in the brain.

PHARMACOKINETICS: Absorption: Rapid; absolute bioavailability (55%), T_{max}=1-2 hrs. **Distribution:** V_d=7.5L/kg, plasma protein binding (40%). **Metabolism:** Liver via CYP1A2 (extensive); N-despropylation and hydroxylation. **Elimination:** Urine, $T_{1/2}$=6 hrs.

RESCRIPTOR   RX
delavirdine mesylate (Pfizer)

THERAPEUTIC CLASS: Non-nucleoside reverse transcriptase inhibitor

INDICATIONS: Treatment of HIV-1 infection in combination with other antiretrovirals.

DOSAGE: *Adults:* Usual: 400mg tid. May disperse 100mg tab in ≥3 oz of water (200mg tab is not dispersible). Take with acidic beverage (eg, orange juice) if achlorhydria.
Pediatrics: ≥16yrs: Usual: 400mg tid. May disperse 100mg tab in ≥3 oz of water (200mg tab is not dispersible). Take with acidic beverage (eg, orange juice) if achlorhydria.

HOW SUPPLIED: Tab: 100mg, 200mg

CONTRAINDICATIONS: Contraindicated with drugs that are highly dependent on CYP3A for clearance (eg, astemizole, terfenadine, dihdroergotamine, egonovine, ergotamine, methylergonovine, cisapride, pimozide, alprazolam, midazolam, triazolam).

WARNINGS/PRECAUTIONS: Caution with hepatic dysfunction. D/C if severe rash develops. May cause immune reconstitution syndrome. May confer cross-resistance to other NNRTIs. May cause body fat redistribution/accumulation.

ADVERSE REACTIONS: Headache, fatigue, nausea, diarrhea, vomiting, increased ALT and AST, rash, maculopapular rash, pruritus, erythema, insomnia, upper respiratory infection.

INTERACTIONS: See Contraindications. Antacids decrease absorption; separate doses by 1 hr. H_2 antagonists reduce absorption; avoid chronic use. CYP3A inducers (eg, carbamazepine, phenobarbital, phenytoin, rifabutin, rifampin) may decrease plasma levels; avoid concomitant use. Increased plasma levels of drugs metabolized by CYP3A and 2C9 and amprenavir. Certain nonsedating antihistamines, sedative hypnotics, antiarrhythmics, CCBs, ergot agents, amphetamines, cisapride, and sildenafil (max of 25mg/48hrs of sildenafil) may result in potentially serious and/or life-threatening adverse events. Reduced effects of both delavirdine and didanosine; separate doses by 1 hr. Monitor LFTs with saquinavir. Increases indinavir plasma levels; reduce indinavir dose to 600mg tid.

PREGNANCY: Category C, not for use in nursing.

MECHANISM OF ACTION: HIV-1 non-nucleoside reverse transcriptase inhibitor (NNRTI). Binds directly to reverse transcriptase (RT) and blocks RNA-dependent and DNA-dependent DNA polymerase activities.

PHARMACOKINETICS: Absorption: Rapid. C_{max} =35μM, T_{max} =1 hr, AUC=180μM•hr. Bioavailability (85%). **Distribution:** Plasma protein binding (98%). **Metabolism:** Hepatic (N-desalkylation, pyridine hydroxylation) via CYP3A (major), 2D6. **Elimination:** Urine (<5%). $T_{1/2}$ =5.8 hrs.

RESERPINE
reserpine (Various)

RX

THERAPEUTIC CLASS: Rauwolfia alkaloid

INDICATIONS: Treatment of mild essential hypertension and adjunct treatment of severe hypertension. Relief of symptoms in agitated psychotic states.

DOSAGE: *Adults:* HTN: Initial: 0.5mg/day for 1-2 weeks. Maint: reduce to 0.1-0.25mg/day. Psychotic Disorders: Initial: 0.5mg/day. Range: 0.1-1mg/day.

HOW SUPPLIED: Tab: 0.1mg, 0.25mg

CONTRAINDICATIONS: Active or history of mental depression, active peptic ulcer, ulcerative colitis, current electroconvulsive therapy.

WARNINGS/PRECAUTIONS: Caution with renal insufficiency. May cause depression; d/c at 1st sign. Caution with history of peptic ulcer, ulcerative colitis, or gallstones.

ADVERSE REACTIONS: GI effects, dry mouth, hypersecretion, arrhythmia, syncope, edema, dyspnea, muscle aches, dizziness, depression, nervousness, impotence, gynecomastia, rash.

INTERACTIONS: Avoid MAOIs or use extreme caution. Prolonged effect of direct-acting sympathomimetics (eg, epinephrine, isoproterenol). May inhibit effects of indirect-acting sympathomimetics (eg, ephedrine, tyramine). Risk of arrhythmia with quinidine or digoxin. Titrate carefully with other antihypertensives. Decreased effect with TCAs.

PREGNANCY: Category C, not for use in nursing.

MECHANISM OF ACTION: Rauwolfia alkaloid: antihypertensive. Depletes stores of catecholamine and 5-hydroxytryptamine in many organs including brain and adrenal medulla, resulting in decreased HR and lowering of arterial BP.

PHARMACOKINETICS: Absorption: (0.5mg) T_{max} =2.5 hrs, C_{max} =1.1ng/mL; Absolute bioavailability (50%). **Distribution:** Plasma protein binding (95%); Found in breast milk. **Metabolism:** Complete. **Elimination:** Urine (1% unchanged); $T_{1/2}$ =200 hrs.

RESTASIS
cyclosporine (Allergan)

RX

THERAPEUTIC CLASS: Topical immunomodulator

INDICATIONS: To increase tear production in patients with suppressed tear production due to ocular inflammation associated with keratoconjunctivitis sicca.

DOSAGE: *Adults:* 1 drop bid, q12h. Concomitant Artificial Tears: Space by 15 min.

Pediatrics: ≥16 yrs: 1 drop bid, q12h. Concomitant Artificial Tears: Space by 15 min.

HOW SUPPLIED: Emul: 0.05% [0.4mL 32ˢ]

CONTRAINDICATIONS: Active ocular infections.

WARNINGS/PRECAUTIONS: Not studied in patients with a history of herpes keratitis. Not to be given while wearing contact lenses; lenses may be reinserted 15 minutes following administration.

ADVERSE REACTIONS: Ocular burning, conjunctival hyperemia, discharge, epiphora, eye pain, foreign body sensation, pruritus, stinging, visual disturbance (eg, blurring).

PREGNANCY: Category C, caution in nursing

MECHANISM OF ACTION: Topical immunomodulator; not established. Systemically acts as an immunosuppressive agent.

PHARMACOKINETICS: Distribution: Following systemic administration, found in human breast milk.

RESTORIL   CIV
temazepam (Mallinckrodt)

THERAPEUTIC CLASS: Benzodiazepine

INDICATIONS: Short-term treatment of insomnia (7-10 days).

DOSAGE: *Adults:* Usual: 7.5-30mg qhs. Transient Insomnia: 7.5mg qhs. Elderly/Debilitated: Initial: 7.5mg qhs.

HOW SUPPLIED: Cap: 7.5mg, 15mg, 22.5mg, 30mg

CONTRAINDICATIONS: Pregnancy.

WARNINGS/PRECAUTIONS: Caution in elderly, debilitated, severely depressed, those with suicidal tendencies, hepatic/renal impairment, pulmonary insufficiency. Avoid abrupt discontinuation. If no improvement after 7-10 days, may indicate primary psychiatric and/or medical condition.

ADVERSE REACTIONS: Headache, dizziness, drowsiness, fatigue, nervousness, nausea, lethargy, hangover.

INTERACTIONS: Additive CNS depressant effects with alcohol and CNS depressants. May be synergistic with diphenhydramine.

PREGNANCY: Category X, caution in nursing.

MECHANISM OF ACTION: Benzodiazepine hypnotic agent.

PHARMACOKINETICS: Absorption: Well-absorbed. C_{max}=666-982ng/mL, T_{max}=approximately 1.5 hrs. **Distribution:** Plasma protein binding (96%, unchanged), crosses placenta. **Metabolism:** Conjugation (major metabolites): O-conjugate . **Elimination:** Urine (80-90%).$T_{1/2}$=8.8 hrs.

RETAVASE   RX
reteplase (PDL)

THERAPEUTIC CLASS: Thrombolytic agent

INDICATIONS: To improve ventricular function following acute myocardial infarction (AMI), reduce the incidence of congestive heart failure (CHF) and reduce the mortality associated with AMI.

DOSAGE: *Adults:* 10 U IV over 2 min. Repeat in 30 min.

HOW SUPPLIED: Inj: 10.4 U

CONTRAINDICATIONS: Active internal bleeding, history of CVA, recent intracranial or intraspinal surgery or trauma, intracranial neoplasm, arteriovenous malformation, aneurysm, bleeding diathesis, severe uncontrolled HTN.

WARNINGS/PRECAUTIONS: Weigh benefits/risks with recent major surgery, previous puncture of noncompressible vessels, cerebrovascular disease, recent GI or GU bleeding, recent trauma, HTN, left heart thrombus, acute pericarditis, subacute bacterial endocarditis, hemostatic defects, severe hepatic or renal dysfunction, pregnancy, diabetic hemorrhagic retinopathy or other hemorrhagic ophthalmic conditions, septic thrombophlebitis or occluded AV cannula at a seriously infected site, elderly, any other bleeding condition that is difficult to manage. Cholesterol embolism and internal/superficial bleeding reported. Arrhythmias may occur with reperfusion. Avoid IM injection, noncompressible arterial puncture, and internal jugular or subclavian venous puncture. Cholesterol embolism and internal/superficial bleeding reported.

ADVERSE REACTIONS: Bleeding, allergic reactions, dyspnea, hypotension.

INTERACTIONS: Increased risk of bleeding with heparin, vitamin K antagonists, and drugs that alter platelet function (eg, ASA, NSAIDs, dipyridamole, abciximab) before or after therapy. Weigh benefits/risks with oral anticoagulants.

PREGNANCY: Category C, caution in nursing.

MECHANISM OF ACTION: Thrombolytic agent; recombinant plasminogen activator that catalyzes the cleavage of endogenous plasminogen to generate plasmin. Plasmin in turn degrades the fibrin matrix of the thrombus, thereby exerting its thrombolytic action.

PHARMACOKINETICS: Metabolism: Liver. **Elimination:** Renal; $T_{1/2}$= 13-16 min.

RETIN-A RX
tretinoin (Ortho Neutrogena)

OTHER BRAND NAMES: Retin-A Micro (Ortho Neutrogena)

THERAPEUTIC CLASS: Retinoid

INDICATIONS: Topical treatment of acne vulgaris.

DOSAGE: *Adults:* Cleanse area thoroughly, then apply qhs. May temporarily d/c or reduce dosing frequency if irritation occurs.
Pediatrics: ≥12 yrs: (Gel: 0.04%, 0.1%) Cleanse area thoroughly, then apply qhs. May temporarily d/c or reduce dosing frequency if irritation occurs.

HOW SUPPLIED: (Retin-A) Cre: 0.025%, 0.05%, 0.1% [20g, 45g]; Gel: 0.01%, 0.025% [15g, 45g]; Sol: 0.05% [28mL]; (Retin-A Micro) Gel: 0.04%, 0.1% [20g, 45g]

WARNINGS/PRECAUTIONS: Avoid eyes, lips, paranasal creases, mucous membranes, and sunburned skin. Acne exacerbation during 1st weeks of therapy may occur. D/C if sensitivity or irritation occurs. Severe irritation with eczematous skin. Causes photosensitivity. Extreme weather (eg, cold, wind) may irritate skin.

ADVERSE REACTIONS: Local skin reactions (red, edematous, blistered, crusted), photosensitivity, temporary skin pigmentation changes.

INTERACTIONS: Caution with topical agents with strong drying effects, high concentration of alcohol, astringents, spices, or lime. Caution with sulfur, resorcinol, or salicylic acid; allow effects of these agents to subside before application of tretinoin.

PREGNANCY: Category C, caution in nursing.

MECHANISM OF ACTION: Retinoic acid derivative; not established. Responsible for decreasing cohesiveness of follicular epithelial cells with decreased microcomedo formation. Also stimulates mitotic activity and increases turnover of follicular epithelial cells, causing extrusion of the comedones.

RETROVIR RX
zidovudine (GlaxoSmithKline)

> Associated with hematologic toxicity (eg, neutropenia, severe anemia), especially with advanced HIV disease. Prolonged use associated with symptomatic myopathy. Lactic acidosis and severe, possibly fatal hepatomegaly with steatosis reported.

THERAPEUTIC CLASS: Nucleoside analogue

INDICATIONS: Treatment of HIV infection in combination with other antiretrovirals. Prevention of maternal-fetal HIV transmission.

DOSAGE: *Adults:* (Tab) 600mg/day in divided doses. (Inj) 1mg/kg IV over 1 hr 5-6 times/day. Prevention of Maternal-Fetal HIV Transmission: >14 weeks pregnancy: 100mg PO five times/day until start of labor. During labor and delivery: 2mg/kg IV over 1 hr followed by 1mg/kg/hr IV infusion until clamping of umbilical cord. End-Stage Renal Disease/Dialysis: 100mg PO q6-8h or 1mg/kg IV q6-8h. Significant Anemia/Neutropenia: May require dose interruption and adjunctive epoetin therapy. Less Severe Anemia/Neutropenia: Reduce daily dose.
Pediatrics: 6 weeks-12 yrs: 160mg/m² PO q8h. Max: 200mg PO q8h. Prevention of Maternal-Fetal HIV Transmission: Neonates: 2mg/kg PO q6h (or 1.5mg/kg IV over 30 min q6h) starting within 12 hrs after birth and continue through 6 weeks of age. End-Stage Renal Disease/Dialysis: 100mg PO q6-8h or 1mg/kg IV q6-8h. Significant Anemia/Neutropenia: May require dose interruption and adjunctive epoetin therapy. Pronounced Anemia: Reduce daily dose. Mild to Moderate Hepatic Impairment: Monitor for hematologic toxicity and reduce dose if needed.

HOW SUPPLIED: Cap: 100mg; Inj: 10mg/mL; Syrup: 50mg/5mL [240mL]; Tab: 300mg

WARNINGS/PRECAUTIONS: Adverse reactions increase with disease progression. Caution with compromised bone marrow or in elderly. Monitor for hematologic toxicity; reduce dose or stop therapy. Myopathy and myositis with pathological changes associated with prolonged use. Caution with obesity and liver disease; increased risk of lactic acidosis and hepatomegaly with steatosis. Increased risk of toxicity with prolonged exposure to nucleosides, in women, obesity, advanced HIV disease, severe hepatic impairment. Possible redistribution or accumuation of body fat. Hepatic decompensation has occurred in HIV/HCV co-infected patients receiving combination antiretroviral therapy for HIV and interferon alfa with or without ribavirin; monitor for treatment associated toxicities. Immune reconstitution syndrome has been reported with combination antiretroviral therapy.

ADVERSE REACTIONS: Headache, nausea, malaise, anorexia, vomiting, asthenia, constipation, anemia, neutropenia.

INTERACTIONS: Increased risk of hematologic toxicities with ganciclovir, interferon-alpha, bone marrow suppressives and cytotoxic drugs. Possible increased levels with phenytoin, atovaquone, fluconazole, methadone, probenecid, valproic acid. Possible decreased levels with nelfinavir, ritonavir, rifampin. Avoid with stavudine, ribavirin, doxorubicin, other combination products containing zidovudine. Prolonged exposure to antiretroviral nucleoside analogues increases risk of lactic acidosis and hepatomegaly with steatosis. May decrease phenytoin levels.

PREGNANCY: Category C, not for use in nursing.

MECHANISM OF ACTION: Pyrimidine nucleoside analogue; inhibits reverse transcriptase via DNA chain termination.

PHARMACOKINETICS: Absorption: (Tab, Cap, Syrup): Rapid. Bioavailability (64%). T_{max}=0.5-1.5 hrs. (IV) C_{max}=1.06mcg/mL. **Distribution:** V_d=1.6L/kg; plasma protein binding (<38%). **Metabolism:** Hepatic. Metabolite (3'-azido-3'-deoxy-5'-*O*-β-*D*-glucopyranuronosylthymidine (GZDV). **Elimination:** (Tab, Cap, Syrup): Zidovudine: Urine (14%). GZDV: Urine (74%); $T_{1/2}$=0.5-3 hrs. (IV): Zidovudine: Urine (18%). GZDV: Urine (60%); $T_{1/2}$=1.1 hrs.

REVATIO   RX
sildenafil citrate (Pfizer)

THERAPEUTIC CLASS: Phosphodiesterase type 5 inhibitor

INDICATIONS: Treatment of pulmonary arterial hypertension (WHO Group I) to improve exercise ability.

DOSAGE: *Adults:* 20mg tid 4-6 hours apart.

HOW SUPPLIED: Tab: 20mg

CONTRAINDICATIONS: Organic nitrates taken regularly and/or intermittently.

WARNINGS/PRECAUTIONS: Caution with MI, stroke, or life-threatening arrhythmia within last 6 months; with resting hypotension (BP<90/50), fluid depletion, severe left ventricular outflow obstruction, autonomic dysfunction, or HTN (BP>170/110); unstable angina due to cardiac failure or CAD; anatomical penile deformation; predisposition to priapism; and retinitis pigmentosa. Avoid in patients with veno-occlusive disease. Decrease in supine BP reported. If erection persists >4 hrs, seek immediate medical assistance; penile tissue damage and permanent loss of potency could result if priapism not treated immediately.

ADVERSE REACTIONS: Epistaxis, headache, flushing, dyspepsia, insomnia, erythema, dyspnea, rhinitis, diarrhea, myalgia, pyrexia, gastritis, sinusitis, paresthesia.

INTERACTIONS: See Contraindications. Reports of bleeding (epistaxis) with vitamin K antagonists. Increased levels with CYP3A4 inhibitors (eg, cimetidine, ketoconazole, itraconazole, erythromycin, saquinavir) and protease inhibitors (eg, ritonavir). CYP2C9 inhibitors may decrease sildenafil clearance. Decreased levels with CYP3A4 inducers (eg, bosentan; more potent inducers such as barbiturates, carbamazepine, phenytoin, efavirenz, nevirapine, rifampin, rifabutin). Co-administration with bosentan resulted in a decrease in AUC of sildenafil and increase in AUC of bosentan. Additional supine BP reduction with amlodipine reported. Simultaneous administration with α-blockers may lead to symptomatic hypotension.

PREGNANCY: Category B, caution in nursing.

MECHANISM OF ACTION: It inhibits cGMP specific phosphodiesterase type-5 (PDE5) in the smooth muscle of the pulmonary vasculature, where PDE5 is responsible for degradation of cGMP. It increases cGMP within pulmonary vascular smooth muscle cells, resulting in relaxation.

PHARMACOKINETICS: Absorption: Rapid; absolute bioavailability (40%), T_{max}=30-120 min. **Distribution:** V_d=105L, plasma protein binding (96%). **Metabolism:** Liver via CYP3A4 (major route) and CYP2C9 (minor route); through N-desmethylation. **Elimination:** Feces (80%; metabolites), urine (13%). $T_{1/2}$=4 hrs.

ReVia
naltrexone HCL (Duramed)   **RX**

THERAPEUTIC CLASS: Opioid antagonist

INDICATIONS: Treatment of alcohol dependence and to block effects of exogenously administered opioids.

DOSAGE: *Adults:* Alcoholism: 50mg qd up to 12 weeks. Opioid Dependence: Initial: 25mg qd. Maint: 50mg qd. Naloxone Challenge Test: 0.2mg IV, observe for 30 sec, then 0.6mg IV, observe for 20 min; or 0.8mg SQ, observe for 20 min.

HOW SUPPLIED: Tab: 50mg

CONTRAINDICATIONS: Acute hepatitis, hepatic failure, patients failing naloxone challenge or opioid-dependent, concomitant opioid analgesics, acute opioid withdrawal, positive urine screen for opioids, phenanthrene sensitivity.

WARNINGS/PRECAUTIONS: Hepatotoxic with excessive doses; margin of separation between safe dose and hepatotoxic dose is 5-fold or less. Only treat patients opioid-free for 7-10 days. Attempting to overcome opiate blockade is very dangerous. More sensitive to lower doses of opioids after naltrexone is discontinued. Safety in ultra-rapid opiate detoxification is not known. Increased risk of suicide in substance abuse patients. Severe opioid withdrawal syndromes reported with accidental ingestion in opioid-dependent patients. Monitor closely during blockade reversal. Caution in renal or hepatic impairment. Perform naloxone challenge test if question of opioid dependence.

ADVERSE REACTIONS: Nausea, headache, dizziness, nervousness, fatigue, restlessness, insomnia, vomiting, anxiety, somnolence.

INTERACTIONS: Caution with other drugs. Do not use with disulfiram unless benefits outweigh risk of hepatotoxicity. Lethargy and somnolence reported with thioridazine. Antagonizes opioid-containing cough and cold, antidiarrheal, and analgesic agents.

PREGNANCY: Category C, caution in nursing.

MECHANISM OF ACTION: Opioid antagonist; markedly attenuates or completely blocks (reversibly) the subjective effects of IV administered opioids.

PHARMACOKINETICS: Absorption: Rapid and complete. Bioavailability (5-40%), T_{max}=1 hr. **Distribution:** V_d=1350L, plasma protein binding (21%). **Metabolism:** Liver , 6β-naltrexol (major metabolite). **Elimination:** Urine 2% (unchanged), 43% (conjugated), (naltrexone, β-naltrexol) $T_{1/2}$=4 hrs, 13 hrs.

REVLIMID RX
lenalidomide (Celgene)

> Potential for human birth defects, hematological toxicity (neutropenia and thrombocytopenia), deep venous thrombosis (DVT) and pulmonary embolism (PE). Lenalidomide is an analogue of thalidomide. Thalidomide is a known human teratogen that causes severe life-threatening human birth defects. If taken during pregnancy, may cause birth defects or death to an unborn baby. Avoid pregnancy due to potential toxicity and to avoid fetal exposure. Only available under a special restricted distribution program called Revassist ᴿᴹ. Associated with significant neutropenia and thrombocytopenia in patients with del 5q MDS. CBC should be monitored weekly for the first 8 weeks of therapy and at least monthly thereafter. May require dose interruption and/or reduction and the use of blood product support and/or growth factors. Increased risk of DVT and PE in patients with multiple myeloma. Observe for signs and symptoms of thromboembolism.

THERAPEUTIC CLASS: Thalidomide Analog

INDICATIONS: Transfusion-dependent anemia due to Low- or Intermediate-1-risk myelodysplastic syndromes associated with a deletion 5q cytogenetic abnormality with or without additional cytogenetic abnormalities. In combination with dexamethasone for the treatment of multiple myeloma in patients who have received at least one prior therapy.

DOSAGE: *Adults:* ≥18 yrs: Myelodysplastic Syndromes: 10mg daily with water. Multiple Myeloma: 25mg daily with water. Administer as single dose on Days 1-21 of repeated 28-day cycles. Do not break, chew, or open capsules. Adjust dose based on platelet and/or neutrophil counts.

HOW SUPPLIED: Cap: 5mg, 10mg, 15mg, 25mg

CONTRAINDICATIONS: Pregnancy.

WARNINGS/PRECAUTIONS: Risk of adverse reactions may be greater in patients with impaired renal function.

ADVERSE REACTIONS: Thrombocytopenia, neutropenia, pruritus, rash, diarrhea, constipation, nausea, nasopharyngitis, fatigue, arthralgia, cough, pyrexia, peripheral edema, insomnia, asthenia.

INTERACTIONS: Co-administration increased digoxin C_{max} by 14%; monitoring suggested.

PREGNANCY: Category X, not for use in nursing.

MECHANISM OF ACTION: Thalidomide analogue; not established, inhibits secretion of pro-inflammatory cytokines and increases secretion of anti-inflammatory cytokines from peripheral blood mononuclear cells, inhibits cell proliferation, and inhibits growth of multiple myeloma cells by inducing cell cycle arrest and apoptosis.

PHARMACOKINETICS: Absorption: T_{max}=0.625-1.5 hrs (healthy), 0.5-4.0 hrs (multiple myeloma). **Distribution**: Plasma protein binding (30%). **Elimination**: Urine; $T_{1/2}$=3 hrs.

REYATAZ RX
atazanavir sulfate (Bristol-Myers Squibb)

THERAPEUTIC CLASS: Protease inhibitor

INDICATIONS: Treatment of HIV-1 infection in combination with other antiretrovirals.

DOSAGE: *Adults:* Therapy-Naive: 400mg qd. Therapy-experienced: 300mg with ritonavir 100mg qd. Concomitant Efavirenz: Give atazanavir 300mg and ritonavir 100mg with efavirenz 600mg qd. Concomitant Buffered Didanosine: Give atazanavir 2 hrs before or 1 hr after didanosine. Concomitant Tenofovir: Give atazanavir 300mg with ritonavir 100mg and tenofovir 300mg. Moderate Hepatic Insufficiency (Child-Pugh Class B): 300mg qd. Take with food.

HOW SUPPLIED: Cap: 100mg, 150mg, 200mg, 300mg

CONTRAINDICATIONS: Concomitant administration with midazolam, triazolam, dihydroergotamine, ergotamine, ergonovine, methylergonovine, cisapride, pimozide.

WARNINGS/PRECAUTIONS: Prolongs PR-interval; caution with pre-existing conduction system disease. New-onset DM, exacerbation of pre-existing DM, hyperglycemia, hyperbilirubinemia, increased bleeding with hemophilia Types A and B, Stevens-Johnson syndrome, erythema multiforme reported. Caution with hepatic impairment; avoid with severe hepatic insufficiency. D/C with severe rash. Possible redistribution/accumulation of body fat. Immune reconstitution syndrome reported with combination therapy. Nephrolithiasis reported.

ADVERSE REACTIONS: Headache, nausea, jaundice, abdominal pain, vomiting, diarrhea, rash, myalgia, peripheral neurologic symptoms, insomnia, jaundice/scleral icterus.

INTERACTIONS: Avoid with rifampin, irinotecan, midazolam, triazolam, bepridil, ergot-derivatives, cisapride, lovastatin, simvastatin, pimozide, indinavir, proton-pump inhibitors, St. John's wort. Avoid nevirapine, voriconazole, other protease inhibitors with atazanavir/ritonavir therapy. May increase levels of drugs metabolized by CYP3A or UGT1A1. CYP3A inducers may decrease levels. CYP3A inhibitors, voriconazole may increase levels. Decreased levels with buffered didanosine, tenofovir, efavirenz, antacids/buffered medications (give atazanavir 2 hrs before or 1 hr after), H_2-receptor antagonists (space dosing by 12 hrs). Increase levels of saquinavir, diltiazem (reduce dose by 50%), amiodarone, lidocaine (systemic), quinidine, warfarin, TCAs, rifabutin (reduce dose up to 75%), CCBs, oral contraceptives (use lowest possible dose), sildenafil/tadalafil/vardenafil (reduce dose), atorvastatin, cyclosporine, sirolimus, tacrolimus, clarithromycin (reduce dose by 50%; consider alternative therapy for infections other than *M.avium* complex). Increased levels with ritonavir (give atazanavir 300mg/day with ritonavir 100mg/day with food). Caution with high doses of ketoconazole, itrazonazole with atazanavir/ritonavir therapy. Atazanavir/ritonavir therapy may significantly increase plasma fluticasone propionate exposure resulting in significantly decreased serum cortisol concentrations.

PREGNANCY: Category B, not for use in nursing.

MECHANISM OF ACTION: HIV-1 protease inhibitor: Inhibits virus-specific processing of viral Gag-Pol polyproteins in HIV-1 infected cells, preventing formation of mature virions.

PHARMACOKINETICS: Absorption: Rapid. T_{max}=2.5 hrs. **Distribution:** Plasma protein binding (86%). **Metabolism:** Hepatic (biotransformation: mono- and dioxygenation) via CYP3A. **Elimination:** $t_{1/2}$=7 hrs. Urine (7%), feces (20%).

RHINOCORT AQUA   RX
budesonide (AstraZeneca)

THERAPEUTIC CLASS: Corticosteroid

INDICATIONS: Management of seasonal or perennial allergic rhinitis.

DOSAGE: *Adults*: 1 spray per nostril qd. Max: 4 sprays/nostril/day.
Pediatrics: >12 yrs: 1 spray per nostril qd. Max: 4 sprays/nostril/day. 6-12 yrs: 1 spray per nostril qd. Max: 2 sprays/nostril/day.

HOW SUPPLIED: Spray: 32mcg/spray [8.6g]

WARNINGS/PRECAUTIONS: Risk of adrenal insufficiency and withdrawal symptoms when replacing systemic corticosteroids with a topical corticosteroids. Caution with active or quiescent TB, ocular herpes simplex, or untreated bacterial, fungal and systemic viral infections. Avoid with recent nasal trauma, surgery or septum ulcers. Risk of more severe/fatal course of infections (eg, chickenpox, measles) and for *Candida* infections of the nose and pharynx. Potential for growth velocity reduction in pediatrics. Should not delay or interfere infant feeding.

ADVERSE REACTIONS: Nasal irritation, pharyngitis, cough, epistaxis.

INTERACTIONS: Oral ketoconazole and cimetidine increase plasma levels. CYP3A inhibitors (eg, itraconazole, clarithromycin, erythromycin) may decrease metabolism and increase systemic exposure. Concomitant systemic corticosteroids increases risk of hypercorticism and/or HPA axis suppression.

PREGNANCY: Category B, caution in nursing.

MECHANISM OF ACTION: Glucocorticosteroid; not established, suspected to have a wide range of inhibitory activities against multiple cell types (eg, mast cells, eosinophils, neutrophils, macrophages, lymphocytes) and mediators (eg, histamine, leukotrienes, ecosanoids, cytokines) involved in allergic mediated inflammation.

PHARMACOKINETICS: Absorption: Well absorbed, T_{max}=0.7 hr. **Distribution:** V_d=approximately 2-3L/Kg, plasma protein binding (85-90%). **Metabolism:** Liver (extensive), 16α-hydroxyprednisolone and 6β-hydroxybudesonide (major metabolites) via CYP3A4-catalyzed biotransformation. **Elimination:** Urine and feces, $T_{1/2}$(the 22R form)=2-3 hrs.

RIDAURA   RX
auranofin (Prometheus)

| May cause gold toxicity. |

THERAPEUTIC CLASS: Gold agent

INDICATIONS: Management of rheumatoid arthritis in patients with inadequate response to NSAIDs.

DOSAGE: *Adults:* Usual: 6mg qd or 3mg bid. If response not adequate after 6 months, increase to 3mg tid. If inadequate response with 9mg/day after 3 months, d/c. Max: 9mg/day. Transferring from Injectable Gold: D/C injectable agent and start with 6mg qd.

HOW SUPPLIED: Cap: 3mg

CONTRAINDICATIONS: History of gold induced disorders: anaphylactic reactions, necrotizing enterocolitis, pulmonary fibrosis, exfoliative dermatitis, bone marrow aplasia, or severe hematologic disorders.

WARNINGS/PRECAUTIONS: Gold toxicity manifests as a falling Hgb, leukopenia <4000 WBC/cu mm, granulocytes <1500/cu mm, decrease in platelets <150,000/cu mm, proteinuria, hematuria, pruritus, rash, stomatitis, or persistent diarrhea. Thrombocytopenia and proteinuria reported. Caution in renal/hepatic disease, inflammatory bowel disease, skin rash or a history of bone marrow depression. GI reactions, dermatitis, stomatitis, nephrotic syndrome, and blood dyscrasias reported.

ADVERSE REACTIONS: Diarrhea, nausea, constipation, anorexia, flatulence, dyspepsia, rash, conjunctivitis, exfoliative dermatitis, anemia, proteinuria, hematuria, elevated liver enzymes.

INTERACTIONS: Increased phenytoin levels.

PREGNANCY: Category C, not for use in nursing.

MECHANISM OF ACTION: Gold agent: mechanism not established. May modify disease activity in rheumatoid arthritis.

PHARMACOKINETICS: Absorption: 25% absorbed. **Distribution:** Plasma protein binding (60%). **Metabolism:** Rapid. **Elimination:** Urine (60% of absorbed gold), feces; $T_{1/2}$=26 days (plasma); $T_{1/2}$=80 days (body).

RIFADIN
rifampin (Sanofi-Aventis) RX

THERAPEUTIC CLASS: Rifamycin derivative

INDICATIONS: Treatment of all forms of TB. Treatment of asymptomatic carriers of *Neisseria meningitidis* to eliminate meningococci from nasopharynx.

DOSAGE: *Adults:* TB: 10mg/kg PO/IV qd. Max: 600mg/day. Meningococcal Carriers: 600mg bid for 2 days. Take 1 hr before or 2 hrs after a meal with a full glass of water.
Pediatrics: TB: 10-20mg/kg PO/IV qd. Max: 600mg/day. Meningococcal Carriers: ≥1 month: 10mg/kg q12h for 2 days. Max: 600mg/dose. <1 month: 5mg/kg q12h for 2 days. Take 1 hr before or 2 hrs after a meal with a full glass of water.

HOW SUPPLIED: Cap: 150mg, 300mg; Inj: 600mg

WARNINGS/PRECAUTIONS: May produce liver dysfunction. May cause hyperbilirubinemia. Not for treatment of meningococcal disease. May produce reddish coloration of the urine, sweat, sputum, and tears. May permanently stain soft contact lenses.

ADVERSE REACTIONS: GI distress, thrombocytopenia, visual disturbances, menstrual disturbances, edema of face and extremities, elevated BUN and serum uric acid levels.

INTERACTIONS: May accelerate elimination of drugs metabolized by CYP450 (eg, anticonvulsants, antiarrhythmics, anticoagulants, azole antifungals, barbiturates, β-blockers, CCBs, chloramphenicol, clarithromycin, corticosteroids, cyclosporine, cardiac glycosides, clofibrate, oral or systemic contraceptives, dapsone, diazepam, doxycycline, fluoroquinolones, haloperidol, oral hypoglycemics, levothyroxine, methadone, narcotics, nortriptyline, progestins, quinine, tacrolimus, theophylline, TCAs, and zidovudine). Give antacids at least 1 hr before rifampin. Increased hepatotoxicity with halothane or isoniazid. Increased serum levels with probenecid and cotrimoxazole. Caution with other hepatotoxic agents. Concomitant ketoconazole decreases both drug serum levels. Decreased levels of enalapril, atovaquone. Increased levels with atovaquone.

PREGNANCY: Category C, not for use in nursing.

MECHANISM OF ACTION: Rifamycin derivative; has bacterial activity against intracellular and extracellular *Mycobacterium tuberculosis.* Inhibits DNA-dependent RNA polymerase activity in susceptible cells. Interacts with bacterial RNA polymerase; does not inhibit the mammalian enzyme.

PHARMACOKINETICS: Absorption: Readily absorbed from GI tract. (PO, 600mg) C_{max}=7mcg/mL. (IV, 300mg, 600mg) C_{max}=9.0mcg/mL, 17.5mcg/mL. **Distribution:** (IV, 300mg, 600mg): V_d=0.66L/kg, 0.64L/kg; distributed in body fluids and cerebrospinal fluid; plasma protein binding 80%. **Metabolism:** Via deacetylation; 25-desacetyl-rifampin (major metabolite). **Elimination:** Urine (30%), bile; (600mg, 900mg) $T_{1/2}$=3.35 hrs, 5.08hrs.

RIFAMATE
rifampin - isoniazid (Sanofi-Aventis) RX

> Isoniazid associated with severe and sometimes fatal hepatitis. Monitor LFTs on a monthly basis.

THERAPEUTIC CLASS: Isonicotinic acid hydrazide/rifamycin derivative

INDICATIONS: For pulmonary TB. Not for initial therapy or prevention.

DOSAGE: *Adults:* 2 caps qd. Take 1 hr before or 2 hrs after meals. Give with pyridoxine in the malnourished, those predisposed to neuropathy (eg, alcoholics, diabetics), and adolescents.

HOW SUPPLIED: Cap: (Isoniazid-Rifampin) 150mg-300mg

CONTRAINDICATIONS: Previous isoniazid-associated hepatic injury, severe adverse reactions to isoniazid (eg, drug fever, chills, and arthritis), acute liver disease.

WARNINGS/PRECAUTIONS: Monitor LFTs before therapy, periodically thereafter. Not for intermittent therapy. Urine, feces, saliva, sputum, sweat, and tears may be colored red-orange; may stain soft contact lenses permanently. Caution with chronic liver disease or severe renal dysfunction. Perform periodic ophthalmoscopic exams.

ADVERSE REACTIONS: Headache, drowsiness, fatigue, ataxia, dizziness, confusion, visual disturbances, weakness, GI effects, peripheral neuropathy, pyridoxine deficiency, anorexia, nausea, renal or hepatic insufficiency, blood dyscrasias.

INTERACTIONS: Anticoagulants may need dose increase. May decrease activity of methadone, oral hypoglycemics, digitoxin, quinidine, disopyramide, dapsone, and corticosteroids. Higher incidence of isoniazid hepatitis with daily alcohol ingestion. Risk of phenytoin toxicity. Caution with other hepatotoxic agents and phenytoin. May decrease effects of oral contraceptives; use alternative measures.

PREGNANCY: Safety in pregnancy not known, caution in nursing.

MECHANISM OF ACTION: Isonicotinic acid hydrazide/rifamycin derivative. Isoniazid: Rifampin: Exhibits bacterial activity against intracellular and extracellular *Mycobacterium tuberculosis*. Inhibits DNA-dependent RNA polymerase activity in susceptible cells; interacts with bacterial RNA polymerase but does not inhibit the mammalian enzyme. Inhibits mycoloic acid synthesis and acts against actively growing tubercle bacilli.

PHARMACOKINETICS: Absorption: Rifampin: C_{max}=10mcg/mL, T_{max}=$1^1/_2$-3 hrs. Isoniazid: T_{max}=1-2 hrs. **Distribution:** Isoniazid: Diffuses into body fluids; crosses placental barrier and into milk. **Metabolism:** Isoniazid: Acetylation and dehydrazination. **Elimination:** Rifampin: $T_{1/2}$=3 hrs; bile, urine.

Rifater   RX
pyrazinamide - rifampin - isoniazid (Sanofi-Aventis)

> Isoniazid associated with severe and sometimes fatal hepatitis. Monitor LFTs on a monthly basis.

THERAPEUTIC CLASS: Isonicotinic acid hydrazide/rifamycin derivative/nicotinamide analogue

INDICATIONS: For initial phase of pulmonary TB treatment.

DOSAGE: *Adults:* ≤44kg: 4 tabs single dose qd. 45-54kg: 5 tabs single dose. ≥55kg: 6 tabs single dose. Give pyridoxine in malnourished, if predisposed to neuropathy (eg, alcoholics, diabetics), and adolescents. Take 1 hr before or 2 hrs after meals with full glass of water. Treatment usually lasts 2 months. *Pediatrics:* ≥15 yrs: ≤44kg: 4 tabs single dose qd. 45-54kg: 5 tabs qd single dose. ≥55kg: 6 tabs qd single dose. Give pyridoxine in malnourished, if predisposed to neuropathy (eg, alcoholics, diabetics), and adolescents. Take 1 hr before or 2 hrs after meals with full glass of water. Treatment usually lasts 2 months.

HOW SUPPLIED: Tab: (Isoniazid-Pyrazinamide-Rifampin) 50mg-300mg-120mg

CONTRAINDICATIONS: Severe hepatic damage, adverse reactions to isoniazid (eg, drug fever, chills, arthritis), acute liver disease, acute gout.

WARNINGS/PRECAUTIONS: Liver dysfunction, hyperbilirubinemia, and hyperuricemia with acute gouty arthritis reported. Monitor LFTs (every 2-4 weeks), serum uric acid. Perform regular ophthalmologic exams. Caution with DM, severe renal dysfunction. May produce reddish coloration of urine, sweat, sputum, and tears. May permanently stain soft contact lenses.

ADVERSE REACTIONS: GI effects, cutaneous reactions, musculoskeletal pain, hepatitis, CNS and cardiorespiratory effects.

INTERACTIONS: Rifampin may accelerate metabolism of anticonvulsants (eg, phenytoin), antiarrhythmics (eg, disopyramide, mexiletine, quinidine, tocainide), anticoagulants, antifungals (eg, fluconazole, itraconazole, keto-conazole), barbiturates, β-blockers, CCBs (eg, diltiazem, nifedipine, vera-pamil), chloramphenicol, ciprofloxacin, corticosteroids, cyclosporine, cardiac glycosides, clofibrate, oral contraceptives, dapsone, diazepam, haloperidol, oral hypoglycemics (eg, sulfonylureas), methadone, narcotic analgesics, nor-triptyline, progestins, theophylline. Antacids may reduce rifampin absorption. Avoid foods containing tyramine and histamine (eg, cheese, red wine, tuna). Anticoagulants may need dose increase. Higher incidence of isoniazid hepati-tis with daily alcohol ingestion. Avoid halothane. INH inhibits certain CYP450 enzymes; monitor with anticonvulsants, benzodiazepines, haloperidol, keto-conazole, warfarin. Decreased levels with corticosteroids. Exaggerates CNS effects of meperidine, cycloserine, disulfiram. Excess catecholamine stimula-tion with L-dopa.

PREGNANCY: Category C, not for use in nursing.

MECHANISM OF ACTION: Rifampin: Inhibits DNA-dependent RNA poly-merase activity in susceptible *Mycobacterium tuberculosis* organism. Interacts with bacterial RNA polymerase, but does not inhibit the mammalian enzyme. Isoniazid: Kills growing tubercle bacilli by inhibiting the biosynthesis of mycolic acids which are major component of the cell wall of *Mycobacterium tuberculosis*. Pyrazinamide: Inhibits growth of *Mycobacterial tuberculosis*.

PHARMACOKINETICS: Absorption: Isoniazid: Bioavailability (100.6%), C_{max}=3.09mcg/mL, T_{max}=1-2 hrs. Rifampin: Bioavailability (88.8 %), C_{max}=11.04mcg/mL. Pyrazinamide: Bioavailability (96.8%), C_{max}=28.02mcg/mL. **Distribution:** Isoniazid: Passes through placental barrier and into milk. Pyrazinamide: Plasma protein binding (10%), distributed in liver, lungs, and CSF; found in breast milk. Rifampin: Protein binding (80%). **Metabolism:** Isoniazid: Acetylation and dehydrazination. Pyrazinamide: Liver, via hydroxy-lation; pyrazinoic acid (major active metabolite). Rifampin: Via deacetylation; 25-desacetyl-rifampin (major metabolite). **Elimination:** Rifampin: Urine (30%), bile; $T_{1/2}$=3.35 hrs. Pyrazinamide: Urine (70%), 4-14% (unchanged); $T_{1/2}$=9-10 hrs. Isoniazid: Urine (50-70%); T1/2=1-4 hrs.

RILUTEK RX
riluzole (Sanofi-Aventis)

THERAPEUTIC CLASS: Benzothiazole

INDICATIONS: Treatment of amyotrophic lateral sclerosis (ALS).

DOSAGE: *Adults:* 50mg q12h. Take 1 hr before or 2 hrs after meals.

HOW SUPPLIED: Tab: 50mg

WARNINGS/PRECAUTIONS: Caution in elderly, and hepatic or renal dysfunc-tion. Perform baseline LFT's before therapy, every month during 1st 3 months, every 3 months, every 3 months for next 9 months, then periodically thereaf-ter. Neutropenia reported; obtain WBC count with febrile illness.

ADVERSE REACTIONS: Asthenia, nausea, dizziness, decreased lung function, diarrhea, abdominal pain, pneumonia, vomiting, vertigo, paresthesia, anorexia, somnolence.

INTERACTIONS: Caution with potentially hepatotoxic drugs (eg, allopurinol, methyldopa, sulfinpyrazine). CYP1A2 inhibitors (eg, caffeine, phenacetin, theophylline, amitriptyline, quinolones) may decrease elimination. CYP1A2 inducers (eg, cigarette smoke, charcoal-broiled food, rifampicin, omeprazole) may increase elimination. Drugs metabolized by CYP1A2 (eg, theophylline, caffeine, tacrine) may interact with riluzole.

PREGNANCY: Category C, not for use in nursing.

MECHANISM OF ACTION: Not established; thought to inhibit the effect on glutamate release, inactivate voltage-dependent sodium channels, and interfere with intracellular events that follow transmitter binding at excitatory amino acid receptors.

PHARMACOKINETICS: Absorption: Well absorbed; absolute bioavailability (60%). **Distribution:** Plasma protein binding (96%). **Metabolism:** Liver via CYP450-dependent hydroxylation and glucuronidation. **Elimination:** $T_{1/2}$=12 hrs. Urine (85%) glucuronides, (2%, unchanged), feces (5%).

RISPERDAL

RX

risperidone (Janssen)

> Elderly patients with dementia-related psychosis treated with atypical antipsychotic drugs are at an increased risk of death; most appeared to be cardiovascular (eg, heart failure, sudden death) or infectious (eg, pneumonia) in nature. Risperidone is not approved for the treatment of patients with dementia-related psychosis.

OTHER BRAND NAMES: Risperdal M-Tab (Janssen)

THERAPEUTIC CLASS: Benzisoxazole derivative

INDICATIONS: Acute and maintenance treatment of schizophrenia in adults. Treatment of schizophrenia in adolescents 13-17 yrs. Short-term treatment of acute manic or mixed episodes associated with bipolar I disorder as monotherapy (adults and adolescents 10-17 yrs) or in combination with lithium or valproate (adults). Treatment of irritability associated with autistic disorder in children and adolescents 5-16 yrs, including symptoms of aggression towards others, deliberate self-injuriousness, temper tantrums, and quickly changing moods.

DOSAGE: *Adults:* Schizophrenia: Initial: 2mg/day given once or twice daily. Titrate: Adjust dose at intervals not <24 hrs, in increments of 1-2mg/day, as tolerated, to recommended dose of 4-8mg/day. Range: 4-16mg/day. Max: 16mg/day. Bipolar Disorder: Initial: 2-3mg qd. Titrate: Adjust dose at intervals not <24 hrs and in increments/decrements of 1mg/day. Range: 1-6mg/day. Max: 6mg/day. Elderly/Debilitated/Hypotension/Severe Renal or Hepatic Impairment: Initial: 0.5mg bid. Titrate: Adjust dose in increments not >0.5mg bid. Increases to doses >1.5mg bid should occur at intervals of ≥1 week. Periodically reassess to determine maintenance treatment.
Pediatrics: Schizophrenia: 13-17 yrs: Initial: 0.5mg qd in morning or evening. Titrate: Adjust dose, if needed, in increments of 0.5 or 1mg/day and at intervals not <24 hrs, as tolerated, to recommended dose of 3mg/day. Max: 6mg/day. Bipolar Disorder: 10-17 yrs: Initial: 0.5mg qd in morning or evening. Titrate: Adjust dose, if needed, in increments of 0.5 or 1mg/day and at intervals not <24 hrs, as tolerated, to recommended dose of 2.5mg/day. Max: 6mg/day. Irritability with Autistic Disorder: 5-16 yrs: Initial: <20kg: 0.25mg/day; ≥20kg: 0.5mg/day. Titrate: After at least 4 days, may increase dose by 0.5mg/day (<20kg) or 1mg/day (≥20kg). Maint: Minimum of 14 days. Inadequate Response: Increase at ≥2-wk intervals: <20kg: Increase by 0.25mg/day; ≥20kg: Increase by 0.5mg/day. Caution in patients <15kg. Max: <20kg: 1mg/day; ≥20kg: 2.5mg/day; >45kg: 3mg/day.

HOW SUPPLIED: Sol: 1mg/mL [30mL]; Tab: 0.25mg, 0.5mg, 1mg, 2mg, 3mg, 4mg; Tab, Disintegrating: (M-Tab) 0.5mg, 1mg, 2mg, 3mg, 4mg

CONTRAINDICATIONS: Anaphylactic reactions and angioedema.

WARNINGS/PRECAUTIONS: Neuroleptic malignant syndrome and/or tardive dyskinesia may occur. Monitor for hyperglycemia; perform fasting blood glucose testing if symptoms develop or with risk factors for DM. Cerebrovascular events (eg, stroke, TIA) reported in elderly with dementia-related psychosis. Not approved for the treatment of dementia-related psychosis. May induce orthostatic hypotension, elevate prolactin levels, have an antiemetic effect. Caution in elderly, renal/hepatic impairment, history of seizures, cardio- or cerebrovascular disease, suicidal tendencies, risk of aspiration pneumonia, conditions predisposing to hypotension (eg, hypovolemia, dehydration) or affecting metabolism or hemodynamic responses. May impair judgement, thinking, or motor skills; caution when operating hazardous machinery. May disrupt body temperature regulation; caution in patients exposed to temperature extremes. Re-evaluate periodically. Patients with Parkinson's disease or dementia with Lewy bodies who receive antipsychotics are reported to have an increased sensitivity to antipsychotic medications.

ADVERSE REACTIONS: Somnolence, increased appetite, fatigue, vomiting, coughing, urinary incontinence, constipation, fever, parkinsonism, abdominal pain, anxiety, nausea, dizziness, tremor, dyspepsia.

INTERACTIONS: Caution with other CNS drugs or alcohol. May potentiate antihypertensives, antagonize levodopa and dopamine agonists, or increase valproate levels. Cimetidine and ranitidine may increase bioavailability. CYP3A4 inducers (eg, carbamazepine, phenytoin, rifampin, phenobarbital) may decrease levels. Clozapine, fluoxetine, and paroxetine may increase levels. Increased mortality with furosemide in elderly patients.

PREGNANCY: Category C, not for use in nursing.

MECHANISM OF ACTION: Benzisoxazole derivatives; suspected to inhibit both dopamine Type 2(D_2) and serotonin Type 2 (5HT_2).

PHARMACOKINETICS: Absorption: Absolute bioavailability (70%). T_{max}=1 hr; (risperidone) T_{max}=3hrs; 9-hydroxyrisperidone (extensive metabolizers). **Distribution:** V_d=1-2L/kg; plasma protein binding (risperidone: 90%) (9-hydroxyrisperidone: 77%); found in breast milk. **Metabolism:** Liver (extensive). Hydroxylation, N-dealkylation; CYP 2D6: 9-hydroxyrisperidone (major metabolite). **Elimination:** Urine (70%), feces (14%); $T_{1/2}$=20 hrs.

RISPERDAL CONSTA   RX
risperidone (Janssen)

> Elderly patients with dementia-related psychosis treated with atypical antipsychotic drugs are at an increased risk of death; most appeared to be cardiovascular (eg, heart failure, sudden death) or infectious (eg, pneumonia) in nature. Risperidone is not approved for the treatment of patients with dementia-related psychosis.

THERAPEUTIC CLASS: Benzisoxazole derivative

INDICATIONS: Treatment of schizophrenia.

DOSAGE: *Adults:* 25mg IM every 2 weeks. Max: 50mg every 2 weeks. Give 1st injection with oral dosage form or other oral antipsychotic. Continue for 3 weeks, then d/c oral. Titrate: Increase at intervals of no more than every 4 weeks. Hepatic or Renal Impairment/Certain Drug Interactions/Poor Tolerability to Psychotropic Meds: Initial: 12.5mg.

HOW SUPPLIED: Inj: 12.5mg, 25mg, 37.5mg, 50mg

WARNINGS/PRECAUTIONS: Neuroleptic malignant syndrome and/or tardive dyskinesia may occur. Monitor for hyperglycemia; perform fasting blood glucose testing if symptoms develop or with risk factors for DM. Cerebrovascular events (eg, stroke, TIA) reported in elderly with dementia-related psychosis. Not approved for the treatment of dementia-related psychosis. May induce orthostatic hypotension, elevate prolactin levels, have an antiemetic effect. Caution in elderly, renal/hepatic impairment, history of seizures, cardio- or cerebrovascular disease, suicidal tendencies, risk of aspiration pneumonia, conditions predisposing to hypotension (eg, hypovolemia, dehydration) or affecting metabolism or hemodynamic responses. May impair judgement, thinking, or motor skills; caution when operating hazardous machinery. May disrupt body temperature regulation; caution in patients exposed to temperature extremes. Re-evaluate periodically. Patients who receive antipsychotics are reported to have an increased sensitivity to antipsychotic medications. Must inject into the gluteal muscle; avoid injection into blood vessel.

ADVERSE REACTIONS: Insomnia, somnolence, headache, dizziness, constipation, dyspepsia, rhinitis, diarrhea, akathisia, parkinsonism, hallucinations, somnolence, weight increase, dry mouth, fatigue.

INTERACTIONS: Caution with other CNS drugs or alcohol. May potentiate antihypertensives, antagonize levodopa and dopamine agonists, or increase valproate levels. Cimetidine and ranitidine may increase bioavailability. CYP3A4 inducers (eg, carbamazepine, phenytoin, rifampin, phenobarbital) may decrease levels. Clozapine, fluoxetine, and paroxetine may increase levels. Increased mortality with furosemide in elderly patients.

PREGNANCY: Category C, not for use in nursing.

R

MECHANISM OF ACTION: Benzisoxazole derivative; suspected to inhibit both dopamine type 2(D_2) and serotonin type 2 ($5HT_2$).

PHARMACOKINETICS: Distribution: Human breast milk, V_d=1-2L/kg. Plasma protein binding: Risperidone (approximately 90%), 9-hydroxyrisperidone (77%). **Metabolism**: Liver (extensive). Hydroxylation, N-dealkylation; CYP 2D6: 9-hydroxyrisperidone (major metabolite). **Elimination**: Urine (70%), feces (14%). $T_{1/2}$=3-6 days.

RITALIN `CII`
methylphenidate HCL (Novartis)

OTHER BRAND NAMES: Ritalin LA (Novartis) - Ritalin SR (Novartis)

THERAPEUTIC CLASS: Sympathomimetic amine

INDICATIONS: (Cap; Extended-Release, Tab; Tab, Extended-Release) Treatment of attention deficit disorders. (Tab; Tab, Extended-Release) Treatment of narcolepsy.

DOSAGE: *Adults:* (Tab) 10-60mg/day given bid-tid 30-45 min ac. Take last dose before 6 pm if insomnia occurs. (Tab, ER) May use in place of immediate release (IR) when the 8 hr dose corresponds to the titrated 8 hr IR dose. Swallow whole; do not chew or crush. (Cap, ER) Initial: 20mg qam. Titrate: Adjust weekly by 10mg. Max: 60mg qam.
Pediatrics: ≥6 yrs: (Tab) Initial: 5mg bid before breakfast and lunch. Titrate: Increase gradually by 5-10mg weekly. Max: 60mg/day. (Tab, ER) May use in place of immediate release (IR) when the 8 hr dose corresponds to the titrated 8 hr IR dose. Swallow whole; do not chew or crush. (Cap, ER) Initial: 20mg qam. Titrate: Adjust weekly by 10mg. Max: 60mg qam. Previous Methylphenidate Use: May use as qd in place of IR dosed bid or daily dose of methylphenidate-SR. Swallow whole or sprinkle over spoonful of applesauce. Do not crush, chew, or divide. Reduce dose or d/c if paradoxical aggravation of symptoms occurs. D/C if no improvement after appropriate dose adjustment over 1 month.

HOW SUPPLIED: Cap, Extended-Release (Ritalin LA): 10mg, 20mg, 30mg, 40mg; Tab (Ritalin): 5mg, 10mg*, 20mg*; Tab, Extended-Release (Ritalin SR): 20mg *scored

CONTRAINDICATIONS: Marked anxiety, tension, and agitation; glaucoma; motor tics or family history or diagnosis of Tourette's syndrome; during or within 14 days of MAOI use.

WARNINGS/PRECAUTIONS: Monitor growth in children. Not for depression or fatigue. May exacerbate symptoms of behavior disturbance and thought disorder in psychotic children. Care should be taken in using stimulants to treat patients with comorbid bipolar disorder because of concern for possible induction of mixed/manic episode in such patients. Stimulants at usual doses can cause treatment emergent psychotic or manic symptoms (hallucinations, delusional thinking, mania) in children and adolescents without prior history of psychotic illness. Aggressive behavior or hostility reported in clinical trials and the postmarketing experience of some medications indicated for the treatment of ADHD. May lower seizure threshold, especially with prior history of seizures or with prior EEG abnormalities; d/c if seizures occur. Caution with HTN and other underlying conditions that may be compromised such as heart failure, recent MI, or hyperthyroidism. Visual disturbances may occur (rare). Monitor CBC, differential, and platelets with prolonged use. Caution with emotionally-unstable patients or prior history of drug dependence or alcoholism; chronic use may lead to tolerance and psychological dependence. Monitor during withdrawal. Periodically d/c to assess condition. Avoid with known structural cardiac abnormalities or other serious cardiac problems.

ADVERSE REACTIONS: Nervousness, insomnia, hypersensitivity reactions, anorexia, nausea, dizziness, palpitations, headache, dyskinesia, drowsiness, BP and pulse changes, tachycardia, angina, arrhythmia, abdominal pain.

INTERACTIONS: See Contraindications. May decrease hypotensive effect of guanethidine. Caution with β_2-agonist (eg, clonidine) and pressor agents.

Potentiates anticoagulants, anticonvulsants (eg, phenobarbital, diphenylhydantoin, primidone), phenylbutazone, TCAs (eg, imipramine, clomipramine, desipramine); monitor plasma drug levels or PT/INR. (Cap, Extended-Release) Antacids or acid suppressants may alter release characteristics of cap.

PREGNANCY: Category C, caution in nursing.

MECHANISM OF ACTION: Sympathomimetic amine; CNS stimulant, blocks reuptake of norepinephrine and dopamine into presynaptic neuron and increases release of monoamines into extraneuronal space.

PHARMACOKINETICS: Absorption: Children: (Tab, ER) T_{max}=4.7 hrs; (Tab) 1.9 hrs. **Metabolism:** α-phenyl-2-piperidine acetic acid (major metabolite). **Elimination:** Urine (78-97%), feces (1-3%); $T_{1/2}$=3.5 hrs (adults), 2.5 hrs (children).

RITUXAN   RX
rituximab (Genentech/Biogen Idec)

Serious, sometimes fatal, infusion reactions reported. Acute renal failure reported in the setting of tumor lysis syndrome (TLS) following treatment of non-Hodgkin's lymphoma. Severe mucocutaneous reactions reported. JC virus infection resulting in progressive multifocal leukoencephalopathy (PML) reported.

THERAPEUTIC CLASS: Monoclonal antibody/CD20-blocker

INDICATIONS: Treatment of non-Hodgkin's lymphoma (NHL) in patients with: 1) relapsed or refractory, low-grade or follicular, CD20-positive, B-cell NHL as a single agent; 2) previously untreated follicular, CD20-positive, B-cell NHL in combination with CVP chemotherapy; 3) nonprogressing (including stable disease), low-grade, CD20-positive, B-cell NHL, as a single agent, after 1st-line CVP chemotherapy; 4) previously untreated diffuse large B-cell, CD20-positive NHL in combination with CHOP or other anthracycline-based chemotherapy regimens. In combination with methotrexate to reduce signs and symptoms and to slow the progression of structural damage in adult patients with moderately to severely active rheumatoid arthritis (RA) who have had inadequate response to one or more TNF-antagonist therapies.

DOSAGE: *Adults:* Administer only as IV infusion. Relapsed or Refractory, Low-Grade or Follicular, CD20-Positive, B-cell NHL: 375mg/m² IV once weekly for 4 or 8 doses. Retreatment for Relapsed or Refractory, Low-Grade or Follicular, CD20-Positive, B-cell NHL: 375mg/m² IV once weekly for 4 doses. Previously Untreated, Follicular, CD20-Positive, B-cell NHL: 375mg/m² IV on Day 1 of each CVP chemotherapy cycle for up to 8 doses. Nonprogressing, Low-Grade, CD20-Positive, B-cell NHL: Following completion of 6-8 cycles of CVP chemotherapy, 375mg/m² IV once weekly for 4 doses at 6 months intervals to maximum 16 doses. Diffuse Large B-cell NHL: 375mg/m² IV given on Day 1 of each chemotherapy cycle for up to 8 infusions. RA: Give with methotrexate. Administer two-1000mg IV infusions separated by 2 weeks. Give methylprednisolone 100mg IV (or equivalent) 30 min prior to each infusion to reduce incidence and severity of infusion reactions. Do not administer as IV push or bolus.

HOW SUPPLIED: Inj: 10mg/mL

WARNINGS/PRECAUTIONS: Interrupt if severe reaction develops; may resume at a 50% rate reduction when symptoms subside. HBV reactivation with fulminant hepatitis, hepatic failure, and death reported; d/c if viral hepatitis develops. Additional serious viral infections, either new, reactivated, or exacerbated, reported. Hypersensitivity reactions may respond to infusion rate adjustment and medical management. D/C if serious arrhythmias occur. Caution with pre-existing cardiac conditions. Use with extreme caution in combination with cisplatin; renal failure may occur. Severe renal toxicity reported; d/c if serum creatinine rises or oliguria occurs. Monitor CBC and platelets regularly; more frequently with cytopenias. Abdominal pain, bowel obstruction, and perforation reported.

ADVERSE REACTIONS: Fever, chills, infection, asthenia, nausea, lymphopenia, leukopenia, neutropenia, headache, abdominal pain, night sweats, rash, pruritus, pain.

INTERACTIONS: Renal toxicity reported with cisplatin. Vaccination with live virus vaccines not recommended. Observe closely for signs of infection if biologic agents and/or DMARDs are used concomitantly.

PREGNANCY: Category C, not for use in nursing.

MECHANISM OF ACTION: Human monoclonal IgG$_1$ kappa antibody/CD20 antigen blocker; binds to CD20 antigen on B lymphocytes and recruits immune effector functions to mediate B-cell lysis, possibly by complement-dependent cytotoxicity and antibody-dependent, cell-mediated cytotoxicity.

PHARMACOKINETICS: Absorption: NHL: C_{max}=486mcg/mL. RA: C_{max}=183mcg/mL (2x500mg), 370mcg/mL (2x1000mg). **Distribution:** RA: V_d=4.3L. **Elimination:** NHL: $T_{1/2}$=22 days. RA: $T_{1/2}$=19 days.

Robaxin RX
methocarbamol (Schwarz)

OTHER BRAND NAMES: Robaxin-750 (Schwarz) - Robaxin Injection (Baxter)

THERAPEUTIC CLASS: Muscular analgesic (central-acting)

INDICATIONS: Adjunct for relief of acute, painful musculoskeletal conditions.

DOSAGE: *Adults:* (PO) Initial: (500mg tab) 1500mg qid for 2-3 days. Maint: 1000mg qid. Initial: (750mg tab) 1500mg qid for 2-3 days. Maint: 750mg q4h or 1500mg tid. Max: 6g/d for 2-3 days; 8g/d if severe. (Inj) Moderate Symptoms: 10mL IV/IM. IV Max Rate: 3mL undiluted drug/min. IM Max: 5mL into each gluteal region. Severe/Post-Op Condition: Max: 20-30mL/day up to 3 consecutive days. If feasible, continue with PO. Tetanus: 10-20mL up to 30mL. May repeat q6h until NG tube can be inserted. Continue with crushed tabs. Max: 24g/day PO.
Pediatrics: Tetanus: Initial: 15mg/kg or 500mg/m². Repeat q6h prn. Max: 1.8g/m² for 3 consecutive days. Administer by injection into tubing or IV infusion.

HOW SUPPLIED: Inj: 100mg/mL [10mL]; Tab: 500mg, 750mg

CONTRAINDICATIONS: (Inj) Renal pathology with injection due to propylene glycol content.

WARNINGS/PRECAUTIONS: May impair mental/physical abilities required for operating machinery or driving a motor vehicle. May cause color interference in certain screening tests for 5-hydroxy-indoleacetic acid (5-HIAA) and vanillylmandelic acid (VMA). Caution in epilepsy with the injection. Injection rate should not exceed 3mL/min. Avoid extravasation with injection. Avoid use of injection particularly during early pregnancy.

ADVERSE REACTIONS: Lightheadedness, dizziness, drowsiness, nausea, urticaria, pruritus, rash, conjunctivitis, nasal congestion, blurred vision, headache, fever, seizures, syncope, flushing.

INTERACTIONS: Additive adverse effects with alcohol and other CNS depressants. May inhibit effect of pyridostigmine; caution in patients with myasthemia gravis receiving anticholinergics.

PREGNANCY: Category C, caution in nursing.

MECHANISM OF ACTION: Carbamate derivative of guaifenesin; not established, suspected to have CNS depressant with sedative and musculoskeletal relaxant properties.

PHARMACOKINETICS: Distribution: Plasma protein binding (46-50%). **Distribution:** Found in breast milk. **Metabolism:** Via dealkylation, hydroxylation, and conjugation pathways. **Elimination:** Urine; $T_{1/2}$=1-2 hrs.

ROBINUL   RX
glycopyrrolate (Sciele)

OTHER BRAND NAMES: Robinul Forte (Sciele)

THERAPEUTIC CLASS: Anticholinergic

INDICATIONS: Adjunct treatment of peptic ulcer.

DOSAGE: *Adults:* Usual: (Tab) 1mg tid (am, pm and hs); may increase to 2mg qhs if needed. Maint: 1mg bid. (Forte) 2mg bid-tid. Max: 8mg/day.
Pediatrics: ≥12 yrs: Usual: (Tab) 1mg tid (am, pm & hs); may increase to 2mg qhs if needed. Maint: 1mg bid. (Forte) 2mg bid-tid. Max: 8mg/day.

HOW SUPPLIED: Tab: 1mg*, (Forte) 2mg* *scored

CONTRAINDICATIONS: Glaucoma, obstructive uropathy, GI tract obstruction, paralytic ileus, intestinal atony of elderly or debilitated, unstable cardiovascular status in acute hemorrhage, severe ulcerative colitis, toxic megacolon complicating ulcerative colitis, myasthenia gravis.

WARNINGS/PRECAUTIONS: May produce drowsiness and blurred vision; avoid operating machinery. Risk of heat prostration with high environmental temperature. Diarrhea may be early symptom of incomplete intestinal obstruction especially with ileostomy or colostomy. Caution in elderly, autonomic neuropathy, hepatic/renal disease, ulcerative colitis, hyperthyroidism, coronary heart disease, CHF, tachyarrhythmias, tachycardia, HTN, prostatic hypertrophy, hiatal hernia associated with reflux esophagitis.

ADVERSE REACTIONS: Blurred vision, dry mouth, urinary retention and hesitancy, increased ocular tension, tachycardia, decreased sweating, xerostomia, loss of taste, headache.

PREGNANCY: Safety in pregnancy is not known; not for use in nursing.

MECHANISM OF ACTION: Anticholinergic; inhibits action of acetylcholine on structures innervated by postganglionic cholinergic nerves and smooth muscles that respond to acetylcholine but lack cholinergic innervation. Diminishes volume and free acidity of gastric secretions and controls excessive pharyngeal, tracheal, and bronchial secretion.

ROBINUL INJECTION   RX
glycopyrrolate (Baxter)

THERAPEUTIC CLASS: Anticholinergic

INDICATIONS: Preoperative antimuscarinic to reduce salivary tracheobronchial, and pharyngeal secretions; decrease gastric sections; and block cardiac vagal inhibitory reflexes during anesthesia induction and intubation. Intra-operatively to counteract drug-induced or vagal traction reflexes associated with arrhythmias. To protect against peripheral muscarinic effects of cholinergic agents. Adjunct therapy for treatment of peptic ulcer when rapid anticholinergic effect is desired or when oral medication is not tolerated.

DOSAGE: *Adults:* Preanesthesia: 0.002mg/lb IM 30-60 min before anesthesia induction or at time of preanesthetic narcotic/sedative. Intraoperatively: 0.1mg IV, repeat prn every 2-3 min. Reverse Neuromuscular Blockade: 0.2mg IV for each 1mg neostigmine or 5mg pyridostigmine. Peptic Ulcer: 0.1mg IV/IM q4h, tid-qid. May use 0.2mg if needed.
Pediatrics: Preanesthesia: 1 month-12 yrs: 0.002mg/lb IM 30-60 min before anesthesia induction or at time of preanesthetic narcotic/sedative. 1 month-2 yrs: May require up to 0.004mg/lb. Intraoperatively: 0.002mg/lb IV. Max: 0.1mg single dose. May repeat prn every 2-3 min. Reverse Neuromuscular Blockade: 0.2mg IV for each 1mg neostigmine or 5mg pyridostigmine. Peptic Ulcer: ≥12 yrs: 0.1mg IV/IM q4h, tid-qid. May use 0.2mg if needed.

HOW SUPPLIED: Inj: 0.2mg/mL

CONTRAINDICATIONS: Newborns (<1 month) due to benzyl alcohol content. For long treatment duration: Glaucoma, obstructive uropathy, obstructive disease of GI tract, paralytic ileus, intestinal atony of elderly or debilitated,

R

unstable cardiovascular status in acute hemorrhage, severe ulcerative colitis, toxic megacolon complicating ulcerative colitis, myasthenia gravis.

WARNINGS/PRECAUTIONS: Caution with CAD, CHF, arrhythmias, HTN, hyperthyroidism, elderly, autonomic neuropathy, hepatic or renal disease, ulcerative colitis, or hiatal hernia. May produce drowsiness and blurred vision; caution when operating machinery. Risk of fever and heat stroke due to decreased sweating in high environmental temperature. Diarrhea may be early symptom of incomplete intestinal obstruction.

ADVERSE REACTIONS: Drowsiness, blurred vision, dry mouth, urinary retention and hesitancy, increased ocular tension, tachycardia, palpation, decreased sweating, loss of taste.

INTERACTIONS: Increased anticholinergic side effects with other anticholinergics, phenothiazines, antiparkinson drugs, TCAs. Increased severity of GI lesions with potassium chloride in a wax matrix.

PREGNANCY: Category B, caution in nursing.

MECHANISM OF ACTION: Anticholinergic; inhibits action of acethylcholine on structures innervated by postganglionic cholinergic nerves and on smooth muscles that respond to acethycholine but lack cholinergic innervation. Diminishes volume and free acidity of gastric secretions and controls excessive pharyngeal, tracheal, and bronchial secretions.

PHARMACOKINETICS: Absorption: (6mcg/kg, IV) AUC=8.64mcg/L•hr; (8mcg/kg, IM) C_{max}=3.47mcg/L, T_{max}=27.48 min, AUC=6.64mcg/L•hr. **Distribution:** V_d=0.42L/kg. **Elimination:** (IV) Urine (85%), bile; $T_{1/2}$=0.83 hrs. (IM) Urine, bile; $T_{1/2}$=0.55-1.25 hrs.

ROCALTROL   RX
calcitriol (Roche Labs)

THERAPEUTIC CLASS: Vitamin D analog

INDICATIONS: Predialysis: Management of secondary hyperparathyroidism and resultant metabolic bone disease with moderate to severe chronic renal failure (CrCl 15-55mL/min). Dialysis: Management of hypocalcemia and resultant metabolic bone disease. Hypoparathyroidism: Management of hypocalcemia and manifestations of postsurgical hypoparathyroidism, idiopathic hypoparathyroidism, and pseudohypoparathyroidism.

DOSAGE: *Adults:* Predialysis: Initial: 0.25mcg/day. Max: 0.5mcg/day. Hypoparathyroidism: Initial: 0.25mcg/day every am. Titrate: May increase at 2-4 week intervals to 0.5-2mcg/day. Elderly: Start at low end of dosing range. Dialysis: Initial: 0.25mcg/day. Titrate: May increase by 0.25mcg/day every 4-8 weeks to 0.5-1mcg/day. Monitor serum calcium levels twice weekly during titration. Normal to slightly reduced serum calcium, give 0.25mcg every other day. Discontinue with hypercalcemia; when calcium levels return to normal continue therapy and decrease dose by 0.25 mcg.
Pediatrics: Predialysis: ≥3 yrs: Initial: 0.25mcg/day. Max: 0.5mcg/day. <3yrs: Initial: 10-15ng/kg/day. Hypoparathyroidism: ≥6 yrs: Initial: 0.25mcg/day every am. Titrate: May increase at 2-4 week intervals to 0.5-2mcg/day. 1-5yrs: Initial: 0.25mcg/day every am. Titrate: May increase at 2-4 week intervals up to 0.75mcg/day. Monitor serum calcium levels twice weekly during titration. Discontinue with hypercalcemia; when calcium levels return to normal continue therapy and decrease dose by 0.25 mcg.

HOW SUPPLIED: Cap: 0.25mcg, 0.5mcg; Sol: 1mcg/mL [15mL]

CONTRAINDICATIONS: Hypercalcemia or vitamin D toxicity.

WARNINGS/PRECAUTIONS: Use non-aluminum phosphate binders and low phosphate diet to control serum phosphate. Chronic hypercalcemia can cause calcification of soft tissues. Monitor calcium levels twice a week initially. Avoid dehydration. Monitor serum creatinine. Maintain adequate calcium intake of at least 600mg/day. Caution in elderly. If treatment switched from ergocalciferol, may take several months for ergocalciferol level to decrease to baseline. May increase inorganic phosphate levels; ectopic calcification reported with renal failure. Monitor phosphorus, magnesium, alkaline phosphatase, and 24-hour urine periodically.

ADVERSE REACTIONS: Weakness, nausea, vomiting, dry mouth, constipation, muscle and bone pain, metallic taste, polyuria, polydipsia, weight loss, pancreatitis, photophobia, pruritus, decreased libido.

INTERACTIONS: Avoid vitamin D products and derivatives during therapy. Hypermagnesemia may occur with magnesium-containing antacids, especially in chronic renal dialysis. Caution with digoxin; hypercalcemia may precipitate arrhythmias. Reduced intestinal absorption with cholestyramine. May need to increase dose if given with phenytoin or phenobarbital. Caution with thiazides; risk of hypercalcemia. Ketoconazole may effect metabolism. Corticosteroids antagonize activity. Changes in diet or uncontrolled intake of calcium preparations can cause hypercalcemia. Adjust dose phosphate-binding agents.

PREGNANCY: Category C, not for use in nursing.

MECHANISM OF ACTION: Synthetic vitamin D analog. Regulates absorption of calcium from the GI tract and its utilization in the body.

PHARMACOKINETICS: Absorption: Rapidly absorbed (intestine). $C_{max}=131\pm17pg/mL$; $T_{max}=3-6$ hrs. **Distribution:** Plasma protein binding (99.9%); crosses placenta; found in breast milk. **Metabolism:** Liver via hydroxylation. 1,25R(OH)$_2$-26, 23S-lactone D_3 lactone (major metabolite). **Elimination:** Urine (16%), feces (49%); $T_{1/2}=5-8$ hrs. Refer to prescribing guidelines for pediatric parameters.

Rocephin   RX
ceftriaxone sodium (Roche Labs)

THERAPEUTIC CLASS: Cephalosporin (3rd generation)

INDICATIONS: Treatment of lower respiratory tract, skin and skin structure, bone and joint, intra-abdominal and urinary tract infections, acute otitis media, uncomplicated gonorrhea, pelvic inflammatory disease, bacterial septicemia, and meningitis caused by susceptible strains of microorganisms. Surgical prophylaxis during surgical procedures classified as contaminated or potentially contaminated.

DOSAGE: *Adults:* Usual: 1-2g/day IV/IM given qd-bid. Max: 4g/day. Gonorrhea: 250mg IM single dose. Surgical Prophylaxis: 1g IV 1/2-2 hrs before surgery. Avoid diluents containing calcium.
Pediatrics: Skin Infections: 50-75mg/kg/day IV/IM given qd-bid. Max: 2g/day. Otitis Media: 50mg/kg (up to 1g) IM single dose. Serious Infections: 50-75mg/kg/day IM/IV given q12h. Max: 2g/day. Meningitis: Initial: 100mg/kg (up to 4g), then 100mg/kg/day given qd-bid for 7-14 days. Max: 4g/day. Avoid diluents containing calcium.

HOW SUPPLIED: Inj: 250mg, 500mg, 1g, 2g, 10g

CONTRAINDICATIONS: Avoid use in hyperbilirubinemic neonates esp. prematures. Avoid concurrent use with calcium-containing solutions/products in newborns.

WARNINGS/PRECAUTIONS: Cross-sensitivity to PCNs and other cephalosporins may occur. *Clostridium difficile*-associated diarrhea reported. May result in overgrowth of nonsusceptible organisms. Altered PT, transient BUN, and serum creatinine elevations may occur. Do not exceed 2g/day and monitor blood levels with both hepatic dysfunction and significant renal disease. Caution with history of GI disease. D/C if gallbladder disease develops. May alter PT; monitor with impaired vitamin K synthesis or low vitamin K stores.

ADVERSE REACTIONS: Injection site reactions, eosinophilia, thrombocytosis, diarrhea, SGOT and SGPT elevations.

INTERACTIONS: See Contraindications. Do not administer calcium containing products within 48 hrs of last administration of drug.

PREGNANCY: Category B, caution in nursing.

MECHANISM OF ACTION: Broad-spectrum cephalosporin; bactericidal activity results from inhibition of cell wall synthesis.

PHARMACOKINETICS: Absorption: (Adults) Complete; T_{max}=2-3 hrs. (Pediatrics) Bacterial meningitis: C_{max}=216mcg/mL (50mg/kg), 275mcg/mL (75mg/mL). Middle ear fluid: C_{max}=35mcg/mL; T_{max}=24 hrs. **Distribution:** (Adults) V_d=5.78-13.5L. (Pediatrics) Bacterial meningitis: V_d=338mL/kg (50mg/kg), 373mL/kg (75mg/kg). **Elimination:** Urine (33-67%), feces. (Adults) $T_{1/2}$=5.8-8.7 hrs. (Pediatrics) Bacterial meningitis: $T_{1/2}$=4.6 hrs (50mg/kg), 4.3 hrs (75mg/kg); Middle ear fluid: $T_{1/2}$=25 hrs.

ROMAZICON   RX

flumazenil (Roche Labs)

THERAPEUTIC CLASS: Benzodiazepine antagonist

INDICATIONS: Complete or partial reversal of sedative effects of benzodiazepines (BZDs) given with general anesthesia, or diagnostic and therapeutic procedures, and for the management of BZD overdose in adults. For reversal of BZD-induced conscious sedation in pediatrics (1-17 yrs old).

DOSAGE: *Adults:* Reversal of Conscious Sedation/General Anesthesia: Give IV over 15 seconds. Initial: 0.2mg. May repeat dose after 45 seconds and again at 60 second intervals up to a max of 4 additional times until reach desired level of consciousness. Max Total Dose: 1mg. In event of resedation, repeated doses may be given at 20-min intervals. Max: 1mg/dose (0.2mg/min) and 3mg/hr. BZD Overdose: Give IV over 30 seconds. Initial: 0.2mg. May repeat with 0.3mg after 30 seconds and then 0.5mg at 1-min intervals until reach desired level of consciousness. Max Total Dose: 3mg. In event of resedation, repeated doses may be given at 20-min intervals. Max: 1mg/dose (0.5mg/min); 3mg/hr. *Pediatrics:* >1yr: Give IV over 15 seconds. Initial: 0.01mg/kg (up to 0.2mg). May repeat dose after 45 seconds and again at 60-second intervals up to a max of 4 additional times until reach desired level of consciousness. Max Total Dose: 0.05mg/kg or 1mg, whichever is lower.

HOW SUPPLIED: Inj: 0.1mg/mL

CONTRAINDICATIONS: Patients given BZDs for life-threatening conditions (eg, control of ICP or status epilepticus), signs of serious cyclic antidepressant overdose.

WARNINGS/PRECAUTIONS: Caution in overdoses involving multiple drug combinations. Risk of seizures, especially with long-term BZD-induced sedation, cyclic antidepressant overdose, concurrent major sedative-hypnotic drug withdrawal, recent therapy with repeated doses of parenteral BZDs, myoclonic jerking or seizure prior to flumazenil administration. Monitor for resedation, respiratory depression, or other residual BZD effects (up to 2 hrs). Avoid use in the ICU; increased risk of unrecognized BZD dependence. Caution with head injury, alcoholism, and other drug dependencies. Does not reverse respiratory depression/hypoventilation or cardiac depression. May provoke panic attacks with history of panic disorder. Adjust subsequent doses in hepatic dysfunction. Not for use as treatment for BZD dependence or for management of protracted abstinence syndromes. May trigger dose-dependent withdrawal syndromes. Extravasation may occur; administer IV into a large vein.

ADVERSE REACTIONS: Nausea, vomiting, dizziness, injection site pain, increased sweating, headache, abnormal or blurred vision, agitation.

INTERACTIONS: Avoid use until neuromuscular blockade effects are reversed. Toxic effects (eg, convulsions, cardiac dysrhythmias) may occur with mixed drug overdose (eg, cyclic antidepressants).

PREGNANCY: Category C, caution in nursing.

MECHANISM OF ACTION: Benzodiazepine receptor antagonist; inhibits activity at the benzodiazepine recognition site on the GABA/benzodiazepine receptor complex.

PHARMACOKINETICS: Absorption: C_{max}=24ng/mL; AUC=15ng•hr/mL. **Distribution:** V_d=1L/kg (steady state); plasma protein binding (50%). **Metabolism:** Complete (99%). **Elimination**: Urine (90-95%), feces (5-10%); $T_{1/2}$=54 min.

RONDEC   RX
pseudoephedrine HCL - carbinoxamine maleate (Biovail)

OTHER BRAND NAMES: Rondec Oral Drops (Biovail) - Rondec-TR (Biovail)

THERAPEUTIC CLASS: Antihistamine/decongestant

INDICATIONS: (Drops) Seasonal/perennial allergic and vasomotor rhinitis. (Tab, Tab, Extended-Release) Relief of upper respiratory symptoms associated with allergic rhinitis and the common cold.

DOSAGE: *Adults:* (Tab) 1 tab qid; (Tab, Extended-Release) 1 tab bid. *Pediatrics:* (Sol) Give qid. 12-24 months: 1mL. 6-12 months: 3/4mL. 3-6 months: 1/2mL. 1-3 months: 1/4mL. (Tab) ≥6 yrs:1 tab qid. (Tab, Extended-Release) ≥12 yrs: 1 tab bid.

HOW SUPPLIED: (Carbinoxamine-Pseudoephedrine) Sol: 1mg-15mg/mL [30mL]; Tab: 4mg-60mg; Tab, Extended-Release: (Rondec TR) 8mg-120mg

CONTRAINDICATIONS: Severe HTN or CAD, MAOIs, narrow-angle glaucoma, urinary retention, peptic ulcer, during asthma attack.

WARNINGS/PRECAUTIONS: Caution in asthma, DM, HTN, heart disease, hyperthyroidism, increased IOP, prostatic hypertrophy, elderly. May cause excitability, especially in children.

ADVERSE REACTIONS: Sedation, dizziness, diplopia, vomiting, diarrhea, dry mouth, headache, nervousness, nausea, convulsions, CNS stimulation, cardiac arrhythmias, respiratory difficulty, increased HR or BP.

INTERACTIONS: May enhance effects of TCAs, benzodiazepines, barbiturates, alcohol, other CNS depressants. Increased sympathomimetic effects with MAOIs, β-blockers. May reduce antihypertensive effects of reserpine, veratrum alkaloids, methyldopa, mecamylamine.

PREGNANCY: Category C, safety in nursing not known.

MECHANISM OF ACTION: Carbinoxamine: H₁ antihistaminic activity with mild anticholinergic and sedative effects. Pseudoephedrine: Sympathomimetic; acts as decongestant to respiratory tract mucous membranes.

PHARMACOKINETICS: Elimination: Carbinoxamine: Urine; $T_{1/2}$=10-20 hrs. Pseudoephedrine: Urine; $T_{1/2}$=6-8 hrs.

RONDEC SYRUP   RX
pseudoephedrine HCL - brompheniramine maleate (Biovail)

THERAPEUTIC CLASS: Antihistamine/decongestant

INDICATIONS: Symptomatic relief of seasonal and perennial allergic rhinitis and vasomotor rhinitis.

DOSAGE: *Adults:* 5mL qid.
Pediatrics: ≥6 yrs: 5mL qid. 2-6 yrs: 2.5mL qid.

HOW SUPPLIED: (Brompheniramine-Pseudoephedrine) Syrup: 4mg-45mg/5mL

CONTRAINDICATIONS: Severe HTN or CAD, MAOIs, narrow-angle glaucoma, urinary retention, peptic ulcer, during asthma attack.

WARNINGS/PRECAUTIONS: Caution in asthma, DM, HTN, heart disease, hyperthyroidism, increased IOP, prostatic hypertrophy, elderly. May cause excitability, especially in children.

ADVERSE REACTIONS: Sedation, dizziness, diplopia, vomiting, diarrhea, dry mouth, headache, nervousness, nausea, convulsions, CNS stimulation, cardiac arrhythmias, respiratory difficulty, increased HR or BP.

INTERACTIONS: May enhance effects of TCAs, benzodiazepines, barbiturates, alcohol, other CNS depressants. Increased sympathomimetic effects with MAOIs, β-blockers. May reduce antihypertensive effects of reserpine, veratrum alkaloids, methyldopa, mecamylamine.

PREGNANCY: Category C, safety in nursing not known.

R

MECHANISM OF ACTION: Brompheniramine: H_1 antihistaminic activity and mild anticholinergic and sedative effects. Pseudoephedrine: Sympathomimetic; acts as decongestant to respiratory tract mucous membranes.

PHARMACOKINETICS: Absorption: Brompheniramine: T_{max}=5 hrs. **Metabolism:** Brompheniramine: Liver. **Elimination:** Brompheniramine: Urine. Pseudoephedrine: Urine; $T_{1/2}$=6-8 hrs.

RONDEC-DM DROPS   RX
dextromethorphan hbr - pseudoephedrine HCL - carbinoxamine maleate
(Biovail)

THERAPEUTIC CLASS: Antihistamine/decongestant/antitussive

INDICATIONS: Relief of coughs and upper respiratory symptoms associated with allergy or the common cold.

DOSAGE: *Pediatrics:* Give qid. 12-24 months: 1mL. 6-12 months: 3/4mL. 3-6 months: 1/2mL. 1-3 months: 1/4mL.

HOW SUPPLIED: (Carbinoxamine-Dextromethorphan-Pseudoephedrine) Sol: 1mg-4mg-15mg/mL [30mL]

CONTRAINDICATIONS: Severe HTN or CAD, during or within 2 weeks of MAOIs, narrow-angle glaucoma, urinary retention, peptic ulcer, during asthma attack.

WARNINGS/PRECAUTIONS: Caution with HTN, DM, heart disease, asthma, hyperthyroidism, increased IOP, prostatic hypertrophy and in atopic children, elderly, sedated, debilitated, or confined to supine positions. May cause excitability especially in children.

ADVERSE REACTIONS: Sedation, drowsiness, dizziness, diplopia, nausea, vomiting, diarrhea, dry mouth, headache, nervousness, convulsions, CNS stimulation, arrhythmias, increased HR or BP, tremors.

INTERACTIONS: Avoid during or within 2 weeks of MAOIs. May enhance effects of TCAs, barbiturates, alcohol, other CNS depressants. May reduce antihypertensive effects of reserpine, veratrum alkaloids, methyldopa, mecamylamine. Increased sympathomimetic effect with MAOIs, β-blockers. Additive cough-suppressant effect with narcotic antitussives.

PREGNANCY: Category C, safety in nursing not known.

MECHANISM OF ACTION: Carbinoxamine: H_1 antihistamine activity with mild anticholinergic and sedative effects. Pseudoephedrine: Sympathomimetic amine; acts as decongestant to repiratory tract mucous membranes. Dextromethorphan: Nonnarcotic/antitussive; acts in the medulla oblongata to elevate the cough threshold.

PHARMACOKINETICS: Elimination: Carbinoxamine: Urine; $T_{1/2}$=10-20 hrs. Pseudoephedrine: Urine; $T_{1/2}$=6-8 hrs. Dextromethophran: Urine (conjugated metabolites).

RONDEC-DM SYRUP   RX
dextromethorphan hbr - pseudoephedrine HCL - brompheniramine
maleate (Biovail)

OTHER BRAND NAMES: Cardec DM (Alpharma) - Carbofed DM (Hi-Tech)

THERAPEUTIC CLASS: Antihistamine/decongestant/antitussive

INDICATIONS: Relief of coughs and upper respiratory symptoms, including nasal congestion, associated with allergy or the common cold.

DOSAGE: *Adults:* 5mL qid.
Pediatrics: >6 yrs: 5mL qid. 2-6 yrs: 2.5mL qid.

HOW SUPPLIED: Syrup: (Brompheniramine-Dextromethorphan-Pseudoephedrine) 4mg-15mg-45mg/5mL [120mL, 480mL]

CONTRAINDICATIONS: Severe HTN or CAD, narrow-angle glaucoma, urinary retention, peptic ulcer, acute asthma attack, with MAOI therapy.

WARNINGS/PRECAUTIONS: Caution with HTN, DM, ischemic heart disease, hyperthyroidism, BPH, asthma, and increased IOP. May produce CNS stimulation with convulsion, cardiovascular collapse and hypotension. Excitability reported especially in children. Do not exceed recommended doses. Caution in atopic children, elderly, sedated/debilitated, and patients confined to supine positions.

ADVERSE REACTIONS: Sedation, drowsiness, dizziness, diplopia, nausea, vomiting, diarrhea, dry mouth, headache, arrhythmias, increased heart rate, tremors, nervousness, insomnia, heartburn, dysuria, polyuria, increased BP.

INTERACTIONS: May enhance effects of TCAs, barbiturates, alcohol, other CNS depressants. May diminish antihypertensive effects of reserpine, veratrum alkaloids, methyldopa, mecamylamine. Increased sympathomimetic effect with β-blockers and MAOIs. Additive cough-suppressant effect with narcotic antitussives. Do not use within 14 days of MAOI therapy.

PREGNANCY: Category C, caution in nursing.

MECHANISM OF ACTION: Brompheniramine: H_1 antihistamine activity; mild anticholinergic and sedative effects. Pseudoephedrine: Oral sympathomimetic amine; acts as decongestant to respiratory tract mucous membranes. Dextromethorphan: Nonnarcotic antitussive with effectiveness equal to codeine; acts in medulla oblongata to elevate the cough threshold.

PHARMACOKINETICS: Absorption: Brompheniramine: T_{max}=5 hrs. **Metabolism:** Brompheniramine: Liver. **Elimination:** Brompheniramine: Urine. Pseudoephedrine: Urine; $T_{1/2}$=6-8 hrs. Dextromethorphan: Urine (conjugated metabolites).

ROSAC
sulfacetamide sodium - sulfur (Stiefel)   RX

THERAPEUTIC CLASS: Sulfonamide/sulfur combination

INDICATIONS: Topical control of acne vulgaris, acne rosacea, and seborrheic dermatitis.

DOSAGE: *Adults:* Apply a thin film qd-tid. *Pediatrics:* ≥12 yrs: Apply a thin film qd-tid.

HOW SUPPLIED: Cre: (Sulfacetamide-Sulfur) 10%-5% [45g]

CONTRAINDICATIONS: Kidney disease.

WARNINGS/PRECAUTIONS: D/C if irritation or hypersensitivity reaction occurs. Avoid contact with eyes. Caution if denuded or abraded skin. May cause reddening and scaling of epidermis.

ADVERSE REACTIONS: Local irritation.

PREGNANCY: Category C, caution in nursing.

MECHANISM OF ACTION: Sulfonamide/sulfur combination. Sulfacetamide: Acts as a competitive antagonist to para-aminobenzoic acid (PABA), an essential component for bacterial growth. Sulfur: Not established. Inhibits the growth of *Propionibacterium acnes* and the formation of free fatty acids.

PHARMACOKINETICS: Absorption: Sulfacetamide: (PO) Readily absorbed. **Distribution:** Small amounts of orally administered sulfonamides have been found in breast milk. **Elimination:** Sulfacetamide: Urine (unchanged).

ROSULA
sulfacetamide sodium - sulfur (Doak)   RX

THERAPEUTIC CLASS: Sulfonamide/sulfur combination

INDICATIONS: Topical treatment of acne vulgaris, acne rosacea, and seborrheic dermatitis.

R

DOSAGE: *Adults:* (Gel) Apply thin film qd-tid. (Cleanser) Wash for 10-20 seconds qd-bid.
Pediatrics: ≥12 yrs: (Gel) Apply thin film qd-tid. (Cleanser) Wash for 10-20 seconds qd-bid.

HOW SUPPLIED: (Sulfacetamide-Sulfur) Gel: 10%-5% [45mL]; Cleanser: 10%-5% [355mL]

CONTRAINDICATIONS: Kidney disease.

WARNINGS/PRECAUTIONS: D/C if irritation or hypersensitivity reaction occurs. Avoid contact with eyes, lips, and mucous membranes. Caution with denuded or abraded skin. Can cause reddening and scaling of epidermis.

ADVERSE REACTIONS: Local irritation.

PREGNANCY: Category C, caution in nursing.

MECHANISM OF ACTION: Sulfonamide/sulfur combination. Sulfacetamide: Acts as a competitive antagonist to para-aminobenzoic acid (PABA), an essential component for bacterial growth. Sulfur: Not established. Inhibits the growth of *Propionibacterium acnes* and the formation of free fatty acids.

PHARMACOKINETICS: Absorption: (PO) Readily absorbed. **Elimination:** Urine (unchanged).

ROSULA NS   RX
sulfacetamide sodium - urea (Doak)

THERAPEUTIC CLASS: Sulfonamide

INDICATIONS: Topical treatment of bacterial infections of the skin including *P.acne* and seborrheic dermatitis.

DOSAGE: *Adults:* Apply to affected area qd-bid.
Pediatrics: ≥12 yrs: Apply to affected area qd-bid.

HOW SUPPLIED: Swab: (Sulfacetamide-Urea) 10%-10% [30ˢ]

CONTRAINDICATIONS: Kidney disease

WARNINGS/PRECAUTIONS: D/C if irritation or hypersensitivity reaction occurs. Avoid contact with eyes, lips, and mucous membranes. Caution with denuded or abraded skin. Cases of Stevens-Johnson syndrome and drug-induced systemic lupus erythematosus reported.

ADVERSE REACTIONS: Local hypersensitivity, instances of Stevens-Johnson syndrome.

INTERACTIONS: Incompatible with silver preparations.

PREGNANCY: Category C, caution in nursing.

MECHANISM OF ACTION: Sulfonamide: Sulfacetamide; possesses bacteriostatic activity against susceptible gram-positive and gram-negative microorganisms, including *P. acne.* Acts as a competitive antagonist to para-aminobenzoic acid (PABA), an essential component for bacterial growth.

PHARMACOKINETICS: Absorption: Sulfacetamide: (PO) Readily absorbed. **Elimination:** Urine (unchanged).

ROTATEQ   RX
rotavirus vaccine, live (Merck)

THERAPEUTIC CLASS: Vaccine

INDICATIONS: Prevention of rotavirus gastroenteritis in infants and children caused by the serotypes G1, G2, G3, and G4 when administered as a 3-dose series to infants between the ages of 6-32 weeks. The first dose should be administered between 6-12 weeks of age.

DOSAGE: *Pediatrics:* Administer series of 3 doses orally starting at 6-12 weeks of age, with subsequent doses administered at 4-10 week intervals. Third dose should not be given after 32 weeks of age. Do not mix with any other vaccines or solutions. Do not reconstitute or dilute.

HOW SUPPLIED: Sus: 2mL

WARNINGS/PRECAUTIONS: Consider delaying use with febrile illness. Vaccination may not result in complete protection in all recipients. May increase risk of intussusception.

ADVERSE REACTIONS: Bronchiolitis, gastroenteritis, pneumonia, fever, UTI.

INTERACTIONS: Immunosuppressive therapies including irradiation, anti-metabolites, alkylating agents, cytotoxic drugs, and corticosteroids (used in greater than physiologic doses) may reduce the immune response to vaccines.

PREGNANCY: Safety in pregnancy and nursing not known.

MECHANISM OF ACTION: Immunologic mechanism not established; may replicate in small intestine and induce immunity against rotavirus gastroenteritis.

ROWASA   RX
mesalamine (Solvay)

INDICATIONS: Treatment of active mild to moderate distal ulcerative colitis, proctosigmoiditis or proctitis.

DOSAGE: *Adults:* Use 1 enema rectally qhs for 3-6 weeks. Retain for 8 hrs. Empty bowel prior to administration.

HOW SUPPLIED: Enema: 4g/60mL

WARNINGS/PRECAUTIONS: D/C if acute intolerance syndrome develops (eg, cramping, bloody diarrhea, abdominal pain, headache); consider sulfasalazine hypersensitivity. If rechallenge is considered, perform under careful observation. Caution with sulfasalazine hypersensitivity. Carefully monitor with renal dysfunction. Contains potassium metabisulfite; caution with sulfite sensitivity especially in asthmatics. Pancolitis, pericarditis (rare) reported.

ADVERSE REACTIONS: Abdominal problems, headache, flatulence, flu, fever, nausea, malaise/fatigue.

PREGNANCY: Category B, not for use in nursing.

MECHANISM OF ACTION: Unknown, possibly diminishes inflammation by blocking cyclooxygenase and inhibiting prostaglandin production in the colon.

PHARMACOKINETICS: Absorption: Colon: poor. Extent dependent on retention time. **Metabolism:** Acetylation, N-acetyl-5-ASA (Metabolite). **Elimination:** Urine and feces, $T_{1/2}$=0.5-1.5 hrs.

ROXANOL   CII
morphine sulfate (Xanodyne)

> Highly concentrated, check dose carefully.

OTHER BRAND NAMES: Roxanol-T (Xanodyne)

THERAPEUTIC CLASS: Opioid analgesic

INDICATIONS: Relief of severe acute and chronic pain.

DOSAGE: *Adults:* Usual: 10-30mg q4h. During first effective pain relief, dose should be maintained for at least 3 days before any dose reduction, if respiratory activity and other vital signs are adequate. Elderly/Very Ill/Respiratory Problems/Severe Renal and Hepatic Impairment: Lower doses may be required.

HOW SUPPLIED: Sol, Concentrate: 20mg/mL (Roxanol) [30mL, 120mL, 240mL], (Roxanol-T) [30mL, 120mL]

CONTRAINDICATIONS: Respiratory insufficiency or depression, severe CNS depression, attack of bronchial asthma, heart failure secondary to chronic lung disease, cardiac arrhythmias, increased intracranial or cerebrospinal pressure, head injuries, brain tumor, acute alcoholism, delirium tremens, convulsive disorders, after biliary tract surgery, suspected surgical abdomen, surgical anastomosis, concomitantly with MAOIs or within 14 days of such treatment.

WARNINGS/PRECAUTIONS: May cause tolerance, psychological, and physical dependence; withdrawal may occur on abrupt discontinuation. Caution with head injury, increased ICP, acute asthmatic attack, COPD, cor pulmonale, decreased respiratory reserve, pre-existing respiratory depression, hypoxia, hypercapnia, elderly, debilitated, severe hepatic/renal impairment, hypothyroidism, Addison's disease, prostatic hypertrophy, or urethral stricture. May cause orthostatic hypotension in ambulatory patients, severe hypotension with depleted blood volume. May obscure diagnosis/clinical course of acute abdominal conditions. May impair mental/physical abilities.

ADVERSE REACTIONS: Respiratory depression, lightheadedness, dizziness, sedation, nausea, vomiting, sweating, constipation.

INTERACTIONS: See Contraindications. Potentiated by alkalizing agents and antagonized by acidifying agents. Analgesic effect potentiated by chlorpromazine, methocarbamol. Enhanced depressant effects with other CNS depressants such as anesthetics, hypnotics, barbiturates, phenothiazines, chloral hydrate, glutethimide, sedatives, MAOIs (eg, procarbazine), antihistamines, β-blockers (eg, propranolol), alcohol, furazolidone, other narcotics, tranquilizers, and TCAs. May increase anticoagulant activity of coumarin and other anticoagulants.

PREGNANCY: Category C, caution in nursing.

MECHANISM OF ACTION: Opioid analgesic; acts as agonist interacting with stereospecific and saturable binding sites or receptors in the brain and other tissues. Major effects are on CNS and bowel.

PHARMACOKINETICS: Absorption: T_{max}=60 mins. **Distribution:** Crosses placenta; found in breast milk.

ROXICET CII
oxycodone HCL - acetaminophen (Roxane)

THERAPEUTIC CLASS: Opioid analgesic

INDICATIONS: Relief of moderate to moderately severe pain.

DOSAGE: *Adults:* Usual: 5mg-325mg (1 tab or 5mL sol) q6h prn. Titrate: May need to exceed usual dose based on individual response, pain severity, and tolerance.

HOW SUPPLIED: (Oxycodone-APAP) Sol: 5mg-325mg/5mL [5mL; 500mL]; Tab: 5mg-325mg

WARNINGS/PRECAUTIONS: May cause drug dependence and tolerance; potential for abuse. Risk of respiratory depression. Capacity to elevate CSF pressure may be exaggerated with head injury, other intracranial lesions, or a pre-existing increase in ICP. May obscure the diagnosis or clinical course with head injuries or with acute abdominal conditions. Caution with severe hepatic impairment, renal dysfunction, hypothyroidism, Addison's disease, prostatic hypertrophy, urethral stricture, the elderly or debilitated.

ADVERSE REACTIONS: Lightheadedness, dizziness, sedation, nausea, vomiting, euphoria, dysphoria, constipation, skin rash, pruritus.

INTERACTIONS: Additive CNS depression with narcotic analgesics, general anesthetics, phenothiazines, tranquilizers, sedatives-hypnotics, alcohol, and other CNS depressants; reduce dose of one or both agents.

PREGNANCY: Category C, caution in nursing.

MECHANISM OF ACTION: Oxycodone: Opioid analgesic; pure opioid agonist. Principle therapeutic effect is analgesia. Other effects include anxiolysis, euphoria, and feelings of relaxation. Effects mediated by CNS receptors (eg, mu and kappa) for endogenous opioid-like compounds (eg, endorphins, enkephalins). APAP: Non-opiate, non-salicylate. Site and mechanism for analgesic effect not established. Antipyretic effect occurs through inhibition of endogenous pyrogen action on the hypothalmic heat-regulating centers.

PHARMACOKINETICS: Absorption: Oxycodone: Absolute bioavailability (87%). APAP: Rapid absorption. **Distribution:** Oxycodone: Plasma protein binding (45%); (IV) V_d=211.9 L; found in breast milk. APAP: Plasma protein binding (20-50%) (variable); found in most body fluids, breast milk. **Metabolism:** Oxycodone: N-dealkylation to norcodone (metabolite); CYP2D6 (O-emethylation) to oxymorphone (metabolite). APAP: Liver via CYP450 (conjugation), NAPQI (toxic metabolite). **Excretion:** Oxycodone: Urine (parent compound and metabolites); $T_{1/2}$=3.51 hrs. APAP: Urine (90-100%).

Roxicodone   CII
oxycodone HCL (Xanodyne)

THERAPEUTIC CLASS: Opioid analgesic

INDICATIONS: Relief of moderate to moderately severe pain.

DOSAGE: *Adults:* Initial: Opioid-Naive: 5mg to 15mg q4-6h prn. Titrate: Based on individual response. For chronic pain or severe chronic pain, use ATC dosing schedule at lowest effective dose.

HOW SUPPLIED: Sol: 5mg/5mL [5mL, 40s; 500mL], (Intensol) 20mg/mL [30mL]; Tab: 5mg*, 15mg*, 30mg* *scored

CONTRAINDICATIONS: Significant respiratory depression (in unmonitored settings or the absence of resuscitative equipment), acute or severe bronchial asthma, hypercarbia, paralytic ileus.

WARNINGS/PRECAUTIONS: Potential for physical dependence. May markedly exaggerate respiratory depressant effects in head injuries and increased ICP. May mask symptoms of acute abdominal conditions. Caution with history of drug abuse, the elderly, debilitated, hypothyroidism, Addison's disease, BPH, urethral stricture, severe hepatic and renal impairment. May cause severe hypotension. May impair mental/physical abilities.

ADVERSE REACTIONS: Respiratory depression/arrest, circulatory depression, cardiac arrest, hypotension, shock, nausea, constipation, vomiting, headache, pruritus, insomnia, dizziness, asthenia, somnolence.

INTERACTIONS: Additive CNS depression with narcotic analgesics, phenothiazines, tranquilizers, sedative-hypnotics, alcohol, and other CNS depressants; reduce dose. Mixed agonist/antagonist analgesics may reduce analgesic effect and/or cause withdrawal. May enhance effect of neuromuscular blockers. Avoid within 14 days of MAOIs. Severe hypotension may occur with concurrent administration of phenothiazines or other agents which compromise vasomotor tone.

PREGNANCY: Category B, not for use in nursing.

MECHANISM OF ACTION: Opioid analgesic; pure opioid agonist whose principal therapeutic effect is analgesia. Precise mechanism of analgesic effect has not been established. Specific CNS opioid receptors for endogenous compounds with opioid-like activity are found in the brain and spinal cord and play a role in analgesic effects.

PHARMACOKINETICS: Absorption: Various doses led to altered parameters. **Distribution:** Plasma protein binding (45%), (IV): V_d=2.6L/kg; found in breast milk. **Metabolism:** Hepatic (extensively); noroxycodone (major metabolite); CYP2D6 to oxymorphone (metabolite) and glucuronides. **Elimination:** Urine (parent compound and metabolites); $T_{1/2}$=3.5-4 hrs.

Rozerem   RX
ramelteon (Takeda)

THERAPEUTIC CLASS: Melatonin receptor agonist

INDICATIONS: Treatment of insomnia characterized by difficulty with sleep onset.

DOSAGE: *Adults:* 8mg within 30 min of bedtime. Do not take with or after high fat meal.

R

HOW SUPPLIED: Tab: 8mg

WARNINGS/PRECAUTIONS: Sleep disturbances may be presenting manifestations of a physical and/or psychiatric disorder, initiate therapy only after careful evaluation. Do not use in severe hepatic impairment. Variety of abnormal thinking and behavioral changes reported to occur in association with use of hypnotics. In primarily depressed patients, worsening of depression, including suicidal ideation, reported in association with use of hypnotics. May impair physical/mental abilities. Not recommended in patients with severe sleep apnea or severe COPD. Caution with alcohol. May affect reproductive hormones.

ADVERSE REACTIONS: Headache, somnolence, fatigue, dizziness, nausea, exacerbated insomnia, upper respiratory tract infection.

INTERACTIONS: Do not use with strong CYP1A2 inhibitors (fluvoxamine). Decreased efficacy with strong CYP inducers (rifampin). Caution with less strong CYP1A2 inhibitors, strong CYP3A4 inhibitors (ketoconazole), strong CYP2C9 inhibitors (fluconazole). Additive effect with alcohol.

PREGNANCY: Category C, not for use in nursing.

MECHANISM OF ACTION: Melatonin receptor agonist; activity at receptors believed to contribute to sleep-promoting properties.

PHARMACOKINETICS: Absorption: Rapid; absolute bioavailabilty (1.8%); T_{max}=0.75 hr. **Distribution:** Plasma protein binding (82%); V_d=73.6 L(IV). **Metabolism:** Oxidation via CYP1A2 (major), CYP3A4 (minor). M-II (active metabolite). **Elimination:** Urine, feces (<0.1%); $T_{1/2}$=1-2.6 hrs, 2-5 hrs (M-II).

RYNATAN RX
chlorpheniramine tannate - phenylephrine tannate (MedPointe)

THERAPEUTIC CLASS: Antihistamine/sympathomimetic

INDICATIONS: Symptomatic relief of coryza and nasal congestion with the common cold, sinusitis, allergic rhinitis, and other upper respiratory tract conditions.

DOSAGE: *Adults:* 1-2 tabs q12h.

HOW SUPPLIED: Tab: (Chlorpheniramine-Phenylephrine) 9mg-25mg

CONTRAINDICATIONS: Newborns, nursing mothers.

WARNINGS/PRECAUTIONS: Caution with HTN, cardiovascular disease, hyperthyroidism, DM, narrow angle glaucoma, prostatic hypertrophy, and elderly. May impair mental alertness. May cause mild stimulation or sedation in children.

ADVERSE REACTIONS: Drowsiness, sedation, dryness of mucous membranes, GI effects.

INTERACTIONS: Increased anticholinergic and sympathomimetic effects with MAOIs; avoid during or within 14 days of use. Additive CNS effects with alcohol or other CNS depressants (eg, sedative, hypnotics, tranquilizers).

PREGNANCY: Category C, not for use in nursing.

RYNATUSS RX
chlorpheniramine tannate - carbetapentane tannate - phenylephrine tannate - ephedrine tannate (MedPointe)

OTHER BRAND NAMES: Rynatuss Pediatric (MedPointe)

THERAPEUTIC CLASS: Antitussive/antihistamine/bronchodilator/sympathomimetic combination

INDICATIONS: Symptomatic relief of cough associated with respiratory tract conditions such as the common cold, bronchial asthma, acute and chronic bronchitis.

DOSAGE: *Adults:* 1-2 tabs q12h.
Pediatrics: >6 yrs: 5-10mL q12h. 2-6 yrs: 2.5-5mL q12h.

HOW SUPPLIED: (Carbetapentane-Chlorpheniramine-Ephedrine-Phenylephrine) Sus: (Rynatuss Pediatric) 30mg-4mg-5mg-5mg/5mL [240mL 480mL]; Tab: (Rynatuss) 60mg-5mg-10mg-10mg* *scored

CONTRAINDICATIONS: Newborns, nursing mothers.

WARNINGS/PRECAUTIONS: Caution with HTN, cardiovascular disease, hyperthyroidism, DM, narrow angle glaucoma, elderly or prostatic hypertrophy. Suspension contains FD&C Yellow No. 5 which may cause allergic-type reactions.

ADVERSE REACTIONS: Drowsiness, sedation, dryness of mucous membranes, GI effects.

INTERACTIONS: Avoid MAOI use within 14 days. Additive CNS effects with alcohol or other CNS depressants.

PREGNANCY: Category C, not for use in nursing.

RYTHMOL   RX
propafenone HCL (Reliant)

THERAPEUTIC CLASS: Class IC antiarrhythmic

INDICATIONS: To prolong the time to recurrence of paroxysmal atrial fibrillation/flutter (PAF) and paroxysmal supraventricular tachycardia (PSVT) associated with disabling symptoms in patients without structural heart disease. Treatment of life-threatening documented ventricular arrhythmias.

DOSAGE: *Adults:* Initial: 150mg q8h. Titrate: May increase at minimum 3-4 day intervals to 225mg q8h, then to 300mg q8h if needed. Max: 900mg/day. Elderly/Marked Myocardial Damage: Increase more gradually during initial phase. Hepatic Dysfunction: Reduce dose by 20-30%.

HOW SUPPLIED: Tab: 150mg*, 225mg*, 300mg* *scored

CONTRAINDICATIONS: Uncontrolled CHF, cardiogenic shock, bradycardia, marked hypotension, bronchospastic disorders, electrolyte imbalance, and sinoatrial, atrioventricular (AV) and intraventricular disorders of impulse generation and/or conduction (eg, sick sinus node syndrome, AV block) in the absence of an artificial pacemaker.

WARNINGS/PRECAUTIONS: Avoid with non-life-threatening ventricular arrhythmias, bronchospastic disorders. May cause new or worsened arrhythmias. Caution with hepatic or renal dysfunction. Slows AV conduction and causes 1st-degree AV block. D/C if CHF worsens. Agranulocytosis, myasthenia gravis exacerbation, positive ANA titers reported. May alter pacing and sensing thresholds of artificial pacemakers.

ADVERSE REACTIONS: Taste disturbances, nausea, vomiting, dizziness, constipation, headache, fatigue, blurred vision, blood dyscrasias.

INTERACTIONS: Inhibitors of CYP2D6 (eg, desipramine, paroxetine, ritonavir, sertraline), CYP1A2 (eg, amiodarone), CYP3A4 (eg, ketoconazole, ritonavir, saquinavir, erythromycin, grapefruit juice) may increase levels; monitor closely. May increase levels of drugs metabolized by CYP2D6 (eg, desipramine, imipramine, haloperidol, venlafaxine). May increase CNS side effects of lidocaine. May increase levels of digoxin, propranolol, warfarin; monitor closely. Cimetidine may increase plasma levels. Rifampin, orlistat may decrease plasma levels.

PREGNANCY: Category C, not for use in nursing.

MECHANISM OF ACTION: Class 1C antiarrhythmic drug with local anesthetic effects and direct stablizing action on myocardium. It reduces upstroke velocity (phase 0) of the monophasic action potential in purkinje fiber and to a lesser extent myocardial fibers, and reduces the fast inward current carried by Na ions. It reduces spontaneous automaticity and depresses triggered activity.

PHARMACOKINETICS: Absorption: Complete, absolute bioavailability (150mg) 3.4%, (300mg) 10.6%. T_{max}=3.5 hrs. **Metabolism:** Liver (rapid, extensive) via CYP3A4, 1A2 and 2D6. 5-hyrdoxypropafenone and N-depropylpropafenone (active metabolites). **Elimination:** $T_{1/2}$=2-10 hrs.

RYTHMOL SR   RX
propafenone HCL (Reliant)

THERAPEUTIC CLASS: Class IC antiarrhythmic

INDICATIONS: To prolong the time to recurrence of symptomatic atrial fibrillation in patients without structural heart disease.

DOSAGE: *Adults:* Initial: 225mg q12h. Titrate: May increase at minimum 5 day intervals to 325mg q12h, then to 425mg q12h if needed. Hepatic Impairment/QRS Widening/2nd- or 3rd-degree AV Block: Reduce dose.

HOW SUPPLIED: Cap, Extended-Release: 225mg, 325mg, 425mg

CONTRAINDICATIONS: CHF, cardiogenic shock, bradycardia, marked hypotension, bronchospastic disorders, electrolyte imbalance, and sinoatrial, atrioventricular (AV) and intraventricular disorders of impulse generation or conduction (eg, sick sinus node syndrome, AV block) unless paced.

WARNINGS/PRECAUTIONS: Avoid with non-life-threatening ventricular arrhythmias, bronchospastic disease, AV and intraventricular conduction defects unless paced. May cause new or worsened arrhythmias, provoke overt CHF. Caution with hepatic or renal dysfunction. 1st-degree AV block, agranulocytosis, myasthenia gravis exacerbation, positive ANA titers reported. May alter pacing and sensing thresholds of artificial pacemakers.

ADVERSE REACTIONS: Dizziness, chest pain, palpitations, taste disturbance, dyspnea, nausea, constipation, anxiety, fatigue, upper respiratory tract infection, influenza, 1st-degree heart block, vomiting.

INTERACTIONS: Avoid with drugs that prolong QT interval (eg, some phenothiazines, cisapride, bepridil, TCAs, oral macrolides, other antiarrhythmics), Class Ia and III antiarrhythmics (eg, quinidine, amiodarone). Inhibitors of CYP2D6 (eg, desipramine, paroxetine, ritonavir, sertraline), CYP1A2 (eg, amiodarone), CYP3A4 (eg, ketoconazole, ritonavir, saquinavir, erythromycin, grapefruit juice) may increase levels; monitor closely. May increase levels of drugs metabolized by CYP2D6 (eg, desipramine, imipramine, haloperidol, venlafaxine). May increase CNS side effects of lidocaine. May increase levels of digoxin, propranolol, warfarin; monitor closely. Cimetidine may increase plasma levels. Rifampin, orlistat may decrease plasma levels.

PREGNANCY: Category C, caution in nursing.

MECHANISM OF ACTION: Class 1 C antiarrhythmic drug with local anesthetic effects and direct stablizing action on myocardium. Reduces upstroke velocity (phase 0) of the monophasic action potential in purkinje fiber and to a lesser extent myocardial fibers, and reduces the fast inward current carried by Na ions. Reduces spontaneous automaticity and depresses triggered activity.

PHARMACOKINETICS: Absorption: T_{max}=3-8 hrs. **Distribution:** Plasma protein binding (≥95%). V_d=252L. **Metabolism:** Rapid, extensive, via CYP2D6, 3A4 and 1A2 through hydroxylation. 5-hydroxypropafenone and N-depropylpropafenone (active metabolites). **Elimination:** Urine, (50% metabolites). $T_{1/2}$=2-10 hrs.

SAIZEN   RX
somatropin (EMD Serono)

THERAPEUTIC CLASS: Human growth hormone

INDICATIONS: Long-term treatment of children with growth failure due to inadequate secretion of endogenous growth hormone. For replacement of endogenous growth hormone in adults who have growth hormone deficiency either alone, or associated with multiple hormone deficiencies, as a result of pituitary disease, hypothalamic disease, surgery, radiation therapy or trauma;

or in patients who were growth hormone deficient during childhood as a result of congenital, genetic, acquired or idiopathic causes.

DOSAGE: *Adults:* Initial: ≤0.005mg/kg/day SQ. Titrate: May increase after 4 weeks to ≤0.01mg/kg/day depending on patient tolerance. Without Consideration of Body Weight: Initial: 0.2mg/day (0.15-0.3mg/day) SQ. Titrate: May increase by increments of 0.1-0.2mg/day every 1-2 months. Consider dose reduction in elderly.
Pediatrics: Individualize dose. Usual: 0.06mg/kg IM/SQ 3x/week. If epiphyses are fused, d/c therapy.

HOW SUPPLIED: Inj: 4mg, 5mg, 8.8mg

CONTRAINDICATIONS: Acute critical illness due to complications following open heart or abdominal surgery, accidental trauma or acute respiratory failure. Active proliferative or severe non-proliferative diabetic retinopathy. Active malignancy, or evidence of progression or recurrence of intracranial tumor. Prader-Willi syndrome when severely obese or have severe respiratory impairment, and in pediatric patients with closed epiphyses. Avoid reconstitution with bacteriostatic water if sensitive to benzyl alcohol.

WARNINGS/PRECAUTIONS: Benzyl alcohol associated with toxicity in newborns; if sensitivity occurs, may reconstitute with SWFI. Insulin resistance reported; use caution with DM or family history of DM. Hypothyroidism may occur; bone maturation should be carefully followed. Increased incidence of slipped capital femoral epiphysis may develop with endocrine disorders; monitor for limping or hip/knee pain. Intracranial hypertension (IH) reported; d/c treatment if papilledema observed. Patients with Turner syndrome, chronic renal insufficiency or Prader-Willi syndrome may have increased risk for IH. If idiopathic IH confirmed, may restart therapy at lower dose after signs/symptoms resolve. Alternate injection sites to reduce development of tissue atrophy. Monitor for any malignant transformation of skin lesions.

ADVERSE REACTIONS: Arthalgia, headache, influenza-like symptoms, peripheral edema, back pain, myalgia, rhinitis, dizziness, upper respiratory tract infection, paraesthesia, hypoaesthesia, insomnia, nausea, generalized edema, depression.

INTERACTIONS: Diminished effects with concomitant glucocorticoid; adjust dose of accordingly. May alter clearance of CYP450 substrates (eg, corticosteroids, sex steroids, anticonvulsants, cyclosporine). May increase dose if taking oral estrogen replacement concomitantly. Adjust dose of insulin/oral antidiabetics when initiating therapy.

PREGNANCY: Category B, caution in nursing.

MECHANISM OF ACTION: Human growth hormone; stimulates skeletal growth, increases number and size of skeletal muscle cells, influences size and function of internal organs and increases red cell mass, stimulates protein synthesis, modulates carbohydrate metabolism, and mobilizes lipids.

PHARMACOKINETICS: Absorption: Absolute bioavailability (70-90%). **Distribution:** V_d=12.0L. **Metabolism:** Liver, kidneys. **Elimination:** $T_{1/2}$=1.75 hrs (SC), 3.4 hrs (IM), 0.6 hrs (IV).

SANCTURA **XR**   RX
trospium chloride (Espirit/Indevus)

OTHER BRAND NAMES: Sanctura (Espirit/Indevus)
THERAPEUTIC CLASS: Muscarinic antagonist
INDICATIONS: Treatment of overactive bladder with symptoms of urge urinary incontinence, urgency, and urinary frequency.
DOSAGE: *Adults:* (Tab) 20mg bid. (Cap, Extended-Release) 60mg qd in am. Take at least 1 hour before meals or on empty stomach. (Tab) CrCl <30mL/min: 20mg qhs. Elderly ≥75 yrs: May titrate to 20mg qd based upon tolerability.
HOW SUPPLIED: Cap, Extended-Release: 60mg; Tab: 20mg

S

CONTRAINDICATIONS: Active or risk of urinary retention, gastric retention, uncontrolled narrow-angle glaucoma.

WARNINGS/PRECAUTIONS: (Tab,Cap) Caution with significant bladder outflow obstruction, GI obstructive disorders, ulcerative colitis, intestinal atony, myasthenia gravis, moderate or severe hepatic dysfunction. Reduce dose with severe renal insufficiency. Consider risks vs benefits with controlled narrow-angle glaucoma. (Cap) Not recommended for use with severe renal impairment (CrCl <30mL/min). Consumption of alcohol within 2 hrs is not recommended.

ADVERSE REACTIONS: Dry mouth, constipation, headache, rash.

INTERACTIONS: Increased adverse effects with other anticholinergics. May alter GI absorption of other drugs due to GI motility effects. Monitor closely with other drugs eliminated by active renal tubular secretion (eg, procain-amide, pancuronium, morphine, vancomycin, metformin, tenofovir).

PREGNANCY: Category C, caution in nursing.

MECHANISM OF ACTION: Antispasmodic, antimuscarinic agent: reduces tonus of smooth muscle in bladder by antagonizing effect of acetylcholine on muscarinic receptors.

PHARMACOKINETICS: Absorption: (Tab) Absolute bioavailability (9.6%), T_{max}=5.3 hrs, C_{max}=3.5ng/mL, AUC=36.4ng•hr/mL; (Cap, Extended-Release) T_{max}=5 hrs, C_{max}=2ng/mL, AUC=18ng•hr/mL. **Distribution:** Plasma protein binding (50-85%); V_d=>600L. **Metabolism:** Ester hydrolysis. **Elimination:** Feces (major), urine. (Tab) $T_{1/2}$=18.3 hrs; (Cap, Extended-Release) $T_{1/2}$=36 hrs.

SANDIMMUNE   RX
cyclosporine (Novartis)

> Give with adrenal corticosteroids but not with other immunosuppressives. Increased susceptibility to infection and development of lymphoma. Sandimmune and Neoral are not bioequivalent. Monitor blood levels to avoid toxicity.

THERAPEUTIC CLASS: Cyclic polypeptide immunosuppressant

INDICATIONS: Prophylaxis of organ rejection in kidney, liver, and heart allogeneic transplants with concomitant adrenal corticosteroids. Treatment of chronic rejection in patients previously treated with other immunosuppressives.

DOSAGE: *Adults:* Initial: PO: 15mg/kg single dose 4-12 hrs before transplant; continue same dose qd for 1-2 weeks. Usual: Taper by 5% per week until 5-10mg/kg/day. May mix oral solution with milk, chocolate milk, or orange juice. IV: 1/3 PO dose. Initial: 5-6mg/kg/day single dose; begin 4 to 12 hrs prior to transplantation. Maint: Continue single daily dose until PO forms are tolerated. Due to risk of anaphylaxis, only use injection if unable to take oral agents.
Pediatrics: Initial: PO: 15mg/kg single dose 4-12 hrs before transplant; continue same dose qd for 1-2 weeks. Usual: Taper by 5% per week until 5-10mg/kg/day. May mix oral solution with milk, chocolate milk, or orange juice. IV: 1/3 PO dose. Initial: 5-6mg/kg/day single dose; begin 4 to 12 hrs prior to transplantation. Maint: Continue single daily dose until PO forms are tolerated. Due to risk of anaphylaxis, only use injection if unable to take oral agents.

HOW SUPPLIED: Cap: 25mg, 100mg; Inj: 50mg/mL; Sol: 100mg/mL [50mL]

CONTRAINDICATIONS: Hypersensitivity to Cremophor EL (polyoxyethylated castor oil).

WARNINGS/PRECAUTIONS: May cause hepatotoxicity and nephrotoxicity. Convulsions, elevated serum creatinine, and BUN levels reported. Thrombocytopenia and microangiopathic hemolytic anemia may develop. Monitor for hyperkalemia. Increases risk for development of lymphomas and other malignancies. Observe for 30 minutes after the start of infusion and frequently thereafter. Caution with malabsorption.

ADVERSE REACTIONS: Renal dysfunction, tremor, hirsutism, HTN, gum hyperplasia, glomerular capillary thrombosis, cramps, acne, convulsions, headache, diarrhea, hepatotoxity, abdominal discomfort, paresthesia, flushing.

INTERACTIONS: Ciprofloxacin, gentamicin, tobramycin, vancomycin, SMZ/TMP, amphotericin B, ketoconazole, melphalan, diclofenac, azapropazon, sulindac, naproxen, colchicine, cimetidine, ranitidine, tacrolimus, bezafirate, fenofibrate may potentiate renal dysfunction. Diltiazem, nicardipine, colchicine, fluconazole, itraconazole, ketoconazole, verapamil, azithromycin, clarithromycin, erythromycin, quinupristin/dalfopristin, allopurinol, amiodarone, bromocriptine, danazol, imatinib, metoclopramide, oral contraceptives, HIV protease inhibitors may increase levels. St. John's wort, grapefruit juice, carbamazepine, phenobarbital, phenytoin, rifampin, sulfinpyrazone, octreotide, orlistat, terbinafine, ticlopidine, and naficillin may decrease levels. Avoid with potassium-sparing diuretics. Caution with ACEIs, angiotensin II blockers, NSAIDs. Digitalis toxicity reported. Myotoxicity with statins, frequent gingival hyperplasia with nifedipine, and convulsions with high dose methylprednisolone reported. Increased levels of sirolimus; give 4 hrs after cyclosporine. Avoid live vaccines during therapy.

PREGNANCY: Category C, not for use in nursing.

MECHANISM OF ACTION: Cyclic polypeptide immunosuppressant; not fully established. May cause specific and reversible inhibition of immunocompetent lymphocytes in the G_0- or G_1-phase of the cell cycle. T lymphocytes are preferentially inhibited with T-helper cell as main target while also possibly suppressing T-suppressor cells. Also inhibits lymphokine production and release (eg, interleukin-2, T-cell growth factor).

PHARMACOKINETICS: Absorption: Incomplete and variable. Absolute bioavailability (30%)(PO); C_{max}=1ng/mL/mg; T_{max}=3.5 hrs. **Distribution:** Plasma protein binding (90%). **Metabolism:** Extensively metabolized via hydroxylation, cyclic ether formation, and N-demethylation. **Elimination:** Urine (6%); $T_{1/2}$=19 hrs.

SANDOSTATIN   RX
octreotide acetate (Novartis)

THERAPEUTIC CLASS: Somatostatin analog

INDICATIONS: To reduce blood levels of growth hormone and IGF-I in acromegaly inadequately responding to or cannot be treated with surgical resection, pituitary irradiation, and maximum dose bromocriptine mesylate. Symptomatic treatment of metastatic carcinoid tumors, where it suppresses or inhibits severe diarrhea and flushing episodes. Treatment of profuse watery diarrhea associated with VIP (Vasoactive Intestinal Peptide)-secreting tumors.

DOSAGE: *Adults:* Give SQ/IV. Acromegaly: Initial: 50mcg tid. Titrate: Adjust dose based on IGF-I levels every 2 weeks. Usual: 100mcg tid. Max: 500mcg tid. Reduce dose if no additional benefit with dose increase. Re-evaluate IGF-I or growth hormone levels every 6 months. Withdraw yearly for 4 weeks to assess disease activity after irradiation. Carcinoid Tumors: Initial: 100-600mcg/day given bid-qid (mean dose 300mcg/day) for 2 weeks. Max: 750mcg/day. VIPomas: Initial: 200-300mcg/day (range 150-750mcg) given bid-qid for 2 weeks. Max: 450mcg/day.

HOW SUPPLIED: Inj: 50mcg/mL, 100mcg/mL, 200mcg/mL, 500mcg/mL, 1000mcg/mL

WARNINGS/PRECAUTIONS: May inhibit gallbladder contractility and decrease bile secretions; increased risk of gallstones. May alter balance between insulin, glucagon, and growth hormone and lead to hypoglycemia or hyperglycemia. Hypothyroidism may result due to TSH suppression; monitor thyroid function at baseline and periodically. Cardiac conduction and other cardiovascular abnormalities may occur. Pancreatitis reported. Depressed vitamin B_{12} levels and abnormal Schilling's test reported. May need dose adjustment in renal failure.

ADVERSE REACTIONS: Gallbladder and cardiac abnormalities, diarrhea, nausea, vomiting, abdominal distention, flatulence, constipation, headache, dizziness, hypo- and hyperglycemia, hyperthyroidism.

INTERACTIONS: May decrease cyclosporine effects. May need dose adjustments of insulin, oral hypoglycemics, β-blockers, CCBs, or agents that control fluid and electrolyte balance. Not compatible in TPN solutions. Increased availability of bromocriptine.

PREGNANCY: Category B, caution in nursing.

MECHANISM OF ACTION: Somatostatin analog; exerts similiar actions to natural hormone somatostatin, but is more potent in inhibiting growth hormone, glucagon and insulin. Like somatostatin, it also supresses LH response to GnRH, decreases splanchnic blood flow, and inhibits release of serotonin, gastrin, vasoactive intestinal peptide, secretin, motilin and pancreatic polypeptide.

PHARMACOKINETICS: Absorption: C_{max}=5.2ng/mL; T_{max}=0.4 hrs; Acromegaly: C_{max}=2.8ng/mL, T_{max}=0.7 hr. **Distribution:** V_d=13.6L; Plasma protein binding (65%); Acromegaly: V_d=21.6±8.5L, plasma protein binding (41.2%). **Elimination:** Urine (32%, unchanged); $T_{1/2}$=1.7-1.9 hrs.

SANDOSTATIN LAR   RX
octreotide acetate (Novartis)

THERAPEUTIC CLASS: Somatostatin analog

INDICATIONS: Maintenance therapy of acromegaly. Long-term treatment of severe diarrhea and flushing associated with metastatic carcinoid tumors. Long-term treatment of profuse watery diarrhea associated with VIP (Vasoactive Intestinal Peptide)-secreting tumors. Use in patients who have responded to and tolerated Sandostatin Injection.In patients with carcinoid treatment and VIPomas, the effect of Sandostatin Injection and Sandostatin Lar Depot on tumor size, rate of growth and development of metastases, has not been determined.

DOSAGE: *Adults:* Administer intragluteally. Acromegaly: Initial: 20mg IM every 4 weeks for 3 months. Titrate: If GH ≤2.5ng/mL, IGF-1 normal, and clinical symptoms controlled then maintain dose. If GH >2.5, IGF-1 elevated, and/or clinical symptoms uncontrolled then increase to 30mg every 4 weeks. If GH ≤1, IGF-1 normal, and clinical symptoms controlled then reduce to 10mg every 4 weeks. Max: 40mg every 4 weeks. Withdraw yearly for 8 weeks to assess disease activity after pituitary irradiation. Carcinoid Tumors/VIPomas: Initial: 20mg IM every 4 weeks for 2 months. Continue with Sandostatin® injection SQ for at least 2 weeks. Titrate: If symptoms not controlled, increase to 30mg every 4 weeks. If symptoms controlled at 20mg, reduce to 10mg. Max: 30mg every 4 weeks. For exacerbation of symptoms, give Sandostatin Injection SQ. for at least 2 weeks. Patients must be considered responders and tolerate the injection before switching to the depot. Renal Failure Requiring Dialysis: Reduce dose.

HOW SUPPLIED: Inj, Depot: 10mg, 20mg, 30mg

WARNINGS/PRECAUTIONS: May inhibit gallbladder contractility and decrease bile secretions; increased risk of gallstones. May alter balance between insulin, glucagon and growth hormone and lead to hypoglycemia or hyperglycemia. Hypothyroidism may result due to TSH suppression; monitor thyroid function at baseline and periodically. Cardiac conduction and other cardiovascular abnormalities may occur. Monitor zinc levels periodically with TPNs. Pancreatitis reported. Depressed vitamin B_{12} levels and abnormal Schilling's test reported. May need dose adjustment in renal failure.

ADVERSE REACTIONS: Diarrhea, nausea, vomiting, abdominal discomfort, flatulence, constipation, hyperglycemia, injection site pain, upper respiratory infection, flu-like symptoms, fatigue, dizziness, headache, malaise, fever.

INTERACTIONS: May decrease cyclosporine levels. May need dose adjustments of insulin, oral hypoglycemics, β-blockers, CCBs, or agents that control fluid and electrolyte balance. May increase availability of bromocriptine.

Caution with drugs that have a low therapeutic index and metabolized by CYP3A4 (eg, quinidine, terfenadine).

PREGNANCY: Category B, caution in nursing.

MECHANISM OF ACTION: Somatostatin analog: long acting. Exerts similiar actions to natural hormone somatostatin. More potent than somatostatin in inhibiting growth hormone, glucagon, and insulin. Also suppresses LH response to GnHR, decreases splanchnic blood flow and inhibits release of serotonin, gastrin, vasoactive intestinal peptide, secretin, motolin and pancreatic polypeptide.

PHARMACOKINETICS: Absorption: Rapidly and completely absorbed; C_{max}=5.2.ng/mL, 2.8ng/mL (acromegaly); T_{max}=1 hrs. (acromegaly). **Distribution:** $V_{d (mean)}$=13.6L, 21.6L (acromegaly); Plasma protein binding (65%), (acromegaly) (41.2%). **Elimination:** Urine (32%, unchanged); $T_{1/2}$=1.7 hrs.

SANTYL COLLAGENASE   RX
collagenase (Healthpoint)

THERAPEUTIC CLASS: Debriding agent

INDICATIONS: For debriding chronic dermal ulcers and severely burned areas.

DOSAGE: *Adults:* Clean and debride wound. Apply ointment qd; use more frequently if dressings becomes soiled. If needed, apply topical antibiotic agent before ointment.

HOW SUPPLIED: Oint: 250 U/g [15g, 30g]

WARNINGS/PRECAUTIONS: Use on skin with optimal pH (6-8); lower or higher pH may diminish efficacy. Monitor debilitated patients for systemic bacterial infections; may increase risk of bacteremia. Apply carefully within area of wound.

INTERACTIONS: Avoid soaks containing metal ions or acidic solutions due to the metal ion and low pH. Diminished effects with certain detergents/antiseptics containing heavy metal ions (eg, mercury, silver).

PREGNANCY: Safety in pregnancy and nursing not known.

MECHANISM OF ACTION: Debridement ointment; possesses ability to digest collagen in necrotic tissue. Contributes to the formation of granulation tissue and subsequent epithelization of dermal ulcers and severely burned areas.

SARAFEM   RX
fluoxetine HCL (Warner Chilcott/Lilly)

> Antidepressants increased the risk of suicidal thinking and behavior (suicidality) in short-term studies in children and adolescents with Major Depressive Disorder (MDD) and other psychiatric disorders. Sarafem is not approved for use in pediatric patients.

THERAPEUTIC CLASS: Selective serotonin reuptake inhibitor

INDICATIONS: Treatment of premenstrual dysphoric disorder.

DOSAGE: *Adults:* Continuous: Initial: 20mg qd. Maint: 20mg/day up to 6 months. Max: 60mg/day. Intermittent: Initial: 20mg qd; start 14 days before menses onset through 1st full day of menses. Maint: 20mg/day up to 3 months. Max: 60mg/day. Hepatic Impairment/Concurrent Disease/Concomitant Medications: Lower dose or less frequent dosing.

HOW SUPPLIED: Cap: 10mg, 20mg

CONTRAINDICATIONS: During or within 14 days of MAOI therapy. During or within 5 weeks of thioridazine use. Concurrent use with pimozide.

WARNINGS/PRECAUTIONS: Monitor for clinical worsening and/or suicidality. Vasculitis reported. D/C if rash or allergic reaction develops. May increase risk of bleeding events with concomitant use of aspirin, NSAIDs, warfarin, etc. Hyponatremia reported. Caution in patients with history of seizures. May impair thinking, judgment, or motor skills. May alter glycemic control. Changes in weight and appetite reported. Caution with cirrhosis. Serotonin syndrome may occur; caution with concomitant use of serotonergic drugs. Rash/ urticaria, pulmonary and anaphylactoid events reported.

ADVERSE REACTIONS: Headache, asthenia, pain, flu syndrome, insomnia, dizziness, nervousness, rhinitis, pharyngitis, anorexia, dry mouth, diarrhea, tremor, anxiety.

INTERACTIONS: See Contraindications. May increase benzodiazepine, thioridazine, TCAs, haloperidol, clozapine, phenytoin, and carbamazepine levels. Lithium levels may increase/decrease. Do not use with or within 14 days of MAOIs. May shift concentrations with plasma-bound drugs (eg, coumadin, digitoxin). Caution with concomitant use with other SSRIs, SNRIs, triptans, or tryptophan.

PREGNANCY: Category C, not for use in nursing.

MECHANISM OF ACTION: SSRI; not established, presumed to be linked to inhibition of CNS neuronal uptake of serotonin.

PHARMACOKINETICS: Absorption: C_{max}=15-55ng/mL; T_{max}=6-8 hrs.
Distribution: Plasma protein binding (94.5%). **Metabolism:** CYP2D6 (demethylation); norfluoxetine (active metabolite). **Elimination:** $T_{1/2}$=1-3 days (acute), 4-6 days (chronic); 4-16 days (norfluoxetine).

SCULPTRA   RX
poly-L-lactic acid (Dermik)

THERAPEUTIC CLASS: Injectable implant

INDICATIONS: Restoration and/or correction of the signs of facial fat loss (lipoatrophy) in people with HIV.

DOSAGE: *Adults:* Reconstitute with 3-5mL of SWFI. Wait at least 2 hrs; agitate until uniform translucent suspension obtained. Inject into deep dermis or SC layer of skin using 26 G sterile needle. Limit to 0.1-0.2mL per injection; may require about 20 injections to cover target area. Use within 72 hrs of reconstitution.

HOW SUPPLIED: Inj: [3mL]

WARNINGS/PRECAUTIONS: Avoid with active skin inflammation or infection in/near target area. Injection procedure reactions reported. Should not be introduced into vasculature; may cause infarction or embolism. Use in deep dermis or SC layer; avoid superficial injections.

ADVERSE REACTIONS: Bruising, edema, discomfort, hematoma, inflammation, erythema, injection site SC papule.

PREGNANCY: Safety in pregnancy and nursing is not known.

MECHANISM OF ACTION: Intended for restoration and/or correction of signs of fat loss in patients with human immunodeficiency virus.

SEASONALE   RX
ethinyl estradiol - levonorgestrel (Duramed)

THERAPEUTIC CLASS: Estrogen/progestogen combination

INDICATIONS: Prevention of pregnancy.

DOSAGE: *Adults:* Sunday start regimen. 1 tablet qd for 91 days, then repeat.

HOW SUPPLIED: (Ethinyl Estradiol-Levonorgestrel) Tab: 0.03mg/0.15mg

CONTRAINDICATIONS: Thrombophlebitis, DVT or thromboembolic disorders, pregnancy, cerebrovascular or CAD, valvular heart disease with complications, uncontrolled HTN, DM with vascular involvement, headaches with focal neurological symptoms, major surgery with prolonged immobilization, undiagnosed abnormal genital bleeding, cholestatic jaundice of pregnancy or jaundice with prior pill use, hepatic adenomas or carcinomas, active liver disease, breast cancer, endometrial carcinoma, or other estrogen-dependent neoplasia.

WARNINGS/PRECAUTIONS: Cigarette smoking increases risk of serious CV side effects. This risk increases with age (especially >35 yrs) and heavy smoking. Increased risk of MI, vascular disease, thromboembolism, stroke, HTN, and gallbladder disease. Retinal thrombosis, hepatic neoplasia, carcinoma of breast and reproductive organs reported. May cause glucose intolerance, fluid retention, breakthrough bleeding, and spotting. May increase BP, elevate LDL levels or cause other lipid changes. May cause or exacerbate migraine. May develop visual changes with contact lens. Increased risk of morbidity and mortality with certain inherited thrombophilias, HTN, hyperlipidemia, obesity, and diabetes. D/C if jaundice, significant depression, recurrent/persistent new headache patterns, or ophthalmic irregularities develop. Perform annual physical exam. Not for use before menarche or with uncontrolled HTN. May affect certain endocrine, LFTs, and blood components. Weigh benefit of fewer planned menses against inconvenience of increased intermenstrual bleeding or spotting.

ADVERSE REACTIONS: Nausea, vomiting, breakthrough bleeding, spotting, amenorrhea, migraine, depression, vaginal candidiasis, edema, weight changes.

INTERACTIONS: Reduced effects, increased breakthrough bleeding with rifampin, barbiturates, phenylbutazone, phenytoin, carbamazepine, felbamate, oxcarbazepine, griseofulvin, topiramate, St. John's wort, and possibly with ampicillin and tetracyclines. Atorvastatin, ascorbic acid, acetaminophen, CYP3A4 inhibitors (eg, itraconazole, ketoconazole) may increase hormone levels. Protease inhibitors may increase or decrease levels. May increase levels of cyclosporine, prednisolone, theophylline. May decrease levels of acetaminophen. Increases clearance of temazepam, salicylic acid, morphine, clofibric acid.

PREGNANCY: Category X, not for use in nursing.

MECHANISM OF ACTION: Estrogen/progestogen combination oral contraceptive: Suppresses gonadotropins and primarily inhibits ovulation. Causes changes in cervical mucus (increases difficulty of sperm entry into uterus) and in endometrium (reduces likelihood of implantation).

PHARMACOKINETICS: Absorption: Levonorgestrel: Rapid and complete, absolute bioavailability (100%), C_{max}=5.6ng/mL, T_{max}=1.4 hrs, AUC=60.8ng•hr/mL; Ethinyl estradiol: Rapid, absolute bioavailability (43%), C_{max}=145ng/mL, T_{max}=1.6 hrs, AUC=1307pg•hr/mL. **Distribution:** Levonorgestrel: V_d=1.8L/kg, plasma protein binding (97.5-99%); Ethinyl estradiol: V_d=4.3L/kg, plasma protein binding (95-97%). **Metabolism:** Levonorgestrel: Sulfate and glucuronide conjugates. Ethinyl estradiol: First-pass metabolism, hepatic via CYP3A4 (hydroxylation), methylation, conjugation. **Elimination:** Levonorgestrel: Urine (45%), feces (32%); $T_{1/2}$=30 hrs. Ethinyl estradiol: Urine, feces; $T_{1/2}$=15 hrs.

SEASONIQUE   RX
ethinyl estradiol - levonorgestrel (Duramed)

THERAPEUTIC CLASS: Estrogen/progestogen combination

INDICATIONS: Prevention of pregnancy.

DOSAGE: *Adults:* 1 tablet qd for 91 days, then repeat. During first cycle of medication, start on 1st Sunday after onset of menstruation. Begin next and all subsequent 91-day courses without interruption on same day of week (Sunday) upon which first course began, following the same schedule.

HOW SUPPLIED: (Ethinyl Estradiol-Levonorgestrel) Tab: 0.03mg-0.15mg; (Ethinyl Estradiol) Tab: 0.01mg

CONTRAINDICATIONS: Thrombophlebitis, DVT or thromboembolic disorders, cerebrovascular or CAD, valvular heart disease with thrombogenic complications, uncontrolled HTN, DM with vascular involvement, headaches with focal neurological symptoms, major surgery with prolonged immobilization, breast cancer, endometrial cancer or other estrogen-dependent neoplasia, undiagnosed abnormal genital bleeding, cholestatic jaundice of pregnancy or jaundice with prior pill use, hepatic adenomas or carcinomas, active liver disease, or pregnancy.

WARNINGS/PRECAUTIONS: Cigarette smoking increases risk of serious CV side effects. This risk increases with age (especially >35 yrs) and heavy smoking. Increased risk of MI, vascular disease, thromboembolism, stroke, HTN, and gallbladder disease. Retinal thrombosis, hepatic neoplasia, carcinoma of breast and reproductive organs reported. May cause glucose intolerance, fluid retention, breakthrough bleeding, and spotting. May increase BP, elevate LDL levels or cause other lipid changes. May cause or exacerbate migraine. May develop visual changes with contact lens. Increased risk of morbidity and mortality with certain inherited thrombophilias, HTN, hyperlipidemia, obesity, and diabetes. D/C if jaundice, significant depression, recurrent/persistent new headache patterns, or ophthalmic irregularities develop. Perform annual physical exam. Not for use before menarche or with uncontrolled HTN. May affect certain endocrine, LFTs, and blood components. Weigh benefit of fewer planned menses against inconvenience of increased intermenstrual bleeding or spotting.

ADVERSE REACTIONS: Nausea, vomiting, breakthrough bleeding, spotting, amenorrhea, migraine, depression, vaginal candidiasis, edema, weight changes.

INTERACTIONS: Reduced effects, increased breakthrough bleeding, and menstrual irregularities with rifampin, barbiturates, phenylbutazone, phenytoin, carbamazepine, felbamate, oxcarbazepine, topiramate, hypericum perforatum, griseofulvin, ampicillin, and tetracyclines. Increased levels with atorvastatin, ascorbic acid, APAP, and CYP3A4 (eg, itraconazole, ketoconazole) inhibitors. Anti-HIV protease inhibitors may increase or decrease levels. May increase plasma levels of cyclosporine, prednisolone, and theophylline. May decrease levels of APAP. Increased clearance of temazepam, salicylic acid, morphine, and clofibric acid.

PREGNANCY: Category X, not for use in nursing.

MECHANISM OF ACTION: Estrogen/progestogen combination oral contraceptive. Acts by suppression of gonadotropins. Primarily inhibits ovulation. Also responsible for causing changes in cervical mucus (which increase difficulty of sperm entry into uterus) and in endometrium (which reduce likelihood of implantation).

PHARMACOKINETICS: Absorption: Rapid; T_{max}=2 hrs; Levonorgestrel: Absolute bioavailability (100%). Ethinyl estradiol: Absolute bioavailability (43%). Oral administration of variable doses resulted in different parameters. **Distribution:** Levonorgestrel: V_d=1.8L/kg; plasma protein binding (97.5-99%). Ethinyl estradiol: V_d=4.3L/kg; plasma protein binding (95-97%). **Metabolism:** Levonogestrel: Sulfate and glucuronide conjugates. Ethinyl estradiol: 1st pass metabolism in gut wall, Hepatic, via CYP3A4 (hydroxylation), methylation, conjugation. **Elimination:** Levonorgestrel: Urine (45%), feces (32%); $T_{1/2}$=34 hrs. Ethinyl estradiol: Urine, feces; $T_{1/2}$=18 hrs.

SECONAL SODIUM

CII

secobarbital sodium (Ranbaxy)

THERAPEUTIC CLASS: Barbiturate

INDICATIONS: Hypnotic, for the short-term treatment of insomnia (may lose effectiveness after 2 weeks); Preanesthetic.

DOSAGE: *Adults:* Hypnotic: 100mg hs; Preoperatively: 200-300mg, 1-2 hrs before surgery; Elderly/Debilitated/Renal or Hepatic Dysfunction: Reduce dose. *Pediatrics:* Preoperatively: 2-6mg/kg. Max: 100mg.

HOW SUPPLIED: Cap: 100mg

CONTRAINDICATIONS: History of manifest or latent porphyria, marked impairment of liver function, or respiratory disease in which dyspnea or obstruction is evident.

WARNINGS/PRECAUTIONS: May be habit-forming; avoid abrupt cessation after prolonged use. Tolerance, psychological and physical dependence may occur with continued use. Use with caution, if at all, in patients who are mentally depressed, have suicidal tendencies, or have a history of drug abuse.

In patients with hepatic damage, use with caution and initially reduce dose. Caution when administering to patients with acute or chronic pain. May impair mental and/or physical abilities. Avoid alcohol.

ADVERSE REACTIONS: Agitation, confusion, hyperkinesia, ataxia, CNS depression, somnolence, bradycardia, hypotension, nausea, vomiting, constipation, headache, hypersensitivity reactions, liver damage.

INTERACTIONS: May increase metabolism and decrease response to oral anticoagulants and enhance metabolism of exogenous corticosteroids. May interfere with absorption of griseofulvin, decreasing its blood level. May shorten half-life of doxycycline for up to 2 weeks after being discontinued. Variable effect on phenytoin and increased levels with sodium valproate and valproic acid; monitor blood levels and adjust dose appropriately. May cause additive depressant effects with other CNS depressants (eg, sedatives/hypnotics, antihistamines, tranquilizers, alcohol). Prolonged effects with MAOIs. May decrease effect of estradiol; alternative contraceptive methods should be suggested.

PREGNANCY: Category D, caution in nursing.

MECHANISM OF ACTION: Barbiturates, nonselective CNS depressants; depress sensory cortex, decrease motor activity, alter cerebellar function, and produce drowsiness, sedation, and hypnosis.

PHARMACOKINETICS: Absorption: Rapidly absorbed. **Distribution:** Crosses placenta, found in breast milk. **Metabolism:** Liver. **Elimination:** Urine and feces; $T_{1/2}$=28 hrs.

SECTRAL   RX
acetabulol HCL (ESP Pharma)

THERAPEUTIC CLASS: Selective beta$_1$-blocker

INDICATIONS: Management of hypertension, ventricular arrhythmias.

DOSAGE: *Adults:* HTN: Initial: 400mg/day, given qd-bid. Usual: 200-800mg/day. Max: 1200mg/day. Ventricular Arrhythmia: Initial: 200mg bid. Maint: Increase gradually to 600-1200mg/day. Elderly: Lower daily doses. Max: 800mg/day. CrCl <50mL/min: Decrease daily dose by 50%. CrCl <25mL/min: Decrease daily dose by 75%.

HOW SUPPLIED: Cap: 200mg, 400mg

CONTRAINDICATIONS: Persistently severe bradycardia, 2nd- and 3rd-degree heart block, overt cardiac failure, cardiogenic shock.

WARNINGS/PRECAUTIONS: Withdrawal before surgery is controversial. Caution with bronchospastic disease, peripheral or mesenteric vascular disease, aortic or mitral valve disease, left ventricular dysfunction, heart failure controlled by digitalis and/or diuretics, hepatic or renal dysfunction. May mask hypoglycemia or hyperthyroidism symptoms. Avoid abrupt discontinuation. May develop antinuclear antibodies (ANA).

ADVERSE REACTIONS: Fatigue, dizziness, headache, constipation, diarrhea, dyspepsia, flatulence, nausea, dyspnea, urinary frequency, insomnia.

INTERACTIONS: Possible additive effects with catecholamine-depleting drugs. NSAIDs may reduce effects. Exaggerated hypertensive responses with alpha stimulants. May antagonize epinephrine. May potentiate insulin-induced hypoglycemia.

PREGNANCY: Category B, not for use in nursing.

MECHANISM OF ACTION: Cardioselective β-adrenoreceptor blocking agent: causes reduction in HR and systolic BP.

PHARMACOKINETICS: Absorption: Well-absorbed; Absolute bioavailability (40%); T_{max}=2.5 hrs. **Distribution:** Plasma protein binding (26%); Crosses placental barrier, secreted in breast milk. **Metabolism:** Diacetolol (major metabolite). **Elimination:** Renal (30-40%), nonrenal (50-60%). (Sectral, Diacetolol) $T_{1/2}$=(3-4, 8-13 hrs.)

SELENIUM SULFIDE TOPICAL RX
selenium sulfide (Various)

THERAPEUTIC CLASS: Antiseborrheic/antifungal

INDICATIONS: Treatment of tinea versicolor, seborrheic dermatitis of the scalp, and dandruff.

DOSAGE: *Adults:* Tinea Versicolor: Apply qd and lather with small amount of water. Rinse off after 10 min. Use for 7 days. Seborrheic Dermatitis/Dandruff: Massage into wet scalp, rinse off after 2-3 min and repeat. Usual: 2 applications/week for 2 weeks. Maint: Use weekly, every 2 weeks, or every 3-4 weeks.

HOW SUPPLIED: Lot: 2.5% [120mL]

WARNINGS/PRECAUTIONS: Avoid with inflammation, exudation, or broken skin. Avoid eyes, genital area, and skinfolds; may cause irritation. Not for treatment of tinea versicolor in pregnant women.

ADVERSE REACTIONS: Skin irritation, increased loss of hair, hair discoloration, oiliness or dryness of scalp.

PREGNANCY: Category C, safety in nursing is not known.

SELZENTRY RX
maraviroc (Pfizer)

> Hepatotoxicity reported; may be preceded by evidence of allergic reaction. Evaluate patients immediately with signs or symptoms of hepatitis or allergic reaction (eg, pruritic rash, eosinophilia, elevated IgE).

THERAPEUTIC CLASS: CCR5 co-receptor antagonist

INDICATIONS: Combination antiretroviral treatment of adults infected with only CCR5-tropic HIV-1 detectable, who have evidence of viral replication and HIV-1 strains resistant to multiple antiretroviral agents.

DOSAGE: *Adults:* >16 yrs: Give in combination with other antiretroviral medications. With Strong CYP3A Inhibitors (with or without CYP3A inducers) Including PIs (except tipranavir/ritonavir), Delavirdine: 150mg bid. With NRTIs, Tipranavir/Ritonavir, Nevirapine, Other Drugs That Are Not Strong CYP3A Inhibitors/Inducers: 300mg bid. With CYP3A Inducers (without strong CYP3A inhibitor): 600mg bid.

HOW SUPPLIED: Tab: 150mg, 300mg

WARNINGS/PRECAUTIONS: D/C if signs or symptoms of hepatitis or with increased liver transaminases combined with rash or other systemic symptoms. Caution with pre-existing liver dysfunction or co-infection with viral hepatitis B or C. Caution with increased risk for CV events especially with history of postural hypotension or on concomitant medication to lower BP. Immune reconstitution syndrome reported. May increase risk of developing infections; monitor closely for evidence of infections.

ADVERSE REACTIONS: Cough, pyrexia, upper respiratory tract infections, rash, musculoskeletal symptoms, abdominal pain, dizziness, diarrhea, edema, esophageal candidiasis, sleep disorders, rhinitis, urinary abnormalities.

INTERACTIONS: Coadministration with CYP3A inhibitors, including protease inhibitors (except tipranavir/ritonavir) and delaviridine, will increase levels. Coadministration with CYP3A inducers, including efavirenz, may decrease levels. Concomitant use with St. John's wort is not recommended.

PREGNANCY: Category B, not for use in nursing.

MECHANISM OF ACTION: CCR5 co-receptor antagonist; selectively binds to human chemokine receptor CCR5 present on cell membranes, preventing interaction of HIV-1 gp120 and CCR5 necessary for CCR5-tropic HIV-1 to enter cells.

PHARMACOKINETICS: Absorption: (1-1200mg) T_{max}=0.5-4 hrs. (100mg, 300mg) Absolute bioavailability (23%, 33%). **Distribution:** Plasma protein binding (76%); V_d=194L. **Metabolism:** CYP3A; secondary amine

(N-dealkylation metabolite). **Elimination:** T$_{1/2}$=14-18 hrs; urine: 20% (8% unchanged), feces: 76% (25% unchanged).

SENOKOT   OTC
senna (Purdue Products)

THERAPEUTIC CLASS: Stimulant laxative

INDICATIONS: To relieve functional constipation. Senokot-S also contains a stool softener.

DOSAGE: *Adults:* Take at bedtime. (Senokot/Senokot-S) 2 tabs qd. Max: 4 tabs bid. (SenokotXTRA) 1 tab qd. Max: 2 tabs bid. (Granules) 5mL qd. Max: 15mL bid. Granules may be eaten plain, mixed with liquids, or sprinkled on food.
Pediatrics: Take at bedtime. (Senokot/Senokot-S) ≥12 yrs: 2 tabs qd. Max: 4 tabs bid. 6-12 yrs: 1 tab qd. Max: 2 tabs bid. 2-6 yrs: 1/2 tab qd. Max: 1 tab bid. (SenokotXTRA) ≥12 yrs: 1 tab qd. Max: 2 tabs bid. 6-12 yrs: 1/2 tab qd. Max: 1 tab bid. (Granules) ≥12 yrs: 1 tsp qd. Max: 2 tsp bid. 6-12 yrs: 1/2 tsp qd. Max: 1 tsp bid. 2-6 yrs: 1/4 tsp qd. Max: 1/2 tsp bid. Granules may be eaten plain, mixed with liquids, or sprinkled on food.

HOW SUPPLIED: Granules: 15mg/dose; Tab (Sennoside A and B): (Senokot) 8.6mg, (SenokotXTRA) 17mg; (Docusate Sodium-Sennoside A and B) (Senokot-S) 50mg-8.6mg

WARNINGS/PRECAUTIONS: Do not use with abdominal pain, nausea, or vomiting. Should not be used for longer than 1 week. Rectal bleeding or failure to have a bowel movement after use may indicate serious condition.

INTERACTIONS: Avoid mineral oil with Senokot-S.

PREGNANCY: Safety in pregnancy and nursing not known.

SENSIPAR   RX
cinacalcet HCL (Amgen)

THERAPEUTIC CLASS: Calcimimetic agent

INDICATIONS: Secondary hyperparathyroidism in patients with chronic kidney disease on dialysis. Hypercalcemia in parathyroid carcinoma.

DOSAGE: *Adults:* Take with food. Swallow whole. Secondary Hyperparathyroidism: Initial: 30mg qd. Titrate: Increase no more frequently than every 2-4 weeks through sequential doses of 60, 90, 120, and 180mg qd to target iPTH of 150-300pg/mL. Parathyroid Carcinoma: Initial: 30mg bid. Titrate: Increase every 2-4 weeks through sequential doses of 30mg bid, 60mg bid, 90mg bid, and 90mg tid-qid prn to normalize serum Ca levels. Adjust based on serum Ca levels (see PI). May be used alone or in combination with vitamin D sterols and/or phosphate binders.

HOW SUPPLIED: Tab: 30mg, 60mg, 90mg

WARNINGS/PRECAUTIONS: Monitor closely for hypocalcemia, especially with history of seizure disorder. Do not initiate with serum Ca <8.4mg/dL. Measure serum Ca and phosphorus within 1 week and iPTH 1-4 weeks after initiation or dose adjustment. After maintenance dose reached, measure serum Ca and phosphorus monthly and iPTH every 1-3 months. Adynamic bone disease may develop with iPTH levels <100pg/mL; reduce dose or d/c therapy if iPTH <150pg/mL. Caution with moderate/severe hepatic impairment.

ADVERSE REACTIONS: Nausea, vomiting, diarrhea, myalgia, dizziness, HTN, asthenia, anorexia, chest pain (non-cardiac), access infection.

INTERACTIONS: Drugs metabolized by CYP2D6 (eg, flecainide, vinblastine, thioridazine, most TCAs) may require dose adjustment. Increased amitriptyline, nortriptyline levels in CYP2D6 extensive metabolizers. Increased levels with strong CYP3A4 inhibitors (eg, ketoconazole, erythromycin, itraconazole); may require dose adjustments.

PREGNANCY: Category C, not for use in nursing.

S

MECHANISM OF ACTION: Calcimimetic agent. Lowers PTH levels by increasing the sensitivity of the calcium-sensing receptor to extracellular calcium.

PHARMACOKINETICS: Absorption: T_{max}=2-6 hrs. **Distribution:** V_d=1000L. Plasma protein binding (93-97%); found in breast milk. **Metabolism:** Rapid and extensively metabolized. Liver via CYP450 enzymes 3A4, 2D6, and 1A2. Oxidation, conjugation, and glucuronidation. **Elimination**: $T_{1/2}$ = 30 to 40 hrs; urine (80%), feces (15%).

SENSORCAINE WITH EPINEPHRINE   RX
bupivacaine HCL - epinephrine (Abraxis)

OTHER BRAND NAMES: Sensorcaine-MPF w/Epinephrine (Abraxis)

THERAPEUTIC CLASS: Local anesthetic

INDICATIONS: Production of local or regional anesthesia for surgery, oral surgery procedures, diagnostic and therapeutic procedures, and for obstetrical procedures. Only 0.25% and 0.5% are indicated for obstetrical anesthesia.

DOSAGE: *Adults:* Individualize dose. Dosage varies depending on procedure, area to be anesthetized, vascularity of tissues, number of neural segments to be blocked, depth and duration of anesthesia, degree of muscle relaxation required, and patient tolerance and physical condition. Single Dose Max: 225mg. May repeat once every 3 hrs. Total Daily Dose Max: 400mg. Epidural Anesthesia: 0.5% or 0.75% in 3-5mL increments. In obstetrics, use only 0.25% or 0.5%. Use 3-5mL increments of 0.5% solution not to exceed 50-100mg at any dosing interval. Repeat doses should be preceded by test dose containing epinephrine if not contraindicated. Young/Elderly/Debilitated/Cardiac or Liver Disease: Reduce dose.
Pediatrics: ≥12 yrs: Individualize dose. Dosage varies depending on procedure, area to be anesthetized, vascularity of tissues, number of neural segments to be blocked, depth and duration of anesthesia, degree of muscle relaxation required, and patient tolerance and physical condition. Single Dose Max: 225mg. May repeat once every 3 hrs. Total Daily Dose Max: 400mg. Epidural Anesthesia: 0.5% or 0.75% in 3-5mL increments. In obstetrics, use only 0.25% or 0.5%. Use 3-5mL increments of 0.5% solution not to exceed 50-100mg at any dosing interval. Repeat doses should be preceded by test dose containing epinephrine if not contraindicated.

HOW SUPPLIED: Inj: (Bupivacaine-Epinephrine) 0.25%/1:200,000, 0.5%/1:200,000; (MPF) 0.25%/1:200,000, 0.5%/1:200,000, 0.75%/1:200,000

CONTRAINDICATIONS: Obstetrical paracervical block anesthesia.

WARNINGS/PRECAUTIONS: The 0.75% strength is not recommended for obstetrical anesthesia. Acidosis, cardiac arrest, death reported from delay in toxicity management. Local anesthetic solutions containing antimicrobial preservatives should not be used for epidural or caudal anesthesia. Not recommended for IV regional anesthesia. Bupivacaine with epinephrine solutions contain sodium metabisulfite which may cause allergic-type reactions in susceptible people. Monitor cardiovascular and respiratory vital signs and state of consciousness after each injection. Caution when local anesthetic solutions containing a vasoconstrictor are used in areas of the body supplied by end arteries or having otherwise compromised blood supply; ischemic injury or necrosis may result with hypertensive vascular disease. Caution with hepatic disease and impaired cardiovascular function. Monitor circulation and respiration with injections into head and neck area. Respiratory arrest following local anesthetic injection during retrobulbar blocks has been reported.

ADVERSE REACTIONS: Restlessness, anxiety, dizziness, tinnitus, blurred vision, tremors, convulsions, NV, chills, hypotension, bradycardia, ventricular arrhythmias, urticaria, pruritus, erythema, edema.

INTERACTIONS: Avoid use with any other local anesthetics. Anesthetic solutions containing epinephrine or norepinephrine with MAOIs or TCAs may produce severe, prolonged HTN; avoid concurrent use or monitor closely if concurrent use is necessary. Concurrent administration of vasopressors and ergot-type oxytocic drugs may cause severe, persistent HTN or CVA. Phenothiazines and butyrophenones may reduce or reverse the pressor effect

S

of epinephrine. Serious dose-related cardiac arrhythmias may occur with use during or following administration of potent inhalation anesthetics.

PREGNANCY: Category C, not for use in nursing.

MECHANISM OF ACTION: Long-acting amide-type local anaesthetic; causes a reversible blockade of impulse propagation along nerve fibres by preventing the inward movement of sodium ions through the cell membrane of the nerve fibres.

PHARMACOKINETICS: Absorption: Complete and biphasic. C_{max}=1-4mg/L; T_{max}=20-45 minutes. **Distribution:** V_d=73L; plasma protein binding (96%); crosses placenta; found in breast milk. **Metabolism:** Liver (extensive), through aromatic hydroxylation and N-dealkylation, via: CYP3A4 to PPX and 4-hydroxy-bupivacaine.**Elimination:** Urine (1%, unchanged); $T_{1/2}$=2.7 hrs (adults), $T_{1/2}$=8 hrs (neonates).

SENSORCAINE-MPF RX
bupivacaine HCL (Abraxis)

OTHER BRAND NAMES: Sensorcaine - Inactive (Abraxis)

THERAPEUTIC CLASS: Local anesthetic

INDICATIONS: Production of local or regional anesthesia for surgery, oral surgery procedures, diagnostic and therapeutic procedures, and for obstetrical procedures. Only 0.25% and 0.5% are indicated for obstetrical anesthesia.

DOSAGE: *Adults:* Individualize dose. Dosage varies depending on procedure, area to be anesthetized, vascularity of tissues, number of neural segments to be blocked, depth and duration of anesthesia, degree of muscle relaxation required, and patient tolerance and physical condition. Single Dose Max: 175mg. May repeat once every 3 hrs. Total Daily Dose Max: 400mg. Epidural Anesthesia: 0.5% or 0.75% in 3-5mL increments. In obstetrics, use only 0.25% or 0.5%. Use 3-5mL increments of 0.5% solution not to exceed 50-100mg at any dosing interval. Repeat doses should be preceded by test dose containing epinephrine if not contraindicated. Young/Elderly/Debilitated/Cardiac or Liver Disease: Reduce dose.
Pediatrics: ≥12 yrs: Individualize dose. Dosage varies depending on procedure, area to be anesthetized, vascularity of tissues, number of neural segments to be blocked, depth and duration of anesthesia, degree of muscle relaxation required, and patient tolerance and physical condition. Single Dose Max: 175mg. May repeat once every 3 hrs. Total Daily Dose Max: 400mg. Epidural Anesthesia: 0.5% in 3-5mL increments. In obstetrics, use only 0.25% or 0.5%. Use 3-5mL increments of 0.5% solution not to exceed 50-100mg at any dosing interval. Repeat doses should be preceded by test dose containing epinephrine if not contraindicated.

HOW SUPPLIED: Inj: 0.25%, 0.5%; (MPF) 0.25%, 0.5%, 0.75%

CONTRAINDICATIONS: Obstetrical paracervical block anesthesia.

WARNINGS/PRECAUTIONS: The 0.75% strength is not recommended for obstetrical anesthesia. Acidosis, cardiac arrest, death reported from delay in toxicity management. Local anesthetic solutions containing antimicrobial preservatives should not be used for epidural or caudal anesthesia. Not recommended for IV regional anesthesia. Monitor cardiovascular and respiratory vital signs and state of consciousness after each injection. Caution with hepatic disease and impaired cardiovascular function. Monitor circulation and respiration with injections into head and neck area. Respiratory arrest following local anesthetic injection during retrobulbar blocks has been reported.

ADVERSE REACTIONS: Restlessness, anxiety, dizziness, tinnitus, blurred vision, tremors, convulsions, nausea, vomiting, chills, hypotension, bradycardia, ventricular arrhythmias, urticaria, pruritus, erythema, edema.

INTERACTIONS: Avoid use with any other local anesthetics.

PREGNANCY: Category C, not for use in nursing.

MECHANISM OF ACTION: A long-acting amide-type local anaesthetic; causes a reversible blockade of impulse propagation along nerve fibers by preventing the inward movement of sodium ions through the cell membrane of the nerve fibers.

PHARMACOKINETICS: Absorption: Complete and biphasic. C_{max}=1-4mg/L; T_{max}= 20-45 min. **Distribution:** V_d=73L; plasma protein binding (96%); crosses placenta, found in breast milk. **Metabolism:** Liver (extensive), through aromatic hydroxylation and N-dealkylation, via CYP3A4 to PPX and 4-hydroxy-bupivacaine. **Elimination:** Urine (1%, unchanged); $T_{1/2}$=2.7 hrs (adults), 8 hrs (neonates).

SEPTOCAINE WITH EPINEPHRINE   RX
articaine HCL - epinephrine (Septodont)

THERAPEUTIC CLASS: Anesthetic agent

INDICATIONS: For local, infiltrative, or conductive anesthesia in both simple and complex dental and periodontal procedures.

DOSAGE: *Adults:* Submucosal Infiltration: 0.5-2.5mL. Nerve Block: 0.5-3.4mL. Oral Surgery: 1-5.1mL. Max: 7mg/kg (0.175mL/kg) or 3.2mg/lb (0.0795mL/lb). *Pediatrics:* ≥4 yrs: Submucosal Infiltration/Nerve Block/Oral Surgery: up to 7mg/kg (0.175mL/kg) or 3.2mg/lb (0.0795mL/lb).

HOW SUPPLIED: Inj: (Articaine-Epinephrine) 4%-1:100,000/1.7mL, 4%-1:200,000/1.7mL.

CONTRAINDICATIONS: Hypersensitivity to sodium metabisulfite.

WARNINGS/PRECAUTIONS: Avoid intravascular injection; aspirate needle before use. Intravascular injection is associated with convulsions, followed by CNS or cardiorespiratory depression and coma progressing to respiratory arrest. Epinephrine can cause local tissue necrosis or systemic toxicity. Contains sodium metabisulfite which can cause allergic reactions. Exaggerated vasoconstrictive response may occur with peripheral vascular disease and hypertensive vascular disease. CNS or cardiovascular effects may occur with systemic absorption. Local anesthetics are capable of producing methemoglobinemia, with signs of cyanosis, fatigue, and weakness.

ADVERSE REACTIONS: Face edema, headache, infection, pain, gingivitis, swelling, paresthesia, trismus.

INTERACTIONS: MAOIs or TCAs may produce severe, prolonged HTN. Phenothiazines and butyrphenones may reduce or reverse pressor effect of epinephrine.

PREGNANCY: Category C, caution in nursing.

MECHANISM OF ACTION: Anaesthetic used in dental procedures.

SEPTRA   RX
sulfamethoxazole - trimethoprim (King)

OTHER BRAND NAMES: Sulfatrim Pediatric (Alpharma) - Septra DS (King)

THERAPEUTIC CLASS: Sulfonamide/tetrahydrofolic acid inhibitor

INDICATIONS: Treatment of urinary tract infections (UTI), acute otitis media, acute exacerbations of chronic bronchitis (AECB), *Pneumocystis carinii* pneumonia (PCP), traveler's diarrhea, and shigellosis caused by susceptible strains of microorganisms.

DOSAGE: *Adults:* UTI/Shigellosis: 800mg-160mg PO q12h for 10-14 days (UTI) or 5 days (shigellosis). AECB: 800mg-160mg PO q12h for 14 days. Traveler's Diarrhea: 800mg-160mg PO q12h for 5 days. PCP Treatment: 15-20mg/kg TMP and 75-100mg/kg SMX per 24 hrs given PO q6h for 14-21 days. PCP Prophylaxis: 800mg-160mg PO qd. Renal Impairment: CrCl 15-30mL/min: 50% usual dose. CrCl <15mL/min: Not recommended.
Pediatrics: ≥2 months: UTI/Otitis Media/Shigellosis: 4mg/kg TMP and 20mg/kg SMX q12h for 10 days (UTI/otitis media) or 5 days (shigellosis). PCP Treatment: 15-20mg/kg TMP and 75-100mg/kg SMX per 24 hrs given q6h for 14-21 days. PCP Prophylaxis: 150mg/m²/day TMP and 750mg/m²/day

SMX PO given bid, on 3 consecutive days per week. Max: 320mg TMP and 1600mg SMX per day. Renal Impairment: CrCl 15-30mL/min: 50% usual dose. CrCl <15mL/min: Not recommended.

HOW SUPPLIED: (Sulfamethoxazole [SMX]-Trimethoprim [TMP]) Sus: (Sulfatrim Pediatric, Septra) 200mg-40mg/5mL [100mL, 473mL]; Tab: (Septra) *400mg-80mg**; Tab, DS: (Septra DS) *800mg-160mg** *scored

CONTRAINDICATIONS: Megaloblastic anemia due to folate deficiency, pregnancy at term, nursing, infants <2 months old.

WARNINGS/PRECAUTIONS: Fatal hypersensitivity reactions (eg, Stevens-Johnson syndrome, toxic epidermal necrolysis, fulminant hepatic necrosis, agranulocytosis, aplastic anemia) may occur. Cough, SOB, and pulmonary infiltrates reported. Avoid with group A β-hemolytic streptococcal infections. *Clostridium difficile*-associated diarrhea reported. Caution with hepatic/renal impairment, elderly, folate deficiency (eg, chronic alcoholics, anticonvulsants, malabsorption, malnutrition), bronchial asthma, and other allergies. In G6PD deficiency, hemolysis may occur. Increased incidence of adverse events in AIDS patients. Maintain adequate fluid intake.

ADVERSE REACTIONS: Anorexia, nausea, vomiting, rash, urticaria, cough, SOB, cholestatic jaundice, agranulocytosis, anemia, hyperkalemia, renal failure, interstitial nephritis, hyponatremia, convulsions.

INTERACTIONS: Increase risk of thrombocytopenia with purpura with diuretics (especially thiazides) in the elderly. Caution with warfarin; may prolong PT. Increased effects of phenytoin, methotrexate. Concomitant ACE inhibitor therapy may cause hyperkalemia.

PREGNANCY: Category C, not for use in nursing.

MECHANISM OF ACTION: Sulfamethoxazole: Inhibits bacterial synthesis of dihydrofolic acid by competing with para-aminobenzoic acid (PABA). Trimetophrim: Blocks production of tetrahydrofolic acid from dihydrofolic acid by binding to and reversibly inhibiting required enzyme, dihydrofolate reductase; thus drug blocks 2 consecutive steps in biosynthesis of nucleic acids and proteins essential to many bacteria.

PHARMACOKINETICS: Absorption: Rapid; T_{max}=1-4 hrs. **Distribution:** Trimethoprim: Plasma protein binding (44%); Sulfamethoxazole: Plasma protein binding (70%). Crosses placenta, found in breast milk. **Metabolism:** Sulfamethoxazole: N_4 acetylation. Trimethoprim: 1-and 3-oxide, 3'-and 4'-hydroxy derivative (principal metabolites). **Elimination:** Urine, trimethoprim (66.8%), sulfamethoxazole (84.5%; 30% as free and remaining as N_4 acetylated metabolite); $T_{1/2}$=10 hr (sulfamethoxazole), 8-10 hr (trimethoprim).

SEREVENT
salmeterol xinafoate (GlaxoSmithKline)

RX

Long-acting β₂-adrenergic agonists, such as salmeterol, may increase the risk of asthma-related deaths.

THERAPEUTIC CLASS: Beta₂-agonist

INDICATIONS: Long-term maintenance treatment of asthma and COPD. Prevention of bronchospasm with reversible obstructive airway disease (including nocturnal asthma) when regular treatment with inhaled short-acting β₂-agonists is required. Prevention of exercise-induced bronchospasm (EIB).

DOSAGE: *Adults:* Asthma/COPD: 1 inh bid, am and pm (12 hrs apart). EIB Prevention: 1 inh 30 min before exercise (do not give preventive doses if already on bid dose).
Pediatrics: ≥4 yrs: Asthma: 1 inh bid, am and pm (12 hrs apart). EIB Prevention: 1 inh 30 min before exercise (do not give preventive doses if already on bid dose).

HOW SUPPLIED: Disk: 50mcg [28, 60 blisters]

WARNINGS/PRECAUTIONS: Avoid with significantly worsening or acutely deteriorating asthma. Not for acute treatment or substitute for oral/inhaled corticosteroids. Monitor for increasing use of inhaled β₂ agonists. QTc interval prolongation reported when exceeded recommended dose. D/C if paradoxical bronchospasm occurs. Immediate hypersensitivity and upper airway symptom reactions reported. Caution with cardiovascular disorder (eg, coronary insufficiency, arrhythmia, HTN), convulsive disorders, thyrotoxicosis, if usually unresponsive to sympathomimetic amines. May cause hypokalemia.

ADVERSE REACTIONS: Nasal/sinus congestion, pallor, rhinitis, headache, tracheitis/bronchitis, influenza, throat irritation.

INTERACTIONS: Caution with non-potassium-sparing diuretics. Extreme caution within 14 days of using MAOIs or TCAs. Avoid with β-blockers. Caution with >8 inhalations of short-acting β$_2$-agonists.

PREGNANCY: Category C, not for use in nursing.

MECHANISM OF ACTION: β$_2$-adrenergic agonist; increases cAMP levels causing relaxation of bronchial smooth muscles and inhibits the release of mediators of immediate hypersensitivity from mast cells.

PHARMACOKINETICS: Absorption: C$_{max}$=167pg/mL; T$_{max}$=20 min. **Distribution**: Plasma protein binding (96%). **Metabolism**: Liver (aliphatic oxidation) via CYP3A4. (Metabolite) α-hydroxysalmeterol. **Elimination**: T$_{1/2}$=5.5 hrs.

SEROMYCIN   RX
cycloserine (Lilly)

THERAPEUTIC CLASS: Cell wall synthesis inhibitor

INDICATIONS: Adjunct treatment of active pulmonary and extrapulmonary TB (including renal disease) when primary agents (eg, streptomycin, isoniazid, rifampin, ethambutol) are inadequate. May be effective for treatment of acute UTI caused by susceptible strains of microorganisms when conventional therapy has failed.

DOSAGE: *Adults:* Initial: 250mg bid (q12h) for 2 weeks. Usual: 500mg-1g daily in divided doses; monitor by blood levels. Max: 1g/day.

HOW SUPPLIED: Cap: 250mg

CONTRAINDICATIONS: Epilepsy, depression, severe anxiety, psychosis, severe renal insufficiency, excessive concurrent alcohol use.

WARNINGS/PRECAUTIONS: D/C or reduce dose if allergic reaction or symptoms of CNS toxicity (eg, convulsions, somnolence, depression, confusion, headache, psychosis) occur. Increased risk of toxicity with blood levels >30mcg/mL. Narrow therapeutic index; caution in dosing. Increased risk of convulsions in chronic alcoholics. Monitor hematology, blood levels, renal and liver functions. Monitor cultures and susceptibility prior to therapy. Vitamin B$_{12}$ and/or folic acid deficiency, megaloblastic anemia and sideroblastic anemia; institute appropriate therapy.

ADVERSE REACTIONS: Drowsiness, headache, tremor, skin rash, vertigo.

INTERACTIONS: Contraindicated with excessive alcohol use. Increased neurotoxicity with ethionamide. Increased incidence of CNS effects with isoniazid.

PREGNANCY: Category C, not for use in nursing.

MECHANISM OF ACTION: Antibacterial agent; inhibits cell wall synthesis in susceptible strains of gram-positive and gram-negative bacteria and in Mycobacterium tuberculosis.

PHARMACOKINETICS: Absorption: Readily absorbed. T$_{max}$=4-8 hrs. **Distribution:** Found in CSF, breast milk, fetal blood, pleural fluid. **Elimination:** Urine (65%).

SEROPHENE   RX
clomiphene citrate (EMD Serono)

THERAPEUTIC CLASS: Ovulatory stimulant

INDICATIONS: Treatment of ovulatory dysfunction in women desiring pregnancy.

DOSAGE: *Adults:* Initial: 50mg/day for 5 days. Start any time if no recent uterine bleeding. If progestin-induced bleeding is intended, or if spontaneous uterine bleeding occurs, start on the 5th day of the cycle. If ovulation does not occur, increase to 100mg qd for 5 days, 30 days after the 1st course. Max: 100mg qd for 5 days and 3 courses of therapy.

HOW SUPPLIED: Tab: 50mg

CONTRAINDICATIONS: Pregnancy, liver disease or history of liver dysfunction, abnormal uterine bleeding of undetermined origin, ovarian cysts or enlargement not due to polycystic ovarian syndrome, uncontrolled thyroid or adrenal dysfunction, organic intracranial lesion (eg, pituitary tumor).

WARNINGS/PRECAUTIONS: Increased incidence of visual symptoms with increasing total dose or therapy duration; d/c treatment and perform complete ophthalmological evaluation. Ovarian hyperstimulation syndrome reported; monitor for abdominal pain, nausea, vomiting, diarrhea, weight gain. Increased chance of multiple pregnancy. Perform pelvic exam before initiating therapy and before each course. Prolonged use may increase risk of borderline/invasive ovarian tumor.

ADVERSE REACTIONS: Ovarian enlargement, vasomotor flushes, nausea, vomiting, breast discomfort, abdominal-pelvic discomfort/distention/bloating, visual symptoms, headache, abnormal uterine bleeding.

PREGNANCY: Category X, caution in nursing.

MECHANISM OF ACTION: Ovulatory stimulant; increases release of pituitary gonadotropins; initiates steroidogenesis and folliculogenesis, resulting in growth of ovarian follicle and increase in circulating levels of estradiol, thus culminating in a preovulatory gonadotropin surge and subsequent follicular rupture. Following ovulation, plasma progesterone and estradiol rise and fall as they would in normal ovulatory cycle.

PHARMACOKINETICS: Absorption: Readily absorbed. **Elimination**: Urine (approximately 8%), feces (42%).

SEROQUEL   RX
quetiapine fumarate (AstraZeneca)

> Elderly patients with dementia-related psychosis treated with atypical antipsychotic drugs are at an increased risk of death; most appeared to be cardiovascular (eg, heart failure, sudden death) or infectious (eg, pneumonia) in nature. Quetiapine is not approved for the treatment of patients with dementia-related psychosis. Antidepressants increased the risk of suicidal thinking and behavior (suicidality) in short-term studies in children, adolescents, and young adults with Major Depressive Disorder (MDD) and other psychiatric disorders. Quetiapine is not approved for use in pediatric patients.

THERAPEUTIC CLASS: Dibenzapine derivative

INDICATIONS: Treatment of schizophrenia. Treatment of depressive episodes associated with bipolar disorder. Treatment of acute manic episodes associated with bipolar I disorder, as monotherapy or adjunct therapy to lithium or divalproex. Maintenance treatment of bipolar I disorder as adjunct therapy to lithium or divalproex.

DOSAGE: *Adults:* Bipolar Depressive Episodes: Give once daily hs. Day 1: 50mg/day. Day 2: 100mg/day. Day 3: 200mg/day. Day 4: 300mg/day. Bipolar Mania: Monotherapy/Adjunctive: Give bid. Initial: 100mg/day on Day 1. Titrate: Increase to 400mg/day on Day 4 in increments of up to 100mg/day in bid divided doses. Adjust doses up to 800mg/day by Day 6 in increments ≤200mg/day. Max: 800mg/day. Maintenance for Bipolar I Disorder: Give bid. 400-800mg/day. Schizophrenia: Initial: 25mg bid. Titrate: Increase by 25-50mg bid-tid on the 2nd and 3rd day to 300-400mg/day given bid-tid by the 4th day. Adjust doses by 25-50mg bid at intervals of at least 2 days. Maint: Lowest effective dose. Max: 800mg/day. Hepatic Impairment: Initial: 25mg/day. Titrate: Increase by 25-50mg/day to effective dose. Elderly/Debilitated/Predisposition to Hypotension: Consider slower rate of dose titration and lower target dose.

HOW SUPPLIED: Tab: 25mg, 50mg, 100mg, 200mg, 300mg, 400mg

S

WARNINGS/PRECAUTIONS: NMS reported. May develop tardive dyskinesia. Hyperglycemia reported; monitor regularly for worsening of glucose control. May induce orthostatic hypotension. Caution with cardiovascular disease, cerebrovascular disease, conditions which predispose to hypotension (eg, dehydration, hypovolemia), history of seizures. Monitor for cataracts at initiation, then every 6 months. Possible hypothyroidism. Hepatic enzyme, cholesterol and triglyceride elevations reported. May impair judgment, thinking and motor skills. Priapism reported. May disrupt body's ability to reduce core temperature. Caution in patients at risk for aspiration, elderly, debilitated. Depression may worsen in patients or suicidal thoughts and behaviors may also arise.

ADVERSE REACTIONS: Headache, dizziness, postural hypotension, dry mouth, dyspepsia, tachycardia, somnolence, constipation.

INTERACTIONS: Caution with other CNS drugs. Increased cognitive and motor effects of alcohol. May antagonize effects of levodopa and dopamine agonists. May enhance effects of antihypertensives. Phenytoin or other hepatic enzyme inducers (eg, carbamazepine, barbiturates, glucocorticoids) may reduce levels. Caution with inhibitors of CYP3A (eg, itraconazole, ketoconazole, fluconazole, erythromycin). Increased clearance with thioridazine. May reduce oral clearance of lorazepam.

PREGNANCY: Category C, not for use in nursing.

MECHANISM OF ACTION: Benzothiapine derivative; believed to inhibit both serotonin Type2(5HT$_2$) and dopamine Type 2(D$_2$) receptors in the brain.

PHARMACOKINETICS: Absorption: Rapid, T$_{max}$=1.5 hrs. **Distribution:** Plasma protein binding (83%), V$_d$=10±4L/kg. **Metabolism:** Liver (extensive) via sulfoxidation and oxidation; CYP 450(3A4). **Elimination:** Urine (73%), feces (20%), (<1%) unchanged.

SEROQUEL XR   RX
quetiapine fumarate (AstraZeneca)

> Elderly patients with dementia-related psychosis treated with atypical antipsychotic drugs are at an increased risk of death; most deaths appeared to be cardiovascular (eg, heart failure, sudden death) or infectious (eg, pneumonia) in nature. Seroquel XR is not approved for the treatment of patients with dementia-related psychosis. Antidepressants increased the risk of suicidal thinking and behavior (suicidality) in short-term studies in children, adolescents, and young adults with Major Depressive Disorder (MDD) and other psychiatric disorders. Seroquel XR is not approved for use in pediatric patients. Seroquel XR is not approved for treatment of depression.

THERAPEUTIC CLASS: Dibenzapine derivative

INDICATIONS: Maintenance treatment of schizophrenia in adult patients.

DOSAGE: *Adults:* Give qd, preferably in evening. Initial: 300mg/day. Titrate: Within range of 400-800mg/day depending on response and tolerance. Dose increases may be made at intervals as short as 1 day and in increments up to 300mg/day. Take without food or with light meal. Elderly/Hepatic Impairment: Start on Seroquel immediate-release 25mg/day; may increase in increments of 25-50mg/day depending on response and tolerance. May switch to Seroquel XR when effective dose reached.

HOW SUPPLIED: Tab, Extended-Release: 200mg, 300mg, 400mg

WARNINGS/PRECAUTIONS: Monitor DM patients regularly for hyperglycemia. NMS reported. May develop tardive dyskinesia. May induce orthostatic hypotension. Caution with cardiovascular or cerebrovascular disease, conditions which predispose to hypotension (eg, dehydration, hypovolemia, and treatment with antihypertensives), history of seizures. Leukopenia, neutropenia, and agranulocytosis reported. Monitor for cataracts at initiation, then every 6 months. Possible hypothyroidism. Hepatic enzyme, cholesterol, and triglyceride elevations reported. May impair judgement, thinking, and motor skills. Priapism reported. May disrupt body's ability to reduce core temperature. Caution in patients at risk for aspiration, elderly, debilitated. Depression may worsen in patients or suicidal thoughts and behaviors may also arise.

ADVERSE REACTIONS: Dry mouth, constipation, dyspepsia, sedation, somnolence, dizziness, orthostatic hypotension.

INTERACTIONS: Caution with other CNS drugs. May increase cognitive and motor effects of alcohol. May antagonize effects of levodopa and dopamine agonists. May enhance effects of antihypertensives. Phenytoin or other hepatic enzyme inducers (eg, carbamazepine, barbiturates, glucocorticoids) may reduce levels. Caution with inhibitors of CYP3A (eg, itraconazole, ketoconazole, fluconazole, erythromycin). May reduce oral clearance of lorazepam.

PREGNANCY: Category C, not for use in nursing.

MECHANISM OF ACTION: Quetiapine fumarate belongs to benzothiazepine derivatives, believed to inhibit both serotonine Type2(5HT$_2$), dopamine Type 2(D$_2$) receptors in the brain.

PHARMACOKINETICS: Absorption: Rapid, AUC=46-56%, C$_{max}$=21-27%, T$_{max}$=6 hrs. **Distribution:** V$_d$=10±4 L/kg. Plasma protein bound (83%). **Metabolism:** Liver (extensive) via sulfoxidation and oxidation;CYP 450(3A4), N-desalkyl quetiapine (major metabolite). **Elimination:** Urine (73%), <1% (unchanged), feces (20%).

Serostim   RX
somatropin (EMD Serono)

THERAPEUTIC CLASS: Human growth hormone

INDICATIONS: Treatment of AIDS wasting or cachexia.

DOSAGE: *Adults:* >55kg: 6mg SQ qhs. 45-55kg: 5mg SQ qhs. 35-44kg: 4mg SQ qhs. <35kg: 0.1mg/kg SQ qhs. Dose Reductions Due to Side Effects: Reduce total daily dose or number of doses/week. Rotate injection sites. Re-evaluate for infection if weight loss continues after 2 weeks of therapy.

HOW SUPPLIED: Inj: 4mg, 5mg, 6mg, 8.8mg

CONTRAINDICATIONS: Acute critical illness due to complications after open heart or abdominal surgery, accidental trauma, acute respiratory failure.

WARNINGS/PRECAUTIONS: Monitor malnutrition, malabsorption and hypogonadism; may contribute to catabolism. Maintain nucleoside analogue therapy throughout treatment. Carpal tunnel syndrome reported. Perform periodic funduscopic exams.

ADVERSE REACTIONS: Musculoskeletal discomfort, increased tissue turgor, edema, arthralgia, extremity pain, hypoesthesia, myalgia, hyperglycemia, arthrosis, diarrhea, headache, paraesthesia, insomnia, upper respiratory tract infection.

PREGNANCY: Category B, caution in nursing.

MECHANISM OF ACTION: Human growth hormone; anabolic and anticatabolic agent exerting influence by interacting with specific receptors on variety of cell types.

PHARMACOKINETICS: Absorption: Absolute bioavailabilty (70-90%). **Distribution:** V$_d$=12.0L. **Metabolism:** Kidneys (major), liver (minor). **Elimination:** T$_{1/2}$=4.28 hrs.

Silvadene   RX
silver sulfadiazine (King)

OTHER BRAND NAMES: SSD (Par)

THERAPEUTIC CLASS: Sulfonamide

INDICATIONS: Adjunct for prevention and treatment of wound sepsis in patients with 2nd- and 3rd-degree burns.

DOSAGE: *Adults:* Apply under sterile conditions qd-bid to thickness of approximately 1/16 inch. Re-apply if removed by patient activity. Continue until wound is healed.

HOW SUPPLIED: Cre: 1% [20g, 50g, 85g, 400g, 1000g]

CONTRAINDICATIONS: Late pregnancy, premature infants, newborns during first 2 months of life.

WARNINGS/PRECAUTIONS: Potential cross-sensitivity with other sulfon-amides. Hemolysis may occur in G6PD deficient patients. Drug accumulation with hepatic and renal dysfunction. Monitor renal function and serum sulfa levels with extensive burns.

ADVERSE REACTIONS: Transient leukopenia, skin necrosis, erythema multi-forme, skin discoloration, burning sensation, rash, interstitial nephritis, fungal superinfection, systemic sulfonamide reactions.

INTERACTIONS: May inactivate topical proteolytic enzymes. Leukopenia increased with cimetidine.

PREGNANCY: Category B, contraindicated in late pregnancy, and not for use in nursing.

MECHANISM OF ACTION: Topical antimicrobial of sulfonamide class; acts on cell membrane and cell wall of many gram-negative and gram-positive bacte-ria and yeast to produce bactericidal effect.

SIMCOR   RX
simvastatin - niacin (Abbott)

THERAPEUTIC CLASS: HMG-CoA reductase inhibitor/Nicotinic acid

INDICATIONS: Adjunct to diet for the reduction of elevated total-C, LDL-C, Apo B, non-HDL-C, TG or to increase HDL-C with primary hypercholester-olemia, mixed dyslipidemia (Types IIa and IIb) and for reduction of elevated TG with hypertriglyceridemia when treatment with monotherapy components is inadequate.

DOSAGE: *Adults:* Patients not currently on niacin extended-release or switch-ing from immediate-release niacin: Initial: 500mg/20mg qd hs, with a low fat snack. Titrate: Adjust dose at ≥4 weeks. After Week 8, titrate to response and tolerance. Maint: 1000mg/20mg to 2000mg/40mg qd. Max: 2000mg/40mg qd. Do not break, crush or chew before swallowing.

HOW SUPPLIED: Tab, Extended Release: (Niacin-Simvastatin) 500mg/20mg, 750mg/20mg, 1000mg/20mg

CONTRAINDICATIONS: Active liver disease (unexplained persistent eleva-tions of serum transaminases), active peptic ulcer disease, arterial bleeding, pregnancy/nursing.

WARNINGS/PRECAUTIONS: Do not substitute for equivalent dose of imme-diate-release niacin. Myopathy and rhabdomyolysis reported; monitor serum creatine kinase (CK) periodically. D/C therapy if myopathy is suspected or diagnosed, if transaminase levels increase ≥3 ULN persist, or a few days prior to major surgery or when any major medical or surgical condition supervenes. Increased risk with higher doses, advanced age (≥65 yrs), hypothyroidism, renal impairment. Caution with heavy alcohol use, or history of liver disease; monitor LFTs prior to therapy, every 12 weeks for the first 6 months and peri-odically thereafter. Severe hepatic toxicity may occur in patients substituting sustained-release niacin for immediate-release niacin at equivalent doses. May increase serum glucose levels in diabetic or potentially diabetic patients, particularly the first few months of therapy; adjust diet and/or hypoglycemic therapy or d/c if necessary. May reduce platelet count. Caution with those predisposed to gout.

ADVERSE REACTIONS: Flushing, headache, backpain, diarrhea, nausea, pruritus.

INTERACTIONS: Avoid use with concomitant CYP3A4 inhibitors includ-ing itraconazole, ketoconazole, and other antifungal azoles, erythromycin, clarithromycin, telithromycin, HIV protease inhibitors, nefazodone, grapefruit juice (>1 quart/day), cyclosporine, danazol, and fibrates; increased risk of myopathy/rhabdomyolysis. Max 20mg/day with amiodarone or verapamil. Concurrent use with propanolol decreases simvastatin levels. Potentiates effects of coumarin anticoagulants; monitor PT/INR. May increase digoxin levels; monitor appropriately. Concomitant use with aspirin decreases niacin levels. Colestipol and cholestyramine may increase niacin-binding capacity.

S

Potentiates adverse effects with nutritional supplements containing large doses of niacin or related compounds.

PREGNANCY: Category X, not for use in nursing.

MECHANISM OF ACTION: Niacin: Nicotinic acid; not well established. May partially inhibit release of free fatty acids from adipose tissue, and increases lipoprotein lipase activity, which increases rate of chylomicron triglyceride removal from plasma. Decreases rate of hepatic synthesis of VLDL and LDL. Simvastatin: HMG-CoA reductase inhibitor; lipid-lowering agent. Inhibits conversion of HMG-CoA to mevalonate. Also reduces VLDL, TG, and increases HDL.

PHARMACOKINETICS: Absorption: Niacin: T_{max}=4.6-4.9 hrs. Simvastatin: T_{max}=1.9-2.0 hrs. Simvastatin acid (active metabolite): C_{max}=3.29ng/mL, T_{max}= 6.56 hrs, AUC =30.81 ng.hr/mL. **Metabolism:** Rapid and extensive first-pass metabolism. **Elimination:** Niacin: Urine (54%). Simvastatin: Feces (60%), urine (13%), $T_{1/2}$ =4.2-4.9 hrs; (simvastatin acid) $T_{1/2}$ =4.6-5.0 hrs.

SIMULECT RX
basiliximab (Novartis)

Manage patient in facility with adequate lab and supportive resources. Prescribing physician should be experienced with immunosuppressives and transplantation. Physician should have complete information requisite for patient follow-up.

THERAPEUTIC CLASS: Monoclonal antibody/IL-2R alpha (CD25) blocker

INDICATIONS: Prophylaxis of acute organ rejection in renal transplantation.

DOSAGE: *Adults:* 20mg within 2 hrs prior to transplant, repeat 4 days after transplant. Withhold 2nd dose if graft loss or complications occur. *Pediatrics:* ≥35kg: 20mg within 2 hrs prior to transplant, repeat 4 days after transplant. <35kg: 10mg within 2 hrs prior to transplant, repeat 4 days after transplant. Withhold 2nd dose if graft loss or complications occur.

HOW SUPPLIED: Inj: 10mg, 20mg

WARNINGS/PRECAUTIONS: Only administer under qualified medical supervision. Increased risk of developing lymphoproliferative disorder and opportunistic infections. Anaphylaxis and other severe hypersensitivity reactions (eg, hypotension, cardiac failure, bronchospasm, respiratory failure, etc) reported and may necessitate discontinuation. Anti-idiotype antibodies may develop.

ADVERSE REACTIONS: GI effects, peripheral edema, fever, viral infection, hyperkalemia, hypokalemia, hyperglycemia, hypercholesterolemia, hypophosphatemia, hyperuricemia, UTI, dyspnea, upper respiratory infection, acne, HTN, headache, tremor, insomnia, anemia.

PREGNANCY: Category B, not for use in nursing.

MECHANISM OF ACTION: Monoclonal antibody/IL-2Rα (CD25) blocker; acts as an IL-2 receptor antagonist by binding to the IL-2 receptor complex and inhibiting IL-2 binding. Specifically targeted against IL-2Rα, which is selectively expressed on the surface of activated T-lymphocytes. Binding to IL-2Rα causes competitive inhibition of IL-2-mediated activation of lymphocytes, a critical pathway in the cellular immune response involved in allograft rejection.

PHARMACOKINETICS: Absorption: C_{max}=7.1ng/mL (adult). **Distribution:** V_d=8.6L (adult); 4.8L (1-11 yrs); 7.8L (12-16 yrs). **Elimination:** $T_{1/2}$=7.2 days (adult); 9.5 days (1-11 yrs); 9.1 days (12-16 yrs).

SINEMET CR RX
levodopa - carbidopa (Bristol-Myers Squibb)

OTHER BRAND NAMES: Sinemet (Bristol-Myers Squibb)

THERAPEUTIC CLASS: Dopa-decarboxylase inhibitor/dopamine precursor

INDICATIONS: Treatment of symptoms of idiopathic Parkinson's disease, postencephalitic parkinsonism, and symptomatic parkinsonism.

DOSAGE: *Adults:* ≥18 yrs: Initial: (25mg-100mg tab) 1 tab tid. Titrate: Increase by 1 tab qd or every other day until 8 tabs/day. 10mg-100mg tab: Initial: 1 tab tid-qid. Titrate: Increase 1 tab qd or every other day until 2 tabs qid. 70-100mg/day carbidopa required. Max: 200mg/day carbidopa. (Tab, Extended-Release) No Prior Levodopa Use: Initial: 1 tab 50mg-200mg bid at intervals >6 hrs. Titrate: Increase or decrease dose or interval accordingly. Adjust dose every 3 days. Usual: 400-1600mg/day levodopa, given in 4-8 hr intervals while awake. Conversion to Extended-Release Tabs: See PI.

HOW SUPPLIED: Tab: (Carbidopa-Levodopa) 10mg-100mg*, 25mg-100mg*, 25mg-250mg*; Tab, Extended-Release: (Carbidopa-Levodopa) 25mg-100mg, 50mg-200mg*. *scored

CONTRAINDICATIONS: MAOIs during or within 14 days of use, narrow-angle glaucoma, suspicious, undiagnosed skin lesions, history of melanoma.

WARNINGS/PRECAUTIONS: D/C levodopa 12 hrs before initiating therapy. Dyskinesias and mental disturbances may occur. Caution with severe cardiovascular or pulmonary disease, bronchial asthma, renal or hepatic disease, endocrine disease, chronic wide-angle glaucoma, peptic ulcer, and MI with residual arrhythmias. NMS reported during dose reduction or withdrawal. Dark color may appear in saliva, urine, or sweat. May cause false (+) ketonuria or false (-) glucosuria (glucose-oxidase method).

ADVERSE REACTIONS: Dyskinesias, nausea, cardiac irregularities, hypotension, dark saliva, GI bleeding, psychotic episodes, NMS, confusion, agitation, dizziness, somnolence, dream abnormalities.

INTERACTIONS: See Contraindications. Risk of postural hypotension with antihypertensives, selegiline. HTN and dyskinesia may occur with TCAs. Reduced effects with dopamine D_2 antagonists (eg, phenothiazines, butyrophenones, risperidone), isoniazid. Antagonized by phenytoin, papaverine, metoclopramide. Reduced bioavailability with iron salts, high-protein diets.

PREGNANCY: Category C, caution in nursing.

MECHANISM OF ACTION: Dopa-decarboxylase inhibitor; Carbidopa: inhibits decarboxylation of peripheral levodopa. Levodopa: rapidly decarboxylated to dopamine in extracerebral tissue so that only portion of a given dose is transported unchanged to the CNS.

PHARMACOKINETICS: Absorption: Levodopa: T_{max}=2 hrs (Sinemet CR). C_{max}=1151ng/mL (Sinemet CR), absolute availability: 70-75% (Sinemet CR), Carbidopa: absolute bioavailability: (approximately 58%) (sinemet CR). **Elimination:** Levodopa and carbidopa: $T_{1/2}$1.5 hrs.

SINGULAIR   RX
montelukast sodium (Merck)

THERAPEUTIC CLASS: Leukotriene receptor antagonist

INDICATIONS: Prophylaxis and chronic treatment of asthma (≥12 months). Relief of symptoms of seasonal allergic rhinitis (≥2 yrs) and perennial allergic rhinitis (≥6 months). Prevention of exercise-induced bronchoconstriction (EIB) (≥15 yrs).

DOSAGE: *Adults:* Asthma: 10mg qpm. Allergic Rhinitis: 10mg qd. EIB: 10mg 2 hrs before exercise. Do not take additional dose within 24 hrs of previous dose.
Pediatrics: Asthma:≥15 yrs: 10mg qpm. 6-14 yrs: 5mg qpm. 2-5 yrs: 4mg qpm. 6-23 months: 4mg qpm. Seasonal/Perennial Allergic Rhinitis: ≥15 yrs: 10mg qd. 6-14 yrs: 5mg qd. 2-5 yrs: 4mg qd. Perennial Allergic Rhinitis: 6-23 months: 4mg qd. EIB: ≥15 yrs: 10mg 2 hrs before exercise. Do not take additional dose within 24 hrs of previous dose. Granules may be mixed with applesauce, carrots, rice, or ice cream; give within 15 min of opening pkt.

HOW SUPPLIED: Granules: 4mg/pkt; Tab, Chewable: 4mg, 5mg; Tab: 10mg

WARNINGS/PRECAUTIONS: Not for treatment of acute asthma attacks. Do not abruptly substitute for inhaled or oral corticosteroids. Eosinophilic conditions reported (rare).

ADVERSE REACTIONS: (Adults, Pediatrics) Headache, abdominal pain, dyspepsia, cough, flu. (Pediatrics) Pharyngitis, flu, fever, sinusitis, nausea, diarrhea, dyspepsia, otitis, viral infection, laryngitis.

INTERACTIONS: Monitor with potent CYP450 inducers (eg, phenobarbital, rifampin).

PREGNANCY: Category B, caution in nursing.

MECHANISM OF ACTION: Leukotriene receptor antagonist; binds to cysteinyl leukotriene receptors found on airway smooth muscle cells and macrophages and other pro-inflammatory cells (eg, eosinophils); inhibits physiologic actions of leukotrienes.

PHARMACOKINETICS: Absorption: Rapid. (10mg) Bioavailability (64%) T_{max}=3-4 hrs. (5mg) T_{max}=2-2.5 hrs. Bioavailability (73%, fasted), (63%, fed). Fasted 2-5 yrs: (4mg Chewable) T_{max}=2 hrs. (4mg Granules) T_{max}=2.3 hrs (fasted), 6.4 hrs (fed). **Distribution:** V_d=8-11L; plasma protein binding (99%). **Metabolism:** Liver (extensive); CYP3A4, 2C9. **Elimination:** Biliary (major); $T_{1/2}$=2.7-5.5 hrs.

SKELAXIN   RX
metaxalone (King)

THERAPEUTIC CLASS: Muscular analgesic (central-acting)

INDICATIONS: Adjunct for acute, painful musculoskeletal conditions.

DOSAGE: *Adults:* 800mg tid-qid.
Pediatrics: >12 yrs: 800mg tid-qid.

HOW SUPPLIED: Tab: 800mg* *scored

CONTRAINDICATIONS: Tendency for drug-induced, hemolytic, and other anemias. Significant renal or hepatic impairment.

WARNINGS/PRECAUTIONS: Caution with pre-existing liver damage. Monitor hepatic function. False-positive Benedict's test reported.

ADVERSE REACTIONS: Nausea, vomiting, GI upset, drowsiness, dizziness, headache, nervousness, leukopenia, hemolytic anemia, jaundice.

INTERACTIONS: May enhance the effects of alcohol, barbiturates and other CNS depressants.

PREGNANCY: Not for use in pregnancy or nursing.

MECHANISM OF ACTION: Centrally acting muscular analgesic; not established; activity may be due to general depression of CNS.

PHARMACOKINETICS: Absorption: (400mg) C_{max}=983ng/mL, T_{max}=3.3 hrs, AUC=7479ng•hr/mL; (800mg) C_{max}=1816ng/mL, T_{max}=3.0 hrs, AUC=15044ng•hr/mL. **Distribution:** Extensive in tissues; V_d=800L. **Metabolism:** Liver. **Elimination:** Urine (metabolites); $T_{1/2}$=9 hrs.

SKELID   RX
tiludronate disodium (Sanofi-Aventis)

THERAPEUTIC CLASS: Bisphosphonate

INDICATIONS: Treatment of Paget's disease when serum alkaline phosphatase is ≥2x ULN, or if symptomatic, or if at risk for future complications.

DOSAGE: *Adults:* 400mg qd for 3 months. After therapy, wait 3 months to assess response. Take with 6-8oz of water. Take 2 hrs after food.

HOW SUPPLIED: Tab: 200mg

WARNINGS/PRECAUTIONS: May cause GI disorders (eg, dysphagia, esophagitis, esophageal or gastric ulcers). Maintain adequate vitamin D and calcium intake. Avoid in severe renal failure. May cause osteonecrosis, primarily in jaw, and musculoskeletal pain.

ADVERSE REACTIONS: Pain, headache, dizziness, paresthesia, diarrhea, nausea, dyspepsia, vomiting, rhinitis, upper respiratory infection.

INTERACTIONS: Increased bioavailability with indomethacin; space dosing by 2 hrs. Decreased bioavailability with calcium supplements, ASA, and aluminum- or magnesium-containing antacids; space dosing by 2 hrs.

PREGNANCY: Category C, caution in nursing.

MECHANISM OF ACTION: Bisphosphonate; acts primarily on bone to inhibit osteoclastic activity, with a probable reduction in the enzymatic and transport processes that lead to resorption of the mineralized matrix. Inhibits osteoclasts through inhibiting protein-tyrosine-phosphatase and through inhibition of the osteoclastic proton pump.

PHARMACOKINETICS: Absorption: Rapidly absorbed; C_{max}=3mg/L; T_{max}=2 hrs. **Distribution:** Plasma protein binding (90%). **Elimination:** Urine (60%); $T_{1/2}$= 150 hrs.

SODIUM CHLORIDE IRRIGATION   RX
sodium chloride (Baxter)

THERAPEUTIC CLASS: Irrigation solution

INDICATIONS: For use as an arthroscopic irrigation fluid with endoscopic instruments during arthroscopic procedures requiring distention and irrigation of the knee, shoulder, elbow, or other bone joints.

DOSAGE: *Adults:* Irrigate as needed. May warm in overpouch to near body temperature in water bath or oven heated to not more than 45° C.

HOW SUPPLIED: Sol: 1000mL, 3000mL, 5000mL

CONTRAINDICATIONS: Not for injection by usual parenteral routes. An electrolyte solution should not be used for irrigation during electrosurgical procedures.

WARNINGS/PRECAUTIONS: Not for injection. Caution in CHF, severe renal insufficiency, and conditions where edema and sodium retention exists. Use opened containers promptly to reduce potential for bacterial contamination. Discard unused portion. Irrigation solutions must be regarded as systemic drugs since irrigating fluids can enter systemic ciruclation in large volumes.

ADVERSE REACTIONS: Infection, distension or disruption of tissues.

INTERACTIONS: Caution with corticosteroids or corticotropin; some of the fluid may be absorbed systemically.

PREGNANCY: Safety in pregnancy and nursing is not known.

SOLAGE   RX
mequinol - tretinoin (Galderma)

THERAPEUTIC CLASS: Retinoid

INDICATIONS: Solar lentigines.

DOSAGE: *Adults:* Apply to solar lentigines bid, morning and evening, at least 8 hrs apart. Avoid surrounding skin. Do not shower or bathe treated area for at least 6 hrs after application. Wait 30 min before applying cosmetics.

HOW SUPPLIED: Sol: (Mequinol-Tretinoin) 2%-0.01% [30mL]

CONTRAINDICATIONS: Women of childbearing potential and pregnancy.

WARNINGS/PRECAUTIONS: Caution with history/family history of vitiligo. Severe irritation with eczematous skin. Avoid/minimize exposure to sunlight/ sunlamps or wear protective clothing. Avoid eyes, mouth, paranasal creases and mucous membranes. D/C if sensitivity, irritation, or systemic adverse reaction develops. Larger amounts will not lead to better or faster results and may increase adverse effects. Extreme weather may increase skin irritation. Caution when using with permanent wave solutions, electrolysis, hair depilatories or waxes.

ADVERSE REACTIONS: Erythema, burning/stinging/tingling, desquamation, pruritus, skin irritation, dry skin, hypopigmentation of treated lesions or surrounding skin.

INTERACTIONS: Avoid with photosensitizers (eg, thiazides, tetracyclines, fluoroquinolones, phenothiazines, sulfonamides); may cause augmented phototoxicity. Caution with other topicals products with a strong drying effect, high concentrations of alcohol, astringents, spices or lime, medicated soaps/shampoos.

PREGNANCY: Category X, caution in nursing.

MECHANISM OF ACTION: Has not been established; acts as competitive inhibitor of the formation of melanin precursors.

PHARMACOKINETICS: Absorption: C_{max}=9.92ng/mL and T_{max}=2 hrs.

SOLAQUIN FORTE   RX
hydroquinone (Valeant)

THERAPEUTIC CLASS: Depigmenting agent

INDICATIONS: For the gradual bleaching of hyperpigmented skin conditions (eg, chloasma, melasma, freckles, senile lentigines).

DOSAGE: *Adults:* Apply bid.
Pediatrics: ≥12 yrs: Apply bid.

HOW SUPPLIED: Cre: 4% [28.4g]; Gel: 4% [28.4g]

WARNINGS/PRECAUTIONS: Avoid sun exposure on bleached skin. Solaquin Forte contains sunscreen. May produce unwanted cosmetic effects if not used as directed. Test for skin sensitivity. D/C if no lightening effect after 2 months. Contains sodium metabisulfite, may cause serious allergic type reactions. Limit treatment to small areas of body at one time. Avoid contact with eyes.

ADVERSE REACTIONS: Cutaneous hypersensitivity (contact dermatitis).

PREGNANCY: Category C, caution in nursing.

MECHANISM OF ACTION: Reversible depigmentaion of the skin by inhibition of enzymatic oxidation of tyrosine to 3,4-dihydroxyphenylalanine (dopa) and suppression of other melanocyte metabolic processes.

SOLARAZE   RX
diclofenac sodium (Bioglan)

THERAPEUTIC CLASS: NSAID

INDICATIONS: Treatment of actinic keratoses.

DOSAGE: *Adults:* Apply generously to lesions bid for 60-90 days.

HOW SUPPLIED: Gel: 3% [50g,100g]

CONTRAINDICATIONS: Known hypersensitivity to benzyl alcohol, polyethylene glycol monomethyl ether 350, hyaluronate sodium.

WARNINGS/PRECAUTIONS: Anaphylactoid reactions may occur. Caution with ASA triad, GI ulceration or bleeding, severe renal/hepatic impairment. Do not apply to open skin wounds, infections, or exfoliative dermatitis. Avoid the eyes and sun/sunlamp exposure during therapy. Interrupt therapy if severe reactions occur.

ADVERSE REACTIONS: Contact dermatitis, dry skin, edema, exfoliation, pain, paresthesia, pruritis, rash.

INTERACTIONS: Minimize oral administration of NSAIDs. Safety of the concomitant use of sunscreens, cosmetics, or other topical medications is unknown.

PREGNANCY: Category B, not for use in nursing.

MECHANISM OF ACTION: Anti-inflammatory agent; has not been established.

PHARMACOKINETICS: Absorption: AUC=9ng•hr/mL. C$_{max}$=4ng/mL. T$_{max}$=4.5 hrs. **Distribution:** V$_d$=550mL/kg. **Metabolism:** Metabolized via conjugation, hydroxylation and glucuronidation. **Elimination:** Urine; T$_{1/2}$=1-2 hrs.

SOLIRIS   RX
eculizumab (Alexion)

> Increases risk of meningococcal infections. Vaccinate 2 weeks prior to receiving first dose; re-vaccinate according to current guidelines. Monitor for early signs of meningococcal infections, evaluate, and treat if necessary.

THERAPEUTIC CLASS: Monoclonal antibody/Protein C5 blocker

INDICATIONS: Treatment of paroxysmal nocturnal hemoglobinuria (PNH) to reduce hemolysis.

DOSAGE: *Adults:* Initial: 600mg every 7 days for first 4 weeks, then 900mg as 5th dose 7 days later, then 900mg every 14 days thereafter. Administer by IV infusion over 35 min.

HOW SUPPLIED: Inj: 10mg/mL [30mL]

CONTRAINDICATIONS: Patients with unresolved serious *Neisseria meningitis* infection and patients not vaccinated against it.

WARNINGS/PRECAUTIONS: Caution in patients with any systemic infection. After discontinuation, monitor for signs and symptoms of intravascular hemolysis and serum LDH levels.

ADVERSE REACTIONS: Meningococcal infections, headache, nasopharyngitis, back pain, nausea, fatigue, cough, herpes simplex infections, sinusitis, respiratory tract infection, constipation, myalgia, pain in extremities, influenza-like illness.

PREGNANCY: Category C, caution in nursing.

MECHANISM OF ACTION: Monoclonal antibody/protein C5 blocker; binds to the complement C5 with high affinity, thereby inhibiting its cleavage to C5a and C5b and preventing the generation of the terminal complement C5b-9. Inhibits terminal complement-mediated intravascular hemolysis in PNH patient.

PHARMACOKINETICS: Absorption: C$_{max}$=194mcg/mL. **Distribution:** V$_d$=7.7L. **Elimination:** T$_{1/2}$=272 hrs.

SOLODYN   RX
minocycline HCL (Medicis)

THERAPEUTIC CLASS: Tetracycline derivative

INDICATIONS: Treatment of inflammatory lesions of non-nodular moderate to severe acne vulgaris in patients ≥12 yrs.

DOSAGE: *Adults:* 1mg/kg qd for 12 weeks. Reduce dose with renal impairment. *Pediatrics:* ≥12 yrs: 1mg/kg qd for 12 weeks. Reduce dose with renal impairment.

HOW SUPPLIED: Tab, Extended-Release: 45mg, 90mg, 135mg.

WARNINGS/PRECAUTIONS: May cause fetal harm during pregnancy. Use during tooth development (last half of pregnancy, infancy, <8yrs) may cause permanent discoloration of the teeth or enamel hypoplasia; avoid use during this period. May decrease bone growth in premature infants. May cause pseudomembranous colitis. Renal toxicity, hepatotoxicity, photosensitivity, increased BUN, superinfection, pseudotumor cerebri may occur. Caution in renal impairment; may lead to azotemia, hyperphosphatemia, and acidosis. Long-term use has been associated with lupus-like syndrome, autoimmune hepatitis and vasculitis. May cause serum sickness. May induce hyperpigmentation.

ADVERSE REACTIONS: Headache, fatigue, dizziness, pruritus, malaise, mood alteration, Stevens-Johnson syndrome, photosensitivity.

INTERACTIONS: May require downward regulation of anticoagulant therapy. May interfere with bactericidal action of penicillin; avoid concurrent. May decrease efficacy of oral contraceptives. Impaired absorption with antacids containing aluminum, calcium or magnesium, and iron-containing preparations. Fatal renal toxicity with methoxyflurane reported.

PREGNANCY: Category D, not for use in nursing.

MECHANISM OF ACTION: Tetracycline derivative; inhibits bacterial protein synthesis.

PHARMACOKINETICS: Absorption: C_{max}=2.63mcg/mL; T_{max}=3.5-4 hrs; AUC=33.32mcg•hr/mL.

SOLTAMOX   RX
tamoxifen citrate (Savient)

> For women with ductal carcinoma in situ (DCIS) and women at high risk for breast cancer. Fatal uterine malignancies (eg, endometrial adenocarcinoma, uterine sarcoma), stroke, and PE reported with use in risk reduction setting. Discuss benefits/risks of events with this patient population. Benefits of tamoxifen outweigh risks in women already diagnosed with breast cancer.

THERAPEUTIC CLASS: Antiestrogen

INDICATIONS: Treatment of metastatic breast cancer in women and men. Treatment of node-positive and axillary node-negative breast cancer in women following mastectomy, axillary dissection and breast irradiation. To reduce risk of invasive breast cancer in women with DCIS. Reduction of breast cancer incidence in high risk women. Use for up to 5 yrs.

DOSAGE: *Adults:* Breast Cancer Treatment: 20-40mg qd. Divide dosages >20mg into AM and PM doses. Breast Cancer Risk Reduction/DCIS: 20mg qd for 5 yrs.

HOW SUPPLIED: Sol: 10mg/5mL

CONTRAINDICATIONS: Reduction in breast cancer incidence in high risk women and women with DCIS who require coumarin-type anticoagulant therapy or have a history of DVT, PE.

WARNINGS/PRECAUTIONS: Hypercalcemia reported in patients with bone metastases. Increased incidence of uterine malignancies (eg, endometrial cancer, uterine sarcoma) and endometrial changes including hyperplasia and polyps reported. Increased incidence of thromboembolic events (eg, DVT, PE). Malignant and non-malignant effects on the liver and ocular disturbances reported. Leukopenia, anemia, thrombocytopenia, neutropenia, pancytopenia reported. Promptly evaluate abnormal vaginal bleeding if receiving or previously received tamoxifen. Patients receiving or previously received tamoxifen should have annual gynecological exam. Do not become pregnant within 2 months of therapy. May cause fetal harm during pregnancy. Does not cause infertility even with menstrual irregularity.

ADVERSE REACTIONS: (Females) Hot flashes, increased bone and tumor pain, vaginal discharge, irregular menses; (Males) loss of libido, impotence.

INTERACTIONS: Increases effects of coumarin-type anticoagulant; monitor PT. Increased risk of thromboembolic events with cytotoxic agents. Increased levels with bromocriptine. May decrease letrozole levels. Decreased levels with rifampin and aminoglutethimide. Decreased plasma levels of major metabolite, N-desmethyl tamoxifen with medroxyprogesterone.

PREGNANCY: Category D, not for use in nursing.

MECHANISM OF ACTION: Nonsteroidal antiestrogen; competes with estrogen for binding sites in target tissues.

PHARMACOKINETICS: Absorption: C_{max}=40mg/mL; T_{max}=5 hrs. N-desmethyl tamoxifen: C_{max}=15ng/mL. **Metabolism:** N-desmethyl tamoxifen (major metabolite). **Elimination:** Feces (primary); $T_{1/2}$=5-7 days.

SOLU-CORTEF   RX
hydrocortisone sodium succinate (Pharmacia & Upjohn)

THERAPEUTIC CLASS: Corticosteroid

INDICATIONS: Steroid-responsive disorders.

DOSAGE: *Adults:* Initial: 100-500mg IV/IM, depending on condition severity. May repeat dose at 2, 4, or 6 hrs based on clinical response. High dose therapy usually not >48-72 hrs; may use antacids prophylactically.
Pediatrics: Use lower adult doses. Determine dose by severity of condition and response. Dose should not be <25mg/day.

HOW SUPPLIED: Inj: 100mg, 250mg, 500mg, 1g

CONTRAINDICATIONS: Premature infants, systemic fungal infections.

WARNINGS/PRECAUTIONS: May need to increase dose before, during, and after stressful situations. May mask signs of infection or cause new infections. Prolonged use may produce glaucoma, optic nerve damage, secondary ocular infections. Increases BP, salt/water retention, potassium and calcium excretion. More severe/fatal course of infections reported with chickenpox, measles. Enhanced effect with hypothyroidism or cirrhosis. Caution with Strongyloides, latent TB, ocular herpes simplex, HTN, diverticulitis, fresh intestinal anastomoses, ulcerative colitis, osteoporosis, myasthenia gravis, renal insufficiency, peptic ulcer disease. Kaposi's sarcoma reported. Monitor for psychic disturbances. Acute myopathy with high doses. Avoid abrupt withdrawal. Monitor growth and development of children on prolonged therapy. Hypernatremia may occur with high dose therapy >48-72 hrs.

ADVERSE REACTIONS: Fluid and electrolyte disturbances, HTN, osteoporosis, muscle weakness, cushingoid state, menstrual irregularities, vertigo, headache, impaired wound healing, DM, ulcerative esophagitis, peptic ulcer, pancreatitis, increased sweating, increases intracranial pressure, carbohydrate intolerance, glaucoma, cataracts.

INTERACTIONS: Reduced efficacy and increased clearance with hepatic enzyme inducers (eg, phenobarbital, phenytoin, and rifampin). Increases clearance of chronic high dose ASA. Caution with ASA in hypoprothrombinemia. Effects on oral anticoagulants are variable; monitor PT/INR. Increased insulin and oral hypoglycemic requirements in DM. Avoid live vaccines with immunosuppressive doses. Possible decreased vaccine response with killed or inactivated vaccines with immunosuppressive doses. Decreased clearance with ketoconazole and troleandomycin.

PREGNANCY: Safety in pregnancy and nursing not known.

MECHANISM OF ACTION: Anti-inflammatory glucocorticoid; causes profound and varied metabolic effects and modifies the body's immune responses to diverse stimuli.

PHARMACOKINETICS: Absorption: (IM) Rapidly absorbed. T_{max}=1 hr.
Distribution: Found in breast milk. **Elimination:** $T_{1/2}$=12 hrs.

SOLU-MEDROL   RX
methylprednisolone sodium succinate (Pharmacia & Upjohn)

THERAPEUTIC CLASS: Glucocorticoid

INDICATIONS: Steroid-responsive disorders.

DOSAGE: *Adults:* Usual: Initial: 10-40mg IV over several min. May repeat IV/IM dose at intervals based on clinical response. High-Dose Therapy: 30mg/kg IV over at least 30 min, may repeat q4-6h for 48 hrs. High dose therapy usually not >48-72 hrs. Give antacids prophylactically. Multiple Sclerosis: (4mg methylprednisolone=5mg prednisolone): 200mg/day prednisolone for 1 week, then 80mg every other day for 1 month.
Pediatrics: Use lower adult doses. Determine dose by severity of condition and response. Dose should not be <0.5mg/kg q24h.

HOW SUPPLIED: Inj: 40mg, 125mg, 500mg, 1g, 2g

CONTRAINDICATIONS: Premature infants (due to benzyl alcohol diluent) and systemic fungal infections.

WARNINGS/PRECAUTIONS: May need to increase dose before, during, and after stressful situations. May mask signs of infection or cause new infections. Prolonged use may produce cataracts, glaucoma, secondary ocular infections. Increases BP, salt/water retention, calcium/potassium excretion. More severe/fatal course of infections reported with chickenpox, measles. Caution with latent TB, hypothyroidism, cirrhosis, ocular herpes simplex, HTN, diverticulitis, fresh intestinal anastomoses, ulcerative colitis, osteoporosis, myasthenia gravis, renal insufficiency, peptic ulcer disease. Kaposi's sarcoma reported. Growth and development of children on prolonged therapy should be monitored. Monitor for psychic disturbances. Avoid abrupt withdrawal. Reports of cardiac arrhythmias, circulatory collapse, cardiac arrest following rapid administration of large IV doses. Effectiveness not established for the treatment of sepsis syndrome and septic shock. Bradycardia reported with high doses.

ADVERSE REACTIONS: Fluid and electrolyte disturbances, HTN, osteoporosis, muscle weakness, cushingoid state, menstrual irregularities, insomnia, impaired wound healing, DM, ulcerative esophagitis, excessive sweating, increases intracranial pressure, carbohydrate intolerance, glaucoma, cataracts, nausea.

INTERACTIONS: Reduced efficacy with hepatic enzyme inducers (eg, phenobarbital, phenytoin, and rifampin). Increases clearance of chronic high dose ASA. Caution with ASA in hypoprothrombinemia. Effects on oral anticoagulants are variable; monitor PT/INR. Increased insulin and oral hypoglycemic requirements in DM. Avoid live vaccines with immunosuppressive doses. Possible decreased vaccine response with killed or inactivated vaccines with immunosuppressive doses. Mutual inhibition of metabolism with cyclosporine; convulsions reported. Decreased clearance with ketoconazole and troleandomycin.

PREGNANCY: Safety in pregnancy and nursing not known.

MECHANISM OF ACTION: Anti-inflammatory glucocorticoid; causes profound and varied metabolic effects and modifies the body's immune responses to diverse stimuli.

SOMA   RX
carisoprodol (MedPointe)

THERAPEUTIC CLASS: Skeletal muscle relaxant (central-acting)

INDICATIONS: Relief of discomfort associated with acute, painful musculoskeletal conditions.

DOSAGE: *Adults:* ≤65 yrs: 250-350mg tid and hs for 2-3 weeks.
Pediatrics: ≥16 yrs: 250-350mg tid and hs for 2-3 weeks.

HOW SUPPLIED: Tab: 250mg, 350mg

CONTRAINDICATIONS: Acute intermittent porphyria and hypersensitivity to a carbamate.

WARNINGS/PRECAUTIONS: May have sedative properties. Cases of drug abuse, dependence and withdrawal reported. Caution in addiction-prone patients. First-dose idiosyncratic reactions reported (rare). Occasionally within period of 1st-4th dose, allergic reactions have occured. Rare reports of seizures in postmarketing surveillance. Caution with liver or renal dysfunction. Seizures reported.

ADVERSE REACTIONS: Drowsiness, dizziness, headache, nausea, vomiting, tachycardia, postural hypotension, agitation, irritability, insomnia, seizures.

INTERACTIONS: Additive effects with alcohol, other CNS depressants, and psychotropic drugs. Concomitant use with meprobamate not recommended. Coadministration with CYP2C19 inhibitors (eg, omeprazole, fluvoxamine); may increase levels and CYP2C19 inducers (eg, St.Johns wort, rifampin); may decrease levels.

PREGNANCY: Category C, caution in nursing.

S

MECHANISM OF ACTION: Skeletal muscle relaxant; not clearly identified; suspected to relieve discomfort associated with acute painful musculoskeletal conditions.

PHARMACOKINETICS: Absorption: Carisoprodol: (250mg) C_{max}=1.2mcg/mL, T_{max}1.5 hrs, AUC=4.5mcg•hr/mL; (350mg) C_{max}=1.8mcg/mL, T_{max}=1.7 hrs, AUC=7.0mcg•hr/mL. Meprobamate: (250mg) C_{max}=1.8mcg/mL, T_{max} = 3.6 hrs, AUC=32mcg•hr/mL; (350mg) C_{max}=2.5mcg/mL, T_{max}=4.5 hr, AUC=46mcg•hr/mL. **Distribution:** Found in breast milk. **Metabolism:** Liver via CYP2C19. Meprobamate (metabolite). **Elimination:** Urine, carisoprodol: $T_{1/2}$=1.7 hrs (250mg), 2.0 hrs (350mg). Meprobamate: $T_{1/2}$=9.7 hrs (250mg), 9.6 hrs (350mg).

SOMA CMPD/CODEINE
CIII

codeine phosphate - carisoprodol - aspirin (MedPointe)

THERAPEUTIC CLASS: Central muscle relaxant/analgesic

INDICATIONS: Adjunct for relief of pain, muscle spasm, and limited mobility associated with acute, painful musculoskeletal conditions.

DOSAGE: *Adults:* 1-2 tabs qid.
Pediatrics: ≥12 yrs: 1-2 tabs qid.

HOW SUPPLIED: Tab: (Carisoprodol-Codeine-Aspirin) 200mg-16mg-325mg

CONTRAINDICATIONS: Acute intermittent porphyria, bleeding disorders.

WARNINGS/PRECAUTIONS: First-dose idiosyncratic reactions reported (rare). Contains sodium metabisulfate; may cause allergic type reactions. Caution with liver or renal dysfunction, elderly, peptic ulcer, gastritis, addiction-prone patients and anticoagulant therapy. Caution in individuals who are ultra rapid metabolizers of codeine.

ADVERSE REACTIONS: Drowsiness, dizziness, vertigo, ataxia, nausea, vomiting, gastritis, occult bleeding, constipation, diarrhea, miosis, allergic-skin rash, postural hypotension.

INTERACTIONS: Enhances methotrexate toxicity and hypoglycemia with oral antidiabetics. Corticosteroids and antacids decrease plasma levels. Increases GI bleeding risk with alcohol. Potentiated by urine acidifiers (eg, ammonium chloride). Antagonizes uricosuric effects of probenecid, sulfinpyrazone. Additive effects with alcohol, other CNS depressants, psychotropic drugs. Increases bleeding risk with anticoagulants.

PREGNANCY: Category C, not for use in nursing.

MECHANISM OF ACTION: Carisoprodol: Centrally acting muscle relaxant: does not directly relax tense skeletal muscle. Action in relieving acute muscle spasm not established; may be related to its sedative properties. ASA: Inhibits prostaglandin biosynthesis producing anti-inflammatory, analgesic, and anti-pyretic properties. Codeine: Centrally acting narcotic-analgesic.

PHARMACOKINETICS: Absorption: ASA: Rapid. **Distribution:** Carisoprodol, ASA, and Codeien: Found in breast milk. **Metabolism:** Carisoprodol: Liver. ASA: Hydrolyzed to salicylic acid. Codeine: Liver. **Elimination:** Carisoprodol: Urine; $T_{1/2}$=2.4 hr (parent), 10 hr (metabolite). ASA: Urine; $T_{1/2}$=15 min. Codeine: Urine (5-15% unchanged). $T_{1/2}$=2.5-4 hr.

SOMA COMPOUND
RX

carisoprodol - aspirin (MedPointe)

THERAPEUTIC CLASS: Central muscle relaxant/analgesic

INDICATIONS: Adjunct for pain, muscle spasm and limited mobility associated with acute, painful musculoskeletal conditions.

DOSAGE: *Adults:* 1-2 tabs qid.
Pediatrics: ≥12 yrs: 1-2 tabs qid.

HOW SUPPLIED: Tab: (Carisoprodol-ASA) 200mg-325mg

CONTRAINDICATIONS: Acute intermittent porphyria, bleeding disorders.

WARNINGS/PRECAUTIONS: First-dose idiosyncratic reactions reported (rare). Caution with liver or renal dysfunction, elderly, peptic ulcer, gastritis, addiction-prone patients and anticoagulant therapy.

ADVERSE REACTIONS: Drowsiness, dizziness, vertigo, ataxia, nausea, vomiting, gastritis, occult bleeding, constipation, diarrhea.

INTERACTIONS: Enhances methotrexate toxicity and hypoglycemia with oral antidiabetics. Corticosteroids and antacids decrease plasma levels. Increases GI bleeding risk with alcohol. Potentiated by urine acidifiers (eg, ammonium chloride). Antagonizes uricosuric effects of probenecid, sulfinpyrazone. Additive effects with alcohol, other CNS depressants, psychotropic drugs. Increases bleeding risk with anticoagulants.

PREGNANCY: Category C, not for use in nursing.

MECHANISM OF ACTION: Carisoprodol: Centrally acting muscle relaxant; does not directly relax tense skeletal muscle. Action in relieving acute muscle spasm not established; may be related to its sedative properties. ASA: Inhibits prostaglandin biosynthesis producing anti-inflammatory, analgesic, and antipyretic properties.

PHARMACOKINETICS: Absorption: ASA: Rapid. **Distribution:** Carisoprodol, ASA: Found in breast milk. **Metabolism:** Carisoprodol: Liver. ASA: Hydrolyzed to salicylic acid. **Elimination:** Carisoprodol: Urine. ASA: Urine; $T_{1/2}$=15 min.

SOMATULINE DEPOT RX
lanreotide (Ipsen/Tercica)

THERAPEUTIC CLASS: Somatostatin analog

INDICATIONS: Long term treatment of acromegalic patients who have had inadequate response to surgery and/or radiotherapy, or for whom surgery and/or radiotherapy is not an option.

DOSAGE: Adults: Initial: 90mg deep SQ at 4 week intervals for 3 months. Titrate: Adjust dose based on IGF and GH levels. GH >1 to ≤2.5ng/mL, IGF-1 Normal and Controlled Clinical Symptoms: 90mg every 4 weeks. GH >2.5ng/mL, IGF-1 Elevated and/or Clinical Symptoms Uncontrolled: 120mg every 4 weeks. GH ≤1ng/mL, IGF-1 Normal and Clinical Symptoms Controlled: 60mg every 4 weeks. Moderate to Severe Renal/Hepatic Impairment: Initial: 60mg deep SQ at 4 week intervals for 3 months.

HOW SUPPLIED: Inj: 60mg, 90mg, 120mg

WARNINGS/PRECAUTIONS: May reduce gallbladder motility and lead to gallstone formation; monitor periodically. Hypo- and/or hyperglycemia may occur; monitor glucose levels. Decreased thyroid function reported. May decrease HR; caution with bradycardia.

ADVERSE REACTIONS: Diarrhea, abdominal pain, nausea, constipation, flatulence, vomiting, loose stools, cholethiasis, injection site reactions.

INTERACTIONS: May decrease cyclosporine levels. May reduce intestinal absorption of concomitant drugs. Dose adjustments for concomitant antidiabetic treatment and drugs that induce bradycardia may be needed. Caution with drugs metabolized by CYP3A4 (eg, quinidine, terfenadine) and have low therapeutic index. Drugs metabolized by liver may need dose reduction.

PREGNANCY: Category C, caution in nursing.

MECHANISM OF ACTION: Somatostatin analog. Acts mainly at the human somatostatin receptors (SSTR) 2 and 5 to inhibit growth hormone. Like somatostatin, lanreotide is an inhibitor of various endocrine, neuroendocrine, exocrine, and paracrine functions.

PHARMACOKINETICS: Absorption: SQ administration of variable doses resulted in different parameters. **Elimination:** Urine (<0.5%), feces (<5% unchanged). Biliary excretion.

SOMAVERT

RX

pegvisomant (Pharmacia & Upjohn)

THERAPEUTIC CLASS: Growth hormone receptor antagonist

INDICATIONS: Treatment of acromegaly in those who have had an inadequate response to surgery and/or radiation therapy, and/or other medical therapies, or for whom these therapies are not appropriate.

DOSAGE: *Adults:* LD: 40mg SQ. Maint: 10mg SQ qd. Titrate: Adjust dose by 5mg increments/decrements, based on IGF-I levels, every 4-6 weeks. Max: 30mg/day. LFTs ≥3x/<5x ULN (without symptoms of liver dysfunction): Monitor LFTs weekly. LFTs ≥5x ULN/Transaminase Elevations ≥3x ULN: D/C immediately and evaluate. Do not initiate if baseline LFTs >3x ULN until cause is determined.

HOW SUPPLIED: Inj: 10mg, 15mg, 20mg

WARNINGS/PRECAUTIONS: May expand and cause serious complications of tumors that secrete GH; monitor with periodic imaging scans of the sella turcica. May increase glucose tolerance and risk of hypoglycemia in diabetics. May result in functional GH deficiency. AST/ALT elevations reported; obtain baseline ALT, AST, TBIL, and ALP levels prior to initiation. Monitor LFTs monthly for first 6 months, quarterly for next 6 months, then biannually; monitor more frequently if elevations occur. D/C if liver injury confirmed. Monitor IGF-I levels 4-6 weeks after initiation or dose adjustments; every 6 months after levels are normalized. Interferes with the measurement serum GH levels by commercially available GH assays; do not adjust dosage based on serum GH levels.

ADVERSE REACTIONS: Infection, abnormal LFTs, pain, injection site reactions, back pain, diarrhea, nausea, flu syndrome, chest pain, dizziness, paresthesia, HTN, sinusitis, peripheral edema.

INTERACTIONS: May need to reduce dosage of insulin and/or hypoglycemic agents. Concomitant opioids may increase dosage requirements of pegvisomant.

PREGNANCY: Category B; caution in nursing.

MECHANISM OF ACTION: Growth hormone receptor antagonist: selectively binds to growth hormone (GH) receptors on cell surfaces, where it blocks binding of endogenous GH and interferes with GH signal transduction. This decreases serum concentrations of insulin such as growth factor-I (IGF-I), as well as other GH-responsive proteins, including IGF binding protein-3 (IGFBP-3), and acid labile subunit (ALS).

PHARMACOKINETICS: Absorption: Absolute bioavailability (57%). **Distribution:** V_d=7L. **Elimination:** Urine (<1%); $T_{1/2}$=6 days.

SONATA

zaleplon (King)

THERAPEUTIC CLASS: Pyrazolopyrimidine (non-benzodiazepine)

INDICATIONS: Short-term treatment of insomnia.

DOSAGE: *Adults:* Insomnia: 10mg qhs. Low Weight Patients: Start with 5mg hs. Max: 20mg/day. Elderly/Debilitated/Concomitant Cimetidine: 5mg qhs. Max: 10mg/day. Mild to Moderate Hepatic Dysfunction: 5mg qhs. Take immediately prior to bedtime.

HOW SUPPLIED: Cap: 5mg, 10mg

WARNINGS/PRECAUTIONS: Monitor elderly/debilitated closely. Abnormal thinking and behavioral changes reported. Avoid abrupt withdrawal. Abuse potential exists. Caution in respiratory disorders, depression, conditions affecting metabolism or hemodynamic responses, and mild-to-moderate hepatic insufficiency. Not for use in severe hepatic impairment. May cause impaired coordination even the following day. Re-evaluate if no improvement of insomnia after 7-10 days of therapy. Contains tartrazine.

ADVERSE REACTIONS: Headache, asthenia, nausea, dizziness, amnesia, somnolence, eye pain, dysmenorrhea, abdominal pain.

INTERACTIONS: Potentiates CNS depression with psychotropics (eg, thioridazine, imipramine), anticonvulsants, antihistamines, alcohol and other CNS depressants. CYP3A4 inducers (eg, rifampin, phenytoin, carbamazepine and phenobarbital) decreases levels. Potentiated by cimetidine.

PREGNANCY: Category C, not for use in nursing.

MECHANISM OF ACTION: Pyrazolopyrimidine class; interacts with GABA-benzodiazepine receptor complex.

PHARMACOKINETICS: Absorption: Rapid and complete. T_{max}=1 hr. Absolute bioavailability (approximately 30%) (IV). **Distribution:** V_d=1.4L/kg. Plasma protein binding (60%). **Metabolism:** Extensive, liver via aldehyde oxidase. **Elimination:** Urine (70%) in 48 hrs , (71%) in urine, (17% in feces) in 6 days, $T_{1/2}$=1 hrs, < 1% (unchanged).

SORIATANE   RX

acitretin (Stiefel)

> Avoid in pregnancy or becoming pregnant ≤3 yrs after discontinuation of therapy; use 2 reliable forms of contraception. Only use in females of reproductive potential with severe psoriasis unresponsive or contraindicated to other therapies, if receive warnings of therapy hazards and risk of contraception failure, if negative pregnancy test within 1 week before therapy, will begin therapy on the 2nd or 3rd day of next menstrual cycle, are capable of complying with contraceptive measures and are reliable. Repeat pregnancy testing and contraception counseling on a regular basis. The patient must have a negative result from a urine or serum pregnancy test. before receiving Soriatane prescription. It is not known whether residual acitretin in seminal fluid poses risk to fetus with male patients during or after therapy. Females should avoid ethanol during and 2 months after therapy. Severe birth defects reported.

THERAPEUTIC CLASS: Retinoid

INDICATIONS: Treatment of severe psoriasis, including erythrodermic and generalized pustular types.

DOSAGE: *Adults:* Initial: 25-50mg single dose qd with main meal. Individualize dose based on intersubject variation in pharmacokinetics, clinical efficacy, and incidence of side effects. Maint: 25-50mg qd. Terminate therapy when lesions resolve. May treat relapses as outlined for initial therapy.

HOW SUPPLIED: Cap: 10mg, 25mg

CONTRAINDICATIONS: See Black Box Warnings. Pregnancy.

WARNINGS/PRECAUTIONS: Risk of hepatotoxicity, hyperostosis, pancreatitis, and pseudotumor cerebri. D/C if visual difficulties occur; decreased night vision and reduced tolerance to contact lenses reported. Bony abnormalities of the vertebral column, knees, and ankles reported. Increases TG and cholesterol and decreases HDL; perform lipid tests before therapy every 1-2 weeks until establish lipid response. Caution with severe hepatic/renal impairment. Transient worsening of psoriasis may occur initially. Do not donate blood during and for 3 yrs after therapy. Avoid sun lamps and excessive sun exposure. Depression and/or psychiatric symptoms (eg, aggressive feelings, thoughts of self-harm) reported. Thinning of the skin observed.

ADVERSE REACTIONS: Ophthalmologic effects, cheilitis, rhinitis, dry mouth, epistaxis, alopecia, dry skin, rash, skin peeling, nail disorder, pruritus, paresthesia, paronychia, skin atrophy, sticky skin, xerophthalmia, arthralgia, rash, acute myocardial infarction, stroke, vulvo-vaginitis.

INTERACTIONS: Caution with oral hypoglycemics. May increase risk of hepatotoxicity with methotrexate. Interferes with microdosed progestin "minipill" oral contraceptives. Females should avoid ethanol during and 2 months after therapy. Possible additive toxic effects with vitamin A doses that exceed minimum RDAs.

PREGNANCY: Category X, not for use in nursing.

MECHANISM OF ACTION: Retinoid antipsoriatic; has not been established.

S

PHARMACOKINETICS: Absorption: C_{max}=416ng/mL. T_{max}=2-5 hrs.
Distribution: Plasma protein binding (99.9%). Found in breast milk.
Metabolism: Extensive; via isomerization to cis-acitretin; metabolized with the parent drug into chain-shortened breakdown metaboilites and conjugates.
Elimination: Chain-shortened breakdown metabolites and conjugates; feces (34-54%), and urine (16-53%). Acitretin; $T_{1/2}$=49 hrs. and cis-acitretin; $T_{1/2}$=63 hrs.

SPECTRACEF

RX

cefditoren pivoxil (Cornerstone)

THERAPEUTIC CLASS: Cephalosporin (3rd generation)

INDICATIONS: Treatment of acute bacterial exacerbations of chronic bronchitis (ABECB), pharyngitis/tonsillitis, community-acquired pneumonia (CAP), and uncomplicated skin and skin structure infections (SSSI) caused by susceptible strains of microorganisms.

DOSAGE: *Adults:* ABECB: 400mg bid for 10 days. Pharyngitis/Tonsillitis/ SSSI: 200mg bid for 10 days. CAP: 400mg bid for 14 days. CrCl 30-49mL/min: 200mg bid. CrCl <30mL/min: 200mg qd. Take with meals.
Pediatrics: ≥12 yrs: ABECB: 400mg bid for 10 days. Pharyngitis/Tonsillitis/ SSSI: 200mg bid for 10 days. CAP: 400mg bid for 14 days. CrCl 30-49mL/min: 200mg bid. CrCl <30mL/min: 200mg qd. Take with meals.

HOW SUPPLIED: Tab: 200mg

CONTRAINDICATIONS: Milk protein hypersensitivity, carnitine deficiency.

WARNINGS/PRECAUTIONS: Cross sensitivity to PCNs and other cephalosporins may occur. Pseudomembranous colitis reported. Not recommended for prolonged antibiotic therapy. Prolonged therapy may cause superinfection. May decrease PT.

ADVERSE REACTIONS: Diarrhea, nausea, vaginal moniliasis, headache.

INTERACTIONS: Avoid concomitant antacids and H_2 receptor antagonists. Increased plasma levels with probenecid.

PREGNANCY: Category B, caution in nursing.

MECHANISM OF ACTION: 3rd generation cephalosporin; inhibits cell wall synthesis via affinity for penicillin-binding proteins (PBPs).

PHARMACOKINETICS: Absorption: C_{max}=1.8mcg/mL (200mg, fasting), 3.1mcg/mL (200mg, high-fat meal), 4.4mcg/mL (400mg, high-fat meal); T_{max}=1.5-3 hrs (fasting). Absolute bioavailability: 14% (fasting), 16.1 (low-fat meal). **Distribution:** V_d=9.3L; plasma protein binding: 88%; found in breast milk. **Metabolism:** Hydrolysis, via esterases to cefditoren (active component). **Elimination:** Urine; $T_{1/2}$=1.6 hrs.

SPIRIVA

RX

tiotropium bromide (Boehringer Ingelheim/Pfizer)

THERAPEUTIC CLASS: Anticholinergic bronchodilator

INDICATIONS: Long-term, once-daily, maintenance treatment of bronchospasm associated with chronic obstructive pulmonary disease (COPD), including chronic bronchitis and emphysema.

DOSAGE: *Adults:* Inhale contents of one capsule (18mcg) qd, with HandiHaler device.

HOW SUPPLIED: Cap, Inhalation: 18mcg

CONTRAINDICATIONS: Hypersensitivity to atropine or its derivatives (eg, ipratropium).

WARNINGS/PRECAUTIONS: Not for initial treatment of acute episodes. D/C if hypersensitivity (eg, angioedema) or paradoxical bronchospasm occurs. Caution with narrow-angle glaucoma, prostatic hyperplasia, bladder-neck obstruction. Monitor with moderate to severe renal impairment (CrCl ≤50mL/min). Contents of caps are for oral inhalation only and must not be swallowed.

ADVERSE REACTIONS: Dry mouth, arthritis, cough, flu-like symptoms, sinusitis, constipation, abdominal pain, UTI, moniliasis, rash, dizziness, dysphagia, hoarseness, intestinal obstruction-ileus paralytic, increased IOP, oral candidiasis, tachycardia, throat irritation.

INTERACTIONS: Avoid with other anticholinergics (eg, ipratropium).

PREGNANCY: Category C, caution in nursing.

MECHANISM OF ACTION: Anticholinergic; inhibits M_3-receptors on smooth muscle leading to bronchodilation.

PHARMACOKINETICS: Absorption: Absolute bioavailability (19.5%). T_{max}=5 mins. **Distribution:** V_d=32L/kg. Plasma protein binding (72%). **Metabolism:** Liver (oxidation, conjugation) via CYP2D6, 3A4. **Elimination:** $T_{1/2}$=5-6 days. (Inhalation): urine (14%); (IV): urine (74%).

SPORANOX   RX
itraconazole (Janssen/Ortho Biotech)

> Contraindicated with cisapride, pimozide, quinidine, dofetilide, or levacetylmethadol. Serious cardiovascular events (eg, QT prolongation, torsade de pointes, ventricular tachycardia, cardiac arrest, and/or sudden death) reported with cisapride, pimozide, quinidine, and other CYP3A4 inhibitors. Do not use caps for onychomycosis with ventricular dysfunction.

THERAPEUTIC CLASS: Azole antifungal

INDICATIONS: (Cap) Onychomycosis of the toenail and fingernail in immunocompetent patients. Confirm diagnosis before therapy. (Cap) Treatment of blastomycosis and histoplasmosis. Treatment of aspergillosis if refractory to or intolerant to amphotericin B. (Sol) Treatment of oropharyngeal and esophageal candidiasis. (Sol) Empiric therapy of febrile, neutropenic patients with suspected fungal infections (ETFN).

DOSAGE: *Adults:* Cap: Take with full meal. If patient has achlorhydria or taking gastric acid suppressors, give with cola beverage. Onychomycosis: Toenail: 200mg qd for 12 consecutive weeks. Fingernail: 200mg bid for 1 week, skip 3 weeks, then repeat. Blastomycosis/Histoplasmosis: 200mg qd. May increase by 100mg increments if no improvement. Max: 400mg/day. Give bid if dose >200mg/day. Aspergillosis: 200-400mg/day. Life-Threatening Infections: LD: 200mg tid for 1st 3 days. Continue for at least 3 months and until infection subsides. Sol: Take on empty stomach. Swish 10mL at a time for several seconds, then swallow. Candidiasis: Oropharyngeal: 200mg/day for 1-2 weeks. If refractory to fluconazole, give 100mg bid (response in 2-4 weeks; may relapse shortly after d/c). Esophageal: 100-200mg/day for at least 3 weeks. Continue for 2 weeks after symptoms resolve.

HOW SUPPLIED: Cap: 100mg; Sol: 10mg/mL [150mL]

CONTRAINDICATIONS: (Cap, Sol) Concomitant cisapride, oral midazolam, pimozide, quinidine, dofetilide, triazolam, and HMG-CoA reductase inhibitors metabolized by CYP3A4 (eg, lovastatin, simvastatin). (Cap) Treatment of onychomycosis if pregnant or contemplating pregnancy, ventricular dysfunction (eg, CHF).

WARNINGS/PRECAUTIONS: Rare cases of hepatotoxicity reported. Monitor LFTs; d/c if hepatic dysfunction develops. Avoid with liver disease. D/C if neuropathy or CHF occurs. Sol and caps not interchangeable. Consider alternative therapy if unresponsive in patients with cystic fibrosis. Avoid with ventricular dysfunction. Caution with ischemic/valvular disease, pulmonary disease, renal failure, other edematous disorders. Avoid injection if CrCl <30mL/min.

ADVERSE REACTIONS: Nausea, diarrhea, vomiting, abdominal pain, fever, cough, rash, increased sweating, headache, hypokalemia.

INTERACTIONS: See Contraindications. Increased levels with cisapride, pimozide, quinidine, dofetilide, oral midazolam, triazolam, HMG-CoA reductase inhibitors; concurrent use contraindicated. Increases levels of rifabutin, immunosuppressants, protease inhibitors, alfentanil, buspirone,

S

methylprednisolone, trimetrexate, carbamazepine, HMG-CoA reductase inhibitors, digoxin, warfarin, busulfan, docetaxel, vinca alkaloids, astemizole, alprazolam, diazepam, oral midazolam, triazolam, dihydropyridine CCBs, verapamil, oral hypoglycemics. CYP3A4 inducers (eg, carbamazepine, phenobarbital, phenytoin, isoniazid, rifabutin, rifampin, nevirapine) decrease itraconazole levels. CYP3A4 inhibitors (eg, erythromycin, clarithromycin, indinavir, ritonavir) may increase itraconazole levels. Severe hypoglycemia with oral hypoglycemics. Additive negative inotropic effects with CCBs. Edema reported with dihydropyridine CCBs; adjust dose. Decreased absorption of caps with antacids or gastric secretion suppressors.

PREGNANCY: Category C, not for use in nursing.

MECHANISM OF ACTION: Azole antifungal agent: Inhibits the CYP450-dependent synthesis of ergosterol, which is a vital component of fungal cell membranes.

PHARMACOKINETICS: Absorption: Absolute bioavailabilty: 55%. Oral administration of variable doses resulted in different parameters. **Metabolism:** Liver via CYP3A4; hydroxyitraconazole (major metabolite). **Distribution:** Plasma protein binding (99.8%). **Elimination:** Urine (40%), feces (3-18%) (inactive metabolites)

SPRYCEL
RX

dasatinib (Bristol-Myers Squibb)

THERAPEUTIC CLASS: Tyrosine kinase inhibitor

INDICATIONS: Treatment of chronic, accelerated, or myeloid or lymphoid blast phase chronic myeloid leukemia (CML) with resistance or intolerance to prior therapy including imatinib. Treatment of Philadelphia chromosome-positive acute lymphoblastic leukemia (Ph+ ALL) with resistance or intolerance to prior therapy.

DOSAGE: *Adults:* Chronic Phase CML: 100mg qd. Accelerated Phase CML/Myeloid or Lymphoid Blast Phase CML/Ph+ ALL: 70mg bid. Swallow whole; do not crush. Concomitant Strong CYP3A4 Inducers: Consider dose increase. Concomitant Strong CYP3A4 Inhibitors: Consider dose decrease to 20mg daily. Refer to PI for dose modifications for neutropenia and thrombocytopenia.

HOW SUPPLIED: Tab: 20mg, 50mg, 70mg

WARNINGS/PRECAUTIONS: Severe thrombocytopenia, neutropenia, and anemia reported; monitor CBC weekly for first 2 months, then monthly thereafter. Severe CNS hemorrhages including fatalities, GI hemorrhage, and other hemorrhage cases reported; caution in patients on medications that inhibit platelet function or anticoagulants. Pleural and pericardial effusion reported. Severe ascites, generalized edema, severe pulmonary edema reported. QT prolongation reported; caution in patients at risk (eg, hypokalemia or hypomagnesemia, congenital long QT syndrome, concomitant antiarrhythmics or other QT prolonging agents, cumulative high-dose anthracycline therapy); correct hypokalemia or hypomagnesemia prior to administration. Caution with hepatic impairment. Fetal harm may occur; avoid pregnancy.

ADVERSE REACTIONS: Fluid retention events, diarrhea, nausea, headache, abdominal pain, vomiting, bleeding events, pyrexia, pleural effusion, neutropenia, thrombocytopenia, dyspnea, anemia, skin rash, fatigue, myelosuppression, QT prolongation.

INTERACTIONS: Increased levels with CYP3A4 inhibitors (eg, ketoconazole, itraconazole, erythromycin, clarithromycin, ritonavir, atazanavir, indinavir, nefazodone, nelfinavir, saquinavir, telithromycin). Decreased levels with CYP3A4 inducers (eg, dexamethasone, phenytoin, carbamazepine, rifampicin, phenobarbital, St. John's wort). Avoid antacids; if necessary, administer 2 hrs prior to or 2 hrs after dose. Concomitant use of H_2 blockers or PPIs not recommended. Caution with CYP3A4 substrates with narrow therapeutic windows (eg, alfentanil, astemizole, terfenadine, cisapride, cyclosporine, fentanyl, pimozide, quinidine, sirolimus, tacrolimus, or ergot alkaloids such as ergotamine and dihydroergotamine).

PREGNANCY: Category D, not for use in nursing.

MECHANISM OF ACTION: Tyrosine kinase inhibitor; inhibits BCR-ABL and SRC family kinases.

PHARMACOKINETICS: Absorption: T_{max}=0.5-6 hrs. **Distribution:** V_d=2505L; plasma protein binding (96%). **Metabolism:** Extensive via CYP3A4. **Elimination:** $T_{1/2}$=3-5 hrs; urine (4%), feces (85%).

Stadol NS
butorphanol tartrate (Bristol-Myers Squibb)

CIV

THERAPEUTIC CLASS: Opioid agonist-antagonist analgesic

INDICATIONS: Management of pain when the use of an opioid analgesic is appropriate.

DOSAGE: *Adults:* ≥18 yrs: Initial: 1 spray (1mg) in 1 nostril, may repeat after 60-90 min (after 90-120 min in elderly or renal/hepatic disease) and may repeat in 3-4 hrs after 2nd dose; or may use 1 spray in each nostril, may repeat after 3-4 hrs. Renal/Hepatic Disease: Increase dose interval to no less than 6 hrs.

HOW SUPPLIED: Nasal Spray: 10mg/mL [2.5mL]

CONTRAINDICATIONS: Hypersensitivity to benzethonium chloride.

WARNINGS/PRECAUTIONS: Not for use in narcotic-dependent patients. May result in physical dependence or tolerance. Avoid abrupt cessation. D/C if severe HTN occurs. Caution with hepatic or renal disease, acute MI, ventricular dysfunction, or coronary insufficiency. May impair ability to operate machinery. Increased respiratory depression with CNS disease or respiratory impairment. Severe risks with head injury.

ADVERSE REACTIONS: Somnolence, dizziness, nausea, vomiting, nasal congestion, insomnia.

INTERACTIONS: Increased CNS depression and respiratory depression with alcohol, barbiturates, tranquilizers, and antihistamines. May be potentiated by erythromycin, theophylline and other drugs that affect hepatic metabolism. Decreased absorption rate with nasal vasoconstrictors (eg, oxymetazoline). Diminished analgesic effect if administered shortly after sumatriptan nasal spray.

PREGNANCY: Category C, caution in nursing.

MECHANISM OF ACTION: Opioid agonist-antagonist analgesic; has activity at receptors of mu-opioid type, and agonist at kappa-opioid receptors.

PHARMACOKINETICS: Absorption: Absolute bioavailability (60-70%); C_{max}=0.9-1.04ng/mL; T_{max}=30-60 mins. **Distribution:** Plasma protein binding (80%); V_d= 305-901L; crosses placenta, found in breast milk. **Metabolism:** Liver. Hydroxybutorphanol (major metabolite). **Elimination:** Urine (5%), feces. Hydroxybutorphanol: Urine (49%); $T_{1/2}$=18 hrs.

S

Stalevo
entacapone - levodopa - carbidopa (Novartis)

RX

THERAPEUTIC CLASS: Dopa-decarboxylase inhibitor/dopamine precursor/ COMT inhibitor

INDICATIONS: Treatment of idiopathic Parkinson's disease to substitute for equivalent doses of previously administered carbidopa/levodopa and entacapone or for those experiencing signs and symptoms of end-of-dose "wearing off" and are taking up to 600mg/day levodopa without experiencing dyskinesias.

DOSAGE: *Adults:* Currently Taking Carbidopa/Levodopa and Entacapone: May switch directly to corresponding strength of levodopa/carbidopa. Currently Taking Carbidopa/Levodopa but not Entacapone: First titrate individually with carbidopa/levodopa product and entacapone product then transfer to corresponding dose. Max: 8 tabs/day.

HOW SUPPLIED: Tab: (Carbidopa/Levodopa/Entacapone): Stalevo 50: 12.5mg/50mg/200mg; Stalevo 100: 25mg/100mg/200mg; Stalevo 150: 37.5mg/150mg/200mg; Stalevo 200: 50mg/200mg/200mg

CONTRAINDICATIONS: MAOIs during or within 14 days of use, narrow-angle glaucoma, undiagnosed skin lesions, history of melanoma.

WARNINGS/PRECAUTIONS: Dyskinesia, mental disturbances, hypotension/syncope, hallucinations, rhabdomyolysis, hyperpyrexia, confusion, and fibrotic complications reported. Caution with biliary obstruction, severe cardiovascular or pulmonary disease, bronchial asthma, renal, hepatic or endocrine disease, chronic wide-angle glaucoma, history of MI with residual arrhythmias, peptic ulcer. Neuroleptic malignant syndrome reported with dose reductions or withdrawal. Avoid rapid withdrawal or abrupt dose reduction. May cause dark color to appear in saliva, urine, or sweat. May cause false (+) ketonuria, false (-) glucosuria (glucose-oxidase method), elevated LFTs, abnormal BUN, positive Coombs test. May depress prolactin secretion and increase growth hormone levels.

ADVERSE REACTIONS: Dyskinesia, hyperkinesia, hypokinesia, dizziness, nausea, diarrhea, abdominal pain, constipation, vomiting, urine discoloration, back pain, fatigue.

INTERACTIONS: See Contraindications. Increased HR, arrhythmias, and BP changes with drugs metabolized by COMT (eg, isoproterenol, epinephrine, norepinephrine, dopamine, dobutamine, alpha-methyldopa, apomorphine, isoetherine, bitolterol). Probenecid, cholestyramine, and some antibiotics (eg, erythromycin, rifampicin, ampicillin, chloramphenicol) may interfere with biliary excretion. Risk of postural hypotension with antihypertensives, selegiline. HTN and dyskinesia may occur with TCAs. Reduced effect with phenytoin, papaverine, metoclopramide, isoniazid, dopamine D_2 antagonists (eg, phenothiazines, butyrophenones, risperidone). Reduced bioavailability with iron salts. Caution with highly protein-bound drugs (eg, warfarin, salicylic acid, phenylbutazone, diazepam).

PREGNANCY: Category C, caution in nursing.

MECHANISM OF ACTION: Antiparkinson's agent; levodopa: crosses blood-brain barrier, and presumably converted to dopamine in the brain. Carbidopa: inhibits the decarboxylation of peripheral levodopa, making more levodopa available for brain transport. Entacapone: Sustains plasma levels of levodopa, resulting in more constant dopaminergic stimulation in the brain.

PHARMACOKINETICS: Absorption: Levodopa: rapidly absorbed. (PO) administration of variable doses resulted in different parameters. Entacapone: rapidly absorbed. T_{max}=0.8-1.2 hrs. C_{max}=1200-1500ng/mL; AUC=1250-1750ng•hr/mL. Carbidopa: slightly absorbed. T_{max}=2.5-3.4 hrs. C_{max}=40-225ng/mL; AUC=170-1200ng•hr/mL. **Distribution:** Levodopa: plasma protein binding (10-30%). Entacapone: (98%). Carbidopa: (approximately 36%). **Metabolism:** Levodopa: extensive (decarboxylation by dopa decarboxylase and O-methylation by catechol-O-methyltransferase. Entacapone: Completely metabolized. Carbidopa: main metabolites: (α-methyl-3-methoxy-4-hydroxyphenylpropionic acid, and α-methyl-3,4-dihydroxyphenylpropionic acid. **Elimination:** Levodopa: $T_{1/2}$=1.7 hrs. Entacapone: $T_{1/2}$=0.8-1 hr. Feces (90%), urine (10%). Carbidopa: $T_{1/2}$=1.6-2 hrs. Urine (30%, unchanged).

STARLIX   RX
nateglinide (Novartis)

THERAPEUTIC CLASS: Meglitinide

INDICATIONS: Adjunct to diet and exercise, as monotherapy, to improve glycemic control in type 2 diabetics who have not been chronically treated with other antidiabetic agents. May be used in combination with metformin or a thiazolidinedione (TZD).

DOSAGE: *Adults:* Initial/Maint: 120mg tid before meals (with or without metformin or TZD). Take 1-30 min before meals. May use 60mg tid (with or without metformin or TZD) in patients near goal HbA$_{1c}$. Skip dose if meal is skipped.

HOW SUPPLIED: Tab: 60mg, 120mg

CONTRAINDICATIONS: Type 1 diabetes, diabetic ketoacidosis.

WARNINGS/PRECAUTIONS: Caution in moderate to severe hepatic impairment. Transient loss of glucose control with trauma, surgery, fever, and infection; may need insulin therapy. Secondary failure may occur in prolonged therapy. Hypoglycemia risk in elderly, debilitated, malnourished, strenuous exercise, and with adrenal or pituitary insufficiency. Autonomic neuropathy may mask hypoglycemia.

ADVERSE REACTIONS: Upper respiratory infection, flu symptoms, dizziness, arthropathy, diarrhea, hypoglycemia, back pain, jaundice, cholestatic hepatitis, elevated liver enzymes.

INTERACTIONS: Potentiated hypoglycemia with alcohol, NSAIDs, salicylates, MAOIs, and non-selective β-blockers. Risk of hyperglycemia with thiazides, corticosteroids, thyroid products and sympathomimetics. May potentiate tolbutamide. Peak plasma levels reduced with liquid meals. β-blockers may mask hypoglycemic effects. Caution with highly protein-bound drugs.

PREGNANCY: Category C, not for use in nursing.

MECHANISM OF ACTION: Meglitinide; lowers blood glucose levels by stimulating insulin secretion from the pancreas.

PHARMACOKINETICS: Absorption: Absolute bioavailability (73%); C_{max} =1 hr. **Distribution:** Plasma protein binding (98%); V_d =10L. **Metabolism:** CYP2C9, 3A4; hydroxylation, glucuronide conjugation. **Elimination:** Urine (75%), feces; $T_{1/2}$ =1.5 hrs.

STRATTERA RX
atomoxetine HCL (Lilly)

> Increased risk of suicidal ideation in short-term studies in children or adolescents with ADHD. Closely monitor for suicidality, clinical worsening, or unusual changes in behavior. Close observation/communication with prescriber by families and caregivers is advised.

THERAPEUTIC CLASS: Selective norepinephrine reuptake inhibitor

INDICATIONS: Treatment of attention-deficit hyperactivity disorder (ADHD).

DOSAGE: *Adults:* Initial: 40mg/day given qam or evenly divided doses in the am and late afternoon/early evening. Titrate: Increase after minimum of 3 days to target dose of about 80mg/day. After 2-4 weeks, may increase to max of 100mg/day. Max: 100mg/day. Hepatic Insufficiency: Moderate (Child-Pugh Class B): Reduce initial and target doses to 50% of normal dose. Severe (Child-Pugh Class C): Reduce initial and target doses to 25% of normal dose. Concomitant CYP450 2D6 inhibitor (eg, paroxetine, fluoxetine, quinidine): Initial: 40mg/day. Titrate: Only increase to 80mg/day if symptoms fail to improve after 4 weeks.
Pediatrics: ≥6 yrs: ≤70kg: Initial: 0.5mg/kg/day given qam or evenly divided doses in the am and late afternoon or early evening. Titrate: Increase after minimum of 3 days to target dose of about 1.2mg/kg/day. Max: 1.4mg/kg/day or 100mg, whichever is less. >70kg: Initial: 40mg/day given qam or evenly divided doses in the am and late afternoon/early evening. Titrate: Increase after minimum of 3 days to target dose of about 80mg/day. After 2-4 weeks, may increase to max of 100mg/day. Max: 100mg/day. Hepatic Insufficiency: Moderate (Child-Pugh Class B): Reduce initial and target doses to 50% of the normal dose. Severe (Child-Pugh Class C): Reduce initial and target doses to 25% of normal dose. Concomitant CYP450 2D6 inhibitor (eg, paroxetine, fluoxetine, quinidine): ≥6 yrs: ≤70kg: Initial: 0.5mg/kg/day. Titrate: Only increase to 1.2mg/kg/day if symptoms fail to improve after 4 weeks. >70kg: Initial: 40mg/day. Titrate: Only increase to 80mg/day if symptoms fail to improve after 4 weeks.

HOW SUPPLIED: Cap: 10mg, 18mg, 25mg, 40mg, 60mg, 80mg, 100mg

CONTRAINDICATIONS: During or within 14 days of MAOI use; narrow angle glaucoma.

WARNINGS/PRECAUTIONS: Monitor for clinical worsening and/or suicidality. Allergic reactions, orthostatic hypotension and syncope reported. Monitor growth. May increase BP and HR; caution with HTN, tachycardia, cardiovascular or cerebrovascular disease. May increase urinary retention and urinary hesitation. Rare cases of priapism reported. May cause severe liver injury in rare cases; monitor liver enzymes and d/c with jaundice or liver injury. Reports of MI, stroke and sudden death in adults. Avoid with known structural cardiac abnormalities or other serious cardiac problems. Physical exam and evaluation of patient history is necessary. Stimulants at usual doses can cause treatment emergent psychotic or manic symptoms (eg, hallucinations, delusional thinking, mania) in children and adolescents without prior history of psychotic illness. Monitor for appearance or worsening of aggressive behavior or hostility.

ADVERSE REACTIONS: (Adults) Dry mouth, headache, insomnia, nausea, decreased appetite, constipation, dysmenorrhea, erectile disturbance, urinary retention. (Pediatrics) Upper abdominal pain, headache, vomiting, decreased appetite, irritability, dizziness, somnolence.

INTERACTIONS: See Contraindications. May potentiate the cardiovascular effects of albuterol or other β_2 agonists. Caution with pressor agents. Increased levels in extensive metabolizers with CYP2D6 inhibitors (eg, paroxetine, fluoxetine, quinidine); atomoxetine may need dose adjustment.

PREGNANCY: Category C, caution in nursing.

MECHANISM OF ACTION: Selective norepinephrine reuptake inhibitor; inhibits the presynaptic norepinephrine transporter, as determined in *ex vivo* uptake.

PHARMACOKINETICS: Absorption: (PO) rapid; T_{max}=1-2 hrs. **Distribution:** Plasma protein binding (98%). **Metabolism:** Via CYP2D6; 4-hydroxyatomoxetine (major metabolite). **Elimination:** Urine (>80%), feces (<17%); $T_{1/2}$=5 hrs;

STREPTOMYCIN   RX
streptomycin sulfate (Various)

> Risk of severe neurotoxic reactions (eg, vestibular and cochlear disturbances) increased significantly with renal dysfunction or pre-renal azotemia. Optic nerve dysfunction, peripheral neuritis, arachnoiditis, and encephalopathy may occur. Monitor renal function; reduce dose with renal impairment and/or nitrogen retention. Do not exceed peak serum level of 20-25mcg/mL with kidney damage. Avoid other neurotoxic and/or nephrotoxic drugs (eg, neomycin, kanamycin, gentamicin, cephaloridine, paromomycin, viomycin, polymyxin B, colistin, tobramycin, cyclosporine). Respiratory paralysis can occur, especially if given soon after anesthesia or muscle relaxants. Reserve parenteral form when adequate lab and audiometric testing is available.

THERAPEUTIC CLASS: Aminoglycoside

INDICATIONS: Treatment of moderate to severe infections such as mycobacterium tuberculosis (TB) and non-TB infections (eg, plague, tularemia, chancroid, granuloma inguinale, *H.influenzae* and *K.pneumoniae* infections, UTI, gram-negative bacillary bacteremia, endocardial infections).

DOSAGE: *Adults:* IM only. TB: 15mg/kg/day (Max: 1g), or 25-30mg/kg twice weekly (Max: 1.5g), or 25-30mg/kg three times weekly (Max: 1.5g). Do not exceed a total dose of 120g over the course of therapy unless no other therapeutic options exist. Elderly (>60 yrs): Reduce dose. Treat for minimum of 1 year if possible. Tularemia: 1-2g/day in divided doses for 7-14 days until afebrile for 5-7 days. Plague: 1g bid for minimum of 10 days. Streptococcal Endocarditis: With PCN, 1g bid for week 1, then 500mg bid for week 2. Elderly (>60 yrs): 500mg bid for 2 weeks. Enterococcal Endocarditis: With PCN, 1g bid for 2 weeks, then 500mg bid for 4 weeks. Renal Impairment: Reduce dose. Moderate/Severe Infections: 1-2g/day in divided doses q6-12h. Max: 2g/day. *Pediatrics:* IM only. TB: 20-40mg/kg/day (Max: 1g), or 25-30mg/kg twice weekly (Max: 1.5g), or 25-30mg/kg three times weekly (Max: 1.5g). Do not exceed a total dose of 120g over the course of therapy unless no other therapeutic options exist. Treat for minimum of 1 year if possible. Moderate/Severe Infections: 20-40mg/kg/day (8-20mg/lb/day) in divided doses q6-12h.

HOW SUPPLIED: Inj: 1g

WARNINGS/PRECAUTIONS: Vestibular and auditory dysfunction may occur. Contains sodium metabisulfite. Can cause fetal harm in pregnancy. Caution with dose selection in renal impairment. Alkalinize urine to minimize or prevent renal irritation with prolonged therapy. CNS depression (eg, stupor, flaccidity) reported in infants with higher than recommended doses. If syphilis is suspected when treating venereal infections, perform dark field exam before initiate treatment, and monthly serologic tests for at least 4 months. Overgrowth of nonsusceptible organisms may occur. Terminate therapy when toxic symptoms appear, when impending toxicity is feared, when organisms become resistant, or when full treatment effect has been obtained. Contains sodium metabisulfite, a sulfite that may cause allergic type reactions including anaphylaxis.

ADVERSE REACTIONS: Vestibular ototoxicity (nausea, vomiting, vertigo), paresthesia of face, rash, fever, urticaria, angioneurotic edema, eosinophilia, nephrotoxicity (rare).

INTERACTIONS: See Black Box Warning. Increased ototoxicity with ethacrynic acid, furosemide, mannitol and possibly other diuretics.

PREGNANCY: Category D, not for use in nursing.

MECHANISM OF ACTION: Aminoglycoside agent; interferes with normal protein synthesis.

PHARMACOKINETICS: Absorption: C_{max}=25-50mcg/mL, T_{max}=1 hr. **Distribution:** Passes through placenta; found in breast milk. **Elimination:** Urine (29-89%).

STRIANT

CIII

testosterone (Columbia Labs)

THERAPEUTIC CLASS: Androgen

INDICATIONS: Testosterone replacement therapy in males with primary or hypogonadotrophic hypogonadism.

DOSAGE: *Adults:* 30mg q12h to gum region, just above the incisor tooth on either side of mouth. Rotate sites with each application. Hold system in place for 30 seconds.

HOW SUPPLIED: Tab, Buccal: 30mg [6 blister packs, 10 buccal systems/blister]

CONTRAINDICATIONS: Women. Breast or prostate carcinoma in men. Hypersensitivity to soy products.

WARNINGS/PRECAUTIONS: Caution in elderly; increased risk of prostatic hyperplasia/carcinoma. Risk of edema with pre-existing cardiac, renal, or hepatic disease; d/c if edema occurs. May potentiate sleep apnea, especially with obesity or chronic lung diseases. Monitor Hgb, Hct, LFTs, PSA, cholesterol, lipids, serum testosterone.

ADVERSE REACTIONS: Gum/mouth irritation, bitter taste, gum pain/tenderness, headache, gynecomastia.

INTERACTIONS: May elevate oxyphenbutazone levels. May decrease blood glucose and, therefore, insulin requirements. Corticosteroids may enhance edema formation; caution with cardiac or hepatic disease.

PREGNANCY: Category X, not for use in nursing.

MECHANISM OF ACTION: Endogenous androgen; responsible for normal growth and development of male sex organs and maintenance of secondary sex characteristics.

PHARMACOKINETICS: Absorption: T_{max}=10-12 hrs. **Metabolism:** Estradiol, dihydrotestosterone (metabolites). **Elimination:** Urine, feces; $T_{1/2}$=10-100 min.

S

STROMECTOL

RX

ivermectin (Merck)

THERAPEUTIC CLASS: Avermectins derivative

INDICATIONS: Treatment of strongyloidiasis of the intestinal tract due to *Strongyloides stercoralis*, and onchocerciasis due to *Onchocerca volvulus*. Has no activity against adult *Onchocerca volvulus* parasites.

DOSAGE: *Adults:* Strongyloidiasis: 200mcg/kg single dose. Onchocerciasis: 150mcg/kg single dose. For mass distribution in international treatment programs, the usual dosing interval is 12 months. Usual dosing interval for re-treatment for individual patients can be as short as 3 months. Take on empty stomach with water. To verify eradication of infection perform follow-up stool exams.
Pediatrics: ≥15kg: Strongyloidiasis: 200mcg/kg single dose. Onchocerciasis: 150mcg/kg single dose. For mass distribution in international treatment programs, the usual dosing interval is 12 months. Usual dosing interval for re-treatment for individual patients can be as short as 3 months. Take on empty stomach with water. To verify eradication of infection perform follow-up stool exams.

HOW SUPPLIED: Tab: 3mg, 6mg* *scored

WARNINGS/PRECAUTIONS: May cause cutaneous and/or systemic reactions of varying severity (the Mazzotti reaction) and ophthalmological reactions. Patients with hyperreactive onchodermatitis (sowda) may be more likely to experience severe advisers reactions, especially edema and aggravation of onchodermatitis. Risk of serious or even fatal encephalopathy with onchocerciasis and *Loa loa* infection. Pretreatment assessment for loiasis and careful posttreatment follow-up should be performed in patients who were exposed to *Loa loa*-endemic areas of West or Central Africa.

ADVERSE REACTIONS: Diarrhea, nausea, dizziness, pruritis, decrease in leukocyte count, arthralgia/synovitis, axillary/cervical/inguinal lymph node enlargement, rash, fever, peripheral edema, tachycardia

PREGNANCY: Category C, caution in nursing.

MECHANISM OF ACTION: Avermectin derivative; binds selectively and with high affinity to glutamate-gated chloride ion channels, which occur in invertebrate nerve and muscle cells. This leads to increase in permeability of cell membrane to chloride ions with hyperpolarization of nerve and muscle cell, resulting in paralysis and death of parasite.

PHARMACOKINETICS: Absorption: Administration of variable doses resulted in different parameters. **Metabolism:** Liver. **Elimination:** Feces, urine (≤1%). $T_{1/2}$=18 hrs.

STROVITE FORTE

RX

multiple vitamin - minerals (Everett)

THERAPEUTIC CLASS: Vitamin/mineral

INDICATIONS: For prophylactic or therapeutic nutritional supplementation in physiologically stressful conditions.

DOSAGE: *Adults:* 1 tab qd.

HOW SUPPLIED: Tab: Biotin 0.15mg-Calcium Pantothenate 25mg-Chromium 0.05mg-Copper 3mg-Folic Acid 1mg-Iron 10mg-Magnesium 50mg-Molybdenum 0.02mg-Niacin 100mg-Selenium 0.05mg-Vitamin A 4000 IU-Vitamin B_1 20mg-Vitamin B_2 20mg-Vitamin B_6 25mg-Vitamin B_{12} 0.05mg-Vitamin C 500mg-Vitamin D 400 IU-Vitamin E 60 IU-Zinc 15mg* *scored

WARNINGS/PRECAUTIONS: Accidental overdose of iron-containing products is a leading cause of fatal poisoning in children <6 yrs. Not for the treatment of pernicious anemia and other megaloblastic anemias where vitamin B_{12} is deficient.

ADVERSE REACTIONS: GI intolerance, allergic and idiosyncratic reactions.

INTERACTIONS: Vitamin B₆ may decrease efficacy of levodopa; avoid concomitant use.

MECHANISM OF ACTION: A vitamin/mineral nutritional supplement.

SUBLIMAZE
fentanyl citrate (Akorn)   **CII**

THERAPEUTIC CLASS: Opioid analgesic

INDICATIONS: For analgesic action of short duration during the anesthetic periods, premedication, induction and maintenance, and in the immediate postoperative period (recovery room) as the need arises. For use as a narcotic analgesic supplement in general or regional anesthesia. For administration with a neuroleptic as an anesthetic premedication, for the induction of anesthesia and as an adjunct in the maintenance of general and regional anesthesia. For use as an anesthetic agent with oxygen in selected high risk patients, such as those undergoing open heart surgery or certain complicated neurological or orthopedic procedures.

DOSAGE: *Adults:* ≥12 yrs: Individualize dose. Premedication: 50-100mcg IM 30-60 min prior to surgery. Adjunct to General Anesthesia: Low-Dose: Total Dose: 2mcg/kg for minor surgery. Maint: 2mcg/kg. Moderate Dose: Total Dose: 2-20mcg/kg for major surgery. Maint: 2-20mcg/kg or 25-100mcg IM or IV if surgical stress or lightening of analgesia. High-Dose: Total Dose: 20-50mcg/kg for open heart surgery, complicated neurosurgery, or orthopedic surgery. Maint: 20-50mcg/kg. Adjunct to Regional Anesthesia: 50-100mcg IM or slow IV over 1-2 min. Post-op: 50-100mcg IM, repeat q 1-2 hrs as needed. General Anesthetic: 50-100mcg/kg with oxygen and a muscle relaxant, up to 150mcg/kg may be used.
Pediatrics: 2-12 yrs: Individualize dose. Induction/Maint: 2-3mcg/kg.

HOW SUPPLIED: Inj: 50mcg/mL

WARNINGS/PRECAUTIONS: Should only be administered by persons specifically trained in the use of IV anesthetics and management of the respiratory effects of potent opioids. An opioid antagonist, resuscitative and intubation equipment and oxygen should be readily available. Fluids and other countermeasures to manage hypotension should be available with tranquilizers. Initial dose reduction recommended with narcotic analgesia for recovery. May cause muscle rigidity particularly with muscles used for respiration. Adequate facilities should be available for postoperative monitoring and ventilation. Caution in respiratory depression susceptible patients (eg, comatose patients with head injury or brain tumor). Reduce dose for elderly and debilitated patients. Caution with obstructive pulmonary disease, decreased respiratory reserve, liver and kidney dysfunction, cardiac bradyarrhythmias. Monitor vital signs routinely.

ADVERSE REACTIONS: Respiratory depression, apnea, rigidity, bradycardia, HTN, hypotension, dizziness, blurred vision, nausea, emesis, diaphoresis, pruritus, urticaria, laryngospasms, anaphylaxis, euphoria, miosis, bradycardia, and bronchoconstriction.

INTERACTIONS: Severe and unpredictable potentiation by MAOIs has been reported. Appropriate monitoring and availability of vasodilators and β-blockers for the treatment of hypertension is indicated. Additive or potentiating effects with other CNS depressants (eg, barbiturates, tranquilizers, narcotics, general anesthetics). Reduce dose of other CNS depressants. Reports of cardiovascular depression with nitrous oxide. Alteration of respiration with certain forms of conduction anesthesia (eg, spinal anesthesia, some peridural anesthesia). Decreased pulmonary arterial pressure and hypotension with tranquilizers. Elevated BP, with and without pre-existing hypertension, slower normalcy of EEG patterns with neuroleptics. Extreme caution with neuroleptics in presence of risk factors for development of prolonged QT syndrome and torsade de pointes; ECG monitoring indicated.

PREGNANCY: Category C, caution with nursing.

MECHANISM OF ACTION: Opioid analgesic; produces analgesic and sedative effects. Alters respiratory rate and aveolar ventilation, which may last longer than analgesic effects.

PHARMACOKINETICS: Distribution: V_d=4L/kg; found in skeletal muscle and fat. **Metabolism:** Liver. **Elimination:** Urine (75%, <10% unchanged), feces (10%); $T_{1/2}$=219 min.

SUBOXONE
buprenorphine - naloxone (Reckitt Benckiser)

`CIII`

OTHER BRAND NAMES: Subutex (Reckitt Benckiser)

THERAPEUTIC CLASS: Partial opioid agonist/opioid antagonist

INDICATIONS: Opioid dependence.

DOSAGE: *Adults:* Give either agent SL as a single daily dose in the range of 12-16mg/day. Hold tabs under tongue until dissolved; swallowing tabs reduces bioavailability. Induction: Subutex: Give at least 4 hrs after last short-acting opioid (eg, heroin) use or preferably when early signs of opioid withdrawal appear. Maint: Suboxone: Range: 4mg-24mg/day. Target dose: 16mg/day. Titrate: Adjust by 2mg or 4mg to a level that maintains treatment and suppresses opioid withdrawal effects. Hepatic Impairment: Adjust dose and observe for precipitated opioid withdrawal. Concomitant CNS Depressants: Consider dose reduction.
Pediatrics: ≥16 yrs: Give either agent SL as a single daily dose in the range of 12-16mg/day. Hold tabs under tongue until dissolved; swallowing tabs reduces bioavailability. Induction: Subutex: Give at least 4 hrs after last short-acting opioid (eg, heroin) use or preferably when early signs of opioid withdrawal appear. Maint: Suboxone: Range: 4mg-24mg/day. Target dose: 16mg/day. Titrate: Adjust by 2mg or 4mg to a level that maintains treatment and suppresses opioid withdrawal effects. Hepatic Impairment: Adjust dose and observe for precipitated opioid withdrawal. Concomitant CNS Depressants: Consider dose reduction.

HOW SUPPLIED: Suboxone (Buprenorphine-Naloxone) Tab, SL: 2mg-0.5mg, 8mg-2mg. Subutex (Buprenorphine) Tab, SL: 2mg, 8mg

WARNINGS/PRECAUTIONS: Significant respiratory depression reported with buprenorphine; caution with compromised respiratory function. Naloxone may not be effective in reversing any respiratory depression produced by buprenorphine. Cytolytic hepatitis and hepatitis with jaundice reported. Obtain LFTs prior to initiation and periodically thereafter. Acute and chronic hypersensitivity reactions reported. May increase CSF pressure; caution with head injury, intracranial lesions. May cause miosis, changes in level of consciousness, and orthostatic hypotension. Caution with elderly, debilitated, myxedema, hypothyroidism, acute alcoholism, Addison's disease, CNS depression or coma, toxic psychoses, prostatic hypertrophy, urethral stricture, delirium tremens, kyphoscoliosis, biliary tract dysfunction or severe hepatic/renal/pulmonary impairment. Suboxone may cause opioid withdrawal symptoms. May obscure diagnosis of acute abdominal conditions. May produce dependence.

ADVERSE REACTIONS: Headache, infection, pain (general, abdomen, back), withdrawal syndrome, constipation, nausea, insomnia, sweating, asthenia, anxiety, depression, rhinitis.

INTERACTIONS: May need dose reduction with CYP3A4 inhibitors (eg, azole antifungals, macrolides and HIV protease inhibitors). General anesthetics, other narcotic analgesics, benzodiazepines, phenothiazines, other tranquilizers, sedative/hypnotics or other CNS depressants (including alcohol) may increase risk of CNS depression; consider dose reduction of one or both agents. Monitor closely with CYP3A4 inducers (eg, phenobarbital, carbamazepine, phenytoin, rifampicin).

PREGNANCY: Category C, not for use in nursing.

MECHANISM OF ACTION: Buprenorphine: Partial agonist at the mu-opioid receptor, antagonist at the kappa-opioid receptor. Naloxone: Inhibits mu-opioid receptor activity.

S

PHARMACOKINETICS: Absorption: (Suboxone 16mg) C_{max}=5.95ng/mL, AUC=34.89 hr•ng/mL. (Subtex 16mg) C_{max}=5.47ng/mL, AUC=32.63 hr•ng/mL. Refer to PI for more detailed information. **Distribution:** Plasma protein binding 96% (buprenorphine), 45% (naloxone). **Metabolism:** Buprenorphine: Through N-dealkylation and glucuronidation pathways; norbuprenorphine (active metabolite). Naloxone: Through glucuronidation, N-dealkylation, and reduction. **Elimination:** Urine (30%), feces (69%), $T_{1/2}$=37 hrs (Buprenorphine), 1.1 hrs (Naloxone).

SUDAFED OTC
pseudoephedrine HCL (McNeil)

THERAPEUTIC CLASS: Decongestant

INDICATIONS: For the temporary relief of nasal congestion due to common cold, hay fever, or other upper respiratory allergies and nasal congestion associated with sinusitis.

DOSAGE: *Adults:* Tab, ER: 120mg q12h or 240mg q24h. Max: 240mg/24h. *Pediatrics:* >12 yrs: Liquid/Tab/Tab, Chew: 60mg q4-6h. Max 240mg/24hrs. Tab, ER: 120mg q12h or 240mg q24h. Max: 240mg/24hrs. 6 to <12 yo: (Liquid/Tab/Tab, Chew) 30mg q4-6h. Max: 4 doses/24hrs. 2 to <6 yo: (Liquid/Tab/Tab, Chew) 15mg q4-6h. Max: 4 doses/24hrs.

HOW SUPPLIED: Liq: 15mg/5mL; Tab: 30mg, 60mg; Tab, Chewable: 15mg; Tab, Extended-Release: 120mg, 240mg

WARNINGS/PRECAUTIONS: Do not exceed recommended dosage. If nervousness, dizziness, or sleeplessness occurs, d/c use. Avoid with heart disease, high BP, thyroid disease, diabetes, or difficulty in urination due to prostate enlargement.

INTERACTIONS: Do not take with MAOI or 14 days after discontinuation.

PREGNANCY: Not rated in pregnancy or nursing.

MECHANISM OF ACTION: Relieves nasal congestion associated with sinusitis. Reduces swelling of nasal passages and relieves sinus pressure.

SUFENTA CII
sufentanil citrate (Akorn)

THERAPEUTIC CLASS: Opioid analgesic

INDICATIONS: Analgesic adjunct in the maintenance of balanced general anesthesia in patients who are intubated and ventilated. Primary anesthetic agent of the induction and maintenance of anesthesia with 100% oxygen in patients undergoing major surgical procedures who are intubated or ventilated, such as cardiovascular surgery or neurosurgical procedures in the sitting position, to provide favorable myocardial and cerebral oxygen balance or when extended postoperative ventilation is anticipated. For epidural administrations an analgesic combined with low dose bupivacaine, usually 12.5mg per administration during labor and vaginal delivery.

DOSAGE: *Adults:* ≥12 yrs: Individualize dose. Premedication: Based on patients needs. Analgesic: Total Dose: 1-8mcg/kg. Maint: Incremental: 10-50mcg. Infusion: Based on induction dose not to exceed 1mcg/kg/hr. Anesthetic: Total Dose: 8-30mcg/kg. Maint: Incremental 0.5-10mcg/kg. Infusion: Based on induction dose not to exceed 30mcg/kg. Epidural: 10-15mcg with 10mL bupivacaine 0.125% with or without epinephrine. May repeat for a total of 3 doses in not less than 1 hour intervals.
Pediatrics: Individualize dose. 10-25mcg/kg with 100% oxygen. Maint: 25-50mcg supplemental doses.

HOW SUPPLIED: Inj: 50mcg/mL

WARNINGS/PRECAUTIONS: Should only be administered by persons specifically trained in the use of IV and epidural anesthetics and management of the respiratory effects of potent opioids. An opioid antagonist, resuscitative and

S

intubation equipment and oxygen should be readily available. Prior to catheter insertion, the physician should be familiar with patient conditions (such as infection at the injection site, bleeding diathesis, anticoagulation therapy) which call for special evaluation of the benefit versus risk potential. May cause muscle rigidity of the neck and extremities. Adequate facilities should be available for postoperative monitoring and ventilation. Monitor vital signs routinely. Reduce dose for elderly and debilitated patients. Caution with pulmonary disease, decreased respiratory reserve, liver and kidney dysfunction, cardiac bradyarrhythmias. Reports of bradycardia responsive to atropine. May obscure clinical course of patients with head injuries.

ADVERSE REACTIONS: Respiratory depression, skeletal muscle rigidity, bradycardia, HTN, hypotension, chest wall rigidity, somnolence, pruritus, nausea, vomiting.

INTERACTIONS: Reports of cardiovascular depression with nitrous oxide. High doses of pancuronium may produce increase in heart rate. Reports of bradycardia and hypotension with other muscle relaxants. Greater incidence and degree of bradycardia and hypotension with chronic CCB and β-blocker therapy. Additive or potentiating effects with other CNS depressants (eg, barbiturates, tranquilizers, narcotics, general anesthetics). Reduce dose of either agent. Decrease in mean arterial pressure and systemic vascular resistance with benzodiazepines.

PREGNANCY: Category C, caution in nursing.

MECHANISM OF ACTION: An opioid analgesic.

PHARMACOKINETICS: Distribution: Plasma protein binding (healthy males: 93%, mothers: 91%, neonates: 79%). **Elimination:** $T_{1/2}$=164 min (adults), 97 min (neonates).

Sular   RX
nisoldipine (Sciele)

THERAPEUTIC CLASS: Calcium channel blocker (dihydropyridine)

INDICATIONS: Treatment of hypertension.

DOSAGE: *Adults:* Initial: 20mg qd. Titrate: Increase by 10mg weekly or longer. Maint: 20-40mg qd. Max: 60mg/day. Elderly (>65 yrs)/Hepatic Dysfunction: Initial: Do not exceed 10mg/day. Do not chew, divide, or crush tabs.

HOW SUPPLIED: Tab, Extended-Release: 10mg, 20mg, 30mg, 40mg

WARNINGS/PRECAUTIONS: May increase angina or MI with severe obstructive CAD. May cause hypotension; monitor BP initially or with titration. Caution with heart failure or compromised ventricular function, especially with concomitant β-blockers. Caution with severe hepatic dysfunction or in elderly.

ADVERSE REACTIONS: Peripheral edema, headache, dizziness, pharyngitis, vasodilation, sinusitis, palpitations.

INTERACTIONS: Increased AUC and Cmax with cimetidine. Avoid phenytoin or CYP3A4 inducers. Decreased bioavailability with quinidine. High-fat meals increase peak drug levels. Avoid high-fat meals, grapefruit juice.

PREGNANCY: Category C, not for use in nursing.

MECHANISM OF ACTION: Dihydropyridine class of calcium channel antagonist (calcium ion antagonist or slow channel blocker) that inhibits transmembrane influx of calcium into vascular smooth muscle and cardiac muscle. Inhibition of Ca+ channel results in dilation of arterioles and decreased peripheral vascular resistance.

PHARMACOKINETICS: Absorption: Well absorbed. Absolute bioavailability (5%). T_{max} =6-12 hrs. **Metabolism:** CYP3A4 via hydroxylation. **Elimination:** $T_{1/2}$=7-12 hrs. Urine: (unchanged).

SULFACET-R
sulfacetamide sodium - sulfur (Dermik)

RX

THERAPEUTIC CLASS: Sulfonamide/sulfur combination

INDICATIONS: Topical treatment of acne vulgaris, acne rosacea, and seborrheic dermatitis.

DOSAGE: *Adults:* Shake well before use. Apply qd-tid. Expires after 4 months. *Pediatrics:* ≥12 yrs: Shake well before use. Apply qd-tid. Expires after 4 months.

HOW SUPPLIED: Lot: (Sulfacetamide-Sulfur) 10%-5% [25g]

CONTRAINDICATIONS: Kidney disease.

WARNINGS/PRECAUTIONS: D/C if irritation or hypersensitivity reaction occurs. Avoid eye contact. Contains sulfites. Caution with denuded or abraded skin. May cause reddening and scaling of epidermis.

ADVERSE REACTIONS: Local irritation.

PREGNANCY: Category C, caution in nursing.

MECHANISM OF ACTION: Sulfonamide/sufur combination. Sulfacetamide: Acts as a competitive antagonist to para-aminobenzoic acid (PABA), an essential component for bacterial growth. Sulfur: Not established. Inhibits the growth of *P. acnes* and the formation of free fatty acids.

PHARMACOKINETICS: Absorption: (PO) Readily absorbed. **Distribution:** Orally administered sulfonamides are found in breast milk. **Elimination:** Urine (unchanged).

SULFAMYLON
mafenide acetate (Mylan Bertek)

RX

THERAPEUTIC CLASS: Sulfonamide

INDICATIONS: (Cre) Adjunctive therapy for 2nd- and 3rd-degree burns. (Sol) Adjunctive therapy for excised burn wounds.

DOSAGE: *Adults:* (Cre) Clean and debride wound, then apply qd-bid. Cre should cover wound at all times. Continue application until healing progressing well or site ready for grafting. (Sol) Cover grafted area with mesh gauze and wet with solution using irrigation syringe/tubing q4h or prn to keep wet. If irrigation tube is not used, moisten gauze q6-8h or prn to keep wet. May use solution up to 5 days with same dressing.
Pediatrics: (Cre) Clean and debride wound, then apply qd-bid. Cre should cover wound at all times. Continue application until healing progressing well or site ready for grafting. (Sol) 3 months-16 yrs: Cover grafted area with mesh gauze and wet with solution using irrigation syringe/tubing q4h or prn to keep wet. If irrigation tube is not used, moisten gauze q6-8h or prn to keep wet. May use solution up to 5 days with same dressing.

HOW SUPPLIED: Cre: 85mg/g [60g, 120g, 453.6g]; Sol: 50g/pkt [1ˢ, 5ˢ]

WARNINGS/PRECAUTIONS: Fatal hemolytic anemia with DIC related to G6PD deficiency reported. Cream contains sodium metabisulfite. Monitor acid-base balance with pulmonary or renal dysfunction; risk of metabolic acidosis due to carbonic anhydrase inhibition. Fungal colonization may occur. D/C if hypersensitivity occurs, and for 24-48 hrs if acidosis occurs. Caution with acute renal failure.

ADVERSE REACTIONS: Facial edema, rash, burning sensation, pruritus, erythema, swelling, hyperventilation, tachypnea, acidosis.

INTERACTIONS: Possible cross sensitivity to other sulfonamides.

PREGNANCY: Category C, not for use in nursing.

MECHANISM OF ACTION: Sulfonamide; not established. Exerts broad bacteriostatic action against susceptible gram-negative and gram-positive organisms.

S

PHARMACOKINETICS: Absorption: T_{max}=2 hrs (cream), 4 hrs (solution). **Elimination:** Kidneys.

SULFOXYL LOTION REGULAR   RX
benzoyl peroxide - sulfur (Stiefel)

OTHER BRAND NAMES: Sulfoxyl Lotion Strong (Stiefel)

THERAPEUTIC CLASS: Antibacterial/keratolytic

INDICATIONS: Treatment of acne vulgaris.

DOSAGE: *Adults:* Apply qd for the first week, and bid thereafter. Shake well. Recommended to initiate Sulfoxyl Regular first, then Sulfoxyl Strong when patients demonstrate accommodation to Regular strength.

HOW SUPPLIED: Lot: (Benzoyl Peroxide-Sulfur) (Regular) 5%-2% [59mL]; (Strong) 10%-5% [59mL]

WARNINGS/PRECAUTIONS: Contact sensitization reactions may occur. For external use only; avoid eye contact or mucosal membranes. Avoid contact with hair, fabrics, or carpeting due to benzoyl peroxide's bleaching effect.

ADVERSE REACTIONS: Excessive erythema, peeling.

PREGNANCY: Category C, caution in nursing.

MECHANISM OF ACTION: Antibacteria/keratolytic; not established, suspected to exert beneficial effects through its antimicrobial activity and mild keratolytic action.

SULINDAC   RX
sulindac (Various)

> NSAIDs may cause an increased risk of serious cardiovascular thrombotic events, MI, stroke and serious GI adverse events including bleeding, ulceration, and perforation of the stomach or intestines. Contraindicated for the treatment of perioperative pain in the setting of coronary artery bypass graft (CABG) surgery.

OTHER BRAND NAMES: Clinoril (Merck)

THERAPEUTIC CLASS: NSAID (indene derivative)

INDICATIONS: Acute or long-term use for osteoarthritis (OA), rheumatoid arthritis (RA), ankylosing spondylitis (AS), acute painful shoulder, and acute gouty arthritis.

DOSAGE: *Adults:* OA/RA/AS: Initial: 150mg bid. Acute Painful Shoulder/Acute Gouty Arthritis: 200mg bid for 7-14 days. Max: 400mg/day. Give with food.

HOW SUPPLIED: Tab: 150mg, 200mg* *scored

CONTRAINDICATIONS: ASA or other NSAID allergy that precipitates acute asthmatic attack, urticaria, or rhinitis. Treatment of perioperative pain in the setting of CABG surgery.

WARNINGS/PRECAUTIONS: May lead to onset of new HTN or worsening of pre-existing HTN; monitor BP closely. Fluid retention and edema reported; caution with fluid retention or heart failure. Renal papillary necrosis and other renal injury reported after long-term use. Not recommended for use with advanced renal disease; if therapy must be initiated, monitor renal function. Anaphylactoid reactions may occur. May cause serious skin adverse events (eg, exfoliative dermatitis, Stevens-Johnson syndrome, and toxic epidermal necrolysis). Avoid in late pregnancy; may cause premature closure of ductus arteriosis. May cause elevations of LFTs; d/c if abnormal LFTs persist/worsen, liver disease develops, or systemic manifestations occur. Caution in elderly. Anemia may occur; monitor Hgb/Hct with long-term use. May inhibit platelet aggregation and prolong bleeding time; monitor with coagulation disorders. Caution with asthma and avoid with ASA-sensitive asthma. Keep patients well-hydrated and caution with renal lithiasis. Pancreatitis reported; if pancreatitis suspected, d/c and do not restart. Adverse eye findings reported. Monitor closely with poor liver function and consider dose reduction.

Increased risk of aseptic meningitis in patients with systemic lupus erythematosus (SLE) and mixed connective tissue disease. Risk of GI ulceration, bleeding, and perforation.

ADVERSE REACTIONS: GI pain, dyspepsia, nausea, vomiting, diarrhea, constipation, rash, dizziness, headache, tinnitus, edema.

INTERACTIONS: Avoid DMSO, ASA, and other NSAIDs. May increase methotrexate and cyclosporine toxicities. Probenecid may increase plasma levels. Diflunisal may decrease plasma levels. May diminish antihypertensive effect of ACE inhibitors and reduce natriuretic effect of diuretics. May elevate plasma lithium levels. Increased risk of GI bleeding with warfarin.

PREGNANCY: Category C, not for use in nursing.

MECHANISM OF ACTION: NSAID; suspected to inhibit prostaglandin synthetase; exerts anti-inflammatory, analgesic, and antipyretic actions.

PHARMACOKINETICS: Absorption: PO administration of variable doses resulted in different parameters. **Distribution:** Penetrates placental and blood brain barrier. Plasma protein binding: Sulindac (93.1%), sulindac sulfone (95.4%), sulindac sulfide (97.9%). **Metabolism:** Via oxidation and reduction. **Elimination:** Urine (50%), feces 25% (metabolites); $T_{1/2}$ (sulindac, sulindac sulfide)=7.8, 16.4 hrs.

SUMYCIN RX
tetracycline HCL (Par)

THERAPEUTIC CLASS: *Streptomyces* derived bacteriostatic agent

INDICATIONS: Treatment of respiratory tract, urinary tract, and skin and skin structure infections, lymphogranuloma, psittacosis, trachoma, uncomplicated urethral/endocervical/rectal infection caused by *Chlamydia*, nongonococcal urethritis, chancroid, plague, cholera, brucellosis, and others. When PCN is contraindicated, treatment of uncomplicated gonorrhea, syphilis, listeriosis, anthrax, *Clostridium* species, and others. Adjunct therapy for amebicides and severe acne.

DOSAGE: *Adults:* Mild-Moderate: 250mg qid or 500mg bid. Severe: 500mg qid. Continue for 24-48 hrs after symptoms subside (minimum 10 days with Group A β-hemolytic streptococci). Severe Acne: Initial: 1g/day in divided doses. Maint: After improvement, 125-500mg/day. Brucellosis: 500mg qid for 3 weeks plus streptomycin 1g IM bid for 1 week, then qd for 1 week. Syphilis: 30-40g equally divided over 10-15 days. Gonorrhea: 500mg q6h for 7 days. *Chlamydia:* 500mg qid for at least 7 days. Renal Dysfunction: Reduce dose or extend dose interval.
Pediatrics: >8 yrs: Usual: 25-50mg/kg divided bid-qid. Continue for 24-48 hrs after symptoms subside (minimum 10 days with Group A β-hemolytic streptococci). Severe Acne: Initial: 1g/day in divided doses. Maint: After improvement, 125-500mg/day. Renal Dysfunction: Reduce dose or extend dose interval.

HOW SUPPLIED: Sus: 125mg/5mL; Tab: 250mg, 500mg

WARNINGS/PRECAUTIONS: May cause fetal harm with pregnancy, permanent tooth discoloration during tooth development (last half of pregnancy and children <8 yrs). May increase BUN. Photosensitivity, enamel hypoplasia reported. Superinfection with prolonged use. Suspension contains sodium metabisulfite. Bulging fontanels in infants and benign intracranial HTN in adults reported. Monitor renal/hepatic and hematopoietic function with long-term use. Caution with history of asthma, hay fever, urticaria, and allergy.

ADVERSE REACTIONS: GI effects, photosensitivity, increased BUN, hypersensitivity reactions, blood dyscrasias, dizziness, headache.

INTERACTIONS: May decrease PT; adjust anticoagulants. May interfere with bactericidal agents (eg, penicillin). May decrease effects of oral contraceptives. Take 1 hr before or 2 hrs after dairy products. Aluminum-, calcium-, iron- and magnesium-containing products impair absorption. Fatal renal toxicity reported with concurrent methoxyflurane.

PREGNANCY: Category D, not for use in nursing.

S

MECHANISM OF ACTION: Tetracycline agent; inhibits bacterial protein synthesis.

PHARMACOKINETICS: Absorption: Adequate/incomplete. **Distribution:** Plasma protein binding (65%); excellent penetration into most bodily fluids and tissues; crosses placental barrier and enters fetal circulation and amniotic fluid; found in breast milk. **Elimination:** Urine, feces.

SUPARTZ RX
sodium hyaluronate (Smith & Nephew)

THERAPEUTIC CLASS: Hyaluronan

INDICATIONS: Treatment of pain in osteoarthritis of the knee in patients who have failed to respond adequately to conservative non-pharmacologic therapy and simple analgesics (eg, APAP).

DOSAGE: *Adults:* Administer 2.5mL by intra-articular injection once a week for a total of 5 injections. Some patients may experience benefit with 3 injections given at weekly intervals. Use strict aseptic technique.

HOW SUPPLIED: Inj: 2.5mL

CONTRAINDICATIONS: Avoid with knee infections or skin diseases in the area of the injection site.

WARNINGS/PRECAUTIONS: Avoid disinfectants containing quaternary ammonium salts for skin preparation; hyaluronic acid can precipitate in their presence. Transient pain and/or swelling of the injected joint may occur. Safety and effectiveness in joints other than the knee or concomitantly with other intra-articular injectables have not been established. Caution in patients who are allergic to avian proteins, feathers, and egg products. Avoid any strenuous activities or prolonged (eg, more than 1 hr) weight-bearing activities within 48 hours following the intra-articular injection. Remove any joint effusion before injecting. Safety and effectiveness have not been demonstrated in children.

ADVERSE REACTIONS: Arthralgia, arthropathy, arthrosis, arthritis, back pain, pain (non-specific), injection site reaction, headache, injection site pain.

PREGNANCY: Safety in pregnancy and nursing not known.

MECHANISM OF ACTION: Hyaluronan.

SUPPRELIN LA RX
histrelin acetate (Indevus)

THERAPEUTIC CLASS: Gonadotropin-releasing hormone analog

INDICATIONS: Treatment of children with central precocious puberty.

DOSAGE: *Pediatrics:* ≥2 yrs: 50mg every 12 months. Inject SQ into inner aspect of upper arm. Remove after 12 months of therapy.

HOW SUPPLIED: Implant: 50mg

CONTRAINDICATIONS: Women who are or may become pregnant.

WARNINGS/PRECAUTIONS: Transient increase in estradiol in females and testosterone in both sexes with initial therapy. Proper surgical technique is critical during implant insertion and removal. Monitor LH, FSH, and estradiol or testosterone at 1 month post-implantation, then every 6 months. Assess height and bone age every 6-12 months.

ADVERSE REACTIONS: Implant site reactions, wound infection, dysmenorrhea, epistaxis, erythema, gynecomastia, headache, weight increase.

PREGNANCY: Category X, not for use in nursing.

MECHANISM OF ACTION: Gonadotropin secretion inhibitor; reversible down-regulation of GnRH receptor in pituitary gland and desensitization of pituitary gonadotropes, resulting in decreased levels of LH and FSH.

PHARMACOKINETICS: Absorption: C_{max}=0.43ng/mL.

SUPRANE
desflurane (Baxter)
RX

THERAPEUTIC CLASS: Inhalation anesthetic

INDICATIONS: Induction and/or maintenance of anesthesia for inpatient and outpatient surgery in adults. Maintenance of anesthesia in infants and children after induction of anesthesia with other agents and tracheal intubation.

DOSAGE: *Adults:* Individualize dose. MAC Values: 70 yrs: 5.2 with oxygen 100% or 1.7 with nitrous oxide 60%. 45 yrs: 6 with oxygen 100% or 2.8 with nitrous oxide 60%. 25 yrs: 7.3 with oxygen 100% or 4 with nitrous oxide 60%. With Fentanyl or Midazolam: 31-65 yrs: No Fentanyl: 6.3. With 3mcg/kg Fentanyl: 3.1. With 6mcg/kg Fentanyl: 2.3. No Midazolam: 5.9. With Midazolam 25mcg/kg: 4.9. With Midazolam 50mcg/kg: 4.9. 18-30 yrs: No Fentanyl: 6.4. With Fentanyl 3mcg/kg: 3.5. With Fentanyl 6mcg/kg: 3. No Midazolam: 6.9.
Pediatrics: Individualize dose. MAC Values: 7 yrs: 8.1 with oxygen 100%. 4 yrs: 8.6 with oxygen 100%. 3 yrs: 6.4 with nitrous oxide 60%. 2 yrs: 9.1 with oxygen 100%. 9 months: 10 with oxygen 100% or 7.5 with nitrous oxide 60%. 10 weeks: 9.4 with oxygen 100%. 2 weeks: 9.2 with oxygen 100%.

HOW SUPPLIED: Liq: [240mL]

CONTRAINDICATIONS: Known or suspected susceptibility to malignant hyperthermia.

WARNINGS/PRECAUTIONS: Not recommended for induction of general anesthesia via mask in infants or children. Produces dose-dependent decreases in BP. Concentrations >1 MAC may increase HR. Administer at 0.8 MAC or less, in conjunction with barbiturate induction and hyperventilation. Maintain normal hemodynamics with CAD. May cause sensitivity hepatitis in patients who have been sensitized by previous exposure to halogenated anesthetics. May trigger malignant hyperthermia. May produce a dose-dependent increase in CSF pressure when administered to patients with intracranial space occupying lesions. Not recommended for maintenence of anesthesia in non-intubated children.

ADVERSE REACTIONS: Coughing, breathholding, apnea, laryngospasm, oxyhemoglobin desaturation, increased secretions, bronchospasm, nausea, vomiting.

INTERACTIONS: Decreased MAC with benzodiazepines and opioids. May decrease the required dose of neuromuscular blocking agents.

PREGNANCY: Category B, caution in nursing.

MECHANISM OF ACTION: Inhalation anesthetic agent.

SUPRAX
cefixime (Lupin)
RX

THERAPEUTIC CLASS: Cephalosporin (3rd generation)

INDICATIONS: Otitis media, pharyngitis, tonsillitis, acute bronchitis, acute exacerbation of chronic bronchitis, uncomplicated UTIs, and cervical/urethral gonorrhea caused by susceptible strains.

DOSAGE: *Adults:* Usual: 400mg qd. Gonorrhea: 400mg single dose. CrCl 21-60mL/min/Hemodialysis: Give 75% of standard dose. CrCl <20mL/min/CAPD: Give 50% of standard dose.
Pediatrics: >12 yrs or >50kg: (Tab/Sus) Usual: 400mg qd. ≥6 months: (Sus) 8mg/kg qd or 4mg/kg bid. Treat for at least 10 days with *S. pyogenes*. CrCl 21-60mL/min/Hemodialysis: Give 75% of standard dose. CrCl <20mL/min/CAPD: Give 50% of standard dose.

HOW SUPPLIED: Tab: 400mg; Sus:100mg/5mL [50mL, 75mL, 100mL]

WARNINGS/PRECAUTIONS: Caution with PCN or other allergy, GI disease (eg, colitis). Anaphylactic/anaphylactoid reactions, pseudomembranous colitis reported. May cause false (+) direct Coombs test or false (+) reaction for urinary glucose using Benedict's/Fehling's solution or Clinitest®.

S

ADVERSE REACTIONS: Diarrhea, abdominal pain, nausea, dyspepsia, flatulence, superinfection.

INTERACTIONS: May increase carbamazepine levels. Increased PT with anticoagulants (eg, warfarin).

PREGNANCY: Category B, not for use in nursing.

MECHANISM OF ACTION: 3rd-generation cephalosporin; inhibits cell-wall synthesis.

PHARMACOKINETICS: Absorption: 40-50% absorbed. C_{max}=2mcg/mL (200mg tab), 3.7mcg/mL (400mg tab), 3mcg/mL (200mg sus), 4.6mcg/mL (400mg sus); T_{max}=2-6 hrs (200mg tab, 400mg tab/sus), 2-5 hrs (200mg sus). **Distribution:** Serum protein binding (65%). **Elimination:** Urine (50%, unchanged); $T_{1/2}$=3-4 up to 9 hrs.

SURMONTIL
RX
trimipramine maleate (Odyssey)

> Antidepressants increased the risk of suicidal thinking and behavior (suicidality) in short-term studies in children, adolescents, and young adults with Major Depressive Disorder (MDD) and other psychiatric disorders. Trimipramine is not approved for use in pediatric patients.

THERAPEUTIC CLASS: Tricyclic antidepressant

INDICATIONS: Relief of symptoms of depression.

DOSAGE: *Adults:* Outpatient: Initial: 75mg/day in divided doses. Titrate: Increase to 150mg/day. Maint: 50-150mg/day. Max: 200mg/day. Hospitalized Patients: Initial: 100mg/day in divided doses. Titrate: Increase gradually to 200mg/day. If no improvement after 2-3 weeks, may increase up to 250-300mg/day. Elderly: Initial: 50mg/day. Titrate: Increase gradually to 100mg/day. Take hs for at least 3 months.
Pediatrics: Adolescents: Initial: 50mg/day. Titrate: Increase gradually to 100mg/day. Take hs for at least 3 months.

HOW SUPPLIED: Cap: 25mg, 50mg, 100mg

CONTRAINDICATIONS: Acute recovery period post-MI, within 14 days of MAOI therapy.

WARNINGS/PRECAUTIONS: Caution with cardiovascular disease, increased IOP, urinary retention, narrow-angle glaucoma, hyperthyroidism, seizure disorder, liver dysfunction. May impair ability to operate machinery. May alter glucose levels. May activate psychosis in schizophrenia. Manic or hypomanic episodes may occur. May increase hazards with electroshock therapy.

ADVERSE REACTIONS: Hypotension, HTN, arrhythmia, confusion, insomnia, incoordination, GI complaints, allergic reactions, gynecomastia, blood dyscrasias, dry mouth, blurred vision, urinary retention.

INTERACTIONS: Cimetidine inhibits elimination. Alcohol may exaggerate effects. May potentiate catecholamine or anticholinergic effects. Potentiated by CYP2D6 inhibitors (eg, quinidine) and substrates (eg, other antidepressants, phenothiazines, propafenone, fleccainide). Caution with SSRIs; wait 5 weeks after fluoxetine withdrawal before initiating therapy. Avoid MAOIs.

PREGNANCY: Category C, safety in nursing not known.

MECHANISM OF ACTION: Tricyclic antidepressant with anxiety-reducing sedative component to its action.

SUSTIVA
RX
efavirenz (Bristol-Myers Squibb)

THERAPEUTIC CLASS: Non-nucleoside reverse transcriptase inhibitor

INDICATIONS: Treatment of HIV-1 infection in combination with other antiretrovirals.

DOSAGE: *Adults:* Initial: 600mg qd. Take on an empty stomach, preferably at bedtime.

Pediatrics: ≥3 yrs: 10 to <15kg: 200mg qd. 15 to <20kg: 250mg qd. 20 to <25kg: 300mg qd. 25 to <32.5kg: 350mg qd. 32.5 to <40kg: 400mg qd. ≥40kg: 600mg qd. Take on an empty stomach, preferably at bedtime.

HOW SUPPLIED: Cap: 50mg, 100mg, 200mg; Tab: 600mg

CONTRAINDICATIONS: Concomitant astemizole, bepridil, cisapride, midazolam, pimozide, triazolam, ergot derivatives, or standard doses of voriconazole.

WARNINGS/PRECAUTIONS: Not for monotherapy. Severe skin rash reported. Avoid pregnancy; use barrier contraception with other contraception methods and obtain (-) pregnancy test before therapy. Monitor LFTs with known or suspected hepatitis B or C. Monitor cholesterol and triglycerides. High fat meals may increase absorption. Possible redistribution or accumulation of body fat. Serious psychiatric and CNS adverse experiences (dizziness, insomnia, impaired concentration, somnolence, abnormal dreams, hallucinations) reported.

ADVERSE REACTIONS: CNS symptoms (eg, dizziness, insomnia, impaired concentration, somnolence, abnormal dreams), psychiatric symptoms (eg, severe depression), rash, GI effects.

INTERACTIONS: Avoid astemizole, cisapride, midazolam, triazolam, voriconazole, St. John's wort, or ergot derivatives. St. John's wort decreases efavirenz to suboptimal levels; increases risk of resistance. Significantly decreased levels of voriconazole. CYP3A4 inducers (eg, phenobarbital, rifampin, rifabutin) may decrease plasma levels. Increased levels of ethinyl estradiol. Decreased levels of clarithromycin; consider alternative. Decreased levels of indinavir and rifabutin; adjust doses. Increased levels of ritonavir and efavirenz with concomitant use; monitor LFTs. Decreased levels of saquinavir, sertraline. May decrease methadone levels; monitor for signs of withdrawal. May affect warfarin levels. May decrease itraconazole, ketoconazole, amprenavir levels. Decreased levels of anticonvulsants (eg, phenytoin, phenobarbital, carbamazepine) and efavirenz; monitor anticonvulsant levels.

PREGNANCY: Category D, not for use in nursing.

MECHANISM OF ACTION: Non-nucleoside reverse transcriptase inhibitor.

PHARMACOKINETICS: Absorption: C_{max}=12.9µM, T_{max}=3-5 hrs; AUC=184µM•h. **Distribution:** Plasma protein binding (99.5-99.75%). **Metabolism:** CYP3A4,2B6 (hydroxylation, glucuronidation). **Elimination:** Urine, feces; $T_{1/2}$=40-55 hrs.

SUTENT   RX
sunitinib malate (Pfizer)

THERAPEUTIC CLASS: Multikinase inhibitor

INDICATIONS: Treatment of gastrointestinal stromal tumor (GIST) after disease progression on or intolerance to imatinib mesylate. Treatment of advanced renal cell carcinoma (RCC).

DOSAGE: *Adults:* 50mg once daily; 4 weeks on, 2 weeks off. Dose increase/reduction in 12.5mg increments is recommended. Concomitant Strong CYP3A4 Inhibitors: Consider dose reduction to minimum of 37.5mg daily. Concomitant CYP3A4 Inducer: Consider dose increase to maximum of 87.5mg daily.

HOW SUPPLIED: Cap: 12.5mg, 25mg, 50mg

WARNINGS/PRECAUTIONS: Cases of decreased left ventricular ejection fraction (LVEF) reported. Patients with cardiac risk factors should be carefully monitored for signs and symptoms of CHF; baseline and periodic evaluation of LVEF should be considered. D/C if clinical manifestations of CHF occur. Prolongation of QT interval and torsade de pointes observed; consider monitoring ECG and electrolytes (magnesium, potassium). Cases of hemorrhagic events reported. Serious, sometimes fatal GI complications including GI perforation have occurred with intra-abdominal malignancies. Cases of HTN reported; monitor for HTN and treat as needed with standard antihypertensive therapy. Temporary suspension recommended if severe HTN occurs. Adrenal toxicity reported; monitor for adrenal insufficiency with stress, trauma, or severe infection. Myelosuppression, hypothyroidism, increases in serum lipase/

amylase, and pancreatitis reported. Monitor CBCs, platelet count, thyroid function, and serum chemistries beginning each treatment cycle. May cause fetal harm; avoid pregnancy.

ADVERSE REACTIONS: Fatigue, asthenia, diarrhea, nausea, mucositis/stomatitis, vomiting, dyspepsia, abdominal pain, HTN, rash, hand-foot syndrome, skin discoloration, altered taste, anorexia, bleeding.

INTERACTIONS: Concomitant CYP3A4 inhibitors (eg, ketoconazole) may increase plasma concentrations; consider dose reduction. CYP3A4 inducers (eg, rifampin) may decrease plasma concentrations; consider dose increase. Avoid concurrent St. John's wort; may decrease plasma concentrations unpredictably.

PREGNANCY: Category D, not for use in nursing.

MECHANISM OF ACTION: Multikinase inhibitor; inhibits multiple receptor tyrosine kinase, implicated in tumor growth, pathologic angiogenesis, and metastatic cancer progression.

PHARMACOKINETICS: Absorption: T_{max}=6-12 hrs. **Distribution:** Plasma protein binding (95%); V_d=2230L. **Metabolism:** CYP3A4. **Elimination:** Feces (61%), renal (16%); $T_{1/2}$=40-60 hrs, 80-110 hrs (metabolite).

SYMBICORT   RX
budesonide fumarate dihydrate - formoterol (AstraZeneca)

> Long-acting β₂-adrenergic agonists (formoterol) may increase the risk of asthma-related death.

THERAPEUTIC CLASS: Corticosteroid/beta₂ agonist

INDICATIONS: Long-term maintenance treatment of asthma in patients ≥12 yrs.

DOSAGE: *Adults:* Current Medium-High Dose Inhaled CS: 2 inh bid of 160/4.5. Current Low to Medium Doses Inhaled CS: 2 inh bid of 80/4.5. No Current Inhaled CS: 2 inh bid of 80/4.5 or 160/4.5 depending on asthma severity. Max: 640mcg/18mcg (2 inh bid of 160/4.5). Patients not responding to the starting dose after 1-2 weeks of therapy with 80/4.5, replace with 160/4.5 for better asthma control. Rinse mouth after use.
Pediatrics: ≥12 yrs: Current Medium-High Dose Inhaled CS: 2 inh bid of 160/4.5. Current Low to Medium Doses Inhaled CS: 2 inh bid of 80/4.5. No Current Inhaled CS: 2 inh bid of 80/4.5 or 160/4.5 depending on asthma severity. Max: 640mcg/18mcg (2 inh bid of 160/4.5). Patients not responding to the starting dose after 1-2 weeks of therapy with 80/4.5, replace with 160/4.5 for better asthma control. Rinse mouth after use.

HOW SUPPLIED: MDI: (Budesonide-Formoterol) 80mcg-4.5mcg/inh, 160mcg-4.5mcg/inh [10.2g]

CONTRAINDICATIONS: Primary treatment of status asthmaticus or other acute asthma attacks.

WARNINGS/PRECAUTIONS: Do not use in patients with significantly worsening or acutely deteriorating asthma. Not for acute treatment of symptoms. Monitor for increasing use of inhaled, short-acting β₂-agonists. Deaths due to adrenal insufficiency have occured with transfer from systemic corticosteroids to inhaled corticosteroids. Resume oral corticosteroids during stress or severe asthma attack. Transferring from oral to inhalation therapy may unmask allergic conditions (eg, rhinitis, conjunctivitis, eczema). Observe for adrenal insufficiency, systemic corticosteroid withdrawal effects, and growth suppression (children). More susceptible to infections. Not for acute bronchospasm. Do not use any additional inhaled long-acting β₂-agonist for prevention of exercise induced bronchospasm or the maintenance treatment of asthma. D/C if paradoxical bronchospasm occurs. Immediate hypersensitivity and upper airway symptom reactions reported. Caution with cardiovascular disorder (eg, coronary insufficiency, arrhythmia, HTN), seizures, thyroid and hepatic problems, diabetes, osteoporosis. QTc interval prolongation reported.

ADVERSE REACTIONS: Nasopharyngitis, headache, upper respiratory tract infections, sinusitis, back pain, nasal/sinus congestion, oral candidiasis, influenza, rhinitis, pharyngolaryngeal pain, vomiting.

INTERACTIONS: Oral ketoconazole increases plasma levels. CYP3A4 inhibitors (eg, itraconazole, clarithromycin, erythromycin) may inhibit metabolism and increase systemic exposure. Caution with non-K$^+$-sparing diuretics. Extreme caution within 14 days of using MAOIs or TCAs. Avoid with β-blockers.

PREGNANCY: Category C, not for use in nursing.

MECHANISM OF ACTION: Budesonide: Corticosteroid; shown to have inhibitory effects on multiple cell types (mast cells, eosinophils, neutrophils, macrophages and lymphocytes) and mediators (histamine, eicosanoids, leukotrienes and cytokines) involved in inflammatory and asthmatic response. Formoterol: β$_2$-adrenergic agonist; stimulates intracellular adenyl cyclase, which catalyzes conversion of ATP to cAMP, to produce relaxation of bronchial smooth muscle and inhibition of release of mediators of immediate hypersensitivity from cells (mast cells).

PHARMACOKINETICS: Absorption: Budesonide: Rapid (lungs). C_{max}=4.5nmol/L, T_{max}=20 min. Formoterol: Rapid (GI). C_{max}=136pmol, T_{max}=5-10 min. **Distribution:** Budesonide: V_d=3L/kg; plasma protein binding (85-90%). Formoterol: Plasma protein binding (RR enantiomer, 46%), (SS enantiomer, 58%). **Metabolism:** Budesonide: Liver (biotransformation) via CYP3A4. Formoterol: Liver (direct glucuronidation and O-demethylation) via CYP2D6, 2C. **Elimination:** Budesonide: $T_{1/2}$=2-3 hrs. Formoterol: Urine (8%).

SYMBYAX   RX
fluoxetine HCL - olanzapine (Lilly)

> Antidepressants increased the risk of suicidal thinking and behavior (suicidality) in short-term studies in children, adolescents, and young adults with Major Depressive Disorder (MDD) and other psychiatric disorders. Symbyax is not approved for use in pediatric patients. Elderly patients with dementia-related psychosis treated with atypical antipsychotic drugs are at an increased risk of death; most appeared to be cardiovascular (eg, heart failure, sudden death) or infectious (eg, pneumonia) in nature. Symbyax is not approved for the treatment of patients with dementia-related psychosis.

THERAPEUTIC CLASS: Thienobenzodiazepine/selective serotonin reuptake inhibitor

INDICATIONS: Treatment of depressive episodes associated with bipolar disorder.

DOSAGE: *Adults:* ≥18 yrs: Initial: 6-25mg qd in evening. Titrate: Adjust dose based on efficacy and tolerability. Max: 18mg/75mg. Hypotension Risk/Hepatic Impairment/Slow Metabolizers: Initial: 3-25mg to 6-25mg qd in evening. Titrate: Increase cautiously. Re-evaluate periodically.

HOW SUPPLIED: Cap: (Olanzapine-Fluoxetine): 3mg-25mg, 6mg-25mg, 6mg-50mg, 12mg-25mg, 12mg-50mg

CONTRAINDICATIONS: During or within 14 days of MAOI use; during or within 5 weeks of discontinuation of thioridazine use; concomitant pimozide use.

WARNINGS/PRECAUTIONS: Monitor for clinical worsening and/or suicidality. Monitor for hyperglycemia, worsening of glucose control with DM, FBG levels with diabetes risk. Not for use with dementia-related psychosis. Risk of orthostatic hypotension, NMS, tardive dyskinesia, hyperprolactinemia, hyponatremia, seizures. Caution with cardio- or cerebrovascular disease, hypotension risk (eg, dehydration, hypovolemia), history of seizures or conditions that lower seizure threshold, elderly (especially with dementia), hepatic impairment, risk of aspiration pneumonia, conditions that affect metabolism or hemodynamic responses, prostatic hypertrophy, narrow-angle glaucoma, history of paralytic ileus, suicidal tendencies. D/C if unexplained allergic reaction occurs. Elevated transaminases, bleeding episodes reported. Monitor for symptoms of mania/hypomania. May cause disruption of body temperature regulation. Serotonin syndrome reported; caution with MAOIs, other serotonergic drugs.

S

Caution when prescribing olanzapine and fluoxetine products concomitantly. May impair judgement, thinking, or motor skills.

ADVERSE REACTIONS: Asthenia, somnolence, weight gain, edema, increased appetite, peripheral edema, pharyngitis, abnormal thinking, tremor, diarrhea, dry mouth, amblyopia, twitching, arthralgia, abnormal ejaculation.

INTERACTIONS: See Contraindications. Risk of orthostatic hypotension with antihypertensives, benzodiazepines, alcohol. May antagonize levodopa, dopamine agonists. Increased clearance with carbamazepine, omeprazole, rifampin, other inducers of CYP1A2 or glucuronyl transferase. Increase in clozapine, haloperidol, phenytoin levels. Caution with other CNS-drugs, sumatriptan, tryptophan, other highly protein bound drugs (eg, warfarin, digitoxin), hepatotoxic drugs, other olanzapine- or fluoxetine-containing products. Decreased clearance with fluvoxamine, fluoroquinolones, other CYP1A2 inhibitors. Monitor lithium levels. May increase TCA levels; may require reduction in TCA dose. Increased risk of bleeding with NSAIDs, ASA, warfarin. Inhibits drugs metabolized by CYP2D6 (eg, flecainide, vinblastine, TCAs); initiate at lower end of dosage range.

PREGNANCY: Category C, not for use in nursing.

MECHANISM OF ACTION: Not established; proposed to activate serotonin, norepinephrine, and dopamine, enhancing antidepressant effect. Olanzepine: Thienobenzodiazepine; psychotropic agent with high affinity binding to $5HT_{2a/2c}$, $5HT_6$, D_{1-4}, H_1, and adrenergic (alpha)$_1$-receptors. Fluoxetine: Selective serotonin reuptake inhibitor; inhibits serotonin transport; weak inhibitor of norepinephrine and dopamine transporters.

PHARMACOKINETICS: Absorption: Olanzepine: Well absorbed; T_{max}=approx. 6 hrs. Fluoxetine: C_{max}=15-55ng/mL ,T_{max}=6-8 hrs. **Distribution:** Olanzepine: Plasma protein binding (93%), V_d=1000L. Fluoxetine: Plasma protein binding (94.5%). **Metabolism:** Olanzapine: Extensively metabolized, via glucuronidation and CYP450 mediated oxidation, 10-N-glucuronide and 4'-N-desmethyl olanzapine (major metabolites). Fluoxetine: Liver (extensive); CYP 2D6 pathway, norfluoxetine (active metabolite). **Elimination:** Olanzapine: $T_{1/2}$=21-54 hrs. Urine (57%), feces (30%). Fluoxetine: Kidneys. (Acute administration) $T_{1/2}$=1-3 days; (chronic administration) $T_{1/2}$=4-6 days.

SYMLIN   RX
pramlintide acetate (Amylin)

> Use with insulin. Risk of insulin-induced severe hypoglycemia, particularly with type 1 DM. Severe hypoglycemia usually occurs within 3 hrs of injection. Serious injuries may occur if severe hypoglycemia occurs while operating a motor vehicle, heavy machinery, or other high-risk activities. Appropriate patient selection, careful patient instruction, and insulin dose adjustments are necessary to reduce this risk.

OTHER BRAND NAMES: SymlinPen (Amylin)

THERAPEUTIC CLASS: Synthetic amylin analog

INDICATIONS: Adjunct treatment in patients with type 1 or type 2 DM who use mealtime insulin therapy and who have failed to achieve desired glucose control despite optimal insulin therapy. May be used with or without sulfonylurea and/or metformin in type 2 DM.

DOSAGE: *Adults:* Before initiating therapy reduce insulin dose by 50%. Monitor blood glucose frequently. Adjust insulin dose once target dose of pramlintide is maintained. Type 2 DM: Initial: 60mcg SQ immediately prior to meals. Titrate: 120mcg as tolerated. Type 1 DM: Initial: 15mcg SQ immediately prior to meals. Titrate: Increase by 15mcg increments to 30mcg or 60mcg as tolerated.

HOW SUPPLIED: Inj: 600mcg/mL [5mL]; Pen injector: 1000mcg/mL [1.5mL, 2.7mL]

CONTRAINDICATIONS: Confirmed diagnosis of gastroparesis; hypoglycemia unawareness.

WARNINGS/PRECAUTIONS: Do not mix with insulin; administer as separate injections.

ADVERSE REACTIONS: Nausea, headache, anorexia, vomiting, abdominal pain, fatigue, dizziness, coughing, pharyngitis.

INTERACTIONS: Do not administer with agents that alter gastrointestinal motility (eg, anticholinergic agents such as atropine), and agents that slow intestinal absorption of nutrients (eg, α-glucosidase inhibitors). Administer analgesics and other oral agents that require rapid onset 1 hr before or 2 hrs after injection.

PREGNANCY: Category C, caution in nursing.

MECHANISM OF ACTION: Amylinomimetic agent that modulates gastric emptying, prevents postprandial rise in plasma glucagon, and produces satiety, which leads to a decreased caloric intake.

PHARMACOKINETICS: Absorption: Absolute bioavailability (30-40%); SQ administration of variable doses resulted in different parameters. **Distribution**: Not extensively bound to blood cells or albumin (40% unbound). **Metabolism**: Kidneys (primarily). Des-lys pramlintide (primary active metabolite). **Elimination**: $T_{1/2}$=48 min.

SYMMETREL   RX
amantadine HCL (Endo)

THERAPEUTIC CLASS: Dopamine agonist

INDICATIONS: Prophylaxis and treatment of uncomplicated influenza A infections. Treatment of parkinsonism and drug-induced extrapyramidal reactions.

DOSAGE: *Adults:* Influenza A Virus Prophylaxis/Treatment: 200mg qd or 100mg bid. Elderly: ≥65 yrs: 100mg qd. Parkinsonism: Initial: 100mg bid. Serious Associated Illness/Concomitant High Dose Antiparkinson Agent: Initial: 100mg qd. Titrate: May increase to 100mg bid after 1 to several weeks. Max: 400mg/day. Drug-Induced Extrapyramidal Reactions: 100mg bid. Titrate: May increase to 300mg/day in divided doses. CrCl 30-50mL/min: 200mg on Day 1, then 100mg qd. CrCl 15-29mL/min: 200mg on Day 1, then 100mg every other day. CrCl <15mL/min/Hemodialysis: 200mg every 7 days. *Pediatrics:* Influenza A Virus Prophylaxis/Treatment: 9-12 yrs: 100mg bid. 1-9 yrs: 4.4-8.8mg/kg/day. Max: 150mg/day.

HOW SUPPLIED: Syrup: 50mg/5mL; Tab: 100mg

WARNINGS/PRECAUTIONS: Deaths reported from overdose. Suicide attempts, NMS reported. Caution with CHF, peripheral edema, orthostatic hypotension, renal or hepatic dysfunction, recurrent eczematoid rash, uncontrolled psychosis or severe psychoneurosis. Avoid in untreated angle closure glaucoma. Do not d/c abruptly in Parkinson's disease. May increase seizure activity.

ADVERSE REACTIONS: Nausea, dizziness, insomnia, depression, anxiety, hallucinations, confusion, anorexia, dry mouth, constipation, ataxia, livedo reticularis, peripheral edema, orthostatic hypotension, agranulocytosis.

INTERACTIONS: Caution with CNS stimulants. Anticholinergic agents may potentiate the anticholinergic side effects. Increased tremor in elderly Parkinson's patients with thioridazine. Increased plasma levels with trimethoprim-sulfamethoxazole, quinine, or quinidine. Avoid use of Attenuated Influenza Vaccine within 2 weeks before or 48 hours after.

PREGNANCY: Category C, not for use in nursing.

MECHANISM OF ACTION: Antiviral; appears to prevent release of infectious viral nucleic acid into host cell by interfering with function of transmembrane domain of viral M2 protein, preventing virus assembly during replication.

PHARMACOKINETICS: Absorption: (Tab) C_{max}=0.51mcg/mL, T_{max}=2-4 hrs. (Syrup) C_{max}=0.24mcg/mL, T_{max}=2-4 hrs. **Distribution:** (IV) V_d=3-8L/Kg; plasma protein binding (67%).

S

SYNAGIS
RX
palivizumab (MedImmune)

THERAPEUTIC CLASS: Monoclonal antibody/RSV F-protein blocker

INDICATIONS: Prevention of serious lower respiratory tract disease caused by respiratory syncytial virus (RSV) in pediatrics at high risk of RSV.

DOSAGE: *Pediatrics:* 15mg/kg IM; give 1st dose before start of RSV season (November-April), then monthly throughout season. Give monthly also if develop RSV infection. Safety and efficacy established in infants with bronchopulmonary dysplasia (BPD) and infants with history of prematurity (≤35 weeks gestational age).

HOW SUPPLIED: Inj: 50mg, 100mg

WARNINGS/PRECAUTIONS: Anaphylactoid reactions reported. Caution with thrombocytopenia or any coagulation disorder due to IM injection. Safety and efficacy not demonstrated for treatment of established RSV disease.

ADVERSE REACTIONS: Upper respiratory infection, otitis media, rash, cough, diarrhea, vomiting, liver function abnormality, fever, rhinitis, hernia, gastroenteritis, wheezing.

PREGNANCY: Category C, safety in nursing not known.

MECHANISM OF ACTION: Monoclonal antibody; exhibits neutralizing and fusion-inhibitory activity against RSV.

PHARMACOKINETICS: Elimination: $T_{1/2}$=20 days.

SYNALAR
RX
fluocinolone acetonide (Medicis)

THERAPEUTIC CLASS: Corticosteroid

INDICATIONS: Corticosteroid responsive dermatoses.

DOSAGE: *Adults:* Apply bid-qid. May use occlusive dressings for psoriasis or recalcitrant conditions; d/c dressings if infection develops.
Pediatrics: Apply bid-qid. May use occlusive dressings for psoriasis or recalcitrant conditions; d/c dressings if infection develops.

HOW SUPPLIED: Cre, Oint: 0.025% [15g, 60g]; Sol: 0.01% [20mL, 60mL]

WARNINGS/PRECAUTIONS: May produce reversible HPA axis suppression, manifestations of Cushing's syndrome, hyperglycemia, and glucosuria. Caution when applied to large surface areas or under occlusive dressings. Use appropriate antifungal or antibacterial agent with dermatological infections; d/c if infection does not clear. Peds may be more susceptible to systemic toxicity. Avoid eyes. D/C if irritation occurs.

ADVERSE REACTIONS: Burning, itching, irritation, dryness, folliculitis, hypertrichosis, acneiform eruptions, premolar dermatitis, hypopigmentation, allergic dermatitis, skin maceration, secondary infection, skin atrophy.

PREGNANCY: Category C, caution with nursing.

MECHANISM OF ACTION: Corticosteroid; possesses anti-inflammatory, antipruritic, and vasoconstrictive actions. Anti-inflammatory activity not established.

PHARMACOKINETICS: Absorption: Percutaneous; occlusion, inflammation, and other disease states may increase absorption. **Distribution:** Systemically administered corticosteroids are found in breast milk. **Metabolism:** Liver. **Excretion:** Kidneys, bile.

SYNAREL
RX
nafarelin acetate (G.D. Searle)

THERAPEUTIC CLASS: Gonadotropin-releasing hormone analog

INDICATIONS: Management of endometriosis, including pain relief and reduction of lesions. Treatment of central precocious puberty (CPP) (gonadotropin-dependent precocious puberty) in children of both sexes.

DOSAGE: (Endometriosis) *Adults:* ≥18 yrs: 1 spray (200mcg) into one nostril qam and 1 spray into other nostril qpm. Initiate therapy between days 2-4 of menstrual cycle. Increase to 1 spray per nostril qam and qpm after 2 months (800mcg/day) if amenorrhea has not occurred. Treat for 6 months.
(CPP) *Pediatrics:* Usual: 2 sprays (400mcg) per nostril qam and qpm. Total Daily Dose: 1600mcg. Increase to 3 sprays into alternating nostrils tid (1800mcg daily) if needed 30 seconds should elapse between sprays. Continue until resumption of puberty is desired.

HOW SUPPLIED: Spray: 200mcg/inh [8mL]

CONTRAINDICATIONS: Pregnancy, women who may become pregnant, nursing, undiagnosed abnormal vaginal bleeding.

WARNINGS/PRECAUTIONS: (Endometriosis) Ovarian cysts reported in adult women. Caution if risk factors for decreased bone mineral content present. Avoid sneezing during or after administration. Use nonhormonal methods of contraception. (CPP) Determine diagnosis before initiating therapy. Monitor regularly. Assess growth and bone age velocity within 3 to 6 months of initiation. Avoid sneezing during or after administration.

ADVERSE REACTIONS: (Endometriosis) Hot flashes, decreased libido, vaginal dryness, headache, emotional lability, myalgia, acne, nasal irritation, reduced breast size, insomnia, edema, seborrhea, weight gain, depression, hirsutism. (CPP) Acne, breast enlargement, vaginal bleeding, emotional lability, transient increase in pubic hair, rhinitis, body odor, seborrhea, white or brownish vaginal discharge.

INTERACTIONS: Avoid topical decongestants within 2 hrs after dosing.

PREGNANCY: Category X, not for use in nursing.

MECHANISM OF ACTION: Gonadotropin-releasing hormone analog. Initially, stimulates the release of the pituitary gonadotropins, LH and FSH, resulting in a temporary increase in gonadal steroidogenesis. Repeated dosing abolishes the stimulatory effects on the pituitary glands. Decreased secretions of gonadal steroids cause gonadal steroid-dependent tissues and functions to become quiescent.

PHARMACOKINETICS: Absorption: Rapidly absorbed. Children: C_{max}=2.2ng/mL (400µg), 6.6ng/mL (600µg); T_{max}=10-45 min. Adult women: C_{max}=0.6ng/mL (200µg), 1.8ng/mL (400µg); T_{max}=10-40 min. Bioavailability: 2.8% (400µg). **Distribution:** Plasma protein binding (80%); found in breast milk. **Metabolism:** Tyr-D(2)-Nal-Leu-Arg-Pro-Gly-NH$_2$(5-10) (major metabolite). **Elimination:** Urine (44-55%) (3% unchanged), feces (18.5-44.2%).

SYNERA   RX
tetracaine - lidocaine (Endo)

THERAPEUTIC CLASS: Acetamide local anesthetic

INDICATIONS: For use on intact skin to provide local dermal analgesia for superficial venous access and superficial dermatological procedures such as excision, electrodessication, and shave biopsy of skin lesions.

DOSAGE: *Adults:* Venipuncture or IV Cannulation: Apply to intact skin for 20-30 min prior to procedure. Superficial Dermatological Procedures: Apply to intact skin for 30 min prior to procedure.
Pediatrics: ≥3 yrs: Venipuncture or IV Cannulation: Apply to intact skin for 20-30 min prior to procedure. Superficial Dermatological Procedure: Apply to intact skin for 30 min prior to procedure.

HOW SUPPLIED: Patch: (Lidocaine-Tetracaine) 70mg-70mg

CONTRAINDICATIONS: PABA hypersensitivity.

WARNINGS/PRECAUTIONS: Serious adverse events may occur in children or pets if ingested. Caution in acutely ill or debillitated. Risk of allergic/anaphylactoid reactions (urticaria, angioedema, bronchospasm, shock). Increased risk of toxicity in severe hepatic disease. Avoid broken or inflamed skin, eye contact, larger area or longer duration than recommended.

ADVERSE REACTIONS: Erythema, blanching, edema, urticaria, angioedema, bronchospasm, shock.

INTERACTIONS: Additive toxic effect with concomitant Class I antiarrhythmics (eg, tocainide, mexiletine). Consider total amount absorbed from all formulations with other local anesthetics.

PREGNANCY: Category B, caution in nursing.

MECHANISM OF ACTION: Lidocaine: Amide-type local anesthetic; blocks Na^+ channels required for initiation and conduction of neuronal impulses. Tetracaine: Ester-type local anesthetic; blocks Na^+ channels required for initiation and conduction of neuronal impulses.

PHARMACOKINETICS: Absorption: C_{max}=1.7ng/mL (lidocaine), <0.9ng/mL (tetracaine); T_{max}=1.7 hrs. (lidocaine). **Distribution:** Lidocaine: V_d=0.8-1.3 L/kg; plasma protein binding (75%). Crosses placenta. **Metabolism:** Lidocaine: CYP1A2, CYP3A4 (N-deethylation). Monoethylglycinexylidide, glycinexylidide (active metabolites). Tetracaine: Plasma esterases (hydrolysis). **Elimination:** Lidocaine: Urine; $T_{1/2}$=1.8 hrs.

SYNERCID   RX
dalfopristin - quinupristin (King)

THERAPEUTIC CLASS: Streptogramin

INDICATIONS: Treatment of serious or life-threatening infections associated with vancomycin-resistant *Enterococcus faecium* (VREF) bacteremia and complicated skin and skin structure infections (cSSSI) caused by *Staphylococcus aureus* (methicillin-susceptible) or *Streptococcus pyogenes*.

DOSAGE: *Adults:* ≥16 yrs: VREF: 7.5mg/kg IV q8h. Duration depends on site and severity of infection. cSSSI: 7.5mg/kg IV q12h for at least 7 days. Hepatic Cirrhosis (Child Pugh A or B): May need dose reduction.
Pediatrics: ≥16 yrs: VREF: 7.5mg/kg IV q8h. Duration depends on site and severity of infection. cSSSI: 7.5mg/kg IV q12h for at least 7 days. Hepatic Cirrhosis (Child Pugh A or B): May need dose reduction.

HOW SUPPLIED: Inj: (Dalfopristin-Quinupristin) 350mg-150mg per 500mg vial

WARNINGS/PRECAUTIONS: Pseudomembranous colitis reported. Flush vein with 5% dextrose after infusion to minimize venous irritation. Arthralgia, myalgia, and bilirubin elevation reported.

ADVERSE REACTIONS: Infusion site reactions (inflammation, pain, edema), nausea, diarrhea, rash.

INTERACTIONS: Significant inhibiton of CYP3A4; caution with drugs metabolized by this enzyme system (eg, cyclosporin A, tacrolimus, midazolam, nifedipine, verapamil, diltiazem, astemizole, terfenadine, delaviridine, nevirapine, indinavir, ritonavir, vinca alkaloids, docetaxel, paclitaxel, diazepam, HMG-CoA reductase inhibitors, methylprednisolone, carbamazepine, quinidine, lidocaine, disopyramide). Monitor cyclosporine levels. Avoid drugs metabolized by CYP3A4 that prolong QTc interval. May inhibit gut metabolism of digoxin.

PREGNANCY: Category B, caution in nursing.

MECHANISM OF ACTION: Bacteriostatic agent; acts on bacterial ribosome. Dalfopristin: Inhibits the early phase of protein synthesis. Quinipristin: Inhibits the late phase of protein synthesis.

PHARMACOKINETICS: Absorption: Quinipristin: C_{max}=3.2mcg/mL, AUC=7.2mcg•hr/mL; Dalfopristin: C_{max}=7.96mcg/mL, AUC=10.57mcg•hr/mL. **Distribution:** Quinipristin: V_d=0.45L/kg, plasma protein binding (moderate); Dalfopristin: V_d=0.24L/kg, plasma protein binding (moderate). **Metabolism:** Quinipristin: 2 conjugated metabolites (1 with glutathione; 1 with cysteine); Dalfopristin: 1 nonconjugated metabolite; active metabolites. **Elimination:** Urine: 15% (quinipristin), 19% (dalfopristin), feces (75-77%); $T_{1/2}$=0.85 hrs. (quinipristin), 0.7 hrs. (dalfopristin).

SYNTHROID   RX
levothyroxine sodium (Abbott)

THERAPEUTIC CLASS: Thyroid replacement hormone

INDICATIONS: Hypothyroidism. As a pituitary TSH suppressant in the treatment and prevention of euthyroid goiters, including thyroid nodules, lymphocytic thyroiditis, and multinodular goiter. Adjunct to surgery and radioiodine therapy for thyrotropin-dependent well-differentiated thyroid cancer.

DOSAGE: *Adults:* Hypothyroidism: Usual: 1.7mcg/kg/day PO. Titrate: May increase by 12.5-25mcg every 6-8 weeks until euthyroid. >200mcg/day (seldom). Elderly/Cardiovascular Disease: Initial: 12.5-50mcg qd PO. Titrate: Increase by 12.5-25mcg every 3-6 weeks until euthyroid. Give 1/2 of oral dose for IV/IM. Pregnancy: May require increased doses. Subclinical Hypothyroidism: Lower doses required.
Pediatrics: Hypothyroidism: 0-3 months: 10-15mcg/kg/day. 3-6 months: 8-10mcg/kg/day. 6-12 months: 6-8mcg/kg/day. 1-5 yrs: 5-6mcg/kg/day. 6-12 yrs: 4-5mcg/kg/day. >12 yrs (growth/puberty complete): 2-3mcg/kg/day. Cardiac Risk: Lower starting dose. Infants with Serum T_4 <5mcg/dL: Initial: 50mcg/day. Chronic/Severe Hypothyroidism: Children: Initial: 25mcg/day. Titrate: Increase by 25mcg for 2 weeks then every 2-4 weeks until euthyroid. May crush tab and sprinkle over food (applesauce) or mix with 5-10mL water, formula (non-soy), or breast milk.

HOW SUPPLIED: Tab: 25mcg*, 50mcg*, 75mcg*, 88mcg*, 100mcg*, 112mcg*, 125mcg*, 137mcg*, 150mcg*, 175mcg*, 200mcg*, 300mcg* *scored

CONTRAINDICATIONS: Untreated thyrotoxicosis, uncorrected adrenal insufficiency.

WARNINGS/PRECAUTIONS: Do not use in the treatment of obesity; larger doses in euthyroid patients can cause serious or even life threatening toxicity. Caution with cardiovascular disorders, angina, CAD, HTN and the elderly. May aggravate DM, diabetes insipidus, or adrenal cortical insufficiency. Treatment of myxedema coma may require glucocorticoids. May lower seizure threshold.

ADVERSE REACTIONS: Craniosynostosis in infants, transient hair loss, pseudotumor cerebri in pediatrics (rare), hypersensitivity reactions, seizures (rare).

INTERACTIONS: Increased risk of coronary insufficiency with sympathomimetics and CAD. May potentiate oral anticoagulant effects; adjust dose and monitor PT/INR. Lithium blocks release of T_4 and T_3. Antidiabetic agents may need adjustment. Decreased absorption with cholestyramine resin, colestipol, ferrous sulfate, aluminum hydroxide, sodium polystyrene sulfonate, soybean flour (infant formula), sucralfate. Altered protein binding with clofibrate, estrogens, androgens/anabolic hormones, asparaginase, 5-FU, furosemide, glucocorticoids, meclofenamic acid, mefenamic acid, methadone, perphenazine, phenytoin, phenylbutazone, tamoxifen, salicylates. Altered thyroid hormone or TSH levels with aminoglutethimide, p-aminosalicylic acid, amiodarone, androgens/anabolic hormones, complex anions (eg, thiocyanate, perchlorate, pertechnetate), antithyroid drugs, β-adrenergic blockers, carbamazepine, chloral hydrate, diazepam, dopamine/dopamine agonists, ethionamide, glucocorticoids, heparin, hepatic enzyme inducers, insulin, iodinated cholestographic agents, iodine-containing compounds, levodopa, lovastatin, lithium, 6-mercaptopurine, metoclopramide, mitotane, nitroprusside, phenobarbital, phenytoin, resorcinol, rifampin, somatostatin analogs, sulfonamides, sulfonylureas, thiazide diuretics. Adrenocorticoid clearance is decreased with hypothyroidism and increased with hyperthyroidism. May potentiate anticoagulants. Cytokines, amiodarone may induce hypo- or hyperthyroidism. Increased risk of arrhythmias with maprotiline. HTN and tachycardia reported with ketamine. Sympathomimetics may increase risk of coronary insufficiency with CAD. Adverse effects of both drugs with TCAs. Decreased clearance of theophylline with hypothyroidism. Impaired β-blocker effects. Decreased digitalis effects. Decreased uptake of iodine-containing radiolabeled ions. Altered levels of theophylline may occur. Use with somatrem/somatropin may accelerate epiphyseal closure. Additive effects of both agents with TCAs.

S

Avoid mixing crushed tabs with foods/formula with large amounts of iron, soybean or fiber.

PREGNANCY: Category A, caution in nursing.

MECHANISM OF ACTION: Thyroid hormone; not understood, suspected to control DNA transcription and protein synthesis.

PHARMACOKINETICS: Distribution: Plasma protein binding (99%); found in breast milk. **Metabolism:** Deiodination and conjugation in the liver (mainly), kidneys, and other tissues. **Elimination:** Urine, feces; (approximately 20% unchanged). (T_4) $T_{1/2}$=6-7days, and (T_3) $T_{1/2}$≤2days.

SYNVISC   RX
hylan G-F 20 (Wyeth)

THERAPEUTIC CLASS: Hylan polymer

INDICATIONS: Treatment of osteoarthritis (OA) knee pain inadequately responsive to conservative nonpharmacologic therapy and simple analgesics.

DOSAGE: *Adults:* Usual: Intra-articular injection once weekly (one week apart) for total of three injections.

HOW SUPPLIED: Inj: 8mg/mL

CONTRAINDICATIONS: Knee joint infections, hyaluronan hypersensitivity, skin diseases or infections in injection site area.

WARNINGS/PRECAUTIONS: Avoid with skin disinfectants containing quaternary ammonium salts; hyaluronan can precipitate in their presence. Do not inject extra-articularly or into synovial tissue and capsule. Intravascular injections may cause systemic adverse events. Caution with allergies to avian proteins, feathers, and egg products. Avoid with severely inflamed knee joints. Remove synovial fluid or effusion, if present, before injecting. Follow strict aseptic administration. Caution with lymphatic or venous stasis. Avoid strenuous activity or prolonged weight-bearing activities after injection. Packaging contains dry natural rubber latex.

ADVERSE REACTIONS: Injection site pain, knee swelling/effusion, rash, calf cramps, ankle edema, muscle pain.

INTERACTIONS: Do not inject anesthetics or other drugs into knee joint during therapy.

PREGNANCY: Safety in pregnancy and nursing not known.

MECHANISM OF ACTION: Hylan polymer.

TACLONEX   RX
betamethasone dipropionate - calcipotriene (Warner Chilcott)

THERAPEUTIC CLASS: Vitamin D_3 analogue/corticosteroid

INDICATIONS: Topical treatment of psoriasis vulgaris for up to 4 weeks.

DOSAGE: *Adults:* ≥18yrs: Apply to affected area(s) qd for up to 4 weeks. Max: 100g/week. Treatment of >30% BSA not recommended. Do not apply to face, axillae, or groin.

HOW SUPPLIED: Oint: (Calcipotriene-Betamethasone) 0.005%-0.064% [15g, 30g, 60g]

CONTRAINDICATIONS: Known or suspected disorders of calcium metabolism; erythrodermic, exfoliative, and pustular psoriasis.

WARNINGS/PRECAUTIONS: Hypercalcemia reported; if elevation of serum calcium outside normal range occurs, d/c treatment until normal calcium levels restored. May produce reversible hypothalamic-pituitary-adrenal axis suppression, manifestations of Cushing's syndrome, hyperglycemia, and glucosuria. D/C if irritation develops. Avoid in presence of pre-existing skin atrophy at treatment site.

ADVERSE REACTIONS: Pruritus, headache.

PREGNANCY: Category C, caution in nursing.

MECHANISM OF ACTION: Calcipotriene: Synthetic vitamin D$_3$ analog. Betamethasone: Coriticosteroid; uncertain, posesses anti-inflammatory, anti-pruritic, and vasoconstrictive properties.

PHARMACOKINETICS: Metabolism: Calcipotriene: Liver (rapid). Betamethasone: Liver. **Elimination:** Betamethasone: Biliary and renal excretion.

TALACEN
pentazocine HCL - acetaminophen (Sanofi-Aventis)

THERAPEUTIC CLASS: Opioid agonist-antagonist analgesic

INDICATIONS: Relief of mild to moderate pain.

DOSAGE: *Adults:* 1 tab q4h prn. Max: 6 tabs/day.

HOW SUPPLIED: Tab: (Pentazocine-APAP) 25mg-650mg* *scored

WARNINGS/PRECAUTIONS: Contains sodium metabisulfite. Caution with head injury, increased ICP, acute CNS manifestations, MI, certain respiratory conditions, renal/hepatic dysfunction, biliary surgery, seizure disorders, and alcohol use. Potential for physical and psychological dependence.

ADVERSE REACTIONS: Nausea, vomiting, constipation, abdominal distress, anorexia, diarrhea, dizziness, lightheadedness, hallucinations, sedation, euphoria, headache, confusion, disorientation, sweating, tachycardia.

INTERACTIONS: Increased CNS depressant effects with alcohol. Withdrawal symptoms with narcotics.

PREGNANCY: Category C, caution in nursing.

MECHANISM OF ACTION: Pentazocine: acts as analgesic and sedative. APAP: acts as analgesic and antipyretic.

PHARMACOKINETICS: Absorption: Pentazocine: Well-absorbed; T$_{max}$=1.7 hrs. APAP: Rapid and complete; T$_{max}$=0.5-2.5 hrs. **Distribution:** Pentazocine: Crosses placental barrier. APAP: Plasma protein binding (8-43%). **Metabolism:** Pentazocine: Liver. APAP: Liver via conjugation. **Elimination:** Pentazocine: Renal excretion, T$_{1/2}$= 3.6 hrs. APAP: Urine=80% (conjugated drug), 3% (unchanged) T$_{1/2}$= 2.8 hrs.

TALWIN NX
pentazocine HCL - naloxone HCL (Sanofi-Aventis)

> For oral use only. Severe, potentially lethal reactions may result from misuse by injection alone, or in combination with other agents.

THERAPEUTIC CLASS: Opioid agonist-antagonist analgesic

INDICATIONS: Relief of moderate to severe pain.

DOSAGE: *Adults:* Usual: 1 tab q3-4h. May increase to 2 tabs q3-4h. Max: 12 tabs/day.
Pediatrics: ≥12 yrs: Usual: 1 tab q3-4h. May increase to 2 tabs q3-4h. Max: 12 tabs/day.

HOW SUPPLIED: Tab: (Pentazocine-Naloxone) 50mg-0.5mg* *scored

WARNINGS/PRECAUTIONS: Caution with elderly, drug dependence, head injury, increased ICP, certain respiratory conditions, acute CNS manifestations, renal or hepatic dysfunction, biliary surgery, and MI.

ADVERSE REACTIONS: Hypotension, tachycardia, hallucinations, dizziness, sedation, euphoria, sweating, nausea, vomiting, constipation, diarrhea, anorexia, facial edema, dermatitis, visual problems, chills, insomnia, urinary retention, paresthesia.

INTERACTIONS: Increased CNS depressant effects with alcohol. Withdrawal symptoms with narcotics.

PREGNANCY: Category C, caution in nursing.

MECHANISM OF ACTION: Pentazocine: Acts as analgesic and sedative. Naloxone: Acts as antagonist to pentazocine and pure antagonist to narcotic analgesics.

PHARMACOKINETICS: Absorption: Pentazocine: GI tract (well absorbed), T_{max}=1-3 hrs. **Distribution:** Pentazocine: Crosses placenta. **Metabolism:** Pentazocine: Liver. **Elimination:** Pentazocine: Urine, $T_{1/2}$=2-3 hrs.

TAMBOCOR   RX
flecainide acetate (Graceway)

THERAPEUTIC CLASS: Class IC antiarrhythmic

INDICATIONS: Prevention of paroxysmal supraventricular tachycardias (PSVT), paroxysmal atrial fibrillation/flutter (PAF) associated with disabling symptoms in patients without structural heart disease. Prevention of life-threatening ventricular arrhythmias such as sustained ventricular tachycardia (VT).

DOSAGE: *Adults:* PSVT/PAF: Initial: 50mg q12h. Titrate: May increase by 50mg bid every 4 days. Max: 300mg/day. Sustained VT: Initial: 100mg q12h. Titrate: May increase by 50mg bid every 4 days. Max: 400mg/day. CrCl ≤35mL/min: Initial: 100mg qd or 50mg bid. Reduce dose by 50% with amiodarone. *Pediatrics:* <6 months: Initial: 50mg/m²/day given bid-tid. ≥6 months: Initial: 100mg/m²/day given bid-tid. Max: 200mg/m²/day. Reduce dose by 50% with amiodarone.

HOW SUPPLIED: Tab: 50mg, 100mg*, 150mg* *scored

CONTRAINDICATIONS: Right bundle branch block associated with left hemiblock (without a pacemaker), pre-existing 2nd- or 3rd-degree AV block, cardiogenic shock.

WARNINGS/PRECAUTIONS: Avoid with non-life-threatening ventricular arrhythmias. Increased mortality and non-cardiac arrests reported. Ventricular proarrhythmic effects may occur with atrial fibrillation/flutter. May cause or worsen CHF, arrhythmias. Slows cardiac conduction; dose related increases in PR, QRS, and QT intervals reported. Conduction changes may cause sinus pause, sinus arrest, bradycardia, 2nd- or 3rd-degree AV block. Extreme caution with sick sinus syndrome. May increase endocardial pacing thresholds and suppress ventricular escape with pacemakers. Correct hypokalemia or hyperkalemia before therapy. Monitor with significant hepatic impairment. Initiate treatment of sustained VT in the hospital.

ADVERSE REACTIONS: Arrhythmias, hepatic dysfunction, cardiac arrest, CHF, flushing, anxiety, vomiting, diarrhea, tinnitus.

INTERACTIONS: Additive negative inotropic effects with β-blockers (eg, propranolol). Potentiated by cimetidine, amiodarone, CYP2D6 inhibitors (eg, quinidine). Increases digoxin levels. Increased elimination with phenytoin, phenobarbital, carbamazepine. Diltiazem, nifedipine, verapamil, disopyramide not recommended.

PREGNANCY: Category C, safety in nursing unknown.

MECHANISM OF ACTION: Class IC antiarrhythmic agent with local anesthetic activity; decreases intracardiac conduction in all parts of the heart with greatest effect on His-Purkinje system (H-V conduction).

PHARMACOKINETICS: Absorption: Complete. T_{max}=3 hrs. **Metabolism:** Extensive, via CYP2D6. Meta-O-dealkylated flecainide (active metabolite). **Elimination:** Urine (30% unchanged), feces (5%); $T_{1/2}$=20 hrs, 29 hrs (at birth), 11-12 hrs (3 months), 6 hrs (1 yr), 8 hrs (1-12 yrs), and 11-12 hrs (12-15 yrs).

TAMIFLU   RX
oseltamivir phosphate (Roche Labs)

THERAPEUTIC CLASS: Neuraminidase inhibitor

INDICATIONS: Treatment of uncomplicated acute illness due to influenza in adults and children ≥1 yr who have been symptomatic for no more than 2 days. Prophylaxis of influenza in adults and children ≥1 yr.

DOSAGE: *Adults:* Prophylaxis: Begin within 2 days of exposure to infection. 75mg qd for at least 10 days, up to 6 weeks with community outbreak. CrCl 10-30mL/min: 75mg every other day or 30mg qd. Treatment: Begin therapy within 2 days of symptom onset. 75mg bid for 5 days. CrCl 10-30mL/min: 75mg qd for 5 days.
Pediatrics: Prophylaxis: ≥13 yr: Begin within 2 days of exposure to infection. 75mg qd for at least 10 days, up to 6 weeks with community outbreak. ≥1 yr: (Sus) ≤15kg: 30mg qd. >15-23kg: 45mg qd. >23-40kg: 60mg qd. >40kg: 75mg qd. Duration: 10 days. Treatment: ≥13 yrs: Begin therapy within 2 days of symptom onset. 75mg bid for 5 days. ≥1 yr: (Sus) ≤15kg: 30mg bid. >15-23kg: 45mg bid. >23-40kg: 60mg bid. >40kg: 75mg bid. Duration: 5 days.

HOW SUPPLIED: Cap: 30mg, 45mg, 75mg; Sus: 12mg/mL [25mL]

WARNINGS/PRECAUTIONS: Efficacy not known with chronic cardiac disease, respiratory disease, and immunocompromised. Not a substitute for influenza vaccine. Adjust dose with renal dysfunction. Postmarketing neuropsychiatric events (self-injury and delirium) reported. Caution with kidney disease, heart disease, respiratory disease, or any serious health condition. Sorbitol in Tamiflu may cause upset stomach and diarrhea in patients with history of fructose intolerance.

ADVERSE REACTIONS: Nausea, vomiting, diarrhea, cough, headache, fatigue, abdominal pain, bronchitis, dizziness.

INTERACTIONS: Avoid administration of attenuated influenza vaccine within 2 weeks before or 48 hours after; may inhibit replication of live vaccine virus.

PREGNANCY: Category C, caution in nursing.

MECHANISM OF ACTION: Neuraminidase inhibitor. Inhibits influenza virus neuraminidase, affecting release of viral particles.

PHARMACOKINETICS: Absorption: (GI tract). Oseltamivir: C_{max}=65.2ng/mL. AUC_{0-12h}=112ng•hr/mL Oseltamivir carboxylate (metabolite). C_{max}=348ng/mL. AUC_{0-12h}=2719ng•hr/mL. **Distribution:** Oseltamivir carboxylate: (IV): V_d=23-26L. Plasma protein binding (3%). Oseltamivir: Plasma protein binding (42%). **Metabolism:** Oseltamivir: Hepatic (esterases). Metabolite: (Oseltamivir carboxylate). **Elimination:** Oseltamivir carboxylate: Renal (>99%). Feces (<20%).

TAMOXIFEN   RX
tamoxifen citrate (Various)

> For women with ductal carcinoma in situ (DCIS) and women at high risk for breast cancer; fatal uterine malignancies (eg, endometrial adenocarcinoma, uterine sarcoma), stroke, and PE reported with use in risk reduction setting. Discuss benefits/risks of events with this patient population. Benefits of tamoxifen outweigh risks in women already diagnosed with breast cancer.

THERAPEUTIC CLASS: Antiestrogen

INDICATIONS: Treatment of metastatic breast cancer in women and men. Treatment of node-positive and axillary node-negative breast cancer in women following mastectomy, axillary dissection and breast irradiation. To reduce risk of invasive breast cancer in women with DCIS. Reduction of breast cancer incidence in high risk women. Use for up to 5 yrs.

DOSAGE: *Adults:* Breast Cancer Treatment: 20-40mg qd. Divide dosages >20mg into AM and PM doses. Breast Cancer Risk Reduction/DCIS: 20mg qd for 5 yrs.

HOW SUPPLIED: Tab: 10mg, 20mg

CONTRAINDICATIONS: Reduction in breast cancer incidence in high risk women and women wtih DCIS who require coumarin-type anticoagulant therapy or have a history of DVT, PE.

WARNINGS/PRECAUTIONS: Hypercalcemia reported in patients with bone metastases. Increased incidence of uterine malignancies (eg, endometrial cancer, uterine sarcoma) and endometrial changes including hyperplasia and polyps reported. Increased incidence of thromboembolic events (eg, DVT, PE). Malignant and non-malignant effects on the liver and ocular disturbances reported. Leukopenia, anemia, thrombocytopenia, neutropenia, pancytopenia reported. Promptly evaluate abnormal vaginal bleeding if receiving or previously received tamoxifen. Patients receiving or previously received tamoxifen should have annual gynecological exam. Do not become pregnant within 2 months of therapy. May cause fetal harm during pregnancy. Does not cause infertility even with menstrual irregularity.

ADVERSE REACTIONS: Hot flashes, increased bone and tumor pain, vaginal discharge, fatigue/asthenia, mood disturbances, nausea/vomiting, irregular menses; (men) loss of libido, impotence.

INTERACTIONS: Increases effects of coumarin-type anticoagulant; monitor PT. Increased risk of thromboembolic events with cytotoxic agents. Increased levels with bromocriptine. May decrease letrozole levels. Decreased levels with rifampin and aminoglutethimide. Decreased plasma levels of major metabolite, N-desmethyl tamoxifen with medroxyprogesterone. Avoid administering with anastrozole.

PREGNANCY: Category D, not for use in nursing.

MECHANISM OF ACTION: Non-steroidal antiestrogen; competes with estrogen for binding sites in target tissues.

PHARMACOKINETICS: Absorption: C_{max}=40ng/mL; T_{max}=5 hrs. N-desmethyl tamoxifen: C_{max}=15ng/mL. **Metabolism:** N-desmethyl tamoxifen (major metabolite). **Elimination:** Feces (primary); $T_{1/2}$=5-7 days.

TAPAZOLE   RX
methimazole (King)

THERAPEUTIC CLASS: Thyroid hormone synthesis inhibitor

INDICATIONS: Treatment of hyperthyroidism. To ameliorate hyperthyroidism prior to subtotal thyroidectomy or radioactive iodine therapy. Also indicated when thyroidectomy is contraindicated or not advisable.

DOSAGE: *Adults:* Initial: Mild Hyperthyroidism: 5mg q8h. Moderately Severe Hyperthyroidism: 30-40mg/day, in divided doses q8h. Severe Hyperthyroidism: 20mg q8h. Maint: 5-15mg/day.
Pediatrics: Initial: 0.4mg/kg/day, in divided doses q8h. Maint: 1/2 of initial dose.

HOW SUPPLIED: Tab: 5mg*, 10mg* *scored

CONTRAINDICATIONS: Nursing mothers.

WARNINGS/PRECAUTIONS: Can cause fetal harm. Agranulocytosis, leukopenia, thrombocytopenia, aplastic anemia may occur; monitor bone marrow function. D/C with agranulocytosis, aplastic anemia, or exfoliative dermatitis. D/C with liver abnormality (eg, hepatitis) including transaminases >3x ULN. Monitor thyroid function periodically. May cause hypoprothrombinemia and bleeding; monitor PT.

ADVERSE REACTIONS: Rash, urticaria, nausea, vomiting, arthralgia, paresthesia, myalgia, neuritis, vertigo, edema, altered taste, hair loss, lymphadenopathy, lupuslike syndrome, insulin autoimmune syndrome.

INTERACTIONS: May potentiate anticoagulants. β-blockers, digitalis, theophylline may need dose reduction when patient becomes euthyroid. Caution with other drugs that cause agranulocytosis.

PREGNANCY: Category D, contraindicated in nursing.

MECHANISM OF ACTION: Inhibits synthesis of thyroid hormones.

PHARMACOKINETICS: Absorption: Readily absorbed (GI tract). **Distribution:** Crosses placenta and found in breast milk. **Elimination:** Urine.

TARCEVA   RX
erlotinib (Genentech/OSI)

THERAPEUTIC CLASS: Epidermal growth factor receptor tyrosine kinase inhibitor

INDICATIONS: Treatment of patients with locally advanced or metastatic non-small cell lung cancer (NSCLC) after failure of at least one prior chemotherapy regimen. First-line treatment of patients with locally advanced, unresectable or metastatic pancreatic cancer in combination with gemcitabine.

DOSAGE: *Adults:* NSCLC: 150mg at least 1 hr before or 2 hrs after ingestion of food. Pancreatic Cancer: 100mg at least 1 hr before or 2 hrs after ingestion of food, in combination with gemcitabine. Continue until disease progression or unacceptable toxicity. Acute Onset of New or Progressive Pulmonary Symptoms: D/C therapy. Severe Diarrhea/Severe Skin Reactions: May require dose reduction or temporary interruption of therapy. Strong CYP3A4 Inhibitors: Consider dose reduction. When dose reduction is necessary, reduce dose in 50mg decrements.

HOW SUPPLIED: Tab: 25mg, 100mg, 150mg

WARNINGS/PRECAUTIONS: Serious interstitial lung disease (ILD), including fatalities, reported; d/c if ILD diagnosed. May increase risk of MI and cerebrovascular accident. Asymptomatic increases in liver transaminases observed. Consider dose reduction or interruption if changes in liver function are severe. Elevations in INR and infrequent reports of bleeding reported. Monitor closely with concomitant anticoagulants. Cases of acute renal failure and renal insufficiency with or without hypokalemia reported. Caution in patients at risk of dehydration; monitor renal function and serum electrolytes periodically. May cause fetal harm; avoid pregnancy. May cause MI/ischemia.

ADVERSE REACTIONS: Rash, diarrhea, anorexia, fatigue, dyspnea, cough, nausea, infection, vomiting, edema, pyrexia, constipation, abdominal pain, decreased weight, bone pain.

INTERACTIONS: Co-treatment with potent CYP3A4 inhibitor ketoconazole increases erlotinib AUC by 2/3. Caution when administering or taking erlotinib with ketoconazole and other strong CYP3A4 inhibitors such as atazanavir, clarithromycin, indinavir, itraconazole, nefazodone, nelfinavir, ritonavir, saquinavir, telithromycin, troleandomycin, voriconazole, and grapefruit or grapefruit juice. CYP3A4 inducer rifampicin decreases erlotinib AUC by 2/3 to 4/5.

PREGNANCY: Category D, not for use in nursing.

MECHANISM OF ACTION: Human epidermal growth factor receptor tyrosine kinase inhibitor; inhibits intracellular phosphorylation of tyrosine kinase associated with epidermal growth factor receptor, which is expressed on cell surface of normal and cancer cells.

PHARMACOKINETICS: Absorption: Absolute bioavailability (60%); T_{max} =4 hrs. **Distribution:** Plasma protein binding (93%); V_d =232L. **Metabolism:** CYP3A4 (major); CYP1A2, 1A1 (minor). **Elimination:** $T_{1/2}$ =36 hrs, feces (1%), urine (0.3%).

TARGRETIN CAPSULES   RX
bexarotene (Eisai)

> Retinoids are associated with birth defects. Avoid in pregnancy.

THERAPEUTIC CLASS: Retinoid

INDICATIONS: Treatment of manifestations of cutaneous T-cell lymphoma (CTCL) in patients refractory to at least one prior systemic therapy.

DOSAGE: *Adults:* Initial: 300mg/m² /day with a meal. If toxicity occurs, adjust to 200mg/m² /day, then to 100mg/m² /day or temporarily suspend. Readjust upward if toxicity controlled. If no response after 8 weeks and 300mg/m² /day is tolerated, increase to 400mg/m² /day with careful monitoring.

HOW SUPPLIED: Cap: 75mg

945

CONTRAINDICATIONS: Pregnancy.

WARNINGS/PRECAUTIONS: May induce lipid and LFT abnormalities, pancreatitis, hypothyroidism, leukopenia, cataracts. Perform fasting lipid levels before therapy, then weekly until lipid response to bexarotene (2-4 weeks), then at 8-week intervals. May need dose reduction or suspension if elevated triglycerides develop. Obtain baseline LFTs, then monitor at 1, 2, and 4 weeks after initial therapy, then periodically if stable. Obtain WBC with differential at baseline, periodically thereafter. Minimize exposure to sunlight and artificial UV light. Great caution with hepatic dysfunction. Avoid if risk factors present for pancreatitis. Obtain thyroid function tests at baseline and monitor during treatment.

ADVERSE REACTIONS: Lipid abnormalities, anemia, nausea, headache, asthenia, infection, abdominal pain, chills, fever, flu syndrome, hypothyroidism, rash, dry skin, leukopenia, peripheral edema.

INTERACTIONS: Limit vitamin A intake to ≤15,000 IU/day. CYP3A4 inhibitors (eg, ketoconazole, itraconazole, erythromycin, gemfibrozil, grapefruit juice) may increase levels and inducers (eg, rifampin, phenytoin, phenobarbital) may decrease levels. Avoid gemfibrozil. May increase metabolism of tamoxifen, hormonal contraceptives. May enhance hypoglycemia with insulin, sulfonylureas, or insulin sensitizers.

PREGNANCY: Category X, not for use in nursing.

MECHANISM OF ACTION: Retinoid: mechanism not established in CTCL. Selectively binds and activates retinoid X receptor subtypes.

PHARMACOKINETICS: Absorption: T_{max}=2 hrs. **Distribution:** Plasma protein binding (>99%) **Metabolism:** Via oxidation by CYP450 3A4 to 6- and 7-hydroxy-bexarotene and 6- and 7-oxo-bexarotene (metabolites) **Elimination:** Hepatobiliary system; $T_{1/2}$=7 hrs.

TARGRETIN GEL   RX
bexarotene (Eisai)

THERAPEUTIC CLASS: Retinoid

INDICATIONS: Topical treatment of cutaneous lesions associated with cutaneous T-cell lymphoma (CTCL) (Stage IA and IB) refractory to, intolerant to, or persistent after other therapies.

DOSAGE: *Adults:* Initial: Apply once every other day for 1 week. Titrate: Increase weekly to qd, then bid, then tid, and finally qid. Max: Apply qid. Allow to dry before covering with clothing. Reduce frequency if application site toxicity occurs. D/C temporarily if severe irritation occurs.

HOW SUPPLIED: Gel: 1% [60g]

CONTRAINDICATIONS: Pregnancy.

WARNINGS/PRECAUTIONS: Avoid normal skin, mucosal surfaces. Minimize exposure to sunlight and artificial UV light. Caution with retinoid hypersensitivity. Possible altered kinetics in renal and hepatic dysfunction.

ADVERSE REACTIONS: Dermatitis, pruritus, rash, sweating, asthenia, skin disorder, pain, headache, edema, paresthesia, cough, pharyngitis.

INTERACTIONS: Avoid DEET-containing products (eg, insect repellents). Limit vitamin A intake to ≤15,000 IU/day. Increased levels possible with ketoconazole, itraconazole, erythromycin, gemfibrozil, and grapefruit juice.

PREGNANCY: Category X, not for use in nursing.

MECHANISM OF ACTION: Retinoids.

PHARMACOKINETICS: Absorption: C_{max}=5-55ng/mL. **Distribution:** Plasma protein binding (>99%). **Metabolism:** Liver iva oxidation by CYP450, 3A4.

TARKA   RX
verapamil HCL - trandolapril (Abbott)

> ACE inhibitors can cause death/injury to developing fetus during 2nd and 3rd trimesters. Stop therapy if pregnancy detected.

THERAPEUTIC CLASS: ACE inhibitor/calcium channel blocker (nondihydropyridine)

INDICATIONS: Treatment of hypertension. Not for initial therapy.

DOSAGE: *Adults:* Replacement Therapy: 1 tab qd with food. Severe Hepatic Dysfunction: Give 30% of normal dose.

HOW SUPPLIED: Tab: (Trandolapril-Verapamil) 2mg-180mg, 1mg-240mg, 2mg-240mg, 4mg-240mg

CONTRAINDICATIONS: Severe ventricular dysfunction, hypotension, cardiogenic shock, sick sinus syndrome or 2nd- or 3rd-degree AV block (except with functioning ventricular pacemaker), A-Fib/Flutter with an accessory bypass tract, history of ACE inhibitor-associated angioedema.

WARNINGS/PRECAUTIONS: Monitor for hypotension with surgery or anesthesia. Risk of hyperkalemia with renal insufficiency, DM. D/C if jaundice develops. Avoid with moderate to severe cardiac failure and ventricular dysfunction if taking a β-blocker. May cause angioedema, cough, fetal/neonatal morbidity, hypotension, AV block, anaphylactoid reactions, transient bradycardia, PR-interval prolongation. Monitor LFTs periodically. Give 30% of normal dose with severe hepatic dysfunction. Caution with CHF, hypertrophic cardiomyopathy, renal or hepatic dysfunction. Decrease dose in those with decreased neuromuscular transmission. Monitor WBC with collagen-vascular disease and/or renal disease.

ADVERSE REACTIONS: AV block, constipation, cough, dizziness, fatigue, headache, increased hepatic enzymes, chest pain, upper respiratory tract infection/congestion.

INTERACTIONS: May increase alcohol blood levels and prolong effects. Additive effects on HR, AV conduction, and contractility with β-blockers. Potentiates other antihypertensives. May increase digoxin, carbamazepine, theophylline, and cyclosporine levels. Avoid disopyramide within 48 hrs before or 24 hrs after verapamil. Additive negative inotropic effects and AV conduction prolongation with flecainide. Avoid quinidine with hypertrophic cardiomyopathy. Monitor lithium. Increased clearance with phenobarbital. Rifampin may reduce oral bioavailability. May potentiate neuromuscular blockers; both agents may need dose reduction. Risk of hyperkalemia with K⁺-sparing diuretics, K⁺ supplements. Caution with inhalation anesthetics.

PREGNANCY: Category C (1st trimester) and D (2nd and 3rd trimesters), not for use in nursing.

MECHANISM OF ACTION: ACE inhibitor; inhibition results in decreased plasma angiotensin II, which leads to decreased vasopressor activity and decreased aldosterone secretion. Calcium channel blocker; inhibits calcium ion influx into cardiac muscle and smooth muscle.

PHARMACOKINETICS: Absorption: Verapamil: absolute bioavailability (20-35%), T_{max}=4-15 hrs. Trandolopril: Absolute bioavailability (~10%), T_{max}=0.5-2 hrs. **Distribution:** Verapamil: Plasma protein binding (90%). Trandolapril: Plasma protein binding (80%). **Metabolism:** Verapamil: Liver. **Elimination:** Verapamil: Urine 70% (metabolite), 3-4% (unchanged), feces 16% (metabolite). Trandolapril: Urine 33% (metabolite), 1% (unchanged), feces 66% (metabolite).

TASIGNA   RX
nilotinib (Novartis)

> Prolongs QT interval. Sudden deaths reported. Avoid with hypokalemia, hypomagnesemia, or
> long QT syndrome. Correct hypokalemia or hypomagnesemia prior to administration and monitor
> periodically. Avoid drugs known to prolong the QT interval and strong CYP3A4 inhibitors. Avoid
> food 2 hours before and 1 hour after taking dose. Caution with hepatic impairment. Monitor QTc
> at baseline, 7 days after initiation, and periodically thereafter, as well as following any dose
> adjustments.

THERAPEUTIC CLASS: Kinase inhibitor

INDICATIONS: Treatment of chronic phase and accelerated phase
Philadelphia chromosome positive chronic myelogenous leukemia (CML) in
adult patients resistant or intolerant to prior therapy that included imatinib.

DOSAGE: *Adults:* 400mg PO bid, approximately 12 hours apart. Swallow
whole with water. Avoid food for at least 2 hours before and 1 hour after dosing. Adjust dose based on hematologic and non-hematologic toxicities, and
drug interactions (see PI).

HOW SUPPLIED: Cap: 200mg

CONTRAINDICATIONS: Hypokalemia, hypomagnesemia, or long QT
syndrome.

WARNINGS/PRECAUTIONS: Myelosuppression associated with neutropenia,
thrombocytopenia, and anemia may occur; perform CBC every 2 weeks for
first 2 months, then monthly. Myelosuppression may be reversed by reducing
or withholding dose. May increase serum lipase; monitor periodically and use
caution with history of pancreatitis. May elevate bilirubin, AST/ALT, and alkaline phosphatase; monitor LFTs periodically. May cause hypophosphatemia,
hypokalemia, hyperkalemia, hypocalcemia, hyponatremia; correct electrolyte
abnormalities prior to initiation and monitor periodically during therapy. Caps
contain lactose; avoid with rare hereditary problems of galactose intolerance,
severe lactase deficiency, or of glucose-galactose malabsorption.

ADVERSE REACTIONS: Rash, pruritus, nausea, fatigue, headache, constipation, diarrhea, vomiting, thrombocytopenia, neutropenia, leukopenia, pneumonia, intracranial hemorrhage, elevated lipase, pyrexia.

INTERACTIONS: See Black Box Warning. May increase levels of drugs eliminated by CYP3A4, CYP2C8, CYP2C9, CYP2D6, and UGT1A1 enzymes; caution
when co-administering with substrates for these enzymes that have a narrow
therapeutic index. Avoid warfarin (metabolized by CYP2C9 and CYP3A4) if
possible. May induce CYP2B6, CYP2C8, and CYP2C9 enzymes and thereby
decrease levels of drugs eliminated by these enzymes. May increase levels
of drugs that are substrates of Pgp; caution when co-administering. Since
nilotinib undergoes metabolism by CYP3A4, concomitant administration of
strong inhibitors (ketoconazole) or inducers (rifampicin) of CYP3A4 may increase or decrease nilotinib levels significantly; avoid concomitant use. Drugs
that inhibit Pgp may increase nilotinib levels; caution when co-administering.
Avoid St. John's wort and grapefruit products.

PREGNANCY: Category D, not for use in nursing.

TASMAR   RX
tolcapone (Valeant)

> Risk of fatal, acute fulminant liver failure. Withdraw if patients fail to show benefit within
> 3 weeks of initiation. D/C if hepatotoxicity develops, and do not consider retreatment. Perform
> LFTs before therapy, then every 2 weeks for 1st year, every 4 weeks for next 6 months, then ev-
> ery 8 weeks thereafter. Perform LFTs before increase dose to 200mg tid. Avoid with liver disease
> or if LFTs ≥2x ULN. Caution with severe dyskinesia or dystonia.

THERAPEUTIC CLASS: COMT inhibitor

INDICATIONS: Adjunct to levodopa/carbidopa for the treatment of symptoms
of idiopathic Parkinson's disease.

DOSAGE: *Adults:* Initial: 100mg tid. Use 200mg tid only if clinical benefit is justified. May need to decrease levodopa dose.

HOW SUPPLIED: Tab: 100mg, 200mg

CONTRAINDICATIONS: Liver disease, patients withdrawn from therapy due to drug-induced hepatocellular injury. History of non-traumatic rhabdomyolysis, hyperpyrexia or confusion related to medication.

WARNINGS/PRECAUTIONS: Hypotension/syncope, rhabdomyolysis, hallucinations, confusion, diarrhea, hematuria reported. Fibrotic complications can occur. Avoid with liver dysfunction. Caution with severe renal dysfunction. Closely monitor when discontinuing therapy.

ADVERSE REACTIONS: Dyskinesia, nausea, dystonia, excessive dreaming, anorexia, muscle cramps, orthostatic complaints, diarrhea, confusion, hallucination, vomiting, constipation, fatigue, increased sweating, xerostomia, urine discoloration, hepatotoxicity.

INTERACTIONS: Dobutamine, apomorphine and isoproterenol may need a dose reduction. Avoid non-selective MAOIs (eg, phenelzine, tranylcypromine). May increase risk of orthostatic hypotension and dyskinesia with levodopa. Caution with tolbutamide, desipramine, warfarin.

PREGNANCY: Category C, caution in nursing.

MECHANISM OF ACTION: Cathecol-*O*-methyltransferase inhibitor; suspected to alter the plasma pharmacokinetics of levodopa, leading to more sustained plasma levels of drug.

PHARMACOKINETICS: Absorption: (PO) Rapidly absorbed. T_{max}=2 hrs. C_{max}=3mcg/mL (100mg, 200mg); C_{max}=6mcg/mL (100mg, 200mg). Absolute bioavailability (65%). **Distribution:** V_d=9L. Plasma protein binding (>99.9%). **Metabolism:** Liver (glucuronidation) via CYP450 enzymes 3A4, 2A6. **Elimination:** Urine=60% (0.5% unchanged) and feces=40%. $T_{1/2}$=2-3 hrs.

TAXOL   RX

paclitaxel (Bristol-Myers Squibb)

> Anaphylaxis, severe hypersensitivity reactions reported. Pretreat with corticosteroids, diphenhydramine, and H_2 antagonists. Do not rechallenge if severe hypersensitivity reaction occurs. Monitor CBC frequently.

THERAPEUTIC CLASS: Antimicrotubule agent

INDICATIONS: First-line (with cisplatin) treatment of advanced ovarian carcinoma and non-small cell lung cancer. Subsequent treatment in advanced ovarian carcinoma. Treatment of breast cancer after failure with combination chemotherapy for metastatic disease or relapse within 6 months of adjuvant chemotherapy. Adjuvant treatment of node-positive breast cancer administered sequentially to doxorubicin-containing chemotherapy. Second-line treatment of AIDS-related Kaposi's sarcoma.

DOSAGE: *Adults:* IV: Ovarian Carcinoma: Previously Untreated: 175mg/m² over 3 hrs or 135mg/m² over 24 hrs every 3 weeks followed by cisplatin. Previous Treatment: 135mg/m² or 175mg/m² over 3 hrs every 3 weeks. Breast Cancer: 175mg/m² over 3 hrs every 3 weeks for 4 courses. Non-Small Cell Lung Cancer: 135mg/m² over 24 hrs every 3 weeks followed by cisplatin. Kaposi's Sarcoma: 135mg/m² over 3 hrs every 3 weeks or 100mg/m² over 3 hrs every 2 weeks. Reduce dose of subsequent courses by 20% if neutrophils <500 cells/mm³ for ≥1 week or severe peripheral neuropathy occurs. Premedicated prior to administration to prevent severe hypersensitivity reactions; dexamethasone 20mg PO 12 and 6 hrs before, diphenhydramine 50mg IV 30-60 min prior, and cimetidine 300mg or ranitidine 50mg IV 30-60 min before.

HOW SUPPLIED: Inj: 6mg/mL

CONTRAINDICATIONS: Hypersensitivity to drugs formulated in Cremophor® EL (eg, cyclosporine for injection concentrate, teniposide for injection concentrate), solid tumor patients with baseline neutrophils <1500 cells/mm³, AIDS-related Kaposi's sarcoma patients with baseline neutrophils <1000 cells/mm³.

WARNINGS/PRECAUTIONS: Severe conduction abnormalities, injection site reactions, peripheral neuropathy (more common in elderly) reported. Bone marrow suppression is dose dependent, dose limiting, and more common in elderly. Can cause fetal harm. Hypotension, bradycardia, and HTN may occur during administration. Toxicity enhanced with elevated liver enzymes. Contains dehydrated alcohol.

ADVERSE REACTIONS: Neutropenia, leukopenia, thrombocytopenia, anemia, infections, bleeding, bradycardia, hypotension, peripheral neuropathy, myalgia/arthralgia, nausea, vomiting, diarrhea, mucositis, alopecia.

INTERACTIONS: Increases doxorubicin levels. Caution with CYP450 2C8 and 3A4 substrates or inhibitors (eg, ritonavir, saquinavir, indinavir, nelfinavir). Myelosuppression more profound with cisplatin.

PREGNANCY: Category D, not for use in nursing.

MECHANISM OF ACTION: Antimicrotubule; promotes assembly of microtubules from tubulin dimers and stabilizes microtubules by preventing depolymerization inhibiting microtubule network essential for vital interphase and mitotic cellular functions.

PHARMACOKINETICS: Absorption: IV administration of multiple doses resulted in different parameters. **Distribution:** V_d=227-688L/m^2; plasma protein binding (89-98%). **Metabolism:** CYP2C8 (major), CYP3A4 (minor). 6α-hydroxy paclitaxel (metabolite). **Elimination:** Urine (1.3-12.6%), feces.

TAXOTERE   RX
docetaxel (Sanofi-Aventis)

> Increased treatment-related mortality reported with hepatic dysfunction, high-dose therapy, and in non-small cell lung carcinoma previously treated with platinum-based chemotherapy with docetaxel 100mg/m^2. Avoid if neutrophils <1500 cells/mm^3, bilirubin >ULN, or SGOT/SGPT >1.5x ULN with alkaline phosphatase >2.5x ULN. Severe hypersensitivity reactions reported.

THERAPEUTIC CLASS: Antimicrotubule agent

INDICATIONS: Treatment of locally advanced or metastatic breast cancer and non-small cell lung cancer (NSCLC) after failure of prior chemotherapy. In combination with doxorubicin and cyclophosphamide for the adjuvant treatment of operable, node-positive breast cancer. In combination with cisplatin for treatment of unresectable, locally advanced or metastatic NSCLC in those previously untreated with chemotherapy. In combination with prednisone for treatment of androgen independent (hormone refractory) metastatic prostate cancer. In combination with cisplatin and fluorouracil for the treatment of advanced gastric adenocarcinoma, including adenocarcinoma of the gastroesophageal junction, in patients who have not received prior chemotherapy for advanced disease. In combination with cisplatin and fluorouracil for the induction treatment of patients with locally advanced squamous cell carcinoma of the head and neck (SCCHN).

DOSAGE: *Adults:* Premedicate with oral corticosteroids. Adjust dose based on febrile neutropenia, neutrophil count, cutaneous reactions, peripheral neuropathy, neurosensory signs/symptoms, or GI toxicities (see PI). Breast Cancer: 60-100mg/m^2 IV over 1 hr every 3 weeks. Adjuvant Treatment Operable Node-Positive Breast CA: 75mg/m^2 1 hr after doxorubicin 50mg/m^2 and cyclophosphamide 500mg/m^2 every 3 weeks for 6 courses. NSCLC: 75mg/m^2 IV over 1 hr every 3 weeks. Prostate Cancer: 75mg/m^2 every 3 weeks over 1 hr with prednisone 5mg bid. Gastric Adenocarcinoma: Premedicate with antiemetics and appropriate hydration. 75mg/m^2 IV over 1 hr, followed by cisplatin 75mg/m^2 IV over 1-3 hrs (both on Day 1 only), followed by fluorouracil 750mg/m^2/day IV over 24 hrs for 5 days, starting at end of cisplatin infusion. Repeat treatment every 3 weeks. SCCHN: Induction followed by Radiotherapy: 75mg/m^2 IV over 1 hr, followed by cisplatin 75mg/m^2 IV over 1 hr, on Day 1, followed by fluorouracil as a continuous IV infusion at 750mg/m^2/day for 5 days. Administer every 3 weeks for 4 cycles. Induction followed by Chemoradiotherapy: 75mg/m^2 IV over 1 hr on Day 1, followed by cisplatin 100mg/m^2 IV over 30 min to 3 hrs, followed by fluorouracil 1000mg/m^2/day

T

as a continuous IV infusion from Day 1 to Day 4. Administer every 3 weeks for 3 cycles.

HOW SUPPLIED: Inj: 20mg/0.5mL, 80mg/2mL

CONTRAINDICATIONS: Neutrophils <1500 cells/mm³, hypersensitivity to polysorbate 80.

WARNINGS/PRECAUTIONS: Toxic deaths, febrile neutropenia, neutropenia, localized erythema of extremities with edema and desquamation, severe neurosensory symptoms, severe asthenia reported. Monitor for hypersensitivity reactions. Can cause fetal harm. Caution in elderly. Monitor CBC frequently; avoid subsequent cycles until neutrophils recover to >1500 cells/mm³ and platelets recover to >100,000 cells/mm³.

ADVERSE REACTIONS: Arthralgia, myalgia, alopecia, stomatitis, nausea, vomiting, diarrhea, nail changes, cutaneous and neurosensory reactions, fluid retention, hypersensitivity reaction, leukopenia, thrombocytopenia, anemia, neutropenia, fever.

INTERACTIONS: Caution with agents that induce, inhibit, or are metabolized by CYP450 3A4 (eg, ketoconazole, erythromycin, terfenadine, astemizole, cyclosporine).

PREGNANCY: Category D, not for use in nursing.

MECHANISM OF ACTION: Antimicrotubule agent; disrupts microtubular network in cells that is essential for mitotic and interphase cellular functions. Binds to free tubulin and promotes assembly of tubulin into stable microtubules while simultaneously inhibiting their disassembly.

PHARMACOKINETICS: Distribution: V_d=113L; Plasma protein binding (94%). **Metabolism:** CYP3A4. **Elimination:** Urine, feces (80%); $T_{1/2}$=11.1 hrs.

TAZICEF RX
ceftazidime (Hospira)

THERAPEUTIC CLASS: Cephalosporin (3rd generation)

INDICATIONS: Treatment of lower respiratory tract (eg, pneumonia), skin and skin structure (SSSI), bone and joint, gynecologic, intra-abdominal, CNS (eg, meningitis), and urinary tract infections (UTI), bacterial septicemia, and sepsis caused by susceptible strains of microorganisms.

DOSAGE: *Adults:* Usual: 1g IV q8-12h. Uncomplicated UTI: 250mg IV q12h. Complicated UTI: 500mg IV q8-12h. Bone and Joint Infections: 2g IV q12h. Uncomplicated Pneumonia/SSSI: 500mg-1g IV q8h. Gynecological/Intra-Abdominal/Meningitis/Severe Life-Threatening Infection: 2g IV q8h. Lung Infection caused by *Pseudomonas* in Cystic Fibrosis (normal renal function): 30-50mg/kg IV q8h. Max: 6g/day. Renal Impairment: CrCl 31-50mL/min: 1g q12h. CrCl 16-30mL/min: 1g q24h. CrCl 6-15mL/min: 500mg q24h. CrCl <5mL/min: 500mg q48h. For severe infections (6g/day), increase renal impairment dose by 50% or increase dosing interval. Apply reduced dosage recommendations after initial 1g LD is given. Hemodialysis: Give 1g LD before and 1g after each hemodialysis period. Intra-Peritoneal Dialysis/Continuous Ambulatory Peritoneal Dialysis: Give 1g LD followed by 500mg q24h, or add to fluid at 250mg/2L.
Pediatrics: Neonates (0-4 weeks): 30mg/kg IV q12h. 1 month-12 yrs: 30-50mg/kg IV q8h. Max: 6g/day. Higher doses for patients with cystic fibrosis or when treating meningitis. Renal Impairment: CrCl 31-50mL/min: 1g q12h. CrCl 16-30mL/min: 1g q24h. CrCl 6-15mL/min: 500mg q24h. CrCl <5mL/min: 500mg q48h. Hemodialysis: Give 1 g before and 1 g after each hemodialysis. For severe infections (6g/day), increase renal impairment dose by 50% or increase dosing interval. Apply reduced dosage recommendations after initial 1g LD is given. Hemodialysis: Give 1g LD before and 1g after each hemodialysis period. Intra-Peritoneal Dialysis/Continuous Ambulatory Peritoneal Dialysis: Give 1g followed by 500mg q24h, or add to fluid at 250mg/2L.

HOW SUPPLIED: Inj: 1g, 2g, 6g

WARNINGS/PRECAUTIONS: Monitor renal function; potential for nephrotoxicity. May result in overgrowth of nonsusceptible organisms. Possible cross-sensitivity between PCNs, cephalosporins, and other β-lactams. Pseudomembranous colitis reported. Elevated levels with renal insufficiency can lead to seizures, encephalopathy, asterixis, and neuromuscular excitability. Possible decrease in PT; caution with renal or hepatic impairment, poor nutritional state; monitor PT and give vitamin K if needed. Caution with colitis and other GI diseases. Distal necrosis may occur after inadvertent intra-arterial administration. Continue for 2 days after signs/symptoms of infection resolve; may require longer therapy with complicated infections. Caution in elderly.

ADVERSE REACTIONS: Phlebitis and inflammation at injection site, pruritus, rash, fever, diarrhea, nausea, vomiting.

INTERACTIONS: Nephrotoxicity reported with aminoglycosides or potent diuretics (eg, furosemide). Avoid with chloramphenicol; may decrease effect of β-lactam antibiotics.

PREGNANCY: Category B, caution in nursing.

MECHANISM OF ACTION: 3rd-generation cephalosporin; inhibits enzymes responsible for cell wall synthesis.

PHARMACOKINETICS: Absorption: C_{max}=90mcg/mL (1g IV), 39mcg/mL (1g IM); see PI for detailed info. **Distribution:** Plasma protein binding (<10%); found in breast milk. **Elimination:** Urine (80-90% unchanged); $T_{1/2}$=1.9 hrs (IV).

TAZORAC   RX
tazarotene (Allergan)

THERAPEUTIC CLASS: Retinoid

INDICATIONS: (Gel 0.05%, 0.1%) Stable plaque psoriasis of up to 20% body surface area involvement. (Gel 0.1%) Acne vulgaris of mild to moderate severity.

DOSAGE: *Adults:* Psoriasis: Start with 0.05% Gel, increase to 0.1% if tolerated. Apply thin film to psoriatic lesions qpm. Acne: Cleanse and dry skin. Apply thin film of 0.1% Gel to acne lesions qpm.
Pediatrics: ≥12 yrs: Psoriasis: Start with 0.05% Gel, increase to 0.1% if tolerated. Apply thin film to psoriatic lesions qpm. Acne: Cleanse and dry skin. Apply thin film of 0.1% Gel to acne lesions qpm.

HOW SUPPLIED: Gel: 0.05%, 0.1% [30g, 100g]

CONTRAINDICATIONS: Women who are or may become pregnant.

WARNINGS/PRECAUTIONS: Use adequate birth control measures. Avoid mouth, eyes, eyelids, exposure to sunlight or sunlamps, or eczematous skin. D/C if pruritus, burning, skin redness, or peeling. Weather extremes (eg, wind, cold) may be irritating.

ADVERSE REACTIONS: Pruritus, burning/stinging, erythema, worsening of psoriasis, irritation, skin pain, desquamation, dry skin, rash, fissuring, localized edema, skin discoloration.

INTERACTIONS: Avoid topical agents that have a strong drying effect. Caution with photosensitizers (eg, thiazides, tetracyclines, fluoroquinolones, phenothiazines, sulfonamides).

PREGNANCY: Category X, caution in nursing.

MECHANISM OF ACTION: Retinoic acid derivative; binds to all 3 members of the retinoic acid receptor RAR (RARα, RARβ, and RAR$_{gamma}$). Treatment of psoriasis not established. Suppresses expression of MRP8, a marker of inflammation; induces expression of a gene which may be a growth suppressor in keratinocytes, and may inhibit epidermal hyperproliferation in treated plaques. Treatment of acne not established; may be due to anti-hyperproliferative, normalizing-of-differentiation, and anti-inflammatory actions.

PHARMACOKINETICS: Absorption: Percutaneous; C_{max}=18.9ng/mL; AUC_{0-24hr}=172ng•hr/mL. **Distribution:** Plasma protein binding (>99%). **Metabolism:** Esterase hydrolysis to form tazarotenic acid (active metabolite). **Excretion:** Urine, feces; $T_{1/2}$=18 hrs.

TEGRETOL

carbamazepine (Novartis)

> Serious and fatal dermatologic reactions, including toxic epiderml necrolysis (TEN), Stevens-Johnson syndrome (SJS), and presence of HLA-B*1502 allele reported. Aplastic anemia and agranulocytosis reported. Obtain complete pretreatment hematological testing as a baseline. D/C if evidence of bone marrow depression develops.

OTHER BRAND NAMES: Tegretol-XR (Novartis)

THERAPEUTIC CLASS: Carboxamide

INDICATIONS: Treatment of partial seizures with complex symptomatology, general tonic-clonic seizures, and mixed seizure patterns of these or other partial or generalized seizures. Treatment of trigeminal or glossopharyngeal neuralgia pain.

DOSAGE: *Adults:* Epilepsy: Initial: (Immediate- or Extended-Release Tabs) 200mg bid or (Sus) 100mg qid. Titrate: (Immediate-Release Tabs/Sus) Increase weekly by 200mg/day given tid-qid. (Extended-Release Tabs) Increase weekly by 200mg/day given bid. Maint: 800-1200mg/day. Max: 1200mg/day. Trigeminal Neuralgia: Initial (Day 1): (Immediate- or Extended-Release Tabs) 100mg bid or (Sus) 50mg qid. Titrate: May increase by 100mg q12h (Tabs) or 50mg qid (Sus). Maint: 400-800mg/day. Max: 1200mg/day. Re-evaluate every 3 months. Extended-Release tabs should be swallowed whole and not crushed or chewed.
Pediatrics: Epilepsy: >12 yrs: Initial: (Immediate- or Extended-Release Tabs) 200mg bid or (Sus) 100mg qid. Titrate: (Immediate-Release Tabs/Sus) Increase weekly by 200mg/day given tid-qid. (Extended-Release Tabs) Increase weekly by 200mg/day given bid. Max: 12-15 yrs: 1000mg/day. >15 yrs: 1200mg/day. 6-12 yrs: Initial: (Immediate- or Extended-Release Tabs) 100mg bid or (Sus) 50mg qid. Titrate: (Immediate-Release Tabs/Sus) Increase weekly by 100mg/day given tid-qid. (Extended-Release Tabs) Increase weekly by 100mg/day given bid. Maint: 400-800mg/day. Max: 1000mg/day. 6 months-6 yrs: Initial: (Immediate-Release Tabs) 10-20mg/kg/day given bid-tid or (Sus) 10-20mg/kg/day given qid. Titrate: (Immediate-Release Tabs/Sus) Increase weekly tid-qid. Max: 35mg/kg/day. Extended-Release tabs should be swallowed whole and not crushed or chewed.

HOW SUPPLIED: Sus: 100mg/5mL [450mL]; Tab: (Tegretol) 200mg*; Tab, Chewable: 100mg*; Tab, Extended-Release: (Tegretol-XR) 100mg, 200mg, 400mg *scored

CONTRAINDICATIONS: History of bone marrow depression, MAOI use within 14 days, hypersensitivity to TCAs. Co-administration with nefazodone.

WARNINGS/PRECAUTIONS: Lyell's syndrome, Stevens-Johnson syndrome, multi-organ hypersensitivity reactions, and presence of HLA-B*1502 reported. Caution with history of adverse hematologic reaction to any drug, increased IOP, the elderly, mixed seizure disorder with atypical absence seizure. Fetal harm with pregnancy. May activate latent psychosis. Caution with cardiac (eg, conduction disturbance including second and third degree AV block), hepatic, or renal damage. Perform eye exam and monitor LFTs and renal function at baseline and periodically. Suspension produces higher peak levels than the tablet. Avoid in hepatic porphyria (eg, acute intermittent porphyria, variegate porphyria, porphyria cutanea tarda). Withdraw gradually to minimize the potential of increased seizure frequency.

ADVERSE REACTIONS: Dizziness, drowsiness, unsteadiness, nausea, vomiting, bone marrow depression, rash, urticaria, photosensitivity reactions, CHF, edema, HTN, hypotension, Stevens-Johnson syndrome, toxic epidermal necrolysis.

INTERACTIONS: Do not give suspension with other medicinal liquids or diluents. Metabolism is inhibited by CYP3A4 inhibitors (eg, cimetidine, macrolides) and induced by CYP3A4 inducers (eg, rifampin, phenytoin). Decreases oral contraceptive effectiveness. Increases plasma levels of clomipramine, phenytoin and primidone. Decreases levels of APAP, alprazolam, clonazepam, clozapine, dicumarol, doxycycline, ethosuximide, haloperidol, lamotrigine, methsuximide, oral contraceptives, phensuximide, phenytoin, theophylline, tiagabine, topiramate, valproate, and warfarin. Increased risk of neurotoxic side effects with lithium. Avoid MAOIs.

PREGNANCY: Category D, not for use in nursing.

MECHANISM OF ACTION: Anticonvulsant; reduces polysynaptic response and blocks past-tetanic potentiation.

PHARMACOKINETICS: Absorption: T_{max}=1.5 hrs (oral); T_{max}=4-5 hrs(conventional tab); T_{max} = 3-12 hrs (XR tab). **Distribution:** Plasma protein binding (76%). Found in placenta and breast milk. **Metabolism:** Liver via cytochrome P450 3A4. Carbamazepine-10,11-epoxide (metabolite). **Elimination:** Urine (3% unchanged); $T_{1/2}$=25-65 hrs (single dose); $T_{1/2}$=12-17 hrs (multiple doses).

TEKTURNA   RX
aliskiren (Novartis)

> When used in pregnancy, drugs that act directly on the renin-angiotensin system can cause injury and even death to the developing fetus. D/C therapy when pregnancy is detected.

THERAPEUTIC CLASS: Renin inhibitor

INDICATIONS: Treatment of hypertension. May be used alone or with other antihypertensives.

DOSAGE: *Adults:* Usual: 150mg qd. Titrate: May increase to 300mg/day if needed. High-fat meals decrease absorption.

HOW SUPPLIED: Tab: 150mg, 300mg

WARNINGS/PRECAUTIONS: Caution with greater than moderate renal dysfunction (SCr >1.7mg/dL (women) or >2mg/dL (men) and/or GFR <30mL/min), history of dialysis, nephrotic syndrome, or renovascular hypertension. May increase serum K^+, especially when used in combination with ACE inhibitors in diabetics. Angioedema of face, extremities, lips, tongue, glottis, and/or larynx reported; d/c and monitor until complete resolution of signs and symptoms. Hypotension rarely seen.

ADVERSE REACTIONS: Diarrhea, headache, nasopharyngitis, dizziness, fatigue, upper respiratory tract infection, back pain, cough.

INTERACTIONS: Coadministration with atorvastatin may increase Cmax up to 50% after multiple dosing. Coadministration of irbesartan may reduce Cmax up to 50% after multiple dosing. Coadministration of ketoconazole 200mg bid may result in an approximate 80% increase in plasma level. Coadministration with furosemide may reduce AUC and Cmax by 30% and 50%, respectively. Concomitant use with cyclosporine is not recommended. Concomitant use with K^+-sparing diuretics, K^+ supplements, salt substitutes containing K^+, or other drugs that increase K^+ levels may lead to increases in serum K^+; caution with concomitant use.

PREGNANCY: Category C (1st trimester) and D (2nd and 3rd trimesters); not for use in nursing.

MECHANISM OF ACTION: Potent renin inhibitor; lowers BP by directly inhibiting renin, decreasing plasma renin activity, and inhibiting conversion of angiotensinogen to angiotensin I.

PHARMACOKINETICS: Absorption: Poor, T_{max}=1-3 hrs., bioavailability (2.5%), accumulation $T_{1/2}$=24 hrs. **Metabolism:** via CYP3A4 enzyme. **Elimination:** Urine (25% of absorbed dose as parent drug).

TEKTURNA HCT   RX
aliskiren - hydrochlorothiazide (Novartis)

> Drugs that act directly on the renin-angiotensin system can cause injury and even death to the developing fetus. D/C therapy when pregnancy is detected.

THERAPEUTIC CLASS: Renin inhibitor/thiazide diuretic

INDICATIONS: Treatment of hypertension as add-on therapy or replacement therapy. Not for initial therapy.

DOSAGE: Adults: Initial: Not Controlled on Monotherapy: 150mg/12.5mg qd. Titrate: May increase to 150mg/25mg, 300mg/12.5mg qd if uncontrolled after 2-4 weeks. Max: 300mg/25mg. Avoid with CrCl ≤30mL/min.

HOW SUPPLIED: Tab: (Aliskiren-HCTZ) 150mg-12.5mg, 150mg-25mg, 300mg-12.5mg, 300mg-25mg

CONTRAINDICATIONS: Anuria, sulfonamide hypersensitivity.

WARNINGS/PRECAUTIONS: Angioedema of head and neck may occur; d/c therapy and monitor until signs and symptoms resolve. May cause symptomatic hypotension in volume- and/or salt-depleted patients; correct condition prior to therapy. Avoid with CrCl <30mL/min. Caution with hepatic impairment, or history of allergy or bronchial asthma. May exacerbate or activate SLE. Monitor serum electrolytes periodically to detect possible electrolyte imbalance.

ADVERSE REACTIONS: Dizziness, influenza, diarrhea, cough, vertigo, asthenia, arthralgia.

INTERACTIONS: (Aliskiren) Ketoconazole and atorvastatin may increase plasma levels. Irbesartan may reduce levels. Co-administration may diminish furosemide levels. (HCTZ) Potentiation of orthostatic hypotension may occur with alcohol, barbiturates, and narcotics. Dosage adjustment of insulin or oral hypoglycemic agents may be required. Potentiates effects of other antihypertensives. Cholestyramine and colestipol resins may impair absorption. Corticosteroids and ACTH deplete electrolytes. May decrease response to pressor amines (eg, norepinephrine). May increase responsiveness to skeletal muscle relaxants (eg, tubocurarine). Increased risk of lithium toxicity; avoid concurrent use. NSAIDs may reduce diuretic effects; monitor closely.

PREGNANCY: Category D, not for use in nursing.

MECHANISM OF ACTION: Aliskiren: Direct renin inhibitor. HCTZ: Thiazide diuretic, affects renal tubular mchanisms of electrolyte reabsorption, directly increasing excretion of sodium and chloride in approximately equivalent amounts.

PHARMACOKINETICS: Absorption: Aliskiren: T_{max}=1 hr. HCTZ: T_{max}=2.5 hrs. **Metabolism**: Aliskiren: CYP3A4 enzyme. HCTZ: Not metabolized. **Elimination**: Aliskiren: Urine (25% of absorbed dose as parent drug). HCTZ: Urine, $t_{1/2}$=5.8-18.9 hrs.

TEMODAR   RX
temozolomide (Schering)

THERAPEUTIC CLASS: Alkylating agent (imidazotetrazine derivative)

INDICATIONS: Treatment of glioblastoma multiforme. Treatment of refractory anaplastic astrocytoma.

DOSAGE: *Adults:* Adjust according to nadir neutrophil and platelet counts of previous cycle and at time of initiating next cycle. Glioblastoma Multiforme: 75mg/m² qd for 42 days with focal radiotherapy. Maint: Cycle 1 (28 days): 150mg/m² qd for 5 days. Cycle 2-6 (28 days): If Cycle 1 toxicity Grade ≤2, ANC ≥1.5 x 10⁹/L and platelets ≥100 x 10⁹/L, increase to 200mg/m²/day for 5 consecutive days per 28-day cycle. Do not increase dose in subsequent cycles if dose not escalated at Cycle 2. Anaplastic Astrocytoma: Initial: 150mg/m² qd for 5 consecutive days per 28-day cycle. If ANC ≥1.5 x 10⁹/L and platelets ≥100 x 10⁹/L for both the nadir and Day 29 (Day 1 of next cycle), may increase to 200mg/m²/day for 5 consecutive days per 28-day cycle. Start next cycle when ANC >1.5 x 10⁹/L and platelets >100 x 10⁹/L . If ANC <1 x 10⁹/L or platelets <50 x 10⁹/L during any cycle, reduce next cycle by 50mg/m², but not <100mg/m². Swallow whole with water.

HOW SUPPLIED: Cap: 5mg, 20mg, 100mg, 140mg, 180mg, 250mg

CONTRAINDICATIONS: Hypersensitivity to DTIC (dacarbazine).

WARNINGS/PRECAUTIONS: Before therapy, must have ANC ≥1.5 x 10^9/L and platelets ≥100 x 10^9/L. Myelosuppression may occur; obtain CBC on Day 22 (21 days after 1st dose) or within 48 hrs of that day, repeat weekly until ANC >1.5 x 10^9/L and platelets >100 x 10^9/L. Greater risk of myelosuppression in women and elderly. May cause fetal harm during pregnancy. Very rare cases of myelodysplastic syndrome and secondary malignancies, including myeloid leukemia have been observed. Do not open capsules. Caution in elderly, or severe renal/hepatic impairment.

ADVERSE REACTIONS: Anorexia, alopecia, headache, fatigue, myelosuppression (thrombocytopenia, neutropenia), nausea, vomiting, convulsions, hemiparesis, asthenia, fever, peripheral edema, constipation, dizziness, diarrhea.

INTERACTIONS: Valproic acid may decrease clearance.

PREGNANCY: Category D, not for use in nursing.

MECHANISM OF ACTION: Alkylating agent (imidazotetrazine derivative); exerts action by alkylation of DNA.

PHARMACOKINETICS: Absorption: Rapid and complete, T_{max}=1 hr. **Distribution:** Plasma protein binding (15%), V_d=0.4L/kg. **Metabolism:** Via hydroxylation; 3-methyl-(triazen-1-yl)imidazole-4-carboxamide (major metabolite) **Elimination:** $T_{1/2}$=1.8 hrs; urine and feces.

TEMOVATE RX
clobetasol propionate (GlaxoSmithKline)

OTHER BRAND NAMES: Temovate Scalp (GlaxoSmithKline) - Temovate-E (GlaxoSmithKline)

THERAPEUTIC CLASS: Corticosteroid

INDICATIONS: Corticosteroid responsive dermatoses. Temovate-E is also used to treat moderate to severe plaque-type psoriasis.

DOSAGE: *Adults:* Apply bid. Max: 50g/week or 50mL/week. Moderate-Severe Psoriasis: (Temovate-E) Apply bid for up to 4 weeks. May use on 5-10% of BSA. Max: 50g/week. Limit treatment to 2 consecutive weeks. Avoid with occlusive dressings.
Pediatrics: ≥12 yrs: Apply bid. Max: 50g/week or 50mL/week. Moderate-Severe Psoriasis: ≥16 yrs: (Temovate-E) Apply bid for up to 4 weeks. May use on 5-10% of BSA. Max: 50g/week. Limit treatment to 2 consecutive weeks. Avoid with occlusive dressings.

HOW SUPPLIED: (Temovate) Cre, Oint: 0.05% [15g, 30g, 45g, 60g]; Gel: 0.05% [15g, 30g, 60g]; Sol: 0.05% [25mL]; (Temovate-E) Cre: 0.05% [15g, 30g, 60g]; (Temovate Scalp) Sol: 0.05% [25mL, 50mL]

CONTRAINDICATIONS: (Scalp Sol) Primary scalp infections.

WARNINGS/PRECAUTIONS: Not for use on face, groin, or axillae, or for treatment of rosacea or perioral dermatitis. May produce reversible HPA axis suppression, manifestations of Cushing's syndrome, hyperglycemia, and glucosuria. Use appropriate antifungal or antibacterial agent with dermatological infections; d/c if infection does not clear. Peds may be more susceptible to systemic toxicity. Avoid eyes. D/C if irritation occurs.

ADVERSE REACTIONS: Burning, stinging, pruritus, skin atrophy, cracking/fissuring of the skin, erythema, folliculitis, numbness of fingers, telangiectasia, tingling (Sol), folliculitis (Sol).

PREGNANCY: Category C, caution in nursing.

MECHANISM OF ACTION: Corticosteroid; possesses anti-inflammatory, antipruritic, and vasoconstrictive properties. Anti-inflammatory effects not established. Suspected to act by induction of phospholipase A_2 inhibitory proteins, lipocortins. Lipocortins control biosynthesis of potent inflammation mediators (eg, prostaglandins, leukotrienes) by inhibiting release of their common precursor, arachidonic acid.

PHARMACOKINETICS: Absorption: Occlusion, inflammation, other disease states may increase absorption. Use of occlusive dressings ≤24 hrs does not increase penetration; use of occlusive dressings for 96 hrs markedly enhances penetration.

TENEX   RX
guanfacine HCL (Dr. Reddy's)

THERAPEUTIC CLASS: Alpha$_2$-agonist

INDICATIONS: Treatment of hypertension.

DOSAGE: *Adults:* 1mg qhs. Titrate: May increase to 2mg qhs after 3-4 weeks. Max: 3mg/day.

HOW SUPPLIED: Tab: 1mg, 2mg

WARNINGS/PRECAUTIONS: Caution with severe coronary insufficiency, recent MI, cerebrovascular disease, chronic renal or hepatic failure. Avoid abrupt discontinuation. Dose-related drowsiness and sedation.

ADVERSE REACTIONS: Dry mouth, somnolence, asthenia, dizziness, constipation, impotence, headache.

INTERACTIONS: Additive sedation with other CNS depressants. Caution with CYP450 inducers (eg, phenobarbital, phenytoin) in renal dysfunction.

PREGNANCY: Category B, caution with nursing.

MECHANISM OF ACTION: α2-adrenoceptor agonist; reduces sympathetic nerve impulses from the vasomotor center to the heart and blood vessels, resulting in decreased peripheral vascular resistance and reduction in heart rate.

PHARMACOKINETICS: Absorption: Absolute bioavailability (80%); T_{max}=2.6 hrs. **Distribution:** Plasma protein binding (70%); V_d=6.3L/kg. **Elimination:** Urine (50%, unchanged); $T_{1/2}$=17 hrs.

TENORETIC   RX
chlorthalidone - atenolol (AstraZeneca)

THERAPEUTIC CLASS: Selective beta$_1$-blocker/monosulfamyl diuretic

INDICATIONS: Treatment of hypertension. Not for initial therapy.

DOSAGE: *Adults:* Initial: 50mg-25mg tab qd. May increase to 100mg-25mg tab qd. CrCl 15-35mL/min: Max: 50mg atenolol/day. CrCl <15mL/min: Max: 25mg qd.

HOW SUPPLIED: Tab: (Atenolol-Chlorthalidone) 50mg-25mg*, 100mg-25mg *scored

CONTRAINDICATIONS: Sinus bradycardia, >1st-degree heart block, cardiogenic shock, overt cardiac failure, anuria, sulfonamide hypersensitivity.

WARNINGS/PRECAUTIONS: Withdrawal before surgery is not recommended. Caution with bronchospastic disease, conduction abnormalities, left ventricular dysfunction, heart failure controlled by digitalis and/or diuretics, renal dysfunction. Can cause heart failure with prolonged use. May mask hypoglycemia or hyperthyroidism symptoms. Avoid abrupt discontinuation. Avoid with untreated pheochromocytoma. Possible fetal harm in pregnancy. May aggravate peripheral arterial circulatory disorders. Enhanced effects in postsympathectomy patient. Neonates born to mothers receiving atenolol may be at risk of hypoglycemia and bradycardia.

ADVERSE REACTIONS: Bradycardia, hypotension, dizziness, fatigue, nausea, depression, dyspnea, blood dyscrasias.

INTERACTIONS: Additive effects with catecholamine-depleting drugs (eg, reserpine), CCBs, and digitalis. Bradycardia, heart block, and left ventricular end diastolic pressure can rise with verapamil or diltiazem. Exacerbates rebound HTN with clonidine withdrawal. Prostaglandin synthase inhibitors (eg, indomethacin) may decrease hypotensive effects. Caution with anesthetic agents. May block epinephrine effects. May decrease arterial response to norepinephrine. Increases risk of lithium toxicity. Possible hypokalemia with corticosteroids or ACTH. May alter insulin requirements.

T

PREGNANCY: Category D, caution in nursing.

MECHANISM OF ACTION: Atenolol: Cardioselective β-adrenoreceptor blocking agent; causes reduction in HR and systolic BP. Chlorthalidone: Monosulfamyl diuretic; acts on distal convoluted tubule and produces diuresis with increased excretion of Na^+ and chloride.

PHARMACOKINETICS: Absorption: Atenolol: Rapid, incomplete (50%). T_{max}= 2-4 hrs. Chlorthalidone: Onset of action within 2 hrs. **Distribution**: Atenolol: Plasma protein binding (6-16%). **Elimination:** Atenolol: $T_{1/2}$= approximately 6-7 hrs. Renal excretion. **Distribution:** Plasma protein binding (75%). **Elimination:** Urine (unchanged), $T_{1/2}$=40-60 hrs.

TENORMIN   RX
atenolol (AstraZeneca)

> Avoid abrupt discontinuation of therapy in coronary artery disease. Severe exacerbation of angina and occurrence of MI and ventricular arrhythmias reported in angina patients following abrupt discontinuation of therapy with β-blockers.

THERAPEUTIC CLASS: Selective beta$_1$-blocker

INDICATIONS: Management of hypertension. Long-term management of angina pectoris. To reduce cardiovascular mortality in hemodynamically stable patients with definite or suspected AMI.

DOSAGE: *Adults:* HTN: Initial: 50mg qd. Titrate: May increase after 1-2 weeks. Max: 100mg qd. Angina: Initial: 50mg qd. Titrate: May increase to 100mg after 1 week. Max: 200mg qd. AMI: Initial: 5mg IV over 5 min, repeat 10 min later. If tolerated, give 50mg PO 10 min after the last IV dose, followed by another 50mg PO 12 hrs later. Maint: 100mg qd or 50mg bid for 6-9 days. Renal Impairment/Elderly: HTN: Initial: 25mg qd. HTN/Angina/AMI: Max: CrCl 15-35mL/min: 50mg/day. CrCl <15mL/min: 25mg/day. Hemodialysis: 25-50mg after each dialysis.

HOW SUPPLIED: Tab: 25mg, 50mg*, 100mg *scored

CONTRAINDICATIONS: Sinus bradycardia, >1st-degree heart block, cardiogenic shock, overt cardiac failure.

WARNINGS/PRECAUTIONS: Withdrawal before surgery is not recommended. Caution with bronchospastic disease, conduction abnormalities, left ventricular dysfunction, heart failure controlled by digitalis and/or diuretics, renal or hepatic dysfunction. Can cause heart failure with prolonged use, hyperuricemia, hypercalcemia, hypokalemia, hypophosphatemia. May mask hypoglycemia or hyperthyroidism symptoms. Avoid abrupt discontinuation. Avoid with untreated pheochromocytoma. Possible fetal harm in pregnancy. May aggravate peripheral arterial circulatory disorders. May manifest latent DM. Monitor for fluid or electrolyte imbalance. May develop antinuclear antibodies (ANA). Neonates born to mothers receiving atenolol may be at risk of hypoglycemia and bradycardia.

ADVERSE REACTIONS: Bradycardia, hypotension, dizziness, fatigue, nausea, depression, dyspnea.

INTERACTIONS: Additive effects with catecholamine-depleting drugs (eg, reserpine), CCBs, and digitalis. Bradycardia, heart block, and left ventricular end diastolic pressure can rise with verapamil or diltiazem. Exacerbates rebound HTN with clonidine withdrawal. Prostaglandin synthase inhibitors (eg, indomethacin) may decrease hypotensive effects. Caution with drugs that depress myocardium (eg, anesthesia). May block epinephrine effects.

PREGNANCY: Category D, caution in nursing.

MECHANISM OF ACTION: Cardioselective β-adrenoreceptor blocking agent; causes reduction in HR and systolic BP.

PHARMACOKINETICS: Absorption: Rapid, incomplete (50%). T_{max}= 2-4 hrs. **Distribution**: Plasma protein binding (6-16%). **Elimination:** $T_{1/2}$= 6-7 hrs. Renal excretion.

TERAZOL 3
terconazole (Ortho-McNeil)

RX

THERAPEUTIC CLASS: Azole antifungal

INDICATIONS: Treatment of vulvovaginal candidiasis.

DOSAGE: *Adults:* 1 applicatorful or sup vaginally qhs for 3 nights.

HOW SUPPLIED: Cre: 0.8% [20g]; Sup: 80mg [3^s]

WARNINGS/PRECAUTIONS: D/C if sensitization, irritation, fever, chills, or flu-like symptoms occur. Confirm diagnosis by KOH smears and/or cultures; reconfirm if no response. Do not use diaphragm with suppository.

ADVERSE REACTIONS: Sup: Localized burning, pruritus, genital pain, headache. Cre: Dysmenorrhea, headache, pruritus, burning, abdominal pain.

PREGNANCY: Category C, not for use in nursing.

MECHANISM OF ACTION: Terconazol (antifungal agent); suspected to exert activity by disruption of normal fungal cell membrane permeability.

PHARMACOKINETICS: Absorption: C_{max}=5.9ng/mL, T_{max}=6.6 hrs. **Distribution:** Plasma protein binding (94.9%).

TERAZOL 7
terconazole (Ortho-McNeil)

RX

THERAPEUTIC CLASS: Azole antifungal

INDICATIONS: Treatment of vulvovaginal candidiasis.

DOSAGE: *Adults:* 1 applicatorful vaginally qhs for 7 nights.

HOW SUPPLIED: Cre: 0.4% [45g]

WARNINGS/PRECAUTIONS: D/C if sensitization, irritation, fever, chills, or flu-like symptoms occur. Confirm diagnosis by KOH smears and/or cultures; reconfirm if no response.

ADVERSE REACTIONS: Headache, body pain, burning, itching, irritation.

PREGNANCY: Category C, not for use in nursing.

MECHANISM OF ACTION: Terconazol (antifungal agent); uncertain; suspected to exert activity by disruption of normal fungal cell membrane permeability.

PHARMACOKINETICS: Absorption: C_{max}=5.9ng/mL, T_{max}=6.6 hrs. **Distribution:** Plasma protein binding (94.9%).

TERBUTALINE
terbutaline sulfate (Various)

RX

THERAPEUTIC CLASS: Beta$_2$-agonist

INDICATIONS: Prevention and reversal of bronchospasm in asthma, and reversible bronchospasm in bronchitis and emphysema.

DOSAGE: *Adults:* (PO) Usual: 5mg tid. May reduce to 2.5mg tid. Max: 15mg/24hrs. (Inj) Usual: 0.25mg SQ into lateral deltoid area. May repeat within 15-30 min if no improvement. Max: 0.5mg/4hrs.
Pediatrics: (PO) 12-15 yrs: Usual: 2.5mg tid. Max: 7.5mg/24hrs. (Inj) ≥12 yrs: Usual: 0.25mg SQ into lateral deltoid area. May repeat within 15-30 min if no improvement. Max: 0.5mg/4hrs.

HOW SUPPLIED: Inj: 1mg/mL [1mL]; Tab: 2.5mg*, 5mg* *scored

CONTRAINDICATIONS: Hypersensitivity to sympathomimetic amines.

WARNINGS/PRECAUTIONS: Caution with ischemic heart disease, HTN, arrhythmias, hyperthyroidism, DM, seizures. Not approved for tocolysis. Hypersensitivity and exacerbation of bronchospasm reported. Monitor for transient hypokalemia.

T

ADVERSE REACTIONS: Nervousness, tremor, headache, somnolence, palpitations, dizziness, tachycardia, nausea.

INTERACTIONS: Avoid other sympathomimetic agents (except aerosol bronchodilators). Extreme caution with MAOIs and TCAs during or within 14 days of treatment. Decreased effects with β-blockers. Possible ECG changes and hypokalemia with loop or thiazide diuretics.

PREGNANCY: Category B, caution in nursing.

MECHANISM OF ACTION: β_2-adrenergic agonist; stimulates intracellular adenyl cyclase, which catalyzes conversion of ATP to cAMP, to produce relaxation of bronchial smooth muscle and inhibition of release of mediators of immediate hypersensitivity from cells (mast cells).

PHARMACOKINETICS: Absorption: (SC) C_{max}=9.6ng/mL; T_{max}=0.5 hrs; AUC=29.4h•ng/mL. (Tab) C_{max}=8.3ng/mL; T_{max}=2 hrs; AUC=54.6h•ng/mL. (Sol) C_{max}=8.6ng/mL; T_{max}=1.5 hrs; AUC=53.1h•ng/mL. **Metabolism:** Sulfate conjugate (metabolite). **Elimination:** SC: Urine (60%); $T_{1/2}$=5.7 hrs. (PO) Urine (30-50%), feces; $T_{1/2}$=3.4 hrs (asthmatics).

TESSALON   RX
benzonatate (Forest)

THERAPEUTIC CLASS: Non-narcotic antitussive

INDICATIONS: Symptomatic relief of cough.

DOSAGE: *Adults:* Usual: 100-200mg tid as needed. Max: 600mg/day.
Pediatrics: >10 yrs: Usual: 100-200mg tid as needed. Max: 600mg/day.

HOW SUPPLIED: Cap: 100mg, 200mg

WARNINGS/PRECAUTIONS: Severe hypersensitivity reactions; confusion and hallucinations reported in combination with other prescribed drugs. Swallow capsules without sucking/chewing to avoid local anesthesia adverse effects.

ADVERSE REACTIONS: Sedation, headache, dizziness, confusion, hallucinations, constipation, nausea, GI upset, pruritus.

PREGNANCY: Category C, caution in nursing.

MECHANISM OF ACTION: Non-narcotic/antitussive agent; acts peripherally by anesthetizing stretch receptors located in respiratory passages, lungs, and pleura by dampening their activity, thereby reducing cough reflex at its source.

TESTIM   CIII
testosterone (Auxilium)

THERAPEUTIC CLASS: Androgen

INDICATIONS: Testosterone replacement in males with primary or hypogonadotropic hypogonadism.

DOSAGE: *Adults:* ≥18 yrs: Apply 5g qd, preferably in the am, to clean, dry, intact skin of shoulders and/or upper arms. Allow to dry prior to dressing. Titrate: May increase to 10g qd if response not achieved or serum concentration is below normal range. Do not apply to genitals or abdomen. To maintain serum testosterone levels, do not wash site of application for at least 2 hrs.

HOW SUPPLIED: Gel: 1% [5g (50mg)/tube, 30s]

CONTRAINDICATIONS: Breast or prostate carcinoma in men. Not for use by women. Pregnant and nursing women should avoid skin contact with application sites on men. Hypersensitivity to soy products.

WARNINGS/PRECAUTIONS: Caution in elderly; increased risk of prostatic hypertrophy/carcinoma. Risk of edema with pre-existing cardiac, renal, or hepatic disease; d/c if edema occurs, diuretic therapy may be required. Risk of gynecomastia. May potentiate sleep apnea especially with obesity or chronic lung diseases. Transfer of testosterone can occur with skin to skin contact. Risk of virilization of female partner. Advise patients to report persistent penis erections, changes in skin color, ankle swelling, unexplained nausea and vomitting, or breathing disturbances. Monitor serum testosterone, LFTs, Hgb, Hct, PSA, cholesterol, lipids. Prolonged use associated with serious hepatic effects (peliosis hepatitis, hepatic neoplasms, choleostatic hepatitis, jaundice).

ADVERSE REACTIONS: Application site reactions, benign prostatic hyperplasia, decreased DBP, increased BP, gynecomastia, headache, Hct/Hgb increases, hot flushes, insomnia, increased lacrimation, mood swings, smell disorder.

INTERACTIONS: May elevate oxyphenbutazone levels. May decrease blood glucose and insulin requirements. May increase clearance of propranolol. Corticosteroids may enhance edema; caution with cardiac or hepatic disease.

PREGNANCY: Category X, not for use in nursing.

MECHANISM OF ACTION: Endogenous androgen; responsible for normal growth and development of male sex organs and for maintenance of secondary sex characteristics.

PHARMACOKINETICS: Metabolism: Skin, liver, male urogenital tract via 5α-reductase; estradiol and dihydrotestosterone (metabolites). **Elimination:** Urine, feces; T$_{1/2}$=10-100 min.

TESTRED
methyltestosterone (Valeant)

`CIII`

THERAPEUTIC CLASS: Androgen

INDICATIONS: Testosterone replacement therapy in males with primary hypogonadism or hypogonadotrophic hypogonadism. To stimulate puberty in males with delayed puberty. Secondary treatment of advancing inoperable metastatic (skeletal) breast cancer in females 1-5 yrs postmenopausal.

DOSAGE: *Adults:* Dose based on age, sex and diagnosis. Adjust dose according to clinical response and adverse events. Male Replacement Therapy: 10-50mg/day. Breast Carcinoma: 50-200mg/day.
Pediatrics: Dose based on age, sex and diagnosis. Adjust dose according to clinical response and adverse events. Delayed Puberty: Use lower range of 10-50mg/day for 4-6 months. Caution in children.

HOW SUPPLIED: Cap: 10mg

CONTRAINDICATIONS: Pregnancy. Males with breast or prostate carcinoma.

WARNINGS/PRECAUTIONS: D/C if hypercalcemia occurs in breast cancer; monitor calcium levels. Monitor for virilization in females. Risk of compromised stature in children; monitor bone growth every 6 months. Risk of hepatic damage with long-term use. D/C if jaundice, cholestatic hepatitis occurs. Risk of edema; caution with pre-existing cardiac, renal or hepatic disease. Caution in the elderly; increased risk of prostatic hypertrophy and prostatic carcinoma. Should not be used for enhancement of athletic performance. Monitor LFTs, Hct, and Hgb periodically.

ADVERSE REACTIONS: Amenorrhea, virilization, menstrual irregularities, gynecomastia, excessive frequency/duration of penile erections, male pattern baldness, increased/decreased libido, oligospermia, hirsutism, acne, fluid and electrolyte disturbances, nausea, hypercholesterolemia, clotting factor suppression, polycythemia, altered LFTs, priapism, anxiety, depression.

INTERACTIONS: Potentiates oral anticoagulants and oxyphenbutazone. May decrease blood glucose and insulin requirements in diabetics.

PREGNANCY: Category X, not for use in nursing.

MECHANISM OF ACTION: Endogenous androgen (derivative of testosterone); responsible for normal growth and development of male sex organs and maintenance of secondary sex characteristics.

PHARMACOKINETICS: Metabolism: Gut, liver. **Elimination:** Urine, feces; T$_{1/2}$=10-100 min.

TETANUS & DIPHTHERIA TOXOIDS ADSORBED   RX
diphtheria toxoid - tetanus toxoid (Sanofi Pasteur)

THERAPEUTIC CLASS: Toxoid combination

INDICATIONS: Active immunization against tetanus and diphtheria (Td).

DOSAGE: *Adults:* 0.5mL IM in the vastus lateralis or deltoid. Repeat 4-8 weeks later. Give 3rd dose 6-12 months after 2nd dose. Booster: 0.5mL IM every 10 yrs.
Pediatrics: >7 yrs: 0.5mL IM in the vastus lateralis or deltoid. Repeat 4-8 weeks later. Give 3rd dose 6-12 months after 2nd dose. Booster: 0.5mL IM every 10 yrs.

HOW SUPPLIED: Inj: 5LFU-2LFU/0.5mL

CONTRAINDICATIONS: Neurological or systemic allergic reaction to previous dose. Defer during febrile illness, acute infection, or an outbreak of poliomyelitis. Thimerosal hypersensitivity.

WARNINGS/PRECAUTIONS: Suboptimal response may occur in immunocompromised patients. Avoid booster more frequently than every 10 yrs especially with Arthus-type hypersensitivity reactions or temperature >39.4°C after a previous dose of tetanus toxoid. Caution with IM injection in thrombocytopenia or any coagulation disorder. Increased risk of local/systemic reactions to boosters doses. Have epinephrine available.

ADVERSE REACTIONS: Injection site reaction, fever, malaise, hypotension, nausea, arthralgia.

INTERACTIONS: Immunosuppressive therapy may reduce response to active immunization. Caution with anticoagulants.

PREGNANCY: Category C, safety in nursing not known.

MECHANISM OF ACTION: Toxoid combination; activates neutralizing antibodies to diphtheria and tetanus toxins for protection against diphtheria and tetanus.

PHARMACOKINETICS: Absorption: Complete.

TEVETEN   RX
eprosartan mesylate (Abbott/Kos)

> Can cause death/injury to developing fetus during 2nd and 3rd trimesters. Stop therapy if pregnancy detected.

THERAPEUTIC CLASS: Angiotensin II receptor antagonist

INDICATIONS: Treatment of hypertension, alone or with other antihypertensives.

DOSAGE: *Adults:* Initial: 600mg qd. Usual: 400-800mg/day, given qd-bid. Moderate to Severe Renal Impairment: Max: 600mg/day.

HOW SUPPLIED: Tab: 400mg, 600mg

WARNINGS/PRECAUTIONS: Can cause fetal injury/death. Correct volume or salt depletion before therapy. Changes in renal function may occur; caution with renal artery stenosis, severe CHF.

ADVERSE REACTIONS: Upper respiratory infection, rhinitis, pharyngitis, cough.

INTERACTIONS: Risk of hypotension with diuretics.

PREGNANCY: Category C (1st trimester) and D (2nd and 3rd trimesters), not for use in nursing.

MECHANISM OF ACTION: Angiotensin II receptor antagonist; blocks vasoconstrictor and aldosterone-secreting effects of angiotensin II by selectively blocking binding of angiotensin II to AT_1 receptor found in many tissues.

PHARMACOKINETICS: Absorption: Absolute bioavailability: (approximately 13%). T_{max}=1-2 hrs. **Distribution:** Plasma protein binding (approximately 98%), V_{ss}=308L. **Elimination:** Feces (90%), urine (7%), (600mg); $T_{1/2}$=20 hrs.

TEVETEN HCT

RX

eprosartan mesylate - hydrochlorothiazide (Abbott/Kos)

> Can cause death/injury to developing fetus during 2nd and 3rd trimesters. Stop therapy if pregnancy detected.

THERAPEUTIC CLASS: Angiotensin II receptor antagonist/thiazide diuretic

INDICATIONS: Treatment of hypertension. Not for initial therapy.

DOSAGE: *Adults:* Usual (Not Volume Depleted): 600mg-12.5mg qd. Titrate: May increase to 600mg-25mg qd if needed. Renal Impairment: Max: 600mg/day (eprosartan).

HOW SUPPLIED: Tab: (Eprosartan-HCTZ) 600mg-12.5mg, 600mg-25mg

CONTRAINDICATIONS: Anuria, sulfonamide hypersensitivity.

WARNINGS/PRECAUTIONS: Hypersensitivity reactions reported. Fetal/neonatal morbidity and death reported. Monitor for hypotension in volume/salt depletion. Caution with CHF, renal or hepatic dysfunction. May exacerbate or activate SLE. Monitor electrolytes periodically. Hypercalcemia, hypomagnesemia, hyperuricemia, hyperglycemia may occur. Enhanced effects in post-sympathectomy patient.

ADVERSE REACTIONS: Dizziness, headache, back pain, fatigue, myalgia, upper respiratory tract infection, sinusitis, viral infection.

INTERACTIONS: Increased risk of hyperkalemia with K+-sparing diuretics, K+ supplements, or K+-containing salt substitutes. Potentiated orthostatic hypotension with alcohol, barbiturates, and narcotics. May need to adjust insulin and antidiabetic drugs. Impaired absorption with cholestyramine, colestipol. Corticosteroids and ACTH deplete electrolytes. May decrease response to pressor amines (eg, norepinephrine). Potentiated effect with other antihypertensives. May increase responsiveness to nondepolarizing skeletal muscle relaxants (eg, tubocurarine). Risk of lithium toxicity; avoid use. NSAIDs may decrease diuretic/antihypertensive effects.

PREGNANCY: Category C (1st trimester) and D (2nd and 3rd trimesters), not for use in nursing.

MECHANISM OF ACTION: Eprosartan: Angiotensin II receptor antagonist; blocks vasoconstrictor and aldosterone-secreting effects of angiotensin II by selectively blocking binding of angiotensin II to AT_1 receptor in vascular smooth muscle and adrenal gland. HCTZ: Thiazide diuretic; affects renal tubular mechanism of electrolyte reabsorption, directly increasing excretion of sodium and chloride.

PHARMACOKINETICS: Absorption: Eprosartan: Absolute bioavailability (13%); T_{max}=1-2 hrs. **Distribution:** Eprosartan: Plasma protein binding (approximately 98%); V_{ss}=308L. HCTZ: Crosses placenta and excreted in breast milk. **Elimination:** Eprosartan: Feces (90%), urine (7%); (600mg) $T_{1/2}$=20 hrs. HCTZ: Urine (61%, unchanged); $T_{1/2}$=5.6-14.8 hrs.

TEV-TROPIN

RX

somatropin (Gate)

THERAPEUTIC CLASS: Human growth hormone

INDICATIONS: Long-term treatment of children who have growth failure due to an inadequate secretion of normal endogenous growth hormone.

DOSAGE: *Pediatrics:* 0.1mg/kg (0.3 IU/kg) SQ 3x week.

HOW SUPPLIED: Inj: 5mg

CONTRAINDICATIONS: Prader-Willi syndrome (PWS) with severe obesity or severe respiratory impairment. Growth failure due to PWS. Acute critical illness due to complications following open heart or abdominal surgery, multiple accidental traumas, acute respiratory failure; closed epiphyses; progression of an underlying intracranial lesion; active neoplasia, benzyl alcohol sensitivity.

WARNINGS/PRECAUTIONS: Reports of fatalities in pediatric patients with PWS. In PWS, evaluate for upper airway obstruction prior to initiation; monitor weight, for sleep apnea, signs of upper airway obstruction (eg, suspend therapy with onset of or increased snoring), respiratory infections (treat early and aggressively if occur). Monitor GHD secondary to intracranial lesion for progression/recurrence; glucose intolerance; hypothyroidism; intracranial hypertension (perform fundoscopic exam at start and periodically). Slipped capital femoral epiphysis may occur. Monitor for malignant transformation of any skin lesion. When injected SQ in same site over long period of time, may cause tissue atrophy; rotate injection site.

ADVERSE REACTIONS: Headaches, injection site reactions (pain, bruise), leukemia.

INTERACTIONS: Decreased effects with glucocorticoids.

PREGNANCY: Category C, caution with nursing.

MECHANISM OF ACTION: Human growth hormone; stimulates linear growth synthesis, metabolizes lipids, reduces body fat stores by increasing cellular protein, and increases plasma fatty acids.

PHARMACOKINETICS: Absorption: C_{max}=80ng/mL. T_{max}=7 hrs. **Elimination:** (IV): $T_{1/2}$=0.42 hrs. (SQ) $T_{1/2}$=2.7 hrs.

THALITONE RX
chlorthalidone (King)

THERAPEUTIC CLASS: Monosulfamyl diuretic

INDICATIONS: Management of hypertension. Adjunct therapy in edema associated with CHF, hepatic cirrhosis, corticosteroid and estrogen therapy, renal dysfunction.

DOSAGE: *Adults:* HTN: Initial: 15mg qd. Titrate: May increase to 30mg qd, then to 45-50mg qd. Edema: Initial: 30-60mg/day or 60mg every other day, up to 90-120mg/day. Maint: May be lower than initial; adjust to patient. Take in the morning with food.

HOW SUPPLIED: Tab: 15mg

CONTRAINDICATIONS: Anuria, sulfonamide hypersensitivity.

WARNINGS/PRECAUTIONS: Caution in severe renal disease, liver dysfunction, allergy history, asthma. May exacerbate or activate SLE. Monitor for fluid and electrolyte imbalance. Hyperuricemia, hypomagnesemia, hypokalemia, hypercalcemia, hypophosphatemia, and hyperglycemia may occur. May manifest latent DM.

ADVERSE REACTIONS: Pancreatitis, jaundice, diarrhea, vomiting, constipation, nausea, blood dyscrasias, rash, photosensitivity, dizziness, headache, electrolyte disturbance, impotence.

INTERACTIONS: Potentiates action of other antihypertensive drugs. May increase responsiveness to tubocurarine. May decrease arterial effectiveness of norepinephrine. Antidiabetic agents may need adjustment. Risk of lithium toxicity. Orthostatic hypotension aggravated by alcohol, barbiturates, or narcotics.

PREGNANCY: Category B, not for use in nursing.

MECHANISM OF ACTION: Monosulfamyl diuretic; acts on the distal convoluted tubule and produces diuresis with increased excretion of sodium and chloride.

PHARMACOKINETICS: Distribution: Plasma protein binding (approx. 75%). **Elimination:** Urine (unchanged), $T_{1/2}$=40-60 hrs.

THALOMID   RX
thalidomide (Celgene)

Severe, life-threatening human birth defects if taken during pregnancy. Women of childbearing potential should have a pregnancy test before starting therapy, then weekly for 1st month, and monthly thereafter. Males must use latex condoms during sexual contact with females of child-bearing potential. Effective contraception must be used 4 weeks before, during, and 4 weeks after therapy. Only prescribers and pharmacists registered with the S.T.E.P.S.® distribution program can prescribe and dispense. The use of thalidomide in multiple myeloma results in an increased risk of venous thromboembolic events (eg, DVT, PE).

THERAPEUTIC CLASS: Immunomodulatory agent

INDICATIONS: Acute treatment of the cutaneous manifestations of moderate to severe erythema nodosum leprosum (ENL). Maintenance therapy for prevention and suppression of the cutaneous manifestations of ENL recurrence. In combination with dexamethasone for the treatment of newly diagnosed multiple myeloma.

DOSAGE: *Adults:* Acute ENL: Initial: 100-300mg qhs with water at least 1 hr after evening meal. <50kg: Start therapy at lower end of dosing range. Severe Cutaneous ENL: Initial: 400mg qhs with water at least 1 hr after evening meal. Use with corticosteroids in moderate to severe neuritis with severe ENL. Taper steroid where neuritis is ameliorated. Duration of therapy is usually 2 weeks. Taper Dose: Decrease by 50mg every 2-4 weeks. Maintenance Therapy for Prevention/Suppression of ENL Recurrence: Use minimum dose to control reaction. Taper Dose: Every 3-6 months, attempt to decrease dose by 50mg every 2-4 weeks. Multiple Myeloma: 200mg qhs at least 1 hr after evening meal. Give with dexamethasone in 28 day treatment cycles.
Pediatrics: ≥12 yrs: Acute ENL: Initial: 100-300mg qhs with water at least 1 hr after evening meal. <50kg: Start therapy at lower end of dosing range. Severe Cutaneous ENL: Initial: 400mg qhs with water at least 1 hour after evening meal. Use with corticosteroids in moderate to severe neuritis with severe ENL. Taper steroid where neuritis is ameliorated. Duration of therapy is usually 2 weeks. Taper Dose: Decrease by 50mg every 2-4 weeks. Maintenance Therapy for Prevention/Suppression of ENL Recurrence: Use minimum dose to control reaction. Taper Dose: Every 3-6 months, attempt to decrease dose by 50mg every 2-4 weeks. Multiple Myeloma: 200mg qhs at least 1 hr after evening meal. Give with dexamethasone in 28-day treatment cycles.

HOW SUPPLIED: Cap: 50mg, 100mg, 200mg

CONTRAINDICATIONS: Women of childbearing potential unless alternative therapies are considered inappropriate and if precautions are taken to avoid pregnancy. Sexually mature males unless they comply with the S.T.E.P.S.® program and mandatory contraceptive measures.

WARNINGS/PRECAUTIONS: See Black Box Warning. If hypersensitivity reaction occurs such as rash, fever, or tachycardia, d/c drug. Stevens-Johnson syndrome and toxic epidermal necrolysis reported. May cause severe birth defects. Drowsiness and somnolence reported, caution when operating machinery. May cause neuropathy, monitor for symptoms. If symptoms of neuropathy arise, d/c immediately. Do not initiate if ANC <750/mm³. Measure viral load of HIV patients after 1st and 3rd month of therapy and every 3 months thereafter.

ADVERSE REACTIONS: Drowsiness, somnolence, peripheral neuropathy, dizziness, orthostatic hypotension, neutropenia, increased HIV viral load, rash, constipation, hypocalcemia, thrombosis/embolism, dyspnea.

INTERACTIONS: Enhanced sedation with barbiturates, alcohol, chlorpromazine, and reserpine. Caution with drugs associated with peripheral neuropathy.

PREGNANCY: Category X, not for use in nursing.

MECHANISM OF ACTION: Immunomodulatory agent; not fully established. Possesses immunomodulatory, anti-inflammatory, and anti-angiogenic properties. Immunologic effects may be caused by suppression of excessive TNF-α production and down-modulation of selected cell surface adhesion molecules involved in leukocyte migration. Also causes suppression of macrophage involvement in prostaglandin synthesis and modulation of interleukin-10 and

T

12 production by peripheral blood mononuclear cells. In multiple myeloma, increased circulating natural killer cells and plasma levels of interleukin-2 and INF-gamma are also seen.

PHARMACOKINETICS: Absorption: Slow; T_{max}=2.9-5.7 hrs. **Distribution:** Plasma protein binding (55-66%); found in semen. **Metabolism:** Non-enzymatic hydrolysis. **Elimination:** Urine (<0.7% unchanged); $T_{1/2}$=5-7 hrs.

THEO-24   RX
theophylline (UCB Pharma)

THERAPEUTIC CLASS: Xanthine bronchodilator

INDICATIONS: Treatment of symptoms and reversible airflow obstruction associated with chronic asthma and other chronic lung diseases.

DOSAGE: *Adults:* Initial: 300-400mg/day. Titrate: After 3 days increase to 400-600mg/day if tolerated. May increase to >600mg/day if needed and tolerated after 3 more days. Renal/Liver Dysfunction/Elderly/CHF: Max: 400mg/day. May give in divided doses q12h in fast metabolizers. Swallow tab whole with full glass of water, do not crush. Dose should be titrated based on serum levels.
Pediatrics: 12-15 yrs: <45kg: Initial: 12-14mg/kg/day. Max: 300mg/day. Titrate: After 3 days increase to 16mg/kg/day. Max: 400mg/day. May increase to 20mg/kg/day if tolerated and needed after 3 more days. Max: 600mg/day. 12-15 yrs (>45kg): Follow adult dose schedule. Renal/Liver Dysfunction/CHF: Max: 16mg/kg/day or 400mg/day. May give in divided doses q12h in fast metabolizers. Swallow tab whole with full glass of water, do not crush. Dose should be titrated based on serum levels.

HOW SUPPLIED: Cap, Extended-Release: 100mg, 200mg, 300mg, 400mg

WARNINGS/PRECAUTIONS: Extreme caution in PUD, seizure disorders, and/or cardiac arrhythmias (except bradycardia). Caution in neonates, children <1 yr, and the elderly. Caution in pulmonary edema, CHF, fever ≥102°F for 24 hrs, cor-pulmonale, hypothyroidism, liver disease, reduced renal function, sepsis, shock, and HTN. If toxicity develops (eg, repetitive vomiting) monitor serum levels and adjust dosage.

ADVERSE REACTIONS: Diarrhea, nausea, vomiting, abdominal pain, nervousness, headache, insomnia, seizures, dizziness, tachycardia, arrhythmias, restlessness, tremor, transient diuresis.

INTERACTIONS: Potentiated by propranolol, allopurinol, erythromycin, cimetidine, interferon, ciprofloxacin, clarithromycin, disulfiram, enoxacin, methotrexate, β-adrenergic blockers, oral contraceptives, fluvoxamine, CCBs, corticosteroid, thyroid hormones, thiabendazole, ticlopidine, troleadomycin, carbamazepine, pentoxifylline, diuretics, tacrine, and isoniazid. Diminishes the effects of adenosine, diazepam, lithium, lorazepam, midazolam, and pancuronium. Synergistic CNS effects with ephedrine. Diminished effects with aminoglutethimide, phenytoin, phenobarbital, carbamazepine, rifampin, barbiturates, hydantoins, ketoconazole, diuretics sympathomimetics, and isoproterenol.

PREGNANCY: Category C, caution in nursing.

MECHANISM OF ACTION: Methylxanthine; not established, suspected to act by relaxation of smooth muscle and suppression of response of airways to stimuli.

PHARMACOKINETICS: Absorption: Rapid, complete; C_{max} =18.1mcg/mL. **Distribution:** V_d=0.45L/kg; plasma protein binding (40%); crosses placenta; excreted in breast milk. **Metabolism:** Liver (N-demethylation); metabolite: Caffeine. Liver (demethylation) via CYP1A2; metabolite: 3-methylxanthine. Liver (hydroxylation) via CYP2E1 and 3A3. **Elimination:** (Neonates) Urine (50%). (>3mo) Urine (10%).

THERACYS   RX
bcg live (Sanofi Pasteur)

> Contains live, attenuated mycobacteria. Potential risk for transmission; prepare, handle, and dispose of as a biohazard material. Nosocomial infections reported in immunosuppressed. Fatal reactions reported with intravesical BCG.

THERAPEUTIC CLASS: Attenuated live BCG culture

INDICATIONS: Treatment and prophylaxis of carcinoma *in situ* of the bladder. Prophylaxis of primary or recurrent stage Ta and/or T1 papillary tumors following transurethral resection (TUR).

DOSAGE: *Adults:* Begin 7-14 days after biopsy or resection. Induction: 81mg intravesically weekly for 6 weeks. Maint: 81mg at 3, 6, 12, 18, and 24 months. Avoid fluids for 4 hrs before treatment. Empty badder before administration. Retain in bladder for 2 hrs, then void. During the 1st 15 min following instillation, patient should lie prone.

HOW SUPPLIED: Inj: 81mg

CONTRAINDICATIONS: Immunocompromised patients, congenital or acquired immune deficiency patients (eg, AIDS, cancer, immunosuppressives), concurrent febrile illness, UTI, gross hematuria, active TB. Wait 7-14 days after biopsy, TUR or traumatic catheterization.

WARNINGS/PRECAUTIONS: Not a vaccine for prevention of cancer. Risk of infectious complications; avoid with actively bleeding urinary mucosa; delay treatment for ≥1 week after TUR, biopsy, traumatic catheterization, or gross hematuria. Possible increased risk of severe local reactions with small bladder capacity. May cause tuberculin sensitivity. BCG infection of aneurysms and prosthetic devices (including arterial grafts, cardiac devices, and artificial joints) reported. Stopper of vial contains natural rubber latex which may cause allergic reactions. Evaluate for serious infectious complication if fever ≥101.3°F, or acute localized inflammation (eg, epididymitis, prostatitis, orchitis) persists >2-3 days. Febrile episodes with flu-like symptoms >72 hrs, fever ≥103°F, systemic manifestations increasing in intensity with repeated instillations, or persistent abnormal LFTs suggest systemic BCG infection and may require antituberculous therapy. D/C if fever persists or if acute febrile illness consistent with BCG infection occur. Administer ≥2 antimycobacterials while diagnostic evaluation is conducted. Sensitive to INH, rifampin, and ethambutol; not sensitive to pyrazinamide. Caution with groups at risk of HIV. Not recommended for stage TaG1 papillary tumors, unless judged to be at high risk of tumor recurrence. Persons with immunologic deficiency should not handle agent.

ADVERSE REACTIONS: Malaise, fever, chills, uveitis, conjunctivitis, iritis, keratitis, granulomatous choreoretinitis, arthritis, arthralgia, urinary symptoms, skin rash.

INTERACTIONS: Immunosuppressants, bone-marrow depressants, and radiation may interfere with immune response; avoid concomitant use. Antimicrobials may interfere with efficacy. Avoid antituberculosis drugs (eg, INH) to prevent or treat the local, irritative toxicities of BCG Live.

PREGNANCY: Category C, not for use in nursing.

MECHANISM OF ACTION: Attenuated live BCG culture, suspected to have an antitumor effect that appears to be T-lymphocyte dependent.

THIOGUANINE   RX
thioguanine (GlaxoSmithKline)

THERAPEUTIC CLASS: Purine analog

INDICATIONS: For remission induction, remission consolidation, and maintenance therapy of acute nonlymphocytic leukemias.

DOSAGE: *Adults:* Monotherapy: 2mg/kg/day. After 4 weeks, may increase to 3mg/kg/day if no improvement and leukocyte or platelet depression. Usual

therapy is with other agents in combination.
Pediatrics: Monotherapy: 2mg/kg/day. After 4 weeks, may increase to 3mg/kg/day if no improvement and leukocyte or platelet depression. Usual therapy is with other agents in combination.

HOW SUPPLIED: Tab: 40mg* *scored

CONTRAINDICATIONS: Prior resistance to this drug.

WARNINGS/PRECAUTIONS: Dose-related bone-marrow suppression. Increased sensitivity to myelosuppression with thiopurine methyltransferase (TPMT) deficiency. D/C temporarily at 1st sign of abnormally large fall in any formed elements of the blood. Withhold therapy with toxic hepatitis or biliary stasis. Monitor Hgb, Hct, platelets, WBCs, and differential frequently. Monitor LFTs weekly at start of therapy, monthly thereafter.

ADVERSE REACTIONS: Myelosuppression, hyperuricemia, hepatotoxicity, nausea, vomiting, anorexia, stomatitis.

INTERACTIONS: May be cross-resistant with mercaptopurine. Caution with TPMT inhibitors such as aminosalicylate derivatives (eg, olsalazine, mesalazine, sulfasalazine); increased sensitivity to myelosuppression. May need dose reduction with other drugs whose primary toxicity is myelosuppression. Esophageal varices reported with busulfan. Veno-occlusive liver disease reported with combination chemotherapy.

PREGNANCY: Category D, not for use in nursing.

MECHANISM OF ACTION: Purine analog; competes with hypoxanthine and guanine for the enzyme hypoxanthine-guanine phosphoribosyltransferase (HGPTase).

PHARMACOKINETICS: Absorption: (30%) Incomplete and variable. [2-amino-6-methylthiopurine (MTG)] T_{max}= 6-8 hrs. **Metabolism:** Rapid via methylation to MTG (active) and inactive compounds. **Elimination:** Urine, (MTG) $T_{1/2}$=12-22 hrs.

THIORIDAZINE   RX
thioridazine HCL (Various)

> Prolongation of QTc interval reported in a dose related manner. Associated with torsade de pointes and sudden death; reserve for patients who fail to respond to or cannot tolerate other antipsychotics.

THERAPEUTIC CLASS: Piperidine phenothiazine

INDICATIONS: Management of schizophrenia in patients not responsive to or intolerant to other antipsychotics.

DOSAGE: *Adults:* Initial: 50-100mg tid. Titrate: Increase gradually. Usual: 200-800mg/day given bid-qid. Max: 800mg/day.
Pediatrics: Initial: 0.6mg/kg/day given in divided doses. Titrate: Increase gradually. Max: 3mg/kg/day.

HOW SUPPLIED: Tab: 10mg, 15mg, 25mg, 50mg, 100mg, 150mg, 200mg

CONTRAINDICATIONS: Severe CNS depression, comatose states, severe hypo- or hypertensive heart disease. Drugs that prolong QTc interval, congenital long QT syndrome, cardiac arrhythmias, drugs that inhibit CYP450 2D6 (eg, fluoxetine, paroxetine), patients with reduced activity of CYP450 2D6.

WARNINGS/PRECAUTIONS: Perform baseline ECG and measure baseline potassium level; monitor periodically thereafter. May develop tardive dyskinesia. NMS, seizures, leukopenia, agranulocytosis reported. Caution with activities requiring alertness. May elevate prolactin levels.

ADVERSE REACTIONS: Tardive dyskinesia, ECG changes, drowsiness, dry mouth, blurred vision, peripheral edema, galactorrhea, nausea, vomiting, gynecomastia, impotence, constipation, diarrhea.

INTERACTIONS: See Contraindications. May potentiate CNS depressants, alcohol, atropine, and phosphorus insecticides. Propranolol, fluvoxamine, pindolol increases thioridazine plasma levels; avoid concomitant use. Avoid CYP2D6 inhibitors (eg, fluoxetine, paroxetine); increased risk of arrhythmias.

PREGNANCY: Safety in pregnancy and nursing not known.

MECHANISM OF ACTION: Phenothiazine; associated with minimal extrapyramidal stimulation.

THROMBIN-JMI   RX
thrombin (bovine origin) (King)

THERAPEUTIC CLASS: Topical Thrombin

INDICATIONS: An aid to hemostasis whenever oozing blood and minor bleeding from capillaries and small venules is accessible. In various types of surgery, may be used in conjuction with an Absorbable Gelatin Sponge, USP for hemostasis.

DOSAGE: *Adults:* Spray topically on surface of bleeding tissue. Reconstitute with sterile isotonic saline at a recommended concentration of 1,000-2,000 IU/mL. Profuse bleeding: Use 1,000 IU/mL. General use (eg, plastic surgery, dental extractions, skin grafting): 100 IU/mL. Intermediate strengths may be prepared by diluting in appropriate isotonic saline volume if needed. Oozing surfaces: Use dry form. May be used with FlowSeal™ NT.

HOW SUPPLIED: Powder: 5,000 IU, 20,000 IU; Kit: Powder: 20,000 IU [Spray; Syringe Spray]

CONTRAINDICATIONS: Sensitivity to material of bovine origin.

WARNINGS/PRECAUTIONS: The use of topical bovine thrombin preparations has occasionally been associated with abnormalities in hemostasis ranging from asymptomatic alterations in laboratory determinations, such as prothrombin time (PT) and partial thromboplastin time (PTT), to severe bleeding or thrombosis which rarely have been fatal. Consultation with an expert is recommended if patient exhibits abnormal coagulation laboratory values, abnormal bleeding, or abnormal thrombosis. Should not be injected or allowed to enter large blood vessels. Extensive intravascular clotting and even death may result.

ADVERSE REACTIONS: Inhibitory antibodies which interfere with hemostasis may develop.

PREGNANCY: Category C, safety in nursing is not known

MECHANISM OF ACTION: Topical thrombin; clots the fibrinogen of the blood directly.

THYMOGLOBULIN   RX
anti-thymocyte globulin (rabbit) (Genzyme)

> Only for use by physicians experienced in immunosuppressive therapy management of renal transplant.

THERAPEUTIC CLASS: Immunoglobulin

INDICATIONS: Treatment of renal transplant acute rejection in conjunction with concomitant immunosuppression.

DOSAGE: *Adults:* 1.5mg/kg qd for 7-14 days. Administer by IV infusion over a minimum of 6 hrs into a high-flow vein for 1st infusion, and over at least 4 hrs for subsequent infusions. If WBC 2000-3000cells/mm³ or platelets 50,000-75,000cells/mm³: Reduce dose by 50%. If WBC <2000cells/mm³ or platelets <50,000cells/mm³: Stop therapy.

HOW SUPPLIED: Inj: 25mg

CONTRAINDICATIONS: Acute viral illness, or history of allergy/anaphylaxis to rabbit protein.

WARNINGS/PRECAUTIONS: Medical surveillance required during infusion. Possible thrombocytopenia or neutropenia from cross-reactive antibodies; reversible with dose adjustment. Infusion-related fever and chills may occur; premedicate with corticosteroids, APAP, and/or an antihistamine, and/ or slowing infusion rate to minimize effects. Prolonged use or overdosage

T

in association with other immunosuppressives may cause over-immunosuppression resulting in severe infections and increased incidence of lymphoma, post-transplant lymphoproliferative disease, or other malignancies; antiviral, antibacterial, antiprotozoal, and/or antifungal prophylaxis is recommended. Monitor lymphocyte and WBC count.

ADVERSE REACTIONS: Fever, chills, leukopenia, pain, headache, abdominal pain, diarrhea, HTN, nausea, thrombocytopenia, peripheral edema, dyspnea, asthenia, hyperkalemia, tachycardia, malaise, dizziness, CMV, sepsis, GI/oral moniliasis, herpes simplex, UTI.

INTERACTIONS: Possible over-immunosuppression with standard immunosuppressive regimen; decrease maintenance immunosuppression therapy during period of antibody therapy. May stimulate antibody production which cross-reacts with rabbit immune globulins.

PREGNANCY: Category C, caution in nursing.

MECHANISM OF ACTION: Gamma immune globulin: Has not been established; contains cytotoxic antibodies directed against antigens expressed on human T-lymphocytes.

PHARMACOKINETICS: Elimination: $T_{1/2}$=2-3 days

THYROGEN

RX

thyrotropin alfa (Genzyme)

THERAPEUTIC CLASS: Recombinant human thyroid stimulating hormone

INDICATIONS: Adjunctive diagnostic tool for serum thyroglobulin testing with or without radioiodine imaging in thyroid cancer. Adjunctive treatment for radioiodine ablation of thyroid tissue remnants in patients who have undergone a near-total or total thyroidectomy for well-differentiated thyroid cancer and who do not have evidence of metastatic thyroid cancer.

DOSAGE: *Adults:* 0.9mg IM q24h for 2 doses into buttock. Radioiodine Imaging or Remnant Ablation: Administer radioiodine 24 hrs following final injection. Perform diagnostic scanning 48 hrs after radioiodine administration. Serum Thyroglobulin (Tg) Testing: Obtain serum sample 72 hrs after final injection.
Pediatrics: ≥16 yrs: 0.9mg IM q24h for 2 dose into buttock. Radioiodine Imaging or Remnant Ablation: Administer radioiodine 24 hrs following final injection. Perform diagnostic scanning 48 hrs after radioiodine administration. Serum Thyroglobulin (Tg) Testing: Obtain serum sample 72 hrs after final injection.

HOW SUPPLIED: Inj: 1.1mg

WARNINGS/PRECAUTIONS: Tg antibodies may confound the Tg assay and render Tg levels uninterpretable; may need to evaluate patients further with, eg, a confirmatory thyroid hormone withdrawal scan. Caution if previously treated with bovine TSH, particularly if hypersensitivity reactions occurred. Caution with history of heart disease and significant residual thyroid tissue. May prolong elevation of TSH levels in dialysis-dependent ESRD patients. IM use only. Caution in elderly.

ADVERSE REACTIONS: Headache, nausea, asthenia, hypercholesterolemia, paresthesia, influenza-like symptoms.

INTERACTIONS: Pretreatment with glucocorticoids may be considered in patients whom local tumor expansion may compromise vital anatomic structures.

PREGNANCY: Category C, caution in nursing.

MECHANISM OF ACTION: Recombinant human thyroid stimulating hormone; binds to TSH receptors on normal thyroid epithelial cells or thyroid cancer tissues and stimulates iodine reuptake and organification, and synthesis and secretion of thyroglobulin, T_3, T_4.

PHARMACOKINETICS: Absorption: (0.9mg IM) C_{max}=116mU/L, T_{max}=3-24 hrs. **Elimination:** $T_{1/2}$=25 hrs.

THYROLAR RX
liotrix (Forest)

THERAPEUTIC CLASS: Thyroid replacement hormone

INDICATIONS: Hypothyroidism. As a pituitary TSH suppressant in the treatment or prevention of euthyroid goiters. Diagnostic agent in suppression tests to differentiate suspected hyperthyroidism or thyroid gland autonomy. Management of thyroid cancer.

DOSAGE: *Adults:* Hypothyroidism: Usual: 12.5mcg-50mcg to 25mcg-100mcg qd. Elderly/Coronary Artery Disease: Initial: 6.25mcg-25mcg qd. Chronic Myxedema: 3.1mcg-12.5mcg qd. Titrate: Increase by 3.1mcg-12.5mcg/d q 2-3 weeks. Reduce dose if angina occurs. Myxedema Coma: 400mcg IV levothyroxine sodium (100mcg/mL rapidly) followed by 100-200mcg/day IV. Switch to PO when stable. Thyroid Suppression: 1.56mg/kg/d levothyroxine (T$_4$) for 7-10 days.
Pediatrics: Hypothyroidism: >12 yrs: 18.75mcg-75mcg qd. 6-12 yrs: 12.5mcg-50mcg to 18.75mcg-75mcg qd. 1-5 yrs: 9.35mcg-37.5mcg to 12.5mcg-50mcg qd. 6-12 months: 6.25mcg-25mcg to 9.35mcg-37.5mcg qd. 0-6 months: 3.1mcg-12.5mcg to 6.25mcg-25mcg qd.

HOW SUPPLIED: (T3-T4) Tab: (1/4) 3.1mcg-12.5mcg, (1/2) 6.25mcg-25mcg, (1) 12.5mcg-50mcg, (2) 25mcg-100mcg, (3) 37.5mcg-150mcg

CONTRAINDICATIONS: Untreated thyrotoxicosis, uncorrected adrenal cortical insufficiency.

WARNINGS/PRECAUTIONS: Do not use in the treatment of obesity; larger doses in euthyroid patients can cause serious or even life-threatening toxicity. Caution with angina pectoris and elderly; use lower doses. May aggravate diabetes mellitus or insipidus and adrenal cortical insufficiency. Excessive doses may cause craniosynostosis. Extreme caution with long-standing myxedema especially with cardiovascular impairment.

INTERACTIONS: May increase insulin or oral hypoglycemic requirements. Decreased absorption with cholestyramine and colestipol; space dosing by 4-5 hrs. Altered effect of oral anticoagulants; monitor PT/INR. Estrogens increase thyroxine-binding globulin; increase in thyroid dose may be needed. Serious or life-threatening side effects can occur with sympathomimetic amines. Androgens, corticosteroids, estrogens, iodine-containing preparations, and salicylates may interfere with thyroid lab tests.

PREGNANCY: Category A, caution in nursing.

MECHANISM OF ACTION: Thyroid hormone; not understood, suspected to enhance oxygen consumption by most tissues of the body, increase basal metabolic rate and metabolism of carbohydrates, lipids, and proteins.

TIAZAC RX
diltiazem HCL (Forest)

OTHER BRAND NAMES: Taztia XT (Andrx)

THERAPEUTIC CLASS: Calcium channel blocker (nondihydropyridine)

INDICATIONS: Hypertension. Chronic stable angina.

DOSAGE: *Adults:* HTN: Initial: 120-240mg qd. Titrate: Adjust at 2-week intervals. Usual: 120-540mg qd. Max: 540mg qd. Angina: Initial: 120-180mg qd Titrate: Increase over 7-14 days. Max: 540mg qd.

HOW SUPPLIED: Cap, Extended-Release: (Taztia XT, Tiazac) 120mg, 180mg, 240mg, 300mg, 360mg; (Tiazac) 420mg

CONTRAINDICATIONS: Sick sinus syndrome and 2nd- or 3rd-degree AV block (except with functioning pacemaker), severe hypotension (<90mm Hg systolic), acute MI, pulmonary congestion.

WARNINGS/PRECAUTIONS: Caution in renal, hepatic, or ventricular dysfunction. Monitor LFTs and renal function with prolonged use. D/C if persistent

T

rash occurs. Symptomatic hypotension may occur. Acute hepatic injury reported.

ADVERSE REACTIONS: Headache, peripheral edema, vasodilation, dizziness, rash, dyspepsia.

INTERACTIONS: Increased levels of buspirone, quinidine, carbamazepine, midazolam, triazolam, lovastatin, and propranolol. Increased levels of diltiazem with cimetidine. Monitor digoxin, cyclosporine. Potentiates cardiac contractility, conductivity, and automaticity; and vascular dilation with anesthetics. Additive cardiac conduction effects with digitalis or β-blockers. Avoid rifampin and other CYP3A4 inducers. Potential additive effects with agents known to affect cardiac contractility and/or conduction.

PREGNANCY: Category C, not for use in nursing.

MECHANISM OF ACTION: Calcium channel blocker; inhibits cellular influx of calcium ions during membrane depolarization of cardiac and vascular smooth muscle.

PHARMACOKINETICS: Absorption: Well-absorbed. Absolute bioavailability (~40%). **Distribution:** Plasma protein binding (70-80%). **Metabolism:** Hepatic; desacetyldiltiazem, desmethyldiltiazem (major metabolites). **Elimination:** Urine, bile; $T_{1/2}$=3.0-4.5 hrs.

Tice BCG RX
bcg live (Organon)

> Contains live, attenuated mycobacteria. Potential risk for transmission; prepare, handle, and dispose of as a biohazard material. Nosocomial infections reported. Fatal reactions reported with intravesical BCG.

THERAPEUTIC CLASS: Attenuated live BCG culture

INDICATIONS: Treatment and prophylaxis of carcinoma *in situ* of the bladder. Prophylaxis of primary or recurrent stage Ta and/or T1 papillary tumors following transurethral resection (TUR). Not indicated for papillary tumors of stages higher than T1.

DOSAGE: *Adults:* Allow 7-14 days after biopsy before initiating therapy. Administer 1 vial (50mg) intravesically weekly for 6 weeks; may repeat schedule once if tumor remission not achieved. Then, continue monthly for 6-12 months. Retain in bladder for 2 hrs, then void. During bladder retention, reposition patient every 15 min to maximize bladder surface exposure.

HOW SUPPLIED: Inj: 50mg

CONTRAINDICATIONS: Immunocompromised patients, congenital or acquired immune deficiency patients (eg, AIDS, cancer, immunosuppressives), concurrent febrile illness, UTI, gross hematuria, active TB. Wait 7-14 days after biopsy, TUR or traumatic catheterization.

WARNINGS/PRECAUTIONS: Not a vaccine for prevention of cancer. Risk of infectious complications; avoid with actively bleeding urinary mucosa; delay treatment for ≥1 week after TUR, biopsy, traumatic catheterization, or gross hematuria. Possible increased risk of severe local reactions with small bladder capacity. May cause tuberculin sensitivity. Evaluate for serious infectious complication if fever ≥101.3°F, or acute localized inflammation (eg, epididymitis, prostatitis, orchitis) persists >2-3 days. Febrile episodes with flu-like symptoms >72 hrs, fever ≥103°F, systemic manifestations increasing in intensity with repeated instillations, or persistent abnormal LFTs suggest systemic BCG infection and may require antituberculous therapy. D/C if fever persists or if acute febrile illness consistent with BCG infection occur. Administer ≥2 antimycobacterials while diagnostic evaluation is conducted. Sensitive to INH, rifampin, and ethambutol; not sensitive to pyrazinamide. Caution with groups at risk of HIV. Not recommended for stage TaG1 papillary tumors, unless judged to be at high risk of tumor recurrence.

ADVERSE REACTIONS: Malaise, fever, chills, urinary symptoms, cramps/pain, rigors, nausea, vomiting, arthritis, myalgia.

INTERACTIONS: Immunosuppressants, bone-marrow depressants, and radiation may interfere with immune response; avoid concomitant use. Antimicrobials may interfere with efficacy; postpone BCG therapy. Avoid antituberculosis drugs (eg, INH) to prevent or treat the local, irritative toxicities of BCG Live.

PREGNANCY: Category C, not for use in nursing.

MECHANISM OF ACTION: Attenuated live BCG culture, suspected to have an antitumor effect that appears to be T-lymphocyte dependent.

TICLID   RX
ticlopidine HCL (Roche Labs)

> Can cause life-threatening hematological adverse reactions, including neutropenia/agranulocy-tosis, thrombotic thrombocytopenic purpura (TTP), and aplastic anemia. Monitor for evidence of neutropenia or TTP during first 3 months; d/c if any seen.

THERAPEUTIC CLASS: Platelet aggregation inhibitor

INDICATIONS: To reduce risk of thrombotic stroke in stroke patients or those with stroke precursors who are ASA intolerant, allergic, or failed ASA therapy. Adjunct to ASA to reduce incidence of subacute stent thrombosis in patients undergoing successful coronary artery stent implantation.

DOSAGE: *Adults:* Take with food. Stroke: 250mg bid. Coronary Artery Stenting: 250mg bid with ASA up to 30 days after stent implant.

HOW SUPPLIED: Tab: 250mg

CONTRAINDICATIONS: Hematopoietic disorders (eg, neutropenia, thrombocytopenia), history of TTP or aplastic anemia, hemostatic disorders, active pathological bleeding, severe liver impairment.

WARNINGS/PRECAUTIONS: Monitor for hematologic toxicity before treatment, then every 2 weeks for 1st 3 months, and 2 weeks after discontinuation. Monitor more frequently if signs of hematological adverse reactions; d/c if neutrophils <1200/mm³, aplastic anemia or TTP occurs. D/C 10-14 days before surgery. Caution in trauma, surgery, bleeding disorders. May need dose adjustment with renal or hepatic impairment. May elevate LFTs, TG, and cholesterol.

ADVERSE REACTIONS: Diarrhea, rash, nausea, GI pain, rash, dyspepsia, neutropenia.

INTERACTIONS: Adjust dose with drugs metabolized by CYP450 with low therapeutic ratios or with hepatic impairment. Potentiates ASA and NSAIDs effect on platelet aggregation. Antacids reduce plasma levels. Cimetidine reduces clearance. Decreases digoxin plasma levels. Significant decrease of theophylline plasma clearance. Caution with phenytoin, propranolol. D/C anti-coagulants or fibrinolytics. Increased bioavailability with food.

PREGNANCY: Category B, not for use in nursing.

MECHANISM OF ACTION: Platelet aggregation inhibitor; interferes with platelet membrane function by inhibiting ADP-induced platelet fibrinogen binding and subsequent platelet-platelet interactions. Effect on platelet function is irreversible. Responsible for prolonging bleeding time.

PHARMACOKINETICS: Absorption: Rapid; T_{max}=2 hrs. **Distribution:** Plasma protein binding (98%). **Metabolism:** Liver (extensive). **Elimination:** Urine (60%), feces (23%). Single dose: $T_{1/2}$=12.6 hrs. Multiple doses: $T_{1/2}$=4-5 days.

TIGAN   RX
trimethobenzamide HCL (King)

THERAPEUTIC CLASS: Emetic response modifier

INDICATIONS: Treatment of postoperative nausea and vomiting and for nausea associated with gastroenteritis.

DOSAGE: *Adults:* (Cap) 300mg tid-qid. (Inj) 200mg IM tid-qid.

HOW SUPPLIED: Cap: 300mg; Inj: 100mg/mL

CONTRAINDICATIONS: Injection in children.

WARNINGS/PRECAUTIONS: Caution in children; may cause EPS, which may be confused with CNS signs of undiagnosed primary disease (eg, Reye's syndrome) and may unfavorably alter the course of Reye's syndrome due to hepatotoxic potential. Caution with acute febrile illness, encephalitides, gastroenteritis, dehydration, electrolyte imbalance, and in elderly; CNS reactions reported. May produce drowsiness.

ADVERSE REACTIONS: Hypersensitivity reactions, parkinson-like symptoms, hypotension (inj), blood dyscrasias, blurred vision, coma, convulsions, mood depression, diarrhea, disorientation, dizziness, drowsiness, headache, jaundice, muscle cramps, opisthotonos.

INTERACTIONS: Caution with CNS agents (eg, phenothiazines, barbiturates, belladonna derivatives) in acute febrile illness, encephalitides, gastroenteritis, dehydration, and electrolyte imbalance. Adverse drug interactions reported with alcohol.

PREGNANCY: Safety in pregnancy and nursing not known.

MECHANISM OF ACTION: Mechanism not established; thought to involve chemoreceptor trigger zone, an area in medulla oblongata through which emetic impulses are conveyed to vomiting center (direct impulses to vomiting center apparently not similarity inhibited).

PHARMACOKINETICS: Absorption: T_{max}=30 min (IM 200mg). **Elimination:** $T_{1/2}$=7-9 hrs.

TIKOSYN   RX
dofetilide (Pfizer)

> To minimize risk of arrhythmia, place patients initiated or reinitiated on therapy for minimum of 3 days in a facility that can provide CrCl, ECG monitoring, and cardiac resuscitation. Dofetilide is available only to hospitals and prescribers who have received appropriate dofetilide dosing and treatment initiation education.

THERAPEUTIC CLASS: Class III antiarrhythmic

INDICATIONS: Conversion to and maintenance of normal sinus rhythm in atrial fibrillation/flutter.

DOSAGE: *Adults:* CrCl: >60mL/min: 500mcg bid. CrCl 40-60mL/min: 250mcg bid. CrCl 20 to <40mL/min: 125mcg bid. Determine QTc interval 2-3 hrs after 1st dose and adjust dose if QTc >500msec or if >15% increase from baseline. QTc/Renal Dose Adjustment: Reduce 500mcg bid to 250mcg bid. Reduce 250mcg bid to 125mcg bid. Reduce 125mcg bid to 125mcg qd. D/C anytime after 2nd dose if QTc >500 msec (550msec with ventricular conduction abnormalities).

HOW SUPPLIED: Cap: 125mcg, 250mcg, 500mcg

CONTRAINDICATIONS: Long QT syndromes, baseline QT interval or QTc >440msec (500msec with ventricular conduction abnormalities), severe renal impairment (CrCl <20mL/min). Concomitant verapamil, cimetidine, trimethoprim, ketoconazole, and inhibitors of renal cation transport system (eg, megestrol, prochlorperazine).

WARNINGS/PRECAUTIONS: Can cause serious ventricular arrhythmia. Calculate CrCl before 1st dose; adjust dose based on CrCl. Caution in severe hepatic impairment. Maintain normal K^+ levels.

ADVERSE REACTIONS: Headache, chest pain, dizziness, arrhythmia, conduction disturbances, dyspnea, nausea, insomnia.

INTERACTIONS: See Contraindications. Hypokalemia or hypomagnesemia may occur with K^+-depleting diuretics. CYP3A4 inhibitors (eg, macrolides, protease inhibitors, grapefruit juice, etc) may potentiate dofetilide. Avoid verapamil, cimetidine, trimethoprim, ketoconazole, and inhibitors of renal cationic secretion. Caution with drugs actively secreted by cationic secretion (eg, amiloride, triamterene, metformin). Not recommended with drugs that prolong the QT interval. Hold Class I and III antiarrhythmics for at least 3 half-lives before initiating dofetilide. Reduce amiodarone to <0.3mcg/mL or withdraw at least 3 months before initiating dofetilide.

PREGNANCY: Category C, not for use in nursing.

MECHANISM OF ACTION: Class III antiarrhythmic; blocks cardiac ion channel carrying rapid component of delayed rectifier K⁺ current, I_{Kr}.

PHARMACOKINETICS: Absorption: Bioavailability (>90%). T_{max}=2-3 hrs. **Distribution:** Plasma protein binding (60-70%). V_d=3L/kg. **Metabolism:** Liver via CYP3A4 though N-dealkylation and N-oxidation pathways. **Elimination:** T_{max}=10 hrs. Urine, (80%, unchanged) and (20% metabolites).

TIMENTIN   RX
ticarcillin disodium - clavulanate potassium (GlaxoSmithKline)

THERAPEUTIC CLASS: Broad-spectrum penicillin/beta-lactamase inhibitor

INDICATIONS: Treatment of lower respiratory tract, bone and joint, skin and skin structure, urinary tract (UTI), gynecologic, and intra-abdominal infections, and septicemia caused by susceptible strains of microorganisms.

DOSAGE: *Adults:* ≥60kg: UTI/Systemic Infection: 3g-100mg (3.1g vial) IV q4-6h. Gynecologic Infections: Moderate: 200mg/kg/day ticarcillin IV given q6h. Severe: 300mg/kg/day ticarcillin IV given q4h. <60kg: Usual: 200-300mg/kg/day ticarcillin IV given q4-6h. Renal Impairment (based on ticarcillin): LD: 3.1g. Maint: CrCl >60mL/min: 3.1g q4h. CrCl 30-60mL/min: 2g IV q4h. CrCl 10-30mL/min: 2g IV q8h. CrCl <10mL/min: 2g IV q12h (2g IV q24h with hepatic dysfunction). Peritoneal Dialysis: 3.1g IV q12h. Hemodialysis: 2g IV q12h, and 3.1g after each dialysis.
Pediatrics: ≥3 months: ≥60kg: Mild to Moderate: 3g-100mg (3.1g vial) IV q6h. Severe: 3g-100mg (3.1g vial) IV q4h. <60 kg: Mild to Moderate: 50mg/kg ticarcillin IV q6h. Severe: 50mg/kg ticarcillin IV q4h. Renal Impairment (based on ticarcillin): LD: 3.1g vial. Maint: CrCl >60mL/min: 3.1g q4h. CrCl 30-60mL/min: 2g IV q4h. CrCl 10-30mL/min: 2g IV q8h. CrCl <10mL/min: 2g IV q12h (2g IV q24h with hepatic dysfunction). Peritoneal Dialysis: 3.1g IV q12h. Hemodialysis: 2g IV q12h, and 3.1g after each dialysis.

HOW SUPPLIED: Inj: (Ticarcillin-Clavulanate) 3g-100mg, 3g-100mg/100mL, 30g-1g

WARNINGS/PRECAUTIONS: Serious, sometimes fatal, hypersensitivity reactions reported with PCN therapy. *Clostridium difficile*-associated diarrhea reported. Prolonged use may result in overgrowth of nonsusceptible organisms. Risk of convulsions with high doses especially with renal impairment. Monitor renal, hepatic, hematopoietic functions, and serum K⁺ with prolonged therapy. Caution with fluid and electrolyte imbalance; hypokalemia reported. Clotting time, platelet aggregation, and PT abnormalities may occur especially with renal impairment; d/c therapy. Continue therapy for at least 2 days after signs/symptoms disappear. Caution in elderly patients with impaired renal function.

ADVERSE REACTIONS: Hypersensitivity reactions, headache, giddiness, taste/smell disturbances, stomatitis, flatulence, nausea, vomiting, diarrhea, hematologic disturbances, hepatic/renal function tests abnormalities, local reactions.

INTERACTIONS: May inactivate aminoglycoside if mixed together in parenteral solution. Increased serum levels and prolonged half-life with probenecid. May reduce efficacy of combined oral estrogen/progesterone contraceptives.

PREGNANCY: Category B, caution in nursing.

MECHANISM OF ACTION: Ticarcillin: Broad-spectrum antibiotic with bactericidal activity against many gram-positive and gram-negative aerobic and anaerobic bacteria. Clavulanic acid: β-lactam, which possesses ability to inactivate wide range of β-lactamase enzymes.

PHARMACOKINETICS: Absorption: Ticarcillin: C_{max}=330mcg/mL, AUC=485mcg•hr/mL. Clavulanic acid: C_{max}=8mcg/mL, AUC=8.2mcg•hr/mL. **Distribution:** Ticarcillin: Plasma protein binding (45%). Clavulanic acid: Plasma protein binding (25%). **Elimination:** Ticarcillin: Urine (unchanged 60-70%);

T

T$_{1/2}$=1.1 hrs, 4.4 hrs (neonates), 1 hr (infants/ children). Clavulanic acid: Urine (35-45% unchanged); T$_{1/2}$=1.1hrs, 1.9 hrs (neonates), 0.9 hr (infants/children).

TIMOLOL GFS

RX

timolol maleate (Falcon)

THERAPEUTIC CLASS: Nonselective beta-blocker

INDICATIONS: Treatment of elevated IOP in patients with open-angle glaucoma or ocular hypertension.

DOSAGE: *Adults:* Initial: 1 drop 0.25-0.5% qd. Evaluate IOP 4 weeks after starting treatment. Max: 1 drop 0.5% qd. Dose other ophthalmic drugs 10 min prior to gel-forming drops.

HOW SUPPLIED: Sol, Gel Forming: 0.25%, 0.5% [2.5mL, 5mL]

CONTRAINDICATIONS: Bronchial asthma, history of bronchial asthma, severe COPD, sinus bradycardia, 2nd- or 3rd-degree AV block, overt cardiac failure, cardiogenic shock.

WARNINGS/PRECAUTIONS: May be absorbed systemically. Caution with cardiac failure, DM, and cerebrovascular insufficiency. May mask symptoms of hypoglycemia and hyperthyroidism. Avoid with COPD, bronchospastic disease. Not for use alone in angle-closure glaucoma. May potentiate muscle weakness. D/C if cardiac failure develops. Withdrawal before surgery is controversial.

ADVERSE REACTIONS: Ocular burning, ocular stinging, transient blurred vision.

INTERACTIONS: May potentiate systemic/ophthalmic β-blockers and catecholamine-depleting drugs (eg, reserpine). Oral/IV calcium antagonists can cause AV conduction disturbances, left ventricular failure, or hypotension. Digitalis can cause additive effects in prolonging AV conduction time. Quinidine may potentiate β-blockade. May antagonize epinephrine. Give other ophthalmic drugs 10 minutes before use.

PREGNANCY: Category C, not for use in nursing.

MECHANISM OF ACTION: Nonselective β-adrenergic receptor blocker; reduces IOP. Actions may also be related to reduced aqueous formation.

PHARMACOKINETICS: Absorption: C$_{max}$≤5ng/mL. **Distribution:** Found in breast milk.

TIMOLOL MALEATE

RX

timolol maleate (Various)

THERAPEUTIC CLASS: Nonselective beta-blocker

INDICATIONS: Treatment of hypertension. To reduce cardiovascular mortality and risk of reinfarction with previous MI. Migraine prophylaxis.

DOSAGE: *Adults:* HTN: Initial: 10mg bid. Maint: 20-40mg/day. Wait at least 7 days between dose increases. Max: 60mg/day given bid. MI: 10mg bid. Migraine: Initial: 10mg bid. Maint: 20mg qd. Max: 30mg/day in divided doses. May decrease to 10mg qd. D/C if inadequate response after 6-8 weeks with max dose.

HOW SUPPLIED: Tab: 5mg, 10mg*, 20mg* *scored

CONTRAINDICATIONS: Active or history of bronchial asthma, severe COPD, sinus bradycardia, 2nd- and 3rd-degree AV block, overt cardiac failure, cardiogenic shock.

WARNINGS/PRECAUTIONS: Caution with well-compensated cardiac failure, DM, mild to moderate COPD, bronchospastic disease, dialysis, hepatic/renal impairment, or cerebrovascular insufficiency. Exacerbation of ischemic heart disease with abrupt cessation. May mask hyperthyroidism or hypoglycemia symptoms. Withdrawal before surgery is controversial. May potentiate weakness with myasthenia gravis. Can cause cardiac failure. Caution and consider monitoring renal function in elderly.

ADVERSE REACTIONS: Fatigue, headache, nausea, arrhythmia, pruritus, dizziness, dyspnea, asthenia, bradycardia, dizziness.

INTERACTIONS: Possible additive effects and hypotension and/or marked bradycardia with catecholamine-depleting drugs. NSAIDs may reduce antihypertensive effects. Quinidine may potentiate β-blockade. AV conduction time prolonged with digitalis and either diltiazem or verapamil. Hypotension, AV conduction disturbances, left ventricular failure reported with oral calcium antagonists. Caution with IV calcium antagonists, insulin, oral hypoglycemics. Avoid calcium antagonists with cardiac dysfunction. May exacerbate rebound HTN following clonidine withdrawal. May block effects of epinephrine.

PREGNANCY: Category C, not for use in nursing.

MECHANISM OF ACTION: β1 and β2 adrenergic receptor blocking agent: reduces cardiac output and plasma renin activity.

PHARMACOKINETICS: Absorption: (PO) Completely absorbed (90%); T_{max}=2 hrs. **Metabolism:** Partially, by liver. **Excretion:** Kidneys; $T_{1/2}$= 4 hrs.

TIMOPTIC RX
timolol maleate (Merck)

OTHER BRAND NAMES: Timoptic-XE (Merck) - Timoptic Ocudose (Preservative Free) (Merck)

THERAPEUTIC CLASS: Nonselective beta-blocker.

INDICATIONS: Treatment of elevated IOP in patients with open-angle glaucoma or ocular hypertension.

DOSAGE: *Adults:* (Sol) Initial: 1 drop 0.25% bid. May increase to a max of 1 drop 0.5% bid. Maint: If adequate control, may attempt 1 drop 0.25-0.5% qd. (Sol, Gel Forming) Initial: 1 drop 0.25-0.5% qd. Max: 1 drop 0.5% qd. Dose other ophthalmic drugs 10 min prior to gel-forming drops.

HOW SUPPLIED: Sol: (Timoptic) 0.25%, 0.5% [5mL, 10mL]; Sol: (Timoptic Ocudose) 0.25%, 0.5% [0.2mL 60s]; Sol, Gel Forming: (Timoptic-XE) 0.25%, 0.5% [5mL]

CONTRAINDICATIONS: Bronchial asthma, history of bronchial asthma, severe COPD, sinus bradycardia, 2nd- or 3rd-degree AV block, overt cardiac failure, cardiogenic shock.

WARNINGS/PRECAUTIONS: Severe cardiac and respiratory reactions reported. Caution with cardiac failure and cerebrovascular insufficiency; d/c if cardiac failure develops. May mask symptoms of hypoglycemia or hyperthyroidism; caution with DM or thyrotoxicosis. Avoid with COPD, bronchospastic disease. Not for use alone in angle-closure glaucoma. May potentiate muscle weakness. Withdrawal before surgery is controversial.

ADVERSE REACTIONS: Ocular: burning, stinging, blurred vision, pain, conjunctivitis, discharge, foreign body sensation, itching, tearing. Systemic: headache dizziness, upper respiratory infections.

INTERACTIONS: May potentiate systemic/ophthalmic β-blockers and catecholamine-depleting drugs (eg, reserpine). Oral/IV calcium antagonists may cause AV conduction disturbances, left ventricular failure, or hypotension. Digitalis may cause additive effects in prolonging AV conduction time. Potentiated systemic β-blockade reported with concomitant CYP2D6 inhibitors. Quinidine may potentiate systemic β-blockade. May antagonize epinephrine. May exacerbate rebound hypertension following clonidine withdrawal. Give other ophthalmic drugs 10 minutes before use.

PREGNANCY: Category C, not for use in nursing.

MECHANISM OF ACTION: Nonselective β-blocker; reduces elevated and normal IOP.

PHARMACOKINETICS: Absorption: C_{max}=0.46ng/mL (morning dosing), 0.35ng/mL (afternoon dosing). **Distribution:** Found in breast milk.

TINDAMAX
RX

tinidazole (Mission)

> Avoid unnecessary use. Reserve only for indicated conditions. Although none reported, potential risk of carcinogenicity exists and has been observed in rats and mice treated chronically with metronidazole, a structurally related drug with similar biologic effects.

THERAPEUTIC CLASS: Antiprotozoal agent

INDICATIONS: Treatment of trichomoniasis caused by *Trichomonas vaginalis*, giardiasis caused by *Giardia duodenalis*, intestinal amebiasis and amebic liver abscess caused by *Entamoeba histolytica*, and bacterial vaginosis in non-pregnant women.

DOSAGE: *Adults:* Take with food. Trichomoniasis/Giardiasis: 2g single dose. Amebiasis: Intestinal: 2g qd for 3 days. Amebic Liver Abscess: 2g qd for 3-5 days. Hemodialysis: Give additional dose equivalent to one-half of recommended dose at the end of dialysis. For trichomoniasis, treat sexual partner with the same dose. Bacterial Vaginosis: 2g qd for 2 days or 1g qd for 5 days. *Pediatrics:* >3 yrs: Take with food. Giardiasis: 50mg/kg single dose. Amebiasis: Intestinal: 50mg/kg qd for 3 days. Amebic Liver Abscess: 50mg/kg qd for 3-5 days. Max (for all): 2g/day. May crush tabs in cherry syrup.

HOW SUPPLIED: Tab: 250mg*, 500mg* *scored

CONTRAINDICATIONS: Treatment during 1st trimester of pregnancy, nursing mothers during therapy and 3 days following last dose.

WARNINGS/PRECAUTIONS: Seizures, peripheral neuropathy reported. D/C if abnormal neurological signs occur. Caution with hepatic impairment, blood dyscrasias, or CNS diseases. May develop vaginal candidiasis. May develop drug resistance if presribed in absence of proven or strongly suspected bacterial infection.

ADVERSE REACTIONS: Metallic/bitter taste, nausea, anorexia, flatulence, urinary tract infection, pelvic pain, vulvo-vaginal discomfort, vaginal odor, menorrhagia, upper respiratory infection, convulsions, peripheral neuropathy.

INTERACTIONS: Avoid alcohol during and for 3 days after use and within 2 weeks of disulfiram. May potentiate oral anticoagulants. May reduce clearance of phenytoin (IV), fluorouracil. May increase levels of lithium, cyclosporine, tacrolimus, fluorouracil. Separate dosing with cholestyramine. Phenobarbital, rifampin, phenytoin, other hepatic enzyme inducers may decrease levels. Cimetidine, ketoconazole, other hepatic enzyme inhibitors may increase levels. Antagonized by oxytetracycline.

PREGNANCY: Category C, not for use in nursing.

MECHANISM OF ACTION: Antiprotozoal: Antibacterial agent; nitro group of tinidazole is reduced by cell extracts of *Trichomonas*. Free nitro radical generated as a result of this reduction may be responsible for antiprotozoal activity.

PHARMACOKINETICS: Absorption: Rapid, complete. (Fasted) C_{max}=47.7mcg/mL, T_{max}=1.6 hrs, AUC=901.6mcg/hr/mL. **Distribution:** V_d= 50L; plasma protein binding (12%); crosses blood-brain and placental barrier; found in breast milk. **Metabolism:** Mainly via oxidation, hydroxylation, conjugation; CYP3A4 mainly involved. **Elimination:** Urine (20-25% unchanged), feces (12%); $T_{1/2}$=12-14 hrs.

TNKASE
RX

tenecteplase (Genentech)

THERAPEUTIC CLASS: Thrombolytic agent

INDICATIONS: To reduce mortality with AMI.

DOSAGE: *Adults:* Administer as single IV bolus over 5 seconds. <60kg: 30mg. 60 to <70kg: 35mg. 70 to <80kg: 40mg. 80 to <90kg: 45mg. ≥90kg: 50mg. Max: 50mg/dose.

HOW SUPPLIED: Inj: 50mg

CONTRAINDICATIONS: Active internal bleeding, history of CVA, intracranial or intraspinal surgery or trauma within 2 months, intracranial neoplasm, arteriovenous malformation, aneurysm, bleeding diathesis, severe uncontrolled HTN .

WARNINGS/PRECAUTIONS: Weigh benefits/risks with recent major surgery, cerebrovascular disease, recent GI or GU bleeding, recent trauma, HTN, left heart thrombus, acute pericarditis, subacute bacterial endocarditis, hemostatic defects, severe hepatic dysfunction, pregnancy, diabetic hemorrhagic retinopathy or other hemorrhagic ophthalmic conditions, septic thrombophlebitis or occluded AV cannula at a seriously infected site, elderly, any other bleeding condition that is difficult to manage. Cholesterol embolism and internal/superficial bleeding reported. Arrhythmias may occur with reperfusion. Avoid IM injection, noncompressible arterial puncture, and internal jugular or subclavian venous puncture. Caution with readministration.

ADVERSE REACTIONS: Bleeding.

INTERACTIONS: Increased risk of bleeding with heparin, vitamin K antagonists, and drugs that alter platelet function (eg, ASA, NSAIDs, dipyridamole, GP IIb/IIIa inhibitors) before or after therapy. Weigh benefits/risks with oral anticoagulants, GP IIb/IIIa inhibitors.

PREGNANCY: Category C, caution in nursing.

MECHANISM OF ACTION: Thrombolytic agent; modified form of human tissue plasminogen activator (tPA) that binds to fibrin and converts plasminogen to plasmin.

PHARMACOKINETICS: Metabolism: Liver. **Elimination:** $T_{1/2}$=90-130 min.

TOBI   RX
tobramycin (Chiron)

THERAPEUTIC CLASS: Aminoglycoside

INDICATIONS: Management of cystic fibrosis patients with *P.aeruginosa.*

DOSAGE: *Adults:* Inhale via nebulizer 300mg q12h for 28 days, then stop for 28 days. Resume therapy for next 28 day on/28 day off cycle.
Pediatrics: ≥6 yrs: Inhale via nebulizer 300mg q12h for 28 days, then stop for 28 days. Resume therapy for next 28 day on/28 day off cycle.

HOW SUPPLIED: Sol: 60mg/mL (300mg/amp)

WARNINGS/PRECAUTIONS: Caution with muscular disorders (eg, myasthenia gravis, Parkinson's disease), and renal, auditory, vestibular, or neuromuscular dysfunction. May cause hearing loss, bronchospasm. Can cause fetal harm in pregnancy. D/C if nephrotoxicity occurs until serum level <2mcg/mL.

ADVERSE REACTIONS: Voice alteration, taste perversion, tinnitus.

INTERACTIONS: Avoid neurotoxic or ototoxic drugs. Hearing loss reported with previous or concomitant systemic aminoglycosides. Avoid ethacrynic acid, furosemide, urea, and mannitol.

PREGNANCY: Category D, not for use in nursing.

MECHANISM OF ACTION: Aminoglycoside antibiotic; inhibits protein synthesis in bacterial cell.

PHARMACOKINETICS: Absorption: C_{max}=1237mcg/g (sputum), 0.95mcg/mL (serum). **Distribution:** Crosses placenta. **Elimination:** Glomerular filtration, sputum expectoration (unchanged). $T_{1/2}$=approximately 2 hrs (IV).

TOBRADEX   RX
tobramycin - dexamethasone (Alcon)

THERAPEUTIC CLASS: Aminoglycoside/corticosteroid

INDICATIONS: Ocular inflammation associated with infection or risk of infection.

DOSAGE: *Adults:* (Sus) 1-2 drops q4-6h. May increase to 1-2 drops q2h for first 24-48 hrs. (Oint) Apply 1/2 inch in conjunctival sac up to tid-qid. Max: 20mL or 8g for initial RX.
Pediatrics: ≥2 yrs: (Sus) 1-2 drops q4-6h. May increase to 1-2 drops q2h for first 24-48 hrs. (Oint) Apply 1/2 inch in conjunctival sac up to tid-qid. Max: 20mL or 8g for initial RX.

HOW SUPPLIED: Oint: (Tobramycin-Dexamethasone) 0.3-0.1% [3.5g]; Sus: 0.3-0.1% [2.5mL, 5mL, 10mL]

CONTRAINDICATIONS: Viral diseases of the cornea and conjunctiva including epithelial herpes simplex keratitis, vaccinia, and varicella. Mycobacterial infection and fungal diseases of the eye.

WARNINGS/PRECAUTIONS: Not for injection into the eye. Prolonged use may result in glaucoma, optic nerve damage, visual acuity and fields of vision defects, cataracts, secondary ocular infections (eg, fungal infections).

ADVERSE REACTIONS: Conjunctival erythema, hypersensitivity, lid itching and swelling, secondary infection.

PREGNANCY: Category C, caution in nursing.

MECHANISM OF ACTION: Tobramycin: Aminoglycoside antibiotic; inhibits synthesis of proteins in bacterial cells. Dexamethasone: Corticoid; suppresses inflammatory response and probably delays or slows healing.

TOBRAMYCIN RX
tobramycin sulfate (Various)

> Potential ototoxicity, nephrotoxicity, and neurotoxicity. Monitor peak and trough serum levels to avoid toxicity. Avoid prolonged serum levels >12mcg/mL. Rising trough levels (>2mcg/mL) may indicate tissue accumulation. Tissue accumulation, excessive peak levels, advanced age, and cumulative dose may contribute to ototoxicity and nephrotoxicity. Monitor urine, BUN, SrCr, and CrCl periodically. Obtain serial audiograms. D/C or adjust dose with renal, vestibular, or auditory dysfunction. Caution in premature and neonatal infants, advanced age, and dehydration. Avoid other neurotoxic or nephrotoxic agents, particularly other aminoglycosides, cephaloridine, viomycin, polymyxin B, colistin, cisplatin, and vancomycin. Avoid potent diuretics (eg, ethacrynic acid, furosemide). Risk of fetal harm during pregnancy.

THERAPEUTIC CLASS: Aminoglycoside

INDICATIONS: Treatment of serious lower respiratory tract, CNS (eg, meningitis), intra-abdominal, bone, skin and skin structure, and complicated/recurrent urinary tract infections, and septicemia.

DOSAGE: *Adults:* IM/IV: Serious Infections: 3mg/kg/day given q8h. Life-Threatening Infections: Up to 5mg/kg/day given tid-qid. Reduce to 3mg/kg/day as soon as clinically indicated. Max: 5mg/kg/day unless serum levels monitored. Treat for 7-10 days; may need longer course in difficult and complicated infections. Severe Cystic Fibrosis: Initial: 10mg/kg/day given qid. Measure levels to determine subsequent doses. Renal Impairment: LD: 1mg/kg, followed by reduced doses given q8h or normal doses given at prolonged intervals based on either CrCl or SrCr. Do not use either method during dialysis. Obese Patients: Calculate dose based on estimated LBW plus 40% of excess as basic weight on which to figure mg/kg. ADD-Vantage vials not for IM use.
Pediatrics: >1 week: IM/IV: 6-7.5mg/kg/day given tid-qid (eg, 2-2.5mg/kg q8h or 1.5-1.89mg/kg q6h). ≤1 week: Up to 2mg/kg q12h. Treat for 7-10 days; may need longer course in difficult and complicated infections. Severe Cystic Fibrosis: Initial: 10mg/kg/day given qid. Measure levels to determine subsequent doses. Renal Impairment: LD: 1mg/kg, followed by reduced doses given q8h or normal doses given at prolonged intervals based on either CrCl or SrCr. Do not use either method during dialysis. Obese Patients: Calculate dose based on estimated LBW plus 40% of excess as basic weight on which to figure mg/kg. ADD-Vantage vials not for IM use.

HOW SUPPLIED: Inj: 10mg/mL, 40mg/mL, 1.2g

CONTRAINDICATIONS: History of serious toxic reactions to aminoglycosides.

WARNINGS/PRECAUTIONS: Increased risk of ototoxicity, nephrotoxicity, and neurotoxicity if treatment >10 days. Contains sodium bisulfite. D/C if allergic reaction occurs. Monitor serum calcium, magnesium, and sodium. For peak levels, measure about 30 min after IV infusion or 1 hr after IM inj. For trough levels, measure at 8 hrs or just before next dose. Prolonged or secondary apnea may occur with massive transfusions of citrated blood. Caution with muscular disorders (eg, myasthenia gravis, parkinsonism). Increased risk of neurotoxicity and nephrotoxicity after absorption from body surfaces with local irrigation or application. Not for intraocular and/or subconjunctival use. Overgrowth of nonsusceptible organisms may occur.

ADVERSE REACTIONS: Neurotoxicity (eg, dizziness, tinnitus, hearing loss, numbness, skin tingling, muscle twitching, convulsions), nephrotoxicity (eg, rising BUN/nonprotein nitrogen/serum creatinine, oliguria, cylindruria, increased proteinuria), blood dyscrasias, fever, rash, exfoliative dermatitis, urticaria, nausea, vomiting, diarrhea, headache, lethargy, injection site pain, confusion, disorientation, increased serum transaminases.

INTERACTIONS: See Black Box Warning. Increased nephrotoxicity with cephalosporins. Do not premix with other drugs; administer separately. Possibility of prolonged or secondary apnea in anesthetized patients receiving neuromuscular blockers (eg, succinylcholine, tubocurarine, decamethonium).

PREGNANCY: Category D, safety not known in nursing.

MECHANISM OF ACTION: Aminoglycoside antibiotic; inhibits synthesis of proteins in bacterial cells.

PHARMACOKINETICS: Absorption: (IM) Rapidly absorbed. C$_{max}$=4mcg/mL. T$_{max}$=30-90 min. **Distribution:** Crosses placenta, distributed in body fluids. **Elimination:** Renal, biliary; T$_{1/2}$=2 hrs.

TOBREX   RX
tobramycin (Alcon)

THERAPEUTIC CLASS: Aminoglycoside

INDICATIONS: External infections of the eye and its adnexa.

DOSAGE: *Adults:* Mild to Moderate Infection: Apply half-inch oint bid-tid or 1-2 drops q4h. Severe Infection: Apply half-inch oint q3-4h or 2 drops hourly until improvement, reduce frequency prior to discontinuation.

HOW SUPPLIED: Oint: 0.3% [3.5g]; Sol: 0.3% [5mL]

WARNINGS/PRECAUTIONS: Oint may retard corneal wound healing.

ADVERSE REACTIONS: Hypersensitivity, lid itching, swelling, conjunctival erythema, superinfection.

INTERACTIONS: Cross-sensitivity to other aminoglycoside antibiotics may occur.

PREGNANCY: Category B, not for use in nursing.

MECHANISM OF ACTION: Aminoglycoside antibiotic: inhibits synthesis of proteins in bacterial cells.

TOFRANIL   RX
imipramine HCL (Mallinckrodt)

> Antidepressants increased the risk of suicidal thinking and behavior (suicidality) in short-term studies in children, adolescents, and young adults with Major Depressive Disorder (MDD) and other psychiatric disorders. Imipramine HCl is not approved for use in pediatric patients except for patients with nocturnal enuresis.

THERAPEUTIC CLASS: Tricyclic antidepressant

INDICATIONS: Treatment of depression. Temporary adjunct in childhood enuresis in ≥6 yrs.

DOSAGE: *Adults:* Depression: Initial: (Inpatient) 100mg/day in divided doses. Titrate: Increase to 200mg/day; up to 250-300mg/day after 2 weeks if needed. (Outpatient) 75mg/day. Titrate: Increase to 150mg/day. Maint: 50-150mg/day. Max: 200mg/day. Elderly/Adolescents: Initial: 30-40mg/day. Max: 100mg/day.

Pediatrics: Depression: Adolescents: Initial: 30-40mg/day. Max: 100mg/day. Enuresis: ≥6 yrs: Initial: 25mg/day 1 hour before bedtime. Titrate: 6-12 yrs: If inadequate response in 1 week, increase to 50mg before bedtime. ≥12 yrs: Increase to 75mg before bedtime after 1 week if needed. Max: 2.5mg/kg/day.

HOW SUPPLIED: Tab: 10mg, 25mg, 50mg

CONTRAINDICATIONS: Within 14 days of MAOI therapy, or during acute recovery period following MI.

WARNINGS/PRECAUTIONS: Caution with elderly, serious depression, cardio-vascular disease, hyperthyroidism, urinary retention, narrow-angle glaucoma, increased IOP, seizure disorders, renal and hepatic impairment. May activate psychosis in schizophrenia; reduce dose. Limit electroshock therapy. May alter blood glucose levels. Photosensitivity reported. D/C prior to elective surgery, or with hypomanic or manic episodes. D/C with pathological neutrophil depression.

ADVERSE REACTIONS: Orthostatic hypotension, HTN, confusion, hallucina-tions, numbness, tremors, dry mouth, urticaria, nausea, vomiting, diarrhea, gynecomastia (male), breast enlargement (female), galactorrhea.

INTERACTIONS: See Contraindications. Increased levels with methylpheni-date, CYP2D6 inhibitors (eg, quinidine, cimetidine, SSRIs) and enzyme sub-strates (eg, phenothiazines, other antidepressants, propafenone, flecainide). Wait 5 weeks after discontinuing SSRIs before initiating TCAs. Decreased levels with enzyme inducers (eg, barbiturates, phenytoin). May block effects of clonidine, guanethidine. Additive effects with anticholinergics, CNS depres-sants, alcohol. Caution with drugs that lower BP and thyroid drugs. Paralytic ileus with anticholinergics. Avoid preparations that contain a sympathomi-metic amine (eg, epinephrine, norepinephrine); may potentiate catecholamine effect.

PREGNANCY: Safety in pregnancy not known; not for use in nursing.

MECHANISM OF ACTION: Tricyclic antidepressant; mechanism unknown. Suspected to potentiate adrenergic synapses by blocking uptake of norepi-nephrine at nerve endings.

TOFRANIL-PM RX
imipramine pamoate (Mallinckrodt)

> Antidepressants increased the risk of suicidal thinking and behavior (suicidality) in short-term studies in children, adolescents, and young adults with Major Depressive Disorder (MDD) and other psychiatric disorders. Imipramine pamoate is not approved for use in pediatric patients.

THERAPEUTIC CLASS: Tricyclic antidepressant

INDICATIONS: Treatment of depression.

DOSAGE: *Adults:* (Inpatient) Initial: 100-150mg/day. Titrate: May increase to 200mg/day. After 2 weeks may increase up to 250-300mg/day if needed. (Outpatient) Initial: 75mg/day. Titrate: May increase to 150mg/day. Max: 200mg/day. (Inpatient/Outpatient) Maint: Following remission, maintain at lowest possible dose. Usual: 75-150mg/day. Elderly/Adolescents: Initiate with Tofranil 25-50mg/day. Switch to Tofranil-PM with doses ≥75mg. Max: 100mg/day.

Pediatrics: Adolescents: Initiate with Tofranil 25-50mg/day. Switch to Tofranil-PM with doses ≥75mg. Max: 100mg/day.

HOW SUPPLIED: Cap: 75mg, 100mg, 125mg, 150mg

CONTRAINDICATIONS: Within 14 days of MAOI therapy or during acute recovery period following MI.

WARNINGS/PRECAUTIONS: Caution with elderly, serious depression, cardio-vascular disease, hyperthyroidism, urinary retention, narrow-angle glaucoma, increased IOP, seizure disorders, renal and hepatic impairment. May activate psychosis in schizophrenia; reduce dose. Limit electroshock therapy. May alter blood glucose levels. Photosensitivity reported. D/C prior to elective surgery, or with hypomanic or manic episodes. D/C with pathological neutrophil depression.

ADVERSE REACTIONS: Orthostatic hypotension, HTN, confusion, hallucinations, numbness, tremors, dry mouth, urticaria, nausea, vomiting, diarrhea, gynecomastia (male), breast enlargement (female), galactorrhea.

INTERACTIONS: See Contraindications. Increased levels with methylphenidate, CYP2D6 inhibitors (eg, quinidine, cimetidine, SSRIs) and enzyme substrates (eg, phenothiazines, other antidepressants, propafenone, flecainide). Wait 5 weeks after discontinuing SSRIs before initiating TCAs. Decreased levels with enzyme inducers (eg, barbiturates, phenytoin). Blocks effects of clonidine, guanethidine. Additive effects with anticholinergics, CNS depressants, alcohol. Caution with drugs that lower BP and thyroid drugs. Paralytic ileus with anticholinergics. Avoid preparations that contain a sympathomimetic amine (eg, epinephrine, norepinephrine); may potentiate catecholamine effect.

PREGNANCY: Safety in pregnancy not known; not for use in nursing.

MECHANISM OF ACTION: Tricyclic antidepressant; mechanism unknown. Suspected to potentiate adrenergic synapses by blocking uptake of norepinephrine at nerve endings.

TOLMETIN   RX
tolmetin sodium (Various)

NSAIDs may cause an increased risk of serious cardiovascular thrombotic events, MI, stroke, and serious GI adverse events including bleeding, ulceration and perforation of the stomach or intestines. Contraindicated for the treatment of perioperative pain in the setting of coronary artery bypass graft (CABG) surgery.

OTHER BRAND NAMES: Tolectin 600 (Ortho-McNeil) - Tolectin DS (Ortho-McNeil)

THERAPEUTIC CLASS: NSAID

INDICATIONS: Treatment of acute flares and the long-term management of rheumatoid arthritis (RA) and osteoarthritis (OA). Treatment of juvenile rheumatoid arthritis (JRA).

DOSAGE: *Adults:* OA/RA: Initial: 400mg tid. Usual: 200-600mg tid. Max: 1800mg/day. Take with antacids other than sodium bicarbonate if GI upset occurs.
Pediatrics: JRA: ≥2 yrs: Initial: 20mg/kg/day given tid-qid. Usual: 15-30mg/kg/day. Max: 30mg/kg/day. Take with antacids other than sodium bicarbonate if GI upset occurs.

HOW SUPPLIED: Cap: (DS) 400mg; Tab: 200mg*, 600mg *scored

CONTRAINDICATIONS: ASA or other NSAID allergy that precipitates asthma, rhinitis, urticaria, or allergic-type reactions. Treatment of perioperative pain in the setting of CABG surgery.

WARNINGS/PRECAUTIONS: May cause adverse ocular events. Prolongs bleeding time. Risk of renal toxicity with heart failure, liver dysfunction, and elderly. Caution with compromised cardiac function, HTN, or other conditions predisposing to fluid retention. Borderline LFT elevations may occur. Decreased bioavailability with milk or food. Can cause serious skin adverse reactions such as exfoliative dermatitis, SJS, and TEN, which can be fatal. Avoid with ASA-sensitive asthma and caution with preexisting asthma. Cannot be expected to substitute for corticosteroids or to treat corticosteroid insufficiency. Notable elevations of ALT or AST reported. Rare cases of severe hepatic reactions, including jaundice and fatal fulminant hepatitis, liver necrosis, and hepatic failure. Patients on long-term treatment should have Hgb or Hct checked if exhibit signs or symptoms of anemia.

ADVERSE REACTIONS: Dyspepsia, GI distress, diarrhea, flatulence, vomiting, headache, asthenia, elevated blood pressure, dizziness, edema, weight gain/loss.

T

INTERACTIONS: Increased PT and bleeding with warfarin. May enhance methotrexate toxicity. May diminish the antihypertensive effect of ACEIs. Concomitant administration with ASA not recommended; potential for increased adverse effects. Can reduce the natriuretic effect of furosemide and thiazides. Can produce elevation of plasma lithium levels and reduction in renal lithium clearance.

PREGNANCY: Category C, not for use in nursing.

MECHANISM OF ACTION: NSAID; not established. Suspected to inhibit prostaglandin synthetase; lowers plasma level of PGE.

PHARMACOKINETICS: Absorption: Rapid; C_{max}=40mcg/mL (400 mg); T_{max}=30-60 min. **Elimination:** Urine; $T_{1/2}$=5 hrs.

TOPAMAX   RX
topiramate (Ortho-McNeil)

OTHER BRAND NAMES: Topamax Sprinkle Capsules (Ortho-McNeil)

THERAPEUTIC CLASS: Sulfamate-substituted monosaccharide antiepileptic

INDICATIONS: Monotherapy In patients 10 yrs of age and older with partial onset or primary generalized tonic-clonic seizures. Adjunct therapy in patients 2-16 yrs of age and older with partial onset seizures, primary generalized tonic-clonic seizures, and seizures associated with Lennox-Gastaut syndrome. Migraine prophylaxis in adults.

DOSAGE: *Adults:* Seizures: Monotherapy: Initial: 25mg qam and qpm for 1 week. Titrate: Increase am and pm dose by 25mg every week until 200mg/day, then increase by 50mg every week until 400mg/day. Adjunct Therapy: ≥17 yrs: Initial: 25-50mg/day. Titrate: Increase by 25-50mg/week. Usual: Partial: 100-200mg bid. Tonic-Clonic: 200mg bid. Max: 1600mg/day. Migraine Prophylaxis: Titrate: Week 1: 25mg qpm. Week 2: 25mg bid. Week 3: 25mg qam and 50mg qpm. Week 4: 50mg bid. Usual: 50mg bid. Renal Dysfunction: 50% of usual dose. Swallow caps whole or sprinkle over food. *Pediatrics:* Seizures: Monotherapy: ≥10 yrs: Initial: 25mg qam and qpm for 1 week. Titrate: Increase am and pm dose by 25mg every week until 200mg/day, then increase by 50mg every week until 400mg/day. Adjunct Therapy: 2-16 yrs: Initial: 1-3mg/kg nightly for 1 week. Titrate: Increase by 1-3mg/kg/day every 1-2 weeks. Usual: 2.5-4.5mg/kg bid. Swallow caps whole or sprinkle over food.

HOW SUPPLIED: Cap, Sprinkle: 15mg, 25mg; Tab: 25mg, 50mg, 100mg, 200mg

WARNINGS/PRECAUTIONS: Hyperchloremic, nonanion gap, metabolic acidosis reported; obtain baseline and periodic serum bicarbonate levels. Withdraw gradually. Psychomotor slowing, difficulty with concentration, speech/language problems, paresthesia, acute myopia with secondary angle closure glaucoma, oligohidrosis, hyperthermia, and dose-related depression or mood problems reported. May cause hyperammonemia and encephalopathy if used concomitantly with valproic acid. Risk of kidney stones; maintain adequate fluid intake. Caution with renal or hepatic dysfunction.

ADVERSE REACTIONS: Somnolence, fatigue, dizziness, ataxia, speech disorders, psychomotor slowing, abnormal vision, memory difficulty, paresthesia, diplopia, depression, anorexia, anxiety, mood problems, pancreatitis, hepatic failure.

INTERACTIONS: Phenytoin, carbamazepine, valproic acid decrease levels. Increases phenytoin, decreases valproic acid levels. May decrease AUC of digoxin. May potentiate CNS depression with alcohol, other CNS depressants. Increased risk of kidney stones with carbonic anhydrase inhibitors. May increase metformin levels; monitor diabetics regularly.

PREGNANCY: Category C, caution in nursing.

MECHANISM OF ACTION: Sulfamate-substituted monosaccharide; unknown mechanism. Suspected to block voltage-dependent Na⁺ channels, augment activity of the neurotransmitter gamma-aminobutyrate at some subtypes of the GABA-A receptor, antagonizes the AMPA/kainate subtype of the glutamate receptor, and inhibits the carbonic anhydrase enzyme, particularly isoenzymes II and IV.

PHARMACOKINETICS: Absorption: Rapid; T$_{max}$=2 hrs. **Distribution:** Plasma protein binding (15-41%); found in breast milk. **Metabolism:** Metabolyzed via hydroxylation, hydrolysis, and glucoronidation. **Elimination:** Urine: (70% unchanged); T$_{1/2}$=21 hrs. For pediatric parameters refer to PI.

TOPICORT   RX
desoximetasone (Taro)

OTHER BRAND NAMES: Topicort LP (Taro)

THERAPEUTIC CLASS: Corticosteroid

INDICATIONS: Corticosteroid-responsive dermatoses.

DOSAGE: *Adults:* Apply bid.
Pediatrics: (Cre, Gel) Apply bid. ≥10 yrs: (Oint) Apply bid.

HOW SUPPLIED: Cre: (LP) 0.05% [15g, 60g], 0.25% [15g, 60g. 100g]; Gel: 0.05% [15g, 60g]; Oint: 0.25% [15g, 60g]

WARNINGS/PRECAUTIONS: May produce reversible HPA axis suppression, manifestations of Cushing's syndrome, hyperglycemia, and glucosuria. Caution when applied to large surface areas or under occlusive dressings. Use appropriate antifungal or antibacterial agent with dermatological infections; d/c if infection does not clear or if irritation occurs. Peds may be more susceptible to systemic toxicity. Avoid eyes.

ADVERSE REACTIONS: Burning, itching, irritation, dryness, folliculitis, hypertrichosis, acneiform eruptions, hypopigmentation, perioral dermatitis, allergic contact dermatitis, skin maceration, secondary infection, skin atrophy, striae, miliaria.

PREGNANCY: Category C, caution in nursing.

MECHANISM OF ACTION: Corticosteroid; possesses anti-inflammatory, anti-pruritic, and vasoconstrictive properties. Anti-inflammatory activity not established.

PHARMACOKINETICS: Absorption: Percutaneous; occlusion, inflammation, and other disease states may increase absorption. **Metabolism:** Liver. **Excretion:** Urine (major), bile.

TOPROL-XL   RX
metoprolol succinate (AstraZeneca)

THERAPEUTIC CLASS: Selective beta$_1$-blocker

INDICATIONS: Treatment of hypertension, angina pectoris, and stable symptomatic (NYHA Class II or III) heart failure of ischemic, hypertensive or cardiomyopathic origin.

DOSAGE: *Adults:* HTN: Initial: 25-100mg qd. Titrate: May increase weekly. Max: 400mg/day. Angina: Initial: 100mg qd. Titrate: May increase weekly. Max: 400mg/day. Heart Failure: Initial: (NYHA Class II) 25mg qd for 2 weeks. Severe Heart Failure: 12.5mg qd for 2 weeks. Titrate: Double dose every 2 weeks as tolerated. Max: 200mg/day.
Pediatrics: ≥6 yrs: HTN: 1mg/kg qd. Max: 50mg/day. Dose adjust according to BP response. Doses above 2mg/kg have not been studied.

HOW SUPPLIED: Tab, Extended-Release: 25mg*, 50mg*, 100mg*, 200mg* *scored

CONTRAINDICATIONS: Severe bradycardia, >1st-degree heart block, cardiogenic shock, sick sinus syndrome (unless a pacemaker is present), decompensated cardiac failure.

WARNINGS/PRECAUTIONS: Exacerbation of angina pectoris and MI reported following abrupt withdrawal; taper over 1-2 weeks. Caution with heart failure, bronchospastic disease, DM, hepatic dysfunction, hyperthyroidism,

985

or peripheral vascular disease. May mask symptoms of hyperthyroidism and hypoglycemia. Withdrawal prior to surgery is controversial.

ADVERSE REACTIONS: Bradycardia, shortness of breath, fatigue, dizziness, depression, diarrhea, pruritus, rash, hepatitis, arthralgia.

INTERACTIONS: Additive effects with catecholamine-depleting drugs (eg, reserpine, MAOIs). CYP2D6 inhibitors (eg, quinidine, fluoxetine, paroxetine, propafenone) may increase levels. May exacerbate rebound hypertension following clonidine withdrawal. Caution when used with CCBs of the verapamil and diltiazem type. Concomitant use of digitalis glycosides and β-blockers can increase the risk of bradycardia.

PREGNANCY: Category C, caution with nursing.

MECHANISM OF ACTION: β_1-selective (cardioselective) adrenergic receptor blocking agent; slows sinus rate and decreases AV nodal conduction.

PHARMACOKINETICS: Absorption: Rapid and complete. **Distribution:** Crosses blood-brain barrier. Plasma protein binding (12%). **Metabolism:** Metabolized via CYP2D6. **Elimination:** Liver. $T_{1/2}$=3-7 hrs. Urine.

TORISEL RX
temsirolimus (Wyeth)

THERAPEUTIC CLASS: Kinase inhibitor

INDICATIONS: Treatment of advanced renal cell carcinoma.

DOSAGE: *Adults:* 25mg infused over 30-60 min once a week. Hold if ANC <1,000/mm³, platelet count <75,000/mm³, or NCI CTCAE grade 3 or greater adverse reactions. Once toxicities resolve to grade 2 or less, restart with dose reduced by 5mg/week to a dose no lower than 15mg/week. Concomitant Strong CYP3A4 Inhibitors: Consider dose reduction to 12.5mg/week. If strong inhibitor is discontinued, allow wash out period of about 1 week before dose adjustment. Concomitant Strong CYP3A4 Inducers: Consider dose increase to 50mg/week. If strong inducer is discontinued, return to dose used prior to initiation of strong inducer.

HOW SUPPLIED: Inj: 25mg/mL

WARNINGS/PRECAUTIONS: Hypersensitivity reactions such as anaphylaxis, dyspnea, flushing, and chest pain have been observed. Give H₁ antihistamine before starting infusion. Hyperglycemia, glucose intolerance, and hyperlipemia may occur; monitor glucose and lipid profiles. Infections may result from immunosuppression. Monitor for interstitial lung disease (ILD); if ILD is suspected, d/c and consider use of corticosteroids and/or antibiotics. Bowel perforation may occur; monitor closely. Renal failure, sometimes fatal, reported; monitor renal function. May cause abnormal wound healing; caution during perioperative period. Caution with CNS tumors and/or anticoagulant therapy. Avoid live vaccines and close contact with those who have received live vaccines. Monitor CBC weekly and chemistry panel every 2 weeks. May cause fetal harm; avoid pregnancy during, and for 3 months after, therapy.

ADVERSE REACTIONS: Rash, asthenia, mucositis, nausea, edema, anorexia, anemia, hyperlipemia, hyperglycemia, hypertriglyceridemia, lymphopenia, elevated alkaline phosphatase, AST, serum creatinine , leukopenia, hypophosphatemia, thrombocytopenia.

INTERACTIONS: Strong inducers of CYP3A4/5 (eg, dexamethasone, carbamazepine, phenytoin, phenobarbital, rifampacin) may decrease levels. Strong CYP3A4 inhibitors (eg, atazanavir, clarithromycin, indinavir, itraconazole, ketoconazole) may increase levels. If alternative treatment cannot be administered, dose adjustment should be considered. Concomitant use with sutinib may result in dose-limiting toxicity.

PREGNANCY: Category D, not for use in nursing.

MECHANISM OF ACTION: Kinase inhibitor; binds to intracellular protein and protein-drug complex, inhibits mTOR activity that controls cell division, reduces levels of hypoxia-inducible factors HIF-1 and HIF-2 alpha, and vascular endothelial growth factor.

PHARMACOKINETICS: Absorption: Mean C_{max}=585ng/mL, mean AUC=1627ng•h/mL. **Distribution:** V_d=172L. **Metabolism:** Liver CYP3A4; sirolimus (active metabolite). **Elimination:** Urine (4.6%), feces (78%). $T_{1/2}$(temsirolimus, sirolimus)=(17.3, 54.6 hrs).

TOTECT   RX
dexrazoxane (TopoTarget)

THERAPEUTIC CLASS: Topoisomerase II inhibitor

INDICATIONS: Treatment of extravasation resulting from IV anthracycline chemotherapy.

DOSAGE: *Adults:* IV infusion over 1-2 hrs qd for 3 days. Initiate within first 6 hrs after extravasation. Day 1: 1000mg/m² (Max: 2000mg); Day 2: 1000mg/m² (Max: 2000mg); Day 3: 500mg/m² (Max: 1000mg). CrCl <40 mL/min; reduce dose by 50%.

HOW SUPPLIED: Inj: 500mg

WARNINGS/PRECAUTIONS: Additive cytotoxicity may occur. May cause leukopenia, neutropenia, and thrombocytopenia; hematological monitoring should be performed. May cuse reversible elevations of liver enzymes. Caution in elderly patients with decreased renal function.

ADVERSE REACTIONS: Nausea, vomiting, diarrhea, stomatitis, bone marrow suppression, altered liver function, infusion site burning, pyrexia, injection site pain/phlebitis, fatigue, peripheral edema, alopecia.

INTERACTIONS: Do not use with dimethylsufoxide.

PREGNANCY: Category D, not for use in nursing.

TRACLEER   RX
bosentan (Actelion)

> Potential liver injury; monitor LFTs before therapy, then monthly. Contraindicated in pregnancy; obtain monthly pregnancy tests. Prescribe through Tracleer Access Program.

THERAPEUTIC CLASS: Endothelin receptor antagonist

INDICATIONS: Treatment of pulmonary arterial hypertension in patients with WHO Class III or IV symptoms, to improve exercise ability and decrease rate of clinical worsening.

DOSAGE: *Adults:* Initial: 62.5mg bid. Titrate/Maint: Increase to 125mg bid after 4 weeks. Low Weight (<40kg): Initial/Maint: 62.5mg bid. Adjust if Develop LFT Abnormality: >3 to ≤5x ULN: Reconfirm LFTs. Reduce dose or interrupt therapy. Monitor LFTs every 2 weeks. If LFTs return to pre-treatment levels, reintroduce or continue therapy. >5 to ≤8x ULN: Reconfirm LFTs. Stop treatment and monitor LFTs every 2 weeks. If LFTs return to pre-treatment values, may reintroduce therapy. >8x ULN: Stop treatment, do not reintroduce. *Pediatrics:* >12 yrs: <40kg: Initial/Maint: 62.5mg bid.

HOW SUPPLIED: Tab: 62.5mg, 125mg

CONTRAINDICATIONS: Pregnancy, cyclosporine A, glyburide.

WARNINGS/PRECAUTIONS: May decrease Hgb and Hct; monitor 1 and 3 months after initiation, then every 3 months. Caution in elderly or mild hepatic impairment. Avoid with moderate to severe hepatic impairment, or LFTs >3x ULN. D/C gradually. Patients with severe chronic heart failure had an increased incidence of hospitalization for CHF associated with weight gain and increased leg edema during the first 4-8 weeks of treatment. Consider intervention with diuretic, fluid management, or hospitalization for decompensating heart failure. If signs of pulmonary edema occur, possibility of associated Pulmonary Veno-Occlusive Disease should be considered. D/C therapy..

ADVERSE REACTIONS: Headache, nasopharyngitis, flushing, hepatic dysfunction, lower limb edema, hypotension, palpitations, dyspepsia, edema, fatigue, pruritus, thrombocytopenia.

T

INTERACTIONS: Do not rely on hormonal contraception alone. Cyclosporine A may increase levels. Glyburide may increase risk of elevated LFTs. May reduce statin efficacy; monitor cholesterol levels. May decrease levels of drugs metabolized by CYP450 3A4 (eg, statins) and 2C9. CYP450 3A4 inhibitors (eg, ketoconazole) increase levels.

PREGNANCY: Category X, not for use in nursing.

MECHANISM OF ACTION: Endothelin receptor antagonist; a neurohormone; binds to ET_A and ET_B receptors in the endothelium and vascular smooth muscle. Specific and competitive antagonist at endothelin receptors types with slightly higher affinity for ET_A receptors than ET_B receptors.

PHARMACOKINETICS: Absorption: Absolute bioavailabilty (50%). T_{max}=3-5 hrs. **Distribution:** V_d=18L; plasma protein binding (>98%). **Metabolism:** Liver via (CYP2C9, CYP3A4, and CYP2C19). **Elimination:** Biliary, and urine (<3%); $T_{1/2}$=5 hrs.

TRANDATE RX
labetalol HCL (Prometheus)

THERAPEUTIC CLASS: Nonselective beta-blocker/alpha₁ blocker

INDICATIONS: Management of hypertension.

DOSAGE: *Adults:* PO: Initial: 100mg bid. Titrate: May increase by 100mg bid every 2-3 days. Maint: 200-400mg bid. Severe HTN: 1200-2400mg/day given bid-tid. Titrate: Do not increase by more than 200mg bid. Elderly: Initial: 100mg bid. Titrate: May increase by 100mg bid. Maint: 100-200mg bid.

HOW SUPPLIED: Tab: 100mg*, 200mg*, 300mg* *scored

CONTRAINDICATIONS: Bronchial asthma, overt cardiac failure, greater than first degree heart block, cardiogenic shock, severe bradycardia, other conditions associated with hypotension, history of obstructive airway disease.

WARNINGS/PRECAUTIONS: Caution with hepatic dysfunction. Avoid abrupt withdrawal; may exacerbate ischemic heart disease. Caution with latent cardiac insufficiency, may exacerbate cardiac failure, reduce sinus HR, and slow AV conduction. Avoid in overt CHF. Avoid with bronchospastic disease. Paradoxical HTN in pheochromocytoma reported. D/C prior to surgery. Caution with DM; may mask symptoms of hypoglycemia.

ADVERSE REACTIONS: Dizziness, fatigue, nausea, vomiting, dyspepsia, paresthesia, nasal stuffiness, ejaculation failure, impotence, edema, dyspnea, headache, vertigo, postural hypotension, increased sweating.

INTERACTIONS: Increased tremor with TCAs. Antagonizes effects of β-agonists (bronchodilators). Potentiated by cimetidine; may need to reduce dose. Synergistic effects with halothane. Synergistic antihypertensive effects blunts the reflex tachycardia with nitroglycerin. Caution with calcium antagonists. May need to adjust dose of antidiabetic drugs.

PREGNANCY: Category C, caution in nursing.

MECHANISM OF ACTION: Selective α₁-adrenergic and nonselective β-adrenergic receptor blocking agent.

PHARMACOKINETICS: Absorption: Complete; T_{max}=1-2 hrs. **Distribution:** Plasma protein binding (50%); crosses placenta. **Metabolism:** Liver (conjugation, glucuronidation). **Elimination:** Feces, urine (55-60%); $T_{1/2}$=6-8 hrs

TRANSDERM SCOP RX
scopolamine (Novartis Consumer)

THERAPEUTIC CLASS: Anticholinergic

INDICATIONS: Prevention of nausea and vomiting associated with motion sickness or recovery from anesthesia and surgery.

DOSAGE: *Adults:* Motion Sickness: Apply 1 patch 4 hrs before travel. Replace after 3 days. Post-OP N/V: Apply 1 patch the evening before surgery or 1 hr prior to cesarean section. Keep in place for 24 hrs. Apply patch to a hairless area behind the ear. Do not cut patch in half.

HOW SUPPLIED: Patch: 0.33mg/24 hrs [4^s]

CONTRAINDICATIONS: Angle-closure (narrow angle) glaucoma, hypersensitivity to belladonna alkaloids.

WARNINGS/PRECAUTIONS: Monitor IOP with open-angle glaucoma. Not for use in children. Caution with pyloric obstruction, urinary bladder neck or intestinal obstruction, elderly. Increased CNS effects with liver or kidney dysfunction. May aggravate seizures or psychosis. Idiosyncratic reactions reported (rare). Remove patch before MRI.

ADVERSE REACTIONS: Dry mouth, drowsiness, blurred vision, dilation of pupils, dizziness, disorientation, confusion.

INTERACTIONS: Caution with anticholinergic drugs (eg, other belladonna alkaloids, antihistamines, TCAs, and muscle relaxants). Increased CNS effects with sedatives, tranquilizers, alcohol. May decrease absorption of oral medications due to delayed gastric emptying or decreased gastric motility.

PREGNANCY: Category C, caution in nursing.

MECHANISM OF ACTION: Anticholinergic agent; acts as competitive inhibitor at postganglionic muscarinic receptor sites of parasympathetic nervous system and on smooth muscle that responds to acetylcholine but lacks cholinergic innervation. Acts in the CNS by blocking cholinergic transmission from vestibular nuclei to higher centers in the CNS and from reticular formation to the vomiting center.

PHARMACOKINETICS: Absorption: Well-absorbed; T_{max}=24 hrs, C_{max}=87pg/mL (free), 354pg/mL (total). **Distribution:** Crosses placenta and blood brain barrier. Plasma protein binding (reversibly bound). Found in breast milk. **Metabolism:** Extensively metabolized. **Elimination:** $T_{1/2}$=9.5 hrs. Urine (10%) parent and metabolite, (5%, unchanged).

TRANXENE-SD
clorazepate dipotassium (Ovation) CIV

OTHER BRAND NAMES: Tranxene T-Tab (Ovation) - Tranxene-SD Half Strength (Ovation)

THERAPEUTIC CLASS: Benzodiazepine

INDICATIONS: Management of anxiety disorders. Adjunct therapy for partial seizures. Symptomatic relief of acute alcohol withdrawal.

DOSAGE: *Adults:* Anxiety: Initial: (Tab) 15mg qhs. Usual: 30mg/day in divided doses. Max: 60mg/day. Elderly/Debilitated: Initial: 7.5-15mg/day. (Tab, Extended-Release) 22.5mg q24h, (may substitute for 7.5mg tid) or 11.25mg q24h (may substitute for 3.75mg tid). Do not use Extended-Release for initial therapy. Alcohol Withdrawal: Day 1: (Tab) 30mg, then 30-60mg/day. Day 2: 45-90mg/day. Day 3: 22.5-45mg/day. Day 4: 15-30mg. Give in divided doses. Reduce dose and continue with 7.5-15mg/day; discontinue when stable. Max: 90mg/day. Antiepileptic Adjunct: Initial: (Tab) 7.5mg tid. Titrate: Increase by no more than 7.5mg/week. Max: 90mg/day.
Pediatrics: >9 yrs: Anxiety: Initial: (Tab) 15mg qhs. Usual: 30mg/day in divided doses. Max: 60mg/day. (Tab, Extended-Release) 22.5mg q24h, (may substitute for 7.5mg tid) or 11.25mg q24h (may substitute for 3.75mg tid). Do not use Extended-Release for initial therapy. >12 yrs: Antiepileptic Adjunct: Initial: (Tab) 7.5mg tid. Titrate: Increase by no more than 7.5mg/week. Max: 90mg/day. 9-12 yrs: Initial: 7.5mg bid. Titrate: Increase by no more than 7.5mg/week. Max: 60mg/day.

HOW SUPPLIED: Tab: (Tranxene T-Tab) 3.75mg*, 7.5mg*, 15mg*; Tab, Extended-Release: (Tranxene-SD) 22.5mg, (Tranxene-SD Half Strength) 11.25mg *scored

CONTRAINDICATIONS: Acute narrow-angle glaucoma.

WARNINGS/PRECAUTIONS: Avoid with depressive neuroses or psychotic reactions. Withdrawal symptoms with abrupt withdrawal; taper gradually.

Caution with known drug dependency, renal/hepatic impairment. Suicidal tendencies reported; give lowest effective dose. Monitor LFTs and blood counts periodically with long-term therapy. Use lowest effective dose in elderly.

ADVERSE REACTIONS: Drowsiness, dizziness, GI complaints, nervousness, blurred vision, dry mouth, headache, mental confusion.

INTERACTIONS: Additive CNS depression with CNS depressants, alcohol. Potentiated by barbiturates, narcotics, phenothiazines, MAOIs, other antidepressants. Increased sedation with hypnotics.

PREGNANCY: Safety in pregnancy not known, not for use in nursing.

MECHANISM OF ACTION: Benzodiazepine; antianxiety/hypnotic agent which has CNS depressant effect.

PHARMACOKINETICS: Absorption: Orally absorbed; completely decarboxylated to nordiazepam. **Distribution:** Plasma protein binding (97-98%) **Metabolism:** Hydroxylation. **Elimination:** Urine (62-67%), feces (15-19%); $T_{1/2}$=40-50 hrs.

TRASYLOL   RX
aprotinin (Bayer Healthcare)

> May cause fatal anaphylactic or anaphylactoid reactions; increased risk if re-exposed to aprotinin-containing products. Weigh benefit against risks in primary CABG surgery if second exposure to aprotinin is required. Administer only in operative settings where cardiopulmonary bypass can be rapidly initiated.

THERAPEUTIC CLASS: Broad-spectrum protease inhibitor

INDICATIONS: Prophylactic use to reduce perioperative blood loss and the need for blood transfusion in patients undergoing cardiopulmonary bypass in the course of coronary artery bypass graft (CABG) surgery who are at an increased risk for blood loss and blood transfusion.

DOSAGE: *Adults:* IV: Administer through central line. Do not administer other drugs in same line. Test Dose: 1mL 10 min before LD. Regimen A: LD: 200mL IV over 20-30 min. Pump Prime Dose: Add 200mL to recirculating priming fluid. Constant Infusion Dose: 50mL/hr. Regimen B: Give 1/2 doses of Regimen A.

HOW SUPPLIED: Inj: 10,000 KIU/mL

CONTRAINDICATIONS: Exposure to aprotinin within previous 12 months. Obtain full patient medical history as aprotinin may be a component in fibrant sealant products.

WARNINGS/PRECAUTIONS: D/C if hypersensitivity reactions occur. Take precautions with re-exposure to aprotinin: have emergency anaphylactic treatment available; give test dose and LD only when conditions for rapid cannulation present; delay aprotinin addition into pump prime solution until after LD safely given. Consider giving H_1 and H_2 blockers 15 minutes before test dose. Greater risk of hypersensitivity to aprotinin if history of allergic reactions to other agents. Administer test dose 10 minutes before LD. Administer LD in supine position over 20-30 minutes. Rapid IV administration may cause hypotension. May increase risk of renal dysfunction and possibly cause an increased need for dialysis in the perioperative period.

ADVERSE REACTIONS: Fever, infection, arrhythmia, hypotension, MI, CHF, pericarditis, peripheral edema, GI effects, confusion, insomnia, lung disorder, pleural effusion, atelectasis, dyspnea, pneumothorax, nausea, abnormal LFTs and renal function, urinary retention.

INTERACTIONS: May inhibit effects of fibrinolytic agents. May block acute hypotensive effect of captopril. Concomitant heparin may prolong activated clotting time. Caution with drugs that affect renal function (eg, aminoglycosides).

PREGNANCY: Category B, safety in nursing not known.

MECHANISM OF ACTION: Broad-spectrum protease inhibitor: modulates systemic inflammatory response (SIR) associated with cardiopulmonary bypass surgery, resulting in decreased need for blood transfusion, reduced bleeding, and decreased mediastinal re-exploration for bleeding. Inhibits multiple mediators (kallikrein, plasmin), pro-inflammatory cytokine release, and maintains glycoprotein homeostasis.

PHARMACOKINETICS: Elimination: Urine (25-40%) and (2%, unchanged).

TRAUMEEL INJECTION   RX
botanical/mineral substances (Heel)

THERAPEUTIC CLASS: Homeopathic Complex

INDICATIONS: Treatment of symptoms associated with inflammatory, exudative, and degenerative processes due to acute trauma (eg, contusions, lacerations, fractures, sprains, post-op wounds), repetitive or overuse injuries (eg, tendonitis, bursitis, epicondylitis), and for minor aches and pains associated with such conditions. Treatment of minor aches and minor pain from rheumatoid arthritis, osteoarthritis, gouty arthritis, and ankylosing spondylitis.

DOSAGE: *Adults:* 1 amp qd for acute disorders or 1-2 amps 1-3 times weekly. May administer IV, IM, SQ, or intradermally.
Pediatrics: >6 yrs: 1 amp qd for acute disorders or 1-2 amps 1-3 times weekly. 2-6 yrs: Use 1/2 of the adult dosage. May administer IV, IM, SQ, or intradermally.

HOW SUPPLIED: Inj: 2.2mL amps [10^s]

WARNINGS/PRECAUTIONS: Carefully re-evaluate if pain persists or worsens, if new symptoms occur, or if redness or swelling is present.

ADVERSE REACTIONS: Allergic reactions, anaphylactic reactions.

PREGNANCY: Category C, caution in nursing.

TRAUMEEL TOPICAL   OTC
botanical/mineral substances (Heel)

THERAPEUTIC CLASS: Homeopathic Complex

INDICATIONS: Temporary relief of symptoms associated with inflammatory, exudative, and degenerative processes due to acute trauma (eg, contusions, lacerations, fractures, sprains, post-op wounds), repetitive or overuse injuries (eg, tendonitis, bursitis, epicondylitis), and for temporary relief of minor aches and pains associated with such conditions. Temporary relief of minor aches and pains associated with backache, muscular aches, and minor pain from rheumatoid arthritis, osteoarthritis, gouty arthritis, and ankylosing spondylitis.

DOSAGE: *Adults:* Individualize dose. Apply to affected area(s) 2-3 times daily. Max: 5x/day. May apply using mild compression and/or occlusive bandaging. Avoid applying over large areas, over broken skin, or directly into open wounds.
Pediatrics: Individualize dose. Apply to affected area(s) 2-3 times daily. Max: 5x/day. May apply using mild compression and/or occlusive bandaging. Avoid applying over large areas, over broken skin, or directly into open wounds.

HOW SUPPLIED: Gel: [50g, 250g]; Oint: [50g, 100g]

WARNINGS/PRECAUTIONS: Avoid administration for pain for >10 days for adults or 5 days for children. Persistent or worsening pain, occurrence of new symptoms, or presence of redness or swelling may signify a serious condition. Consult physician before use in children with arthritis pain.

ADVERSE REACTIONS: Allergic reactions, anaphylactic reactions.

PREGNANCY: Category C, caution in nursing.

MECHANISM OF ACTION: Acts to relieve pain, joint pain, sports injuries, and bruising.

T

TRAVATAN   RX
travoprost (Alcon)

OTHER BRAND NAMES: Travatan Z (Alcon)

THERAPEUTIC CLASS: Prostaglandin analog

INDICATIONS: Reduction of elevated IOP in open-angle glaucoma and ocular hypertension if intolerant to or unresponsive to other IOP therapies.

DOSAGE: *Adults:* 1 drop in affected eye(s) qd in pm. Max: Once daily dosing.

HOW SUPPLIED: Sol: (Travatan) 0.004% [2.5mL]; (Travatan Z) 0.004% [2.5mL, 5mL]

WARNINGS/PRECAUTIONS: Contains benzalkonium chloride; remove contact lenses prior to administration, may reinsert after 15 minutes (Travatan). Avoid with active intraocular inflammation. Caution with history of intraocular inflammation (iritis/uveitis), aphakia, pseudophakia with torn posterior lens capsule, risk of macular edema. Increased ocular pigmentation (iris, eyelid, eyelashes) reported; may be permanent. Other eyelash changes reported. Not for the treatment of angle closure, inflammatory or neovascular glaucoma.

ADVERSE REACTIONS: Ocular hyperemia/pruritus/discomfort, foreign body sensation, decreased visual acuity, blepharitis, blurred vision, cataract, dry eye, photophobia, tearing.

INTERACTIONS: Space dosing of other ophthalmics by 5 minutes.

PREGNANCY: Category C, caution in nursing.

MECHANISM OF ACTION: Selective FP prostanoid receptor agonist; believed to reduce IOP by increasing outflow of aqueous humor.

PHARMACOKINETICS: Absorption: C_{max}=0.018ng/mL; T_{max}=30 min. **Metabolism:** Cornea, via esterases to active free acid and systemically to inactive metabolites via β-oxidation and reduction. **Elimination:** Urine (2%); $T_{1/2}$=45 min.

TRAZODONE   RX
trazodone HCL (Various)

> Antidepressants increased the risk of suicidal thinking and behavior (suicidality) in short-term studies in children and adolescents with Major Depressive Disorder (MDD) and other psychiatric disorders. Trazodone is not approved for use in pediatric patients.

THERAPEUTIC CLASS: Triazolopyridine derivative

INDICATIONS: Treatment of depression.

DOSAGE: *Adults:* Initial: 150mg/day in divided doses pc. Titrate: May increase by 50mg/day every 3-4 days. Max: (Outpatient) 400mg/day, (Inpatient) 600mg/day.

HOW SUPPLIED: Tab: 50mg*, 100mg*, 150mg*, 300mg* *scored

WARNINGS/PRECAUTIONS: Avoid during initial recovery phase of MI. Caution in cardiac disease. D/C prior to elective surgery.

ADVERSE REACTIONS: Dry mouth, edema, constipation, blurred vision, fatigue, nervousness, drowsiness, dizziness, headache, insomnia, nausea, vomiting, musculoskeletal pain, hypotension, confusion, priapism.

INTERACTIONS: Potent CYP3A4 inhibitors (eg, ritonavir, ketoconazole, indinavir, itraconazole, nefazodone) may increase levels. Carbamazepine decreases levels. Increases digoxin and phenytoin serum levels. Caution with antihypertensives and MAOIs. May enhance response to alcohol, barbiturates and other CNS depressants. May affect PT in patients on warfarin.

PREGNANCY: Category C, caution in nursing.

MECHANISM OF ACTION: Triazolopyridine derivative; suspected to inhibit serotonin uptake by brain synaptosomes and potentiate behavioral changes.

PHARMACOKINETICS: Absorption: Well absorbed; T_{max}=1 hr. **Metabolism:** Metabolized to m-chlorophenylpiperazine (active metabolite) by CYP450 3A4 enzyme.

TRECATOR   RX
ethionamide (Wyeth)

THERAPEUTIC CLASS: Peptide synthesis inhibitor

INDICATIONS: Treatment of active TB in patients with *M.tuberculosis* resistant to isoniazid or rifampin, or where there is intolerance to other drugs.

DOSAGE: *Adults:* 15-20mg/kg qd with food. May give in divided doses with poor GI tolerance. Max: 1g/day. Alternate Regimen: Initial: 250mg qd then titrate gradually to optimal doses as tolerated, or 250mg qd for 1-2 days, then 250mg bid for 1-2 days, then 1g/day in 3-4 divided doses. Continue therapy until bacteriological conversion has become permanent and maximal clinical improvement occurs.
Pediatrics: ≥12 yrs: 10-20 mg/kg/day in divided doses given bid or tid with food, or 15mg/kg/day as single dose. Continue therapy until bacteriological conversion has become permanent and maximal clinical improvement occurs.

HOW SUPPLIED: Tab: 250mg

CONTRAINDICATIONS: Severe hepatic impairment.

WARNINGS/PRECAUTIONS: Rapid development of resistance if used alone; should be used with at least 1 or 2 other drugs. Perform ophthalmologic exams before and periodically during therapy. Measure serum transaminases prior to initiation and monthly thereafter. Risk of hypoglycemia in diabetics; monitor blood glucose prior to initiation then periodically. Hypothyroidism reported; monitor TFTs.

ADVERSE REACTIONS: Nausea, vomiting , diarrhea, abdominal pain, excessive salivation, metallic taste, stomatitis, anorexia, psychotic disturbances, drowsiness, dizziness, hypersensitivity reactions, increase in serum bilirubin, SGOT or SGPT.

INTERACTIONS: Discontinue all antituberculous medication with elevated serum transaminases until resolved; reintroduce sequentially to determine which drug is responsible. May raise isoniazid levels. May potentiate adverse effects of other antituberculous drugs. Convulsions reported with cycloserine. Risk of psychotic reactions with excessive ethanol ingestion. Give with pyridoxine.

PREGNANCY: Category C, not for use in nursing.

MECHANISM OF ACTION: Peptide synthesis inhibitor; may be bacteriostatic or bactericidal in action.

PHARMACOKINETICS: Absorption: Completely absorbed; C_{max}=2.16mcg/mL, T_{max}=1.02 hrs, AUC=7.67mcg•hr/mL. **Distribution:** V_d=93.5L; plasma protein binding (30%); widely distributed into body tissues. **Metabolism:** Liver (extensive). **Elimination:** Urine ≤1%; $T_{1/2}$=1.92 hrs.

TRELSTAR   RX
triptorelin pamoate (Watson)

OTHER BRAND NAMES: Trelstar LA (Watson) - Trelstar Depot (Watson)

THERAPEUTIC CLASS: Luteinizing hormone releasing hormone agonist

INDICATIONS: Palliative treatment of advanced prostate cancer.

DOSAGE: *Adults:* (Depot) 3.75mg IM every month or (LA) 11.25mg IM every 84 days.

HOW SUPPLIED: Inj: (Depot) 3.75mg, (LA) 11.25mg

CONTRAINDICATIONS: Pregnancy.

WARNINGS/PRECAUTIONS: Anaphylactic shock, angioedema, ureteral obstruction, spinal cord compression, renal impairment reported. May worsen symptoms during 1st few weeks of treatment. Closely monitor patients with metastatic vertebral lesions and/or urinary tract obstruction during 1st few weeks of therapy. Monitor serum testosterone levels, PSA.

ADVERSE REACTIONS: Hot flushes, HTN, headache, skeletal pain, dysuria, leg edema, pain, impotence.

INTERACTIONS: Avoid hyperprolactinemic drugs.

PREGNANCY: Category X, not for use in nursing.

MECHANISM OF ACTION: Luteinizing hormone releasing hormone agonist; potent inhibitor of gonadotropin secretion.

PHARMACOKINETICS: Absorption: (IM) mean C_{max}=28.43, T_{max}=1 hr. **Distribution**: V_d=30-33L. **Elimination**: Liver and kidneys; $T_{1/2}$=3 hrs.

TRENTAL   RX
pentoxifylline (Sanofi-Aventis)

THERAPEUTIC CLASS: Blood viscosity reducer

INDICATIONS: Treatment of intermittent claudication due to chronic occlusive arterial disease of the limbs.

DOSAGE: *Adults:* 400mg tid with meals for at least 8 weeks. Reduce to 400mg bid if digestive and GI side effects occur; discontinue if side effects persist.

HOW SUPPLIED: Tab, Extended-Release: 400mg

CONTRAINDICATIONS: Recent cerebral and/or retinal hemorrhage, intolerance to methylxanthines (eg, caffeine, theophylline, theobromine).

WARNINGS/PRECAUTIONS: Monitor Hgb and Hct with risk factors complicated by hemorrhage (eg, recent surgery, peptic ulceration, cerebral/retinal bleeding). Occasional reports of angina, hypotension, and arrhythmia in patients with concurrent coronary artery and cerebrovascular diseases.

ADVERSE REACTIONS: Bloating, dyspepsia, nausea, vomiting, dizziness, headache.

INTERACTIONS: Increase risk of bleeding with warfarin; monitor PT/INR more frequently. May increase in theophylline levels; risk of theophylline toxicity. May increase effect of antihypertensives.

PREGNANCY: Category C, not for use in nursing.

MECHANISM OF ACTION: Blood viscosity reducer; mechanism not fully established. Increases blood flow to affected microcirculation and enhances tissue oxygenation. Improves erythrocyte flexibility, increases leukocyte deformability, and inhibits neutrophil adhesion and activation.

PHARMACOKINETICS: Absorption: T_{max}= 1 hr. **Distribution:** Found in human breast milk. **Metabolism:** 1st pass; metabolites (major): Metabolite 1(1-[5-hydroxyhexyl]-3,7-dimethylxanthine); metabolite V (1-[3-carboxypropyl]-3,7-dimethylxanthine). **Elimination:** Urine (major), feces (<4%); $T_{1/2}$= 0.4-0.8 hrs.; $T_{1/2}$=0.4-0.8 hrs. (metabolites).

TREXIMET   RX
naproxen sodium - sumatriptan succinate (GlaxoSmithKline)

> Treximet may cause an increased risk of serious cardiovascular thrombotic events, MI, stroke and serious GI adverse events including bleeding, ulceration, and perforation of the stomach or intestines.

THERAPEUTIC CLASS: 5-HT$_1$-agonist/NSAID

INDICATIONS: Acute treatment of migraine attacks with or without aura.

DOSAGE: *Adults:* ≥18 yrs: Initial: 1 tab; may repeat after 2 hrs. Max 2 tabs/24 hrs. Do not split, crush or chew.

HOW SUPPLIED: Tab: (Naproxen-Sumatriptan): 500mg/85mg [9^s]

CONTRAINDICATIONS: History, symptoms, or signs of ischemic cardiac, cerebrovascular, or peripheral vascular syndromes. Other significant CVD;

uncontrolled HTN; hemiplegic or basilar migraine; severe hepatic impairment; MAOIs during or within 2 weeks of use; within 24 hrs of ergotamine-containing agents, ergot-type agents, or other 5-HT$_1$ agonists; allergy to naproxen/asthma, nasal polyps, urticaria, and hypotension associated with NSAIDs.

WARNINGS/PRECAUTIONS: Establish clear diagnosis. Caution in patients with uncontrolled HTN; monitor closely during initiation and throughout course of therapy. Caution in patients with fluid retention and heart failure. Serotonin syndrome may occur. Caution in those with prior history of ulcer disease or GI bleed; impaired renal function; heart failure; liver dysfunction; elderly; taking ACE-inhibitors or diuretics; with diseases that may alter absorption, metabolism, excretion of drugs; history of epilepsy or condition that lower seizure threshold. Not recommended in patients with advanced renal disease. Anaphylactic/anaphylactoid reactions, serious skin reaction such as exfoliative dermatitis, Stevens-Johnson syndrome and toxic epidermal necrosis may occur. Chest, jaw, or neck pain/discomfort reported. May cause vision disturbances. Caution in those with coagulation disorders, or receiving anticoagulants, and preexisting asthma.

ADVERSE REACTIONS: Dizziness, somnolence, paresthesia, nausea, dyspepsia, dry mouth, chest/neck/throat/jaw pain, tightness, pressure.

INTERACTIONS: See Contraindications. Caution when administered concomitantly with methotrexate (MTX) due to elevated and prolonged serum MTX levels. Avoid use with ASA. Use with ACE inhibitors may potentiate renal disease states. Combined use with SSRIs, SNRIs, and triptans may cause serotonin syndrome. May cause lithium toxicity when administered concurrently with lithium. Probencid may extend naproxen plasma half-life. May reduce the antihypertensive effect of propranolol and other β-blockers. Increases GI bleed with warfarin.

PREGNANCY: Category C, not for use in nursing.

MECHANISM OF ACTION: Naproxen: NSAID; inhibits the synthesis of inflammatory mediators and prostaglandin synthetase. Sumatriptan: 5-HT$_1$ receptor agonist; mediates vasoconstricition of human basilar artery and vasculature of human dura mater, which correlates with the relief of migraine headache.

PHARMACOKINETICS: Absorption: Naproxen: Absolute bioavailability (95%), T_{max} =5 hrs; Sumatriptan: Absolute bioavailability (15%), T_{max} =1 hr. **Distribution:** Naproxen: V_d = 0.16L/kg. Plasma protein binding (99%); Sumatriptan: V_d =2.4L/kg. Plasma protein binding (14-21%). **Metabolism:** Naproxen: Extensively metabolized to 6-0-desmethyl naproxen; Sumatriptan: via monoamine oxidase. **Elimination:** Naproxen: Urine (95%), $T_{1/2}$ =19 hrs; Sumatriptan: Renal (60%), feces (40%); $T_{1/2}$ =2 hrs.

TRIAZ   RX
benzoyl peroxide (Medicis)

THERAPEUTIC CLASS: Antibacterial/keratolytic

INDICATIONS: Topical treatment of acne vulgaris.

DOSAGE: *Adults:* (Cleanser) Wash for 10-20 seconds qd-bid. (Gel) Apply qd-bid after washing with cleanser.

HOW SUPPLIED: Gel: 3%, 6%, 9% [42.5g]; Cleanser: 3%, 6%, 9% [170.3g, 340.2g]; Pads: 3%, 6%, 9% [30s]

WARNINGS/PRECAUTIONS: External use only. Avoid contact with eyes, lips, and mucous membranes. Avoid sun exposure and use sunscreen. D/C if severe irritation develops.

ADVERSE REACTIONS: Dryness, contact dermatitis.

PREGNANCY: Category C, caution in nursing.

MECHANISM OF ACTION: Antibacterial/keratolytic; mechanism not fully established. Produces antibacterial activity against *Propionibacterium acnes*. Also found to reduce lipids and free fatty acids, and produce mild desquamation (drying and peeling activity) with simultaneous reduction in comedones and acne lesions.

PHARMACOKINETICS: Absorption: Percutaneous. **Metabolism:** Metabolized to benzoic acid. **Elimination:** Urine (benzoate).

TRICOR   RX
fenofibrate (Abbott)

THERAPEUTIC CLASS: Fibric acid derivative

INDICATIONS: Adjunct to diet, for treatment of hypertriglyceridemia (Types IV and V) and to reduce elevated Total-C, LDL-C, Apo B, TG, and to increase HDL-C in primary hypercholesterolemia or mixed dyslipidemia (Types IIa and IIb).

DOSAGE: *Adults:* Hypercholesterolemia/Mixed Dyslipidemia: Initial: 145mg qd. Hypertriglyceridemia: Initial: 48-145mg/day. Titrate: Adjust if needed after repeat lipid levels at 4-8 week intervals. Max: 145mg/day. Renal Dysfunction/Elderly: Initial: 48mg/day. Take without regards to meals.

HOW SUPPLIED: Tab: 48mg, 145mg

CONTRAINDICATIONS: Preexisting gallbladder disease, unexplained persistent hepatic function abnormality, hepatic or severe renal dysfunction (including primary biliary cirrhosis).

WARNINGS/PRECAUTIONS: Monitor LFTs regularly; d/c if >3x ULN. May cause cholelithiasis; d/c if gallstones found. D/C if myopathy or marked CPK elevation occurs. Decreased Hgb, Hct, WBCs, thrombocytopenia, and agranulocytosis reported; monitor CBC during first 12 months of therapy. Acute hypersensitivity reactions (rare) and pancreatitis reported. Monitor lipids periodically initially; d/c if inadequate response after 2 months on 145mg/day. Minimize dose in severe renal impairment. Caution in elderly.

ADVERSE REACTIONS: Abdominal pain, back pain, headache, abnormal LFTs, respiratory disorder, increased creatinine phosphokinase.

INTERACTIONS: Potentiates coumarin anticoagulants; reduce anticoagulant dose and monitor PT/INR. Avoid HMG-CoA reductase inhibitors unless benefits outweigh risks. Bile acid sequestrants may impede absorption; take at least 1 hr before or 4-6 hrs after the resin. Evaluate benefits/risks with immunosuppressants (eg, cyclosporine) and other nephrotoxic agents.

PREGNANCY: Category C, not for use in nursing.

MECHANISM OF ACTION: Fibric acid derivative; activates peroxisome proliferator activated receptor α (PPARα), increasing lipolysis and elimination of triglyceride-rich particles from plasma by activating lipoprotein lipase and reducing production of apoprotein C-III (lipoprotein lipase inhibitor). The resulting fall in triglycerides produces an alteration in size and composition of LDL particle, from small dense particles to large buoyant particles, which have greater affinity for cholesterol receptors and are catabolized rapidly. Activation of PPARα also induces an increase in synthesis of apoproteins A-I, A-II, and HDL-cholesterol.

PHARMACOKINETICS: Absorption: Well absorbed; T_{max}=6-8 hrs. **Distribution:** Plasma protein binding (99%). **Metabolism:** Hydrolysis, conjugation; fenofibric acid (active metabolite). **Elimination:** Urine (60%), feces (25%); $T_{1/2}$=20 hrs.

TRIFLUOPERAZINE   RX
trifluoperazine HCL (Various)

THERAPEUTIC CLASS: Piperazine phenothiazine

INDICATIONS: Management of psychotic disorders (eg, schizophrenia) and for short-treatment of generalized non-psychotic anxiety (not as initial therapy).

DOSAGE: *Adults:* Psychotic Disorders: Initial: 2-5mg PO bid. Usual: 15-20mg/day. Max: 40mg/day or more if needed. Non-Psychotic Anxiety: 1-2mg bid. Max: 6mg/day or >12 weeks. Elderly: Lower dose and increase more gradually.

Pediatrics: Psychotic Disorders: 6-12 yrs: Initial: 1mg PO qd-bid. Titrate: Increase gradually until symptoms controlled. Usual: 15mg/day.

HOW SUPPLIED: Tab: 1mg, 2mg, 5mg, 10mg

CONTRAINDICATIONS: Comatose or greatly depressed states due to CNS depressants, bone marrow depression, blood dyscrasias, hepatic damage.

WARNINGS/PRECAUTIONS: May develop tardive dyskinesia, neuroleptic malignant syndrome. May elevate prolactin levels; caution with prolactin-dependent tumors. May mask drug toxicity and drug overdose due to antiemetic effects. May obscure diagnosis and treatment of intestinal obstruction, brain tumor, and Reye's syndrome. Risk of hypotension; avoid large doses and IV use with cardiovascular disease. Caution with glaucoma, angina, and elderly. May cause retinopathy; d/c if retinal changes occur. Evaluate therapy periodically with prolonged use. May interfere with thermoregulatory mechanism; caution in extreme heat. Solution contains sodium bisulfite. Jaundice, hepatic damage reported. May cause false-positive PKU test.

ADVERSE REACTIONS: EPS, motor restlessness, dystonias, pseudo-parkinsonism, tardive dyskinesia, convulsions, dryness of mouth, headache, nausea, blood dyscrasias.

INTERACTIONS: Additive CNS depression with other CNS depressants (eg, sedatives, narcotics, anesthetics, tranquilizers, alcohol). May decrease effects of guanethidine, oral anticoagulants. Propranolol may increase levels of both drugs. Thiazide diuretics may potentiate orthostatic hypotension. May lower seizure threshold; adjust anticonvulsants. May cause phenytoin toxicity. May potentiate -adrenergic blockade. Risk of encephalopathic syndrome with lithium. Avoid with Amipaque®; discontinue 48 hrs before myelography, resume 24 hrs post procedure.

PREGNANCY: Safety in pregnancy not known. Not for use in nursing.

TRIGLIDE RX
fenofibrate (Sciele)

THERAPEUTIC CLASS: Fibric acid derivative

INDICATIONS: Adjunct to diet for treatment of hypertriglyceridemia (Types IV and V) and for the reduction of LDL-C, Total-C, TG, and Apo B in primary hypercholesterolemia or mixed dyslipidemia (Types IIa and IIb).

DOSAGE: *Adults:* Hypercholesterolemia/Mixed Hyperlipidemia: 160mg qd. Hypertriglyceridemia: Initial: 50-160mg/day. Titrate: Adjust if needed after repeat lipid levels at 4-8 week intervals. Max: 160mg/day. Renal Dysfunction/Elderly: Initial: 50mg/day. Take without regards to meals.

HOW SUPPLIED: Tab: 50mg, 160mg

CONTRAINDICATIONS: Severe renal dysfunction, hepatic dysfunction (including primary biliary cirrhosis and unexplained persistent liver function abnormality), pre-existing gallbladder disease.

WARNINGS/PRECAUTIONS: Monitor LFTs regularly; d/c if >3x ULN. May cause cholelithiasis; d/c if gallstones found. D/C if myopathy or marked CPK elevation occurs. Decreased Hgb, Hct, WBCs, thrombocytopenia, and agranulocytosis reported; monitor CBCs during first 12 months of therapy. Acute hypersensitivity reactions (rare) and pancreatitis reported. Monitor lipids periodically initially; d/c if inadequate response after 2 months on 160mg/day. Minimize dose in severe renal impairment. Caution in elderly.

ADVERSE REACTIONS: Abdominal pain, back pain, headache, abnormal LFTs, respiratory disorder, increased creatinine phosphokinase/SGPT/SGOT.

INTERACTIONS: May potentiate coumarin anticoagulants; reduce anticoagulant dose and monitor PT/INR. Avoid HMG-CoA reductase inhibitors unless benefits outweigh risks. Bile acid sequestrants may impede absorption; take at least 1 hr before or 4-6 hrs after the resin. Evaluate benefits/risks with immunosuppressants (eg, cyclosporine) and other nephrotoxic agents; use lowest effective dose.

PREGNANCY: Category C, not for use in nursing.

MECHANISM OF ACTION: Fibric acid derivative; activates peroxisome proliferators activated receptor α (PPARα). Causes increase in lipolysis and elimination of triglyceride-rich particles from plasma by activating lipoprotein lipase and reducing production of apoprotein C-III. Decreases in triglycerides then produce an alteration in size and composition of LDL particles, from small and dense to large, buoyant particles. Larger particles have a greater affinity for cholesterol receptors and are catabolized rapidly. Activation of PPARα also induces an increase in the synthesis of apoproteins A-1, A-II, and HDL cholesterol.

PHARMACOKINETICS: Absorption: Well absorbed; T_{max} =3 hrs. **Distribution:** Plasma protein binding (99%). **Metabolism:** Hydrolysis to fenofibric acid (active metabolite); Conjugation. **Elimination:** Urine (60%), feces (25%); $T_{1/2}$=16 hrs (metabolite).

TRIHEXYPHENIDYL HCL   RX
trihexyphenidyl HCL (Various)

THERAPEUTIC CLASS: Anticholinergic/antispasmodic

INDICATIONS: Adjunct treatment for all forms of parkinsonism. To control extrapyramidal disorders caused by CNS drugs.

DOSAGE: *Adults:* Idiopathic Parkinsonism: 1mg on Day 1. Titrate: Increase by 2mg every 3-5 days. Usual: 6-10mg/day. Max: 15mg/day. Drug-Induced Parkinsonism: Initial: 1mg. If extrapyramidal manifestations not controlled in a few hrs, increase dose until achieve control. Usual: 5-15mg/day. Concomitant Levodopa: Trihexyphenidyl dose may need reduction. Usual: 3-6mg/day. Divide total daily dose into 3 doses. May divide doses >10mg/day into 4 doses. Take with meals and at bedtime.

HOW SUPPLIED: Sol: 2mg/5mL; Tab: 2mg, 5mg

CONTRAINDICATIONS: Narrow angle glaucoma.

WARNINGS/PRECAUTIONS: Monitor IOP. Caution with exposure in hot weather (esp. alcoholics), glaucoma, obstructive disease of GI or GU tract, prostatic hypertrophy, HTN, and cardiac, liver, or kidney disorders. Angle-closure glaucoma reported with long-term treatment. Neuroleptic Malignant Syndrome (NMS) reported with dose reduction or discontinuation. Avoid in tardive dyskinesia except in Parkinson's Disease. Use low initial dose with history of idiosyncrasy to other drugs or arteriosclerosis. Avoid abrupt withdrawal.

ADVERSE REACTIONS: Dry mouth, blurred vision, dizziness, nausea, nervousness, constipation, drowsiness, urinary hesitancy/retention, tachycardia, pupil dilation, increased intraocular tension, vomiting.

INTERACTIONS: Additive effects with cannabinoids, barbiturates, opiates, alcohol, and other CNS depressants. MAOIs and TCAs may intensify anticholinergic effects. Increased risk of tardive dyskinesia with neuroleptics. May need to reduce concomitant levodopa dose.

PREGNANCY: Safety in pregnancy not known, caution in nursing.

MECHANISM OF ACTION: Synthetic antispasmodic drug used as an adjunct therapy to control extrapyramidal disorders.

TRILEPTAL   RX
oxcarbazepine (Novartis)

THERAPEUTIC CLASS: Dibenzazepine

INDICATIONS: Monotherapy or adjunct therapy in adults and children 4-16 yrs with partial seizures.

DOSAGE: *Adults:* Monotherapy: Initial: 300mg bid. Titrate: Increase by 300mg/day every 3rd day. Maint: 1200mg/day. Adjunct Therapy: Initial: 300mg bid. Titrate: Increase weekly by a maximum of 600mg/day. Maint: 600mg bid. Conversion to Monotherapy: Initial: 300mg bid while reducing

other AEDs. Titrate: Increase weekly by 600mg/day. Withdraw other AEDs over 3-6 weeks. Maint: 2400mg/day. Renal Impairment: CrCl <30mL/min: Initial: 300mg qd. Titrate: Increase gradually.
Pediatrics: 4-16yrs: Monotherapy: Initial: 4-5mg/kg bid. Titrate: Increase by 5mg/kg/day every 3rd day. Maint (mg/day): 20kg: Initial: 600mg. Max: 900mg. 25-30kg: Initial: 900mg. Max: 1200mg. 35-40kg: Initial: 900mg. Max: 1500mg. 45kg: Initial: 1200mg. Max: 1500mg. 50-55kg: Initial: 1200mg. Max: 1800mg. 60-65kg: Initial: 1200mg. Max: 2100mg. 70kg: Initial: 1500mg. Max: 2100mg. Adjunct Therapy: Initial: 4-5mg/kg bid. Max: 600mg/day. Titrate: Increase over 2 weeks. Maint (mg/day): 20-29kg: 900mg. 29.1-39kg: 1200mg. >39kg: 1800mg. Conversion to Monotherapy: Initial: 4-5mg/kg bid while reducing other AEDs. Titrate: Increase weekly by max of 10mg/kg/day to target dose. Withdraw other AEDs over 3-6 weeks. Renal Impairment: CrCl <30mL/min: Initial: 300mg qd. Titrate: Increase gradually.

HOW SUPPLIED: Sus: 300mg/5mL [250mL]; Tab: 150mg*, 300mg*, 600mg* *scored

WARNINGS/PRECAUTIONS: Risk of hyponatremia. Cross sensitivity with carbamazepine. Avoid abrupt withdrawal. Adjust dose in renal impairment. Reports of serious dermatologic reactions (eg, Stevens-Johnson syndrome, toxic epidermal necrolysis). CNS effects reported (eg, psychomotor slowing, concentration difficulty, speech or language problems, somnolence or fatigue, coordination abnormalities). Reports of multi-organ hypersensitivity reactions in close temporal association to initiation of therapy. Rare cases of anaphylaxis and angioedema involving the larynx, glottis, lips and eyelids reported.

ADVERSE REACTIONS: Dizziness, somnolence, diplopia, nausea, vomiting, asthenia, nystagmus, ataxia, abnormal vision, tremor, abnormal gait, headache.

INTERACTIONS: Additive sedative effect with alcohol. Verapamil, carbamazepine, phenytoin, phenobarbital, valproic acid may decrease levels. Decreased plasma levels of felodipine and oral contraceptives. Increased plasma levels of phenytoin, phenobarbital.

PREGNANCY: Category C, not for use in nursing.

MECHANISM OF ACTION: Dibenzazepine; mechanism unknown. Oxcarbazepine and 10-monohydroxy metabolite (MHD) suspected to exert antiseizure effects through blockade of voltage-sensitive Na^+ channels, resulting in stabilization of hyperexcited neural membranes, inhibition of repetitive neuronal firing, and diminution of propagation of synaptic impulses. Also, increased K^+ conductance and modulation of high-voltage activated calcium channels may contribute to anticonvulsant activity.

PHARMACOKINETICS: Absorption: Completely absorbed. T_{max}=4.5 hrs (Tab), 6 hrs (Sus). **Distribution:** V_d=49L (MHD). Plasma protein binding (40%) (metabolite). Found in breast milk. **Metabolism:** Liver; reduced to MHD (active metabolite), then conjugated. **Elimination:** Urine (>95%), feces (<4%). $T_{1/2}$=2 hrs (parent drug), 9 hrs (MHD). In pediatrics, MHD clearance decreases as age/weight increase, approaching that of adults.

Tri-Levlen

RX   T

ethinyl estradiol - levonorgestrel (Bayer Healthcare)

THERAPEUTIC CLASS: Estrogen/progestogen combination

INDICATIONS: Prevention of pregnancy.

DOSAGE: *Adults:* Start 1st Sunday after menses begin or 1st day of menses. 21-day: 1 tab qd for 21 days, stop 7 days, then repeat. 28-day: 1 tab qd for 28 days, then repeat.

HOW SUPPLIED: Tab: (Ethinyl Estradiol-Levonorgestrel) 0.03mg-0.05mg, 0.04mg-0.075mg, 0.03mg-0.125mg

CONTRAINDICATIONS: Thrombophlebitis, DVT or thromboembolic disorders, pregnancy, cerebrovascular or coronary artery disease, undiagnosed abnormal genital bleeding, cholestatic jaundice of pregnancy or jaundice with prior pill use, hepatic adenomas or carcinomas, breast cancer or other estrogen-dependent neoplasia.

WARNINGS/PRECAUTIONS: Cigarette smoking increases risk of serious cardiovascular side effects. This risk increases with age (especially >35 yrs) and heavy smoking. Increased risk of MI, vascular disease, thromboembolism, stroke and gallbladder disease. Retinal thrombosis, hepatic neoplasia, carcinoma of breast and reproductive organs reported. May cause glucose intolerance. May increase BP, elevate LDL levels or cause other lipid changes, fluid retention, breakthrough bleeding, and spotting. May cause or exacerbate migraine. May develop visual changes with contact lens. Increased risk of MI with HTN, hyperlipidemia, obesity, and diabetes. D/C if develop jaundice, significant depression or ophthalmic irregularities. Perform annual physical exam. Use before menarche is not indicated. May affect certain endocrine, LFTs and blood components.

ADVERSE REACTIONS: Nausea, vomiting, breakthrough bleeding, spotting, amenorrhea, migraine, depression, vaginal candidiasis, edema, weight changes.

INTERACTIONS: Reduced effects, increased breakthrough bleeding, and menstrual irregularities with rifampin, barbiturates, phenylbutazone, phenytoin, and possibly with griseofulvin, ampicillin, and tetracyclines. Increases or decreases levels of cyclosporine and theophylline.

PREGNANCY: Category X, not for use in nursing.

MECHANISM OF ACTION: Oral contraceptive combination; suppresses gonadotropins, inhibits ovulation, increases difficulty of sperm entry into uterus by producing changes in cervical mucus, and reduces likelihood of implantation by producing changes in endometrium.

PHARMACOKINETICS: Distribution: Found in breast milk.

TRI-LUMA RX
fluocinolone acetonide - hydroquinone - tretinoin (Galderma)

THERAPEUTIC CLASS: Corticosteroid/depigmenting agent/keratolytic

INDICATIONS: Short-term treatment of moderate to severe melasma of the face.

DOSAGE: *Adults:* Gently wash face and neck with mild cleanser. Apply thin film to hyperpigmented areas of melasma including 1/2 inch of normal skin surrounding lesion, at least 30 min before bedtime.

HOW SUPPLIED: Cre: (Fluocinolone-Hydroquinone-Tretinoin) 0.01%-4%-0.05% [30g]

WARNINGS/PRECAUTIONS: Contains sodium metabisulfite. D/C if ochronosis, sensitivity, or irritation occurs. Cutaneous hypersensitivity reported. May produce reversible HPA axis suppression, manifestations of Cushing's syndrome, hyperglycemia, and glucosuria. Avoid eyes, nose, angles of mouth, occlusive dressings, or sunlight/UV exposure. Extreme weather (eg, cold, wind) may irritate skin.

ADVERSE REACTIONS: Erythema, desquamation, burning, dryness, pruritus, acne, paresthesia, telangiectasia.

INTERACTIONS: Avoid medicated/abrasive soaps or cleansers, soaps/cosmetics with drying effects, products with high concentration of alcohol/astringent, and other irritants or keratolytic agents. Caution with other photosensitizers. Use non-hormonal birth control.

PREGNANCY: Category C, caution in nursing.

MECHANISM OF ACTION: Fluocinolone: Corticosteroid; acts as anti-inflammatory agent. Hydroquinone: Depigmenting agent; interrupts 1 or more steps in tyrosine-tyrosinase pathway in melanin systhesis. Tretinoin: Keratolytic.

PHARMACOKINETICS: Absorption: Hydroquinone: C_{max}=25.55-86.52ng/mL. Tretinoin: (gp I) C_{max}=2,01-5.34ng/mL, (gpII) C_{max}=2-4.99ng/mL. **Distribution:** Corticosteroid; (found in breast milk).

TRI-NORINYL RX
ethinyl estradiol - norethindrone (Watson)

THERAPEUTIC CLASS: Estrogen/progestogen combination

INDICATIONS: Prevention of pregnancy.

DOSAGE: *Adults:* 1 tab qd for 28 days, then repeat. Start 1st Sunday after menses begin or 1st day of menses.

HOW SUPPLIED: Tab: (Ethinyl Estradiol-Norethindrone) 0.035mg-0.5mg, 0.035mg-1mg

CONTRAINDICATIONS: Thrombophlebitis, DVT or thromboembolic disorders, pregnancy, cerebrovascular or coronary artery disease, undiagnosed abnormal genital bleeding, cholestatic jaundice of pregnancy or jaundice with prior pill use, hepatic adenomas or carcinomas, breast cancer or other estrogen-dependent neoplasia.

WARNINGS/PRECAUTIONS: Cigarette smoking increases risk of serious cardiovascular side effects. This risk increases with age (especially >35 yrs) and heavy smoking. Increased risk of MI, vascular disease, thromboembolism, stroke and gallbladder disease. Retinal thrombosis, hepatic neoplasia, carcinoma of breast and reproductive organs reported. May cause glucose intolerance. May increase BP, elevate LDL levels or cause other lipid changes, fluid retention, breakthrough bleeding, and spotting. May cause or exacerbate migraine. May develop visual changes with contact lens. Increased risk of MI with HTN, hyperlipidemia, obesity, and diabetes. D/C if jaundice, significant depression or ophthalmic irregularities develop. Perform annual physical exam. Use before menarche is not indicated. May affect certain endocrine, LFTs and blood components.

ADVERSE REACTIONS: Nausea, vomiting, breakthrough bleeding, spotting, amenorrhea, migraine, depression, vaginal candidiasis, edema, weight changes.

INTERACTIONS: Reduced effects, increased breakthrough bleeding, and menstrual irregularities with rifampin, barbiturates, phenylbutazone, phenytoin, and possibly with griseofulvin, ampicillin, and tetracyclines.

PREGNANCY: Category X, not for use in nursing.

MECHANISM OF ACTION: Combination oral contraceptive; acts by suppression of gonadotropins, primary mechanism is inhibition of ovulation; other alterations include changes in cervical mucus (which increases the difficulty of sperm entry into the uterus) and endometrium (which may reduce likelihood of implantation).

TRIPEDIA RX
pertussis vaccine, acellular - diphtheria toxoid - tetanus toxoid (Sanofi Pasteur)

THERAPEUTIC CLASS: Vaccine/toxoid combination

INDICATIONS: Active immunization against diphtheria, tetanus, and pertussis in pediatrics 6 weeks to 7 yrs of age (prior to 7th birthday). Combined with ActHIB for active immunization in pediatrics 15-18 months previously immunized against diphtheria, tetanus, and pertussis with 3 doses of whole-cell pertussis DTP or acellular pertussis vaccine and 3 or fewer doses of ActHIB® within 1st year of life for prevention of *H. influenzae* type b, diphtheria, tetanus, and pertussis.

DOSAGE: *Pediatrics:* <7 yrs: Primary Series: 3 doses of 0.5mL IM at 4-8 week intervals. 1st dose usually at 2 months, but can give at 6 weeks up to 7th birthday. Booster: 4th dose (0.5mL IM) at 15-20 months, at least 6 months after 3rd dose, 5th dose at 4-6 yrs; prior to school entry. May give to complete 4th or 5th dose of primary series of 3 doses of whole-cell pertussis DTP (4th dose at 15-20 months and 5th dose before school if 4th dose not given on or before 4th birthday). May combine with ActHIB® for 4th dose at 15-18 months.

T

HOW SUPPLIED: Inj: (Diphtheria-Pertussis-Tetanus) 6.7LFU-46.8mcg-5LFU/0.5mL

CONTRAINDICATIONS: Hypersensitivity to thimersal and gelatin, immediate anaphylactic reaction associated with previous dose, encephalopathy not due to an identifiable cause within 7 days of prior pertussis immunization. Defer during poliomyelitis outbreak or acute febrile illness.

WARNINGS/PRECAUTIONS: Caution if within 48 hrs of previous whole-cell DTP or acellular DTP vaccine, fever ≥105°F not due to another identifiable cause, collapse or shock-like state, or inconsolable crying lasting ≥3 hrs occurs, or if convulsions occur within 3 days. For high seizure risk, give APAP at time of vaccination and q4-6h for 24 hrs. Caution if neurologic or CNS disorders. Avoid with coagulation disorders. Have epinephrine available. Suboptimal response may occur in immunocompromised patients.

ADVERSE REACTIONS: Local erythema and swelling, irritability, drowsiness, anorexia, fever.

INTERACTIONS: Avoid with anticoagulants. Immunosuppressive therapy (eg, irradiation, antimetabolites, alkylating agents, cytotoxic drugs, corticosteroids) may decrease response. Do not combine through reconstitution with any vaccine for infants <15 months.

PREGNANCY: Category C, safety in nursing not known.

MECHANISM OF ACTION: Active immunization against diphtheria, tetanus, and pertussis (whooping cough).

TRIPHASIL   RX
ethinyl estradiol - levonorgestrel (Wyeth)

OTHER BRAND NAMES: Enpresse (Barr)

THERAPEUTIC CLASS: Estrogen/progestogen combination

INDICATIONS: Prevention of pregnancy.

DOSAGE: *Adults:* 1 tab qd for 28 days, then repeat. Start 1st Sunday after menses begin or 1st day of menses.

HOW SUPPLIED: Tab: (Ethinyl Estradiol-Levonorgestrel) 0.03mg-0.05mg, 0.04mg-0.075mg, 0.03mg-0.125mg

CONTRAINDICATIONS: Thrombophlebitis, DVT or thromboembolic disorders, pregnancy, cerebrovascular or coronary artery disease, undiagnosed abnormal genital bleeding, cholestatic jaundice of pregnancy or jaundice with prior pill use, hepatic adenomas or carcinomas, breast cancer or other estrogen-dependent neoplasia, thrombogenic valvulopathies, thrombogenic rhythm disorders, diabetes with vascular involvement, uncontrolled HTN, endometrium carcinoma, active liver disease if liver function has not returned to normal.

WARNINGS/PRECAUTIONS: Cigarette smoking increases risk of serious cardiovascular side effects; risk increases with age (especially >35 yrs) and heavy smoking. Increased risk of MI, vascular disease, thromboembolism, stroke and gallbladder disease. Retinal thrombosis, hepatic neoplasia, carcinoma of breast and reproductive organs reported. May cause glucose intolerance. May increase BP, elevate LDL levels or cause other lipid changes, fluid retention, breakthrough bleeding, and spotting. May cause or exacerbate migraine. May develop visual changes with contact lens. Diarrhea and vomiting may decrease hormone absorption. Increased risk of MI with HTN, hyperlipidemia, obesity, and diabetes. D/C if jaundice, significant depression or ophthalmic irregularities develop. Perform annual physical exam. Use before menarche is not indicated. May affect certain endocrine, LFTs and blood components.

ADVERSE REACTIONS: Nausea, vomiting, breakthrough bleeding, spotting, amenorrhea, migraine, depression, vaginal candidiasis, edema, weight changes.

INTERACTIONS: Reduced effects, increased breakthrough bleeding, and menstrual irregularities with rifampin, rifabutin, barbiturates, phenylbutazone, phenytoin, griseofulvin, topiramate, some protease inhibitors, modafinil, ampicillin, other penicillins, tetracyclines and possibly with St. John's wort.

Troleadomycin may increase risk of intrahepatic cholestasis. Increased levels with ascorbic acid, APAP, CYP3A4 inhibitors (eg, indinavir, fluconazole, troleandomycin), and atorvastatin. May alter levels of cyclosporine, theophylline, and corticosteroids.

PREGNANCY: Category X, not for use in nursing.

MECHANISM OF ACTION: Combination oral contraceptive; acts by suppression of gonadotropins. Inhibits ovulation and produces changes in cervical mucus (increasing difficulty of sperm entry into uterus) and endometrium (reducing likelihood of implantation).

PHARMACOKINETICS: Absorption: (LNG): Rapid and complete. (50/30mcg LNG/EE single dose): C_{max}=1.7ng/mL, T_{max}=1.3 hr, AUC=17ng•hr/mL; (EE) Rapid and complete, (50/30mcg LNG/EE single dose): C_{max}=141pg/mL, T_{max}=1.5 hr, AUC=1126pg•hr/mL. **Distribution**: Found in breast milk, (EE) plasma protein binding (97%). **Metabolism**: (LNG) reduction, hydroxylation, conjugation; (EE) in liver via CYP3A4 through hydroxylation (major), methylation, glucuronidation. **Elimination**: (LNG) $T_{1/2}$=approximately 36 hrs., urine (40%-68%), feces (16-48%); (EE); $T_{1/2}$=18 hrs., in urine and feces.

TRISENOX   RX
arsenic trioxide (Cephalon)

> Administer under supervision of a physician experienced in the management of acute leukemia. Acute promyelocytic leukemia (APL) differentiation syndrome reported. Can cause QT interval prolongation and complete AV block. Monitor ECG, serum electrolytes, and creatinine before and during therapy.

THERAPEUTIC CLASS: DNA fragmentation agent

INDICATIONS: For induction of remission and consolidation of APL refractory to or relapsed from retinoid and anthracycline chemotherapy, and has t(15;17) translocation or PML/RAR-alpha gene expression.

DOSAGE: *Adults:* Induction: 0.15mg/kg IV qd until bone marrow remission. Max: 60 doses. Consolidation: 0.15mg/kg IV qd for 25 doses over 5 weeks. Begin 3-6 weeks after complete induction therapy.
Pediatrics: ≥5 yrs: Induction: 0.15mg/kg IV qd until bone marrow remission. Max: 60 doses. Consolidation: 0.15mg/kg IV qd for 25 doses over 5 weeks. Begin 3-6 weeks after complete induction therapy.

HOW SUPPLIED: Inj: 1mg/mL

WARNINGS/PRECAUTIONS: Hyperleukocytosis, QT interval prolongation, torsade de pointes, and complete AV block reported. Caution with renal failure. Monitor electrolyte, hematologic, and coagulation profiles at least twice weekly, and more frequently in unstable patients during induction. Obtain ECG weekly, and more frequently for unstable patients. May cause fetal harm; avoid pregnancy.

ADVERSE REACTIONS: Fatigue, pyrexia, edema, chest pain, injection site pain, nausea, vomiting, abdominal pain, constipation, hypokalemia, hypomagnesemia, hyperglycemia, increased ALT, headache, insomnia, dyspnea.

INTERACTIONS: Caution with agents that prolong the QT interval (eg, certain antiarrhythmics, thioridazine) or lead to electrolyte abnormalities (eg, diuretics, amphotericin B).

PREGNANCY: Category D, not for use in nursing.

MECHANISM OF ACTION: DNA fragmentation agent; suspected to cause morphological changes in cells and DNA fragmentation characteristic of apoptosis, and damage or degradation of fushion protein PML/RAR-Alpha.

PHARMACOKINETICS: Metabolism: Liver via reduction and methylation. **Elimination:** Urine.

T

TRIVORA   RX
ethinyl estradiol - levonorgestrel (Watson)

OTHER BRAND NAMES: Enpresse (Barr)

THERAPEUTIC CLASS: Estrogen/progestogen combination

INDICATIONS: Prevention of pregnancy.

DOSAGE: *Adults:* 1 tab qd for 28 days, then repeat. Start 1st Sunday after menses begin or 1st day of menses.

HOW SUPPLIED: Tab: (Ethinyl Estradiol-Levonorgestrel) 0.03mg-0.05mg, 0.04mg-0.075mg, 0.03mg-0.125mg

CONTRAINDICATIONS: Thrombophlebitis, deep vein thrombophlebitis, thromboembolic disorders, pregnancy, cerebrovascular or coronary artery disease, undiagnosed abnormal genital bleeding, cholestatic jaundice of pregnancy or jaundice with prior pill use, hepatic carcinoma, benign liver tumor, breast cancer, endometrial cancer, or other estrogen-dependent neoplasia.

WARNINGS/PRECAUTIONS: Cigarette smoking increases risk of serious cardiovascular side effects. This risk increases with age (especially >35 yrs) and heavy smoking. Increased risk of MI, vascular disease, thromboembolism, stroke, and gallbladder disease. Retinal thrombosis, hepatic neoplasia reported. May cause glucose intolerance. May increase BP, elevate LDL levels or cause other lipid changes, fluid retention, breakthrough bleeding, and spotting. May cause or exacerbate migraine. May develop visual changes with contact lens. Morbidity and mortality risk increased with HTN, hyperlipidemia, obesity, and diabetes. D/C if jaundice, significant depression or ophthalmic irregularities develop. Perform annual physical exam. Use before menarche is not indicated. May affect certain endocrine, LFTs, and blood components.

ADVERSE REACTIONS: Nausea, vomiting, breakthrough bleeding, spotting, amenorrhea, migraine, depression, vaginal candidiasis, edema, weight changes.

INTERACTIONS: Reduced effects, increased breakthrough bleeding, and menstrual irregularities with rifampin, barbiturates, phenylbutazone, phenytoin, and possibly with griseofulvin, ampicillin, and tetracyclines.

PREGNANCY: Category X, not for use in nursing.

MECHANISM OF ACTION: Combination oral contraceptive: acts by suppression of gonadotropins, primary mechanism is inhibition of ovulation. Other alterations include changes in cervical mucus (increasing difficulty of sperm entry into uterus) and endometrium (reducing likelihood of implantation).

PHARMACOKINETICS: Absorption: Triphasic pharmacokinetic parameters varied according to variable dosing. Levonorgestrel: Rapidly and completely absorbed. Absolute bioavailability (100%). Ethinyl: Rapid and almost completely absorbed. Absolute bioavailabilty (38-48%). **Distribution:** Found in breast milk. Levonorgestrel: SHBG binding (60%). Ethinyl: Albumin binding (97%). **Metabolism:** Levonorgestrel: Via hydroxylation and conjugation. Ethinyl: Liver via CYP3A4 enzyme through hydroxylation, methylation and glucuronidation. **Elimination:** Levonorgestrel: Urine (40-68%), feces (16-48%); $T_{1/2}$=36 hrs. Ethinyl: Urine, feces; $T_{1/2}$=18 hrs.

TRIZIVIR   RX
abacavir sulfate - zidovudine - lamivudine (GlaxoSmithKline)

> Fatal hypersensitivity reactions reported; discontinue if hypersensitivy reaction suspected and do not restart. Hematologic toxicities, lactic acidosis, and severe hepatomegaly with steatosis (including fatal cases) reported. Severe exacerbations of hepatitis B in patients co-infected with HIV upon discontinuation; monitor hepatic function.

THERAPEUTIC CLASS: Nucleoside analog combination

INDICATIONS: Treatment of HIV-1 infection alone or in combination with other antiretrovirals.

DOSAGE: *Adults:* >40kg and CrCl >50mL/min: 1 tab bid.
Pediatrics: Adolescents: >40kg and CrCl >50mL/min: 1 tab bid.

HOW SUPPLIED: Tab: (Abacavir-Lamivudine-Zidovudine) 300mg-150mg-300mg

WARNINGS/PRECAUTIONS: Hypersensitivity; d/c if suspected and register patients by calling 1-800-270-0425. Caution with bone marrow compromise. Prolonged use associated with myopathy and myositis with pathological changes. Avoid with mild to moderate hepatic impairment or liver cirrhosis. Recurrent hepatitis upon discontinuation of lamivudine reported in hepatitis B patients. Lamivudine-resistant hepatitis B virus reported.

ADVERSE REACTIONS: Nausea, vomiting, diarrhea, loss of appetite, insomnia, fever, chills, fatigue.

INTERACTIONS: Ethanol decreases elimination. Ganciclovir, interferon-alpha, and other bone marrow suppressants or cytotoxic agents may increase hematologic toxicity. Antagonistic effects with stavudine. Increased lamivudine exposure with trimethoprim 160mg/sulfamethoxazole 800mg. Avoid zalcitabine. Hepatic decompensation reported in patients on combination antiretroviral therapy for HIV and interferon alfa with or without ribavarin; monitor closely for treatment-associated toxicities.

PREGNANCY: Category C, not for use in nursing.

MECHANISM OF ACTION: Abacavir: Carbocyclic nucleoside analogue; inhibits HIV-1 reverse transcriptase (RT) by competing with natural substrate dGTP and incorporating into viral DNA. Lamivudine/Zidovudine: Nucleoside analogue; inhibits RT via DNA chain termination.

PHARMACOKINETICS: Absorption: Abacavir: Rapid; bioavailability (86%). Lamivudine: Rapid; bioavailability (86%). Zidovudine: Rapid; bioavailability (64%). **Distribution:** Abacavir: V_d=0.86L/kg; plasma protein binding (50%). Lamivudine: V_d=1.3L/kg; plasma protein binding (low). Zidovudine: V_d=1.6L/kg; plasma protein binding (low). **Metabolism:** Abacavir: Hepatic, via alcohol dehydrogenase and glucuronyl transferase. Lamivudine: Metabolite (trans-sulfoxide). Zidovudine: Hepatic, via glucuronyl transferase. Major metabolite: (3'-azido-3'-deoxy-5'-O-β-D-glucopyranuronosylthymidine (GZDV). **Elimination:** Abacavir: $T_{1/2}$=1.45 hrs. Lamivudine: (IV): Urine (70%); $T_{1/2}$=5-7 hrs. Zidovudine: Urine (14%); (GZDV): Urine (74%); $T_{1/2}$=0.5-3 hrs.

TRUSOPT   RX
dorzolamide HCL (Merck)

THERAPEUTIC CLASS: Carbonic anhydrase inhibitor

INDICATIONS: Treatment of open-angle glaucoma and ocular hypertension.

DOSAGE: *Adults:* 1 drop tid. Space dosing other ophthalmic drugs by 10 min.
Pediatrics: 1 drop tid. Space dosing other ophthalmic drugs by 10 min.

HOW SUPPLIED: Sol: 2% [5mL, 10mL]

WARNINGS/PRECAUTIONS: Systemically absorbed. Avoid with sulfonamide allergy or severe renal impairment. Caution with hepatic impairment. Not studied in acute angle-closure glaucoma. Local ocular adverse effects (conjunctivitis, lid reactions) reported with chronic use. Bacterial keratitis reported with contaminated containers.

ADVERSE REACTIONS: Ocular burning, stinging, discomfort, superficial punctate keratitis, bitter taste, blurred vision, eye redness, tearing, dryness, photophobia, ocular allergic reactions, lid reactions, conjunctivitis.

INTERACTIONS: Caution with high-dose salicylates. Acid-base disturbances with oral carbonic anhydrase inhibitors. Avoid oral carbonic anhydrase inhibitors due to additive effects. Wait 10 minutes before using another ophthalmic drug.

PREGNANCY: Category C, not for use in nursing.

MECHANISM OF ACTION: Carbonic anhydrase inhibitor; catalyzes reversible reaction involving hydration of carbon dioxide and dehydration of carbonic acid; also decreases aqueous humor secretion in ciliary processes of the eye by slowing the formation of bicarbonate ions with subsequent reduction in Na$^+$ and fluid transport, which results in reduction in IOP.

PHARMACOKINETICS: Distribution: Plasma protein binding (33%). **Metabolism:** Metabolites: N-desethyl. **Elimination:** Urine (unchanged, metabolite).

TRUVADA   RX
tenofovir disoproxil fumarate - emtricitabine (Gilead)

> Lactic acidosis and severe hepatomegaly with steatosis, including fatal cases, reported with nucleoside analogs alone or with concomitant antiretrovirals. Severe acute exacerbations of hepatitis B reported in patients coinfected with HBV and HIV upon discontinuation of emtricitabine or tenofovir disoproxil fumarate (DF).

THERAPEUTIC CLASS: Nucleoside analog combination

INDICATIONS: Treatment of HIV-1 infection in combination with other antiretrovirals.

DOSAGE: *Adults:* ≥18 years: CrCl ≥50mL/min: 1 tab qd. CrCl 30-49mL/min: 1 tab q48h.

HOW SUPPLIED: Tab: (Emtricitabine-Tenofovir Disoproxil Fumarate) 200mg-300mg

WARNINGS/PRECAUTIONS: Obesity and prolonged nucleosides exposure may be risk factors for lactic acidosis and severe hepatomegaly with steatosis. Avoid in patients with CrCl <30mL/min or patients requiring hemodialysis. Tenofovir DF may cause renal impairment. Monitor CrCl and phosphorous in patients at risk or with a history of renal dysfunction and those receiving concomitant nephrotoxic agents. May decrease in bone mineral density; monitor bone density in patients with history of pathologic bone fracture or at risk for osteopenia. Possible redistribution/accumulation of body fat. Hepatic function should be monitored closely for at least several months in patients who are coinfected with HIV and HBV and d/c Viread.

ADVERSE REACTIONS: Dizziness, diarrhea, nausea, anxiety, fever, vomiting, headache, asthenia, abdominal pain, depression, flatulence, rash, paresthesia, dyspepsia, insomnia, neuropathy, increased cough, rhinitis.

INTERACTIONS: May increase levels of didanosine; use caution when coadministering, monitor for didanosine-associated adverse effects, and d/c if these adverse effects develop. Atazanavir and lopinavir/ritonavir may increase tenofovir DF-concentrations; monitor for emtricitabine/tenofovir DF associated adverse effects. Atazanavir without ritonavir should not be coadministered with emtricitabine/tenofovir DF. Drugs that reduce renal function or compete for active tubular secretion may increase serum levels of emtricitabine, tenofovir DF, and/or other renally eliminated drugs (eg, adefovir, dipivoxil, cidofovir, acyclovir, valacyclovir, ganciclovir, valganciclovir). Avoid coadministration with other drugs containing lamivudine. Avoid with concurrent or recent use of nephrotoxic agents. Do not coadminister with Atripla, Emtriva or Viread.

PREGNANCY: Category B, not for use in nursing.

MECHANISM OF ACTION: Emtricitabine: nucleoside analog of cytidine. Inhibits activity of HIV-1 reverse transcriptase (RT) by competing with natural substrate deoxycytidine 5'-triphosphate and incorporating into nascent viral DNA, resulting in chain termination. Tenofovir disoproxil: acyclic nucleoside phosphonate diester analog of adenosine monophosphate. Inhibits activity of HIV-1 RT by competing with natural substrate deoxydenosine 5'-triphosphate and incorporating into DNA, by DNA chain termination.

PHARMACOKINETICS: Absorption: Emtricitabine: T_{max}=1-2 hrs, C_{max}=1.8mcg/mL, Bioavailability (92%), AUC=10mcg•h/mL. Tenofovir disoproxil: C_{max}=0.3mcg/mL, T_{max}=1 hr, Bioavailability (25%), AUC=2.29mcg•h/mL. **Distribution:** Emtricitabine: Plasma protein binding (<4%). Tenofovir disoproxil: Plasma protein binding (<0.7%). **Elimination:** Emtricitabine: Urine (86%). $T_{1/2}$=10 hrs. Tenofovir disoproxil: (IV); Urine (70-80%). $T_{1/2}$=17 hrs.

TUSSEND

CIII

pseudoephedrine HCL - chlorpheniramine maleate - hydrocodone bitartrate
(King)

THERAPEUTIC CLASS: Cough suppressant

INDICATIONS: Relief of cough and congestion of the respiratory tract. Relief of hay fever symptoms.

DOSAGE: *Adults:* 1 tab or 10mL q4-6h. Max: 4 doses/24 hrs.
Pediatrics: >12 yrs: 1 tab or 10mL q4-6h. Max: 4 doses/24 hrs. 6-12 yrs: 1/2 tab or 5mL q4-6h. Max: 4 doses/24 hrs.

HOW SUPPLIED: (Hydrocodone-Chlorpheniramine-Pseudophedrine) Syrup: 2.5mg-2mg-30mg/5mL; Tab: 5mg-4mg-60mg

CONTRAINDICATIONS: Severe CAD, MAOI therapy, narrow-angle glaucoma, urinary retention, peptic ulcer, during an asthma attack, nursing mothers and infants. Hypersensitivity to other sympathomimetic amines.

WARNINGS/PRECAUTIONS: Caution with HTN, ischemic heart disease, DM, asthma, increased IOP, elderly/debilitated, severe impairment of hepatic or renal function, hyperthyroidism, or prostatic hypertrophy. Caution with head injury, intracranial lesions or pre-existing increase in ICP. May obscure diagnosis/clinical course with acute abdominal conditions. May impair mental and physical abilities.

ADVERSE REACTIONS: Lightheadedness, dizziness, sedation, nausea, vomiting, constipation, urethral spasm, urinary retention.

INTERACTIONS: See Contraindications. Narcotics, antipsychotics, antianxiety agents, alcohol, and other CNS depressants may potentiate CNS depression. Increased effect of antidepressant or hydrocodone with MAOIs or TCAs. Anticholinergics may produce paralytic ileus. Digitalis glycosides may increase risk of cardiac arrhythmias. Decreased hypotensive effects of guanethidine, mecamylamine, methyldopa, reserpine, and veratrum alkaloids. TCAs may antagonize the effects of pseudoephedrine. Risk of hypertensive crises with pseudoephedrine and MAOIs, indomethacin, or with β-adrenergic blockers and methyldopa.

PREGNANCY: Category C, not for use in nursing.

TUSSEND EXPECTORANT

CIII

pseudoephedrine HCL - hydrocodone bitartrate - guaifenesin (King)

THERAPEUTIC CLASS: Cough suppressant/expectorant/decongestant

INDICATIONS: For exhausting, nonproductive cough accompanying respiratory tract congestion associated with the common cold, influenza, sinusitis and bronchitis.

DOSAGE: *Adults:* 10mL q4-6h. Max: 10mL qid prn. May take with meals. *Pediatrics:* 6-12 yrs: 5mL q4-6h. Max: 5mL qid prn. May take with meals.

HOW SUPPLIED: Sol: (Hydrocodone-Guaifenesin-Pseudophedrine) 2.5mg-100mg-30mg/5mL

CONTRAINDICATIONS: Severe HTN, severe CAD, MAOI therapy and nursing women. Hypersensitivity to sympathomimetics and phenanthrene derivatives.

WARNINGS/PRECAUTIONS: Caution with severe respiratory impairment , HTN, DM, ischemic heart disease, hyperthyroidism, increased IOP, prostatic hypertrophy, and in elderly or debilitated patients. May impair mental and physical abilities. May produce drug dependence of the morphine type.

ADVERSE REACTIONS: GI upset, nausea, drowsiness, constipation, tachycardia, palpitations, headache, dizziness.

INTERACTIONS: Hydrocodone may potentiate effects of narcotics, general anesthetics, tranquilizers, sedatives and hypnotics, alcohol, and other CNS depressants. Increased effect of antidepressant or hydrocodone with MAOIs or TCAs. Decreased hypotensive effects of mecamylamine, methyldopa,

T

reserpine, and veratrum alkaloids. MAOIs and β-adrenergic blockers potentiate the sympathomimetic effect of pseudoephedrine.

PREGNANCY: Category C, not for use in nursing.

Tussi-12   RX
chlorpheniramine tannate - carbetapentane tannate (Wallace)

THERAPEUTIC CLASS: Antitussive/antihistamine

INDICATIONS: Symptomatic relief of cough.

DOSAGE: *Adults:* 1-2 tabs q12h.
Pediatrics: >6 yrs: 5-10mL q12h. 2-6 yrs: 2.5-5mL q12h.

HOW SUPPLIED: (Carbetapentane-Chlorpheniramine) Sus: 30mg-4mg/5mL [118mL]; Tab: 60mg-5mg* *scored

CONTRAINDICATIONS: Newborns, nursing mothers.

WARNINGS/PRECAUTIONS: Caution with HTN, CVD, hyperthyroidism, DM, elderly, narrow angle glaucoma, or prostatic hypertrophy. Excitation in children may occur. Suspension contains tartrazine.

ADVERSE REACTIONS: Drowsiness, sedation, dryness of mucous membranes, GI effects.

INTERACTIONS: Avoid with or within 14 days of discontinuation of MAOIs. Additive CNS effects with alcohol, CNS depressants.

PREGNANCY: Category C, not for use in nursing.

MECHANISM OF ACTION: Carbetapentane: Produces antitussive actions. Phenylephrine: Produces decongestant effect.

Tussionex Pennkinetic   CIII
hydrocodone polistirex - chlorpheniramine polistirex (UCB)

THERAPEUTIC CLASS: Opioid antitussive/antihistamine

INDICATIONS: Relief of cough and upper respiratory symptoms associated with allergy and cold.

DOSAGE: *Adults:* ≥12 yrs: 5mL q12h. Max: 10mL/24 hrs.
Pediatrics: 6-11 yrs: 2.5mL q12h. Max: 5mL/24 hrs.

HOW SUPPLIED: Sus: (Hydrocodone-Chlorpheniramine) 10mg-8mg/5mL

CONTRAINDICATIONS: Should not be used in children less than 6 years of age due to the risk of fatal respiratory depression.

WARNINGS/PRECAUTIONS: May produce dose-related respiratory depression. Caution with pulmonary disease, post-surgery, head injury, intracranial lesions or pre-existing increase in ICP, narrow angle glaucoma, asthma, BPH, elderly, debilitated, impaired hepatic/renal functions, hypothyroidosis, Addison's disease or urethral stricture. May mask acute abdominal conditions and the clinical course of head injuries. May cause obstructive bowel disease. Consider risk/benefit ratio in pediatrics, especially with croup. Impairment of mental and physical performance.

ADVERSE REACTIONS: Sedation, drowsiness, lethargy, anxiety, dysphoria, euphoria, dizziness, psychotic dependence, rash, pruritus, nausea, vomiting, ureteral spasm, urinary retention, respiratory depression, dryness of the pharynx, tightness of the chest.

INTERACTIONS: Additive CNS depression with narcotics, antipsychotics, antianxiety agents, and alcohol. Increased effect of antidepressant or hydrocodone with MAOIs or TCAs. Concurrent anticholinergics may cause paralytic ileus.

PREGNANCY: Category C, not for use in nursing.

MECHANISM OF ACTION: Hydrocodone: Opioid antitussive/antihistamine; not established. Suspected to act directly on cough center. Chlorpheniramine: H$_1$-receptor antagonist; possesses anticholinergic and sedative activity.

Prevents released histamine from dilating capillaries and causing edema of the respiratory mucosa.

PHARMACOKINETICS: Absorption: Hydrocodone: C_{max}=22.8ng/mL, T_{max}=3.4 hrs. Chlorpheniramine: C_{max}=58.4ng/mL, T_{max}=6.3 hrs. **Elimination**: Hydrocodone: $T_{1/2}$=4 hrs. Chlorpheniramine: $T_{1/2}$=16 hrs.

TWINJECT   RX
epinephrine (Verus)

THERAPEUTIC CLASS: Sympathomimetic catecholamine

INDICATIONS: Emergency treatment of severe allergic reactions (type 1) including anaphylaxis to insect stings or bites, allergens, foods, drugs, diagnostic testing substances, as well as idiopathic or exercise-induced anaphylaxis.

DOSAGE: *Adults:* Administer SQ or IM into thigh. 15-30kg: (Twinject 0.15mg) 0.15mg. May repeat if needed. ≥30kg: (Twinject 0.3mg) 0.3mg. May repeat if needed.
Pediatrics: Administer SQ or IM into thigh. 15-30kg: (Twinject 0.15mg) 0.15mg. May repeat if needed. ≥30kg: (Twinject 0.3mg) 0.3mg. May repeat if needed.

HOW SUPPLIED: Inj: (Twinject 0.15mg, Twinject 0.3mg) 1mg/mL

WARNINGS/PRECAUTIONS: Inject into anterolateral aspect of thigh; avoid injecting into hands, feet, or buttock. Avoid IV use. Contains sodium bisulfite. Caution with cardiac arrhythmias, coronary artery or organic heart disease, or HTN. May precipitate/aggravate angina pectoris or produce ventricular arrhythmias with coronary insufficiency or ischemic heart disease. Light-sensitive; store in tube provided.

ADVERSE REACTIONS: Anxiety, apprehensiveness, restlessness, tremor, weakness, dizziness, sweating, palpitations, pallor, nausea, vomiting, headache, respiratory difficulties, HTN.

INTERACTIONS: Monitor for cardiac arrhythmias with cardiac glycosides or diuretics. Effects may be potentiated by TCAs, MAOIs, levothyroxine, and certain antihistamines (notably chlorpheniramine, tripelennamine, diphenhydramine). Cardiostimulating and bronchodilating effects antagonized by β-adrenergic blockers (eg, propranolol). Vasoconstricting and hypertensive effects antagonized by α-adrenergic blockers (eg, phentolamine). Ergot alkaloids and phenothiazines may reverse pressor effects.

PREGNANCY: Category C, safety in nursing not known.

MECHANISM OF ACTION: Acts on α- and β-adrenergic receptors.

TWINRIX   RX
hepatitis A vaccine (inactivated) - hepatitis B (recombinant) (GlaxoSmithKline)

THERAPEUTIC CLASS: Vaccine

INDICATIONS: Active immunization against hepatitis A virus and hepatitis B virus in patients ≥18yrs of age.

DOSAGE: *Adults:* ≥18 yrs: 3-Dose Schedule: 1mL IM in deltoid region at 0, 1, and 6 months. Alternative 4-Dose Schedule: 1 ml IM in deltoid region on Days 0, 7, and 21-30, followed by booster dose at 12 months.

HOW SUPPLIED: Inj: (Hepatitis A-Hepatitis B) 720 ELISA U-20mcg/mL

CONTRAINDICATIONS: Hypersensitivity to monovalent hepatitis A or B vaccines.

WARNINGS/PRECAUTIONS: Anaphylaxis reported (rare). Hepatitis A and B have long incubation periods, so vaccine may be ineffective with unrecognized hepatitis. May not prevent disease if protective antibody titers are not achieved. Delay vaccine with moderate to severe acute illness. Caution with thrombocytopenia or bleeding disorders. Suboptimal response may occur in immunocompromised patients. Have epinephrine (1:1000) available.

ADVERSE REACTIONS: Injection site reactions (soreness, redness, swelling, induration), respiratory infection, headache, fatigue, diarrhea, nausea, fever.

INTERACTIONS: Caution with anticoagulants. Immunosuppressive therapy may reduce response.

PREGNANCY: Category C, caution in nursing.

MECHANISM OF ACTION: Produces immune response against hepatitis A and all subtypes of hepatitis B virus.

TYGACIL   RX
tigecycline (Wyeth)

THERAPEUTIC CLASS: Glycylcycline

INDICATIONS: Treatment of complicated skin and skin structure infections (cSSSI) and complicated intra-abdominal infections (cIAI) caused by susceptible strains of microorganisms.

DOSAGE: *Adults:* 100mg IV over 30-60 min then 50mg q12h over 30-60 min for 5-14 days. Severe Hepatic Impairment (Child-Pugh C): 100mg IV over 30-60 min then 25mg q12h.

HOW SUPPLIED: Inj: 50mg/5mL

WARNINGS/PRECAUTIONS: Structurally similar to tetracyclines and may have similar adverse effects: photosensitivity, pseudotumor cerebri, pancreatitis, and antianabolic action (may lead to increased BUN, azotemia, acidosis, and hyperphosphatemia). Caution with known hypersensitivity to tetracyclines. May cause fetal harm and permanent tooth discoloration (yellow-gray-brown) when administered during tooth development (last half of pregnancy to 8 yrs). *Clostridium difficile*-associated diarrhea reported. Caution when used for cIAI secondary to clinical apparent intestinal perforations.

ADVERSE REACTIONS: Nausea, vomiting, diarrhea, abdominal pain, infection, fever, headache, HTN, thrombocythemia, anemia, hypoproteinemia, increased lactic dehydrogenase, increased SGOT, increased SGPT.

INTERACTIONS: Decreased effectiveness of oral contraceptives. Monitor PT with warfarin.

PREGNANCY: Category D, caution in nursing.

MECHANISM OF ACTION: Glycylcycline; inhibits protein translation in bacteria by binding to the 30S ribosomal subunit and blocking entry of amino-acyl tRNA molecules into A site of ribosome.

PHARMACOKINETICS: Absorption: IV infusion of variable doses resulted in different parameters. **Distribution:** Plasma protein binding (71-89%), V_{ss}=7-9L/kg. **Metabolism:** Liver. **Elimination:** Bile (primary), urine; $T_{1/2}$(100mg)=27.1 hrs.

TYKERB   RX
lapatinib (GlaxoSmithKline)

THERAPEUTIC CLASS: Kinase inhibitor

INDICATIONS: Treatment of patients with advanced or metastatic breast cancer, in combination with capecitabine, whose tumors overexpress HER2 and recieved prior therapy including an anthracycline, a taxane, and trastuzumab.

DOSAGE: *Adults:* Usual: 1250mg qd on Days 1-21 continuously with capecitabine 2000mg/m²/day (administered orally in 2 doses 12 hrs apart) on Days 1-14 in a repeating 21-day cycle. Give at least 1 hr before or after a meal (however, give capecitabine with food). ≥Grade 2 LVEF: D/C dose. If LVEF recovers and asymptomatic after 2 weeks, restart at 1000mg/day. Hepatic Impairment (Child-Pugh Class C): Consider dose reduction to 750mg/day. Concomitant Strong CYP3A4 Inhibitors: Avoid use. Concomitant Strong CYP3A4 Inducers: Avoid use and if must coadminister titrate gradually from 1250mg/day up to 4500mg/day based on tolerability. ≥Grade 2 NCI CTC Toxicity: D/C or interrupt dose and restart with 1250mg/day when toxicity <Grade 1. Restart at 1000mg/day if toxicity recurs.

HOW SUPPLIED: Tab: 250mg

WARNINGS/PRECAUTIONS: Decreased left ventricular ejection fraction reported; confirm normal LVEF prior to therapy and evaluate during treatment. Reduce dose in patients with severe hepatic impairment. Severe diarrhea reported; manage with antidiarrheals, replace electrolytes. Prolongs the QT interval in some patients; consider ECG and electrolyte monitoring. Fetal harm may occur if administered to pregnant women; women should not become pregnant during therapy. Has been associated with interstitial lung disease and pneumonitis in monotherapy or in combination with other chemotherapies.

ADVERSE REACTIONS: Diarrhea, nausea, vomiting, stomatitis, dyspepsia, palmar-plantar erythrodysesthesia, rash, dry skin, mucosal inflammation, pain in extremity, back pain, dyspnea, insomnia.

INTERACTIONS: May increase exposure to concomitant drugs metabolized by CYP3A4 or CYP2C8. Avoid coadministration with strong CYP3A4 inhibitors and inducers; if unavoidable, consider dose reduction with concomitant CYP3A4 inhibitors, and gradual dose increase with concomitant CYP3A4 inducers. Levels may increase if given with a P-glycoprotein inhibitor.

PREGNANCY: Category D, not for use in nursing.

MECHANISM OF ACTION: Kinase inhibitor; acts by inhibiting intracellular tyrosine kinase domains of both Epidermal Growth Factor Receptor (EGFR) and Human Epidermal Receptor Type 2 (HER2) receptors.

PHARMACOKINETICS: Absorption: Incomplete and variable. C_{max}=2.43mcg/mL, AUC=36.2mcg•hr/mL. T_{max}=4 hrs. **Distribution**: Plasma protein binding (>99%). **Metabolism**: CYP3A4, CYP3A5. **Elimination**: $T_{1/2}$ (single dose, repeated dose)=14.2 hrs, 24 hrs. Feces (27%), urine (<2%).

TYLENOL   OTC
acetaminophen (McNeil Consumer)

OTHER BRAND NAMES: Tylenol 8 Hour (McNeil Consumer) - Tylenol Arthritis Pain (McNeil Consumer) - Tylenol Regular Strength (McNeil Consumer) - Tylenol Junior (McNeil Consumer) - Tylenol Infants' (McNeil Consumer) - Tylenol Extra Strength (McNeil Consumer) - Tylenol Children's (McNeil Consumer)

THERAPEUTIC CLASS: Analgesic

INDICATIONS: Temporary relief of minor aches and pains. Temporary reduction of fever.

DOSAGE: *Adults:* ≥12 yrs: (Regular Strength) 650mg q4-6h prn. Max: 3900mg/day. (Extra Strength GoTabs, EZ Tabs, Rapid Release Gels, Caplets, Cool Caplets) 1000mg q4-6h prn. Max: 4000mg/day. (Arthritis Pain, 8 Hour) 2 caplets or geltabs q8h with water. Max: 6 caplets or geltabs/day.
Pediatrics: Max: 5 doses/day. 0-3 months (6-11 lbs): 40mg q4h prn. 4-11 months (12-17 lbs): 80mg q4h prn. 12-23 months (18-23 lbs): 120mg q4h prn. 2-3 yrs (24-35 lbs): 160mg q4h prn. 4-5 yrs (36-47 lbs): 240mg q4h prn. 6-8 yrs (48-59 lbs): 320mg q4h prn. 9-10 yrs (60-71 lbs): 400mg q4h prn. 11 yrs (72-95 lbs): 480mg q4h prn. 12 yrs (≥96 lbs): 640mg q4h prn. Older Children: Regular Strength: 6-11 yrs: 325mg q4-6h prn. Max: 1625mg/day.

HOW SUPPLIED: Caplets: (Arthritis Pain, 8 Hour) 650mg; Drops: (Infants') 80mg/0.8mL [15mL, 30mL]; Geltabs: (Arthritis Pain) 650mg; Sol: (Extra Strength) 500mg/15mL; Sus: (Children's) 160mg/5mL; Tab: (Regular Strength) 325mg; (Extra Strength EZ Tabs, GoTabs, Caplets, Cool Caplets, Rapid Release Gels) 500mg; Tab, Chewable: (Children's) 80mg, (Junior) 160mg

WARNINGS/PRECAUTIONS: May cause liver damage.

INTERACTIONS: Increased risk of hepatotoxicity with excessive alcohol use (≥3 drinks/day).

PREGNANCY: Safety in pregnancy or nursing not known.

TYLENOL WITH CODEINE

CIII

codeine phosphate - acetaminophen (Ortho-McNeil)

OTHER BRAND NAMES: Acetaminophen w/Codeine Elixir (Various)

THERAPEUTIC CLASS: Opioid analgesic

INDICATIONS: Relief of mild to moderately severe pain.

DOSAGE: *Adults:* (Tab) Usual: 15-60mg codeine/dose and 300-1000mg APAP/dose up to q4h prn. Max: 60mg codeine/dose, 360mg codeine/day, and 4g APAP/day. (Elixir): 15mL q4h prn.
Pediatrics: (Elixir): Usual: 7-12 yrs: 10mL tid-qid. 3-6 yrs: 5mL tid-qid.

HOW SUPPLIED: (Codeine-APAP) Elixir: (CV) 12-120mg/5mL; Tab: (#3, CIII) 30-300mg, (#4, CIII) 60-300mg

WARNINGS/PRECAUTIONS: Respiratory depressant effects may be exacerbated with head injury or increased ICP. May obscure head injuries, acute abdominal conditions. Caution in the elderly, debilitated, severe hepatic or renal dysfunction, hypothyroidism, Addison's disease, prostatic hypertrophy, or urethral stricture. Potential for physical dependence, tolerance. Tabs contain sulfites.

ADVERSE REACTIONS: Lightheadedness, dizziness, sedation, shortness of breath, nausea, vomiting, allergic reactions, euphoria, dysphoria, constipation, abdominal pain, pruritus.

INTERACTIONS: Additive CNS depression with narcotic analgesics, antipsychotics, antianxiety agents, alcohol, other CNS depressants. Anticholinergics may produce paralytic ileus.

PREGNANCY: Category C, caution in nursing.

MECHANISM OF ACTION: Codeine: Narcotic analgesic and antitussive; produces centrally-acting analgesic effects. APAP: Non-opiate, non-salicyclate analgesic and antipyretic.

PHARMACOKINETICS: Absorption: Codeine: Rapidly absorbed. APAP: Rapidly absorbed. **Distribution:** Codeine: Found in liver, spleen, kidneys; crosses blood brain barrier; found in fetal tissue and breast milk. APAP: Found in breast milk. **Metabolism:** APAP: Liver (conjugation). **Elimination:** Codeine: Urine (90%) (parent compound and metabolites); $T_{1/2}$=2.9 hrs. APAP: Urine (85%); $T_{1/2}$=1.25-3 hrs.

TYLOX

CII

oxycodone HCL - acetaminophen (Ortho-McNeil)

OTHER BRAND NAMES: Roxilox (Roxane)

THERAPEUTIC CLASS: Opioid analgesic

INDICATIONS: Moderate to moderately severe pain.

DOSAGE: *Adults:* Usual: 1 cap q6h prn.

HOW SUPPLIED: Cap: (Oxycodone-APAP) 5mg-500mg

WARNINGS/PRECAUTIONS: Contains sulfites. Monitor with head injury; may increase respiratory depressant effects and CSF pressure. Caution in elderly, debilitated, severe hepatic or renal dysfunction, hypothyroidism, Addison's disease, prostatic hypertrophy, or urethral stricture. Potential for physical dependence, tolerance. Inappropriate for intractable/severe pain.

ADVERSE REACTIONS: Dizziness, sedation, nausea, vomiting, euphoria, dysphoria, constipation, abdominal pain, pruritus.

INTERACTIONS: Additive CNS depression with alcohol, tranquilizers, sedative-hypnotics, narcotic analgesics, general anesthetics, phenothiazines, antipsychotics, antianxiety agents, other CNS depressants. May produce paralytic ileus with anticholinergics.

PREGNANCY: Category C, caution in nursing.

MECHANISM OF ACTION: Oxycodone: narcotic analgesic. Produces similiar action to morphine, prominently in CNS and smooth muscle organs. Produces analgesia and sedative effects. APAP: nonopiate, nonsalicylate analgesic and antipyretic.

TYSABRI   RX
natalizumab (Biogen Idec/Elan)

> Increases risk of progressive multifocal leukoencephalopathy (PML), an opportunistic viral infection of the brain that usually leads to death or severe disability. Because of risk of PML, natalizumab is available only through a special restricted distribution program called the TOUCH™ Prescribing Program. Natalizumab must be administered only to patients who are enrolled in and meet all conditions of the TOUCH™ Prescribing Program. Monitor patients for any new signs or symptoms that may be suggestive of PML. Dosing should be withheld immediately at 1st sign or symptom suggestive of PML.

THERAPEUTIC CLASS: Monoclonal antibody/VCAM-1 blocker

INDICATIONS: Treatment of patients with relapsing forms of multiple sclerosis (MS) to delay the accumulation of physical disability and reduce the frequency of clinical exacerbations. Treatment for inducing and maintaining clinical response and remission in adult patients with moderately to severely active Crohn's disease (CD) with evidence of inflammation who have had an inadequate response to, or are unable to tolerate, conventional CD therapies and TNF-α inhibitors.

DOSAGE: *Adults:* MS/CD: 300mg IV infusion over 1 hr every 4 weeks. (CD) D/C therapy if no therapeutic benefit by 12 weeks, if patient cannot be tapered off corticosteroids within 6 months, or in patients who require additional steroid use that exceeds 3 months within a calendar year to control their CD.

HOW SUPPLIED: Inj: 300mg/15mL

CONTRAINDICATIONS: Progressive multifocal leukoencephalopathy (PML).

WARNINGS/PRECAUTIONS: Possible hypersensitivity reactions, including anaphylaxis. Concurrent use with antineoplastic, immunosuppressive, or immunomodulating agents may further increase the risk of infections. Liver injury reported. Induces increases in circulating lymphocytes, monocytes, eosinophils, basophils, and nucleated RBCs.

ADVERSE REACTIONS: Headache, fatigue, UTI, depression, lower respiratory tract infection, arthralgia, abdominal discomfort, rash, gastroenteritis, vaginitis, allergic reaction, urinary urgency/frequency, irregular menstruation/dysmenorrhea, dermatitis, abnormal LFTs.

INTERACTIONS: Avoid with concomitant immunosuppresants (eg, 6-mercaptopurine, azathioprine, cyclosporine, or methotrexate) or inhibitors of TNF-α. Taper corticosteroids in CD patients before starting therapy.

PREGNANCY: Category C, caution in nursing.

MECHANISM OF ACTION: Monoclonal antibody; specific mechanism not defined. Binds to α4-subunit of α4β1 and α4β7 integrins expressed on surface of all leukocytes except neutrophils. Inhibits α4-mediated adhesion of leukocytes to their counter-receptor(s).

PHARMACOKINETICS: Absorption: (MS) C_{max}=110mcg/mL; (CD) C_{max}=101mcg/mL. **Distribution:** (MS) V_d=5.7L; (CD) V_d=5.2L. **Elimination:** (MS) $T_{1/2}$=11 days; (CD) $T_{1/2}$=10 days.

TYZEKA   RX
telbivudine (Idenix)

> Lactic acidosis and severe hepatomegaly with steatosis reported. Discontinuation may result in severe acute exacerbations of hepatitis; monitor hepatic function closely for at least several months following discontinuation of therapy.

THERAPEUTIC CLASS: Nucleoside analogue

INDICATIONS: Treatment of chronic hepatitis B.

DOSAGE: *Adults:* CrCl ≥50mL/min: 600mg qd. CrCl 30-49mL/min: 600mg every 48 hrs. CrCl <30mL/min (not requiring dialysis): 600mg every 72 hrs. ESRD: 600mg every 96 hrs.
Pediatrics: ≥16 yrs: CrCl ≥50mL/min: 600mg qd. CrCl 30-49mL/min: 600mg every 48 hrs. CrCl <30mL/min (not requiring dialysis): 600mg every 72 hrs. ESRD: 600mg every 96 hrs.

HOW SUPPLIED: Tab: 600mg

WARNINGS/PRECAUTIONS: Myopathy reported; interrupt therapy if myopathy suspected and d/c if myopathy diagnosed. Monitor renal function.

ADVERSE REACTIONS: Upper respiratory tract infection, fatigue, malaise, abdominal pain, nasopharyngitis, headache, elevated blood CPK, cough, nausea, vomiting, influenza, flu-like symptoms, diarrhea, loose stools, pharyngolaryngeal pain.

INTERACTIONS: Drugs that alter renal function may alter plasma concentrations of telbivudine.

PREGNANCY: Category B, not for use in nursing.

MECHANISM OF ACTION: Thymidine nucleoside analogue; inhibits HBV DNA polymerase by competing with thymidine 5'-triphosphate and inhibits viral replication by incorporating into viral DNA causing DNA chain termination.

PHARMACOKINETICS: Absorption: C_{max}=3.69mcg/mL, T_{max}=2 hrs, AUC=26.1mcg•h/mL. **Distribution:** Plasma protein binding (3.3%). **Elimination:** Urine; $T_{1/2}$=40-49 hrs.

ULTANE   RX
sevoflurane (Abbott)

THERAPEUTIC CLASS: Inhalation anesthetic

INDICATIONS: For induction and maintenance of general anesthesia in adult and pediatric patients for inpatient and outpatient surgery.

DOSAGE: *Adults:* Individualize dose. MAC Values: 80 yrs: 1.4% sevoflurane in oxygen or 0.7% sevoflurane in 65% nitrous oxide/35% oxygen. 60 yrs: 1.7% sevoflurane in oxygen or 0.9% sevoflurane in 65% nitrous oxide/35% oxygen. 40 yrs: 2.1% sevoflurane in oxygen or 1.1% sevoflurane in 65% nitrous oxide/35% oxygen. 25 yrs: 2.6% sevoflurane in oxygen or 1.4% sevoflurane in 65% nitrous oxide/35% oxygen.
Pediatrics: Individualize dose. MAC Values: 3-12 yrs: 2.5% sevoflurane in oxygen. 6 months-<3 yrs: 2.8% sevoflurane in oxygen or 2% sevoflurane in 65% nitrous oxide/35% oxygen. 1-<6 months: 3% sevoflurane in oxygen. 0-1 month: 3.3% sevoflurane in oxygen.

HOW SUPPLIED: Liq: [250mL]

CONTRAINDICATIONS: Susceptibility to malignant hyperthermia.

WARNINGS/PRECAUTIONS: Potential for renal injury. May be associated with glycosuria and proteinuria. May cause malignant hyperthermia. May cause perioperative hyperkalemia resulting in cardiac arrhythmias. May decrease BP. Rare cases of seizures reported. Transient changes in postoperative LFTs and very rare cases of post-operative hepatic dysfunction or hepatitis reported. Concomitant use of desiccated CO_2 absorbents (eg, potassium hydroxide) not recommended, may result in rare cases of extreme heat, smoke, and/or spontaneous fire in anesthesia breathing circuit; replace CO_2 absorbent routinely.

ADVERSE REACTIONS: Bradycardia, hypotension, agitation, laryngospasm, airway obstruction, breathholding, cough, tachycardia, shivering, somnolence, dizziness, increased salivation, nausea, vomiting.

INTERACTIONS: Decreased anesthetic requirement with nitrous oxide. May increase both the intensity and duration of neuromuscular blockade induced by nondepolarizing muscle relaxants.

PREGNANCY: Category B, caution in nursing.

MECHANISM OF ACTION: Inhalational anesthetic agent; used for induction and maintenance of general anesthesia.

PHARMACOKINETICS: Absorption: T_{max}=2 hr. **Metabolism**: Via CYP2E1 to Hexafluoroisopropanol (HFIP) inactive. **Elimination:** Lungs and urine (3.5% as inorganic fluoride). $T_{1/2}$= 15-23 hrs (Flouride Ion), 33 hrs (Flouride Ion in renal impairement)

ULTIVA
remifentanil HCL (Abbott) `CII`

THERAPEUTIC CLASS: Opioid analgesic

INDICATIONS: As an analgesic agent for use during the induction and maintenance of general anesthesia. For continuation as an analgesic into the immediate postoperative period in adults under the direct supervision of an anesthesia practitioner in a postoperative anesthesia care unit or intensive care setting. As an analgesic component of monitored anesthesia care in adults.

DOSAGE: *Adults:* Continuous IV Infusion: Induction: 0.5-1mcg/kg/min. Maint: 0.4mcg/kg with nitrous oxide 66%; 0.25mcg/kg with isoflurane (0.4-1.25 MAC); 0.25 with propofol (100-200mcg/kg/min). Post-Op Continuation: 0.1mcg/kg/min. CABG: Induction/Maint/Continuation: 1mcg/kg/min. Elderly (>65 yrs): Use 50% of adult dose. Titrate carefully.
Pediatrics: Anesthesia Maint: Continuous IV Infusion: 1-12 yrs: 0.25mcg/kg/min with halothane (0.3-1.5 MAC), sevoflurane (0.3-1.5 MAC, or isoflurane (0.4-1.5 MAC). Range: 0.05-1.3mcg/kg/min. Birth-2 months: 0.4mcg/kg/min. Range: 0.4-1mcg/kg/min.

HOW SUPPLIED: Inj: 1mg, 2mg, 5mg

CONTRAINDICATIONS: Epidural or intrathecal administration, hypersensitivity to fentanyl analogs.

WARNINGS/PRECAUTIONS: Administer only with infusion device. IV bolus administration should be used only during the maintenance of general anesthesia. Interruption of infusion will result in rapid offset of effect. Use associated with apnea and respiratory depression. Not for use in diagnostic or therapeutic procedures outside the monitored anesthesia care setting. Resuscitative and intubation equipment, oxygen, and opioid antagonist must be readily available. May cause skeletal muscle rigidity and is related to the dose and speed of administration. Do not administer into the same IV tubing with blood due to potential inactivation by nonspecific esterases in blood products. Continuously monitor vital signs and oxygenation. Bradycardia, hypotension, intraoperative awareness reported. Not recommended as sole agent for induction of anesthesia.

ADVERSE REACTIONS: Nausea, vomiting, hypotension, muscle rigidity, bradycardia, shivering, fever, dizziness, visual disturbances, respiratory depression, apnea.

INTERACTIONS: Synergism with thiopental, propafol, isoflurane, midazolam; reduce doses of these drugs by up to 75%.

PREGNANCY: Category C, caution in nursing.

MECHANISM OF ACTION: Opioid analgesic.

PHARMACOKINETICS: Distribution: V_d=100mL/kg, 350mL/kg (initial, steady-state), plasma protein binding (70%). **Metabolism**: Hydrolysis via nonspecific blood and tissue esterases to carboxylic acid metabolite. **Elimination**: $T_{1/2}$=10-20 min.

`U`

ULTRACET `RX`
tramadol HCL - acetaminophen (Ortho-McNeil)

THERAPEUTIC CLASS: Central acting analgesic
INDICATIONS: Short-term management of acute pain.

DOSAGE: *Adults:* 2 tabs q4-6h prn for 5 days or less. Max: 8 tabs/24 hrs. CrCl <30mL/min: Max: 2 tabs q12h.

HOW SUPPLIED: Tab: (Tramadol-APAP) 37.5mg-325mg

CONTRAINDICATIONS: Acute intoxication with any of the following: alcohol, hypnotics, narcotics, centrally-acting analgesics, opioids or psychotropic drugs.

WARNINGS/PRECAUTIONS: Seizures and anaphylactic reactions reported. May complicate acute abdominal conditions. Caution with risk of respiratory depression, increased ICP, or head injury. Avoid abrupt withdrawal. Caution in elderly. Avoid use in opioid-dependent patients and with hepatic impairment.

ADVERSE REACTIONS: Constipation, diarrhea, nausea, somnolence, anorexia, increased sweating, dizziness.

INTERACTIONS: See Contraindications. Caution and reduce dose with CNS depressants (eg, alcohol, opioids, anesthetics, phenothiazines, tranquilizers, sedatives, hypnotics). May need dose adjustment with carbamazepine. Possible digoxin toxicity and altered warfarin effects. Caution with quinidine. CYP2D6 inhibitors (eg, fluoxetine, paroxetine, amitriptyline) may potentiate tramadol. May potentiate seizure risk with MAOIs, SSRIs, naloxone (with overdose), TCAs, tricyclics (eg, cyclobenzaprine, promethazine), neuroleptics, opioids and drugs that lower seizure threshold. Avoid other APAP-containing products and alcohol.

PREGNANCY: Category C, not for use in nursing.

MECHANISM OF ACTION: Tramadol: Centrally acting synthetic opioid analgesic; mechanism not fully understood. Binds to μ-opioid receptors and inhibits reuptake of norepinephrine and serotonin. APAP: Non-opiate, non-salicylate analgesic.

PHARMACOKINETICS: Absorption: Tramadol: Bioavailability (75%), T_{max}=2 hrs, 3 hrs (M1). APAP: Small intestines; T_{max}=1 hr. **Distribution:** (IV) Tramadol: V_d=2.4L/kg (male), 2.9L/kg (female); Plasma protein binding (20%). APAP: V_d=0.9L/kg; Plasma protein binding (20%). **Metabolism:** Tramadol: CYP2D6, 3A4 (N-and O-demethylation, glucuronidation or sulfation); M1 (active metabolite). APAP: CYP2E1, 1A2, 3A4 (conjugation, sulfation, oxidation). **Elimination:** Tramadol: $T_{1/2}$=5-6 hrs, 7 hrs (M1); urine (30%). APAP: $T_{1/2}$=2-3 hrs; urine (<9%).

ULTRAM   RX
tramadol HCL (Ortho-McNeil)

OTHER BRAND NAMES: Ultram ER (PRICARA)

THERAPEUTIC CLASS: Central acting analgesic

INDICATIONS: Management of moderate to moderately severe pain.

DOSAGE: *Adults:* ≥17 yrs: (Tab) Initial: 25mg qam. Titrate: May increase by 25mg every 3 days to 25mg qid, then may increase by 50mg every 3 days to 50mg qid. Usual: 50-100mg q4-6h as needed. Max: 400mg/day. Elderly: Start at low end of dosing range. >75 yrs: Max: 300mg/day. CrCl <30mL/min: Dose q12h. Max: 200mg/day. Cirrhosis: 50mg q12h. ≥18 yrs: (Tab, ER) Initial: 100mg qd. Titrate: May increase by 100mg every 5 days. Max: 300mg/day. Elderly: Start at low end of dosing range. Avoid in CrCl <30mL/min and severe hepatic impairment (Child-Pugh Class C).

HOW SUPPLIED: Tab: 50mg*; Tab, Extended-Release: 100mg, 200mg, 300mg *scored

CONTRAINDICATIONS: Acute intoxication with any of the following: alcohol, hypnotics, narcotics, centrally-acting analgesics, opioids or psychotropic drugs.

WARNINGS/PRECAUTIONS: Seizures and anaphylactoid reactions reported. Do not use in opioid-dependent patients. Caution if at risk for respiratory depression, or with increased ICP or head trauma. May complicate acute abdominal conditions. Do not d/c abruptly. Adjust dose with renal or hepatic impairment.

ADVERSE REACTIONS: Dizziness, nausea, constipation, headache, somnolence, vomiting, nervousness, sweating, asthenia, dyspepsia, dry mouth, diarrhea, CNS stimulation, pruritus.

INTERACTIONS: See Contraindications. Caution and reduce dose with CNS depressants (eg, alcohol, opioids, anesthetics, phenothiazines, tranquilizers, sedatives, hypnotics). Avoid with carbamazepine. Possible digoxin toxicity and altered warfarin effects. Caution with quinidine. CYP2D6 inhibitors (eg, fluoxetine, paroxetine, amitriptyline) may potentiate tramadol. May potentiate seizure risk with MAOIs, SSRIs, naloxone (with overdose), TCAs, tricyclics (eg, cyclobenzaprine, promethazine), neuroleptics, opioids and drugs that lower seizure threshold.

PREGNANCY: Category C, not for use in nursing.

MECHANISM OF ACTION: Centrally acting synthetic opioid analgesic; mechanism not fully understood. Shown to inhibit reuptake of norepinephrine and serotonin.

PHARMACOKINETICS: Absorption: Rapid, complete. Bioavailability (75%). T_{max}=2 hrs. (drug), 3 hrs (M1). **Distribution:** V_d=2.6L/kg (male), 2.9L/kg (female). Plasma protein binding (20%). **Metabolism:** Liver (extensive); through N-and O-demethylation and glucuronidation or sulfation pathways via CYP3A4, 2D6. M1 (active metabolite). **Elimination:** Urine: (30% unchanged), (60% as metabolite). $T_{1/2}$=6.3 hrs (drug), 7.4 hrs (M1).

ULTRAVATE   RX
halobetasol propionate (Ranbaxy)

THERAPEUTIC CLASS: Corticosteroid

INDICATIONS: Corticosteroid-responsive dermatoses.

DOSAGE: *Adults:* Apply qd-bid. Rub in gently. Limit treatment to 2 weeks. Max: 50g/week.
Pediatrics: ≥12 yrs: Apply qd-bid. Rub in gently. Limit treatment to 2 weeks. Max: 50g/week.

HOW SUPPLIED: Cre, Oint: 0.05% [15g, 50g]

WARNINGS/PRECAUTIONS: Avoid face, groin, or axillae. Not for treatment of rosacea or perioral dermatitis. May produce reversible HPA axis suppression, manifestations of Cushing's syndrome, hyperglycemia, and glucosuria. Caution when applied to large surface areas or under occlusive dressings. Use appropriate antifungal or antibacterial agent with dermatological infections; d/c if infection does not clear. Pediatrics may be more susceptible to systemic toxicity. Avoid eyes. D/C if irritation occurs. Re-assess if no improvement after 2 weeks.

ADVERSE REACTIONS: Stinging, burning, itching, irritation, dryness, folliculitis, hypertrichosis, acneiform eruptions, hypopigmentation, perioral dermatitis, allergic contact dermatitis, skin maceration, secondary infection, skin atrophy, striae, miliaria.

PREGNANCY: Category C, caution in nursing.

MECHANISM OF ACTION: Corticosteroid; possesses anti-inflammatory, antipruritic, and vasoconstrictive properties. Anti-inflammatory activity not established; suspected to act by induction of phospholipase A_2 inhibitory proteins called lipocortins. Lipocortins control biosynthesis of potent inflammation mediators (eg, prostaglandins, leukotrienes) by inhibiting release of their common precursor, arachidonic acid.

PHARMACOKINETICS: Absorption: Percutaneous; occlusion, inflammation, and other disease states may increase absorption. **Distribution:** Systemically administered corticosteroids appear in breast milk.

U

UNASYN   RX
ampicillin sodium - sulbactam sodium (Pfizer)

THERAPEUTIC CLASS: Semisynthetic penicillin/beta-lactamase inhibitor

INDICATIONS: Treatment of skin and skin structure (SSSI), intra-abdominal, and gynecological infections caused by susceptible microorganisms.

DOSAGE: *Adults:* 1.5-3g (ampicillin+sulbactam) IM/IV q6h. Max: 4g sulbactam/day. Renal Impairment: CrCl ≥30mL/min: 1.5-3g q6-8h. CrCl 15-29mL/min: 1.5-3g q12h. CrCl 5-14mL/min: 1.5-3g q24h.
Pediatrics: ≥1 yr: 300mg/kg/day (ampicillin+sulbactam) IV in equally divided doses q6h. Max: 4g sulbactam/day. ≥40kg: Dose according to adult recommendations.

HOW SUPPLIED: Inj: (Ampicillin-Sulbactam) 1g-0.5g, 2g-1g, 10g-5g

WARNINGS/PRECAUTIONS: Serious, sometimes fatal, hypersensitivity reactions reported with PCN therapy. *Clostridium difficile*-associated diarrhea reported. Increased risk of skin rash with mononucleosis; use alternate agent.

ADVERSE REACTIONS: Injection site pain, thrombophlebitis, diarrhea.

INTERACTIONS: Probenecid increases and prolongs blood levels. Increased incidence of rash with allopurinol. Do not reconstitute with aminoglycosides; may inactivate aminoglycosides.

PREGNANCY: Category B, caution in nursing.

MECHANISM OF ACTION: Ampicillin: Broad-spectrum antibacterial agent; inhibits cell-wall mucopeptide biosynthesis. Sulbactam: Broad-spectrum antibacterial agent; good inhibitory activity against clinically important plasmid mediated β-lactamases most frequently responsible for transferred drug resistance.

PHARMACOKINETICS: Absorption: IV/IM administration of variable doses resulted in different parameters. **Distribution**: Plasma protein binding: 28% (ampicillin); 38% (sulbactam). **Elimination:** Urine (75-80% unchanged), $T_{1/2}$=1 hr.

UNIPHYL   RX
theophylline (Purdue Pharmaceutical)

THERAPEUTIC CLASS: Xanthine bronchodilator

INDICATIONS: Treatment of the symptoms and reversible airflow obstruction associated with chronic asthma and other chronic lung disease (eg, emphysema, chronic bronchitis).

DOSAGE: *Adults:* Initial: 300-400mg qd for 3 days with meals. Titrate: Increase to 400-600mg qd. After 3 days and if needed/tolerated, increase dose according to blood levels. Tab may be split in half; do not chew or crush. Renal Dysfunction/Elderly (>60 yrs): Max: 400mg/day. Conversion from Immediate-Release Theophylline: Give same daily dose as once daily.
Pediatrics: 12-15 yrs: (<45kg): Initial: 12-14mg/kg/day up to 300mg qd for 3 days with meals. Titrate: Increase to 16mg/kg/day up to 400mg qd. After 3 days if needed/tolerated increase to 20mg/kg/day up to 600mg qd. (>45kg): Follow adult dose schedule. Tab may be split in half; do not chew or crush. Conversion from Immediate-Release Theophylline: ≥12 yrs: Give same daily dose as once daily. Renal Dysfunction: Max: 400mg qd.

HOW SUPPLIED: Tab, Extended-Release: 400mg*, 600mg* *scored

WARNINGS/PRECAUTIONS: Extreme caution in peptic ulcer disease, seizure disorders and/or cardiac arrhythmias (except bradycardia). Caution in neonates, children <1 yr, and the elderly. Caution in pulmonary edema, CHF, fever ≥102°F for 24 hrs, cor-pulmonale, hypothyroidism, liver disease, reduced renal function, sepsis, shock, and HTN. If toxicity develops (eg, repetitive vomiting) monitor serum levels and adjust dosage.

ADVERSE REACTIONS: Vomiting, headache, insomnia, diarrhea, restlessness, tremors, hematemesis, hypokalemia, hyperglycemia, tachycardia, hypotension/shock, nervousness, disorientation, arrhythmias, seizures.

INTERACTIONS: Diminished effects with charcoal broiled food, phenytoin, carbamazepine, phenobarbital, hydantoins, rifampin, ritonavir, aminoglutethimide, barbiturates, ketoconazole, sulfinpyrazone, INH, loop diuretics, sympathomimetics, high protein/low carbohydrate diet, St. John's wort. Potentiated by propranolol, allopurinol, erythromycin, troleandomycin, ciprofloxacin, quinolone antibiotics, oral contraceptives, CCBs, corticosteroids, disulfiram, ephedrine, influenza virus vaccine, interferon, macrolides, mexiletine, thiabendazole, thyroid hormones, carbamazepine, loop diuretics.

PREGNANCY: Category C, caution in nursing.

MECHANISM OF ACTION: Methylxanthine; acts via smooth muscle relaxation and suppression of airway response to stimuli. Bronchodilatation suggested to be mediated by inhibiting isozymes of phosphodiesterase. Also increases the force of contraction of diaphragmatic muscles due to enhancement of calcium uptake through adenosine-mediated channel.

PHARMACOKINETICS: Absorption: Rapid, complete; (800 qam, fed) C_{max}=12.1mcg/mL, C_{min}=4.5mcg/mL, T_{max}=8.8 hrs, AUC=203mcg•hr/mL. (600 qd, fed) C_{max}=12.91mcg/mL, C_{min}=5.52mcg/mL, T_{max}=8.62 hrs, AUC=209mcg•hr/mL. Bioavailability Ratio 600/400: 98.8%. **Distribution:** V_d= 0.45L/kg; plasma protein binding (40%). **Metabolism:** Extensive; CYP1A2, 2E1, 3A3; Caffeine and 3-methylxanthine (active metabolites). **Elimination:** Urine (10% unchanged), $T_{1/2}$=8 hrs.

UNIRETIC   RX
moexipril HCL - hydrochlorothiazide (Schwarz)

> ACE inhibitors can cause death/injury to developing fetus during 2nd and 3rd trimesters. Stop therapy if pregnancy detected.

THERAPEUTIC CLASS: ACE inhibitor/thiazide diuretic

INDICATIONS: Treatment of hypertension. Not for initial therapy.

DOSAGE: *Adults:* Initial (if not controlled on moexipril/HCTZ monotherapy): Switch to 7.5mg-12.5mg tab, 15mg-12.5mg tab, or 15mg-25mg tab qd. Titrate: May increase after 2-3 weeks. Initial (if controlled on 25mg HCTZ/day with hypokalemia): 3.75mg-6.25mg (1/2 of 7.5mg-12.5mg tab). If excessive reduction with 7.5mg-12.5mg tab, may switch to 3.75mg-6.25mg. Replacement Therapy: Substitute combination for titrated components. Take 1 hr before meals.

HOW SUPPLIED: Tab: (Moexipril-HCTZ) 7.5mg-12.5mg*, 15mg-12.5mg*, 15mg-25mg* *scored

CONTRAINDICATIONS: History of ACE inhibitor-associated angioedema, anuria, sulfonamide hypersensitivity.

WARNINGS/PRECAUTIONS: D/C if angioedema, jaundice, or if marked LFT elevation occurs. Intestinal angioedema reported. Risk of hyperkalemia with DM, renal dysfunction. Persistent nonproductive cough reported. Monitor WBCs in renal and collagen vascular disease. Anaphylactoid reactions reported. Fetal/neonatal morbidity and death reported. Monitor for hypotension in high-risk patients (eg, surgery/anesthesia, volume/salt depletion). Caution in elderly, CHF, renal or hepatic dysfunction. More reports of angioedema in blacks than nonblacks. May exacerbate or activate SLE. Monitor electrolytes. Avoid if CrCl ≤40mL/min/1.73m². May increase cholesterol, TG. Hypercalcemia, hypomagnesemia, hyperuricemia may occur.

ADVERSE REACTIONS: Cough, dizziness, fatigue.

INTERACTIONS: Increase risk of hyperkalemia with K⁺-sparing diuretics, K⁺ supplements, or K⁺-containing salt substitutes. Potentiates orthostatic hypotension with alcohol, barbiturates, and narcotics. Adjust antidiabetic drugs. Reduced absorption with cholestyramine, colestipol. Corticosteroids, ACTH deplete electrolytes. May decrease response to pressor amines. Potentiates other antihypertensives. May increase responsiveness to skeletal muscle

U

relaxants. Risk of lithium toxicity. NSAIDs reduce effects. Increased absorption of HCTZ with guanabenz and propantheline.

PREGNANCY: Category C (1st trimester) and D (2nd and 3rd trimesters), not for use in nursing.

MECHANISM OF ACTION: Moexipril: ACE inhibitor; inhibition results in decreased plasma angiotensin II, leading to decreased vasopressor activity and decreased aldosterone secretion. HCTZ: Thiazide diuretic; affects renal tubular mechanism of electrolyte reabsorption, directly increasing excretion of Na^+ and chloride.

PHARMACOKINETICS: Absorption: Moexipril: Incomplete, T_{max}=0.8 hrs. **Distribution:** Moexiprilat: V_d=2.8L/kg; Plasma protein binding (50%). HCTZ: V_d=1.5-4.2L/kg; Plasma protein binding (21-24%). **Metabolism:** Moexiprilat (active metabolite). **Elimination**: Moexipril: Urine (24%), feces (20%); $T_{1/2}$=2-9 hrs (Moexiprilat). HCTZ: Renal excretion;,$T_{1/2}$=5.6-14.8 hrs.

UNISOM OTC
doxylamine succinate (Chattem)

THERAPEUTIC CLASS: Antihistamine

INDICATIONS: As a sleep aid 30 minutes before retiring.

DOSAGE: *Adult:* 1 tab 30 min prior to going to bed. Max: 1 tab qhs.
Pediatrics: >12 yrs: 1 tab 30 min prior to going to bed. Max: 1 tab qhs.

HOW SUPPLIED: Tab: 25mg

CONTRAINDICATIONS: Pregnancy, nursing, asthma, glaucoma, prostate enlargement.

WARNINGS/PRECAUTIONS: Caution in emphysema, chronic bronchitis, glaucoma, and difficulty in urination due to BPH. Caution with alcohol. Re-evaluate therapy if sleeplessness persists >2 weeks.

ADVERSE REACTIONS: Anticholinergic effects.

PREGNANCY: Not for use in pregnancy or nursing.

MECHANISM OF ACTION: Antihistamine; helps reduce difficulty falling asleep.

UNITHROID RX
levothyroxine sodium (Lannett)

THERAPEUTIC CLASS: Thyroid replacement hormone

INDICATIONS: Hypothyroidism. As a pituitary TSH suppressant in the treatment and prevention of euthyroid goiters, including thyroid nodules, lymphocytic thyroiditis, and multinodular goiter. Adjunct to surgery and radioiodine therapy for thyrotropin-dependent well-differentiated thyroid cancer.

DOSAGE: *Adults:* Take in AM at least 1/2-1 hr before food. Hypothyroid: Usual: 1.7mcg/kg/day. >200mcg/day (seldom). >50 yrs/<50 yrs with Cardiac Disease: Initial: 25-50mcg/day. Titrate: Increase by 12.5-25mcg/day every 6-8 weeks until euthyroid. Elderly with Cardiac Disease: Initial: 12.5-25mcg/day. Titrate: Increase by 12.5-25mcg/day every 4-6 weeks until euthyroid. Severe Hypothyroidism: Initial: 12.5-25mcg/day. Titrate: Increase by 25mcg/day every 2-4 weeks until euthyroid. Pregnancy: May increase dose requirements. Subclinical Hypothyroidism: Lower doses required.
Pediatrics: Take in AM at least 1/2-1 hr before food. Hypothyroidism: 0-3 months: 10-15mcg/kg/day. 3-6 months: 8-10mcg/kg/day. 6-12 months: 6-8mcg/kg/day. 1-5 yrs: 5-6mcg/kg/day. 6-12 yrs: 4-5mcg/kg/day. >12 yrs: 2-3mcg/kg/day. Growth/Puberty Complete: 1.7mcg/kg/day. Cardiac Risk: Initial: Use lower dose. Titrate: Increase dose every 4-6 weeks until euthyroid. Infants with Serum T_4 <5mcg/dL: Initial: 50mcg/day. Chronic/Severe Hypothyroidism: Children: Initial: 25mcg/day. Titrate: Increase by 25mcg/day every 2-4 weeks until desired effect. Minimize Hyperactivity in Older Children: Initial: Give 1/4 of full replacement dose. Titrate: Increase by same amount weekly until full dose achieved. May crush tab and mix with 5-10mL water.

HOW SUPPLIED: Tab: 25mcg*, 50mcg*, 75mcg*, 88mcg*, 100mcg*, 112mcg*, 125mcg*, 150mcg*, 175mcg*, 200mcg*, 300mcg* *scored

CONTRAINDICATIONS: Untreated thyrotoxicosis, acute MI, uncorrected adrenal insufficiency.

WARNINGS/PRECAUTIONS: Do not use in the treatment of obesity; larger doses in euthyroid patients can cause serious or even life threatening toxicity. Caution with cardiovascular disease, CAD, adrenal insufficiency, autonomous thyroid tissue, hypothalamic/pituitary hormone deficiencies, and the elderly with risk of occult cardiac disease. Carefully titrate dose to avoid over or under treatment. Decreased bone mineral density with long term use. With adrenal insufficiency supplement with glucocorticoids before therapy.

INTERACTIONS: Sympathomimetics may increase risk of coronary insufficiency with CAD. Upward dose adjustments needed for insulin and oral hypoglycemic agents. Decreased absorption with soybean flour (infant formula), cotton seed meal, walnuts, and fiber. May potentiate oral anticoagulant effects; adjust dose and monitor PT/INR. May decrease levels and effects of digitalis glycosides. Cholestyramine, colestipol, ferrous sulfate, aluminum hydroxide, sodium polystyrene, soybean flour, sucralfate may decrease absorption. Reduced TSH secretion with dopamine/dopamine agonists, glucocorticoids, octreotide. Decreased thyroid hormone secretion with aminoglutethimide, amiodarone, iodine (including iodine-containing radiographic contrast agents), lithium, methimazole, PTU, sulfonamides, tolbutamide. Increased thyroid hormone secretion with amiodarone, iodide (including iodine-containing radiographic contrast agents). Decreased T_4 absorption with antacids (aluminum & magnesium hydroxides), simethicone, bile acid sequestrants (cholestyramine, colestipol), calcium carbonate, cation exchange resins (eg, Kayexalate), ferrous sulfate, sucralfate. Increased serum TBG concentration with clofibrate, estrogens, heroin/methadone, 5-FU, mitotane, tamoxifen. Decreased serum TBG concentration with androgens/anabolic steroids, asparaginase, glucocorticoids, nicotinic acid (slow-release). Protein-binding site displacement with furosemide, heparin, hydantoins, NSAIDs, salicylates. Increased hepatic metabolism with carbamazepine, hydantoins, phenobarbital, rifampin. Decreased conversion of T_4 to T_3 levels with amiodarone, β-adrenergic antagonists (propranolol >160mg/day), glucocorticoids (dexamethasone >4mg/day), PTU. Additive effects of both agents with antidepressants. Interferon-(alpha) may cause development of antithyroid microsomal antibodies causing transient hypothyroidism, hyperthyroidism, or both. Interleukin-2 has been associated with transient painless thyroiditis. Excessive use with growth hormones may accelerate epiphyseal closure. Ketamine use may produce marked HTN and tachycardia. May reduce uptake of iodine-containing radiographic contrast agents. Altered levels of thyroid hormone and/or TSH level with choral hydrate, diazepam, ethionamide, lovastatin, metoclopramide, 6-mercaptopurine, nitroprusside, para-aminosalicylate sodium, perphenazine, resorcinol (excessive topical use), thiazide diuretics.

PREGNANCY: Category A, caution in nursing.

MECHANISM OF ACTION: Thyroid hormone; not understood, suspected to control DNA transcription and protein synthesis.

PHARMACOKINETICS: Distribution: Plasma protein binding (99%), found in breast milk. **Metabolism**: Liver via sequential deiodination (major pathway), conjugation in liver (mainly), kidneys, other tissues. **Elimination**: Urine, feces (20% unchanged), (T_4) $T_{1/2}$=6-7 days, (T_3) $T_{1/2}$≤2days.

U

UNIVASC   RX
moexipril HCL (Schwarz)

> ACE inhibitors can cause death/injury to developing fetus during 2nd and 3rd trimesters. Stop therapy if pregnancy detected.

THERAPEUTIC CLASS: ACE inhibitor

INDICATIONS: Treatment of hypertension.

DOSAGE: *Adults:* If possible, d/c diuretic 2-3 days prior to therapy. Take 1 hr before meals. Initial: 7.5mg qd, 3.75mg with concomitant diuretic therapy. Maint: 7.5-30mg/day given qd-bid. Resume diuretic if BP not controlled. Max: 60mg/day. CrCl ≤40mL/min: Initial: 3.75mg qd. Max: 15mg/day.

HOW SUPPLIED: Tab: 7.5mg*, 15mg* *scored

CONTRAINDICATIONS: History of ACE inhibitor-associated angioedema.

WARNINGS/PRECAUTIONS: D/C if angioedema, jaundice, or if marked LFT elevation occurs. Intestinal angioedema reported. Risk of hyperkalemia with DM, renal dysfunction. Persistent nonproductive cough reported. Monitor WBCs in renal and collagen vascular disease. Anaphylactoid reactions reported. Fetal/neonatal morbidity and death reported. Monitor for hypotension in high risk patients (heart failure, surgery/anesthesia, prolonged diuretic therapy, volume and/or salt depletion, etc.). Caution with CHF, renal dysfunction, and renal artery stenosis. Less effective on BP in blacks and more reports of angioedema than nonblacks.

ADVERSE REACTIONS: Cough, dizziness, diarrhea, flu syndrome, fatigue, pharyngitis, flushing, rash, myalgia.

INTERACTIONS: May increase lithium levels. Hypotension risk with diuretics. Increased risk of hyperkalemia with K$^+$-sparing diuretics, K$^+$-containing salt substitutes, or K$^+$ supplements.

PREGNANCY: Category C (1st trimester) and D (2nd and 3rd trimesters), not for use in nursing.

MECHANISM OF ACTION: ACE inhibitor; inhibition results in decreased plasma angiotensin II, which leads to decreased vasopressor activity and decreased aldosterone secretion.

PHARMACOKINETICS: Absorption: Incomplete; T_{max}=90 min (moexiprilat). **Distribution:** Moexiprilat: Plasma protein binding (80%); V_d=183L. **Metabolism:** Moexiprilat (active metabolite). **Elimination:** Moexiprilat: $T_{1/2}$=2-9 hrs; Urine (7%), feces (52%).

URECHOLINE   RX
bethanechol chloride (Merck/Odyssey)

THERAPEUTIC CLASS: Cholinergic agent

INDICATIONS: Treatment of acute postoperative and postpartum nonobstructive urinary retention and for neurogenic atony of the urinary bladder with retention.

DOSAGE: *Adults:* Initial: 5-10mg. Titrate: May repeat every hr until satisfactory response or 50mg given. Usual: 10-50mg tid-qid. Max: 200mg/day.

HOW SUPPLIED: Tab: 5mg*, 10mg*, 25mg*, 50mg* *scored

CONTRAINDICATIONS: GI or bladder wall strength or integrity is in question or with mechanical obstruction, if increased muscular activity of GI tract or urinary bladder may be harmful, bladder neck obstruction, spastic GI disturbances, acute inflammatory lesions of GI tract, peritonitis, marked vagotonia, hyperthyroidism, peptic ulcer, bronchial asthma, bradycardia, hypotension, vasomotor instability, CAD, epilepsy, parkinsonism.

WARNINGS/PRECAUTIONS: If sphincter fails to relax, urine may be forced up ureter into kidney pelvis; may increase risk of reflux infection.

ADVERSE REACTIONS: Malaise, abdominal cramps/discomfort, nausea, belching, diarrhea, salivation, urinary urgency, headache, fall in BP with reflex tachycardia, vasomotor response, flushing, sweating, bronchial constriction, lacrimation.

INTERACTIONS: Caution with ganglionic blockers; a critical fall in BP may occur.

PREGNANCY: Category C, not for use in nursing.

MECHANISM OF ACTION: Cholinergic agent: Stimulates parasympathetic nervous system; increases detrusor muscle tone, producing strong contractions to initiate micturition and emptying of bladder; stimulates gastric motility, increases gastric tone and restores rhythmic peristalsis impairment.

URISED

RX

hyoscyamine sulfate - atropine sulfate - benzoic acid - methenamine - phenyl salicylate - methylene blue (PolyMedica)

THERAPEUTIC CLASS: anticholinergic/antiseptic/antibacterial/analgesic

INDICATIONS: Relief of lower urinary tract discomfort due to hypermotility. Treatment of formaldehyde-susceptible cystitis, urethritis, trigonitis.

DOSAGE: *Adults:* Usual: 2 tabs qid with plenty of fluid. *Pediatrics:* ≥6 yrs: Individualize dose. Take with plenty of fluid.

HOW SUPPLIED: Tab: Atropine 0.03mg-Benzoic Acid 4.5mg-Hyoscyamine 0.03mg-Methenamine 40.8mg-Methylene Blue 5.4mg-Phenyl Salicylate 18.1mg

CONTRAINDICATIONS: Glaucoma, pyloric or duodenal obstruction, urinary bladder neck obstruction, or cardiospasm.

WARNINGS/PRECAUTIONS: Caution with cardiovascular disorders. May precipitate acute urinary retention in prostatic hypertrophy.

ADVERSE REACTIONS: Rash, dry mouth, flushing, difficult micturition, rapid pulse, dizziness, blurred vision, urine/feces discoloration.

INTERACTIONS: Avoid alkalinizing agents/foods. Sulfonamides may precipitate in the urine; avoid concomitant use.

PREGNANCY: Category C, caution in nursing.

MECHANISM OF ACTION: Methenamine: Hydrolyses in acidic urine releasing formaldehyde, which provides mild antiseptic action. Methylene Blue/Benzoic acid: Has mild but effective antiseptic activity. Phenyl Salicylate: Has mild analgesic and antipyretic with weak antiseptic. Hyoscyaminea/Atropine: Stimulates parasympatholytic action; leads to relaxing of smooth muscle spasm.

PHARMACOKINETICS: Absorption: Rapid (Methenamine, Phenyl Salicylate, Methylene Blue and Benzoic acid). **Metabolism:** Methenamine: Hydrolyses in acidic urine to formaldehyde. **Elimination:** Urine.

URISPAS

RX

flavoxate HCL (Ortho-McNeil)

THERAPEUTIC CLASS: Smooth muscle antispasmodic

INDICATIONS: Relief of dysuria, urgency, nocturia, suprapubic pain, frequency and incontinence.

DOSAGE: *Adults:* 100-200mg tid-qid. Reduce dose with improvement. *Pediatrics:* ≥12 yrs: 100-200mg tid-qid. Reduce dose with improvement.

HOW SUPPLIED: Tab: 100mg

CONTRAINDICATIONS: Pyloric or duodenal obstruction, obstructive intestinal lesions or ileus, achalasia, GI hemorrhage, and obstructive uropathies of the lower urinary tract.

WARNINGS/PRECAUTIONS: Caution with glaucoma and while operating machinery where alertness is required. Drowsiness, blurred vision may occur.

ADVERSE REACTIONS: Drowsiness, dry mouth, nausea, vomiting, tachycardia, palpitations, leukopenia, vertigo, nervousness, confusion, fatigue, headache, hyperpyrexia, urticaria, blurred vision.

PREGNANCY: Category B, caution in nursing.

MECHANISM OF ACTION: Urinary tract spasmolytic; counteracts smooth muscle spasm of urinary tract and exerts effect directly on muscle.

U

URO KP NEUTRAL RX
disodium phosphate - dipotassium phosphate - sodium phosphate (Esprit)

THERAPEUTIC CLASS: Phosphate supplement

INDICATIONS: Prevention of recurrent calcium oxalate stones; increases urinary phosphate and pyrophosphate.

DOSAGE: *Adults:* 1-2 tab qid with a full glass of water.

HOW SUPPLIED: Tab: (Phosphorous-Potassium-Sodium) 258mg-49.4mg-262.4mg

CONTRAINDICATIONS: Infected phosphate stones. Severe renal impairment (<30% of normal). Hyperphosphatemia.

WARNINGS/PRECAUTIONS: Caution with potassium and/or sodium adjustments. May experience laxative effect during first few days of therapy; reduce daily dose or d/c if severe. Caution with cardiac disease (eg, digitalized patients), severe adrenal insufficiency (eg, Addison's disease), acute dehydration, severe renal insufficiency/impairment or chronic renal disease, extensive tissue breakdown (eg, severe burns), myotonia congenita, cardiac failure, liver cirrhosis or severe hepatic disease, peripheral or pulmonary edema, hypernatremia, HTN, toxemia of pregnancy, hypoparathyroidism, acute pancreatitis. High serum phosphate may increase incidence of extraskeletal calcification. May be beneficial in rickets; use with caution. Monitor renal function and serum electrolytes.

ADVERSE REACTIONS: Diarrhea, nausea, stomach pain, vomiting, bone and joint pain.

INTERACTIONS: Antacids containing aluminum, magnesium or calcium may prevent absorption. Hypernatremia with concurrent diazoxide, guanethidine, hydralazine, methyldopa, rauwolfia alkaloids, mineralocorticoids. Calcium products and/or vitamin D may antagonize effects in hypercalcemia treatment. Hyperkalemia with concurrent potassium sparing diuretics or potassium-containing products.

PREGNANCY: Category C, caution in nursing.

MECHANISM OF ACTION: Phosphate supplement: Source of dietary phosphorus used to decrease urinary calcium levels, increase urinary pyrophosphate inhibitor; may be another effect that has not been established.

UROCIT-K RX
potassium citrate (Mission)

THERAPEUTIC CLASS: Urinary tract alkalinizer

INDICATIONS: Management of renal tubular acidosis (RTA) with calcium stones, hypocitraturic calcium oxalate nephrolithiasis of any etiology, and uric acid lithiasis with or without calcium stones.

DOSAGE: *Adults:* Initial: Severe Hypocitraturia (urinary citrate <150mg/day): 20mEq tid or 15mEq qid. Mild-Moderate Hypocitraturia (urinary citrate ≥150mg/day): 10mEq tid. Max: 100mEq/day. Measure urinary pH and 24-hr urinary citrate after 1st dose before titration.

HOW SUPPLIED: Tab, Extended-Release: 5mEq, 10mEq

CONTRAINDICATIONS: Hyperkalemia, conditions with predisposition to hyperkalemia (eg, chronic renal failure, uncontrolled DM, acute dehydration, strenuous exercise, adrenal insufficiency, extensive tissue breakdown, K⁺-sparing agents), delayed gastric emptying, esophageal compression, intestinal obstruction or stricture, anticholinergics, UTI, renal insufficiency, and PUD.

WARNINGS/PRECAUTIONS: Avoid with impaired mechanisms for excreting K⁺ (eg, chronic renal failure, severe myocardial damage, or heart failure). Do not crush, chew, or suck tablet. GI mucosal lesions reported; d/c with severe vomiting, abdominal pain, or GI bleeding. Monitor serum electrolytes, serum creatinine and CBC every 4 months. D/C with hyperkalemia, urinary citrate and/or pH, increased serum creatinine, or decreased Hct or Hgb. Limit salt intake.

ADVERSE REACTIONS: Abdominal discomfort, vomiting, diarrhea, nausea.

INTERACTIONS: Avoid K+-sparing diuretics. Increased GI irritation with drugs that slow GI transit time (eg, anticholinergics).

PREGNANCY: Category C, caution in nursing.

MECHANISM OF ACTION: Potassium supplement; urinary tract alkalinizer; appears to increase urinary citrate principally by modifying renal handling of citrate rather than by increasing filtered load of citrate. Raises urinary pH and citrate; causes transient reduction in urinary Ca.

UROGESIC BLUE   RX
hyoscyamine sulfate - methenamine - sodium biphosphate - phenyl salicylate - methylene blue (Edwards)

THERAPEUTIC CLASS: anticholinergic/antibacterial/antiseptic/analgesic/Acidifier

INDICATIONS: Treatment of symptoms of irritative voiding. Relief of lower urinary tract discomfort.

DOSAGE: *Adults:* 1 tab qid with plenty of fluid.
Pediatrics: >6 yrs: Individualize dose. Take with plenty of fluid.

HOW SUPPLIED: Tab: Hyoscyamine 0.12mg-Methenamine, 81.6mg-Methylene Blue, 10.8mg-Phenyl Salicylate, 36.2mg-Sodium Biphosphate 40.8mg

CONTRAINDICATIONS: Consider risk-benefit with: cardiac disease, GI tract obstructive disease, glaucoma, myasthenia gravis, obstructive uropathy.

WARNINGS/PRECAUTIONS: D/C if rapid pulse, dizziness, or blurred vision occurs. Delay in gastric emptying may obscure gastric ulcer therapy. Caution in elderly.

ADVERSE REACTIONS: Rapid pulse, flushing, blurred vision, dizziness, shortness of breath, difficult micturition, acute urinary retention, dry mouth, NV, urine/feces discoloration.

INTERACTIONS: May decrease absorption of other oral agents (dose 2 hrs after ketoconazole). Reduced effectiveness with urinary alkaliners, thiazide diuretics, antacids/antidiarrheals (space dosing by 1 hr). Antimuscarinic effects potentiated with other antimuscarinics, MAOIs. Caution with antimyasthenics. Increased risk of constipation with opioids. Sulfonamides may precipitate in the urine.

PREGNANCY: Category C, safety in nursing not known.

MECHANISM OF ACTION: Hyoscyamine: Parasympatholytic; relaxes smooth muscle and produces antispasmodic effect. Methenamine: Hydrolyses in acidic urine releasing formaldehyde which provides bactericidal and bacteriostatic action. Methylene Blue: Has mild but effective antiseptic activity. Phenyl Salicylate: Mild analgesic. Sodium biphosphate: Helps to maintain acidic pH in urine for methenamine degredation.

PHARMACOKINETICS: Absorption: Well absorbed (Hyoscyamine, Methenamine, and Methylene Blue). **Metabolism:** Hyoscyamine: Hepatic. Methenamine: Hydrolysis to formaldehyde. **Elimination:** Hyoscyamine: Urine (13-50% unchanged); $T_{1/2}$=12 hrs. Methenamine: Urine (70-90% unchanged); $T_{1/2}$=24 hrs.

UROXATRAL   RX
alfuzosin HCL (Sanofi-Aventis)

THERAPEUTIC CLASS: Alpha₁-blocker

INDICATIONS: Treatment of signs and symptoms of benign prostatic hyperplasia.

DOSAGE: *Adults:* 10mg qd, taken immediately after same meal each day.

HOW SUPPLIED: Tab, Extended-Release: 10mg

CONTRAINDICATIONS: Moderate or severe hepatic insufficiency. Concomitant potent CYP3A4 inhibitors (eg, ketoconazole, itraconazole, ritonavir).

WARNINGS/PRECAUTIONS: Monitor for postural hypotension, syncope. Rule out prostate cancer. D/C with new or worsening angina. Caution with severe renal insufficiency. Caution in patients with congenital or aquired QT prolongation.

ADVERSE REACTIONS: Dizziness, upper respiratory tract infection, headache, fatigue, urticaria, angioedema, pruritis, rhinitis, tachycardia, chest pain, priapism, diarrhea, flushing, edema, angina pectoris.

INTERACTIONS: Increased levels with potent CYP3A4 inhibitors (eg, ketoconazole, itraconazole, ritonavir); concomitant use is contraindicated. Avoid use with other α-blockers. Increased levels with cimetidine, diltiazem, atenolol. Possibility of significant hypotension with other antihypertensives. Caution with medications which prolong the QT interval.

PREGNANCY: Category B, not for use in nursing.

MECHANISM OF ACTION: Post-synaptic α_1-adrenoreceptor antagonist; inhibits adrenoreceptors in lower urinary tract causing smooth muscle in bladder neck and prostate to relax resulting in improved urine flow and decreased symptoms of BPH.

PHARMACOKINETICS: Absorption: Absolute bioavailability (49%), T_{max}=8 hrs, C_{max}=13.6ng/mL, AUC=194ng•hr/mL. **Distribution**: V_d=3.2L/kg, plasma protein binding (82-90%). **Metabolism**: CYP3A4 (Oxidation, O-demethylation, N-dealkylation). **Elimination**: Urine (11%), $T_{1/2}$=10 hrs.

URSO 250   RX
ursodiol (Axcan Scandipharm)

OTHER BRAND NAMES: Urso Forte (Axcan Scandipharm)

THERAPEUTIC CLASS: Bile acid

INDICATIONS: Treatment of primary biliary cirrhosis.

DOSAGE: *Adults:* Usual: 13-15mg/kg/day given bid-qid with food.

HOW SUPPLIED: Tab: (Urso 250) 250mg, (Urso Forte) *500mg* *scored*

WARNINGS/PRECAUTIONS: Administer appropriate specific treatment with variceal bleeding, hepatic encephalopathy, ascites, or when in need of urgent liver transplant.

ADVERSE REACTIONS: Diarrhea, leukopenia, peptic ulcer, hyperglycemia, skin rash, increased creatinine.

INTERACTIONS: Decreased absorption with bile acid sequestering agents (eg, cholestyramine, colestipol), aluminum-based antacids. Estrogens, oral contraceptives, clofibrate and perhaps other cholesterol-lowering agents may counteract effectiveness.

PREGNANCY: Category B, caution in nursing.

MECHANISM OF ACTION: Bile acid.

PHARMACOKINETICS: Absorption: Passive diffusion, incomplete. **Distribution**: Plasma protein binding (70%). **Metabolism**: Liver via conjugation. **Elimination**: Feces (major), urine (<1%).

VAGIFEM   RX
estradiol (Novo Nordisk)

> Estrogens increase the risk of endometrial cancer.

THERAPEUTIC CLASS: Estrogen

INDICATIONS: Treatment of atrophic vaginitis.

DOSAGE: *Adults:* Initial: Insert 1 tab vaginally qd for 2 weeks. Maint: Insert 1 tab twice weekly. Attempt to d/c or taper at 3-6 month intervals.

HOW SUPPLIED: Tab, Vaginal: 25mcg

CONTRAINDICATIONS: Breast carcinoma or other estrogen dependent neoplasia, abnormal genital bleeding, pregnancy, porphyria, thrombophlebitis, thromboembolic disorders. History of thrombophlebitis, thrombosis, or thromboembolic disorders associated with estrogen use.

WARNINGS/PRECAUTIONS: Risk of gallbladder disease, thromboembolism, thrombotic disease. Elevated BP and hepatic adenomas reported. Monitor for hypercalcemia in breast cancer and bone metastases. Caution in asthma, epilepsy, migraine, cardiac or renal dysfunction due to fluid retention. Excessive uterine bleeding and mastodynia reported. Caution in liver dysfunction, metabolic bone disease associated with hypercalcemia, diabetes. May cause hypercoagulability and hyperlipoproteinemia. Caution in young patients.

ADVERSE REACTIONS: Vaginal spotting, vaginal discharge, allergic reactions, headache, abdominal pain, respiratory infection, genital moniliasis, back pain, rash.

PREGNANCY: Category X, caution in nursing.

MECHANISM OF ACTION: Estrogen (estradiol); binds and activates estrogen receptors, regulating growth, differentiation and functioning of different tissues within and outside reproductive system.

PHARMACOKINETICS: Absorption: C_{max}=50pg/mL. **Metabolism:** Liver; estrone, estriol (metabolites). **Elimination:** Urine.

VAGISTAT-1
tioconazole (Novartis)   OTC

THERAPEUTIC CLASS: Azole antifungal

INDICATIONS: Treatment of recurrent vaginal yeast infections.

DOSAGE: *Adults:* Insert applicatorful intravaginally hs single dose. *Pediatrics:* ≥12 yrs: Insert applicatorful intravaginally hs single dose.

HOW SUPPLIED: Oint: 6.5% [4.6g]

WARNINGS/PRECAUTIONS: Do not use if abdominal pain, fever (>100°F), chills, nausea, vomiting, diarrhea, or foul smelling discharge. Do not use with tampons. Do not rely on condoms or diaphragm to prevent STDs or pregnancy until 3 days after last use.

PREGNANCY: Not for use in pregnancy, safety in nursing not known.

MECHANISM OF ACTION: Azole Antifungal.

VALCYTE
valganciclovir HCL (Roche Labs)   RX

Granulocytopenia, anemia, and thrombocytopenia reported. Carcinogenic, teratogenic, and may cause aspermatogenesis based on animal studies.

THERAPEUTIC CLASS: Synthetic guanine derivative nucleoside analogue

INDICATIONS: Treatment of cytomegalovirus (CMV) retinitis in AIDS patients. Prevention of CMV disease in kidney, heart, and kidney-pancreas transplant patients at high risk (Donor CMV seropositive/recipient CMV seronegative).

DOSAGE: *Adults:* Treatment of CMV retinitis: Initial: 900mg bid for 21 days. Maint: 900mg qd. Prevention of CMV disease: 900mg qd starting within 10 days of transplantation until 100 days posttransplantation. CrCl 40-59mL/min: Initial: 450mg bid. Maint: 450mg qd. CrCl 25-39mL/min: Initial: 450mg qd. Maint: 450mg every 2 days. CrCl 10-24mL/min: Initial: 450mg every 2 days. Maint: 450mg twice weekly. CrCl <10mL/min: Not recommended. Take with food.

HOW SUPPLIED: Tab: 450mg

CONTRAINDICATIONS: Hypersensitivity to ganciclovir.

WARNINGS/PRECAUTIONS: Avoid if the neutrophils <500cells/mcL, platelet count <25,000/mcL or hemoglobin >8g/dL. Severe leukopenia, neutropenia, anemia, thrombocytopenia, pancytopenia, bone marrow depression, and aplastic anemia observed. Adjust dose in renal impairment. Do not substitute with ganciclovir caps. May cause temporary or permanent inhibition of spermatogenesis.

ADVERSE REACTIONS: Diarrhea, nausea, vomiting, graft rejection, abdominal pain, pyrexia, headache, neutropenia, leukopenia, anemia, insomnia, peripheral neuropathy, HTN.

INTERACTIONS: Greater risk for neutropenia and anemia with zidovudine. Monitor for toxicity with probenecid. Increased levels of metabolites of both drugs with mycophenolate mofetil. Increased risk of didanosine toxicity. Caution with myelosuppressive drugs or irradiation.

PREGNANCY: Category C, not for use in nursing.

MECHANISM OF ACTION: Guanine derivative; inhibits viral DNA synthesis, resulting in inhibition of human CMV replication.

PHARMACOKINETICS: Absorption: AUC=29.1mcg•h/mL; C_{max}=5.61mcg/mL; Absolute bioavailability (59.4%); T_{max}=1-3 hrs. **Distribution:** (Ganciclovir) Plasma protein binding (1-2%); V_d=0.703L/kg. **Metabolism:** Intestinal wall, liver (hydrolysis). **Elimination:** Renal; $T_{1/2}$=4.08 hrs.

VALIUM CIV
diazepam (Roche Labs)

THERAPEUTIC CLASS: Benzodiazepine

INDICATIONS: Management of anxiety disorders and short-term relief of anxiety symptoms. Symptomatic relief of acute alcohol withdrawal. Adjunct therapy in skeletal muscle spasm and convulsive disorders.

DOSAGE: *Adults:* Anxiety: 2-10mg bid-qid. Alcohol Withdrawal: 10mg tid-qid for 24 hours. Maint: 5mg tid-qid prn. Skeletal Muscle Spasm: 2-10mg tid-qid: Seizure Disorders: 2-10mg bid-qid. Elderly/Debilitated: 2-2.5mg qd-bid initially; may increase gradually as needed and tolerated.
Pediatrics: ≥6 months: 1-2.5mg tid-qid initially; may increase gradually as needed and tolerated.

HOW SUPPLIED: Tab: 2mg*, 5mg*, 10mg* *scored

CONTRAINDICATIONS: Acute narrow angle glaucoma, untreated open angle glaucoma, patients <6 months.

WARNINGS/PRECAUTIONS: Monitor blood counts and LFTs in long-term use. Neutropenia and jaundice reported. Increase in grand mal seizures reported. Avoid abrupt withdrawal. Caution with kidney or hepatic dysfunction.

ADVERSE REACTIONS: Drowsiness, fatigue, ataxia, paradoxical reactions, minor EEG changes.

INTERACTIONS: Phenothiazines, narcotics, barbiturates, MAOIs, and other antidepressants may potentiate effects. Delayed clearance with cimetidine. Avoid alcohol and other CNS-depressants. Risk of seizure with flumazenil.

PREGNANCY: Not for use during pregnancy, safety in nursing not known.

MECHANISM OF ACTION: Benzodiazepine; exerts anxiolytic, sedative, muscle-relaxant, anticonvulsant and amnestic effect. Facilitates GABA, an inhibitory neurotransmitter in CNS.

PHARMACOKINETICS: Absorption: T_{max}=0.25-2.5 hrs. **Distribution:** V_d=0.8-1.0 L/kg, plasma protein binding (98%), crosses blood-brain and placental barrier, appears in breast milk. **Metabolism:** Via N-desmethylation, hydroxylation, glucuronidation to N-desmethyldiazepam, temazepam, oxazepam by CYP3A4, CYP2C19 enzymes. **Elimination:** Urine; $T_{1/2}$=48 hrs, $T_{1/2}$(N-desmethyldiazepam)=100 hrs.

VALSTAR   RX
valrubicin (Indevus)

THERAPEUTIC CLASS: Anthracycline

INDICATIONS: Intravesical therapy of BCG-refractoray carcinoma *in-situ* (CIS) of the urinary bladder in patients for whom immediate cystectomy would be associated with unacceptable morbidity or mortality.

DOSAGE: *Adults:* 800mg intravesically once weekly for 6 weeks. Delay administration for at least 2 weeks after transurethral resection and/or fulguration.

HOW SUPPLIED: Inj: 40mg/mL

CONTRAINDICATIONS: Concurrent UTI, small bladder capacity (unable to tolerate a 75mL instillation). Hypersensitivity to anthracyclines or Cremophor® EL (polyoxyethyleneglycol triricinoleate).

WARNINGS/PRECAUTIONS: Avoid in patients with a perforated bladder or to those in whom the integrity of the bladder mucosa has been compromised. Caution with severe irritable bladder symptoms. Bladder spasm and spontaneous discharge of the intravesical instillate may occur; clamping of urinary catheter is not advised and, if performed, should be executed under medical supervision and with caution.

ADVERSE REACTIONS: Local bladder symptoms: urinary frequency, dysuria, urinary urgency, bladder spasm, hematuria, bladder pain, urinary incontinence, cystitis, nocturia, local burning symptoms, urethral pain. Systemic symptoms: UTI, nausea, abdominal pain.

PREGNANCY: Category C, not for use in nursing.

VALTREX   RX
valacyclovir HCL (GlaxoSmithKline)

THERAPEUTIC CLASS: Nucleoside analogue

INDICATIONS: Treatment of herpes zoster (shingles) and herpes labialis (cold sores). Treatment or suppression of genital herpes in immunocompetent patients and for the suppression of recurrent genital herpes in HIV-infected patients.

DOSAGE: *Adults:* Herpes Zoster: 1g q8h for 7 days. Start within 48-72 hrs after onset of rash. CrCl 30-49mL/min: 1g q12h. CrCl 10-29mL/min: 1g q24h. CrCl <10mL/min: 500mg q24h. Genital Herpes: Initial: 1g q12h for 10 days. Start within 48-72 hrs after onset of symptoms. CrCl 10-29mL/min: 1g q24h. CrCl <10mL/min: 500mg q24h. Recurrent Episodes: Treatment: 500mg bid for 3 days. Start within 24 hrs after onset of symptoms. CrCl ≤29mL/min: 500mg q24h. Suppressive Therapy with Normal Immune Function:1g q24h. CrCl ≤29mL/min: 500mg q24h. Alternative: (≤9 episodes/yr) 500mg q24h. CrCl ≤29mL/min: 500mg q48h. Suppressive Therapy with HIV and CD4 ≥100cells/mm³: 500mg q12h. CrCl ≤29mL/min: 500mg q24h. Herpes Labialis: 2g q12h for 1 day. Start at earliest symptom of cold sore. CrCl 30-49mL/min: 1g q12h. CrCl 10-29mL/min: 500mg q12h. <10mL/min: 500mg single dose. Administer therapy for 1 day. Initiate at earliest symptoms of a cold sore. *Pediatrics:* Post-Pubertal: Herpes Zoster: 1g q8h for 7 days. Start within 48-72 hrs after onset of rash. CrCl 30-49mL/min: 1g q12h. CrCl 10-29mL/min: 1g q24h. CrCl <10mL/min: 500mg q24h. Genital Herpes: Initial: 1g q12h for 10 days. Start within 48-72 hrs after onset of symptoms. CrCl 10-29mL/min: 1g q24h. CrCl <10mL/min: 500mg q24h. Recurrent Episodes: Treatment: 500mg bid for 3 days. Start within 24 hrs after onset of symptoms. CrCl ≤29mL/min: 500mg q24h. Suppressive Therapy with Normal Immune Function:1g q24h. CrCl ≤29mL/min: 500mg q24h. Alternative: (≤9 episodes/yr) 500mg q24h. CrCl ≤29mL/min: 500mg q48h. Suppressive Therapy with HIV and CD4 ≥100cells/mm³: 500mg q12h. CrCl ≤29mL/min: 500mg q24h. Herpes Labialis: 2g q12h for 1 day. Start at earliest symptom of cold sore. CrCl 30-49mL/min: 1g q12h. CrCl 10-29mL/min: 500mg q12h. <10mL/min: 500mg single dose. Administer therapy for 1 day. Initiate at earliest symptoms of a cold sore.

V

HOW SUPPLIED: Tab: 500mg, 1g

CONTRAINDICATIONS: Acyclovir hypersensitivity.

WARNINGS/PRECAUTIONS: Thrombotic thrombocytopenic purpura/hemolytic uremic syndrome reported with advanced HIV disease, allogenic bone marrow or renal transplants. Reduce dose with renal dysfunction. Possible renal and CNS toxicity in elderly.

ADVERSE REACTIONS: Nausea, headache, vomiting, dizziness, abdominal pain.

INTERACTIONS: Renal and CNS toxicity with nephrotoxic drugs.

PREGNANCY: Category B, caution in nursing.

MECHANISM OF ACTION: Nucleoside analogue; inhibits replication of herpes viral DNA by inhibiting viral DNA polymerase, incorporating and terminating growing viral DNA chain, and inactivating viral DNA polymerase.

PHARMACOKINETICS: Absorption: Rapid (GI tract). Oral administration of variable doses resulted in different parameters. **Distribution:** Plasma protein binding (13.5-17.9%). **Metabolism:** Hepatic/Intestinal (1st pass). **Elimination:** Urine (45.6%), feces (47.12%); $T_{1/2}$=2.5-3.3 hrs.

VALTROPIN RX
somatropin (LG Life)

THERAPEUTIC CLASS: Human growth hormone

INDICATIONS: Treatment of pediatric patients who have growth failure due to inadequate secretion of endogenous growth hormone. Treatment of growth failure associated with Turner syndrome in pediatric patients who have open epiphyses. Long-term replacement therapy in adults with growth hormone deficiency (GHD) of either adult or childhood onset etiology

DOSAGE: *Adults:* Individualize dose. Initial: 0.33mg/day SQ 6 days a week. Dosage may be increased to individual patient requirement to maximum of 0.66mg/day after 4 weeks. Alternative Dosing: 0.2mg/day (Range: 0.15-0.3mg/day). May increase gradually every 1-2 months by 0.1-0.2mg/day based on individual patient requirements.
Pediatrics: Individualize dose. Divide weekly dose into equal amounts given either daily or 6 days a week by SQ injection. GHD: 0.17-0.3mg/kg of body weight/week. Turner Syndrome: Up to 0.375mg/kg of body weight/week.

HOW SUPPLIED: Inj: 5mg

CONTRAINDICATIONS: Pediatrics with closed epiphyses. Active proliferative and severe non-proliferative diabetic retinopathy. Presence of active malignancy. Acute critical illness due to complications following open heart surgery, abdominal surgery, or multiple accidental trauma, or those with acute respiratory failure. Patients with Prader-Willi syndrome who are severely obese or have severe respiratory impairment.

WARNINGS/PRECAUTIONS: Known sensitivity to supplied diluent (metacresol). Caution in pediatric pateints with Prader-Willi syndrome with 1 or more risk factors (severe obesity, history of upper airway destruction or sleep apnea, or unidentified respiratory infection). May decrease insulin sensitivity. Patients with GHD secondary to intracranial lesion should be monitered closely for progression or recurrence of underlying disease process. Intracranial HTN reported. Monitor closely with DM, glucose intolerance, hypopituitarism. Fundoscopic exam recommended at initiation and periodically during course of therapy. Monitor carefully for any malignant transformation of skin lesions.

ADVERSE REACTIONS: Headache, pyrexia, cough, respiratory tract infection, diarrhea, vomiting, pharyngitis.

INTERACTIONS: Growth-promoting effects may be inhibited by glucocorticoids. May alter clearance of compounds metabolized by CP450 liver enzymes (eg, corticosteroids, sex steroids, anticonvulsants, cyclosporine); monitor closely. May need insulin adjustment.

PREGNANCY: Category B, caution in nursing.

MECHANISM OF ACTION: Human growth hormone; stimulates linear growth synthesis, metabolizes lipids, reduces body fat stores by increasing cellular protein, and increases plasma fatty acids.

PHARMACOKINETICS: Absorption: C_{max}=43.97ng/mL, T_{max}=4 hrs, AUC=369.9ng•hr/mL. **Metabolism:** Liver, kidneys (protein catabolism). **Elimination:** $T_{1/2}$=3.03 hrs.

VANAMIDE RX
urea (Dermik)

THERAPEUTIC CLASS: Debriding/Healing Agent

INDICATIONS: Debridement and promotion of normal healing of surface lesions, particularly where healing is retarded by local infection, necrotic tissue, fibrinous or purulent debris, or eschar.

DOSAGE: *Adults*: Apply until absorbed. May cover with adhesive bandage or gauze. Keep dry and occlusive for 3-7 days.

HOW SUPPLIED: Cre: 40% [85g, 199g]

WARNINGS/PRECAUTIONS: Avoid contact with eyes. D/C if redness or irritation occurs.

ADVERSE REACTIONS: Transient stinging, burning, itching, irritation.

PREGNANCY: Safety in pregnancy or nursing not known.

MECHANISM OF ACTION: Keratolytic and emollient agent. Mechanism of action via topical route of administration not established. Responsible for dissolving the intercellular matrix, thereby softening hyperkeratotic areas by enhancing shedding of scales.

VANCOCIN ORAL RX
vancomycin HCL (Viro Pharma)

THERAPEUTIC CLASS: Tricyclic glycopeptide antibiotic

INDICATIONS: Treatment of enterocolitis caused by *Staphylococcus aureus* and antibiotic-associated pseudomembranous colitis caused by *C.difficile*.

DOSAGE: *Adults:* 500mg-2g/day given tid-qid for 7-10 days. *Pediatrics:* 40mg/kg/day given tid-qid for 7-10 days. Max: 2g/day.

HOW SUPPLIED: Cap: 125mg, 250mg

WARNINGS/PRECAUTIONS: Not effective for other types of infection. Caution with inflammatory disorders of intestinal mucosa, renal impairment; increased risk of systemic absorption. Ototoxicity reported. Monitor auditory function.

ADVERSE REACTIONS: Nephrotoxicity, ototoxicity, reversible neutropenia, anaphylactoid reactions (hypotension, wheezing, "Red Man Syndrome," pruritus), superinfection.

INTERACTIONS: Monitor renal function with aminoglycosides.

PREGNANCY: Category B, not for use in nursing.

MECHANISM OF ACTION: Tricyclic glycopeptide antibiotic; inhibits cell-wall biosynthesis, altering bacterial cell membrane permeabilty and RNA synthesis.

PHARMACOKINETICS: Absorption: Poor. **Elimination:** Urine, feces.

VANCOMYCIN INJECTION RX
vancomycin HCL (Various)

THERAPEUTIC CLASS: Tricyclic glycopeptide antibiotic

INDICATIONS: Treatment of serious or severe infections caused by susceptible strains of methicillin-resistant (β-lactam resistant) staphylococci.

Indicated for PCN-allergic patients, for patients who cannot receive or have failed to respond to other drugs, and for infections caused by vancomycin-susceptible organisms that are resistant to other antimicrobials. Indicated for initial therapy when methicillin-resistant staphylococci are suspected, but after susceptibility data are available, therapy should be adjusted accordingly. Effective in the treatment of staphylococcal endocarditis; effectiveness has been documented in other infections due to staphylococci, including septicemia, bone infections, lower respiratory tract infections, and skin and skin-structure infections. Reported to be effective alone or in combination with an aminoglycoside for endocarditis caused by *S.viridans* or *S.bovis*. Reported to be effective only in combination with an aminoglycoside for endocarditis caused by enterococci (eg, *E.faecalis*). Reported to be effective for treatment of diphtheroid endocarditis. Successfully used in combination with either rifampin, an aminoglycoside, or both in early-onset prosthetic valve endocarditis caused by *S.epidermidis* or diphtheroids. Parenteral form may be administered orally for treatment of antibiotic-associated pseudomembranous colitis produced by *C.difficile* and for staphylococcal enterocolitis.

DOSAGE: *Adults*: Inj: Usual: 500mg IV q6h or 1g IV q12h. Administer at not >10mg/min or over at least 60 min, whichever is longer. Max Conc: 5mg/mL. Max Rate: 10mg/min. Renal Impairment: Initial: Not <15mg/kg. Dosage per day in mg is about 15x the GFR in mL/min (refer to table in PI). Elderly: Require greater dose reductions than expected. Functionally Anephric: Initial: 15mg/kg, then 1.9mg/kg/24 hrs. Marked Renal Impairment: 250-1000mg every several days. Anuria: 1000mg every 7-10 days. PO: 500-2000mg/day in 3-4 divided doses for 7-10 days. Max: 2000mg/day. May dilute in 1oz of water. *Pediatrics*: Inj: Usual: 10mg/kg IV q6h. Infants/Neonates: Initial: 15mg/kg, then 10mg/kg q12h for neonates in 1st week of life and q8h thereafter until 1 month of age. Administer over at least 60 min. Renal Impairment: Initial: Not <15mg/kg. Dosage per day in mg is about 15x the GFR in mL/min (refer to table in PI). Premature Infants: Require greater dose reduction. ADD-Vantage vials should not be used in neonates, infants, and pediatrics who require doses <500mg. PO: 40mg/kg/day in 3-4 divided doses for 7-10 days. Max: 2000mg/day. May dilute in 1oz of water.

HOW SUPPLIED: Inj: 500mg, 1g, 5g, 500mg/100mL, 1g/200mL

WARNINGS/PRECAUTIONS: Rapid bolus administration may cause hypotension and cardiac arrest (rare); administer in diluted solution over ≥60 min. Frequency of infusion-related events may increase with concomitant use of anesthetic agents. Ototoxicity reported; monitor auditory function. Caution with renal insufficiency and adjust dose with renal dysfunction. Pseudomembranous colitis reported. Alters the normal flora of the colon and may permit overgrowth of clostridia. Prolonged use may result in overgrowth of nonsusceptible organisms. Reversible neutropenia reported; monitor leukocyte count. Administer via IV route; pain, avoid IM route. Thrombophlebitis may occur; rotate injection sites. Safety and efficacy of administration via the intraperitoneal and intrathecal (intralumbar and intraventricular) routes has not been established. Administration via intraperitoneal route during CAPD has resulted in a syndrome of chemical peritonitis. Adjust dosing schedules in elderly.

ADVERSE REACTIONS: Infusion-related events, hypotension, wheezing, pruritus, pain, chest and head muscle spasm, dyspnea, urticaria, "Red Man Syndrome," nephrotoxicity, pseudomembranous colitis, ototoxicity, neutropenia, phlebitis.

INTERACTIONS: Concomitant use of anesthetic agents has been associated with erythema, histamine-like flushing, and anaphylactoid reactions. Concurrent and/or sequential systemic or topical use of other potentially neurotoxic and/or nephrotoxic drugs (eg, amphotericin B, aminoglycosides, bacitracin, polymyxin B, colistin, viomycin, cisplatin) requires careful monitoring.

PREGNANCY: Category C, not for use in nursing.

MECHANISM OF ACTION: Tricyclic glycopeptide antibiotic; inhibits cell-wall biosynthesis, alters bacterial cell membrane permeability and RNA synthesis.

PHARMACOKINETICS: **Absorption:** (1g at 2 hrs) C_{max} =23mcg/mL; (500mg at 2 hrs) C_{max} = 19mcg/mL. **Distribution:** Serum protein binding (55%). **Elimination:** Urine (75% in 24 hrs); $T_{1/2}$=4-6 hrs.

VANDAZOLE RX
metronidazole (Upsher-Smith)

THERAPEUTIC CLASS: Imidazole antibacterial

INDICATIONS: Treatment of bacterial vaginosis in non-pregnant women.

DOSAGE: *Adults:* One applicator full intravaginally qd-bid for 5 days. For once daily dosing, administer at bedtime.

HOW SUPPLIED: Gel: 0.75% [70g]

CONTRAINDICATIONS: Hypersensitivity to other nitroimidazole derivatives.

WARNINGS/PRECAUTIONS: Caution with CNS or severe hepatic disease. D/C if abnormal neurologic signs appear. Avoid vaginal intercourse or use of other vaginal products during therapy. May develop *Candida* vaginitis. May interfere with lab tests (ALT, SGPT, AST, SGOT, LDH, triglycerides, and glucose hexokinase).

ADVERSE REACTIONS: Fungal infection, headache, pruritus, abdominal pain, nausea, dysmenorrhea.

INTERACTIONS: May potentiate warfarin and other courmarin anticoagulants. May elevate lithium levels. Cimetidine may prolong half-life and reduce clearance. Caution with alcohol; disulfiram-like reaction possible. Avoid within 2 weeks of discontinuing disulfiram therapy.

PREGNANCY: Category B, not for use in nursing.

VANIQA RX
eflornithine HCL (SkinMedica)

THERAPEUTIC CLASS: Ornithine decarboxylase inhibitor

INDICATIONS: Reduction of unwanted facial hair in women. Usage is limited to the face and areas under the chin.

DOSAGE: *Adults:* Apply to affected areas bid, at least 8 hrs apart. Rub in thoroughly. May wash area after 4 hrs. May apply 5 min after other hair removal techniques. May apply sunscreen or cosmetics after cream dries. *Pediatrics:* ≥12 yrs: Apply to affected areas bid, at least 8 hrs apart. Rub in thoroughly. May wash area after 4 hrs. May apply 5 min after other hair removal techniques. May apply sunscreen or cosmetics after cream dries.

HOW SUPPLIED: Cre: 13.9% [30g]

WARNINGS/PRECAUTIONS: D/C if hypersensitivity or continued irritation occurs. Transient stinging/burning with abraded/broken skin. Condition may return to pretreatment levels 8 weeks after discontinuation.

ADVERSE REACTIONS: Acne, stinging/tingling skin, burning/dry skin, pseudofolliculitis barbae, alopecia.

PREGNANCY: Category C, caution in nursing.

MECHANISM OF ACTION: Ornithine decarboxylase inhibitor; inhibits cell division and synthetic functions that effect the rate of hair growth (animal study).

PHARMACOKINETICS: Absorption: C_{max}=10ng/mL; AUC=92ng•hr/mL. **Elimination:** Urine (unchanged); $T_{1/2}$=8 hrs.

V

VANOS RX
fluocinonide (Medicis)

THERAPEUTIC CLASS: Corticosteroid

INDICATIONS: Corticosteroid-responsive dermatoses.

DOSAGE: *Adults:* Apply thin layer to affected area qd-bid. Max: 60g/week. Do not exceed 2 weeks.
Pediatrics: ≥12 yrs: Appy thin layer to affected area qd-bid. Max: 60g/week. Do not exceed 2 weeks.

HOW SUPPLIED: Cre: 0.1% [30g, 60g]

WARNINGS/PRECAUTIONS: May produce reversible HPA axis suppression, manifestations of Cushing's syndrome, hyperglycemia, and glucosuria. Caution when applied to large surface areas or under occlusive dressings. Use appropriate antifungal or antibacterial agent with dermatological infections. D/C if infection does not clear or irritation develops. Do not use for more than 2 weeks at a time.

ADVERSE REACTIONS: Headache, application site burning, nasopharyngitis, nasal congestion, unspecified application site reaction.

PREGNANCY: Category C, not for use in nursing.

MECHANISM OF ACTION: Corticosteroid; possesses anti-inflammatory, antipruritic, and vasoconstrictive properties. Anti-inflammatory activity not established; suspected to act by induction of phospholipase A_2 inhibitory proteins, lipocortins. Lipocortins control biosynthesis of potent inflammation mediators (eg, prostaglandins, leukotrienes) by inhibiting release of their common precursor, arachidonic acid.

PHARMACOKINETICS: Absorption: Percutaneous; inflammation and/or other disease states may increase absorption. **Distribution:** Systemically administered corticosteroids appear in breast milk.

VANTAS   RX
histrelin acetate (Indevus)

THERAPEUTIC CLASS: Luteinizing hormone releasing hormone agonist

INDICATIONS: Palliative treatment of advanced prostate cancer.

DOSAGE: *Adults:* 50mg every 12 months. Inject SQ into inner aspect of the upper arm. Refrain from wetting the inserted arm for 24 hours. Refrain from heavy lifting or strenuous exercise of the inserted arm for 7 days after implant insertion. Must remove after 12 months of therapy.

HOW SUPPLIED: Implant: 50mg

CONTRAINDICATIONS: Women and pediatric patients.

WARNINGS/PRECAUTIONS: Transient increase in serum testosterone and worsening of symptoms of prostate cancer with initial therapy. Urethral obstruction and spinal cord compression reported. Anaphylactic reactions may occur.

ADVERSE REACTIONS: Hot flashes, fatigue, implant site reaction, testicular atrophy, renal impairment, gynecomastia, constipation, erectile dysfunction.

PREGNANCY: Category X, not for use in nursing.

MECHANISM OF ACTION: LH-RH agonist; acts as potent inhibitor of gonadotropin secretion, desensitizes responsiveness of pituitary gonadotropin, causing reduction in testicular steroidogenesis.

PHARMACOKINETICS: Absorption: C_{max}=1.1ng/mL; T_{max}=12 hrs. **Distribution:** V_d=58.4L. **Elimination:** $T_{1/2}$=3.92 hrs.

VANTIN   RX
cefpodoxime proxetil (Pharmacia & Upjohn)

THERAPEUTIC CLASS: Cephalosporin (3rd generation)

INDICATIONS: Treatment of acute otitis media, pharyngitis/tonsillitis, community-acquired pneumonia (CAP), acute bacterial exacerbation of chronic bronchitis (ABECB), acute uncomplicated urethral and cervical gonorrhea, acute uncomplicated anorectal infections in women, uncomplicated skin and skin structure infections (SSSI), acute maxillary sinusitis, and uncomplicated urinary tract infections (UTI) caused by susceptible strains of microorganisms.

DOSAGE: *Adults:* Take tabs with food. Pharyngitis/Tonsillitis: 100mg q12h for 5-10 days. CAP: 200mg q12h for 14 days. ABECB: 200mg q12h for 10 days. Uncomplicated Gonorrhea (Men/Women)/Rectal Gonococcal Infections (Women): 200mg single dose. SSSI: 400mg q12h for 7-14 days. Sinusitis: 200mg q12h for 10 days. UTI: 100mg q12h for 7 days. CrCl <30mL/min: Increase interval to q24h. Hemodialysis: Dose 3 times weekly after dialysis. *Pediatrics:* ≥12 yrs: Take tabs with food. Pharyngitis/Tonsillitis: 100mg q12h for 5-10 days. CAP: 200mg q12h for 14 days. ABECB: 200mg q12h for 10 days. Uncomplicated Gonorrhea (Men/Women)/Rectal Gonococcal Infections (Women): 200mg single dose. SSSI: 400mg q12h for 7-14 days. Sinusitis: 200mg q12h for 10 days. UTI: 100mg q12h for 7 days. 2 months-12 yrs: Otitis Media: 5mg/kg q12h for 5 days. Max: 200mg/dose. Pharyngitis/Tonsillitis: 5mg/kg q12h for 5-10 days. Max: 100mg/dose. Sinusitis: 5mg/kg q12h for 10 days. Max: 200mg/dose. CrCl <30mL/min: Increase interval to q24h. Hemodialysis: Dose 3 times weekly after dialysis.

HOW SUPPLIED: Sus: 50mg/5mL [50mL, 75mL, 100mL], 100mg/5mL [50mL, 75mL, 100mL]; Tab: 100mg, 200mg

WARNINGS/PRECAUTIONS: Cross-sensitivity to PCNs and other cephalosporins may occur. *Clostridium difficile*-associated diarrhea reported. Positive direct Coombs' tests reported. Caution with renal impairment; dose reduction may be needed. May result in overgrowth of nonsusceptible organisms.

ADVERSE REACTIONS: Diarrhea, nausea.

INTERACTIONS: Decreased plasma levels and absorption with antacids and H_2-blockers. Delayed peak plasma levels with anticholinergics. Probenecid inhibits renal excretion. Closely monitor renal function with nephrotoxic agents. Caution with potent diuretics.

PREGNANCY: Category B, not for use in nursing.

MECHANISM OF ACTION: Cephalosporin; inhibits cell wall synthesis.

PHARMACOKINETICS: Absorption: C_{max}(100mg)=1.4mcg/mL, T_{max}=2-3 hrs. **Distribution:** Plasma protein binding (22-31%). **Metabolism:** Via desterification. **Elimination:** Urine; $T_{1/2}$= 2.09-2.84 hrs.

VAPRISOL   RX
conivaptan HCL (Astellas)

THERAPEUTIC CLASS: Arginine vasopressin antagonist

INDICATIONS: Treatment of euvolemic hyponatremia in hospitalized patients.

DOSAGE: *Adults:* IV use only. Use large veins and change infusion site every 24 hrs. Loading Dose: 20mg IV over 30 min. Follow with 20mg continuous IV over 24 hrs. Following initial day of treatment, administer for an additional 1-3 days in continuous infusion of 20mg/day. Titrate: May increase to 40mg/day if needed. Total duration of infusion should not exceed 4 days.

HOW SUPPLIED: Inj: 5mg/mL

CONTRAINDICATIONS: Hypovolemic hyponatremia. Concurrent potent CYP3A4 inhibitors (eg, ketoconazole, itraconazole, clarithromycin, ritonavir, and indinavir).

WARNINGS/PRECAUTIONS: Safety in CHF not established. Monitor sodium concentration and neurologic status during administration; d/c if rapid rise in serum sodium. Caution with hepatic or renal impairment. Rotate infusion site every 24 hrs.

ADVERSE REACTIONS: Infusion site reactions, erythema/pain/phlebitis at infusion site, anemia, constipation, diarrhea, dry mouth, nausea, vomiting, peripheral edema, pyrexia, thirst, hypokalemia, headache, cardiac failure, atrial dyrthythmias, and sepsis.

INTERACTIONS: See Contraindications. CYP3A4 inhibitors may increase levels. May increase levels of drugs primarily metabolized by CYP3A4 and digoxin.

PREGNANCY: Category C, caution in nursing.

MECHANISM OF ACTION: Nonpeptide dual antagonist of arginine vasopressin (AVP) V_{1A} and V_2 receptors.

PHARMACOKINETICS: Absorption: C_{max}=619ng/mL. **Distribution:** >99% protein bound; crosses the placenta. **Metabolism:** CYP3A4; Four metabolites formed (minimal effect). **Elimination:** Urine (12%), feces (83%). $T_{1/2}$=5 hrs.

Vaqta RX
hepatitis A vaccine (inactivated) (Merck)

THERAPEUTIC CLASS: Vaccine

INDICATIONS: Active immunization against hepatitis A virus in persons 12 months of age and older. Give primary immunization at least 2 weeks before expected exposure.

DOSAGE: *Adults:* ≥19 yrs: 1mL (50 U) IM followed by a booster of 1mL (50 U) 6-18 months later.
Pediatrics: 1-18 yrs: 0.5mL (25 U) IM followed by a booster of 0.5mL (25 U) 6-18 months later.

HOW SUPPLIED: Inj: 25 U/0.5mL, 50 U/mL

WARNINGS/PRECAUTIONS: Have epinephrine (1:1000) available. May not prevent hepatitis A with unrecognized infection. Caution with bleeding disorders. Defer use with acute infection or febrile illness. Suboptimal response may occur in immunocompromised patients.

ADVERSE REACTIONS: Injection-site pain, tenderness, erythema, swelling, warmth, fever.

INTERACTIONS: Immunosuppressive therapy may reduce response to active immunization.

PREGNANCY: Category C, caution in nursing.

MECHANISM OF ACTION: Vaccine; produces an antibody response against hepatitis A virus.

Varivax RX
varicella virus vaccine live (Merck)

THERAPEUTIC CLASS: Vaccine

INDICATIONS: Vaccination against varicella.

DOSAGE: *Adults:* 0.5mL SQ at elected date, repeat 4-8 weeks later.
Pediatrics: 12 months-12 yrs: 0.5mL SQ. ≥13 yrs: 0.5mL SQ at elected date, repeat 4-8 weeks later.

HOW SUPPLIED: Inj: 1350PFU/0.5mL

CONTRAINDICATIONS: Pregnancy (avoid pregnancy for 3 months after vaccine); gelatin hypersensitivity; anaphylactoid reactions to neomycin, blood dyscrasias, leukemia, lymphomas, malignant neoplasms affecting bone marrow or lymphatic system, febrile infection, active untreated TB, immunosuppressive therapy, immunosuppressant doses of corticosteroids, immunodeficiency states.

WARNINGS/PRECAUTIONS: Children and adolescents with ALL in remission can receive the vaccine under an investigational protocol. Defer vaccine for at least 5 months after blood or plasma transfusions, or administration of immune globulin or varicella zoster immune globulin. Defer vaccine with family history of congenital, hereditary immunodeficiency until immune system evaluated. Rarely, vaccine virus transmission through varicella-like rash can occur; avoid close association with susceptible high-risk individuals for up to six weeks (eg, immunocompromised patients, pregnant women without history of chickenpox, newborns of mothers without documented history of chickenpox). Have epinephrine available.

ADVERSE REACTIONS: Fever, local reactions, pain, varicella-like rashes.

INTERACTIONS: Avoid immune globulins for 2 months after vaccination. Avoid salicylates for 6 weeks after vaccination. Contraindicated with immuno-suppressive therapy or immunosuppressant doses of corticosteroids.

PREGNANCY: Category C, contraindicated in pregnancy and caution in nursing.

MECHANISM OF ACTION: Vaccine; cell-mediated immune response stimulation against varicella zoster virus (VZV) infection.

VASERETIC   RX
enalapril maleate - hydrochlorothiazide (Merck)

> ACE inhibitors can cause death/injury to developing fetus during 2nd and 3rd trimesters. Stop therapy if pregnancy detected.

THERAPEUTIC CLASS: ACE inhibitor/thiazide diuretic

INDICATIONS: Treatment of hypertension. Not for initial therapy.

DOSAGE: *Adults:* Initial (if not controlled with enalapril/HCTZ monotherapy): 5mg-12.5mg tab or 10mg-25mg tab qd. Titrate: May increase after 2-3 weeks. Max: 20mg enalapril/50mg HCTZ per day. Replacement Therapy: Substitute combination for titrated components.

HOW SUPPLIED: Tab: (Enalapril-HCTZ) 5mg-12.5mg, 10mg-25mg

CONTRAINDICATIONS: History of ACE inhibitor-associated angioedema and hereditary or idiopathic angioedema. Anuria, sulfonamide hypersensitivity.

WARNINGS/PRECAUTIONS: D/C if angioedema, jaundice, or if marked LFT elevation occurs. Risk of hyperkalemia with DM, renal dysfunction. Persistent nonproductive cough reported. Monitor WBCs in renal and collagen vascular disease. Anaphylactoid reactions reported. Fetal/neonatal morbidity and death reported. Monitor for hypotension in high-risk patients (surgery/ anesthesia, hyponatremia, severe volume/salt depletion, etc). Caution with CHF, renal or hepatic dysfunction, obstruction to left ventricle outflow tract, elderly, renal artery stenosis. More reports of angioedema in blacks than nonblacks. May exacerbate or activate SLE. Monitor serum electrolytes. Avoid if CrCl ≤30mL/min/1.73m^2. May increase cholesterol, TG, uric acid levels, and blood glucose. Intestinal angioedema reported.

ADVERSE REACTIONS: Dizziness, cough, fatigue, orthostatic effects, diarrhea, nausea, muscle cramps, asthenia, impotence.

INTERACTIONS: Increase risk of hyperkalemia with K$^+$-sparing diuretics, K$^+$ supplements, or K$^+$-containing salt substitutes. Potentiates orthostatic hypotension with alcohol, barbiturates, and narcotics. Adjust insulin and antidiabetic drugs. Impaired absorption with cholestyramine, colestipol. Corticosteroids and ACTH deplete electrolytes. May decrease response to pressor amines. Potentiates other antihypertensives. May increase responsiveness to skeletal muscle relaxants. Risk of lithium toxicity. NSAIDs may reduce antihypertensive effect and worsen renal dysfunction.

PREGNANCY: Category C (1st trimester) and D (2nd and 3rd trimesters), not for use in nursing.

MECHANISM OF ACTION: Enalapril: ACE inhibitor; inhibition results in decreased plasma angiotensin II, which leads to decreased vasopressor activity and decreased aldosterone secretion. HCTZ: Thiazide diuretic; affects renal tubular mechanism of electrolyte reabsorption directly increasing excretion of Na$^+$ and chloride.

PHARMACOKINETICS: Absorption: T$_{max}$ (enalapril, enalaprilat)=(1, 3-4 hrs). **Distribution:** HCTZ: Crosses placental barrier. **Metabolism:** Via hydrolysis; Enalaprilat (metabolite). **Elimination:** Urine, feces; T$_{1/2}$ (enalaprilat)=11 hrs. HCTZ: Kidneys; T$_{1/2}$= 5.6-14.8 hrs.

V

VASOCON-A   OTC
naphazoline HCL - antazoline phosphate (Novartis Ophthalmics)

THERAPEUTIC CLASS: Antihistamine/decongestant

INDICATIONS: Temporary relief of minor allergic symptoms of the eye, including itching and redness due to pollen and animal hair.

DOSAGE: *Adults:* 1-2 drops prn. Max: 4 doses/day.
Pediatrics: >6 yrs: 1-2 drops prn. Max: 4 doses/day.

HOW SUPPLIED: Sol: (Antazoline-Naphazoline) 0.5%-0.05% [15mL]

WARNINGS/PRECAUTIONS: Do not use if solution changes color or becomes cloudy. D/C if develop eye pain, vision changes, redness or irritaton continues, or if condition worsens or persists >72hrs. Supervision required with heart disease, HTN, or narrow angle glaucoma.

PREGNANCY: Safety in pregnancy and nursing not known.

VASOTEC   RX
enalapril maleate (Merck)

> ACE inhibitors can cause death/injury to developing fetus during 2nd and 3rd trimesters. Stop therapy if pregnancy detected.

THERAPEUTIC CLASS: ACE inhibitor

INDICATIONS: Treatment of hypertension. Treatment of symptomatic CHF usually in combination with diuretics and digitalis. To decrease overt heart failure development and hospitalization in stable asymptomatic left ventricular dysfunction.

DOSAGE: *Adults:* HTN: If possible, d/c diuretic 2-3 days prior to therapy. Initial: 5mg qd, 2.5mg qd with concomitant diuretic. Usual: 10-40mg/day given qd or bid. Resume diuretic if BP not controlled. CrCl ≤30mL/min: Initial: 2.5mg/day. Dialysis: 2.5mg/day on dialysis days. Heart Failure: Initial: 2.5mg/day. Usual: 2.5-20mg given bid. Max: 40mg/day. Left Ventricular Dysfunction: Initial: 2.5mg bid. Titrate: Increase to 20mg/day. Hyponatremia or SrCr 1.6mg/dL with Heart Failure: Initial: 2.5mg qd. Titrate: Increase to 2.5mg bid, then 5mg bid. Max: 40mg/day.
Pediatrics: HTN: 1 month-16 yrs: Initial: 0.08mg/kg (up to 5mg) qd. Titrate: Adjust according to response. Max: 0.58mg/kg/dose (or 40mg/dose). Avoid if GFR <30mL/min/1.73m². (To prepare 200mL of 1mg/mL sus: Add 50mL of Bicitra® to polyethylene terephthalate bottle with ten 20mg tabs and shake for at least 2 min. Let stand for 60 min, then shake again for 1 min. Add 150mL of Ora-Sweet SF™ and shake, then refrigerate. Can store up to 30 days.)

HOW SUPPLIED: Tab: 2.5mg*, 5mg*, 10mg, 20mg *scored

CONTRAINDICATIONS: History of ACE inhibitor associated angioedema and hereditary or idiopathic angioedema.

WARNINGS/PRECAUTIONS: D/C if angioedema, jaundice, or if marked LFT elevation occurs. Risk of hyperkalemia with DM, renal dysfunction. Persistent nonproductive cough reported. Monitor WBCs in renal or collagen vascular disease. Anaphylactoid reactions reported. Fetal/neonatal morbidity and death reported. Monitor for hypotension in high-risk patients (heart failure, surgery/anesthesia, hyponatremia, high-dose diuretic therapy, severe volume and/or salt depletion, etc). Caution with CHF, obstruction to left ventricle outflow tract, renal dysfunction, and renal artery stenosis. Less effective on BP in blacks and more reports of angioedema than nonblacks. Intestinal angioedema reported.

ADVERSE REACTIONS: Fatigue, orthostatic effects, asthenia, diarrhea, nausea, headache, dizziness, cough, rash, hypotension, vomiting.

INTERACTIONS: May increase lithium levels. Hypotension risk with diuretics. May further decrease renal dysfunction with NSAIDs. Increase risk of hyperkalemia with K⁺-sparing diuretics, K⁺-containing salt substitutes or K⁺

V

supplements. Augmented effect by antihypertensives that cause renin release (eg, thiazides). NSAIDs may diminish antihypertensive effect.

PREGNANCY: Category C (1st trimester) and D (2nd and 3rd trimesters), not for use in nursing.

MECHANISM OF ACTION: ACE inhibitor; inhibition results in decreased plasma angiotensin II, which leads to decreased vasopressor activity and decreased aldosterone secretion.

PHARMACOKINETICS: Absorption: T_{max}=1, 3-4 hrs (enalapril, enalaprilat). **Metabolism:** Via hydrolysis, enalaprilat (metabolite). **Elimination:** Urine, feces; $T_{1/2}$=11 hrs (enalaprilat).

VASOTEC I.V. RX
enalaprilat (Merck)

> ACE inhibitors can cause death/injury to developing fetus during 2nd and 3rd trimesters. Stop therapy if pregnancy detected.

THERAPEUTIC CLASS: ACE inhibitor

INDICATIONS: Treatment of hypertension when oral therapy is not practical.

DOSAGE: *Adults:* Administer IV over 5 min. Usual: 1.25mg q6h for no longer than 48 hrs. Max: 20mg/day. Concomitant Diuretic/CrCl ≤30mL/min: Initial: 0.625mg, may repeat after 1 hr. Maint: 1.25mg q6h. Risk of Excessive Hypotension: Initial: 0.625mg over 5 min to 1 hr. PO/IV Conversion: Give 5mg/day PO for 1.25mg IV q6h and 2.5mg/day PO for 0.625mg q6h IV.

HOW SUPPLIED: Inj: 1.25mg/mL

CONTRAINDICATIONS: History of ACE inhibitor associated angioedema and hereditary or idiopathic angioedema.

WARNINGS/PRECAUTIONS: D/C if angioedema, jaundice, or if marked LFT elevation occurs. Risk of hyperkalemia with DM, renal dysfunction. Persistent nonproductive cough reported. Monitor WBCs in renal or collagen vascular disease. Anaphylactoid reactions reported. Fetal/neonatal morbidity and death reported. Monitor for hypotension in high risk patients (heart failure, surgery/anesthesia, hyponatremia, high dose diuretic therapy, severe volume and/or salt depletion, etc). Caution with CHF, obstruction to left ventricle outflow tract, renal dysfunction, and renal artery stenosis. Less effective on BP in blacks and more reports of angioedema than nonblacks.

ADVERSE REACTIONS: Hypotension, headache, angioedema, myocardial infarction, fatigue, dizziness, fever, rash, constipation, cough.

INTERACTIONS: May increase lithium levels. Hypotension risk with diuretics. May further decrease renal dysfunction with NSAIDs. Increase risk of hyperkalemia with K^+-sparing diuretics, K^+-containing salt substitutes or K^+ supplements. Augmented effect by antihypertensives that cause renin release (eg, thiazides). NSAIDs may diminish antihypertensive effect.

PREGNANCY: Category C (1st trimester) and D (2nd and 3rd trimesters), not for use in nursing.

MECHANISM OF ACTION: ACE inhibitor; inhibition results in decreased plasma angiotensin II, which leads to decreased vasopressor activity and decreased aldosterone secretion.

PHARMACOKINETICS: Absorption: (PO) Poorly absorbed. **Elimination:** Urine (90% unchanged); $T_{1/2}$=11 hrs.

V

VECTIBIX RX
panitumumab (Amgen)

> Dermatologic toxicities and severe infusion reactions reported; d/c if severe dermatologic or infusion reaction occurs.

THERAPEUTIC CLASS: Monoclonal antibody/EGFR-blocker

INDICATIONS: Treatment of EGFR-expressing, metastatic colorectal carcinoma with disease progression on or following fluoropyrimidine-, oxaliplatin-, and irinotecan-containing chemotherapy regimens.

DOSAGE: *Adults:* 6mg/kg IV infusion over 60 min every 14 days. Infuse doses >1000mg over 90 min. Reduce infusion rate by 50% with mild or moderate (Grade 1 or 2) infusion reaction for duration of that infusion. Immediately and permanently d/c infusion with severe (Grade 3 or 4) infusion reactions. Withhold for dermatologic toxicities that are ≥Grade 3 or considered intolerable. If toxicity does not improve to ≤Grade 2 within 1 month, permanently d/c. If dermatologic toxicity improves to ≤Grade 2 and symptoms improve after withholding no more than 2 doses, treatment may be resumed at 50% of original dose. If toxicities recur, permanently d/c. If toxicities do not recur, subsequent doses may be increased by increments of 25% of original dose until recommended dose of 6mg/kg is reached.

HOW SUPPLIED: Inj: 20mg/mL

WARNINGS/PRECAUTIONS: See Black Box Warning. Toxicity involving GI mucosa, eye, and nail reported. Pulmonary fibrosis reported; d/c with interstitial lung disease, pneumonitis, or lung infiltrates. Diarrhea may occur; incidence and severity may increase when used in combination with irinotecan. Use with leucovorin not recommended. Hypomagnesemia and hypocalcemia reported; monitor electrolytes during and for 8 weeks following therapy. Sunlight may exacerbate any skin reactions that may occur; use sunscreen and/or hats and limit sun exposure during therapy. Detection of EGFR protein expression is necessary for selection of appropriate patients. Avoid in combination with chemotherapy with or without bevacizumab.

ADVERSE REACTIONS: Rash, hypomagnesemia, paronychia, fatigue, abdominal pain, nausea, diarrhea, constipation, vomiting, erythema, acneiform dermatitis, pruritus, skin exfoliation, skin fissures, cough.

PREGNANCY: Category C, not for use in nursing.

MECHANISM OF ACTION: IgG2 kappa monoclonal antibody; binds specifically to epidermal growth factor receptor (EGFR) on both normal and tumor cells, and competitively inhibits binding of ligands for EGFR.

PHARMACOKINETICS: Absorption: C_{max}=213mcg/mL, AUC=1306mcg•day/mL. **Elimination:** $T_{1/2}$=7.5 days.

VELCADE   RX
bortezomib (Millennium)

THERAPEUTIC CLASS: Proteasome inhibitor

INDICATIONS: Treatment of multiple myeloma and mantle cell lymphoma in patients who have received at least 1 prior therapy.

DOSAGE: *Adults:* Initial 1.3mg/m²/dose IV bolus twice weekly for 2 weeks (Days 1, 4, 8, and 11) followed by a 10-day rest period (Days 12-21). At least 72 hrs should elapse between consecutive doses. Grade 3 Non-Hematological/Grade 4 Hematological Toxicities (excluding neuropathy): Withhold therapy until symptoms of toxcitiy resolve. Reinitiate at 25% reduced dose. Peripheral Neuropathy: Grade 1 with pain or Grade 2 (interfering with function but not activities of daily living): Reduce dose to 1mg/m². Grade 2 with pain or Grade 3 (interfering with activities of daily living): Withhold dose until toxicity resolves. Reinitiate at 0.7mg/m² once weekly. Grade 4 (permanent sensory loss interfering with funtion): D/C therapy.

HOW SUPPLIED: Inj: 3.5mg

CONTRAINDICATIONS: Hypersensitivity to boron or mannitol.

WARNINGS/PRECAUTIONS: Avoid pregnancy. May cause or worsen peripheral neuropathy along with reports of severe sensory and motor peripheral neuropathy. Thrombocytopenia and neutropenia reported; monitor CBC and platelets frequently. May cause orthostatic/postural hypotension; caution with history of syncope or dehydration. May cause acute development or exacerbation of CHF and/or new onset of decreased left ventricular ejection fraction. Rare reports of acute diffuse infiltrative pulmonary disease of unknown etiology such as pneumonitis, interstitial pneumonia, lung infiltration and ARDS. May cause nausea, diarrhea, constipation, and vomiting; use of antiemetic and antidiarrheal medications may be necessary. Rare reports of Reversible Posterior Leukoencephalopathy syndrome. May cause tumor lysis syndrome. Hepatic impairment may decrease clearance. Closely monitor if CrCl <13mL/min or on hemodialysis. Patients on oral antidiabetic agents may require close monitoring of blood glucose levels. Monitor CBC frequently. Dosing adjustments not necessary for patients with renal impairment. Should be administered after dialysis procedure.

ADVERSE REACTIONS: Asthenic disorders, diarrhea, nausea, constipation, peripheral neuropathy, vomiting, pyrexia, thrombocytopenia, psychiatric disorders, anorexia/decreased appetite, paresthesia/dysesthesia, anemia, headache, cough, dyspnea.

INTERACTIONS: Caution with concomitant use of medications associated with peripheral neuropathy (eg, amiodarone, antivirals, isoniazid, nitrofurantoin, statins) or hypotension. Oral antidiabetic agents may require dosage adjustment. Caution with CYP3A4 inducers and inhibitors; may alter levels.

PREGNANCY: Category D, not for use in nursing.

MECHANISM OF ACTION: Proteasome inhibitor; inhibits chymotrypsin-like activity of 26S proteosome cell.

PHARMACOKINETICS: Absorption: (Twice weekly: 1mg/m²; 1.3mg/m²) C_{max}=67-106ng/mL; 89-120ng/mL. **Distribution:** V_d=498-1884L/m²; plasma protein binding (83%). **Metabolism:** Oxidation via CYP3A4, 2C19, 1A2; 2D6, 2C9 (minor). Deboronation (major). **Elimination:** (1mg/m²; 1.3mg/m²) $T_{1/2}$=40-193 hrs; 76-108 hrs.

VENOFER   RX
iron sucrose (American Regent)

THERAPEUTIC CLASS: Iron supplement

INDICATIONS: Treatment of iron deficiency anemia in the following patients: non-dialysis dependent chronic kidney disease (NDD-CKD) patients receiving and not receiving erythropoietin, hemodialysis dependent chronic kidney disease (HDD-CKD) patients receiving an erythropoietin; peritoneal dialysis dependent chronic kidney disease (PDD-CKD) patients receiving an erythropoietin.

DOSAGE: *Adults:* HDD-CKD: 100mg IV inj over 2-5 min or 100mg infusion over at least 15 min per consecutive HD session for a total cumulative dose of 1000mg. NDD-CKD: 1000mg over a 14-day period as a 200mg slow IV inj undiluted over 2-5 min on 5 different occasions within the 14-day period. PDD-CKD: 1000mg slow IV infusion in 3 divided doses within a 28-day period (2 infusions of 300mg over 1.5 hrs 14 days apart, then 400mg infusion over 2.5 hrs 14 days later).

HOW SUPPLIED: Inj: 20mg/mL

CONTRAINDICATIONS: Iron overload, anemia not caused by iron deficiency.

WARNINGS/PRECAUTIONS: Fatal hypersensitivity reactions characterized by anaphylactic shock, collapse, hypotension, and dyspnea reported. Caution with administration; hypotension may occur. Monitor hematologic and hematinic parameters periodically.

ADVERSE REACTIONS: Headache, fever, pain, asthenia, malaise, hypotension, chest pain, HTN, hypervolemia, nausea, vomiting, elevated LFTs, dizziness, cramps, musculoskeletal pain, dyspnea, cough, pruritus, application site reaction.

INTERACTIONS: Avoid oral iron preparations.

PREGNANCY: Category B, caution in nursing.

MECHANISM OF ACTION: Hematinic.

PHARMACOKINETICS: Distribution: Liver, spleen, and bone marrow; V_d=10.0L (non-steady state), 7.9L (steady state). **Metabolism:** Dissociation via reticuloendothelial system. **Elimination:** $T_{1/2}$=6 hrs; urine (5%).

VENTAVIS   RX
iloprost (Actelion)

THERAPEUTIC CLASS: Systemic and pulmonary arterial vasulcar bed dilator

INDICATIONS: Treatment of pulmonary arterial hypertension (WHO Group I) in patients with NYHA Class III or IV symptoms.

DOSAGE: *Adults:* Initial: 2.5mcg via Prodose AAD System. Maint: 5mcg. Max: 45mcg/day. Should be taken 6 to 9 times per day.

HOW SUPPLIED: Sol, Inhalation: 20mcg/2mL

WARNINGS/PRECAUTIONS: Risk of syncope and hypotension. If signs of pulmonary edema occur when inhaled iloprost is administered, the treamtent should be immediately stopped. Avoid oral ingestion and contact with skin or eyes. Administration only via I-neb® AAD or Prodose® AAD System.

ADVERSE REACTIONS: Vasodilation, increased cough, headache, trismus, insomnia, nausea, hypotension, vomiting, flu syndrome, back pain, syncope, palpitations, muscle cramps, increased GGT, increased alk phos.

INTERACTIONS: Iloprost has the potential to increase the hypotensive effect of vasodilators and antihypertensive agents. Increased risk of bleeding with anticoagulants.

PREGNANCY: Category C, not recommended in nursing.

MECHANISM OF ACTION: Synthetic prostacyclin PGI_2 analogue; dilates systemic and pulmonary arterial vascular beds. Affects platelet aggregation.

PHARMACOKINETICS: Absorption: C_{max}=150pg/mL. **Distribution:** V_d=0.7-0.08L/kg; Plasma protein binding (60%). **Metabolism:** β-oxidation. Tetranor-iloprost (main metabolite). **Elimination:** Urine (68%), feces (12%).

VENTOLIN HFA   RX
albuterol sulfate (GlaxoSmithKline)

THERAPEUTIC CLASS: $Beta_2$-agonist

INDICATIONS: Prevention and treatment of bronchospasm with reversible obstructive airway disease. Prevention of Exercise-Induced Bronchospasm (EIB).

DOSAGE: *Adults:* Bronchospasm: 2 inh q4-6h or 1 inh q4h. EIB: 2 inh 15-30 min before activity.
Pediatrics: ≥4 yrs: Bronchospasm: 2 inh q4-6h or 1 inh q4h. EIB: 2 inh 15-30 min before activity.

HOW SUPPLIED: MDI: 90mcg/inh [18g]

WARNINGS/PRECAUTIONS: D/C if paradoxical bronchospasm or cardiovascular events occur. Avoid excessive use. Caution with coronary insufficiency, arrhythmias, HTN, DM, hyperthyroidism, seizures, sensitivity to sympathomimetics. Hypersensitivity reactions may occur. May cause transient hypokalemia.

ADVERSE REACTIONS: Throat irritation, viral respiratory infections, upper respiratory inflammation, cough, musculoskeletal pain.

INTERACTIONS: Avoid other short-acting sympathomimetic bronchodilators; caution with oral sympathomimetics. Extreme caution with MAOIs, TCAs during or within 2 weeks of discontinuation. May cause severe bronchospasm with β-blockers. Decreases digoxin levels. ECG changes and/or hypokalemia with nonpotassium-sparing diuretics.

PREGNANCY: Category C, not for use in nursing.

MECHANISM OF ACTION: $β_2$-adrenergic bronchodilator; stimulates adenyl cyclase, the enzyme that catalyzes formation of cAMP from ATP. Increased cAMP levels associated with relaxation of bronchial smooth muscle and inhibition of release of mediators of immediate hypersensitivity.

PHARMACOKINETICS: Absorption: C_{max}=3ng/mL, T_{max}=0.42 hrs.

VERAMYST
fluticasone furoate (GlaxoSmithKline)
RX

THERAPEUTIC CLASS: Corticosteroid

INDICATIONS: Treatment of the symptoms of seasonal and perennial allergic rhinitis in patients ≥2 yrs.

DOSAGE: *Adults:* Initial: 2 sprays per nostril qd. Maint: 1 spray per nostril qd. *Pediatrics:* ≥12 yrs: Initial: 2 sprays per nostril qd. Maint: 1 spray per nostril qd. 2-11 yrs: Initial: 1 spray per nostril qd. Titrate: If inadequate response, may increase to 2 sprays per nostril.

HOW SUPPLIED: Spray: 27.5mcg/spray [10g]

WARNINGS/PRECAUTIONS: Excessive use may cause hypercorticism and adrenal suppression. Risk of adrenal insufficiency and withdrawal symptoms when replacing systemic corticosteroids with topical corticosteroids. Caution with active or quiescent TB, ocular herpes simplex, or untreated bacterial, fungal, and systemic viral infections. Risk for more severe/fatal course of infections (eg, chickenpox, measles); avoid exposure in patients who have not had disease or have not been properly immunized. Epistaxis and nasal ulcerations may occur. Candida infection of nose reported. Avoid with recent nasal trauma, ulcers, or surgery. May result in glaucoma and cataracts. Potential for growth velocity reduction in pediatrics.

ADVERSE REACTIONS: Headache, epistaxis, nasopharyngitis, pyrexia, pharynolaryngeal pain, cough, nasal ulceration, back pain.

INTERACTIONS: Ketoconazole or other potent CYP3A4 inhibitors may increase serum fluticasone levels; co-administer with caution. Increased levels with ritonavir; avoid use.

PREGNANCY: Category C, caution in nursing.

MECHANISM OF ACTION: Corticosteroid; unknown. Anti-inflammatory agent with wide range of effects on multiple cell types (eg, mast cells, eosinophils, neutrophils, macrophages, lymphocytes) and mediators (eg, histamine, eicosanoids, cytokines, leukotrienes) involved in inflammation.

PHARMACOKINETICS: Absorption: Incomplete absorption, absolute bioavailability (0.5%). **Distribution:** Plasma protein binding (99%). **Metabolism:** Hepatic (extensive) via CYP3A4. **Elimination:** Feces.

VERDESO
desonide (Stiefel)
RX

THERAPEUTIC CLASS: Corticosteroid

INDICATIONS: Mild to moderate atopic dermatitis.

DOSAGE: *Adults:* Apply thin layer to affected area(s) bid. Max Duration: 4 consecutive weeks. Not to dispense directly on face; use hands to gently massage. Avoid occlusive dressings.
Pediatrics: ≥3 months: Apply thin layer to affected area(s) bid. Max Duration: 4 consecutive weeks. Not to dispense directly on face; use hands to gently massage. Avoid occlusive dressings.

HOW SUPPLIED: Foam: 0.05% [50g, 100g]

WARNINGS/PRECAUTIONS: May produce reversible HPA axis suppression, manifestations of Cushing's syndrome, hyperglycemia, and glucosuria. D/C if irritation occurs. Caution when applied to large surface areas. Pediatrics may be more susceptible to systemic toxicity. Use appropriate antifungal or antibacterial with concomitant skin infections; d/c if infection does not clear.

ADVERSE REACTIONS: Application site burning, upper respiratory tract infection, cough.

PREGNANCY: Category C, caution in nursing.

MECHANISM OF ACTION: Corticosteroid; possesses anti-inflammatory, antipruritic, and vasoconstrictive properties. Anti-inflammatory activity not

V

established. Suspected to act by induction of phospholipase A_2 inhibitory proteins, lipocortins. Lipocortins control biosynthesis of potent mediators of inflammation (eg, prostaglandins, leukotrienes) by inhibiting release of their common precursor, arachidonic acid.

PHARMACOKINETICS: Absorption: Percutaneous; occlusion, inflammation, and other disease states may increase absorption. **Distribution:** Systemically administered corticosteroids found in breast milk. **Metabolism:** Liver. **Elimination:** Kidneys (major), bile.

VERELAN   RX
verapamil HCL (Schwarz)

THERAPEUTIC CLASS: Calcium channel blocker (nondihydropyridine)

INDICATIONS: Management of hypertension.

DOSAGE: *Adults:* Usual: 240mg qam. Titrate: May increase by 120mg qam. Max: 480mg qam. Elderly/Small People: Initial: 120mg qam. Titrate: May increase to 180mg qam, then 240mg qam, then 360mg qam, then 480mg qam. May sprinkle on applesauce; do not crush or chew.

HOW SUPPLIED: Cap, Extended-Release: 120mg, 180mg, 240mg, 360mg

CONTRAINDICATIONS: Severe ventricular dysfunction, hypotension, cardiogenic shock, sick sinus syndrome or 2nd- or 3rd-degree AV block (except with functioning ventricular pacemaker), A-Fib/Flutter with an accessory bypass tract.

WARNINGS/PRECAUTIONS: Avoid with moderate to severe cardiac failure, and ventricular dysfunction if taking a β-blocker. May cause hypotension, AV block, transient bradycardia, PR interval prolongation. Monitor LFTs periodically; hepatocellular injury reported. Give 30% of normal dose with severe hepatic dysfunction. Caution with hypertrophic cardiomyopathy, renal or hepatic dysfunction. Decrease dose in those with decreased neuromuscular transmission

ADVERSE REACTIONS: Constipation, dizziness, nausea, hypotension, headache, peripheral edema, infection, flu syndrome, fatigue, bradycardia, AV block.

INTERACTIONS: Additive negative effects on HR, AV conduction, and contractility with β-blockers. Potentiates other antihypertensives. May increase digoxin, carbamazepine, theophylline, cyclosporine, and alcohol levels. Avoid disopyramide within 48 hrs before or 24 hrs after verapamil. Additive negative inotropic effects and AV conduction prolongation with flecainide. Avoid quinidine with hypertrophic cardiomyopathy. Monitor lithium levels. Increased clearance with phenobarbital. Rifampin may reduce oral bioavailability. May potentiate neuromuscular blockers; both agents may need dose reduction. Caution with inhalation anesthetics. Increased bleeding time with ASA. Increased efficacy of doxorubicin. Reduced absorption with COPP and VAC cytotoxic drug regimens. May decrease clearance of paclitaxel. CYP3A4 inhibitors (eg, erythromycin, ritonavir) or grapefruit juice may increase levels. CYP3A4 inducers (eg, rifampin) may lower levels.

PREGNANCY: Category C, not for use in nursing.

MECHANISM OF ACTION: Dihydropyridine calcium antagonist (calcium ion antagonist or slow-channel blocker); inhibits transmembrane influx of calcium ions into vascular smooth muscle and cardiac muscle.

PHARMACOKINETICS: Absorption: T_{max} = 7-9 hrs; administration of variable doses resulted in different parameters. **Distribution:** Plasma protein binding (90%). **Metabolism:** Liver, norverapamil (metabolite). **Elimination:** Urine, feces; $T_{1/2}$=12 hrs.

VERELAN PM   RX
verapamil HCL (Schwarz)

THERAPEUTIC CLASS: Calcium channel blocker (nondihydropyridine)

INDICATIONS: Management of hypertension.

DOSAGE: *Adults:* Usual: 200mg qhs. Titrate: May increase to 300mg qhs, then 400mg qhs. Renal or Hepatic Dysfunction/Elderly/Small People: Initial: 100mg qhs. Max: 400mg qhs. May sprinkle on applesauce; do not crush or chew.

HOW SUPPLIED: Cap, Extended-Release: 100mg, 200mg, 300mg

CONTRAINDICATIONS: Severe ventricular dysfunction, hypotension, cardiogenic shock, sick sinus syndrome or 2nd- or 3rd-degree AV block (except with functioning ventricular pacemaker), A-Fib/Flutter with an accessory bypass tract.

WARNINGS/PRECAUTIONS: Avoid with moderate to severe cardiac failure, and ventricular dysfunction if taking a β-blocker. May cause hypotension, AV block, transient bradycardia, PR interval prolongation. Monitor LFTs periodically; hepatocellular injury reported. Give 30% of normal dose with severe hepatic dysfunction. Caution with hypertrophic cardiomyopathy, renal or hepatic dysfunction. Decrease dose in those with decreased neuromuscular transmission.

ADVERSE REACTIONS: Constipation, dizziness, nausea, hypotension, headache, peripheral edema, infection, flu syndrome, fatigue, bradycardia, AV block.

INTERACTIONS: Additive negative effects on HR, AV conduction, and contractility with β-blockers. Potentiates other antihypertensives. May increase digoxin, carbamazepine, theophylline, cyclosporine, and alcohol levels. Avoid disopyramide within 48 hrs before or 24 hrs after verapamil. Additive negative inotropic effects and AV conduction prolongation with flecainide. Avoid quinidine with hypertrophic cardiomyopathy. Monitor lithium levels. Increased clearance with phenobarbital. Rifampin may reduce oral bioavailability. May potentiate neuromuscular blockers; both agents may need dose reduction. Caution with inhalation anesthetics. Increased bleeding time with ASA. Increased efficacy of doxorubicin. Reduced absorption with COPP and VAC cytotoxic drug regimens. May decrease clearance of paclitaxel. CYP3A4 inhibitors (eg, erythromycin, ritonavir) or grapefruit juice may increase levels. CYP3A4 inducers (eg, rifampin) may decrease levels.

PREGNANCY: Category C, not for use in nursing.

VESANOID   RX
tretinoin (Roche Labs)

> Administer under strict supervision of experienced physician and institution. Risk of retinoic acid-APL syndrome and leukocytosis. High risk of teratogenic effects.

THERAPEUTIC CLASS: Retinoid

INDICATIONS: Induction of remission in acute promyelocytic leukemia (APL) in those resistant to anthracycline therapy or those where anthracycline-based therapy is contraindicated.

DOSAGE: *Adults:* 45mg/m^2/day in 2 divided doses. D/C 30 days after achieving complete remission or after 90 days of therapy, whichever occurs 1st. *Pediatrics:* ≥1 yrs: 45mg/m^2/day in 2 divided doses. D/C 30 days after achieving complete remission or after 90 days of therapy, whichever occurs 1st.

HOW SUPPLIED: Cap: 10mg

CONTRAINDICATIONS: Sensitivity to parabens.

WARNINGS/PRECAUTIONS: May cause abortion or fetal abnormalities. Females should use contraception during and 1 month after therapy. Confirm APL diagnosis. Pseudotumor cerebri reported, especially in pediatrics.

V

Reversible hypercholesterolemia, hypertriglyceridemia reported. Elevated LFTs reported; d/c if >5x ULN. Monitor for signs of respiratory compromise or leukocytosis. Check hematologic profile, coagulation profile, LFTs, and cholesterol frequently.

ADVERSE REACTIONS: Malaise, shivering, hemorrhage, infections, peripheral edema, pain, chest discomfort, edema, disseminated intravascular coagulation, weight change, injection site reactions, dyspnea, pleural effusion, respiratory insufficiency, pneumonia.

INTERACTIONS: Possible interactions with drugs that affect CYP450 system. Aggravated symptoms of hypervitaminosis A with vitamin A. Cases of fatal thrombotic complications with antifibrinolytic agents (eg, tranexamic acid, aminocaproic acid). Increased risk of pseudotumor cerebri/intracranial HTN with tetracyclines.

PREGNANCY: Category D, not for use in nursing.

MECHANISM OF ACTION: Retinoid; not known. Induces cytodifferentiation and decreases proliferation of APL cells.

PHARMACOKINETICS: Absorption: C_{max}=394ng/mL, T_{max}=1-2 hrs; AUC=537ng•h/mL. **Distribution:** Plasma protein binding (>95%). **Metabolism**: Oxidation via CYP450. **Elimination:** $T_{1/2}$=0.5-2 hrs.

VESICARE RX
solifenacin succinate (Astellas/GlaxoSmithKline)

THERAPEUTIC CLASS: Muscarinic antagonist

INDICATIONS: Treatment of overactive bladder with symptoms of urge urinary incontinence, urgency, and urinary frequency.

DOSAGE: *Adults:* Usual: 5mg qd. Max: 10mg qd. Renal Impairment (CrCl< 30mL/min)/ Moderate Hepatic Impairment (Child-Pugh B)/ Potent CYP3A4 Inhibitors: Max: 5mg qd. Do not use in severe hepatic impairment (Child-Pugh C).

HOW SUPPLIED: Tab: 5mg, 10mg

CONTRAINDICATIONS: Urinary retention, gastric retention, uncontrolled narrow-angle glaucoma.

WARNINGS/PRECAUTIONS: Caution with bladder outflow obstruction, decreased gastrointestinal motility, and narrow-angle glaucoma. Caution with renal and hepatic impairment.

ADVERSE REACTIONS: Dry mouth, constipation, nausea, dyspepsia, UTI, blurred vision.

INTERACTIONS: Do not exceed 5mg daily dose when administered with therapeutic doses of ketoconazole or other potent CYP3A4 inhibitors.

PREGNANCY: Category C, not for use in nursing.

MECHANISM OF ACTION: Muscarinic receptor antagonist; inhibits muscarinic receptors resulting in decreased urinary smooth muscle contraction and salivary secretion.

PHARMACOKINETICS: Absorption: T_{max}=3-8 hrs. Absolute bioavailabilty (90%). **Distribution:** Plasma protein binding (98%); V_d=600L. **Metabolism:** CYP3A4 (N-oxidation; 4R-hydroxylation), 4R-hydroxy solifenacin (active metabolite). **Elimination**: $T_{1/2}$=45-68 hrs. Urine (<15%), feces.

VEXOL RX
rimexolone (Alcon)

THERAPEUTIC CLASS: Corticosteroid

INDICATIONS: Management of postoperative inflammation. Treatment of anterior uveitis.

DOSAGE: *Adults:* Postoperative Inflammation: 1-2 drops qid beginning 24 hrs postoperative; continue for 2 weeks thereafter. Anterior Uveitis: 1-2 drops every hourr while awake for 1st week, then 1 drop q2h while awake in 2nd week, then taper dose until resolved.

HOW SUPPLIED: Sus: 1% [5mL, 10mL]

CONTRAINDICATIONS: Viral diseases of the cornea and conjunctiva including epithelial herpes simplex keratitis, vaccinia, and varicella. Mycobacterial infection and fungal diseases of the eye. Acute purulent untreated infections.

WARNINGS/PRECAUTIONS: Not for injection into the eye. Prolonged use may result in ocular HTN/glaucoma, optic nerve damage, visual acuity and vision field defects, cataracts, secondary ocular infections (eg, fungal infections). Monitor IOP after 10 days of therapy. Re-evaluate if no response after 2 days.

ADVERSE REACTIONS: Elevated IOP, secondary ocular infections, blurred vision, ocular pain, discharge, hyperemia, pruritus, foreign body sensation, discomfort.

PREGNANCY: Category C, not for use in nursing.

MECHANISM OF ACTION: Ophthalmic corticosteroid; anti-inflammatory; inhibits edema, cellular infiltration, capillary dilatation, fibroblastic proliferation, deposition of collagen and scar formation associated with inflammation.

PHARMACOKINETICS: Absorption: C_{max}=130pg/mL. **Metabolism:** Liver (extensive). **Elimination**: Feces (drug and metabolites).

VFEND RX
voriconazole (Pfizer)

THERAPEUTIC CLASS: Azole antifungal

INDICATIONS: Treatment of invasive aspergillosis, esophageal candidiasis. Treatment of candidemia in nonneutropenic patients and the following *Candida* infections: disseminated infections in skin and infections in abdomen, kidney, bladder wall, and wounds. Treatment of serious fungal infections caused by *Scedosporium apiospermum* and *Fusarium* spp. including *Fusarium solani* in patients intolerant of, or refractory to, other therapy.

DOSAGE: *Adults:* (Inj) LD: 6mg/kg IV q12h x 2 doses. Maint: 4mg/kg IV q12h. Switch to PO when appropriate. (PO) Maint: ≥40kg: 200mg q12h; 300mg q12h if inadequate response. <40kg: 100mg q12h; 150 mg q12h if inadequate response. Esophageal Candidiasis: (PO) ≥40kg: 200mg q12h. <40kg: 100mg q12h. Treat for minimum of 14 days and at least 7 days following resolution of symptoms. Intolerant: (Inj/PO) Maint: IV: 3mg/kg q12h. PO: Reduce by 50mg steps to minimum of 200mg q12h for >40kg or 100mg q12h for <40kg. Concomitant Phenytoin: Maint: IV: 5mg/kg q12h. PO: ≥40kg: 400mg q12h. <40kg: 200mg q12h. Concomitant Efavirenz: Maint: 400mg q12h and efavirenz should be decreased to 300mg q24h. Mild to Moderate Hepatic Cirrhosis: Maint: 1/2 of maint dose. CrCl <50mL/min: Use PO. Give PO 1 hr before or 1 hr after a meal. Base duration on severity of underlying disease, recovery from immunosuppression, and clinical response.

HOW SUPPLIED: Inj: 200mg; Sus: 40mg/mL; Tab: 50mg, 200mg

CONTRAINDICATIONS: Concomitant CYP3A4 substrates (terfenadine, astemizole, cisapride, pimozide, quinidine), sirolimus, rifampin, carbamazepine, long-acting barbiturates, high-dose ritonavir (400mg q12h), efavirenz (standard voriconazole doses; adjusted doses may be administered), rifabutin, ergot alkaloids.

WARNINGS/PRECAUTIONS: Monitor visual function with treatment >28 days. Hepatic reactions (clinical hepatitis, cholestasis, fulminant hepatic failure) reported; monitor LFTs at initiation and during therapy. D/C if liver dysfunction occurs. Tabs contain lactose; avoid with galactose intolerance, Lapp lactase deficiency, or glucose-galactose malabsorption. Anaphylactoid-type reactions reported with infusion. Avoid strong, direct sunlight. Monitor renal function. May prolong QT interval; caution with proarrhythmic conditions. Correct electrolyte disturbances before starting therapy. If rash develops, monitor closely and consider discontinuation of voriconazole.

V

ADVERSE REACTIONS: Visual disturbances, fever, chills, rash, headache, nausea, vomiting, sepsis, peripheral edema, abdominal pain, respiratory disorder, increased LFTs and alkaline phosphatase.

INTERACTIONS: See Contraindications. Avoid with low-dose ritonavir (100mg q12h). May increase levels of CYP3A4 inhibitors; monitor for adverse events and toxicity with HIV protease inhibitors, NNRTIs, benzodiazepines, HMG-CoA reductase inhibitors, dihydropyridine CCBs, and vinca alkaloids. May increase levels of CYP2C9 inhibitors; monitor phenytoin, warfarin, hypoglycemics, tacrolimus (reduce tacrolimus to 1/3 of initial dose), and cyclosporine (reduce cyclosporine to 1/2 of initial dose). Omeprazole is CYP2C19/3A4 inhibitor; reduce omeprazole by 1/2 if voriconazole ≥40mg. Proton pump inhibitors that are CYP2C19 substrates may increase levels. Phenytoin may decrease levels. Oral contraceptives containing ethinyl estradiol and norethindrone may increase levels. May increase levels of oral contraceptives containing ethinyl estradiol and norethindrone. May increase levels of methadone; may prolong QT interval; dose reduction may be needed. Do not infuse into same line or cannula with other drug infusions or parenteral nutrition. Do not infuse simultaneously with blood products or electrolyte supplements.

PREGNANCY: Category D, not for use in nursing.

MECHANISM OF ACTION: Triazole antifungal agent; inhibits fungal CYP450 mediated 14α-lanosterol demethylation, an essential step in fungal ergosterol biosynthesis. Accumulation of 14-α methyl-sterols correlates with subsequent loss of ergosterol in fungal cell wall and may be responsible for antifungal activity of voriconazole.

PHARMACOKINETICS: Absorption: Administration of different doses led to varying parameters. T_{max}=1-2 hrs. **Distribution:** V_d=4.6L/kg; Plasma protein binding (58%). **Metabolism:** Hepatic, via CYP2C19, CYP2C9, CYP3A4; N-oxide (major metabolite). **Elimination:** <2% excreted unchanged in urine.

Viadur   RX
leuprolide acetate (Bayer Healthcare)

THERAPEUTIC CLASS: Synthetic gonadotropin releasing hormone analog

INDICATIONS: Palliative treatment of advanced prostate cancer.

DOSAGE: *Adults:* Insert 1 implant SQ in upper arm every 12 months.

HOW SUPPLIED: Implant: 65mg

CONTRAINDICATIONS: Women, pregnancy, pediatrics.

WARNINGS/PRECAUTIONS: Transient worsening of symptoms may occur during 1st few weeks of therapy. Closely monitor patients with metastatic vertebral lesions and/or urinary tract obstruction during 1st few weeks of therapy. Monitor serum testosterone, PSA. Ureteral obstruction and spinal cord decompression reported.

ADVERSE REACTIONS: Headache, asthenia, hot flashes, ecchymosis, peripheral edema, depression, sweating, gynecomastia, nocturia, urinary frequency, testis atrophy, breast pain, urinary retention/frquency, local bruising/burning.

PREGNANCY: Category X, safety in nursing not known.

MECHANISM OF ACTION: LH-RH agonist; acts as potent inhibitor of gonadotropin secretion resulting in suppressing ovarian and testicular steroidogenesis.

PHARMACOKINETICS: Absorption: C_{max}=16.9ng/mL; T_{max}=4 hrs. **Distribution:** V_d=27L; Plasma protein binding (43-49%). **Metabolism:** (Major metabolite): M-I. **Elimination:** $T_{1/2}$=3 hrs.

Viagra   RX
sildenafil citrate (Pfizer)

THERAPEUTIC CLASS: Phosphodiesterase type 5 inhibitor

INDICATIONS: Treatment of erectile dysfunction (ED).

DOSAGE: *Adults:* Usual: 50mg 1 hr (range 0.5-4 hrs) prior to sexual activity at frequency of up to once daily. Titrate: May decrease to 25mg qd or increase to 100mg qd. Max: 100mg qd. Elderly/Hepatic Impairment/CrCl <30mL/min/Concomitant CYP450 3A4 Inhibitors (eg, ketoconazole, itraconazole, erythromycin, saquinavir): Initial: 25mg qd. Concomitant Ritonavir: Max: 25mg q48h. Concomitant α-blocker: Avoid doses >25mg sildenafil within 4 hours of an α-blocker.

HOW SUPPLIED: Tab: 25mg, 50mg, 100mg

CONTRAINDICATIONS: Organic nitrates taken regularly and/or intermittently.

WARNINGS/PRECAUTIONS: Caution with MI, stroke or life-threatening arrhythmia within last 6 months; with resting hypotension (BP<90/50) or HTN (BP>170/110); unstable angina due to cardiac failure or CAD; anatomical penile deformation; predisposition to priapism; and retinitis pigmentosa. Avoid in men where sexual activity is inadvisable due to underlying CV status. Decrease in supine BP reported. Rare reports of nonarteritic anterior ischemic optic neuropathy (NAION) with PDE5 inhibitors. Caution when PDE5 inhibitors are given concomitantly with α-blockers. PDE5 inhibitors and α-adrenergic blocking agents are both vasodilators with BP-lowering effects; additive effect on BP may be anticipated. Cases of sudden decrease or loss of hearing reported. D/C if experienced these symptoms.

ADVERSE REACTIONS: Headache, flushing, dyspepsia, nasal congestion, UTI, abnormal vision (eg, color tinge, increased light sensitivity, blurred vision), diarrhea, cardiovascular events, sudden decrease or loss of hearing.

INTERACTIONS: See Contraindications. Increased levels with CYP3A4 inhibitors (eg, cimetidine, ketoconazole, itraconazole, erythromycin, saquinavir) and protease inhibitors (eg, ritonavir). CYP2C9 inhibitors may decrease sildenafil clearance. CYP3A4 inducers (eg, rifampin) may decrease levels. Potentiates hypotensive effects of nitrates. Additional supine BP reduction with amlodipine reported. Simultaneous administration with α-blockers may lead to symptomatic hypotension; sildenafil dose should not exceed 25mg and should not be taken within 4 hrs of taking an α-blocker. Avoid with other ED treatments.

PREGNANCY: Category B, not for use in nursing.

MECHANISM OF ACTION: Phosphodiesterase type 5 inhibitor; enhances effect of nitric oxide by inhibiting phosphodiesterase type 5, which is responsible for the degradation of cGMP in corpus cavernosum.

PHARMACOKINETICS: Absorption: Rapid; Absolute bioavailability (40%). **Distribution**: V_d=105L; Plasma protein binding (96%). **Metabolism**: Liver, via CYP450 3A4 (major), 2C9 (minor); N-desmethyl. **Elimination**: $T_{1/2}$=4 hrs; feces (80% metabolites), urine (13%).

VIBRAMYCIN   RX
doxycycline hyclate (Pfizer)

OTHER BRAND NAMES: Vibra-Tabs (Pfizer)

THERAPEUTIC CLASS: Tetracycline derivative

INDICATIONS: Treatment of the following infections caused by susceptible microorganisms: Rocky Mountain spotted fever; typhus fever and the typhus group; Q fever; rickettsialpox; tick fevers; respiratory tract infections; lymphogranuloma venereum; psittacosis (ornithosis); trachoma; inclusion conjunctivitis; uncomplicated urethral, endocervical, or rectal infections; nongonococcal urethritis; relapsing fever; chancroid; plague; tularemia; cholera; *Camphylobacter fetus* infections; brucellosis; bartonellosis; granuloma inguinale; respiratory tract and urinary tract infections; anthrax. Treatment of infections caused by *Escherichia coli, Enterobacter aerogenes, Shigella* species, *Acinetobacter* species. When penicillin is contraindicated, treatment of the following infections caused by susceptible microorganisms: uncomplicated gonorrhea, syphilis, yaws, listeriosis, Vincent's infection, actinomycosis, infections caused by *Clostridium* species. Adjunct in acute intestinal amebiasis and severe acne. Prophylaxis of malaria.

DOSAGE: *Adults:* Usual: 100mg q12h on Day 1, then 100mg qd or 50mg q12h. Severe Infection: 100mg q12h. Treat for 10 days with strep infection. Uncomplicated Gonococcal Infection (Except Anorectal in Men): 100mg bid for 7 days or 300mg followed by 300mg in 1 hr. Uncomplicated Urethral/Endocervical/Rectal Infection and Nongonococcal Urethritis: 100mg bid for 7 days. Syphilis: 100mg bid for 2 weeks. Syphilis for >1 yr: 100mg bid for 4 weeks. Acute Epididymo-orchitis: 100mg bid for at least 10 days. Inhalation Anthrax (Post-Exposure): 100mg bid for 60 days. Malaria Prophylaxis: 100mg qd. Begin 1-2 days before travel and continue for 4 weeks after leaving malarious area.

Pediatrics: >8 yrs: ≤100 lbs: 1mg/lb bid on Day 1, then 1mg/lb qd or 0.5mg/lb bid. Severe Infections: Maint: 2mg/lb. >100 lbs: Usual: 100mg q12h on Day 1, then 100mg qd or 50mg q12h. Severe Infection: 100mg q12h. Treat for 10 days with strep infection. Inhalation Anthrax (Post-Exposure): <100 lbs: 1mg/lb bid for 60 days. ≥100 lbs: 100mg bid for 60 days. Malaria Prophylaxis: >8 yrs: 2mg/kg qd. Max: 100mg/day. Begin 1-2 days before travel and continue for 4 weeks after leaving malarious area.

HOW SUPPLIED: Cap: (Doxycycline Hyclate) 50mg, 100mg; Syrup: (Doxycycline Calcium) 50mg/5mL; Sus: (Doxycycline Monohydrate) 25mg/5mL [60mL]; Tab: (Vibra-Tabs) 100mg

WARNINGS/PRECAUTIONS: May cause fetal harm with pregnancy. Permanent tooth discoloration during tooth development (last half of pregnancy, infancy, and children <8 yrs) reported. *Clostridium difficile*-associated diarrhea reported. May increase BUN. Photosensitivity, enamel hypoplasia reported. Superinfection with prolonged use. Syrup contains sodium metabisulfite. Bulging fontanels in infants and benign intracranial HTN in adults reported. Monitor renal/hepatic and hematopoietic function with long-term use. Take adequate fluids with caps or tabs to reduce esophageal irritation. Take with food or milk if GI irritation occurs.

ADVERSE REACTIONS: GI effects (eg, anorexia, nausea, vomiting, diarrhea), photosensitivity, increased BUN, hypersensitivity reactions, hemolytic anemia, thrombocytopenia, neutropenia, eosinophilia.

INTERACTIONS: May decrease PT, adjust anticoagulants. May interfere with bactericidal agents (eg, penicillin). May decrease effects of oral contraceptives. Aluminum-, calcium-, iron-, and magnesium-containing products and bismuth subsalicylate impair absorption. Decreased half-life with barbiturates, carbamazepine, and phenytoin. Fatal renal toxicity with methoxyflurane.

PREGNANCY: Category D, not for use in nursing.

MECHANISM OF ACTION: Tetracycline derivative; thought to inhibit protein synthesis.

PHARMACOKINETICS: Absorption: (PO) completely absorbed, C_{max}=2.6 mcg/mL, T_{max}=2 hrs. **Distribution:** Crosses placenta. **Elimination:** Urine, feces.

VICODIN   `CIII`
hydrocodone bitartrate - acetaminophen (Abbott)

OTHER BRAND NAMES: Vicodin HP (Abbott) - Vicodin ES (Abbott)

THERAPEUTIC CLASS: Opioid analgesic

INDICATIONS: Relief of moderate to moderately severe pain.

DOSAGE: *Adults:* Usual: Vicodin: 1-2 tabs q4-6h prn. Max: 8 tabs/day. Vicodin HP: 1 tab q4-6h prn. Max: 6 tabs/day. Vicodin ES: 1 tab q4-6h prn. Max: 5 tabs/day.

HOW SUPPLIED: (Hydrocodone-APAP) Tab: Vicodin: 5mg-500mg*; Vicodin HP: 10mg-660mg*; Vicodin ES: 7.5mg-750mg* *scored

WARNINGS/PRECAUTIONS: Caution in elderly, debilitated, severe hepatic or renal dysfunction, hypothyroidism, Addison's disease, prostatic hypertrophy, urethral stricture, pulmonary disease and postoperative use. May obscure acute abdominal conditions or head injuries. May produce dose-related respiratory depression. Monitor for tolerance. Suppresses cough reflex.

ADVERSE REACTIONS: Lightheadedness, dizziness, sedation, nausea, vomiting, constipation, rash, respiratory depression.

INTERACTIONS: Additive CNS depression with other narcotic analgesics, antihistamines, antipsychotics, antianxiety agents, alcohol and other CNS depressants. Increased effect of antidepressant or hydrocodone with MAOIs or TCAs.

PREGNANCY: Category C, not for use in nursing.

MECHANISM OF ACTION: Hydrocodone: opioid analgesic; Precise mechanism not known;.suspected to relate to existence of opiate receptors in CNS. APAP: nonopiate, nonsalicylate analgesic and antipyretic. Analgesic action involves peripheral influences, specific mechanism not established. Antipyretic activity mediated through hypothalmic heat-regulating centers. Inhibits prostaglandin synthetase.

PHARMACOKINETICS: Absorption: Hydrocodone: C_{max}=23.6ng/mL; T_{max}=1.3 hrs. APAP: Rapidly absorbed. **Distribution:** APAP: Found in breast milk. **Metabolism:** Hydrocodone: O-demethylation, N-demethylation and 6-keto reduction. APAP: Liver (conjugation). **Elimination:** Hydrocodone: $T_{1/2}$=3.8 hrs. APAP: Urine (85%) (parent compound and metabolites); $T_{1/2}$=1.25-3 hrs.

VICOPROFEN CIII
hydrocodone bitartrate - ibuprofen (Abbott)

OTHER BRAND NAMES: Reprexain (Centrix)

THERAPEUTIC CLASS: Opioid analgesic

INDICATIONS: Short-term (generally <10 days) management of acute pain.

DOSAGE: *Adults:* Usual: 1 tab q4-6h prn. Max: 5 tabs/day. Elderly: Use lowest dose or longest interval.
Pediatrics: ≥16 yrs: Usual: 1 tab q4-6h prn. Max: 5 tabs/day.

HOW SUPPLIED: (Hydrocodone-Ibuprofen) Tab: (Vicoprofen) 7.5mg-200mg; (Reprexain) 5mg-200mg, 7.5mg-200mg *scored

CONTRAINDICATIONS: ASA or other NSAID allergy that precipitates asthma, urticaria, or other allergic reaction.

WARNINGS/PRECAUTIONS: May produce dose-related respiratory depression. May obscure acute abdominal conditions or head injuries. Avoid with ASA triad, late pregnancy, advanced renal disease, ASA-sensitive asthma. Caution in elderly, debilitated, dehydration, renal disease, intrinsic coagulation defects, severe hepatic dysfunction, asthma, hypothyroidism, Addison's disease, prostatic hypertrophy, urethral stricture, heart failure, HTN, ulcer disease, pulmonary disease, postoperative use. May be habit-forming. Suppresses cough reflex. Risk of GI ulceration, bleeding, perforation. Anemia, fluid retention, edema, severe hepatic reactions reported. Possible risk of aseptic meningitis, especially in SLE patients. Increased risk of serious cardiovascular thrombotic events, MI and stroke. Fluid retention and edema observed. Skin reactions (eg, exfoliative dermatitis, TEN, SJS) can occur.

ADVERSE REACTIONS: Headache, somnolence, dizziness, constipation, dyspepsia, nausea, vomiting, infection, edema, nervousness, anxiety, pruritus, diarrhea, asthenia, abdominal pain, insomnia, dry mouth, sweating.

INTERACTIONS: Additive CNS depression with other narcotics, antihistamines, antipsychotics, antianxiety agents, alcohol, CNS depressants. Increased effect of antidepressant or hydrocodone with MAOIs or TCAs. May produce paralytic ileus with anticholinergics. May decrease effects of furosemide and thiazide diuretics, ACE-inhibitors. Avoid ASA. Risk of serious GI bleeding with warfarin. May enhance methotrexate toxicity. Monitor for lithium toxicity.

PREGNANCY: Category C, not for use in nursing.

MECHANISM OF ACTION: Hydrocodone: Opioid analgesic and antitussive. Not known; suspected to be related to existence of opiate receptors in CNS. Produces actions similiar to codeine; most occur in CNS and smooth muscle. Ibuprofen: Non-steroidal anti-inflammatory agent. Not established; suspected

V

to inhibit cyclooxygenase activity and prostaglandin synthesis. Peripherally acting analgesic; has no known effects on opiate receptors. Possesses anti-pyretic activity.

PHARMACOKINETICS: Absorption: Hydrocodone: C_{max}=27ng/mL; T_{max}=1.7 hrs. Ibuprofen: C_{max}=30mcg/mL; T_{max}=1.8 hrs. **Distribution:** Ibuprofen: Plasma protein binding (99%). **Metabolism:** Hydrocodone: CYP2D6, via O-demethylation to hydromorphone (active metabolite); CYP3A4 via N-demethylation; 6-keto reduction. Ibuprofen: Interconversion from R-isomer to S-isomer; (+)-2-4'-(2-hydroxy-2-methyl-propyl) phenyl propionic acid and (+)-2-4-(2-carboxypropyl) phenyl propionic acid (primary metabolites). **Elimination:** Hydrocodone: Urine (primary); $T_{1/2}$=4.5 hrs. Ibuprofen: Urine (50-60% metabolites, 15% unchanged, conjugate), $T_{1/2}$=2.2 hrs.

VIDAZA   RX
azacitidine (Pharmion)

THERAPEUTIC CLASS: Pyrimidine nucleoside analog

INDICATIONS: Treatment of myelodysplastic syndrome subtypes: refractory anemia or refractory anemia with ringed sideroblasts (if accompanied by neutropenia or thrombocytopenia or requiring transfusions), refractory anemia with excess blasts, refractory anemia with excess blasts in transformation, and chronic myelomonocytic leukemia.

DOSAGE: *Adults:* Initial: 75mg/m² SQ or IV (administer over 10-40 min) daily for 7 days. Repeat cycle every 4 weeks. May increase to 100mg/m² after 2 cycles if no beneficial effect and no toxicity. Treat ≥4 cycles. Adjust dose based on hematology lab values, renal function, and serum electrolytes.

HOW SUPPLIED: Inj: 100mg

CONTRAINDICATIONS: Advanced malignant hepatic tumors.

WARNINGS/PRECAUTIONS: May cause fetal harm. Avoid pregnancy in women of childbearing potential. Neutropenia and thrombocytopenia may occur; monitor CBC periodically (at minimum, before each cycle). May cause hepatotoxicity; caution with liver disease. Renal abnormalities reported; reduce dose or hold for unexplained reductions in serum bicarbonate <20mEq/L or elevations of BUN or serum creatinine occur. Monitor for toxicity with renal impairment.

ADVERSE REACTIONS: (SQ) Nausea, anemia, thrombocytopenia, vomiting, pyrexia, leukopenia, diarrhea, fatigue, injection site erythema, constipation, neutropenia, ecchymosis, cough, dyspnea, weakness. (IV) Petechiae, rigors, weakness, hypokalemia.

PREGNANCY: Category D, not for use in nursing.

MECHANISM OF ACTION: Pyrimidine analogue; believed to cause hypomethylation of DNA and direct cytotoxicity on abnormal hematopoietic cells in bone marrow.

PHARMACOKINETICS: Absorption: (SQ) Rapid; C_{max}=750ng/mL; T_{max}=0.5 hr; Bioavailability (89%). **Distribution:** (IV) V_d=76L. **Elimination:** (SQ) $T_{1/2}$=41 min.

VIDEX   RX
didanosine (Bristol-Myers Squibb)

> Fatal/nonfatal pancreatitis, lactic acidosis, and severe hepatomegaly with steatosis reported. Suspend therapy if suspect pancreatitis and discontinue if pancreatitis confirmed. Fatal lactic acidosis reported in pregnant women receiving concomitant stavudine.

OTHER BRAND NAMES: Videx EC (Bristol-Myers Squibb)

THERAPEUTIC CLASS: Nucleoside analogue

INDICATIONS: Treatment of HIV-1 infection in combination with other antiretrovirals (use Videx EC when management requires once daily dosing or alternative didanosine formulation).

DOSAGE: *Adults:* ≥60kg: (Cap) 400mg qd; (Sol) 200mg bid or 400mg qd. <60kg: (Cap) 250mg qd; (Sol) 125mg bid or 250mg qd. CrCl 30-59mL/min: ≥60kg: (Cap) 200mg qd; (Sol) 200mg qd. <60kg: (Cap) 125mg qd; (Sol) 150mg qd or 75mg bid. CrCl 10-29mL/min: ≥60kg: (Cap) 125mg qd; (Sol) 150mg qd. <60kg: (Cap) 125mg qd; (Sol) 100mg qd. CrCl <10mL/min: ≥60kg: (Cap) 125mg qd; (Sol) 100mg qd. <60kg: (Sol) 75mg qd. Concomitant Viread: CrCl ≥60mL/min :≥60kg: 250mg qd; <60kg: 200mg qd. Take on empty stomach at least 30 min before or 2 hrs after meals. Swallow caps whole. *Pediatrics:* 2 weeks-8 months: (Sol) 100mg/m^2 bid. >8 months: 120mg/m^2 bid.

HOW SUPPLIED: Sol: 2g, 4g [120mL], 240mL]; Cap, Delayed-Release: (Videx EC) 125mg, 200mg, 250mg, 400mg

WARNINGS/PRECAUTIONS: Risk of toxicity with CrCl <60mL/min; reduce dose. Retinal changes and optic neuritis reported; perform periodic retinal exams. Peripheral neuropathy reported. Caution with hepatic dysfunction. May cause asymptomatic hyperuricemia. Twice daily dosing is preferred over once daily dosing. Chewable tabs contain phenylalanine. Caution with sodium restricted diets; buffered powder solution contains 1380mg sodium. Monitor for lactic acidosis in pregnancy if used with stavudine. Possible redistribution or accumulation of fat. Immune reconstitution syndrome has been reported in patients treated with combination antiretroviral therapy. Fatal and non-fatal pancreatitis reported; increased risk in combination with stavudine, with or without hydroxyurea.

ADVERSE REACTIONS: Pancreatitis, lactic acidosis, hepatomegaly, visual changes, diarrhea, neuropathy, abdominal pain, headache, nausea, vomiting, rash, elevated LFTs.

INTERACTIONS: Extreme caution with drugs that may cause pancreatitis. Increase risk of peripheral neuropathy with neurotoxic agents (eg, stavudine). Aluminum- and magnesium-containing antacids may potentiate adverse events. Space dose by 2 hrs of drugs whose absorption can be affected by stomach acidity (eg, ketoconazole, itraconazole). Increased serum levels with oral ganciclovir. Space dose by 2 hrs after or 6 hrs before ciprofloxacin. Avoid allopurinol. Decreased serum levels with methadone. Caution with tenofovir or ribavirin; monitor closely for didanosine-related toxicities and suspend therapy if signs of pancreatitis, symptomatic hyperlactatemia, or lactic acidosis develop.

PREGNANCY: Category B, not for use in nursing.

MECHANISM OF ACTION: Antiviral agent; inhibits activity of HIV-1 reverse transcriptase both by competing with natural substrate deoxyadenosine 5-triphosphate and by incorporation into viral DNA, causing termination of viral DNA chain elongation.

PHARMACOKINETICS: Absorption: Rapid. T_{max}=0.25-1.5 hrs. **Distribution:** V_d=1.08+/-0.22L/kg, <5% protein bound. **Elimination:** $T_{1/2}$=1.5+/-0.4 hrs. Refer to PI for pediatric guidelines.

VIGAMOX   RX
moxifloxacin HCL (Alcon)

THERAPEUTIC CLASS: Fluoroquinolone

INDICATIONS: Treatment of bacterial conjunctivitis.

DOSAGE: *Adults:* 1 drop tid for 7 days.
Pediatrics: ≥1 yr: 1 drop tid for 7 days.

HOW SUPPLIED: Sol: 0.5% [3mL]

WARNINGS/PRECAUTIONS: Not for injection. Do not inject subconjunctivally or into the anterior chamber of the eye. Superinfection may result with prolonged use. Fatal hypersensitivity reactions reported after first dose of systemic quinolone therapy. Avoid contact lenses when symptoms are present.

ADVERSE REACTIONS: Conjunctivitis, decreased visual acuity, dry eye, keratitis, ocular discomfort/hyperemia, ocular pain/pruritus, subconjunctival hemorrhage, tearing.

PREGNANCY: Category C, caution in nursing.

MECHANISM OF ACTION: Fluoroquinolone antibiotic; inhibits topoisomerase II (DNA gyrase) and topoisomerase IV. DNA gyrase is essential enzyme involved in replication, transcription, and repair of bacterial DNA. Topoisomerase IV is enzyme known to play key role in partitioning of chromosomal DNA during bacterial cell division.

PHARMACOKINETICS: Absorption: C_{max}=2.7ng/mL; AUC=45ng•hr/mL. **Distribution:** Presumed to be excreted in breast milk.

VINBLASTINE RX
vinblastine sulfate (Various)

> For IV use only; fatal if given intrathecally. Considerable irritation if leakage occurs into surrounding tissue. If this occurs, d/c and restart in another vein. Heat and hyaluronidase minimize discomfort and cellulitis.

THERAPEUTIC CLASS: Vinca alkaloid

INDICATIONS: Palliative treatment of generalized Hodgkin's disease (Stages III and IV), lymphocytic lymphoma, histiocytic lymphoma, advanced mycosis fungoides, advanced testis carcinoma, Kaposi's sarcoma, Letterer-Siwe disease, and resistant choriocarcinoma and unresponsive breast carcinoma.

DOSAGE: *Adults:* Dose at intervals of ≤7 days. 1st Dose: 3.7mg/m². 2nd Dose: 5.5mg/m². 3rd Dose: 7.4mg/m². 4th Dose: 9.25mg/m². 5th Dose: 11.1mg/m². Max: 18.5mg/m². Do not increase dose after that dose which reduces WBC to 3000 cells/mm³. Maint: Use dose of 1 increment smaller than this dose at weekly intervals. Reduce to 50% dose if direct serum bilirubin >3mg/100mL. Only dose if WBC ≥4000 cells/mm³.
Pediatrics: Letterer-Swine Disease as Single Agent: Initial: 6.5mg/m². Hodgkin's Disease in Combination Therapy: Initial: 6mg/m². Testicular Germ Cell Carcinoma in Combination Therapy: Initial: 3mg/m².

HOW SUPPLIED: Inj: 1mg/mL [10mL]

CONTRAINDICATIONS: Significant granulocytopenia (unless result of disease being treated), bacterial infections.

WARNINGS/PRECAUTIONS: Avoid pregnancy. Acute shortness of breath, severe bronchospasm, aspermia, stomatitis, neurologic toxicity reported. Increased toxicity with hepatic insufficiency. Monitor for infection with WBC <2000 cells/mm³. Avoid with malignant-cell infiltration of bone marrow, or in older persons with cachexia or ulcerated skin. Small daily amounts for long periods is not advised. Avoid eye contamination. Monitor WBCs. May cause fetal harm during pregnancy. Caution with ischemic cardiac disease.

ADVERSE REACTIONS: Leukopenia (granulocytopenia), anemia, thrombocytopenia, alopecia, constipation, anorexia, nausea, vomiting, abdominal pain, diarrhea, HTN, paresthesis.

INTERACTIONS: May increase phenytoin metabolism/elimination, or decrease phenytoin absorption. Caution with CYP3A inhibitors (eg, erythromycin, doxorubicin, etoposide), or with hepatic dysfunction; may cause earlier onset and/or an increased severity of side effects. Increased risk of acute shortness of breath and severe bronchospasm with mitomycin-C.

PREGNANCY: Category D, not for use in nursing.

MECHANISM OF ACTION: Vinca alkaloid; inhibits microtubule formation in mitotic spindle, resulting in cell division arrest.

PHARMACOKINETICS: Metabolism: CYP3A. **Elimination:** $T_{1/2}$=24.8 hrs.

VINCRISTINE RX
vincristine sulfate (Various)

> Properly position IV needle or catheter before injection; considerable irritation with extravasation. Use hyaluronidase and heat to minimize discomfort and cellulitis with extravasation. Fatal with intrathecal use. For IV use only.

THERAPEUTIC CLASS: Vinca alkaloid

INDICATIONS: For treatment of acute leukemia. As an adjunct in the treatment of Hodgkin's disease, non-Hodgkin's malignant lymphomas, rhabdomyosarcoma, neuroblastoma, and Wilms' tumor.

DOSAGE: *Adults:* Usual: 1.4mg/m² IV at weekly intervals. Bilirubin >3mg/dL: 50% dose reduction. If given together with L-asparaginase, give 12-24 hrs before the enzyme.
Pediatrics: Usual: 2mg/m2 IV at weekly intervals. ≤10kg: Initial: 0.05mg/kg IV once weekly. Bilirubin >3mg/dL: 50% dose reduction. If given together with L-asparaginase, give 12-24 hrs before the enzyme.

HOW SUPPLIED: Inj: 1mg/mL

CONTRAINDICATIONS: Demyelinating form of Charcot-Marie-Tooth syndrome.

WARNINGS/PRECAUTIONS: Acute uric acid nephropathy may occur. May require additional agents with CNS leukemia. Neurotoxicity is dose-limiting toxicity. Perform CBC before each dose. Determine serum uric acid levels frequently during 1st 3-4 weeks. Acute shortness of breath, severe bronchospasm reported. Monitor with pre-existing neuromuscular disease. Avoid eye contamination. May cause fetal harm during pregnancy.

ADVERSE REACTIONS: Alopecia, abdominal cramps, weight loss, nausea, vomiting, diarrhea, constipation, paralytic ileus, HTN, hypotension, polyuria, dysuria, urinary retention, sensory impairment, paresthesia, neuritic pain, motor difficulties, rash, fever.

INTERACTIONS: Reduced levels of phenytoin and increased seizures reported. Increased risk of acute shortness of breath and severe bronchospasm with mitomycin-C. Monitor with other neurotoxic agents. Discontinue drugs known to cause urinary retention for 1st few days after administration. Give 12-24 hrs before L-asparaginase therapy to minimize toxicity. Do not give with radiation therapy through ports that include the liver. Do not dilute in solutions that raise or lower the pH outside the range of 3.5-5.5.

PREGNANCY: Category D, not for use in nursing.

MECHANISM OF ACTION: Antineoplastic agent; inhibits microtubule formation in mitotic spindle, resulting in arrest of dividing cells at metaphase stage.

PHARMACOKINETICS: Distribution: Crosses blood-brain barrier. **Metabolism:** Liver, via CYP450 isoenzyme 3A **Elimination:** Feces (80%), urine (10-20%); $T_{1/2}$=85 hrs.

VIOKASE RX
protease - amylase - lipase (Axcan Scandipharm)

THERAPEUTIC CLASS: Pancreatic enzyme supplement

INDICATIONS: Treatment of pancreatic exocrine insufficiency (eg, cystic fibrosis, chronic pancreatitis, pancreatectomy, and pancreatic ductal obstruction).

DOSAGE: *Adults:* (Powder) Cystic Fibrosis: 0.7g (1/4 tsp) with meals. (Tab) Cystic Fibrosis/Pancreatitis: 8,000-32,000 U Lipase with meals. Pancreatectomy/Pancreatic Duct Obstruction: 8,000-16,000 U Lipase q2h. *Pediatrics:* (Powder) Cystic Fibrosis: 0.7g (1/4 tsp) with meals. (Tab) Cystic Fibrosis/Pancreatitis: 8,000-32,000 U Lipase with meals. Pancreatectomy/Pancreatic Duct Obstruction: 8,000-16,000 U Lipase q2h.

V

HOW SUPPLIED: (Amylase-Lipase-Protease) Powder: 70,000 U-16,800 U-70,000 U/0.7g [240g]; Tab: (Viokase 8) 30,000 U-8,000 U-30,000 U; (Viokase 16) 60,000 U-16,000 U-60,000 U

CONTRAINDICATIONS: Pork protein hypersensitivity.

WARNINGS/PRECAUTIONS: May have allergic reactions if previously sensitized to trypsin, pancreatin or pancrelipase. Irritating to oral mucosa if held in mouth. Inhalation of powder can cause an asthma attack. High doses can cause hyperuricemia and hyperuricosuria.

ADVERSE REACTIONS: Irritation to nasal mucosa and respiratory tract with inhaled powder.

PREGNANCY: Category C, caution in nursing.

MECHANISM OF ACTION: Panrealipase; pancreatic enzyme concentrate of porcine origin. Natural digestive enzyme; acts to hydrolyze fats into fatty acid and glycerol, split protein into amino acids, and convert carbohydrates to dextrins and short chain sugars.

VIRACEPT   RX
nelfinavir mesylate (Pfizer)

THERAPEUTIC CLASS: Protease inhibitor

INDICATIONS: Treatment of HIV infection in combination with other antiretrovirals.

DOSAGE: *Adults:* 1250mg bid or 750mg tid. Concomitant rifabutin: Reduce rifabutin dose by one-half and nelfinavir 1250mg bid is preferred dose. Take with a meal or light snack. May crush or dissolve whole tab in water or mix in food and consume immediately. May store mixture under refrigeration up to 6 hrs.
Pediatrics: 2-13 yrs: 20-30mg/kg tid. Take with a meal or light snack. May mix powder with non-acidic liquid (eg, water, milk, formula, etc.); consume immediately. May store up to 6 hrs under refrigeration.

HOW SUPPLIED: Sus: (powder) 50mg/g [144g]; Tab: 250mg, 625mg

CONTRAINDICATIONS: Concomitant pimozide, triazolam, midazolam, ergot derivatives, amiodarone or quinidine.

WARNINGS/PRECAUTIONS: Powder contains phenylalanine. New-onset DM, exacerbation of DM and hyperglycemia reported. Register pregnant patients (800-258-4263). Caution with hepatic dysfunction. Increased bleeding reported. Possible redistribution or accumulation of fat.

ADVERSE REACTIONS: Diarrhea, nausea, flatulence, rash, redistribution of body fat, jaundice, hypersensitivity reactions, bilirubinemia, hyperglycemia, metabolic acidosis.

INTERACTIONS: See Contraindications. Avoid pimozide, triazolam, midazolam, ergot derivatives, amiodarone or quinidine; potential for life-threatening adverse events. Avoid rifampin. Avoid lovastatin or simvastatin; caution with other HMG-CoA reductase inhibitors. May increase sildenafil or other PDE5 inhibitor levels and adverse effects. Avoid St. John's wort; may decrease levels of nelfinavir. May increase levels of drugs metabolized by CYP450 3A (eg, dihydropyridine CCBs, immunosuppressants, etc). Use alternative or additional contraception with oral contraceptives. May increase levels of cyclosporine, tacrolimus, sirolimus, atorvastatin, cerivastatin, fluticasone, azithromycin. Carbamazepine, phenobarbital may decrease levels of nelfinavir. May decrease levels of phenytoin, methadone. Give didanosine 1 hr before or 2 hrs after nelfinavir. Omeprazole decreases levels of nelfinavir; concomitant use with proton pump inhibitors may lead to loss of virologic response and development of resistance.

PREGNANCY: Category B, not for use in nursing.

MECHANISM OF ACTION: HIV-1 protease inhibitor; prevents cleavage of *gag* and *gag-pol* polyprotein resulting in production of immature, non-infectious virus.

PHARMACOKINETICS: Absorption: (1250mg bid) C_{max}=4mg/L; AUC=52.8mg•h/L. (750mg tid); C_{max}=3mg/L; AUC=43.6mg•h/L. **Distribution:** V_d=2-7L/kg; plasma protein binding (>98%). **Metabolism:** CYP3A, 2C19 (oxidation). **Elimination:** Feces (22%), urine (1-2%); $T_{1/2}$=3.5-5 hrs.

VIRAMUNE RX

nevirapine (Boehringer Ingelheim)

> Severe, life-threatening, in some cases fatal, hepatotoxicity and skin reactions (eg, Stevens-Johnson syndrome, toxic epidermal necrolysis, hypersensitivity) reported. Women, including pregnant women, and/or patients with higher CD4 counts are at higher risk of hepatotoxicity. Permanently d/c following severe hepatitic, skin or hypersensitivity reactions.

THERAPEUTIC CLASS: Non-nucleoside reverse transcriptase inhibitor

INDICATIONS: Treatment of HIV-1 infection in combination with other antiretrovirals.

DOSAGE: *Adults:* 200mg qd for 14 days (lead-in period), then 200mg bid. Do not increase dose if rash occurs, until it resolves. Retitrate if interrupt >7 days. *Pediatrics:* 2 months-8 yrs: 4mg/kg qd for 14 days, then 7mg/kg bid. Max: 400mg/day. ≥8 yrs: 4mg/kg qd for 14 days, then 4mg/kg bid. Max: 400mg/day. Do not increase dose if rash occurs, until it resolves. Retitrate if interrupt >7 days.

HOW SUPPLIED: Sus: 50mg/5mL [240mL]; Tab: 200mg* *scored

WARNINGS/PRECAUTIONS: Avoid with severe hepatic impairment. Caution with moderate impairment and dialysis. Perform laboratory tests (eg, LFTs) at baseline and during first 18 weeks of therapy. Possible redistribution or accumulation of body fat.

ADVERSE REACTIONS: Headache, fever, severe rash, GI effects, fatigue, thrombocytopenia, fatigue, hepatotoxicity, granulocytopenia (pediatrics), rhabdomyolysis.

INTERACTIONS: Avoid use of prednisone for prevention of therapy-associated rash. Decreased levels of clarithromycin; consider alternative. Decreased levels of efavirenz, indinavir, nelfinavir, saquinavir. May decrease effectiveness of oral contraceptives and other hormonal contraceptives; use alternate or additional method of contraception. Increased levels with fluconazole. Avoid with ketoconazole, St. John's wort, rifampin. Decreased levels of lopinavir; adjust lopinavir/ritonavir doses. May decrease levels of methadone; monitor for signs of withdrawal. Increased levels of rifabutin. Possible decreased levels with antiarrhythmics (eg, amiodarone, disopyramide, lidocaine), anticonvulsants (eg, carbamazepine, clonazepam, ethosuximide), itraconazole, CCBs (eg, diltiazem, nifedipine, verapamil), cyclophosphamide, ergotamine, immunosuppressants (eg, cyclosporine, tacrolimus, sirolimus), cisapride, fentanyl. Monitor with warfarin.

PREGNANCY: Category B, not for use in nursing.

MECHANISM OF ACTION: Non-nucleoside reverse transcriptase inhibitor; binds directly to reverse transcriptase and blocks RNA-dependent DNA polymerase activities by causing disruption of the enzyme's catalytic site.

PHARMACOKINETICS: Absorption: Absolute bioavailability: 93+/- 9% (tab), 91+/-8% (sol); C_{max}=2+/-0.4 Mcg/mL; T_{max}=4 hrs. **Distribution:** V_d=1.21±0.09L/Kg; plasma protein binding (60%); readily crosses placenta; found in breast milk. **Metabolism:** Liver; oxidative metabolism, via CYP3A4 and CYP2B6 (extensively); glucuronide metabolites. **Elimination:** Urine (<3% excreted as parent drug); $T_{1/2}$=45 hrs.

V

VIRAZOLE RX
ribavirin (Valeant)

> Sudden deterioration of respiratory function associated with initiation in infants. Monitor respiratory function carefully. Not for use in adults. Use with mechanical ventilator assistance with staff familiar with mode of administration and specific type of ventilator.

THERAPEUTIC CLASS: Nucleoside analogue

INDICATIONS: Treatment of hospitalized infants and young children with severe lower respiratory tract infections due to respiratory syncytial virus.

DOSAGE: *Pediatrics:* Continuous aerosol administration of 20mg/mL in the drug reservoir of the SPAG-2 unit for 12-18 hrs/day for 3-7 days.

HOW SUPPLIED: Sol, Inhalation: 6g

CONTRAINDICATIONS: Women who are or may become pregnant during exposure to drug.

WARNINGS/PRECAUTIONS: Monitor respiratory function and fluid status according to SPAG-2 manual. Accumulation of drug precipitate can result in mechanical ventilator dysfunction and associated increased pulmonary pressures.

ADVERSE REACTIONS: Worsening of respiratory status, bronchospasm, pulmonary edema, hypoventilation, cyanosis, dyspnea, bacterial pneumonia, pneumothorax, apnea, atelectasis, ventilator dependence, cardiac arrest, hypotension, bradycardia.

INTERACTIONS: Digoxin toxicity reported.

PREGNANCY: Category X, safety in nursing not known.

MECHANISM OF ACTION: Nucleoside analogue; mechanism unknown. Suspected to be analogue of guanosine or xanthosine.

PHARMACOKINETICS: Elimination: $T_{1/2}$=9.5 hrs.

VIREAD RX
tenofovir disoproxil fumarate (Gilead)

> Lactic acidosis and severe hepatomegaly with steatosis, including fatal cases, reported with nucleoside analogs alone or with concomitant antiretrovirals. Not approved for treatment of chronic hepatitis B virus (HBV) infection and safety and efficacy have not been established in patients coinfected with HBV and HIV. Severe acute exacerbations of hepatitis B have been reported in patients coinfected with HBV and HIV and have discontinued Viread. Monitor hepatic function closely for at least several months if coinfected with HBV and HIV and d/c Viread. If appropriate, initiate anti-hepatitis B therapy.

THERAPEUTIC CLASS: Nucleoside analogue

INDICATIONS: Treatment of HIV-1 infection in combination with other antiretrovirals.

DOSAGE: *Adults:* 300mg qd without regard to food.

HOW SUPPLIED: Tab: 300mg

WARNINGS/PRECAUTIONS: Obesity and prolonged nucleoside exposure may be risk factors for lactic acidosis and severe hepatomegaly with steatosis. Caution if risk factors for hepatic disease present or with hepatic insufficiency. Monitor hepatic function with both clinical and laboratory follow-up for at least several months in patients who are coinfected with HIV and HBV and d/c Viread. All patients should have CrCl calculated prior to and during therapy. Dose adjust and monitor renal function when CrCl <50mL/min. May cause renal impairment. Monitor serum creatinine and phosphorous in patients at risk or with a history of renal dysfunction and those receiving concomitant nephrotoxic agents. Bone monitoring should be considered for HIV patients at risk for osteopenia. Cases of osteomalacia reported. Possible fat redistribution and accumulation of body fat.

ADVERSE REACTIONS: Nausea, diarrhea, vomiting, flatulence, asthenia, headache, abdominal pain, anorexia.

INTERACTIONS: Increases levels of didanosine; use caution when coadministering, monitor for didanosine-associated adverse effects (suppression of CD4 cell counts), and discontinue if these adverse events develop. Renally eliminated drugs (eg, cidofovir, acyclovir, valacyclovir, ganciclovir, valganciclovir) may increase levels of itself or tenofovir. Indinavir/ritonavir, and drugs that decrease renal function may increase tenofovir plasma levels. May decrease lamivudine, indinavir, lopinavir, and ritonavir plasma levels. Avoid with concurrent or recent use of nephrotoxic agents. Avoid use with Truvada or Atripla.

PREGNANCY: Category B, not for use in nursing.

MECHANISM OF ACTION: Nucleotide analog reverse transcriptase inhibitor; inhibits activity of HIV-1 reverse transcriptase by competing with natural substrate deoxyadenosine 5'-triphosphate and, after incorporation into DNA, by DNA termination.

PHARMACOKINETICS: Absorption: C_{max}=296±90ng/mL; AUC=2287±685ng•hr/mL; T_{max}=1.0±0.4 hrs. **Distribution:** Serum protein bound (<7.2%); V_d=1.3±0.6L/kg (after 1mg/kg dose); V_d=1.2±0.4L/kg (after 3mg/kg dose). **Elimination:** Urine (70-80%, unchanged); $T_{1/2}$=17 hrs.

VIROPTIC RX
trifluridine (King)

THERAPEUTIC CLASS: Fluorinated pyrimidine nucleoside antiviral

INDICATIONS: Treatment of primary keratoconjunctivitis and recurrent epithelial keratitis due to herpes simplex virus, types 1 and 2.

DOSAGE: *Adults:* 1 drop q2h while awake until re-epithelialization. Max: 9 drops/day. Following Re-epithelialization: 1 drop q4h while awake for 7 days; minimum of 5 drops/day. If no improvement after 7 days or if complete re-epithelialization has not occurred after 14 days, consider other therapy. Avoid using >21 days.
Pediatrics: ≥6 yrs: 1 drop q2h while awake until re-epithelialization. Max: 9 drops/day. Following Re-epithelialization: 1 drop q4h while awake for 7 days; minimum of 5 drops/day. If no improvement after 7 days or if complete re-epithelialization has not occurred after 14 days, consider other therapy. Avoid using >21 days.

HOW SUPPLIED: Sol: 1% [7.5mL]

WARNINGS/PRECAUTIONS: Only use with a clinical diagnosis of herpetic keratitis. May cause transient, mild local irritation of the conjunctiva and cornea when instilled.

ADVERSE REACTIONS: Burning, stinging, palpebral edema, superficial punctate keratopathy, epithelial keratopathy, hypersensitivity reaction, stromal edema, irritation, keratitis sicca, hyperemia, increased IOP.

PREGNANCY: Category C, caution in nursing.

MECHANISM OF ACTION: Fluorinated pyrimidine nucleoside antiviral; unknown, suspected to interfere with DNA synthesis.

PHARMACOKINETICS: Absorption: Penetrates intact cornea. **Metabolism:** 5-carboxy-2'-deoxyuridine (major metabolite).

VISICOL RX
sodium phosphate (Salix)

THERAPEUTIC CLASS: Bowel cleanser

INDICATIONS: For cleansing the colon in preparation for colonoscopy in adults ≥18 yrs..

DOSAGE: *Adults:* ≥18 yrs: Drink only clear liquids 12 hrs before dose. Evening Before Exam: 3 tabs with 8 oz clear liquids every 15 min for total of 20 tabs (last dose is 2 tabs). Repeat on day of exam 3-5 hrs before procedure. May retreat after 7 days.

HOW SUPPLIED: Tab: (Sodium Phosphate Monobasic Monohydrate-Sodium Phosphate Dibasic Anhydrous) 1.102g-0.398g* *scored

CONTRAINDICATIONS: Patients with biopsy-proven acute phosphate nephropathy.

WARNINGS/PRECAUTIONS: Fatalities reported from electrolyte imbalances and arrhythmias if administered with other sodium phosphate-containing products. May induce QT prolongation, colonic mucosal aphthous ulcerations and exacerbate IBS. Caution with severe renal insufficiency (creatinine clearance less than 30 mL/minute), CHF, ascites, unstable angina, acute bowel obstruction, bowel perforation, toxic megacolon, gastric retention, ileus, pseudo-obstruction of the bowel, severe chronic constipation, acute colitis, gastric bypass, stapling surgery, or hypomotility syndrome. Correct electrolyte disturbance before use. Caution within 3 months of acute MI or cardiac surgery. Do not use additional enema or laxative. Reports of generalized tonic-clonic seizures and/or loss of consciousness in patients with no prior history of seizures.

ADVERSE REACTIONS: Nausea, vomiting, abdominal bloating, dizziness, headache, abdominal pain.

INTERACTIONS: May reduce absorption of other drugs. Caution with sodium phosphate-containing products, agents that prolong QT interval or affect electrolyte levels.

PREGNANCY: Category C, safety in nursing not known.

MECHANISM OF ACTION: Osmotic laxative; causes large amounts of water to be drawn into colon, promoting colon evacuation.

VISTIDE   RX
cidofovir (Gilead)

> Renal impairment is a major toxicity; prehydrate with IV normal saline (NS) and administer probenecid with each dose. Monitor serum creatinine (SCr) and urine protein within 48 hrs prior to each dose. Modify dose with renal function changes. Contraindicated with nephrotoxic agents. Neutropenia reported; monitor neutrophils. Carcinogenic, teratogenic, and hypospermatic in animal studies.

THERAPEUTIC CLASS: Viral DNA synthesis inhibitor

INDICATIONS: Treatment of cytomegalovirus (CMV) retinitis in AIDS patients.

DOSAGE: *Adults:* IV: Induction: 5mg/kg once weekly for 2 weeks. Maint: 5mg/kg once every 2 weeks. Reduce maint from 5mg/kg to 3mg/kg for an increase in SCr of 0.3-0.4mg/dL above baseline. D/C with increase in SCr ≥0.5mg/kg above baseline or ≥3+ proteinuria. Administer probenecid 2g PO 3 hrs before cidofovir, then 1g at 2 hrs and 8 hrs after completion of cidofovir infusion. Administer at least 1L 0.9% NS immediately before infusion. If tolerated, give 2nd liter at start of or immediately after infusion.

HOW SUPPLIED: Inj: 75mg/mL

CONTRAINDICATIONS: SCr >1.5mg/dL, CrCl ≤55mL/min, or urine protein ≥100mg/dL (≥2+ proteinuria) with therapy initiation. Nephrotoxic agents (discontinue at least 7 days before therapy), severe hypersensitivity to probenecid or other sulfa-containing agents, direct intraocular use.

WARNINGS/PRECAUTIONS: Dose-dependent nephrotoxicity. Monitor IOP, visual acuity, ocular symptoms, uveitis/iritis, and renal function periodically. Monitor WBC with differential before each dose. Avoid during pregnancy. Adequate contraception for both sexes during and following treatment is advised. May cause male infertility. Potentially carcinogenic.

ADVERSE REACTIONS: Nausea, vomiting, neutropenia, proteinuria, decreased IOP/ocular hypotony, anterior uveitis/iritis, metabolic acidosis, nephrotoxicity, pneumonia, dyspnea, infection, fever, creatinine ≥2mg/dL, decreased sodium bicarbonate.

INTERACTIONS: Avoid nephrotoxic agents (aminoglyosides, amphotericin B, foscarnet, IV pentamidine, vancomycin, and NSAIDs); discontinue nephrotoxic agents at least 7 days before therapy. Temporarily discontinue zidovudine or decrease zidovudine by 50% with probenecid.

PREGNANCY: Category C, not for use in nursing.

MECHANISM OF ACTION: Viral DNA synthesis inhibitor; suppresses CMV replication by selective inhibition of viral DNA synthesis.

PHARMACOKINETICS: Administration: Variable doses resulted in altered parameters. **Absorption:** 5mg/kg: AUC=28.3 mcg•mL/hr (without probenecid), AUC=40.8+/-+9.0 mcg•mL/hr (with probenecid); C_{max}=11.5mcg/mL (without probenecid), C_{max}=19.6+/-7.2 mcg/mL (with probenecid); 3mg/kg: AUC=20.0+/-2.3mcg•mL/hr (without probenecid), AUC=25.7+/-8.5mcg•mL/hr (with probenecid); C_{max}=7.3+/-1.4 mcg/mL (without probenecid), C_{max}=9.8+/-3.7mcg/mL (with probenecid). **Distribution:** V_d=537±126mL/kg (without probenecid), V_d = 410+/-102mL/kg (with probenecid); Plasma protein binding (≤6%). **Elimination:** 80-100% excreted unchanged in urine.

VISUDYNE   RX
verteporfin (Novartis Ophthalmics)

THERAPEUTIC CLASS: Photosensitizing agent

INDICATIONS: Treatment of age-related macular degeneration with subfoveal choroidal neovascularization.

DOSAGE: *Adults:* 6mg/m^2 IV over 10 min at 3mL/min. Photoactivation with laser light therapy with nonthermal diode laser 15 min after start IV infusion. Re-evaluate every 3 months and repeat if choroidal neovascular leakage detected on fluorescein angiography.

HOW SUPPLIED: Inj: 15mg

CONTRAINDICATIONS: Porphyria.

WARNINGS/PRECAUTIONS: Avoid direct sunlight or bright indoor light for 5 days. Avoid extravasation. If extravasation occurs, protect area from direct light until swelling and discoloration fade. Protect from intense light if surgery within 48 hrs after therapy. Do not retreat if severe vision decrease of 4 lines or more occurs within 1 week after therapy. Only use compatible lasers. Caution with moderate to severe hepatic dysfunction. Reduced effects with increasing age.

ADVERSE REACTIONS: Headache, injection site reactions, visual disturbances, asthenia, HTN, eczema, constipation, nausea, anemia, arthralgia, vertigo, pharyngitis.

INTERACTIONS: CCBs, polymyxin B, and radiation therapy may enhance rate of uptake by vascular endothelium. Increased photosensitivity with tetracyclines, sulfonamides, phenothiazines, sulfonylureas, thiazide diuretics, and griseofulvin. Decreased effects with dimethyl sulfoxide, β-carotene, ethanol, formate, mannitol, and drugs that decrease clotting, vasoconstriction, or platelet aggregation (eg, thromboxane A$_2$ inhibitors).

PREGNANCY: Pregnancy C, not for use in nursing.

MECHANISM OF ACTION: Photosensitizing agent; transported into plasma by lipoproteins. Activated by light in presence of oxygen; light activation causes local damage to neovascular endothelium, subsequently leading to vessel occlusion. Damaged endothelium releases procoagulant and vasoactive factors through lipo-oxygenase and cyclo-oxygenase pathways, resulting in platelet aggregation, fibrin clot formation, and vasoconstriction.

PHARMACOKINETICS: Absorption: Dose proportional. **Distribution:** Found in breast milk. **Metabolism:** Liver and plasma esterases; diacid metabolite. **Elimination:** $T_{1/2}$=5-6 hrs; Feces (major), urine (≤0.01%).

V

VITAFOL-PN
RX
multiple vitamin - minerals (Everett)

THERAPEUTIC CLASS: Prenatal vitamin

INDICATIONS: Vitamin and mineral supplementation for before, during, and after pregnancy.

DOSAGE: *Adults:* 1 tab qd.

HOW SUPPLIED: Tab: Calcium 125mg-Folic Acid 1mg-Iron 65mg-Magnesium 25mg-Niacin 15mg-Vitamin A 1700 IU-Vitamin B_1 1.6mg-Vitamin B_2 1.8mg-Vitamin B_6 2.5mg-Vitamin B_{12} 0.005mg-Vitamin C 60mg-Vitamin D 400 IU-Vitamin E 30 IU-Zinc 15mg

CONTRAINDICATIONS: Untreated and uncomplicated pernicious anemia, hemachromatosis, pyridoxine responsive anemia, liver cirrhosis, cobalt sensitivity, iron storage disease or the potential for this disease due to chronic hemolytic anemia.

WARNINGS/PRECAUTIONS: Accidental overdose of iron-containing products is a leading cause of fatal poisoning in children <6 yrs. Folic acid may partially correct hematological damage due to vitamin B_{12} deficiency of pernicious anemia, while neurological damage progresses. Prolonged use of iron salts may cause iron storage disease.

ADVERSE REACTIONS: GI disturbances, allergic sensitization, black tarry stools.

VITAPLEX
RX
multiple vitamin (Amide)

INDICATIONS: For nutritional supplementation in conditions requiring water-soluble vitamins.

DOSAGE: *Adults:* 1 tab qd.

HOW SUPPLIED: Tab: Folic Acid 0.5mg-Niacin 100mg-Pantothenic Acid 18mg-Vitamin B_1 15mg-Vitamin B_2 15mg-Vitamin B_6 4mg-Vitamin B_{12} 5mcg-Vitamin C 500mg

WARNINGS/PRECAUTIONS: Not for treatment of pernicious anemia or other megoblastic anemias, or severe specific deficiencies.

ADVERSE REACTIONS: Allergic and idiosyncratic reactions.

INTERACTIONS: May decrease efficacy of levodopa.

MECHANISM OF ACTION: Multivitamin/multimineral nutritional supplement.

VITAPLEX PLUS
RX
multiple vitamin - minerals (Amide)

THERAPEUTIC CLASS: Vitamin/Mineral Supplements

INDICATIONS: For prophylactic or therapeutic nutritional supplementation in physiologically stressful conditions.

DOSAGE: *Adults:* 1 tab qd.

HOW SUPPLIED: Tab: Biotin 0.15mg-Chromium 0.1mg-Copper 3mg-Folic Acid 0.8mg-Iron 27mg-Magnesium 50mg-Manganese 5mg-Niacin 100mg-Pantothenic Acid 25mg-Vitamin A 5000IU-Vitamin B_1 20mg-Vitamin B_2 20mg-Vitamin B_6 25mg-Vitamin B_{12} 50mcg-Vitamin C 500mg-Vitamin E 30IU-Zinc 22.5mg

WARNINGS/PRECAUTIONS: Not for treatment of pernicious anemia or other megoblastic anemias, or severe specific deficiencies.

ADVERSE REACTIONS: Allergic and idiosyncratic reactions, GI intolerance.

INTERACTIONS: May decrease efficacy of levodopa.

MECHANISM OF ACTION: Multivitamin/mineral nutritional supplement.

V

VITRASERT   RX
ganciclovir (Bausch & Lomb)

THERAPEUTIC CLASS: Nucleoside analogue

INDICATIONS: Treatment of cytomegalovirus (CMV) retinitis in AIDS patients.

DOSAGE: *Adults:* Each implant releases 4.5mg over 5-8 months. Remove and replace when there is evidence of progression of retinitis.
Pediatrics: ≥9 yrs: Each implant releases 4.5mg over 5-8 months. Remove and replace when there is evidence of progression of retinitis.

HOW SUPPLIED: Implant: 4.5mg

CONTRAINDICATIONS: Hypersensitivity to acyclovir, patients with contraindication for intraocular surgery (eg, external infection, severe thrombocytopenia).

WARNINGS/PRECAUTIONS: For intravitreal implantation only. Monitor for extraocular CMV disease. Implant does not treat systemic CMV. Complications from surgery include vitreous loss or hemorrhage, cataract formation, retinal detachment, uveitis, endophthalmitis, decrease in visual acuity. Immediate decrease in visual acuity will last 2-4 weeks postop. Maintain sterility of the surgical field, implant. Handle implant by suture tab to avoid damage to polymer coating. Handling and disposal of the implant should follow guidelines for antineoplastics.

ADVERSE REACTIONS: Visual acuity loss, vitreous hemorrhage, retinal detachments, cataract formation/lens opacities, macular abnormalities, IOP spikes, optic disk/nerve changes, uveitis, hyphemas.

PREGNANCY: Category C, not for use in nursing.

MECHANISM OF ACTION: Nucleoside analogue antiviral; inhibits replication of herpes viruses.

VIVACTIL   RX
protriptyline HCL (Various)

> Antidepressants increased the risk of suicidal thinking and behavior (suicidality) in short-term studies in children, adolescents, and young adults with Major Depressive Disorder (MDD) and other psychiatric disorders. Protriptyline is not approved for use in pediatric patients.

THERAPEUTIC CLASS: Tricyclic antidepressant

INDICATIONS: Treatment of symptoms of depression in those under close medical supervision.

DOSAGE: *Adults:* Usual: 15-40mg/day taken tid-qid. Titrate: May increase to 60mg/day. Max: 60mg/day. Elderly: Initial: 5mg tid. Titrate: Increase gradually if needed. Monitor cardiovascular system with doses >20mg/day.
Pediatrics: Adolescents: Initial: 5mg tid. Titrate: Increase gradually if needed.

HOW SUPPLIED: Tab: 5mg, 10mg

CONTRAINDICATIONS: Within 14 days of MAOI therapy, cisapride, acute recovery period following MI.

WARNINGS/PRECAUTIONS: Caution with history of seizures, urinary retention, increased IOP, cardiovascular disorders, hyperthyroidism, elderly. May aggravate psychotic symptoms in schizophrenia, manic symptoms in manic-depressive psychosis, and anxiety/agitation in overactive/agitated patients. D/C several days before elective surgery. Both elevation and lowering of blood sugar levels reported.

ADVERSE REACTIONS: Tachycardia, hypotension, confusion, anxiety, insomnia, nightmares, seizures, EPS, dizziness, headache, anticholinergic effects, rash, photosensitivity, blood dyscrasias, GI effects, impotence, decreased libido, flushing.

INTERACTIONS: See Contraindications. Risk of hyperpyrexia with anticholinergics and neuroleptics. Reduced hepatic metabolism with cimetidine. Enhanced seizure risk with tramadol. Enhanced response to alcohol,

V

barbiturates, other CNS depressants. Use with CYP2D6 enzyme inhibitors (eg, quinidine, cimetidine, other antidepressants, phenothiazines, propafenone, flecainide, SSRIs) require lower doses for either TCA or other drug. Hyperpyretic crises, severe convulsions, and deaths reported with MAOIs. May block antihypertensive effect of guanethidine, or similarly acting compounds.

PREGNANCY: Safety in pregnancy and nursing not known.

MECHANISM OF ACTION: Unknown.

VIVELLE   RX
estradiol (Novartis)

> Estrogens increase risk of endometrial cancer in postmenopausal women. Estrogens, with or without progestins, should not be used for the prevention of cardiovascular disease. Increased risks of MI, stroke, invasive breast cancer, PE, and DVT in postmenopausal women (50-79 yrs of age) reported. Increased risk of developing probable dementia in postmenopausal women ≥65 yrs of age reported.

OTHER BRAND NAMES: Vivelle-Dot (Novartis)

THERAPEUTIC CLASS: Estrogen

INDICATIONS: Treatment of moderate to severe vasomotor symptoms and/or vulvar/vaginal atrophy associated with menopause. Treatment of hypo-estrogenism due to hypogonadism, castration, or primary ovarian failure. Prevention of postmenopausal osteoporosis.

DOSAGE: *Adults:* Vasomotor Symptoms/Vulvar/Vaginal Atrophy: Initial: 0.0375mg/day twice weekly. Titrate: Adjust after at least 1 month. D/C or taper at 3-6 month intervals. Wait 1 week after withdrawal of oral therapy before initiating therapy. Osteoporosis Prevention: Minimum Effective Dose: 0.025mg/day twice weekly. Apply to clean, dry area of the trunk; avoid breasts and waistline. Rotate sites; allow 1 week between same site. Without intact uterus, may give continuously; with intact uterus, may give cyclically (3 weeks on, 1 week off) with a progestin.

HOW SUPPLIED: Patch: (Vivelle) 0.05mg/day, 0.1mg/day [8ˢ, 48ˢ]; (Vivelle-Dot) 0.025mg/day, 0.0375mg/day, 0.05mg/day, 0.075mg/day, 0.1mg/day [8ˢ, 24ˢ]

CONTRAINDICATIONS: Pregnancy, undiagnosed abnormal genital bleeding, breast cancer, estrogen dependent neoplasia, DVT/PE, active or recent (eg, within past year) arterial thromboembolic disease (eg, stroke, MI), liver dysfunction or disease.

WARNINGS/PRECAUTIONS: May increase risk of cardiovascular events (eg, MI, stroke), venous thrombosis, and PE; d/c immediately if any of these events occur or are suspected. May increase risk of breast/endometrial cancer and gallbladder disease. May lead to severe hypercalcemia with breast cancer and bone metastases; monitor and d/c if hypercalcemia occurs. Retinal vascular thrombosis reported; monitor and d/c if papilledema or retinal vascular lesions occur. Consider addition of a progestin if no hysterectomy. May elevate BP; monitor at regular intervals. May cause elevations of plasma triglycerides with pre-existing hypertriglyceridemia. Caution with history of cholestatic jaundice associated with past estrogen use or with pregnancy; d/c with recurrence. May lead to increased thyroid-binding globulin levels; monitor thyroid function. May cause fluid retention; caution with cardiac/renal dysfunction. Caution with severe hypocalcemia. May increase risk of ovarian cancer. May exacerbate endometriosis, asthma, DM, epilepsy, migraine, porphyria, SLE, and hepatic hemangiomas; use with caution.

ADVERSE REACTIONS: Altered vaginal bleeding, vaginal candidiasis, breast tenderness/enlargement, nausea, vomiting, melasma, headache, weight changes, edema, altered libido.

INTERACTIONS: CYP3A4 inducers (eg, St. John's wort, phenobarbital, carbamazepine, rifampin) may decrease levels which may decrease therapeutic effects and/or change uterine bleeding profile. CYP3A4 inhibitors (eg, erythromycin, clarithromycin, ketoconazole, itraconazole, ritonavir, grapefruit juice) may increase levels which may result in side effects.

PREGNANCY: Contraindicated in pregnancy, caution in nursing.

MECHANISM OF ACTION: Estrogen; responsible for development and maintenance of female reproductive system, and secondary sexual characteristics by modulating pituitary secretion of gonadotropins, LH and FSH.

PHARMACOKINETICS: Absorption: Transdermal administration of variable doses resulted in different parameters. **Metabolism:** Liver, estrone (metabolite), estriol (major urinary metabolite). **Elimination:** Urine; $T_{1/2}$=4.4 hrs, 5.9-7.7 hrs (Dot).

VIVITROL   RX
naltrexone (Cephalon)

THERAPEUTIC CLASS: Opioid antagonist

INDICATIONS: Treatment of alcohol dependence.

DOSAGE: *Adults:* Administer 380mg IM gluteal inj every 4 weeks or once a month using alternating buttocks.

HOW SUPPLIED: Inj, Extended-Release: 380mg

CONTRAINDICATIONS: Concomitant opioid analgesics, physiologic opioid dependence, acute opiate withdrawal, positive urine screen for opioids.

WARNINGS/PRECAUTIONS: Hepatotoxic with excessive doses; margin of separation between safe dose and hepatotoxic dose is 5-fold or less. May cause eosinophilic pneumonia. Only treat patients opioid-free for 7-10 days. Perform naloxone challenge test if risk of precipitating withdrawal. Attempting to overcome the opiate blockade using opioids is very dangerous. More sensitive to lower doses of opioids after naltrexone is discontinued. In emergency situation, suggested plan for pain management is regional analgesia, conscious sedation with a benzodiazepine, or use of non-opioid analgesics or general anesthesia. Monitor for development of depression or suicidal thinking. Caution in renal or hepatic impairment. Administration will not eliminate or diminish alcohol withdrawal symptoms.

ADVERSE REACTIONS: Nausea, vomiting, diarrhea, abdominal pain, upper respiratory tract infection, pharyngitis, insomnia, anxiety, depression, injection site reactions, arthralgia, muscle cramps, dizziness, syncope, appetite disorder, retinal artery occlusion.

INTERACTIONS: See Contraindications.

PREGNANCY: Category C, not for use in nursing.

MECHANISM OF ACTION: Opioid antagonist; high affinity for μ opioid receptor.

PHARMACOKINETICS: Absorption: T_{max}=2 hrs. **Distribution:** Plasma protein binding (21%). **Metabolism:** Extensive, via dihydrodiol dehydrogenase, 6β-naltrexol (primary metabolite). **Elimination:** Urine; $T_{1/2}$=5-10 days.

VOLTAREN GEL   RX
diclofenac sodium (Novartis Consumer)

> NSAIDs may cause an increased risk of serious cardiovascular thrombotic events, MI, stroke and serious GI adverse events including bleeding, ulceration, and perforation of the stomach or intestines. Contraindicated for the treatment of perioperative pain in the setting of coronary artery bypass graft (CABG) surgery.

THERAPEUTIC CLASS: NSAID

INDICATIONS: Relief of the pain of osteoarthritis of joints amenable to topical treatment, such as knees and hands. Not evaluated for use on spine, hip, or shoulder.

DOSAGE: *Adults:* Measure onto enclosed dosing card to appropriate 2g or 4g line. Lower Extremities: Apply 4g to affected foot, knee, or ankle qid. Max: 16g/day to any single joint. Upper Extremities: Apply 2g to affected hand, elbow, or wrist qid. Max: 8g/day to any single joint. Total dose should not

V

exceed 32g/day over all affected joints. Avoid showering or bathing for at least 1 hour after application. Avoid open wounds, eyes, mucous membranes, external heat, and/or occlusive dressings. Avoid wearing clothing or gloves for at least 10 min after application.

HOW SUPPLIED: Gel: 1%

CONTRAINDICATIONS: ASA or other NSAID allergy that precipitates asthma, urticaria, or allergic-type reactions. Treatment of perioperative pain in the setting of CABG surgery.

WARNINGS/PRECAUTIONS: May lead to onset of new HTN or worsening of pre-existing HTN; monitor BP closely. Fluid retention and edema reported; caution with fluid retention or heart failure. Renal papillary necrosis and other renal injury reported after long-term use. Not recommended for use with advanced renal disease; if therapy must be initiated, monitor renal function. Anaphylactoid reactions may occur. May cause serious skin adverse events (eg, exfoliative dermatitis, Stevens-Johnson syndrome, and toxic epidermal necrolysis). Avoid in late pregnancy; may cause premature closure of ductus arteriosis. May cause elevations of LFTs; d/c if liver disease develops or systemic manifestations occur. Caution in elderly. Anemia may occur; with long-term use, monitor Hgb/Hct if signs or symptoms of anemia develop. May inhibit platelet aggregation and prolong bleeding time; monitor with coagulation disorders. Caution with asthma and avoid with ASA-sensitive asthma. Patients should minimize or avoid exposure to natural or artificial sunlight on treated areas. Monitor for signs or symptoms of GI bleeding.

ADVERSE REACTIONS: Application-site reactions, including dermatitis.

INTERACTIONS: Avoid with other diclofenac products. Increased adverse effects with ASA; avoid use. May enhance methotrexate toxicity; caution when coadministering. May increase nephrotoxicity of cyclosporine; caution when coadministering. May diminish antihypertensive effect of ACE-inhibitors. May reduce natriuretic effect of furosemide and thiazides; monitor for renal failure. May increase lithium levels; monitor for toxicity. Synergistic effects on GI bleeding with warfarin. Avoid concomitant use with other topical products, including topical medications, sunscreens, lotions, moisturizers, and cosmetics, on the same skin site.

PREGNANCY: Category C, not for use in nursing.

MECHANISM OF ACTION: NSAID; inhibits cyclooxygenase, resulting in reduced formation of prostaglandins, thromboxanes, and prostacylin.

PHARMACOKINETICS: Absorption: (4g) C_{max}=15ng/mL; T_{max}=14 hrs; AUC=233ng•h/mL. (12g)C_{max}=53.8ng/mL; T_{max}=10 hrs; AUC=807ng•h/mL.

VOLTAREN OPHTHALMIC RX
diclofenac sodium (Novartis Ophthalmics)

THERAPEUTIC CLASS: NSAID

INDICATIONS: Treatment of postoperative inflammation following cataract surgery. Temporary relief of pain and photophobia in corneal refractive surgery.

DOSAGE: *Adults:* Cataract Surgery: 1 drop qid, start 24 hrs after surgery and continue for 2 weeks. Corneal Refractive Surgery: 1-2 drops within 1 hr prior to, and within 15 min after surgery. Continue qid for up to 3 days.

HOW SUPPLIED: Sol: 0.1% [2.5mL, 5mL]

WARNINGS/PRECAUTIONS: May delay wound healing. Caution with bleeding tendencies. Monitor for 1 yr after use in corneal refractive procedures. May increase bleeding of ocular tissues. No significant increase in tumor incidence. No differences in safety and effectiveness observed between elderly and younger adult patients.

ADVERSE REACTIONS: Transient burning/stinging, keratitis, elevated IOP, lacrimation, abnormal vision, conjunctivitis, eyelid swelling, discharge, iritis, itching.

INTERACTIONS: Caution with agents that prolong bleeding time (eg, NSAIDs). Potential for cross-sensitivity to acetylsalicylic acid, phenylacetic acid derivatives, and other NSAIDs.

PREGNANCY: Category C, safety in nursing not known.

MECHANISM OF ACTION: NSAID; anti-inflammatory and analgesic that inhibits the enzyme cyclo-oxygenase, which is essential for biosynthesis of prostaglandins.

PHARMACOKINETICS: Absorption: C_{max}<10ng/mL; T_{max}=4 hrs.

VOLTAREN-XR

RX

diclofenac sodium (Novartis)

> NSAIDs may cause an increased risk of serious cardiovascular thrombotic events, MI, stroke and serious GI adverse events including bleeding, ulceration, and perforation of the stomach or intestines. Contraindicated for the treatment of perioperative pain in the setting of coronary artery bypass graft (CABG) surgery.

OTHER BRAND NAMES: Voltaren (Novartis)

THERAPEUTIC CLASS: NSAID (benzeneacetic acid derivative)

INDICATIONS: (Voltaren) Relief of signs and symptoms of osteoarthritis (OA), rheumatoid arthritis (RA), and ankylosing spondylitis (AS). (Voltaren-XR) Relief of signs and symptoms of OA and RA.

DOSAGE: *Adults:* (Voltaren) OA: 50mg bid-tid or 75mg bid. Max: 150mg/day. RA: 50mg tid-qid or 75mg bid. Max: 200mg/day. AS: 25mg qid and 25mg qhs prn. Max: 125mg/day. (Voltaren-XR) OA: 100mg qd. RA: 100mg qd-bid.

HOW SUPPLIED: Tab, Delayed-Release: (Voltaren) 25mg, 50mg, 75mg; Tab, Extended-Release: (Voltaren-XR) 100mg

CONTRAINDICATIONS: ASA or other NSAID allergy that precipitates asthma, urticaria, or allergic-type reactions. Treatment of perioperative pain in the setting of CABG surgery.

WARNINGS/PRECAUTIONS: May lead to onset of new HTN or worsening of pre-existing HTN; monitor BP closely. Fluid retention and edema reported; caution with fluid retention or heart failure. Caution with considerable dehydration. Renal papillary necrosis and other renal injury reported after long-term use. Not recommended for use with advanced renal disease; if therapy must be initiated, monitor renal function. Anaphylactoid reactions may occur. May cause serious skin adverse events (eg, exfoliative dermatitis, Stevens-Johnson syndrome, and toxic epidermal necrolysis). Avoid in late pregnancy; may cause premature closure of ductus arteriosis. May cause elevations of LFTs; d/c if liver disease develops or systemic manifestations occur. Caution in elderly. Anemia may occur; with long-term use, monitor Hgb/Hct if signs or symptoms of anemia develop. May inhibit platelet aggregation and prolong bleeding time; monitor with coagulation disorders. Caution with asthma and avoid with ASA-sensitive asthma. Risk of GI ulceration, bleeding, and perforation.

ADVERSE REACTIONS: Fluid retention, dizziness, rash, nausea, abdominal cramps, LFT abnormalities, constipation, diarrhea, heartburn, tinnitus, GI ulceration, flatulence, dyspepsia, anemia, abnormal renal function.

INTERACTIONS: Avoid with other diclofenac products. Increased adverse effects with ASA; avoid use. May enhance methotrexate toxicity; caution when co-administering. May increase nephrotoxicity of cyclosporine; caution when co-administering. May diminish antihypertensive effect of ACE-inhibitors. May reduce natriuretic effect of furosemide and thiazides; monitor for renal failure. May increase lithium levels; monitor for toxicity. Synergistic effects on GI bleeding with warfarin.

PREGNANCY: Category C, not for use in nursing.

MECHANISM OF ACTION: NSAID; mechanism not completely known. Suspected to inhibit prostaglandin synthetase.

PHARMACOKINETICS: Absorption: Absolute bioavailability (55%); T_{max}=5.3 hrs. **Distribution:** V_d=1.4L/kg; Plasma protein binding (99%). **Metabolism:** Liver

V

(glucuronidation and sulfation). **Elimination:** Urine (65%), bile (35%); $T_{1/2}$=2.3 hrs.

VoSpire ER

RX

albuterol sulfate (Odyssey)

THERAPEUTIC CLASS: Beta$_2$-agonist

INDICATIONS: Treatment of bronchospasm in reversible obstructive airway disease.

DOSAGE: *Adults:* Usual: 4-8mg q12h. Low Body Weight: Initial: 4mg q12h. Titrate: May increase to 8mg q12h. Max: 32mg/day in divided doses. Swallow whole with liquids; do not chew or crush.
Pediatrics: >12 yrs: Usual: 4-8mg q12h. Low Body Weight: Initial: 4mg q12h. Titrate: May increase to 8mg q12h. Max: 32mg/day in divided doses. 6-12 yrs: Usual: 4mg q12h. Max: 24mg/day in divided doses. Swallow whole with liquids; do not chew or crush.

HOW SUPPLIED: Tab, Extended-Release: 4mg, 8mg

WARNINGS/PRECAUTIONS: Hypersensitivity reactions reported. Caution with cardiovascular disorders, especially coronary insufficiency, arrhythmias and HTN. Increased doses may signify need for concomitant corticosteroids. Can produce paradoxical bronchospasm. Caution with DM, hyperthyroidism, seizures. May produce transient hypokalemia. Erythema multiforme and Stevens-Johnson (rare) reported in children.

ADVERSE REACTIONS: Tremor, headache, nervousness, tachycardia, palpitations, nausea, vomiting, muscle cramps.

INTERACTIONS: Avoid oral sympathomimetic agents. Extreme caution within 14 days of MAOI or TCA therapy. Monitor digoxin. May worsen ECG changes and/or hypokalemia with nonpotassium-sparing diuretics. Antagonized by β-blockers.

PREGNANCY: Category C, not for use in nursing.

MECHANISM OF ACTION: β$_2$-adrenergic bronchodilator; stimulates adenyl cylase, enzyme that catalyzes formation of cAMP from ATP. Increased cAMP levels associated with relaxation of bronchial smooth muscle and inhibition of release of mediators of immediate hypersensitivity.

PHARMACOKINETICS: Absorption: C_{max}=13.7ng/mL, T_{max}=6 hrs, AUC=134ng•hr/mL. **Elimination:** $T_{1/2}$=9.3 hrs.

Vumon

RX

teniposide (Bristol-Myers Squibb)

> Cytotoxic. Severe myelosuppression, with resulting infection or bleeding, and/or hypersensitivity reactions may occur.

THERAPEUTIC CLASS: Type II topoisomerase inhibitor

INDICATIONS: With other anticancer agents, for induction therapy of refractory childhood acute lymphoblastic leukemia.

DOSAGE: *Pediatrics:* 165mg/m^2 with cytarabine 300mg/m^2 IV twice weekly for 8-9 doses; or 250mg/m^2 with vincristine 1.5mg/m^2 IV weekly for 4-8 weeks and prednisone 40mg/m^2 PO for 28 days. Down Syndrome: Initial: Half usual dose. Maint: Increase based on degree of myelosuppression/mucositis.

HOW SUPPLIED: Inj: 10mg/mL [5mL]

CONTRAINDICATIONS: Hypersensitivity to Cremophor EL (polyoxyethylated castor oil).

WARNINGS/PRECAUTIONS: Monitor CBC, hepatic and renal function before and during therapy. Avoid rapid IV infusion. May cause fetal harm. Dose-limiting bone marrow suppression. D/C if significant hypotension occurs. Hypersensitivity (HS) reactions manifested by chills, fever, urticaria, tachycardia, bronchospasm, dyspnea, HTN, and hypotension may occur. If re-treating patient with earlier HS reaction, pretreat with corticosteroid and antihistamine. Continuously observe for at least 60 minutes after starting infusion and frequently thereafter. Use gloves when handling or preparing solution. Reduce dose or d/c if severe reactions occur.

ADVERSE REACTIONS: Myelosuppression, leukopenia, neutropenia, thrombocytopenia, anemia, mucositis, diarrhea, nausea, vomiting, infection, alopecia, bleeding, hypersensitivity reactions, rash, fever.

INTERACTIONS: Risk of CNS depression with antiemetics and high dose teniposide. Tolbutamide, sodium salicylate, and sulfamethizole displace protein-bound teniposide; may potentiate toxicity. Increased plasma clearance of methotrexate.

PREGNANCY: Category D, not for use in nursing.

MECHANISM OF ACTION: Podophyllotoxin derivative; acts in late S or early G_2 phase, preventing cells from entering mitosis; inhibits toposiomerase II, causing breaks in DNA and DNA-protein crosslinks.

PHARMACOKINETICS: Absorption: $C_{max} \geq 40mcg/mL$; $T_{max}=1$-2 hrs. **Distribution:** $V_d=3.1L/m^2$; plasma protein binding (>99%). **Elimination:** Urine (4-12%); $T_{1/2}=5$ hrs.

VYTONE   RX
iodoquinol - hydrocortisone (Dermik)

THERAPEUTIC CLASS: Corticosteroid/Anti-infective

INDICATIONS: "Possibly" Effective: Contact or atopic dermatitis, impetiginized eczema, nummular eczema, endogenous chronic infectious dermatitis, stasis dermatitis, pyoderma, nuchal eczema and chronic eczematoid otitis externa, acne urticata, localized or disseminated neurodermatitis, lichen simplex chronicus, anogenital pruritus (vulvae, scroti, ani), folliculitis, bacterial dermatoses, mycotic dermatoses such as tinea (capitis, cruris, corporis, pedis), monliasis, intertrigo.

DOSAGE: *Adults:* Apply to affected area(s) tid-qid.
Pediatrics: ≥12 yrs: Apply tid-qid.

HOW SUPPLIED: Cre: (Hydrocortisone-Iodoquinol) 1%-1% [30g]

WARNINGS/PRECAUTIONS: For external use only. Avoid eyes. D/C if irritation develops. May stain skin, hair, or fabrics. Risk of systemic absorption with treatment of extensive areas or use of occlusive dressings. Increased risk of systemic absorption in children. Iodoquinol may interfere with thyroid tests. False-positive phenylketonuria test reported.

ADVERSE REACTIONS: Burning, itching, irritation, dryness, folliculitis, hypertrichosis, acneiform eruptions, hypopigmentation, perioral dermatitis, allergic dermatitis, skin maceration, secondary infection, skin atrophy, striae, miliaria.

PREGNANCY: Category C, caution in nursing.

MECHANISM OF ACTION: Hydrocortisone: Corticosteroid; possesses anti-inflammatory, antipruritic, and vasoconstrictive properties; anti-inflammatory activity not established. Iodoquinol: Antifungal and antibacterial agent.

PHARMACOKINETICS: Absorption: Hydrocortisone: Percutaneous absorption; inflammation, other disease states, and use of occlusive dressings may increase absorption. **Metabolism:** Hydrocortisone: Liver. **Elimination:** Hydrocortisone: Urine (metabolites and parent compound).

VYTORIN   RX
simvastatin - ezetimibe (Merck/Schering-Plough)

THERAPEUTIC CLASS: Cholesterol absorption inhibitor/HMG-CoA reductase inhibitor

INDICATIONS: When treatment with both components is appropriate, used as an adjunct to diet for the reduction of elevated total-C, LDL-C, Apo B, TG, non-HDL-C, and to increase HDL-C in primary hypercholesterolemia (heterozygous familial and non-familial) or mixed hyperlipidemia. For the reduction of elevated total-C, LDL-C in homozygous familial hypercholesterolemia as an adjunct to other lipid-lowering treatments or if such treatments are unavailable.

DOSAGE: *Adults:* Take once daily in the evening. Initial: 10mg/20mg qd. Less Aggressive LDL-C Reductions: Initial: 10mg/10mg qd. LDL-C Reduction >55%: Initial: 10mg/40mg qd. Titrate: Adjust at ≥2 weeks. Homozygous Familial Hypercholesterolemia: 10mg/40mg or 10mg/80mg qd. Severe Renal Insufficiency: Avoid unless tolerant of ≥5mg of simvastatin; monitor closely. Concomitant Bile Acid Sequestrant: Take either ≥2 hrs before or ≥4 hrs after bile acid sequestrant. Concomitant Cyclosporine: Avoid unless tolerant of ≥5mg of simvastatin. Max: 10mg/10mg/day. Concomitant Amiodarone/ Verapamil: Max: 10mg/20mg/day.

HOW SUPPLIED: Tab: (ezetimibe-simvastatin) 10mg/10mg, 10mg/20mg, 10mg/40mg, 10mg/80mg

CONTRAINDICATIONS: Active liver disease, unexplained persistent elevations in serum transaminases, pregnancy, lactation.

WARNINGS/PRECAUTIONS: Rhabdomyolysis (rare), myopathy reported. D/C therapy if myopathy is suspected or diagnosed, if AST or ALT ≥3x ULN persist, a few days prior to major surgery or when any major medical or surgical condition supervenes. Monitor LFTs prior to therapy and thereafter when clinically indicated. With 10mg/80mg dose, monitor LFTs prior to titration, 3 months after titration and periodically thereafter for 1st yr. Caution with heavy alcohol use, severe renal insufficiency, or history of hepatic disease. Avoid use in moderate or severe hepatic insufficiency.

ADVERSE REACTIONS: Headache, upper respiratory tract infection, myalgia, CK and transaminase elevations, urticaria, arthralgia.

INTERACTIONS: Avoid use with concomitant itraconazole, ketoconazole, erythromycin, clarithromycin, telithromycin, HIV protease inhibitors, nefazodone, grapefruit juice (>1 quart/day); increased risk of myopathy/ rhabdomyolysis. Max 10/10mg daily with gemfibrozil, cyclosporin, danazol. Max 10/20mg daily with amiodarone, verapamil. Caution with other fibrates, ≥1g/day of niacin. Incremental LDL-C reductions with concomitant cholestyramine. Monitor digoxin, warfarin.

PREGNANCY: Category X, not for use in nursing.

MECHANISM OF ACTION: Ezetimibe: Cholesterol absorption inhibitor. Reduces blood cholesterol by inhibiting absorption of cholesterol by small intestine. Molecular target is sterol transporter, Niemann-Pick C1-Like 1 (NPC1L1), which is involved in intestinal uptake of cholesterol and phytosterols. Simvastatin: HMG-CoA reductase inhibitor. Inhibits conversion of HMG-CoA to mevalonate. Also reduces VLDL, TG, and increases HDL-C.

PHARMACOKINETICS: Distribution: Ezetimibe: Plasma protein binding (>90%). Simvastatin: Plasma protein binding (95%); crosses blood-brain barrier. **Metabolism:** Ezetimibe: Small intestine, liver via glucuronide conjugation, ezetimibe-glucuronide (active metabolite). Simvastatin: Hydrolysis; β-hydroxyacid; 6'-hydroxy; 6'hydroxymethyl, and 6'-exomethylene (major active metabolites) . **Elimination:** Ezetimibe: Feces (78%), urine (11%). Simvastatin: Feces (60%), urine (13%).

VYVANSE
lisdexamfetamine dimesylate (Shire) | CII

> High abuse potential; prolonged periods of administration may lead to dependence. Misuse of amphetamine may cause sudden death and serious cardiovascular events.

THERAPEUTIC CLASS: Sympathomimetic amine

INDICATIONS: Treatment of ADHD.

DOSAGE: *Adults:* Individualize dose. Usual: 30mg qam. Titrate: If needed, may increase in increments of 10mg or 20mg at weekly intervals. Max: 70mg/day. Swallow caps or dissolve contents in glass of water; do not store once dissolved. Re-evaluate periodically.

Pediatrics: 6-12 yrs: Individualize dose. Usual: 30mg qam. Titrate: If needed, may increase in increments of 10mg or 20mg at weekly intervals. Max: 70mg/day. Swallow caps or dissolve contents in glass of water; do not store once dissolved. Re-evaluate periodically.

HOW SUPPLIED: Cap: 20mg, 30mg, 40mg, 50mg, 60mg, 70mg

CONTRAINDICATIONS: Advanced arteriosclerosis, symptomatic CVD, moderate to severe HTN, hyperthyroidism, glaucoma, agitated states, history of drug abuse, during or within 14 days of MAOI use.

WARNINGS/PRECAUTIONS: Avoid use with structural cardiac abnormalities, cardiomyopathy, serious heart rhythm abnormalities, or other serious cardiac problems; sudden death reported. Assess presence of cardiac disease through cardiac evaluation. Caution with HTN, heart failure, recent MI, or ventricular arrhythmia; monitor BP and HR. May exacerbate symptoms of behavior disturbance and thought disorder in psychotic patients. Caution with comorbid bipolar disorder; concern for possible induction of mixed/manic episode. Treatment emergent psychotic or manic symptoms (eg, hallucinations, delusional thinking, or mania, without prior history of psychotic illness) may occur; d/c treatment if needed. Aggressive behavior or hostility reported; monitor condition as it worsens. Monitor growth in children. Stimulants may lower the convulsive threshold; d/c in the presence of seizures. Difficulties with accommodation and blurring of vision reported. May exacerbate motor or phonic tics and Tourette's syndrome.

ADVERSE REACTIONS: Ventricular hypertrophy, tic, vomiting, psychomotor hyperactivity, insomnia, rash, upper abdominal pain, decreased appetite, dizziness, dry mouth, irritability, weight loss, nausea, headache, affect lability.

INTERACTIONS: Urinary acidifying agents (eg, ammonium chloride, sodium acid phosphate) and methenamine decrease efficacy. Inhibits adrenergic blockers, antihistamines, and antihypertensives (veratrum alkaloids). Potentiated effects of both agents with TCAs. MAOIs and furazolidone metabolite may cause hypertensive crisis. Antagonized by chlorpromazine, haloperidol, and lithium carbonate. May delay absorption of ethosuximide, phenobarbital, and phenytoin. Potentiates meperidine, norepinephrine, phenobarbital, and phenytoin. Potentiated by propoxyphene overdose; fatal convulsions may occur.

PREGNANCY: Category C, not for use in nursing.

MECHANISM OF ACTION: Dextroamphetamine; blocks reuptake of norepinephrine and dopamine into presynaptic neuron and increases release of these monoamines into extraneuronal space.

PHARMACOKINETICS: Absorption: Rapidly absorbed; T_{max}=1 hr. **Metabolism:** 1st-pass intestinal and/or hepatic metabolism to dextroamphetamine and L-lysine. **Elimination:** Urine, feces; $T_{1/2} \le$ 1hr.

WelChol   RX
colesevelam HCL (Daiichi Sankyo)

THERAPEUTIC CLASS: Bile acid sequestrant

INDICATIONS: Adjunct to diet and exercise to reduce elevated LDL-cholesterol in primary hyperlipidemia as monotherapy or with an HMG-CoA reductase inhibitor and to improve glycemic control in adults with type 2 diabetes mellitus (DM).

DOSAGE: *Adults:* Hyperlipidemia/Type 2 DM: 3 tabs bid or 6 tabs qd. Take with liquids and a meal.

HOW SUPPLIED: Tab: 625mg

CONTRAINDICATIONS: Bowel obstruction, hypertriglyceridemia-induced pancreatitis, serum TG concentrations >500mg/dL.

WARNINGS/PRECAUTIONS: Monitor lipids, including TG and non-HDL-cholesterol levels prior to initiation of treatment and periodically thereafter. Caution in TG levels >300mg/dL, dysphagia or swallowing disorders, gastroparesis, GI motility disorders, major GI tract surgery, bowel obstruction, and those susceptible to vitamin K or fat soluble vitamin deficiencies. Coadministered drugs should be given at least 4 hrs prior to treatment; monitor drug levels. Not for use in treatment of type 1 DM or for diabetic ketoacidosis.

ADVERSE REACTIONS: Asthenia, constipation, dyspepsia, pharyngitis, myalgia, nausea, hypoglycemia, bowel obstruction, dysphagia, esophageal obstruction, fecal impaction, hypertriglyceridemia, pancreatitis, increased transaminases.

INTERACTIONS: Increases TG levels when used with insulin or sulfonylureas. Decreases levels of glyburide, levothyroxine, and oral contraceptives containing ethinyl estradiol and norethindrone. Colesevelam decreases phenytoin levels. Concomitant use with warfarin decreases International Normalized Ratio (INR); monitor INR. Elevates TSH in patients receiving thyroid hormone replacement therapy.

PREGNANCY: Category B, caution in nursing.

MECHANISM OF ACTION: Bile acid sequestrant; non-absorbed, lipid-lowering polymer that binds bile acids in intestine, impeding their reabsorption. Consequently, compensatory effects lead to increased LDL-C clearance from blood, resulting in decreased serum LDL-C levels.

PHARMACOKINETICS: Absorption: Not hydrolyzed by digestive enzymes and not absorbed. **Distribution:** Limited to GI tract. **Metabolism:** Not metabolized systemically. **Excretion:** Urine.

WELLBUTRIN SR   RX
bupropion HCL (GlaxoSmithKline)

> Antidepressants increased the risk of suicidal thinking and behavior (suicidality) in short-term studies in children, adolescents, and young adults with Major Depressive Disorder (MDD) and other psychiatric disorders. Bupropion is not approved for use in pediatric patients.

OTHER BRAND NAMES: Wellbutrin (GlaxoSmithKline)

THERAPEUTIC CLASS: Aminoketone

INDICATIONS: Treatment of MDD.

DOSAGE: *Adults:* ≥18 yrs: (Tab, Extended-Release) Initial: 150mg qd, may increase to 150mg bid after 3 days. Usual: 150mg bid. Max: 200mg bid. Separate doses by at least 8 hrs. Severe Hepatic Cirrhosis: 100mg/day or 150mg every other day. Mild-Moderate Hepatic Cirrhosis/Renal Impairment: Reduce frequency and/or dose. (Tab) Initial: 100mg bid, may increase to 100mg tid after 3 days. Usual: 100mg tid. Max: 450mg/day, given in divided doses of not more than 150mg each. Severe Hepatic Cirrhosis: Max: 75mg qd.

HOW SUPPLIED: Tab: 75mg, 100mg; Tab, Extended-Release: 100mg, 150mg, 200mg

CONTRAINDICATIONS: Seizure disorder, bulimia or anorexia nervosa, within 14 days of MAOIs, other forms of bupropion, abrupt discontinuation of alcohol or sedatives.

WARNINGS/PRECAUTIONS: Dose-related risk of seizures. D/C and do not restart if seizure occurs. Extreme caution with history of seizure, cranial trauma, severe hepatic cirrhosis. Agitation, insomnia, psychosis, confusion and other neuropsychiatric signs reported. Caution with bipolar disorder, recent MI, unstable heart disease, renal impairment. Altered appetite/weight, allergic reactions, HTN reported. Monitor for clinical worsening and/or suicidality, especially at initiation of therapy or dose changes.

ADVERSE REACTIONS: Headache, dry mouth, nausea, insomnia, dizziness, pharyngitis, infection, abdominal pain, constipation, diarrhea, tinnitus, agitation, anxiety, rash, anorexia.

INTERACTIONS: See Contraindications. Extreme caution with drugs that lower seizure threshold (eg, antidepressants, antipsychotics, theophylline, systemic steroids). Increased seizure risk with opioid, cocaine, or stimulant addiction, OTC stimulants or anorectics, oral hypoglycemics, insulin, excessive use or abrupt discontinuation of alcohol or sedatives. Caution with levodopa, amantadine, and drugs that are metabolized by CYP2D6 (eg, SSRIs, TCAs, antipsychotics, β-blockers, type 1C antiarrhythmics); use low initial dose and gradually titrate. Avoid other bupropion-containing drugs. Monitor HTN with transdermal nicotine. Caution with CYP2B6 substrates or inhibitors (eg, orphenadrine, cyclophosphamide, thiotepa). Carbamazepine, phenytoin, cimetidine, and phenobarbital may induce metabolism of bupropion. Minimize or avoid alcohol.

PREGNANCY: Category C, not for use in nursing.

MECHANISM OF ACTION: Aminoketone antidepressant; suspected to inhibit neuronal uptake of norepinephrine and dopamine.

PHARMACOKINETICS: Absorption: T_{max}=3 hrs (bupropion, hydroxybupropion). **Distribution**: Plasma protein binding (84%). **Metabolism**: Hydroxylation, hydroxybupropion (CYP2B6); Reduction of carbonyl group, threohydrobupropion, erythrohydrobupropion. **Elimination**: Urine (87%), feces (10%), (0.5% unchanged); Mean $T_{1/2}$=21 hrs, 20 hrs, 33 hrs, 37 hrs (bupropion, hydroxybupropion, erythrohydrobupropion, threohydrobupropion, respectively).

WELLBUTRIN XL   RX
bupropion HCL (GlaxoSmithKline)

> Antidepressants increased the risk of suicidal thinking and behavior (suicidality) in short-term studies in children, adolescents, and young adults with Major Depressive Disorder (MDD) and other psychiatric disorders. Bupropion is not approved for use in pediatric patients.

THERAPEUTIC CLASS: Aminoketone

INDICATIONS: Treatment of MDD and prevention of seasonal major depressive episodes in patients diagnosed with seasonal affective disorder (SAD).

DOSAGE: *Adults:* ≥18 yrs: Give in AM. Swallow whole. MDD: Initial: 150mg qd. May increase to 300mg qd on Day 4. Usual: 300mg qd. Max: 450mg qd. SAD: Start in autumn; stop in early spring. Initial: 150mg qd. May increase to 300mg after 1 week. Usual/Max: 300mg qd. Taper dose for 2 weeks prior to discontinuation. Mild-Moderate Hepatic Cirrhosis/Renal Impairment: Reduce frequency and/or dose. Severe Hepatic Cirrhosis: Max: 150mg every other day.

HOW SUPPLIED: Tab, Extended-Release: 150mg, 300mg

CONTRAINDICATIONS: Seizure disorder, bulimia or anorexia nervosa, within 14 days of MAOIs, other forms of bupropion, abrupt discontinuation of alcohol or sedatives.

WARNINGS/PRECAUTIONS: Dose-related risk of seizures. D/C and do not restart if seizure occurs. Extreme caution with history of seizure, cranial trauma, severe hepatic cirrhosis. Agitation, insomnia, psychosis, confusion and other neuropsychiatric signs reported. Caution with bipolar disorder, recent MI, unstable heart disease, renal impairment. Altered appetite/weight, allergic reactions, HTN reported. Monitor for clinical worsening and/or suicidality, especially at initiation of therapy or dose changes.

ADVERSE REACTIONS: Headache, dry mouth, nausea, insomnia, dizziness, pharyngitis, abdominal pain, agitation, diarrhea, palpitations, myalgia, anxiety, tinnitus, constipation, sweating, rash.

INTERACTIONS: See Contraindications. Extreme caution with drugs that lower seizure threshold (eg, antidepressants, antipsychotics, theophylline, systemic steroids). Increased seizure risk with opioid, cocaine, or stimulant addiction, OTC stimulants or anorectics, oral hypoglycemics, insulin, excessive use or abrupt discontinuation of alcohol or sedatives. Caution with levodopa, amantadine, and drugs that are metabolized by CYP2D6 (eg, SSRIs, TCAs, antipsychotics, β-blockers, type 1C antiarrhythmics); use low initial dose and gradually titrate. Monitor HTN with transdermal nicotine. Caution with CYP2B6 substrates or inhibitors (eg, orphenadrine, cyclophosphamide, thiotepa). Carbamazepine, phenytoin, cimetidine, and phenobarbital may induce metabolism of bupropion. Minimize or avoid alcohol.

PREGNANCY: Category C, not for use in nursing.

W

MECHANISM OF ACTION: Aminoketone antidepressant; suspected to inhibit neuronal uptake of norepinephrine and dopamine.

PHARMACOKINETICS: Absorption: T_{max}=2 hrs. **Distribution**: Plasma protein binding (84%). **Metabolism**: Extensive to hydroxybupropion (CYP2B6) via hydroxylation; threohydrobupropion, eythrohydrobupropion via reduction of carbonyl group. **Elimination**: Urine (87%), feces (10%), (0.5% unchanged). $T_{1/2}$= 21 hrs, 20 hrs, 33 hrs, 37 hrs (bupropion, hydroxybupropion, erythrohydrobupropion, threohydrobupropion respectively).

WESTCORT RX
hydrocortisone valerate (Ranbaxy)

THERAPEUTIC CLASS: Corticosteroid

INDICATIONS: Corticosteroid-responsive dermatoses.

DOSAGE: *Adults:* Apply bid-tid. May use occlusive dressings for psoriasis or recalcitrant conditions; d/c dressings if infection develops.
Pediatrics: Apply bid-tid. May use occlusive dressings for psoriasis or recalcitrant conditions; d/c dressings if infection develops.

HOW SUPPLIED: Cre, Oint: 0.2% [15g, 45g, 60g]

WARNINGS/PRECAUTIONS: May produce reversible HPA axis suppression, manifestations of Cushing's syndrome, hyperglycemia, and glucosuria. Caution when applied to large surface areas or under occlusive dressings. Use appropriate antifungal or antibacterial agent with dermatological infections; d/c if infection does not clear. Pediatrics may be more susceptible to systemic toxicity. Avoid eyes. D/C if irritation occurs.

ADVERSE REACTIONS: Burning, itching, dryness, irritation, folliculitis, hypertrichosis, acneiform eruptions, hypopigmentation, allergic contact dermatitis, skin maceration, secondary infection, skin atrophy, striae, miliaria.

PREGNANCY: Category C, caution in nursing.

MECHANISM OF ACTION: Corticosteroid; possesses anti-inflammatory, antipruritic, and vasoconstrictive properties. Anti-inflammatory effects not established; suspected to act by induction of phospholipase A_2 inhibitory proteins, lipocortins. Lipocortins control biosynthesis of potent inflammation mediators (eg, prostaglandins, leukotrienes) by inhibiting release of their common precursor, arachidonic acid.

PHARMACOKINETICS: Absorption: Percutaneous; inflammation and other disease states may increase absorption. Use of occlusive dressings for ≤24 hrs not shown to increase penetration; use for ≥96 hrs markedly enhances penetration. **Distribution:** Systemically administered corticosteroids found in breast milk.

WINRHO SDF RX
rho (D) immune globulin (Baxter)

INDICATIONS: Treatment of non-splenectomized, Rh_o(D) positive children with chronic or acute immune thrombocytopenic purpura (ITP), adults with chronic ITP, or children and adults with ITP secondary to HIV infection. To prevent Rh isoimmunization in Rh_o (D) negative mothers who had not been previously sensitized to Rh_o (D) factor. To suppress Rh isoimmunization in non-sensitized, Rh_o(D) negative women within 72 hours after spontaneous or induced abortions, amniocentesis, chorionic villus sampling, ruptured tubal pregnancy, abdominal trauma or transplacental hemorrhage or in the normal course of pregnancy, unless fetus or father is known to be Rh_o(D) negative. To suppress Rh isoimmunization in Rh_o(D) negative female children and adults transfused with Rh_o(D) positive blood products.

DOSAGE: Adults: ITP: Initial: 50mcg/kg IV as a single dose or in 2 divided doses on separate days. Hgb <10g/dL: 25-40mcg/kg. Subsequent/Maint: 25-60mcg/kg. Hgb 8-10g/dL: 25-40mcg/kg. Hgb >10g/dL: 50-60mcg/kg. Hgb <8g/dL: Use caution. Rh Suppression: Pregnancy: Give as IM or IV.

28 Weeks Gestation: 300mcg. If early in pregnancy, give at 12 week intervals. Postpartum: With Rh Positive Baby: 120mcg at birth, but no later than 72 hours after. Rh Status of Baby Unknown at 72 Hours: Administer to mother at 72 hours after birth. May give up to 28 days after birth. Abortion/Amniocentesis or Other Manipulation After 34 Weeks Gestation: 120mcg dose within 72 hours. Amniocentesis Before 34 Weeks Gestation/Post Chorionic Villus Sampling: 300mcg dose immediately after procedure. Repeat every 12 weeks. Threatened Abortion: 300mcg as soon as possible. Transfusion: Exposure to Rh_o(D) Positive Blood: 9mcg/mL blood given as 600mcg q8h IV or 12mcg/mL blood given as 1200mcg q12h IM. Exposure to Rh_o(D) Positive RBCs: 18mcg/mL cells given as 600mcg q8h IV or 24mcg/mL cells given as 1200mcg q12h IM.

Pediatrics: ITP: Initial: 50mcg/kg IV as a single dose or in 2 divided doses on separate days. Hgb <10g/dL: 25-40mcg/kg. Subsequent/Maint: 25-60mcg/kg. Hgb 8-10g/dL: 25-40mcg/kg. Hgb >10g/dL: 50-60mcg/kg. Hgb <8g/dL: Use caution. Transfusion: Exposure to Rh_o(D) Positive Blood: 9mcg/mL blood given as 600mcg q8h IV or 12mcg/mL blood given as 1200mcg q12h IM. Exposure to Rh_o(D) Positive RBCs: 18mcg/mL cells given as 600mcg q8h IV or 24mcg/mL cells given as 1200mcg q12h IM.

HOW SUPPLIED: Inj: 120mcg (600 IU), 300mcg (1500 IU), 1000mcg (5000 IU)

CONTRAINDICATIONS: When used to prevent Rh alloimmunization, should not be adminstered to Rh_o(D) positive individuals including babies; Rh_o(D) negative women who are Rh immunized as evidenced by standard manual Rh antibody screening test; individuals with a history of anaphylactic or other severe systemic reaction to immune globulins. When used to treat patients with ITP, should not be administered to Rh_o(D) negative individuals; splenectomized individuals; individuals with known hypersensitivity to plasma products.

WARNINGS/PRECAUTIONS: May transmit disease. Avoid use in Rh_o(D) negative, Rh_o(D) negative who are Rh immunized, or spelenectomized patients. Not for replacement therapy for immuneglobulin deficiency syndromes. Caution with IgA deficiency; anaphylactic reactions may occur. (ITP): Monitor for intravascular hemolysis, clinically compromising anemia, renal insufficiency. If transfused, use Rh_o(D) negative RBCs. Caution if platelets from Rh_o(D) positive donors are transfused.

ADVERSE REACTIONS: Headache, chills, fever, decreased Hgb, back pain, intravascular hemolysis.

INTERACTIONS: May interfere with response to live vaccines; delay immunization for 3 months.

PREGNANCY: Category C, safety in nursing not known.

MECHANISM OF ACTION: Gamma globulin; not established. For ITP, thought to aid in formation of anti-Rh_o(D) (anti-D)-coated RBC complexes resulting in Fc receptor blockade, sparing antibody-coated platelets.

PHARMACOKINETICS: Absorption: (IV, IM) C_{max}=36-48ng/mL, 18-19ng/mL. (IV, IM) T_{max}=2 hrs, 5-10 days. **Elimination:** (IV, IM) $T_{1/2}$=24 days; 30 days.

XALATAN

RX

latanoprost (Pharmacia & Upjohn)

THERAPEUTIC CLASS: Prostaglandin analog

INDICATIONS: Reduction of elevated IOP in open-angle glaucoma or ocular hypertension.

DOSAGE: *Adults:* Usual: 1 drop in affected eye(s) qd in the evening. Max: Once daily dosing. Space dosing with other ophthalmic drugs by at least 5 min.

HOW SUPPLIED: Sol: 0.005% [2.5mL, 2.5mL x 3]

CONTRAINDICATIONS: Hypersensitivity to benzalkonium chloride.

WARNINGS/PRECAUTIONS: Changes to pigmented tissues, growth of eyelashes, and macular edema reported. May change eye color. Caution with history of intraocular inflammation, aphakic patients, pseudophakic patients with

X

a torn posterior lens capsule, patients at risk of macular edema. Avoid with active intraocular inflammation. Do not administer with contact lenses.

ADVERSE REACTIONS: Eyelash changes (increased length, thickness, pigmentation, number of lashes), eyelid skin darkening, intraocular inflammation, iris pigmentation changes, macular edema.

INTERACTIONS: Administer at least 5 minutes apart from other topical ophthalmic agents.

PREGNANCY: Category C, caution in nursing.

MECHANISM OF ACTION: Selective FP prostanoid receptor agonist; believed to reduce IOP by increasing outflow of aqueous humor.

PHARMACOKINETICS: Absorption: C_{max}=2 hrs. **Distribution:** V_d=0.16L/kg. **Metabolism:** Cornea, via esterases to active free acid; Liver, via fatty acid β-oxidation to 1,2-dinor and 1,2,3,4-tetranor (metabolites). **Elimination:** Urine (88-98%).

XANAX   `CIV`
alprazolam (Pharmacia & Upjohn)

THERAPEUTIC CLASS: Benzodiazepine

INDICATIONS: Anxiety disorders and short-term relief of anxiety symptoms. Panic disorder with or without agoraphobia.

DOSAGE: *Adults:* Anxiety: Initial: 0.25-0.5mg tid. Titrate: May increase every 3-4 days. Max: 4mg/day. Elderly/Advanced Liver Disease/Debilitated: Initial: 0.25mg bid-tid. Titrate: Increase gradually as tolerated. Panic Disorder: Initial: 0.5mg tid. Titrate: Increase by no more than 1mg/day every 3-4 days; slower titration if ≥4mg/day. Usual: 1-10mg/day. Decrease dose slowly (no more than 0.5mg every 3 days).

HOW SUPPLIED: Tab: 0.25mg*, 0.5mg*, 1mg*, 2mg* *scored

CONTRAINDICATIONS: Acute narrow angle glaucoma, untreated open angle glaucoma, concomitant ketoconazole or itraconazole.

WARNINGS/PRECAUTIONS: Risk of dependence. Withdrawal symptoms, including seizures, reported with dose reduction or abrupt discontinuation; avoid abrupt withdrawal. Caution with impaired renal, hepatic, or pulmonary function, severe depression, obesity, elderly, and debilitated. May cause fetal harm. Hypomania/mania reported with depression. Weak uricosuric effect. Periodically reassess usefulness.

ADVERSE REACTIONS: Drowsiness, light-headedness, depression, headache, confusion, insomnia, dry mouth, constipation, diarrhea, nausea/vomiting, tachycardia/palpitations, blurred vision, nasal congestion.

INTERACTIONS: See Contraindications. Increases plasma levels of imipramine, desipramine. Additive CNS depressant effects with psychotropics, anticonvulsants, antihistamines, ethanol. Potentiated by fluoxetine, fluvoxamine, nefazodone, cimetidine, oral contraceptives. Propoxyphene decreases plasma levels. Caution with diltiazem, isoniazid, macrolides, grapefruit juice, sertraline, paroxetine, ergotamine, cyclosporine, amiodarone, nicardipine, nifedipine and other CYP3A inhibitors. Avoid azole antifungals.

PREGNANCY: Category D, not for use in nursing.

MECHANISM OF ACTION: Benzodiazepine; exact mechanism unknown. Suspected to bind at stereo specific receptors at several sites within the CNS.

PHARMACOKINETICS: Absorption: (PO) Readily absorbed; T_{max}=1-2 hrs; C_{max}(0.5-3mg)=8-37ng/mL. **Distribution:** Plasma protein binding (80%). **Metabolism:** Liver via CYP3A4; 4-hydroxyalprazolam and α-hydroxyalprazolam (metabolites). **Elimination:** Mean $T_{1/2}$=11.2 hrs; urine.

XANAX XR
alprazolam (Pharmacia & Upjohn)

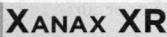 CIV

THERAPEUTIC CLASS: Benzodiazepine

INDICATIONS: Panic disorder with or without agoraphobia.

DOSAGE: *Adults:* ≥18 yrs: Initial: 0.5-1mg qd, preferably in the am. Titrate: Increase by no more than 1mg/day every 3-4 days. Maint: 1-10mg/day. Usual: 3-6mg/day. Decrease dose slowly (no more than 0.5mg every 3 days). Elderly/ Advanced Liver Disease/Debilitated: Initial: 0.5mg qd.

HOW SUPPLIED: Tab, Extended-Release: 0.5mg, 1mg, 2mg, 3mg

CONTRAINDICATIONS: Acute narrow angle glaucoma, untreated open angle glaucoma, concomitant ketoconazole or itraconazole.

WARNINGS/PRECAUTIONS: Risk of dependence. Withdrawal symptoms, including seizures, reported with dose reduction or abrupt discontinuation; avoid abrupt withdrawal. Caution with impaired renal, hepatic, or pulmonary function, severe depression, obesity, elderly, and debilitated. May cause fetal harm. Hypomania/mania reported with depression. Weak uricosuric effect. Periodically reassess usefulness.

ADVERSE REACTIONS: Sedation, somnolence, memory impairment, dysarthria, abnormal coordination, fatigue, depression, constipation, mental impairment, ataxia, dry mouth, decreased libido, increased/decreased appetite.

INTERACTIONS: See Contraindications. Increases plasma levels of imipramine, desipramine. Additive CNS depressant effects with psychotropics, anticonvulsants, antihistamines, ethanol. Potentiated by fluoxetine, fluvoxamine, nefazodone, cimetidine, oral contraceptives. Decreased levels with CYP3A inducers (eg, carbamazepine) or propoxyphene. Caution with diltiazem, isoniazid, macrolides, grapefruit juice, sertraline, paroxetine, ergotamine, cyclosporine, amiodarone, nicardipine, nifedipine and other CYP3A inhibitors. Avoid azole antifungals.

PREGNANCY: Category D, not for use in nursing.

MECHANISM OF ACTION: Benzodiazepine; exact mechanism unknown. Suspected to bind at stereo specific receptors at several sites within the CNS.

PHARMACOKINETICS: Absorption: Readily absorbed; Absolute bioavailability (90%); T_{max}=1-2 hrs; C_{max}(0.5-3mg)=8-37ng/mL. **Distribution:** Plasma protein binding (80%). **Metabolism:** Liver, via CYP3A4; 4-hydroxyalprazolam and α-hydroxyalprazolam (metabolites). **Elimination:** Urine (unchanged and metabolites); $T_{1/2}$=10.7-15.58 hrs.

XELODA
capecitabine (Roche Labs)

RX

> Altered coagulation parameters and/or bleeding, including death, reported with coumarin-derivative anticoagulants (eg, warfarin). Monitor PT/INR frequently to adjust anticoagulant dose.

THERAPEUTIC CLASS: Fluoropyrimidine carbamate

INDICATIONS: First-line treatment of metastatic colorectal carcinoma when fluoropyrimidine therapy alone is preferred. Adjuvant treatment in patients with Dukes' C colon cancer who have undergone complete resection of the primary tumor when treatment with fluoropyrimidine therapy alone is preferred. Treatment of metastatic breast cancer in combination with docetaxel after failure of prior anthracycline-containing chemotherapy. Treatment of metastatic breast cancer in patients resistant to paclitaxel and anthracycline-containing chemotherapy or resistant to paclitaxel and for whom further anthracycline therapy is not indicated.

DOSAGE: *Adults:* Take with water within 30 min after meals. Usual/ Concomitantly w/ docetaxel: 1250mg/m² bid for 2 weeks, then 1 week off. Give as 3-week cycles. For adjuvant treatment of Dukes' C colon cancer give as 3-week cycles for a total of 8 cycles (24 weeks). CrCl 30-50mL/min: Reduce to 75% of starting dose. Interrupt and/or reduce dose if toxicity occurs. Readjust according to adverse effects (see PI for details).

HOW SUPPLIED: Tab: 150mg, 500mg

CONTRAINDICATIONS: Hypersensitivity to 5-FU, dihydropyrimidine dehydrogenase (DPD) deficiency, severe renal impairment (CrCl <30mL/min).

WARNINGS/PRECAUTIONS: Reduce dose with moderate renal dysfunction. Carefully monitor for adverse events with mild to moderate renal dysfunction. Carefully monitor with severe diarrhea fluid/electrolyte balance; may need dose adjustment. Patients ≥80 yrs may experience increased Grade 3 and 4 adverse events (see full prescribing info). Possible fetal harm with pregnancy. Monitor for hand-and-foot syndrome. Cardiotoxicity reported; more common with history of CAD. Carefully monitor with mild to moderate hepatic dysfunction due to hepatic metastases. Hyperbilirubinemia, neutropenia, thrombocytopenia, and decrease in hemoglobin reported.

ADVERSE REACTIONS: Diarrhea, hand and foot syndrome, pyrexia, anemia, nausea, fatigue, vomiting, dermatitis, neutropenia, thrombocytopenia, stomatitis, anorexia, hyperbilirubinemia, abdominal pain, paresthesia.

INTERACTIONS: May increase phenytoin levels; reduce phenytoin dose. Leucovorin may increase levels and toxicity of 5-FU. Altered coagulation parameters and/or bleeding reported with anticoagulants (eg, coumarin, phenprocoumon); monitor PT/INR frequently. Caution with CYP2C9 substrates. Aluminum and/or magnesium antacids may increase levels.

PREGNANCY: Category D, not for use in nursing.

MECHANISM OF ACTION: Fluoropyrimidine carbamate (prodrug of 5-FU) antineoplastic; binds to thymidylate synthetase, forming covalently bound ternary complex that inhibits formation of thymidylate from 2-deoxyuridylate, inhibits DNA synthesis, and interferes with RNA processing and protein synthesis.

PHARMACOKINETICS: Absorption: T_{max}=1.5 hrs. **Distribution:** Plasma protein binding (<60%). **Metabolism:** Extensive enzymatic conversion to 5-FU; hydrogenated to less toxic metabolite via dihydropyrimidine dehydrogenase. 5-FU (metabolite). **Elimination:** Urine (3%).

XENICAL RX
orlistat (Roche Labs)

THERAPEUTIC CLASS: Lipase inhibitor

INDICATIONS: For weight loss and weight maintenance and to reduce risk of weight regain after weight loss in obese patients with initial BMI ≥30kg/m² or ≥27kg/m² in presence of other risk factors.

DOSAGE: *Adults:* 120mg tid with each main meal containing fat. Take during or up to 1 hr after meals. Use with reduced-calorie diet with about 30% of calories from fat. Omit dose if meal is missed or contains no fat. Separate multivitamin (containing fat-soluble vitamins) by at least 2 hrs.
Pediatrics: ≥12 yrs: 120mg tid with each main meal containing fat. Take during or up to 1 hr after meals. Use with reduced-calorie diet with about 30% of calories from fat. Omit dose if meal is missed or contains no fat. Separate multivitamin (containing fat-soluble vitamins) by at least 2 hrs.

HOW SUPPLIED: Cap: 120mg

CONTRAINDICATIONS: Chronic malabsorption syndrome, cholestasis.

WARNINGS/PRECAUTIONS: Exclude organic causes of obesity. Caution with history of hyperoxaluria or calcium oxalate nephrolithiasis. GI effects may increase with a high-fat diet (>30%). Weight loss may improve metabolic control; monitor dosage of antidiabetic agents. Increased risk of cholelithiasis due to substantial weight loss.

ADVERSE REACTIONS: Oily spotting, flatus with discharge, fecal urgency, fatty/oily stool, oily evacuation, increased defecation, fecal incontinence.

INTERACTIONS: Monitor warfarin and cyclosporine (separate cyclosporine dose by 2 hrs). May decrease absorption of fat-soluble vitamins and β-carotene; supplement with fat-soluble multivitamin.

PREGNANCY: Category B, not for use in nursing.

MECHANISM OF ACTION: Lipase inhibitor; inhibits absorption of dietary fats. Acts in lumen of stomach and small intestine by forming covalent bond with active serine residue site of gastric and pancreatic lipases, inactivating enzymes making them unavailable to hydrolyze dietary fats.

PHARMACOKINETICS: Distribution: Plasma protein binding (>99%). **Metabolism:** GI wall. **Elimination:** Feces (83%); T$_{1/2}$=1-2 hrs.

XIBROM   RX
bromfenac (Ista)

THERAPEUTIC CLASS: NSAID

INDICATIONS: Treatment of postoperative inflammation after cataract extraction.

DOSAGE: *Adults:* 1 drop bid in affected eye(s), start 24 hours post-op and continue for 2 weeks.

HOW SUPPLIED: Sol: 0.09% [5mL]

WARNINGS/PRECAUTIONS: Contains sodium sulfite; may cause allergic-type reactions including anaphylactic symptoms and life-threatening or less severe asthmatic episodes. Potential cross-sensitivity to acetylsalicylic acid, phenylacetic acid derivatives, and other NSAIDs. May cause increased bleeding of ocular tissues; slow or delay healing; keratitis. Continued use may lead to sight-threatening epithelial breakdown, corneal thinning, corneal erosion, corneal ulceration, corneal perforation; d/c if this occurs. Caution in complicated ocular surgeries, corneal denervation, corneal epithelial defects, DM, ocular surface diseases (eg, dry eye syndrome), RA, repeat ocular surgeries within a short period of time, bleeding tendencies, or receiving other medication which may prolong bleeding time.

ADVERSE REACTIONS: Abnormal sensation in eye, conjunctival hyperemia, eye irritation (burning/stinging), eye pain, eye pruritus, eye redness, headache, iritis.

INTERACTIONS: Concomitant use of topical NSAIDs and topical steroids may increase potential for healing problems. Caution with other medications which may prolong bleeding time.

PREGNANCY: Category C, caution in nursing.

MECHANISM OF ACTION: NSAID; thought to block prostaglandin synthesis by inhibiting cyclooxygenase 1 and 2.

XIFAXAN   RX
rifaximin (Salix)

THERAPEUTIC CLASS: Semisynthetic rifampin analog

INDICATIONS: Traveler's diarrhea caused by noninvasive strains of *E.coli*

DOSAGE: *Adults:* 1 tab tid for 3 days.
Pediatrics: ≥12 yrs: 1 tab tid for 3 days.

HOW SUPPLIED: Tab: 200mg

WARNINGS/PRECAUTIONS: Avoid in diarrhea complicated by fever or blood in the stool or diarrhea due to pathogens other than *E.coli*. D/C if diarrhea symptoms worsen or persist >24-48 hrs; consider alternative antibiotic therapy. Pseudomembranous colitis reported.

ADVERSE REACTIONS: Flatulence, headache, abdominal pain, rectal tenesmus, defecation urgency, nausea, constipation, pyrexia.

PREGNANCY: Category C; not for use in nursing.

MECHANISM OF ACTION: Antibacterial agent; binds to β-subunit of bacterial DNA-dependent RNA polymerase, resulting in inhibition of bacterial RNA synthesis.

PHARMACOKINETICS: Absorption: C_{max}=4.3ng/mL; T_{max}=1.25 hrs. **Metabolism:** CYP3A4. **Elimination:** Feces (97%), urine (0.32%).

XIGRIS   RX
drotrecogin alfa (Lilly)

THERAPEUTIC CLASS: Activated protein C

INDICATIONS: For reduction of mortality in severe sepsis (associated with acute organ dysfunction) in patients at a high risk of death.

DOSAGE: *Adults:* 24mcg/kg/hr IV for 96 hrs.

HOW SUPPLIED: Inj: 5mg, 20mg

CONTRAINDICATIONS: Active internal bleeding, hemorrhagic stroke within 3 months, intracranial or intraspinal surgery or severe head trauma within 2 months, trauma with an increased risk of life-threatening bleeding, epidural catheter, intracranial neoplasm or mass lesion, evidence of cerebral herniation.

WARNINGS/PRECAUTIONS: Increased risk of bleed with platelets <30,000 x 10^6/L (even if platelets increased by transfusions), PT/INR >3, GI bleed within 6 weeks, ischemic stroke within 3 months, intracranial arteriovenous malformation or aneurysm, known bleeding diathesis, chronic severe hepatic disease, or condition where bleeding is a significant hazard or difficult to manage due to location. If bleeding occurs, stop infusion. D/C 2 hrs before invasive surgical procedures or procedures with risk of bleeding. Avoid noncompressible puncture sites.

ADVERSE REACTIONS: Bleeding.

INTERACTIONS: Caution with drugs that affect hemostasis; increased risk of bleed with therapeutic heparin, thrombolytic therapy within 3 days, and oral anticoagulants, ASA >650mg, platelet inhibitors or glycoprotein IIb/IIIa inhibitors within 7 days.

PREGNANCY: Category C, not for use in nursing.

MECHANISM OF ACTION: Activated protein C; exerts antithrombotic effect by inhibiting Factors Va and VIIIa.

XOLAIR   RX
omalizumab (Genentech)

Anaphylaxis, presenting as bronchospasm, hypotension, syncope, urticaria, and/or angioedema of the throat or tongue has been reported. Monitor patients closely for an appropriate time period after administration.

THERAPEUTIC CLASS: Monoclonal antibody/IgE-blocker

INDICATIONS: Moderate-severe persistent asthma in those who have a positive skin test or *in vitro* reactivity to a perennial aeroallergen and whose symptoms are inadequately controlled with inhaled corticosteroids.

DOSAGE: *Adults:* 150-375mg SQ every 2 or 4 weeks based on body weight and pretreatment serum total IgE level. Max: 150mg/site. 30-90kg & IgE ≥30-100 IU/mL: 150mg every 4 weeks. >90-150kg & IgE ≥30-100 IU/mL OR 30-90kg & IgE >100-200 IU/mL OR 30-60kg & IgE >200-300 IU/mL: 300mg every 4 weeks. >90-150kg & IgE >100-200 IU/mL OR >60-90kg & IgE >200-300 IU/mL OR 30-70kg & IgE >300-400 IU/mL: 225mg every 2 weeks. >90-150kg & IgE >200-300 IU/mL OR >70-90kg & IgE >300-400 IU/mL OR 30-70kg & IgE >400-500 IU/mL OR 30-60kg & IgE >500-600 IU/mL: 300mg every 2 weeks. >70-90kg & IgE >400-500 IU/mL OR >60-70kg & IgE >500-600 IU/mL OR 30-60kg & IgE >600-700 IU/mL: 375mg every 2 weeks.
Pediatrics: ≥12 yrs: 150-375mg SQ every 2 or 4 weeks based on body weight

and pretreatment serum total IgE level. Max: 150mg/site. 30-90kg & IgE ≥30-100 IU/mL: 150mg every 4 weeks. >90-150kg & IgE ≥30-100 IU/mL OR 30-90kg & IgE >100-200 IU/mL OR 30-60kg & IgE >200-300 IU/mL: 300mg every 4 weeks. >90-150kg & IgE >100-200 IU/mL OR >60-90kg & IgE >200-300 IU/mL OR 30-70kg & IgE >300-400 IU/mL: 225mg every 2 weeks. >90-150kg and IgE >200-300 IU/mL OR >70-90kg & IgE >300-400 IU/mL OR 30-70kg & IgE >400-500 IU/mL OR 30-60kg & IgE >500-600 IU/mL: 300mg every 2 weeks. >70-90kg & IgE >400-500 IU/mL OR >60-70kg & IgE >500-600 IU/mL OR 30-60kg & IgE >600-700 IU/mL: 375mg q2 weeks.

HOW SUPPLIED: Inj: 150mg [5mL]

WARNINGS/PRECAUTIONS: Malignant neoplasms reported. Not for use in treatment of acute bronchospasm or status asthmaticus. Systemic or inhaled corticosteroids should not be abruptly discontinued when initiating therapy.

ADVERSE REACTIONS: Anaphylaxis, malignancies, injection site reactions, viral infections, upper respiratory infection, sinusitis, headache, pharyngitis, pain, arthralgia.

PREGNANCY: Category B, caution in nursing.

MECHANISM OF ACTION: Monoclonal antibody/IgE blocker; inhibits binding of IgE to high-affinity IgE receptor on surface of mast cells and basophils and limits degree of release of mediators of allergic response.

PHARMACOKINETICS: Absorption:(SQ) Absolute bioavailability (62%); T_{max}=7-8 days. **Distribution:** V_d=78mL/kg; crosses placental barrier. **Elimination:** $T_{1/2}$=26 days.

XOPENEX   RX
levalbuterol HCL (Sepracor)

THERAPEUTIC CLASS: Beta$_2$-agonist

INDICATIONS: Prevention and treatment of bronchospasm with reversible obstructive airway disease.

DOSAGE: *Adults:* Initial: 0.63mg tid, q6-8h. Severe Asthma: 1.25mg tid, q6-8h. Administer by nebulizer.
Pediatrics: ≥12 yrs: Initial: 0.63mg tid, q6-8h. Severe Asthma: 1.25mg tid, q6-8h. 6-11 yrs: 0.31mg tid. Max: 0.63mg tid. Administer by nebulizer.

HOW SUPPLIED: Sol: 0.31mg/3mL, 0.63mg/3mL, 1.25mg/3mL [3mL, 24ˢ]

WARNINGS/PRECAUTIONS: Hypersensitivity reactions reported. D/C immediately if paradoxical bronchospasm occurs. May produce ECG changes; caution with cardiovascular disorders, coronary insufficiency, arrhythmias, and HTN. Caution with convulsive disorders, hyperthyroidism, and diabetes. May produce transient hypokalemia.

ADVERSE REACTIONS: Tachycardia, migraine, dyspepsia, leg cramps, nervousness, dizziness, tremor, rhinitis, increased cough, chest pain, HTN, hypotention, diarrhea, dry mouth, anxiety, insomnia, paresthesia, wheezing.

INTERACTIONS: Avoid other sympathomimetic agents. Extreme caution with MAOIs and TCAs. Monitor digoxin. ECG changes and/or hypokalemia with nonpotassium-sparing diuretics. Antagonized by β-blockers.

PREGNANCY: Category C, not for use in nursing.

MECHANISM OF ACTION: β$_2$-adrenergic bronchodilator; stimulates adenyl cylase, the enzyme that catalyzes formation of cAMP from ATP. Increased cAMP levels associated with relaxation of bronchial smooth muscle and inhibition of release of mediators of immediate hypersensitivity.

PHARMACOKINETICS: Absorption: C_{max}(1.25, 5mg)=1.1, 4.5ng/ml; T_{max}(1.25, 5mg)=0.2, 0.2 hrs. **Metabolism:** GI tract by SULT1A3. **Elimination:** Renal (80-100%), urine (25-46% unchanged), feces (≤20%); $T_{1/2}$(1.25, 5mg)=3.3, 4 hrs.

X

XOPENEX HFA RX
levalbuterol tartrate (Sepracor)

THERAPEUTIC CLASS: Beta$_2$-agonist

INDICATIONS: Prevention and treatment of bronchospasm with reversible obstructive airway disease.

DOSAGE: *Adults:* 2 inh (90mcg) q4-6h or 1 inh (45mcg) q4h may be sufficient. *Pediatrics:* ≥4 yrs: 2 inh (90mcg) q4-6h or 1 inh (45mcg) q4h may be sufficient.

HOW SUPPLIED: MDI: 45mcg/inh [15g]

WARNINGS/PRECAUTIONS: D/C immediately if paradoxical bronchospasm occurs. May produce ECG changes; caution with cardiovascular disorders, coronary insufficiency, arrhythmias, and HTN. Caution with convulsive disorders, hyperthyroidism, and diabetes. May produce transient hypokalemia.

ADVERSE REACTIONS: Asthma, pharyngitis, rhinitis, pain, vomiting.

INTERACTIONS: Avoid other sympathomimetic agents. Extreme caution with MAOIs and TCAs. Monitor digoxin. ECG changes and/or hypokalemia with nonpotassium-sparing diuretics. Antagonized by β-blockers.

PREGNANCY: Category C, not for use in nursing.

MECHANISM OF ACTION: β$_2$-adrenergic bronchodilator; stimulates adenyl cyclase, the enzyme that catalyzes formation of cAMP from ATP. Increased cAMP levels associated with relaxation of bronchial smooth muscle and inhibition of release of mediators of immediate hypersensitivity.

PHARMACOKINETICS: Absorption: C_{max}=0.199ng/mL (≥12 yrs), 0.163ng/mL (4-11 yrs); T_{max}=0.54 hrs (≥12 yrs), 0.76 hrs (4-11 yrs); AUC=0.695ng•hr/mL (≥12 yrs), 0.579ng•hr/mL (4-11 yrs). **Metabolism:** GI tract by SULT1A3. **Elimination:** Renal (80-100%), urine (25-46% unchanged), feces (≤20%).

XYLOCAINE INJECTION RX
lidocaine HCL (Abraxis)

OTHER BRAND NAMES: Xylocaine-MPF (Abraxis)

THERAPEUTIC CLASS: Local anesthetic

INDICATIONS: For production of local or regional anesthesia by infiltration techniques such as percutaneous injection and IV regional anesthesia by peripheral nerve block techniques such as brachial plexus and intercostal and by central neural techniques such as lumbar and caudal epidural blocks.

DOSAGE: *Adults:* Dosage varies depending on procedure, depth, and duration of anesthesia, degree of muscular relaxation, and patient physical condition. Max: 4.5mg/kg or total dose of 300mg. Epidural/Caudal Anesthesia: Max: Intervals not less than 90 min. Paracervical Block: Max: 200mg/90 min. Regional Anesthesia: IV: Max: 4mg/kg. Children/Elderly/Debilitated/Cardiac or Liver Disease: Reduce dose. *Pediatrics:* >3 yrs: Max: 1.5-2mg/lb. Regional Anesthesia: IV: Max: 3mg/kg.

HOW SUPPLIED: Inj: 0.5%, 1%, 2%; (MPF) 0.5%, 1%, 1.5%, 2%

WARNINGS/PRECAUTIONS: Acidosis, cardiac arrest, death reported from delay in toxicity management. Local anesthetic solutions containing antimicrobial preservatives should not be used for epidural or spinal anesthesia. Use lowest effective dose. During epidural anesthesia, administer initial test dose and monitor for CNS and cardiovascular toxicity as well as for signs of unintended intrathecal administration. Reduce dose with debilitated, elderly, acutely ill, and children. Extreme caution when using lumbar and caudal epidural anesthesia with existing neurological disease, spinal deformities, septicemia, and severe HTN. Monitor cardiovascular and respiratory vital signs and state of consciousness after each injection. Caution with hepatic disease, cardiovascular disorders. Monitor circulation and respiration with injections into head and neck area.

X

ADVERSE REACTIONS: Lightheadedness, nervousness, euphoria, confusion, dizziness, drowsiness, tinnitus, blurred vision, vomiting, heat/cold sensations, twitching, tremors, convulsions, respiratory depression, bradycardia, hypotension, urticaria, edema, anaphylactoid reactions.

PREGNANCY: Category B, caution in nursing.

MECHANISM OF ACTION: Anesthetic; stabilizes neuronal membrane by inhibiting ionic fluxes required for initiation and conduction of impulses, thereby effecting local anesthetic action.

PHARMACOKINETICS: Absorption: Complete. **Distribution:** Crosses blood-brain and placental barriers. **Metabolism:** Liver (rapid), oxidative N-alkylation (major pathway), yields monoethylglycinexylidide and glycinexylidide (metabolites). **Elimination:** Urine, 90% (metabolites) and ≤10% (unchanged); $T_{1/2}$=1.5-2.0 hrs.

XYREM

CIII

sodium oxybate (Orphan Medical)

> Sodium oxybate is GHB (gamma hydroxybutyrate), a known drug of abuse. Do not use with alcohol or other CNS depressants. Associated with confusion, depression, and other neuropsychiatric events. Available only through the Xyrem Success Program, call 1-866-XYREM88.

THERAPEUTIC CLASS: CNS Depressant

INDICATIONS: Treatment of excessive daytime sleepiness and cataplexy in patients with narcolepsy.

DOSAGE: *Adults:* Initial: 2.25g qhs, then take 2.25g 2.5-4 hrs later. Titrate: Increase by 0.75g/dose every 1-2 weeks. Range: 6-9g/night. Max: 9g/night. Hepatic Insufficiency: Initial: Decrease by 50%. Titrate dose increments to effect. Take 1st dose at bedtime while in bed and the 2nd dose while sitting in bed. Dilute each dose with 2 ounces of water.
Pediatrics: ≥16 yrs: Initial: 2.25g qhs, then take 2.25g 2.5-4 hrs later. Titrate: Increase by 0.75g/dose every 1-2 weeks. Range: 6-9g/night. Max: 9g/night. Hepatic Insufficiency: Initial: Decrease by 50%. Titrate dose increments to effect. Take 1st dose at bedtime while in bed and the 2nd dose while sitting in bed. Dilute each dose with 2 ounces of water.

HOW SUPPLIED: Sol: 500mg/mL [180mL]

CONTRAINDICATIONS: Sedative hypnotic agents, succinic semialdehyde dehydrogenase deficiency.

WARNINGS/PRECAUTIONS: Rapid onset of CNS depressant effects; ingest only at bedtime and while in bed. Avoid engaging in activities requiring mental alertness for 6 hrs after ingestion. Daily sodium intake ranges from 0.5g (with 3g dose) to 1.6g (with 9g dose); caution in heart failure, HTN, or renal impairment. Caution with compromised respiratory function, hepatic insufficiency, history of depressive illness or suicide attempts, elderly. Evaluate patients who develop through disorders or behavior abnormalities. Sleepwalking reported. Rule out worsening sleep apnea or nocturnal seizures if incontinence develops.

ADVERSE REACTIONS: Headache, nausea, dizziness, pain, somnolence, pharyngitis, infection, flu syndrome, diarrhea, urinary incontinence, vomiting, rhinitis, asthenia, sinusitis, nervousness, back pain, confusion, sleepwalking, depression, dyspepsia, abdominal pain, abnormal dreams, insomnia.

INTERACTIONS: Avoid alcohol, sedative hypnotics, or other CNS depressants. Food decreases bioavailability.

PREGNANCY: Category B, caution in nursing.

MECHANISM OF ACTION: CNS depressant agent; effect on cataplexy not established, causes CNS depression.

PHARMACOKINETICS: Absorption: Rapid (incomplete); absolute bioavailabiltiy (25%). C_{max}=78mcg/mL (1st peak), 142mcg/mL (2nd peak); T_{max}=0.5-1.25 hr. **Distribution:** V_d=190-384mL/kg; plasma protein binding (<1%). **Metabolism:** Liver via CYP450. **Elimination:** By transformation to CO_2 eliminated by expiration. Urine (<5%), feces; $T_{1/2}$=0.5-1 hr.

X

XYZAL   RX
levocetirizine dihydrochloride (UCB)

THERAPEUTIC CLASS: H_1-antagonist

INDICATIONS: Relief of symptoms associated with seasonal and perennial allergic rhinitis. Treatment of uncomplicated skin manifestations of chronic idiopathic urticaria.

DOSAGE: *Adults:* 5mg qd in evening. Adjust dose with decreased renal function.
Pediatrics: ≥12 yrs: 5mg qd in evening. Adjust dose with decreased renal function. 6-11 yrs: 2.5mg (1/2 tab) qd in evening.

HOW SUPPLIED: Sol: 2.5mg/5mL; Tab: 5mg* *scored

CONTRAINDICATIONS: End stage renal disease (CrCl <10mL/min) or hemodialysis. Pediatrics 6-11 yrs with renal impairment.

WARNINGS/PRECAUTIONS: May impair mental/physical abilities.

ADVERSE REACTIONS: Somnolence, fatigue, dry mouth, headache, nasopharyngitis, abdominal pain, cough, epistaxis, asthenia, pharyngitis.

INTERACTIONS: Avoid alcohol and CNS depressants. Possible decreased clearance with large doses of theophylline.

PREGNANCY: Category B, not for use in nursing.

MECHANISM OF ACTION: Antihistamine; inhibits H_1-receptor.

PHARMACOKINETICS: Absorption: Rapid, extensive; C_{max}=270ng/mL (single dose), 308ng/mL (multiple doses); T_{max}=0.9 hrs. **Distribution:** V_d=0.4L/kg; plasma protein binding (91-92%). Found in breast milk. **Metabolism:** Through aromatic oxidation, N and O- dealkylation and taurine conjugation pathways, via CYP3A4. **Elimination:** Urine (58.4%), feces (12.9%); $T_{1/2}$=8 hrs.

YASMIN   RX
drospirenone - ethinyl estradiol (Bayer Healthcare)

THERAPEUTIC CLASS: Estrogen/progestogen combination

INDICATIONS: Prevention of pregnancy.

DOSAGE: *Adults:* 1 tab qd for 28 days, then repeat. Start 1st Sunday after menses begin or 1st day of menses.

HOW SUPPLIED: Tab: (Ethinyl Estradiol-Drospirenone) 0.03mg-3mg

CONTRAINDICATIONS: Renal or adrenal insufficiency, hepatic dysfunction, thrombophlebitis, thromboembolic disorders, history of deep vein thrombophlebitis, cerebrovascular or CAD, breast carcinoma, endometrial carcinoma, estrogen-dependent neoplasia, undiagnosed abnormal genital bleeding, cholestatic jaundice of pregnancy or jaundice with prior pill use, liver tumor, active liver disease, pregnancy, heavy smoking (≥15 cigarettes daily) and >35 yrs.

WARNINGS/PRECAUTIONS: Cigarette smoking increases risk of serious CV side effects; risk increases with age (especially >35 yrs) and heavy smoking. Increased risk of MI, thromboembolism, thrombotic disease, cerebrovascular events, and gallbladder disease. Monitor K^+ levels during first cycle with conditions predisposing to hyperkalemia. Retinal thrombosis, hepatic neoplasia, carcinoma of breast and reproductive organs reported. May cause glucose intolerance. May increase BP, elevate LDL levels or cause other lipid changes, fluid retention, breakthrough bleeding and spotting. May cause or exacerbate migraine. May develop visual changes with contact lens. Increased risk of MI with HTN, hyperlipidemia, obesity and DM. D/C if jaundice, significant depression or ophthalmic irregularities develop. Use before menarche is not indicated.

ADVERSE REACTIONS: Nausea, vomiting, breakthrough bleeding, spotting, amenorrhea, migraine, depression, vaginal candidiasis, edema, weight changes.

INTERACTIONS: Reduced effects, increased breakthrough bleeding, and menstrual irregularities with rifampin, phenobarbital, phenytoin, carbamazepine, possibly with griseofulvin, ampicillin, tetracycline, St. John's wort, and phenylbutazone. Increased levels with atorvastatin, ascorbic acid and APAP. Risk of hyperkalemia with ACE inhibitors, angiotensin-II receptor antagonists, K$^+$-sparing diuretics, heparin, aldosterone antagonists, and NSAIDs; monitor K$^+$ levels during 1st cycle. May increase levels of cyclosporine, prednisolone, and theophylline. May decrease APAP levels and increase clearance of temazepam, salicylic acid, morphine, and clofibric acid.

PREGNANCY: Category X, not for use in nursing.

MECHANISM OF ACTION: Combination oral contraceptive; acts by suppression of gonadotropins. Inhibits ovulation and produces changes in cervical mucus (increasing difficulty of sperm entry into uterus) and endometrium (reducing likelihood of implantation).

PHARMACOKINETICS: Absorption: Drospirenone (DRSP): Absolute bioavailability (76%); (Cycle 13/Day 21) C_{max}=78.7ng/mL; T_{max}=1.6 hrs; AUC=968ng•h/mL. Ethinyl estradiol (EE): Absolute bioavailability (40%); (Cycle 13/Day 21) C_{max}=90.5pg/mL; T_{max}=1.6 hrs; AUC=469.5pg•h/mL. **Distribution:** DRSP: V_d=4L/kg; Serum protein binding (97%). EE: V_d=4-5L/kg; Serum albumin binding (98.5%). **Metabolism:** DRSP: Liver, via CYP3A4 (minor). EE: Hydroxylation (via CYP3A4), conjugation (glucuronidation and sulfation). **Elimination:** DRSP: $T_{1/2}$=30 hrs; Urine, feces. EE: $T_{1/2}$=24 hrs; Urine, feces.

YAZ RX
drospirenone - ethinyl estradiol (Berlex)

THERAPEUTIC CLASS: Estrogen/progestogen combination

INDICATIONS: Prevention of pregnancy. Treatment of symptoms of premenstrual dysphoric disorder (PMDD). Treatment of moderate acne vulgaris in women ≥14 yrs.

DOSAGE: *Adults:* 1 tab qd for 28 days (24 active plus 4 inert pills), then repeat. Start 1st Sunday after menses begin or 1st day of menses.
Pediatrics: ≥14 yrs: Acne: 1 tab qd for 28 days (24 active plus 4 inert pills), then repeat. Start 1st Sunday after menses begin or 1st day of menses.

HOW SUPPLIED: Tab: (Ethinyl Estradiol-Drospirenone) 0.02mg-3mg

CONTRAINDICATIONS: Renal or adrenal insufficiency, hepatic dysfunction, thrombophlebitis, thromboembolic disorders, history of deep vein thrombophlebitis, valvular heart disease with thrombogenic complications, severe HTN, DM with vascular involvement, HA with focal neurological symptoms, major surgery with prolonged immobilization, cerebrovascular or CAD, breast carcinoma, endometrial carcinoma, estrogen-dependent neoplasia, undiagnosed abnormal genital bleeding, cholestatic jaundice of pregnancy or jaundice with prior pill use, liver tumor, active liver disease, pregnancy, heavy smoking (>15 cigarettes daily) and >35 yrs.

WARNINGS/PRECAUTIONS: Cigarette smoking increases risk of serious CV side effects. Risk increases with age (especially >35 yrs) and with heavy smoking. Increased risk of MI, thromboembolism, thrombotic disease, cerebrovascular events, and gallbladder disease. Monitor K$^+$ levels during first cycle with conditions predisposing to hyperkalemia. Retinal thrombosis, hepatic neoplasia, carcinoma of breast and reproductive organs reported. May cause glucose intolerance. May increase BP, elevate LDL levels or cause other lipid changes, fluid retention, breakthrough bleeding and spotting. May cause or exacerbate migraine. May develop visual changes with contact lens. Increased risk of MI with HTN, hyperlipidemia, obesity and DM. D/C if jaundice, significant depression or ophthalmic irregularities develop. Use before menarche is not indicated.

ADVERSE REACTIONS: Nausea, vomiting, breakthrough bleeding, spotting, amenorrhea, migraine, mental depression, vaginal candidiasis, edema, weight changes, depression decrease in serum folate levels, aggravation of varicose veins, uritcaria, angioedema; severe reactions with respiratory and circulatory symptoms, dysmenorrhea.

INTERACTIONS: Reduced effects, increased breakthrough bleeding, and menstrual irregularities with rifampin, phenobarbital, phenytoin, carbamazepine, possibly with griseofulvin, ampicillin, tetracycline, St. John's wort, and phenylbutazone. Increased levels with atorvastatin, ascorbic acid and APAP. Risk of hyperkalemia with ACE inhibitors, angiotensin-II receptor antagonists, potassium-sparing diuretics, heparin, aldosterone antagonists, and NSAIDs; monitor K+ levels during 1st cycle. Increased levels of cyclosporine, prednisolone, and theophylline. May decrease APAP levels and increase clearance of temazepam, salicylic acid, morphine, and clofibric acid.

PREGNANCY: Category X, not for use in nursing.

MECHANISM OF ACTION: Estrogen/progestogen oral contraceptive; acts by suppressing gonadotropins, inhibiting ovulation, and causing other alterations, including changes in the cervical mucus (which increases difficulty of sperm entry into uterus) and the endometrium (which reduces likelihood of implantation).

PHARMACOKINETICS: Absorption: Drospirenone (DRSP): Absolute bioavailability (76%); (Cycle 1/Day 21) C_{max}=70.3ng/mL; T_{max}=1.5 hrs; AUC=763ng•h/mL. Ethinyl estradiol (EE): Absolute bioavailability (40%); (Cycle 1/Day 21) C_{max}=45.1pg/mL; T_{max}=1.5 hrs; AUC=220pg•h/mL. **Distribution:** DRSP: V_d=4L/kg; serum protein binding (97%). EE: V_d=4-5L/kg; serum albumin binding (98.5%). **Metabolism:** DRSP: Liver, via CYP3A4 (minor). EE: Hydroxylation (via CYP3A4), conjugation (glucuronidation and sulfation). **Elimination:** DRSP: Urine, feces; $T_{1/2}$=30 hrs. EE: Urine, feces; $T_{1/2}$=24 hrs.

ZADITOR OTC
ketotifen fumarate (Novartis Ophthalmics)

THERAPEUTIC CLASS: H_1-antagonist and mast cell stabilizer

INDICATIONS: Temporary prevention of itching of the eye due to allergic conjunctivitis.

DOSAGE: *Adults:* 1 drop q8-12h.
Pediatrics: ≥3 yrs: 1 drop q8-12h.

HOW SUPPLIED: Sol: 0.025% [5mL]

WARNINGS/PRECAUTIONS: Not for contact lens irritation. Do not wear a contact lens if eye is red. If eyes are not red, wait 10 minutes after instillation before inserting contacts. Soft contact lens can absorb benzalkonium chloride.

ADVERSE REACTIONS: Rhinitis, allergic reactions, burning, stinging, conjunctivitis, dry eye, eye pain, eyelid disorder, itching, keratitis, lacrimation disorder, mydriasis, photophobia, headache, rash.

PREGNANCY: Category C, caution in nursing.

ZANAFLEX RX
tizanidine HCL (Acorda)

THERAPEUTIC CLASS: Centrally acting alpha$_2$-adrenergic agonist

INDICATIONS: Short-term treatment of spasticity.

DOSAGE: *Adults:* Initial: 4mg single dose q6-8h. Titrate: Increase by 2-4mg. Usual: 8mg single dose q6-8h. Max: 3 doses/24h or 36mg/day.

HOW SUPPLIED: Cap: 2mg, 4mg, 6mg; Tab: 2mg*, 4mg* *scored

CONTRAINDICATIONS: Concomitant use with fluvoxamine, ciprofloxacin or potent inhibitors of CYP1A2.

WARNINGS/PRECAUTIONS: May prolong QT interval. May cause liver damage; monitor baseline LFTs and at 1, 3, and 6 months. Retinal degeneration and corneal opacities reported. Caution with renal impairment or elderly. May cause hypotension, caution with antihypertensives; avoid ciprofloxacin and fluvoxamine. Use with extreme cautions in patients with hepatic impairment. May cause sedation and hallucinations. Avoid concomitant use with

Z

oral contraceptives. When discontinuing, taper dose to avoid withdrawal and rebound HTN, tachycardia, and hypertonia.

ADVERSE REACTIONS: Dry mouth, somnolence, asthenia, dizziness, UTI, urinary frequency, flu-like syndrome, rhinitis.

INTERACTIONS: See Contraindications. Potentiated depressant effect with alcohol. Potentiated by oral contraceptives. Avoid α-adrenergic agonists. Avoid with CYP1A2 inhibitors.

PREGNANCY: Category C, caution in nursing.

MECHANISM OF ACTION: Centrally acting α_2-adrenergic agonist: reduces spasticity by increasing presynaptic inhibition of motor neurons.

PHARMACOKINETICS: Absorption: Complete; Fasting: T_{max}=1 hr; Fed: T_{max}=1.25 hrs, C_{max} increased by 30%; Absolute bioavailability (40%). **Distribution:** V_d=2.4L/kg; Plasma protein binding (30%); Excreted in human milk. **Metabolism:** CYP1A2. **Elimination:** Urine (60%), feces (20%); $T_{1/2}$=2.5 hrs.

ZANTAC   RX
ranitidine HCL (GlaxoSmithKline)

THERAPEUTIC CLASS: H_2-blocker

INDICATIONS: (PO) Short-term treatment of active duodenal (DU) and benign gastric ulcers (GU). Maintenance therapy for duodenal and gastric ulcers. Treatment of pathological hypersecretory conditions (eg, Zollinger-Ellison) and GERD. Treatment and maintenance of erosive esophagitis. (Inj) Hospitalized patients with pathological hypersecretory conditions or intractable duodenal ulcer. Short-term alternate to oral therapy.

DOSAGE: *Adults:* (PO) DU/GU: 150mg bid or (DU) 300mg after evening meal or qhs. Maint: 150mg qhs. GERD: 150mg bid. Erosive Esophagitis: 150mg qid. Maint: 150mg bid. Hypersecretory Conditions: 150mg bid. May give up to 6g/day with severe disease. (Inj) Usual: 50mg IV/IM q6-8 hrs or 6.25mg/hr continuous IV. Max: 400mg/day. Zollinger-Ellison: Initial: 1mg/kg/hr. Titrate: May increase after 4 hrs by 0.5mg/kg/hr increments. Max: 2.5mg/kg/hr or 220mg/hr. CrCl <50mL/min: 50mg IV q18-24 hrs or 150mg PO q24h. Give more frequent (q12h) if necessary. Hemodialysis: Give dose at end of treatment. Dissolve each 150mg effervescent tab in 6-8oz of water before administration.
Pediatrics: 1 month-16 yrs: (PO) DU/GU: 2-4mg/kg bid. Max: 300mg/day. Maint: 2-4mg/kg qd. Max: 150mg/day. GERD/Erosive Esophagitis: 2.5-5mg/kg bid. (Inj) DU: 2-4mg/kg/day IV given q6-8 hrs. Max: 50mg q6-8 hrs. CrCl <50mL/min: 50mg IV q18-24 hrs or 150mg PO q24h. Give more frequent (q12h) if necessary. Hemodialysis: Give dose at end of treatment. Dissolve each 25mg effervescent tab in 5mL of water before administration.

HOW SUPPLIED: Inj: 1mg/mL, 25mg/mL; Syrup: 15mg/mL; Tab: 150mg, 300mg; Tab, Effervescent: 25mg

WARNINGS/PRECAUTIONS: Do not exceed recommended infusion rates; bradycardia reported with rapid infusion. Caution with liver and renal dysfunction. Monitor SGPT if on IV therapy for ≥5 days at dose >100mg qid. Avoid use with history of acute porphyria. Symptomatic response does not preclude the presence of gastric malignancy. May cause false (+) urine protein test. Granules and effervescent tablets contain phenylalanine.

ADVERSE REACTIONS: Headache, constipation, diarrhea, nausea, abdominal discomfort, vomiting, hepatitis, blood dyscrasias, rash, injection site reactions (IV/IM).

INTERACTIONS: Increases plasma levels of triazolam. Monitor anticoagulants.

PREGNANCY: Category B, caution with nursing.

MECHANISM OF ACTION: H_2-blocker; competitive, reversible inhibitor of histamine action at histamine H_2-receptors, including those found on gastric cells.

PHARMACOKINETICS: Absorption: (PO, 150mg) C_{max}=440-545ng/mL, T_{max}=2-3 hrs; (IM) Rapid; C_{max}= 576ng/mL, T_{max}=15 min. **Distribution**: V_d = 1.4L/kg;

Z

plasma protein binding (15%); found in breast milk. **Metabolism**: Liver, N-oxide (principal metabolite). **Elimination**: Urine, (PO 30% unchanged); (IV 70% unchanged); (PO) $T_{1/2}$=2.5-3 hrs, (IV) $T_{1/2}$=2-2.5 hrs. Refer to PI for pediatric parameters.

ZANTAC OTC
ranitidine HCL (Boehringer Ingelheim)

OTC

OTHER BRAND NAMES: Zantac 150 (Boehringer Ingelheim) - Zantac 75 (Boehringer Ingelheim)

THERAPEUTIC CLASS: H_2-blocker

INDICATIONS: For prevention and relief of heartburn associated with acid indigestion and sour stomach brought on by certain foods and beverages.

DOSAGE: *Adults:* Treatment/Relief of Heartburn: 75-150mg with water. Heartburn Prevention: 75-150mg 30-60 min before eating food or drinking beverages that cause heartburn. Max: 300mg/24 hrs.
Pediatrics: ≥12 yrs: Treatment/Relief of Heartburn: 75-150mg with water. Heartburn Prevention: 75-150mg 30-60 min before eating food or drinking beverages that cause heartburn. Max: 300mg/24 hrs.

HOW SUPPLIED: Tab: 75mg, 150mg

WARNINGS/PRECAUTIONS: Do not use if trouble or pain swallowing food, vomiting with blood, or bloody or black stools; with other acid reducers; or in patients with kidney disease. D/C if heartburn continues/worsens or use for >14 days.

INTERACTIONS: Avoid other acid reducers.

PREGNANCY: Safety in pregnancy and nursing not known.

MECHANISM OF ACTION: H_2-blocker; competitive, reversible inhibitor of histamine action at histamine H_2-receptors, including those found on gastric cells.

PHARMACOKINETICS: Apsorption: C_{max}=440-545ng/mL, T_{max}=2-3 hrs (IV). **Distribution:** V_d=1.4L/kg; serum protein binding (15%). **Metabolism:** Liver. **Elimination:** Urine 80% (unchanged); $T_{1/2}$=2.5-3 hrs (PO).

ZARONTIN
ethosuximide (Parke-Davis)

RX

THERAPEUTIC CLASS: Succinimide

INDICATIONS: Control of absence (petit mal) epilepsy.

DOSAGE: *Adults:* 500mg qd. Titrate: May increase daily dose by 250mg every 4-7 days. Max: 1.5g/day.
Pediatrics: Initial: 3-6 yrs: 250mg qd. ≥6 yrs: 500mg qd. Titrate: May increase daily dose by 250mg every 4-7 days. Usual: 20mg/kg/day. Max: 1.5g/day.

HOW SUPPLIED: Cap: 250mg; Syrup: 250mg/5mL

WARNINGS/PRECAUTIONS: Extreme caution in liver and renal dysfunction. Monitor blood counts, liver and renal function periodically. SLE, blood dyscrasias reported. Adjust dose slowly and avoid abrupt withdrawal. May increase grand mal seizures in mixed types of epilepsy when used alone. Caution with mental/physical activities.

ADVERSE REACTIONS: Anorexia, nausea, vomiting, abdominal pain, blood dyscrasias, drowsiness, headache, urticaria, SLE, myopia.

INTERACTIONS: May increase phenytoin levels. Valproic acid may alter levels.

PREGNANCY: Safety in pregnancy and nursing not known.

MECHANISM OF ACTION: Succinimide anticonvulsant; suppresses paroxysmal 3 cycles/second spike and wave activity associated with lapses of consciousness, which is common in absence (petit mal) seizures. Frequency of attacks is reduced through depression of motor cortex and elevation of the CNS threshold to convulsive stimuli.

PHARMACOKINETICS: **Distribution:** Crosses placenta, found in breast milk.

ZAROXOLYN   RX
metolazone (Celltech)

> **Do not interchange rapid and complete bioavailability metolazone formulations for other slow and incomplete bioavailability metolazone formulations; they are not therapeutically equivalent.**

THERAPEUTIC CLASS: Quinazoline diuretic

INDICATIONS: Treatment of hypertension and of salt and water retention in edema accompanying CHF or renal disease.

DOSAGE: *Adults:* Edema: 5-20mg qd. HTN: 2.5-5mg qd. Elderly: Start at low end of dosing range.

HOW SUPPLIED: Tab: 2.5mg, 5mg, 10mg

CONTRAINDICATIONS: Anuria, hepatic coma or precoma.

WARNINGS/PRECAUTIONS: Risk of hypokalemia, orthostatic hypotension, hypercalcemia, hyperuricemia, azotemia and rapid onset hyponatremia. Cross-allergy with sulfonamide-derived drugs, thiazides, or quinethazone. Sensitivity reactions may occur with 1st dose. Monitor electrolytes. May cause hyperglycemia and glycosuria in diabetics. Caution in elderly or severe renal impairment. May exacerbate or activate SLE.

ADVERSE REACTIONS: Chest pain/discomfort, orthostatic hypotension, syncope, neuropathy, necrotizing angiitis, hepatitis, jaundice, pancreatitis, blood dyscrasias, joint pain.

INTERACTIONS: Furosemide and other loop diuretics prolong fluid and electrolyte loss. Adjust dose of other antihypertensives. Potentiates hypotensive effects of alcohol, barbiturates, and narcotics. Lithium, digitalis toxicity. Corticosteroids and ACTH increase hypokalemia and salt and water retention. Enhanced neuromuscular blocking effects of curariform drugs. Salicylates and NSAIDs decrease effects. Decreased arterial response to norepinephrine. Decrease in methenamine efficacy. Adjust anticoagulants, antidiabetics.

PREGNANCY: Category B, not for use in nursing.

MECHANISM OF ACTION: Quinazoline diuretic; acts primarily to inhibit Na$^+$ reabsorption at cortical diluting site and, to a lesser extent, in proximal convoluted tubule.

PHARMACOKINETICS: Absorption: T_{max}=8 hrs. **Elimination:** Urine (unchanged).

ZEBETA   RX
bisoprolol fumarate (Duramed)

THERAPEUTIC CLASS: Selective beta$_1$-blocker

INDICATIONS: Management of hypertension.

DOSAGE: *Adults:* Initial: 2.5-5mg qd. Max: 20mg/day. Hepatic Dysfunction or CrCl <40mL/min: Initial: 2.5mg qd; caution with dose titration.

HOW SUPPLIED: Tab: 5mg*, 10mg *scored

CONTRAINDICATIONS: Cardiogenic shock, overt cardiac failure, 2nd- or 3rd-degree AV block, marked sinus bradycardia.

WARNINGS/PRECAUTIONS: Avoid abrupt withdrawal. May mask hypoglycemia or hyperthyroidism symptoms. Caution with compensated cardiac failure, DM, bronchospastic disease, hepatic/renal impairment, or peripheral vascular disease. May precipitate cardiac failure. Both digitalis glycosides and β-blockers slow atrioventricular conduction and decrease HR. Concomitant use can increase risk of bradycardia.

ADVERSE REACTIONS: Diarrhea, URI, fatigue.

INTERACTIONS: May block epinephrine effects. Caution with clonidine withdrawal. Excessive reduction of sympathetic activity with catecholamine-depleting drugs. Avoid other β-blockers. Caution with CCBs (eg, verapamil, diltiazem), antiarrhythmics (eg, disopyramide), and anesthetics that depress myocardial function. Rifampin increases clearance. Antidiabetic agents may need adjustment.

PREGNANCY: Category C, caution in nursing.

MECHANISM OF ACTION: Synthetic β₁-selective (cardioselective) adrenoreceptor blocking agent; inhibits β₂-adrenoreceptors, chiefly in bronchial and vascular musculature.

PHARMACOKINETICS: Absorption: Absolute bioavailability 80%; T_{max} = 2-4 hrs. **Distribution:** Plasma protein binding (30%). **Elimination:** $T_{1/2}$=9-12 hrs; urine, feces (≤2%).

ZEGERID RX
sodium bicarbonate - omeprazole (Santarus)

THERAPEUTIC CLASS: Proton pump inhibitor

INDICATIONS: (Cap, Powder) Short-term treatment of erosive esophagitis diagnosed by endoscopy, active duodenal ulcer, and active benign gastric ulcer. Treatment of heartburn and other symptoms associated with GERD. Maintain healing of erosive espophagitis. (Powder, 40mg-1680mg) Reduction of risk of upper GI bleeding in critically ill patients.

DOSAGE: *Adults:* Cap/Powder: Duodenal Ulcer: 20mg qd for 4-8 weeks. Gastric Ulcer: 40mg qd for 4-8 weeks. GERD: 20mg qd for up to 4 weeks without esophageal lesions and for 4-8 weeks with erosive esophagitis. Maintenance of Healing Erosive Esophagitis: 20mg qd. Powder (40mg-1680mg): Risk Reduction of Upper GI Bleeding in Critically Ill Patients: Initial: 40mg, followed by 40mg after 6-8 hrs. Maint: 40mg qd for 14 days. Take 1 hr before a meal. Add pkt contents to 2 tablespoons of water; do not use other liquids or foods. Stir powder well and drink immediately. Swallow caps whole with water.

HOW SUPPLIED: (Omeprazole-Sodium Bicarbonate) Cap: 20mg-1100mg, 40mg-1100mg; Powder: 20mg-1680mg/pkt [30ˢ], 40mg-1680mg/pkt [30ˢ].

WARNINGS/PRECAUTIONS: Atrophic gastritis reported with long-term use. Symptomatic response does not preclude the presence of gastric malignancy. Due to sodium bicarbonate content, avoid with metabolic alkalosis, hypocalcemia and use caution with a sodium-restricted diet, Bartter's syndrome, hypokalemia, respiratory alkalosis. Long-term use of bicarbonate with calcium or milk may cause milk-alkali syndrome.

ADVERSE REACTIONS: Abdominal pain, headache, nausea, vomiting.

INTERACTIONS: May prolong elimination of diazepam, warfarin, phenytoin, and drugs metabolized by oxidation. May increase PT and INR if given concomitantly with warfarin. May alter absorption of pH-dependent drugs (eg, ketoconazole, ampicillin esters, and iron salts). Monitor when given with drugs metabolized by CYP450 (eg, cyclosporine, disulfiram, benzodiazepines). Clarithromycin may increase levels. May increase levels of tacrolimus, clarithromycin. May reduce levels of atazanavir.

PREGNANCY: Category C, not for use in nursing.

MECHANISM OF ACTION: Omeprazole: Proton-pump inhibitor; suppresses gastric acid secretion by specific inhibition of the H^+/K^+ ATPase enzyme at secretory surface of gastric parietal cell. Sodium Bicarbonate: Acts as antacid.

PHARMACOKINETICS: Absorption: Omeprazole: Rapid absorption; T_{max}=30 min; (Sus) Absolute bioavailability (30-40%); C_{max}=1954ng/mL. (Cap) C_{max}=1526ng/mL. **Distribution:** Omeprazole: Plasma protein binding (95%); found in breast milk. **Metabolism:** Omeprazole: Hydroxyomeprazole and corresponding carboxylic acid (metabolites). **Elimination:** Omeprazole: Urine (77% as metabolites), feces; $T_{1/2}$=1 hr.

ZELAPAR RX
selegiline HCL (Valeant)

THERAPEUTIC CLASS: Monoamine oxidase inhibitor (Type B)

INDICATIONS: Adjunct in the management of Parkinson's disease in patients exhibiting a deteriorated response to levodopa/carbidopa therapy.

DOSAGE: *Adults:* 1.25mg every AM without liquid for 6 weeks. Titrate: After 6 weeks, may increase to 2.5mg if desired benefit not achieved. Max: 2.5mg/day.

HOW SUPPLIED: Tab, Orally Disintigrating: 1.25mg

CONTRAINDICATIONS: Concomitant meperidine, tramadol, methadone, propoxyphene dextromethorphan, and other MAOIs.

WARNINGS/PRECAUTIONS: Do not exceed 2.5mg/day; risk of non-selective MAO inhibition. Greater risk of orthostatic hypotension and dizziness in geriatric patients. Decrease levodopa/carbidopa to prevent exacerbation of levodopa side effects. Perform periodic dermatologic screening. May increase frequency of mild oropharyngeal abnormality. Caution with renal or hepatic impairment. Neuroleptic malignant syndrome reported in association with rapid dose reduction, withdrawal of, or changes in antiparkinsonian therapy.

ADVERSE REACTIONS: Nausea, dizziness, pain, headache, insomnia, rhinitis, skin disorders, dyskinesia, backache, dyspepsia, stomatitis, constipation, hallucinations, pharyngitis, rash.

INTERACTIONS: See Contraindications. Serious, sometimes fatal, reactions have been precipitated with meperidine, tramadol, methadone, and propoxyphene; avoid concomitant use. Episodes of psychosis or bizarre behavior reported with dextromethorphan; avoid concomitant use. Severe toxicity reported with SSRIs or TCAs; avoid concurrent use and allow 2 weeks between discontinuation of selegiline and initiation of TCAs or SSRIs. Allow 5 weeks for fluoxetine due to a longer half-life. Caution with sympathomimetics and CYP3A4 inducers (eg, phenytoin, carbamazepine, nafcillin, phenobarbital, and rifampin).

PREGNANCY: Category C, not for use in nursing.

MECHANISM OF ACTION: Irreversible MAO inhibitor; blocks catabolism of dopamine and increases net amount of dopamine available.

PHARMACOKINETICS: Absorption: (1.25mg, 2.5mg, 5mg) T_{max}=(10-15 min, 10-15 min, 40-90 min); Mean C_{max}(1.25mg, 2.5mg, 5mg)=(3.34, 4.47, 1.12ng/mL). **Distribution:** Plasma protein binding (85%). **Metabolism:** Liver (1st-pass metabolism). **Elimination:** $T_{1/2}$=10 hrs (steady state); urine.

ZEMAIRA RX
alpha1-proteinase inhibitor (human) (CSL Behring)

THERAPEUTIC CLASS: Alpha$_1$-Proteinase Inhibitor

INDICATIONS: Chronic augmentation and maintenance therapy in individuals with alpha$_1$-proteinase inhibitor (A$_1$-PI) deficiency and clinical evidence of emphysema.

DOSAGE: *Adults:* 60mg/kg IV once weekly.

HOW SUPPLIED: Inj: 1000mg

CONTRAINDICATIONS: IgA deficiencies with known antibodies against IgA.

WARNINGS/PRECAUTIONS: May contain infectious agents (eg, viruses). Infusion rates and clinical status should be monitored closely during infusion. May cause increase in plasma volume.

ADVERSE REACTIONS: Asthenia, injection site pain, dizziness, headache, paresthesia, pruritus.

PREGNANCY: Category C, caution in nursing.

MECHANISM OF ACTION: α$_1$-antitrypsin; A$_1$-PI is the primary antiprotease where it inhibits neutrophil elastase.

Z

ZEMPLAR IV
paricalcitol (Abbott)

RX

THERAPEUTIC CLASS: Vitamin D analog

INDICATIONS: Prevention and treatment of secondary hyperparathyroidism associated with chronic kidney disease Stage 5.

DOSAGE: *Adults:* Initial: 0.04-0.1mcg/kg bolus no more frequently than every other day during dialysis. Max: 0.24mcg/kg (16.8mcg). Titrate: May increase by 2-4mcg at 2-4 week intervals. Monitor serum Ca and phosphorus more frequently during dose adjustments. Reduce or interrupt dose if elevated Ca level or Ca x P product >75, may reinitiate at lower dose once normalized. May need dose decrease as PTH levels decrease (see PI).
Pediatrics: ≥5 yrs: (Inj) Initial: 0.04-0.1mcg/kg bolus no more frequently than every other day during dialysis. Max: 0.24mcg/kg (16.8mcg). Titrate: May increase by 2-4mcg at 2-4 week intervals. Monitor serum Ca and phosphorus more frequently during dose adjustments. Reduce or interrupt dose if elevated Ca level or Ca x P product >75, may reinitiate at lower dose once normalized. May need dose decrease as PTH levels decrease (see PI).

HOW SUPPLIED: Inj: 2mcg/mL, 5mcg/mL

CONTRAINDICATIONS: Vitamin D toxicity, hypercalcemia.

WARNINGS/PRECAUTIONS: Overdose may cause progressive hypercalcemia. Should supplement with calcium and restrict phosphorus. May need phosphate-binding compounds to control serum phosphorus levels. Avoid concomitant phosphate or vitamin D-related compounds.

ADVERSE REACTIONS: Nausea, vomiting, edema, chills, flu, GI bleeding, lightheadedness, pneumonia, pain, allergic reaction, headache, HTN, diarrhea, arthritis, rash.

INTERACTIONS: Digitalis toxicity potentiated by hypercalcemia. Avoid excessive use of aluminum containing compounds.

PREGNANCY: Category C, caution in nursing.

MECHANISM OF ACTION: Synthetic vitamin D analog; binds to vitamin D receptor, which results in selective activation of vitamin D pathways. Shown to reduce parathyroid hormone levels by inhibiting PTH synthesis and secretion.

PHARMACOKINETICS: Absorption: C_{max} =1.680ng/mL (hemodialysis), 1.832ng/mL (peritoneal dialysis); AUC= 14.51ng•h/mL (hemodialysis), 16.01ng•h/mL (peritoneal dialysis). **Distribution:** V_d=23.8L (healthy), 31L (hemodialysis), and 35L (peritoneal dialysis); plasma protein binding (≥99.8%). **Metabolism:** Hepatic, via hydroxylation and glucuronidation; CYP24, CYP3A4, UGT1A4. **Elimination:** Hepatobiliary excretion (primary), urine (19%), feces (63%); $T_{1/2}$=13.9 hrs (hemodialysis), 15.4 hrs (peritoneal dialysis).

ZEMPLAR ORAL
paricalcitol (Abbott)

RX

THERAPEUTIC CLASS: Vitamin D analog

INDICATIONS: Prevention and treatment of secondary hyperparathyroidism associated with Stage 3 and 4 chronic kidney disease.

DOSAGE: *Adults:* Initial: Baseline iPTH Level ≤500pg/mL: 1mcg qd or 2mcg tiw. Baseline iPTH Level >500pg/mL: 2mcg qd or 4mcg tiw. May need dose adjustment based on iPTH level relative to baseline (see PI).

HOW SUPPLIED: Cap: 1mcg, 2mcg, 4mcg

CONTRAINDICATIONS: Vitamin D toxicity, hypercalcemia.

WARNINGS/PRECAUTIONS: May cause over suppression of PTH, hypercalcemia, hypercalciuria, hyperphosphatemia, and adynamic bone disease. Overdose may cause progressive hypercalcemia.

ADVERSE REACTIONS: Pain, allergic reactions, headache, infection, hypotension, HTN, diarrhea, nausea, vomiting, constipation, edema, arthritis, dizziness, vertigo, rhinitis, rash.

INTERACTIONS: Digitalis toxicity potentiated by hypercalcemia. Caution with strong CYP3A inhibitors (ketoconazole, atazanavir, clarithromycin, indinavir, itraconazole, nefazodone, nelfinavir, ritonavir, saquinavir, telithromycin, voriconazole). Drugs that may impair intestinal absorption of fat-soluble vitamins (cholestyramine) may intefere with absorption.

PREGNANCY: Category C, not for use in nursing.

MECHANISM OF ACTION: Synthetic vitamin D analog; binds to vitamin D receptor (VDR), which results in selective activation of vitamin D responsive pathways. Shown to reduce parathyroid hormone levels by inhibiting PTH synthesis and secretion.

PHARMACOKINETICS: Absorption: Well absorbed; Absolute bioavailability (72%); C_{max}=0.630ng/mL; T_{max}=3 hrs; AUC=5.25ng•h/mL. **Distribution:** Plasma protein binding (≥99.8%); V_d=34L (healthy); 44-46L (CKD stage 3 and 4). **Metabolism:** Hepatic, via hydroxylation and glucuronidation; Extensively metabolized by CYP24, as well as CYP3A4, UGT1A4. 24(R)-hydroxy paracalcitol (minor metabolite). **Elimination:** Hepatobiliary excretion (primary); Urine (18%), feces (70%); $T_{1/2}$=17 hrs (CKD Stage 3), 20 hrs (CKD Stage 4).

ZENAPAX RX
daclizumab (Roche Labs)

THERAPEUTIC CLASS: Immunosuppressive agent

INDICATIONS: For prophylaxis of acute organ rejection in renal transplants, in combination with cyclosporine and corticosteroids.

DOSAGE: *Adults:* 1mg/kg IV over 15 min for 5 doses. Administer 1st dose no more than 24 hrs prior to transplant and remaining 4 doses at 14-day intervals. *Pediatrics:* ≥11 months: 1mg/kg IV over 15 min for 5 doses. Administer 1st dose no more than 24 hrs prior to transplant and remaining 4 doses at 14-day intervals.

HOW SUPPLIED: Inj: 25mg/5mL

WARNINGS/PRECAUTIONS: Increased risk of lymphoproliferative disorder and opportunistic infections. Anaphylactic reactions reported. Caution in elderly. Re-administration after initial course of therapy has not been studied in humans.

ADVERSE REACTIONS: Constipation, nausea, vomiting, diarrhea, abdominal pain, pyrosis, dyspepsia, abdominal distention, epigastric pain.

PREGNANCY: Category C, not for use in nursing.

MECHANISM OF ACTION: IL-2 receptor antagonist; binds with high affinity to the Tac subunit of the high affinity IL-2 receptor complex and inhibits IL-2 binding.

PHARMACOKINETICS: Absorption: C_{max}=7.6µg/mL (adult); 5.0µg/mL (pediatric). **Elimination:** $T_{1/2}$=20 days (adult), 13 days (pediatric).

ZERIT RX
stavudine (Bristol-Myers Squibb)

> Lactic acidosis and severe, fatal hepatomegaly reported. Fatal and non-fatal pancreatitis reported with didanosine.

THERAPEUTIC CLASS: Synthetic thymidine nucleoside analogue

INDICATIONS: Treatment of HIV-1 infection in combination with other antiretrovirals.

DOSAGE: *Adults:* ≥60kg: 40mg q12h. <60kg: 30mg q12h. Interrupt therapy if develop peripheral neuropathy, resume at 1/2 dose when neuropathy resolves. D/C permanently if neuropathy recurs after resumption. Suspend therapy if

lactic acidosis or hepatotoxicity occurs. CrCl 26-50mL/min: ≥60kg: 20mg q12h. <60kg: 15mg q12h. CrCl 10-25mL/min: ≥60kg: 20mg q24h. <60kg: 15mg q24h.
Pediatrics: ≥60kg: 40mg q12h. 30-59 kg: 30mg q12h. ≥14 days and <30kg: 1mg/kg q12h. Birth-13 days: 0.5mg/kg q12h. Interrupt therapy if develop peripheral neuropathy, resume with 1/2 dose when neuropathy resolves. D/C permanently if neuropathy recurs after resumption. Suspend therapy if lactic acidosis or hepatotoxicity occurs. Renal Impairment: Reduce dose and/or increase interval.

HOW SUPPLIED: Cap: 15mg, 20mg, 30mg, 40mg; Sus: 1mg/mL [200mL]

WARNINGS/PRECAUTIONS: Obesity and prolonged nucleoside exposure may increase risk to lactic acidosis and hepatomegaly. Caution with risk factors for hepatic disease. Peripheral neuropathy reported. Monitor for lactic acidosis in pregnancy if used with didanosine. D/C if motor weakness develops.

ADVERSE REACTIONS: Peripheral neuropathy, rash, elevated LFTs and amylase, headache, diarrhea, nausea, vomiting.

INTERACTIONS: Avoid zidovudine. Increased risk of neuropathy with neurotoxic drugs (eg, didanosine). Increased risk of hepatotoxicity with didanosine and hydroxyurea. Motor weakness reported with other antiretrovirals.

PREGNANCY: Category C, not for use in nursing.

MECHANISM OF ACTION: Thymidine nucleoside analogue; inhibits activity of HIV-1 reverse transcriptase by competing with natural substrate thymidine triphosphate and by DNA chain termination following incorporation into viral DNA. Inhibits cellular DNA polymerases β and gamma and markedly reduces synthesis of mitochondrial DNA.

PHARMACOKINETICS: Absorption: Rapidly absorbed; C_{max}=536±146ng/mL; T_{max}=1 hr; AUC=2568±454ng.h/mL. **Distribution**: V_d=46±21L (adults); V_d=0.73+/-0.32L/kg (age 5 weeks to 15 yrs). **Elimination**: Renal (40%); $T_{1/2}$=1.15±0.35 hrs (IV, adult), 1.6±0.23 hrs (PO, adult); $T_{1/2}$=1.11+/-0.28 hrs (IV, age 5 weeks to 15 yrs); $T_{1/2}$= 0.96+/-0.26 hrs (PO, age 5 weeks to 15 yrs).

ZESTORETIC   RX
lisinopril - hydrochlorothiazide (AstraZeneca)

> ACE inhibitors can cause death/injury to developing fetus during 2nd and 3rd trimesters. Stop therapy if pregnancy detected.

THERAPEUTIC CLASS: ACE inhibitor/thiazide diuretic

INDICATIONS: Treatment of hypertension. Not for initial therapy.

DOSAGE: *Adults:* Initial (If Not Controlled with Lisinopril/HCTZ monotherapy): 10mg-12.5mg tab or 20mg-12.5mg tab daily. Titrate: May increase after 2-3 weeks. Initial (If Controlled on 25mg HCTZ/Day with Hypokalemia): 10mg-12.5mg tab. Replacement Therapy: Substitute combination for titrated components.

HOW SUPPLIED: Tab: (Lisinopril-HCTZ) 10mg-12.5mg, 20mg-12.5mg, 20mg-25mg

CONTRAINDICATIONS: History of ACE inhibitor-associated angioedema, hereditary or idiopathic angioedema, anuria, sulfonamide hypersensitivity.

WARNINGS/PRECAUTIONS: D/C if angioedema, jaundice, or marked LFT elevation occur. Risk of hyperkalemia with DM, renal dysfunction. Persistent nonproductive cough reported. Monitor WBCs in renal and collagen vascular disease. Anaphylactoid reactions during membrane exposure reported. Fetal/neonatal morbidity and death reported. Monitor for hypotension in high-risk patients (eg, surgery/anesthesia, volume/salt depletion). Caution with CHF, renal or hepatic dysfunction. More reports of angioedema in blacks than nonblacks. May exacerbate or activate SLE. Monitor electrolytes. Avoid if CrCl ≤30mL/min/1.7m². May increase cholesterol, TG. Hypercalcemia, hypomagnesemia, hyperuricemia may occur. Caution with left ventricle outflow obstruction.

Z

ADVERSE REACTIONS: Dizziness, headache, cough, fatigue, orthostatic effects, diarrhea, nausea, muscle cramps, angioedema, cutaneous pseudolymphoma.

INTERACTIONS: Increases risk of hyperkalemia with K^+-sparing diuretics, K^+ supplements, or K^+-containing salt substitutes. Potentiates orthostatic hypotension with alcohol, barbiturates, and narcotics. Adjust antidiabetic drugs. Reduced absorption with cholestyramine, colestipol. Corticosteroids, ACTH deplete electrolytes. May decrease response to pressor amines. Potentiates other antihypertensives. May increase responsiveness to skeletal muscle relaxants. Risk of lithium toxicity. NSAIDs reduce effects and worsen renal dysfunction. Nitritoid reactions with gold.

PREGNANCY: Category C (1st trimester) and D (2nd and 3rd trimesters), not for use in nursing.

MECHANISM OF ACTION: Lisinopril: ACE inhibitor. Inhibition results in decreased plasma angiotensin II, which leads to decreased vasopressor activity and decreased aldosterone secretion. HCTZ: thiazide diuretic. Affects renal tubular mechanism of electrolyte reabsorption, directly increasing excretion of Na^+ and chloride.

PHARMACOKINETICS: Absorption: Lisinopril: T_{max}=7 hrs. **Distribution:** HCTZ: Crosses placenta. **Elimination:** Lisinopril: Urine (unchanged); $T_{1/2}$= 12 hrs. HCTZ: Kidneys; $T_{1/2}$= 5.6-14.8 hrs.

ZESTRIL   RX
lisinopril (AstraZeneca)

> ACE inhibitors can cause death/injury to developing fetus during 2nd and 3rd trimesters. D/C if pregnancy is detected.

THERAPEUTIC CLASS: ACE inhibitor

INDICATIONS: Treatment of HTN. Adjunct therapy in heart failure if inadequately controlled by diuretics and digitalis. Adjunct therapy in stable patients within 24 hrs of AMI to improve survival.

DOSAGE: *Adults:* HTN: If possible, d/c diuretic 2-3 days prior to therapy. Initial: 10mg qd, 5mg qd with diuretic. Usual: 20-40mg qd. Resume diuretic if BP not controlled. Max: 80mg/day. CrCl 10-30mL/min: Initial: 5mg/day. Max: 40mg/day. CrCl <10mL/min: Initial: 2.5mg/day. Max: 40mg/day. Heart Failure: Initial: 5mg qd. Usual: 5-40mg qd. May increase by 10mg every 2 weeks. Max: 40mg/day. Hyponatremia or CrCl ≤30mL/min: Initial: 2.5mg qd. AMI: Initial: 5mg within 24 hrs, then 5mg after 24 hrs, then 10mg after 48 hrs, then 10mg qd. Use 2.5mg during first 3 days with low SBP. Maint: 10mg qd for 6 weeks, 2.5-5mg with hypotension. D/C with prolonged hypotension. Elderly: Caution with dose adjustment.
Pediatrics: ≥6 yrs: HTN: Initial: 0.07mg/kg qd up to 5mg total. Dose adjust according to response. Max: 0.61mg/kg or 40mg.

HOW SUPPLIED: Tab: 2.5mg, 5mg, 10mg, 20mg, 30mg, 40mg

CONTRAINDICATIONS: History of ACE inhibitor-associated angioedema, hereditary or idiopathic angioedema.

WARNINGS/PRECAUTIONS: D/C if angioedema, jaundice, or marked LFT elevation occur. Risk of hyperkalemia, hypoglycemia with DM, renal dysfunction. Persistent nonproductive cough reported. Monitor WBCs in renal and collagen vascular disease. Anaphylactoid reactions during membrane exposure reported. Fetal/neonatal morbidity and death reported. Monitor for hypotension in high-risk patients (heart failure with SBP <100mmHg, surgery/anesthesia, hyponatremia, high-dose diuretic therapy, severe volume and/or salt depletion, etc). Caution with CHF, aortic stenosis/hypertrophic cardiomyopathy, renal dysfunction, and renal artery stenosis. Less effective on BP in blacks and more reports of angioedema than nonblacks.

ADVERSE REACTIONS: Hypotension, diarrhea, headache, dizziness, hyperkalemia, chest pain, cough, cutaneous pseudolymphoma.

Z

INTERACTIONS: May increase lithium levels. Hypotension risk with diuretics. Concomitant use with antidiabetic medications may increase risk of hypoglycemia. Increase risk of hyperkalemia with K^+-sparing diuretics, K^+-containing salt substitutes, or K^+ supplements. Indomethacin may reduce effects. Nitritoid reactions with gold.

PREGNANCY: Category C (1st trimester) and D (2nd and 3rd trimesters), not for use in nursing.

MECHANISM OF ACTION: ACE inhibitor; inhibition results in decreased plasma angiotensin II, which leads to decreased vasopressor activity and aldosterone secretion.

PHARMACOKINETICS: Absorption: T_{max}=7 hrs. **Elimination:** Urine (unchanged); $T_{1/2}$=12 hrs.

ZETIA   RX
ezetimibe (Merck/Schering-Plough)

THERAPEUTIC CLASS: Cholesterol absorption inhibitor

INDICATIONS: Adjunct to diet, as monotherapy or with concomitant HMG-CoA reductase inhibitors, to reduce total-C, LDL-C, and Apo B levels in primary (heterozygous familial and nonfamilial) hypercholesterolemia. Adjunct to diet, with concomitant fenofibrate, to reduce elevated total-C, LDL-C, Apo B, and non-HDL-C in mixed hyperlipidemia. Adjunct to other lipid-lowering treatments or if such treatments are unavailable, with concomitant atorvastatin or simvastatin, to reduce total-C and LDL-C in homozygous familial hypercholesterolemia. Adjunct to diet, to reduce sitosterol and campesterol levels in homozygous familial sitosterolemia.

DOSAGE: *Adults:* 10mg qd. May give with HMG-CoA reductase inhibitor (with primary hypercholesterolemia) or fenofibrate (with mixed hyperlipidemia) for incremental effect. Concomitant Bile Sequestrant: Give either ≥2 hrs before or ≥4 hrs after bile acid sequestrant.

HOW SUPPLIED: Tab: 10mg

CONTRAINDICATIONS: When used with a statin, refer to the HMG-CoA reductase inhibitor monographs.

WARNINGS/PRECAUTIONS: Monitor LFTs with concurrent statin therapy. Not recommended with moderate or severe hepatic insufficiency.

ADVERSE REACTIONS: Back pain, arthralgia, diarrhea, sinusitis, abdominal pain, myalgia.

INTERACTIONS: Incremental LDL-C reduction may be reduced with concomitant cholestyramine. Fibrates may increase cholesterol excretion into the bile; concurrent use is not recommended. Increased levels with fenofibrate and gemfibrozil. Monitor cyclosporine levels with concomitant use of cyclosporine. Monitor INR when administered with warfarin.

PREGNANCY: Category C, contraindicated in nursing.

MECHANISM OF ACTION: Cholesterol absorption inhibitor; inhibits absorption of cholesterol by small intestine. Targets the sterol transporter, Neimann-Pick C1-like 1 (NPC1L1), which is involved in intestinal uptake of cholesterol and phytosterol; inhibited uptake leads to decrease of intestinal cholesterol to the liver, causing reduction of hepatic cholesterol stores and increase in clearance of cholesterol from the blood.

PHARMACOKINETICS: Absorption: Ezetimibe: C_{max}=3.4-5.5ng/mL; T_{max}=4-12 hrs; Ezetemibe-glucuronide (active metabolite): C_{max}=45-71ng/mL; T_{max}=1-2 hrs. **Distribution:** Plasma protein binding (>90%). **Metabolism:** Small intestine, liver via glucuronide conjugation; Ezetimibe-glucuronide (major active metabolite). **Elimination:** Feces (78%), urine (11%); $T_{1/2}$=22 hrs.

ZEVALIN   RX
ibritumomab tiuxetan (Biogen Idec)

> Discontinue if severe infusion reactions occurs. Severe and prolonged cytopenias reported; avoid if ≥25% lymphoma marrow involvement and/or impaired bone marrow reserve. Severe, some fatal, cutaneous and mucocutaneous reactions reported. Do not exceed the maximum dose. Avoid patients with altered biodistribution.

THERAPEUTIC CLASS: Monoclonal antibody

INDICATIONS: Treatment of relapsed or refractory low grade, follicular, or transformed B-cell non-Hodgkin's lymphoma, including rituximab refractory follicular non-Hodgkin's lymphoma.

DOSAGE: *Adults:* Day 1: Rituximab 250mg/m² IV single infusion. Within 4 hrs, give 5mCi of In-111 ibritumomab IV. Assess biodistribution by conducting 1st image at 2-24 hrs, 2nd image at 48-72 hrs, and optional 3rd image at 90-120 hrs. If biodistribution acceptable, Day 7-9: Rituximab 250mg/m² IV. Within 4 hrs, give Y-90 Ibritumomab 0.4mCi/kg (or 0.3mCi/kg if platelets 100,000-149,000 cells/mm³). Max: Y-90 ibritumomab 32mCi.

HOW SUPPLIED: Inj: 3.2mg/2mL

CONTRAINDICATIONS: Type I hypersensitivity or anaphylactic reactions to murine proteins or to any component of this product including rituximab, yttrium chloride, and indium chloride.

WARNINGS/PRECAUTIONS: Use with rituximab, Contains albumin; remote risk of transmission of viral disease and CJD. Single course treatment only. Minimize radiation exposure during and after radiolabeling. Monitor CBC and platelets weekly until levels recover. Increased risk of hypersensitivity reactions with HAMA from prior murine protein use. Caution with transfusion. Secondary leukemia and mylodysplastic syndrome reproted. Monitor closely for evidence of extravasation. Immediately terminate infusion if signs or symptoms of extravasation occured.

ADVERSE REACTIONS: Neutropenia, thrombocytopenia, anemia, nausea, vomiting, abdominal pain, diarrhea, increased cough, dyspnea, dizziness, arthralgia, anorexia, anxiety, ecchymosis, infusion site erythema, ulceration following extravasation, radiation injury, tissue complications.

INTERACTIONS: Increased risk of bleeding and hemorrhage with drugs that interfere with platelet function or coagulation; monitor for thrombocytopenia more frequently. Safety of immunization with live viral vaccines not studied.

PREGNANCY: Category D, not for use in nursing.

MECHANISM OF ACTION: Monoclonal antibody; binds specifically to CD20 antigen, which is expressed on pre-B and mature B lymphocytes, and on B-cell non-Hodgkin's lymphomas.

PHARMACOKINETICS: Elimination: Urine (7.5%); $T_{1/2}$=30 hrs.

ZIAC   RX
bisoprolol fumarate - hydrochlorothiazide (Duramed)

THERAPEUTIC CLASS: Selective beta₁-blocker/thiazide diuretic

INDICATIONS: Management of hypertension.

DOSAGE: *Adults:* Initial: 2.5mg-6.25mg tab qd. Maint: May increase every 14 days. Max: 20mg bisoprolol-12.5mg HCTZ/day. Renal/Hepatic Dysfunction: Caution in dosing/titrating.

HOW SUPPLIED: Tab: (Bisoprolol-HCTZ) 2.5mg-6.25mg, 5mg-6.25mg, 10mg-6.25mg

CONTRAINDICATIONS: Cardiogenic shock, overt cardiac failure, 2nd- or 3rd-degree AV block, marked sinus bradycardia, anuria, sulfonamide hypersensitivity.

WARNINGS/PRECAUTIONS: Caution with compensated cardiac failure, DM, bronchospastic disease, hepatic/renal impairment, or peripheral vascular

Z

disease. Avoid abrupt withdrawal. Photosensitivity reactions, hypokalemia, hypercalcemia, hypophosphatemia reported. May activate/exacerbate SLE. Enhanced effects in post-sympathectomy patients. May mask hyperthyroidism or hypoglycemia symptoms. Monitor for fluid/electrolyte imbalance. May precipitate hyperuricemia, acute gout, cardiac failure.

ADVERSE REACTIONS: Cough, diarrhea, myalgia, headache, dizziness, fatigue, upper respiratory infection.

INTERACTIONS: Alcohol, barbiturates, or narcotics may potentiate orthostatic hypotension. Adjust dose of antidiabetic drugs. Potentiates other antihypertensives. Avoid other β-blockers. Impaired absorption with cholestyramine, colestipol. Corticosteroids, ACTH intensify electrolyte depletion. May decrease response to pressor amines. May increase response to nondepolarizing muscle relaxants. Risk of lithium toxicity. NSAIDs may reduce effects. May block epinephrine effects. Excessive reduction of sympathetic activity with catecholamine-depleting drugs. Caution with clonidine withdrawal. Increased clearance with rifampin. Caution with CCBs, myocardial depressants, anesthesia, and antiarrhythmics. Digitalis glycosides and β-blockers slow atrioventricular conduction and decrease HR; concomitant use can increase the risk of bradycardia.

PREGNANCY: Category C, not for use in nursing.

MECHANISM OF ACTION: Bisoprolol: $β_1$-selective, cardioselective, adreno-receptor-blocking agent; decreases HR, increases sinus node recovery time, prolongs AV-node refractory periods, and prolongs AV-nodal conduction with rapid atrial stimulation. HCTZ: Thiazide diuretic; affects renal tubular mechanisms of electrolyte reabsorption and increases excretion of Na^+ and chloride.

PHARMACOKINETICS: Absorption: Bisoprolol: Absolute bioavailability (80%); (2.5mg) C_{max}=9ng/mL, T_{max}=3 hrs. HCTZ: Well-absorbed; C_{max}=30ng/mL, T_{max}=2.5 hrs. **Distribution**: Bisoprolol: Plasma protein binding (30%). HCTZ: Plasma protein binding (40-68%). **Elimination:** Bisoprolol: $T_{1/2}$= 7-15 hrs; Urine (55% unchanged). HCTZ: $T_{1/2}$=4-10 hrs; Urine (60% unchanged).

ZIAGEN   RX
abacavir sulfate (GlaxoSmithKline)

> Fatal hypersensitivity reactions, lactic acidosis, severe hepatomegaly with steatosis, including fatal cases reported. D/C if hypersensitivity reaction is suspected and do not restart.

THERAPEUTIC CLASS: Synthetic carbocyclic nucleoside analogue

INDICATIONS: Treatment of HIV-1 infection in combination with other antiretrovirals.

DOSAGE: *Adults:* >16 yrs: 300mg bid or 600mg qd.
Pediatrics: 3 months-16 yrs: 8mg/kg bid. Max: 300mg bid.

HOW SUPPLIED: Sol: 20mg/mL [240mL]; Tab: 300mg

WARNINGS/PRECAUTIONS: Register abacavir hypersensitive patients at 800-270-0425. Caution with liver disease; lactic acidosis and severe hepatomegaly with steatosis, including fatal cases, reported. Not for monotherapy when antiretroviral regimens are changed. Immune reconstitution syndrome reported. Should not be coadministered with Epzicom or Trizivir.

ADVERSE REACTIONS: Hypersensitivity reactions (eg, fever, rash, fatigue, GI symptoms), nausea, vomiting, diarrhea, loss of appetite, insomnia, chills, headache, fatigue.

INTERACTIONS: Decreased elimination with ethanol.

PREGNANCY: Category C, not for use in nursing.

MECHANISM OF ACTION: Carbocyclic nucleoside analogue; inhibits HIV-1 reverse transcriptase (RT) by competing with natural substrate dGTP and incorporating into viral DNA.

PHARMACOKINETICS: Absorption: Rapid; absolute bioavailabilty (83%); (BID dosing): C_{max} = 3mcg/mL, AUC_{0-12h}=6.02mcg•hr/mL; (QD dosing): C_{max} = 4.26mcg/mL, AUC=11.95mcg•hr/mL. **Distribution:** (IV) V_d=0.86L/kg; plasma

Z

protein binding (50%). **Metabolism:** Hepatic, via alcohol dehydrogenase and glucuronyl transferase. **Elimination:** Urine (1.2%). (QD dosing): $T_{1/2}$=1.54 hrs.

ZIANA   RX
clindamycin phosphate - tretinoin (Medicis)

THERAPEUTIC CLASS: Lincosamide derivative/retinoid

INDICATIONS: Topical treatment of acne vulgaris.

DOSAGE: *Adults:* Apply pea-sized amount to entire face qd at bedtime. Avoid eyes, mouth, angles of nose, or mucous membranes. Not for oral, ophthalmic, or intravaginal use.
Pediatrics: ≥12 yrs: Apply pea-sized amount to entire face qd at bedtime. Avoid eyes, mouth, angles of nose, or mucous membranes. Not for oral, ophthalmic, or intravaginal use.

HOW SUPPLIED: Gel: (Clindamycin-Tretinoin) 1.2%-0.025% [2g, 30g, 60g]

CONTRAINDICATIONS: Regional enteritis, ulcerative colitis, or history of antibiotic-associated colitis.

WARNINGS/PRECAUTIONS: May cause severe colitis; d/c if significant diarrhea occurs. Avoid exposure to sunlight and sunlamps; wear sunscreen daily.

ADVERSE REACTIONS: Nasopharyngitis, erythema, scaling, itching, burning.

INTERACTIONS: Caution with concomitant topical medications, medicated/abrasive soaps and cleansers, soaps/cosmetics with strong drying effect, products with high concentrations of alcohol, astringents, spices, or lime. Avoid with erythromycin-containing products. Caution with neuromuscular blocking agents.

PREGNANCY: Category C, not for use in nursing.

MECHANISM OF ACTION: Clindamycin: Lincosamide antibiotic; binds to 50S ribosomal subunits of susceptible bacteria and prevents elongation of peptide chains by interfering with peptidyl transfer, thereby suppressing bacterial protein synthesis. Found to have activity against *P.acnes*. Tretinoin: Retinoid; mechanism not established. Suspected to decrease cohesiveness of follicular epithelial cells with decreased micromedo formation. Also responsible for stimulating miotic activity and increasing turnover of follicular epithelial cells, causing extrusion of comedones.

PHARMACOKINETICS: Absorption: Tretinoin: Percutaneous (minimal). **Distribution:** Orally and parenterally administered clindamycin found in breast milk. **Metabolism:** Tretinoin: 13-cis-retinoic acid and 4-oxo-13-cis-retinoic acid (metabolites).

ZINACEF   RX
cefuroxime (GlaxoSmithKline)

THERAPEUTIC CLASS: Cephalosporin (2nd generation)

INDICATIONS: Treatment of septicemia; meningitis; gonorrhea; lower respiratory tract, urinary tract, skin and skin structure (SSSI), and bone and joint infections caused by susceptible strains of microorganisms. For preoperative and perioperative surgical prophylaxis.

DOSAGE: *Adults:* Usual: 750mg-1.5g q8h for 5-10 days. Uncomplicated Pneumonia and UTI/SSSI/Disseminated Gonococcal Infections: 750mg q8h. Severe/Complicated Infections: 1.5g q8h. Bone and Joint Infections: 1.5g q8h. Life-Threatening Infections/Infections With Susceptible Organisms: 1.5g q6h. Meningitis: Max: 3g q8h. Uncomplicated Gonococcal Infection: 1.5g IM single dose at 2 different sites with 1g PO probenecid. Surgical Prophylaxis: 1.5g IV 0.5-1 hr before incision, then 750mg IM/IV q8h with prolonged procedure. Open Heart Surgery (Perioperative): 1.5g IV at induction of anesthesia and q12h thereafter, for total of 6g. Renal Impairment: CrCl 10-20mL/min: 750mg q12h. CrCl <10mL/min: 750mg q24h. Hemodialysis: Give further dose at end of dialysis.

Z

Pediatrics: >3 months: Usual: 50-100mg/kg/day in divided doses q6-8h. Severe Infections: 100mg/kg/day (not to exceed max adult dose). Bone and Joint Infections: 150mg/kg/day in divided doses q8h (not to exceed max adult dose). Meningitis: 200-240mg/kg/day IV in divided doses q6-8h. Renal Dysfunction: Modify dosing frequency consistent with adult recommendations.

HOW SUPPLIED: Inj: 750mg, 1.5g, 7.5g, 750mg/50mL, 1.5g/50mL

WARNINGS/PRECAUTIONS: Cross-sensitivity to PCNs and other cephalosporins may occur. *Clostridium difficile*-associated diarrhea reported, ranging in severity from mild diarrhea to fatal colitis. Monitor renal function. May result in overgrowth of nonsusceptible organisms. Caution with history of GI disease, particularly colitis. Hearing loss in peds being treated for meningitis. Risk of decreased prothrombin activity with renal or hepatic impairment, poor nutritional state, or protracted course of therapy. False (+) urine glucose with copper reduction tests and false (-) with ferricyanide test.

ADVERSE REACTIONS: Thrombophlebitis, GI symptoms, decreased Hgb and Hct, eosinophilia. Transient rise in SGOT, SGPT, alkaline phosphatase, bilirubin, and LDH.

INTERACTIONS: Possible nephrotoxicity with concomitant aminoglycosides. Caution with potent diuretics; may adversely affect renal function. May decrease prothrombin activity; caution with anticoagulants. May reduce efficacy of combined estrogen/progesterone oral contraceptives.

PREGNANCY: Category B, caution in nursing.

MECHANISM OF ACTION: 2nd-generation cephalosporin; inhibits cell wall synthesis.

PHARMACOKINETICS: Absorption: C_{max}(750mg IM, IV)=27mcg/mL, 50mcg/mL, T_{max}(750mg IM, IV)=45 min, 15 min. **Distribution:** Plasma protein binding (50%). **Elimination**: Urine; $T_{1/2}$=80 min.

ZINECARD   RX
dexrazoxane (Pharmacia & Upjohn)

THERAPEUTIC CLASS: EDTA derivative

INDICATIONS: To reduce the incidence and severity of cardiomyopathy associated with doxorubicin in women with metastatic breast cancer who received a cumulative doxorubicin dose of 300mg/m^2 and who will continue doxorubicin therapy.

DOSAGE: *Adults:* IV: 10:1 ratio of dexrazoxane:doxorubicin (eg, 500mg/m^2 dexrazoxane:50mg/m^2 doxorubicin). Hepatic Impairment: Reduce dose proportionally. Give by slow IV push or rapid IV infusion. Give doxorubicin within 30 min after start of infusion.

HOW SUPPLIED: Inj: 250mg, 500mg

CONTRAINDICATIONS: Chemotherapy regimens not containing an anthracycline.

WARNINGS/PRECAUTIONS: Not for use with initiation of doxorubicin therapy. Monitor cardiac function. May cause secondary malignancies. Obtain frequent CBCs. Caution with moderate or severe renal insufficiency; reduce dose by 50% if CrCl <40mL/min.

ADVERSE REACTIONS: Alopecia, nausea, vomiting, fatigue, malaise, anorexia, stomatitis, fever, infection, diarrhea, pain on injection, sepsis, neurotoxicity, streaking/erythema.

INTERACTIONS: Avoid use during the initiation of FAC (fluorouracil, doxorubicin, cyclophosphamide) therapy. Additive myelosuppression with other chemotherapies.

PREGNANCY: Category C, not for use in nursing.

MECHANISM OF ACTION: EDTA derivative; suspected to interfere with iron-mediated free radical generation.

Z

PHARMACOKINETICS: Absorption: C_{max}(500mg/m²)=36.5mcg/ml. **Distribution**: V_d=25L/m². **Elimination:** Urine (42%).

ZITHROMAX   RX
azithromycin (Pfizer)

THERAPEUTIC CLASS: Macrolide

INDICATIONS: Treatment of the following infections caused by susceptible microorganisms: (PO) Acute bacterial exacerbations of COPD, acute bacterial sinusitis (ABS), community-acquired pneumonia (CAP), pharyngitis/tonsillitis, uncomplicated skin and skin structure, urethritis/cervicitis, genital ulcer disease (men), acute otitis media. Prevention (alone) or treatment (with ethambutol) of disseminated *Mycobacterium avium* complex (MAC) disease in advanced HIV infection. (IV) CAP and pelvic inflammatory disease (PID).

DOSAGE: *Adults:* PO: CAP/Pharyngitis/Tonsillitis (2nd-line therapy)/SSSI: 500mg on Day 1, then 250mg qd on Days 2-5. COPD: 500mg qd for 3 days or 500 mg on Day 1, then 250ng qd on Days 2-5. ABS: 500mg qd for 3 days. Genital Ulcer Disease and Nongonococcal Urethritis/Cervicitis: 1g single dose. Gonococcal Urethritis/Cervicitis: 2g single dose. MAC Prophylaxis: 1200mg once weekly. MAC Treatment: 600mg qd with ethambutol 15mg/kg/day. IV: CAP: 500mg qd for at least 2 days, then 500mg PO qd to complete 7-10 day course. PID: 500mg qd for 1-2 days, then 250mg PO qd to complete 7 day course.
Pediatrics: Sus: Otitis Media: ≥6 months: 30mg/kg single dose; 10mg/kg qd for 3 days; or 10mg/kg qd on Day 1, then 5mg/kg qd on Days 2-5. ABS: ≥6 months: 10mg/kg qd for 3 days. CAP: ≥6 months: 10mg/kg qd on Day 1, then 5mg/kg qd on Days 2-5. Sus/Tab: Pharyngitis/Tonsillitis: ≥2 yrs: 12mg/kg qd for 5 days. 1g sus not for pediatric use.

HOW SUPPLIED: Inj: 500mg; Sus: 100mg/5mL [15mL], 200mg/5mL [15mL, 22.5mL, 30mL], 1g/pkt [3ˢ, 10ˢ]; Tab: 250mg [Z-PAK, 6 tabs], 500mg [TRI-PAK, 3 tabs], 600mg

WARNINGS/PRECAUTIONS: D/C if allergic reaction occurs. Oral therapy only for CAP of mild severity. Hypersensitivity reactions may recur after initial successful symptomatic treatment. *Clostridium difficile*-associated diarrhea reported. Caution with renal/hepatic dysfunction. 1g sus not for pediatric use.

ADVERSE REACTIONS: Diarrhea/loose stools, nausea, abdominal pain, taste/smell perversion.

INTERACTIONS: Monitor theophylline, terfenadine, cyclosporine, hexobarbital, phenytoin, warfarin. May increase digoxin, carbamazepine levels. Potentiates triazolam. Aluminum- and magnesium-containing antacids may reduce PO levels. Acute ergot toxicity may occur with ergotamine or dihydroergotamine. Monitor for side effects (eg, liver enzyme abnormalities, hearing impairment) with nelfinavir.

PREGNANCY: Category B, caution in nursing.

MECHANISM OF ACTION: Macrolide; inhibits protein synthesis by binding 50S ribosomal subunits of susceptible organisms.

PHARMACOKINETICS: Absorption: Administration of variable doses resulted in different parameters. **Distribution:** Plasma protein binding (7-51%). **Elimination:** Biliary (major), urine; $T_{1/2}$=68 hrs.

ZMAX   RX
azithromycin (Pfizer)

THERAPEUTIC CLASS: Macrolide

INDICATIONS: Treatment of mild to moderate acute bacterial sinusitis due to *Haemophilus influenzae*, *Moraxella catarrhalis*, or *Streptococcus pneumoniae*. Treatment of community-acquired pneumonia due to *Chlamydophila pneumoniae*, *Haemophilus influenzae*, *Mycoplasma pneumoniae*, or *Streptococcus pneumoniae* in patients appropriate for oral therapy.

Z

DOSAGE: *Adults:* 2g single dose. Take on empty stomach (1 hr before or 2 hrs after a meal).

HOW SUPPLIED: Sus, Extended-Release: 2g

CONTRAINDICATIONS: Hypersensitivity to macrolide or ketolide antibiotics.

WARNINGS/PRECAUTIONS: Rare reports of angioedema, anaphylaxis, and dermatologic reactions including Stevens-Johnson syndrome and toxic epidermal necrolysis. D/C if allergic reaction occurs. Hypersensitivity reactions may recur after initial successful symptomatic treatment. *Clostridium difficile*-associated diarrhea reported. Caution with renal/hepatic dysfunction and patients with increased risk for prolonged cardiac repolarization.

ADVERSE REACTIONS: Diarrhea/loose stools, nausea, abdominal pain, headache, vomiting, taste/smell perversion.

INTERACTIONS: Monitor for azithromycin side effects (eg, liver enzyme abnormalities, hearing impairment) with nelfinavir. Monitor cyclosporine, hexobarbital, phenytoin, warfarin concentrations. May increase digoxin levels. Acute ergot toxicity may occur with ergotamine or dihydroergotamine.

PREGNANCY: Category B, caution in nursing.

MECHANISM OF ACTION: Macrolide antibiotic; inhibits protein synthesis by binding 50S ribosomal subunits of susceptible organisms.

PHARMACOKINETICS: Absorption: Oral administration of variable doses resulted in different parameters. **Distribution:** Plasma protein binding (7-51%); V_d=31.1L/kg. **Elimination:** Bile (major route), urine. $T_{1/2}$=59 hrs.

ZOCOR   RX
simvastatin (Merck)

THERAPEUTIC CLASS: HMG-CoA reductase inhibitor

INDICATIONS: May initiate with diet in patients with, or at high risk for, coronary heart disease (CHD). In high risk patients with CHD, diabetes, peripheral vessel disease, history of stroke or other cerebrovascular disease to reduce risk of total mortality by reducing CHD deaths, risk of non-fatal MI and stroke, need for revascularization procedures. To reduce elevated total-C, LDL-C, Apo B, TG, and increase HDL-C in primary hypercholesterolemia (heterozygous familial and nonfamilial) and mixed dyslipidemia (Types IIa and IIb). To treat hypertriglyceridemia (Type IV) and primary dysbetalipoproteinemia (Type III). To reduce total-C, LDL-C in homozygous familial hypercholesterolemia as adjunct to other lipid-lowering agents or if such treatments are unavailable. To reduce total-C, LDL-C, Apo B in adolescents 10-17 yrs old, at least 1 yr postmenarche, with heterozygous familial hypercholesterolemia. To reduce elevated LDL-C, TG in Type IIb hyperlipidemia.

DOSAGE: *Adults:* Initial: 20-40mg qpm. Usual: 5-80mg/day. Titrate: Adjust at ≥4-week intervals. High Risk for CHD Events: Initial: 40mg/day. Homozygous Familial Hypercholesterolemia: 40mg qpm or 80mg/day given as 20mg bid plus 40mg qpm. Concomitant Cyclosporine: Initial: 5mg/day. Max: 10mg/day. Concomitant Gemfibrozil (try to avoid): Max: 10mg/day. Concomitant Amiodarone/Verapamil: Max: 20mg/day. Severe Renal Insufficiency: 5mg/day; monitor closely.
Pediatrics: Heterozygous Familial Hypercholesterolemia: 10-17 yrs (at least 1 yr postmenarchal): Initial: 10mg qpm. Usual: 10-40mg/day. Titrate: Adjust at ≥4-week intervals. Max: 40mg/day.

HOW SUPPLIED: Tab: 5mg, 10mg, 20mg, 40mg, 80mg

CONTRAINDICATIONS: Active liver disease, unexplained persistent elevations of serum transaminases, pregnancy, nursing mothers.

WARNINGS/PRECAUTIONS: Caution with heavy alcohol use, severe renal insufficiency or history of hepatic disease. Monitor LFT's prior to therapy, periodically thereafter for 1st yr, or until 1 yr after last dose elevation (additional test at 3 months for 80mg dose). D/C if AST or ALT ≥3x ULN persist, if myopathy is suspected or diagnosed, a few days prior to major surgery. Rhabdomyolysis (rare), myopathy reported.

Z

ADVERSE REACTIONS: Abdominal pain, headache, CK and transaminase elevations, constipation, upper respiratory infection, hepatic failure.

INTERACTIONS: Avoid use with concomitant itraconazole, ketoconazole, erythromycin, clarithromycin, telithromycin, HIV protease inhibitors, nefazodone, grapefruit juice (>1 quart/day); increased risk of myopathy/rhabdomyolysis. Max 10mg/day with gemfibrozil, cyclosporine, danazol. Max 20mg/day with amiodarone, verapamil. Caution with other fibrates, ≥1g/day of niacin. Monitor digoxin, warfarin.

PREGNANCY: Category X, not for use in nursing.

MECHANISM OF ACTION: HMG-CoA reductase inhibitor; lipid-lowering agent.

PHARMACOKINETICS: Absorption: T_{max}=1.3-2.4 hrs. **Distribution:** Plasma protein binding (95%); crosses blood-brain barrier. **Metabolism:** Liver (1st pass); β-hydroxyacid; 6'hydroxy. 6'-hydroxymethyl, 6'-exomethylene (active metabolites). **Elimination:** Feces (60%), urine (13%).

ZODERM   RX
benzoyl peroxide (Doak)

THERAPEUTIC CLASS: Antibacterial/keratolytic

INDICATIONS: Acne vulgaris.

DOSAGE: *Adults*: (Cleanser) Wash and rinse affected area qd-bid. (Cre, Gel) Apply to cleansed area qd-bid.

HOW SUPPLIED: Cleanser: 4.5%, 6.5%, 8.5% [400mL]; Cre, Gel: 4.5%, 6.5%, 8.5% [125mL]

WARNINGS/PRECAUTIONS: Avoid eyes, mouth, mucous membranes, sun exposure. D/C if severe irritation occurs. May bleach fabrics or hair.

ADVERSE REACTIONS: Allergic contact dermatitis, dryness.

PREGNANCY: Category C, caution in nursing.

MECHANISM OF ACTION: Antibacterial/keratolytic agent; not established. Possesses antibacterial activity against *Propionibacterium acnes*. In addition, has shown to cause a reduction in lipids and free fatty acids, and mild desquamation (drying and peeling activity) with simultaneous reduction in comedones and acne lesions.

PHARMACOKINETICS: Absorption: Percutaneous. **Metabolism:** Metabolized to benzoic acid. **Elimination:** Urine (benzoate).

ZOFRAN   RX
ondansetron (GlaxoSmithKline)

THERAPEUTIC CLASS: 5-HT$_3$-antagonist

INDICATIONS: (Inj) Prevention of nausea and vomiting associated with initial and repeat courses of emetogenic cancer chemotherapy, including high-dose cisplatin. Prevention of postoperative nausea and/or vomiting. (Sol/Tab) Prevention of nausea and vomiting associated with: highly emetogenic cancer chemotherapy, including cisplatin ≥50mg/m²; initial and repeat courses of moderately emetogenic cancer chemotherapy; and radiotherapy in patients receiving either total body irradiation, single high-dose fraction to the abdomen, or daily fractions to the abdomen. Prevention of postoperative nausea and/or vomiting.

DOSAGE: *Adults:* Prevention of Chemotherapy-Induced Nausea/Vomiting: (Inj) 32mg single dose or three 0.15mg/kg doses, 1st dose 30 min before chemotherapy, then 4 and 8 hrs after 1st dose. Prevention of Nausea/Vomiting Associated With Highly Emetogenic Cancer Chemotherapy: (Tab) 24mg single dose tab 30 min before chemotherapy. Prevention of Nausea/Vomiting Associated With Moderately Emetogenic Cancer Chemotherapy: (Sol/Tab) 8mg bid, 1st dose 30 min before chemotherapy, then 8 hrs later, then bid for 1-2 days after chemotherapy. Prevention of Post-Op Nausea/Vomiting: (Inj) 4mg IM/IV immediately before anesthesia or post-op after surgery if nausea

Z

or vomiting occurs. (Sol/Tab) 16mg 1 hr before anesthesia. Prevention of Nausea/Vomiting Associated with Radiation Therapy: (Sol/Tab) Usual: 8mg tid. Total Body Irradiation: 8mg 1-2 hrs before therapy daily. Single High-Dose Therapy To Abdomen: 8mg 1-2 hrs before therapy then q8h after 1st dose for 1-2 days after completion of therapy. Daily Fractionated Therapy To Abdomen: 8mg 1-2 hrs before therapy then q8h after 1st dose. Severe Hepatic Dysfunction (Child-Pugh ≥10): Max: 8mg/day IV single dose infused over 15 min, start 30 min before chemotherapy or 8mg/day PO.
Pediatrics: Prevention of Chemotherapy-Induced Nausea/Vomiting: (Inj) 6 months-18 yrs: Three 0.15mg/kg doses, 1st dose 30 min before chemotherapy, then 4 and 8 hrs after the 1st dose. (Sol/Tab) Prevention of Nausea/Vomiting Associated With Moderately Emetogenic Cancer Chemotherapy: ≥12 yrs: 8mg bid, 1st dose 30 min before chemotherapy, then 8mg 8 hrs later, then bid for 1-2 days. 4-11 yrs: 4mg tid, 1st dose 30 min before chemotherapy, then 4 and 8 hrs after 1st dose, then tid for 1-2 days. Prevention of Post-Op Nausea/Vomiting: (Inj) >12 yrs: 4mg IM/IV immediately before anesthesia or post-op after surgery if nausea or vomiting occurs. 1 month-12 yrs: ≤40kg: 0.1mg/kg single dose. >40kg: 4mg single dose. Severe Hepatic Dysfunction: Max: 8mg/day IV single dose infused over 15 min, start 30 min before chemotherapy or 8mg/day PO.

HOW SUPPLIED: Inj: 2mg/mL, 32mg/50mL; Sol: 4mg/5mL [50mL]; Tab: 4mg, 8mg, 24mg; Tab, Disintegrating: 4mg, 8mg

WARNINGS/PRECAUTIONS: Hypersensitivity reactions reported in those hypersensitive to other 5-HT$_3$ receptor antagonists. Transient ECG changes including QT interval prolongation reported with IV administration. May mask progressive ileus or gastric distension. Orally disintegrating tabs contain phenylalanine; caution in phenylketonurics.

ADVERSE REACTIONS: Headache, diarrhea, dizziness, drowsiness, malaise/fatigue, constipation, LFT abnormalities.

INTERACTIONS: Ondansetron is metabolized by CYP450 enzymes; inducers or inhibitors of these enzymes may change the clearance and half-life of ondansetron.

PREGNANCY: Category B, caution in nursing.

MECHANISM OF ACTION: Serotonin 5-HT$_3$ receptor blocker; not established. Blocks 5-HT$_3$ receptors from serotonin which may stimulate vagal afferents through 5-HT$_3$ receptors which initiate vomiting reflex.

PHARMACOKINETICS: Absorption: IV and oral administration of variable ages resulted in different parameters. **Distribution:** Plasma protein binding (70-76%). **Metabolism:** Hydroxylation, conjugation. **Elimination:** Urine.

ZOLADEX 1-MONTH RX

goserelin acetate (AstraZeneca)

THERAPEUTIC CLASS: Synthetic gonadotropin releasing hormone analog

INDICATIONS: Palliative treatment of advanced prostate cancer and advanced breast cancer in pre-and perimenopausal women. Adjunct to and during radiotherapy and in combination with flutamide for management of locally confined Stage T2b-T4 (Stage B2-C) prostate cancer. Management of endometriosis, including pain relief and reduction of endometriotic lesions. Use as an endometrial thinning agent prior to ablation for dysfunctional uterine bleeding.

DOSAGE: *Adults:* Inject SQ into anterior abdominal wall below navel line. Advanced Prostate/Breast Cancers: 3.6mg every 28 days. Stage B2-C Prostate Cancer: 3.6mg starting 8 weeks before radiotherapy then 10.8mg formulation 28 days after 1st injection or 3.6mg at 28 day intervals for 4 doses (2 before and 2 during radiotherapy). Endometriosis: 3.6mg every 28 days for up to 6 months. Endometrial Thinning: 3.6mg then surgery 4 weeks later, or 3.6mg for 2 doses (4 weeks apart) followed by surgery 2-4 weeks after 2nd dose.

HOW SUPPLIED: Implant: 3.6mg

Z

CONTRAINDICATIONS: Pregnancy, nursing.

WARNINGS/PRECAUTIONS: Exclude pregnancy before initiating therapy. Premenopausal women should use nonhormonal contraception during and 12 weeks post-therapy. Worsening of symptoms of prostate and breast cancer with initial therapy. Ureteral obstruction and spinal cord compression reported with prostate cancer. Temporary increases in bone pain may occur. Ovarian cysts reported. Hypercalcemia reported in prostate and breast cancer patients with bone metastases. May increase cervical resistance. Hypersensitivity, antibody formation and acute anaphylactic reactions may occur.

ADVERSE REACTIONS: (Males) Hot flashes, sexual dysfunction, decreased erections, lower urinary tract symptoms, lethargy, pain (worsened in the first 30 days), edema, URI, rash, sweating, diarrhea, nausea. (Females, Endometriosis Treatment) Hot flashes, vaginitis, emotional lability, decreased libido, sweating, depression, headache, acne, breast atrophy. (Breast Cancer Treatment) Hot flashes, tumor flare, nausea, edema, malaise/fatigue/lethargy, vomiting.

INTERACTIONS: Ovarian hyperstimulation syndrome reported when used concomitantly with other gonadotropins.

PREGNANCY: Category X (endometriosis and endometrial thinning), Category D (breast cancer), not for use in nursing.

MECHANISM OF ACTION: Synthetic analog of luteinizing hormone-releasing hormone (LHRH); acts as potent inhibitor of pituitary gonadotropin secretion. In males, causes initial increase in serum LH and FSH levels, causing increase in testosterone. In females, causes decrease in serum estradiol levels consistent with postmenopausal state, reduction of ovarian size and function, reduction in size of uterus and mammary gland, and regression of sex hormone-responsive tumors.

PHARMACOKINETICS: Absorption: C_{max}=2.84ng/mL (male), 1.46ng/mL (female); T_{max}=12-15 days (male), 8-22 days (female); AUC=27.8ng•hr/mL (male), 18.5ng•hr/mL (female). **Distribution:** V_d=44.1L (male), 20.3L (female); Plasma protein binding (27.3%). **Metabolism:** Liver. **Elimination:** Urine: 90% (20%, unchanged); $T_{1/2}$=4.2 hrs (male), 2.3 hrs (female).

ZOLADEX 3-MONTH   RX
goserelin acetate (AstraZeneca)

THERAPEUTIC CLASS: Synthetic gonadotropin releasing hormone analog

INDICATIONS: Palliative treatment of advanced prostate cancer. Adjunct to radiotherapy and flutamide for management of locally confined Stage T2b-T4 (Stage B2-C) prostate cancer.

DOSAGE: *Adults:* Inject SQ into anterior abdominal wall below navel line. Advanced Prostate Cancer: 10.8mg every 12 weeks. Stage B2-C Prostate Cancer: 3.6mg depot formulation 8 weeks before radiotherapy then 10.8mg 28 days after 1st injection.

HOW SUPPLIED: Implant: 10.8mg

CONTRAINDICATIONS: Pregnancy, 10.8mg implant is not indicated in women.

WARNINGS/PRECAUTIONS: Worsening of symptoms of prostate cancer with initial therapy. Ureteral obstruction and spinal cord compression reported. Temporary increase in bone pain may occur. Hypersensitivity, antibody formation and acute anaphylactic reactions may occur.

ADVERSE REACTIONS: Hot flashes, sexual dysfunction, decreased erections, osteoporosis, pain, asthenia, gynecomastia.

PREGNANCY: Category X, not for use in nursing.

MECHANISM OF ACTION: Synthetic analog of luteinizing hormone-releasing hormone (LHRH); acts as potent inhibitor of pituitary gonadotropin secretion. In males, causes initial increase in serum LH and FSH levels, causing increase in testosterone. In females, causes decrease in serum estradiol levels consistent with postmenopausal state, reduction of ovarian size and

Z

function, reduction in size of uterus and mammary gland, and regression of sex hormone-responsive tumors.

PHARMACOKINETICS: Absorption: C_{max}=8.85ng/mL; T_{max}=1.8 hrs. **Distribution:** Mean V_d=44.1 L; Plasma protein binding (27%). **Metabolism:** Hydrolysis of C-terminal amino acids. **Elimination:** Urine (90%, 20% unchanged); $T_{1/2}$=4.16 hrs.

ZOLINZA   RX
vorinostat (Merck)

THERAPEUTIC CLASS: Histone deacetylase inhibitor

INDICATIONS: Treatment of cutaneous manifestations in patients with cutaneous T-cell lymphoma who have progressive, persistent, or recurrent disease on or following two systemic therapies.

DOSAGE: *Adults:* 400mg PO qd with food. Intolerant to Therapy: May reduce dose to 300mg PO qd with food. If necessary, may further reduce dose to 300mg PO qd with food for 5 consecutive days each week.

HOW SUPPLIED: Cap: 100mg

WARNINGS/PRECAUTIONS: Pulmonary embolism and DVT reported; monitor for signs and symptoms. Dose-related thrombocytopenia and anemia may occur; consider dose modification or discontinuation. GI disturbances reported. Hyperglycemia observed; monitor glucose levels. QTc prolongation reported; monitor electrolytes and ECGs at baseline and periodically during treatment. Monitor CBC and chemistry tests every 2 weeks during first 2 months of therapy and monthly thereafter.

ADVERSE REACTIONS: Diarrhea, fatigue, nausea, thrombocytopenia, anorexia, dysgeusia, decreased weight, muscle spasms, alopecia, dry mouth, increased SrCr, chills, vomiting, constipation, dizziness.

INTERACTIONS: Prolongation of PT and INR observed with coumarin-derivative anticoagulants; monitor closely. Severe thrombocytopenia and GI bleeding reported with concomitant use of other histone deacetylase inhibitors (eg, valproic acid); monitor platelet count every 2 weeks for the first two months of therapy.

PREGNANCY: Category D, not for use in nursing.

MECHANISM OF ACTION: Histone decetylase inhibitor; inhibits activity of histone deacetylases (HDAC) allowing for accumulation of acetyl groups on the histone lysine residues, resulting in open chromatin structure and transcriptional activation.

PHARMACOKINETICS: Absorption: Fasted: C_{max}=1.2μM, T_{max}=1.5 hrs, AUC=4.2μM•hr. Fed: C_{max}=1.2μM, T_{max}=4 hrs, AUC=6.0μM•hr. **Distribution:** Plasma protein binding (71%). **Metabolism:** Liver, via glucuronidation and β-oxidation. **Elimination:** Urine (unchanged); $T_{1/2}$=2 hrs.

ZOLOFT   RX
sertraline HCL (Pfizer)

> Antidepressants increased the risk of suicidal thinking and behavior (suicidality) in short-term studies in children, adolescents, and young adults with Major Depressive Disorder (MDD) and other psychiatric disorders. Sertraline HCl is not approved for use in pediatric patients except for patients with obsessive compulsive disorder (OCD).

THERAPEUTIC CLASS: Selective serotonin reuptake inhibitor

INDICATIONS: Treatment of MDD, social anxiety disorder (SAD), OCD, panic disorder with or without agoraphobia, premenstrual dysphoric disorder (PMDD) and posttraumatic stress disorder (PTSD).

DOSAGE: *Adults:* MDD/OCD: 50mg qd. Titrate: Adjust dose at 1 week intervals. Max: 200mg/day. Panic Disorder/PTSD/SAD: Initial: 25mg qd. Titrate: Increase to 50mg qd after 1 week. Adjust dose at 1 week intervals. Max: 200mg/day. PMDD: Initial: 50mg qd continuous or limited to luteal phase of

Z

cycle. Titrate: Increase 50mg/cycle if needed up to 150mg/day for continuous or 100mg/day for luteal phase dosing. If 100mg/day is established for luteal phase dosing, a 50mg/day titration step for 3 days should take place at the beginning of each luteal phase dosing period. Hepatic Impairment: Use lower or less frequent doses. Dilute sol with 4oz water, ginger ale, lemon/lime soda, lemonade or orange juice. Take immediately after mixing.

Pediatrics: OCD: Initial: 6-12 yrs: 25mg qd. 13-17 yrs: 50mg qd. Titrate: Adjust dose at 1 week intervals. Max: 200mg/day. Hepatic Impairment: Use lower or less frequent doses. Dilute sol with 4oz water, ginger ale, lemon/lime soda, lemonade or orange juice. Take immediately after mixing.

HOW SUPPLIED: Sol: 20mg/mL [60mL]; Tab: 25mg*, 50mg*, 100mg* *scored

CONTRAINDICATIONS: Concomitant use with MAOIs or pimozide. Concomitant disulfiram with solution.

WARNINGS/PRECAUTIONS: Activation of mania/hypomania reported. Monitor weight loss. Caution with conditions that could affect metabolism or hemodynamic responses, seizure disorder. Dose adjust with liver dysfunction. Altered platelet function and hyponatremia reported. Weak uricosuric effects reported. Caution with latex sensitivity; solution dropper dispenser contains rubber. Monitor for clinical worsening and/or suicidality, especially at initiation of therapy or dose changes. Avoid abrupt withdrawal. Monitor for discontinuation symptoms.

ADVERSE REACTIONS: Ejaculation failure, dry mouth, increased sweating, somnolence, tremor, anorexia, dizziness, headache, vomiting, diarrhea, dyspepsia, nausea, agitation, insomnia, nervousness, abnormal vision.

INTERACTIONS: See Contraindications. Increased levels with cimetidine. Avoid with alcohol, pimozide or MAOIs. Decreases clearance of tolbutamide. Rare reports of weakness, hyperreflexia, incoordination with an SSRI and sumatriptan. May potentiate drugs metabolized by CYP2D6 (eg, TCAs, Type 1C antiarrhythmics). Caution with CNS drugs (eg, diazepam). Monitor lithium. Caution with TCAs; may need dose adjustment. May shift concentrations with plasma protein-bound drugs (eg, warfarin, digitoxin). Monitor PT with warfarin. Caution with OTC products. May induce metabolism of cisapride. Caution with drugs that interfere with hemostasis (eg, non-selective NSAIDs, ASA, warfarin) due to increased risk of bleeding.

PREGNANCY: Category C, caution in nursing.

MECHANISM OF ACTION: SSRI; inhibits CNS neuronal uptake of serotonin.

PHARMACOKINETICS: Absorption: T_{max}=4.5-8.4 hrs. **Distribution:** Plasma protein binding (98%). **Metabolism:** Liver (extensive). **Elimination:** Feces 12-14% (unchanged), urine (minor); $T_{1/2}$=26 hrs.

ZOMETA   RX
zoledronic acid (Novartis)

THERAPEUTIC CLASS: Bisphosphonate

INDICATIONS: Treatment of hypercalcemia of malignancy. Treatment of multiple myeloma and bone metastases from solid tumors, in conjunction with antineoplastic therapy.

DOSAGE: *Adults:* Hypercalcemia of Malignancy: Max: 4mg IV over no less than 15 min. Retreatment (if necessary): Wait at least 7 days from initial dose. Multiple Myeloma/Bone Metastases: 4mg IV over 15 min every 3-4 weeks. CrCl 50-60mL/min: 3.5mg; CrCl 40-49mL/min: 3.3mg; CrCl 30-39mL/min: 3mg. Measure SrCr prior to each dose. Withhold dose with renal deterioration; resume when SrCr returns to within 10% of baseline. Take with oral calcium 500mg/day and vitamin D 400 IU/day.

HOW SUPPLIED: Inj: 4mg/5mL

CONTRAINDICATIONS: Urticaria, angioedema, anaphylactic shock.

WARNINGS/PRECAUTIONS: Caution with hepatic insufficiency, ASA-sensitive asthma, and the elderly. Risk of renal toxicity/failure. In severe renal impairment, avoid with bone metastases and use caution with hypercalcemia

Z

of malignancy. Rehydrate before use with hypercalcemia of malignancy. Monitor serum creatinine before each dose, and serum calcium, electrolytes, phosphate, magnesium, and Hct/Hgb regularly. May cause fetal harm during pregnancy. Osteonecrosis of the jaw reported in cancer patients treated with bisphosphonates; avoid invasive dental procedures during therapy. Severe and occasionally incapacitating bone, joint, and/or muscle pain reported.

ADVERSE REACTIONS: Fever, chills, bone pain, arthralgia, myalgia, nausea, vomiting, diarrhea, constipation, injection site reactions, conjunctivitis, hypomagnesemia, abnormal serum creatinine, hypophosphatemia, hypokalemia, anorexia, anemia, insomnia, anxiety, dyspnea.

INTERACTIONS: Additive effect/risk of hypocalcemia with aminoglycosides and loop diuretics. Caution with other nephrotoxic drugs. Increased risk of renal dysfunction with thalidomide in multiple myeloma patients.

PREGNANCY: Category D, not for use in nursing.

MECHANISM OF ACTION: Bisphosphonate; inhibits bone resorption through osteoclastic activity and induces osteoclast apoptosis. Also blocks osteoclastic resorption of mineralized bone and cartilage through binding to bone.

PHARMACOKINETICS: Absorption: IV administration of different doses resulted in different parameters. **Distribution:** Plasma protein binding: 28-53%. **Elimination:** Urine; $T_{1/2}$=146 hrs.

ZOMIG
zolmitriptan (AstraZeneca)

RX

OTHER BRAND NAMES: Zomig Nasal Spray (AstraZeneca) - Zomig-ZMT (AstraZeneca)

THERAPEUTIC CLASS: 5-HT$_{1D/1B}$-agonist

INDICATIONS: Acute treatment of migraine attacks with or without aura.

DOSAGE: *Adults:* ≥18 yrs: (Spray) 5mg single dose; may repeat once after 2 hrs. Max: 10mg/24 hrs. Safety of treating >4 headaches/30 days unknown. (Tab) Initial: 2.5mg or lower (2.5mg tab may be broken in 1/2), may repeat after 2 hrs. Max: 10mg/24 hrs. Safety of treating >3 headaches in 30 days is unknown. (ZMT) Dissolve on tongue without water. Hepatic Impairment: Use low dose and monitor blood pressure.

HOW SUPPLIED: Nasal Spray: 5mg [0.1mL, 6^s]; Tab: 2.5mg*; 5mg; Tab, Disintegrating: (ZMT) 2.5mg, 5mg *scored

CONTRAINDICATIONS: Ischemic heart disease, coronary artery vasospasm (eg, Prinzmetal's angina), uncontrolled HTN, other significant cardiovascular disease, hemiplegic or basilar migraine, MAOI use during or within 14 days, other 5-HT$_1$ agonist or ergot-type agent use within 24 hrs.

WARNINGS/PRECAUTIONS: Confirm migraine diagnosis. Supervise 1st dose and monitor cardiac function in those at risk of CAD (eg, HTN, hypercholesterolemia, smoker, obesity, diabetes, CAD family history, postmenopausal women, males >40 yrs). Serious adverse cardiac events, cerebrovascular events, vasospastic reactions reported with 5-HT$_1$ agonists. Disintegrating tabs contain phenylalanine. Caution with hepatic dysfunction. Reconsider diagnosis before 2nd dose, if no response seen after 1st dose.

ADVERSE REACTIONS: Paresthesia, asthenia, warm/cold sensation, neck/throat/jaw pain, dry mouth, nausea, dizziness, somnolence, unusual taste (nasal spray).

INTERACTIONS: Ergot-agents may prolong vasospastic reactions. Avoid MAOIs, during or within 14 days of therapy. Serotonin syndrome reported with combined use of an SSRI or SNRI. Half-life and AUC doubled with cimetidine. Avoid 5-HT$_{1B/1D}$ agonists within 24 hrs.

PREGNANCY: Category C, caution in nursing.

MECHANISM OF ACTION: 5-HT$_{1D/1B}$ agonist; binds with high affinity to 5-HT$_{1D/1B}$ receptors on intracranial vessels (including arteriovenous anastomoses) and sensory nerves of trigeminal system, which results in cranial vessel constriction and inhibition of pro-inflammatory neuropeptide release.

Z

PHARMACOKINETICS: Absorption: Well-absorbed; absolute bioavailability (40%); T_{max}=3 hrs (ODT/Nasal Spray), 1.5 hrs (Tab). **Distribution:** (Oral) V_d=7L/kg, (Nasal Spray) V_d=8.4L/kg. Plasma protein binding (25%). **Metabolism:** N-desmethyl (active metabolite). **Elimination:** Urine (65%, 8% unchanged), feces (30% oral); $T_{1/2}$=3 hrs (Nasal Spray).

ZONALON   RX
doxepin HCL (Bioglan)

THERAPEUTIC CLASS: H_1/H_2-receptor blocker

INDICATIONS: Short-term management of moderate pruritus in atopic dermatitis, and lichen simplex chronicus.

DOSAGE: *Adults:* Apply qid up to 8 days. Wait at least 3-4 hrs between applications. Avoid occlusive dressings.

HOW SUPPLIED: Cre: 5% [30g, 45g]

CONTRAINDICATIONS: Untreated narrow-angle glaucoma, urinary retention.

WARNINGS/PRECAUTIONS: Significant drowsiness reported when applied to >10% of BSA; may need to reduce amount or area covered, or number of applications. Avoid eyes.

ADVERSE REACTIONS: Drowsiness, dry mouth, dry lips, thirst, headache, fatigue, dizziness, emotional changes, taste changes.

INTERACTIONS: Discontinue MAOIs at least 2 weeks before therapy. Alcohol may potentiate sedation. Caution with drugs metabolized by CYP2D6 (eg, other antidepressants, phenothiazines, carbamazepine, flecainide, encainide, propafenone, quinidine). Poor metabolizers may have increased plasma levels. Possible serum level fluctuations with cimetidine. Hypoglycemia reported when oral doxepin was added to tolazamide therapy.

PREGNANCY: Category B, not for use in nursing.

MECHANISM OF ACTION: H_1 and H_2 histamine receptor blocker; exact mechanism by which it exerts its antipruritic effect has not been established.

PHARMACOKINETICS: Absorption: Percutaneous. **Distribution:** Distributed to the lungs, heart, brain, and liver. After oral administration, found in breast milk. **Metabolism:** Hepatic, desmethyldoxepin (active metabolite). **Elimination:** Urinary, $T_{1/2}$=28-52 hrs.

ZONEGRAN   RX
zonisamide (Eisai)

THERAPEUTIC CLASS: Sulfonamide anticonvulsant

INDICATIONS: Adjunctive therapy in the treatment of partial seizures.

DOSAGE: *Adults:* Initial: 100mg qd for 2 weeks. Titrate: May increase to 200mg/day for at least 2 weeks. May then increase to 300mg/day, then to 400mg/day for at least 2-week intervals. Max: 400mg/day.
Pediatrics: ≥16 yrs: Initial: 100mg qd for 2 weeks. Titrate: May increase to 200mg/day for at least 2 weeks. May then increase to 300mg/day, then to 400mg/day for at least 2-week intervals. Max: 400mg/day.

HOW SUPPLIED: Cap: 25mg, 100mg

CONTRAINDICATIONS: Sulfonamide hypersensitivity.

WARNINGS/PRECAUTIONS: Sulfonamide hypersensitivity reactions (eg, Stevens-Johnson syndrome, toxic epidermal necrolysis, fulminant hepatic necrosis, blood dyscrasias), cognitive/neuropsychiatric effects, kidney stones, sudden death reported. D/C with unexplained rash. Increased risk of oligohidrosis and hyperthermia in pediatrics; monitor for decreased sweating and increased body temperature. Advise females to use contraceptives to prevent pregnancy. Caution with renal/hepatic impairment. Avoid abrupt withdrawal. May cause cognitive/neuropsychiatric adverse events. Caution while driving, operating machinery, or performing hazardous tasks. Taper and

Z

d/c if CPK levels elevated or if patient manifests clinical signs and symptoms of pancreatitis.

ADVERSE REACTIONS: Headache, abdominal pain, anorexia, nausea, dizziness, ataxia, confusion, difficulty concentrating, memory difficulties, agitation/irritability, depression, insomnia, somnolence, fatigue, tiredness.

INTERACTIONS: Liver enzyme inducers increase metabolism and clearance and decrease half-life. Caution with drugs that predispose patients to heat-related disorders (eg, carbonic anhydrase inhibitors, anticholinergic drugs).

PREGNANCY: Category C, not for use in nursing.

MECHANISM OF ACTION: Sulfonamide; mechanism unknown. Found to block Na^+ channels and reduce voltage-dependent, transient inward currents (T-type Ca^{2+} currents), which then stabilize neuronal membranes and suppress neuronal hypersynchronization. Facilitates both dopaminergic and serotonergic neurotransmission.

PHARMACOKINETICS: Absorption: C_{max}=2-5mcg/mL; T_{max}=2 to 6 hrs. **Distribution:** V_d=1.45L/kg; plasma protein binding (40%). **Metabolism:** Liver, via acetylation and reduction by CYP3A4; N-acetyl zonisamide, 2-sulfamoylacetyl phenol (metabolites). **Elimination**: Urine (62%), feces (3%); $T_{1/2}$=63 hrs.

ZORBTIVE RX
somatropin (EMD Serono)

THERAPEUTIC CLASS: Human growth hormone

INDICATIONS: Treatment of Short Bowel Syndrome in patients receiving specialized nutritional support.

DOSAGE: *Adults:* 0.1mg/kg qd SC for 4 weeks. Max: 8mg qd. Rotate injection site.

HOW SUPPLIED: Inj: 8.8mg

CONTRAINDICATIONS: Acute critical illness due to complications following open heart or abdominal surgery, multiple accidental trauma, or acute respiratory failure; active neoplasia (either newly diagnosed or recurrent); benzyl alcohol sensitivity.

WARNINGS/PRECAUTIONS: Associated with acute pancreatitis. New onset impaired glucose intolerance, new onset type 2 DM, exacerbation of pre-existing DM, ketoacidosis, diabetic coma reported; closely monitor with risk factors for glucose intolerance. Perform funduscopic evaluations periodically. Increased tissue turgor, musculoskeletal discomfort, and carpal tunnel syndrome may occur.

ADVERSE REACTIONS: Peripheral/facial edema, chest/back pain, fever, flu-like disorder, malaise, flatulence, abdominal pain, nausea, vomiting, viral infection, dizziness, headache, rash.

PREGNANCY: Category B, caution in nursing.

MECHANISM OF ACTION: Human growth hormone; anabolic and anticatabolic agent, Exerts influence by interacting with specific receptors. On gut, actions may be direct or mediated via local or systemic production of IGF-1; also enhances transmucosal transport of water, electrolytes, and nutrients.

PHARMACOKINETICS: Absorption: (SQ); Absolute bioavailability (70-90%). **Distribution:** V_d=12.0L. **Metabolism:** Liver, kidneys. **Elimination:** Urine; (SQ): $T_{1/2}$=3.94 hrs. (IV): $T_{1/2}$=0.58 hrs.

ZOSTAVAX RX
zoster vaccine live (Merck)

THERAPEUTIC CLASS: Vaccine

INDICATIONS: Prevention of herpes zoster in individuals ≥60.

DOSAGE: *Adults:* ≥60 yrs: Inject SQ immediately after reconstitution with supplied diluent.

HOW SUPPLIED: Inj: 19,400 PFU/0.65mL

CONTRAINDICATIONS: Anaphylactic/anaphylactoid reactions to gelatin or neomycin. Primary or acquired immunodeficiency states (eg, leukemia); lymphomas or other malignant neoplasms affecting the bone marrow or lymphatic system; AIDS or other clinical manifestations HIV infections. Immunosuppressive therapy, including high-dose corticosteroids. Active untreated tuberculosis. Pregnancy.

WARNINGS/PRECAUTIONS: More extensive vaccine-associated rash or disseminated disease with immunosuppression. Anaphlactic/anaphylactoid reaction may occur. Deferral of vaccination should be considered in acute illness.

ADVERSE REACTIONS: Erythema, pain, tenderness, swelling, pruritus.

INTERACTIONS: See Contraindications.

PREGNANCY: Category C, caution in nursing.

MECHANISM OF ACTION: Vaccine; stimulates immune system to produce antibodies that may protect against herpes zoster infection (shingles).

ZOSYN RX
piperacillin sodium - tazobactam (Wyeth)

THERAPEUTIC CLASS: Broad-spectrum penicillin/beta-lactamase inhibitor

INDICATIONS: Treatment of appendicitis, peritonitis, uncomplicated/complicated skin and skin structure infections, postpartum endometritis, pelvic inflammatory disease, moderate severity of community acquired pneumonia (CAP), and moderate to severe nosocomial pneumonia caused by susceptible strains of microorganisms.

DOSAGE: *Adults:* Usual: 3.375g q6h for 7-10 days. CrCl 20-40mL: 2.25g q6h. CrCl <20mL/min: 2.25g q8h. Hemodialysis/CAPD: 2.25g q12h. Give 1 additional 0.75g dose after each dialysis period. Nosocomial Pneumonia: 4.5g q6h for 7-14 days plus aminoglycoside. CrCl 20-40mL/min: 3.375g q6h. CrCl <20mL/min: 2.25g q6h. Hemodialysis/CAPD: Max: 2.25g q8h. Give 1 additional 0.75g dose after each dialysis period.
Pediatrics: Appendicitis/Peritonitis: ≤40kg: ≥9 months: 100mg piperacillin-12.5mg tazobactam/kg q8h. 2-9 months: 80mg piperacillin-10mg tazobactam/kg q8h. ≥40kg: Use adult dose.

HOW SUPPLIED: Inj: (Piperacillin-Tazobactam) 40mg-5mg/mL, 60mg-7.5mg/mL, 2g-0.25g, 3g-0.375g, 4g-0.5g, 2g-0.25g/50mL, 3g-0.375g/50mL, 4g-0.5g/100mL, 36g-4.5g

CONTRAINDICATIONS: History of allergic reactions to cephalosporins.

WARNINGS/PRECAUTIONS: Serious, fatal hypersensitivity reactions may occur with PCN allergy. *Clostridium difficile*-associated diarrhea reported. D/C if bleeding manifestations occur. May experience neuromuscular excitability or convulsions with higher doses. Contains 2.79mEq/g Na; caution with restricted salt intake. Increased incidence of rash and fever in cystic fibrosis. Monitor electrolyte periodically with low K⁺ reserves. Therapy may lead to emergence of resistant organisms that can cause superinfections. Caution with renal impairment (CrCl <40mL/min).

ADVERSE REACTIONS: Diarrhea, headache, constipation, nausea, insomnia, rash, vomiting, dyspepsia, pruritus.

INTERACTIONS: May inactivate aminoglycosides. Probenecid prolongs half-life. Monitor coagulation parameters with heparin, oral anticoagulants, or drugs that affect blood coagulation system or thrombocyte function. May prolong neuromuscular blockade of vecuronium.

PREGNANCY: Category B, caution in nursing.

MECHANISM OF ACTION: Piperacillin: Broad spectrum penicillin; exerts bactericidal activity by inhibiting septum formation and cell wall synthesis of susceptible bacteria. Tazobactam: β-lactamase enzyme inhibitor.

PHARMACOKINETICS: Absorption: (2.25g, 3.375g, 4.5g of piperacillin): C_{max}=134mcg/mL, 242mcg/mL, 298mcg/mL. (2.25g, 3.375g, 4.5g of tazobactam): C_{max} = 15mcg/mL, 24mcg/mL, 34mcg/mL. **Distribution:** V_d=0.243L/

Z

kg; plasma protein binding (30%); wide distribution into tissues and bodily fluids; crosses placental barrier; found in breast milk. **Elimination:** Kidneys; Piperacilin: Urine (68% unchanged); Tazobactam: Urine (80% unchanged, 20% as single metabolite); $T_{1/2}$=0.7-1.2 hrs.

ZOVIRAX CREAM

RX

acyclovir (Biovail)

THERAPEUTIC CLASS: Nucleoside analogue

INDICATIONS: Treatment of recurrent herpes labialis (cold sores).

DOSAGE: *Adults:* Apply 5x/day for 4 days. Initiate with 1st sign/symptom. *Pediatrics:* ≥12 yrs: Apply 5x/day for 4 days. Initiate with 1st sign/symptom.

HOW SUPPLIED: Cre: 5% [2g, 5g]

WARNINGS/PRECAUTIONS: Cutaneous use only; not for use in the eye, mouth or nose.

ADVERSE REACTIONS: Dry lips, desquamation, dryness of skin, cracked lips, burning skin, pruritus, flakiness of skin, stinging on skin.

PREGNANCY: Category B, caution in nursing.

MECHANISM OF ACTION: Synthetic purine nucleoside analogue; possesses inhibitory activity against herpes simplex virus types 1 and 2, and varicella-zoster virus. Stops replication of herpes viral DNA by competitive inhibition of viral DNA polymerase, incorporation into and termination of growing viral DNA chain, and inactivation of viral DNA polymerase.

PHARMACOKINETICS: Absorption: Minimal systemic absorption.

ZOVIRAX INJECTION

RX

acyclovir sodium (GlaxoSmithKline)

THERAPEUTIC CLASS: Nucleoside analogue

INDICATIONS: Treatment of neonatal herpes simplex infections and herpes simplex encephalitis. Treatment of varicella-zoster (shingles), initial and recurrent mucosal and cutaneous herpes simplex in immunocompromised patients. Treatment of severe initial clinical episodes of herpes genitalis in immunocompetent patients.

DOSAGE: *Adults:* Initiate with 1st sign/symptom. Max: 20mg/kg q8h for any patient. Mucosal/Cutaneous Herpes Simplex Infections: 5mg/kg q8h for 7 days. Herpes Genitalis: 5mg/kg q8h for 5 days. Herpes Simplex Encephalitis: 10mg/kg q8h for 10 days. Varicella Zoster: 10mg/kg q8h for 7 days. Obese Patients: Dose according to IBW. CrCl 25-50mL/min: Give 100% of recommended dose q12h. CrCl 10-25: Give 100% of recommended dose q24h. CrCl 0-10mL/min: Give 50% of recommended dose q24h. Elderly: Reduce dose and monitor renal function.
Pediatrics: Initiate with 1st sign/symptom. Max: 20mg/kg q8h for any patient. Mucosal/Cutaneous Herpes Simplex: ≥12 yrs: 5mg/kg q8h for 7 days. <12 yrs: 10mg/kg q8h for 7 days. Herpes Genitalis: ≥12 yrs: 5mg/kg q8h for 5 days. Herpes Simplex Encephalitis: ≥12 yrs: 10mg/kg q8h for 10 days. 3 months-12 yrs: 20mg/kg q8h for 10 days. Neonatal Herpes Simplex: Birth-3 months: 10mg/kg q8h for 10 days. Varicella Zoster: ≥12 yrs: 10mg/kg q8h for 7 days. <12 yrs: 20mg/kg q8h for 7 days. Obese Patients: Dose according to IBW. CrCl 25-50mL/min: Give 100% of recommended dose q12h. CrCl 10-25: Give 100% of recommended dose q24h. CrCl 0-10mL/min: Give 50% of recommended dose q24h.

HOW SUPPLIED: Inj: 500mg, 1000mg

CONTRAINDICATIONS: Hypersensitivity to valacyclovir.

WARNINGS/PRECAUTIONS: Do not administer topically, IM, PO, SQ, or in the eye. Adjust dose in renal impairment and the elderly. Renal failure and death reported. Thrombotic thrombocytopenic purpura/hemolytic uremic syndrome in immunocompromised patients reported. Patient must be adequately hydrated. Caution with underlying neurologic abnormalities, electrolyte abnormalities, significant hypoxia, and serious renal or hepatic abnormalities. Infusion must not be given over <1 hr.

ADVERSE REACTIONS: Injection site inflammation, phlebitis, transient serum creatinine and BUN elevations, nausea, vomiting.

INTERACTIONS: Increased serum levels with probenecid. Avoid with nephrotoxic drugs.

PREGNANCY: Category B, caution in nursing.

MECHANISM OF ACTION: Synthetic purine nucleoside analogue; possesses inhibitory activity against herpes simplex virus types 1 and 2, and varicella-zoster virus. Stops replication of herpes viral DNA by competitive inhibition of viral DNA polymerase, incorporation into and termination of growing viral DNA chain, and inactivation of viral DNA polymerase.

PHARMACOKINETICS: Absorption: C_{max}=9.8mcg/mL (5mg/kg), 22.9mcg/mL (10mg/kg). **Distribution:** Plasma protein binding (9-33%); found in breast milk. **Metabolism:** 9-carboxymethoxymethylguanine (major metabolite). **Elimination:** Urine (62-91% unchanged) (14.1% metabolite). Refer to PI for detailed info regarding renal function and pediatrics.

ZOVIRAX OINTMENT RX
acyclovir (Biovail)

THERAPEUTIC CLASS: Nucleoside analogue

INDICATIONS: Management of initial genital herpes and in limited non-life-threatening mucocutaneous herpes simplex infections in immunocompromised patients.

DOSAGE: *Adults:* Apply to all lesions q3h, 6x/day for 7 days. Apply with finger cot or rubber glove to prevent autoinoculation and transmission. Initiate with 1st sign/symptom.

HOW SUPPLIED: Oint: 5% [15g]

WARNINGS/PRECAUTIONS: Not for use for the prevention of recurrent HSV infections. Cutaneous use only; avoid eyes.

ADVERSE REACTIONS: Pain with application, transient burning and stinging, pruritus.

PREGNANCY: Category B, not for use in nursing.

MECHANISM OF ACTION: Synthetic purine nucleoside analogue; possesses inhibitory activity against herpes simplex virus types 1 and 2, and varicella-zoster virus. Stops replication of herpes viral DNA by competitive inhibition of viral DNA polymerase, incorporation into and termination of growing viral DNA chain, and inactivation of viral DNA polymerase.

PHARMACOKINETICS: Absorption: Minimal systemic absorption.

ZOVIRAX ORAL RX
acyclovir (GlaxoSmithKline)

THERAPEUTIC CLASS: Nucleoside analogue

INDICATIONS: Acute treatment of herpes zoster (shingles). Treatment of initial and recurrent episodes of genital herpes. Treatment of chickenpox (varicella).

DOSAGE: *Adults:* Herpes Zoster: 800mg q4h, 5x/day for 7-10 days. Start within 72 hrs after onset of rash. Genital Herpes: Initial: 200mg q4h, 5x/day for 10 days. Chronic Therapy: 400mg bid or 200mg 3-5x/day up to 12 months, then re-evaluate. Intermittent Therapy: 200mg q4h, 5x/day for 5 days. Start with 1st sign/symptom of recurrence. Chickenpox: 800mg qid for 5 days. CrCl 10-25mL/min: For a dose of 800mg q4h, give 800mg q8h. CrCl 0-10mL/min: For a dose of 200mg q4h, give 200mg q12h. For a dose of 400mg q12h, give 200mg q12h. For a dose of 800mg q4h, give 800mg q12h. Elderly:

Reduce dose.
Pediatrics: ≥2 yrs: ≤40kg: Chickenpox: 20mg/kg qid for 5 days. >40kg: 800mg qid for 5 days.

HOW SUPPLIED: Cap: 200mg; Sus: 200mg/5mL; Tab: 400mg, 800mg

CONTRAINDICATIONS: Hypersensitivity to valacyclovir.

WARNINGS/PRECAUTIONS: Adust dose in renal impairment, elderly. Renal failure and death reported. Thrombotic thrombocytopenic purpura/hemolytic uremic syndrome in immunocompromised patients reported.

ADVERSE REACTIONS: Nausea, vomiting, diarrhea, headache, malaise, renal dysfunction.

INTERACTIONS: Probenecid increased levels of IV formulation. Caution with potentially nephrotoxic agents.

PREGNANCY: Category B, caution in nursing.

MECHANISM OF ACTION: Synthetic purine nucleoside analogue; possesses inhibitory activity against herpes simplex virus types 1 and 2, and varicella-zoster virus. Stops replication of herpes viral DNA by competitive inhibition of viral DNA polymerase, incorporation into and termination of growing viral DNA chain, and inactivation of viral DNA polymerase.

PHARMACOKINETICS: Absorption: Absolute bioavailability (10-20%). Oral administration of variable doses resulted in different parameters. **Distribution:** Plasma protein binding (9-33%) **Elimination:** $T_{1/2}$=2.5-3.3 hrs.

ZYBAN   RX
bupropion HCL (GlaxoSmithKline)

> Antidepressants increased the risk of suicidal thinking and behavior (suicidality) in short-term studies in children, adolescents, and young adults with Major Depressive Disorder (MDD) and other psychiatric disorders. Bupropion is not approved for use in pediatric patients.

THERAPEUTIC CLASS: Aminoketone

INDICATIONS: Aid to smoking cessation treatment.

DOSAGE: *Adults:* ≥18 yrs: Initial: 150mg qd for 3 days. Usual: 150mg bid; separate dose intervals by at least 8 hrs. Max: 300mg/day. Initiate treatment while patient is still smoking. Patients should set a "target quit date" within the first 2 weeks. Treat for 7 to 12 weeks; d/c at 7 weeks if no progress seen. Renal/Hepatic Dysfunction: Reduce dose. Severe Hepatic Cirrhosis: 150mg every other day.

HOW SUPPLIED: Tab, Extended-Release: 150mg

CONTRAINDICATIONS: Seizure disorder, bulimia or anorexia nervosa, within 14 days of MAOIs, other forms of bupropion, abrupt discontinuation of alcohol or sedatives.

WARNINGS/PRECAUTIONS: Dose-related risk of seizures. D/C and do not restart if seizure occurs. Extreme caution with history of seizure, cranial trauma, severe hepatic cirrhosis. Caution with recent MI, unstable heart disease, renal impairment. Agitation, insomnia, psychosis, confusion and other neuropsychiatric phenomena reported. Allergic reactions, HTN reported. May precipitate manic episodes in bipolar disorder.

ADVERSE REACTIONS: Anxiety, dizziness, anorexia, myalgia, pruritus, dry mouth, insomnia, nausea, constipation, tremor, dream abnormality, rash, confusion.

INTERACTIONS: Extreme caution with drugs that lower seizure threshold (eg, antidepressants, antipsychotics, theophylline, systemic steroids). Increased seizure risk with opioid, cocaine, or stimulant addiction, OTC stimulants or anorectics, oral hypoglycemics or insulin, excessive use or abrupt discontinuation of alcohol or sedatives. Caution with levodopa, amantadine, and drugs that are metabolized by CYP2D6 (eg, SSRIs, TCAs, antipsychotics, β-blockers, type 1C antiarrhythmics); use low initial dose and gradually titrate. Avoid other bupropion-containing drugs and MAOIs. Monitor HTN with transdermal nicotine. Caution with CYP2B6 substrates or inhibitors (eg, orphenadrine,

Z

cyclophosphamide). Carbamazepine, phenytoin, cimetidine, and phenobarbital may induce metabolism of bupropion. Minimize or avoid alcohol.

PREGNANCY: Pregnancy B, not for use in nursing.

MECHANISM OF ACTION: Mechanism unknown; suspected to inhibit neuronal uptake of norepinephrine and dopamine.

PHARMACOKINETICS: Absorption: C_{max}=136ng/mL; T_{max}=3 hrs. **Distribution:** Plasma protein binding (84%); V_d=1,950L; found in breast milk. **Metabolism:** Extensive, through hydroxylation and reduction pathways. Hydroxybupropion, threohydrobupropion, and erythrohydrobupropion (active metabolites). **Elimination:** Urine; $T_{1/2}$=21 hrs.

ZYDONE   CIII
hydrocodone bitartrate - acetaminophen (Endo)

THERAPEUTIC CLASS: Opioid analgesic

INDICATIONS: Relief of moderate to moderately severe pain.

DOSAGE: *Adults:* (5/400): 1-2 tabs q4-6h prn. Max: 8 tabs/day. (7.5/400, 10/400): 1 tab q4-6h prn. Max: 6 tabs/day.

HOW SUPPLIED: Tab: (Hydrocodone-APAP) 5mg-400mg, 7.5mg-400mg, 10mg-400mg

WARNINGS/PRECAUTIONS: May produce dose-related respiratory depression. May obscure diagnosis of acute abdominal conditions or head injuries. Caution in elderly, debilitated, severe hepatic or renal dysfunction, hypothyroidism, Addison's disease, prostatic hypertrophy, urethral stricture, pulmonary disease, and postoperative use. May be habit-forming. May impair mental/physical abilities. Suppresses cough reflex.

ADVERSE REACTIONS: Lightheadedness, dizziness, sedation, nausea, vomiting.

INTERACTIONS: Additive CNS depression with opioids, antihistamines, antipsychotics, antianxiety agents, or other CNS depressants (including alcohol). Increased effect of antidepressant or hydrocodone with MAOIs or TCAs.

PREGNANCY: Category C, not for use in nursing.

MECHANISM OF ACTION: Hydrocodone: Opioid analgesic and antitussive; not established. Possibly related to existence of opiate receptors in CNS. Most actions involve CNS and smooth muscle. APAP: Non-opiate, non-salicylate analgesic and antipyretic. Mechanism of analgesic effect not established; involves peripheral influences. Antipyretic activity mediated through hypothalamic heat-regulating centers. Inhibits prostaglandin synthetase.

PHARMACOKINETICS: Absorption: Hydrocodone: C_{max}=23.6ng/mL; T_{max}=1.3 hrs. APAP: Rapidly absorbed. **Distribution:** APAP: Found in breast milk. **Metabolism:** Hydrocodone: O-demethylation, N-demethylation and 6-keto reduction. APAP: Liver (conjugation). **Elimination:** Hydrocodone: $T_{1/2}$=3.8 hrs. APAP: Urine (85%); $T_{1/2}$=1.25-3 hrs.

ZYFLO CR   RX
zileuton (Critical Therapeutics)

THERAPEUTIC CLASS: Leukotriene inhibitor

INDICATIONS: Prophylaxis and chronic treatment of asthma.

DOSAGE: *Adults:* 1200mg bid within 1 hr after am and pm meals. Max: 2400mg/day.
Pediatrics: ≥12 yrs: 1200mg bid within 1 hr after am and pm meals. Max: 2400mg/day.

HOW SUPPLIED: Tab: Extended-Release: 600mg *scored

CONTRAINDICATIONS: Active liver disease or transaminase elevations (≥3x ULN).

Z

WARNINGS/PRECAUTIONS: Not for treatment of acute attacks. Evaluate liver function prior to therapy and periodically thereafter. D/C if signs of liver disease occur.

ADVERSE REACTIONS: Headache, ALT elevation, dyspepsia, pain, nausea, asthenia, myalgia, sinusitis, pharyngolaryngeal pain.

INTERACTIONS: Monitor drugs metabolized by CYP450 3A4. Increases theophylline levels; reduce theophylline by 50% and monitor levels. Potentiates warfarin, propranolol.

PREGNANCY: Category C, not for use in nursing.

MECHANISM OF ACTION: Leukotriene inhibitor; anti-asthmatic agent, inhibits leukotriene (LTB_4, LTC_4, LTD_4, and LTE_4) formation by inhibiting the enzyme 5-lipoxygenase.

PHARMACOKINETICS: Absorption: T_{max}=4.3 hrs. **Distribution:** V_d=1.2L/kg; plasma protein binding (93%). **Metabolism:** Liver, via oxidation by CYP1A2, CYP2C9, CYP3A4; glucoronidation. **Elimination:** Urine, feces; $T_{1/2}$=3.2 hrs.

Zylet   RX
loteprednol etabonate - tobramycin (Bausch & Lomb)

THERAPEUTIC CLASS: Aminoglycoside/corticosteroid

INDICATIONS: Treatment of steroid-responsive inflammatory ocular conditions for which a corticosteroid is indicated and where superficial bacterial ocular infection or a risk of bacterial ocular infection exists.

DOSAGE: *Adults:* Initial: 1-2 drops q4-6h. May increase to 1-2 drops q1-2h for first 24-48 hours. Max: 20mL for initial Rx.

HOW SUPPLIED: Sus: 2.5mL, 5mL, 10mL

CONTRAINDICATIONS: Viral diseases of the cornea and conjunctiva including epithelial herpes simplex keratitis (dendritic keratitis), vaccinia, and varicella, and also in mycobacterial infection of the eye and fungal diseases of ocular structures.

WARNINGS/PRECAUTIONS: Not for injection into the eye. Prolonged use may result in glaucoma, optic nerve damage, visual acuity and fields of vision defects, cataracts, secondary ocular infections. May exacerbate the severity of many viral infections of the eye (including herpes simplex). May delay healing and increase incidence of bleb formation after cataract surgery.

ADVERSE REACTIONS: Injection and superficial punctate keratitis, increased IOP, burning, stinging, headache, secondary infection, vision disorders, discharge, itching, lacrimation disorder, photophobia, corneal deposits, ocular discomfort, eyelid disorder.

PREGNANCY: Category C, caution in nursing.

MECHANISM OF ACTION: Loteprednol: Corticosteroid; mechanism not fully understood. Thought to act by induction of phospholipase A_2 inhibitory proteins, lipocortins. Tobramycin: Aminoglycoside antibiotic; inhibits synthesis of proteins in bacterial cells.

Zyloprim   RX
allopurinol (Prometheus)

THERAPEUTIC CLASS: Xanthine oxidase inhibitor

INDICATIONS: Management of symptoms of primary and secondary gout. Management of hyperuricosuria and hyperuricemia due to chemotherapy. Management of recurrent calcium oxalate calculi in those with hyperuricosuria (uric acid excretion >800mg/day in males and >750mg/day in females).

DOSAGE: *Adults:* Gout: Initial: 100mg/day. Titrate: Increase by 100mg/week until serum uric acid level is ≤6mg/dL. Mild Gout: Usual: 200-300mg/day. Moderately Severe Gout: Usual: 400-600mg/day. Max: 800mg/day. Recurrent Calcium Oxalate Stones: Usual: 200-300mg/day. Prevention of Uric Acid

Nephropathy with Chemotherapy: Usual: 600-800mg/day for 2-3 days with high fluid intake. CrCl 10-20mL/min: 200mg/day. CrCl <10mL/min: Max: 100mg/day. CrCl <3mL/min: Also increase dosing intervals. Take after meals. Divide dose if >300mg.
Pediatrics: Hyperuricemia with Malignancies: 6-10 yrs: 300mg/day. <6 yrs: 150mg/day. Evaluate response after 48 hrs. Take after meals.

HOW SUPPLIED: Tab: 100mg*, 300mg* *scored

WARNINGS/PRECAUTIONS: D/C if skin rash occurs. Severe hypersensitivity reactions, hepatotoxicity, and bone marrow depression reported. Monitor LFTs during early stages of therapy with liver disease. Caution with activities that require alertness. Caution with renal impairment. Renal failure reported with hyperuricemia secondary to neoplastic diseases. Fluid intake should yield ≥2L of urinary output/day. Maintain neutral or slightly alkaline urine. Acute gout attacks increase during early stages of therapy; give colchicine.

ADVERSE REACTIONS: Acute gout attacks, rash, diarrhea, SGOT/SGPT increase, alkaline phosphatase increase, nausea.

INTERACTIONS: Increased toxicity with thiazide diuretics or renal impairment; monitor renal function. Reduce mercaptopurine or azathioprine to 1/3 or 1/4 of usual dose. Potentiates dicumarol, chlorpropamide and cyclosporine. Decreased effects with uricosurics. Increased skin rash with ampicillin, amoxicillin. Enhanced bone marrow suppression with cytotoxic agents (eg, cyclophosphamide). Caution with sulfinpyrazone.

PREGNANCY: Category C, caution in nursing.

MECHANISM OF ACTION: Xanthine oxidase inhibitor; acts on purine catabolism; reduces production of uric acid by inhibiting biochemical reactions immediately preceding its formation.

PHARMACOKINETICS: Absorption: C_{max}=3mcg/mL, T_{max}=1.5 hrs; Oxipurinol: C_{max}=6.5mcg/mL, T_{max}=4.5 hrs. **Metabolism:** Oxidation, oxipurinol (metabolite). **Elimination:** Kidneys, feces (20%); $T_{1/2}$=1-2 hrs. Oxipurinol: $T_{1/2}$=15 hrs.

ZYMAR   RX
gatifloxacin (Allergan)

THERAPEUTIC CLASS: Fluoroquinolone

INDICATIONS: Treatment of bacterial conjunctivitis.

DOSAGE: *Adults:* 1 drop q2h while awake, up to 8x/day for 2 days; then 1 drop up to qid while awake for 5 days.
Pediatrics: ≥1 yr: 1 drop q2h while awake, up to 8x/day for 2 days; then 1 drop up to qid while awake for 5 days.

HOW SUPPLIED: Sol: 0.3% [5mL]

WARNINGS/PRECAUTIONS: Not for injection. Do not inject subconjunctivally or into the anterior chamber of the eye. Superinfection may result with prolonged use. Fatal hypersensitivity reactions reported after 1st dose of systemic quinolone therapy. Avoid contact lenses when symptoms are present.

ADVERSE REACTIONS: Conjunctival irritation, increased lacrimation, keratitis, papillary conjunctivitis, chemosis, conjunctival hemorrhage, dry eye, eye discharge/irritation/pain, red eye, eyelid edema, headache, reduced visual acuity, taste disturbance.

INTERACTIONS: Systemic quinolone therapy may increase theophylline levels, interfere with caffeine metabolism, enhance warfarin effects, and elevate serum creatinine with cyclosporine.

PREGNANCY: Category C, caution in nursing.

MECHANISM OF ACTION: Fluoroquinolone antibiotic; inhibits topoisomerase II (DNA gyrase) and topoisomerase IV. DNA gyrase is essential enzyme involved in replication, transcription, and repair of bacterial DNA. Topoisomerase IV is enzyme known to play key role in partitioning of chromosomal DNA during bacterial cell division.

Z

ZYMASE   RX
protease - amylase - lipase (Organon)

THERAPEUTIC CLASS: Pancreatic enzyme supplement

INDICATIONS: Treatment of conditions with pancreatic enzyme deficiency with resultant inadequate fat digestion (eg, chronic pancreatitis, pancreatectomy, cystic fibrosis, steatorrhea).

DOSAGE: *Adults:* 1-2 caps with each meal or snack. Contents of cap may be mixed with liquids or soft foods that do not require chewing.
Pediatrics: 1-2 caps with each meal or snack. Contents of cap may be mixed with liquids or soft foods that do not require chewing.

HOW SUPPLIED: Cap, Delayed-Release: (Amylase-Lipase-Protease) 24,000 U-12,000 U-24,000 U

CONTRAINDICATIONS: Pork protein hypersensitivity.

WARNINGS/PRECAUTIONS: Do not chew or crush contents of capsules. High doses can cause hyperuricemia and hyperuricosuria.

PREGNANCY: Safety in pregnancy and nursing not known.

ZYPREXA   RX
olanzapine (Lilly)

> Elderly patients with dementia-related psychosis treated with atypical antipsychotic drugs are at an increased risk of death; most appeared to be cardiovascular (eg, heart failure, sudden death) or infectious (eg, pneumonia) in nature. Olanzapine is not approved for the treatment of patients with dementia-related psychosis.

OTHER BRAND NAMES: Zyprexa IntraMuscular (Lilly) - Zyprexa Zydis (Lilly)

THERAPEUTIC CLASS: Thienobenzodiazepine

INDICATIONS: (PO) Treatment of schizophrenia. Treatment of acute mixed or manic episodes in bipolar I disorder. Short-term treatment of acute manic episodes associated with bipolar I disorder in combination with lithium or valproate. (Inj) Agitation associated with schizophrenia, bipolar I mania.

DOSAGE: *Adults:* (PO) Schizophrenia: Initial/Usual: 5-10mg qd. Titrate: Adjust by 5mg daily at weekly intervals. Max: 20mg/day. Bipolar Disorder: Initial: 10-15mg qd. Titrate: May increase/decrease dose by 5mg daily. Max: 20mg/day. With Lithium or Valproate: Initial/Usual: 10mg qd. Max: 20mg/day. Debilitated/Hypotension Risk/Slow metabolizers/Sensitivity to Olanzapine Effects: Initial: 5mg qd. Titrate: Increase cautiously. (IM) Agitation: Initial: 10mg IM. Usual: 2.5-10mg IM. Max: 3 doses of 10mg q 2-4h. Elderly: 5mg IM. Debilitated/Hypotension Risk/Sensitivity to Olanzapine Effects: 2.5mg IM. May initiate PO therapy when clinically appropriate.

HOW SUPPLIED: Inj: 10mg; Tab: 2.5mg, 5mg, 7.5mg, 10mg, 15mg, 20mg; Tab, Disintegrating: (Zydis) 5mg, 10mg, 15mg, 20mg

WARNINGS/PRECAUTIONS: Monitor for hyperglycemia, worsening of glucose control with DM, FBG levels with diabetes risk. Risk of NMS, tardive dyskinesia, orthostatic hypotension, seizures. Caution in hepatic impairment, prostatic hypertrophy, narrow-angle glaucoma, history of paralytic ileus, elderly patients with dementia, cardio- or cerebrovascular disease, hypotension risk (eg, hypovolemia, dehydration), risk for aspiration pneumonia, suicidal tendencies. May cause alterations in lipid levels and weight gain; monitor regularly. May cause cognitive and motor impairment. Elevated transaminases, hyperprolactinemia reported. May cause disruption of body temperature regulation. Re-evaluate periodically.

ADVERSE REACTIONS: Postural hypotension, constipation, dry mouth, weight gain, somnolence, dizziness, personality disorder, akathisia, asthenia, dyspepsia, tremor, increased appetite, ecchymosis, rhinitis, joint pain.

INTERACTIONS: May potentiate antihypertensives. Decreased levels with activated charcoal. Increased clearance with carbamazepine. Increased levels with fluvoxamine; lower olanzapine dose. Caution with other CNS drugs, alcohol. May antagonize levodopa, dopamine agonists. Inducers of CYP1A2 or glucuronyl transferase (eg, omeprazole, rifampin) may increase clearance. Inhibitors of CYP1A2 may decrease clearance.

PREGNANCY: Category C, not for use in nursing.

MECHANISM OF ACTION: Thienobenzodiazepine psychotropic agent; mechanism unknown. Selective monoaminergic antagonist with high affinity binding to selective serotonin, dopamine, histamine, muscurinic, and α-adrenergic receptors.

PHARMACOKINETICS: Absorption: Well-absorbed. (PO): T_{max}=6 hrs; (IM): T_{max}=15-45 min; **Distribution:** Plasma protein binding (93%); V_d=1000L. **Metabolism**: Via CYP450 mediated oxidation and direct glucoronidation; 10-N-glucuronide, 4'-N-desmethyl (major metabolites). **Elimination:** Urine (57%, 7% unchanged), feces (30%); $T_{1/2}$=21-54 hrs.

ZYRTEC

RX

cetirizine HCL (Pfizer)

THERAPEUTIC CLASS: H_1-antagonist

INDICATIONS: Seasonal or perennial allergic rhinitis. Chronic idiopathic urticaria.

DOSAGE: *Adults:* 5-10mg qd. Hepatic Impairment/Hemodialysis/CrCl <31mL/min: 5mg qd.
Pediatrics: ≥12 yrs: 5-10mg qd. 6-11 yrs: 5-10mg qd. 2-5 yrs: 2.5mg qd. Max: 5mg qd or 2.5mg q12h. Perennial Allergic Rhinitis/Urticaria: 6 months-23 months: 2.5mg qd. 12 months-23 months: May increase to max 5mg/day given as 2.5mL q12h. Hepatic Impairment/Hemodialysis/CrCl <31mL/min: ≥12 yrs: 5mg qd. 6-11 yrs: Use lower the recommended dose. <6 yrs: Not recommended.

HOW SUPPLIED: Syrup: 1mg/mL [120mL, 480mL]; Tab: 5mg, 10mg; Tab, Chewable: 5mg, 10mg

CONTRAINDICATIONS: Hydroxyzine hypersensitivity.

WARNINGS/PRECAUTIONS: Adjust dose with hepatic or renal impairment. May impair mental/physical abilities.

ADVERSE REACTIONS: Somnolence, fatigue, dry mouth, headache, pharyngitis, abdominal pain, cough, epistaxis, diarrhea, bronchospasm.

INTERACTIONS: Avoid alcohol and CNS depressants. Possible decreased clearance with large doses of theophylline.

PREGNANCY: Category B, not for use in nursing.

ZYRTEC-D

OTC

pseudoephedrine HCL - cetirizine HCL (Pfizer)

THERAPEUTIC CLASS: Antihistamine/decongestant

INDICATIONS: Relief of nasal and non-nasal symptoms associated with seasonal or perennial allergic rhinitis.

DOSAGE: *Adults:* 1 tab bid. Hepatic Impairment/Renal Dysfunction (CrCl <31mL/min): 1 tab qd. Swallow tabs whole.
Pediatrics: ≥12 yrs: 1 tab bid. Hepatic Impairment/Renal Dysfunction (CrCl <31mL/min): 1 tab qd. Swallow tabs whole.

HOW SUPPLIED: Tab, Extended-Release: (Cetirizine-Pseudoephedrine) 5mg-120mg

CONTRAINDICATIONS: Narrow angle glaucoma, urinary retention, MAOIs during or within 14 days of use, severe HTN, severe CAD, hypersensitivity to adrenergics.

WARNINGS/PRECAUTIONS: Caution with HTN, DM, ischemic heart disease, increased IOP, hyperthyroidism, renal impairment, or prostatic hypertrophy.

Z

May produce CNS stimulation with convulsions or cardiovascular collapse. May impair mental/physical abilities.

ADVERSE REACTIONS: Insomnia, dry mouth, fatigue, somnolence.

INTERACTIONS: Avoid MAOIs during or within 14 days of use.

PREGNANCY: Category C, not for use in nursing.

MECHANISM OF ACTION: Cetirizine: Antihistamine/decongestant; selectively inhibits H1-receptors. Pseudoephedrine: orally active sympathomimetic amine; exerts a decongestant effect on the nasal mucosa.

PHARMACOKINETICS: Absorption: Cetirizine: C_{max}=114 ng/mL (single dose), 178ng/mL (multiple doses); T_{max}=2.2 hrs. Pseudoephedrine: C_{max}=309 ng/mL, 526ng/mL (multiple doses); T_{max}=4.4 hrs. **Distribution:** Found in breast milk. Cetirizine: Plasma protein binding (93%). Pseudoephedrine: V_d=2.6-3.3 L/kg. **Metabolism:** Cetirizine: Oxidative-O-dealkylation. Pseudoephedrine: N-demethylation; (1%-7%) metabolized to norpseudoephedrine. **Elimination:** Cetirizine: $T_{1/2mean}$=7.9 hrs; urine (70%), feces (10%). Pseudoephedrine: $T_{1/2}$=6hrs.

ZYVOX RX
linezolid (Pharmacia & Upjohn)

THERAPEUTIC CLASS: Oxazolidinone class antibacterial

INDICATIONS: Treatment of vancomycin-resistant *Enterococcus faecium* (VRE) infections, nosocomial pneumonia caused by *Staphylococcus aureus* (methicillin-susceptible and -resistant strains) or *Streptococcus pneumoniae* (including multi drug-resistant strains [MDRSP]), complicated skin and skin structure infections (SSSI) including diabetic foot infections without concomitant osteomyelitis caused by *Staphylococcus aureus* (methicillin-susceptible and -resistant strains), *Streptococcus pyogenes*, or *Streptococcus agalactiae*, uncomplicated SSSI caused by *Staphylococcus aureus* (methicillin-susceptible only) or *Streptococcus pyogenes*, community-acquired pneumonia (CAP) caused by *Streptococcus pneumoniae* (MDRSP), including concurrent bacteremia, or *Staphylococcus aureus* (methicillin-susceptible strains only).

DOSAGE: *Adults:* Complicated SSSI/CAP/Nosocomial Pneumonia: 600mg IV/PO q12h for 10-14 days. VRE: 600mg IV/PO q12h for 14-28 days. Uncomplicated SSSI: 400mg PO q12h for 10-14 days.
Pediatrics: Complicated SSSI/CAP/Nosocomial Pneumonia: Treat for 10-14 days. ≥12 yrs: 600mg IV/PO q12h. Birth-11 yrs: 10mg/kg IV/PO q8h. VRE: Treat for 14-28 days: ≥12 yrs: 600mg IV/PO q12h; Birth-11 yrs: 10mg/kg IV/PO q8h. Uncomplicated SSSI: Treat for 10-14 days: ≥12 yrs: 600mg PO q12h; 5-11 yrs: 10mg/kg PO q12h; <5 yrs: 10mg/kg PO q8h. Neonates <7 days: Initiate with dosing regimen of 10mg/kg q12h; may increase to 10mg/kg q8h if suboptimal response. All neonatal patients should receive 10mg/kg q8h by 7 days of life.

HOW SUPPLIED: Inj: 2mg/mL [100mL, 200mL, 300mL]; Sus: 100mg/5mL [150mL]; Tab: 400mg, 600mg

WARNINGS/PRECAUTIONS: Myelosuppression including anemia, thrombocytopenia, pancytopenia, and leukopenia reported; monitor CBC weekly. *Clostridium difficile*-associated diarrhea reported. Oral sus contains phenylalanine. Peripheral and optic neuropathy reported; monitor visual function if on extended periods (≥3 months). Lactic acidosis and convulsions reported. May promote overgrowth of nonsusceptible organisms.

ADVERSE REACTIONS: Diarrhea, headache, nausea, vomiting.

INTERACTIONS: Potential interaction with adrenergic and serotonergic agents. May enhance pressor response to sympathomimetics, vasopressors, and dopaminergic agents; caution with dopamine, epinephrine, pseudoephedrine, and phenylpropanolamine. Serotonin syndrome may occur with concomitant serotonergic agents, including antidepressants such as SSRIs. Avoid large quantities of tyramine-containing foods or beverages.

PREGNANCY: Category C, caution in nursing.

MECHANISM OF ACTION: Oxazolidinone antibacterial; inhibits bacterial protein synthesis; binds to a site on the bacterial 23S ribosomal RNA of the 50S subunit and prevents formation of functional 70S initiation complex, which is an essential component of the bacterial translation process.

PHARMACOKINETICS: Absorption: Rapid/extensive; absolute bioavailability (100%); T_{max}=1-2 hrs. **Distribution:** V_d=40-50L; plasma protein binding (31%); distributes to well-perfused tissues. **Metabolism:** Via oxidation; aminoethoxyacteic acid (A), hydroxyethyl glycine (B) (inactive metabolites). **Elimination:** Urine (30% as parent drug, 40% as B, 10% as A) and feces (6% as B, 3% as A).

Z

Indices

BRAND/GENERIC INDEX

Organized alphabetically, this index includes the brand and generic names of each drug in the Product Information section. Brand-name drug entries are capitalized; generic names are not. If more than one brand name is associated with a generic, each brand can be found under the generic entry.

J

K

THERAPEUTIC CLASS INDEX

Organized alphabetically, this index includes the therapeutic class of each drug in the Product Information section. Therapeutic class headings are based on information provided in the drug monographs. The drug entries listed under each bold therapeutic class are organized alphabetically by brand name or monograph title (shown in capitalized letters), followed by the generic name in parentheses.

A

M

RECOMBINANT HUMAN LUTEINIZING HORMORE

RECOMBINANT HUMAN PARATHYROID HORMONE

RECOMBINANT HUMAN THYROID STIMULATING HORMONE

RECOMBINANT URATE-OXIDASE ENZYME

RENIN INHIBITOR

RENIN INHIBITOR/THIAZIDE DIURETIC

RETINOID

REVERSIBLE CHOLINESTERASE INHIBITOR

RIBONUCLEOTIDE REDUCTASE INHIBITOR

RIFAMYCIN DERIVATIVE

S

SALICYLATE

SCABICIDE/ANTIPRURITIC

SELECTIVE ALPHA₂ AGONIST

SELECTIVE BETA₁-BLOCKER

SELECTIVE BETA₁-BLOCKER/ MONOSULFAMYL DIURETIC

SELECTIVE BETA₁-BLOCKER/THIAZIDE DIURETIC

SELECTIVE COSTIMULATION MODULATOR

SELECTIVE ESTROGEN RECEPTOR MODULATOR

SELECTIVE NOREPINEPHRINE REUPTAKE INHIBITOR

SELECTIVE SEROTONIN REUPTAKE INHIBITOR

SEMISYNTHETIC AMPICILLIN DERIVATIVE

SEMISYNTHETIC ANSAMYCIN (RNA POLYMERASE INHIBITOR)

SEMISYNTHETIC PENICILLIN DERIVATIVE

Appendix: Reference Tables

ABBREVIATIONS, ACRONYMS, AND SYMBOLS

ABBREVIATIONS	DESCRIPTIONS
- (eg, 6-8)	to (eg, 6 to 8)
/	per
<	less than
>	greater than
≤	less than or equal to
≥	greater than or equal to
α	alpha
β	beta
5-FU	5-fluorouracil
5-HT	5-hydroxytriptamine (serotonin)
ABECB	acute bacterial exacerbation of chronic bronchitis
aa	of each
ACTH	adrenocorticotrophic hormone
ad	right ear
ADHD	attention-deficit/hyperactivity disorder
A-fib	atrial fibrillation
A-flutter	atrial flutter
AIDS	acquired immunodeficiency syndrome
ALT	alanine transaminase (SGPT)
am	morning
AMI	acute myocardial infarction
ANA	antinuclear antibodies
ANC	absolute neutrophil count
APAP	acetaminophen
as	left ear
ASA	aspirin
AST	aspartate transaminase (SGOT)
au	each ear
AUC	area under the curve
AV	atrioventricular
bid	twice daily
BMI	body mass index
BP	blood pressure
BPH	benign prostatic hypertrophy
BSA	body surface area
BUN	blood urea nitrogen
CABG	coronary artery bypass graft
CAD	coronary artery disease
Cap	capsule
CAP	community-acquired pneumonia
CBC	complete blood count
CF	cystic fibrosis
CHF	congestive heart failure
cm	centimeter
CMV	cytomegalovirus
C_{max}	peak plasma concentration
CNS	central nervous system
COPD	chronic obstructive pulmonary disease
CrCl	creatinine clearance
Cre	cream
CRF	chronic renal failure

(Continued)

ABBREVIATIONS	DESCRIPTIONS
CSF	cerebrospinal fluid
CVA	cerebrovascular accident
CVD	cardiovascular disease
CYP450	cytochrome P450
d/c	discontinue
DHEA	dehydroepiandrosterone
DM	diabetes mellitus
DVT	deep vein thrombus
ECG	electrocardiogram
EEG	electroencephalogram
eg	for example
EPS	extrapyramidal symptom
ESRD	end-stage renal disease
FSH	follicle-stimulating hormone
g	gram
GABA	gamma-aminobutyric acid
GAD	general anxiety disorder
GERD	gastroesophageal reflux disease
GFR	glomerular filtration rate
GI	gastrointestinal
GnRH	gonadotropin-releasing hormone
GVHD	graft versus host disease
HCG	human chorionic gonadotropin
Hct	hematocrit
HCTZ	hydrochlorothiazide
HDL	high density lipoprotein
Hgb	hemoglobin
HIV	human immunodeficiency virus
HMG-CoA	3-hydroxy-3-methylglutaryl-coenzyme A
HR	heart rate
hr or hrs	hour or hours
hs	bedtime
HSV	herpes simplex virus
HTN	hypertension
IBD	inflammatory bowel disease
IBS	irritable bowel syndrome
ICH	intracranial hemorrhage
ICP	intracranial pressure
IM	intramuscular
INH	isoniazid
Inj	injection
INR	international normalized ratio
IOP	intraocular pressure
IU	international units
IV	intravenous/intravenously
K+	potassium
kg	kilogram
KIU	kallikrein inhibitor unit
L	liter
lbs	pounds
LD	loading dose
LDL	low density lipoprotein
LFT	liver function test
LH	luteinizing hormone

(Continued)

ABBREVIATIONS	DESCRIPTIONS
LHRH	luteinizing-hormone releasing hormone
Lot	lotion
Loz	lozenge
LVH	left ventricular hypertrophy
M	molar
MAC	mycobacterium avium complex
Maint	maintenance
MAOI	monoamine oxidase inhibitor
Max	maximum
mcg	microgram
mEq	milli-equivalent
mg	milligram
MI	myocardial infarction
min	minute (usually as mL/min)
mL	milliliter
mm	millimeter
mM	millimolar
MRI	magnetic resonance imaging
MS	multiple sclerosis
msec	millisecond
MTX	methotrexate
Na	sodium
NaCl	sodium chloride
NG	nasogastric
NKA	no known allergies
NMS	neuroleptic malignant syndrome
NPO	nothing by mouth
NSAID	nonsteroidal anti-inflammatory drug
NV	nausea and vomiting
OA	osteoarthritis
OCD	obsessive-compulsive disorder
od	right eye
Oint	ointment
os	left eye
ou	each eye
PAT	paroxysmal atrial tachycardia
pc	after meals
PCN	penicillin
PCP	*Pneumocystis Carinii* pneumonia
PD	Parkinson's disease
PID	pelvic inflammatory disease
pkt, pkts	packet, packets
pm	evening
po	orally
PONV	postoperative nausea and vomiting
pr	rectally
prn	as needed
PSA	prostate-specific antigen
PSVT	paroxysmal supraventricular tachycardia
PT	prothrombin time
PTSD	post-traumatic stress disorder
PTT	partial thromboplastin time
PTU	propylthiouracil
PUD	peptic ulcer disease

ABBREVIATIONS	DESCRIPTIONS
PVD	peripheral vascular disease
q4h, q6h, q8h, etc.	every four hours, every six hours, every eight hours, etc.
qd	once daily
qh	every hour
qid	four times daily
qod	every other day
qs	a sufficient quantity
qs ad	a sufficient quantity up to
RA	rheumatoid arthritis
RBC	red blood cells
RDIs	reference daily intakes
RDS	respiratory distress syndrome
REM	rapid eye movement
SAH	subarachnoid hemorrhage
SBP	systolic blood pressure
sec	second(s)
SGOT	serum glutamic-oxaloacetic transaminase (AST)
SGPT	serum glutamic-pyruvic transaminase (ALT)
SIADH	syndrome of inappropriate antidiuretic hormone secretion
SLE	systemic lupus erythematosus
SOB	shortness of breath
Sol	solution
SQ, SC	subcutaneous
SrCr	serum creatinine
SSRI	selective serotonin reuptake inhibitor
SSSI	skin and skin structure infection
STD	sexually transmitted disease
Sup	suppository
Sus	suspension
SVT	supraventricular tachycardia
$T_{1/2}$	half-life
Tab	tablet
Tab, SL	sublingual tablet
TB	tuberculosis
TBG	thyroxine binding globulin
tbl	tablespoon
TCA	tricyclic antidepressant
TD	tardive dyskinesia
TFT	thyroid function test
TG	triglyceride
tid	three times daily
T_{max}	time to maximum concentration
TNF	tumor necrosis factor
TPN	total parenteral nutrition
TSH	thyroid stimulating hormone
tsp	teaspoonful
TTP	thrombotic thrombocytopenic purpura

(Continued)

ABBREVIATIONS	DESCRIPTIONS
U	unit
ud	as directed
ULN	upper limit of normal
URTI/URI	upper respiratory tract infection
UTI	urinary tract infection
UV	ultraviolet
WBC	white blood cell count
Vd	volume of distribution
VTE	venous thromboembolism
X	times (eg, >2X ULN)
yr or yrs	year or years

ABBREVIATIONS	DESCRIPTIONS
U	unit
UD	as directed
ULN	upper limit of normal
URI/URTI	upper respiratory tract infection
UTI	urinary tract infection
UV	ultraviolet
WBC	white blood cell count
Vd	volume of distribution
VTE	venous thromboembolism
X	times (e.g., X DUH)
yr or yrs	year or years

CALCULATIONS AND FORMULAS

WEIGHTS AND MEASURES

METRIC MEASURES

1 kilogram (kg)	1000 g
1 gram (g)	1000 mg
1 milligram (mg)	0.001 g
1 microgram (mcg or μg)	0.001 mg; 1 x 10⁻⁶ g
1 liter (L)	1000 mL
1 milliliter (mL)	0.001 L; 1 cc (cubic centimeter)

APOTHECARY MEASURES (AP)

1 scruple	20 grains (gr)
1 drachm	3 scruples; 60 gr
1 ounce (oz)	8 drachms; 24 scruples; 480 gr
1 pound (lb)	12 oz; 96 drachms; 288 scruples; 5760 gr

U.S. FLUID MEASURES

1 fluidrachm	60 minim
1 fluidounce	8 fluidrachm; 480 minim
1 pint (pt)	16 fl oz; 7680 minim
1 quart (qt)	2 pt; 32 fl oz
1 gallon (gal)	4 qt; 128 fl oz

AVOIRDUPOIS WEIGHT (AV)

1 ounce	437.5 gr
1 pound	16 oz

CONVERSION FACTORS

1 gram	15.4 gr
1 grain	64.8 mg
1 ounce (Av)	28.35 g; 437.5 gr
1 ounce (Ap)	31.1 g; 480 gr
1 pound (Av)	453.6 g; 2.68 lb (Ap); 2.20 lb (Av)
1 fluidounce	29.57 mL
1 fluidrachm	3.697 mL
1 minim	0.06 mL

COMMON MEASURES

1 teaspoonful	5 mL; ⅙ fl oz
1 tablespoonful	15 mL; ½ fl oz
1 wineglassful	60 mL; 2 fl oz
1 teacupful	120 mL; 4 fl oz
1 gallon	3800 mL; 128 fl oz
1 quart	960 mL; 32 fl oz
1 pint	480 mL; 16 fl oz (exactly 473.2 mL)
8 fluid ounces	240 mL
4 fluid ounces	120 mL
2.2 lb	1 kg

DOSE EQUIVALENTS

WEIGHT (METRIC)	WEIGHT (APOTHECARY)
30 g	1 ounce
15 g	4 drams
10 g	2 ½ drams
7.5 g	2 drams
6 g	90 grains
5 g	75 grains
4 g	60 grains; 1 dram
3 g	45 grains
2 g	30 grains; ½ dram
1.5 g	22 grains
1 g	15 grains
750 mg	12 grains
600 mg	10 grains
500 mg	7 ½ grains
400 mg	6 grains
300 mg	5 grains
250 mg	4 grains

(Continued)

DOSE EQUIVALENTS (Continued)

WEIGHT (METRIC)	WEIGHT (APOTHECARY)
200 mg	3 grains
150 mg	2 $^1/_2$ grains
125 mg	2 grains
100 mg	1 $^1/_2$ grains
75 mg	1 $^1/_4$ grains
60 mg	1 grain
50 mg	$^3/_4$ grain
40 mg	$^2/_3$ grain
30 mg	$^3/_8$ grain
25 mg	$^3/_8$ grain
20 mg	$^1/_3$ grain
15 mg	$^1/_5$ grain
12 mg	$^1/_5$ grain
10 mg	$^1/_6$ grain
8 mg	$^1/_8$ grain
6 mg	$^1/_{10}$ grain
5 mg	$^1/_{12}$ grain
4 mg	$^1/_{15}$ grain
3 mg	$^1/_{20}$ grain
2 mg	$^1/_{30}$ grain
1.5 mg	$^1/_{40}$ grain
1.2 mg	$^1/_{50}$ grain
1 mg	$^1/_{60}$ grain

LIQUID MEASURES (METRIC)	LIQUID MEASURES (APOTHECARY)
1000 mL	1 quart
750 mL	1 $^1/_2$ pints
500 mL	1 pint
230 mL	8 fluid ounces
200 mL	7 fluid ounces
100 mL	3 $^1/_2$ fluid ounces
50 mL	1 $^3/_4$ fluid ounces
30 mL	1 fluid ounces
15 mL	4 fluid drams
10 mL	2 $^1/_2$ fluid drams
8 mL	2 fluid drams
5 mL	1 $^1/_4$ fluid drams
4 mL	1 fluid dram
3 mL	45 minims
2 mL	30 minims
1 mL	15 minims
0.75 mL	12 minims
0.6 mL	10 minims
0.5 mL	8 minims
0.3 mL	5 minims
0.25 mL	4 minims
0.2 mL	3 minims
0.1 mL	1 $^1/_2$ minims
0.06 mL	1 minim
0.05 mL	$^3/_4$ minim
0.03 mL	$^1/_2$ minim

MILLIEQUIVALENT (mEq) AND MILLIMOLE (mmol)

CALCULATIONS

moles = $\dfrac{\text{weight of a substance (grams)}}{\text{molecular weight of that substance (grams)}}$	**OR**	= $\dfrac{\text{equivalent}}{\text{valence of ion}}$
millimoles = $\dfrac{\text{weight of a substance (milligrams)}}{\text{molecular weight of that substance (milligrams)}}$	**OR**	= $\dfrac{\text{milliequivalents}}{\text{valence of ion}}$ **OR** = moles x 1000
equivalents = moles x valence of ion		
milliequivalents = millimoles x valence of ion	**OR**	= equivalents x 1000

(Continued)

CONVERSIONS

mg/100mL to mEq/L	$mEq/L = \dfrac{(mg/100mL) \times 10 \times valence}{atomic\ weight}$
mEq/L to mg/100mL	$mg/100mL = \dfrac{(mEq/L) \times atomic\ weight}{10 \times valence}$
mEq/L to volume percent of a gas	$volume\ \% = \dfrac{(mEq/L) \times 22.4}{10}$

ACID-BASE ASSESSMENT

DEFINITIONS

PIO_2	Oxygen partial pressure of inspired gas (mmHg); 150 mmHg in room air at sea level
FiO_2	Fractional pressure of oxygen in inspired gas (0.21 in room air)
PAO_2	Alveolar oxygen partial pressure
$PACO_2$	Alveolar carbon dioxide partial pressure
PaO_2	Arterial oxygen partial pressure
$PaCO_2$	Arterial carbon dioxide partial pressure
R	Respiratory exchange quotient (typically 0.8, increases with high carbohydrate diet, decreases with high fat diet)

HENDERSON-HASSELBALCH EQUATION

$pH = 6.1 + \log [HCO_3^- / (0.03)\ (pCO_2)]$

ALVEOLAR GAS EQUATION

$PIO_2 = FiO_2 \times$ (total atmospheric pressure - vapor pressure of H_2O at 37°C)
$\quad = FiO_2 \times$ (760 mmHg - 47 mmHg)

$PaO_2 = PIO_2 - PaCO_2/R$

ALVEOLAR/ARTERIAL OXYGEN GRADIENT

$PAO_2 - PaO_2$

ACID-BASE DISORDERS

Disorder	pH	HCO₃⁻	PCO₂	Compensation
Metabolic acidosis	< 7.35	Primary decrease	Compensatory decrease	1.2-mmHg decrease in PCO_2 for every 1-mmol/L decrease in HCO_3^- or $PCO_2 = (1.5 \times HCO_3^-) + 8\ (\pm 2)$ or $PCO_2 = HCO_3^- + 15$ or PCO_2 = last 2 digits of pH x 100
Metabolic alkalosis	> 7.45	Primary increase	Compensatory increase	0.6-0.75 mmHg increase in PCO_2 for every 1-mmol/L increase in HCO_3^-. PCO_2 should not rise above 60 mm Hg in compensation.
Respiratory acidosis	< 7.35	Compensatory increase	Primary increase	*Acute:* 1-2 mmol decrease in HCO_3^-. for every 10-mmHg decrease in PCO_2 *Chronic:* 3-4 mmol increase in HCO_3^-. for every 10-mmHg increase in PCO_2
Respiratory alkalosis	> 7.45	Compensatory decrease	Primary decrease	*Acute:* 1-2 mmol increase in HCO_3^-. for every 10-mmHg increase in PCO_2 *Chronic:* 4-5 mmol decrease in HCO_3^-. for every 10-mmHg decrease in PCO_2

ACID-BASE EQUATION

H^+ (in mEq/L) = (24 x $PaCO_2$) divided by HCO_3^-

(Continued)

OTHER CALCULATIONS

ANION GAP

Anion gap = Na^+ - (Cl^- + HCO_3^- measured)

AA GRADIENT

Aa gradient [(713) (FiO_2 - ($PaCO_2$ divided by 0.8))] - PaO_2

OSMOLALITY

Definition:
Osmolality is a measure of the total number of particles in a solution.

U.S. units (sodium as mEq/L, BUN (blood urea nitrogen) and glucose as (mg/dL)
   Plasma osmolality (mOsm/kg) = $2([Na^+] + [K^+]) + ([BUN]/2.8) + ([glucose]/18)$
SI units (all variables in mmol/L):
   Plasma osmolality (mOsm/kg) = $2[Na^+] + [urea] + [glucose]$
   Normal range plasma osmolality: 280 - 303 mOsm/kg

Corrected Sodium
Corrected Na+ = measured Na^+ + [1.5 x (glucose - 150 divided by 100)]*
*Do not correct for glucose <150.

Total Serum Calcium Corrected for Albumin Level
[(Normal albumin - patient's albumin) x 0.8] + patient's measured total calcium

Water Deficit
Water deficit = 0.6 x body weight [1 - (140 divided by Na^+)]*
*Body weight is estimated weight in kg; Na^+ is serum or plasma sodium.

Bicarbonate Deficit
HCO_3^- deficit = [0.4 x weight (kg)] x (HCO_3^- desired - HCO_3^- measured)

CHILD-PUGH SCORE

The Child-Pugh classification used to assess the prognosis of chronic liver disease, mainly cirrhosis. Child-Pugh is also used to determine the required strength of treatment and the necessity of liver transplantation.

Score:
   The score employs five clinical measures of liver disease. Each measure is scored 1-3, with
   3 indicating most severe derangement.

Measure	1 point	2 points	3 points	Units
Bilirubin (total)*	<34 (<2)	34-50 (2-3)	>50 (>3)	mol/L (mg/dL)
Serum albumin	>3	528-35	<28	mg/L
INR*	<1.7	1.71-2.20	> 2.20	no unit
Ascites	None	Suppressed with medication	Refractory	no unit
Hepatic encephalopathy	None	Grade I-II (or suppressed with medication)	Grade III-IV (or refractory)	no unit

* In primary sclerosing cholangitis and primary biliary cirrhosis, the bilirubin references are changed to reflect the fact that these diseases feature high conjugated bilirubin levels. The upper limit for 1 point is 68 mol/L (4 mg/dL) and the upper limit for 2 points is 170 mol/L (10 mg/dL).

** Some older reference works substitute PT prolongation for INR.

Interpretation:
   Chronic liver disease is classified into Child-Pugh class A to C, employing the added score from above.

Points	Class	One year survival	Two year survival
5-6	A	100%	85%
7-9	B	81%	57%
10-15	C	45%	35%

CREATININE CLEARANCE

Clinically, creatinine clearance is a useful measure for estimating the glomerular filtration rate (GFR) of the kidneys.

Factors	Abbreviations
Creatinine clearance	Cl_{Cr}
Plasma creatinine concentration	P_{Cr}
Serum creatinine concentration	S_{Cr}
Urine creatinine concentration	U_{Cr}
Urine flow rate	V
Plasma creatinine concentration	P_{Cr}

(Continued)

CREATININE CLEARANCE *(Continued)*

Calculations:

$$Cl_{Cr} = \frac{U_{Cr} \times V}{P_{Cr}}$$

Example:
Patient with P_{Cr} 1 mg/dL, U_{Cr} 60 mg/dL, and V of 0.5 dL/hr.

$$Cl_{Cr} = \frac{60 \text{ mg/dL} \times 0.5 \text{ dL/hr}}{1 \text{ mg/dL}} = 30 \text{ dL/hr}$$

Cockcroft-Gault formula: Estimates creatinine clearance (mL/min).

Male:

$$Cl_{Cr} = \frac{(140 - age) \times mass \text{ (kg)}}{72 \times S_{Cr} \text{ (mg/dL)}}$$

Example:
Male patient, 67 years of age, weight 75 kg, and S_{Cr} 1 mg/dL.

$$Cl_{Cr} = \frac{(140 - 67) \times 75}{72 \times 1} = 76 \text{ mL/min}$$

Female:

$$Cl_{Cr} = \frac{(140 - age) \times mass \text{ (kg)} \times 0.85 \text{ if female}}{72 \times S_{Cr} \text{ (mg/dL)}}$$

Example:
Female patient, 67 years of age, weight 75 kg, and S_{Cr} 1 mg/dL.

$$Cl_{Cr} = \frac{(140 - 67) \times 75}{72 \times 1} \times 0.85 = 64.6 \text{ mL/min}$$

Note: Using actual body weight (ABW) in obese patients can significantly overestimate creatinine clearance. Adjusted ideal body weight (IBW) can provide more approximate estimate. Adjusted IBW = IBW + 0.4 (ABW - IBW).

BASAL ENERGY EXPENDITURE (BEE)

Basal energy expenditure: the amount of energy required to maintain the body's normal metabolic activity (ie, respiration, maintenance of body temperature, etc).

H = height (cm), W = weight (kg), A = age (years)

Male:
BEE = 66.67 + 13.75W + 5H - 6.76A

Female:
BEE = 665.1 + 9.56W + 1.85H - 4.68A

BODY MASS INDEX (BMI)

$$BMI = \frac{weight \text{ (kg)}}{[height \text{ (m)}]^2}$$

BODY SURFACE AREA (BSA)

$$BSA \text{ (m}^2) = \sqrt{\frac{height \text{ (in)} \times weight \text{ (lb)}}{3131}}$$ **OR** $$BSA \text{ (m}^2) = \sqrt{\frac{height \text{ (cm)} \times weight \text{ (kg)}}{3600}}$$

IDEAL BODY WEIGHT (IBW)

Adults (18 years and older; IBW is in kg):
  IBW (male) = 50 + (2.3 x height [inches] over 5 feet)
  IBW (female) = 45.5 + (2.3 x height [inches] over 5 feet)

Children (IBW is in kg; height is in cm):
  1-18 years of age:
  $$IBW = \frac{(height^2 \times 1.65)}{100}$$

  5 feet and taller:
  IBW (male) = 39 + (2.27 x height [inches] over 5 feet)
  IBW (female) = 42.2 + (2.27 x height [inches] over 5 feet)

(Continued)

POUNDS/KILOGRAM CONVERSION

1 pound = 0.45359 kilogram				1 kilogram = 2.2 pounds			
lb	kg	lb	kg	lb	kg	lb	kg
1	0.45	105	47.63	210	95.25	315	142.88
5	2.27	110	49.89	215	97.52	320	145.15
10	4.54	115	52.16	220	99.79	325	147.42
15	6.80	120	54.43	225	102.06	330	149.68
20	9.07	125	56.70	230	104.33	335	151.95
25	11.34	130	58.97	235	106.59	340	154.22
30	13.61	135	61.23	240	108.86	345	156.49
35	15.88	140	63.50	245	111.13	350	158.76
40	18.14	145	65.77	250	113.40	355	161.02
45	20.41	150	68.04	255	115.67	360	163.29
50	22.68	155	70.31	260	117.93	365	165.56
55	24.95	160	72.57	265	120.20	370	167.83
60	27.22	165	74.84	270	122.47	375	170.10
65	29.48	170	77.11	275	124.74	380	172.36
70	31.75	175	79.38	280	127.01	385	174.63
75	34.02	180	81.65	285	129.27	390	176.90
80	36.29	185	83.91	290	131.54	395	179.17
85	38.56	190	86.18	295	133.81	400	181.44
90	40.82	195	88.45	300	136.08	405	183.70
95	43.09	200	90.72	305	138.34	405	183.70
100	45.36	205	92.99	310	140.61	415	188.24

TEMPERATURE CONVERSION

Fahrenheit to Celsius = (°F - 32) x 5/9 = °C				Celsius to Fahrenheit = (°C x 9/5) + 32 = °F			
°F	°C	°F	°C	°C	°F	°C	°F
0.0	-17.8	92.0	33.3	0.0	32.0	49.0	120.2
5.0	-15.0	93.0	33.9	5.0	41.0	50.0	122.0
10.0	-12.2	94.0	34.4	10.0	50.0	51.0	123.8
15.0	-9.4	95.0	35.0	15.0	59.0	85.0	185.0
20.0	-6.7	96.0	35.6	20.0	68.0	52.0	125.6
25.0	-3.9	97.0	36.1	25.0	77.0	53.0	127.4
30.0	-1.1	98.0	36.7	30.0	86.0	54.0	129.2
35.0	1.7	98.6	37.0	35.0	95.0	55.0	131.0
40.0	4.4	99.0	37.2	36.0	96.8	56.0	132.8
45.0	7.2	100.0	37.8	37.0	98.6	57.0	134.6
50.0	10.0	101.0	38.3	38.0	100.4	58.0	136.4
55.0	12.8	102.0	38.9	39.0	102.2	59.0	138.2
60.0	15.6	103.0	39.4	40.0	104.0	60.0	140.0
65.0	18.3	104.0	40.0	41.0	105.8	65.0	149.0
70.0	21.1	105.0	40.6	42.0	107.6	70.0	158.0
75.0	23.9	106.0	41.1	43.0	109.4	75.0	167.0
80.0	26.7	107.0	41.7	44.0	111.2	80.0	176.0
85.0	29.4	108.0	42.2	45.0	113.0	90.0	194.0
90.0	32.2	109.0	42.8	46.0	114.8	95.0	203.0
91.0	32.8	110.0	43.3	47.0	116.6	100.0	212.0
				48.0	118.4	105.0	221.0

(Continued)

PEDIATRIC DOSAGE ESTIMATION FORMULAS

The following formulas can be used to estimate the approximate pediatric dosage of a medication. These formulas are based on the adult dose and either the child's age or weight. These formulas should be used with caution as the response to any drug is not always directly proportional to the age or weight of the child relative to the usual adult dose. Dosage will also vary based on the formula used. Care should be taken when using any of these methods to calculate the child's dosage. Some products have FDA approved pediatric indications and dosages, always refer to full prescribing information first before calculating a pediatric dosage.

BASED ON WEIGHT

Augsberger's Rule:

$\dfrac{[(1.5 \times \text{weight [kg]}) + 10]}{100} \times$ adult dose = approximate child's dose

Example: If the child's weight is 15 kg (33 lb) and the adult dose is 50 mg then the child's dose is 16.25 mg.
$\dfrac{[(1.5 \times 15 \text{ kg}) + 10]}{100} \times 50$ mg = 0.325 x 50 mg = 16.25 mg

Clark's Rule:

(weight [lb]/150) x adult dose = approximate child's dose

Example: If the child's weight is 15 kg (33 lb) and the adult dose is 50 mg then the child's dose is 11 mg.

(33/150) x 50 mg = 0.22 x 50 mg = 11 mg

Based on Age

Augsberger's Rule:

$\dfrac{[(4 \times \text{age [years]}) + 20]}{100} \times$ adult dose = approximate child's dose

Example: If the child's age is 8 years and the adult dose is 50 mg then the child's dose is 26 mg.
[(4 x 8) + 20)/100] x 50 mg = 0.52 X 50 mg = 26 mg

Dilling's Rule:

(age [years]/20) x adult dose = approximate child's dose

Example: If the child's age is 8 years and the adult dose is 50 mg then the child's dose is 20 mg.
(8/20) x 50 mg = 0.40 x 50 mg = 20 mg

Cowling's Rule:

$\dfrac{[\text{age at next birthday (years)}]}{24} \times$ adult dose = approximate child's dose

Example: If the child is going to turn 8 years old in few months and the adult dose is 50 mg then the child's dose is 16.7 mg. (8/24) x 50 mg = 0.33 x 50 mg = 16.7 mg

Younge's Rule:

$\dfrac{[\text{age (years)}]}{\text{age} + 12} \times$ adult dose = approximate child's dose

Example: If the child's age is 8 years and the adult dose is 50 mg then the child's dose is 20 mg.
[8/(8+12)] x 50 mg = 0.4 x 50 mg = 20 mg

Fried's Rule (younger than 1 year):

$\dfrac{[\text{age (months)}]}{150} \times$ adult dose = approximate infant's dose

Example: If the child's age is 10 months and the adult dose is 50 mg then the child's dose is 3.33 mg.
(10/150) x 50 mg = 0.067 x 50 mg = 3.33 mg

PEDIATRIC DOSAGE ESTIMATION FORMULAS

The following formulas can be used to estimate the approximate pediatric dosage of a medication. These formulas are based on the adult dose and either the child's age or weight. These formulas should be used with caution as the response to any drug is not always directly proportional to either the weight of the child, since the usual adult dose. Dosages will also vary based on the formula used. Care should be taken when using these formulas to calculate the child's dosage. Some products have FDA-approved pediatric doses and are recommended. Always refer to the prescribing information first before administering a pediatric dose.

BASED ON WEIGHT

Augsberger's Rule

$$\frac{(1.5 \times weight\ (kg) + 10) \times adult\ dose}{100} = approximate\ child's\ dose$$

Example: If the child's weight is 25 kg (55 lb) and the adult dose is 500 mg, then for this child, dose is 156.25 mg

$$\frac{(1.5 \times 25) + 10) \times 500\ mg}{100} = \frac{0.48 \times 50\ mg}{100} = 0.23\ mg$$

Clark's Rule

$$\frac{weight\ (lb)/150 \times adult\ dose}{} = approximate\ child's\ dose$$

Example: If the child's weight is 15.9 kg (35 lb) and the adult dose is 500 mg, then the child's dose is 117 mg

$$(35/150) \times 500\ mg = 0.23 \times 500\ mg = 117\ mg$$

Based on Age

Augsberger's Rule

$$\frac{(4 \times age\ (years) + 20) \times adult\ dose}{100} = approximate\ child's\ dose$$

Example: If the child's age is 8 years, and the adult dose is 500 mg, then for this child's dose is 26 mg

$$\frac{(4 \times 8) + 20) \times 50\ mg}{100} = \frac{0.52 \times 50\ mg}{100} = 26\ mg$$

Dilling's Rule

$$\frac{age\ (years)/20 \times adult\ dose}{} = approximate\ child's\ dose$$

Example: If the child's age is 8 years, and the adult dose is 50 mg, then the child's dose is 20 mg

$$(8/20) \times 50\ mg = 0.4 \times 50\ mg = 20\ mg$$

Cowling's Rule

$$\frac{age\ at\ next\ birthday\ (years) \times adult\ dose}{24} = approximate\ child's\ dose$$

Example: If the child is going to turn 8 years old in her months, and the adult dose is 50 mg, then the child's dose is 16.7 mg

$$\frac{8 \times 50\ mg}{24} = 0.33 \times 50\ mg = 16.7\ mg$$

Young's Rule

$$\frac{age\ (years)}{age\ (years) + 12} \times adult\ dose = approximate\ child's\ dose$$

Example: If the child's age is 8 years and the adult dose is 50 mg, then the child's dose is 20 mg

$$(8/(8+12)) \times 50\ mg = 0.4 \times 50\ mg = 20\ mg$$

Fried's Rule (infants < 1 year)

$$\frac{age\ (months) \times adult\ dose}{150} = approximate\ infant's\ dose$$

Example: If the infant is age 10 months and the adult dose is 50 mg, then the infant's child's dose is 3.33 mg

$$(10/150) \times 50\ mg = 0.07 \times 50\ mg = 3.35\ mg$$

DRUG INFORMATION CENTERS

ALABAMA

BIRMINGHAM

Drug Information Service
University of Alabama
UAB Hospital Pharmacy

Drug Information-JT1720
619 S. 19th St.
Birmingham, AL 35249-6860
Mon.-Fri. 7 AM-4 PM
      205-934-2162
www.health.uab.edu/pharmacy

Global Drug
Information Service
Samford University
McWhorter School
of Pharmacy

800 Lakeshore Dr.
Birmingham, AL 35229-7027
Mon. 8 AM-9 PM
Tues.-Fri. 8 AM-4:30 PM
      205-726-2519 or 2891
www.samford.edu/schools/
pharmacy/dic/index.html

HUNTSVILLE

Huntsville Hospital Drug
Information Center

101 Sivley Rd.
Huntsville, AL 35801
Mon.-Fri. 8 AM-4:30 PM
      256-265-8284

ARIZONA

TUCSON

Arizona Poison and Drug
Information Center

1259 N. Martin Ave.
Drachman Hall B308
Tucson, AZ 85724
7 days/week, 24 hours
      520-626-6016
      800-222-1222 **(Emergency)**
www.pharmacy.arizona.edu

ARKANSAS

LITTLE ROCK

Arkansas Drug Information Center

4301 W. Markham St.
Slot 522-2
Little Rock, AR 72205
Mon.-Fri. 8:30 AM-5 PM
      501-686-6161
      (Little Rock area only -
      for healthcare
      professionals only)
      888-228-1233
      (AR only - **for healthcare**
      professionals only)

CALIFORNIA

LOS ANGELES

Los Angeles Regional
Drug Information Center
LAC & USC Medical Center

1200 N. State St.
Trailer 25
Los Angeles, CA 90033
Mon.-Fri. 8 AM-4 PM
Closed 12 PM to 1 PM
      323-226-7741

SAN DIEGO

Drug Information Service
University of California
San Diego Medical Center

200 West Arbor Dr.
MC 8925
San Diego, CA 92103-8925
Mon.-Fri. 9 AM-5 PM
      619-543-6971
      (for healthcare
      professionals only)

STANFORD

Drug Information Center
University of California
Stanford Hospital and Clinics

300 Pasteur Dr.
Room H-0301
Stanford, CA 94305
Mon.-Fri. 8 AM-4 PM
      650-723-6422

COLORADO

DENVER

Rocky Mountain Poison
and Drug Center

990 Bannock St.
(Physical address)
777 Bannock St.
(Mailing address)
Denver, CO 80264
      303-739-1100
      800-222-1222 **(Emergency)**
www.rmpdc.org

CONNECTICUT

FARMINGTON

Drug Information Service
University of Connecticut
Health Center

263 Farmington Ave.
Farmington, CT 06030
Mon.-Fri. 10 AM-2 PM
      860-679-2783

HARTFORD

Drug Information Center
Hartford Hospital

PO Box 5037
80 Seymour St.
Hartford, CT 06102
Mon.-Fri. 8:30 AM-5 PM
      860-545-2221
      860-545-2961 (After 5 PM)
www.hartfordhospital.org

NEW HAVEN

Drug Information Center
Yale-New Haven Hospital

20 York St.
New Haven, CT 06540-3202
Mon.-Fri. 9 AM-5 PM
      203-688-2248
www.ynhh.org

DISTRICT OF COLUMBIA

Drug Information Service
Howard University Hospital

2041 Georgia Ave. NW
Room BB06
Washington, DC 20060
Mon.-Fri. 8:30 AM-4 PM
      202-865-7413
www.huhosp.org/patientpublic/
pharmacy.htm

FLORIDA

FT. LAUDERDALE

Nova Southeastern University
College of Pharmacy
Drug Information Center

3200 S. University Dr.
Ft. Lauderdale, FL 33328
Mon.-Fri. 9 AM-5 PM
      954-262-3103
http://pharmacy.nova.edu

GAINESVILLE

Drug Information &
Pharmacy Resource Center
Shands Hospital at
University of Florida

PO Box 100316
Gainesville, FL 32610-0316
Mon.-Fri. 9 AM-5 PM
      352-265-0408
      (for healthcare
      professionals only)
http://shands.org/professional/drugs

JACKSONVILLE

Drug Information Service Shands Jacksonville

655 W. 8th St.
Jacksonville, FL 32209
Mon.-Fri. 8:30 AM-5 PM
    904-244-4185
    (for healthcare professionals only)
Mon.-Fri. 9:30 AM-4 PM
    904-244-4700
    (for consumers)

http://jax.shands.org/
education/pharmacy/contact.asp

ORLANDO

Orlando Regional Drug Information Service Orlando Regional Healthcare System

1414 Kuhl Ave., MP 192
Orlando, FL 32806
Mon.-Fri. 8 AM-4 PM
    321-841-8717

TALLAHASSEE

Drug Information Education Center Florida Agricultural and Mechanical University College of Pharmacy and Pharmaceutical Sciences

Tallahassee, FL 32307
Mon.-Fri. 9 AM-5 PM
    850-561-2688

WEST PALM BEACH

Drug Information Center Nova Southeastern University, West Palm Beach

3970 RCA Blvd.
Suite 7006A
Palm Beach Gardens, FL 33410
Mon.-Fri. 9 AM-5 PM
    561-622-0658
    (for healthcare professionals only)

GEORGIA
ATLANTA

Emory University Hospital Dept. of Pharmaceutical Services-Drug Information

1364 Clifton Rd. NE
Atlanta, GA 30322
Mon.-Fri. 9 AM-4 PM
    404-712-4644
    (for healthcare professionals only)

Drug Information Service Northside Hospital

1000 Johnson Ferry Rd. NE
Atlanta, GA 30342
Mon.-Fri. 9 AM-4 PM
    404-851-8676 (GA only)

COLUMBUS

Columbus Regional Drug Information Center

710 Center St.
Columbus, GA 31902
Mon.-Fri. 8 AM-5 PM
    706-571-1934
    (for healthcare professionals only)

IDAHO
POCATELLO

Drug Information Center Idaho State University School of Pharmacy

970 S. 5th St.
Campus Box 8092
Pocatello, ID 83209
Mon.-Thur. 8:30 AM-5 PM
Fri. 8:30 AM-3 PM
    208-282-4689
    800-334-7139 (ID only)
http://pharmacy.isu.edu

ILLINOIS
CHICAGO

Drug Information Center Northwestern Memorial Hospital

Feinberg Pavilion, LC 700
251 E. Huron St.
Chicago, IL 60611
Mon.-Fri. 8:30 AM-5 PM
    312-926-7573

Drug Information Center University of Illinois at Chicago

833 S. Wood St.
MC 886
Chicago, IL 60612-7231
Mon.-Fri. 8 AM-4 PM
    312-996-3681
    (for healthcare professionals only)
Mon.-Fri. 9 AM-12 PM
    312-996-5332
    (for consumers)
www.uic.edu/pharmacy/
services/di/index.html

HARVEY

Drug Information Center Ingalls Memorial Hospital

1 Ingalls Dr.
Harvey, IL 60426
Mon.-Fri. 8 AM-7 PM

Sat. 9 AM-3:30 PM
    708-333-4300

HINES

Drug Information Service Hines Veterans Administration Hospital

Pharmacy Services
MC119
PO Box 5000
Hines, IL 60141-5000
Mon.-Fri. 8 AM-4:30 PM
    708-202-8387, ext. 23780

PARK RIDGE

Drug Information Center Advocate Lutheran General Hospital

1775 Dempster St.
Park Ridge, IL 60068
Mon.-Fri. 7:30 AM-4 PM
    847-723-8128
    (for healthcare professionals only)

INDIANA
INDIANAPOLIS

Drug Information Center St. Vincent Hospital and Health Services

2001 W. 86th St.
Indianapolis, IN 46260
Mon.-Fri. 8 AM-4 PM
    317-338-3200
    (for healthcare professionals only)

Drug Information Service Clarian Health Partners

Pharmacy Department I-65
at 21st St.
Room CG04
Indianapolis, IN 46202
Mon.-Fri. 8 AM-4:30 PM
    317-962-1750

MUNCIE

Drug Information Center Ball Memorial Hospital

2401 University Ave.
Muncie, IN 47303
Mon.-Fri. 8 AM-4:30 PM
    765-747-3033

IOWA
DES MOINES

Regional Drug Information Center Mercy Medical Center-Des Moines

1111 Sixth Ave.
Des Moines, IA 50314
Mon.-Fri. 8 AM-4:30 PM
    515-247-3286
    (regional service; in-house service answered 7 days/ week, 24 hours)

IOWA CITY

Drug Information Center
University of Iowa
Hospitals and Clinics

200 Hawkins Dr.
Iowa City, IA 52242
Mon.-Fri. 8 AM-4:30 PM
319-356-2600

KANSAS

KANSAS CITY

Drug Information Center
University of Kansas
Medical Center

3901 Rainbow Blvd.
Kansas City, KS 66160
Mon.-Fri. 8:30 AM-4:30 PM
913-588-2328

KENTUCKY

LEXINGTON

University of Kentucky
Central Pharmacy
Chandler Medical Center

800 Rose St.
C-114
Lexington, KY 40536-0293
7 days/week, 24 hours
859-323-5642
859-323-6289

LOUISIANA

MONROE

Louisiana Drug and Poison
Information Center
University of Louisiana at Monroe
College of Pharmacy

Sugar Hall
Monroe, LA 71209-6430
Mon.-Thur. 8 AM-4:30 PM
Fri. 8 AM-11:30 AM
318-342-1710

NEW ORLEANS

Xavier University Drug
Information Center
Tulane University
Hospital and Clinic

1440 Canal St.
Suite 808
New Orleans, LA 70112
Mon.-Fri. 9 AM-5 PM
504-588-5670

MARYLAND

ANDREWS AFB

Drug Information Services

79 MDSS/SGQP
1050 W. Perimeter Rd.
Suite D1-119
Andrews AFB, MD 20762-6660
Mon.-Fri. 7:30 AM-5 PM
240-857-4565

BALTIMORE

Drug Information Service
Johns Hopkins Hospital

600 N. Wolfe St.
Carnegie 180
Baltimore, MD 21287-6180
Mon.-Fri. 8:30 AM-5 PM
410-955-6348

Drug Information Service
University of Maryland

School of Pharmacy
Hall Room 760
20 North Pine St.
Baltimore, MD 21201
Mon.-Fri. 8:30 AM-5 PM
410-706-7568
(consumers only)
410-706-0898
(for healthcare
professionals only)
www.pharmacy.umaryland.
edu/umdi

EASTON

Drug Information
Pharmacy Dept.
Memorial Hospital

219 S. Washington St.
Easton, MD 21601
7 days/week, 7 AM-5:30 PM
410-822-1000, ext. 5645

MASSACHUSETTS

BOSTON

Drug Information Services
Brigham and Women's Hospital

75 Francis St.
Boston, MA 02115
Mon.-Fri. 7 AM-3 PM
617-732-7166

WORCESTER

Drug Information Pharmacy
UMass Memorial
Medical Center
Healthcare Hospital

55 Lake Ave. North
Worcester, MA 01655
Mon.-Fri. 8:30 AM-5 PM
508-856-3456
508-856-2775 (24-hour)

MICHIGAN

ANN ARBOR

Drug Information Service Dept. of
Pharmacy Services
University of Michigan
Health System

1500 East Medical Center Dr.
UH B2D301
Box 0008
Ann Arbor, MI 48109-0008
Mon.-Fri. 8 AM-5 PM
734-936-8200

DETROIT

Drug Information Center
Dept. of Pharmacy Services
Detroit Receiving Hospital and
University Health Center

4201 St. Antoine Blvd.
Detroit, MI 48201
Mon.-Fri. 9 AM-5 PM
313-745-4556
www.dmcpharmacy.org

LANSING

Drug Information Services
Sparrow Hospital

1215 East Michigan Ave.
Lansing, MI 48912
7 days/week, 24 hours
517-364-2444

PONTIAC

Drug Information Center
St. Joseph Mercy Oakland

44405 Woodward Ave.
Pontiac, MI 48341
Mon.-Fri. 8 AM-4:30 PM
248-858-3055

ROYAL OAK

Drug Information Services
William Beaumont Hospital

3601 West 13 Mile Rd.
Royal Oak, MI 48073-6769
Mon.-Fri. 8 AM-4:30 PM
248-898-4077

SOUTHFIELD

Drug Information Service
Providence Hospital

16001 West 9 Mile Rd.
Southfield, MI 48075
Mon.-Fri. 8 AM-4 PM
248-849-3125

MISSISSIPPI

JACKSON

Drug Information Center
University of Mississippi
Medical Center

2500 N. State St.
Jackson, MS 39216
Mon.-Fri. 8 AM-4:30 PM
601-984-2060

MISSOURI

KANSAS CITY

University of Missouri-Kansas City
Drug Information Center

2464 Charlotte St.
Suite 1220
Kansas City, MO 64108
Mon.-Fri. 9 AM-4 PM
816-235-5490
http://druginfo.umkc.edu/

SPRINGFIELD

Drug Information Center
St. John's Hospital

1235 E. Cherokee St.
Springfield, MO 65804
Mon.-Fri. 8 AM-4:30 PM
417-820-3488

ST. JOSEPH

Regional Medical Center Pharmacy

5325 Faraon St.
St. Joseph, MO 64506
7 days/week, 24 hours
816-271-6141

MONTANA

MISSOULA

Drug Information Service
University of Montana School of
Pharmacy and Allied Health
Sciences

32 Campus Dr.
1522 Skaggs Bldg.
Missoula, MT 59812-1522
Mon.-Fri. 8 AM-5 PM
406-243-5254
800-501-5491
www.health.umt.edu/dis

NEBRASKA

OMAHA

Drug Informatics Service
School of Pharmacy
Creighton University

2500 California Plaza
Health Science Library
Room 204
Omaha, NE 68178
Mon.-Fri. 8:30 AM-4:30 PM
402-280-5101
http://druginfo.creighton.edu

NEW JERSEY

NEWARK

New Jersey Poison Information and
Education System

140 Bergen St.
Newark, NJ 07107
Mon.-Fri. 8 AM- 5 PM
973-972-9280
800-222-1222 **(Emergency)**
www.njpies.org

NEW BRUNSWICK

Drug Information Service
Robert Wood Johnson
University Hospital

Pharmacy Department
1 Robert Wood Johnson Pl.
New Brunswick, NJ 08901
Mon.-Fri. 8:30 AM-4:30 PM
732-937-8842

NEW MEXICO

ALBUQUERQUE

New Mexico Poison Center
University of New Mexico
Health Sciences Center

MSC09 5080
1 University of New Mexico
Albuquerque, NM 87131
7 days/week, 24 hours
505-272-4261
800-222-1222 **(Emergency)**
http://hsc.unm.edu/pharmacy/
poison

NEW YORK

BROOKLYN

International Drug
Information Center
Long Island University
Arnold & Marie Schwartz
College of Pharmacy &
Health Sciences

75 DeKalb Ave.
RM-HS509
Brooklyn, NY 11201
Mon.-Fri. 9 AM-5 PM
718-488-1064
www.liu.edu

NEW HYDE PARK

Drug Information Center
St. John's University at Long
Island Jewish Medical Center

270-05 76th Ave.
New Hyde Park, NY 11040
Mon.-Fri. 8 AM-3 PM
718-470-DRUG (3784)

NEW YORK CITY

Drug Information Center
Memorial Sloan-Kettering
Cancer Center

1275 York Ave.
RM S-702
New York, NY 10021
Mon.-Fri. 9 AM-5 PM
212-639-7552

Drug Information Center
Mount Sinai Medical Center

1 Gustave Levy Pl.
New York, NY 10029
Mon.-Fri. 9 AM-5 PM
212-241-6619
(for in-house healthcare
professionals only)

ROCHESTER

Finger Lakes
Poison and Drug
Information Center
University of Rochester

601 Elmwood Ave.
Rochester, NY 14642
Mon.-Fri. 8 AM-5 PM
585-275-3718

NORTH CAROLINA

BUIES CREEK

Drug Information Center
School of Pharmacy
Campbell University

PO Box 1090
Buies Creek, NC 27506
Mon.-Fri. 8:30 AM-4:30 PM
910-893-1200,
ext. 2701
800-760-9697 (Toll free),
ext. 2701
800-327-5467 (NC only)

CHAPEL HILL

University of North
Carolina Hospitals
Drug Information Center
Dept. of Pharmacy

101 Manning Dr.
Chapel Hill, NC 27514
Mon.-Fri. 8 AM-4:30 PM
919-966-2373

DURHAM

Drug Information Center
Duke University Health
Systems

DUMC Box 3089
Durham, NC 27710
Mon.-Fri. 8 AM-5 PM
919-684-5125

GREENVILLE

Eastern Carolina Drug
Information Center
Pitt County
Memorial Hospital
Dept. of Pharmacy Service

PO Box 6028
2100 Stantonsburg Rd.
Greenville, NC 27835
Mon.-Fri. 8 AM-5 PM
252-847-4257

WINSTON-SALEM

Drug Information
Service Center
Wake-Forest University
Baptist Medical Center

Medical Center Blvd.
Winston-Salem, NC 27157
Mon.-Fri. 8 AM-5 PM
336-716-2037
(for healthcare
professionals only)

OHIO

ADA

**Drug Information Center
Raabe College of Pharmacy
Ohio Northern University**

Ada, OH 45810
Mon.-Thurs. 8:30 AM-5 PM
Fri. 8:30 AM-4 PM
419-772-2307
www.onu.edu/pharmacy/druginfo

CINCINNATI

**Drug and Poison
Information Center
Children's Hospital
Medical Center**

3333 Burnet Ave.
Cincinnati, OH 45229
Mon.-Fri. 9 AM-5 PM
513-636-5063
(administration)
513-636-5111
(7 days/week, 24 hours)

CLEVELAND

**Drug Information Service
Cleveland Clinic Foundation**

9500 Euclid Ave.
Cleveland, OH 44195
Mon.-Fri. 8:30 AM-4:30 PM
216-444-6456
(for healthcare
professionals only)

Columbus

**Drug Information Center
Ohio State University Hospital
Dept. of Pharmacy**

Doan Hall 368
410 W. 10th Ave.
Columbus, OH 43210-1228
Mon.-Fri. 8 AM-4:30 PM
614-293-8679
(for in-house healthcare
professionals only)

**Drug Information Center
Riverside Methodist Hospital**

3535 Olentangy River Road
Columbus, OH 43214
7 days/week, 24 hours
614-566-5425

TOLEDO

**Drug Information Services
St. Vincent Mercy Medical Center**

2213 Cherry St.
Toledo, OH 43608-2691
Mon.-Fri. 7 AM-5 PM
419-251-4227
www.rx.medctr.ohio-state.edu

OKLAHOMA

OKLAHOMA CITY

**Drug Information Service
Integris Health**

3300 Northwest Expressway
Oklahoma City, OK 73112
Mon.-Fri. 8 AM-4:30 PM
405-949-3660

**Drug Information Center
OU Medical Center**

1200 Everett Dr.
Oklahoma City, OK 73104
Mon.-Fri. 8 AM-4:30 PM
405-271-6226
Fax: 405-271-6281

TULSA

**Drug Information Center
Saint Francis Hospital**

6161 S. Yale Ave.
Tulsa, OK 74136
Mon.-Fri. 8 AM-4:30 PM
918-494-6339
(for healthcare
professionals only)

PENNSYLVANIA

PHILADELPHIA

**Drug Information Center
Temple University Hospital
Dept. of Pharmacy**

3401 N. Broad St.
Philadelphia, PA 19140
Mon.-Fri. 8 AM-4:30 PM
215-707-4644

**Drug Information Service
Dept. of Pharmacy
Thomas Jefferson
University Hospital**

111 S. 11th St.
Philadelphia, PA 19107-5089
Mon.-Fri. 8 AM-5 PM
215-955-8877

**University of Pennsylvania
Health System Drug Information
Service Hospital of the University
of Pennsylvania
Dept. of Pharmacy**

3400 Spruce St.
Philadelphia, PA 19104
Mon.-Fri. 8:30 AM-4 PM
215-662-2903

PITTSBURGH

**Pharmaceutical
Information Center
Mylan School of Pharmacy
Duquesne University**

431 Mellon Hall
Pittsburgh, PA 15282
Mon.-Fri. 8 AM-4 PM
412-396-4600

UPLAND

**Drug Information Center
Crozer-Chester Medical Center
Dept. of Pharmacy**

1 Medical Center Blvd.
Upland, PA 19013
Mon.-Fri. 8 AM-4:30 PM
610-447-2851
(for in-house healthcare
professionals only)

PUERTO RICO

PONCE

**Centro Informacion
Medicamentos
Escuela de Medicina de Ponce**

PO Box 7004
Ponce, PR 00732-7004
Mon.-Fri. 8 AM-4:30 PM
787-840-2575

SAN JUAN

**Centro de Informacion de
Medicamentos-CIM
Escuela de Farmacia-RCM**

PO Box 365067
San Juan, PR 00936-5067
Mon.-Fri. 8 AM-4:30 PM
787-758-2525, ext. 1516

SOUTH CAROLINA

CHARLESTON

**Drug Information Service
Medical University of
South Carolina**

150 Ashley Ave.
Rutledge Tower Annex
Room 604
PO Box 250584
Charleston, SC 29425-0810
Mon.-Fri. 9 AM-5:30 PM
843-792-3896
800-922-5250

SPARTANBURG

**Drug Information Center
Spartanburg Regional
Healthcare System**

101 E. Wood St.
Spartanburg, SC 29303
Mon.-Fri. 8 AM-4:30 PM
864-560-6910

TENNESSEE

KNOXVILLE

**Drug Information Center
University of Tennessee
Medical Center at Knoxville**

1924 Alcoa Highway
Knoxville, TN 37920-6999
Mon.-Fri. 8 AM-4:30 PM
865-544-9124

MEMPHIS

**South East Regional Drug
Information Center
VA Medical Center**

1030 Jefferson Ave.
Memphis, TN 38104
Mon.-Fri. 6:30 AM-4 PM
901-523-8990, ext. 6720

**Drug Information Center
University of Tennessee**

875 Monroe Ave.
Suite 109
Memphis, TN 38163
Mon.-Fri. 8 AM-5 PM
901-448-5556

TEXAS
AMARILLO

**Drug Information Center
Texas Tech Health
Sciences Center**

School of Pharmacy
1300 Coulter Rd.
Amarillo, TX 79106
Mon.-Fri. 8 AM-5 PM
806-356-4008

GALVESTON

**Drug Information Center
University of Texas
Medical Branch**

301 University Blvd.
Galveston, TX 77555-0701
Mon.-Fri. 8 AM-5 PM
409-772-2734

HOUSTON

**Drug Information Center
Ben Taub General Hospital
Texas Southern University/HCHD**

1504 Taub Loop
Houston, TX 77030
Mon.-Fri. 8:30 AM-5 PM
713-873-3710

LACKLAND A.F.B.

**Drug Information Center
Dept. of Pharmacy
Wilford Hall Medical Center**

2200 Bergquist Dr.
Suite 1
Lackland A.F.B., TX 78236
7 days/week, 24 hours
210-292-5414

LUBBOCK

**Drug Information and Consultation
Service
Covenant Medical Center**

3615 19th St.
Lubbock, TX 79410
7 days/week, 24 hours
806-725-0408

SAN ANTONIO

**Drug Information Service
University of Texas Health Science
Center at San Antonio
Dept. of Pharmacology**

7703 Floyd Curl Drive
San Antonio, TX 78229-3900
Mon.-Fri. 8 AM-4 PM
210-567-4280

TEMPLE

**Drug Information Center
Scott and White Memorial Hospital**

2401 S. 31st St.
Temple, TX 76508
Mon.-Fri. 8 AM-5 PM
254-724-4636

UTAH
SALT LAKE CITY

**Drug Information Service
University of Utah Hospital**

421 Wakara Way
Suite 204
Salt Lake City, UT 84108
Mon.-Fri. 7:30 AM-5 PM
801-581-2073

VIRGINIA
HAMPTON

**Drug Information Center
Hampton University School
of Pharmacy**

Hampton Harbors Annex
Hampton, VA 23668
Mon.-Fri. 9 AM-4 PM
757-728-6693

WEST VIRGINIA
MORGANTOWN

**West Virginia Center for
Drug and Health Information
West Virginia University
Robert C. Byrd
Health Sciences Center**

1124 HSN, PO Box 9520
Morgantown, WV 26506
Mon.-Fri. 8:30 AM-5 PM
304-293-6640
800-352-2501 (WV)
www.hsc.wvu.edu/SOP

WYOMING
LARAMIE

**Drug Information Center
University of Wyoming**

1000 East University Ave.
Dept. 3375
Laramie, WY 82071
Mon.-Fri. 8:30 AM-4:30 PM
307-766-6988

POISON CONTROL CENTERS

The American Association of Poison Control Centers (AAPCC) uses a single, nationwide emergency number to automatically link callers with their regional poison center. This toll-free number, **800-222-1222**, also works for **teletype lines (TTY)** for the hearing-impaired and **telecommunication devices (TTD)** for individuals who are deaf. However, a few local poison centers and the ASPCA/Animal Poison Control Center are not part of this nationwide system and continue to use separate numbers.

Most of the centers listed below are certified by the AAPCC. Certified centers are marked by an asterisk after the name. Each has to meet certain criteria. It must, for example, serve a large geographic area; it must be open 24 hours a day and provide direct-dial or toll-free access; it must be supervised by a medical director; and it must have registered pharmacists or nurses available to answer questions from the public.

Within each state, centers are listed alphabetically by city. Some state poison centers also list their original emergency numbers (including TTY/TDD), which only work within that state. For these listings, callers may use either the state number or the nationwide 800 number.

ALABAMA

BIRMINGHAM

Regional Poison Control Center, The Children's Hospital of Alabama (*)

1600 7th Ave. South
Birmingham, AL 35233-1711
Business: 205-939-9201
Emergency: 800-222-1222
www.chsys.org

TUSCALOOSA

Alabama Poison Center (*)

2503 Phoenix Dr.
Tuscaloosa, AL 35405
Business: 205-345-0600
Emergency: 800-222-1222
                    800-462-0800 (AL)
www.alapoisoncenter.org

ALASKA

JUNEAU

Alaska Poison Control System

Section of Community
Health and EMS
410 Willoughby Ave.
Room 103
Box 110616
Juneau, AK 99811-0616
Business: 907-465-3027
Emergency: 800-222-1222
www.chems.alaska.gov

(PORTLAND, OR)

Oregon Poison Center (*)
Oregon Health Sciences University

3181 SW Sam Jackson Park Rd.
CB550
Portland, OR 97239
Business: 503-494-8968
Emergency: 800-222-1222
www.oregonpoison.com

ARIZONA

PHOENIX

Banner Poison Control Center (*)
Banner Good Samaritan
Medical Center

901 E. Willetta St.
Room 2701
Phoenix, AZ 85006
Business: 602-495-4884
Emergency: 800-222-1222
www.bannerpoisoncontrol.com

TUCSON

Arizona Poison and Drug Information Center

1295 N. Martin Ave.
Drachman Hall B308
Tucson, AZ 85724
Business: 520-626-7899
Emergency: 800-222-1222

ARKANSAS

LITTLE ROCK

Arkansas Poison and Drug Information Center College of Pharmacy - UAMS

4301 West Markham St.
Mail Slot 522-2
Little Rock, AR 72205-7122
Business: 501-686-6161
Emergency: 800-222-1222
                    800-376-4766 (AR)
TDD/TTY: 800-641-3805

ASPCA/Animal Poison Control Center

1717 South Philo Rd.
Suite 36
Urbana, IL 61802
Business: 217-337-5030
Emergency: 888-426-4435
                    800-548-2423
www.napcc.aspca.org

CALIFORNIA

FRESNO/MADERA

California Poison Control System-Fresno/Madera Div. (*)
Children's Hospital of Central California

9300 Valley Children's Place
MB 15
Madera, CA 93638-8762
Business: 559-622-2300
Emergency: 800-222-1222
                    800-876-4766 (CA)
TDD/TTY: 800-972-3323
www.calpoison.org

SACRAMENTO

California Poison Control System-Sacramento Div.(*)
UC Davis Medical Center

Room HSF 1024
2315 Stockton Blvd.
Sacramento, CA 95817
Business: 916-227-1400
Emergency: 800-222-1222
                    800-876-4766 (CA)
TDD/TTY: 800-972-3323
www.calpoison.org

SAN DIEGO

California Poison Control System-San Diego Div. (*)
UC San Diego Medical Center

200 West Arbor Dr.
San Diego, CA 92103-8925
Business: 858-715-6300
Emergency: 800-222-1222
                    800-876-4766 (CA)
TDD/TTY: 800-972-3323
www.calpoison.org

SAN FRANCISCO

California Poison Control System-San Francisco Div. (*)
San Francisco General Hospital
University of California
San Francisco

Box 1369
San Francisco, CA 94143-1369
Business: 415-502-6000
Emergency: 800-222-1222
                    800-876-4766 (CA)
TDD/TTY: 800-972-3323
www.calpoison.org

COLORADO

DENVER

Rocky Mountain Poison and Drug Center (*)

777 Bannock St.
Mail Code 0180
Denver, CO 80204-4507
Business: 303-739-1100
Emergency: 800-222-1222
TDD/TTY: 303-739-1127 (CO)
www.RMPDC.org

CONNECTICUT

FARMINGTON

Connecticut Regional Poison Control Center (*)
University of Connecticut Health Center

263 Farmington Ave.
Farmington, CT 06030-5365
Business: 860-679-4540
Emergency: 800-222-1222
TDD/TTY: 866-218-5372
http://poisoncontrol.uchc.edu

DELAWARE

(PHILADELPHIA, PA)

The Poison Control Center (*)
Children's Hospital of Philadelphia

34th St. & Civic Center Blvd.
Philadelphia, PA 19104-4303
Business: 215-590-2003
Emergency: 800-222-1222
TDD/TTY: 215-590-8789
www.poisoncontrol.chop.edu

DISTRICT OF COLUMBIA

WASHINGTON, DC

National Capital Poison Center (*)

3201 New Mexico Ave., NW
Suite 310
Washington, DC 20016
Business: 202-362-3867
Emergency: 800-222-1222
www.poison.org

FLORIDA

JACKSONVILLE

Florida Poison Information Center-Jacksonville (*)
SHANDS Hospital

655 West 8th St.
Jacksonville, FL 32209
Business: 904-244-4465
Emergency: 800-222-1222
http://fpicjax.org

MIAMI

Florida Poison Information Center-Miami (*)
University of Miami–Department of Pediatrics

PO Box 016960 (R-131)
Miami, FL 33101
Business: 305-585-5250
Emergency: 800-222-1222
www.miami.edu/poison-center

TAMPA

Florida Poison Information Center-Tampa (*)
Tampa General Hospital

PO Box 1289
Tampa, FL 33601-1289
Business: 813-844-7044
Emergency: 800-222-1222
www.poisoncentertampa.org

GEORGIA

ATLANTA

Georgia Poison Center (*)
Hughes Spalding Children's Hospital, Grady Health System

80 Jesse Hill Jr. Dr., SE
PO Box 26066
Atlanta, GA 30303-3050
Business: 404-616-9237
Emergency: 800-222-1222
               404-616-9000
               (Atlanta)
TDD: 404-616-9287
www.georgiapoisoncenter.org

HAWAII

(DENVER, CO)

Rocky Mountain Poison and Drug Center (*)

777 Bannock St.
Mail Code 0180
Denver, CO 80204-4507
Business: 303-739-1100
Emergency: 800-222-1222
www.RMPDC.org

IDAHO

(DENVER, CO)

Rocky Mountain Poison and Drug Center (*)

777 Bannock St.
Mail Code 0180
Denver, CO 80204-4507
Business: 303-739-1100
Emergency: 800-222-1222
www.RMPDC.org

ILLINOIS

CHICAGO

Illinois Poison Center (*)

222 South Riverside Plaza
Suite 1900
Chicago, IL 60606
Business: 312-906-6136
Emergency: 800-222-1222
TDD/TTY: 312-906-6185
www.illinoispoisoncenter.org

INDIANA

INDIANAPOLIS

Indiana Poison Control Center (*)
Clarian Health Partners Methodist Hospital

I-65 at 21st St.
Indianapolis, IN 46206-1367
Business: 317-962-2335
Emergency: 800-222-1222
               800-382-9097
               317-962-2323
               (Indianapolis)
TTY: 317-962-2336
www.clarian.org/poisoncontrol

IOWA

SIOUX CITY

Iowa Statewide Poison Control Center Iowa Health System and the University of Iowa Hospitals and Clinics

401 Douglas St.
Suite 402
Sioux City, IA 51101
Business: 712-279-3710
Emergency: 800-222-1222
               712-277-2222 (IA)
www.iowapoison.org

KANSAS

KANSAS CITY

University of Kansas Poison Control Medical Center

3901 Rainbow Blvd.
Room B-400
Kansas City, KS 66160-7231
Business   913-588-6638
Emergency: 800-222-1222
               800-332-6633 (KS)
TDD: 913-588-6639
www.kumc.com/bodyside.cmf?2144

KENTUCKY

LOUISVILLE

**Kentucky Regional
Poison Center (*)**

PO Box 35070
Louisville, KY 40232-5070
Business: 502-629-7264
Emergency: 800-222-1222
www.krpc.com

LOUISIANA

MONROE

**Louisiana Drug and Poison
Information Center (*)
University of Louisiana at Monroe**

700 University Ave.
Monroe, LA 71209-6430
Business: 318-342-3648
Emergency: 800-222-1222
          800-256-9822
          (LA only)

www.lapcc.org

MAINE

PORTLAND

**Northern New England
Poison Center**

Maine Medical Center
22 Bramhall St.
Portland, ME 04102
Business: 207-662-0111
Emergency: 800-222-1222
          207-871-2879 (ME)
TDD/TTY: 207-662-4900 (ME)
www.nnepc.org

MARYLAND

BALTIMORE

**Maryland Poison Center (*)
University of Maryland at Baltimore
School of Pharmacy**

220 Arch St.
Office Level 1
Baltimore, MD 21201
Business: 410-706-7604
Emergency: 800-222-1222
TDD: 410-706-1858
www.mdpoison.com

(WASHINGTON, DC)

**National Capital
Poison Center (*)**

3201 New Mexico Ave., NW
Suite 310
Washington DC 20016
Business: 202-362-3867
Emergency: 800-222-1222
TDD/TTY: 202-362-8563 (MD)
www.poison.org

MASSACHUSETTS

BOSTON

**Regional Center for Poison Control
and Prevention (*)
(Serving Massachusetts and Rhode
Island)**

300 Longwood Ave.
Boston, MA 02115
Business: 617-355-6609
Emergency: 800-222-1222
TDD/TTY: 888-244-5313
www.maripoisoncenter.com

MICHIGAN

DETROIT

**Regional Poison
Control Center (*)
Children's Hospital of Michigan**

4160 John R. Harper
  Professional Office Bldg.
Suite 616
Detroit, MI 48201
Business: 313-745-5335
Emergency: 800-222-1222
TDD/TTY: 800-356-3232
www.mitoxic.org/pcc

GRAND RAPIDS

**DeVos Children's Hospital
Regional Poison Center (*)**

100 Michigan St., NE
Grand Rapids, MI 49503
Business: 616-391-3690
Emergency: 800-222-1222
http://poisoncenter.
    devoschildrens.org

MINNESOTA

MINNEAPOLIS

**Minnesota Poison Control System
(*) Hennepin County Medical Center**

701 Park Ave.
Mail Code RL
Minneapolis, MN 55415
Business: 612-873-3144
Emergency: 800-222-1222
www.mnpoison.org

MISSISSIPPI

JACKSON

**Mississippi Regional Poison Control
Center, University of Mississippi
Medical Center**

2500 North State St.
Jackson, MS 39216
Business: 601-984-1680
Emergency: 800-222-1222

MISSOURI

ST. LOUIS

**Missouri Regional
Poison Center (*)
Cardinal Glennon
Children's Hospital**

7980 Clayton Rd.
Suite 200
St. Louis, MO 63117
Business: 314-772-5200
Emergency: 800-222-1222
TDD/TTY: 314-612-5705
www.cardinalglennon.com

MONTANA

(DENVER, CO)

**Rocky Mountain Poison
and Drug Center (*)**

777 Bannock St.
Mail Code 0180
Denver, CO 80204-4507
Business: 303-739-1100
Emergency: 800-222-1222
TDD/TTY: 303-739-1127
www.RMPDC.org

NEBRASKA

OMAHA

**The Poison Center (*)
Children's Hospital**

8401 W. Dodge St.
Suite 115
Omaha, NE 68114
Business: 402-955-5555
Emergency: 800-222-1222
www.nebraskapoison.com

NEVADA

(DENVER, CO)

**Rocky Mountain Poison
and Drug Center (*)**

777 Bannock St.
Mail Code 0180
Denver, CO 80204-4507
Business: 303-739-1100
Emergency: 800-222-1222
www.RMPDC.org

(PORTLAND, OR)

**Oregon Poison Center (*)
Oregon Health
Sciences University**

3181 SW Sam Jackson Park Rd.
Portland, OR 97201
Business: 503-494-8600
Emergency: 800-222-1222
www.oregonpoison.com

NEW HAMPSHIRE
(PORTLAND, ME)

**Northern New England
Poison Center**

Maine Medical Center
22 Bramhall St.
Portland, ME 04102
Business: 207-662-0111
Emergency: 800-222-1222
www.nnepc.org

NEW JERSEY
NEWARK

**New Jersey Poison Information and
Education System (*)
UMDNJ**

65 Bergen St.
Newark, NJ 07101
Business: 973-972-9280
Emergency: 800-222-1222
TDD/TTY: 973-926-8008
www.njpies.org

NEW MEXICO
ALBUQUERQUE

**New Mexico Poison and
Drug Information Center (*)**

MSC09-5080
1 University of New Mexico
Albuquerque, NM 87131-0001
Business: 505-272-4261
Emergency: 800-222-1222
http://HSC.UNM.edu/pharmacy/
poison

NEW YORK
BUFFALO

**Western New York Regional Poison
Control Center (*) Children's
Hospital of Buffalo**

219 Bryant St.
Buffalo, NY 14222
Business: 716-878-7654
Emergency: 800-222-1222
www.fingerlakespoison.org

MINEOLA

**Long Island Regional Poison
and Drug Information Center (*)
Winthrop University Hospital**

259 First St.
Mineola, NY 11501
Business: 516-663-2650
Emergency: 800-222-1222
TDD: 516-747-3323
                 (Nassau)
                 631-924-8811
                 (Suffolk)
www.lirpdic.org

NEW YORK CITY

**New York City
Poison Control Center (*)
NYC Dept. of Health**

455 First Ave.
Room 123
New York, NY 10016
Business: 212-447-8152
Emergency: 800-222-1222
(English)   212-340-4494
                 212-POISONS
                 (212-764-7667)
Emergency: 212-venenos
(Spanish)   (212-836-3667)
TDD: 212-689-9014

ROCHESTER

**Finger Lakes Regional Poison and
Drug Information Center(*)
University of Rochester
Medical Center**

601 Elmwood Ave.
Box 321
Rochester, NY 14642
Business: 585-273-4155
Emergency: 800-222-1222
TTY: 585-273-3854

SYRACUSE

**Central New York
Poison Center (*)
SUNY Upstate Medical University**

750 East Adams St.
Syracuse, NY 13210
Business: 315-464-7078
Emergency: 800-222-1222
www.cnypoison.org

NORTH CAROLINA
CHARLOTTE

**Carolinas Poison Center (*)
Carolinas Medical Center**

PO Box 32861
Charlotte, NC 28232
Business: 704-512-3795
Emergency: 800-222-1222
www.ncpoisoncenter.org

NORTH DAKOTA
BISMARK

**ND Department of Health
Injury Prevention Program**

600 E. Boulevard Ave.
Bismark, ND 58505
Business: 612-873-3144
Emergency: 800-222-1222
www.ndpoison.org

OHIO
CINCINNATI

**Cincinnati Drug and Poison
Information Center (*)
Regional Poison Control System**

3333 Burnet Ave.
Vernon Place, 3rd Floor
Cincinnati, OH 45229
                 513-636-5063
Emergency: 800-222-1222
TDD/TTY: 800-253-7955
www.cincinnatichildrens.org/dpic

CLEVELAND

**Greater Cleveland
Poison Control Center**

11100 Euclid Ave.
MP 6007
Cleveland, OH 44106-6007
Business: 216-844-1573
Emergency: 800-222-1222
                 216-231-4455 (OH)

COLUMBUS

Central Ohio Poison Center (*)

700 Children's Dr.
Room L032
Columbus, OH 43205-2696
Business: 614-722-2635
Emergency: 800-222-1222
TTY: 614-228-2272
www.bepoisonsmart.com

OKLAHOMA
OKLAHOMA CITY

**Oklahoma Poison
Control Center (*)
Children's Hospital at OU Medical
Center**

940 Northeast 13th St.
Room 3510
Oklahoma City, OK 73104
Business: 405-271-5062
Emergency: 800-222-1222
www.oklahomapoison.org

OREGON
PORTLAND

**Oregon Poison Center (*)
Oregon Health Sciences University**

3181 S.W. Sam Jackson Park Rd.,
CB550
Portland, OR 97239
Business: 503-494-8968
Emergency: 800-222-1222
www.ohsu.edu/poison

PENNSYLVANIA

PHILADELPHIA

The Poison Control Center (*)
Children's Hospital of Philadelphia

34th Street & Civic Center Blvd.
Philadelphia, PA 19104-4399
Business: 215-590-2003
Emergency: 800-222-1222
               215-386-2100 (PA)
TDD/TTY: 215-590-8789
www.poisoncontrol.chop.edu

PITTSBURGH

Pittsburgh Poison Center (*)
Children's Hospital of Pittsburgh

3705 Fifth Ave.
Pittsburgh, PA 15213
Business: 412-390-3300
Emergency: 800-222-1222
               412-681-6669
www.chp.edu/clinical/03a_
   poison.php

RHODE ISLAND

(BOSTON, MA)

Regional Center for Poison Control
and Prevention (*)

(Serving Massachusetts and Rhode
Island)

300 Longwood Ave.
Boston, MA 02115
Business: 617-355-6609
Emergency: 800-222-1222
TDD/TTY: 888-244-5313
www.maripoisoncenter.com

SOUTH DAKOTA

(MINNEAPOLIS, MN)

Hennepin Regional Poison Center
(*) Hennepin County Medical Center

701 Park Ave.
Minneapolis, MN 55415
Business: 612-873-3144
Emergency: 800-222-1222
www.mnpoison.org

SIOUX FALLS

Provides education only—Does not
manage exposure cases.

Sioux Valley Poison Control
Center (*)

1305 W. 18th St.
Box 5039
Sioux Falls, SD 57117-5039
Business: 605-328-6670
www.sdpoison.org

TENNESSEE

NASHVILLE

Tennessee
Poison Center (*)

1161 21st Ave. South
501 Oxford House
Nashville, TN 37232-4632
Business: 615-936-0760
Emergency: 800-222-1222
www.poisonlifeline.org

TEXAS

AMARILLO

Texas Panhandle
Poison Center (*)
Northwest Texas Hospital

1501 S. Coulter Dr.
Amarillo, TX 79106
Business: 806-354-1630
Emergency: 800-222-1222
www.poisoncontrol.org

DALLAS

North Texas Poison Center (*)
Texas Poison Center Network
Parkland Health and Hospital
System

5201 Harry Hines Blvd.
Dallas, TX 75235
Business: 214-589-0911
Emergency: 800-222-1222
www.poisoncontrol.org

EL PASO

West Texas Regional
Poison Center (*)
Thomason Hospital

4815 Alameda Ave.
El Paso, TX 79905
Business   915-534-3800
Emergency: 800-222-1222
www.poisoncontrol.org

GALVESTON

Southeast Texas
Poison Center (*)
The University of Texas
Medical Branch

3.112 Trauma Bldg.
301 University Blvd.
Galveston, TX 77555-1175
Business: 409-772-9142
Emergency: 800-222-1222
www.poisoncontrol.org

SAN ANTONIO

South Texas Poison Center (*)
The University of Texas Health
Science Center–San Antonio

7703 Floyd Curl Dr., MSC 7849
San Antonio, TX 78229-3900
Business: 210-567-5762
Emergency: 800-222-1222
www.poisoncontrol.org

TEMPLE

Central Texas Poison Center (*)
Scott & White Memorial Hospital

2401 South 31st St.
Temple, TX 76508
Business: 254-724-7401
Emergency: 800-222-1222
www.poisoncontrol.org

UTAH

SALT LAKE CITY

Utah Poison Control Center (*)

585 Komas Dr.
Suite 200
Salt Lake City, UT 84108
Business: 801-587-0600
Emergency: 800-222-1222
http://uuhsc.utah.edu/poison

VERMONT

(PORTLAND, ME)

Northern New England
Poison Center

Maine Medical Center
22 Bramhall St.
Portland, ME 04102
Business: 207-662-7220
Emergency: 800-222-1222
www.nnepc.org

VIRGINIA

CHARLOTTESVILLE

Blue Ridge Poison Center (*)
University of Virginia Health System

PO Box 800774
Charlottesville, VA 22908-0774
Business: 434-924-0347
Emergency: 800-222-1222
www.healthsystem.virginia.edu.brpc

RICHMOND

Virginia Poison Center (*)
Virginia Commonwealth University

PO Box 980522
Richmond, VA 23298-0522
Business: 804-828-4780
Emergency: 800-222-1222
               804-828-9123
www.vcu.edu/mcved/vpc

WASHINGTON

SEATTLE

Washington Poison Center (*)

155 NE 100th St.
Suite 400
Seattle, WA 98125-8011
Business: 206-517-2359
Emergency: 800-222-1222
www.wapc.org

WEST VIRGINIA

CHARLESTON

**West Virginia
Poison Center (*)**

3110 MacCorkle Ave. SE
Charleston, WV 25304
Business: 304-347-1212
Emergency: 800-222-1222
www.wvpoisoncenter.org

WISCONSIN

MILWAUKEE

Wisconsin Poison Center

Suite CC 660
PO Box 1997
Milwaukee, WI 53201
Business: 414-266-2952
Emergency: 800-222-1222
TDD/TTY: 414-266-2542
www.wisconsinpoison.org

WYOMING

(OMAHA, NE)

**The Poison Center (*)
Nebraska Regional Poison Center**

8401 W. Dodge St.
Suite 115
Omaha, NE 68114
Business: 402-955-5555
Emergency: 800-222-1222
www.nebraskapoison.com

PROFESSIONAL ORGANIZATIONS FOR OB/GYNs

Advancing Minimally Invasive Gynecology Worldwide
6757 Katella Ave.
Cypress, CA 90630-5105
714-503-6200
www.aagl.org

American Board of Obstetrics and Gynecology, Inc.
2915 Vine St.
Dallas, TX 75204
214-871-1619
www.abog.org

American College of Nurse-Midwives
8403 Colesville Rd., Suite 1550
Silver Spring, MD 20910
240-485-1800
www.midwife.org

American College of Obstetrians and Gynecologists
409 12th St., SW
PO Box 96920
Washington, DC 20090-6920
202-638-5577
www.acog.org

American College of Osteopathic Obstetricians and Gynecologists
8851 Camp Bowie West, Suite 120
Fort Worth, TX 76116
817-377-0421
www.acoog.com

American Society for Colposcopy and Cervical Pathology
20 West Washington St., Suite 1
Hagerstown, MD 21740
301-733-3840
www.asccp.org

American Society of Forensic Obstetricians and Gynecologists
University of Alabama School of Medicine
850 5th Ave., East
Tuscaloosa, AL 35401
205-348-4487
www.asfog.org

American Society for Reproductive Medicine
1209 Montgomery Highway
Birmingham, AL 35216-2809
205-978-5000
www.asrm.org

American Urogynecologic Society
2025 M St., NW, Suite 800
Washington, DC 20036
202-367-1167
www.augs.org

Association of Physician Assistants in Obstetrics and Gynecology
702-A Eisenhower Dr.
Kimberly, WI 54136
800-545-0636
www.paobgyn.org

Association of Professors of Gynecology and Obstetrics
2130 Priest Bridge Dr., Suite #7
Crofton, MD 21114
410-451-9560
www.apgo.org

Association of Reproductive Health Professionals
1901 L St., NW, Suite 300
Washington, DC 20036
202-466-3825
www.arhp.org

Association of Women's Health, Obstetric & Neonatal Nurses
2000 L St., NW, Suite 740
Washington, DC 20036
202-261-2400
www.awhonn.org

Central Association of Obstetricians and Gynecologists
PO Box 3010
Minot, ND 58702-3010
701-838-8323
www.caog.org

Endometriosis Association
8585 N. 76th Pl.
Milwaukee, WI 53223
414-355-2200
www.endometriosisassn.org

EngenderHealth
440 Ninth Ave.
New York, NY 10001
212-561-8000
www.engenderhealth.org

Gynecologic Surgery Society
2440 M St., NW, Suite 801
Washington, DC 20037
202-293-2046
www.gynecologicsurgerysociety.org

Infectious Diseases Society for Obstetrics and Gynecology
409 12th St., SW
PO Box 96920
Washington, DC 20090-6920
202-863-2570
www.idsog.org

InterNational Council on Infertility Information Dissemination
PO Box 6836
Arlington, VA 22206
703-379-9178
www.inciid.org

International Pelvic Pain Society
Two Woodfield Lake
1100 E. Woodfield Rd., Suite 520
Schaumburg, IL 60173
847-517-8712
www.pelvicpain.org

International Society of Perinatal Obstetricians
Wayne State University
15801 Providence Dr.,10E
Southfield, MI 48075
www.internationalspo.org

Jacobs Institute of Women's Health
The George Washington University
SPHHS Dept. of Health Policy
2021 K St., NW, Suite 800
Washington, DC 20006
202-530-2376
www.jiwh.org

March of Dimes
1275 Mamaroneck Ave.
White Plains, NY 10605
914-997-4488
www.marchofdimes.com

National Association of Childbearing Centers
3123 Gottschall Rd.
Perkiomenville, PA 18074
215-234-8068
www.birthcenters.org

National Center for Education in Maternal and Child Health
Georgetown University
2115 Wisconsin Ave., NW, Suite 601
Washington, DC 20007-2292
202-784-9770
www.ncemch.org/default.html

National Cervical Cancer Coalition
6520 Platt Ave., #693
West Hills, CA 91307
800-685-5531
www.nccc-online.org

National Fetal and Infant Mortality Review Program
American College of Obstetricians and Gynecologists
409 12th St., SW
PO Box 96920
Washington, D.C. 20090-6920
202-638-5577
www.nfimr.org

National Perinatal Association
2090 Linglestown Rd., Suite 107
Harrisburg, PA 17110
888-971-3295
www.nationalperinatal.org

National Vulvodynia Association
PO Box 4491
Silver Spring, MD 20914-4491
301-299-0775
www.nva.org

National Women's Health Information Center
Office on Women's Health
Department of Health and Human Services
200 Independence Ave., SW
Room 712E
Washington, DC 20201
202-690-7650
www.4woman.gov

North American Menopause Society
PO Box 94527
Cleveland, OH 44101
440-442-7550
www.menopause.org

North American Society for Psychosocial Obstetrics and Gynecology
409 12th St., SW
Washington, DC 20024-2188
202-863-2570
www.naspog.org

OBGYN.net - The Universe of Women's Health
1050 George St., Suite 14L
New Brunswick, NJ 08901
732-828-6382
www.obgyn.net

Physicians for Reproductive Choice and Health
55 West 39th St., Suite 1001
New York, NY 10018-3889
646-366-1890
131 Steuart St., Suite 300
San Francisco, CA. 94105
415-947-0680
www.prch.org

Reproductive Health Gateway
111 Market Pl., Suite 310
Baltimore, MD 21202
410-659-6266
www.infoforhealth.org

Reproductive Health Technologies Project
1020 19th St., NW, Suite 875
Washington, DC 20036
202-530-4401
www.rhtp.org

Society for Gynecologic Investigation
409 12th St., SW
Washington, DC 20024-2188
202-863-2544
www.sgionline.org

Society for Maternal-Fetal Medicine (formerly SPO)
409 12th St., SW
Washington, DC 20024
202-863-2476
www.smfm.org

Society of Gynecologic Oncologists
230 West Monroe St., Suite 710
Chicago, IL 60606
312-235-4060
www.sgo.org

Society of Gynecologic Surgeons
7800 Wolf Trail Cove
Germantown, TN 38138
901-682-2079
www.sgsonline.org

Society for Obstetric Anesthesia & Perinatology
520 N. Northwest Highway
Park Ridge, IL 60068-2573
847-825-5586
www.soap.org

Society for Sex Therapy and Research
409 12th St., SW
PO Box 96920
Washington, DC 20090-6920
202-863-1644
www.sstarnet.org

The Endocrine Society
8401 Connecticut Ave., Suite 900
Chevy Chase, MD 20815
301-941-0200
www.endo-society.org

The Hormone Foundation
8401 Connecticut Ave., Suite 900
Chevy Chase, MD 20815-5817
1-800-HORMONE
www.hormone.org

Western Association of Gynecologic Oncologists
409 12th St., SW
Washington, DC 20024-2188
202-863-1648
www.wagogynonc.org

ANTIPYRETIC PRODUCTS

BRAND	INGREDIENT/STRENGTH	DOSE
ACETAMINOPHEN		
Anacin Aspirin Free Extra Strength Tablets	Acetaminophen 500mg	**Adults & Peds:** ≥12 yrs: 2 tabs q6h. **Max:** 8 tabs q24h.
Feverall Childrens' Suppositories	Acetaminophen 120mg	**Peds: 3-6 yrs:** 1-2 supp. q4-6h. **Max:** 6 supp q24h.
Feverall Infants' Suppositories	Acetaminophen 80mg	**Peds: 3-11 months:** 1 supp q6h. **12-36 months:** 1 supp q4h. **Max:** 6 supp q24h.
Feverall Jr. Strength Suppositories	Acetaminophen 325mg	**Peds: 6-12 yrs:** 1 supp q4-6h. **Max:** 6 supp q24h.
Tylenol 8 Hour Caplets	Acetaminophen 650mg	**Adults & Peds:** ≥12 yrs: 2 tabs q8h prn. **Max:** 6 tabs q24h.
Tylenol 8 Hour Geltabs	Acetaminophen 650mg	**Adults & Peds:** ≥12 yrs: 2 tabs q8h prn. **Max:** 6 tabs q24h.
Tylenol Arthritis Caplets	Acetaminophen 650mg	**Adults:** 2 tabs q8h prn. **Max:** 6 tabs q24h.
Tylenol Arthritis Geltabs	Acetaminophen 650mg	**Adults:** 2 tabs q8h prn. **Max:** 6 tabs q24h.
Tylenol Children's Meltaways Tablets	Acetaminophen 80mg	**Peds: 2-3 yrs (24-35 lbs):** 2 tabs. **4-5 yrs (36-47 lbs):** 3 tabs. **6-8 yrs (48-59 lbs):** 4 tabs. **9-10 yrs (60-71 lbs):** 5 tabs. **11 yrs (72-95 lbs):** 6 tabs. May repeat q4h. **Max:** 5 doses q24h.
Tylenol Children's Suspension	Acetaminophen 160mg/5mL	**Peds: 2-3 yrs (24-35 lbs):** 1 tsp (5mL). **4-5 yrs (36-47 lbs):** 1.5 tsp (7.5mL). **6-8 yrs (48-59 lbs):** 2 tsp (10mL). **9-10 yrs (60-71 lbs):** 2.5 tsp (12.5mL). **11 yrs (72-95 lbs):** 3 tsp (15mL). May repeat q4h. **Max:** 5 doses q24h.
Tylenol Extra Strength Caplets	Acetaminophen 500mg	**Adults & Peds:** ≥12 yrs: 2 tabs q4-6h prn. **Max:** 8 tabs q24h.
Tylenol Extra Strength Cool Caplets	Acetaminophen 500mg	**Adults & Peds:** ≥12 yrs: 2 tabs q4-6h prn. **Max:** 8 tabs q24h.
Tylenol Extra Strength Gelcaps	Acetaminophen 500mg	**Adults & Peds:** ≥12 yrs: 2 caps q4-6h prn. **Max:** 8 caps q24h.
Tylenol Extra Strength Geltabs	Acetaminophen 500mg	**Adults & Peds:** ≥12 yrs: 2 tabs q4-6h prn. **Max:** 8 tabs q24h.
Tylenol Extra Strength Liquid	Acetaminophen 1000mg/30mL	**Adults & Peds:** ≥12 yrs: 2 tbl (30mL) q4-6h prn. **Max:** 8 tbl (120mL) q24h.
Tylenol Extra Strength Tablets	Acetaminophen 500mg	**Adults & Peds:** ≥12 yrs: 2 tabs q4-6h prn. **Max:** 8 tabs q24h.
Tylenol Infants' Suspension	Acetaminophen 80mg/0.8mL	**Peds: 2-3 yrs (24-35 lbs):** 1.6 mL q4h prn. **Max:** 5 doses (8mL) q24h.
Tylenol Junior Meltaways Tablets	Acetaminophen 160mg	**Peds: 6-8 yrs (48-59 lbs):** 2 tabs. **9-10 yrs (60-71 lbs):** 2.5 tabs. **11 yrs (72-95 lbs):** 3 tabs. **12 yrs (≥96 lbs):** 4 tabs. May repeat q4h. **Max:** 5 doses q24h.
Tylenol Regular Strength Tablets	Acetaminophen 325mg	**Adults & Peds:** ≥12 yrs: 2 tabs q4-6h prn. **Max:** 12 tabs q24h. **Peds: 6-11 yrs:** 1 tab q4-6h. **Max:** 5 tabs q24h.

(Continued)

BRAND	INGREDIENT/STRENGTH	DOSE
NONSTEROIDAL ANTI-INFLAMMATORY DRUGS (NSAIDs)		
Advil Children's Chewable Tablets	Ibuprofen 50mg	**Peds: 2-3 yrs (24-35 lbs):** 2 tabs q6-8h. **4-5 yrs (36-47 lbs):** 3 tabs q6-8h. **6-8 yrs (48-59 lbs):** 4 tabs q6-8h. **9-10 yrs (60-71 lbs):** 5 tabs q6-8h. **11 yrs (72-95 lbs):** 6 tabs q6-8h. **Max:** 4 doses q24h.
Advil Children's Suspension	Ibuprofen 100mg/5mL	**Peds: 2-3 yrs (24-35 lbs):** 1 tsp (5mL). **4-5 yrs (36-47 lbs):** 1.5 tsp (7.5mL). **6-8 yrs (48-59 lbs):** 2 tsp (10mL). **9-10 yrs (60-71 lbs):** 2.5 tsp (12.5mL). **11 yrs (72-95 lbs):** 3 tsp (15mL). May repeat q6-8h. **Max:** 4 doses q24h.
Advil Gel Caplets	Ibuprofen 200mg	**Adults & Peds: ≥12 yrs:** 1-2 caps q4-6h. **Max:** 6 caps q24h.
Advil Infants' Concentrated Drops	Ibuprofen 50mg/1.25mL	**Peds: 6-11 months (12-17 lbs):** 1.25mL. **12-23 months (18-23 lbs):** 1.875mL. May repeat q6-8h. **Max:** 4 doses q24h.
Advil Junior Strength Chewable Tablets	Ibuprofen 100mg	**Peds: 6-8 yrs (48-59 lbs):** 2 tabs. **9-10 yrs (60-71 lbs):** 2.5 tabs. **11 yrs (72-95 lbs):** 3 tabs. May repeat q6-8h. **Max:** 4 doses q24h.
Advil Junior Strength Swallow Tablets	Ibuprofen 100mg	**Peds: 6-10 yrs (48-71 lbs):** 2 tabs **11 yrs (72-95 lbs):** 3 tabs. May repeat q6-8h. **Max:** 4 doses q24h.
Advil Liqui-Gels	Ibuprofen 200mg	**Adults & Peds: ≥12 yrs:** 1-2 caps q4-6h. **Max:** 6 caps q24h.
Advil Tablets	Ibuprofen 200mg	**Adults & Peds: ≥12 yrs:** 1-2 tabs q4-6h. **Max:** 6 tabs q24h.
Aleve Caplets	Naproxen Sodium 220mg	**Adults & Peds: ≥12 yrs:** 1 tab q8-12h. May take 1 additional tab within 1 hour of first dose. **Max:** 3 tabs q24h.
Aleve Liquid Gels	Naproxen Sodium 220mg	**Adults & Peds: ≥12 yrs:** 1 cap q8-12h. May take 1 additional tab within 1 hour of first dose. **Max:** 3 caps q24h.
Aleve Smooth Gels	Naproxen Sodium 220mg	**Adults & Peds: ≥12 yrs:** 1 cap q8-12h. May take 1 additional tab within 1 hour of first dose. **Max:** 3 caps q24h.
Aleve Tablets	Naproxen Sodium 220mg	**Adults & Peds: ≥12 yrs:** 1 tab q8-12h. May take 1 additional tab within 1 hour of first dose. **Max:** 3 caps q24h.
Motrin Children's Suspension	Ibuprofen 100mg/5mL	**Peds: 2-3 yrs (24-35 lbs):** 1 tsp (5mL). **4-5 yrs (36-47 lbs):** 1.5 tsp (7.5mL). **6-8 yrs (48-59 lbs):** 2 tsp (10mL). **9-10 yrs (60-71 lbs):** 2.5 tsp (12.5mL). **11 yrs (72-95 lbs):** 3 tsp (15mL). May repeat q6-8h. **Max:** 4 doses q24h.
Motrin IB Caplets	Ibuprofen 200mg	**Adults & Peds: ≥12 yrs:** 1-2 tabs q4-6h. **Max:** 6 tabs q24h.
Motrin IB Tablets	Ibuprofen 200mg	**Adults & Peds: ≥12 yrs:** 1-2 tabs q4-6h. **Max:** 6 tabs q24h.
Motrin Infants' drops	Ibuprofen 50mg/1.25mL	**Peds: 6-11 months (12-17 lbs):** 1.25mL. **12-23 months (18-23 lbs):** 1.875mL. May repeat q6-8h. **Max:** 4 doses q24h.

(Continued)

BRAND	INGREDIENT/STRENGTH	DOSE
NONSTEROIDAL ANTI-INFLAMMATORY DRUGS (NSAIDs) *(Continued)*		
Motrin Junior Strength Caplets	Ibuprofen 100mg	**Peds: 6-8 yrs (48-59 lbs):** 2 tabs. **9-10 yrs (60-71 lbs):** 2.5 tabs. **11 yrs (72-95 lbs):** 3 tabs. May repeat q6-8h. **Max:** 4 doses q24h.
Motrin Junior Strength Chewable Tablets	Ibuprofen 100mg	**Peds: 6-8 yrs (48-59 lbs):** 2 tabs. **9-10 yrs (60-71 lbs):** 2.5 tabs. **11 yrs (72-95 lbs):** 3 tabs. May repeat q6-8h. **Max:** 4 doses q24h.
SALICYLATES		
Anacin 81 Tablets	Aspirin 81mg	**Adults & Peds: ≥12 yrs:** 2 tabs q6h. **Max:** 8 tabs q24h.
Aspergum Chewable Tablets	Aspirin 227mg	**Adults & Peds: ≥12 yrs:** 2 tabs q4h. **Max:** 16 tabs q24h.
Bayer Aspirin Extra Strength Caplets	Aspirin 500mg	**Adults & Peds: ≥12 yrs:** 1-2 tabs q4-6h. **Max:** 8 tabs q24h.
Bayer Genuine Aspirin Caplets	Aspirin 325mg	**Adults & Peds: ≥12 yrs:** 1-2 tabs q4h or 3 tabs q6h. **Max:** 12 tabs q24h.
Bayer Aspirin Safety Coated Caplets	Aspirin 325mg	**Adults & Peds: ≥12 yrs:** 1-2 tabs q4h or 3 tabs q6h. **Max:** 12 tabs q24h.
Bayer Children's Aspirin Chewable Tablets	Aspirin 81mg	**Adults & Peds: ≥12 yrs:** 4-8 tabs q4h. **Max:** 48 tabs q24h.
Bayer Low Dose Aspirin Tablets	Aspirin 81mg	**Adults & Peds: ≥12 yrs:** 4-8 tabs q4h. **Max:** 48 tabs q24h.
Ecotrin Low Strength Tablets	Aspirin 81mg	**Adults:** 4-8 tabs q4h. **Max:** 48 tabs q24h.
Ecotrin Enteric Regular Strength Tablets	Aspirin 325mg	**Adults & Peds: ≥12 yrs:** 1-2 tabs q4h. **Max:** 12 tabs q24h.
Ecotrin Maximum Strength Tablets	Aspirin 500mg	**Adults & Peds: ≥12 yrs:** 2 tabs q6h. **Max:** 8 tabs q24h.
Halfprin 162mg Tablets	Aspirin 162mg	**Adults & Peds: ≥12 yrs:** 2-4 tabs q4h. **Max:** 24 tabs q24h.
Halfprin 81mg Tablets	Aspirin 81mg	**Adults & Peds: ≥12 yrs:** 4-8 tabs q4h. **Max:** 48 tabs q24h.
St. Joseph Aspirin Chewable Tablets	Aspirin 81mg	**Adults & Peds: ≥12 yrs:** 4-8 tabs q4h. **Max:** 48 tabs q24h.
St. Joseph Enteric Safety-Coated Tablets	Aspirin 81mg	**Adults & Peds: ≥12 yrs:** 4-8 tabs q4h. **Max:** 48 tabs q24h.
SALICYLATES, BUFFERED		
Bayer Extra Strength Plus Caplets	Aspirin Buffered with Calcium Carbonate 500mg	**Adults & Peds: ≥12 yrs:** 1-2 tabs q4-6h. **Max:** 8 tabs q24h.
Bufferin Extra Strength Tablets	Aspirin Buffered with Calcium Carbonate/ Magnesium Oxide/Magnesium Carbonate 500mg	**Adults & Peds: ≥12 yrs:** 2 tabs q6h. **Max:** 8 tabs q24h.
Bufferin Tablets	Aspirin Buffered with Calcium Carbonate/ Magnesium Oxide/Magnesium Carbonate 325mg	**Adults & Peds: ≥12 yrs:** 2 tabs q4h. **Max:** 12 tabs q24h.

HEADACHE/MIGRAINE PRODUCTS

BRAND	INGREDIENT/STRENGTH	DOSE
ACETAMINOPHEN		
Anacin Extra Strength Aspirin Free Tablets	Acetaminophen 500mg	**Adults & Peds:** ≥**12 yrs:** 2 tabs q6h. **Max:** 8 tabs q24h.
Tylenol 8 Hour Caplets	Acetaminophen 650mg	**Adults & Peds:** ≥**12 yrs:** 2 tabs q8h prn. **Max:** 6 tabs q24h.
Tylenol 8 Hour Geltabs	Acetaminophen 650mg	**Adults & Peds:** ≥**12 yrs:** 2 tabs q8h prn. **Max:** 6 tabs q24h.
Tylenol Arthritis Caplets	Acetaminophen 650mg	**Adults:** 2 tabs q8h prn. **Max:** 6 tabs q24h.
Tylenol Arthritis Geltabs	Acetaminophen 650mg	**Adults:** 2 tabs q8h prn. **Max:** 6 tabs q24h.
Tylenol Children's Meltaway Tablets	Acetaminophen 80mg	**Peds: 2-3 yrs (24-35 lbs):** 2 tabs **4-5 yrs (36-47 lbs):** 3 tabs. **6-8 yrs (48-59 lbs):** 4 tabs. **9-10 yrs (60-71 lbs):** 5 tabs. **11 yrs (72-95 lbs):** 6 tabs. May repeat q4h. **Max:** 5 doses q24h.
Tylenol Children's Suspension	Acetaminophen 160mg/5mL	**Peds: 2-3 yrs (24-35 lbs):** 1 tsp (5mL). **4-5 yrs (36-47 lbs):** 1.5 tsp (7.5mL). **6-8 yrs (48-59 lbs):** 2 tsp (10mL). **9-10 yrs (60-71 lbs):** 2.5 tsp (12.5mL). **11 yrs (72-95 lbs):** 3 tsp (15mL). May repeat q4h. **Max:** 5 doses q24h.
Tylenol Extra Strength Caplets	Acetaminophen 500mg	**Adults & Peds:** ≥**12 yrs:** 2 tabs q4-6h prn. **Max:** 8 tabs q24h.
Tylenol Extra Strength Cool Caplets	Acetaminophen 500mg	**Adults & Peds:** ≥**12 yrs:** 2 tabs q4-6h prn. **Max:** 8 tabs q24h.
Tylenol Extra Strength Rapid Release Gels	Acetaminophen 500mg	**Adults & Peds:** ≥**12 yrs:** 2 caps q4-6h prn. **Max:** 8 caps q24h.
Tylenol Extra Strength Rapid Blast Liquid	Acetaminophen 1000mg/30mL	**Adults & Peds:** ≥**12 yrs:** 2 tbl (30mL) q4-6h prn. **Max:** 8 tbl (120mL) q24h.
Tylenol Extra Strength EZ Tabs	Acetaminophen 500mg	**Adults & Peds:** ≥**12 yrs:** 2 tabs q4-6h prn. **Max:** 8 tabs q24h.
Tylenol Extra Strength Go Tabs	Acetaminophen 500mg	**Adults & Peds:** ≥**12 yrs:** 2 tabs q4-6h prn. **Max:** 8 tabs q24h.
Tylenol Infants' Suspension	Acetaminophen 80mg/0.8mL	**Peds: 2-3 yrs (24-35 lbs):** 1.6 mL q4h prn. **Max:** 5 doses (8mL) q24h.
Tylenol Junior Meltaways Tablets	Acetaminophen 160mg	**Peds: 6-8 yrs (48-59 lbs):** 2 tabs. **9-10 yrs (60-71 lbs):** 2.5 tabs. **11 yrs (72-95 lbs):** 3 tabs. **12 yrs (≥96 lbs):** 4 tabs. May repeat q4h. **Max:** 5 doses q24h.
Tylenol Regular Strength Tablets	Acetaminophen 325mg	**Adults & Peds:** ≥**12 yrs:** 2 tabs q4-6h prn. **Max:** 12 tabs q24h. **Peds: 6-11 yrs:** 1 tab q4-6h. **Max:** 5 tabs q24h.
ACETAMINOPHEN COMBINATIONS		
Excedrin Extra Strength Caplets	Acetaminophen/Aspirin/Caffeine 250mg-250mg-65mg	**Adults & Peds:** ≥**12 yrs:** 2 tabs q6h. **Max:** 8 tabs q24h.
Excedrin Extra Strength Geltabs	Acetaminophen/Aspirin/Caffeine 250mg-250mg-65mg	**Adults & Peds:** ≥**12 yrs:** 2 tabs q6h. **Max:** 8 tabs q24h.
Excedrin Extra Strength Tablets	Acetaminophen/Aspirin/Caffeine 250mg-250mg-65mg	**Adults & Peds:** ≥**12 yrs:** 2 tabs q6h. **Max:** 8 tabs q24h.
Excedrin Migraine Caplets	Acetaminophen/Aspirin/Caffeine 250mg-250mg-65mg	**Adults:** 2 tabs prn. **Max:** 2 tabs q24h.
Excedrin Migraine Geltabs	Acetaminophen/Aspirin/Caffeine 250mg-250mg-65mg	**Adults:** 2 tabs prn. **Max:** 2 tabs q24h.

(Continued)

BRAND	INGREDIENT/STRENGTH	DOSE
ACETAMINOPHEN COMBINATIONS *(Continued)*		
Excedrin Migraine Tablets	Acetaminophen/Aspirin/Caffeine 250mg-250mg-65mg	**Adults:** 2 tabs prn. **Max:** 2 tabs q24h.
Excedrin Sinus Headache Caplets	Acetaminophen/Phenylephrine HCl 325mg-5mg	**Adults & Peds:** ≥12 yrs: 2 tabs q4h. **Max:** 12 tabs q24h.
Excedrin Sinus Headache Tablets	Acetaminophen/Phenylephrine HCl 325mg-5mg	**Adults & Peds:** ≥12 yrs: 2 tabs q4h. **Max:** 12 tabs q24h.
Excedrin Tension Headache Caplets	Acetaminophen/Caffeine 500mg-65mg	**Adults & Peds:** ≥12 yrs: 2 tabs q6h. **Max:** 8 tabs q24h.
Excedrin Tension Headache Geltabs	Acetaminophen/Caffeine 500mg-65mg	**Adults & Peds:** ≥12 yrs: 2 tabs q6h. **Max:** 8 tabs q24h.
Excedrin Tension Headache Tablets	Acetaminophen/Caffeine 500mg-65mg	**Adults & Peds:** ≥12 yrs: 2 tabs q6h. **Max:** 8 tabs q24h.
Goody's Extra Strength Headache Powders	Acetaminophen/Aspirin/Caffeine 260mg-520mg-32.5mg	**Adults & Peds:** ≥12 yrs: 1 powder q4-6h. **Max:** 4 powders q24h.
Sudafed PE Sinus Headache Coated Caplets	Acetaminophen/Phenylephrine HCl 325mg-5mg	**Adults & Peds:** ≥12 yrs: 2 tabs q4h. **Max:** 12 tabs q24h.
Tylenol Sinus Congestion & Pain Daytime Gelcaps	Acetaminophen/Phenylephrine HCl 325mg-5mg	**Adults & Peds:** ≥12 yrs: 2 caps q4h. **Max:** 12 caps q24h.
Tylenol Sinus Congestion & Pain Daytime Rapid Release Gelcaps	Acetaminophen/Phenylephrine HCl 325mg-5mg	**Adults & Peds:** ≥12 yrs: 2 caps q4h. **Max:** 12 caps q24h.
Vanquish Caplets	Acetaminophen/Aspirin/Caffeine 194mg-227mg-33mg	**Adults & Peds:** ≥12 yrs: 2 tabs q6h. **Max:** 8 tabs q24h.
ACETAMINOPHEN/SLEEP AID		
Excedrin PM Caplets	Acetaminophen/Diphenhydramine 500mg-38mg	**Adults & Peds:** ≥12 yrs: 2 tabs qhs.
Excedrin PM Geltabs	Acetaminophen/Diphenhydramine citrate 500mg-38 mg	**Adults & Peds:** ≥12 yrs: 2 tabs qhs.
Excedrin PM Tablets	Acetaminophen/Diphenhydramine citrate 500mg-38 mg	**Adults & Peds:** ≥12 yrs: 2 tabs qhs.
Goody's PM Powder	Acetaminophen/Diphenhydramine 1000mg-76mg/dose	**Adults & Peds:** ≥12 yrs: 1 packet (2 powders) qhs.
Tylenol PM Caplets	Acetaminophen/Diphenhydramine 500mg-25mg	**Adults & Peds:** ≥12 yrs: 2 tabs qhs.
Tylenol PM Rapid Release Gels	Acetaminophen/Diphenhydramine 500mg-25mg	**Adults & Peds:** ≥12 yrs: 2 caps qhs.
Tylenol PM Geltabs	Acetaminophen/Diphenhydramine 500mg-25mg	**Adults & Peds:** ≥12 yrs: 2 tabs qhs.
Tylenol Sinus Night Time Caplets	Acetaminophen/Pseudoephedrine HCl/ Doxylamine Succinate 500mg-30mg-6.25mg	**Adults & Peds:** ≥12 yrs: 2 tbl (30mL) qhs. **Max:** 8 tbl (120mL) q24h.
NONSTEROIDAL ANTI-INFLAMMATORY DRUGS (NSAIDs)		
Advil Caplets	Ibuprofen 200mg	**Adults & Peds:** ≥12 yrs: 1-2 tabs q4-6h. **Max:** 6 tabs q24h.
Advil Children's Chewable Tablets	Ibuprofen 50mg	**Peds: 2-3 yr (24-35 lbs):** 2 tabs q6-8h. **4-5 yr (36-47 lbs):** 3 tabs q6-8h. **6-8 yr (48-59 lbs):** 4 tabs q6-8h. **9-10 yr (60-71 lbs):** 5 tabs q6-8h. **11 yr (72-95 lbs):** 6 tabs q6-8h. **Max:** 4 doses q24h
Advil Children's Suspension	Ibuprofen 100mg/5mL	**Peds: 2-3 yrs (24-35 lbs):** 1 tsp (5mL). **4-5 yrs (36-47 lbs):** 1.5 tsp (7.5mL). **6-8 yrs (48-59 lbs):** 2 tsp (10mL). **9-10 yrs (60-71 lbs):** 2.5 tsp (12.5mL). **11 yrs (72-95 lbs):** 3 tsp (15mL). May repeat q6-8h. **Max:** 4 doses q24h.
Advil Gel Caplets	Ibuprofen 200mg	**Adults & Peds:** ≥12 yrs: 1-2 caps q4-6h. **Max:** 6 caps q24h.
Advil Infants' Concentrated Drops	Ibuprofen 50mg/1.25mL	**Peds: 6-11 months (12-17 lbs):** 1.25mL. **12-23 months (18-23 lbs):** 1.875mL. May repeat q6-8h. **Max:** 4 doses q24h.

(Continued)

BRAND	INGREDIENT/STRENGTH	DOSE
NONSTEROIDAL ANTI-INFLAMMATORY DRUGS (NSAIDs) *(Continued)*		
Advil Junior Strength Swallow Tablets	Ibuprofen 100mg	**Peds: 6-10 yrs (48-71 lbs):** 2 tabs. **11 yrs (72-95 lbs):** 3 tabs. May repeat q6-8h. **Max:** 4 doses q24h.
Advil Junior Strength Chewable Tablets	Ibuprofen 100mg	
Advil Liqui-Gels	Ibuprofen 200mg	**Adults & Peds:** ≥**12 yrs:** 1-2 caps q4-6h. **Max:** 6 caps q24h.
Advil Migraine Capsules	Ibuprofen 200mg	**Adults:** 2 caps prn. **Max:** 2 caps q24h.
Advil Tablets	Ibuprofen 200mg	**Adults & Peds:** ≥**12 yrs:** 1-2 tabs q4-6h. **Max:** 6 tabs q24h.
Aleve Caplets	Naproxen Sodium 220mg	**Adults & Peds:** ≥**12 yrs:** 1 tab q8-12h. May take 1 additional tab within 1 hour of first dose. **Max:** 3 tabs q24h.
Aleve Gelcaps	Naproxen Sodium 220mg	**Adults & Peds:** ≥**12 yrs:** 1 cap q8-12h. May take 1 additional tab within 1 hour of first dose. **Max:** 3 caps q24h.
Aleve Tablets	Naproxen Sodium 220mg	**Adults & Peds:** ≥**12 yrs:** 1 tab q8-12h. May take 1 additional tab within 1 hour of first dose. **Max:** 3 q24h.
Motrin Children's Suspension	Ibuprofen 100mg/5mL	**Peds: 2-3 yrs (24-35 lbs):** 1 tsp (5mL). **4-5 yrs (36-47 lbs):** 1.5 tsp (7.5mL). **6-8 yrs (48-59 lbs):** 2 tsp (10mL). **9-10 yrs (60-71 lbs):** 2.5 tsp (12.5mL). **11 yrs (72-95 lbs):** 3 tsp (15mL). May repeat q6-8h. **Max:** 4 doses q24h.
Motrin IB Caplets	Ibuprofen 200mg	**Adults & Peds:** ≥**12 yrs:** 1-2 tabs q4-6h. **Max:** 6 tabs q24h.
Motrin IB Tablets	Ibuprofen 200mg	**Adults & Peds:** ≥**12 yrs:** 1-2 tabs q4-6h. **Max:** 6 tabs q24h.
Motrin Infants' Drops	Ibuprofen 50mg/1.25mL	**Peds: 6-11 months (12-17 lbs):** 1.25mL. **12-23 months (18-23 lbs):** 1.875mL. May repeat q6-8h. **Max:** 4 doses q24h.
Motrin Junior Strength Chewable Tablets	Ibuprofen 100mg	**Peds: 6-8 yrs (48-59 lbs):** 2 tabs. **9-10 yrs (60-71 lbs):** 2.5 tabs. **11 yrs (72-95 lbs):** 3 tabs. May repeat q6-8h. **Max:** 4 doses q24h.
NSAID COMBINATIONS		
Aleve Sinus & Headache Caplets	Naproxen Sodium/Pseudoephedrine HCl 220 mg-120 mg	**Adults & Peds:** ≥**12 yrs:** 1 tab q12h. **Max:** 2 tabs q24h.
SALICYLATES		
Anacin 81 Tablets	Aspirin 81mg	**Adults & Peds:** ≥**12 yrs:** 2 tabs q6h. **Max:** 8 tabs q24h.
Aspergum Chewable Tablets	Aspirin 227mg	**Adults & Peds:** ≥**12 yrs:** 2 tabs q4h. **Max:** 16 tabs q24h.
Bayer Aspirin Extra Strength Caplets	Aspirin 500mg	**Adults & Peds:** ≥**12 yrs:** 1-2 tabs q4-6h. **Max:** 8 tabs q24h.
Bayer Genuine Aspirin Tablets	Aspirin 325mg	**Adults & Peds:** ≥**12 yrs:** 1-2 tabs q4h or 3 tabs q6h. **Max:** 12 tabs q24h.
Bayer Genuine Aspirin Caplets	Aspirin 325mg	**Adults & Peds:** ≥**12 yrs:** 1-2 tabs q4h or 3 tabs q6h. **Max:** 12 tabs q24h.
Bayer Aspirin Chewable Tablets	Aspirin 81mg	**Adults & Peds:** ≥**12 yrs:** 4-8 tabs q4h. **Max:** 48 tabs q24h.
Bayer Low Dose Aspirin Tablets	Aspirin 81mg	**Adults & Peds:** ≥**12 yrs:** 4-8 tabs q4h. **Max:** 48 tabs q24h.

(Continued)

BRAND	INGREDIENT/STRENGTH	DOSE
SALICYLATES (Continued)		
Doan's Extra Strength Caplets	Magnesium Salicylate Tetrahydrate 580mg	**Adults & Peds:** ≥12 yrs: 2 tabs q6h. **Max:** 8 tabs q24h.
Ecotrin Low Strength Tablets	Aspirin 81mg	**Adults:** 4-8 tabs q4h. **Max:** 48 tabs q24h.
Ecotrin Regular Strength Tablets	Aspirin 325mg	**Adults & Peds:** ≥12 yrs: 1-2 tabs q4h. **Max:** 12 tabs q24h.
Ecotrin Maximum Strength Tablets	Aspirin 500mg	**Adults & Peds:** ≥12 yrs: 2 tabs q6h. **Max:** 8 tabs q24h.
Halfprin 162mg Tablets	Aspirin 162mg	**Adults & Peds:** ≥12 yrs: 2-4 tabs q4h. **Max:** 24 tabs q24h.
Halfprin 81mg Tablets	Aspirin 81mg	**Adults & Peds:** ≥12 yrs: 4-8 tabs q4h. **Max:** 48 tabs q24h.
St. Joseph Chewable	Aspirin 81mg	**Adults & Peds:** ≥12 yrs: 4-8 tabs q4h.
St. Joseph Enteric	Aspirin 81mg	**Adults & Peds:** ≥12 yrs: 4-8 tabs q4h.
SALICYLATES, BUFFERED		
Alka-Seltzer Original Effervescent Tablets	Aspirin/Citric Acid/Sodium Bicarbonate 325mg-1000mg-1916mg	**Adults & Peds:** ≥12 yrs: 2 tabs q4h. **Max:** 8 tabs q24h. ≥**60 yrs: Max:** 4 tabs q24h.
Alka-Seltzer Extra Strength Effervescent Tablets	Aspirin/Citric Acid/Sodium Bicarbonate 500mg-1000mg-1985mg	**Adults & Peds:** ≥12 yrs: 2 tabs q6h. **Max:** 7 tabs q24h. ≥**60 yrs: Max:** 3 tabs q24h.
Ascriptin Maximum Strength Tablets	Aspirin Buffered with Maalox/Calcium Carbonate 500mg	**Adults & Peds:** ≥12 yrs: 2 tabs q4h. **Max:** 8 tabs q24h.
Ascriptin Regular Strength Tablets	Aspirin Buffered with Maalox/Calcium Carbonate 325mg	**Adults & Peds:** ≥12 yrs: 2 tabs q4h. **Max:** 12 tabs q24h.
Bayer Extra Strength Plus Caplets	Aspirin Buffered with Calcium Carbonate 500mg	**Adults & Peds:** ≥12 yrs: 1-2 tabs q4-6h. **Max:** 8 tabs q24h.
Bufferin Extra Strength Tablets	Aspirin Buffered with Calcium Carbonate/Magnesium Oxide/Magnesium Carbonate 500mg	**Adults & Peds:** ≥12 yrs: 2 tabs q6h. **Max:** 8 tabs q24h.
Bufferin Tablets	Aspirin Buffered with Benzoic Acid/Citric Acid 325	**Adults & Peds:** ≥12 yrs: 2 tabs q4h. **Max:** 12 tabs q24h.
SALICYLATE COMBINATIONS		
Alka-Seltzer Morning Relief Effervescent Tablets	Aspirin/Caffeine 500mg-65mg	**Adults & Peds:** ≥12 yrs: 2 tabs q6h. **Max:** 8 tabs q24h. ≥**60 yrs: Max:** 4 tabs q24h.
Anacin Max Strength Tablets	Aspirin/Caffeine 500mg-32mg	**Adults & Peds:** ≥12 yrs: 2 tabs q6h. **Max:** 8 tabs q24h.
Anacin Tablets	Aspirin/Caffeine 400mg-32mg	**Adults & Peds:** ≥12 yrs: 2 tabs q6h. **Max:** 8 tabs q24h.
Bayer Back & Body Pain Caplets	Aspirin/Caffeine 500mg-32.5mg	**Adults & Peds:** ≥12 yrs: 2 tabs q6h. **Max:** 8 tabs q24h.
BC Arthritis Strength Powders	Aspirin/Caffeine/Salicylamide 742mg-38mg-222mg	**Adults & Peds:** ≥12 yrs: 1 powder q3-4h. **Max:** 4 powders q24h.
BC Original Formula Powders	Aspirin/Caffeine/Salicylamide 650mg-33.3mg-195mg	**Adults & Peds:** ≥12 yrs: 1 powder q3-4h. **Max:** 4 powders q24h.
SALICYLATE/SLEEP AID		
Alka-Seltzer PM Pain Reliever & Sleep Aid effervescent Tablets	Aspirin/Diphenhydramine Citrate 325mg-38 mg	**Adults & Peds:** ≥12 yrs: 2 tabs qpm.
Bayer PM Relief Caplets	Aspirin/Diphenhydramine 500mg-38.3mg	**Adults & Peds:** ≥12 yrs: 2 tabs qhs.
Doan's Extra Strength PM Caplets	Magnesium Salicylate Tetrahydrate/Diphenhydramine 580mg-25mg	**Adults & Peds:** ≥12 yrs: 2 tabs qhs.

INSOMNIA PRODUCTS

BRAND	INGREDIENT/STRENGTH	DOSE
DIPHENHYDRAMINE		
Nytol Quick Caps Caplets	Diphenhydramine 25mg	**Adults & Peds:** ≥**12 yrs:** 2 tabs qpm.
Nytol Quick Gels Capsules	Diphenhydramine 50mg	**Adults & Peds:** ≥**12 yrs:** 1 tab qpm.
Simply Sleep Nighttime Sleep Aid Caplets	Diphenhydramine 25mg	**Adults & Peds:** ≥**12 yrs:** 2 tabs qpm.
Sominex Original Formula	Diphenhydramine 25mg	**Adults & Peds:** ≥**12 yrs:** 2 tabs qpm.
Sominex Maximum Strength Formula	Diphenhydramine 50mg	**Adults & Peds:** ≥**12 yrs:** 1 tab qpm.
Unisom Nighttime Sleep-Aid Sleep Gels	Diphenhydramine 50mg	**Adults & Peds:** ≥**12 yrs:** 1 tab qpm.
DIPHENHYDRAMINE COMBINATION		
Alka-Seltzer PM	Aspirin/Diphenhydramine Citrate 325mg-38mg	**Adults & Peds:** ≥**12 yrs:** 2 tabs qpm.
Bayer PM Relief Caplets	Aspirin/Diphenhydramine 500mg-38.3mg	**Adults & Peds:** ≥**12 yrs:** 2 tabs qhs.
Doan's Extra Strength PM Caplets	Magnesium Salicylate Tetrahydrate/ Diphenhydramine 580mg-25mg	**Adults & Peds:** ≥**12 yrs:** 2 tabs qhs.
Excedrin PM Caplets	Acetaminophen/Diphenhydramine 500mg-38mg	**Adults & Peds:** ≥**12 yrs:** 2 tabs qhs.
Excedrin PM Geltabs	Acetaminophen/Diphenhydramine 500mg-38mg	**Adults & Peds:** ≥**12 yrs:** 2 tabs qhs.
Excedrin PM Tablets	Acetaminophen/Diphenhydramine 500mg-38mg	**Adults & Peds:** ≥**12 yrs:** 2 tabs qhs.
Goody's PM Powders	Acetaminophen/Diphenhydramine 1000mg-76mg/dose	**Adults & Peds:** ≥**12 yrs:** 1 packet (2 powders) qhs.
Tylenol PM Caplets	Acetaminophen/Diphenhydramine 500mg-25mg	**Adults & Peds:** ≥**12 yrs:** 2 tabs qhs.
Tylenol PM Rapid Release Gelcaps	Acetaminophen/Diphenhydramine 500mg-25mg	**Adults & Peds:** ≥**12 yrs:** 2 caps qhs.
Tylenol PM Geltabs	Acetaminophen/Diphenhydramine 500mg-25mg	**Adults & Peds:** ≥**12 yrs:** 2 tabs qhs.
Tylenol PM Liquid	Acetaminophen/Diphenhydramine 1000g-50mg/30mL	**Adults & Peds:** ≥**12 yrs:** 2 tbl (30mL) qhs. **Max:** 8 tbl (120mL) q24h.
DOXYLAMINE		
Unisom Nighttime Sleep-Aid Sleep Tabs	Doxylamine Succinate 25mg	**Adults & Peds:** ≥**12 yrs:** 1 tab 30 min before hs.

SMOKING CESSATION PRODUCTS

BRAND	INGREDIENT/STRENGTH	DOSE
Commit Stop Smoking 2mg Lozenges	Nicotine Polacrilex 2mg	**Adults:** If smoking first cigarettte >30 minutes after waking up use 2mg lozenge. **Weeks 1 to 6:** 1 lozenge q1-2h. **Weeks 7 to 9:** 1 lozenge q2-4h. **Weeks 10 to 12:** 1 lozenge q4-8h. **Max:** 5 lozenges/6 hours; 20 lozenges/day. Stop using at the end of 12 weeks.
Commit Stop Smoking 4mg Lozenges	Nicotine Polacrilex 4mg	**Adults:** If smoking first cigarettte within 30 minutes after waking up use 4mg lozenge. **Weeks 1 to 6:** 1 lozenge q1-2h. **Weeks 7 to 9:** 1 lozenge q2-4h. **Weeks 10 to 12:** 1 lozenge q4-8h. **Max:** 5 lozenges/6 hours; 20 lozenges/day. Stop using at the end of 12 weeks.
NicoDerm CQ Step 1 Clear Patch	Nicotine 21mg	**Adults:** If smoking >10 cigarettes/day. **Weeks 1 to 6:** Apply one 21mg patch/day. **Weeks 7 to 8:** Apply one 14mg patch/day. **Weeks 9 to 10:** Apply one 7mg patch/day.
NicoDerm CQ Step 2 Clear Patch	Nicotine 14mg	**Adults:** If smoking <10 cigarettes/day. **Weeks 1 to 6:** Apply one 14mg patch/day. **Weeks 7 to 8:** Apply one 7mg patch/day.
NicoDerm CQ Step 3 Clear Patch	Nicotine 7mg	**Adults:** Apply 1 patch qd Weeks 9 to 10 if smoking >10 cigarettes/day or Weeks 7 to 8 if smoking ≤10 cigarettes/day.
Nicorette 2mg, Original/Mint/Orange Gum	Nicotine Polacrilex 2mg	**Adults:** If smoking <25 cigarettes/day use 2mg gum. **Weeks 1 to 6:** 1 piece q1-2h. **Weeks 7 to 9:** 1 piece q2-4h. **Weeks 10 to 12:** 1 piece q4-8h. **Max:** 24 pieces/day.
Nicorette 4mg, Original/Mint/Orange Gum	Nicotine Polacrilex 4mg	**Adults:** If smoking ≥25 cigarettes/day use 4mg gum. **Weeks 1 to 6:** 1 piece q1-2h. **Weeks 7 to 9:** 1 piece q2-4h. **Weeks 10 to 12:** 1 piece q4-8h. **Max:** 24 pieces/day.
Habitrol Nicotine Transdermal System Patch Step 1	Nicotine 21mg/24hr	**Adults:** If smoking >10 cigarettes/day. **Weeks 1 to 4:** Apply one 21mg patch/day. **Weeks 5 to 6:** Apply one 14mg patch/day. **Weeks 7 to 8:** Apply one 7mg patch/day.
Habitrol Nicotine Transdermal System Patch Step 2	Nicotine 14mg/24hr	**Adults:** If smoking >10 cigarettes/day. **Weeks 1 to 4:** Apply one 21mg patch/day. **Weeks 5 to 6:** Apply one 14mg patch/day. **Weeks 7 to 8:** Apply one 7mg patch/day. If smoking <10 cigarettes/day. **Weeks 1 to 6:** Apply one 14 mg patch/day. **Weeks 7 to 8:** Apply one 7mg patch/day.
Habitrol Nicotine Transdermal System Patch Step 3	Nicotine 7mg/24hr	**Adults:** If smoking >10 cigarettes/day. **Weeks 1 to 4:** Apply one 21mg patch/day. **Weeks 5 to 6:** Apply one 14mg patch/day. **Weeks 7 to 8:** Apply one 7mg patch/day. If smoking <10 cigarettes/day. **Weeks 1 to 6:** Apply one 14mg patch/day. **Weeks 7 to 8:** Apply one 7mg patch/day.

ANTIFUNGAL PRODUCTS

BRAND	INGREDIENT/STRENGTH	DOSE
BUTENAFINE		
Lotrimin Ultra Antifungal Cream	Butenafine HCl 1%	**Adults & Peds ≥12 yrs:** Use bid.
CLOTRIMAZOLE		
FungiCure Anti-Fungal Liquid Spray	Clotrimazole 1%	**Adults & Peds:** Use bid.
Lotrimin AF Antifungal Athlete's Foot Cream	Clotrimazole 1%	**Adults & Peds ≥2 yrs:** Use bid.
Lotrimin AF Antifungal Athlete's Foot Topical Solution	Clotrimazole 1%	**Adults & Peds ≥2 yrs:** Use bid.
Lotrimin AF For Her Antifungal Cream	Clotrimazole 1%	**Adults & Peds ≥2 yrs:** Use bid.
MICONAZOLE		
Clearly Confident Triple Action Fungus Treatment	Miconazole Nitrate 2%	**Adults:** Apply to affected area bid.
Desenex Antifungal Liquid Spray	Miconazole Nitrate 2%	**Adults:** Use bid.
Desenex Antifungal Powder	Miconazole Nitrate 2%	**Adults:** Use bid.
Desenex Antifungal Spray	Miconazole Nitrate 2%	**Adults:** Use bid.
DiabetAid Antifungal Foot Bath Tablets	Miconazole Nitrate 2%	**Adults & Peds ≥2 yrs:** Use prn.
Diabet-X Antifungal Skin Treatment Cream	Miconazole Nitrate 2%	**Adults & Peds ≥2 yrs:** Use prn.
Lotrimin AF Antifungal Aerosol Liquid Spray	Miconazole Nitrate 2%	**Adults & Peds ≥2 yrs:** Use bid.
Lotrimin AF Antifungal Jock Itch Aerosol Powder Spray	Miconazole Nitrate 2%	**Adults & Peds ≥2 yrs:** Use bid.
Lotrimin AF Antifungal Powder	Miconazole Nitrate 2%	**Adults & Peds ≥2 yrs:** Use bid.
Micatin Athlete's Foot Cream	Miconazole Nitrate 2%	**Adults:** Use bid.
Micatin Athlete's Foot Spray Liquid	Miconazole Nitrate 2%	**Adults:** Use bid.
Micatin Athlete's Foot Spray Liquid	Miconazole Nitrate 2%	**Adults:** Use bid.
Micatin Jock Itch Spray Powder	Miconazole Nitrate 2%	**Adults:** Use bid.
Micatin Jock Itch Antifungal Cream	Miconazole Nitrate 2%	**Adults:** Use bid.
Neosporin AF Antifungal Cream	Miconazole Nitrate 2%	**Adults & Peds ≥12 yrs:** Use bid.
Neosporin AF Athlete's Foot Antifungal Spray Liquid	Miconazole Nitrate 2%	**Adults & Peds ≥12 yrs:** Use bid.
Neosporin AF Athlete's Foot Antifungal Spray Powder	Miconazole Nitrate 2%	**Adults & Peds ≥12 yrs:** Use bid.
Neosporin AF Jock Itch Antifungal Cream	Miconazole Nitrate 2%	**Adults & Peds ≥12 yrs:** Use bid.
Zeasorb Super Absorbent Antifungal Powder	Miconazole Nitrate 2%	**Adults & Peds:** Use bid.
TERBINAFINE		
Lamisil AT Antifungal Cream	Terbinafine HCl 1%	**Adults & Peds ≥12 yrs:** Use bid.
Lamisil AT Antifungal Spray Pump	Terbinafine HCl 1%	**Adults & Peds ≥12 yrs:** Use qd or bid.
Lamisil AT Athlete's Foot Cream	Terbinafine HCl 1%	**Adults & Peds ≥12 yrs:** Use bid.
Lamisil AT Athlete's Foot Gel	Terbinafine HCl 1%	**Adults & Peds ≥12 yrs:** Use qd.
Lamisil AT Athlete's Foot Spray Pump	Terbinafine HCl 1%	**Adults & Peds ≥12 yrs:** Use bid.

(Continued)

BRAND	INGREDIENT/STRENGTH	DOSE
TERBINAFINE *(Continued)*		
Lamisil AT for Women Cream	Terbinafine HCl 1%	**Adults & Peds ≥12 yrs:** Use bid.
Lamisil AT Jock Itch Cream	Terbinafine HCl 1%	**Adults & Peds ≥12 yrs:** Use qd.
Lamisil AT Jock Itch Spray Pump	Terbinafine HCl 1%	**Adults & Peds ≥12 yrs:** Use qd.
TOLNAFTATE		
Aftate Antifungal Liquid Spray for Athlete's Foot	Tolnaftate 1%	**Adults:** Use qd-bid
FungiCure Anti-Fungal Gel	Tolnaftate 1%	**Adults & Peds:** Use bid.
Gold Bond Antifungal Foot Swabs	Tolnaftate 1%	**Adults & Peds:** Use bid.
Miracle of Aloe Miracure Anti-Fungal	Tolnaftate 1%	**Adults & Peds ≥12 yrs:** Use bid.
Swabplus Foot Care Fungus Relief Swabs	Tolnaftate 1%	**Adults & Peds:** Use bid.
Tinactin Antifungal Deodorant Powder Spray	Tolnaftate 1%	**Adults & Peds:** Use bid.
Tinactin Antifungal Liquid Spray	Tolnaftate 1%	**Adults & Peds:** Use bid.
Tinactin Antifungal Powder Spray	Tolnaftate 1%	**Adults & Peds:** Use bid.
Tinactin Antifungal Cream	Tolnaftate 1%	**Adults & Peds:** Use bid.
Tinactin Antifungal Absorbent Powder	Tolnaftate 1%	**Adults & Peds:** Use qd-tid.
Tinactin Antifungal Jock Itch Powder Spray	Tolnaftate 1%	**Adults & Peds:** Use qd-tid.
UNDECYLENIC ACID		
Fungi Nail Anti-fungal Solution	Undecylenic Acid 25%	**Adults & Peds:** Use bid.
FungiCure Anti-fungal Liquid	Undecylenic Acid 10%	**Adults & Peds:** Use bid.
Tineacide Antifungal Cream	Undecylenic Acid 10%	**Adults & Peds ≥12 yrs:** Use bid.

CONTACT DERMATITIS PRODUCTS

BRAND	INGREDIENT/STRENGTH	DOSE
ANTIHISTAMINE		
Benadryl Extra Strength Gel	Diphenhydramine HCl 2%	**Adults & Peds ≥2 yrs:** Apply to affected area tid-qid.
ANTIHISTAMINE COMBINATION		
Benadryl Extra Strength Itch-Stopping Cream	Diphenhydramine HCl/Zinc Acetate 2%-0.1%	**Adults & Peds ≥2 yrs:** Apply to affected area tid-qid.
Benadryl Extra Strength Spray	Diphenhydramine HCl/Zinc Acetate 2%-0.1%	**Adults & Peds ≥12 yrs:** Apply to affected area tid-qid.
Benadryl Itch Relief Spray	Diphenhydramine HCl/Zinc Acetate 2%-0.1%	**Adults & Peds ≥2 yrs:** Apply to affected area tid-qid.
Benadryl Itch Relief Stick	Diphenhydramine HCl/Zinc Acetate 2%-0.1%	**Adults & Peds ≥2 yrs:** Apply to affected area tid-qid.
Benadryl Original Cream	Diphenhydramine HCl/Zinc Acetate 1%-0.1%	**Adults & Peds ≥2 yrs:** Apply to affected area tid-qid.
CalaGel Anti-Itch Gel	Diphenhydramine HCl/Zinc Acetate/Benzethonium Chloride 2%-0.215%-0.15%	**Adults & Peds ≥2 yrs:** Apply to affected area tid-qid.
Ivarest Anti-Itch Cream	Diphenhydramine HCl/Calamine 2%-14%	**Adults & Peds ≥2 yrs:** Apply to affected area tid-qid.
ASTRINGENT		
Domeboro Powder Packets	Aluminum Acetate/Aluminum Sulfate	**Adults & Peds:** Dissolve 1-2 packets and apply to affected area for 15-30 min tid.
Ivy-Dry Super Lotion Extra Strength	Zinc Acetate/Benzyl Alcohol/Camphor/Menthol 2%-10%-0.5%-0.25%	**Adults & Peds: ≥6 yrs:** Apply to affected area qd-tid.
ASTRINGENT COMBINATION		
Aveeno Calamine and Pramoxine HCl Anti-Itch Cream	Calamine/Pramoxine HCl 3%-1%	**Adults & Peds ≥2 yrs:** Apply to affected area tid-qid.
Aveeno Anti-Itch Concentrated Lotion	Calamine/Pramoxine HCl/Camphor 3%-1%-0.47%	**Adults & Peds ≥2 yrs:** Apply to affected area qid.
Caladryl Clear Lotion	Zinc Acetate/Pramoxine HCl 0.1%-1%	**Adults & Peds ≥2 yrs:** Apply to affected area tid-qid.
Caladryl Lotion	Calamine/Pramoxine HCl 8%-1%	**Adults & Peds ≥2 yrs:** Apply to affected area tid-qid.
Calamine Lotion (generic)	Calamine/Zinc Oxide	**Adults & Peds:** Apply to affected area prn.
CLEANSER		
Ivy-Dry Scrub	Polyethylene, sodium lauryl sulfoacetate, cetearyl alcohol, nonoxynol-9, camellia sinensis oil, phenoxyethanol, methylparaben, propylparaben, triethanolamine, carbomer, erythorbic acid, aloe barbadensis extract, tocopheryl acetate extract, tetrasodium EDTA	**Adults & Peds:** Wash affected area prn.
Cortaid Poison Ivy Care Toxin Removal Cloths	Water, lauroyl sarcosinate, glycerin, DMDM, hydantoin, methylparaben, tetrasodium EDTA, Aloe barnadenis leaf extract, citric acid	**Adults & Peds:** Wash affected area prn.
CORTICOSTEROID		
Aveeno 1% Hydrocortisone Anti-Itch Cream	Hydrocortisone 1%	**Adults & Peds ≥2 yrs:** Apply to affected area tid-qid.
Cortaid Advanced 12-Hour Anti-Itch Cream	Hydrocortisone 1%	**Adults & Peds ≥2 yrs:** Apply to affected area tid-qid.
Cortaid Intensive Therapy Cooling Spray	Hydrocortisone 1%	**Adults & Peds ≥2 yrs:** Apply to affected area tid-qid.
Cortaid Intensive Therapy Moisturizing Cream	Hydrocortisone 1%	**Adults & Peds ≥2 yrs:** Apply to affected area tid-qid.
Cortaid Maximum Strength Cream	Hydrocortisone 1%	**Adults & Peds ≥2 yrs:** Apply to affected area tid-qid.

(Continued)

BRAND	INGREDIENT/STRENGTH	DOSE
CORTICOSTEROID (Continued)		
Cortaid Maximum Strength Ointment	Hydrocortisone 1%	**Adults & Peds ≥2 yrs:** Apply to affected area tid-qid.
Cortizone-10 Cream	Hydrocortisone 1%	**Adults & Peds ≥2 yrs:** Apply to affected area tid-qid.
Cortizone-10 Maximum Strength Anti-Itch Ointment	Hydrocortisone 1%	**Adults & Peds ≥2 yrs:** Apply to affected area tid-qid.
Cortizone-10 Ointment	Hydrocortisone 1%	**Adults & Peds ≥2 yrs:** Apply to affected area tid-qid.
Cortizone-10 Plus Intensive Healing Formula	Hydrocortisone 1%	**Adults & Peds ≥2 yrs:** Apply to affected area tid-qid.
IvyStat!	Hydrocortisone 1%	**Adults & Peds ≥2 yrs:** Apply to affected area tid-qid.
Dermarest Eczema Lotion	Hydrocortisone 1%	**Adults & Peds ≥2 yrs:** Apply to affected area tid-qid.
COUNTERIRRITANT		
Gold Bond First Aid Quick Spray	Menthol/Benzethonium Chloride 1%-0.13%	**Adults & Peds ≥2 yrs:** Apply to affected area tid-qid.
Gold Bond Medicated Maximum Strength Anti-Itch Cream	Menthol/Pramoxine HCl 1%-1%	**Adults & Peds ≥2 yrs:** Apply to affected area tid-qid.
Ivy Block Lotion	Bentoquatam 5%	**Adults & Peds ≥2 yrs:** Apply q4h for continued protection.
LOCAL ANESTHETIC		
Solarcaine Aloe Extra Burn Relief Gel	Lidocaine HCl 0.5%	**Adults & Peds ≥2 yrs:** Apply to affected area tid-qid.
Solarcaine Aloe Extra Spray	Lidocaine HCl 0.5%	**Adults & Peds ≥2 yrs:** Apply to affected area tid-qid.
Solarcaine First Aid Medicated Spray	Benzocaine/Triclosan 20%-0.13%	**Adults & Peds ≥2 yrs:** Apply to affected area qd-tid.
LOCAL ANESTHETIC COMBINATION		
Bactine First Aid Liquid	Lidocaine HCl/Benzalkonium Chloride 2.5%-0.13%	**Adults & Peds ≥2 yrs:** Apply to affected area qd-tid.
Lanacane Maximum Strength Cream	Benzocaine/Benzethonium Chloride 20%-0.2%	**Adults & Peds ≥2 yrs:** Apply to affected area qd-tid.
Lanacane Maximum Strength Spray	Benzocaine/Benzethonium Chloride 20%-0.2%	**Adults & Peds ≥2 yrs:** Apply to affected area qd-tid.
Lanacane Original Formula Cream	Benzocaine/Benzethonium Chloride 6%-0.2%	**Adults & Peds ≥2 yrs:** Apply to affected area qd-tid.
SKIN PROTECTANT		
Aveeno Skin Relief Moisturizing Cream	Dimethicone 2.5%	**Adults & Peds ≥2 yrs:** Apply to affected area tid-qid.
SKIN PROTECTANT COMBINATION		
Aveeno Itch Relief Lotion	Dimethicone/Menthol	**Adults & Peds ≥2 yrs:** Apply to affected area tid-qid.
Gold Bond Extra Strength Medicated Body Lotion Triple Action Relief	Dimethicone/Menthol 5%-0.5%	**Adults & Peds:** Apply to affected area tid-qid.
Gold Bond Medicated Body Lotion	Dimethicone/Menthol 5%-0.15%	**Adults & Peds:** Apply to affected area prn.
Gold Bond Medicated Extra Strength Powder	Zinc Oxide/Menthol 0.5%-0.8%	**Adults & Peds ≥2 yrs:** Apply to affected area tid-qid.
Vaseline Intensive Care Lotion Advanced Healing	Dimethicone 1%-White Petrolatum	**Adults & Peds:** Apply to affected area prn.

ANTACID AND HEARTBURN PRODUCTS

BRAND	INGREDIENT/STRENGTH	DOSE
ANTACID		
Alka-Seltzer Gold Tablets	Citric Acid/Potassium Bicarbonate/ Sodium Bicarbonate 1000mg-344mg-1050mg	**Adults:** ≥**60 yrs:** 2 tabs q4h prn. **Max:** 6 tabs q24h. **Adults & Peds:** ≥**12 yrs:** 2 tabs q4h prn. **Max:** 8 tabs q24h. **Peds:** ≤**12 yrs:** 1 tab q4h prn. **Max:** 4 tabs q24h.
Alka-Seltzer Heartburn Relief Tablets	Citric Acid/Sodium Bicarbonate 1000mg-1940mg	**Adults:** ≥**60 yrs:** 2 tabs q4h prn. **Max:** 4 tabs q24h. **Adults & Peds:** ≥**12 yrs:** 2 tabs q4h prn. **Max:** 8 tabs q24h.
Alka-Seltzer Tablets, Original	Aspirin/Sodium Bicarbonate/Citric Acid 325mg-1916mg-1000mg	**Adults:** ≥**60 yrs:** 2 tabs q4h prn. **Max:** 4 tabs q24h. **Adults & Peds:** ≥**12 yrs:** 2 tabs q4h prn. **Max:** 8 tabs q24h.
Alka-Seltzer Tablets, Extra-Strength	Aspirin/Sodium Bicarbonate/Citric Acid 500mg-1985mg-1000mg	**Adults:** ≥**60 yrs:** 2 tabs q6h prn. **Max:** 3 tabs q24h. **Adults & Peds:** ≥**12 yrs:** 2 tabs q6h prn. **Max:** 7 tabs q24h.
Brioschi Powder	Sodium Bicarbonate/Tartaric Acid 2.69g-2.43g/dose	**Adults & Peds:** ≥**12 yrs:** 1 capful (6g) dissolved in 4-6 oz water q1h. **Max:** 6 doses q24h.
Gaviscon Extra Strength Liquid	Aluminum Hydroxide/Magnesium Carbonate 254mg-237.5mg/5mL	**Adults:** 2-4 tsp (10-20mL) qid.
Gaviscon Extra Strength Tablets	Aluminum Hydroxide/Magnesium Carbonate 160mg-105mg	**Adults:** 2-4 tabs qid. **Max:** 16 doses q24h.
Gaviscon Regular Strength Chewable Tablets	Aluminum Hydroxide/Magnesium Carbonate 80mg-20mg	**Adults:** 2-4 tabs qid. **Max:** 16 tabs q24h.
Gaviscon Regular Strength Liquid	Aluminum Hydroxide/Magnesium Carbonate 95mg-358mg/15mL	**Adults:** 1-2 tbl (15-30mL) qid.
Gaviscon Acid Breakthrough, Chewable Tablets	Calcium Carbonate 500mg	**Adults:** 2 tabs prn. **Max:** 15 tabs q24h.
Maalox Antacid Barrier Chewable Tablets	Calcium Carbonate 500mg	**Adults:** 2-4 tabs qid. **Max:** 16 tabs q24h.
Maalox Quick Dissolve Regular Strength Chewable Tablets	Calcium Carbonate 600mg	**Adults:** 1-2 tabs prn. **Max:** 12 tabs q24h.
Mylanta, Children's	Calcium Carbonate 400 mg	**Peds: 6-11 yrs (48-95 lbs):** Take 2 tab prn. **Max:** 6 tabs q24h. **Peds: 2-5 yrs (24-47 lbs):** Take 1 tab prn **Max:** 3 tabs q24h.
Mylanta Ultimate Strength Liquid	Aluminum Hydroxide/Magnesium Hydroxide 500mg-500mg/5mL	**Adults & Peds** ≥**12 yrs:** 2-4 tsp (10-20mL) qid (between meals & hs). **Max:** 9 tsp (45mL) q24h for ≤2 weeks.
Mylanta Supreme Antacid Liquid	Calcium Carbonate/Magnesium Hydroxide 400mg-135mg/5mL	**Adults:** 2-4 tsp (10-20mL) qid. **Max:** 18 tsp (90mL) q24h.
Mylanta Ultimate Strength Chewable Tablets	Calcium Carbonate/Magnesium Hydroxide 700mg-300mg	**Adults:** 2-4 tabs qid. (between meals & hs). **Max:** 10 tabs q24h for ≤2 weeks.
Phillips Milk of Magnesia Liquid	Magnesium Hydroxide 400mg/5mL	**Adults & Peds:** ≥**12 yrs:** 30-60mL qd. **Peds: 6-11 yrs:** 15-30mL qd. **2-5 yrs:** 5-15mL qd.
Rolaids Extra Strength Softchews	Calcium Carbonate 1177mg	**Adults:** 2-3 chews q1h prn. **Max:** 6 chews q24h.
Rolaids Extra Strength Tablets	Calcium Carbonate/Magnesium Hydroxide 675mg-135mg	**Adults:** 2-4 tabs q1h prn. **Max:** 10 tabs q24h.
Rolaids Tablets	Calcium Carbonate/Magnesium Hydroxide 550mg-110mg	**Adults:** 2-4 tabs q1h prn. **Max:** 12 tabs q24h.
Titralac Chewable Tablets	Calcium Carbonate 420mg	**Adults:** 2 tabs q2-3h prn. **Max:** 19 tabs q24h.

(Continued)

BRAND	INGREDIENT/STRENGTH	DOSE
ANTACID *(Continued)*		
Tums Chewable Tablets	Calcium Carbonate 500mg	**Adults:** 2-4 tabs q1h prn. **Max:** 15 tabs q24h.
Tums E-X Chewable Tablets	Calcium Carbonate 750mg	**Adults:** 2-4 tabs prn. **Max:** 10 tabs q24h.
Tums E-X Sugar Free Chewable Tablets	Calcium Carbonate 750mg	**Adults:** 2-4 tabs prn. **Max:** 10 tabs q24h.
Tums Kids Chewable Tablets	Calcium Carbonate 750mg	**Peds: >4 yrs (>49 lbs):** Take 1 tab tid. **Max:** 4 tabs q24h. **Peds: 2-4 yrs (24-47 lbs):** Take ½ tab bid. **Max:** 2 tabs q24h.
Tums Smoothies Tablets	Calcium Carbonate 750mg	**Adults:** 2-4 tabs prn. **Max:** 10 tabs q24h.
Tums Ultra 1000 Chewable Tablets	Calcium Carbonate 1000mg	**Adults:** 2-4 tabs prn. **Max:** 7 tabs q24h for ≤2 weeks.
ANTACID/ANTIFLATULENT		
Gas-X with Maalox Capsules	Calcium Carbonate/Simethicone 250mg-62.5mg	**Adults:** 2-4 caps prn. **Max:** 8 caps q24h.
Gas-X Extra Strength with Maalox Capsules	Calcium Carbonate/Simethicone 500mg-125mg	**Adults:** 1-2 caps prn. **Max:** 4 caps q24h.
Gelusil Chewable Tablets	Aluminum Hydroxide/Magnesium Hydroxide/Simethicone 200mg-200mg-20mg	**Adults:** 2-4 tabs qid.
Maalox Max Liquid	Aluminum Hydroxide/Magnesium Hydroxide/Simethicone 400mg-400mg-40mg/5mL	**Adults & Peds:** ≥12 yrs: 2-4 tsp (10-20mL) qid. **Max:** 12 tsp (60mL) q24h.
Maalox Max Chewable Tablets	Calcium Carbonate/Simethicone 100mg-60mg	**Adults:** 1-2 tabs prn. **Max:** 8 tabs q24h.
Maalox Regular Strength Liquid	Aluminum Hydroxide/Magnesium Hydroxide/Simethicone 200mg-200mg-20mg/5mL	**Adults & Peds:** ≥12 yrs: 2-4 tsp (10-20mL) qid. **Max:** 12 tsp (60mL) q24h.
Mylanta Maximum Strength Liquid	Aluminum Hydroxide/Magnesium Hydroxide/Simethicone 400mg-400mg-40mg/5mL	**Adults & Peds:** ≥12 yrs: 2-4 tsp (10-20mL) qid. **Max:** 12 tsp (60mL) q24h.
Mylanta Regular Strength Liquid	Aluminum Hydroxide/Magnesium Hydroxide/Simethicone 200mg-200mg-20mg/5mL	**Adults & Peds:** ≥12 yrs: 2-4 tsp (10-20mL) qid. **Max:** 12 tsp (60mL) q24h.
Rolaids Multi-Symptom Chewable Tablets	Calcium Carbonate/Magnesium Hydroxide/Simethicone 675mg-135mg-60mg	**Adults:** 2 tabs qid prn. **Max:** 8 tabs q24h.
Titralac Plus Chewable Tablets	Calcium Carbonate/Simethicone 420mg-21mg	**Adults:** 2 tabs q2-3h prn. **Max:** 19 tabs q24h.
BISMUTH SUBSALICYLATE		
Maalox Total Stomach Relief Maximum Strength Liquid	Bismuth Subsalicylate 525mg/15mL	**Adults & Peds:** ≥12 yrs: 2 tbl (30mL) q1/2-1h. **Max:** 8 tbl (120mL) q24h.
Pepto Bismol Chewable Tablets	Bismuth Subsalicylate 262mg	**Adults & Peds:** ≥12 yrs: 2 tabs q1/2-1h. **Max:** 8 doses q24h.
Pepto Bismol Caplets	Bismuth Subsalicylate 262mg	**Adults & Peds:** ≥12 yrs: 2 tabs q1/2-1h. **Max:** 8 doses q24h.
Pepto Bismol Liquid	Bismuth Subsalicylate 262mg/15mL	**Adults & Peds:** ≥12 yrs: 2 tbl (30mL) q1/2-1h. **Max:** 8 doses (240mL) q24h.
Pepto Bismol Maximum Strengtth Liquid	Bismuth Subsalicylate 525mg/15mL	**Adults & Peds:** ≥12 yrs: 2 tbl (30mL) q1h. **Peds: 9-12 yrs:** 1 tbl (15mL) q1h. **6-9 yrs:** 2 tsp (10mL) q1h. **3-6 yrs:** 1 tsp (5mL). **Max:** 8 doses (240mL) q24h.

(Continued)

BRAND	INGREDIENT/STRENGTH	DOSE
H₂-RECEPTOR ANTAGONIST		
Pepcid AC Chewable Tablets	Famotidine 10mg	**Adults & Peds:** ≥**12 yrs:** 1 tab qd. **Max:** 2 tabs q24h.
Pepcid AC Gelcaps	Famotidine 10mg	**Adults & Peds:** ≥**12 yrs:** 1 tab qd. **Max:** 2 tabs q24h.
Pepcid AC Maximum Strength EZ Chews	Famotidine 20mg	**Adults & Peds:** ≥**12 yrs:** 1 tab qd. **Max:** 2 tabs q24h.
Pepcid AC Maximum Strength Tablets	Famotidine 20mg	**Adults & Peds:** ≥**12 yrs:** 1 tab qd. **Max:** 2 tabs q24h.
Pepcid AC Tablets	Famotidine 10mg	**Adults & Peds:** ≥**12 yrs:** 1 tab qd. **Max:** 2 tabs q24h.
Tagamet HB Tablets	Cimetidine 200mg	**Adults & Peds:** ≥**12 yrs:** 1 tab qd. **Max:** 2 tabs q24h.
Zantac 150 Tablets	Ranitidine 150mg	**Adults & Peds:** ≥**12 yrs:** 1 tab qd. **Max:** 2 tabs q24h.
Zantac 75 Tablets	Ranitidine 75mg	**Adults & Peds:** ≥**12 yrs:** 1 tab qd. **Max:** 2 tabs q24h.
H₂-RECEPTOR ANTAGONIST/ANTACID		
Pepcid Complete Chewable Tablets	Famotidine/Calcium Carbonate/ Magnesium Hydroxide 10mg-800mg-165mg	**Adults & Peds:** ≥**12 yrs:** 1 tab qd. **Max:** 2 tabs q24h.
PROTON PUMP INHIBITOR		
Prilosec OTC Tablets	Omeprazole 20mg	**Adults:** 1 tab qd x 14 days. May repeat 14 day course q 4 months.

ANTIDIARRHEAL PRODUCTS

BRAND	INGREDIENT/STRENGTH	DOSE
ABSORBENT AGENTS		
Equalactin Chewable Tablets	Calcium Polycarbophil 625mg	**Adults:** ≥12 yrs: 2 tabs q30min prn. **Max:** 8 tabs q24h. **Peds: 6-12 yrs:** 1 tab q30min. **Max:** 4 tabs q24h. **2 to ≤6 yrs:** 1 tab q30min. **Max:** 2 tabs q24h.
Fibercon Caplets	Calcium Polycarbophil 625mg	**Adults:** ≥12 yrs: 2 tabs qd. **Max:** 8 tabs q24h.
Konsyl Fiber Caplets	Calcium Polycarbophil 625mg	**Adults:** ≥12 yrs: 2 tabs qd. **Max:** 8 tabs q24h. **Peds:** 6-12 yrs: 1 tab qd. **Max:** 3 tabs q24h.
ANTIPERISTALTIC AGENTS		
Imodium A-D Caplet	Loperamide HCl 2mg	**Adults:** ≥12 yrs: 2 caplets after first loose stool; 1 caplet after each subsequent loose stool. **Max:** 4 caplets q24h. **Peds: 9-11 yrs (60-95 lbs):** 1 caplet after first loose stool; ½ caplet after each subsequent loose stool. **Max:** 3 caplets q24h. **6-8 yrs (48-59 lbs):** 1 caplet after first loose stool; ½ caplet after each subsequent loose stool. **Max:** 2 caplets q24h.
Imodium A-D E-Z Chews	Loperamide HCl 2mg	**Adults:** ≥12 yrs: 2 caplets after first loose stool; 1 caplet after each subsequent loose stool. **Max:** 4 caplets q24h. **Peds: 9-11 yrs (60-95 lbs):** 1 caplet after first loose stool; ½ caplet after each subsequent loose stool. **Max:** 3 caplets q24h. **6-8 yrs (48-59 lbs):** 1 caplet after first loose stool; 1/2 caplet after each subsequent loose stool. **Max:** 2 caplets q24h.
Imodium A-D Liquid	Loperamide HCl 1mg/7.5mL	**Adults:** ≥12 yrs: 30mL (6 tsp) after first loose stool; 15mL (3 tsp) after each subsequent loose stool. **Max:** 60mL (12 tsp) q24h. **Peds: 9-11 yrs (60-95 lbs):** 15mL (3 tsp) after first loose stool; 7.5mL (1½ tsp) after each subsequent loose stool. **Max:** 45mL (9 tsp) q24h. **6-8 yrs (48-59 lbs):** 15 mL (3 tsp) after first loose stool; 7.5mL (1½ tsp) after each subsequent loose stool. **Max:** 30mL (6 tsp) q24h.
ANTIPERISTALTIC/ANTIFLATULENT AGENTS		
Imodium Advanced Caplet	Loperamide HCl/Simethicone 2mg-125mg	**Adults:** ≥12 yrs: 2 caplets after first loose stool; 1 caplet after each subsequent loose stool. **Max:** 4 caplets q24h. **Peds: 9-11 yrs (60-95 lbs):** 1 caplet after first loose stool; 1/2 caplet after each subsequent loose stool. **Max:** 3 caplets q24h. **6-8 yrs (48-59 lbs):** 1 caplet after first loose stool; ½ caplet after each subsequent loose stool. **Max:** 2 caplets q24h.

(Continued)

BRAND	INGREDIENT/STRENGTH	DOSE
ANTIPERISTALTIC/ANTIFLATULENT AGENTS *(Continued)*		
Imodium Advanced Chewable Tablet	Loperamide HCl/Simethicone 2mg-125mg	**Adults:** ≥12 yrs: 2 caplets after first loose stool; 1 caplet after each subsequent loose stool. **Max:** 4 caplets q24h. **Peds: 9-11 yrs (60-95 lbs):** 1 caplet after first loose stool; ½ caplet after each subsequent loose stool. **Max:** 3 caplets q24h. **6-8 yrs (48-59 lbs):** 1 caplet after first loose stool; ½ caplet after each subsequent loose stool. **Max:** 2 caplets q24h.
BISMUTH SUBSALICYLATE		
Kaopectate Caplets	Bismuth Subsalicylate 262mg	**Adults & Peds:** ≥12 yrs: 2 caplets q½-1h prn. **Max:** 8 doses q24h.
Kaopectate Extra Strength Liquid	Bismuth Subsalicylate 525mg/15mL	**Adults:** ≥12 yrs: 2 tbl (30mL). **Peds: 9-12 yrs:** 1 tbl (15mL) q1h prn. **6-9 yrs:** 2 tsp (10mL) q1h prn. **3-6 yrs:** 1 tsp (5mL) q1h prn. **Max:** 8 doses q24h.
Kaopectate Liquid	Bismuth Subsalicylate 262mg/15mL	**Adults:** ≥12 yrs: 2 tbl (30mL). **Peds: 9-12 yrs:** 1 tbl (15mL) q1h prn. **6-9 yrs:** 2 tsp (10mL) q1h prn. **3-6 yrs:** 1 tsp (5mL) q1h prn. **Max:** 8 doses q24h.
Pepto Bismol Chewable Tablets	Bismuth Subsalicylate 262mg	**Adults & Peds:** ≥12 yrs: 2 tabs q½-1h. **Max:** 8 doses (16 tabs) q24h.
Pepto Bismol Caplets	Bismuth Subsalicylate 262mg	**Adults & Peds:** ≥12 yrs: 2 tabs q½-1h. **Max:** 8 doses (16 caps) q24h.
Pepto Bismol Liquid	Bismuth Subsalicylate 262mg/15mL	**Adults & Peds:** ≥12 yrs: 2 tbl (30mL) q½-1h prn. **Max:** 8 doses (16 tbl) q24h.
Pepto Bismol Maximum Strength	Bismuth Subsalicylate 525mg/15mL	**Adults:** ≥12 yrs: 2 tbl (30mL) q1h prn. **Max:** 4 doses (8 tbl) q24h.

ANTIFLATULANT PRODUCTS

BRAND	INGREDIENT/STRENGTH	DOSE
ALPHA-GALACTOSIDASE		
Beano Food Enzyme Dietary Supplement Drops	Alpha-Galactosidase Enzyme 150 GalU	**Adults:** Add 5 drops before meals.
Beano Food Enzyme Dietary Supplement Tablets	Alpha-Galactosidase Enzyme 150 GalU	**Adults:** Take 3 tabs before meals.
ANTACID/ANTIFLATULENCE		
Gas-X with Maalox Capsules	Calcium Carbonate/Simethicone 250mg-62.5mg	**Adults:** 2-4 caps prn. **Max:** 8 caps q24h.
Gas-X Extra Strength with Maalox Capsules	Calcium Carbonate/Simethicone 500mg-125mg	**Adults:** 1-2 caps prn. **Max:** 4 caps q24h.
Gelusil Chewable Tablets	Aluminum Hydroxide/Magnesium Hydroxide/Simethicone 200mg-200mg-20mg	**Adults:** 2-4 tabs qid.
Maalox Max Liquid	Aluminum Hydroxide/Magnesium Hydroxide/Simethicone 400mg-400mg-40mg/5mL	**Adults & Peds: ≥12 yrs:** 2-4 tsp (10-20mL) qid. **Max:** 12 tsp (60mL) q24h.
Maalox Max Chewable Tablets	Calcium Carbonate/Simethicone 100mg-60mg	**Adults:** 1-2 caps prn. **Max:** 8 tabs q24h.
Maalox Regular Strength Liquid	Aluminum Hydroxide/Magnesium Hydroxide/Simethicone 200mg-200mg-20mg/5mL	**Adults & Peds: ≥12 yrs:** 2-4 tsp (10-20mL) qid. **Max:** 12 tsp (60mL) q24h.
Mylanta Maximum Strength Liquid	Aluminum Hydroxide/Magnesium Hydroxide/Simethicone 400mg-400mg-40mg/5mL	**Adults & Peds: ≥12 yrs:** 2-4 tsp (10-20mL) qid. **Max:** 12 tsp (60mL) q24h.
Mylanta Regular Strength Liquid	Aluminum Hydroxide/Magnesium Hydroxide/Simethicone 200mg-200mg-20mg/5mL	**Adults & Peds: ≥12 yrs:** 2-4 tsp (10-20mL) qid. **Max:** 24 tsp (120mL) q24h.
Rolaids Antacid & Antigas Soft Chews	Calcium Carbonate/Simethicone 1177mg-80mg	**Adults:** 2-3 chews hourly prn.
Titralac Plus Chewable Tablets	Calcium Carbonate/Simethicone 420mg-21mg	**Adults:** 2 tabs q2-3h prn. **Max:** 19 tabs q24h.
SIMETHICONE		
GasAid Maximum Strength Anti-Gas Softgels	Simethicone 125mg	**Adults:** Take 1-2 caps prn and qhs. **Max:** 4 caps q24h.
Gas-X Infant Drops	Simethicone 20mg/0.3mL	**Peds: ≥2 yrs (≥24 lbs):** 0.6mL prn. **Peds: <2 yrs (<24 lbs):** 0.3mL prn. **Max:** 6 doses q24h.
Gas-X Children's Thin Strips	Simethicone 40mg	**Peds: 2-12 yrs:** 1 strip prn and hs. **Max:** 6 strips q24h.
Gas-X Thin Strips	Simethicone 62.5mg	**Adults:** Allow 2-4 strips to dissolve prn. **Max:** 8 strips q24h.
Gas-X Antigas Chewable Tablets	Simethicone 80mg	**Adults:** Take 1-2 caps and qhs. **Max:** 6 caps q24h.
Gas-X Extra Strength Antigas Softgels	Simethicone 125mg	**Adults:** Take 1-2 caps and qhs. **Max:** 4 caps q24h.
Gas-X Maximum Strength Antigas Softgels	Simethicone 166mg	**Adults:** Take 1-2 caps and qhs. **Max:** 3 caps q24h.
Little Tummys Gas Relief Drops	Simethicone 20mg/0.3mL	**Peds: ≥2 yrs (≥24 lbs):** 0.6mL prn (after meals & hs). **Peds: <2 yrs (<24 lbs):** 0.3mL prn (after meals & hs). **Max:** 12 doses q24h.
Mylanta Gas Maximum Strength Softgels	Simethicone 125mg	**Adults:** Chew 1-2 tabs (after meals & hs). **Max:** 4 tabs q24h.
Mylanta Gas Maximum Strength Chewable Tablets	Simethicone 125mg	**Adults:** Chew 1-2 tabs (after meals & hs). **Max:** 4 tabs q24h.
Mylicon Infant's Gas Relief Drops	Simethicone 20mg/0.3mL	**Peds: ≥2 yrs (≥24 lbs):** 0.6mL (after meals & hs). **Peds: <2 yrs (<24 lbs):** 0.3mL (after meals & hs). **Max:** 12 doses q24h.

LAXATIVE PRODUCTS

BRAND	INGREDIENT/STRENGTH	DOSE
BULK-FORMING		
Citrucel Caplets	Methylcellulose 500mg	**Adults:** ≥**12 yrs:** 2 caps qd prn. **Max:** 12 tabs q24h. **Peds: 6-12 yrs:** 1 cap qd prn. **Max:** 6 tabs q24h.
Citrucel Powder	Methylcellulose 2g/tbl	**Adults:** ≥**12 yrs:** 1 tbl (11.5g) qd tid. **Peds: 6-12 yrs:** ½ tbl (5.75g) qd.
Equalactin Chewable Tablet	Calcium Polycarbophil 625mg	**Adults & Peds:** ≥**12 yrs:** 2 tabs qd. **Max:** 8 tabs qd. **Peds: 6-12 yrs:** 1 tab qd. **Max:** 2 tabs qd. **2 to <6 yrs:** 1 tab qd. **Max:** 2 tabs qd.
Fibercon Caplets	Calcium Polycarbophil 625mg	**Adults & Peds:** ≥**12 yrs:** 2 tabs qd. **Max:** 8 tabs qd. **Peds: 6-12 yrs:** 1 tab qd. **Max:** 4 tabs qd. **2 to <6 yrs:** 1 tab qd. **Max:** 2 tabs qd.
Konsyl Easy Mix Powder	Psyllium 6g/tsp	**Adults:** ≥**12 yrs:** 1 tsp qd-tid. **Peds: 6-12 yrs:** ½ tsp qd-tid.
Konsyl Fiber Caplets	Calcium Polycarbophil 625mg	**Adults & Peds:** ≥**12 yrs:** 2 tabs qd. **Max:** 8 tabs qd.
Konsyl Orange Powder	Psyllium 3.4g	**Adults:** ≥**12 yrs:** 1 tsp qd-tid. **Peds: 6-12 yrs:** ½ tsp qd-tid.
Konsyl Original Powder	Psyllium 6g/tsp	**Adults:** ≥**12 yrs:** 1 tsp qd-tid. **Peds: 6-12 yrs:** ½ tsp qd-tid.
Konsyl-D Powder	Psyllium 3.4g/tsp	**Adults:** ≥**12 yrs:** 1 tsp qd-tid. **Peds: 6-12 yrs:** ½ tsp qd-tid.
Metamucil Capsules	Psyllium 0.52g	**Adults & Peds:** ≥**12 yrs:** 5 caps qd-tid.
Metamucil Original Texture Powder	Psyllium 3.4g/tbs	**Adults:** ≥**12 yrs:** 1 tbs qd-tid. **Peds: 6-12 yrs:** ½ tsp qd-tid.
Metamucil Smooth Texture Powder	Psyllium 3.4g/tbs	**Adults:** ≥**12 yrs:** 1 tbs qd-tid. **Peds: 6-12 yrs:** ½ tsp qd-tid.
Metamucil Wafers	Psyllium 3.4 g/dose	**Adults:** ≥**12 yrs:** 2 wafers qd-tid. **Peds: 6-12 yrs:** 1 wafer qd-tid.
HYPEROSMOTICS		
Fleet Children's Babylax Suppositories	Glycerin 2.3g	**Peds: 2-5 yrs:** 1 supp. ud.
Fleet Glycerin Suppositories	Glycerin 2g	**Adults & Peds:** ≥**6 yrs:** 1 supp ud.
Fleet Liquid Glycerin Suppositories	Glycerin 5.6g	**Adults & Peds:** ≥**6 yrs:** 1 supp ud.
Fleet Mineral Oil Enema	Mineral Oil 133mL	**Adults:** ≥**12 yrs:** 1 bottle (133mL). **Peds: 2-12 yrs:** ½ bottle (66.5mL)
HYPEROSMOTIC COMBINATION		
Fleet Pain Relief Pre-Moistened Anorectal Pads	Glycerin/Pramoxine HCl 12%-1%	**Adults & Peds:** ≥**12 yrs:** Apply to affected area up to five times daily.
OSMOTIC		
MiraLAX	Polyethylene Glycol 3350	**Adults & Peds:** ≥**17 yrs:** Stir and dissolve 17g in 4-8 oz of beverage and drink qd. Use no more than 7 days.
SALINES		
Ex-Lax Milk of Magnesia Liquid	Magnesium Hydroxide 400mg/5mL	**Adults & Peds:** ≥**12 yrs:** Take 2-4 tbs hs. **Peds: 6-11 yrs:** 1-2 tbs hs. **2-5 yrs:** 1-3 tbs hs.

(Continued)

BRAND	INGREDIENT/STRENGTH	DOSE
SALINES *(Continued)*		
Fleet Children's Enema	Monobasic Sodium Phosphate/Dibasic Sodium Phosphate 9.5g-3.5g/66mL	**Peds: 5-11 yrs:** 1 bottle (66mL). **2-5 yrs:** ½ bottle (33mL).
Fleet Enema	Monobasic Sodium Phosphate/Dibasic Sodium Phosphate 19g-7g/133mL	**Adults & Peds: ≥12 yrs:** 1 bottle (133mL).
Fleet Phospho-Soda	Monobasic Sodium Phosphate/Dibasic Sodium Phosphate 2.4g-0.9g/5mL	**Adults: ≥12 yrs:** 1 tbl in 8 oz of water. **Max:** 3 tbl. **Peds: 10-11 yrs:** 1 tbl in 8 oz of water. **Max:** 1 tbl. **5-9 yrs:** ½ tbl in 8 oz of water. **Max:** ½ tbl.
Magnesium Citrate Solution	Magnesium Citrate 1.75gm/30mL	**Adults: ≥12 yrs:** 300mL. **Peds: 6-12 yrs:** 90-210mL. **2-6 yrs:** 60-90mL.
Phillips Antacid/Laxative Chewable Tablets	Magnesium Hydroxide 311mg	**Adults: ≥12 yrs:** 6-8 tabs qd. **Peds: 6-11 yrs:** 3-4 tabs qd. **2-5 yrs:** 1-2 tabs qd.
Phillips Soft Chews, Laxative	Magnesium/Sodium 500mg-10 mg	**Adults & Peds: ≥12 yrs:** Take 2-4 tab qd. **Max:** 4 tab q24h.
Phillips Cramp-Free Laxative Caplets	Magnesium 500 mg	**Adults & Peds: ≥12 yrs:** Take 2-4 tabs qd. **Max:** 4 tabs q24h.
Phillips Milk of Magnesia Concentrated Liquid	Magnesium Hydroxide 800mg/5mL	**Adults: ≥12 yrs:** 15-30mL qd. **Peds: 6-11 yrs:** 7.5-15mL qd. **2-5 yrs:** 2.5-7.5mL qd.
Phillips Milk of Magnesia Liquid	Magnesium Hydroxide 400mg/5mL	**Adults: ≥12 yrs:** 30-60mL qd. **Peds: 6-11 yrs:** 15-30mL qd. **2-5 yrs:** 5-15mL qd.
SALINE COMBINATION		
Phillips M-O Liquid	Magnesium Hydroxide/Mineral Oil 300mg-1.25mL/5mL	**Adults: ≥12 yrs:** 30-60mL qd. **Peds: 6-11 yrs:** 5-15mL qd.
STIMULANTS		
Alophen Enteric Coated Stimulant Laxative Pills	Bisacodyl 5mg	**Adults: ≥12 yrs:** Take 1-3 tabs qd. **Peds: 6-12 yrs:** Take 1 tab qd.
Carter's Laxative, Sodium Free Pills	Bisacodyl 5mg	**Adults: qd.12 yrs:** Take 1-3 tabs (usually 2 tabs) qd. **Peds: 6-12 yrs:** Take 1 tab qd.
Castor Oil	Castor Oil	**Adults: ≥12 yrs:** 15-60mL. **Peds: 2-12 yrs:** 5-15mL.
Correctol Stimulant Laxative Tablets For Women	Bisacodyl 5mg	**Adults: ≥12 yrs:** Take 1-3 tabs qd. **Peds: 6-12 yrs:** Take 1 tab qd.
Doxidan Capsules	Bisacodyl 5mg	**Adults: ≥12 yrs:** 1-3 caps (usually 2) qd. **Peds: 6-12 yrs:** 1 cap qd.
Dulcolax Overnight Relief Laxative Tablets	Bisacodyl 5mg	**Adults: ≥12 yrs:** 1-3 tabs (usually 2) qd. **Peds: 6-12 yo:** 1 tab qd.
Dulcolax Suppository	Bisacodyl 10mg	**Adults: ≥12 yrs:** 1 supp qd. **Peds: 6-12 yrs:** ½ supp qd.
Dulcolax Tablets	Bisacodyl 5mg	**Adults: ≥12 yrs:** 1-3 tabs (usually 2) qd. **Peds: 6-12 yrs:** 1 tab qd.
Ex-Lax Maximum Strength Tablets	Sennosides 25mg	**Adults: ≥12 yrs:** 2 tabs qd-bid. **Peds: 6-12 yrs:** 1 tab qd-bid.
Ex-Lax Tablets	Sennosides 15mg	**Adults: ≥12 yrs:** 2 tabs qd-bid. **Peds: 6-12 yrs:** 1 tab qd-bid.
Ex-Lax Ultra Stimulant Laxative Tablets	Bisacodyl 5mg	**Adults: ≥12 yrs:** 1-3 tabs qd. **Peds: 6-12 yrs:** 1 tab qd.
Fleet Bisacodyl Suppositories	Bisacodyl 10mg	**Adults: ≥12 yrs:** 1 supp. qd. **Peds: 6-12 yrs:** ½ supp. qd.

(Continued)

BRAND	INGREDIENT/STRENGTH	DOSE
STIMULANTS *(Continued)*		
Fleet Stimulant Laxative Tablets	Bisacodyl 5mg	**Adults:** ≥12 yrs: 1-3 tabs (usually 2) qd. **Peds: 6-12 yrs:** 1 tab qd.
Nature's Remedy Caplets	Aloe/Cascara Sagrada 100mg-150mg	**Adults:** ≥12 yrs: 2 tabs qd-bid. **Max:** 4 tabs bid. **Peds: 6-12 yrs:** 1 tab qd-bid. **Max:** 2 tabs bid. **2-6 yrs:** ½ tab qd-bid. **Max:** 1 tab bid.
Perdiem Overnight Relief Tablets	Sennosides 15mg	**Adults:** ≥12 yrs: 2 tabs qd-bid. **Peds: 6-12 yrs:** 1 tab qd-bid.
Senokot Tablets	Sennosides 8.6mg	**Adults:** ≥12 yrs: 2 tabs qd. **Max** 4 tabs bid. **Peds: 6-12 yrs:** 1 tab qd. **Max:** 2 tabs bid. **2-6 yrs:** ½ tab qd. **Max:** 1 tab bid.
STIMULANT COMBINATIONS		
Peri-Colace Tablets	Sennosides/Docusate 8.6mg-50mg	**Adults:** ≥12 yrs: 2-4 tabs qd. **Peds: 6-12 yrs:** 1-2 tabs qd. **2-6 yrs:** 1 tab qd.
Senokot S Tablets	Sennosides/Docusate 8.6mg-50mg	**Adults:** ≥12 yrs: 2 tabs qd. **Max:** 4 tabs bid. **Peds: 6-12 yrs:** 1 tab qd. **Max:** 2 tabs bid. **2-6 yrs:** ½ tab qd. **Max:** 1 tab bid.
SURFACTANTS (STOOL SOFTENERS)		
Colace Capsules	Docusate Sodium 100mg	**Adults:** ≥12 yrs: 1-3 caps qd. **Peds: 2-12 yrs:** 1 cap qd.
Colace Capsules	Docusate Sodium 50mg	**Adults:** ≥12 yrs: 1-6 caps qd. **Peds: 2-12 yrs:** 1-3 caps qd.
Colace Liquid	Docusate Sodium 10mg/mL	**Adults:** ≥12 yrs: 5-15mL qd-bid. **Peds: 2-12 yrs:** 5-15mL qd.
Colace Syrup	Docusate Sodium 60mg/15mL	**Adults:** ≥12 yrs: 15-90mL qd. **Peds: 2-12 yrs:** 5-37.5mL qd.
Correctol Stool Softener Laxative Soft-Gels	Docusate Sodium 100mg	**Adults:** ≥12 yrs: Take 2 caps qd. **Peds: 2-12 yrs:** Take 1 cap qd
Docusol Constipation Relief, Mini Enemas	Docusate Sodium 283mg	**Adults:** ≥12 yrs: Take 1-3 units qd. **Peds: 6-12 yrs:** Take 1 unit qd
Dulcolax Stool Softener Capsules	Docusate Sodium 100mg	**Adults:** ≥12 yrs: 1-3 caps qd. **Peds: 2-12 yrs:** 1 cap qd.
Ex-Lax Stool Softener Tablets	Docusate Sodium 100mg	**Adults:** ≥12 yrs: 1-3 caps qd. **Peds: 2-12 yrs:** 1 cap qd.
Kaopectate Liqui-Gels	Docusate Calcium 240mg	**Adults & Peds:** ≥12 yrs: 1 cap qd until normal bowel movement.
Phillips Stool Softener Capsules	Docusate Sodium 100mg	**Adults:** ≥12 yrs: 1-3 caps qd. **Peds: 6-12 yrs:** 1 cap qd.
Kaopectate Liqui-Gels	Docusate Calcium 240mg	**Adults & Peds:** ≥12 yrs: 1 cap qd until normal bowel movement.
Phillips Stool Softener Capsules	Docusate Sodium 100mg	**Adults:** ≥12 yrs: 1-3 caps qd. **Peds: 2-12 yrs:** 1 cap qd.

ALLERGIC RHINITIS PRODUCTS

BRAND	INGREDIENT/STRENGTH	DOSE
ANTIHISTAMINE		
Alavert Oral Disintegrating Tablets	Loratadine 10mg	**Adults & Peds:** ≥6 yrs: 1 tab qd. **Max:** 1 tab q24h.
Alavert 24-Hour Allergy Tablets	Loratadine 10mg	**Adults & Peds:** ≥6 yrs: 1 tab qd. **Max:** 1 tab q24h.
Benadryl Allergy Quick Dissolve Strips	Diphenhydramine HCl 25mg	**Adults & Peds:** ≥12 yrs: Dissolve 1-2 strips on tongue q4-6h. **Max:** 6 doses q24h.
Benadryl Allergy Capsules	Diphenhydramine HCl 25mg	**Adults & Peds:** ≥12 yrs: 1-2 caps q4-6h. **Peds: 6-12 yrs:** 1 cap q4-6h. **Max:** 6 doses q24h.
Benadryl Allergy Chewable Tablets	Diphenhydramine HCl 12.5mg	**Adults & Peds:** ≥12 yrs: 2-4 tabs q4-6h. **Peds: 6-12 yrs:** 1-2 tabs q4-6h. **Max:** 6 doses q24h.
Benadryl Allergy Liquid	Diphenhydramine HCl 12.5mg/5mL	**Adults & Peds:** ≥12 yrs: 2-4 tsp (10-20mL) q4-6h. **Peds: 6-12 yrs:** 1-2 tsp (5-10mL) q4-6h. **Max:** 6 doses q24h.
Benadryl Allergy Ultratab	Diphenhydramine HCl 25mg	**Adults & Peds:** ≥12 yrs: 1-2 tabs q4-6h. **Peds: 6-12 yrs:** 1 tab q4-6h. **Max:** 6 doses q24h.
Benadryl Children's Quick Dissolve Strips	Diphenhydramine HCl 12.5mg	**Adults & Peds:** ≥12 yrs: Dissolve 1 or 2 strips on tongue q4-6h. Allow first strip to dissolve before placing second strip on tongue. **Max:** 6 doses q24h.
Chlor-Trimeton 4-Hour Allergy Tablets	Chlorpheniramine Maleate 4mg	**Adults & Peds:** ≥12 yrs: 1 tab q4-6h. **Max:** 6 tabs q24h. **Peds: 6-12 yrs:** ½ tab q4-6h. **Max:** 3 tabs q24h.
Claritin 24 Hour Allergy Tablets	Loratadine 10mg	**Adults & Peds:** ≥6 yrs: 1 tab qd. **Max:** 1 tab q24h.
Claritin Children's Syrup	Loratadine 5mg/5mL	**Adults & Peds:** ≥6 yrs: 2 tsp qd. **Max:** 2 tsp q24h. **Peds: 2-6 yrs:** 1 tsp qd. **Max:** 1 tsp q24h.
Claritin RediTabs	Loratadine 10mg	**Adults & Peds:** ≥6 yrs: 1 tab qd. **Max:** 1 tab q24h.
Dimetapp ND Children's Allergy Tablets	Loratadine 10mg	**Adults & Peds:** ≥6 yrs: 1 tab qd. **Max:** 1 tab q24h.
Zyrtec Tablets	Cetirizine 10mg	**Adults:** 18 yrs-64 yrs & Peds: ≥6 yrs: 1 tab q24h. **Max:** 1 tab q24h.
Zyrtec Children's Syrup	Cetirizine 5mg/5mL	**Adults** ≥65: 1 tsp q24h. **Peds: 2-6 yrs:** ½ tsp (2.5mL) qd or bid. ≥6 to 12: 1 or 2 tsp (5-10mL) qd. **Max: Adults:** ≥65 & Peds: 2-6 yrs: 1 tsp (5mL) q24h ≥6 to 12yrs: 2 tsp (10mL) qd
Zyrtec Children's Chewables 5mg	Cetirizine 5mg	**Adults & Peds** ≥6 yrs-64 yrs: 1 tab q24h. **Adults** ≥65 yrs: 1 tab q24h. **Max:** 1 tab q24h.
Zyrtec Children's Chewables 10mg	Cetirizine 10mg	**Adults & Peds** ≥6 yrs: 1 tab q24h. **Adults** ≥65 yrs: Ask doctor. **Max:** 1 tab qd
Zyrtec Children's Hive Relief Syrup	Cetirizine 5mg/5mL	**Adults & Peds** ≥6 yrs-64yrs: 1-2 tsp (5-10ml) q24h. **Max:** 2 tsp (10ml) q24h. **Adults** >65: 1 tsp q24h. **Max:** 1 tsp (5ml) q24h.

(Continued)

BRAND	INGREDIENT/STRENGTH	DOSE
ANTIHISTAMINE COMBINATIONS		
Advil Allergy Sinus Caplets	Chlorpheniramine Maleate/ Ibuprofen/Pseudoephedrine 2mg-200mg-30mg	**Adults & Peds:** ≥**12 yrs:** 1 tab q4-6h. **Max:** 6 tabs q24h.
Alavert D-12 Hour Allergy and Sinus Tablets	Loratadine/Pseudoephedrine Sulfate 5mg-120mg	**Adults & Peds:** ≥**12 yrs:** 1 tab q12h. **Max:** 2 tabs q24h.
Benadryl Allergy & Sinus Headache Caplets	Diphenhydramine HCl/ Acetaminophen/Phenylephrine HCl/ 12.5mg-325mg-5mg	**Adults & Peds:** ≥**12 yrs:** 2 caps q4h. **Max:** 12 caps q24h.
Benadryl Severe Allergy & Sinus Headache Caplets	Diphenhydramine HCl/ Acetaminophen/Phenylephrine HCl 25mg-325mg-5mg	**Adults & Peds:** ≥**12 yrs:** 2 tabs q4h. **Max:** 12 tabs q24h.
Benadryl-D Allergy & Sinus Liquid	Diphenhydramine HCl/ Phenylephrine 12.5mg-5mg/5mL	**Adults & Peds:** ≥**12 yrs:** 2 tsp q4h. **Peds: 6-12 yrs:** 1 tsp q4h. **Max:** 6 doses q24h.
Claritin-D 12 Hour Allergy & Congestion Tablets	Loratadine/Pseudoephedrine Sulfate 5mg-120mg	**Adults & Peds:** ≥**12 yrs:** 1 tab q12h. **Max:** 2 tabs q24h.
Claritin-D 24 Hour Allergy & Congestion Tablets	Loratadine/Pseudoephedrine Sulfate 10mg-240mg	**Adults & Peds:** ≥**12 yrs:** 1 tab q24h. **Max:** 1 tab q24h.
Drixoral Cold & Allergy Sustained Action Tablets	Dexbrompheniramine Maleate/Pseudoephedrine HCl 6mg-120mg	**Adults & Peds:** ≥**12 yrs:** 1 tabs q12h. **Max:** 2 tabs q24h.
Dimetapp Elixir Cold & Allergy	Brompheniramine/Phenylephrine 1mg-2.5mg/5ml	**Adults & Peds:** ≥**12 yrs:** 4 tsp (20mL) q4h. **Peds: 6-12 yrs:** 2 tsp (10mL) q4h. **Max:** 6 doses q24h.
Dimetapp Children's Chewable Tablets	Brompheniramine/Phenylephrine 1mg-2.5mg	**Peds:** ≥**6-12 yrs:** 2 tabs q4h. **Max:** 6 doses q24h
Sudafed Sinus & Allergy Tablets	Chlorpheniramine/ Pseudoephedrine 4mg-60mg	**Adults:** ≥**12 yrs:** 1 tab q4-6h. **Peds: 6-12 yrs:** 1/2 tab q4h-6h. **Max:** 4 doses q24h.
Tylenol Allergy Complete Multi-Symptom Cool Burst Caplets	Chlorpheniramine Maleate/ Acetaminophen/Phenylephrine HCl 2mg-325mg-5mg	**Adults & Peds:** ≥**12 yrs:** 2 tabs q4h. **Max:** 12 tabs q24h.
Tylenol Allergy Complete Nighttime Cool Burst Caplets	Diphenhydramine HCl/ Acetaminophen/Phenylephrine HCl 25mg-325mg-5mg	**Adults & Peds:** ≥**12 yrs:** 2 tabs q4h. **Max:** 12 tabs q24h.
Tylenol Severe Allergy Caplets	Diphenhydramine HCl/ Acetaminophen 12.5mg-500mg	**Adults & Peds:** ≥**12 yrs:** 2 tabs q4-6h. **Max:** 8 tabs q24h.
TOPICAL NASAL DECONGESTANTS		
4-Way Fast Acting Nasal Decongestant Spray	Phenylephrine HCl 1%	**Adults & Peds:** ≥**12 yrs:** Instill 2-3 sprays per nostril q4h.
4-Way Mentholated Nasal Decongestant Spray	Phenylephrine HCl 1%	**Adults & Peds:** ≥**12 yrs:** Instill 2-3 sprays per nostril q4h.
Afrin No Drip Extra Moisturizing Nasal Spray	Oxymetazoline HCl 0.05%	**Adults & Peds:** ≥**6 yrs:** Instill 2-3 sprays per nostril q10-12h. **Max:** 2 doses q24h.
Afrin No Drip Sinus Nasal Spray	Oxymetazoline HCl 0.05%	**Adults & Peds:** ≥**6 yrs:** Instill 2-3 sprays per nostril q10-12h. **Max:** 2 doses q24h.
Afrin Original Nasal Spray	Oxymetazoline HCl 0.05%	**Adults & Peds:** ≥**6 yrs:** Instill 2-3 sprays per nostril q10-12h.
Afrin No Drip Original Pump Mist Nasal Spray	Oxymetazoline HCl 0.05%	**Adults & Peds:** ≥**6 yrs:** Instill 2-3 sprays per nostril q10-12h. **Max:** 2 doses q24h.
Afrin No Drip All Night 12 Hour Pump Mist	Oxymetazoline HCl 0.05%	**Adults & Peds:** ≥**6 yrs:** Instill 2-3 sprays per nostril q10-12h.
Benzedrex Inhaler	Propylhexedrine 250mg	**Adults & Peds:** ≥**6 yrs:** Inhale 2 sprays per nostril q2h

(Continued)

BRAND	INGREDIENT/STRENGTH	DOSE
TOPICAL NASAL DECONGESTANTS *(Continued)*		
Dristan 12 Hour Nasal Spray	Oxymetazoline HCl 0.05%	**Adults & Peds: ≥12 yrs:** Instill 2-3 sprays per nostril q10-12h. **Max:** 2 doses q24h.
Neo-Synephrine 12 Hour Extra Moisturizing Nasal Spray	Oxymetazoline HCl 0.05%	**Adults & Peds: ≥6 yrs:** Instill 2-3 sprays per nostril q10-12h. **Max:** 2 doses per 24 hours.
Neo-Synephrine 12 Hour Nasal Decongestant Spray	Oxymetazoline HCl 0.05%	**Adults & Peds: ≥6 yrs:** Instill 2-3 sprays per nostril q10-12h.
Neo-Synephrine Extra Strength Nasal Decongestant Drops	Phenylephrine HCl 1%	**Adults & Peds: ≥12 yrs:** Instill 2-3 drops per nostril q4h.
Neo-Synephrine Extra Strength Nasal Spray	Phenylephrine HCl 1%	**Adults & Peds: ≥6 yrs:** Instill 2-3 sprays per nostril q4h.
Neo-Synephrine Mild Formula Nasal Spray	Phenylephrine HCl 0.25%	**Adults & Peds: ≥6 yrs:** Instill 2-3 sprays per nostril q4h.
Neo-Synephrine Regular Strength Nasal Decongestant Spray	Phenylephrine HCl 0.5%	**Adults & Peds: ≥12 yrs:** Instill 2-3 sprays per nostril q4h.
Nostrilla 12 Hour Nasal Decongestant	Oxymetazoline HCl 0.05%	**Adults & Peds: ≥6 yrs:** Instill 2-3 sprays per nostril q10-12h. **Max:** 2 doses q24h.
Vicks Sinex 12 Hour Ultra Fine Mist For Sinus Relief	Oxymetazoline HCl 0.05%	**Adults & Peds: ≥6 yrs:** Instill 2-3 sprays per nostril q10-12h. **Max:** 2 doses q24h.
Vicks Sinex Long Acting Nasal Spray For Sinus Relief	Oxymetazoline HCl 0.05%	**Adults & Peds: ≥6 yrs:** Instill 2-3 sprays per nostril q10-12h. **Max:** 2 doses per day.
Vicks Sinex Nasal Spray For Sinus Relief	Phenylephrine HCl 0.5%	**Adults & Peds: ≥12 yrs:** Instill 2-3 sprays per nostril q4h.
Zicam Extreme Congestion Relief	Oxymetazoline HCl 0.05%	**Adults & Peds: ≥6 yrs:** Instill 2-3 sprays per nostril q10-12h. **Max:** 2 doses q24h.
Zicam Intense Sinus Relief	Oxymetazoline HCl 0.05%	**Adults & Peds: ≥12 yrs:** Instill 2-3 sprays per nostril q10-12h. **Max:** 2 doses q24h.
TOPICAL NASAL MOISTURIZERS		
4-Way Saline Moisturizing Mist	Water, Boric Acid, Glycerin, Sodium Chloride, Sodium Borate, Eucalyptol, Menthol, Polysorbate 80, Benzalkonium Chloride	**Adults & Peds: ≥2 yrs:** Instill 2-3 sprays per nostril prn.
Ayr Baby's Saline Nose Spray, Drops	Sodium Chloride 0.65%	**Peds:** Instill 2 to 6 drops in each nostril.
Ayr Saline Nasal Gel With Soothing Aloe	Water, Methyl Gluceth 10, Propylene Glycol, Glycerin, Glyceryl Polymethacrylate, Triethanolamine, Aloe Barbadensis Leaf Juice (Aloe Vera Gel), PEG/PPG 18/18 Dimethicone, Carbomer, Poloxamer 184, Sodium Chloride, Xanthan Gum, Diazolidinyl Urea, Methylparaben, Propylpara-ben, Glycine Soja Oil (Soybean), Geraniuim Maculatum Oil, Tocopheryl Acetate, Blue 1	**Adults & Peds: ≥12 yrs:** Apply to nostril prn.

(Continued)

BRAND	INGREDIENT/STRENGTH	DOSE
TOPICAL NASAL MOISTURIZERS *(Continued)*		
Ayr Saline Nasal Gel, No-Drip Sinus Spray	Water, Sodium Carbomethyl Starch, Propylene Glycol, Glycerin, Aloe Barbadensis Leaf Juice (Aloe Vera Gel), Sodium Chloride, Cetyl Pyridinium Chloride, Citric Acid, Disodium EDTA, Glycine Soja (Soybean Oil), Tocopheryl Acetate, Benzyl Alcohol, Benzalkonium Chloride, Geranium Maculatum Oil	**Adults & Peds:** ≥12 yrs: Instill 1 spray in each nostril prn.
Ayr Saline Nasal Mist	Sodium Chloride 0.65%	**Adults & Peds:** ≥12 yrs: Instill 2 sprays per nostril prn.
ENTSOL Mist, Buffered Hypertonic Nasal Irrigation Mist	Purified Water, Sodium Chloride, Sodium Phosphate Dibasic Edetate Disodium, Potassium Phosphate Monobasic, Benzalkonium Chloride	**Adults & Peds:** ≥12 yrs: Instill 1-2 sprays per nostril prn.
ENTSOL Single Use, Pre-Filled Nasal Wash Squeeze Bottle	Purified Water, Sodium Chloride, Sodium Phosphate Dibasic, Potassium Phosphate Monobasic	**Adults & Peds:** ≥12 yrs: Use as directed.
ENTSOL Spray, Buffered Hypertonic Saline Nasal Spray	Purified Water, Sodium Chloride Phosphate Dibasic, Potassium Phosphate Monobasic	**Adults & Peds:** ≥12 yrs: Instill 1 spray per nostril bid, 2-6 times daily
ENTSOL Nasal Gel with Aloe and Vitamin E	Water (Purified), Propylene Glycol, Aloe, Glycerin, Dimethicone Copolyol, Poloxamer 184, Methyl Gluceth 10, Triethanolamine, Carbomer, Sodium Chloride, Vitamin E, Disodium EDTA, Xanthan Gum, Benzalkonium Chloride	**Adults & Peds:** Use prn.
Little Noses Saline Spray/Drops, Non-Medicated	Sodium Chloride 0.65%	**Peds:** 2-6 drops or sprays per nostril as directed.
Ocean Premium Saline Nasal Spray	Sodium Chloride 0.65%	**Adults & Peds:** ≥6 yrs: Instill 2 sprays per nostril prn.
Simply Saline Sterile Saline Nasal Mist	Sodium Chloride 0.9%	**Adults & Peds:** ≥12 yrs: Use prn as directed.
SinoFresh Moisturizing Nasal & Sinus Spray	Purified water, Propylene Glycol, Monobasic Sodium Phosphate, Dibasic Sodium Phosphate, Sodium Chloride, Polysorbate 80, Sorbitol Solution, Essential Oil Blend (Wintergreen Oil, Spearmint Oil, Peppermint Oil, Eucalyptus Oil) Cetylpyridinium Chloride, Benzalkonium Chloride	**Adults & Peds:** ≥12 yrs: Instill 1-3 sprays per nostril bid.
MISCELLANEOUS		
NasalCrom Nasal Allergy Symptom Prevention and Controller, Nasal Spray	Cromolyn Sodium 5.2mg	**Adults & Peds:** ≥2 yrs: Instill 1 spray per nostril q4-6h. **Max:** 6 doses q24h.
Similasan Hay Fever Relief, Non-Drowsy Formula, Nasal Spray	Cardiospermum HPUS 6X, Galphimia Glauca HPUS 6X, Luffa Operculata HPUS 6X, Sabadilla HPUS 6x	**Adults & Peds:** Instill 1 to 3 sprays in each nostril prn.
Zicam Allergy Relief, Homeopathic Nasal Solution, Pump	Luffa Operculata 4x, 12x, 30x, Galphimia Glauca 12x, 30x, Histaminum Hydrochloricum 12x, 30x, 200x, Sulphur 12x, 30x, 200x	**Adults & Peds:** ≥6 yrs: Instill 1 spray per nostril q4h.

IS IT A COLD, THE FLU, OR AN ALLERGY?

	COLD	FLU	AIRBORNE ALLERGY
SYMPTOMS			
Chest discomfort	Mild to moderate	Common; can become severe	Sometimes
Cough	Common (hacking cough)	Sometimes	Sometimes
Duration	3-14 days	Days to weeks	Weeks (eg, 6 weeks for ragweed or grass pollen seasons)
Extreme exhaustion	Never	Early and prominent	Never
Fatigue, weakness	Sometimes	Can last up to 2-3 weeks	Sometimes
Fever	Rare	Characteristic, high (100-102°F); lasts 3-4 days	Never
General aches, pains	Slight	Usual; often severe	Never
Headache	Rare	Prominent	Sometimes
Itchy eyes	Rare or never	Rare or never	Common
Runny nose	Common		Common
Sneezing	Usual	Sometimes	Usual
Sore throat	Common	Sometimes	Sometimes
Stuffy nose	Common	Sometimes	Common
TREATMENT*			
	Antihistamines	Amantadine	Antihistamines
	Decongestants	Rimantadine	Nasal steroids
	Nonsteroidal anti-inflammatories	Oseltamivir	Decongestants
		Zanamavir	
PREVENTION			
	Wash your hands often; avoid close contact with anyone with a cold	Annual vaccination Amantadine Rimantadine Oseltamivir	Avoid allergens such as pollen, house flies, dust mites, mold, pet dander, cockroaches
COMPLICATIONS			
	Sinus infection	Bronchitis	Sinus infections
	Middle ear infection	Pneumonia	Asthma
	Asthma	Can be life-threatening	

Adapted from the National Institute of Allergy and Infectious Diseases, September 2005.

*Used only for temporary relief of cold symptoms.

COUGH-COLD-FLU PRODUCTS

BRAND NAME	ANALGESIC	ANTIHISTAMINE	DECONGESTANT	COUGH SUPPRESSANT	EXPECTORANT	DOSE
ANTIHISTAMINE + DECONGESTANT						
Actifed Cold & Allergy Tablets		Chlorpheniramine Maleate 4mg	Phenylephrine HCl 10mg			**Adults: ≥12 yrs:** 1 tab q4-6h. **Max:** 6 doses q24h. **Peds: 6-12 yrs:** ½ tab q4-6h. **Max:** 2 tabs q24h.
Benadryl Children's Allergy & Cold Fastmelt Tablets		Diphenhydramine HCl 19mg	Pseudoephedrine HCl 30mg			**Adults: ≥12 yrs:** 2 tabs q4h. **Max:** 8 tabs q24h. **Peds: 6-12 yrs:** 1 tab q4h. **Max:** 4 tabs q24h.
Benadryl-D Allergy/Sinus Tablets		Diphenhydramine HCl 25mg	Phenylephrine HCl 10mg			**Adults & Peds: ≥12 yrs:** 1 tab q4h. **Max:** 6 tab q24h.
Children's Benadryl-D Allergy & Sinus Liquid		Diphenhydramine HCl 12.5mg/5mL	Phenylephrine HCl 5mg/5mL			**Adults: ≥12 yrs:** 2 tsp (10mL) q4h. **Peds: 6-12 yrs:** 1 tsp (5mL) q4h. **Max:** 6 doses q24h.
Dimetapp Children's Cold & Allergy Elixir		Brompheniramine Maleate 1mg/5mL	Phenylephrine HCl 2.5mg/5mL			**Adults & Peds: ≥12 yrs:** 2 tabs q4h. **Max:** 8 tabs q24h. **Peds: 6-12 yrs:** 1 tab q4hr. **Max:** 6 doses q24h.
Dimetapp Children's Cold & Allergy Chewable Tablets		Brompheniramine Maleate 1mg	Phenylephrine HCl 2.5mg			**Peds: 6-12 yrs:** 2 tabs q4h. **Max:** 6 doses q24h.
Pedicare Children's NightRest Multi-Symptom Cold Liquid		Diphenhydramine HCl 12.5mg/5mL	Phenylephrine HCl 5mg/5mL			**Peds: 6-12 yrs:** 1 tsp (5mL) q4h. **Max:** 6 doses q24h.
Robitussin Night Time Cough & Cold Liquid		Diphenhydramine HCl 6.25mg/5mL	Phenylephrine HCl 2.5mg/5mL			**Adults & Peds: ≥12 yrs:** 4 tsp (20mL) q4h. **Peds: 6-12 yrs:** 2 tsp (10mL) q4h. **Max:** 6 doses q24h.
Robitussin Pediatric Night Time Cough & Cold Liquid		Diphenhydramine HCl 6.25mg/5mL	Phenylephrine HCl 2.5mg/5mL			**Adults & Peds: ≥12 yrs:** 4 tsp (20mL) q4h. **Peds: 6-12 yrs:** 2 tsp (10mL) q4h. **Max:** 6 doses q24h.
Sudafed Sinus & Allergy Tablets		Chlorpheniramine Maleate 4mg	Pseudoephedrine HCl 60mg			**Adults: ≥12 yrs:** 1 tab q4-6h. **Peds: 6-12 yrs:** ½ tab q4-6h. **Max:** 4 doses q24h.
Sudafed Sinus Nighttime Tablets		Triprolidine HCl 2.5mg	Pseudoephedrine HCl 60mg			**Adults & Peds: ≥12 yrs:** 1 tab q4-6h. **Peds: 6-12 yrs:** ½ tab q4-6h. **Max:** 4 doses q24h.

BRAND NAME	ANALGESIC	ANTIHISTAMINE	DECONGESTANT	COUGH SUPPRESSANT	EXPECTORANT	DOSE
Theraflu Nighttime Cold & Cough Thin Strips		Diphenhydramine HCl 25mg/strips	Phenylephrine HCl 10mg/strip			**Adults: ≥12 yrs:** 1 strip q4h. **Max:** 6 strips q24h.
Triaminic Cold & Allergy Liquid		Chlorpheniramine Maleate 1mg/5mL	Phenylephrine HCl 2.5mg/5mL			**Peds: 6-12 yrs:** 2 tsp (10mL) q4h. **Max:** 6 doses q24h.
Triaminic Nighttime Cough & Cold Liquid		Diphenhydramine HCl 6.25mg/5mL	Phenylephrine HCl 2.5mg/5mL			**Peds: 6-12 yrs:** 2 tsp (10mL) q4h. **Max:** 6 doses q24h.
Triaminic Nighttime Cough & Cold Thin Strips		Diphenhydramine HCl 12.5mg/strip	Phenylephrine HCl 5mg/strip			**Peds: 6-12 yrs:** 1 strip q4h. **Max:** 6 strips q24h.
ANTIHISTAMINE + DECONGESTANT + ANALGESIC						
Actifed Cold & Sinus Caplets	Acetaminophen 500mg	Chlorpheniramine Maleate 2mg	Pseudoephedrine HCl 30mg			**Adults & Peds: ≥12 yrs:** 2 tabs q6h. **Max:** 8 tabs q24h.
Advil Multi-Symptom Cold Caplets	Ibuprofen 200mg	Chlorpheniramine Maleate 2mg	Pseudoephedrine HCl 30mg			**Adults & Peds: ≥12 yrs:** 1 tab q4-6h. **Max:** 6 tabs q24h.
Advil Allergy Sinus Caplets	Ibuprofen 200mg	Chlorpheniramine Maleate 2mg	Pseudoephedrine HCl 30mg			**Adults & Peds: ≥12 yrs:** 1 tab q4-6h. **Max:** 6 tabs q24h.
Advil Allergy Sinus Children's Liquid	Ibuprofen 100mg	Chlorpheniramine Maleate 1mg	Pseudoephedrine HCl 15mg			**Peds: 6-11 yrs (48-95 lbs):** 2 tsp q6h. **Max:** 8 tsp q24h.
Alka-Seltzer Plus Cold Effervescent Tablets	Acetaminophen 325mg	Chlorpheniramine Maleate 2mg	Phenylephrine HCl 5mg			**Adults & Peds: ≥12 yrs:** 2 tabs q4h. **Max:** 8 tabs q24h.
Alka-Seltzer Plus Cold Cherry Burst Formula Effervescent Tablets	Acetaminophen 250mg	Chlorpheniramine Maleate 2mg	Phenylephrine HCl 5mg			**Adults & Peds: ≥12 yrs:** 2 tabs q4h. **Max:** 8 tabs q24h.
Alka-Seltzer Plus Cold Orange Zest Formula Effervescent Tablets	Acetaminophen 250mg	Chlorpheniramine Maleate 2mg	Phenylephrine HCl 5mg			**Adults & Peds: ≥12 yrs:** 2 tabs q4h. **Max:** 8 tabs q24h.
Alka-Seltzer Plus Regular Seltzer Multi-Symptom Cold Relief Effervescent Tablets	Acetaminophen 250mg	Chlorpheniramine Maleate 2mg	Phenylephrine HCl 5mg			**Adults & Peds: ≥12 yrs:** 2 tabs q4h. **Max:** 8 tabs q24h.
Benadryl Allergy & Cold Caplets	Acetaminophen 325mg	Diphenhydramine HCl 12.5mg	Phenylephrine HCl 5mg			**Adults & Peds: ≥12 yrs:** 2 tabs q4h. **Max:** 12 tabs q24h. **Peds: 6-12 yrs:** 1 tab q4h. **Max:** 5 tabs q24h.
Benadryl Allergy & Sinus Headache Caplets	Acetaminophen 325mg	Diphenhydramine HCl 12.5mg	Phenylephrine HCl 5mg			**Adults & Peds: ≥12 yrs:** 2 tabs q4h. **Max:** 12 tabs q24h. **Peds: 6-12 yrs:** 1 tab q4h. **Max:** 5 tabs q24h.

(Continued)

ANTIHISTAMINE + DECONGESTANT + ANALGESIC (Continued)

BRAND NAME	ANALGESIC	ANTIHISTAMINE	DECONGESTANT	COUGH SUPPRESSANT	EXPECTORANT	DOSE
Benadryl Severe Allergy & Sinus Headache Caplets	Acetaminophen 325mg	Diphenhydramine HCl 25mg	Phenylephrine HCl 5mg			**Adults & Peds: ≥12 yrs:** 2 tabs q4h. **Max:** 12 tabs q24h.
Comtrex Day & Night Severe Cold & Sinus Caplets	Acetaminophen 325mg	Chlorpheniramine Maleate 2mg (nighttime dose only)	Phenylephrine HCl 5mg			**Adults & Peds: ≥12 yrs:** *Daytime:* 2 daytime tabs q4h. **Max:** 8 daytime tabs q24h. *Nighttime:* 2 nighttime tabs q24h. **Max:** 4 nighttime tabs q24h.
Contac Cold & Flu Maximum Strength Caplets	Acetaminophen 500mg	Chlorpheniramine Maleate 2mg	Phenylephrine HCl 5mg			**Adults & Peds: ≥12 yrs:** 2 tabs q4-6h **Max:** 8 tabs q24h.
Dristan Cold Multi-Symptom Tablets	Acetaminophen 325mg	Chlorpheniramine Maleate 2mg	Phenylephrine HCl 5mg			**Adults & Peds: ≥12 yrs:** 2 tabs q4h. **Max:** 12 tabs q24h.
Robitussin Cold & Congestion Tablets	Acetaminophen 325mg	Chlorpheniramine Maleate 2mg	Phenylephrine HCl 5mg			**Adults & Peds: ≥12 yrs:** 2 tabs q4h. **Max:** 12 tabs q24h.
Sudafed Sinus PE Nighttime Cold Caplets	Acetaminophen 325mg	Diphenhydramine HCl 25mg	Phenylephrine HCl 5mg			**Adults & Peds: ≥12 yrs:** 2 tabs q4h. **Max:** 12 tabs q24h.
Sudafed PE Nighttime Cold Caplets	Acetaminophen 325mg	Diphenhydramine HCl 12.5mg	Phenylephrine HCl 5mg			**Adults & Peds: ≥12 yrs:** 2 tabs q4h. **Max:** 12 tabs q24h. **Peds: 6-12 yrs:** 1 tab q4h. **Max:** 5 tabs q24h.
Sudafed PE Severe Cold Caplets	Acetaminophen 325mg	Diphenhydramine HCl 12.5mg	Phenylephrine HCl 5mg			**Adults & Peds: ≥12 yrs:** 2 tabs q4h. **Max:** 12 tabs q24h. **Peds: 6-12 yrs:** 1 tab q4h. **Max:** 5 tabs q24h.
Theraflu Cold & Sore Throat Hot Liquid	Acetaminophen 325mg/packet	Pheniramine Maleate 20mg/packet	Phenylephrine HCl 10mg/packet			**Adults & Peds: ≥12 yrs:** 1 packet q4h. **Max:** 6 packets q24h.
Theraflu Nighttime Severe Cold Hot Liquid	Acetaminophen 650mg/packet	Pheniramine Maleate 20mg/packet	Phenylephrine HCl 10mg/packet			**Adults & Peds: ≥12 yrs:** 1 packet q4h. **Max:** 6 packets q24h.
Theraflu Flu & Sore Throat Liquid	Acetaminophen 650mg/packet	Pheniramine Maleate 20mg/packet	Phenylephrine HCl 10mg/packet			**Adults & Peds: ≥12 yrs:** 1 packet q4h. **Max:** 6 packets q24h.
Theraflu Nighttime Warming Relief Syrup	Acetaminophen 325mg/15mL	Diphenhydramine HCl 12.5mg/15mL	Phenylephrine HCl 5mg/15mL			**Adults & Peds: ≥12 yrs:** 2 tbl (30mL) q4h. **Max:** 6 doses (12 tbl) q24h.
Theraflu Flu & Sore Throat Relief Syrup	Acetaminophen 325mg/15mL	Diphenhydramine HCl 12.5mg/15mL	Phenylephrine HCl 5mg/15mL			**Adults & Peds: ≥12 yrs:** 2 tbl (30mL) q4h. **Max:** 6 doses (12 tbl) q24h.
Tylenol Children's Plus Cold Liquid	Acetaminophen 160mg/5mL	Chlorpheniramine Maleate 1mg/5mL	Phenylephrine HCl 2.5mg/5mL			**Peds: 6-11 yrs (48-95 lbs):** 2 tsp (10mL) q4h. **Max:** 5 doses q24h.

BRAND NAME	ANALGESIC	ANTIHISTAMINE	DECONGESTANT	COUGH SUPPRESSANT	EXPECTORANT	DOSE
ANTIHISTAMINE + DECONGESTANT + ANALGESIC *(Continued)*						
Tylenol Children's Plus Cold & Allergy Liquid	Acetaminophen 160mg/5mL	Diphenhydramine HCl 12.5mg/5mL	Phenylephrine HCl 2.5mg/5mL			**Peds: 6-11 yrs (48-95 lbs):** 2 tsp (10mL) q4-6h. **Max:** 4 doses q24h.
Tylenol Children's Plus Cold & Allergy Liquid	Acetaminophen 160mg/5mL	Diphenhydramine HCl 12.5mg/5mL	Pseudoephedrine HCl 15mg/5mL			**Peds: 6-11 yrs (48-95 lbs):** 2 tsp (10mL) q4-6h. **Max:** 4 doses q24h.
Tylenol Sinus Congestion & Pain Nighttime Caplets	Acetaminophen 325mg	Chlorpheniramine Maleate 2mg	Phenylephrine HCl 5mg			**Adults & Peds: ≥12 yrs:** 2 tabs q4h. **Max:** 12 tabs q24h.
Tylenol Allergy Multi-Symptom Caplets	Acetaminophen 325mg	Chlorpheniramine Maleate 2mg	Phenylephrine HCl 5mg			**Adults & Peds: ≥12 yrs:** 2 tabs q4h. **Max:** 12 tabs q24h.
Tylenol Allergy Multi-Symptom Nighttime Caplets	Acetaminophen 325mg	Diphenhydramine HCL 25mg	Phenylephrine HCl 5mg			**Adults & Peds: ≥12 yrs:** 2 tabs q4h. **Max:** 12 tabs q24h.
Vicks NyQuil Sinus Liquicaps	Acetaminophen 325mg	Doxylamine Succinate 6.25 mg	Phenylephrine HCl 5mg			**Adults & Peds: ≥12 yrs:** 2 tabs q4h. **Max:** 6 doses q24h.
COUGH SUPPRESSANT						
Delsym 12 Hour Cough Relief Liquid				Dextromethorphan Polistrex 30mg/5mL		**Adults: ≥12 yrs:** 2 tsp (10mL) q12h. **Max:** 4 doses q24h. **Peds: 6-12 yrs:** 1 tsp (5mL) q12h. **Max:** 2 doses q24h. **2-6 yrs:** ½ tsp (2.5mL) q12h. **Max:** 1 dose q24h.
PediaCare Long-Acting Cough Liquid				Dextromethorphan HBr 7.5mg/5mL		**Peds: 6-12 yrs:** 2 tsp q6-8h. **2-6 yrs:** 1 tsp q6-8h. **Max:** 4 doses q24h.
Robitussin Cough Long-Acting Liquid				Dextromethorphan HBr 15mg/5mL		**Adults & Peds: ≥12 yrs:** 2 tsp (10mL) q6-8h. **Max:** 8 tsp (40mL) q24h.
Robitussin CoughGels Liqui-gels				Dextromethorphan HBr 15mg		**Adults & Peds: ≥12 yrs:** 2 caps q6-8h. **Max:** 8 caps q24h.
Robitussin Pediatric Cough Liquid				Dextromethorphan HBr 7.5mg/5mL		**Adults: ≥12 yrs (≥96 lbs):** 4 tsp (20mL) q6-8h. **Peds: 6-12 yrs (48-95 lbs):** 2 tsp (10mL) q6-8h. **2-6 yrs:** 1 tsp (5mL) q6-8h. **Max:** 4 doses q24h.
Triaminic Long-Acting Cough Liquid				Dextromethorphan HBr 7.5mg/5mL		**Peds: 6-12 yrs:** 2 tsp (10mL) q6-8h. **2-6 yrs:** 1 tsp (5mL) q6-8h. **Max:** 4 doses q24h.

(Continued)

BRAND NAME	ANALGESIC	ANTIHISTAMINE	DECONGESTANT	COUGH SUPPRESSANT	EXPECTORANT	DOSE
COUGH SUPPRESSANT (Continued)						
Triaminic Long Acting Cough Thin Strips				Dextromethorphan 5.5mg/strip		**Peds: 6-12 yrs:** 2 strips q6-8h. **Max:** 8 strips q24h.
Vicks DayQuil Cough Liquid				Dextromethorphan HBr 15mg/15mL		**Adults & Peds: ≥12 yrs:** 2 tbl (30mL) q6-8h. **Peds: 6-12 yrs:** 1 tbl (15mL) q6-8h. **Max:** 4 doses q24h.
Vicks 44 Liquid				Dextromethorphan HBr 30mg/15mL		**Adults & Peds: ≥12 yrs:** 1 tbl (15mL) q6-8h. **Peds: 6-12 yrs:** 1.5 tsp (7.5mL) q6-8h. **Max:** 4 doses q24h.
Vicks BabyRub				Eucalyptus, petrolatum, fragrance, aloe extract, eucalyptus oil, lavender oil, rosemary oil		**Peds:** Gently massage on the chest, neck, and back to help soothe and comfort.
Vicks Casero Cough Suppressant/Topical Analgesic				Camphor 4.7%, Menthol 2.6%, Eucalyptus 1.2%		**Adults & Peds: ≥2 yrs:** Apply 3 times q24h.
Vicks Cough Drops Cherry Flavor				Menthol 1.7mg		**Adults & Peds: ≥5 yrs:** 3 drops q1-2h.
Vicks Cough Drops Original Flavor				Menthol 3.3mg		**Adults & Peds: ≥5 yrs:** 2 drops q1-2h.
Vicks VapoRub Cream				Camphor 5.2%, Menthol 2.8%, Eucalyptus 1.2%		**Adults & Peds: ≥2 yrs:** Apply q8h.
Vicks VapoRub Ointment				Camphor 4.8%, Menthol 2.6%, Eucalyptus 1.2%		**Adults & Peds: ≥2 yrs:** Apply q8h.
Vicks VapoSteam				Camphor 6.2%		**Adults & Peds: ≥2 yrs:** 1 tbl/quart q8h.
COUGH SUPPRESSANT + ANTIHISTAMINE						
Coricidin HBP Cough & Cold Tablets		Chlorpheniramine Maleate 4mg		Dextromethorphan HBr 30mg		**Adults & Peds: ≥12 yrs:** 1 tab q6h. **Max:** 4 tabs q24h.
Dimetapp Long-Acting Cold Plus Cough Elixir		Chlorpheniramine Maleate 1mg/5mL		Dextromethorphan HBr 7.5mg/5mL		**Peds: ≥12 yrs:** 4 tsp (20mL) q6h. **6-12 yrs:** 2 tsp (10 mL) q6h. **Max:** 4 doses q24h.

BRAND NAME	ANALGESIC	ANTIHISTAMINE	DECONGESTANT	COUGH SUPPRESSANT	EXPECTORANT	DOSE
COUGH SUPPRESSANT + ANTIHISTAMINES *(Continued)*						
Robitussin Cough & Cold Long-Acting Liquid		Chlorpheniramine Maleate 2mg/5mL		Dextromethorphan HBr 15mg/5mL		**Adults:** ≥**12 yrs:** 2 tsp (10mL) q6h. **Max:** 4 doses q24h.
Robitussin Pediatric Cough & Cold Long-Acting Liquid		Chlorpheniramine Maleate 1mg/5mL		Dextromethorphan HBr 7.5mg/5mL		**Adults & Peds:** ≥**12 yrs:** 4 tsp (20mL) q6h. **Peds: 6-12 yrs:** 2 tsp (10mL) q6h. **Max:** 4 doses q24h.
Triaminic Softchews Cough & Runny Nose		Chlorpheniramine Maleate 1mg		Dextromethorphan HBr 5mg		**Peds: 6-12 yrs:** 2 tabs q4-6h. **Max:** 6 doses q24h.
Vicks Children's NyQuil Liquid		Chlorpheniramine Maleate 2mg/15mL		Dextromethorphan HBr 15mg/15mL		**Adults:** ≥**12 yrs:** 2 tbl (30mL) q6h. **Peds: 6-11 yrs:** 1 tbl (15mL) q6h. **Max:** 4 doses q24h.
Vicks NyQuil Cough Liquid		Doxylamine Succinate 6.25mg/15mL		Dextromethorphan HBr 15mg/15mL		**Adults & Peds:** ≥**12 yrs:** 2 tbl (30mL) q6h. **Max:** 8 tbl (120mL) q24h.
Vicks Pediatric Formula 44M Cough & Cold Relief		Chlorpheniramine Maleate 2mg/15mL		Dextromethorphan HBr 15mg/15mL		**Adults & Peds:** ≥**12 yrs:** 2 tbl (30mL) q6h. **Peds: 6-12 yrs:** 1 tbl (15mL) q6h. **Max:** 4 doses q24h.
COUGH SUPPRESSANT + ANALGESIC						
Triaminic Cough & Sore Throat Liquid	Acetaminophen 160mg/5mL			Dextromethorphan HBr 5mg/5mL		**Peds: 6-12 yrs:** 2 tsp (10mL) q4h. **2-6 yrs:** 1 tsp (5mL) q4h. **Max:** 5 doses q24h.
Triaminic Softchews Cough & Sore Throat Tablets	Acetaminophen 160mg			Dextromethorphan HBr 5mg		**Peds: 6-12 yrs:** 2 tabs q4h. **2-6 yrs:** 1 tab q4h. **Max:** 5 doses q24h.
Tylenol Children's Plus Cough & Sore Throat Liquid	Acetaminophen 160mg/5mL			Dextromethorphan HBr 5mg/5mL		**Peds: 6-11 yrs: [48-95 lbs]:** 2 tsp (10mL) q4h. **2-5 yrs [24-47 lbs]:** 1 tsp (5mL) q4h. **Max:** 5 doses q24h.
Tylenol Cough & Sore Throat Daytime Liquid	Acetaminophen 1000mg/30mL			Dextromethorphan HBr 30mg/30mL		**Adults & Peds:** ≥**12 yrs:** 2 tbl (30mL) q6h. **Max:** 8 tbl q24h.
COUGH SUPPRESSANT + ANTIHISTAMINES + ANALGESIC						
Alka-Seltzer Plus Flu Effervescent Tablets	Aspirin 500mg	Chlorpheniramine Maleate 2mg		Dextromethorphan HBr 15mg		**Adults & Peds:** ≥**12 yrs:** 2 tabs q6h. **Max:** 8 tabs q24h.
Alka-Seltzer Plus Nighttime Liquid Gels	Acetaminophen 325mg	Doxylamine Succinate 6.25mg		Dextromethorphan HBr 15mg		**Adults & Peds:** ≥**12 yrs:** 2 tabs q6h. **Max:** 12 tabs q24h.

(Continued)

BRAND NAME	ANALGESIC	ANTIHISTAMINE	DECONGESTANT	COUGH SUPPRESSANT	EXPECTORANT	DOSE
COUGH SUPPRESSANT + ANTIHISTAMINES + ANALGESIC (Continued)						
Tylenol Children's Plus Cough & Runny Nose Liquid	Acetaminophen 160mg/5mL	Chlorpheniramine Maleate 1mg/5mL		Dextromethorphan HBr 5mg/5mL		Peds: 6-11 yrs (48-95 lbs): 2 tsp (10mL) q4h. Max: 5 doses q24h.
Coricidin HBP Maximum Strength Flu Tablets	Acetaminophen 500mg	Chlorpheniramine Maleate 2mg		Dextromethorphan HBr 15mg		Adults & Peds: ≥12: 2 tabs q6h. Max: 8 tabs q24h.
Triaminic Flu Cough & Fever Liquid	Acetaminophen 160mg/5mL	Chlorpheniramine Maleate 1mg/5mL		Dextromethorphan HBr 7.5mg/5mL		Peds: 6-12 yrs: 2 tsp (10mL) q6h. Max: 4 doses (20mL) q24h.
Tylenol Nighttime Cough & Sore Throat Cool Burst Liquid	Acetaminophen 1000mg/30mL	Doxylamine 12.5mg/30mL		Dextromethorphan HBr 30mg/30mL		Adults & Peds: ≥12 yrs: 2 tbl (30mL) q6h. Max: 8 tbl (120mL) q24h.
Vicks 44M Liquid	Acetaminophen 162.5mg/5mL	Chlorpheniramine Maleate 1mg/5mL		Dextromethorphan HBr 7.5mg/5mL		Adults & Peds: ≥12 yrs: 4 tsp (20mL) q6h. Max: 16 tsp (80mL) q24h.
Vicks NyQuil Liquicaps	Acetaminophen 325mg	Doxylamine Succinate 6.25mg		Dextromethorphan HBr 15mg		Adults & Peds: ≥12 yrs: 2 caps q6h. Max: 8 caps q24h.
Vicks NyQuil Liquid	Acetaminophen 500mg/15mL	Doxylamine Succinate 6.25mg/15mL		Dextromethorphan HBr 15mg/15mL		Adults & Peds: ≥12 yrs: 2 tbl (30mL) q6h. Max: 8 tbl (120mL) q24h.
COUGH SUPPRESSANT + ANTIHISTAMINES + ANALGESIC + DECONGESTANT						
Alka-Seltzer Plus Cough & Cold Liquid Gels	Acetaminophen 325mg	Chlorpheniramine Maleate 2mg	Phenylephrine HCl 5mg	Dextromethorphan HBr 10mg		Adults & Peds: ≥12 yrs: 2 caps q4h. Max: 12 caps q24h.
Alka-Seltzer Plus Effervescent Tablets	Acetaminophen 250mg	Doxylamine Succinate 6.25mg	Phenylephrine HCl 5mg	Dextromethorphan HBr 10mg		Adults & Peds: ≥12 yrs: 2 tabs q4h. Max: 8 tabs q24h.
Alka-Seltzer Plus Cough & Cold Effervescent Tablets	Acetaminophen 250mg	Chlorpheniramine Maleate 2mg	Phenylephrine HCl 5mg	Dextromethorphan HBr 10mg		Adults & Peds: ≥12 yrs: 2 tabs q4h. Max: 8 tabs q24h
Alka-Seltzer Plus Cough & Cold Liquid	Acetaminophen 162.5mg/5mL	Chlorpheniramine Maleate 1mg/5mL	Phenylephrine HCl 2.5mg/5mL	Dextromethorphan HBr 5mg/5mL		Adults & Peds: ≥12 yrs: 4 tsp q4h. Max: 24 tsp q24h.
Alka-Seltzer Plus Night Cold Liquid	Acetaminophen 162.5mg/5mL	Doxylamine Succinate 3.125/5mL	Phenylephrine HCl 2.5mg/5mL	Dextromethorphan HBr 5mg/5mL		Adults & Peds: ≥12 yrs: 4 tsp q4h. Max: 24 tsp q24h.
Comtrex Nighttime Cold & Cough Caplets	Acetaminophen 325mg	Chlorpheniramine Maleate 2mg	Phenylephrine HCl 5mg	Dextromethorphan HBr 10mg		Adults & Peds: ≥12 yrs: 2 tabs q6h. Max: 8 tabs q24h.
Dimetapp Children's Nighttime Flu Liquid	Acetaminophen 160mg/5mL	Chlorpheniramine Maleate 1mg/5mL	Phenylephrine HCl 2.5mg/5mL	Dextromethorphan HBr 5mg/5mL		Adults: ≥12 yrs: 4 tsp (20mL) q4h. Peds: 6-12 yrs: 2 tsp (10mL) q4h. Max: 5 doses q24h.
Robitussin Nighttime Cold Cough & Flu Liquid	Acetaminophen 160mg/5mL	Chlorpheniramine Maleate 1mg/5mL	Phenylephrine HCl 2.5mg/5mL	Dextromethorphan HBr 5mg/5mL		Adults: ≥12 yrs: 4 tsp (20mL) q4h. Peds: 6-12 yrs: 2 tsp (10mL) q4h. Max: 5 doses q24h.

BRAND NAME	ANALGESIC	ANTIHISTAMINE	DECONGESTANT	COUGH SUPPRESSANT	EXPECTORANT	DOSE
COUGH SUPPRESSANT + ANTIHISTAMINE + ANALGESIC + DECONGESTANT *(Continued)*						
Theraflu Nighttime Severe Cold Caplets	Acetaminophen 325mg	Chlorpheniramine Maleate 2mg	Phenylephrine HCl 5mg	Dextromethorphan HBr 10mg		**Adults & Peds:** ≥12 yrs: 2 tabs q6h. **Max:** 8 tabs q24h.
Tylenol Children's Plus Multisymptom Cold Liquid	Acetaminophen 160mg/5mL	Chlorpheniramine Maleate 1mg/5mL	Phenylephrine HCl 2.5mg/5mL	Dextromethorphan HBr 5mg/5mL		**Peds: 6-11 yrs (48-95 lbs):** 2 tsp (10mL) q4h. **Max:** 5 doses q24h.
Tylenol Children's Plus Flu Liquid	Acetaminophen 160mg/5mL	Chlorpheniramine Maleate 1mg/5mL	Phenylephrine HCl 2.5mg/5mL	Dextromethorphan HBr 5mg/5mL		**Peds: 6-11 yrs (48-95 lbs):** 2 tsp (10mL) q6-8h. **Max:** 4 doses q24h.
Tylenol Children's Plus Flu Liquid	Acetaminophen 160mg/5mL	Chlorpheniramine Maleate 1mg/5mL	Pseudoephedrine HCl 15mg/5mL	Dextromethorphan HBr 7.5mg/5mL		**Peds: 6-11 yrs (48-95 lbs):** 2 tsp (10mL) q6-8h. **Max:** 4 doses q24h.
Tylenol Cold Head Congestion Nighttime Caplets	Acetaminophen 325mg	Chlorpheniramine Maleate 2mg	Phenylephrine HCl 5mg	Dextromethorphan HBr 10mg		**Adults & Peds:** ≥12 yrs: 2 tabs q4h. **Max:** 12 tabs q24h.
Tylenol Cold Multi-Symptom Nighttime Caplets	Acetaminophen 325mg	Chlorpheniramine Maleate 2mg	Phenylephrine HCl 5mg	Dextromethorphan HBr 10mg		**Adults & Peds:** ≥12 yrs: 2 tabs q4h. **Max:** 12 tabs q24h.
Tylenol Cold Multi-Symptom Nighttime Liquid	Acetaminophen 325mg/15mL	Doxylamine 6.25mg/30mL	Phenylephrine HCl 5mg/15mL	Dextromethorphan HBr 10mg/15mL		**Adults & Peds:** ≥12 yrs: 2 tbl (30mL) q4h. **Max:** 12 tbl (180mL) q24h.
Vicks NyQuil D Liquid	Acetaminophen 500mg/15mL	Doxylamine 6.25mg/15mL	Phenylephrine HCl 30mg/15mL	Dextromethorphan HBr 15mg/15mL		**Adults & Peds:** ≥12 yrs: 2 tbl (30mL) q6h. **Max:** 4 doses q24h.
COUGH SUPPRESSANT + ANTIHISTAMINE + DECONGESTANT						
Dimetapp DM Children's Cold & Cough Elixr		Brompheniramine Maleate 1mg/5mL	Phenylephrine HCl 2.5mg/5mL	Dextromethorphan HBr 5mg/5mL		**Adults:** ≥12 yrs: 4 tsp (20mL) q4h. **Peds: 6-12 yrs:** 2 tsp (10mL) q4h. **Max:** 6 doses q24h.
Robitussin Allergy & Cough Liquid		Chlorpheniramine Maleate 2mg/5mL	Phenylephrine HCl 5mg/5mL	Dextromethorphan HBr 10mg/5mL		**Adults:** ≥12 yrs: 2 tsp (10mL) q4h. **Peds: 6-12 yrs:** 1 tsp (5mL) q4h. **Max:** 6 doses q24h.
Theraflu Cold & Cough Hot Liquid		Pheniramine Maleate 20mg/packet	Phenylephrine HCl 10mg/packet	Dextromethorphan HBr 20mg/packet		**Adults & Peds:** ≥12 yrs: 1 packet q4h. **Max:** 6 packets q24h.
COUGH SUPPRESSANT + DECONGESTANT						
Dimetapp Toddler's Decongestant Plus Cough Drops			Phenylephrine HCl 1.25mg/0.8mL	Dextromethorphan HBr 2.5mg/0.8mL		**Peds: 2-6 yrs:** 1.6mL q4h. **Max:** 6 doses q24h.
PediaCare Children's Multi-Symptom Cold Liquid			Phenylephrine HCl 2.5mg/5mL	Dextromethorphan HBr 5mg/5mL		**Peds: 6-12 yrs:** 2 tsp (10mL) q4h. **2-6 yrs:** 1 tsp (5mL) q4h. **Max:** 6 doses q24h.

(Continued)

BRAND NAME	ANALGESIC	ANTIHISTAMINE	DECONGESTANT	COUGH SUPPRESSANT	EXPECTORANT	DOSE
COUGH SUPPRESSANT + DECONGESTANT *(Continued)*						
Sudafed Children's Cold & Cough Liquid			Pseudoephedrine HCl 15mg/5mL	Dextromethorphan HBr 5mg/5mL		**Adults & Peds: ≥12 yrs:** 4 tsp (20mL) q4h. **Peds: 6-12 yrs:** 2 tsp (10mL) q4h. **2-6 yrs:** 1 tsp (5mL) q4h. **Max:** 4 doses q24h.
Theraflu Daytime Cold & Cough Thin Strips			Phenylephrine HCl 10mg/strip	Dextromethorphan HBr 20mg/strip		**Adults & Peds: ≥12 yrs:** 1 strip q4h. **Max:** 6 strips q24h.
Triaminic Daytime Cold & Cough Liquid			Phenylephrine HCl 2.5mg/5mL	Dextromethorphan HBr 5mg/5mL		**Peds: 6-12 yrs:** 2 tsp (10mL) q4h. **2-6 yrs:** 1 tsp (5mL) q4h. **Max:** 6 doses q24h.
Triaminic Daytime Cold & Cough Thin Strips			Phenylephrine HCl 2.5mg/strip	Dextromethorphan HBr 3.67mg/strip		**Peds: 6-12 yrs:** 2 strips q4h. **2-6 yrs:** 1 strip q4h. **Max:** 6 doses q24h.
Vicks 44D Cough & Congestion Relief Liquid			Phenylephrine HCl 10mg/15mL	Dextromethorphan HBr 20mg/15mL		**Adults: ≥12 yrs:** 1 tbl (15mL) q4h. **Peds: 6-12 yrs:** 1.5 tsp (7.5mL) q4h. **Max:** 6 doses q24h.
COUGH SUPPRESSANT + DECONGESTANT + ANALGESIC						
Alka-Seltzer Plus Day Cold Liquid Gels	Acetaminophen 325mg		Phenylephrine HCl 5mg	Dextromethorphan HBr 10mg		**Adults & Peds: ≥12 yrs:** 2 caps q4h. **Max:** 12 caps q24h.
Alka-Seltzer Plus Day & Night Liquid Gels	Acetaminophen 325mg		Phenylephrine HCl 5mg	Dextromethorphan HBr 10mg		**Adults & Peds: ≥12 yrs:** 2 caps q4h. **Max:** 12 caps q24h.
Alka-Seltzer Plus Day & Night Effervescent Tablets	Acetaminophen 250mg		Phenylephrine HCl 5mg	Dextromethorphan HBr 10mg		**Adults & Peds: ≥12 yrs:** 2 tabs q4h. **Max:** 8 tabs q24h.
Alka-Seltzer Plus Day Cold Liquid	Acetaminophen 162.5mg/5mL		Phenylephrine HCl 2.5mg/5mL	Dextromethorphan HBr 5mg/5mL		**Adults & Peds: ≥12 yrs:** 4 tsps q4h. **Max:** 6 doses q24h.
Comtrex Cold & Cough Caplets	Acetaminophen 325mg		Phenylephrine HCl 5mg	Dextromethorphan HBr 10mg		**Adults & Peds: ≥12 yrs:** 2 tabs q4h. **Max:** 12 tabs q24h.
Theraflu Daytime Warming Relief Syrup	Acetaminophen 325mg/15mL		Phenylephrine HCl 5mg/15mL	Dextromethorphan HBr 10mg/15mL		**Adults & Peds: ≥12 yrs:** 2 tbl (30mL) q4h. **Max:** 6 doses (12 tbl) q24h.
Theraflu Daytime Severe Cold Caplets	Acetaminophen 325mg		Phenylephrine HCl 5mg	Dextromethorphan HBr 15mg		**Adults & Peds: ≥12 yrs:** 2 tabs q6h. **Max:** 8 tabs q24h.
Tylenol Cold Head Congestion Daytime Capsules	Acetaminophen 325mg		Phenylephrine HCl 5mg	Dextromethorphan HBr 10mg		**Adults & Peds: ≥12 yrs:** 2 caps q4h. **Max:** 12 caps q24h.
Tylenol Cold Head Congestion Day/Night Pack	Acetaminophen 325mg		Phenylephrine HCl 5mg	Dextromethorphan HBr 10mg		**Adults & Peds: ≥12 yrs:** 2 tabs q4h. **Max:** 12 tabs q24h.

BRAND NAME	ANALGESIC	ANTIHISTAMINE	DECONGESTANT	COUGH SUPPRESSANT	EXPECTORANT	DOSE
COUGH SUPPRESSANT + DECONGESTANT + ANALGESIC *(Continued)*						
Tylenol Cold Multi-Symptom Daytime Capsules	Acetaminophen 325mg		Phenylephrine HCl 5mg	Dextromethorphan HBr 10mg		**Adults & Peds: ≥12 yrs:** 2 caps q4h. **Max:** 12 caps q24h.
Tylenol Cold Multi-Symptom Daytime Cool Burst Liquid	Acetaminophen 325mg/15mL		Phenylephrine HCl 5mg/15mL	Dextromethorphan HBr 10mg/15mL		**Adults & Peds: ≥12 yrs:** 2 tbl (30mL) q4h. **Max:** 6 doses (12 tbl) q24h.
Tylenol Cold Multi-Symptom Day/Night Pack	Acetaminophen 325mg		Phenylephrine HCl 5mg	Dextromethorphan HBr 10mg		**Adults & Peds: ≥12 yrs:** 2 caps q4h. **Max:** 12 caps q24h.
Tylenol Flu Daytime Gelcaps	Acetaminophen 500mg		Pseudoephedrine HCl 30mg	Dextromethorphan HBr 15mg		**Adults & Peds: ≥12 yrs:** 2 caps q6h. **Max:** 8 caps q24h.
Vicks DayQuil Liquicaps	Acetaminophen 325mg		Phenylephrine HCl 5mg	Dextromethorphan HBr 10mg		**Adults & Peds: ≥12 yrs:** 2 caps q4h. **Max:** 6 caps q24h.
Vicks DayQuil Liquid	Acetaminophen 325mg/15mL		Phenylephrine HCl 5mg/15mL	Dextromethorphan HBr 10mg/15mL		**Adults & Peds: ≥12 yrs:** 2 tbl (30mL) q4h. **Max:** 12 tbl (120mL) q24h.
COUGH SUPPRESSANT + DECONGESTANT + EXPECTORANT						
Robitussin CF Liquid			Phenylephrine HCl 5mg/5mL	Dextromethorphan HBr 10mg/5mL	Guaifenesin 100mg/5mL	**Adults: ≥12 yrs:** 2 tsp (10mL) q4h. **Peds: 6-12 yrs:** 1 tsp (5mL) q4h. **2-6 yrs:** ½ tsp (2.5mL) q4h. **Max:** 6 doses q24h.
COUGH SUPPRESSANT + DECONGESTANT + EXPECTORANT + ANALGESIC						
Sudafed Cold & Cough Capsules	Acetaminophen 250mg		Pseudoephedrine HCl 30mg	Dextromethorphan HBr 10mg	Guaifenesin 100mg	**Adults & Peds: ≥12 yrs:** 2 caps q4h. **Max:** 8 caps q24h.
Sudafed PE Cold & Cough Caplets	Acetaminophen 325mg		Phenylephrine HCl 5mg	Dextromethorphan HBr 10mg	Guaifenesin 100mg	**Adults & Peds: ≥12 yrs:** 2 tabs q4h. **Max:** 12 tabs q24h.
Tylenol Cold Multi-Symptom Severe Liquid	Acetaminophen 325mg/15mL		Phenylephrine HCl 5mg/15mL	Dextromethorphan HBr 10mg/15mL	Guaifenesin 200mg/15mL	**Adults & Peds: ≥12 yrs:** 2 tbs q4h. **Max:** 12 tbs q24h.
Tylenol Cold Multi-Symptom Severe Caplets	Acetaminophen 325mg		Phenylephrine HCl 5mg	Dextromethorphan HBr 10mg	Guaifenesin 200mg	**Adults & Peds: ≥12 yrs:** 2 tabs q4h. **Max:** 12 tabs q24h.
Tylenol Cold Head Congestion Severe Caplets	Acetaminophen 325mg		Phenylephrine HCl 5mg	Dextromethorphan HBr 10mg	Guaifenesin 200mg	**Adults & Peds: ≥12 yrs:** 2 tabs q4h. **Max:** 12 tabs q24h.
Tylenol Cold Severe Congestion Daytime Caplets	Acetaminophen 325mg		Pseudoephedrine HCl 30mg	Dextromethorphan HBr 15mg	Guaifenesin 200mg	**Adults & Peds: ≥12 yrs:** 2 tabs q6h. **Max:** 8 tabs q24h.

(Continued)

BRAND NAME	ANALGESIC	ANTIHISTAMINE	DECONGESTANT	COUGH SUPPRESSANT	EXPECTORANT	DOSE
COUGH SUPPRESSANT & EXPECTORANT						
Alka-Seltzer Plus Mucus & Congestion Effervescent Tablets				Dextromethorphan HBr 10mg	Guaifenesin 200mg	**Adults & Peds: ≥12 yrs:** 2 tabs q4h. **Max:** 8 tabs q24h.
Coricidin HBP Chest Congestion & Cough Softgels				Dextromethorphan HBr 10mg	Guaifenesin 200mg	**Adults & Peds: ≥12 yrs:** 1-2 caps q4h. **Max:** 12 caps q24h.
Mucinex DM Extended-Release Tablets				Dextromethorphan HBr 30mg	Guaifenesin 600mg	**Adults & Peds: ≥12 yrs:** 1-2 tabs q12h. **Max:** 4 tabs q24h.
Mucinex Liquid Cherry				Dextromethorphan HBr 5mg	Guaifenesin 100mg	**Peds: 6-12 yrs:** 1-2 tsp q4h. **2-6 yrs:** ½-1 tsp q4h. **Max:** 6 doses q24h.
Robitussin Cough & Congestion Liquid				Dextromethorphan HBr 10mg/5mL	Guaifenesin 200mg/5mL	**Adults: ≥12 yrs:** 2 tsp (10mL) q4h. **Peds: 6-12 yrs:** 1 tsp (5mL) q4h. **2-6 yrs:** ½ tsp (2.5mL) q4h. **Max:** 6 doses q24h.
Robitussin DM Liquid				Dextromethorphan HBr 10mg/5mL	Guaifenesin 100mg/5mL	**Adults: ≥12 yrs:** 2 tsp (10mL) q4h. **Peds: 6-12 yrs:** 1 tsp (5mL) q4h. **2-6 yrs:** ½ tsp (2.5mL) q4h. **Max:** 6 doses q24h.
Robitussin Sugar-Free Cough Liquid				Dextromethorphan HBr 10mg/5mL	Guaifenesin 100mg/5mL	**Adults: ≥12 yrs:** 2 tsp (10mL) q4h. **Peds: 6-12 yrs:** 1 tsp (5mL) q4h. **2-6 yrs:** ½ tsp (2.5mL) q4h. **Max:** 6 doses q24h.
Vicks 44E Liquid				Dextromethorphan HBr 20mg/15mL	Guaifenesin 200mg/15mL	**Adults: ≥12 yrs:** 1 tbl (15mL) q4h. **Peds: 6-12 yrs:** 1.5 tsp (7.5mL) q4h. **Max:** 6 doses q24h.
Vicks 44E Pediatric Liquid				Dextromethorphan HBr 10mg/15mL	Guaifenesin 100mg/15mL	**Adults: ≥12 yrs:** 2 tbl (30mL) q4h. **Peds: 6-12 yrs:** 1 tbl (15mL) q4h. **2-5 yrs:** ½ tbl (7.5mL) q4h. **Max:** 6 doses q24h.
DECONGESTANT						
Contac-D Cold Decongestant Tablets			Phenylephrine HCl 10mg			**Adults & Peds: ≥12 yrs:** 1 tabs q4h. **Max:** 6 tabs q24h.
Dimetapp Toddler's Drops Decongestant			Phenylephrine HCl 1.25mg/0.8mL			**Peds: 2-6 yrs:** 1.6mL q4h. **Max:** 6 doses q24h.

BRAND NAME	ANALGESIC	ANTIHISTAMINE	DECONGESTANT	COUGH SUPPRESSANT	EXPECTORANT	DOSE
DECONGESTANT *(Continued)*						
PediaCare Children's Decongestant Liquid			Phenylephrine HCl 2.5mg/5mL			**Peds: 6-12 yrs:** 2 tsp (10mL) q4h. **2-6 yrs:** 1 tsp (5mL) q4h. **Max:** 6 doses q24h.
Sudafed 12-Hour Tablets			Pseudoephedrine HCl 120mg			**Adults & Peds: ≥12 yrs:** 1 tab q12h. **Max:** 2 tabs q24h.
Sudafed 24-Hour Tablets			Pseudoephedrine HCl 240mg			**Adults & Peds: ≥12 yrs:** 1 tab q24h. **Max:** 1 tab q24h.
Sudafed Children's Chewable Tablets			Pseudoephedrine HCl 15mg			**Adults: ≥12 yrs:** 4 tabs q4-6h. **Peds: 6-12 yrs:** 2 tabs q4-6h. **2-6 yrs:** 1 tab q4-6h. **Max:** 4 doses q24h.
Sudafed Children's Liquid			Pseudoephedrine HCl 15mg/5mL			**Adults: ≥12 yrs:** 4 tsp (20mL) q4-6h. **Peds: 6-12 yrs:** 2 tsp (10mL) q4-6h. **2-6 yrs:** 1 tsp (5mL) q4-6h. **Max:** 4 doses q24h.
Sudafed PE Tablets			Phenylephrine HCl 10mg			**Adults & Peds: ≥12 yrs:** 1 tab q4h. **Max:** 6 tabs q24h.
Sudafed PE Quick Dissolve Strips			Phenylephrine HCl 10mg			**Adults & Peds: ≥12 yrs:** 1 film q4h. **Max:** 6 films q24h.
Sudafed Nasal Decongestant Tablets			Pseudoephedrine HCl 30mg			**Adults: ≥12 yrs:** 2 tabs q4-6h. **Peds: 6-12 yrs:** 1 tab q4-6h. **Max:** 4 doses q24h.
Triaminic Cold with Stuffy Nose Thin Strips			Phenylephrine HCl 2.5mg/strip			**Peds: 6-12 yrs:** 2 strips q4h. **2-6 yrs:** 1 strip q4h. **Max:** 6 doses q24h.
Vicks Sinex 12-Hour Nasal Spray			Oxymetazoline HCl 0.05%			**Adults & Peds: ≥6 yrs:** 2-3 sprays q10-12h. **Max:** 2 doses q24h.
Vicks Sinex Nasal Spray			Phenylephrine HCl 0.5%			**Adults & Peds: ≥12 yrs:** 2-3 sprays q4h. **Max:** 18 sprays q24h.
Vicks Sinex UltraFine Mist			Phenylephrine HCl 0.5%			**Adults & Peds: ≥12 yrs:** 2-3 sprays q4h. **Max:** 18 sprays q24h.
Vicks Sinex 12-Hour UltraFine Mist			Oxymetazoline HCl 0.05%			**Adults & Peds: ≥6 yrs:** 2-3 sprays q10-12h. **Max:** 2 doses q24h.

(Continued)

BRAND NAME	ANALGESIC	ANTIHISTAMINE	DECONGESTANT	COUGH SUPPRESSANT	EXPECTORANT	DOSE
DECONGESTANT *(Continued)*						
Vicks Vapor Inhaler			Levmetamfetamine 50mg			**Adults:** ≥12 yrs: 2 inhalations q2h. **Max:** 24 inhalations q24h. **Peds: 6-12 yrs:** 1 inhalation q2h. **Max:** 12 inhalations q24h.
DECONGESTANT + ANALGESIC						
Advil Children's Cold Liquid	Ibuprofen 100mg/5mL		Pseudoephedrine HCl 15mg/5mL			**Peds: 6-11 yrs (48-95 lbs):** 2 tsp (10mL) q6h. **2-5 yrs (24-47 lbs):** 1 tsp (5mL) q6h. **Max:** 4 doses q24h
Advil Cold & Sinus Caplets	Ibuprofen 200mg		Pseudoephedrine HCl 30mg			**Adults & Peds:** ≥12 yrs: 1-2 tabs q4-6h. **Max:** 6 tabs q24h.
Advil Cold & Sinus Liqui-gels	Ibuprofen 200mg		Pseudoephedrine HCl 30mg			**Adults & Peds:** ≥12 yrs: 1-2 caps q4-6h. **Max:** 6 caps q24h.
Alka-Seltzer Plus Cold & Sinus Tablets	Acetaminophen 250mg		Phenylephrine HCl 5mg			**Adults & Peds:** ≥12 yrs: 2 tabs q4h. **Max:** 8 tab q24h.
Alka-Seltzer Plus Sinus Effervescent Tablets	Acetaminophen 250mg		Phenylephrine HCl 5mg			**Adults & Peds:** ≥12 yrs: 2 tabs q4h. **Max:** 8 tab q24h.
Contac Cold & Flu Day & Night Caplets	Acetaminophen 500mg		Phenylephrine HCl 5mg			**Adults & Peds:** ≥12 yrs: 2 tabs q4-6h. **Max:** 8 tabs q24h.
Contac Cold & Flu Non-Drowsy Maximum Strength Caplets	Acetaminophen 500mg		Phenylephrine HCl 5mg			**Adults & Peds:** ≥12 yrs: 2 tabs q4-6h. **Max:** 8 tabs q24h.
Motrin Children's Cold Suspension	Ibuprofen 100mg/5mL		Pseudoephedrine HCl 15mg/5mL			**Peds: 6-12 yrs (48-95 lbs):** 2 tsp (10mL) q6h. **2-6 yrs (24-47 lbs):** 1 tsp (5mL) q6h. **Max:** 4 doses q24h.
Sinutab Sinus Tablets	Acetaminophen 500mg		Phenylephrine HCl 5mg			**Adults & Peds:** ≥12 yrs: 2 tabs q6h. **Max:** 8 tabs q24h.
Sudafed PE Sinus Headache Caplets	Acetaminophen 325mg		Phenylephrine HCl 5mg			**Adults & Peds:** ≥12 yrs: 2 tabs q4h. **Max:** 12 tabs q24h.
Sudafed Sinus & Cold Liquid Capsules	Acetaminophen 325mg		Pseudoephedrine HCl 30mg			**Adults & Peds:** ≥12 yrs: 2 caps q4-6h. **Max:** 8 caps q24h.
Theraflu Daytime Severe Cold Hot Liquid	Acetaminophen 650mg		Phenylephrine HCl 10mg			**Adults & Peds:** ≥12 yrs: 1 packet q4h. **Max:** 6 packets q24h.

BRAND NAME	ANALGESIC	ANTIHISTAMINE	DECONGESTANT	COUGH SUPPRESSANT	EXPECTORANT	DOSE
DECONGESTANT + ANALGESIC *(Continued)*						
Tylenol Sinus Congestion & Pain Daytime Caplets	Acetaminophen 325 mg		Phenylephrine HCl 5mg			**Adults & Peds: ≥12 yrs:** 2 tabs q4h. **Max:** 12 tabs q24h.
Tylenol Sinus Congestion & Pain Daytime Gelcaps	Acetaminophen 325 mg		Phenylephrine HCl 5mg			**Adults & Peds: ≥12 yrs:** 2 caps q4h. **Max:** 12 caps q24h.
Tylenol Sinus Congestion & Pain Daytime Rapid Release Gelcaps	Acetaminophen 325 mg		Phenylephrine HCl 5mg			**Adults & Peds: ≥12 yrs:** 2 caps q4h. **Max:** 12 caps q24h.
Vicks DayQuil Sinus Liquicaps	Acetaminophen 325 mg		Phenylephrine HCl 5mg			**Adults & Peds: ≥12 yrs:** 2 caps q4h. **Max:** 6 caps q4h.
DECONGESTANT + EXPECTORANT						
Dimetapp Children's Cold & Chest Congestion Syrup			Phenylephrine HCl 5mg/5mL		Guaifenesin 100mg/5mL	**Adults: ≥12 yrs:** 2 tsp (10mL) q4h. **Peds: 6-12 yrs:** 1 tsp (5mL) q4h. 2-6 yrs: ½ tsp (2.5mL) 14 h. **Max:** 6 doses q24h.
Mucinex D Extended-Release Tablets			Pseudoephedrine HCl 60mg		Guaifenesin 600mg	**Adults & Peds: ≥12 yrs:** 2 tabs q12h. **Max:** 4 tabs q24h.
Robitussin PE Head & Chest Liquid			Phenylephrine HCl 5mg/5mL		Guaifenesin 100mg/5mL	**Adults: ≥12 yrs:** 2 tsp (10mL) q4h. **Peds: 6-12 yrs:** 1 tsp (5mL) q4h. **Max:** 6 doses q24h.
Sudafed Non-Drying Sinus Liquid Caps			Pseudoephedrine HCl 30mg		Guaifenesin 200mg	**Adults & Peds: ≥12 yrs:** 2 caps q4h. **Max:** 8 caps q24h.
Sudafed PE Non-Drying Sinus Caplets			Phenylephrine HCl 5mg		Guaifenesin 200mg	**Adults & Peds: ≥12 yrs:** 2 tabs q4h. **Max:** 12 tabs q24h.
Triaminic Chest & Nasal Liquid			Phenylephrine HCl 2.5mg/5mL		Guaifenesin 50mg/5mL	**Adults & Peds: ≥12 yrs:** 1 tsp q 4h. **Max:** 6 doses q24h. **Peds: 6-12 yrs:** 2 tsp (10mL), **2-6 yrs:** 1 tsp (5mL).
DECONGESTANT + EXPECTORANT + ANALGESIC						
Tylenol Sinus Congestion & Severe Pain Caplets	Acetaminophen 325 mg		Phenylephrine HCl 5mg		Guaifenesin 200mg	**Adults & Peds: ≥12 yrs:** 2 tabs q4h. **Max:** 12 tabs q24h.

BRAND NAME	ANALGESIC	ANTIHISTAMINE	DECONGESTANT	COUGH SUPPRESSANT	EXPECTORANT	DOSE
EXPECTORANT						
Mucinex Extended-Release Tablets					Guaifenesin 600mg	**Adults & Peds: ≥12 yrs:** 1-2 tabs q12h. **Max:** 4 tabs q24h.
Mucinex Liquid Grape					Guaifenesin 100mg/5mL	**Peds: 6-12 yrs:** 1-2 tsp q4h. **2-6 yrs:** ½-1 tsp q4h. **Max:** 6 doses 24h.
Mucinex Mini-Melts Bubble Gum Packets					Guaifenesin 100mg	**Adults & Peds: ≥12 yrs:** 2-4 packets q4h. **Peds: 6-12 yrs:** 1-2 packets q4h. **2-6 yrs:** 1 packet q4h. **Max:** 6 doses q24h.
Mucinex Mini-Melts Grape Packets					Guaifenesin 50mg	**Peds: 6-12 yrs:** 2-4 packets q4h. **2-6 yrs:** 1-2 packets q4h. **Max:** 6 doses 24h.
Robitussin Chest Congestion Liquid					Guaifenesin 100mg/5mL	**Adults: ≥12 yrs:** 2-4 tsp (10-20mL) q4h. **Peds: 6-12 yrs:** 1-2 tsp (5-10mL) q4h. **2-6 yrs:** 1/2-1 tsp (2.5-5mL) q4h. **Max:** 6 doses q24h.
Vicks Casero Chest Congestion Relief Liquid					Guaifenesin 100mg/6.25mL	**Adults & Peds: ≥12 yrs:** 2.5 tsp (12.5mL) q4h. **Peds: 6-12 yrs:** 1.25 tsp (6.25mL) q4h. **2-6 yrs:** 3.12mL q4h. **Max:** 6 doses q24h.
EXPECTORANT + ANALGESIC						
Comtrex Deep Chest Cold Caplets	Acetaminophen 325mg				Guaifenesin 200mg	**Adults & Peds: ≥12 yrs:** 2 tabs q4-6h. **Max:** 12 tabs q24h.
Tylenol Chest Congestion Caplets	Acetaminophen 325mg				Guaifenesin 200mg	**Adults & Peds: ≥12 yrs:** 2 tabs q4-6h. **Max:** 12 tabs q24h.

BRAND NAME	ANALGESIC	ANTIHISTAMINE	DECONGESTANT	COUGH SUPPRESSANT	EXPECTORANT	DOSE
EXPECTORANT + ANALGESIC (Continued)						
Tylenol Chest Congestion Liquid	Acetaminophen 500mg/15mL				Guaifenesin 200mg/15mL	**Adults & Peds: ≥12 yrs:** 2 tbl (30mL) q4-6h. **Max:** 8 tbl (120mL) q24h.
Theraflu Flu & Chest Liquid	Acetaminophen 1000mg/packet				Guaifenesin 400mg/packet	**Adults & Peds: ≥12 yrs:** 1 packet q6h. **Max:** 4 packets q24h.
EXPECTORANT + DECONGESTANT + COUGH SUPPRESSANT						
Robitussin Cold & Cough CF Liquid			Phenylephrine HCl 5mg/5mL	Dextromethorphan HBr 10mg/5mL	Guaifenesin 100mg/5mL	**Adults & Peds: ≥12 yrs:** 2 tsp (10mL) q4h. **Peds: 6-12 yrs:** 1 tsp (5mL) q4h. **2-6 yrs:** ½ tsp (2.5mL) q4h. **Max: 6** doses q24h.
Robitussin Pediatric Cold & Cough CF Liquid			Phenylephrine HCl 2.5mg/5mL	Dextromethorphan HBr 5mg/2.5mL	Guaifenesin 100mg/2.5mL	**Peds: 2-6 yrs:** 2.5mL q4h. **Max: 6** doses q24h.
EXPECTORANT + DECONGESTANT + ANALGESIC						
Tylenol Sinus Congestion & Severe Pain Caplets	Acetaminophen 325mg		Phenylephrine HCl 5mg		Guaifenesin 200mg	**Adults & Peds: ≥12 yrs:** 2 tabs q4h. **Max:** 12 tabs q24h.
Tylenol Sinus Severe Congestion Daytime Caplets	Acetaminophen 325mg		Pseudoephedrine HCl 30mg		Guaifenesin 200mg	**Adults & Peds: ≥12 yrs:** 2 tabs q6h. **Max:** 8 tabs q24h.
ANTIHISTAMINE + ANALGESIC						
Coricidin Cold & Flu Tablets	Acetaminophen 325mg	Chlorpheniramine Maleate 2mg				**Adults & Peds: ≥12 yrs:** 2 tabs q4-6h. **Max:** 12 tabs q24h.
Tylenol Sore Throat Nighttime Liquid	Acetaminophen 1000mg/30mL	Diphenhydramine HCl 50mg/30mL				**Adults & Peds: ≥12 yrs:** 2 tbl q4-6h. **Max:** 8 tbl (120mL) q24h.

ACE INHIBITORS

DRUG (BRAND)	PEAK PLASMA LEVEL	FOOD EFFECT ON AMOUNT ABSORBED	HYPERTENSION DOSING*	HEART FAILURE DOSING	RENAL DOSE ADJUSTMENT
Benazepril (Lotensin)	1-2 hrs (fasting); 2-4 hrs (non-fasting**)	None	**Initial:** 10mg qd. **Usual:** 20-40mg/day given qd-bid. **Max:** 80mg/day.	Not FDA approved.	CrCl<30mL/min/1.73m²: **Initial:** 5mg qd. **Max:** 40mg/day.
Captopril (Capoten)	1 hr	Reduced***	**Initial:** 25mg bid-tid. **Usual:** 50mg bid-tid. **Max:** 50mg tid.	**Initial:** 25mg tid. **Usual:** 50-100mg tid. **Max:** 450mg/day.	**Significant Renal Dysfunction:** Lower initial dose and titrate slowly.
Enalapril (Vasotec)	3-4 hrs**	None	**Initial:** 5mg qd. **Usual:** 10-40mg/day given qd-bid. **Max:** 40mg/day.†	**Initial:** 2.5mg qd. **Usual:** 2.5-20mg given bid. **Max:** 40mg/day.	**HTN:** CrCl ≤30mL/min: **Initial:** 2.5mg qd. **Max:** 40mg/day. **Dialysis:** 2.5mg/day on dialysis day. **HF:** SCr 1.6mg/dL: **Initial:** 2.5mg qd. **Max:** 40mg/day.
Fosinopril (Monopril)	3 hrs**	None	**Initial:** 10mg qd. **Usual:** 20-40mg/day. **Max:** 80mg/day.	**Initial:** 10mg qd. **Usual:** 20-40mg qd. **Max:** 40mg/day.	**HTN:** No dosage adjustment needed. **HF:** Moderate to severe renal failure/vigorous diuresis: 5mg qd.
Lisinopril (Prinivil, Zestril)	7 hrs	None	**Initial:** 10mg qd. **Usual:** 20-40mg qd. **Max:** 80mg/day.	(Prinivil) **Initial:** 5mg qd. **Usual:** 5-20mg qd. (Zestril) **Initial:** 5mg qd. **Usual:** 5-40mg qd. **Max:** 40mg/day.	**HTN:** CrCl 10-30mL/min: **Initial:** 5mg qd. **Max:** 40mg/day. CrCl <10mL/min: **Initial:** 2.5mg qd. **Max:** 40mg/day. **HF:** CrCl ≤30mL/min: **Initial:** 2.5mg qd.
Moexipril (Univasc)	1-1.5 hrs**	Reduced***	**Initial:** 7.5mg qd. **Usual:** 7.5-30mg/day given qd-bid. **Max:** 60mg/day.	Not FDA approved.	CrCl ≤40mL/min/1.73m²: **Initial:** 3.75mg qd. **Max:** 15mg/day.
Perindopril (Aceon)	3-7 hrs**	None	**Initial:** 4mg qd. **Usual:** 4-8mg/day given qd-bid. **Max:** 16mg/day.	Not FDA approved.	CrCl >30mL/min: **Initial:** 2mg qd. **Max:** 8mg/day.
Quinapril (Accupril)	2 hrs**	Reduced (after high-fat meals)	**Initial:** 10-20mg qd. **Usual:** 20-80mg/day given qd-bid.	**Initial:** 5mg bid. **Usual:** 10-20mg bid.	CrCl 30-60mL/min: **Initial:** 5mg qd. CrCl 10-30mL/min: **Initial:** 2.5mg qd.
Ramipril (Altace)	2-4 hrs**	None	**Initial:** 2.5mg qd. **Usual:** 2.5-20mg/day given qd-bid.	**Post MI:** **Initial:** 2.5mg bid; 1.25mg bid if hypotensive. Titrate to 5mg bid.	**HTN:** **Initial:** 1.25mg qd. **Max:** 5mg/day. **Post MI:** **Initial:** 1.25mg qd. **Max:** 2.5mg/bid.
Trandolapril (Mavik)	4-10 hrs**	None	**Initial:** 1mg qd in non-black patients. 2mg qd in black patients. **Usual:** 2-4mg/day. **Max:** 8mg/day.	**Post MI:** **Initial:** 1mg qd. Titrate to 4mg qd if tolerated.	CrCl <30mL/min: **Initial:** 0.5mg qd.

* Reduce dose with concomitant diuretic.
** Peak effect of active metabolite.
*** Administer 1 hour before meals captopril and moexipril.
† Refer to monograph for pediatric dosing.

ARBs* AND COMBINATIONS

DRUG	BRAND	USUAL HTN† DOSAGE RANGE	HOW SUPPLIED
ANGIOTENSIN II RECEPTOR BLOCKERS			
Candesartan	Atacand	8–32 mg/day.	**Tab:** 4mg, 8mg, 16mg, 32mg
Eprosartan	Teveten	400–800 mg/day.	**Tab:** 400mg, 600mg
Irbesartan	Avapro	150–300 mg/day.	**Tab:** 75mg, 150mg, 300mg
Losartan	Cozaar	25–100 mg/day.	**Tab:** 25mg, 50mg, 100mg
Olmesartan	Benicar	20–40 mg/day.	**Tab:** 5mg, 20mg, 40mg
Telmisartan	Micardis	20–80 mg/day.	**Tab:** 20mg, 40mg, 80mg
Valsartan	Diovan	80–320 mg/day.	**Tab:** 40mg, 80mg, 160mg, 320mg
COMBINATIONS			
Candesartan-Hydrochlorothiazide	Atacand HCT	16/12.5–32/25 mg/day.	**Tab:** 16mg-12.5mg, 32mg-12.5mg
Eprosartan-Hydrochlorothiazide	Teveten HCT	600/12.5–600/25 mg/day.	**Tab:** 600mg-12.5mg, 600mg-25mg
Irbesartan-Hydrochlorothiazide	Avalide	150/12.5–300/25 mg/day.	**Tab:** 150mg-12.5mg, 300mg-12.5mg, 300mg-25mg
Losartan-Hydrochlorothiazide	Hyzaar	50/12.5–100/25 mg/day.	**Tab:** 50mg-12.5mg, 100mg-12.5mg, 100mg-25mg
Olmesartan-Hydrochlorothiazide	Benicar HCT	20/12.5–40/25 mg/day.	**Tab:** 20mg-12.5mg, 40mg-12.5mg, 40mg-25mg
Telmisartan-Hydrochlorothiazide	Micardis HCT	40/12.5–160/25 mg/day.	**Tab:** 40mg-12.5mg, 80mg-12.5mg, 80mg-25mg
Valsartan-Hydrochlorothiazide	Diovan HCT	80/12.5–320/25 mg/day	**Tab:** 80mg-12.5mg, 160mg-12.5mg, 160mg-25mg, 320mg-12.5mg, 320mg-25mg

*ARBs: Angiotensin II receptor blockers.

†HTN: Hypertension.

Adopted from the Seventh Report of the Joint National Committee on Prevention, Detection, Evaluation, and Treatment of High Blood Pressure (JNC 7); http://www.nhlbi.nih.gov/guidelines/hypertension/jnc7full.htm.

BETA-BLOCKERS

DRUG	BRAND	HOW SUPPLIED	HYPERTENSION DOSING	ANGINA DOSING	POST-MI DOSING
NONSELECTIVE BETA-BLOCKERS					
Nadolol	Corgard	**Tab:** 20mg, 40mg, 80mg, 120mg, 160mg	**Initial:** 40mg qd. **Usual:** 40mg–80mg qd. **Max:** 320mg/day.	**Initial:** 40mg qd. **Usual:** 40mg–80mg qd. **Max:** 240mg/day.	Not FDA approved
Penbutolol sulfate	Levatol	**Tab:** 20mg	**Initial** and **Usual:** 20mg qd.	Not FDA approved	Not FDA approved
Pindolol	Visken	**Tab:** 5mg, 10mg	**Initial:** 5mg, bid **Max:** 60mg/day.	Not FDA approved	Not FDA approved
Propranolol HCl	Inderal	**Tab:** 10mg, 20mg, 40mg, 60mg, 80mg	**Initial:** 40mg bid **Usual:** 120mg–240mg/day. **Max:** 640mg/day.	**Usual:** 80mg–320mg/day.	**Initial:** 40mg bid **Usual:** 180mg–240mg. **Max:** 240mg/day.
	Inderal LA	**Cap, LA:** 60mg, 80mg, 120mg, 160mg	**Initial:** 80mg bid **Usual:** 120mg–160mg qd. **Max:** 640mg/day.	**Initial:** 80mg qd. **Usual:** 160mg qd. **Max:** 320mg	Not FDA approved
	Innopran XL	**Cap, ER:** 80mg, 120mg	**Initial:** 80mg qd. **Max:** 120mg qd.	Not FDA approved	Not FDA approved
Timolol maleate	Various generics	**Tab:** 5mg, 10mg 20mg	**Initial:** 10mg, bid **Usual:** 20mg–40mg/day. **Max:** 60mg/day.	Not FDA approved	**Usual:** 10mg bid (post acute MI).
SELECTIVE BETA₁-BLOCKERS					
Acebutolol	Sectral	**Cap:** 200mg, 40mg, 400mg	**Initial:** 400mg qd. **Usual:** 400mg–800mg/day. **Max:** 1200mg/day.	Not FDA approved	Not FDA approved
Atenolol	Tenormin	**Tab:** 25mg, 50mg, 100mg	**Initial:** 50mg qd. **Max:** 100mg qd.	**Initial:** 50mg qd. **Usual:** 100mg qd. **Max:** 200mg qd.	**Usual:** 50mg bid or 100mg qd for 6–9 days post MI.
Betaxolol HCl	Kerlone	**Tab:** 10mg, 20mg	**Initial:** 10mg qd. **Max:** 40mg qd.	Not FDA approved	Not FDA approved
Bisoprolol fumarate	Zebeta	**Tab:** 5mg, 10mg	**Initial:** 2.5mg–5mg qd. **Usual:** 2.5mg–20mg qd. **Max:** 40mg qd.	Not FDA approved	Not FDA approved
Esmolol	Brevibloc	**Inj:** 10mg/mL [10mL, 250mL], 20mg/mL [5mL, 100mL]	**Initial:** 80mg bolus over 30 sec. **Maint:** 0.15mg/kg/min. May titrate up to 0.3mg/kg/min. **Gradual Control: Initial:** 0.5mg/kg over 1 min. **Maint:** 0.05mg/kg/min for 4 min. If needed, may repeat load and increase to 0.1mg/kg/min.**	Not FDA approved	Not FDA approved

(Continued)

DRUG	BRAND	HOW SUPPLIED	HYPERTENSION DOSING	ANGINA DOSING	POST-MI DOSING
SELECTIVE BETA₁-BLOCKERS *(Continued)*					
Metoprolol succinate	Toprol-XL	**Tab, XL:** 25mg, 50mg, 100mg, 200mg	**Initial:** 25mg–100mg qd. **Max:** 400mg/day.	**Initial:** 100mg qd. **Max:** 400mg/day.	Not FDA approved
Metoprolol tartrate	Lopressor	**Tab:** 50mg, 100mg	**Initial:** 50mg–100mg qd. **Usual:** 100mg–450mg/day. **Max:** 450mg/day.	**Initial:** 50mg bid **Usual:** 100mg–400mg/day. **Max:** 400mg/day.	**Usual:** 100mg bid for 3 months.
	Various generics	**Tab:** 25mg, 50mg 100mg	**Initial:** 50mg–100mg qd. **Usual:** 100mg–450mg/day. **Max:** 450mg/day.	**Initial:** 50mg bid **Usual:** 100mg–400mg/day. **Max:** 400mg/day.	**Usual:** 100mg bid for 3 months.
Nebivolol	Bystolic	**Tab:** 2.5mg, 5mg 10mg	**Initial:** 5mg qd. **Titrate:** May in increase dose if needed at 2-week intervals. **Max:** 40mg. **Hepatic impairment/ CrCl <30mL/min:** 2.5mg qd.	Not FDA approved	Not FDA approved
MIXED ALPHA- AND BETA-BLOCKERS					
Carvedilol	Coreg	**Tab:** 3.125mg, 6.25mg, 12.5mg, 25mg	**Initial:** 6.25mg bid **Max:** 25mg bid	Not FDA approved	Left Ventricular Dysfunction post MI: **Initial:** 6.25mg bid. **Usual:** 25mg bid.
	Coreg CR	**Tab, CR:** 10mg, 20mg, 40mg, 80mg	**Initial:** 20mg qd. **Max:** 80mg/day.	Not FDA approved	Left Ventricular Dysfunction post MI: **Initial:** 10mg–20mg qd. **Usual:** 80mg qd.
Labetalol HCl	Trandate	**Tab:** 100mg, 200mg, 300mg	**Initial:** 100mg, bid **Usual:** 200mg–400mg bid	Not FDA approved	Not FDA approved
COMBINATIONS					
Atenolol/ Chlorthali-done	Tenoretic	**Tab:** 50mg/25mg, 100mg/25mg	**Initial:** 50mg/25mg qd. **Max:** 100mg/25mg/day.	Not FDA approved	Not FDA approved
Nadolol/ Bendroflu-methiazide	Corzide	**Tab:** 40mg/5mg, 80mg/5mg	**Initial:** 40mg/5mg qd. **Max:** 80mg/5mg/day.	Not FDA approved	Not FDA approved
Bisoprolol/ fumarate/ HCTZ*	Ziac	**Tab:** 2.5mg/6.25mg, 5mg/6.25mg, 10mg/6.25mg	**Initial:** 2.5mg/6.25mg qd. **Max:** 20mg/12.5mg/day.	Not FDA approved	Not FDA approved
Metoprolol tartrate/ HCTZ*	Lopressor HCT	**Tab:** 50mg/25mg, 100mg/25mg, 100mg/50mg	**Initial:** 50mg/25mg qd or bid. **Max:** 200mg/50mg/day.	Not FDA approved	Not FDA approved
Propranolol/ HCTZ*	Inderide	**Tab:** 40mg/25mg	**Initial:** 40mg/25mg bid. **Max:** 160mg/50mg/day.	Not FDA approved	Not FDA approved

*Hydrochlorothiazide.

**Brevibloc is used for the treatment of tachycardia and hypertension that occur during induction and tracheal intubation, during surgery, on emergence from anesthesia, and in the postoperative period.

Source: FDA-approved labeling.

CALCIUM CHANNEL BLOCKERS

DRUG	BRAND	HOW SUPPLIED	HYPERTENSION DOSING*	ANGINA DOSING*
DIHYDROPYRIDINES				
Amlodipine besylate	Norvasc	**Tab:** 2.5mg, 5mg, 10mg	**Initial:** 5mg qd. **Max:** 10mg qd.	**Initial/Usual:** 10mg qd.
Felodipine	Plendil	**Tab, ER:** 2.5mg, 5mg, 10mg	**Initial:** 5mg qd. **Usual:** 2.5-10mg qd.	Not FDA approved
Isradipine	DynaCirc CR, generic	**Tab, CR:** 5mg, 10mg **Cap:** 2.5mg, 5mg	**Initial:** 2.5mg bid or 5mg qd. **Max:** 20mg/day.	Not FDA approved
Nicardipine HCl	Cardene	**Cap:** 20mg, 30mg	**Initial:** 20mg tid. **Usual:** 20-40mg tid.	**Initial:** 20mg tid. **Usual:** 20-40mg tid.
	Cardene SR	**Cap, ER:** 30mg, 45mg, 60mg	**Initial:** 30mg bid. **Usual:** 30-60mg bid.	Not FDA approved
Nifedipine	Adalat CC	**Tab, ER:** 30mg, 60mg, 90mg	**Initial:** 30mg qd. **Usual:** 30-60mg qd. **Max:** 90mg/day.	Not FDA approved
	Procardia	**Cap:** 10mg, 20mg	Not FDA approved	**Initial:** 10mg tid. **Usual:** 10-20mg tid. **Max:** 180mg/day.
	Procardia XL	**Tab, ER:** 30mg, 60mg, 90mg	**Initial:** 30-60mg qd. **Max:** 120mg/day.	**Initial:** 30-60mg qd. **Max:** 90-120mg/day.
Nisoldipine	Sular	**Tab, ER:** 10mg, 20mg, 30mg, 40mg	**Initial:** 20mg qd. **Usual:** 20-40mg qd. **Max:** 60mg/day.	Not FDA approved
NON-DIHYDROPYRIDINES				
Diltiazem HCl	Cardizem	**Tab:** 30mg, 60mg, 90mg, 120mg	Not FDA approved	**Initial:** 30mg qid. **Usual:** 180-360mg/day.
	Cardizem CD, Cartia XT	**Cap, ER:** 120mg, 180mg, 240mg, 300mg, (Cardizem CD) 360mg	**Initial:** 180-240mg qd. **Usual:** 240-360mg qd. **Max:** 480mg qd.	**Initial:** 120-180mg qd. **Max:** 480mg/day.
	Cardizem LA	**Tab, ER:** 120mg, 180mg, 240mg, 300mg, 360mg, 420mg	**Initial:** 180-240mg qd. **Max:** 540mg/day.	**Initial:** 180 qd.
	Dilacor XR, Diltia XT	**Cap, ER:** 120mg, 180mg, 240mg	**Initial:** 180-240mg qd. **Usual:** 180-480mg qd. **Max:** 540mg qd.	**Initial:** 120mg qd. **Max:** 480mg/day.
	Tiazac, Taztia XT	**Cap, ER:** 120mg, 180mg, 240mg, 300mg, 360mg, (Tiazac) 420mg	**Initial:** 120-240mg qd. **Usual:** 120-540mg qd. **Max:** 540mg qd.	**Initial:** 120-180mg qd.
Verapamil HCl	Calan**	**Tab:** 40mg, 80mg, 120mg	**Initial:** 80mg tid. **Usual:** 360-480mg/day.	**Usual:** 80-120mg tid.
	Calan SR, Isoptin SR	**Tab, ER:** 120mg, 180mg, 240mg	**Initial:** 180mg qam. **Max:** 480mg/day.	Not FDA approved
	Covera HS	**Tab, ER:** 180mg, 240mg	**Initial:** 180mg qhs. **Max:** 480mg qhs.	**Initial:** 180mg qhs. **Max:** 480mg qhs.
	Isoptin SR	**Tab, ER:** 120mg, 180mg, 240mg	**Initial:** 180mg qam. **Max:** 480mg/day.	Not FDA approved
	Verelan	**Cap, ER:** 120mg, 180mg, 240mg, 360mg	**Usual:** 240mg qam. **Max:** 480mg qam.	Not FDA approved
	Verelan PM	**Cap, ER:** 100mg, 200mg, 300mg	**Usual:** 200mg qhs. **Max:** 400mg qhs.	Not FDA approved

* NOTE: Adult dosing shown is for monotherapy. Dosage needs to be adjusted by titration to individual patient needs. Dosages may need to be reduced in the elderly, or with renal/hepatic impairment. When used in combination with other antihypertensives the dosage of the calcium channel blocker or the concomitant antihypertensives may need to be adjusted due to possible additive effect. Monitor patient closely. For more information refer to monograph listings or drug's FDA-approved labeling.
** For additional indications refer to monograph listings or drug's FDA-approved labeling.

CHOLESTEROL-LOWERING AGENTS

BRAND (GENERIC)	HOW SUPPLIED (MG)*	USUAL DOSAGE RANGE**	T-CHOL (% DECREASE)	LDL (% DECREASE)	HDL (% INCREASE)	TG (% DECREASE)
HMG-CoA REDUCTASE INHIBITORS (STATINS)						
Lipitor (Atorvastatin)	**Tabs:** 10, 20, 40 80	10-80mg/day	29 to 45	39 to 60	5 to 9	19 to 37
Lescol (Fluvastatin)	**Tabs:** 20, 40	20-80mg/day	17 to 27	22 to 36	3 to 6	12 to 18
Lescol XL (Fluvastatin)	**Tabs, ER:** 80	20-80mg/day	17 to 27	22 to 36	3 to 6	12 to 18
Altoprev (Lovastatin)	**Tab, ER:** 20, 40, 60	20-60mg/day	17 to 29	24 to 40	6.6 to 9.5	10 to 19
Mevacor (Lovastatin)	**Tabs:** 10, 20, 40	10-80mg/day given qd or bid	17 to 29	24 to 40	6.6 to 9.5	10 to 19
Pravachol (Pravastatin)	**Tabs:** 10, 20, 40, 80	10-80mg/day	16 to 27	22 to 37	2 to 12	11 to 24
Crestor (Rosuvastatin)	**Tabs:** 5, 10, 20, 40	5-40mg/day	33 to 46	45 to 63	8 to 14	10 to 35
Zocor (Simvastatin)	**Tabs:** 5, 10, 20, 40, 80	5-80mg/day	19 to 36	26 to 47	8 to 16	12 to 33
FIBRATES						
Tricor (Fenofibrate)	**Tab:** 48, 145	48-145mg/day	18.7	20.6	11	28.9
Lofibra (Fenofibrate)	**Tabs:** 54, 160; **Caps:** 67, 134, 200	54-160mg/day, 67-200mg/day	18.7	20.6	11	28.9
Antara (Fenofibrate)	**Caps:** 43, 130	43-130mg/day	18.7	20.6	11	28.9
Triglide (Fenofibrate)	**Tabs:** 50, 160	50-160mg/day	18.7	20.6	11	28.9
Lopid (Gemfibrozil)	**Tab:** 600	1200mg/day in divided doses	n/a	4.1	12.6	Not specified-but decrease
BILE-ACID SEQUESTRANTS						
Colestid (Colestipol)	Granules: 5000/pk; **Tab:** 1000	500-2000mg qhs	Not specified	Not specified	Not specified	Not specified
Questran, Questran Light (Cholestyramine)	**Can:** 268, 378	2-4 packets or scoopfuls daily (8-16 g) divided into two doses	7.2	10.4	n/a	n/a
WelChol (Colesevelam HCl)	**Tabs:** 625	3750mg/day given qd for bid	7 to 10	15 to 18	3	9 to 10
CHOLESTEROL ABSORPTION INHIBITOR						
Zetia (Ezetimibe)	**Tab:** 10	10mg qd	13	18	1	8
NICOTINIC ACID DERIVATIVE						
Nispan (Niacin, Extended-Release)	**Tabs, ER:** 500, 750, 1000	1-2g hs	3 to 10	5 to 14	18 to 22	13 to 28
LIPID-REGULATING AGENT						
Lovaza (Omega-3-Acid Ethyl Esters)	**Cap:** 1000	4g qd	10	44	9	45
COMBINATIONS						
Caduet (Amlodipine/Atorvastatin)	**Tabs:** 2.5/10, 2.5/20, 2.5/40, 5/10, 5/20, 5/40, 5/80, 10/10, 10/20, 10/40, 10/80	5/20mg to 10/80mg	n/a	n/a	n/a	n/a

(Continued)

CHOLESTEROL-LOWERING AGENTS

BRAND (GENERIC)	HOW SUPPLIED (MG)*	USUAL DOSAGE RANGE**	T-CHOL (% DECREASE)	LDL (% DECREASE)	HDL (% INCREASE)	TG (% DECREASE)
COMBINATIONS *(Continued)*						
Vytorin (Ezetimibe/ Simvastatin)	**Tabs:** 10/10, 10/20, 10/40, 10/80	10/10 to 10/80mg/day	31 to 43	45 to 60	6 to 8	23 to 31
Advicor (Niacin ER/ Lovastatin)	**Tabs:** 500/20, 750/20, 1000/20, 1000/40	500/20mg to 2000mg/40mg	Not specified	30 to 42	20 to 30	32 to 44
Simcor (Niacin ER/ Simvastatin)	**Tabs:** 500/20, 750/20, 1000/20	500mg/20mg to 2000mg/40mg	8.8 to 11.1	11.9 to 14.3	20.7 to 29	26.5 to 38.0

* Unless otherwise indicated
** NOTE: Dosage shown is for adults and may need to be adjusted to individual patient needs. For pediatric dosing and additional information please refer to the individual monograph listing or the drug's FDA-approved labeling. According to NCEP-ATP III guidelines, lipid-altering agents should be used in addition to a diet restricted in saturated fat and cholesterol only when the response to diet and other nonpharmacological measures has been inadequate.
Abbreviation: ER: Extended-Release

COAGULATION MODIFIERS

DRUG (BRAND)	HOW SUPPLIED	INDICATIONS	DOSAGE	HEPATIC/RENAL IMPAIRMENT
Thrombolytics				
Alteplase (Activase)	Inj: 50mg, 100mg	To improve ventricular function, reduce incidence of congestive heart failure, and reduce mortality with acute myocardial infarction (AMI). Management of acute ischemic stroke and acute massive pulmonary embolism (PE).	AMI: Accelerated Infusion: >67kg: 15mg IV bolus, then 50mg over next 30 min, and then 35mg over next 60 min. ≤67kg: 15mg IV bolus, then 0.75mg/kg (max 50mg) over next 30 min, then 0.5mg/kg (max 35mg) over next 60 min. Max: 100mg total dose. 3-Hr Infusion: ≥65kg: 60mg in 1st hr (give 6-10mg as IV bolus), then 20mg over 2nd hr, then 20mg over 3rd hr. <65kg: 1.25mg/kg over 3 hrs as described above. Stroke: 0.9mg/kg IV over 1 hr (max 90mg total dose). Administer 10% of total dose as IV bolus over 1 min. PE: 100mg IV over 2 hrs. Start heparin at end or immediately after infusion when PTT or PT ≤2× normal.	
Reteplase (Retavase)	Inj: 10.4 U	To improve ventricular function following acute myocardial infarction (AMI), reduce the incidence of congestive heart failure (CHF) and reduce the mortality associated with AMI.	10 U IV over 2 min. Repeat in 30 min.	
Tenecteplase (TNKase)	Inj: 50mg	To reduce mortality with AMI.	Administer as single IV bolus over 5 seconds. <60kg: 30mg. 60 to <70kg: 35mg. 70 to <80kg: 40mg. 80 to <90kg: 45mg. ≥90kg: 50mg. Max: 50mg/dose.	
Urokinase (Abbokinase)	Inj: 250,000 IU	Lysis of acute massive pulmonary emboli (PE) and PE accompanied by unstable hemodynamics.	LD: 4400 IU/kg IV at 90mL/hr over 10 min. Maint: 4400 IU/kg/hr IV at 15mL/hr for 12 hrs. Flush line after each cycle. For IV use only.	
Platelet aggregation inhibitor				
Abciximab (Reopro)	Inj: 2mg/mL	Adjunct to percutaneous coronary intervention (PCI) for prevention of cardiac ischemic complications in patients undergoing PCI or with unstable angina unresponsive to conventional therapy when PCI is planned within 24 hrs. Intended for use with aspirin and heparin.	PCI: 0.25mg/kg IV bolus given 10-60 min before start PCI, followed by 0.125mcg/kg/min IV infusion (Max: 10mcg/min) for 12 hrs. Unstable Angina: 0.25mg/kg IV bolus followed by 10mcg/min infusion for 18-24 hrs, concluding 1 hr after PCI.	

(Continued)

DRUG (BRAND)	HOW SUPPLIED	INDICATIONS	DOSAGE	HEPATIC/RENAL IMPAIRMENT
Anagrelide (Agrylin)	Cap: 0.5mg, 1mg	Treatment of thrombocythemia secondary to myeloproliferative disorders.	Initial: 0.5mg qid or 1mg bid for at least 1 week. Titrate: Increase by no more than 0.5mg/day per week. Max: 10mg/day or 2.5mg/dose. Adjust lowest effective dose to reduce and maintain platelets <600,000/mcL. Monitor platelets every 2 days during first week, then weekly thereafter until reach maintenance dose. **Pediatrics:** Initial: 0.5mg qd. Titrate: Increase by no more than 0.5mg/day per week. Max:10mg/day or 2.5mg/dose. Adjust to lowest effective dose to reduce and maintain platelets <600,000/mcL. Monitor platelets every 2 days during first week, then weekly thereafter until reach maintenance dose.	Moderate Hepatic Impairment: Initial: 0.5mg qd for at least 1 week. Titrate: Increase by no more than 0.5mg/day per week. Max: 10mg/day or 2.5mg/dose.
Aspirin (Halfprin)	Tab, Delayed-Release: 81mg, 162mg	To reduce the risk of vascular mortality and fatal and nonfatal cardiovascular and cerebrovascular events in patients with a suspected acute MI.	162mg as soon as MI suspected; continue qd for 30 days. May need to continue as prophylaxis for recurrent MI. Crush, chew, or suck the 1st dose.	
Cilostazol (Pletal)	Tab: 50mg, 100mg	Reduction of symptoms with intermittent claudication.	100mg bid, ½ hr before or 2 hrs after breakfast and dinner. Concomitant CYP3A4 and CYP2C19 Inhibitors: Consider 50mg bid.	
Clopidogrel (Plavix)	Tab: 75mg, 300mg	For reduction of thrombotic events in those with recent stroke or MI, established peripheral arterial disease (PAD); or with non-ST-segment elevation acute coronary syndrome (unstable angina/non-Q-wave MI); and patients with ST-segment elevation acute myocardial infarction (STEMI).	MI/Stroke/PAD: 75mg qd. Acute Coronary Syndrome: Take with 75-325mg ASA qd. LD: 300mg. Maint: 75mg qd. STEMI: 75mg, with 75-325mg ASA, qd with or without LD.	
Dipyridamole and aspirin (Persantine)	Tab: 25mg, 50mg, 75mg	Adjunct to coumarin anticoagulants for prevention of postoperative thromboembolic complications of cardiac valve replacement.	75-100mg qid.	
Dipyridamole and aspirin (Aggrenox)	Cap: (Dipyridamole Extended-Release/ ASA) 200mg-25mg	Reduce risk of stroke in patients with transient brain ischemia or complete ischemic stroke due to thrombosis.	1 cap bid (am and pm).	
Eptifibatide (Integrilin)	Sol: 0.75mg/mL, 2mg/mL	Treatment of acute coronary syndrome (ACS) in patients being medically managed or undergoing percutaneous coronary intervention (PCI) including intracoronary stenting.	ACS: 180mcg/kg IV bolus, then 2mcg/kg/min IV infusion until discharge, initiation of CABG, or up to 72 hrs. If undergoing PCI, continue until discharge or 18-24 hrs post-PCI. PCI: 180mcg/kg IV bolus immediately before PCI, then 2mcg/kg/min IV infusion. Give 2nd bolus of 180mcg/kg 10 min after 1st bolus. Continue until discharge or 18-24 hrs post-PCI. See PI for concomitant ASA and heparin doses.	ACS: CrCl <50mL/min: 180mcg/kg IV bolus, then 1mcg/kg/min IV infusion. PCI: CrCl <50mL/min: 180mcg/kg IV bolus immediately before PCI, then 1mcg/kg/min IV infusion. Give 2nd bolus of 180mcg/kg 10 min after 1st bolus.

DRUG (BRAND)	HOW SUPPLIED	INDICATIONS	DOSAGE	HEPATIC/RENAL IMPAIRMENT
Platelet aggregation inhibitor (Continued)				
Ticlopidine (Ticlid)	Tab: 250mg	To reduce risk of thrombotic stroke in stroke patients or those with stroke precursors who are ASA intolerant, allergic, or failed ASA therapy. Adjunct to ASA to reduce incidence of subacute stent thrombosis in patients undergoing successful coronary artery stent implantation.	Take with food. Stroke: 250mg bid. Coronary Artery Stenting: 250mg bid with ASA up to 30 days after stent implant.	
Tirofiban (Aggrastat)	Inj: 0.05mg/mL, 0.25mg/mL	In combination with heparin, for treatment of acute coronary syndrome, in patients being medically managed or undergoing PTCA or atherectomy.	Initial: 0.4mcg/kg/min IV for 30 min. Maint: 0.1mcg/kg/min IV. Continue through angiography and for 12-24 hrs after angioplasty or atherectomy.	CrCl <30mL/min: Administer half of the usual rate of infusion.
Coagulation Factor inhibitor				
Dalteparin	Inj: (Syringe) 2500 IU/0.2mL, 5000 IU/0.2mL, 7500 IU/0.3mL, 10,000 IU/0.4mL, 10,000 IU/1mL, 12,500 IU/0.5mL, 15,000 IU/0.6mL, 18,000 IU/0.72mL; (MDV) 95,000 IU/mL [3.8mL], 95,000 IU/mL [9.5mL]	Prevention of ischemic complications in unstable angina and non-Q-wave MI with concurrent ASA therapy. Prophylaxis of DVT in hip replacement surgery, abdominal surgery in patients who are at high risk for thromboembolic complications, and for those at risk for thromboembolic complications due to severely restricted mobility during acute illness. Extended treatment of symptomatic VTE (proximal DVT and/or PE), to reduce the recurrence of VTE in patients with cancer.	Administer SQ. Unstable Angina/Non-Q-Wave MI: 120 IU/kg up to 10,000 IU q12h with ASA (75-165mg/day) for 5-8 days. Hip Surgery: Pre-Op Start: Initial (if start 2 hrs pre-op): 2500 IU within 2 hrs pre-op, then 2500 IU 4-8 hrs post-op. Initial (if start 10-14 hrs pre-op): 5000 IU 10-14 hrs pre-op, then 5000 IU 4-8 hrs post-op. Maint (for either initial dose): 5000 IU SQ qd for 5-10 days post-op (up to 14 days). Post-Op Start: 2500 IU 4-8 hrs post-op. Maint: 5000 IU qd. Abdominal Surgery: 2500 IU 1-2 hrs pre-op. Maint: 2500 IU qd for 5-10 days post-op. Abdominal Surgery with High Risk: 5000 IU evening before surgery. Maint: 5000 IU qd for 5-10 days post-op. Abdominal Surgery with Malignancy: Initial: 2500 IU 1-2 hrs pre-op, then 2500 IU 12 hrs later. Maint: 5000 IU qd for 5-10 days post-op. Severely Restricted Mobility During Acute Illness: 5000 IU qd for 12-14 days. Symptomatic VTE in Cancer Patients: 200 IU/kg qd for first 30 days, then 150 IU/kg qd for months 2-6. Max: 18,000 IU/day. Platelet Count 50,000-100,000/mm³: Reduce dose by 2500 IU until platelet count >50,000/mm³. Platelet Count <50,000/mm³: D/C therapy until platelet count >50,000/mm³.	Renal Impairment (CrCl <30mL/min): Monitor anti-Xa levels to determine appropriate dose.

(Continued)

DRUG (BRAND)	HOW SUPPLIED	INDICATIONS	DOSAGE	HEPATIC/RENAL IMPAIRMENT
Coagulation Factor inhibitor *(Continued)*				
Enoxaparin (Lovenox)	Inj: (MDV) 300mg/3mL; (Syringe) 30mg/0.3mL, 40mg/0.4mL, 60mg/0.6mL, 80mg/0.8mL, 100mg/mL, 120mg/0.8mL, 150mg/mL	Prevention of DVT in hip or knee replacement surgery, abdominal surgery, or with severely restricted mobility during acute illness. With concomitant warfarin, inpatient treatment of acute DVT with or without PE and outpatient treatment of DVT without PE. Prevention of ischemic complications in unstable angina and non-Q-wave MI with concurrent ASA therapy. Treatment of acute ST-segment elevation MI (STEMI) in patients receiving thrombolysis and being managed medically or with percutaneous coronary intervention (PCI).	Hip/Knee Surgery: 30mg SQ q12h, starting 12-24 hrs post-op, for 7-10 days (up to 12 days) or 40mg SQ qd for hip surgery for 3 weeks. Abdominal Surgery: 40mg SQ qd, starting 2 hrs pre-op, for 7-10 days (up to 14 days). DVT with or without PE treatment: (inpatient/outpatient) 1mg/kg SQ q12h or (inpatient) 1.5mg/kg qd with warfarin (start within 72 hrs) for 7 days (up to 17 days). Acute Illness: 40mg SQ qd for 6-11 days (up to 14 days). Unstable Angina/Non-Q-Wave MI: 1mg/kg SQ q12h with 100-325mg/day of ASA for 2-8 days (up to 12.5 days). Acute STEMI (<75 yrs): 30mg single IV bolus plus a 1mg/kg SQ dose followed by 1mg/kg SQ q12h with ASA. Max: 100mg for 1st 2 doses only. Acute STEMI (≥75 yrs): 0.75mg/kg SQ q12h (no initial bolus) with ASA. Max: 75mg for 1st 2 doses only. When given with thrombolytic, give enoxaparin dose between 15 min before and 30 min after start of fibrinolytic therapy. With PCI, if last enoxaparin SQ dose was given >8 hrs before balloon inflation, an IV bolus of 0.3mg/kg of enoxaparin should be given. DVT with or without PE treatment (inpatient/outpatient)/Unstable Angina/Non-Q-Wave MI: 1mg/kg SQ qd. Acute STEMI: <75 yrs: 30mg single IV bolus plus a 1mg/kg SQ dose followed by 1mg/kg SQ qd. ≥75 yrs: 1mg/kg SQ qd (no initial bolus).	CrCl <30mL/min: Surgery/Acute Illness: 30mg SQ qd.
Fondaparinux (Arixtra)	Inj: (Syringe) 2.5mg/0.5mL, 5mg/0.4mL, 7.5mg/0.6mL, 10mg/0.8mL	Prophylaxis of DVT in patients undergoing hip fracture surgery, including extended prophylaxis; hip replacement surgery; knee replacement surgery; abdominal surgery who are at risk of thromboembolic complications. With concomitant warfarin, treatment of acute PE when initial therapy is administered in hospital and acute DVT.	DVT Prophylaxis: 2.5mg SQ qd, starting 6-8 hrs post-op for 5-9 days (up to 11 days). Hip Fracture Surgery: Extended prophylaxis up to 24 additional days is recommended. DVT/PE Treatment: <50kg: 5mg SQ qd. 50-100kg: 7.5mg SQ qd. >100kg: 10mg SQ qd. Add concomitant warfarin ASAP (usually within 72 hrs) and continue for 5-9 days (up to 26 days) until INR=2-3.	
Heparin	Inj: 1000 U/mL, 2500 U/mL, 5000 U/mL, 7500 U/mL, 10,000 U/mL	Prophylaxis and treatment of venous thrombosis and its extension, PE in atrial fibrillation. Prevention of peripheral arterial embolism. Diagnosis and treatment of acute and chronic consumptive coagulopathies, for prevention of clotting in arterial and cardiac surgery.	Based on 68kg: Initial: 5000 U IV, then 10,000-20,000 U SQ. Maint: 8000-10,000 U q8h or 15,000-20,000 U q12h. Intermittent IV Injection: Initial: 10,000 U. Maint: 5000-10,000 U q4-6h. Continuous IV Infusion: Initial: 5000U. Maint: 20,000-40,000 U/24 hrs. Adjust to coagulation test results. See PI for details in specific disease states. Pediatrics: Initial: 50 U/kg IV drip. Maint: 100 U/kg IV drip q4h or 20,000 U/m2/24 hrs continuously.	

DRUG (BRAND)	HOW SUPPLIED	INDICATIONS	DOSAGE	HEPATIC/RENAL IMPAIRMENT
Coagulation Factor inhibitor *(Continued)*				
Phytonadione (Mephyton)	Tab: 5mg* *scored; Inj: 1mg/0.5 mL; 10mg/mL	For coagulation disorders caused by vitamin K deficiency or interference with vitamin K activity, including anticoagulant-induced prothrombin deficiency caused by coumarin or indanedione derivatives; and hypoprothrombinemia secondary to antibacterials, salicylates, obstructive jaundice, or biliary fistulas.	(Tab): Anticoagulant-Induced Prothrombin Deficiency: Initial: 2.5-10mg up to 25mg (rarely 50mg). May repeat if PT is still elevated 12-48 hrs after initial dose. Hypoprothrombinemia Due to Other Causes: 2.5-25mg or more (rarely up to 50mg). Give bile salts when endogenous bile supply to GIT is deficient. **Adults (IV):** Administer SQ when possible. Anticoagulant-Induced PT Deficiency: Initial: 2.5-10mg up to 25mg (rarely 50mg). May repeat if PT is still elevated 6-8 hrs after initial dose. Hypoprothrombinemia Due to Other Causes: 2.5-25mg or more (rarely up to 50mg); route depends on severity of condition and response. **Pediatrics (IV):** Prophylaxis of Hemorrhagic Disease in Newborn: 0.5-1mg IM within 1 hr of birth. Treatment of Hemorrhagic Disease in Newborn: 1mg SQ/IM (may need higher dose if mother has received oral anticoagulants).	
Tinzaprin (Innohep)	Inj: 20,000 anti-Xa IU/mL	Treatment of acute symptomatic DVT with or without PE with concomitant warfarin.	175 anti-Xa IU/kg SQ qd for at least 6 days and until anticoagulated with warfarin (INR is at least 2 for 2 days). Begin warfarin within 1-3 days of therapy.	
Warfarin (Coumadin, Jantoven)	Inj: (Coumadin) 5mg; Tab: (Coumadin, Jantoven) 1mg*, 2mg*, 2.5mg*, 3mg*, 4mg*, 5mg*, 6mg*, 7.5mg*, 10mg* *scored	Prophylaxis and treatment of venous thrombosis, PE, and thromboembolic disorders associated with atrial fibrillation and/or cardiac valve replacement. To reduce risk of death, recurrent MI, and thromboembolic events after MI.	≥18 yrs: Adjust dose based on PT/INR. Give IV as alternate to PO. Initial: 2-5mg qd. Usual: 2-10mg qd. Venous Thromboembolism (including pulmonary embolism): INR 2-3. Atrial Fibrillation: INR 2-3. Post-MI: Initiate 2-4 weeks post-infarct and maintain INR 2.5-3.5. Mechanical/Bioprosthetic Heart Valve: INR 2-3 for 12 weeks after valve insertion, then INR 2.5-3.5 long term.	
Thrombin inhibitor				
Argatroban	Inj: 100mg/mL	Prophylaxis or treatment of thrombosis in heparin-induced thrombocytopenia (HIT). As an anticoagulant in patients with or at risk for HIT undergoing percutaneous coronary intervention (PCI).	Thrombosis: D/C heparin and obtain baseline aPTT. Initial: 2mcg/kg/min IV. Check aPTT after 2 hrs. Titrate: Increase dose until aPTT is 1.5-3× the initial baseline. Max: 10mcg/kg/min. PCI: Initial: 350mcg/kg bolus with 25mcg/kg/min IV. Check activated clotting time (ACT) 5-10 min after bolus. Proceed with PCI if ACT >300 seconds. See PI for detailed information for dose adjustment.	Thrombosis: Moderate Hepatic Impairment: Initial: 0.5mcg/kg/min

(Continued)

DRUG (BRAND)	HOW SUPPLIED	INDICATIONS	DOSAGE	HEPATIC/RENAL IMPAIRMENT
Thrombin inhibitor *(Continued)*				
Bivalirudin (Angiomax)	Inj: 250mg	Adjunct to aspirin for anticoagulation in patients with unstable angina undergoing percutaneous transluminal coronary angioplasty (PTCA) or percutaneous coronary intervention (PCI). Patients with, or at risk of, HIT/HITTS undergoing PCI.	Initial: 0.75mg/kg IV bolus, then 1.75mg/kg/hr for duration of PCI procedure. Additional bolus of 0.3mg/kg can be given if needed based on ACT. Continuation of infusion for up to 4 hrs post-procedure is optional. After 4 hrs, if needed, an additional 0.2mg/kg IV for up to 20 hrs may be initiated.	Renal Impairment: CrCl <30mL/min: 1mg/kg/hr infusion. Hemodialysis: 0.25mg/kg/hr infusion. Reduction in bolus dose not necessary; monitor anticoagulation.
Lepirudin (Refludan)	Inj: 50mg	Anticoagulant for heparin-induced thrombocytopenia (HIT) and associated thromboembolic disease.	LD: 0.4mg/kg (max 44mg) IV over 15-20 seconds. Initial: 0.15mg/kg (max 16.5mg/hr) continuous infusion for 2-10 days. Adjust dose based on aPTT. Concomitant Thrombolytic Therapy: LD: 0.2mg/kg. Initial: 0.1mg/kg/hr. See PI for monitoring and adjusting therapy details.	Renal Impairment: LD: 0.2mg/kg. Initial: CrCl 45-60 mL/min: 0.075mg/kg/hr. CrCl 30-44mL/min: 0.045mg/kg/hr. CrCl 15-29 mL/min: 0.0225mg/kg/hr. CrCl <15mL/min/Hemodialysis: Avoid or stop infusion.
Miscellaneous				
Aminocaproic Acid (Amicar)	Inj: 250mg/mL [20mL]; Syrup: 1.25g/5mL; Tab: 500mg*, 1000mg* *scored	To enhance hemostasis when fibrinolysis contributes to bleeding.	IV: 16-20mL (4-5g) in 250mL diluent during 1st hr, then 4mL/hr (1g) in 50mL of diluent. PO: 5g during 1st hr, then 5mL (syr) or 1g (tabs) per hr. Continue therapy for 8 hrs or until bleeding is controlled.	
Pentoxifylline (Trental)	Tab, Extended-Release: 400mg	Treatment of intermittent claudication due to chronic occlusive arterial disease of the limbs.	400mg tid with meals for at least 8 weeks. Reduce to 400mg bid if digestive and GI side effects occur; d/c if side effects persist.	
Thrombin (Recombinant) (Recothrom)	Powder: 5000 IU	Aid to hemostasis whenever oozing blood and minor bleeding from capillaries and small venules is accessible and control of bleeding by standard surgical techniques is ineffective or impractical. May be used in conjunction with an absorbable gelatin sponge, USP.	Apply directly on the surface of bleeding tissue or in conjunction with absorbable gelatin sponge. Required amount depends upon the tissue area to be treated. Reconstitute with sterile isotonic saline at a recommended concentration of 1000 IU/mL.	
Topical Thrombin (Thrombin-JMI)	Powder: 5,000 IU, 20,000 IU; Kit: Powder: 20,000 IU [Spray; Syringe Spray]	An aid to hemostasis whenever oozing blood and minor bleeding from capillaries and small venules is accessible. In various types of surgery, may be used in conjunction with an Absorbable Gelatin Sponge, USP for hemostasis.	Spray topically on surface of bleeding tissue. Reconstitute with sterile isotonic saline at a recommended concentration of 1,000-2,000 IU/mL. Profuse Bleeding: Use 1,000 IU/mL. General use (eg, plastic surgery, dental extractions, skin grafting): 100 IU/mL. Intermediate strengths may be prepared by diluting in appropriate isotonic saline volume if needed. Oozing surfaces: Use dry form. May be used with FlowSeal™ NT.	

DIURETICS

DRUG	BRAND	USUAL HYPERTENSION DOSAGE RANGE	HOW SUPPLIED
THIAZIDE DIURETICS			
Chlorothiazide	Diuril	**Sus:** 0.5–1g/day.	**Sus:** 250mg/5mL
	Various generics	**Tab:** 0.5g–1g/day.	**Tab:** 250mg, 500mg
Chlorthalidone	Thalitone	15mg–50mg qd.	**Tab:** 15mg
	Various generics	25mg–100mg qd.	**Tab:** 25mg, 50mg
Hydrochlorothiazide	Microzide	12.5mg–50mg qd.	**Cap:** 12.5mg
	Various generics	12.5mg–50mg qd.	**Cap:** 12.5mg; **Tab:** 12.5mg, 25mg, 50mg
Indapamide	Lozol	1.25mg–5mg qd.	**Tab:** 1.25mg, 2.5mg
Metolazone	Zaroxolyn	2.5mg–5mg qd.	**Tab:** 2.5mg, 5mg, 10mg
LOOP DIURETICS			
Bumetanide	Bumex	0.5mg–2mg qd.	**Tab:** 0.5mg, 1mg, 2mg
Furosemide	Lasix	40mg bid.	**Tab:** 20mg, 40mg, 80mg
Torsemide	Demadex	5mg–10mg qd.	**Tab:** 5mg, 10mg, 20mg, 100mg
POTASSIUM-SPARING DIURETICS			
Amiloride	Various generics	5mg–10mg qd.	**Tab:** 5mg
Spironolactone	Aldactone	50mg–100mg/day.	**Tab:** 25mg, 50mg, 100mg
Triamterene	Dyrenium	100mg–150mg bid.	**Cap:** 50mg, 100mg
ALDOSTERONE-RECEPTOR BLOCKER			
Eplerenone	Inspra	50mg qd or bid.	**Tab:** 25mg, 50mg
COMBINATION DIURETICS			
Amiloride HCl/ Hydrochlorothiazide	Various generics	5/50mg–10/100mg qd.	**Tab:** 5/50mg
Hydrochlorothiazide/ Triamterene	Dyazide	25/37.5–50/75mg qd.	**Cap:** 25/37.5mg
Spironolactone/ Hydrochlorothiazide	Aldactazide	100/100mg qd.	**Tab:** 25/25mg, 50/50mg

LIPID MANAGEMENT

DRUG	BRAND	HOW SUPPLIED (mg)*	USUAL DOSAGE RANGE**	COMMENTS
HMG-CoA REDUCTASE INHIBITORS (STATINS)**				
Atorvastatin	Lipitor	**Tab:** 10, 20, 40, 80	10-80mg/day	CI: Active liver disease, unexplained persistent elevations of serum transaminases, pregnancy, nursing mothers.
Fluvastatin	Lescol	**Cap:** 20, 40	20-80mg/day	Generally LFTs should be monitored prior to therapy, at 12 weeks, with dose elevations, and periodically thereafter.
	Lescol XL	**Tab, ER:** 80		
Lovastatin	Altoprev	**Tab, ER:** 10, 20, 40, 60	20-60mg/day	
	Mevacor	**Tab:** 10, 20, 40	10-80mg/day given qd or bid	Increased risk of myopathy with concomitant use of cyclosporine, fibrates, erythromycin, niacin, or azole antifungals.
Pravastatin	Pravachol	**Tab:** 10, 20, 40, 80	10-80mg/day	
Rosuvastatin	Crestor	**Tab:** 5, 10, 20, 40	5-40mg/day	Use with fibrates and niacin should generally be avoided.
Simvastatin	Zocor	**Tab:** 5, 10, 20, 40, 80	5-80mg/day	
FIBRATES				
Fenofibrate	Antara	**Tab:** 43, 130	43-130mg/day	Use with statins should generally be avoided.
	Triglide	**Tab:** 50, 160	50-160mg/day.	CI: Pre-existing gallbladder disease, hepatic or severe renal dysfunction.
	Tricor	**Tab:** 48, 145	48-145mg/day	
	Lofibra	**Cap:** 67,134, 200 **Tab:** 54, 160	67-200mg/day 54-160mg/day	
Gemfibrozil	Lopid	**Tab:** 600	1200mg/day in divided doses	
BILE-ACID SEQUESTRANTS				
Cholestyramine	Questran Questran Light	4g/pkt or scoop	8-16g/day, given bid	CI: Complete biliary obstruction. Mix with fluid or highly fluid food. (Light): Contains phenylalanine.
Colesevelam HCl	WelChol	**Tab:** 625	3750mg/day given qd or bid	CI: Bowel obstruction. Take with liquids and a meal.
Colestipol	Colestid	**Granules:** 5000/pkt; **Tab:** 1000	500-2000mg qhs	CI: Bowel obstruction. Take with liquids and a meal.
CHOLESTEROL ABSORPTION INHIBITOR				
Ezetimibe	Zetia	**Tab:** 10	10mg qd	Not recommended with moderate or severe hepatic insufficiency or with concurrent use of fibrates.
NICOTINIC ACID DERIVATIVE				
Niacin, extended-release	Niaspan	**Tab, ER:** 500, 750, 1000	1-2g qhs	CI: Hepatic dysfunction, active peptic ulcer disease, arterial bleeding. May pretreat with ASA or NSAIDs 30 minutes before to reduce flushing.
LIPID-REGULATING AGENT				
Omega-3-Acid Ethyl Esters	Lovaza	**Cap:** 1000	4g qd	CI: Caution in patients with known sensitivity or allergy to fish.
COMBINATIONS				
Amlodipine-Atorvastatin	Caduet	**Tab:** (Amlodipine/ Atorvastatin): 2.5/10, 2.5/20, 2.5/40, 5/10, 5/20, 5/40, 5/80, 10/10, 10/20, 10/40, 10/80	5mg/20mg to 10mg/80mg	See Statins.

(Continued)

LIPID MANAGEMENT

DRUG	BRAND	HOW SUPPLIED (mg)*	USUAL DOSAGE RANGE**	COMMENTS
COMBINATIONS *(Continued)*				
Ezetimibe-Simvastatin	Vytorin	**Tab:** (Ezetimibe/Simvastatin): 10/10, 10/20, 10/40, 10/80	10/10 to 10/80mg/day	See Statins. Avoid use in moderate to severe hepatic insufficiency.
Niacin ER-Lovastatin	Advicor	**Tab:** (Niacin ER/Lovastatin) 500/20, 750/20, 1000/20, 1000/40	500mg/20mg to 2000mg/40mg	See Statins and Niacin. Do not substitute for equivalent dose of immediate-release niacin.
Niacin ER-Simvastatin	Simcor	**Tab:** (Niacin ER/Simvastatin) 500/20, 750/20, 1000/20	500mg/20mg to 2000mg/40mg	See Statins and Niacin. Do not substitute for equivalent dose of immediate-release niacin.

* Unless otherwise indicated.

** **NOTE:** Dosages shown are for adults and may need to be adjusted to individual patient needs. For pediatric dosing and additional information please refer to the individual monograph listings or the drug's FDA-approved labeling. According to NCEP-ATP III guidelines, lipid-altering agents should be used in addition to a diet restricted in saturated fat and cholesterol only when the response to diet and other nonpharmacological measures has been inadequate.

Abbreviations: CI: Contraindications; ER: Extended-Release.

PSORIASIS MANAGEMENT: SYSTEMIC THERAPIES

DRUG (BRAND)	HOW SUPPLIED	DOSAGE	SIDE EFFECTS
ANTIMETABOLITE			
Methotrexate	**Inj:** 20mg, 1g, 25mg/mL; **Tab:** 2.5mg, 5mg, 7.5mg, 10mg, 15 mg	**Initial:** 10-25mg weekly until response or use divided oral dose schedule, 2.5mg at 12-hr intervals for 3 doses. **Titrate:** Increase gradually until optimal response. **Maint:** Reduce to lowest effective dose. **Max:** 30mg/wk.	Ulcerative stomatitis, leukopenia, nausea, abdominal distress, malaise, fatigue, chills, fever, dizziness, decreased resistance to infection
IMMUNOSUPPRESSIVES			
Alefacept (Amevive)	**Inj:** (IV) 7.5mg, (IM) 15mg	7.5mg IV bolus or 15mg IM once wkly for 12 wks. May repeat cycle 12 wks after first cycle complete. Adjust dose, D/C, based on CD4+ T-lymphocyte counts.	Lymphopenia, injection-site reactions, influenza-like symptoms, pruritus, hypersensitivity reactions
Cyclosporine (Neoral)	**Cap:** 25mg, 100mg; **Sol:** 100mg/mL [50mL]	**Initial:** 1.25mg/kg bid for 4 wks. **Titrate:** May increase by 0.5mg/kg/day every 2 weeks. **Max:** 4mg/kg/day.	Infection, renal dysfunction, HTN, malignancy risk w/certain psoriasis therapies, hirsutism, muscle cramps, acne, tremor, headache, gingival hyperplasia, diarrhea, nausea, vomiting
MONOCLONAL ANTIBODIES/TNF BLOCKERS			
Adalimumab (Humira)	**Inj:** 20mg/0.4mL, 40mg/0.8mL	**Initial:** 80mg. **Maint:** 40mg every other week starting 1 week after initial dose.	URI, injection-site pain/reactions, headache, rash, sinusitis, nausea, UTI, flu syndrome, abdominal pain, hyperlipidemia, hypercholesterolemia, back pain, hematuria, HTN, immunogenicity
Efalizumab (Raptiva)	**Inj:** 125mg	**Initial:** 0.7mg/kg SQ x 1. **Maint:** 1mg/kg SQ per wk. **Max:** 200mg/dose.	Influenza-like symptoms, URI, acne, psoriasis exacerbation, thrombocytopenia
Infliximab (Remicade)	**Inj:** 100mg	5mg/kg IV infusion; repeat at 2 and 6 weeks. **Maint:** 5mg/kg every 8 weeks.	Infusion reactions, nausea, infections, URI, pruritus, headache, sore throat, potential risk of reactivating TB
PSORALENS			
Methoxsalen* (8-Mop, Oxsoralen-Ultra)	**Cap:** 10mg	Take with food or milk. **Initial:** <30kg: 10mg. 30-50kg: 20mg. 51-65kg: 30mg. 66-80kg: 40mg. 81-90kg: 50mg. 91-115kg: 60mg. >115kg: 70mg. Take 2 hrs before UVA exposure. **Titrate:** May increase by 10mg after 15th treatment under certain conditions. **Max:** Do not treat more often than qod.	Nausea, nervousness, insomnia, depression, pruritus, erythema
RETINOID			
Acitretin (Soriatane)	**Cap:** 10mg, 25mg	**Initial:** 25-50mg qd w/food. Individualize dose based on intersubject variation in pharmacokinetics, clinical efficacy, and incidence of side effects. **Maint:** 25-50mg qd. Terminate therapy when lesions resolve. May treat relapses.	Ophthalmologic effects, cheilitis, rhinitis, dry mouth, epistaxis, alopecia, dry skin, rash, skin peeling, nail disorder, pruritus, paresthesia, paronychia, skin atrophy, sticky skin, xerophthalmia, arthralgia, rash

(Continued)

DRUG (BRAND)	HOW SUPPLIED	DOSAGE	SIDE EFFECTS
TNF-BLOCKING AGENT			
Etanercept (Enbrel)	**Inj:** 25mg [vial], 50mg/mL [syringe]	**Initial:** 50mg SQ twice weekly given 3 or 4 days apart for 3 months. May begin with 25-50mg/wk. **Maint:** 50mg/wk.	Injection site reactions, infections, headache

* Oxsoralen-Ultra and 8-MOP are not interchangeable due to significantly greater bioavailability and earlier photosensitization onset time of Oxsoralen-Ultra.

Sources: FDA-approved product labeling. Luba KM, Stulberg DL. Chronic plaque psoriasis. *Am Fam Physician.* 2006 Feb 15;73(4):636-44. Review.

PSORIASIS MANAGEMENT: TOPICAL THERAPIES

DRUG (BRAND)	HOW SUPPLIED	DOSAGE	SIDE EFFECTS
TOPICAL IMMUNOSUPPRESSANT			
Pimecrolimus (Elidel)	Cre: 1% [30g, 60g, 100g]	Apply bid.	Burning, headache, nasopharyngitis, pyrexia, influenza, pharyngitis, viral infection
TOPICAL STEROIDS			
Clobetasol (Temovate, Temovate-E, Clobex, Embeline E, Olux, Olux-E)	(Temovate) Cre, Oint: 0.05% [15g, 30g, 45g, 60g]; Gel: 0.05% [15g, 30g, 60g]; Sol: 0.05% [25mL]; (Temovate-E) Cre: 0.05% [15g, 30g, 60g]; (Clobex) Lot: 0.05% [30mL, 59mL]; Shampoo: 0.05% [118mL]; Spray: 0.05% [2oz]; (Embeline E) Cre: 0.05% [15g, 30g,60g]; (Olux) Foam: 0.05% [50g, 100g] (Olux-E) Foam: 0.05% [50g, 100g]	Apply bid.	Hypopigmentation, tachyphylaxis, striae, skin atrophy
Fluocinolone (Synalar)	Cre, Oint: 0.025% [15g, 60g]; Sol: 0.01% [20mL, 60mL]	Apply bid-qid.	Dryness, folliculitis, acne, skin atrophy, burning, itching, irritation
Fluocinonide (Lidex, Lidex-E, Vanos)	(Lidex) Cre, Gel, Oint: 0.05% [15g, 30g, 60g]; Sol: 0.05% [60mL]; (Lidex-E) Cre: 0.05% [15g, 30g, 60g]; (Vanos) Cre: 0.1% [30mg, 60mg]	(Lidex, Lidex-E) Apply bid-tid. (Vanos) Apply qd-bid.	Burning, itching, irritation, dryness, folliculitis, acne, hypopigmentation, skin atrophy
Halcinonide (Halog, Halog-E)	(Halog) Cre, Oint: 0.1% [15g, 30g, 60g]; Sol: 0.1% [20mL, 60mL]; (Halog-E) Cre: 0.1% in a hydrophilic vanishing cream [30g, 60g]	(Cre, Oint, Sol) Apply bid-tid. (Cre, hydrophilic base) Apply qd-tid.	Burning, itching, irritation, dryness, folliculitis, hypopigmentation, contact dermatitis, skin maceration
Hydrocortisone (Hytone, Locoid, Pandel, Westcort)	(Hytone 1%) Lot: 1% [30mL, 120mL]; (Locoid) Cre, Oint: 0.1% [15g, 45g]; Sol: 0.1% [20mL, 60mL]; (Pandel) Cre: 0.1% [15g, 45g, 80g]; (Westcort) Cre, Oint: 0.2% [15g, 45g, 60g]	(Hytone 1%, Locoid) Apply tid-qid. (Pandel) Apply qd-bid. (Westcort) Apply bid-tid.	Burning, stinging, moderate paresthesia, itching, dryness, folliculitis, hypopigmentation, skin atrophy
Hydrocortisone/ Pramoxine (Epifoam, Novacort, Pramosone)	(Epifoam) Foam: (Hydrocortisone-Pramoxine) 1%-1% [10g]; (Novacort) Gel: 2%-1% [29g]; (Pramosone) Cre: 1%-1%, 1%-2.5% Lot: 1%-1% [60mL, 120mL, 240mL], 1%-2.5% [60mL, 120mL]; Oint: 1%-1%, 1%-2.5% [30g]	Apply tid-qid.	Burning, itching, irritation, dryness, folliculitis, hypopigmentation, maceration, skin atrophy atrophy
Mometasone (Elocon)	Cre, Oint: 0.1% [15g, 45g]; Lot: 0.1% [30mL, 60mL]	Apply qd.	Burning, pruritus, skin atrophy, rosacea, acneiform reaction, tingling, stinging, furunculosis, folliculitis
Prednicarbate (Dermatop)	Cre, Oint: 0.1% [15g, 60g]	Apply bid.	Burning, itching, irritation, dryness, folliculitis, hypertrichosis, acneiform eruptions, hypopigmentation
Triamcinolone (Kenalog)	(Kenalog) Cre: 0.1% [15g, 60g, 80g], 0.5% [20g]; Lot: 0.025%, 0.1% [60mL]; Oint: 0.1% [15g, 60g]; Spray: 0.147mg/g [63g]	(Kenalog) Cre, Lot, Oint: Apply 0.025% bid-qid. Apply 0.1% or 0.5% bid-tid. Spray: Apply tid-qid.	Burning, itching, irritation, dryness, folliculitis, hypopigmentation, allergic contact dermatitis

(Continued)

DRUG (BRAND)	HOW SUPPLIED	DOSAGE	SIDE EFFECTS
TOPICAL RETINOID			
Tazarotene (Tazorac)	Cre: 0.05%, 0.1% [30g, 60g]; Gel: 0.05%, 0.1% [30g, 100g]	Apply hs.	Pruritus, erythema, irritation, dry skin, rash, skin discoloration
VITAMIN D DERIVATIVES & COMBINATIONS			
Calcipotriene (Dovonex, Dovonex Scalp)	(Dovonex) Cre, Oint: 0.005% [60g, 120g]; (Dovonex Scalp) Sol: 0.005% [60mL]	(Dovonex) Apply bid. (Dovonex Scalp) Apply bid.	Skin irritation, pruritus, burning, hypercalcemia
Calcipotriene/ betamethasone (Taclonex)	Oint: (Calcipotriene-Betamethasone) 0.005%-0.064% [15g, 30g, 60g]	Apply qd.	Pruritus, headache
MISCELLANEOUS AGENTS			
Anthralin (Anthra-Derm)	Cre: 1% [50g]	Apply qd-bid.	Skin irritation, erythema, staining (skin and clothing), odor
Coal Tar (Zetar)	Sol 10%: 2% [3.8oz]	Apply hs.	Skin irritation, folliculitis, odor, staining of clothing
Urea (Carmol 40)	Cre: 40% [28.35g, 85g, 198.6g]; Gel: 40% [15mL]; Lot: 40% [236.6 mL]	Apply bid.	Transient stinging, burning, itching, irritation

Sources:
FDA-approved drug labeling.
Luba KM, Stulberg DL. Chronic plaque psoriasis. *Am Fam Physician*. 2006 Feb 15;73(4):636-44. Review.

TOPICAL CORTICOSTEROIDS

STEROID	DOSAGE FORM(S)	STRENGTH (%)	POTENCY	FREQUENCY
Alclometasone Dipropionate (Aclovate)	Cre, Oint	0.05	Low	bid/tid
Amcinonide (Cyclocort)	Cre, Oint	0.05, 0.005	Medium	bid/tid
Augmented Betamethasone Dipropionate (Diprolene, Diprolene AF)	Cre, Oint	0.05	Very High	qd/bid
	Cre, Lot	0.05	High	qd/bid
Betamethasone Dipropionate	Cre, Lot, Oint	0.05	High	qd/bid
Betamethasone Valerate (Luxiq)	Foam	0.12	Medium	bid
Clobetasol Propionate (Clobevate, Clobex, Cormax, Embeline E, Olux, Olux E, Temovate, Temovate-E)	Cre, Foam (Olux)	0.05	Very High	bid
	Cream (Embeline E), Foam, Gel (Clobevate), Lotion (Clobex), Oint, Shampoo (Clobex), Sol	0.05	Very High	qd (shampoo)
Clocortolone Pivalate (Cloderm)	Cre	0.1	Low	tid
Desonide (Desonate, DesOwen, Verdeso)	Cre, Foam, Gel (Desonate), Lot, Oint	0.05	Low	bid/tid
Desoximetasone (Topicort, Topicort LP)	Cre	0.05	Medium	bid
	Cre, Oint	0.25	High	bid
	Gel	0.05	High	bid
Diflorasone Diacetate (Psorcon)	Oint (Psorcon)	0.05	Very High	qd/qid
Fluocinolone Acetonide (Capex, Derma-Smoothe/FS, Synalar)	Cre, Oint	0.025	Medium	bid/qid
	Sol	0.01	Medium	bid/qid
	Oil (Derma-Smoothe/FS)	0.01	Medium	qd/tid
	Shampoo (Capex)	0.01	Medium	qd
Fluocinonide (Lidex, Lidex-E, Vanos)	Cre, Gel, Oint, Sol	0.05	High	bid/qid
	Cre	0.1	Very High	qd/bid
Flurandrenolide (Cordran, Cordran SP)	Cre, Oint	0.025	Medium	bid/tid
	Cre, Lot, Oint	0.05	Medium	bid/tid
	Tape	4mcg/cm^2	Medium	qd/bid
Fluticasone Propionate (Cutivate)	Cre, Lot	0.05	Medium	qd/bid
	Oint	0.005	Medium	bid
Halcinonide (Halog, Halog-E)	Cre, Oint, Sol	0.1	High	qd/tid
Halobetasol Propionate (Ultravate)	Cre, Oint	0.05	Very High	qd/bid
Hydrocortisone (Anusol HC, Hytone)	Lot	2	Low	tid/qid
	Cre, Lot, Oint	2.5	Low	tid/qid
Hydrocortisone Butyrate (Locoid, Locoid Lipo Cream)	Cre, Lot, Oint, Sol	0.1	Medium	bid/tid
Hydrocortisone Probutate (Pandel)	Cre	0.1	Medium	qd/bid
Hydrocortisone Valerate (Westcort)	Cre, Oint	0.2	Medium	bid/tid
Mometasone Furoate (Elocon)	Cre, Lot, Oint	0.1	Medium	qd
Prednicarbate (Dermatop)	Cre, Oint	0.1	Medium	bid
Triamcinolone Acetonide (Kenalog, Triderm)	Cre, Lot, Oint	0.025	Medium	bid/qid
	Cre, Lot, Oint	0.1	Medium	bid/tid
	Cre, Oint	0.5	High	bid/tid
	Spray	0.147	Medium	tid/qid

INSULIN FORMULATIONS

TYPE OF INSULIN	BRAND	ONSET* (hrs)	PEAK* (hrs)	DURATION* (hrs)	COMMON PITFALLS**
Rapid-acting Insulin Glulisine Insulin Lispro Insulin Aspart	Apidra Humalog Novolog	– <0.25 <0.25	0.5 to 1.7 0.5 to 1.5 0.5 to 1	1 to 3 3 to 5 3 to 5	See individual comments. Hypoglycemia occurs if lag time is too long or the patient exercises within 1 hr of dose; with high-fat meals, the dose should be adjusted downward.
Short-acting Regular Insulin	Humulin R† Novolin R	0.5 to 1 0.5 to 1	2 to 4 2 to 5	4 to 12 8	Lag time is not used appropriately; the insulin should be given 20 to 30 minutes before the patient eats.
Intermediate-acting NPH (Isophane)	Humulin N Novolin R	1 to 3	6 to 12	18 to 24	In many patients, breakfast injection does not last the evening until the evening meal; administration with the evening meal does not meet insulin needs on awakening.
Long-acting Insulin glargine Insulin detemir	Lantus Levemir	1 –	Flat 6 to 8	24 24	Administer once daily at the same time every day. See individual comments.
Combinations Isophane insulin suspension (70%)/regular insulin (30%)	Humulin 70/30 Novolin 70/30	0.5 to 1	4 to 6	24	See individual comments.
Isophane insulin suspension (50%)/regular insulin (50%)	Humulin 50/50	0.5 to 1	3 to 5	24	See individual comments.
Insulin lispro protamine (75%)/insulin lispro (25%)	Humalog Mix 75/25	≤0.25	0.5 to 4	24	See individual comments.
Insulin aspart protamine (70%)/insulin aspart (30%)	Novolog Mix 70/30	≤0.25	1 to 4	24	See individual comments.

*Approximate parameters following SC injection of an average patient dose; insulin concentration: 100U/mL. (Not applicable for inhalation insulin.)

**Source: Hirsch, IB. Type 1 Diabetes Mellitus and the Use of Flexible Insulin Regimens. *Am Fam Physician*. November 1999;60(8):2343-2352,2355-2356.

†Also available 500 U/mL for insulin resistant patients (rapid onset; up to 24 hour duration).

ORAL ANTIDIABETIC AGENTS

DRUG	HOW SUPPLIED	INITIAL* & (MAX) DOSE	USUAL DOSE RANGE*
BIGUANIDES			
Metformin HCl Fortamet, Glumetza, Glucophage	**Tab, ER:** 500mg, 1000mg **Tab:** 500mg, 850mg, 1000mg, **Sol:** 500mg/5ml	500-1000mg qd (2500mg/day). 500mg bid or 850mg qd (2550mg/day).	500-2500mg qd. 1-2g daily in divided doses.
Glucophage XR	**Tab, ER:** 500mg, 750mg	500mg qd (2000mg/day).	500mg-2g qd.
DIPEPTIDYL PEPTIDASE-4 INHIBITOR			
Sitagliptin Januvia	**Tab:** 25mg, 50mg, 100mg	100mg qd.	100mg qd.
GLUCOSIDASE INHIBITORS			
Acarbose (Precose)	**Tab:** 25mg, 50mg, 100mg	25mg tid (300mg/day).	25-100mg tid.
Miglitol (Glyset)	**Tab:** 25mg, 50mg, 100mg	25mg tid (300mg/day).	50-100mg tid.
MEGLITINIDES			
Nateglinide Starlix	**Tab:** 60mg, 120mg	120mg tid (360mg/day).	120mg tid.
Repaglinide Prandin	**Tab:** 0.5mg, 1mg, 2mg	0.5-2mg with each meal (16mg/day).	0.5-4mg with each meal.
SULFONYLUREAS			
Chlorpropamide Diabinese	**Tab:** 100mg, 250mg	50-125mg qd (750mg/day).	100-500mg qd.
Glimepiride Amaryl	**Tab:** 1mg, 2mg, 4mg	1-2mg qd (8mg/day).	1-4mg qd.
Glipizide Glucotrol	**Tab:** 5mg, 10mg	5mg qd (40mg/day).	5-40mg qd or divided if >15mg/day.
Glucotrol XL	**Tab, ER:** 2.5mg, 5mg, 10mg	5mg qd (20mg/day).	5-10mg qd.
Glyburide Diabeta, Micronase	**Tab:** 1.25mg, 2.5mg, 5mg	2.5-5mg qd (20mg/day).	1.25-20mg qd or divided doses.
Glynase PresTab	**Tab:** 1.5mg, 3mg, 6mg	1.5-3mg qd (12mg/day).	0.75-12mg qd divided doses.
THIAZOLIDINEDIONES			
Pioglitazone HCl Actos	**Tab:** 15mg, 30mg, 45mg	15-30mg qd (45mg/day).	15-30mg qd.
Rosiglitazone maleate Avandia	**Tab:** 2mg, 4mg, 8mg	2mg bid or 4mg qd (8mg/day).	4mg bid or 8mg qd.
COMBINATIONS			
Glipizide/ Metformin HCl Metaglip	**Tab:** 2.5mg/250mg, 2.5mg/500mg, 5mg/500mg	2.5mg/250mg qd or 2.5mg/500mg bid (10mg/1g qd or 20mg/2g divided doses)	1-2 tab qd-bid.
Glyburide/ Metformin HCl Glucovance	**Tab:** 1.25mg/250mg, 2.5mg/500mg, 5mg/500mg	1.25mg/250mg qd or bid (20mg/2g/day).	1-2 tabs bid.

(Continued)

DRUG	HOW SUPPLIED	INITIAL* & (MAX) DOSE	USUAL DOSE RANGE*
COMBINATIONS *(Continued)*			
Pioglitazone/ Glimepiride Duetact	**Tab:** 30mg/2mg, 30mg/4mg	30mg/2mg qd or 30mg/4mg qd	1 tab am.
Pioglitazone/ Metformin HCl Actoplus Met	**Tab:** 15mg/500mg, 15mg/850mg	15mg/500mg or 15mg/850mg qd-bid (45mg/2250mg/day).	1 tab qd-bid.
Rosiglitazone/ Glimepiride Avandaryl	**Tab:** 4mg/1mg, 4mg/2mg, 4mg/4mg	4mg/1mg or 4mg/2mg qd (8mg/4mg qd).	1 tab am.
Rosiglitazone/ Metformin HCl Avandamet	**Tab:** 1mg/500mg, 2mg/500mg, 4mg/500mg, 2mg/1g, 4mg/1g	2mg/500mg qd-bid. (8mg/2g/day).	1-2 tabs bid.
Sitagliptin/ Metformin Janumet	**Tab:** 50mg/500mg, 50mg/1000mg	50mg/500mg or 50mg/1000mg bid (100mg/2g qd).	1 tab bid.

*NOTE: Usual dose ranges are derived from the drug's FDA-approved labeling. There is no fixed dosage regimen for the management of diabetes mellitus with any hypoglycemic agent. The initial and maintenance dosing should be conservative, depending on the patient's individual needs, especially in elderly, debilitated or malnourished patients, and with impaired renal or hepatic function. Management of type 2 diabetes should include blood glucose and HbA1c monitoring, nutritional counseling, exercise, and weight reduction as needed. For more detailed information refer to the individual monograph listings or the drug's FDA-approved labeling.

ANTIEMETICS

DRUG (BRAND)	INDICATIONS	HOW SUPPLIED	ADULT DOSING	PEDIATRIC DOSING
Anticholinergic Agent				
Scopolamine (Transderm Scōp)	Prevention of nausea and vomiting associated with motion sickness or recovery from anesthesia and surgery.	Patch: 0.33mg/24 hrs [4⁵]	Apply 1 patch the evening before surgery or 1 hr prior to cesarean section. Keep in place for 24 hrs. Apply patch to a hairless area behind the ear. Do not cut patch in half.	
Antihistamines				
Dimenhydrinate (Dramamine Original Formula)	For prevention and treatment of symptoms associated with motion sickness, nausea, vomiting, and dizziness.	Tab: 50mg	1-2 tabs PO q4-6h. Max: 8 tabs/24 hrs.	**≥12 yrs:** 1-2 tabs PO q4-6h. Max: 8 tabs/24 hrs. **6 to <12 yrs:** ½-1 tab PO q6-8h. Max: 3 tabs/24 hrs. **2 to <6 yrs:** ½ tab PO q6-8h. Max: 1½ tabs/24 hrs.
Meclizine HCl (Antivert)	Management of nausea, vomiting and dizziness associated with motion sickness. Management of vertigo associated with diseases affecting the vestibular system.	Tab: 12.5mg, 25mg, 50mg* *scored	25-50mg 1 hr prior to trip/departure, repeat q24h prn.	**≥12 yrs:** Motion Sickness: 25-50mg 1 hr prior to trip/departure, repeat q24h prn. Vertigo: 25-100mg/day in divided doses.
Promethazine HCl (Phenergan)	Prevention and control of nausea and vomiting in surgery.	Liq: 118ml, Sup: 12.5mg, 25mg, 50mg,Tab: 12.5mg, 25mg, 50mg	12.5-25mg q4h.	**≥2 yrs:** Dose should not exceed half of adult dose. Premedication: Usual: 0.5mg/mL. Do not give IV administration >25mg/mL and at a rate >25mg/min.
Cannabinoids				
Dronabinol (Marinol)	Treatment of nausea and vomiting associated with chemotherapy when conventional treatment has failed.	Cap: 2.5mg, 5mg, 10mg	Initial: 5mg/m² given 1-3 hrs before chemotherapy, then q2-4h after chemotherapy, up to 4-6 doses/day. Titrate: May increase by 2.5mg/m² increments. Max: 15mg/m²/dose.	
Nabilone (Cesamet)	Treatment of the nausea and vomiting associated with chemotherapy when conventional treatment has failed.	Cap: 1mg	Initial: 1 or 2mg bid; given 1-3 hrs before chemotherapy. A dose of 1 or 2mg the night before may be useful. Max: 6mg/day given in divided doses tid.	

(Continued)

DRUG (BRAND)	INDICATIONS	HOW SUPPLIED	ADULT DOSING	PEDIATRIC DOSING
5-HT₃ Antagonists				
Dolasetron mesylate (Anzemet)	(Inj) Prevention of nausea/vomiting associated with emetogenic cancer chemotherapy including high-dose cisplatin. Prevention and treatment of post-op nausea/vomiting (PONV). (Tab) Prevention of nausea/vomiting associated with moderately emetogenic cancer chemotherapy and prevention of PONV.	Inj: 20mg/mL; Tab: 50mg, 100mg	(Inj) Prevention of Chemotherapy-Induced Nausea/Vomiting (CINV): 1.8mg/kg IV single dose or 100mg IV 30 min before chemotherapy. Prevention/Treatment of PONV: 12.5mg IV single dose 15 min before cessation of anesthesia or as soon as nausea/vomiting presents. (Tab) Prevention of CINV: 100mg PO within 1 hr before chemotherapy. Prevention of PONV: 100mg PO within 2 hrs before surgery.	**2-16 yrs:** (Inj) Prevention of CINV: 1.8mg/kg IV single dose 30 min before chemotherapy. Max: 100mg. May mix inj in apple or grape juice and take orally within 1 hr before chemotherapy. Prevention/Treatment of PONV: 0.35mg/kg IV single dose 15 min before cessation of anesthesia or as soon as nausea/vomiting presents. Max: 12.5mg single dose. May mix 1.2mg/kg inj in apple or grape juice and take orally within 2 hrs before surgery. Max: 100mg/dose. (Tab) Prevention of CINV: 1.8mg/kg PO within 1 hr before chemotherapy. Max: 100mg. Prevention of PONV: 1.2mg/kg PO within 2 hrs before surgery. Max: 100mg.
Granisetron hydrochloride (Kytril)	(Inj, Sol, Tab) Prevention of nausea and vomiting associated with chemotherapy. (Sol, Tab) Prevention of nausea and vomiting associated with radiation. (Inj) Prevention and treatment of post-op nausea and vomiting (PONV).	Inj: 0.1mg/mL, 1mg/mL; Sol: 2mg/10mL [30mL]; Tab: 1mg	(Sol/Tab) Prevention of Chemotherapy-Induced Nausea/Vomiting (CINV): 2mg qd up to 1 hr before chemotherapy or 1mg bid (up to 1 hr before chemotherapy and 12 hrs later). (Inj) 10mcg/kg within 30 min before chemotherapy. Prevention with Radiation: (Sol/Tab) 2mg within 1 hr of radiation. Prevention of PONV: (Inj) Administer 1mg over 30 sec before induction of anesthesia or immediately before anesthesia reversal. Treatment of PONV: (Inj) Administer 1mg over 30 sec.	**2-16 yrs:** Prevention of CINV: 10mcg/kg IV within 30 min before chemotherapy.

DRUG (BRAND)	INDICATIONS	HOW SUPPLIED	ADULT DOSING	PEDIATRIC DOSING
5-HT3 Antagonists *(Continued)*				
Ondansetron hydrochloride (Zofran)	(Inj) Prevention of nausea and vomiting associated with initial and repeat courses of emetogenic cancer chemotherapy, including high-dose cisplatin. Prevention of post-op nausea and/or vomiting (PONV). (Sol/Tab) Prevention of nausea and vomiting associated with: highly emetogenic cancer chemotherapy, including cisplatin ≥50mg/m², initial and repeat courses of moderately emetogenic cancer chemotherapy; and radiotherapy in patients receiving either total body irradiation, single high-dose fraction to the abdomen, or daily fractions to the abdomen. Prevention of PONV.	Inj: 2mg/mL, 32mg/50mL; Sol: 4mg/5mL [50mL]; Tab: 4mg, 8mg, 24mg; Tab, Disintegrating: 4mg, 8mg	Prevention of Chemotherapy-Induced Nausea/Vomiting (CINV): (Inj) 32mg single dose or three 0.15mg/kg doses, 1st dose 30 min before chemotherapy, then 4 and 8 hrs after 1st dose. Prevention of CINV, Highly Emetogenic Therapy: (Tab) 24mg single dose tab 30 min before chemotherapy. Prevention of CINV, Moderately Emetogenic Therapy: (Sol/Tab) 8mg bid, 1st dose 30 min before chemotherapy, then 8 hrs later, then bid for 1-2 days after chemotherapy. Prevention of PONV: (Inj) 4mg IM/IV immediately before anesthesia or post-op after surgery if nausea or vomiting occurs. (Sol/Tab) 16mg 1 hr before anesthesia. Prevention of Nausea/Vomiting Associated with Radiation Therapy: (Sol/Tab) Usual: 8mg tid. Total Body Irradiation: 8mg 1-2 hrs before therapy daily. Single High-Dose Therapy To Abdomen: 8mg 1-2 hrs before therapy then q8h after 1st dose for 1-2 days after completion of therapy. Daily Fractionated Therapy To Abdomen: 8mg 1-2 hrs before therapy then q8h after 1st dose. Severe Hepatic Severe Hepatic Dysfunction (Child-Pugh ≥10): Max: 8mg/day IV single dose infused over 15 min, start 30 min before chemotherapy or 8mg/day PO.	Prevention of CINV: (Inj) **6 months-18 yrs:** Three 0.15mg/kg doses, 1st dose 30 min before chemotherapy, then 4 and 8 hrs after the 1st dose. (Sol/Tab) Prevention of CINV, Moderately Emetogenic Therapy: **≥12 yrs:** 8mg bid, 1st dose 30 min before chemotherapy, then 8mg 8 hrs later, then bid for 1-2 days. 4-11 yrs: 4mg tid, 1st dose 30 min before chemotherapy, then 4 and 8 hrs after 1st dose, then tid for 1-2 days. Prevention of PONV: (Inj) **>12 yrs:** 4mg IM/IV immediately before anesthesia or post-op after surgery if nausea or vomiting occurs. **1 month-12 yrs:** ≤40kg: 0.1mg/kg single dose. >40kg: 4mg single dose. Severe Hepatic Dysfunction: Max: 8mg/day IV single dose infused over 15 min, start 30 min before chemotherapy or 8mg/day PO.
Palonosetron hydrochloride (Aloxi)	Prevention of acute nausea and vomiting associated with initial and repeat courses of moderately and highly emetogenic cancer chemotherapy. Prevention of delayed nausea and vomiting associated with initial and repeat courses of moderately emetogenic cancer chemotherapy. Prevention of post-op nausea and vomiting (PONV) for up to 24 hrs following surgery.	Inj: 0.25mg/5mL, 0.075mg/1.5mL	Prevention of Chemotherapy-Induced Nausea/Vomiting: 0.25mg IV single dose 30 min before start of chemotherapy. Repeated dosing within a 7 day interval not recommended. PONV: 0.075mg IV single dose 10 sec before induction of anesthesia.	

(Continued)

DRUG (BRAND)	INDICATIONS	HOW SUPPLIED	ADULT DOSING	PEDIATRIC DOSING
Miscellaneous				
Dextrose glucose 1.87g, Levulose Fructose 1.87g, and Phosphoric Acid 21.5 mg (Emetrol)	For relief of nausea due to upset stomach from intestinal flu, and food or drink indiscretions.	Liq: 118mL	1-2 tblsp PO every 15 min until response is achieved.	**2-12 yrs:** 1-2 tsp PO every 15 min until response is achieved.
Droperidol (Inapsine)	To reduce incidence of nausea and vomiting associated with surgical and diagnostic procedures.	Inj: 2.5mg/mL	Initial (Max): 2.5mg IM/IV. May give additional 1.25mg cautiously to achieve desired effect. Lower initial doses in elderly, debilitated, poor-risk patients.	**2-12 yrs:** Initial (Max): 0.1 mg/kg IM/IV. May give additional doses cautiously. Lower initial doses in debilitated, poor-risk patients.
Metoclopramide	(Inj) Prevention of post-op or chemo-induced nausea/vomiting.	Inj: 5mg/mL; Syr: 5mg/5mL; Tab: 5mg, 10mg* *scored	Antiemetic: (Postoperative) 10-20mg IM near end of surgery. (Chemotherapy-Induced) 1-2mg/kg 30 min before chemotherapy then q2h for two doses, then q3h for three doses. Give 2mg/kg for highly emetogenic drugs for initial 2 doses.	
Trimethobenzamide hydrochloride (Tigan)	Treatment of postoperative nausea and vomiting and for nausea associated with gastroenteritis.	Cap: 300mg; Inj: 100mg/mL; Supp: 200mg (Adult), 100mg (Pediatric).	(Cap) 300mg tid-qid. (Inj) 200mg IM tid-qid. Supp: 200mg tid-qid.	<30 lbs: 100mg pr tid-qid. 30-90 lbs: 100-200mg pr tid-qid.
Phenothiazine Derivative				
Prochlorperazine	Control of severe nausea and vomiting.	Inj: (Edisylate) 5mg/mL; Supp: 25mg; Tab: (Maleate) 5mg, 10mg, 25mg	Nausea/Vomiting: (Tab) Usual: 5-10mg tid-qid. Max: 40mg/day. (Supp) 25mg pr bid. (IM) 5-10mg IM q3-4h prn. Max: 40mg/day. (IV) 2.5-10mg IV (not bolus). Max: 10mg single dose and 40mg/day. Nausea/Vomiting with Surgery: 5-10mg IM 1-2 hrs or 5-10mg IV 15-30 min before anesthesia, or during or after surgery; repeat once if needed.	Nausea/Vomiting: >2 yrs and >20 lbs: (PO/PR) 20-29 lbs: Usual: 2.5mg qd-bid. Max: 7.5mg/day. 30-39 lbs: 2.5mg bid-tid. Max: 10mg/day. 40-85 lbs: 2.5mg tid or 5mg bid. Max: 15mg/day. (IM) 0.06mg/lb, usually single dose for control.

DRUG (BRAND)	INDICATIONS	HOW SUPPLIED	ADULT DOSING	PEDIATRIC DOSING
Substance P/neurokinin 1 Receptor Antagonist				
Aprepitant (Emend)	In combination with other antiemetics for prevention of acute and delayed nausea and vomiting associated with initial and repeat courses of highly emetogenic cancer chemotherapy (eg, high-dose cisplatin) and for moderately emetogenic cancer chemotherapy. For the prevention of postop nausea and vomiting (PONV).	Cap: 40mg, 80mg, 125mg; Tri-Pak: (one 125mg & two 80mg caps)	Prevention of Chemotherapy-Induced Nausea/Vomiting: Day 1: 125mg 1 hr prior to chemotherapy. Days 2 and 3: 80mg qam. Regimen should include a corticosteroid and a 5-HT$_3$ antagonist. Prevention of PONV: 40mg within w3 hrs prior to induction of anesthesia.	
Fosaprepitant Dimeglumine (Emend for injection)	In combination with other antiemetics for prevention of acute and delayed nausea and vomiting associated with initial and repeat courses of highly emetogenic cancer chemotherapy (eg, high-dose cisplatin) and for moderately emetogenic cancer chemotherapy.	Powder (Vial): 115mg/10mL [10mL]	115mg IV over 15 min or 125mg PO 30 min prior to chemotherapy on day 1, 80mg PO days 2 and 3 only of a 3-day regimen, in addition to corticosteroid and 5-HT$_3$ anataganist.	

H₂ ANTAGONISTS AND PPIs COMPARISON

	DRUG	HOW SUPPLIED	Heartburn	PUD	GERD	Zollinger-Ellison	H.pylori	NSAID† Induced	Upper GI‡ Bleeding
H₂ ANTAGONISTS	**CIMETIDINE**								
	Tagamet	**Inj:** 150mg/mL, 300mg/ 50mL; **Sol:** 300mg/5mL **Tab:** 200mg, 300mg, 400mg, 800mg		X	X	X			X
	Tagamet HB*	**Tab:** 200mg	X						
	FAMOTIDINE								
	Pepcid, Pepcid RPD	**Inj:** 0.4mg/mL, 10mg/mL **Sus:** 40mg/5mL; **Tab:** 20mg, 40mg; **Tab, Disintegrating:** (RPD); 20mg, 40mg		X	X	X			
	Pepcid AC*	**Cap:** 10mg **Tab:** 10mg, 20mg **Tab, Chewable:** 10mg	X						
	Pepcid Complete*	**Tab, Chewable:** (Famotidine-Calcium Carbonate-Magnesium Hydroxide) 10mg-800mg-165mg	X						
	NIZATIDINE								
	Axid	**Cap:** 150mg, 300mg **Sol:** 15mg/mL		X	X				
	RANITIDINE								
	Zantac	**Inj:** 1mg/mL, 25mg/mL **Syrup:** 15mg/mL **Tab:** 150mg, 300mg **Tab, Effervescent:** 25mg, 150mg		X	X	X			
	Zantac OTC*	**Tab:** 75mg, 150mg	X						
PROTON PUMP INHIBITORS	**ESOMEPRAZOLE**								
	Nexium	**Cap, Delayed-Release:** 20mg, 40mg; **Inj:** 20mg, 40mg			X	X	X	X	
	LANSOPRAZOLE								
	Prevacid	**Cap, Delayed-Release:** 15mg, 30mg; **Inj:** 30mg **Sus:** 15mg/packet, 30mg/packet **Tab, Disintegrating:** 15mg, 30mg		X	X	X	X	X	
	Prevpac	**Cap:** (Amoxicillin) 500mg **Tab:** (Clarithromycin) 500mg **Cap, Delayed-Release:** (Lansoprazole) 30mg					X		
	Prevacid NapraPAC	**Cap, Delayed-Release:** (Naproxen Lansoprazole): 500mg-15mg						X	
	OMEPRAZOLE								
	Prilosec	**Cap, Delayed-Release:** 10mg, 20mg, 40mg; **Sus, Delayed-Release:** 2.5mg, 10mg granules/packet		X	X	X	X		
	Prilosec OTC*	**Tab:** 20mg	X						
	Zegerid	(Omeprazole-Sodium Bicarbonate); **Cap:** 20mg-1100mg, 40mg-1100mg; **Pow:** 20mg-1680mg/ packet, 40mg-1680mg/packet		X	X				X
	PANTOPRAZOLE								
	Protonix	**Inj:** 40mg; **Sus, Delayed-Release:** 40mg granules/ packet; **Tab, Delayed-Release:** 20mg, 40mg			X	X			
	RABEPRAZOLE								
	Aciphex	**Tab, Delayed-Release:** 20mg		X	X	X	X		

*OTC.   †Prevention of NSAID-induced gastric ulcers.   ‡Prevention of upper GI bleeding in critically ill patients.

DRUG TREATMENTS FOR COMMON STDs*

DISEASE	DRUG	RECOMMENDED DOSAGE
Bacterial Vaginosis		
Nonpregnant Women	Metronidazole (Flagyl) *or*	500mg PO bid x 7d.
	Clindamycin cream (Cleocin) *or*	2%, 1 full applicator intravaginally qhs x 7d.
	Metronidazole gel (MetroGel)	0.75%, 1 full applicator intravaginally qd x 5d.
Alternative Regimens	Clindamycin *or*	300mg PO bid x 7d.
(Nonpregnant Women)	Clindamycin ovules	100g intravaginally qhs x 3d.
Pregnant Women	Metronidazole (CI in 1st	250mg PO tid x 7d or
	trimester) *or* Clindamycin	300mg PO bid x 7d or
		500mg PO bid x 7d.
Chancroid	Azithromycin (Zithromax) *or*	1g PO single dose.
	Ceftriaxone (Rocephin) *or*	250mg IM single dose.
	Ciprofloxacin (Cipro) *or*	500mg PO bid x 3d.
	Erythromycin base	500mg PO tid x 7d.
Chlamydial Infection		
Nonpregnant Women	Azithromycin (Zithromax) *or*	1g PO single dose.
	Doxycycline (Vibramycin)	100mg PO bid x 7d.
Alternative Regimens	Erythromycin base or	500mg PO qid x 7d or
(Nonpregnant/pregnant)		250mg PO qid x 14d (pregnancy)
	Erythromycin Ethylsuccinate or	800mg PO qid x 7d or
		400mg PO qid x 14d (pregnancy)
	Ofloxacin (Floxin) *or*	300mg PO bid x 7d (nonpregnant)
	Levofloxacin (Levaquin)	500mg PO qd x 7d (nonpregnant)
Pregnant Women	Azithromycin (Zithromax) *or*	1g PO single dose.
	Amoxicillin	500mg PO tid x 7d
Epididymitis		
Gonococcal or	Ceftriaxone (Rocephin) *plus*	250mg IM single dose.
Chlamydial Infection	Doxycycline (Vibramycin)	100mg PO bid x 10d.
Enteric Organisms	Ofloxacin (Floxin) *or*	300mg PO bid x 10d.
(>35 yrs or allergic to	Levofloxacin (Levaquin)	500mg PO qd x 10d.
cephalosporins and/or		
tetracyclines)		
Granuloma Inguinale	Doxycycline (Vibramycin)	100mg PO bid for at least 3 weeks.
Alternative Regimens	Ciprofloxacin (Cipro) *or*	750mg PO bid for at least 3 weeks.
	Erythromycin base (during	
	pregnancy) *or*	500mg PO qid for at least 3 weeks.
	Azithromycin (Zithromax)	1g PO once weekly for at least 3 weeks.
	plus (if no improvement)	
	Aminoglycoside (ie, gentamicin)	1mg/kg IV q8h for at least 3 weeks.
	Trimethoprim/Sulfamethoxazole	1 tab (DS) PO bid for at least 3 weeks.
	(Bactrim, Septra)	
Herpes Simplex Virus (HSV)		
First Episode	Acyclovir (Zovirax) *or*	400mg PO tid x 7-10d or 200mg PO 5x/d x 7-10d.
	Famciclovir (Famvir) *or*	250mg PO tid x 7-10d.
	Valacyclovir (Valtrex)	1g PO bid x 7-10d.
Recurrent Episodes	Acyclovir *or*	400mg PO tid x 5d or 800mg PO bid x 5d or
		800mg PO tid x 2d.
	Famciclovir *or*	1g bid x 1d or 125mg PO bid x 5d or
	Valacyclovir	500mg PO bid x 3d or
		1g PO qd x 5d.
Daily Suppressive Therapy	Acyclovir *or*	400mg PO bid.
	Famciclovir *or*	250mg PO bid.
	Valacyclovir	500mg PO qd (<10 episodes/yr) or
		1g PO qd.

(Continued)

DISEASE	DRUG	RECOMMENDED DOSAGE
Human Papillomavirus (HPV) Infection		
External Genital Area	Podofilox (Condylox) *or*	0.5% sol or gel (patient-applied) bid x 3d, wait 4d, repeat as necessary x 4 cycles.
	Imiquimod (Aldara)	5% cre (patient-applied) tiw at bedtime up to 16 wks.
	Cryotherapy *or*	Physician-applied every 1-2 wks.
	Podophyllum resin	10-25% (physician-applied) qwk if necessary.
	Trichloroacetic acid *or*	80-90% (physician-applied) qwk if necessary.
	Bichloroacetic acid *or*	80-90% (physician-applied) qwk if necessary.
	Surgical removal	
HPV Infection		
External Genital Area (cont.)		
Alternative Regimens	Intralesional interferon *or* laser surgery	
Vaginal	Cryotherapy *or*	With liquid nitrogen.
	Trichloroacetic acid *or*	80-90% (physician-applied) qwk if necessary.
	Bichloroacetic acid	80-90% (physician-applied) qwk if necessary.
Urethral Meatus	Cryotherapy *or*	With liquid nitrogen.
	Podophyllum	10-25% (physician-applied) qwk if necessary.
Anal Area	Cryotherapy	With liquid nitrogen.
	Trichloroacetic acid *or*	80-90% (physician-applied) qwk if necessary.
	Bichloroacetic acid *or*	80-90% (physician-applied) qwk if necessary.
	Surgical removal	
Lymphogranuloma Venereum	Doxycycline (Vibramycin)	100mg PO bid x 21d.
Alternative Regimen (including pregnancy)	Erythromycin base	500mg PO qid x 21d.
Nongonococcal Urethritis	Azithromycin (Zithromax) *or*	1g PO single dose.
	Doxycycline (Vibramycin)	100mg PO bid x 7d.
Alternative Regimens	Erythromycin base *or*	500mg PO qid x 7d.
	Erythromycin ethylsuccinate *or*	800mg PO qid x 7d.
	Ofloxacin (Floxin) *or*	300mg PO bid x 7d.
	Levofloxacin (Levaquin)	500mg PO qd x 7d.
Recurrent and Persistent Urethritis	Metronidazole *or*	2g PO single dose.
	Tinidazole *plus*	2g PO single dose.
	Azithromycin	1g PO single dose (if not used for initial episodes).
Pediculosis Pubis	Permethrin cream (NIX)	1% cre: Apply to affected area & wash off after 10 min.
	Pyrethrins with piperonyl butoxide (compounded by pharmacist)	Apply to affected area and wash off after 10 min.
Alternative Regimens	Malathion	0.5% lotion: Apply for 8-12 hours and wash off.
	Ivermectin	250µg/kg repeat in 2 weeks.
Pelvic Inflammatory Disease		
Parenteral Regimen A	Cefotetan (Cefotan) *or*	2g IV q12h.
	Cefoxitin (Mefoxin) *plus*	2g IV q6h.
	Doxycycline (Vibramycin)	100mg IV q12h.
Parenteral Regimen B	Clindamycin (Cleocin) *plus*	900mg IV q8h.
	Gentamicin	LD: 2mg/kg IM/IV. MD: 1.5mg/kg IM/IV q8h (may substitute single daily dosing).
Alternative Regimens	Ampicillin/Sulbactam *plus*	3g IV q6h.
	Doxycycline	100mg PO/IV q12h.
	Levofloxacin *or*	500mg IV qd or
	Ofloxacin *w/ or w/o*	400 mg IV q12h
	Metronidazole	w/ or w/o 500mg IV q8h.
Oral Regimen A	Levofloxacin *or*	500mg PO qd x 14d.
	Ofloxacin *w/ or w/o*	400mg PO bid x 14d.
	Metronidazole	500mg PO bid x 14d.
Alternative Regimen B (also give presumptive therapy for Chlamydia infection: Doxycycline 100mg PO bid x 7d)	Ceftriaxone (Rocephin) *or*	250mg IM single dose.
	Cefoxitin *or*	2g IM single dose plus.
	3rd gen cephalosporin (eg ceftizoxime or cefotaxime)	probenecid 1g PO single dose.
	plus Doxycycline *w/ or w/o*	100mg PO bid x 14d.
	Metronidazole	500mg PO bid x 14d.

(Continued)

DISEASE	DRUG	RECOMMENDED DOSAGE
Proctitis, Proctocolitis & Enteritis	Ceftriaxone (Rocephin) *plus* Doxycycline (Vibramycin)	125mg IM single dose. 100mg PO bid x 7d.
Scabies	Permethrin cream (Elimite)	5% cre: Apply to body from the neck down & wash off after 8-14h; re-evaluate in 1 week.
	Ivermectin	200mcg/kg PO; repeat in 2 weeks.
Alternative Regimens	Lindane (Kwell)	1% lot or cre: Apply 1oz lotion or 30g cream to body from the neck down & wash off after 8h; re-evaluate in 1 wk (not recommended in pregnancy, lactating women or children <2 yrs).
Syphilis Primary & Secondary Disease	Benzathine Penicillin G	**Adults:** 2.4 MU IM single dose. **Pediatrics:** 50,000 U/kg IM single dose. **Max:** 2.4 MU/dose.
Penicillin Allergy	Doxycycline (Vibramycin) *or* Tetracycline	100mg PO bid x 14d. 500mg PO qid x 14d.
Early Latent Disease	Benzathine Penicillin G	**Adults:** 2.4 MU IM single dose. **Pediatrics:** 50,000 U/kg IM single dose. **Max:** 2.4 MU/dose.
Late Latent, Unknown Duration	Benzathine Penicillin G	**Adults:** 2.4 MU IM qwk x 3 doses. **Pediatrics:** 50,000 U/kg IM qwk x 3 doses. **Max:** 2.4 MU/dose.
Tertiary Disease	Benzathine Penicillin G	2.4 MU IM qwk x 3 doses.
Neurosyphilis	Aqueous Crystalline Penicillin G	3-4 MU IV q4h or continuous infusion x 10-14d.
Alternative Regimen	Procaine Penicillin *plus* Probenecid	2.4 MU IM qd x 10-14d. 500mg PO qid x 10-14d.
Trichomoniasis	Metronidazole (Flagyl) Timidazole	2g PO single dose. 2g PO single dose.
Alternative Regimen	Metronidazole	500mg PO bid x 7d.
Pregnant Women	Metronidazole (CI in 1st trimester)	2g PO single dose.
Uncomplicated Gonococcal Infections Cervix, Urethra, and Rectum *Recommended Regimens*	Ceftriaxone or Ciprofloxacin	125mg IM single dose. 500mg PO single dose or
	Ofloxacin	400 mg PO single dose or
	Levofloxacin	250 mg PO single dose or
	Cefixime Plus	400 mg PO single dose.
	If Chlamydial infection is not ruled out: Azithromycin (Zithromax) *or* Doxycycline (Vibramycin)	1g PO single dose. 100mg PO bid x 7d.
Alternative Regimens	Spectinomycin or *Cephalosporin regimens:*	2g IM single dose.
	Ceftizoxime *or*	500mg IM single dose.
	Cefotaxime *or*	500mg IM single dose.
	Cefoxitin plus	2g IM.
	Probenecid	1g PO.
	Quinolone regimens: Gatifloxacin	400mg PO or
	Lomefloxacin	400mg PO or
	Norfloxacin	800mg PO single dose
Pharynx *Recommended Regimens*	Ciprofloxacin or Ceftriaxone *plus*	500mg PO single dose or 125mg IM single dose.
	If Chlamydial infection is not ruled out: Azithromycin (Zithromax) *or* Doxycycline (Vibramycin)	1g PO single dose. 100 mg PO bid x 7d.

(Continued)

DISEASE	DRUG	RECOMMENDED DOSAGE
Vulvovaginal Candidiasis		
Intravaginal Agents	Butoconazole *or*	2% cre, 5g intravaginally x 3d or 5g single dose.
	Butoconazole *or*	2% cre, 5g intravaginally single dose.
	Clotrimazole *or*	1% cre, 5g intravaginally x 7-14d.
	Clotrimazole *or*	100mg vaginal tab qd x 7 days or 2 tabs qd x 3d.
	Miconazole *or*	2% cre, 5g intravaginally qd x 7d.
	Miconazole *or*	200mg vaginal supp qd x 3d.
	Miconazole *or*	100mg vaginal supp qd x 7d.
	Nystatin *or*	100,000-U vaginal tab qd x 14d.
	Tioconazole *or*	6.5% oint, 5g intravaginally single dose.
	Terconazole *or*	0.4% cre, 5g intravaginally x 7d.
	Terconazole *or*	0.8% cre, 5g intravaginally x 3d.
	Terconazole	80mg vaginal supp qd x 3d.
Oral Agent	Fluconazole	150mg tab PO single dose.

*Adapted from: Centers for Disease Control and Prevention. Sexually Transmitted Diseases Treatment Guidelines 2006.
MMWR 2002; 51 (No. RR-6): 1-77.

HIV/AIDS PHARMACOTHERAPY

DRUG	BRAND	HOW SUPPLIED	USUAL DOSE	FOOD EFFECT
CCR5 ANTAGONISTS				
Maraviroc (MVC)	Selzentry	**Tab:** 150mg, 300mg	**Adults: >16 yrs:** Give in combination with other anti-retroviral medications. With Strong CYP3A Inhibitors (with or without CYP3A inducers) Including PIs (excepts tipranavir/ritonavir), Delavirdine: 150mg bid. With NRTIs, Tipranavir/Ritonavir, Nevirapine, Other Drugs That Are Not Strong CYP3A Inhibitors/Inducers: 300mg bid. With CYP3A Inducers (without strong CYP3A inhibitor): 600mg bid.	Take without regard to meals.
HIV INTEGRASE STRAND TRANSFER INHIBITOR				
Raltegravir	Isentress	**Tab:** 400mg	**Adults:** 400mg bid.	Take without regard to meals.
NUCLEOSIDE REVERSE TRANSCRIPTASE INHIBITORS (NRTIs)				
Abacavir (ABC)	Ziagen	**Sol:** 20mg/mL [240mL]; **Tab:** 300mg	**Adults: >16 yrs:** or 600mg qd. **Pediatrics: 3 months-16 yrs:** 8mg/kg bid. **Max:** 300mg bid.	Take without regard to meals.
Didanosine (ddI)	Videx Powder for Oral Sol; Videx EC	**Powder for Sol:** 2g, 4g; **Cap, Delayed Release:** (Videx EC) 125mg, 200mg, 250mg, 400mg	**Adults: ≥60kg: (Cap)** 400mg qd; **(Sol)** 200mg bid or 400mg qd. **<60kg: (Cap)** 250mg qd. **(Sol)** 125mg bid. or 250mg qd. **Pediatrics: 2 weeks-8 months: (Sol)** 100mg/m^2 bid. **>8 months:** 120mg/m^2 bid.	Take on empty stomach at least 30 minutes before or 2 hrs after meals. Swallow caps whole.
Emtricitabine (FTC)	Emtriva	**Cap:** 200mg; **Sol:** 10mg/mL	**Adults: ≥18 yrs: Cap:** 200 mg qd. **Sol:** 240mg (24mL) qd. **Pediatrics: 0-3 mos:** 3mg/kg qd. **3 mos-17 yrs: Cap: >33kg:** 200mg qd. **Sol:** 6mg/kg qd. **Max:** 240mg (24mL).	Take without regard to meals.
Lamivudine	Epivir	**Sol:** 10mg/mL [240mL]; **Tab:** 150mg, 300mg	**Adults:** 150mg bid or 300mg qd. **Pediatrics: 3 months-16 yrs:** 4mg/kg bid. **Max:** 150mg bid.	Take without regard to meals.
Stavudine (d4T)	Zerit	**Cap:** 15mg, 20mg, 30mg, 40mg; **Sol:** 1mg/mL [200mL]	**Adults: ≥60kg:** 40mg q12h. **<60kg:** 30mg q12h. **Pediatrics: ≥60kg:** 40mg q12h. **30-59 kg:** 30mg q12h. **≥14 days and <30kg:** 1mg/kg q12h. **Birth-13 days:** 0.5mg/kg q12h.	Take without regard to meals.
Tenofovir Disoproxil Fumarate (TDF)	Viread	**Tab:** 300mg	**Adults:** 300mg once daily.	Take without regard to meals.
Zalcitabine (ddC)	Hivid	**Tab:** 0.375mg, 0.75mg	**Adults:** 0.75mg q8h. **Pediatrics: >13 yrs:** 0.75mg q8h.	Take without regard to meals.
Zidovudine (AZT, ZDV)	Retrovir	**Cap:** 100mg; **Inj:** 10mg/mL; **Syrup:** 50mg/5mL [240mL]; **Tab:** 300mg	**Adults: (Cap, Tab)** 600mg/day in divided doses. **(Inj)** 1mg/kg IV over 1 hr 5-6 times/day. **Pediatrics: 6 weeks-12 yrs:** 160mg/m^2 PO q8h. **Max:** 200mg PO q8h.	Take without regard to meals.

(Continued)

DRUG	BRAND	HOW SUPPLIED	USUAL DOSE	FOOD EFFECT
NON-NUCLEOSIDE REVERSE TRANSCRIPTASE INHIBITORS (NNRTIs)				
Delavirdine (DLV)	Rescriptor	**Tab:** 100mg, 200mg	**Adults:** Usual: 400mg tid. **Pediatrics:** ≥16 yrs: Usual: 400mg tid.	Take without regard to meals.
Efavirenz (EFV)	Sustiva	**Cap:** 50mg, 100mg, 200mg; **Tab:** 600mg	**Adults: Initial:** 600mg qd at bedtime. **Pediatrics:** ≥3 yrs: 10 to <15kg: 200mg qd. 15 to <20kg: 250mg qd. 20 to <25kg: 300mg qd. 25 to <32.5kg: 350mg qd. 32.5 to <40kg: 400mg qd. ≥40kg: 600mg qd at bedtime.	Take on an empty stomach.
Etravirine (ETR)	Intelence	**Tab:** 100mg	**Adults:** 200mg bid.	Take with meals.
Nevirapine (NVP)	Viramune	**Sus:** 50mg/5mL [240mL]; **Tab:** 200mg* *scored	**Adults:** 200mg qd for 14 days (lead-in period), then 200mg bid. **Pediatrics:** 2 months-8 yrs: 4mg/kg qd for 14 days, then 7mg/kg bid. **Max:** 400mg/day. 8 yrs: 4mg/kg qd for 14 days, then 4mg/kg bid. **Max:** 400mg/day.	Take without regard to meals.
PROTEASE INHIBITORS (PIs)				
Atazanavir (ATV)	Reyataz	**Cap:** 100mg, 150mg, 200mg, 300mg	**Adults: Therapy-naive:** 400mg qd. Therapy Experienced: (ATV 300mg + RTV 100mg) qd.	Take with food; avoid taking with antacids.
Darunavir (DRV)	Prezista	**Tab:** 300mg	**Adults:** (DRV 600mg + RTV 100mg) bid.	Take with food.
Fosamprenavir (fAPV)	Lexiva	**Tab:** 700mg **Sus:** 50mg/1mL [225mL]	**Adults: Therapy-naive:** 1400mg bid OR 1400mg qd + RTV 200mg qd OR 700mg bid + RTV 100mg bid. PI-Experienced: 700mg bid + RTV 100mg bid.	Take without regard to meals.
Indinavir (IDV)	Crixivan	**Cap:** 100mg, 200mg, 333mg, 400mg	**Adults:** 800mg q8h OR (IDV 800mg + RTV 100 or 200mg) q12h.	Take 1 hr before or 2 hr after meals; may take with skim milk or low-fat meal. RTV-boosted, take with or without food.
Nelfinavir (NFV)	Viracept	**Sus:** (powder) 50mg/g [144g] **Tab:** 250mg, 625mg	**Adults:** 1250mg bid or 750mg tid. **Pediatrics:** 2-13 yrs: 45-55mg/kg bid; 25-35mg/kg tid. **Max:** 2500mg/day	Take with meals.
Ritonavir (RTV)	Norvir	**Cap:** 100mg **Sol:** 80mg/mL [240mL]	**Adults: Initial:** 300mg bid. **Titrate:** Increase every 2-3 days by 100mg bid. **Maint:** 600mg bid. **Pediatrics:** >1 month: **Initial:** 250mg/m² po bid. **Titrate:** Increase by 50mg/m² every 2-3 days. **Maint:** 350-400mg/m² po bid or highest tolerated dose. **Max:** 600mg bid.	Take with food, may improve tolerability.
Saquinavir (SQV)	Invirase	**Hard Gel Cap:** 200mg **Tab:** 500mg	**Adults/Pediatrics:** >16 yrs: 1000mg bid with RTV 100mg bid OR 1000mg bid with LPV/RTV 400/100mg bid (no additional RTV).	Take within 2 hrs after a meal when taken with RTV.

(Continued)

DRUG	BRAND	HOW SUPPLIED	USUAL DOSE	FOOD EFFECT
PROTEASE INHIBITORS (PIs) *(Continued)*				
Tipranavir (TPV)	Aptivus	**Cap:** 250mg	**Adults:** (500mg + RTV 200mg) bid.	Take with food.
FUSION INHIBITORS				
Enfuvirtide (T20)	Fuzeon	**Inj:** 90mg/1ml (60s)	**Adults:** 90mg SQ bid. **Pediatrics: 6-16 yrs:** 2mg/kg SQ bid. **Max:** 90mg bid. 11-15.5kg: 27mg bid. 15.6-20.0kg: 36mg bid. 20.1-24.5kg: 45mg bid. 24.6-29.0kg: 54mg bid. 29.1-33.5kg: 63mg bid. 33.6-38.0kg: 72mg bid. 38.1-42.5kg: 81mg bid. ≥42.6kg: 90mg bid.	
COMBINATIONS				
EFV/FTC/TDF	Atripla	**Tab:** (Efavirenz-Emtricitabine-Tenofovir DF) 600mg-200mg-300mg	**Adults: ≥18 yrs:** 1 tab qd.	Take on empty stomach.
3TC/ZDV	Combivir	**Tab:** (Lamivudine-Zidovudine) 150mg-300mg	**Adults:** 1 tab bid. **Pediatrics: ≥12 yrs:** 1 tab bid. Do not give if CrCl ≥50mL/min.	Take without regard to meals.
ABC/3TC	Epzicom	**Tab:** (Abacavir Sulfate-Lamivudine) 600mg-300mg	**Adults: ≥18 yrs:** CrCl >50 mL/min: 1 tab qd.	Take without regard to meals.
LPV/RTV	Kaletra	**Tab:** (Lopinavir-Ritonavir) 200mg-50mg; 100mg-25mg; **Sol:** (Lopinavir-Ritonavir) 80mg-20mg/mL [160mL]	**Adults: Therapy-Naive:** 400/100mg (2 tabs or 5mL) bid or 800/200mg qd (4 tabs or 10mL). **Therapy Experienced:** 400/100mg bid (2 tabs or 5mL).	Take without regard to meals. **Sol:** Take with meal.
ABC/ZDV/3TC	Trizivir	**Tab:** (Abacavir-Lamivudine-Zidovudine) 300mg-150mg-300mg	**Adults:** >40kg and CrCl >50mL/min: 1 tab bid.	Take without regard to meals.
FTC/TDF	Truvada	**Tab:** (Emtricitabine-Tenofovir Disoproxil Fumarate) 200mg-300mg	**Adults: ≥18 yrs:** CrCl ≥50mL/min: 1 tab qd. CrCl 30-49mL/min: 1 tab q48h.	Take without regard to meals.

Sources: FDA Approved Labeling; Guidelines for the Use of Antiretroviral Agents in HIV-1-Infected Adults and Adolescents - October 10, 2006.

HIV/AIDS COMPLICATIONS THERAPY

BRAND	USE	DOSE
ANTIBIOTICS		
Atovaquone (Mepron)	PCP prevention and treatment	**Adults/Pediatrics:** ≥**13yrs:** Prevention: 1500mg qd. Treatment: 750mg bid x 21 days. Take with food.
Azithromycin (Zithromax)	MAC prevention and treatment	**Adults:** Prevention: 1200mg once weekly. Treatment: 600mg qd with ethambutol 15mg/kg/day.
Clarithromycin (Biaxin)	MAC prevention and treatment	**Adults:** 500mg bid. **Pediatrics:** ≥**20 months:** 7.5mg/kg bid, up to 500mg bid.
Rifabutin (Mycobutin)	MAC prevention	**Adults:** 300mg qd; give 150mg bid with food if intolerant to GI side effects.
Sulfamethoxazole/ Trimethoprim (Bactrim, Septra)	PCP prevention and treatment	**Adults/Pediatrics:** Treatment: 15-20mg/kg TMP and 75-100mg/kg SMX divided q6h x 14-21 days. **Adults:** Prevention: 800mg SMX-160mg TMP qd. **Pediatrics:** Prevention: 150mg/m^2 TMP and 750mg/ m^2 SMX divided bid x 3 consecutive days per week.
ANTIFUNGALS		
Amphotericin B (Ambisome)	Aspergillosis, candida, cryptococcal meningitis, visceral leishmaniasis	See complete monograph for full dosing information.
Amphotericin B lipid complex (Abelcet)	Invasive fungal infections	**Adults/Pediatrics:** 5mg/kg at 2.5mg/kg/hr.
Fluconazole (Diflucan)	Candidiasis, cryptococcal meningitis	See complete monograph for full dosing information.
Itraconazole (Sporanox)	Aspergillosis, blastomycosis, candidiasis, histoplasmosis,	See complete monograph for full dosing information.
Voriconazole (VFEND)	Aspergillosis, candidiasis, serious fungal infection	See complete monograph for full dosing information.
ANTIVIRALS		
Cidofovir (Vistide)	CMV retinitis	**Adults:** Induction: 5mg/kg q week x 2 weeks. **Maint:** 5mg/kg q 2 weeks.
Famciclovir (Famvir)	HSV	**Adults:** 500mg bid x 7 days.
Foscarnet (Foscavir)	HSV, CMV retinitis	**Adults:** CMV: Induction: 90mg/kg q12h or 60mg/kg q8h. **Maint:** 90-120mg/kg/day. HSV: 40mg/kg q 8-12h.
Ganciclovir (Cytovene)	CMV retinitis	**Adults:** 1000mg tid or 500mg 6 times/day. Take with food. IV: Induction 5mg/kg q12h x 14-21 days. **Maint:** 5mg/kg x 7 days/week or 6mg/kg qd x 5 days/week.
Ganciclovir (Vitrasert)	CMV retinitis	**Adults/Pediatrics:** ≥**9yrs:** One implant q 5-8 months.
Interferon alfa-2b (Intron A)	Kaposi's sarcoma, HCV	**Adults:** KS: 30MIU/m^2 SC/IM tiw. HCV: 3MIU IM/SC tiw x 18-24 months.
Valganciclovir (Valcyte)	CMV retinitis	**Adults:** Induction: 900mg bid x 21 days. **Maint:** 900mg qd.
CHEMOTHERAPEUTICS		
Daunorubicin (DaunoXome)	Kaposi's sarcoma	**Adults:** 40mg/m2 over 60 minutes q 2 weeks.
Doxorubicin (Doxil)	Kaposi's sarcoma	**Adults:** 20mg/m2 over 30 minutes q 3 weeks.
Paclitaxel (Taxol)	Kaposi's sarcoma	**Adults:** 135mg/m2 over 3h q 3 weeks or 100mg/m2 q 2 weeks.
MISCELLANEOUS		
Alitretinoin (Panretin)	Kaposi's sarcoma	**Adults: Initial:** Apply bid to lesions. **Titrate:** Gradually increase to tid-qid as tolerated.
Dronabinol (Marinol)	Appetite loss	**Adults:** 2.5mg qhs or bid before meal. **Max:** 20mg/day in divided doses.
Megestrol (Megace)	Appetite/weight loss	**Adults: Initial:** 800mg/d. **Usual:** 400-800mg/d.
Somatropin (Serostim)	Weight loss	**Adults:** >55kg: 6mg SQ qhs. 45-55kg: 5mg SQ qhs. 35-44kg: 4mg SQ qhs. <35kg: 0.1mg/kg SQ qhs.

Abbreviations: CMV-Cytomegalovirus, HCV-Hepatitis C Virus, HSV-Herpes Simplex Virus, MAC-Mycobacterium avium, PCP-Pneumocystis carinii pneumonia

Systemic Antibiotics

BRAND NAME (Generic)	DOSAGE FORM/ STRENGTH	INDICATIONS	ADULT DOSE	PEDIATRIC DOSE
AMINOGLYCOSIDES				
Amikacin (amikacin sulfate)	**Inj:** 50mg/mL, 250mg/mL	Short-term treatment of serious infections caused by gram-negative bacteria such as septicemia, and respiratory tract, bone/joint, CNS (including meningitis), skin and soft tissue, and intra-abdominal infections; burns and postoperative infections; complicated and recurrent urinary tract infections (UTI); and staphylococcal disease.	(IM/IV)15mg/kg/day given q8h or q12h. Max: 15mg/kg/day. Heavier Weight Patients: Max: 1.5g/ day. Recurrent Uncomplicated UTI: 250mg bid. Duration: 7-10 days. Stop therapy if no response after 3-5 days. Reduce dose if suspect renal dysfunction. Discontinue if azotemia increases or if a progressive decrease in urinary output occurs.	15mg/kg/day given bid-tid. Newborns: LD: 10mg/kg. MD: 7.5mg/kg q12h. Duration: 7-10 days.
Amikacin Pediatric (amikacin sulfate)	**Inj:** 50mg/mL	Short-term treatment of serious infections caused by gram-negative bacteria such as septicemia, and respiratory tract, bone/joint, CNS (including meningitis), skin and soft tissue, and intra-abdominal infections; burns and postoperative infections; complicated and recurrent urinary tract infections (UTI); and staphylococcal disease.		15mg/kg/day given bid-tid. Newborns: LD: 10mg/kg. MD: 7.5mg/kg q12h. Duration: 7-10 days.
Gentamicin sulfate	**Inj:** 10mg/mL, 40mg/mL	Treatment of bacterial neonatal sepsis, bacterial septicemia, and serious bacterial infections of the CNS (meningitis), urinary tract, respiratory tract, gastrointestinal tract (including peritonitis), skin, bone and soft tissue (including burns) caused by susceptible strains of microorganisms.	(IM/IV) Serious Infections: 3mg/kg/day given q8h. Life-Threatening Infections: 5mg/kg/day tid-qid; reduce to 3mg/kg/day as soon as clinically indicated. Treat for 7-10 days; may need longer course in difficult and complicated infections. Renal Impairment: Reduced dose given q8h or usual dose given at prolonged intervals based on either CrCl or serum creatinine. Dialysis: 1-1.7mg/kg, depending on severity of infection, at end of each dialysis period. Obese Patients: Calculate dose based on estimated lean body mass.	6-7.5mg/kg/day (2-2.5mg/kg given q8h). Infants and Neonates: 7.5mg/kg/day (2.5mg/kg given q8h). Premature and Full-Term Neonates 1 week: 5mg/kg/day (2.5mg/kg given q12h). Treat for 7-10 days; may need longer course in difficult and complicated infections. Renal Impairment: Reduced dose given q8h or usual dose given at prolonged intervals based on either CrCl or serum creatinine. Dialysis: 2mg/kg at end of each dialysis period. Obese Patients: Calculate dose based on estimated lean body mass.

BRAND NAME (Generic)	DOSAGE FORM/ STRENGTH	INDICATIONS	ADULT DOSE	PEDIATRIC DOSE
Tobramycin (tobramycin sulfate)	**Inj:** 10mg/mL, 40mg/mL, 1.2g	Treatment of serious lower respiratory tract, CNS (eg, meningitis), intra-abdominal, bone, skin and skin structure, and complicated/recurrent urinary tract infections; and septicemia.	(IM/IV) Serious Infections: 3mg/kg/day given q8h. Life-Threatening Infections: Up to 5mg/kg/day given tid-qid. Reduce to 3mg/kg/day as soon as clinically indicated. Max: 5mg/kg/day unless serum levels monitored. Treat for 7-10 days; may need longer course in difficult and complicated infections. Severe Cystic Fibrosis: Initial: 10mg/kg/day given qid. Measure levels to determine subsequent doses. Renal Impairment: Initial: 1mg/kg followed by reduced doses given q8h or normal doses given at prolonged intervals based on either CrCl or serum creatinine. Do not use either method during dialysis. Obese Patients: Calculate dose based on estimated lean body weight plus 40% of the excess as the basic weight on which to figure mg/kg. ADD-Vantage vials are not for IM use.	>1 week: (IM/IV) 6-7.5mg/kg/day given tid-qid (eg, 2-2.5mg/kg q8h or 1.5-1.89mg/kg q6h). 1 week: Up to 2mg/kg q12h. Treat for 7-10 days; may need longer course in difficult and complicated infections. Severe Cystic Fibrosis: Initial: 10mg/kg/day given qid. Measure levels to determine subsequent doses. Renal Impairment: LD: 1mg/kg, followed by reduced doses given q8h or normal doses given at prolonged intervals based on either CrCl or serum creatinine. Do not use either method during dialysis. Obese Patients: Calculate dose based on estimated lean body weight plus 40% of the excess as the basic weight on which to figure mg/kg. ADD-Vantage vials are not for IM use.
Streptomycin sulfate	**Inj:** 1g	Treatment of moderate to severe infections such as mycobacterium tuberculosis (TB) and non-TB infections (eg, plague, tularemia, chancroid granuloma inguinale, *H.influenzae* and *K.pneumoniae* infections, UTI, gram-negative bacillary bacteremia, endocardial infections).	IM only. TB: 15mg/kg/day (Max: 1g), or 25-30mg/ kg twice weekly (Max: 1.5g), or 25-30mg/kg three times weekly (Max: 1.5g). Do not exceed a total dose of 120g over the course of therapy unless no other therapeutic options exist. Elderly (>60 yrs): Reduce dose. Treat for minimum of 1 year if possible. Tularemia: 1-2g/day in divided doses for 7-14 days until afebrile for 5-7 days. Plague: 1g bid for minimum of 10 days. Streptococcal Endocarditis: With PCN, 1g bid for week 1, then 500mg bid for week 2. Elderly (>60 yrs): 500mg bid for 2 weeks. Enterococcal Endocarditis: With PCN, 1g bid for 2 weeks, then 500mg bid for 4 weeks. Renal Impairment: Reduce dose. Moderate/Severe Infections: 1-2g/day in divided doses q6-12h. Max: 2g/day.	IM only. TB: 20-40mg/kg/day (Max: 1g), or 25-30 mg/kg twice weekly (Max: 1.5g), or 25-30mg/kg three times weekly (Max: 1.5g). Do not exceed a total dose of 120g over the course of therapy unless no other therapeutic options exist. Treat for minimum of 1 year if possible. Moderate/Severe Infections: 20-40mg/kg/day (8-20mg/lb/day) in divided doses q6-12h.
TOBI (tobramycin)	**Sol:** 60mg/mL (300mg/ampule)	Management of cystic fibrosis patients with *P.aeruginosa.*	Inhale via nebulizer 300mg q12h for 28 days, then stop for 28 days. Resume therapy for next 28-day on/28-day off cycle.	≥6 yrs: Inhale via nebulizer 300mg q12h for 28 days, then stop for 28 days. Resume therapy for next 28-day on/28-day off cycle.

(Continued)

BRAND NAME (Generic)	DOSAGE FORM/ STRENGTH	INDICATIONS	ADULT DOSE	PEDIATRIC DOSE
CARBAPENEMS				
Doribax (doripenem)	Inj: 500mg	Treatment of complicated intra-abdominal and urinary tract infections, including pyelonephritis, caused by susceptible microorganisms.	500 mg IV q8h for 5-14 days (intra-abdominal) or 10 days (UTI). Infuse over 1 hr. Renal impairment: CrCl: >50mL/min: No dose adjustment. CrCl 30-50mL/min: 250mg IV q8h. CrCl >10 to <30mL/min: 250mg IV q12h.	
Invanz (ertapenem sodium)	Inj: 1g	Treatment of complicated intra-abdominal infections; skin and skin structure infections (SSSI), including diabetic foot infections without osteomyelitis; community acquired pneumonia (CAP); complicated urinary tract infections (UTI) including pyelonephritis; acute pelvic infections including postpartum endomyometritis, septic abortion, and post surgical gynecologic infections; prophylaxis of surgical site infection following elective colorectal surgery.	Treatment: 1g IM/IV qd. Duration: Intra-Abdominal Infections: 5-14 days. CAP/UTI: 10-14 days. SSSI: 7-14 days. Pelvic Infection: 3-10 days. May administer IV for up to 14 days and IM for up to 7 days. CrCl ≤30mL/min/1.73m²: 500mg IM/IV qd. Hemodialysis: Give 150mg IM/IV after dialysis only if 500mg dose was given within 6 hrs prior to dialysis. Prophylaxis: 1g IV as single dose given 1 hr prior to surgical incision.	≥13 yrs: 1g IM/IV qd. 3 mo-12 yrs: 15mg/kg IM/IV bid (not to exceed 1g/day). Treatment Duration: Intra-Abdominal Infections: 5-14 days. SSSI: 7-14 days. CAP/UTI: 10-14 days. Pelvic Infections: 3-10 days. May administer IV for up to 14 days and IM for up to 7 days. CrCl ≤30mL/min/1.73 m²: 500mg IM/IV qd.
Merrem (meropenem)	Inj: 500mg, 1g	Treatment of intra-abdominal infections, bacterial meningitis, and complicated skin and skin structure infections (cSSSI) caused by susceptible strains of microorganisms.	Intra-Abdominal: 1g q8h. cSSSI: 500mg q8h. CrCl 26-50mL/min: 1 g q12h. CrCl 10-25mL/min: 500mg q12h. CrCl <10mL/min: 500mg q24h. cSSSI: 500mg q8h. CrCl 26-50mL/min: 500mg q12h. CrCl 10-25mL/min: 250mg q12h. CrCl <10mL/min: 250mg q24h.	3 months >50kg: Intra-Abdominal: 1g q8h. Meningitis: 2g q8h. cSSSI: 500mg q8h. 50kg: Intra-Abdominal: 20mg/kg q8h. Max: 1g q8h. Meningitis: 40mg/kg q8h. Max: 2g q8h. cSSSI: 10mg/kg q8h. Max: 500mg q8h.
CEPHALOSPORINS, FIRST GENERATION				
Cefazolin (cefazolin)	Inj: 500mg, 1g, 10g, 20g	Treatment of respiratory tract, urinary tract (UTI), skin and skin structure, biliary tract, bone and joint, and genital infections, septicemia, and endocarditis caused by susceptible strains of microorganisms. Perioperative prophylaxis for surgical procedures classified as contaminated or potentially contaminated.	Moderate-Severe Infections: 500mg-1g q6-8h. Mild Gram-Positive Cocci Infection: 250-500mg q8h. Acute, Uncomplicated UTI: 1g q12h. Pneumococcal Pneumonia: 500mg q12h. Severe Life-Threatening Infection (eg, Endocarditis, Septicemia): 1-1.5g q6h; Max: 12g/day (rare). Perioperative Prophylaxis: 1g IM/IV 0.5-1 hr before surgery. For Procedures ≥2 hrs: 500mg-1g IM/IV during surgery. Maint: 500mg-1g IM/IV q6-8h for 24 hrs post-op. Continue for 3-5 days post-op for devastating procedures (eg, open-heart surgery and prosthetic arthroplasty). Renal Impairment: CrCl 35-54 mL/min: Full dose q8h. CrCl 11-34 mL/min ½ usual dose q12h. CrCl <10mL/min: ¼ usual dose q18-24h. Apply reduced dosage recommendations after initial LT is given.	Mild-Moderately Severe Infection: 25-50mg/kg/day in 3-4 equal doses. Severe Infection: 100mg/kg/day in divided doses. Renal impairment: CrCl 40-70mL/min: 60% of normal daily dose in equally divided doses q12h. CrCl 20-40mL/min: 25% of normal daily dose in equally divided doses q12h. CrCl 5-20mL/min: 10% of normal daily dose q24h. Apply reduced dosage recommendations after initial LD is given.

BRAND NAME (Generic)	DOSAGE FORM/ STRENGTH	INDICATIONS	ADULT DOSE	PEDIATRIC DOSE
Duricef (cefadroxil monohydrate)	**Cap:** 500mg; **Sus:** 250mg/5mL [50mL, 100mL], 500mg/5mL [50mL, 75mL, 100mL]; **Tab:** 1g	Skin and skin structure infections (SSSI) and urinary tract infections (UTI), pharyngitis, and tonsillitis.	Uncomplicated Lower UTI: 1-2g/day given qd or bid. Other UTI: 1gm bid. SSSI: 1g qd or 500mg bid. Group A ß-hemolytic Strep Pharyngitis/ Tonsillitis: 1g qd or 500mg bid for 10 days. CrCl ≤50mL/min: Initial: 1g. Maint: CrCl 25-50mL/min: 500mg q12h; CrCl 10-25mL/min: 500mg q24h; CrCl 0-10mL/min: 500mg q36h	UTI/SSSI: 15mg/kg q12h. Pharyngitis/Tonsillitis/ Impetigo: 30mg/kg qd or 15mg/kg q12h. Treat ß-hemolytic strep infections for at least 10 days.
Keflex (cephalexin)	**Cap:** 250mg, 333mg 500mg, 750mg; **Sus:** 125mg/5mL, 250mg/5mL [100mL, 200mL]	Treatment of otitis media and skin and skin structure infections (SSSI); bone, genitourinary tract, and respiratory tract infections.	Usual: 25-50mg/kg/day in divided doses. Streptococcal Pharyngitis/SSSI/Uncomplicated Cystitis (>15 yrs): 500mg q12h. Treat cystitis for 7-14 days. Max: 4g/day.	Usual: 25-50mg/kg/day in divided doses. Streptococcal Pharyngitis (>1 yr)/SSSI: May divide dose and give q12h. Otitis Media: 75-100mg/kg/day in divided doses. Administer for ≥10 days in, ß-hemolytic streptococcal infections.
Panixine (cephalexin)	**Tab, Dispersible:** 125mg, 250mg	Skin and skin structure (SSSI), bone genitourinary and respiratory tract infections, otitis media, acute prostatitis.	Usual: 25-50mg/kg/day in divided doses. Streptococcal Pharyngitis/SSSI/Uncomplicated Cystitis (>15 yrs): 500mg q12h. Treat cystitis for 7-14 days. Max: 4g/day.	Usual: 25-50mg/kg/day in divided doses. Streptococcal Pharyngitis (>1 yr)/SSSI: May divide dose and give q12h. Otitis Media: 75-100mg/kg/day in divided doses. Administer for ≥10 days in, ß-hemolytic streptococcal infections.
CEPHALOSPORINS, SECOND GENERATION				
Cefaclor	**Cap:** 250mg, 500mg; **Sus:** 125mg/5mL [75mL, 150mL], 187mg/5mL [50mL], 250mg/5mL [75mL, 150mL], 375mg/5mL [50mL, 100mL]	Treatment of otitis media, pharyngitis, tonsillitis, lower respiratory tract, urinary tract, and skin and skin structure infections caused by susceptible strains of microorganisms.	Usual: 250mg q8h. Severe Infections/Pneumonia: 500mg q8h. Treat ß-hemolytic strep for 10 days.	≥1 mo: Usual: 20mg/kg/day given q8h. Otitis Media/Serious Infections: 40mg/kg/day. Max: 1g/day. May administer q12h for otitis media and pharyngitis. Treat ß-hemolytic strep for 10 days.
Cefaclor ER	**Tab, Extended-Release:** 375mg, 500mg	Acute bacterial exacerbation of chronic bronchitis (ABECB), secondary bacterial infections of acute bronchitis, pharyngitis, tonsillitis, and uncomplicated skin and skin structure infections (SSSI) caused by susceptible strains of microorganisms.	ABECB/Acute Bronchitis: 500mg q12h for 7 days. Pharyngitis/Tonsillitis: 375mg q12h for 10 days. SSSI: 375mg q12h for 7-10 days. Take with meals. Do not crush, cut or chew tab.	≥16 yrs: ABECB/Acute Bronchitis: 500mg q12h for 7 days. Pharyngitis/Tonsillitis: 375mg q12h for 10 days. SSSI: 375mg q12h for 7-10 days. Take with meals. Do not crush, cut or chew tab.

(Continued)

BRAND NAME (Generic)	DOSAGE FORM/ STRENGTH	INDICATIONS	ADULT DOSE	PEDIATRIC DOSE
CEPHALOSPORINS, SECOND GENERATION *(Continued)*				
Cefoxitin (cefoxitin sodium)	**Inj:** 1g, 1g/50mL, 2g, 2g/50mL, 10g	Treatment of lower respiratory tract, urinary tract, intra-abdominal, gynecological, skin and skin structure, and bone and joint infections, and septicemia. For surgical prophylaxis.	Usual: 1-2g IV q6-8h. Uncomplicated Infections: 1g IV q6-8h. Moderate-Severe: 1g IV q4h or 2g IV q6-8h. Gas Gangrene/Other Infections Requiring Higher Dose: 2g IV q4h or 3g IV q6h. Renal Insufficiency: LD: 1-2g IV. Maint: CrCl 30-50mL/ min: 1-2g IV q8-12h. CrCl 10-29mL/min: 1-2g IV q12-24h. CrCl 5-9mL/min: 0.5-1g IV q12-24h. CrCl <5mL/min: 0.5-1g IV q24-48h. Hemodialysis: LD: 1-2g IV after dialysis. Maint: See renal insufficiency doses above. Prophylaxis: Uncontaminated GI Surgery/Hysterectomy: 2g IV 0.5-1 hr prior to surgery, then 2g IV q6h after first dose up to 24 hrs. C-Section: 2g IV single dose after umbilical cord is clamped, or 2g IV after umbilical cordis clamped followed by 2g IV 4 and 8 hrs after initial dose.	≥3 mo: 80-160mg/kg/day divided into 4-6 equal doses. Max: 12g/day. Prophylaxis: Uncontaminated GI Surgery/Hysterectomy: 30-40mg/kg IV 0.5-1 hr prior to surgery, then 30-40mg/kg IV q6h after first dose up to 24 hrs.
Ceftin (cefuroxime axetil)	**Sus:** 125mg/5mL [100mL], 250mg/ 5mL [50mL, 100mL]; **Tab:** 125mg, 250mg, 500mg	(Sus/Tab) Pharyngitis/tonsillitis, acute otitis media, and impetigo. (Tab) Uncomplicated skin and skin structure (SSSI), and urinary tract infection (UTI), gonorrhea, early lyme disease, acute bacterial maxillary sinusitis, acute bacterial exacerbations of chronic bronchitis (ABECB) and secondary bacterial infections of acute bronchitis.	(Tab) Pharyngitis/Tonsillitis/Sinusitis: 250mg bid for 10 days. ABECB/SSSI: 250-500mg bid for 10 days. Acute Bronchitis: 250-500mg bid for 5-10 days. UTI: 125-250mg bid for 7-10 days. Gonorrhea: 1000mg single dose. Lyme Disease: 500mg bid for 20 days.	≥13 yrs: (Tab) Pharyngitis/Tonsillitis/Sinusitis: 250mg bid for 10 days. ABECB/SSSI: 250-500mg bid for 10 days. Acute Bronchitis: 250-500mg bid for 5-10 days. UTI: 125-250mg bid for 7-10 days. Gonorrhea: 1000mg single dose. Lyme Disease: 500mg bid for 20 days. 3 mo-12 yrs: (Sus) Pharyngitis/Tonsillitis: 10mg/kg bid for 10 days. Max: 500mg/day. Otitis Media/Sinusitis/Impetigo: 15mg/kg bid for 10 days. Max: 1000mg/day. (Tab-if can swallow whole) Pharyngitis/Tonsillitis: 125mg bid for 10 days. Otitis Media/Sinusitis: 250mg bid for 10 days.
Cefzil (cefprozil)	**Sus:** 125mg/5mL, 250mg/5mL [50mL, 75mL, 100mL]; **Tab:** 250mg, 500mg	Mild to moderate pharyngitis/tonsillitis, otitis media, acute sinusitis, secondary bacterial infection of acute bronchitis, acute bacterial exacerbation of chronic bronchitis (ABECB), and uncomplicated skin and skin structure infections (SSSI).	≥13 yrs: Pharyngitis/Tonsillitis: 500mg q24h for 10 days. Acute Sinusitis: 250-500mg q12h for 10 days. ABECB/Acute Bronchitis: 500mg q12h for 10 days. SSSI: 250-500mg q12h or 500mg q24h. CrCl <30mL/min: 50% of standard dose.	2-12 yrs: Pharyngitis/Tonsillitis: 7.5mg/kg q12h for 10 days. SSSI: 20mg/kg q24h for 10 days. 6 mos-12 yrs: Otitis Media: 15mg/kg q12h for 10 days. Acute Sinusitis: 7.5-15mg/kg q12h for 10 days. Do not exceed adult dose. CrCl <30mL/min: 50% of standard dose.

BRAND NAME (Generic)	DOSAGE FORM/ STRENGTH	INDICATIONS	ADULT DOSE	PEDIATRIC DOSE
Mefoxin (cefoxitin sodium)	**Inj:** 1g, 1g/50mL, 2g, 2g/50mL, 10g	Treatment of lower respiratory tract, urinary tract, intra-abdominal, gynecological, skin and skin structure, and bone and joint infections, and septicemia. For surgical prophylaxis.	Usual: 1-2g IV q6-8h. Uncomplicated Infections: 1g IV q6-8h. Moderate-Severe: 1g IV q4h or 2g IV q6-8h. Gas Gangrene/Other Infections Requiring Higher Dose: 2g IV q4h or 3g IV q6h. Renal Insufficiency: LD: 1-2g IV. Maint: CrCl 30-50mL/min: 1-2g IV q8-12h. CrCl 10-29mL/min: 1-2g IV q12-24h. CrCl 5-9mL/min: 0.5-1g IV q12-24h. CrCl <5mL/min: 0.5-1g IV q24-48h. Hemodialysis: LD: 1-2g IV after dialysis. Maint: See renal insufficiency doses above. Prophylaxis: Uncontaminated GI Surgery/Hysterectomy: 2g IV q6h after first dose up to 24 hrs. C-Section: 2g IV single dose after umbilical cord is clamped, or 2g IV after umbilical cord is clamped followed by 2g IV 4 and 8 hrs after initial dose.	≥3 mos: 80-160mg/kg/day divided into 4-6 equal doses. Max: 12g/day. Prophylaxis: Uncontaminated GI Surgery/Hysterectomy: 30-40mg/kg IV 0.5-1 hr prior to surgery, then 30-40mg/kg IV q6h after first dose up to 24 hrs.
Zinacef (cefuroxime)	**Inj:** 750mg, 1.5g, 7.5g, 750mg/50mL, 1.5g/50mL	Treatment of septicemia; meningitis; gonorrhea; lower respiratory tract, urinary tract, skin and skin structure (SSSI), and bone and joint infections caused by susceptible strains of microorganisms. For preoperative and perioperative surgical prophylaxis.	Usual: 750mg-1.5g q8h for 5-10 days. Uncomplicated Pneumonia and UTI/SSSI/Disseminated Gonococcal Infections: 750mg q8h. Severe/Complicated Infections: 1.5g q8h. Bone and Joint Infections: 1.5g q8h. Life-Threatening Infections/Infections With Susceptible Organisms: 1.5g q6h. Meningitis: Max: 3g q8h. Uncomplicated Gonococcal Infection: 1.5g IM single dose at 2 different sites with 1g PO probenecid. Surgical Prophylaxis: 1.5g IV 0.5-1 hr before incision, then 750mg IM/IV q8h with prolonged procedure. Open Heart Surgery (Perioperative): 1.5g IV at induction of anesthesia and q12h thereafter, for total of 6g. Renal impairment: CrCl 10-20mL/min: 750mg q12h. CrCl <10mL/min: 750mg q24h. Hemodialysis: Give further dose at end of dialysis.	>3 months: Usual: 50-100 mg/kg/day in divided doses q6-8h. Severe infections: 100mg/kg/day (not to exceed max adult dose). Bone and Joint Infections: 150mg/kg/day in divided doses q8h (not to exceed max adult dose). Meningitis: 200-240mg/kg/day IV in divided doses q6-8h. Renal Dysfunction: Modify dosing frequency consistent with adult recommendations.

(Continued)

BRAND NAME (Generic)	DOSAGE FORM/ STRENGTH	INDICATIONS	ADULT DOSE	PEDIATRIC DOSE
CEPHALOSPORINS, THIRD GENERATION				
Cedax (ceftibuten)	**Cap:** 400mg; **Sus:** 90mg/5mL [30mL, 60mL, 90mL, 120mL]	Acute bacterial exacerbations of chronic bronchitis (ABECB), acute bacterial otitis media, pharyngitis and tonsillitis.	ABECB/Otitis Media/Pharyngitis/Tonsillitis: 400mg qd for 10 days. Max: 400mg/day. CrCl 30-49mL/min: 4.5mg/kg or 200mg qd. CrCl 5-29mL/min: 2.25mg/kg or 100mg qd. Take 2 hrs before or at least 1 hr after a meal.	≥6 mo: Pharyngitis/Tonsillitis/Otitis Media: 9mg/kg qd for 10 days. Max: 400mg. ABECB/Otitis Media/ Pharyngitis/Tonsillitis: ≥12 yrs: 400mg qd for 10 days Max: 400mg/day. CrCl 30-49mL/min: 4.5mg/kg or 200mg qd. CrCl 5-29mL/min: 2.25mg/kg or 100mg qd. Take 2 hrs before or at least 1 hr after a meal.
Cefizox (ceftizoxime)	**Inj:** 1g, 2g, 10g	Treatment of lower respiratory tract, skin and skin structure, intra-abdominal, bone and joint, and urinary tract infections (UTI), gonorrhea, pelvic inflammatory disease (PID), meningitis, and septicemia.	Uncomplicated UTI: 500mg q12h IM/IV. Other Sites: 1g q8-12h IM/IV. Severe/Refractory Infections: 1-2g IM/IV q8-12h. PID: 2g IV q8h. Life Threatening Infections: 3-4g IV q8h. Uncomplicated Gonorrhea: 1g IM as single dose. Renal Impairment: LD: 500mg-1g IM/IV. Less Severe Infection: Maint: CrCl 50-79mL/min: 500mg q8h. CrCl 5-49mL/min: 250-500mg q12h. CrCl 0-4mL/min (Dialysis): 500mg q48h or 250mg q24h. Life Threatening Infection: Maint: CrCl 50-79mL/min: 0.75-1.5g q8h. CrCl 5-49mL/min: 0.5-1g q12h. CrCl 0-4mL/min (Dialysis): 0.5-1g q48h or 0.5g q24h.	≥6 mos: 50mg/kg IM/IV q6-8h, up to 200mg/kg/day. Max: 6g/day for serious infections.
Fortaz (ceftazidime)	**Inj:** 500mg, 1g, 1g/50mL, 2g, 2g/50mL, 6g	Treatment of lower respiratory tract (eg, pneumonia), skin and skin structure (SSSI), bone and joint, gynecologic, CNS (eg, meningitis), intra-abdominal, and urinary tract infections (UTI), and septicemia. For use in sepsis.	≥12 yrs: Usual: 1g IM/IV q8-12h. Uncomplicated UTI: 250 mg IM/IV q12h. Complicated UTI: 500 mg IM/IV q8-12h. Bone and Joint Infection: 2g IV q 12h. Uncomplicated Pneumonia/SSSI: 500mg-1g IM/IV q8h. Gynecological/Intra-Abdominal/Meningitis/ Severe Life-Threatening Infection: 2g IV q8h. Lung Infection caused by Pseudomonas spp. in Cystic Fibrosis (normal renal function): 30-50mg/kg IV q8h. Max: 6g/day. CrCl 31-50mL/min: 1g q12h. CrCl 16-30mL/min: 1g q24h. CrCl 6-15mL/min: 500mg q24h. CrCl <5mL/min: 500mg q48h. For severe infections (6g/day), increase renal impairment dose by 50% or increase dosing interval. Apply reduced dosage recommendations after initial 1g LD is given. Hemodialysis: Give 1g before then 1g after each hemodialysis. Intra-Peritoneal Dialysis/ Continuous Peritoneal Dialysis: Ambulatory Peritoneal Dialysis: Give 1g followed by 500mg q24h.	≥12 yrs: Usual: 1g IM/IV q8-12h. Uncomplicated UTI: 250mg IM/IV q12h. Complicated UTI: 500mg IM/IV q8-12h. Bone and Joint Infection: 2g IV q12h. Uncomplicated Pneumonia/SSSI: 500mg-1g IM/IV q8h. Gynecological/Intra-Abdominal/Meningitis/ Severe Life-Threatening Infection: 2g IV q8h. Lung Infection caused by Pseudomonas spp. in Cystic Fibrosis (normal renal function): 30-50mg/kg IV q8h. Max: 6g/day. CrCl 31-50mL/min: 1g q12h. CrCl 16-30mL/min: 1g q24h. CrCl 6-15mL/min: 500mg q24h. CrCl <5mL/min: 500mg q48h. For severe infections (6g/day), increase renal impairment dose by 50% or increase dosing interval. Apply reduced dosage recommendations after initial 1g LD is given. Hemodialysis: Give 1g before then 1g after each hemodialysis. Intra-Peritoneal Dialysis/Continuous Ambulatory Peritoneal Dialysis: Give 1g followed by 500mg q24h.

BRAND NAME (Generic)	DOSAGE FORM/ STRENGTH	INDICATIONS	ADULT DOSE	PEDIATRIC DOSE
Claforan (cefotaxime sodium)	Inj: 500mg, 1g, 2g, 10g	Treatment of lower respiratory tract, genitourinary, gynecologic, intra-abdominal, skin and skin structure, bone and joint, and CNS infections (eg, meningitis), bacteremia, and septicemia. For surgical prophylaxis.	Gonococcal Urethritis/Cervicitis (Males/Females): 500mg single dose IM. Rectal Gonorrhea: 0.5g (females) or 1g (males) single dose IM. Uncomplicated Infections: 1g IM/IV q12h. Moderate-Severe Infections: 1-2g IM/IV q8h. Septicemia: 2g IV q6-8h. Life-Threatening Infections: 2g IV q4h. Max: 12g/day. Surgical Prophylaxis: 1g IM/IV 30-90 min before surgery. Cesarean Section: 1g IV when umbilical cord is clamped, then 1g IV at 6 and 12 hrs after 1st dose. CrCl <20mL/min/1.73 m²: Give ½ of usual dose.	≥50kg: Use adult dose. Max: 12g/day. 1mo-12 yrs and ≤50kg: 50-180mg/kg/day IM/IV divided in 4-6 doses. 1-4 weeks: 50mg/kg IV q8h. 0-1 week: 50mg/kg IV q12h. CrCl <20mL/min/1.73 m²: Give ½ of usual dose.
Fortaz (ceftazidime)	Inj: 500mg, 1g, 1g/50mL, 2g, 2g/50mL, 6g	Treatment of lower respiratory tract (eg, pneumonia), skin and skin structure (SSSI), bone and joint, gynecologic, CNS (eg, meningitis), intra-abdominal, and urinary tract infections (UTI), and septicemia. For use in sepsis.	Usual: 1g IM/IV q8-12h. Uncomplicated UTI: 250mg IM/IV q12h. Complicated UTI: 500mg IM/ IV q8-12h. Bone and Joint Infection: 2g IV q12h. Uncomplicated Pneumonia/SSSI: 500mg-1g IM/IV q8h. Gynecological/Intra-Abdominal/Meningitis/ Severe Life-Threatening Infection: 2g IV q8h. Lung Infection Caused by Pseudomonas spp. in Cystic Fibrosis (Normal Renal Function): 30-50mg/kg IV q8h. Max: 6g/day. CrCl 31-50mL/min: 1g q12h. CrCl 16-30mL/min: 1g q24h. CrCl 6-15mL/min: 500mg q24h. CrCl <5mL/min: 500mg q48h. For severe infections (6g/day), increase renal impairment dose by 50% or increase dosing interval. Apply reduced dosage recommendations after initial 1g LD is given Hemodialysis: Give 1g before then 1g after each hemodialysis. Intra-Peritoneal Dialysis/Continuous Ambulatory Peritoneal Dialysis: Give 1g followed by 500mg q24h, or add to fluid at 250mg/2L.	1 mo-12 yrs: 30-50mg/kg IV q8h. Max: 6g/day. Neonates (0-4 weeks): 30mg/kg IV q12h. Higher doses for cystic fibrosis or meningitis. CrCl 31-50 mL/min: 1g q12h. CrCl 16-30mL/min: 1g q24h. CrCl 6-15mL/min: 500mg q24h. CrCl <5mL/min: 500mg q48h. For severe infections (6g/day), increase renal impairment dose by 50% or increase dosing interval. Apply reduced dosage recommendations after initial 1g LD is given. Hemodialysis: Give 1g before then 1g after each hemodialysis. Intra-Peritoneal Dialysis/Continuous Ambulatory Peritoneal Dialysis: Give 1g followed by 500mg q24h, or add to fluid at 250mg/2L.

(Continued)

BRAND NAME (Generic)	DOSAGE FORM/ STRENGTH	INDICATIONS	ADULT DOSE	PEDIATRIC DOSE
CEPHALOSPORINS, THIRD GENERATION *(Continued)*				
Omnicef (cefdinir)	**Cap:** 300mg; **Sus:** 125mg/5mL, 250mg/5mL [60mL, 100mL]	Community acquired pneumonia (CAP), acute exacerbations of chronic bronchitis (AECB), acute maxillary sinusitis, pharyngitis/tonsillitis, uncomplicated skin and structure infections (SSSI), and acute bacterial otitis media.	(Cap) SSSI/Cap: 300mg q12h for 10 days. AECB/Pharyngitis/Tonsillitis: 300mg q12h for 5-10 days or 600mg q24h for 10 days. Sinusitis: 300mg q12h or 600mg q24h for 10 days. CrCl <30mL/min: 300mg qd.	(Sus) 6 mo-12 yrs: OtitisMedia/Pharyngitis/Tonsillitis: 7mg/kg q12h for 5-10 days or 14mg/kg q24h for 10 days. Sinusitis: 7mg/kg q12h or 14mg/kg q24h for 10 days. SSSI: 7mg/kg q12h for 10 days. (Cap) ≥13 yrs: CAP/SSSI: 300mg q12h for 10 days. AECB/Pharyngitis/Tonsillitis: 300mg q12h for 5-10 days or 600mg q24h for 10 days. Sinusitis: 300mg q12h or 600mg q24h for 10 days. CrCl <30mL/min/1.73m²: 7mg/kg qd. Max: 300mg qd.
Rocephin (ceftriaxone sodium)	**Inj:** 250mg, 500mg, 1g, 2g, 10g	Treatment of lower respiratory tract infections, skin and skin structure infections, bone and joint infections, intra-abdominal infections, acute otitis media, uncomplicated gonorrhea, pelvic inflammatory disease, UTI, septicemia, and meningitis. For surgical prophylaxis.	Usual: 1-2g/day IV/IM given qd-bid. Max: 4g/day. Gonorrhea: 250mg IM single dose. Surgical Prophylaxis: 1g IV ½-2 hrs before surgery.	Skin Infections: 50-75mg/kg/day IV/IM given qd-bid. Max: 2g/day. Otitis Media: 50mg/kg (up to 1g) IM single dose. Serious Infections: 50-75mg/kg/day IM/IV given q12h. Max: 2g/day. Meningitis: Initial: 100mg/kg (up to 4g), then 100mg/kg/day given qd-bid for 7-14 days. Max: 4g/day.
Spectracef (cefditoren pivoxil)	**Tab:** 200mg	Treatment of acute bacterial exacerbations of chronic bronchitis (ABECB), pharyngitis/tonsillitis, community acquired pneumonia (CAP), and uncomplicated skin and skin-structure infections (SSSI).	ABECB: 400mg bid for 10 days. Pharyngitis/Tonsillitis/SSSI: 200mg bid for 10 days. Cap: 400mg bid for 14 days. CrCl 30-49mL/min: 200mg bid. CrCl<30mL/min: 200mg qd. Take with meals.	≥12 yrs: ABECB: 400mg bid for 10 days. Pharyngitis/Tonsillitis/SSSI: 200mg bid for 10 days. Cap: 400mg bid for 14 days. CrCl 30-49mL/min: 200mg bid. CrCl<30mL/min: 200mg qd. Take with meals.
Suprax (cefixime)	**Sus:** 100mg/5mL [50mL, 75mL, 100mL]	Otitis media, pharyngitis, tonsillitis, acute bronchitis, acute exacerbation of chronic bronchitis, uncomplicated UTIs, and cervical/urethral gonorrhea caused by susceptible strains.	Usual: 400mg qd. Gonorrhea: 400mg single dose. CrCl 21-60mL/min/Hemodialysis: Give 75% of standard dose. CrCl <20mL/min/CAPD: Give 50% of standard dose.	>12 yrs or >50kg: (Tab/Sus) Usual: 400mg qd. ≥6 mos: (Sus) 8mg/kg qd or 4mg/kg bid. Treat for at least 10 days with *S. pyogenes*. CrCl 21-60mL/min/Hemodialysis: Give 75% of standard dose. CrCl <20mL/min/CAPD: Give 50% of standard dose.

BRAND NAME (Generic)	DOSAGE FORM/ STRENGTH	INDICATIONS	ADULT DOSE	PEDIATRIC DOSE
Tazicef (ceftazidime)	Inj: 1g, 2g, 6g	Treatment of lower respiratory tract (eg, pneumonia), skin and skin structure (SSSI), bone and joint, gynecologic, CNS (eg, meningitis), intra-abdominal, and urinary tract infections (UTI), and septicemia. For use in sepsis.	Usual: 1g IM/IV q8-12h. Uncomplicated UTI: 250mg IM/IV q12h. Complicated UTI: 500mg IM/IV q8-12h. Bone and Joint Infection: 2g IV q12h. Uncomplicated Pneumonia/SSSI: 500mg-1g IM/IV q8h. Gynecological/Intra-Abdominal/Meningitis/Severe Life-Threatening Infection: 2g IV q8h. Lung Infection caused by Pseudomonas in Cystic Fibrosis (normal renal function): 30-50mg/kg IV q8h. Max: 6g/day. Renal Impairment: CrCl 31-50mL/min: 1g q12h. CrCl 16-30mL/min: 1g q24h. CrCl 6-15mL/min: 500mg q24h. CrCl <5mL/min: 500mg q48h. For severe renal impairment dose by 50% or increase dosing interval. Apply reduced dosage recommendations after initial 1g LD is given. Hemodialysis: Give 1g before and 1g after each hemodialysis. Intra-Peritoneal Dialysis/Continuous Ambulatory Peritoneal Dialysis: Give 1g followed by 500mg q24h, or add to fluid at 250mg/2L.	Neonates (0-4 weeks): 30mg/kg IV q12h. 1 mo-12 yrs: 30-50mg/kg IV q8h. Max: 6g/day. Higher doses for patients with cystic fibrosis or when treating meningitis. Renal Impairment: CrCl 31-50mL/min: 1g q12h. CrCl 16-30mL/min: 1g q24h. CrCl 6-5mL/min: 500mg q24h. CrCl <5mL/min: 500mg q48h. For severe renal impairment dose by 50% or increase dosing interval. Apply reduced dosage recommendations after initial 1g LD is given. Hemodialysis: Give 1g before and 1g after each hemodialysis. Intra-Peritoneal Dialysis/Continuous Ambulatory Peritoneal Dialysis: Give 1g followed by 500mg q24h, or add fluid at 250mg/2L.
Tazidime (ceftazidime)	Inj: 1g, 2g, 6g	Treatment of lower respiratory tract (eg, pneumonia), skin and skin structure (SSSI), bone and joint, gynecologic, CNS (eg, meningitis), intra-abdominal and urinary tract infections (UTI). For use in sepsis.	Usual: 1g IM/IV q8-12h. Uncomplicated UTI: 250mg IM/IV q12h. Complicated UTI: 500mg IM/IV q8-12h. Bone and Joint Infection: 2g IV q12h. Uncomplicated Pneumonia/Skin and Skin Structure Infection: 500mg-1g IM/IV q8h. Gynecological/Intra-Abdominal/Meningitis/Severe Life-Threatening Infection: 2g IV q8h. Lung Infection caused by Pseudomonas spp. in Cystic Fibrosis (normal renal function): 30-50mg/kg IV q8h. Max: 6g/day. Renal Impairment: CrCl 31-50mL/min: 1g q12h. CrCl 16-30mL/min: 1g q24h. CrCl 6-15mL/min: 500mg q24h. CrCl <5mL/min: 500mg q48h. For severe infections (6g/day), increase renal impairment dose by 50% or increase dosing interval. Apply reduced dosage recommendations after initial 1g LD is given. Hemodialysis: Give 1g before then 1g after each hemodialysis. Intra-Peritoneal Dialysis/Continuous Ambulatory Peritoneal Dialysis: Give 1g followed by 500mg q24h, or add to fluid at 250mg/2L.	Neonates (0-4 weeks): 30mg/kg IV q12h. 1 mo-12 yrs: 30-50mg/kg IV q8h. Max: 6g/day. Higher doses for cystic fibrosis and meningitis. Renal Impairment: CrCl 31-50mL/min: 1g q12h. CrCl 16-30mL/min: 1g q24h. CrCl 6-15mL/min: 500mg q24h. CrCl <5mL/min: 500mg q48h. For severe infections (6g/day), increase renal impairment dose by 50% or increase dosing interval. Apply reduced dosage recommendations after initial 1g LD is given. Hemodialysis: Intra-Peritoneal Dialysis/Continuous Ambulatory Peritoneal Dialysis: Give 1g followed by 500mg q24h, or add to fluid at 250mg/2L.

(Continued)

BRAND NAME (Generic)	DOSAGE FORM/ STRENGTH	INDICATIONS	ADULT DOSE	PEDIATRIC DOSE
CEPHALOSPORIN, THIRD GENERATION *(Continued)*				
Vantin (cefpodoxime proxetil)	**Sus:** 50mg/mL [50mL, 50mL]; 100mg/5mL [50mL, 75mL, 100mL]; **Tab:** 100mg, 200mg	Acute otitis media, pharyngitis/tonsillitis, community acquired pneumonia (CAP), acute bacterial exacerbation of chronic bronchitis (ABECB), acute uncomplicated urethral and cervical gonorrhea, acute uncomplicated ano-rectal infections in women, uncomplicated skin and skin structure infections (SSSI), acute maxillary sinusitis, uncomplicated urinary tract infections (UTI).	Take tabs with food. Pharyngitis/Tonsillitis: 100mg q12h for 5-10 days. Cap: 200mg q12h for 14 days. ABECB: 200mg q12h for 10 days. Uncomplicated Gonorrhea (Men and Women)/Rectal Gonococcal Infections (women): 200mg single dose. SSSI: 400mg q12h for 7-14 days. Sinusitis: 200mg q12h for 10 days. UTI: 100mg q12h for 7 days. CrCl<30mL/min: Increase interval to q24h. Hemodialysis: Dose 3 times weekly after dialysis.	≥12 yrs: Take tabs with food. Pharyngitis/Tonsillitis: 100mg q12h for 5-10 days. Cap: 200mg q12h for 14 days. ABECB: 200mg q12h for 10 days. Uncomplicated Gonorrhea (men and women)/Rectal Gonococcal Infections (women): 200mg single dose. SSSI: 400mg q12h for 7-14 days. Sinusitis: 200mg q12h for 10 days. UTI: 100mg q12h for 7 days. 2 mos-11 yrs: Otitis Media: 5mg/kg q12h for 5 days. Max: 200mg/dose. Pharyngitis/Tonsillitis: 5mg/kg q12h for 5-10 days. Max: 100mg/dose. Sinusitis: 5mg/kg q12h for 10 days. Max:200mg/dose. CrCl<30mL/min: Increase interval to q24h. Hemodialysis: Dose 3 times weekly after dialysis.
CEPHALOSPORIN, FOURTH GENERATION				
Maxipime (cefepime HCl)	**Inj:** 500mg, 1g, 2g	Treatment of uncomplicated/complicated urinary tract (UTI), uncomplicated skin and skin structure (SSSI), and complicated intra-abdominal infections, and pneumonia. Emperic therapy for febrile neutropenia.	Moderate-Severe Pneumonia: 1-2g IV q12h for 10 days. Febrile Neutropenia Emperic Therapy: 2g IV q8h for 7 days or until neutropenia resolved. Mild-Moderate UTI: 0.5-1g IM/IV q12h for 7-10 days. Severe UTI/Moderate-Severe SSSI: 2g IV q12h for 10 days. Complicated Intra-Abdominal Infections: 2g IV q12h for 7-10 days. CrCl<60mL/min: Initial: Same dose as normal renal function. Maint: Refer to prescribing information for dose-adjustment.	2 months-16 yrs: ≤40kg: UTI/SSSI/Pneumonia: 50mg/kg IV q12h. Febrile Neutropenia: 50mg/kg IV q8h. Max: Do not exceed adult dose. CrCl ≤60mL/min: Initial: Same dose as normal renal function. Maint: Refer to prescribing information for dose adjustment.
FLUOROQUINOLONES				
Avelox (moxifloxacin HCl)	**Inj:** 400mg/250mL; **Tab:** 400mg [ABC pack, 5 tabs]	Acute bacterial sinusitis, acute bacterial exacerbation of chronic bronchitis (ABECB), uncomplicated skin and skin structure infections (SSSI), complicated skin and skin structure infections (cSSSI), complicated intra-abdominal infections (cIAI), and community acquired pneumonia (CAP), including multi-drug resistant *S.pneumoniae*.	≥18 yrs: Sinusitis: 400mg PO/IV q24h for 10 days. ABECB: 400mg PO/IV q24h for 5 days. SSSI: 400mg PO/IV q24h for 7 days. cSSSI: 400mg PO/IV q24h for 7-21 days. cIAI: 400mg IV q24h for 5-14 days. Cap: 400mg PO/IV q24h for 7-14 days.	

BRAND NAME (Generic)	DOSAGE FORM/ STRENGTH	INDICATIONS	ADULT DOSE	PEDIATRIC DOSE
Cipro (ciprofloxacin HCl)	**Sus:** 250mg/5mL, 500mg/5mL [100mL]; **Tab:** 250mg, 500mg, 750mg	Treatment of lower respiratory tract (LRTI), complicated intra-abdominal, skin and skin structure (SSSI), bone and joint, and urinary tract infections (UTI), acute exacerbations of chronic bronchitis, acute sinusitis, acute uncomplicated cystitis in females, chronic bacterial prostatitis, infectious diarrhea, typhoid fever, post-exposure inhalational anthrax, uncomplicated cervical and urethral gonorrhea, complicated UTI and pyelonephritis in pediatrics.	≥18 yrs: Acute Sinusitis/Typhoid Fever: 500mg q12h for 10 days. LRTI/SSSI: Mild-Moderate: 500mg q12h for 7-14 days. Severe/Complicated: 750mg q12h for 7-14 days. Cystitis/Acute Uncomplicated UTI: 250mg q12h for 3 days. Mild-Moderate UTI: 250mg q12h for 7-14 days. Severe/Complicated UTI: 500mg q12h for 7-14 days. Chronic Bacterial Prostatitis: 500mg q12h for 28 days. Intra-Abdominal: 500mg q12h (w/ metronidazole) for 7-14 days. Bone and Joint: Mild-Moderate: 500mg q12h for ≥4-6 weeks. Severe/Complicated: 750mg q12h for ≥4-6 weeks. Infectious Diarrhea: 500mg q12h for 5-7 days. Uncomplicated Urethral/Cervical Gonococcal: 250mg single dose. Inhalational Anthrax: 500mg q12h for 60 days. CrCl 30-50mL/min: 250-500mg q12h. CrCl 5-29mL/min: 250-500mg q18h. Hemodialysis/Peritoneal Dialysis: 250-500mg q24h (after dialysis). Administer at least 2 hrs before or 6 hrs after magnesium or aluminum containing antacids, sucralfate, Videx (didanosine) chewable/buffered tablets or pediatric powder, or other products containing calcium, iron or zinc.	<18 yrs: Inhalational Anthrax: 15mg/kg q12h for 60 days. Max: 500mg/dose. 1-17 yrs: Complicated UTI/Pyelonephritis: 10-20mg/kg q12h for 10-21 days. Max: 750mg/dose.

(Continued)

BRAND NAME (Generic)	DOSAGE FORM/ STRENGTH	INDICATIONS	ADULT DOSE	PEDIATRIC DOSE
FLUOROQUINOLONES *(Continued)*				
Cipro IV (ciprofloxacin)	**Inj:** 10mg/mL, 200mg/100mL, 400mg/200mL	Treatment of skin and skin structure (SSSI), bone and joint, complicated intra-abdominal infections, lower respiratory (LRTI), and urinary tract infections (UTI), nosocomial pneumonia, acute sinusitis, chronic bacterial prostatitis, post-exposure inhalational anthrax, empirical therapy for febrile neutropenia, complicated UTI and pyelonephritis in pediatrics	≥18 yrs: IV: UTI: Mild-Moderate: 200mg q12h for 7-14 days. Complicated/Severe: 400mg q12h for 7-14 days. LRTI/SSSI: Mild-Moderate: 400mg q12h for 7-14 days. Complicated/Severe: 400mg q8h for 7-14 days. Bone and Joint: Mild-Moderate: 400mg q12h for ≥4-6 weeks. Complicated/Severe: 400mg q8h for ≥4-6 weeks. Nosocomial Pneumonia: 400mg q8h for 10-14 days. Complicated Intra-Abdominal: 400mg q12h (w/metronidazole) for 7-14 days. Acute Sinusitis: 400mg q12h for 10 days. Chronic Bacterial Prostatitis: 400mg q12h for 28 days. Febrile Neutropenia: 400mg q8h (w/piperacillin 50mg/kg q4h) for 7-14 days. Max: 24g/day. Inhalational Anthrax: 400mg q12h for 60 days. Administer over 60 min. CrCl 5-29mL/min: 200-400mg q18-24h.	<18 yrs: Inhalational Anthrax: 10mg/kg q12h for 60 days. Max: 400mg/dose; 800mg/day. 1-17 yrs: Complicated UTI/Pyleonephritis: 6-10mg/kg q8h for 10-21 days. Max: 400mg/dose.
Cipro XR (ciprofloxacin)	**Tab, Extended-Release:** 500mg, 1000mg	Uncomplicated (acute cystitis) and complicated urinary tract infections (UTI), and acute uncomplicated pyelonephritis due to *E.coli.*	≥18 yrs: Uncomplicated UTI: 500mg qd or 3 days. Complicated UTI: 1000mg qd for 7-14 days. CrCl <30mL/min: 500 mg qd. Acute Uncomplicated Pyelonephritis: 1000mg qd for 7-14 days. CrCl <30mL/min: 500mg qd. Take with fluids. Administer at least 2 hrs before or 6 hrs after magnesium or aluminum containing antacids, sucralfate, Videx (didanosine) chewable/buffered tablets or pediatric powder, metal cations (eg, iron), multivitamins with zinc. Avoid concomitant administration with dairy products alone, or with calcium-fortified products. Space concomitant calcium intake (>800mg) by at least 2 hrs. Do not split, crush, or chew. Swallow tab whole. Dialysis: Give after procedure is completed.	

BRAND NAME (Generic)	DOSAGE FORM/ STRENGTH	INDICATIONS	ADULT DOSE	PEDIATRIC DOSE
Factive (gemifloxacin mesylate)	**Tab:** 320mg	Treatment of community-acquired pneumonia (CAP), including multi-drug resistant *Streptococcus pneumoniae* (MDRSP), and acute bacterial exacerbation of chronic bronchitis (ABECB).	≥18 yrs: ABECB: 320mg qd for 5 days. Cap: 320mg qd for 5 days *S.pneumoniae*, *H.influenzae*, *M. pneumoniae*, or *C.pneumoniae* or 7 days (MDRSP, *K.pneumoniae*, or *M.catarrhalis*. Renal Impairment: CrCl ≤40mL/min or Dialysis: 160mg qd. Take with fluids.	
Floxin (ofloxacin)	**Tab:** 200mg, 300mg, 400mg	Treatment of acute urinary tract (UTI) and uncomplicated skin and skin structure infection (SSSI), acute bacterial exacerbation of chronic bronchitis (ABECB), community acquired pneumonia (CAP), acute uncomplicated urethral and cervical gonorrhea, nongonococcal urethritis and cervicitis, mixed infections of the urethra and cervix, acute pelvic inflammatory disease (PID), uncomplicated cystitis, prostatitis.	≥18 yrs: ABECB/CAP/SSSI: 400mg q12h for 10 days. Cervicitis/Urethritis: 300mg q12h for 7 days. Gonorrhea: 400mg single dose. PID: 400mg q12h for 10-14 days. Uncomplicated Cystitis: 200mg q12h for 3 days (*E.coli* or *K.pneumoniae*) or 7 days (other pathogens). Complicated UTI: 200mg q12h for 10 days. Prostatitis: (*E.coli*) 300mg q12h for 6 weeks. CrCl 20-50mL/min: Dose q24h. CrCl <20mL/min: After regular initial dose, give 50% of normal dose q24h. Severe Hepatic Impairment: Max: 400mg/day.	
Floxin IV (ofloxacin)	**Inj:** 4mg/mL, 40mg/mL	Treatment of acute bacterial exacerbation of chronic bronchitis, community-acquired pneumonia, uncomplicated skin and skin structure infections, acute uncomplicated urethral and cervical gonorrhea, nongonococcal urethritis and cervicitis, urethral and cervical infections, acute pelvic inflammatory disease (PID), uncomplicated cystitis, urinary tract infections (UTI), prostatitis.	Lower Respiratory Tract Infection/Skin Structure Infections: 400mg q12h for 10 days. Cervicitis/Urethritis: 300mg q12h for 7 days. Gonorrhea: 400mg single dose. PID: 400mg q12h for 10-14 days. Uncomplicated Cystitis: 200mg q12h for 3 days. Other Uncomplicated UTIs: 200mg q12h for 7 days. Complicated UTI: 200mg q12h for 10 days. Prostatitis: 300mg q12h for 6 weeks. Renal Impairment: CrCl 20-50mL/min: increase dosing interval to 24 hrs. CrCl<20mL/min: give normal initial dose then 50% of normal dose and increase dosing interval to 24 hrs. Severe Hepatic Impairment: Max: 400mg qdy. Switch to oral form when appropriate. Max: 10 days IV.	

(Continued)

BRAND NAME (Generic)	DOSAGE FORM/ STRENGTH	INDICATIONS	ADULT DOSE	PEDIATRIC DOSE
FLUOROQUINOLONES *(Continued)*				
Levaquin (levofloxacin)	**Inj:** 5mg/mL, 25mg/mL; **Sol:** 25mg/mL; **Tab:** 250mg, 500mg, 750mg [Leva-pak, 5]	Uncomplicated and complicated skin and skin structure (SSSI), and urinary tract infections (UTI), acute bacterial sinusitis, acute bacterial exacerbation of chronic bronchitis (ABECB), community acquired pneumonia (CAP), including multi-drug resistant *Streptococcus pneumoniae*, nosocomial pneumonia, chronic bacterial prostatitis (CBP), and acute pyelonephritis caused by susceptible strains of microorganisms. Prevention of inhalational anthrax following exposure to *Bacillus anthracis*.	≥18 yrs: IV/PO: ABECB: 500mg qd for 7 days. Cap: 500mg qd for 7-14 days or 750mg qd for 5 days. Sinusitis: 500mg qd for 10-14 days or 750mg qd for 5 days. CBP: 500mg qd for 28 days. Uncomplicated SSSI: 500mg qd for 7-10 days. Complicated SSSI/Nosocomial Pneumonia: 750mg qd for 7-14 days. Inhalational Anthrax: 500mg qd for 60 days. Complicated SSSI/Nosocomial Pneumonia/CAP/Sinusitis: CrCl 20-49mL/min: 750mg, then 750mg q48h. CrCl 10-19mL/min/ Hemodialysis/CAPD: 750mg, then 500mg q48h. ABECB/CAP/Sinusitis/Uncomplicated SSSI/CBP/ Inhalational Anthrax:CrCl 20-49mL/min: 500mg, then 250mg q24h. CrCl 10-19mL/min/Hemodialysis/ CAPD: 500mg,then 250mg q48h. Complicated UTI/ Acute Pyelonephritis: 250mg qd for 10 days. CrCl 10-19mL/min: 250mg, then 250mg q48h. Uncomplicated UTI: 250mg qd for 3 days. Take oral solution 1 hr before or 2 hrs after eating.	
Maxaquin (lomefloxacin HCl)	**Tab:** 400mg	Treatment of acute bacterial exacerbation of chronic bronchitis (ABECB) and uncomplicated/complicated urinary tract infections (UTI). Preoperatively for the prevention of infections from transrectal prostate biopsy (TRPB) and in transurethral surgical procedures (TUSP).	≥18 yrs: ABECB: 400mg qd for 10 days. Uncomplicated Cystitis: 400mg qd for 3 days *E.coli* or 10 days *K.pneumoniae, P.mirabilis,* or *S.saprophyticus.* Complicated UTI: 400mg qd for 14 days. Hemodialysis/CrCl>10 to <40mL/min: LD: 400mg. Maint: 200mg qd. Preoperative Prevention: TRPB: 400mg single dose 1-6 hrs before procedure. TUSP: 400mg single dose 2-6 hrs before procedure.	
Proquin XR (ciprofloxacin HCl)	**Tab, Extended-Release:** 500mg	Treatment of uncomplicated urinary tract infections (acute cystitis) caused by *E.coli* and *K.pneumoniae.*	500mg qd with pm meal for 3 days. Administer at least 4 hrs before or 2 hrs after magnesium or aluminum containing antacids, sucralfate, Videx (didanosine) chewable/buffered tablets of pediatric powder, metal cations (eg, iron), multivitamins with zinc. Do not split, crush, or chew. Swallow tab whole.	

BRAND NAME (Generic)	DOSAGE FORM/ STRENGTH	INDICATIONS	ADULT DOSE	PEDIATRIC DOSE
MACROLIDES				
Biaxin (clarithromycin)	**Sus:** 125mg/5mL, 250mg/5mL [50mL, 100mL]; **Tab:** 250mg, 500mg	Adults: Pharyngitis/tonsillitis, acute maxillary sinusitis, acute bacterial exacerbation of chronic bronchitis (ABECB), community acquired pneumonia (CAP), uncomplicated skin and skin structure infections (SSSI), disseminated mycobacterial infections, combination therapy for *H.pylori* infection with duodenal ulcers. MAC prophylaxis in advanced HIV. Pediatrics: Pharyngitis/tonsillitis, CAP, acute maxillary sinusitis; acute otitis media, uncomplicated SSSI, disseminated mycobacterial infections. MAC prophylaxis in advanced HIV.	Pharyngitis/Tonsillitis: 250mg q12h for 10 days. Sinusitis: 500mg q12h for 14 days. ABECB: 250-500mg q12h for 7-14 days. SSSI/Cap: 250mg q12h for 7-14 days. MAC Prophylaxis/Treatment: 500mg bid. *H.pylori:* Triple Therapy: 500mg + amoxicillin 1g + omeprazole 20mg, all q12h for 10 days; or 500mg + amoxicillin 1g + lansoprazole 30mg, all q12h for 10-14 days. Give additional omeprazole 20mg qd for 18 days with active ulcer. Dual Therapy: 500mg q8h + omeprazole 40mg qd for 14 days (give additional omeprazole 20mg qd for 14 days with active ulcer); or 500mg q8h or q12h + raniti-dine bismuth citrate 400mg q12h for 14 days (give additional ranitidine bismuth citrate 400mg bid for 14 days with active ulcer). Avoid Biaxin and ranitidine bismuth citrate combination with CrCl<25mL/min.	≥6 mo: Usual: 7.5mg/kg q12h for 10 days. MAC Prophylaxis/Treatment: ≥20 mo: 7.5mg/kg bid, up to 500mg bid. CrCl <30mL/min: Give 50% dose or double interval.
Biaxin XL (clarithromycin)	**Tab, Extended-Release:** 500mg [PAC 14 tabs]	Treatment of acute maxillary sinusitis, community acquired pneumonia (CAP), and acute bacterial exacerbation of chronic bronchitis (ABECB).	Sinusitis: 1000mg qd for 14 days. ABECB/Cap: 1000mg qd for 7 days. CrCl <30mL/min: Give 50% dose or double interval. Take with food.	
E.E.S. (erythromycin ethylsuccinate)	**Sus:** 200mg/5mL, 400mg/5mL (100mL, 480mL]; **Tab:** 400mg	Mild to moderate upper and lower respiratory tract and skin and skin structure infections, listeriosis, pertussis, diphtheria, erythrasma, intestinal amebiasis, acute pelvic inflammatory disease (PID) *N.gonorrhea,* primary syphilis in PCN allergy, Legionnaires' disease, chlamydial infections (eg, newborn conjunctivitis urethral, endocervical, or rectal, etc), and nongonococcal urethritis. Prophylaxis of endocarditis or rheumatic fever.	Usual: 1600mg/day given q6h, q8h or q12h. Max: 4g/day. Treat strep infections for 10 days. Strept-ococcal Infection Prophylaxis with Rheumatic Heart Disease: 400mg bid. Urethritis *C.trachomatis* or *U. urealyticum:* 800mg tid for 7 days. Primary Syphilis: 48-64g in divided doses over 10-15 days. Intestinal Amebiasis: 400mg qid for 10-14 days. Pertussis: 40-50mg/kg/day in divided doses for 5-14 days. Legionnaires' Disease: 1.6-4g/day in divided doses.	Usual: 30-50mg/kg/day in divided doses q6h, q8h or q12h. Double dose for more severe infections. Treat strep infections for 10 days. Intestinal Amebiasis: 30-50mg/kg/day in divided doses for 10-14 days. Pertussis: 40-50mg/kg/day in divided doses for 5-14 days.

(Continued)

BRAND NAME (Generic)	DOSAGE FORM/ STRENGTH	INDICATIONS	ADULT DOSE	PEDIATRIC DOSE
MACROLIDES *(Continued)*				
ERYC (erythromycin)	**Cap, Delayed-Release:** 250mg	Mild to moderate upper and lower respiratory tract and skin and soft tissue infections, pertussis, diphtheria, erythrasma, intestinal amebiasis, acute pelvic inflammatory disease (PID) (*N. gonorrhea*), *Listeria monocytogenes* infections, primary syphilis in PCN allergy, Legionnaires' disease, chlamydial infections (eg, newborn conjunctivitis, urethral, endocervical, or rectal, etc), and nongonococcal urethritis. Prophylaxis of endocarditis or rheumatic fever in PCN allergy.	Usual: 250mg q6h or 500mg q12h. Max: 4g/day. Chlamydial Urogenital Infection During Pregnancy: 500mg qid for at least 7 days or 250mg qid for 14 days. Urethral/Endocervical/Rectal Chlamydial Infections: 500mg qid for 7 days. Primary Syphilis: 30-40g in divided doses for 10-15 days. Acute PID: 500mg (erythromycin lactobionate) IV q6h for 3 days, then 250mg PO q6h for 7 days. Streptococcal Infection Long-Term Prophylaxis of Rheumatic Fever: 250mg bid. Intestinal Amebiasis: 250mg qid for 10-14 days. Pertussis: 40-50mg/kg/day in divided doses for 5-14 days. Legionnaires' Disease: 1-4g/day in divided doses. Bacterial Endocarditis Prophylaxis: 1g 1 hr before procedure, then 500mg 6 hrs later.	Usual: 30-50mg/kg/day in divided doses without food. Max: 4g/day. Severe Infections: Double dose up to 4g/day. Treat strep infections for 10 days. Intestinal Amebiasis: 30-50mg/kg/day in divided doses for 10-14 days. Bacterial Endocarditis Prophylaxis: 20mg/kg 1 hr before procedure, then 10mg/kg 6 hrs later.
EryPed (erythromycin ethylsuccinate)	**Sus:** 100mg/2.5mL [50mL], 200mg/5mL, 400mg/5mL [5mL, 100mL, 200mL]; **Tab, Chewable:** 200mg	Treatment of mild to moderate upper and lower respiratory tract and skin and skin structure infections, listeriosis, pertussis, diphtheria, erythrasma, intestinal amebiasis, acute pelvic inflammatory disease (PID) *N.gonorrhea*, primary syphilis in PCN allergy, Legionnaires' disease, chlamydial infections (eg, newborn conjunctivitis, urethral, endocervical, or rectal, etc), and nongonococcal urethritis. Prophylaxis of endocarditis or rheumatic fever.	Usual: 1600mg/day given q6h, q8h or q12h. Max: 4g/day. Treat strep infections for 10 days. Streptococcal Infection Prophylaxis with Rheumatic Heart Disease: 400mg bid. Urethritis *C.trachomatis* or *U. urealyticum*: 800mg tid for 7 days. Primary Syphilis:48-64g in divided doses over 10-15 days. Intestinal Amebiasis: 400mg qid for 10-14 days. Pertussis:40-50mg/kg/day in divided doses for 5-14 days. Legionnaires' Disease: 1.6-4g/day in divided doses.	Usual: 30-50mg/kg/day in divided doses q6h, q8h or q12h. Double dose for more severe infections. Treat strep infections for 10 days. Intestinal Amebiasis: 30-50mg/kg/day in divided doses for 10-14 days. Pertussis: 40-50mg/kg/day in divided doses for 5-14 days.

BRAND NAME (Generic)	DOSAGE FORM/ STRENGTH	INDICATIONS	ADULT DOSE	PEDIATRIC DOSE
Ery-Tab (erythromycin)	**Tab, Delayed-Release:** 250mg, 333mg, 500mg	Mild to moderate upper and lower respiratory tract and skin and skin structure infections, listeriosis, pertussis, diphtheria, erythrasma, intestinal amebiasis, acute pelvic inflammatory disease (PID) (*N. gonorrhoeae*), primary syphilis in PCN allergy, Legionnaires' disease, chlamydial infections (eg, newborn conjunctivitis urethral, endocervical, rectal, etc), and nongonococcal urethritis. Prophylaxis of rheumatic fever.	Usual: 250mg qid, 333mg q8h or 500mg q12h without food. Max: 4g/day. Do not take bid when dose is ≥1g/day. Treat strep infections for 10 days. Chlamydial Urogenital Infection During Pregnancy: 500mg qid or 666mg q8h for 7 days, or 500mg q 12h, 333mg q8h or 250mg qid for 14 days. Urethral/Endocervical/Rectal Chlamydial Infections and Nongonococcal Urethritis: 500mg qid or 666mg q8h for at least 7 days. Primary Syphilis: 30-40g in divided doses for 10-15 days. Acute PID: 500mg (erythromycin lactobionate) IV q6h for 3 days, then 500mg PO q12h or 333mg q8h for 7 days. Streptococcal Infection Long-Term Prophylaxis of Rheumatic Fever: 250mg bid. Intestinal Amebiasis: 500mg q12h, 333mg q8h or 250mg q6h for 10-14 days. Pertussis: 40-50mg/kg in divided doses for 5-14 days. Legionnaires' Disease: 1-4g/day in divided doses.	Usual: 30-50mg/kg/day in divided doses without food. Max: 4g/day. Severe Infections: Double dose up to 4g/day. Treat strep infections for 10 days. Chlamydial Conjunctivitis of Newborns and Chlamydial Pneumonia in Infancy: 12.5mg/kg qid for 2 weeks and 3 weeks, respectively. Intestinal Amebiasis: 30-50mg/kg/day in divided doses for 10-14 days. Long-Term Prophylaxis of Rheumatic Fever: 250mg bid. Intestinal Amebiasis: 30-50mg/kg/day in divided doses for 10-14 days. Pertussis: 40-50mg/kg/day in divided doses for 5-14 days. Legionnaire's Disease: 1-4g/day in divided doses.
Erythrocin (erythromycin stearate)	**Tab:** 250mg, 500mg	Mild to moderate upper and lower respiratory tract and skin and skin structure infections, listeriosis, pertussis, diphtheria, erythrasma, intestinal amebiasis, acute pelvic inflammatory disease (PID) (gonorrhea), primary syphilis in PCN allergy, Legionnaires' disease, chlamydial infections (eg, newborn conjunctivitis urethral, endocervical, or rectal, etc), and nongonococcal urethritis. Prophylaxis of rheumatic fever.	Usual: 250mg q6h or 500mg q12h without food. Max: 4g/day. Treat strep infections for 10 days. Streptococcal Infection Prophylaxis of Rheumatic Fever: 250mg bid. Chlamydial Urogenital Infection During Pregnancy: 500mg qid for 7 days or 250mg qid for 14 days. Urethral/Endocervical/Rectal Chlamydial Infections and Nongonococcal Urethritis: 500mg qid for at least 7 days. Acute PID: 500mg (erythromycin lactobionate) IV q6h for 3 days, then 500mg PO q12h for 7 days. Intestinal Amebiasis: 250mg qid in divided doses over 10-15 days. Primary Syphilis: 30-40g in divided doses for 10-14 days. Pertussis: 40-50mg/day in divided doses for 5-14 days. Legionnaires' Disease: 1-4g/day in divided doses.	Usual: 30-50mg/kg/day in divided doses without food. Severe Infections: Double dose up to 4g/day. Treat strep infections for 10 days. Streptococcal Infection Prophylaxis of Rheumatic Fever: 250mg bid. Chlamydial Conjunctivitis of Newborns/Chlamydial Pneumonia in Infancy: 12.5mg/kg qid for 2 weeks and 3 weeks, respectively. Intestinal Amebiasis: 30-50mg/kg/day in divided doses for 10-14 days. Pertussis: 40-50mg/kg/day in divided doses for 5-14 days.

(Continued)

MACROLIDES *(Continued)*

BRAND NAME (Generic)	DOSAGE FORM/ STRENGTH	INDICATIONS	ADULT DOSE	PEDIATRIC DOSE
Erythromycin	**Cap, Delayed-Release:** 250mg	Mild to moderate upper and lower respiratory tract and skin and skin structure infections, listeriosis, pertussis, diphtheria, erythrasma, intestinal amebiasis, primary syphilis in PCN allergy, Legionnaires' disease, chlamydial infections (eg, newborn conjunctivitis urethral, endocervical, rectal, etc), and nongonococcal urethritis. Prophylaxis of endocarditis or rheumatic fever.	Usual: 250mg q6h or 500mg q12h without food. Max: 4g/day. Treat strep infections for 10 days. Streptococcal Infection Prophylaxis of Rheumatic Fever: 250mg bid. Chlamydial Urogenital Infection During Pregnancy: 500mg qid for 7 days or 250mg qid for 14 days. Urethral/Endocervical/Rectal Chlamydial Infections: 500mg qid for at least 7 days. Primary Syphilis: 30-40g in divided doses over 10-15 days. Intestinal Amebiasis: 250mg q6h for 10-14 days. Pertussis: 40-50mg/kg/day in divided doses for 5-14 days. Legionnaires' Disease: 1-4g/day in divided doses. Bacterial Endocarditis Prophylaxis: 1g 1 hr before procedure, then 500mg 6 hrs later.	Usual: 30-50mg/kg/day in divided doses without food. Severe Infections: Double dose up to 4g/day. Streptococcal Infection Prophylaxis of Rheumatic Fever: 250mg bid. Intestinal Amebiasis: 30-50mg/kg/day in divided doses for 10-14 days. Pertussis: 40-50mg/kg/day in divided doses for 5-14 days. Bacterial Endocarditis Prophylaxis: 20mg/kg 1 hr before procedure, then 10mg/kg 6 hrs later.
Erythromycin Base	**Tab:** 250mg	Mild to moderate upper and lower respiratory tract and skin and skin structure infections, listeriosis, pertussis, diphtheria, erythrasma, intestinal amebiasis, acute pelvic inflammatory disease (PID) *(N.gonorrhoeae)*, primary syphilis in PCN allergy, Legionnaires' disease, chlamydial infections (eg, newborn conjunctivitis urethral, endocervical, rectal, etc), and nongonococcal urethritis. Prophylaxis of rheumatic fever.	Usual: 250mg q6h or 500mg q12h without food. Max: 4g/day. Treat strep infections for 10 days. Streptococcal Infection Prophylaxis of Rheumatic Fever: 250mg bid. Chlamydial Urogenital Infection During Pregnancy: 500mg qid for 7 days or 250mg qid for 14 days. Urethral/Endocervical/Rectal Chlamydial Infections and Nongonococcal Urethritis: 500mg qid for at least 7 days. Primary Syphilis: 30-40g in divided doses over 10-15 days. Acute PID: 500mg (erythromycin lactobionate) IV q6h for 3 days, then 500mg PO q12h for 7 days. Intestinal Amebiasis: 250mg qid for 10-14 days. Pertussis: 40-50mg/kg/day in divided doses for 5-14 days. Legionnaires' Disease: 1-4g/day in divided doses.	Usual: 30-50mg/kg/day in divided doses without food. Severe Infections: Double dose up to 4g/day. Treat strep infections for 10 days. Streptococcal Infection Prophylaxis of Rheumatic Fever: 250mg bid. Chlamydial Conjunctivitis of Newborns and Chlamydial Pneumonia in Infancy: 12.5mg/kg qid for 2 weeks and 3 weeks, respectively. Intestinal Amebiasis: 30-50mg/kg/day in divided doses for 10-14 days. Pertussis: 40-50mg/kg/day in divided doses for 5-14 days.
Pediazole (sulfisoxazole acetyl-erythromycin ethylsuccinate)	**Sus:** (Erythromycin Ethylsuccinate-Sulfisoxazole Acetyl) 200 mg-600mg/5mL [100 mL, 150mL, 200mL]	Acute otitis media caused by *H.influenzae.*		>2 mos: Dose based on 50mg/kg/day erythromycin or 150mg/kg/day sulfisoxazole given tid-qid for 10 days. Max: 6g/day sulfisoxazole.

BRAND NAME (Generic)	DOSAGE FORM/ STRENGTH	INDICATIONS	ADULT DOSE	PEDIATRIC DOSE
PCE (erythromycin)	**Tab, Extended-Release:** 333mg, 500mg	Mild to moderate upper and lower respiratory tract and skin structure infections, listeriosis, pertussis, diphtheria, erythrasma, intestinal amebiasis, acute pelvic inflammatory disease (PID) (N.gonorrhoeae), primary syphilis in PCN allergy, Legionnaires' disease, chlamydial infections (eg, newborn conjunctivitis urethral, endocervical, or rectal, etc), and nongonococcal urethritis. Prophylaxis of rheumatic fever.	Usual: 333mg q8h or 500mg q12h without food. Max: 4g/day. Do not take bid when dose is ≥1g/day food. Severe Infections: Double dose up to 4g/day. Treat strep infections for 10 days. Chlamydial Urogenital Infection During Pregnancy: 500mg qid or 666mg q8h for 7 days, or 500mg q12h, 333mg q8h or 250mg qid for 14 days. Urethral/Endocervical/ Rectal Chlamydial Infections and Nongonococcal Urethritis: 500mg qid or 666mg q8h for at least 7 days. Primary Syphilis: 30-40g in divided doses for 10-15 days. Acute PID: 500mg (erythromycin lactobionate) IV q6h for 3 days, then 500mg PO q12h or 333mg q8h for 7 days. Streptococcal Infection or 333mg q8h for 7 days. Streptococcal Infection Long-Term Prophylaxis of Rheumatic Fever: 250mg bid. Intestinal Amebiasis: 500mg q12h, or 333mg q8h or 250mg q6h for 10-14 days. Pertussis: 40-50mg/day in divided doses for 5-14 days. Legionnaires' Disease: 1-4g/day in divided doses.	Usual: 30-50mg/kg/day in divided doses without food. Max: 4g/day. Severe Infections: Double dose up to 4g/day. Treat strep infections for 10 days. Chlamydial Conjunctivitis of Newborns and Chlamydial Pneumonia in Infancy: 12.5mg/kg qid for 2 weeks and 3 weeks, respectively. Intestinal Amebiasis: 30-50mg/kg/day in divided doses for 10-14 days. Long-Term Prophylaxis of Rheumatic Fever: 250mg bid. Pertussis: 40-50mg/kg/day in divided doses for 5-14 days. Legionnaires' Disease: 1-4g/day in divided doses.
Zithromax (azithromycin)	**Inj:** 500mg; **Sus:** 100mg/5mL [15mL], 200mg/5mL [15mL, 22.5mL, 30mL], 1g/pkt [3³ 10⁵]; **Tab:** 250mg [Z-Pak, 6 tabs], [3³ 10⁵]; **Tab:** 250mg [Tri-Pak, 3 tabs], 500mg [Z-Pak, 6 tabs], 600mg	(PO) Treatment of acute bacterial exacerbations of COPD, acute bacterial sinusitis (ABS), community acquired pneumonia (CAP), pharyngitis/tonsillitis, uncomplicated skin and skin structure, urethritis/ cervicitis, genital ulcer disease (men), acute otitis media, prevention of disseminated Mycobacterium avium complex (MAC) disease in advanced HIV infection. (IV) Treatment of CAP and pelvic inflammatory disease (PID).	(PO) COPD/CAP/Pharyngitis/Tonsillitis (second line therapy)/SSSIs: ≥16 yrs: 500mg on day 1, then 250 mg qd on days 2-5. COPD: 500mg qd for 3 days. ABS: 500mg qd for 3 days. Genital Ulcer Disease and Non-Gonococcal Urethritis/Cervicitis: 1g single dose. Urethritis/Cervicitis due to gonorrhea: 2g single dose. MAC Prophylaxis: 1200mg once weekly. MAC Treatment: 600mg qd with ethambutol 15mg/ kg/day. (IV) ≥16 yrs: Cap: 500mg qd for at least 2 days, then 500mg PO to complete 7-10 day course. PID: 500mg qd for 1-2 days, then 250mg PO to complete 7-day course.	(Sus) Otitis Media: ≥6 mo: 30mg/kg single dose; 10mg/kg qd for 3 days; or 10mg/kg qd on day 1, then 5mg/kg qd on days 2-5. ABS: ≥6 mo: 10mg/kg qd for 3 days. Cap: ≥6 mo: 10mg/kg qd on day 1, then 5mg/kg qd on days 2-5. (Sus, Tab) Pharyngitis/ Tonsillitis: ≥2 yrs: 12mg/kg qd for 5 days. 1g suspension is not for pediatric use.
Zmax (azithromycin)	**Sus, Extended-Release:** 2g	Treatment of mild to moderate acute bacterial sinusitis due to Haemophilus influenzae, Moraxella catarrhalis, or Streptococcus pneumoniae. Treatment of community-acquired pneumonia due to Chlamydophila pneumoniae, Haemophilus influenzae, Mycoplasma pneumoniae, or Streptococcus pneumoniae in patients appropriate for oral therapy.	2g single dose. Take on an empty stomach (1 hr before or 2 hrs after a meal).	

(Continued)

BRAND NAME (Generic)	DOSAGE FORM/ STRENGTH	INDICATIONS	ADULT DOSE	PEDIATRIC DOSE
PENICILLINS				
Amoxil (amoxicillin)	**Cap:** 250mg, 500mg; **Sus:** 50mg/mL [15mL, 30mL], 125mg/5mL [80mL, 100mL, 150mL], 200mg/5mL [5mL, 50mL, 75mL, 100mL], 250mg/5mL [80mL, 100mL, 150mL], 400mg/5mL [5mL, 50mL, 75mL, 100mL]; **Tab:** 500mg, 875mg; **Tab, Chewable:** 200mg, 400mg	Infections of the ear, nose, throat, genitourinary tract, skin and skin structure, lower respiratory tract due to susceptible (beta lactamase negative) organisms; gonorrhea (acute uncomplicated). *H.pylori* eradication to reduce the risk of duodenal ulcer recurrence.	Ear/Nose/Throat/SSSI/GU: (Mild/Moderate): 500mg q12h or 250mg q8h. (Severe): 875mg q12h or 500 mg q8h. LRTI: 875mg q12h or 500mg q8h. Gonorrhea: 3g as single dose. *H.pylori:* (Dual Therapy) 1g + 30mg lansoprazole, both tid for 14 days. (Triple Therapy) 1g + 30mg lansoprazole + 500mg clarithromycin, all q12h X 14 days. CrCl 10-30mL/min: 250-500mg q12h. <10mL/min: 250-500mg q24h. Hemodialysis: 250-500mg or 250mg q24h, additional dose during and at the end.	**Neonates:** ≤12 weeks: Max: 30mg/kg/day divided q12h. >3 mo: Ear/Nose/Throat/SSSI/GU: (Mild/Moderate): 25mg/kg/day given q12h or 20mg/kg/day given q8h. (Severe): 45mg/kg/day given q12h or 40 mg/kg/day given q8h. LRTI: 45mg/kg/day given q12h or 40mg/kg/day given q8h. Gonorrhea: (Prepubertal) 50mg/kg with 25mg/kg probenecid as single dose. (Not for <2 yrs). >40kg: Dose as adult.
Ampicillin (ampicillin sodium)	**Inj:** 125mg, 250mg, 500mg, 1g, 2g, 10g	Treatment of respiratory tract, urinary tract, and GI infections, bacterial meningitis, septicemia, endocarditis.	IM/IV: Respiratory Tract: ≥40kg: 250-500mg q8h. <40kg: 25-50mg/kg/day given q6-8h. GI/GU Caused by *N.gonorrhea* (Females): ≥40kg: 500mg q6h. <40kg: 50mg/kg/day given q6-8h. Urethritis Caused by *N.gonorrhea* (Males): 500mg q8-12h for 2 doses; may retreat if needed. Bacterial Meningitis: 150-200mg/kg/day given q3-4h. Septicemia: 150-200mg/kg/day IV for 3 days, continue with IM q3-4h. Treat for minimum of 10 days and 48-72 hrs after being asymptomatic.	Bacterial Meningitis: 150-200mg/kg/day given q3-4h. Septicemia: 150-200mg/kg/day IV given q3-4h for 3 days, continue with IM q3-4h. Treat for minimum of 10 days and 48-72 hrs after being asymptomatic.

BRAND NAME (Generic)	DOSAGE FORM/ STRENGTH	INDICATIONS	ADULT DOSE	PEDIATRIC DOSE
Augmentin (amoxicillin-clavulanate potassium)	(Amoxicillin-Clavulanate) **Sus:** 125-31.25mg/5mL [75mL, 100mL, 150mL] 200-28.5mg/5mL [50mL, 75mL, 100mL]; 250-62.5mg/5mL [75mL, 100mL, 150mL], 400-57mg/5mL [50mL, 75mL, 100mL]; **Tab:** 250-125mg, 500-125mg, 875-125mg; Tab, Chewable: 200-28.5mg, 250-62.5mg, 400-57mg	Treatment of lower respiratory tract (LRTI), skin and skin structure (SSSI), and urinary tract infections (UTI), otitis media (OM), sinusitis.	(Dose based on amoxicillin) 500mg q12h or 250mg q8h. Severe Infections/RTI: 875mg q12h or 500mg q8h. May use 125mg/5mL or 250mg/5mL sus in place of 500mg tab and 200mg/5mL sus or 400mg/5mL sus in place of 875mg tab. CrCl <30mL/min: Do not give 875mg tab. CrCl 10-30mL/min: 250-500mg q12h. CrCl <10mL/min: 250-500mg q24h. Hemodialysis: 250-500mg q24h, give additional dose during and at the end of dialysis.	(Dose based on amoxicillin) ≥40kg: Use adult dose. ≥12 weeks: Sinusitis/OM/LRTI/Severe Infections: (Sus/Tab, Chewable) 45mg/kg/day given q12h or 40mg/kg/day given q8h. Less Severe Infections: 25mg/kg/day given q12h or 20mg/kg/day given q8h. <12 weeks:15mg/kg q12h (use 125mg/5mL sus).
Augmentin ES-600 (amoxicillin-clavulanate potassium)	**Sus:** (Amoxicillin-Clavulanate) 600mg-42.9mg/5mL [50mL, 75mL, 100mL]	Treatment of recurrent or persistent acute otitis media.		(Dose based on amoxicillin) 3 mo-12 yrs: <40kg: 45mg/kg q12h for 10 days.
Augmentin XR (amoxicillin-clavulanate potassium)	**Tab, Extended-Release:** (Amoxicillin-Clavulanate) 1000 mg-62.5mg	Treatment of community acquired pneumonia (CAP) or acute bacterial sinusitis due to confirmed or suspected ß-lactamase producing pathogens.	Sinusitis: 2 tabs q12h for 10 days. Cap: 2 tabs q12h for 7-10 days. Take at the start of a meal.	≥16 yrs: Sinusitis: 2 tabs q12h for 10 days. Cap: 2 tabs q12h for 7-10 days. Take at the start of a meal.
Bicillin C-R (penicillin G benzathine-penicillin G procaine)	**Inj:** (Penicillin G Benzathine-Penicillin G Procaine) 300,000-300,000 U/mL	Treatment of moderately severe to severe upper-respiratory tract (URTI) and skin and soft-tissue infections (SSTI); scarlet fever and erysipelas due to streptococci. Treatment of moderately severe pneumonia and otitis media due to pneumococci.	Group A Strep: URTI/SSTI/Scarlet Fever/Erysipelas: 2.4 MU IM. Treat at a single session using multiple IM sites, or use an alternative schedule and give ½ of the total dose on Day 1 and ½ on Day 3. Pneumococcal Infections (Except Meningitis): 1.2 MU IM, repeat every 2-3 days until temperature is normal for 48 hrs. Administer IM into upper, outer quadrant of buttock.	Group A Strep: URTI/SSTI/Scarlet Fever/Erysipelas: >60 lbs: 2.4 MU IM. 30-60 lbs: 900,000 U-1.2 MU IM. <30 lbs: 600,000 U IM. Treat at a single session using multiple IM sites, or use an alternative schedule and give ½ of the total dose on Day 1 and ½ on Day 3. Pneumococcal Infections (Except Meningitis): 600,000 U IM, repeat every 2-3 days until temperature is normal for 48 hrs. Administer IM into upper, outer quadrant of buttock. Use the midlateral aspect of thigh in neonates, infants, and small children.

(Continued)

BRAND NAME (Generic)	DOSAGE FORM/ STRENGTH	INDICATIONS	ADULT DOSE	PEDIATRIC DOSE
PENICILLINS *(Continued)*				
Bicillin C-R 900/300 (penicillin G benzathine-penicillin G procaine)	**Inj:** (Penicillin G Benzathine-Penicillin G Procaine) 900,000-300,000 U/2mL	Treatment of moderately severe to severe upper-respiratory tract (URT) and skin and soft-tissue infections (SSTI), scarlet fever and erysipelas due to streptococci. Treatment of moderately severe pneumonia and otitis media due to pneumococci.		Group A Strep: URTI/SSTI/Scarlet Fever/Erysipelas: 1.2 MU IM single dose. Pneumococcal Infections (Except Meningitis): 1.2 MU IM every 2-3 days until temperature is normal for 48 hrs. Administer IM into upper, outer quadrant of buttock. Use midlateral aspect of thigh in neonates, infants, and small children.
Bicillin L-A (penicillin G benzathine)	**Inj:** 600,000 U/mL	Treatment of mild to moderate upper respiratory tract infections (URTI) due to streptococci and venereal infections (eg, syphilis, yaws, bejel, pinta). Prophylaxis to prevent recurrence of rheumatic fever or chorea.	Group A Strep: URTI: 1.2 MU IM single dose. Primary/Secondary/Latent Syphilis: 2.4 MU IM single dose. Late Syphilis (Tertiary/Neurosyphilis): 2.4 MU IM every 7 days for 3 doses. Yaws/Bejel/Pinta: 1.2 MU IM single dose. Rheumatic Fever/Glomerulonephritis Prophylaxis: 1.2 MU IM once a mo or 600,000 U IM every 2 weeks. Administer IM into upper, outer quadrant of buttock.	Group A Strep: URTI: Older Pediatrics: 900,000 U IM single dose. <60lbs: 300,000-600,000 U IM single dose. Congenital Syphilis: 2-12 yrs: Adjust dose based on adult schedule. <2 yrs: 50,000 U/kg IM single dose. Rheumatic Fever/Glomerulonephritis Prophylaxis: 1.2 MU IM once a mo or 600,000 U IM every 2 weeks. Administer IM into upper, outer quadrant of buttock. Use the midlateral aspect of thigh in neonates, infants, and small children.
Dicloxacillin (dicloxacillin sodium)	**Cap:** 250mg, 500mg; **Sus:** 62.5mg/5mL [100mL]	Infections caused by penicillinase-producing staphylococci.	Mild-Moderate Infection: 125mg q6h. Severe Infection: 250mg q6h for at least 14 days.	<40kg: Mild-Moderate Infection: 12.5mg/kg/day in divided doses q6h. Severe Infection: 25mg/kg/day in divided doses q6h for at least 14 days.
Geocillin (carbenicillin disodium)	**Tab:** 382mg	Treatment of acute and chronic infections of the upper and lower urinary tract (UTI) and asymptomatic bacteriuria.	UTI: *E.coli, Proteus,* and *Enterobacter:* 1-2 tabs qid. *Pseudomonas, Enterococcus:* 2 tabs qid. Prostatitis: *E.coli, Proteus, Enterococcus* and *Enterobacter:* 2 tabs qid. CrCl 10-20mL/min: Adjust dose.	
Penicillin VK, Veetids (penicillin V potassium)	**Sus:** 125mg/5mL, 250mg/5mL [100mL, 200mL]; **Tab:** 250mg, 500mg	Mild to moderately severe bacterial infections including conditions of the respiratory tract, oropharynx, skin and soft tissue. Prevention of recurrence following rheumatic fever and/or chorea.	Usual: Streptococcal Infections (Scarlet Fever, Erysipelas, Upper Respiratory Tract): 125-250mg q6-8h for 10 days. Pneumococcal Infections (Otitis Media, Respiratory Tract): 250-500mg q6h until afebrile for at least 2 days. Staphylococcus Infections (Skin/Soft Tissue): 250-500mg q6-8h. Fusospirochetosis Infections (Oropharynx): 250-500mg q6-8h. Rheumatic Fever/Chorea Prevention: 125-250mg bid.	≥12 yrs: Usual: Streptococcal Infections (Scarlet fever, Erysipelas, Upper Respiratory Tract): 125-250mg q6-8h for 10 days. Pneumococcal Infections (Otitis media, Respiratory Tract): 250-500mg q6h until afebrile for at least 2 days. Staphylococcus Infections (Skin/Soft Tissue): 250-500mg q6-8h. Fusospirochetosis Infections (Oropharynx): 250-500mg q6-8h. Rheumatic Fever/Chorea Prevention: 125-250mg bid.

BRAND NAME (Generic)	DOSAGE FORM/ STRENGTH	INDICATIONS	ADULT DOSE	PEDIATRIC DOSE
Pfizerpen (penicillin G potassium)	**Inj:** 1 MU, 5 MU, 20 MU	For therapy of severe infections when rapid and high blood levels of penicillin required. Management of streptococcal, pneumococcal, staphylococcal, clostridial, fusospirochetal, listeria, and gram negative bacillary, and pasteurella infections. For anthrax, actinomycosis, diphtheria, erysipeloid, meningitis, endocarditis, bacteremia, rat-bite fever, syphilis, and gonorrheal endocarditis and arthritis. With combined oral therapy, prophylaxis against endocarditis in patients with congenital heart disease, rheumatic, or other acquired valvular heart disease undergoing dental procedures or surgical procedures of upper respiratory tract.	Anthrax/Gonorrheal Endocarditis/Severe Infections (Streptococci, Pneumococci, Staphylococci): Minimum of 5 MU/day. Syphilis: Administer in hospital. Determine dose and duration based on age and weight. Meningococcal Meningitis: 1-2 MU IM q2h or 20-30 MU/day continuous IV. Actinomycosis: 1-6 MU/day for cervicofacial cases; 10-20 MU/day for thoracic and abdominal disease. Clostridial Infections: 20 MU/day (adjunct to antitoxin). Fusospirochetal Severe Infections: 5-10 MU/day for oropharynx, lower respiratory tract, and genital area infection. Rat-bite Fever: 12-15 MU/day for 3-4 weeks. Listeria Endocarditis: 15-20 MU/day for 4 weeks. Pasteurella Bacteremia/Meningitis: 4-6 MU/day for 2 weeks. Erysipeloid Endocarditis: 2-20 MU/day for 4-6 weeks. Gram Negative Bacillary Bacteremia: 20-80 MU/day. Diphtheria (carrier state): 0.3-0.4 MU/day in divided doses for 10-12 days. Endocarditis Prophylaxis: 1 MU IM mixed with 0.6 MU procaine penicillin G 0.5-1 hr before procedure. Renal/Cardiac/Vascular Dysfunction: Consider dose reduction. For streptococcal infection, treat for minimum 10 days.	Listeria Infections: Neonates: 0.5-1 MU/day. Congenital Syphilis: Administer in hospital. Determine dose and duration based on age and weight. Endocarditis Prophylaxis: 30,000 U/kg IM mixed with 0.6 MU procaine penicillin G 0.5-1 hr before procedure. For streptococcal infection, treat for minimum 10 days.
Permapen (penicillin G benzathine)	**Inj:** 600,000 U/mL	Treatment of microorganisms susceptible to low and very prolonged serum levels in upper respiratory tract infections (streptococci group A—without bacteremia), syphilis, yaws, bejel, and pinta. Prophylaxis for rheumatic fever and/or chorea. Follow-up prophylactic therapy for rheumatic heart disease and acute glomerulonephritis.	Streptococcal Infection: 1.2 MU IM single dose. Primary/Secondary/Latent Syphilis: 1 MU IM single dose. Late (Tertiary/Neurosyphilis) Syphilis: 3 MU IM every 7 days for total of 6-9 MU. Yaws/Bejel/ Pinta: 1.2 MU IM single dose. Rheumatic Fever/ Glomerulonephritis Prophylaxis: 1.2 MU IM once moly or 600,000 U IM twice moly. Use upper outer quadrant of buttock. Rotate injection site.	≤12 yrs: Adjust dose according to age and weight and severity of infection. Streptococcal Infection: 900,000 U IM single dose in older children. Congenital Syphilis: <2 yrs: 50,000 U/kg IM single dose. 2-12 yrs: Adjust dose based on adult schedule. Use midlateral aspect of thigh in infants and small children. May divide dose between 2 buttocks in peds <2 yrs. Rotate injection site.

(Continued)

BRAND NAME (Generic)	DOSAGE FORM/ STRENGTH	INDICATIONS	ADULT DOSE	PEDIATRIC DOSE
PENICILLINS (Continued)				
Piperacillin	**Inj:** 2g, 3g, 4g	Treatment of serious intra-abdominal, urinary tract, gynecologic, lower respiratory tract, skin and skin structure, bone and joint, and gonococcal infections, septicemia, and perioperative surgical prophylaxis.	Usual: 3-4g IM/IV q4-6h. Max: 24g/day; IM: 2g/site. Usual: 3-4g IM/IV q4-6h. Max: 24g/day; IM: 2g/site. Serious Infections: 200-300mg/kg/day IV divided q4-6h. Complicated UTI: 125-200mg/kg/day IV divided q6-8h. Uncomplicated UTI/Community Acquired Pneumonia: 100-125mg/kg/day IM/IV divided q6-12h. Uncomplicated Gonorrhea: 2g IM single dose with 1g PO probenecid 1/2 hr before injection. Surgical Prophylaxis: 2g IV 20-30 min just prior to anesthesia (See labeling for follow-up dosing). C-Section: 2g IV after cord is clamped, then 2g IV 4 hrs and 8 hrs after 1st dose. Renal Impairment: Uncomplicated/Complicated UTI: CrCl 20-40mL/min: 3g q12h. Complicated UTI: CrCl 20-40mL/min: 3g q8h. CrCl<20mL/min: 3g q12h. Serious Infection: CrCl 20-40mL/min: 4g q8h. CrCl<20mL/min: 4g q12h. Hemodialysis: Give 1g additional dose after each dialysis. Max: 2g q8h. Usual treatment is for 7-10 days; treat gynecologic infections for 3-10 days; treat *S.pyogenes* infections for at least 10 days.	≥12 yrs: Usual: 3-4g IM/IV q4-6h. Max: 24g/day; IM: 2g/site. Serious Infections: 200-300mg/kg/day IV divided q4-6h. Complicated UTI: 125-200mg/kg/day IV divided q6-8h. Uncomplicated UTI/Community Acquired Pneumonia: 100-125mg/kg/day IM/IV divided q6-12h. Uncomplicated Gonorrhea: 2g IM single dose with 1g PO probenecid 1/2 hr before injection. Surgical Prophylaxis: 2g IV 20-30 minute just prior to anesthesia (See labeling for follow-up dosing). C-section: 2g IV after cord is clamped, then 2g 4 hrs and 8 hrs after 1st dose. Renal Impairment: Uncomplicated/Complicated UTI: CrCl <20mL/min: 3g q12h. Complicated UTI: CrCl 20-40mL/min: 3g q8h. Serious Infection: CrCl 20-40mL/min: 4g q8h. CrCl <20mL/min: 4g q12h. Hemodialysis: Give 1g additional dose after each dialysis. Max: 2g q8h. Usual treatment is for 7-10 days; treat gynecologic infections for 3-10 days; treat *S.pyogenes* nfections for at least 10 days.
Timentin (ticarcillin-clavulanate potassium)	**Inj:** (Ticarcillin-Clavulanate) 3g-100mg-100mg/100mL, 3g-100mg/100mL, 30g-1g	Treatment of lower respiratory tract, bone and joint, skin and skin structure, urinary tract (UTI), gynecologic, and intra-abdominal infections, and septicemia.	≥60kg: UTI/Systemic Infection: 3g-100mg (3.1g vial) IV q4-6h. Gynecologic Infections: Moderate: 200mg/kg/day ticarcillin IV given q6h. Severe: 300mg/kg/day ticarcillin IV given q4h.<60kg: Usual: 200-300mg/kg/day ticarcillin IV given q4-6h. UTI: 3g-200mg (3.2g vial) q8h. Renal Impairment (based on ticarcillin): CrCl 60-30mL/min: 2g IV q4h. CrCl 30-10mL/min: 2g IV q8h. CrCl<10mL/min: 2g IV q12h (2g IV q24h with hepatic dysfunction). Peritoneal Dialysis: 3.1g IV q12h. Hemodialysis: 2g IV q12h, and 3.1g after each dialysis. Apply reduced dosage after initial 3.1g LD is given.	≥3 mo: >60kg: Mild to Moderate: 3g-100mg (3.1g vial) IV q6h. Severe: 3g-100mg (3.1g vial) IV q4h. <60kg: Mild to Moderate: 50mg/kg ticarcillin IV q6h. Severe: 50mg/kg ticarcillin IV q4h. Renal Impairment (based on ticarcillin): CrCl 60-30mL/min: 2g IV q4h. CrCl 30-10mL/min: 2g IV q8h. CrCl<10mL/min: 2g IV q12h (2g IV q24h with hepatic dysfunction). Peritoneal Dialysis: 3.1g IV q12h. Hemodialysis: 2g IV q12h, and 3.1g after each dialysis. Apply reduced dosage after initial 3.1g LD is given.

BRAND NAME (Generic)	DOSAGE FORM/ STRENGTH	INDICATIONS	ADULT DOSE	PEDIATRIC DOSE
Unasyn (ampicillin sodium/ sulbactam sodium)	Inj: (Ampicillin-Sulbactam) 1g-0.5g, 2g-1g, 10g-5g	Treatment of skin and skin structure (SSSI), intra-abdominal, and gynecological infections caused by susceptible microorganisms.	1.5-3g (ampicillin + sulbactam) IM/IV q6h. Max: 4g/day sulbactam. Renal Impairment: CrCl ≥30mL/min: 1.5-3g q6-8h. CrCl 15-29mL/min: 1.5-3g q12h. CrCl 5-14mL/min: 1.5-3g q24h.	≥1 yr: SSSI: 1.5-3g (ampicillin + sulbactam) IM/IV q6h. Max: 4g/day sulbactam.
Veetids (penicillin V potassium)	Sus: 125mg/5mL, 250mg/5mL [100mL, 200mL]; Tab: 250mg, 500mg	Mild to moderately severe bacterial infections including conditions of the respiratory tract, oropharynx, skin and soft tissue. Prevention of recurrence following rheumatic fever and/or chorea.	Streptococcal Infections (Scarlet Fever, Erysipelas, Upper Respiratory Tract): 125-250mg q6-8h for 10 days. Pneumococcal Infections (Otitis media, Respiratory Tract): 250-500mg q6h until afebrile for at least 2 days. Staphylococcus Infections (Skin/Soft Tissue): 250-500mg q6-8h. Fusospirochetosis Infections (Oropharynx): 250-500mg q6-8h. Rheumatic Fever/Chorea Prevention: 125-250mg bid.	Streptococcal Infections (Scarlet fever, Erysipelas, Upper Respiratory Tract): 125-250mg q6-8h for 10 days. Pneumococcal Infections (Otitis media, Respiratory Tract): 250-500mg q6h until afebrile for at least 2 days. Staphylococcus Infections (Skin/Soft Tissue): 250-500mg q6-8h. Fusospirochetosis Infections (Oropharynx): 250-500mg q6-8h. Rheumatic Fever/Chorea Prevention: 125-250mg bid.
Zosyn (piperacillin sodium-tazobactam)	Inj: (Piperacillin-Tazobactam) 40mg-5mg/mL, 60mg-7.5mg/mL, 2g-0.25g, 3g-0.375g, 4g-0.5g, 4g-0.5g/100mL, 36g-4.5g	Treatment of appendicitis, peritonitis, uncomplicated/complicated skin and skin structure infections, postpartum endometritis, pelvic inflammatory disease, moderate severity of community acquired pneumonia, and moderate to severe nosocomial pneumonia.	Usual: 3.375g q6h for 7-10 days. Nosocomial Pneumonia: 4.5g q6h for 7-14 days plus aminoglycoside. CrCl 20-40mL/min: 2.25g q6h. CrCl <20mL/min: 2.25g q8h. Hemodialysis: Max: 2.25g q12h.Give 1 additional 0.75g dose after each dialysis period.	
STREPTOMYCES DERIVATIVES				
Sumycin (tetracycline HCl)	Sus: 125mg/5mL; Tab: 250mg, 500mg	Treatment of respiratory tract, urinary tract, and skin and skin structure infections, lymphogranuloma, psittacosis, trachoma, uncomplicated urethral/endocervical/rectal infection caused by Chlamydia, nongonococcal urethritis, chancroid, plague, cholera, brucellosis, and others. When PCN is contraindicated, treatment of uncomplicated gonorrhea, syphilis, listeriosis, anthrax, Clostridium species, and others. Adjunct therapy for amebicides and severe acne.	Mild-Moderate: 250mg qid or 500mg bid. Severe: 500mg qid. Continue for 24-48 hrs after symptoms subside (minimum 10 days with Group A β-hemolytic streptococci). Severe Acne: Initial: 1g/day in divided doses. Maint: After improvement, 125-500mg/day. Brucellosis: 500mg qid for 3 weeks plus streptomycin 1g IM bid for 1 week, then qd for 1 week. Syphilis: 30-40g equally divided over 10-15 days. Gonorrhea: 500mg q6h for 7 days. Chlamydia: 500mg qid for at least 7 days. Renal Dysfunction: Reduce dose or extend dose interval.	Usual: 25-50mg/kg divided bid-qid. Continue for 24-48 hrs after symptoms subside (minimum 10 days with Group A β-hemolytic streptococci). Severe Acne: Initial: 1g/day in divided doses. Maint: After improve ment. 125-500mg /day. Renal Dysfunction: Reduce dose or extend dose interval.

(Continued)

BRAND NAME (Generic)	DOSAGE FORM/ STRENGTH	INDICATIONS	ADULT DOSE	PEDIATRIC DOSE
STREPTOMYCES DERIVATIVES *(Continued)*				
Lincocin (lincomycin HCl)	Inj: 300mg/mL	Treatment of serious infections due to streptococci, pneumococci, and staphylococci. Reserve for PCN allergy or if PCN is inappropriate.	IM: Serious Infection: 600mg q24h. More Severe Infection: 600mg q12h or more often. IV: Dose depends on severity. Serious Infection: 600mg-1g q8-12h. More Severe Infection: Increase dose. Infuse over ≥1 hr: Life-Threatening Situation: Up to 8g/day has been given. Max: 8g/day. Severe Renal Dysfunction: 25-30% of normal dose.	>1 mo: IM: Serious Infection: 10mg/kg q24h. More Severe Infection: 10mg/kg q12h or more often. IV: 10-20mg/kg/day, depending on severity infused in divided doses as described for adults. Severe Renal Dysfunction: 25-30% of normal dose.
TETRACYCLINE DERIVATIVES				
Declomycin (demeclocycline HCl)	Tab: 150mg, 300mg	Treatment of infections due to *rickettsiae, Mycoplasma pneumoniae, B.recurrentis*; agents of psittacosis, ornithosis, lymphomagranuloma venereum or granuloma inguinale. Treatment of gram-negative infections (eg, respiratory, urinary tract), gram-positive infections (eg, respiratory tract, skin and soft tissue), trachoma, inclusion conjunctivitis. When PCN is contraindicated, treatment of gonorrhea, syphilis, listeriosis, anthrax, *Clostridium* species, and others. Adjunct therapy for amebicides.	Usual: 150mg qid or 300mg bid. Gonorrhea: Initial: 600mg, then 300mg q12h for 4 days. Gonorrhea: 600mg followed by 300mg q12h for 4 days to a total of 3g. Renal/Hepatic Impairment: Reduce dose and/or extend dose intervals. Continue therapy for at least 24-48 hrs after symptoms subside. Treat strep infections for at least 10 days. Take at least 1 hr before or 2 hrs after meals with plenty of fluids.	>8 yrs: Usual: 3-6mg/lb/day given bid-qid. Gonorrhea: 600mg followed by 300mg q12h for 4 days to a total of 3g. Renal/Hepatic Impairment: Reduce dose and/or extend dose intervals. Continue therapy for at least 24-48 hrs after symptoms subside. Treat strep infections for at least 10 days. Take at least 1 hr before or 2 hrs after meals with plenty of fluids.
Doryx (doxycycline hyclate)	Cap: 75mg, 100mg	Treatment of susceptible infections including respiratory, urinary, skin and skin structure, lymphogranuloma, psittacosis, trachoma, uncomplicated urethral/endocervical/rectal, nongonococcal urethritis, rickettsiae, chancroid, plague, cholera, brucellosis, anthrax. When penicillin is contraindicated, treatment of syphilis, listeriosis, *Clostridium* species, and others. Adjunct therapy for amebiasis and severe acne.	Usual: 100mg q12h on 1st day, followed by 100mg qd. Severe Infections/Chronic UTI: 100mg q12h. Uncomplicated Gonococcal Infections (Men, except anorectal infections): 100mg bid for 7 days, or 300mg followed 1 hr by another 300mg dose. Acute Epididymo-Orchitis: 100mg bid for at least 10 days. Primary/Secondary Syphilis: 300mg/day in divided doses for at least 10 days. Nongonococcal Urethritis, Uncomplicated Urethral/Endocervical/Rectal Infection: 100mg bid for at least 7 days. Inhalational Anthrax (post-exposure): 100mg bid for 60 days. Treat Strep infections for 10 days.	>8 yrs: >100 lbs: 100mg q12h on 1st day, followed by 100mg qd. Severe Infections/Chronic UTI: 100mg q12h; ≤100 lbs: 2mg/lb given bid on Day 1, followed by 1mg/lb given qd-bid thereafter. Severe Infections: Up to 2mg/lb. Inhalational Anthrax (post-exposure): >100 lbs: 1mg/lb for 60 days. <100 lbs: 100mg bid for 60 days.

BRAND NAME (Generic)	DOSAGE FORM/ STRENGTH	INDICATIONS	ADULT DOSE	PEDIATRIC DOSE
Dynacin (minocycline HCl)	**Cap:** 50mg, 75mg, 100mg; **Tab:** 50mg, 75mg, 100mg	Treatment of inclusion conjunctivitis, nongonococcal urethritis, and other infections (eg, respiratory tract, endocervical, rectal, urinary tract, skin and skin structure) caused by susceptible strains of microorganisms. Alternative treatment in certain other infections (eg, urethritis, gonococcal, syphilis, anthrax). Adjunctive therapy in acute intestinal amebiasis and severe acne. Treatment of *Mycobacterium marinum* and asymptomatic carriers of *Neisseria meningitidis.*	Usual: 200mg initially, then 100mg q12h; alternative is 100-200mg initially, then 50mg qid. Uncomplicated Gonococcal Infection (Men, Other Than Urethritis and Anorectal Infections): 200mg initially, then 100mg q12h for minimum 4 days. Uncomplicated Gonococcal Urethritis (Men): 100mg q12h for 5 days. Syphilis: Administer usual dose for 10-15 days. Meningococcal Carrier State: 100mg q12h for 5 days. *Mycobacterium marinum:* 100mg q12h for 6-8 weeks. Uncomplicated urethral, endocervical, or rectal infection: 100mg q12h for at least 7 days. Renal Dysfunction: Reduce dose and/or extend dose intervals.	>8 yrs: 4mg/kg initially followed by 2mg/kg q12h. Take with plenty of fluids.
Minocin (minocycline HCl)	**Cap:** 50mg, 100mg;	Treatment of inclusion conjunctivitis, nongonococcal urethritis, and other infections (eg, respiratory tract, endocervical, rectal, urinary tract, skin and skin structure) caused by susceptible strains of microorganisms. Alternative treatment in certain other infections (eg, urethritis, gonococcal, syphilis, anthrax). Adjunctive therapy in acute intestinal amebiasis and severe acne. Treatment of *Mycobacterium marinum* and asymptomatic carriers of *Neisseria meningitidis.*	Usual: 200mg initially, then 100mg q12h; alternative is 100-200mg initially, then 50mg qid. Uncomplicated Gonococcal Infection (Men, other than urethritis and anorectal infections): 200mg initially, then 100mg q12h for minimum 4 days. Uncomplicated Gonococcal Urethritis (Men): 100mg q12h for 5 days. Syphilis: Administer usual dose for 10-15 days. Meningococcal Carrier State: 100mg q12h for 5 days. *Mycobacterium marinum:* 100mg q12h for 6-8 weeks. Uncomplicated Urethral, Endocervical, or Rectal Infection Caused by *Chlamydia trachomatis* or *Ureaplasma urealyticum:* 100mg q12h for at least 7 days. Gonorrhea in Patients Sensitive to PCN: 200mg initially, then 100mg q12h for at least 4 days, with post-therapy cultures within 2-3 days. Take with plenty of fluids. Renal Dysfunction: Max: 200mg/24hrs.	>8 yrs: 4mg/kg initially followed by 2mg/kg q12h. Take with plenty of fluids. Renal Dysfunction: Max: 200mg/24 hrs.

(Continued)

TETRACYCLINE DERIVATIVES (Continued)

BRAND NAME (Generic)	DOSAGE FORM/ STRENGTH	INDICATIONS	ADULT DOSE	PEDIATRIC DOSE
Monodox (doxycycline monohydrate)	Cap: 50mg, 100mg	Treatment of respiratory tract, urinary tract, skin and skin structure, uncomplicated urethral/endocervical/rectal infection caused by C.trachomatis, nongonococcal urethritis caused by C.trachomatis and U.urealyticum, lymphogranuloma, psittacosis, trachoma, chancroid, plague, cholera, brucellosis. Treatment of uncomplicated gonorrhea, syphilis, listeriosis, anthrax, Clostridium species when PCN is contraindicated. Adjunct therapy for amebicides and severe acne.	Usual: 100mg q12h or 50mg q6h for 1 day, then 100 mg/day. Severe Infection: 100mg q12h. Uncomplicated Gonococcal Infections (except anorectal infections in men): 100mg bid for 7 days or 300mg stat, then repeat in 1 hr. Acute Epididymo-Orchitis caused by N.gonorrhea or C.trachomatis: 100mg bid for at least 10 days. Primary/Secondary Syphilis: 300mg/day in divided dose for at least 10 days. Uncomplicated Urethral/Endocervical/Rectal Infection caused by C.trachomatis: 100mg bid for at least 7 days. Nongonococcal Urethritis caused by C.trachomatis and U.urealyticum: 100mg bid for at least 7 days. Take with full glass of water. Take with food if GI upset occurs.	>8 yrs: ≤100 lbs: 2mg/lb divided in 2 doses for 1 day, then 1mg/lb daily in single or 2 divided doses. Severe Infection: May use up to 2mg/lb/day. >100 lbs: 100mg q12h or 50mg q6h for 1 day, then 100mg/day. Severe Infection: 100mg q12h. Take with food if GI upset occurs.
Oracea (doxycycline)	Cap: 40mg	Treatment of only inflammatory lesions (papules and pustules) of rosacea.	40mg qd in am. Take on empty stomach.	
Periostat (doxycycline hyclate)	Tab: 20mg	Adjunct to scaling and root planing to promote attachment level gain and reduces pocket depth in patients with adult periodontitis.	Following scaling and root planing, 20mg bid, 1 hour prior to morning and evening meals for up to 9 mos. Maintain adequate fluid intake with caps to reduce risk of esophageal irritation and ulceration.	
Solodyn (minocycline HCl)	Tab, Extended-Release: 45mg, 90mg, 135mg.	Treatment of inflammatory lesions of non-nodular moderate to severe acne vulgaris in patients ≥12 yrs.	1mg/kg qd for 12 weeks. Reduce dose with renal impairment.	≥12 yrs: 1mg/kg qd for 12 weeks. Reduce dose with renal impairment.
Vibra-tabs (doxycycline hyclate)	Tab: 100mg	Treatment of susceptible infections including respiratory, urinary, skin and skin structure, lymphogranuloma, psittacosis, trachoma, uncomplicated urethral/endocervical/rectal, nongonococcal urethritis, rickettsiae, chancroid, plague, cholera, brucellosis, anthrax. When penicillin is contraindicated, treatment of uncomplicated gonorrhea, syphilis, listeriosis, Clostridium species, and others. Adjunct therapy for amebiasis and severe acne. Prophylaxis of malaria.	Usual: 100mg q12h on day 1, then 100mg qd or 50mg q12h. Severe Infection: 100mg q12h. Treat for 10 days with strep infection. Uncomplicated Gonococcal Infection (Except Anorectal in Men): 100mg bid for 7 days or 300mg followed by 300mg in 1 hr. Uncomplicated Urethral/Endocervical/Rectal Infection and Nongonococcal Urethritis: 100mg bid for 7 days. Syphilis: 100mg bid for 2 weeks. Syphilis for >1 yr: 100mg bid for 4 weeks. Acute Epididymo-orchitis: 100mg bid for at least 10 days. Inhalation Anthrax (Post-Exposure): 100mg bid for 60 days. Malaria Prophylaxis: 100mg qd. Begin 1-2 days before travel and continue for 4 weeks after leaving malarious area.	

BRAND NAME (Generic)	DOSAGE FORM/ STRENGTH	INDICATIONS	ADULT DOSE	PEDIATRIC DOSE
Vibramycin (doxycycline)	**Cap:** (Doxycycline Hyclate) 50mg, 100mg. **Syrup:** (Doxycycline Calcium) 50mg/5mL; **Sus:** (Doxycycline Monohydrate) 25mg/5mL [60mL]	Treatment of susceptible infections including respiratory, urinary, skin and skin structure, lymphogranuloma, psittacosis, trachoma, uncomplicated urethral/endocervical/rectal, nongonococcal urethritis, rickettsiae, chancroid, plague, cholera, brucellosis, anthrax. When penicillin is contraindicated, treatment of uncomplicated gonorrhea, syphilis, listeriosis, Clostridium species, and others. Adjunct therapy for amebiasis and severe acne. Prophylaxis of malaria.	Usual: 100mg q12h on day 1, then 100mg qd or 50mg q12h. Severe Infection: 100mg q12h. Treat for 10 days with strep infection. Uncomplicated Gonococcal Infection (Except Anorectal in Men): 100mg bid for 7 days or 300mg followed by 300mg in 1 hr. Uncomplicated Urethral/Endocervical/Rectal Infection and Nongonococcal Urethritis: 100mg bid for 7 days. Syphilis: 100mg bid for 2 weeks. Syphilis for >1 yr: 100mg bid for 4 weeks. Acute Epididymo-orchitis: 100mg bid for at least 10 days. Inhalation Anthrax (Post-Exposure): 100mg bid for 60 days. Malaria Prophylaxis: 100mg qd. Begin 1-2 days before travel and continue for 4 weeks after leaving malarious area.	>8 yrs: ≤100 lbs: 1mg/lb bid on day 1, then 1mg/lb qd or 0.5mg/lb bid. Severe Infections: Maint: 2mg/lb. >100 lbs: Usual: 100mg q12h on day 1, then 100mg qd or 50mg q12h. Severe Infection: 100mg q12h. Treat for 10 days with strep infection. Inhalation Anthrax (Post-Exposure): <100 lbs: 1mg/lb bid for 60 days. ≥100 lbs: 100mg bid for 60 days. Malaria Prophylaxis: 2mg/kg qd. Max: 100mg/day. Begin 1-2 days before travel and continue for 4 weeks after leaving malarious area.
Vibramycin IV (doxycycline hyclate)	**Inj:** 100mg, 200mg	Treatment of rickettsiae, Mycoplasma pneumoniae, psittacosis, ornithosis, lymphogranuloma venereum, granuloma inguinale, relapsing fever, chancroid, Pasteurella pestis, Pasteurella tularensis, Bartonella bacilliformis, Bacteroides species, Vibrio comma, Vibrio fetus, Brucella species, E.coli, Enterobacter aerogenes, Shigella species, Mima species, Herellea species, Haemophilus influenzae, Klebsiella species, Streptococcus species, Diplococcus pneumoniae, Staphylococcus aureus, anthrax, and trachoma. When PCN is contraindicated; treatment of Neisseria gonorrhoeae, N.meningitidis, syphilis, yaws, Listeria monocytogenes, Clostridium species, Fusobacterium fusiforme and Actinomyces species. Adjunct therapy for amebiasis.	Usual: 200mg IV divided qd-bid on Day 1 then 100-200mg/day IV depending on severity, with 200mg administered in 1 or 2 infusions. Primary/Secondary Syphilis: 300mg/day IV for at least 10 days. Inhalation Anthrax (Post-Exposure): 100mg IV bid. Institute oral therapy as soon as possible and continue therapy for a total of 60 days.	>8 yrs: >100 lbs: Usual: 200mg IV divided qd-bid on Day 1 then 100-200mg/day depending on severity, with 200mg administered in 1 or 2 infusions. ≤100 lbs: 2mg/lb IV divided qd-bid on Day 1 then 1-2mg/lb/day IV divided qd-bid depending on severity. Inhalational Anthrax (Post-Exposure): ≤100 lbs: 1mg/lb IV bid. Institute oral therapy as soon as possible and continue therapy for a total of 60 days.

(Continued)

BRAND NAME (Generic)	DOSAGE FORM/ STRENGTH	INDICATIONS	ADULT DOSE	PEDIATRIC DOSE
MISCELLANEOUS				
Bactrim (trimethoprim-sulfamethoxazole)	(Sulfamethoxazole [SMX]-Trimethoprim [TMP]) **Tab:** 400mg-80mg; **DS:** 800mg-160mg	Treatment of urinary tract infection (UTI), acute otitis media, acute exacerbation of chronic bronchitis (AECB), travelers' diarrhea, Shigellosis, and pneumocystis carinii pneumonia (PCP).	UTI: 800mg SMX-160mg TMP q12h for 10-14 days. Shigellosis: 800mg SMX-160mg TMP q12h for 5 days. AECB: 800mg SMX-160mg TMP q12h for 14 days. PCP Treatment: 15-20mg/kg TMP and 75-100 mg/kg SMX per 24 hrs given q6h for 14-21 days. PCP Prophylaxis: 800mg SMX-160mg TMP qd. Traveler's Diarrhea: 800mg SMX-160mg TMP q12h for 5 days. CrCl: 15-30mL/min: 50% usual dose. CrCl: <15mL/min: Not recommended.	≥2 mo: UTI/Otitis Media: 4mg/kg TMP and 20mg/kg SMX q12h for 10 days. Shigellosis: 8mg/kg TMP and 40mg/kg SMX per 24 hrs given q12h for 5 days. PCP Treatment: 15-20mg/kg TMP and 75-100mg/kg SMX per 24 hrs given q6h for 14 days. PCP Prophylaxis: 150mg/m2/day TMP with 750mg/m2/day SMX given bid, on 3 consecutive days/week. Max: 320mg TMP/1600mg SMX/day. CrCl: 15-30mL/min: 50% usual dose. CrCl: <15mL/min: Not recommended.
Cleocin (clindamycin)	**Cap:** (HCl) 75mg, 150mg, 300mg; **Inj:** (Phosphate) 150mg/ mL, 300mg/50mL, 600mg/50mL, 900mg/ 50mL; **Sus:** (HCl) 75mg/5mL [100g]	Serious infections caused by anaerobes, streptococci, pneumococci and staphylococci.	Serious Infection: 150-300mg PO q6h or 600-1200 mg/day IM/IV given bid-qid. More Severe Infection: 300-450mg PO q6h or 1200-2700mg/day IM/IV given bid-qid. Life-threatening Infections: Up to 4800mg/day IV. Max: 600mg per IM injection. Take oral form with full glass of water. Treat B-hemolytic strep for at least 10 days.	Birth-16 yrs: Serious Infection: 8-16mg/kg/day PO. More Severe Infection: 16-20mg/kg/day PO. 1 mo-16 yrs: 20-40mg/kg/day IM/IV given bid-qid; use higher dose for more severe infection. <1 mo: 15-20mg/ kg/day IM/IV given tid-qid. Take oral form with full glass of water. Treat B-hemolytic strep for at least 10 days.
Coly-Mycin M (colistimethate sodium)	**Inj:** 150mg	Treatment of acute or chronic infections due to certain gram-negative bacilli (eg. Pseudomonas aeruginosa, Enterobacter aerogenes, E.coli, Klebsiella pneumoniae).	Usual: 2.5-5mg/kg/day IV/IM in 2-4 divided doses. Max: 5mg/kg/day. SCr 1.3-1.5mg/dL: 2.5-3.8mg/ kg/day IV/IM in 2 divided doses. SCr 1.6-2.5mg/dL: 2.5-3.8mg/day IV/IM in 2 divided doses. SCr 2.6-4mg/dL: 1.5mg/kg/day IV/IM q36h. Obesity: Base dose on IBW.	Usual: 2.5-5mg/kg/day IV/IM in 2-4 divided doses. Max: 5mg/kg/day. SCr 1.3-1.5mg/dL: 2.5-3.8mg/kg/day IV/IM in 2 divided doses. SCr 1.6-2.5mg/dL: 2.5-3.8mg/day IV/IM in 2 divided doses. SCr 2.6-4mg/day IV/IM q36h. Obesity: Base dose on IBW
Cubicin (daptomycin)	**Inj:** 500mg	Susceptible complicated skin and skin structure infections (cSSSI). Staphylococcus aureus blood stream infections (bacteremia).	≥18 yrs: Administer as IV infusion over 30 minutes. cSSSI: 4mg/kg once every 24 hrs for 7-14 days. S.aureus Bacteremia: 6mg/kg once every 24 hrs for minimum 2-6 weeks. Renal impairment: CrCl <30 mL/min, Hemodialysis or CAPD: (cSSSI) 4mg/kg or (S.aureus bacteremia) 6mg/kg once every 48 hrs.	
Flagyl IV (metronidazole HCl)	**Inj:** 500mg, 500mg (RTU)	Treatment of anaerobic intra-abdominal, skin and skin structure, gynecologic, bone and joint, CNS, lower respiratory tract infections, endocarditis, and septicemia.	LD: 15mg/kg IV. Maint: 6 hrs later, 7.5mg/kg IV q6h for 7-10 days or more. Max: 4g/24 hrs.	

BRAND NAME (Generic)	DOSAGE FORM/ STRENGTH	INDICATIONS	ADULT DOSE	PEDIATRIC DOSE
Hiprex (methenamine hippurate)	Tab: 1g	Prophylaxis or suppression of recurrent urinary tract infections when long-term therapy is necessary. For use only after infection is eradicated by other appropriate antimicrobials.	1g bid.	>12 yrs: 1g bid. 6 to 12 yrs: 0.5g-1g bid.
Ketek (telithromycin)	Tab: 300mg [20s], 400mg [60s, Ketek Pak; 100s]	Treatment of mild to moderate community-acquired pneumonia (CAP).	800mg qd for 7-10 days. Severe Renal Impairment (CrCl <30mL/min): Give after dialysis session on dialysis days. Severe Renal Impairment (CrCl <30mL/min) with Hepatic Impairment: 400mg qd.	
Macrobid (nitrofurantoin monohydrate)	Cap: 100mg	Treatment of acute uncomplicated urinary tract infections (acute cystitis).	100mg every 12 hrs for 7 days. Take with food.	>12 yrs: 100mg every 12 hrs for 7 days. Take with food.
Macrodantin (nitrofurantoin macrocrystals)	Cap: 25mg, 50mg, 100mg	Treatment of urinary tract infection.	50-100mg qid for at least 7 days. Take with food. Long-term Suppressive Use: 50-100mg at bedtime.	≥1 mo: 5-7mg/kg/day given qid for at least 7 days. Take with food. Long-term Suppressive Use: 1mg/kg/day given qd-bid.
Monurol (fosfomycin tromethamine)	Pow: 3g/sachet	Uncomplicated urinary tract infection (acute cystitis) in women.	≥18 yrs: 1 single-dose sachet. Mix with 3-4oz of water before ingesting.	
Primsol (trimethoprim HCl)	Sol: 50mg/5mL	Treatment of acute otitis media in pediatrics and urinary tract infection (UTI) in adults.	UTI: Usual: 100mg q12h or 200mg q24h for 10 days. CrCl: 15-30mL/min: Give 50% of usual dose.	Otitis Media: ≥6 mos: 5mg/kg q12h for 10 days. CrCl: 15-30mL/min: Give 50% of usual dose.
Rifadin (rifampin)	Cap: 150mg, 300mg; Inj: 600mg	Treatment of all forms of tuberculosis (TB). Treatment of asymptomatic carriers of *Neisseria meningitidis* to eliminate meningococci from the nasopharynx.	TB: 10mg/kg PO/IV qd. Max: 600mg/day. Meningococcal Carriers: 600mg bid for 2 days. Take 1 hr before or 2 hrs after a meal with a full glass of water.TB: 10-20mg/kg PO/IV qd. Max: 600mg/day.	Meningococcal Carriers: ≥1 mo: 10mg/kg q12h for 2 days. Max: 600mg/dose. <1 mo: 5mg/kg q12h for 2 days. Take 1 hr before or 2 hrs after a meal with a full glass of water.
Rifamate (isoniazid-rifampin)	Cap: (Isoniazid-Rifampin) 150mg-300mg	For pulmonary tuberculosis (TB). Not for initial therapy or prevention of TB.	2 caps qd. Take 1 hr before or 2 hrs after meals. Give with pyridoxine in the malnourished, those predisposed to neuropathy (eg, alcoholics, diabetics), and adolescents.	

(Continued)

BRAND NAME (Generic)	DOSAGE FORM/ STRENGTH	INDICATIONS	ADULT DOSE	PEDIATRIC DOSE
MISCELLANEOUS *(Continued)*				
Rifater (isoniazid-rifampin-pyrazinamide)	**Tab:** (Isoniazid-Pyrazinamide-Rifampin) 50mg-300mg-120mg	For initial phase of pulmonary tuberculosis treatment	≥44kg: 4 tabs single dose qd. 45-54kg: 5 tabs qd single dose. ≥55kg: 6 tabs single dose. Give pyridoxine in malnourished, if predisposed to neuropathy (eg, alcoholics, diabetics). Take 1 hr before or 2 hrs after meals with full glass of water. Treatment usually lasts 2 months.	≥15 yrs: ≤44kg: 4 tabs single dose qd. 45-54kg: 5 tabs qd single dose. ≥55kg: 6 tabs qd single dose. Give pyridoxine in malnourished, if predisposed to neuropathy (eg, alcoholics, diabetics), and adolescents. Take 1 hr before or 2 hrs after meals with full glass of water. Treatment usually lasts 2 months.
Septra (sulfamethoxazole-trimethoprim)	(Sulfamethoxazole [SMX]-Trimethoprim [TMP]) **Inj:** 80mg-16mg/mL; **Sus:** 200mg-40mg/5mL [100mL, 473mL]; **Tab:** 400mg-80mg; **Tab. DS:** 800mg-160mg	(Inj, Sus, Tab) Treatment of urinary tract infection (UTI), pneumocystis carinii pneumonia (PCP) and enteritis caused by *Shigella*. (Sus, Tab). Treatment of acute exacerbation of chronic bronchitis (AECB), travelers' diarrhea, and acute otitis media.	(Sus, Tab) UTI: 800mg-160mg PO q12h for 10-14 days. Shigellosis/Traveler's Diarrhea: 800mg-160mg PO q12h for 5 days. AECB: 800mg-160mg PO q 12h for 14 days. PCP Treatment: 15-20mg/kg TMP and 75-100mg/kg SMX per 24 hrs given PO q6h for 14-21 days PCP Prophylaxis: 800mg-160mg PO qd. (Inj) Severe UTI: 8-10mg/kg TMP IV given in divided doses q6, 8 or 12h for up to 14 days. PCP Treatment: 15-20mg/kg TMP IV given in divided doses q6-8h for up to 14 days. Shigellosis: 8-10mg/kg TMP IV given in divided doses q6, 8 or 12h for 5 days. (Inj, Sus, Tab) Renal Impairment: CrCl 15-30 mL/min: 50% usual dose. CrCl <15mL/min: Not recommended.	(Sus, Tab) ≥2 mo: UTI/Otitis Media: 4mg/kg TMP and 20mg/kg SMX q12h for 10 days. Shigellosis/Traveler's Diarrhea: 4mg/kg TMP and 20mg/kg SMX q12h for 5 days. PCP Treatment: 15-20mg/kg TMP and 75-100mg/kg SMX/24 hrs given q6h for 14-21 days. PCP Prophylaxis: 150mg/m2/day TMP and 750mg/m2/day SMX PO given bid, on 3 consecutive days per week. Max: 320mg TMP and 1600mg SMX per day. (Inj) Severe UTI: 8-10mg/kg TMP IV given in divided doses q6, 8 or 12h for up to 14 days. PCP Treatment: 15-20mg/kg TMP IV given in divided doses q6-8h for up to 14 days. Shigellosis: 8-10mg/kg TMP IV given in divided doses q6, 8 or 12h for 5 days. (Inj, Sus, Tab) Renal Impairment: CrCl 15-30mL/min: 50% usual dose. CrCl <15mL/min: Not recommended.
Synercid (dalfopristin-quinupristin)	**Inj:** (Dalfopristin-Quinupristin) 350mg-150mg per 500mg vial	Treatment of serious or life-threatening infections associated with vancomycin-resistant *Enterococcus faecium* (VREF) bacteremia and complicated skin and skin structure infections (SSSI) caused by *Staphylococcus aureus* (methicillin susceptible) or *Streptococcus pyogenes*.	VREF: 7.5mg/kg IV q8h. Duration depends on site and severity of infection. Complicated SSSI: 7.5mg/kg IV q12h for at least 7 days. Hepatic Cirrhosis (Child Pugh A or B): May need dose reduction.	≥16 yrs: VREF: 7.5mg/kg IV q8h. Duration depends on site and severity of infection. Complicated SSSI: 7.5mg/kg IV q12h for at least 7 days. Hepatic Cirrhosis (Child Pugh A or B): May need dose reduction.

BRAND NAME (Generic)	DOSAGE FORM/ STRENGTH	INDICATIONS	ADULT DOSE	PEDIATRIC DOSE
Vancocin (vancomycin HCl)	**Inj:** 500mg/100mL; 1g/200mL	Treatment of severe infections caused by susceptible strains of methicillin-resistant staphylococci. Indicated for penicillin-allergic patients, those who cannot receive or have failed to respond to other drugs, and for vancomycin-susceptible organisms that are resistant to other antimicrobials.	Usual: 500mg IV q6h or 1g IV q12h. Mild to Moderate Renal Impairment: Initial: 15mg/kg/day. Maint: 1.9mg/kg/d. Administer 10mg/min or over at least 60 min, whichever is longer. Renal Dysfunction: Initial: 15mg/kg. Dose is about 15x the GFR in mL/min (refer to table in labeling). Elderly: Require greater dose reduction. Functionally Anephric: Initial: 15mg/kg, then 1.9mg/kg24hrs. Marked Renal Dysfunction: 250-1000mg every several days. Anuria: 1000mg every 7-10 days.	Usual: 10mg/kg IV q6h. Infants/Neonates: Initial: 15mg/kg, then 10mg/kg q12h for neonates in the 1st week of life and q8h thereafter until 1 mo of age. Administer over at least 60 min. Renal Dysfunction: Initial: 15mg/kg. Dose is about 15x the GFR in mL/min (refer to table in labeling). Premature Infants: Require greater dose reduction.
Vancocin Oral (vancomycin HCl)	**Cap:** 125mg, 250mg	Staphylococcal enterocolitis and antibiotic-associated pseudomembranous colitis caused by *C.difficile*.	500mg-2g/day given tid-qid for 7-10 days.	40mg/kg/day given tid-qid for 7-10 days. Max: 2g/day.
Zyvox (linezolid)	**Inj:** 2mg/mL [100mL, 200mL, 300mL]; **Sus:** 100mg/5mL; **Tab:** 400mg, 600mg	Vancomycin resistant *Enterococcus faecium* (VRE) infections, nosocomial pneumonia caused by *Staphylococcus aureus* (methicillin-susceptible and -resistant strains) or *Streptococcus pneumoniae* (including multi-drug resistant strains (MDRSP)), complicated skin and skin structure infections (SSSI) including diabetic foot infections without concomitant osteomyelitis caused by *Staphylococcus aureus* (methicillin-susceptible and -resistant strains), *Streptococcus pyogenes*, or *Streptococcus agalactiae*, uncomplicated SSSI caused by *Staphylococcus aureus* (methicillin-susceptible only) or *Streptococcus pyogenes*, community-acquired pneumonia (CAP) caused by *Streptococcus pneumoniae* (MDRSP), including concurrent bacteremia, or *Staphylococcus aureus* (methicillin-susceptible strains only).	Complicated SSSI/CAP/Nosocomial Pneumonia: 600mg IV/PO q12h for 10-14 days. VRE: 600mg IV/PO q12h for 14-28 days. Uncomplicated SSSI: 400mg PO q12h for 10-14 days.	Complicated SSSI/CAP/Nosocomial Pneumonia: Treat for 10-14 days. ≥12 yrs: 600mg IV/PO q12h. Birth-11 yrs: 10mg/kg IV/PO q8h. VRE: Treat for 14-28 days: IV/PO q8h. Uncomplicated SSSI: Treat for 10-14 days: ≥12 yrs: 600mg PO q12h. 5-11 yrs: 10mg/kg PO q12h. <5 yrs: 10mg/kg PO q8h. Neonates <7 days should be initiated with dosing regimen of 10mg/kg q12h; may increase to 10mg/kg q8h if suboptimal response. All neonatal patients should receive 10mg/kg q8h by 7 days of life.

SYSTEMIC ANTIFUNGALS

GENERIC	BRAND	INDICATION	DOSAGE FORM	DOSAGE
Amphotericin B lipid complex injection	Abelcet	Invasive fungal infections in patients who are refractory to or intolerant of conventional amphotericin B therapy.	**Inj:** 5mg/mL	Single infusion 5mg/kg.
Amphotericin B liposome injection	AmBisome	Treatment of patients with *Aspergillus* species, *Candida* species and/or *Cryptococcus* species infections refractory to amphotericin B deoxycholate, cryptococcal meningitis in HIV patients, fungal infection in febrile, neutropenic patients, and treatment of visceral leishmaniasis.	**Inj:** 50mg	3-6mg/kg/day.
Amphotericin B	Amphocin	Progressive, potentially life-threatening fungal infections: Aspergillosis, cryptococcosis, North American blastomycosis, systemic candidiasis, coccidioidomycosis, histoplasmosis, zygomycosis, sporotrichosis, and infections due to *Conidiobolus* and *Basidiobolus* species.	**Inj:** 50mg	**Initial:** 0.25mg/kg. **Titrate:** Increase by 5-10mg/day, depending on cardio-renal status, up to 0.5-0.7mg/kg/day.
Amphotericin B cholesteryl sulfate	Amphotec	Treatment of invasive aspergillosis in patients with renal impairment, unacceptable toxicity, or previous failure to amphotericin deoxycholate.	**Inj:** 50mg, 100mg	3-4mg/kg/day IV at 1mg/kg/hr.
Caspofungin Acetate	Cancidas	Treatment of candidemia, esophageal candidiasis, fungal infections in febrile, neutropenic patients, invasive aspergillosis in patients who are refractory to or intolerant of other therapies.	**Inj:** 50mg, 70mg	70mg loading dose on Day 1 and then 50mg qd.
Griseofulvin	Grifulvin V	Indicated for ringworm.	**Sus:** 125mg/5mL [120mL]; **Tab:** 500mg	0.5-1g qd.
Griseofulvin	Gris-PEG	Indicated for ringworm.	**Tab** (ultramicrosize): 125mg, 250mg	375mg as a single dose or in divided doses.
Terbinafine HCl	Lamisil	Onychomycosis of the toenail or fingernail.	**Tab:** 250mg	250mg po qd for 6 weeks.
Micafungin sodium	Mycamine	Esophageal candidiasis and prophylaxis of *Candida* infection in HSCT patients.	**Inj:** 50mg	**Candidiasis:** 150mg/day for 5 days; **Prophylaxis:** 150mg/day for 20 days.
Voriconazole	Vfend	Invasive aspergillosis, esophageal candidiasis, serious fungal infections caused by *Scedosporium apiospermum* and *Fusarium* spp. including *Fusarium solani*, candidemia in nonneutropenic patients.	**Inj:** 200mg; **Sus:** 40mg/mL [100mL]; **Tab:** 50mg, 200mg	PO 200mg q12h. IV LD: 6mg/kg q12h for first 24h. IV MD: 3-4mg/kg q12h.
Fluconazole	Diflucan	Treatment of vaginal, oropharyngeal, esophageal, and systemic candidiasis. Treatment of peritonitis and UTI caused by *Candida*. Treatment of cryptococcal meningitis. Prophylaxis in patients undergoing BMT.	**Inj:** 200mg/100mL, 400mg/200mL; **Sus:** 50mg/5mL, 200mg/5mL [35mL]; **Tab:** 50mg, 100mg,150mg, 200mg	**Vaginal *Candida*:** 150mg po x 1 day. **All other:** 100-200mg/day. **Max:** 400mg/day.

(Continued)

GENERIC	BRAND	INDICATION	DOSAGE FORM	DOSAGE
Clotrimazole	Mycelex Troche	Oropharyngeal candidiasis. To prevent oropharyngeal candidiasis in immunocompromised conditions.	Loz/Troche: 10mg	1 troche in mouth 5 times/day for 14 days. **Prophylaxis:** 1 troche tid.
Nystatin	Mycostatin	(Cream, Powder) Treatment of cutaneous or mucocutaneous mycoticnfections caused by *Candida*. **(Sus):** Oral candidiasis. **(Tab):** Treatment of non-esophageal mucous membrane GI candidiasis.	**Cream:** 100,000 U/gm, **Powder:** 100,000 U/gm **Sus:** 100,000 U/mL [60mL, 480mL]; **Tab:** 500,000 U	**Powder:** Apply to affected area twice daily or as indicated until healing is complete. **Cream:** Apply to candidal lesions two or three times daily until healing is complete. **Sus:** 4-6mL qid. Retain in mouth as long as possible before swallowing. **Tab:** 500,000-1,000,000 U tid.
Flucytosine	Ancobon	Treatment of septicemia, endocarditis, and urinary tract infections caused by *Candida*. Treatment of meningitis and pulmonary infection caused by *Cryptococcus*.	**Cap:** 250mg, 500mg	50-150mg/kg/day given q6h.
Ketoconazole	Nizoral	Candidiasis, chronic mucocutaneous candidiasis, oral thrush, candiduria, blastomycosis, coccidioidomycosis, histoplasmosis, chromomycosis, and paracoccidioidomycosis. Treatment of patients with severe recalcitrant cutaneous dermatophyte infections.	**Tab:** 200mg	200mg qd. **Max:** 400mg qd.
Itraconazole	Sporanox	Onychomycosis of the toenail and fingernail, blastomycosis and histoplasmosis. Treatment of aspergillosis if refractory to or intolerant to amphoteracin B. (Sol) Treatment of oropharyngeal and esophageal candidiasis.	**Cap:** 100mg; **Inj:** 10mg/mL; **Sol:** 10mg/mL [150mL]	**(Cap) Blastomycosis:** 200mg once daily (2 capsules). **Aspergillosis:** 200-400mg. **Max:** 400mg/day. **(Inj):** 200 mg b.i.d. for four doses, followed by 200 mg once daily for up to 14 days. **(Sol):** Swish (10 mL at a time) for several seconds and swallow.
Anidulafungin	Eraxis	Treatment of candidemia and other forms of *Candida* infections esophageal candidiasis.	**Inj:** 50mg	**Candidemia:** LD 200mg on Day 1, MD 100mg x 14d. **Esophageal Candidiasis:** 100mg qd x 1 day then 50mg qd x 14 days
Posaconazole	Noxafil	Prophylaxis of invasive *Aspergillus* and *Candida*, oropharyngeal candidiasis, including oropharyngeal candidiasis refractory to itraconazole and/or fluconazole.	**Susp:** 40mg/mL [105mL]	**Prophylaxis:** 200mg tid. **Oropharyngeal Candidiasis:** 100mg bid x 1 day, 100mg qd x 13 days.

ANKYLOSING SPONDYLITIS AGENTS

DRUG (BRAND)	HOW SUPPLIED	USUAL DOSE RANGE	MAX DOSE
COX-2 INHIBITOR			
Celecoxib (Celebrex)	**Cap:** 50mg, 100mg, 200mg, 400mg	200mg qd or 100mg bid.	400mg/day with food.
MISCELLANEOUS			
Botanical/Mineral Substances (Traumeel Injection)	**Inj:** 2.2mL amps [10S]	**Adults:** 1 amp qd for acute disorders or 1-2 amps 1-3 times weekly. **Pediatrics:** >6 yrs: 1 amp qd for acute disorders or 1-2 amps 1-3 times weekly. **2-6 yrs:** Use ½ of the adult dosage. May administer IV, IM, SQ, or intradermally.	n/a
MONOCLONAL ANTIBODIES/TNF-RECEPTOR BLOCKERS			
Infliximab (Remicade)	**Inj:** 100mg	5mg/kg as IV infusion repeat at 2 and 6 wks.	20mg/kg.
Adalimumab (Humira)	**Inj:** 40mg/0.8mL	40mg SQ every other wk.	n/a
NSAIDs			
Sulindac (Clinoril)	**Tab:** 150mg, 200mg*	150mg bid with food.	400mg/day with food.
Diclofenac Potassium (Cataflam)	**Tab:** 50mg	50mg tid-qid.	200mg/day.
Diclofenac Sodium (Voltaren)	**Tab, Delayed-Release:** 25mg, 50mg, 75mg **Tab, Extended-Release:** 100mg	25mg qid and 25mg qhs prn.	200mg/day.
Indomethacin (Indocin)	**Cap:** 25mg, 50mg; **Sus:** 25mg/5mL [237mL]	25mg PO bid-tid.	200mg/day.
Naproxen (EC-Naprosyn, Naprosyn)	**Sus:** 25mg/mL; **Tab:** 250mg, 375mg, 500mg; **Tab, Delayed-Release:** 375mg, 500mg	250mg, 375mg, or 500mg bid; 375mg or 500mg bid.	1500mg/day.
Naproxen sodium (Anaprox)	**Tab:** 275mg	750mg-1g qd; 275mg bid or 550mg bid.	1650mg/day.
(Anaprox DS)	**Tab:** 550mg*	750mg-1g qd; 275mg bid or 550mg bid.	1g/day.
(Naprelan)	**Tab, Extended-Release:** 375mg, 500mg	750mg-1g qd; 275mg bid or 550mg bid.	1g/day.
SALICYLATE			
Aspirin (Genuine Bayer Aspirin, Bayer Extra Strength)	**Tab:** 325mg; **Tab, Extra-Strength:** 500mg	Up to 4g/day in divided doses.	4g/day.
(Ecotrin)	**Tab, Delayed-Release:** 81mg, 325mg, 500mg	Up to 4g/day in divided doses.	4g/day.
TNF-RECEPTOR BLOCKER			
Etanercept (Enbrel)	**Inj:** 25mg [vial], 50mg/mL [syringe]	50mg SQ per wk, given as one SQ injection.	50mg/wk.

*Scored.

BONE MINERAL DENSITY CLASSIFICATION/TESTS

World Health Organization (WHO) Definition of Osteoporosis	
Normal	Bone mineral density within 1 standard deviation (SD) of the mean young adult women (T-score ≥ -1.0)
Osteopenia (low bone mass)	Bone mineral density between 1.0 and 2.5 SD below the mean for young adult women ($-2.5 <$ T-score < -1.0)
Osteoporosis	Bone mineral density 2.5 SD or more below the normal mean for young adult women (T-score ≤ -2.5)

Note: The definitions above should not be applied to premenopausal women, men <50 years of age, and children.

Bone mineral density (BMD) tests

- BMD tests provide a measurement of T-score for bone density at hip and spine to:
  - —Establish and confirm a diagnosis of osteoporosis
  - —Predict future fracture risk
  - —Measure response to osteoporosis treatment
- BMD is measured in grams of mineral per square centimeter scanned (g/cm^2) and compared to the expected BMD for the patient's age and sex (Z-score) or compared with "normal adults" of the same sex (T-score).
- The difference between the patient's score and the optimal BMD is expressed in standard deviations (SD) above and below the mean. Usually 1 SD equals about 10-15% of the bone density value in g/cm^2.
- Negative values for T-score, such as -1, -2, or -2.5, indicate low bone mass.
- The greater the negative score, the greater the risk of fracture.

DIETARY CALCIUM INTAKE

Recommended Calcium Intakes*	
Age	**Daily Intake (mg)**
Birth-6 months	210
6 months-1 year	270
1-3 years	500
4-8 years	800
9-13 years	1300
14-18 years	1300
19-30 years	1000
31-50 years	1000
51-70 years	1200
70 years or older	1200
Pregnant or Lactating	
14-18 years	1300
19-50 years	1000
*National Academy of Sciences, 1997.	

Estimating Daily Dietary Calcium Intake

Step 1: Estimate calcium intake from calcium-rich foods.*

Product	Servings/Day	Calcium/Serving (mg)		Calcium (mg)
Milk (8 oz)	_____	× 300	=	_____
Yogurt (8 oz)	_____	× 400	=	_____
Cheese (1 oz, or 1 cubic inch)	_____	× 200	=	_____
Fortified foods or juices	_____	× 80-1000**	=	_____

Step 2: Total from above + 250 mg for nondairy sources = total dietary calcium.

* About 75-80% of the calcium consumed in American diets is from dairy products.
** Calcium content of fortified foods varies.

Factors related to vitamin D that may affect calcium absorption:

- National Osteoporosis Foundation recommends an intake of 800 to 1000 International Units (IU) of vitamin D_3 per day for adults over age 50
- Desired level for the average adult's serum 25(OH)D concentration is 30 ng/mL (75 nmol/L) or higher
- Safe upper limit for vitamin D intake was set at 2000 IU per day in 1997
- Patients with malabsorption (eg, celiac disease) or chronic renal insufficiency, or those who are housebound, chronically ill, or have limited sun exposure, may need vitamin D supplements

Source: National Institute of Arthritis and Musculoskeletal and Skin Diseases (NIAMS), National Institutes of Health.

GOUT AGENTS

DRUG (BRAND)	HOW SUPPLIED	USUAL DOSE RANGE	MAX DOSE
ALKALINIZING AGENT			
Citric acid/ Potassium citrate (Polycitra)	**Packet:** 1002mg-3300mg/pack [100^S]; **Sol:** (Citric Acid-Potassium Citrate) 334mg-550mg/5mL [480mL]	15mL or 1 packet qid, pc and hs. Dilute in 6 oz of water or juice.	
CORTICOSTEROID			
Hydrocortisone acetate	**Inj:** 25mg/mL	**Large joints:** 25-37.5mg. **Small joints:** 10-25mg. **Bursae:** 25-37.5mg. **Tendon Sheaths:** 5-12.5mg. **Soft Tissue Infiltration:** 25-50mg. **Ganglia:** 12.5-25mg.	50mg/injection.
NSAIDs			
Indomethacin (Indocin)	**Cap:** 25mg, 50mg; **Sus:** 25mg/5mL [237mL]	**Acute Gout:** 50mg PO tid until pain is tolerable, then d/c.	
Naproxen (Anaprox)	**Tab:** 275mg	**Acute Gout:** 825mg followed by 275mg q8h.	
(Anaprox DS)	550mg*	**Acute Gout:** 825mg followed by 275mg q8h.	
(Naprelan)	**Tab, Extended-Release:** 375mg, 500mg	**Acute Gout:** 1-1.5g qd x 1 day, then 1g qd until attack subsides.	1g/day.
(Naprosyn)	**Sus:** 25mg/mL; **Tab:** 250mg*, 375mg, 500mg*; **Tab, Delayed-Release:** (EC-Naprosyn) 375mg, 500mg	**Acute Gout:** 750mg followed by 250mg q8h until attack subsides.	1500mg/day.
Sulindac (Clinoril)	**Tab:** 150mg, 200mg*	**Acute Gout:** 200mg bid	400mg/day
PHENANTHRENE DERIVATIVE			
Colchicine	**Inj:** 0.5mg/mL; **Tab:** 0.5mg, 0.6mg	**Acute Gout:** 1-1.2mg, then 0.5-0.6mg/hr until pain relief attack. or diarrhea ensues (wait 3 days between courses). **Prophylaxis:** <1 attack/yr: 0.5-0.6mg/day given 3-4x/wk. >1 attack/yr: 0.5-0.6mg qd.	4-8mg/acute
URICOSURIC AGENTS			
Probenecid	**Tab:** 500mg	**Initial:** 250mg bid x 1 wk. **Titrate:** Increase by 500mg every 4 wks. **Maint:** 500mg bid.	2g/day.
Sulfinpyrazone	**Tab:** 100mg, 200mg	**Initial:** 100-200mg bid x 1 wk. **Maint:** 200mg bid, increase to 300mg if needed.	800mg/day.
XANTHINE OXIDASE INHIBITOR			
Allopurinol (Zyloprim)	**Tab:** 100mg*, 300mg*	**Mild Gout: Usual:** 200-300mg/day. **Moderately-Severe Gout: Usual:** 400-600mg/day.	800mg/day.
COMBINATION			
Colchicine/ Probenecid	**Tab:** (Colchicine-Probenecid) 0.5mg-500mg	1 tab qd x 1 wk, then 1 tab bid. **Titrate:** May increase by 1 tab/day every 4 wks.	4 tabs/day.

*Scored.

OSTEOARTHRITIS AGENTS

DRUG (BRAND)	HOW SUPPLIED	USUAL DOSE RANGE	MAX DOSE
NSAIDs			
Diclofenac sodium (Voltaren)	**Tab, Delayed-Release:** 25mg, 50mg, 75mg;	50mg bid-tid or 75mg bid 100mg qd.	150mg/day.
(Voltaren-XR)	**Tab, Delayed-Release:** 100mg	50mg bid-tid or 75mg bid 100mg qd.	150mg/day.
(Voltaren Gel)	**Gel:** 1%	Measure onto enclosed dosing card to appropriate 2g or 4g line. Lower Extremities: Apply 4g to affected foot, knee, or ankle qid. Upper Extremities: Apply 2g to affected hand, elbow, or wrist qid.	Lower Extremities: 16g/day to any single joint. Upper Extremities: 8g/day to any single joint. 32g/day over all affected joints.
Diflunisal (Dolobid)	**Tab:** 250mg, 500mg	250-500mg bid.	1500mg/day.
Etodolac	**Cap:** 300mg, 400mg, 500mg	300mg bid-tid or 400-500mg bid.	1000mg/day.
(Etodolac XR)	**Tab, Delayed-Release:** 400mg, 500mg, 600mg	400-1000mg qd.	1200mg/day.
Fenoprofen (Nalfon)	**Cap:** 200mg, 300mg; **Tab:** 600mg	300-600mg tid-qid	3200mg/day.
Flurbiprofen (Ansaid)	**Tab:** 50mg, 100mg	200-300mg/day given bid, tid or qid.	300mg/day or 100mg/dose.
Ketoprofen (Oruvail)	**Cap, Extended-Release:** 200mg	200mg qd.	200mg/day.
Ibuprofen (Motrin, Motrin IB)	**Sus:** 100mg/5mL [120mL, 480mL]; **Tab:** 400mg, 600mg, 800mg **Tab:** 200mg	300mg qid or 400mg, 600mg or 800mg tid-qid. (Motrin IB) 200mg q4-6h. 400mg with meals/milk.	3200mg/day. 1200mg/day. (Motrin IB)
Meclofenamate	**Cap:** 50mg, 100mg	200-400mg/day in 3-4 divided doses.	400mg/day.
Meloxicam (Mobic)	**Sus:** 7.5mg/5mL **Tab:** 7.5mg, 15mg	7.5mg qd.	15mg/day.
Nabumetone (Relafen)	**Tab:** 500mg, 750mg	1000mg qd.	2000mg/day.
Naproxen (Naprosyn, EC-Naprosyn)	**Sus:** 25mg/mL **Tab:** 250mg, 375mg, 500mg; **Tab, Delayed-Release:** 375 or 500mg bid	250, 375, or 500mg bid. 375mg, 500mg.	1500mg/day.
Naproxen sodium (Anaprox)	**Tab:** 275mg	750mg-1g qd, 275mg bid or 550mg bid.	1650mg/day.
(Anaprox DS)	**Tab:** 550mg*	750mg-1g qd, 275mg bid or 550mg bid.	1.5g/day.
(Naprelan)	**Tab, Extended-Release:** 375mg, 500mg	750mg-1g qd, 275mg bid or 550mg bid.	1.5g/day.
Oxaprozin (Daypro)	**Tab:** 600mg*	1200mg qd.	1800mg/day in divided doses (not to exceed 26mg/kg/day).
Piroxicam (Feldene)	**Cap:** 10mg, 20mg	20mg qd or 10mg bid.	
Sulindac (Clinoril)	**Tab:** 150mg, 200mg	150mg bid with food.	400mg/day with food.
Tolmetin (Tolectin)	**Cap:** (DS) 400mg; **Tab:** 200mg*, 600mg	400mg tid.	1800mg/day.
COX-2 INHIBITOR			
Celecoxib (Celebrex)	**Cap:** 50mg, 100mg, 200mg, 400mg	200mg qd or 100mg bid.	

(Continued)

OSTEOARTHRITIS AGENTS

DRUG (BRAND)	HOW SUPPLIED	USUAL DOSE RANGE	MAX DOSE
SALICYLATE			
Aspirin (Genuine Bayer Aspirin, Bayer Extra Strength, Ecotrin)	**Tab:** 325mg Tab, Extra Strength: **Tab, Delayed-Release:** 81mg, 325mg, 500mg	Up to 3g/day in 500mg divided doses.	4g/day.
Salsalate (Salflex)	**Tab:** 500mg, 750mg*	1000mg tid or 1500mg bid.	
Choline Magnesium Trisalicylate (Trilisate)	**Liq:** 500mg/5mL; **Tab:** 500mg*, 750mg*, 1000mg*	1500mg bid.	3g/d.
NSAID COMBINATION			
Diclofenac sodium/Misoprostol (Arthrotec)	**Tab:** 50mg-0.2mg, 75mg-0.2mg	50mg tid. Do not crush, chew or divide.	
MISCELLANEOUS			
Botanical/Mineral substances (Traumeel Inj)	**Inj:** 2.2mL amps [10^S]	1 amp qd for acute disorders or 1-2 amps 1-3 times weekly. May administer IV, IM, SQ, or intradermally.	NA
Flavocoxid (Limbrel)	**Cap:** 250mg, 500mg	250-500mg q12h. May increase to 2 or more caps q12h under physician supervision.	500-1000mg/ day.
Hyaluronan (Euflexxa)	**Inj:** 1% [2mL]	Inject 2mL intra-articularly into the knee weekly for 3 wks. Total 3 injections.	3 injections.
(Hyalgan)	**Inj:** 2mL	2mL by intra-articular injection once a wk. Some patients may experience benefit with 3 injections given at weekly intervals.	5 injections.
(Orthovisc)	**Inj:** 30mg/2mL	30mg intra-articularly once a wk. Total 3-4 injections.	3-4 injections.
(Supartz)	**Inj:** 2.5mL	2.5mL by intra-articular injection once a wk. Some patients may experience benefit with 3 injections given at weekly intervals.	5 injections.
Hylan G-F 20 (Synvisc)	**Inj:** 8mg/mL	Intra-articular injection once weekly (one wk apart).	3 injections.

*Scored

OSTEOPOROSIS AGENTS

DRUG (BRAND)	INDICATIONS	HOW SUPPLIED	DOSAGE
BISPHOSPHONATES & COMBINATIONS			
Alendronate Sodium (Fosamax)	Treatment and prevention of osteoporosis in postmenopausal women. Treatment to increase bone mass in men with osteoporosis. Treatment of glucocorticoid-induced osteoporosis.	Sol: 70mg [75mL]; Tab: 5mg, 10mg, 35mg, 40mg, 70mg	Osteoporosis: Treatment: 70mg once weekly or 10mg qd. Prevention: 35mg once weekly or 5mg qd. Glucocorticoid-Induced: 5mg qd; 10mg qd for postmenopausal women not on estrogen. Take at least 30 min before the first food, beverage (other than water), or medication (Take tabs with 6-8 oz plain water or 2oz with oral sol). Do not lie down for at least 30 min and until after 1st food of day.
Alendronate Sodium/ Cholecalciferol (Fosamax Plus D)	Treatment of osteoporosis in postmenopausal women. Treatment to increase bone mass in men with osteoporosis.	Tab: (Alendronate Sodium-Cholecalciferol) 70mg-2800 IU, 70mg-5600 IU	Adults: 1 tab (70mg/5600 IU or 70mg/2800 IU) once weekly. Take at least 30 min before 1st food, beverage (other than water), or medication. Do not lie down for at least 30 min and until after 1st food of day.
Ibandronate Sodium (Boniva)	(Inj) Treatment of osteoporosis in postmenopausal women. (PO) Treatment and prevention of postmenopausal osteoporosis.	Inj: 3mg/3mL; Tab: 2.5mg, 150mg	Inj: 3mg IV over 15-30 sec every 3 months. PO: 2.5mg qd or 150mg once monthly. Swallow whole with 6-8 oz water. Do not lie down for 60 min after dose. Take at least 60 min before 1st food, drink (other than water), medication, or supplementation.
Risedronate Sodium (Actonel)	Prevention and treatment of osteoporosis in postmenopausal women, glucocorticoid-induced osteoporosis in men and women. Increase bone mass in men with osteoporosis.	Tab: 5mg, 30mg, 35mg, 75mg, 150mg	Postmenopausal Osteoporosis Prevention/Treatment: 5mg qd or 35mg once weekly or 75mg on 2 consecutive days each month or 150mg once a month. Glucocorticoid-Induced Osteoporosis: 5mg qd. Increase Bone Mass in Men with Osteoporosis: 35mg once weekly. Take at least 30 min before the first food or drink of the day other than water. Swallow tab in upright position with 6-8 oz of plain water. Do not lie down for 30 min after dose.
Risedronate Sodium/ Calcium Carbonate (Actonel with Calcium)	Treatment and prevention of postmenopausal osteoporosis.	Tab: (Risedronate Sodium) 35mg; Tab: (Calcium Carbonate) 1250mg	Risedronate: 35mg once weekly (Day 1 of 7-day treatment cycle). Take at least 30 min before 1st food or drink of day other than water. Swallow tab in upright position with 6-8oz of plain water. Do not lie down for 30 min after dose. Calcium: 1250mg qd with food on each of remaining 6 days (Days 2-7 of the 7-day treatment cycle).
Zoledronic Acid (Reclast)	Treatment of osteoporosis in postmenopausal women and to reduce incidence of new clinical fractures in patients at high risk of fractures.	Sol: 5mg/100mL [100mL]	5mg IV once a year. Infuse for >15 min at constant rate. Hydrate prior to administration.
HORMONE THERAPY			
Conjugated Estrogens (Premarin Tabs)	Prevention of postmenopausal osteoporosis.	Tab: 0.3mg, 0.45mg, 0.625mg, 0.9mg, 1.25mg	0.3mg qd continuous or cyclically (eg, 25 days on, 5 days off).

DRUG (BRAND)	INDICATIONS	HOW SUPPLIED	DOSAGE
HORMONE THERAPY (Continued)			
Conjugated Estrogens/ Medroxyprogesterone Acetate (Premphase)	For prevention of osteoporosis in women with intact uterus.	Tab: 0.625mg (Estrogens, Conjugated) and 0.625mg-5mg (Estrogens, Conjugated-Medroxyprogesterone)	0.625mg tab qd on Days 1-14 and 0.625mg-5mg tab qd on Days 15-28. Re-evaluate after 3-6 months.
Conjugated Estrogens/ Medroxyprogesterone Acetate (Prempro)	Prevention of postmenopausal osteoporosis in women with intact uterus.	Tab: (Estrogens, Conjugated-Medroxyprogesterone) 0.3mg-1.5mg, 0.45mg-1.5mg, 0.625mg-2.5mg, 0.625mg-5mg	Initial: 0.3mg-1.5mg qd. Adjust dose based on response. Re-evaluate after 3-6 months.
Estradiol (Alora)	Prevention of postmenopausal osteoporosis.	Patch: 0.025mg/ 24 hrs, 0.05mg/ 24 hrs [8^s 24^s], 0.075mg/24 hrs, 0.1mg/24 hrs [8^s]	Apply to lower abdomen, upper quadrant of the buttocks or the hip; avoid breasts and waistline. Osteoporosis: Apply 0.025mg/day twice weekly. Titrate: May increase depending on bone mineral density and adverse events.
Estradiol (Climara)	Prevention of postmenopausal osteoporosis.	Patch: 0.025mg/day, 0.0375mg/day, 0.05mg/day, 0.06mg/day, 0.075mg/day, 0.1mg/day [4^s]	Apply 1 patch weekly to lower abdomen or upper area of buttocks (avoid breasts and waistline). Rotate application sites. Minimum Effective Dose: 0.025mg/day once weekly.
Estradiol (Estrace)	Prevention of osteoporosis.	Tab: 0.5mg*, 1mg*, 2mg* *scored	0.5mg qd cyclically (23 days on and 5 days off).
Estradiol (Estraderm)	Prevention of postmenopausal osteoporosis.	Patch: 0.05mg/24 hrs, 0.1mg/24 hrs [1^s, 8^s, 48^s]	Initial: 0.05mg/day. May give continuously without intact uterus. May give cyclically (3 weeks on, 1 week off) with intact uterus. Apply to clean, dry area on trunk of body. Do not apply to breast or waistline. Replace twice weekly. Rotate application site.
Estradiol (Gynodiol)	Prevention of osteoporosis.	Tab: 0.5mg*, 1mg*, 1.5mg*, 2mg* *scored	0.5mg qd (23 days on and 5 days off).
Estradiol (Menostar)	Prevention of postmenopausal osteoporosis.	Patch: 14mcg/day [4^s]	Apply 1 patch weekly to lower abdomen (avoid breasts, waistline, and areas where sitting would dislodge the patch). Rotate application sites.
Estradiol (Vivelle, Vivelle-Dot)	Prevention of postmenopausal osteoporosis.	Patch: (Vivelle) 0.05mg/day, 0.1mg/day [8^s, 48^s]; (Vivelle-Dot) 0.025mg/day, 0.0375mg/day, 0.05mg/day, 0.075mg/day, 0.1mg/day [8^s, 24^s]	Minimum Effective Dose: 0.025mg/day twice weekly. Apply to clean, dry area of the trunk; avoid breasts and waistline. Rotate sites; allow 1 week between same site. Without intact uterus, may give continuously; with intact uterus, may give cyclically (3 weeks on, 1 week off) with a progestin.
Estradiol/Levonorgestrel (Climara Pro)	Prevention of postmenopausal osteoporosis.	Patch: (Estradiol-Levonorgestrel): 0.045mg-0.015mg/day [4^s]	Apply 1 patch weekly to lower abdomen (avoid breasts and waistline). Rotate application site; allow 1 week between same site. Re-evaluate periodically (3-6 month intervals).
Estradiol/Norethindrone (Activella)	Prevention of postmenopausal osteoporosis in women with intact uterus.	Tab: (Estradiol-Norethindrone) 1mg-0.5mg	1 tab qd.

DRUG (BRAND)	INDICATIONS	HOW SUPPLIED	DOSAGE
HORMONE THERAPY *(Continued)*			
Estradiol/Norgestimate (Prefest)	Prevention of postmenopausal osteoporosis in women with intact uterus.	Tab: (Estradiol) 1mg and (Estradiol-Norgestimate) 1mg-0.09mg	1 estradiol (pink color) tab for three days followed by 1 estradiol-norgestimate (white color) tab for three days. Repeat regimen continuously.
Estropipate (Ogen)	Prevention of postmenopausal osteoporosis.	Tab: 0.625mg* (0.75mg estropipate), 1.25mg* (1.5mg estropipate), 2.5mg* (3mg estropipate) *scored	0.75mg (as estropipate) qd for 25 days of 31-day cycle.
Estropipate (Ortho-Est)	Prevention of osteoporosis.	Tab: 0.625mg* (0.75mg estropipate), 1.25mg* (1.5mg estropipate) *scored	0.75mg (as estropipate) qd for 25 days of a 31-day cycle.
Ethinyl Estradiol/ Norethindrone (Femhrt)	Prevention of postmenopausal osteoporosis in women with intact uterus.	Tab: (Ethinyl Estradiol-Norethindrone) 2.5mcg-0.5mg, 5mcg-1mg	1 tab qd. Assess response by measuring bone mineral density.
MISCELLANEOUS			
Calcitonin-Salmon (Miacalcin)	(Inj) Treatment of postmenopausal osteoporosis. (Spray) Treatment of postmenopausal osteoporosis in females >5 yrs postmenopause.	Inj: 200 IU/mL; Nasal Spray: 200 IU/inh [2mL 2ˢ]	(Inj) 100 IU IM/SQ every other day. If >2mL, use IM injection. (Spray) 200 IU qd intranasally. Alternate nostrils daily. Take with supplemental calcium and vitamin D for postmenopausal osteoporosis.
Calcitonin-Salmon (rDNA origin) (Fortical))	Treatment of postmenopausal osteoporosis in females >5 yrs postmenopause in conjunction with an adequate calcium and vitamin D intake.	Nasal Spray: 200 IU/inh	200 IU qd intranasally. Alternate nostrils daily.
Raloxifene (Evista)	Treatment and prevention of osteoporosis in postmenopausal women.	Tab: 60mg	60mg qd.
Teriparatide (Forteo)	Treatment of postmenopausal women with osteoporosis who are at high risk for fracture. To increase bone mass in men with primary or hypogonadal osteoporosis who are at high risk for fracture.	Inj: 250mcg/mL [3mL pen]	20mcg qd SQ into thigh or abdominal wall. Administer initially under circumstances where patient can sit or lie down if symptoms of orthostatic hypotension occur. Discard pen after 28 days. Use for >2 yrs is not recommended.

OSTEOPOROSIS RISK FACTORS

Nonmodifiable risk factors	
Gender	Women > men
Age	Older age > younger age
Body size	Low body weight (small and thin) > high or overweight
Ethnicity	Caucasian, Asian, or Hispanic/Latino descent > African heritage
Family history	History of fractures or osteoporosis
Sex hormones	Females: delayed puberty, amenorrhea, early menopause, removal of ovaries, low estrogen levels
	Males: low testosterone
Modifiable risk factors	
Lifestyle	Cigarette smoking, excessive alcohol ($\geq$3 drinks/day), excessive caffeine intake
Exercise	Inactive or bedridden
Vitamins	Low intake of calcium, vitamin D, phosphorous, magnesium, vitamin K, vitamin B_6, vitamin B_{12}; excessive intake of vitamin A

Drugs associated with increased risk of osteoporosis*

- Aluminum
- Anticonvulsants
- Cytotoxic drugs
- Depo-Provera
- Glucocorticosteroids and adrenocorticotrophin
- Gonadotrophin-releasing hormone agonists
- Heparin
- Lithium
- Tamoxifen (premenopausal use)
- Thyroxine
- Vitamin D toxicity

Diseases/conditions associated with increased risk of osteoporosis

- Anorexia nervosa
- Celiac disease
- Cushing's syndrome
- Hyperoxia
- Hyperparathyroidism
- Hyperthyroidism
- Hypogonadism
- Insulin-dependent diabetes mellitus
- Leukemia
- Lymphoma
- Multiple myeloma
- Rheumatoid arthritis

*This list does not include all drugs that may increase the risk factors for osteoporosis.
Sources: National Osteoporosis Foundation and World Health Organization.

- Hyperoid
- Hypophosphatasia
- Hyperprolactinemia

RHEUMATOID ARTHRITIS AGENTS

DRUG (Brand)	HOW SUPPLIED	USUAL DOSE RANGE	MAX DOSE
5-AMINOSALICYLIC ACID DERIVATIVE			
Sulfasalazine (Azulfidine EN)	**Tab, Delayed-Release:** 500mg	1g bid.	4g/day.
COPPER CHELATING AGENT			
Penicillamine (Cuprimine, Depen)	**Cap:** (Cuprimine) 250mg; **Tab:** (Depen) 250mg*	500-750mg/day.	1.5g/day.
COX-2 INHIBITOR			
Celecoxib (Celebrex)	**Cap:** 50, 100mg, 200mg, 400mg	100-200mg bid.	400mg/day.
DIHYDROFOLIC ACID REDUCTASE INHIBITOR			
Methotrexate sodium	**Inj:** 25mg/mL; **Tab:** 2.5mg	7.5mg once weekly.	20mg/wk.
GOLD AGENT			
Auranofin (Ridaura)	**Cap:** 3mg	6mg qd or 3mg bid.	9mg/day.
IMMUNOSUPPRESSANTS			
Azathioprine (Imuran)	**Tab:** 50mg*	**Initial:** 1mg/kg/day given qd-bid. **Titrate:** Increase by 0.5mg/kg/day after 6-8 wks, then at 4 wk intervals.	2.5mg/kg/day.
Cyclosporine (Neoral)	**Cap:** 25mg, 100mg; **Sol:** 100mg/mL [50mL]	**Initial:** 1.25mg/kg bid. **Titrate:** Increase by 0.5-0.75mg/kg/day after 8 wks, again after 12 wks. D/C if no benefit by wk 16.	4mg/kg/day.
INTERLEUKIN-1 RECEPTOR ANTAGONIST			
Anakinra (Kineret)	**Inj:** 100mg/0.67mL	100mg SQ qd	
MONOCLONAL ANTIBODIES/CD20-BLOCKER			
Rituximab (Rituxan)	**Inj:** 10mg/mL	Two-1000mg IV infusions separated by 2 wks, with MTX.	
MONOCLONAL ANTIBODIES/TNF-BLOCKERS			
Adalimumab (Humira)	**Inj:** 40mg/0.8mL	40mg SQ every other wk.	40mg w/o MTX.
Infliximab (Remicade)	**Inj:** 100mg	3mg/kg IV infusion repeat at 2 and 6 wks. **Maint:** 3mg/kg every 8 wks.	10mg/kg or every 4 wks.
NONSTEROIDAL ANTI-INFLAMMATORY DRUGS (NSAIDs)			
Diclofenac (Voltaren XR)	**Tab, Delayed-Release:** (Voltaren) 25mg, 50mg, 75mg; **Tab, Extended-Release:** (Voltaren-XR) 100mg	50mg tid-qid or 75mg bid.	200mg/day.
Diflunisal (Dolobid)	**Tab:** 250mg, 500mg	250-500mg bid.	1500mg/day.
Etodolac	**Cap:** 200mg, 300mg, 400mg, 500mg	300mg bid-tid or 400-500mg bid.	1000mg/day.
(Etodolac XR)	**Tab, Extended-Release:** 400mg, 500mg, 600mg	400-1000mg qd.	1200mg/day.
Fenoprofen (Nalfon)	**Cap:** 200mg, 300mg; **Tab:** 600mg	300-600mg tid-qid	3200mg/day.
Flurbiprofen (Ansaid)	**Tab:** 50mg, 100mg	200-300mg/day bid, tid or qid.	300mg/day.

(Continued)

DRUG (Brand)	HOW SUPPLIED	USUAL DOSE RANGE	MAX DOSE
NONSTEROIDAL ANTI-INFLAMMATORY DRUGS (NSAIDs) *(Continued)*			
Ibuprofen (Motrin)	**Sus:** 100mg/5mL; **Tab:** 400mg, 600mg, 800mg	300mg qid or 400mg, 600mg or 800mg tid-qid.	3200mg/day.
(Motrin IB)	**Tab:** 200mg	200mg q4-6h. 400mg if no response.	3200mg/day.
Ketoprofen (Oruvail)	**Cap, Extended-Release:** 200mg	200mg qd.	200mg/day.
Meclofenamate	**Cap:** 50mg, 100mg	200-400mg/day in 3-4 divided doses.	400mg/day.
Meloxicam (Mobic)	**Sus:** 7.5mg/5mL; **Tab:** 7.5mg, 15mg	7.5mg qd.	15mg/day.
Nabumetone (Relafen)	**Tab:** 500mg, 750mg	1000mg qd.	2000mg/day.
Naproxen (Anaprox DS)	**Tab:** 275mg, 550mg*	275mg bid or 550mg bid.	1650mg/day.
(Naprelan)	**Tab, Extended-Release:** 375mg, 500mg	750mg-1g qd.	1.5g/day.
(Naprosyn)	**Sus:** 25mg/mL; **Tab:** 250mg*, 375mg, 500mg*; **Tab, Delayed-Release:** (EC-Naprosyn) 375mg, 500mg	250, 375, or 500mg bid (EC-Naprosyn) 375 or 500mg bid.	1500mg/day.
Oxaprozin (Daypro)	**Tab:** 600mg*	1200mg qd.	1800mg/day.
Piroxicam (Feldene)	**Cap:** 10mg, 20mg	20mg qd or 10mg bid.	20mg/day.
Sulindac (Clinoril)	**Tab:** 150mg, 200mg*	150mg bid.	400mg/day.
Tolmetin (Tolectin)	**Cap:** (DS) 400mg; **Tab:** 200mg*, 600mg	200-600mg tid.	1800mg/day.
NSAID/PROSTAGLANDIN E₁ ANALOGUE			
Diclofenac/Misoprostol (Arthrotec)	**Tab:** (Diclofenac-Misoprostol) 50mg-0.2mg, 75mg-0.2mg	50mg tid-qid.	
SELECTIVE COSTIMULATION MODULATOR			
Abatacept (Orencia)	**Inj:** 250mg	**Initial:** <60kg: 500mg; 60-100kg: 750mg; >100kg: 1g. **Maint:** Give at 2 and 4 wks after initial infusion, then q 4 wks thereafter.	
SALICYLATE			
Aspirin (Bayer Aspirin)	**Tab:** (Genuine Bayer Aspirin) 325mg **Tab:** (Bayer Extra Strength) 500mg	**Initial:** 3g/day in divided doses.	4g/day.
(Ecotrin)	**Tab, Delayed-Release:** 81mg, 325mg, 500mg	3g qd in divided doses.	4g/day.
Choline Magnesium Trisalicylate	1000mg*	1500mg bid.	3g/d.
TNF-RECEPTOR BLOCKER			
Etanercept (Enbrel)	**Inj:** 25mg [vial], 50mg/mL [syringe]	50mg SQ per wk.	

(Continued)

DRUG (Brand)	HOW SUPPLIED	USUAL DOSE RANGE	MAX DOSE
MISCELLANEOUS			
Botanical/Mineral Substances (Traumeel Injection)	**Inj:** 2.2mL amps [10^S]	**Adults:** 1 amp qd for acute disorders or 1-2 amps 1-3 times weekly. **Pediatrics:** >**6 yrs:** 1 amp qd for acute disorders or 1-2 amps 1-3 times weekly. **2-6 yrs:** Use ½ of the adult dosage. May administer IV, IM, SQ, or intradermally.	
Hydroxychloroquine (Plaquenil)	**Tab:** 200mg	**Initial:** 400-600mg qd. **Maint:** After 4-12 wks, 200-400mg qd with food or milk.	
*scored			

ADHD AGENTS

BRAND (GENERIC)	HOW SUPPLIED	ADULT DOSE	PEDIATRIC DOSE
Adderall (Amphetamine plus dextroamphetamine)	Tab: 5mg*, 7.5mg*, 10mg*, 12.5mg*, 15mg*, 20mg*, 30mg* scored		**3-5 yrs:** Initial: 2.5mg qd. Titrate: May increase by 2.5mg weekly. **≥6 yrs:** Initial: 5mg qd-bid. May increase by 5mg weekly. Max (usual): 40mg/day.
Adderall XR* (Amphetamine salt combo)	Cap: 5mg, 10mg, 15mg, 20mg, 25mg, 30mg	Initial: 20mg qam. Currently Using Adderall: Switch to Adderall XR at the same total daily dose, taken once daily. Titrate at weekly intervals as needed.	**≥6 yrs:** Initial: 10mg qam. Titrate: May increase weekly by 5-10mg/day. Max: 30mg/day. **13-17 yrs:** Initial: 10mg/day. Titrate: May increase to 20mg/day after one week. Currently Using Adderall: Switch to Adderall XR at the same total daily dose, taken once daily. Titrate at weekly intervals as needed.
Concerta* (Methylphenidate HCl)	Tab, Extended-Release: 18mg, 27mg, 36mg, 54mg	Methylphenidate-Naive or Receiving Other Stimulant: Initial: 18mg qam. Titrate: Adjust dose at weekly intervals. Previous Methylphenidate Use: Initial: 18mg qam if previous dose 10-15mg/day; 36mg qam if previous dose 20-30mg/day; 54mg qam if previous dose 30-45mg/day. Initial conversion should not exceed 54mg/day. Titrate: Adjust dose at weekly intervals. Max: 72mg/day. Reduce dose or d/c if paradoxical aggravation of symptoms occurs. D/C if no improvement after appropriate dosage adjustments over 1 month.	**≥6 yrs:** Methylphenidate-Naive or Receiving Other Stimulant: Initial: 18mg qam. Titrate: Adjust dose at weekly intervals. Max: **6-12 yrs:** 54mg/day; **13-17 yrs:** 72mg/day not to exceed 2mg/kg/day. Previous Methylphenidate Use: Initial: 18mg qam if previous dose 10-15mg/day; 36mg qam if previous dose 20-30mg/day; 54mg qam if previous dose 30-45mg/day. Initial conversion should not exceed 54mg/day. Titrate: Adjust dose at weekly intervals. Max: 72mg/day. Reduce dose or d/c if paradoxical aggravation of symptoms occurs. D/C if no improvement after appropriate dosage adjustments over 1 month.
Daytrana (Methylphenidate transdermal system)	Patch: 10mg/9 hrs, 15mg/9 hrs, 20mg/9 hrs, 30mg/9 hrs [10§, 30§]	Individualize dose. Apply to hip area 2 hrs before effect is needed and remove 9 hrs after application. Recommended Titration Schedule: Week 1: 10mg/9 hrs. Week 2: 15mg/9 hrs. Week 3: 20mg/9 hrs. Week 4: 30mg/9 hrs.	**≥6 yrs:** Individualize dose. Apply to hip area 2 hrs before effect is needed and remove 9 hrs after application. Recommended Titration Schedule: Week 1: 10mg/9 hrs. Week 2: 15mg/9 hrs. Week 3: 20mg/9 hrs. Week 4: 30mg/9 hrs.
Desoxyn (Methamphetamine HCl)	Tab: 5mg		**≥6 yrs:** Initial: 5mg qd-bid. Titrate: Increase weekly by 5mg/day until optimum response. Usual: 20-25mg/day given bid.
Dexedrine (Dextroamphetamine sulfate)	Cap, Extended-Release: (Spansules) 5mg, 10mg, 15mg; Tab: 5mg* scored		**3-5 yrs:** Initial: 2.5mg qd. Titrate: Increase weekly by 2.5mg/day. **≥6 yrs:** Initial: 5mg qd-bid. Titrate: Increase weekly by 5mg/day. Max: 40mg/day. For tabs, give 1st dose upon awakening and additional every 4-6 hrs. May give caps once daily.

BRAND (GENERIC)	HOW SUPPLIED	ADULT DOSE	PEDIATRIC DOSE
DextroStat (Dextroamphetamine sulfate)	Tab: 5mg*, 10mg* *scored		**3-5 yrs:** Initial: 2.5mg/day. Titrate: Increase weekly by 2.5mg/day until optimum response. **6-16 yrs:** Initial 5mg qd-bid. Titrate: Increase weekly by 5mg/day until optimum response. Give 1st dose upon awakening, and additional doses q4-6h.
Focalin (Dexmethylphenidate HCl)	Tab: 2.5mg, 5mg, 10mg	Take bid at least 4 hrs apart. Methylphenidate Naive: Initial: 2.5mg bid. Titrate: Increase weekly by 2.5-5mg/day. Currently on Methylphenidate: Initial: Take ½ of methylphenidate dose. Max: 20mg/day. Reduce or d/c if paradoxical aggravation of symptoms. D/C if no improvement after appropriate dosage adjustments over 1 month.	**≥6 yrs:** Take bid at least 4 hrs apart. Methylphenidate Naive: Initial: 2.5mg bid. Titrate: Increase weekly by 2.5-5mg/day. Max: 20mg/day. Currently on Methylphenidate: Initial: Take ½ of methylphenidate dose. Max: 20mg/day. Reduce or d/c if paradoxical aggravation of symptoms. D/C if no improvement after appropriate dosage adjustments over 1 month.
Focalin XR* (Dexmethylphenidate HCl)	Cap, Extended-Release: 5mg, 10mg, 15mg, 20mg	Methylphenidate Naive: Initial: 10mg/day. Titrate: May adjust weekly by 10mg/day. Max: 20mg/day. Currently on Methylphenidate: Initial: Take ½ of methylphenidate dose. Max: 20mg/day. Reduce or d/c if paradoxical aggravation of symptoms. D/C if no improvement after appropriate dosage adjustments over 1 month.	**≥6 yrs:** Methylphenidate Naive: Initial: 5mg/day. Titrate: May adjust weekly by 5mg/day. Max: 20mg/day. Currently on Methylphenidate: Initial: Take ½ of methylphenidate dose. Max: 20mg/day. Reduce or d/c if paradoxical aggravation of symptoms. D/C if no improvement after appropriate dosage adjustments over 1 month.
Metadate CD* (Methylphenidate HCl)	Cap, Extended-Release: 10mg, 20mg, 30mg, 40mg, 50mg, 60mg		**≥6 yrs:** Usual: 20mg qam before breakfast. Titrate: Increase weekly by 10-20mg depending on tolerability/efficacy. Max: 60mg/day. Reduce dose or d/c if paradoxical aggravation of symptoms occur. D/C if no improvement after appropriate dose adjustments over 1 month.
Metadate ER** (Methylphenidate HCl)	Tab, Extended-Release: 10mg, 20mg	(Immediate-Release Methylphenidate) 10-60mg/day given bid-tid 30-45 min ac. If insomnia occurs, take last dose before 6 pm.†	**≥6 yrs:** (Immediate-Release Methylphenidate) Initial: 5mg bid before breakfast and lunch. Titrate: Increase gradually by 5-10mg weekly. Max: 60mg/day. Reduce dose or d/c if paradoxical aggravation of symptoms occur. D/C if no improvement after appropriate dose adjustment over 1 month.†
Methylin** (Methylphenidate HCl)	Sol: 5mg/5mL [500mL], 10mg/5mL [500mL]; Tab: 5mg, 10mg, 20mg; Tab, Chewable: 2.5mg, 5mg, 10mg; Tab, Extended-Release: 10mg, 20mg	(Sol/Tab/Tab, Chewable) 10-60mg/day given bid-tid 30-45 min ac. If insomnia occurs, take last dose before 6 pm.†	**≥6 yrs:** (Sol/Tab/Tab, Chewable) Initial: 5mg bid before breakfast and lunch. Titrate: Increase gradually by 5-10mg weekly. Max: 60mg/day. Reduce dose or d/c if paradoxical aggravation of symptoms occur. D/C if no improvement after appropriate dose adjustment over 1 month.†

(Continued)

BRAND (GENERIC)	HOW SUPPLIED	ADULT DOSE	PEDIATRIC DOSE
Ritalin, Ritalin LA*, Ritalin SR** (Methylphenidate HCl)	Cap, Extended-Release (Ritalin LA): 10mg, 20mg, 30mg, 40mg; Tab (Ritalin): 5mg, 10mg*, 20mg*; Tab, Extended-Release (Ritalin SR): 20mg *scored*	(Tab) 10-60mg/day given bid-tid 30-45 min ac. Take last dose before 6 pm if insomnia occurs. (Cap, ER) Initial: 20mg qam. Titrate: Adjust weekly by 10mg. Max: 60mg qam.†	≥6 yrs: (Tab) Initial: 5mg bid before breakfast and lunch. Titrate: Increase gradually by 5-10mg weekly. Max: 60mg/day. (Cap, ER) Initial: 20mg qam. Titrate: Adjust weekly by 10mg. Max: 60mg qam. Previous Methylphenidate Use: May use as qd in place of IR dosed bid or daily dose of methylphenidate-SR. Reduce dose or d/c if paradoxical aggravation of symptoms occurs. D/C if no improvement after appropriate dose adjustment over 1 month.†
Strattera (Atomoxetine HCl)	Cap: 10mg, 18mg, 25mg, 40mg, 60mg, 80mg, 100mg	Initial: 40mg/day given qam or evenly divided doses in the am and late afternoon/early evening. Titrate: Increase after minimum of 3 days to target dose of about 80mg/day. After 2-4 weeks, may increase to max of 100mg/day. Dose adjust in hepatic insufficiency and when used with concomitant CYP450 2D6 inhibitors. See PI for detailed dosing information	≥6 yrs: ≤70kg: Initial: 0.5mg/kg/day given qam or evenly divided doses in the am and late afternoon or early evening. Titrate: Increase after minimum of 3 days to target dose of about 1.2mg/kg/day. Max: 1.4mg/kg/day or 100mg, whichever is less. >70kg: Initial: 40mg/day given qam or evenly divided doses in the am and late afternoon/ early evening. Titrate: Increase after minimum of 3 days to target dose of about 80mg/day. After 2-4 weeks, may increase to max of 100mg/day. Max: 100mg/day. Dose adjust in hepatic insufficiency and when used with concomitant CYP450 2D6 inhibitors. See PI for detailed dosing information.
Vyvanse (Lisdexamfetamine dimesylate)	Cap: 20mg, 30mg, 40mg, 50mg, 60mg, 70mg	Individualize dose. Usual: 30mg qam. Titrate: If needed, may increase in increments of 10mg or 20mg at weekly intervals. Max: 70mg/day. Swallow caps or dissolve contents in glass of water; do not store once dissolved. Re-evaluate periodically.	Individualize dose. 6-12 yrs: Usual: 30mg qam. Titrate: If needed, may increase in increments of 10mg or 20mg at weekly intervals. Max: 70mg/day. Swallow caps or dissolve contents in glass of water; do not store once dissolved. Re-evaluate periodically.

ADHD = attention-deficit/hyperactivity disorder.
*Swallow cap whole or open cap and sprinkle contents on applesauce; do not chew.
**Swallow whole; do not chew, crush, or divide.
†Tab, Extended-Release: May use in place of immediate-release tabs when the 8-hr dose corresponds to the titrated 8-hr immediate-release dose.

ALZHEIMER'S DISEASE AGENTS

DRUG (BRAND)	INDICATIONS	HOW SUPPLIED	DOSAGE	SIDE EFFECTS
Donepezil HCl (Aricept)	Treatment of dementia of the Alzheimer's type.	Tab: 5mg, 10mg; Tab. Disintegrating: 5mg, 10mg	Mild to Moderate Alzheimer's Disease: Initial: 5mg qd. Titrate: May increase to 10mg after 4-6 weeks. Severe Alzheimer's Disease: 10mg qd. Start with 5mg qd and increase to 10mg after 4-6 weeks.	Nausea, diarrhea, insomnia, vomiting, muscle cramps, fatigue, anorexia, dizziness, depression, weight decrease, infection, HTN, back pain, abnormal dreams, ecchymosis
Ergoloid Mesylates (Ergoloid mesylates)	Treatment of symptomatic decline in mental capacity of unknown etiology (eg, Alzheimer's dementia, multi-infarct dementia).	Tab: 1mg; Tab, Sublingual: 1mg	Usual: 1mg tid.	Transient nausea, gastric disturbances
Galantamine HBr (Razadyne, Razadyne ER)	Treatment of mild to moderate dementia of the Alzheimer's type.	Sol: (Razadyne) 4mg/mL [100mL]; Tab: (Razadyne) 4mg, 8mg, 12mg. Cap, Extended-Release: (Razadyne ER) 8mg, 16mg, 24mg	(Sol, Tab) Initial: 4mg bid with am and pm meals. Titrate: Increase to 8mg bid after 4 weeks if tolerated, then increase to 12mg bid after 4 weeks if tolerated. Usual: 16-24mg/day. Max: 24mg/day. (Cap, ER) Initial: 8mg qd with am meal. Titrate: Increase to 16mg qd after 4 weeks, then increase to 24mg qd after 4 weeks if tolerated. Usual: 16-24mg/day. Max: 24mg/day. If therapy is interrupted, restart at lowest dose and increase to current dose. See PI for dose modification in moderate renal/hepatic impairment.	Nausea, vomiting, diarrhea, anorexia, weight loss, fatigue, dizziness, headache, depression, insomnia, abdominal pain, dyspepsia
Memantine HCl (Namenda)	Treatment of moderate to severe dementia of the Alzheimer's type.	Sol: 2mg/mL [360mL]; Tab: 5mg, 10mg; Titration-Pak: 5mg [28ˢ], 10mg [21ˢ]	Initial: 5mg qd. Titrate: Increase at intervals of at least one week to 5mg bid, then 5mg and 10mg as separate doses, then to 10mg bid. Severe Renal Impairment: Reduce dose.	Dizziness, confusion, headache, constipation, coughing, HTN, pain, vomiting, somnolence, hallucinations
Rivastigmine tartrate (Exelon)	Treatment of mild to moderate dementia of the Alzheimer's type.	Cap: 1.5mg, 3mg, 4.5mg, 6mg; Sol: 2mg/mL [120mL]; Patch: 4.6mg/24hrs, 9.5 mg/24 hrs [30ˢ]	Initial: 1.5mg bid. Titrate: May increase by 1.5mg bid every 2 weeks. Max: 12mg/day. If not tolerating, suspend therapy for several doses and restart at same or next lower dose. If interrupted longer than several days, reinitiate with lowest daily dose and titrate as above. (Patch) Initial: Apply 4.6mg/24 hrs patch qd to clean, dry, hairless intact skin. Maint: Increase dose after 4 weeks. Max: 9.5mg/24 hrs if well tolerated. Switching from Capsules/Oral Sol: Total Oral Daily Dose <6mg: Switch to 4.6mg/24 hrs patch. Total Oral Daily Dose 6-12mg: Switch to 9.5mg/24 hrs patch. Apply 1st patch on day following last oral dose.	Nausea, vomiting, abdominal pain, dyspepsia, constipation, somnolence, anorexia, asthenia, headache, dizziness, fatigue, diarrhea, tremor, depression
Tacrine HCl (Cognex)	Treatment of mild to moderate dementia of the Alzheimer's type.	Cap: 10mg, 20mg, 30mg, 40mg	Initial: 10mg qid. Titrate: Increase to 20mg qid after 4 weeks, then increase at 4-week intervals to 30mg qid then to 40mg qid. See PI for dose modification in case of elevated AST/SGPT elevations.	Elevated LFTs, nausea, vomiting, diarrhea, dyspepsia, myalgia, anorexia, ataxia, dizziness

ANTIPARKINSON'S AGENTS

DRUG (BRAND)	INDICATIONS	HOW SUPPLIED	DOSAGE	SIDE EFFECTS
Bromocriptine mesylate (Parlodel)	Treatment of symptoms of Parkinson's disease.	Tab, Snap: 2.5mg*; Cap: 5mg *scored	Initial: 1.25mg bid. Titrate: If needed, increase by 2.5mg/day every 2-4 weeks. Max: 100mg/day. Take with food.	Headache, dizziness, GI effects, orthostatic hypotension, fatigue, arrhythmia, insomnia, hallucinations, abnormal involuntary movements, depression, syncope
Carbidopa (Lodosyn)	For use with Sinemet or levodopa in treatment of symptoms of idiopathic Parkinson's disease, postencephalitic parkinsonism, and symptomatic parkinsonism. For use in patients for whom the dosage of Sinemet provides less than adequate daily dosage (usually 70mg daily) of carbidopa.	Tab: 25mg* *scored	With Sinemet or Levodopa: Determine dose by careful titration. Most patients respond to a 1:10 proportion of carbidopa: levodopa provided carbidopa dose is ≥70mg/day. Max: 200mg/day. Consider amount of carbidopa in Sinemet when calculating dose. See PI for detailed dosing information.	Dyskinesia, psychotic episodes, delusions, hallucinations, paranoid ideation, depression with or without suicidal tendencies, dementia
Carbidopa/levodopa (Sinemet, Sinemet CR)	Treatment of symptoms of idiopathic Parkinson's disease, postencephalitic parkinsonism, and symptomatic parkinsonism.	Tab: (Carbidopa-Levodopa) 10mg-100mg*, 25mg-100mg*, 25mg-250mg*; Tab Extended Release: (Carbidopa-Levodopa) 25mg-100mg, 50mg-200mg* *scored	**(Tab) 25mg-100mg tab:** Initial: 1 tab tid. Titrate: Increase by 1 tab qd or every other day up to 8 tabs/day. **10mg-100mg tab:** Initial: 1 tab tid-qid. Titrate: Increase by 1 tab qd or every other day up to 2 tabs qid. Max: 200mg/day carbidopa required. **(Tab, Extended-Release) No Prior Levodopa Use:** Initial: 1 50mg-200mg tab bid at intervals >6 hrs. Titrate: Increase or decrease dose or interval accordingly. Adjust dose every 3 days. Usual: 400-1600mg/day levodopa, given in 4-8 hr intervals while awake. Conversion to Extended-Release Tabs: See PI.	Dyskinesia, nausea, cardiac irregularities, hypotension, dark saliva, GI bleeding, psychotic episodes, NMS, confusion, agitation, dizziness, somnolence, dream abnormalities
Carbidopa/levodopa (Parcopa)	Treatment of symptoms of idiopathic Parkinson's disease, postencephalitic parkinsonism, and symptomatic parkinsonism.	Tab, Disintegrating: (Carbidopa-Levodopa) 10mg-100mg*, 25mg-100mg*, 25mg-250mg* *scored	**25mg-100mg tab:** Initial: 1 tab tid. Titrate: Increase by 1 tab qd or qod up to 8 tabs/day. **10mg-100mg tab:** Initial: 1 tab tid-qid. Titrate: Increase by 1 tab qd or qod up to 2 tabs qid. 70-100mg/day carbidopa required. Max: 200mg/day carbidopa.	Dyskinesia, choreiform, dystonic and other involuntary movements, nausea

DRUG (BRAND)	INDICATIONS	HOW SUPPLIED	DOSAGE	SIDE EFFECTS
Carbidopa/levodopa/ entacapone (Stalevo)	Treatment of idiopathic Parkinson's disease to substitute for equivalent doses of previously administered carbidopa/levodopa and entacapone, or for those experiencing signs and symptoms of end-of-dose "wearing off" and taking up to 600mg/day levodopa without experiencing dyskinesias.	Tab: (Carbidopa/Levodopa/ Entacapone): Stalevo 50: 12.5mg/50mg/200mg; Stalevo 100: 25mg/100mg/ 200mg; Stalevo 150: 37.5mg/150mg/200mg; Stalevo 200: 50mg/200mg/ 200mg	Currently Taking Carbidopa/Levodopa and Entacapone: May switch directly to corresponding strength of levodopa/carbidopa and entacapone, but not Entacapone: First, titrate individually with carbidopa/levodopa product and entacapone product, then transfer to corresponding dose. Max: 8 tabs/day.	Dyskinesia, hyperkinesia, hypokinesia, dizziness, nausea, diarrhea, abdominal pain, constipation, vomiting, urine discoloration, back pain, fatigue
Diphenhydramine HCl Injection	For parkinsonism when oral therapy is not possible or contraindicated.	Inj: 50mg/mL	Usual: 10-50mg IV or up to 100mg IM if needed. Max: 400mg/day.	Sedation, drowsiness, dizziness, disturbed coordination, epigastric distress, thickening of bronchial secretions
Pramipexole dihydrochloride (Mirapex)	Treatment of signs and symptoms of idiopathic Parkinson's disease.	Tab: 0.125mg, 0.25mg*, 0.5mg*, 0.75mg, 1mg*, 1.5mg** scored	Initial: 0.125mg tid. Titrate: May increase every 5-7 days (eg, Week 2: 0.25mg tid; Week 3: 0.5mg tid; Week 4: 0.75mg tid; Week 5: 1mg tid; Week 6: 1.25mg tid; Week 7: 1.5mg tid). Maint: 0.5-1.5mg tid. Max: 1.5mg tid.†	Nausea, dizziness, somnolence, insomnia, constipation, asthenia, hallucinations, vision abnormalities, peripheral edema, arthritis, dry mouth, postural hypotension, chest pain, malaise
Rasagiline mesylate (Azilect)	Treatment of signs and symptoms of idiopathic Parkinson's disease as initial monotherapy and adjunct therapy to levodopa.	Tab: 0.5mg, 1mg	Monotherapy: 1mg qd. Adjunctive Therapy: Initial: 0.5mg qd. Titrate: May increase to 1mg qd. Adjust dose of levodopa with concomitant use. Concomitant Ciprofloxacin or Other CYP1A2 Inhibitors/Hepatic Impairment: 0.5mg qd.	Headache, arthralgia, depression, fall, flu syndrome, dyskinesia, accidental injury, nausea, weight loss, constipation, postural hypotension, vomiting, dry mouth, rash, somnolence
Ropinirole HCl (Requip)	Treatment of symptoms of idiopathic Parkinson's disease.	Tab: 0.25mg, 0.5mg, 1mg, 2mg, 3mg, 4mg, 5mg	Initial: 0.25mg tid. Titrate: May increase weekly by 0.25mg tid (0.75mg/day) for 4 weeks. After Week 4, may increase weekly by 1.5mg/day up to 9mg/day, then by 3mg/day weekly to 24mg/day. Max: 24mg/day. Withdrawal: Decrease dose to bid for 4 days, then qd for 3 days.	Neuralgia, increased BUN, hallucinations, somnolence, vomiting, headache, sweating, asthenia, edema, fatigue, syncope, orthostatic symptoms
ADJUNCT THERAPY				
Amantadine HCl (Symmetrel)	Treatment of parkinsonism and drug-induced extrapyramidal reactions.	Sol: 50mg/5mL [480mL]; Tab: 100mg	Parkinsonism: Initial: 100mg bid. Serious Associated Illness/ Concomitant High-Dose Antiparkinson Agent: Initial: 100mg qd. Titrate: May increase to 100mg bid.	Nausea, dizziness, insomnia, depression, anxiety, hallucinations, confusion, anorexia, dry mouth, constipation, ataxia

(Continued)

DRUG (BRAND)	INDICATIONS	HOW SUPPLIED	DOSAGE	SIDE EFFECTS
ADJUNCT THERAPY *(Continued)*				
Apomorphine HCl (Apokyn)	Acute, intermittent treatment of hypomobility, "off" episodes (end-of-dose "wearing off" and unpredictable "on/off" episodes) associated with advanced Parkinson's disease.	Inj: 10mg/mL [3mL]	Initial: Test Dose: 2mg SC; monitor BP closely. Titrate: Increase by 1mg every few days; assess efficacy/tolerability. Max: 6mg/day. Renal Impairment: Initial: 1mg SC.	Yawning, dyskinesia, nausea, vomiting, somnolence, dizziness, rhinorrhea, edema, chest pain, increased sweating, flushing, pallor
Benztropine mesylate	Adjunct in all forms of parkin-sonism. Control of drug-induced extrapyramidal disorders.	Inj: 1mg/mL; Tab: 0.5mg, 1mg, 2mg	Parkinsonism: Initial: 0.5-1mg PO/IV/IM qhs. Titrate: May in-crease every 5-6 days by 0.5mg. Usual: 1-2mg PO/IV/IM qhs. Max: 6mg/day. Extrapyramidal Disorders: 1-4mg PO/IV/IM qd-bid. Acute Dystonic Reactions: 1-2mg IM/IV, then 1-2mg PO bid.	Tachycardia, paralytic ileus, constipation, vomiting, nausea, dry mouth, confusion, blurred vision, urinary retention, heat stroke, hyperthermia, fever
Entacapone (Comtan)	Adjunct to levodopa/carbidopa for treatment of idiopathic Parkinson's disease if experience signs of end-of-dose "wearing-off."	Tab: 200mg	200mg with each levodopa/carbidopa dose. Max: 1600mg/day. Withdraw slowly for discontinuation.	Sweating, back pain, dyskinesia, hyper-kinesia, hypokinesia, nausea, diarrhea, abdominal pain, urine discoloration
Hyoscyamine sulfate (Levsin, Levbid, Levsinex)	To reduce rigidity and tremors of Parkinson's disease.	(Levbid) Tab, Extended-Release: 0.375mg. (Levsin) Drops: 0.125mg/mL [15mL]; Elixir: 0.125mg/5mL [473mL]; Inj: 0.5mg/mL; Tab: 0.125mg*; Tab, Sublingual: 0.125mg*. (Levsinex) Cap, Extended-Release: 0.375mg *scored	May also chew or swallow SL tab. (Drops; Elixir; Tab; and Tab, SL) 0.125-0.25mg q4h or prn. Max: 1.5mg/24 hrs. (Cap and Tab, Extended-Release) 0.375-0.75mg q12h; or 1 cap q8h. Max: 1.5mg/24 hrs. Do not crush or chew.	Anticholinergic effects, drowsiness, headache, nervousness
Selegiline HCl (Eldepryl)	Adjunct to levodopa/carbidopa for management of Parkinson's disease.	Cap: 5mg	5mg bid, at breakfast and lunch. Max: 10mg/day. May reduce levodopa/carbidopa by 10-30% after 2-3 days of therapy. May reduce further with continued therapy.	Nausea, dizziness, lightheadedness, fainting, abdominal pain, confusion, hallucinations, dry mouth

DRUG (BRAND)	INDICATIONS	HOW SUPPLIED	DOSAGE	SIDE EFFECTS
Selegiline HCl (Zelapar)	Adjunct in the management of Parkinson's disease in patients exhibiting a deteriorated response to levodopa/carbidopa therapy.	Tab, Orally Disintegrating: 1.25mg	1.25mg qd for 6 weeks. Titrate: After 6 weeks, may increase to 2.5mg qd if desired benefit not achieved. Max: 2.5mg/day.	Nausea, dizziness, pain, headache, insomnia, rhinitis, skin disorders, dyskinesia, backache, dyspepsia, stomatitis, constipation, hallucinations, pharyngitis, rash
Tolcapone (Tasmar)	Adjunct to levodopa/carbidopa for the treatment of symptoms of idiopathic Parkinson's disease.	Tab: 100mg, 200mg	Initial: 100mg tid. Use 200mg tid only if clinical benefit is justified. May need to decrease levodopa dose.	Dyskinesia, nausea, dystonia, excessive dreaming, anorexia, muscle cramps, orthostatic complaints, diarrhea, dizziness, headache
Trihexyphenidyl HCl	Adjunct treatment for all forms of parkinsonism (postencephalitic, arteriosclerotic, and idiopathic). For control of extrapyramidal disorders caused by CNS drugs.	Sol: 2mg/5mL [473mL]; Tab: 2mg*, 5mg* *scored	Idiopathic Parkinsonism: 1mg on Day 1. Titrate: Increase by 2mg every 3-5 days. Usual: 6-10mg/day. Max: 15mg/day. Drug-Induced Parkinsonism: Initial: 1mg. If extrapyramidal manifestations not controlled in a few hrs, increase dose until achieve control. Usual: 5-15mg/day.	Dry mouth, blurred vision, dizziness, nausea, nervousness, constipation, drowsiness, urinary hesitancy/retention, tachycardia, pupil dilation, increased intraocular tension, vomiting, weakness, headache

†For specific dosing information on different creatinine clearance values, see full Prescribing Information.

OPIOID PRODUCTS

GENERIC	BRAND	DOSAGE FORMS	ORAL EQUI-ANALGESIC DOSE	EQUI-ANALGESIC DOSE	USUAL ADULT DOSE	MAX DOSE	INDICATION	DEA SCHEDULE
Codeine		Inj, Oral Sol: (15mg/5mL); Tab: 15mg, 30mg, 60mg	200mg.	130mg.	PO, IM, SC, IV 15-60mg q4-6h.	360mg/24 hrs.	Relief of mild to moderate pain; cough suppression.	Schedule II
Codeine phosphate/ Acetaminophen	Tylenol w/Codeine Tylenol #3 Tylenol #4	Elixir: 12mg-120mg/5mL Tab: 30mg/300mg Tab: 60mg/300mg			15mL q4h prn. 15-60mg codeine/dose and 300-1000mg APAP.	Codeine: 360mg/ 24 hrs. Acetaminophen: 4g/day.	Relief of mild to moderately severe pain.	Schedule V Schedule III Schedule III
Hydrocodone bitartrate/ Acetaminophen	Anexia	Tab: 5mg-325mg, 7.5mg-325mg, 5mg-500mg, 7.5mg-650mg			1-2 tabs q4-6h prn.	8 tabs/day.	Relief of moderate to moderately severe pain.	Schedule III
	Lorcet, Lorcet-HD Lorcet Plus	Cap: (HD) 5mg-500mg; Tab: (Plus) 7.5mg-650mg, (10/650) 10mg-650mg			(Plus)1 cap q4-6h pm pain. (HD) 1-2 caps q4-6h pm pain.	(Plus) Max: 6 tabs/ caps/day. (HD) 8 caps/day.		
	Lortab Elixir Lortab	Sol: 7.5mg-500mg/15mL Tab: 2.5mg/500mg, 5mg/ 500mg, 7.5mg/500mg, 10mg/500mg			1 tbs q4-6h prn (2.5/500, 5/500): 1-2 tabs q4-6h prn. (7.5/500,10/500): 1 tab q4-6h prn.	6 tbs. (2.5/500, 5/500):8 tabs/day. (7.5/500, 10/500): 6 tabs/day.		
	Norco	Tab: 5mg/325mg, 7.5mg/ 325mg, 10mg/325mg			(5/325): 1-2 tabs q4-6h prn. (7.5/325, 10/325): 1 tab q4-6h prn.	(7.5/325,10/325): 6 tabs/day.		
	Vicodin	Tab: 5mg/500mg			1-2 tabs q4-6h prn.	8 tabs/day.		
	Vicodin ES	Tab: 7.5mg/750mg			1 tab q4-6h prn.	5 tabs/day.		
	Vicodin HP	Tab: 10mg/660mg			1 tab q4-6h prn.	6 tabs/day.		
	Zydone	Tab: 5mg/400mg, 7.5mg/ 400mg, 10mg/400mg			(5/400): 1-2 tabs q4-6h prn. (7.5/400, 10/400): 1 tab q4-6h prn.	(5/400): 8 tabs/day (7.5/400, 10/400): 6 tabs/day.		
Hydrocodone bitartrate/ibuprofen	Vicoprofen	Tab: 7.5/200mg			1-2 tabs q4-6h prn.	5 tabs/day.	Short-term (generally <10 days) management of acute pain.	Schedule III

GENERIC	BRAND	DOSAGE FORMS	ORAL EQUI-ANALGESIC DOSE	EQUI-ANALGESIC DOSE	USUAL ADULT DOSE	MAX DOSE	INDICATION	DEA SCHEDULE
Oxycodone HCl	OxyContin	**Tab, ER:** 10mg, 20mg, 40mg, 80mg, 160mg			10mg q12h. Titrate: May increase the q12h dose (not the dosing frequency). May increase the total daily dose by 25-50% of the current dose.		Management of moderate to severe pain when a continuous around the clock analgesic is needed for an extended period. Only for postoperative use in patients already receiving the drug before surgery or those expected to have moderate-severe postoperative pain for an extended period of time.	Schedule II
	OxyFast	**Sol:** 20mg/mL			5mg q6h prn for pain.		Relief of moderate to moderately severe pain.	
	OxyIR	**Cap, IR:** 5mg			5mg q6h prn.			
	Roxicodone	**Sol:** 5mg/5mL; **Liq:** 20mg/mL; **Tab:** 5mg, 15mg, 30mg			Tab: 15mg q4-6h prn; Sol/Liq: 10-30mg q4h prn.			
Oxycodone/ Acetaminophen	Percocet	**Tab:** 2.5mg/325mg, 5mg/325mg, 7.5mg/325mg, 7.5mg/500mg, 10mg/325mg, 10mg/650mg			(2.5/325): 1-2 tabs q6h. (5/325): 1 tab q6h prn. (7.5/500): 1 tab q6h prn. (10-650) 1 tab q6h prn. (7.5/325): 1 tab q6h prn. (10/325): 1 tab q6h prn.	(2.5/325): 12 tabs/day. (5/325):12 tabs/day. (7.5/500): 8 tabs/day. (10-650) 6 tabs/day. (7.5/325):8 tabs/day. (10/325): 6 tabs/day.	Relief of moderate to moderately severe pain.	Schedule II
	Tylox	**Cap:** 5mg/500mg			1 cap q6h prn.			
Oxycodone/Ibuprofen	Combunox	**Tab:** 5mg/400mg			1 tab/dose.	4 tabs/day for 7 days.	Short term (<7 days) management of acute, moderate to severe pain.	Schedule II
Oxycodone HCl/ Aspirin	Percodan	**Tab:** 4.835mg/325mg			1 tab q6h prn	12 tabs/day or ASA 4g/day.	Relief of moderate to moderately severe pain.	Schedule II
Oxymorphone HCl	Opana	**Inj:** 1mg/1mL; **Tab:** 5mg, 10mg			10-20mg q4-6hrs.	20mg/dose	Relief of moderate to severe acute pain.	Schedule II
	Opana ER	**Tab:** 5mg, 7.5mg, 10mg, 15mg, 20mg, 30mg, 40mg			5-20mg q12h.	20mg/dose	(Tab, ER) Relief of moderate to severe pain in patients requiring continuous, around-the-clock opioid treatment for extended period of time.	

(Continued)

GENERIC	BRAND	DOSAGE FORMS	ORAL EQUI-ANALGESIC DOSE	EQUI-ANALGESIC DOSE	USUAL ADULT DOSE	MAX DOSE	INDICATION	DEA SCHEDULE
Meperidine HCl	Demerol	**Syr:** 50mg/5mL, **Tab:** 50mg; **Inj:** 25mg/mL, 50mg/mL, 75mg/mL, 100mg/mL	300mg.	75mg.	Tab: 50-150mg q3-4h prn. Inj: 50-150mg IM/SC q3-4h prn.		Moderate to severe pain. Inj: also for preoperative medication, anesthesia support, and obstetrical analgesia.	Schedule II
Propoxyphene HCl	Darvon	**Cap:** 65mg			65mg q4h prn.	390mg/day.	Relief of mild to moderate pain.	Schedule IV
Propoxyphene napsylate	Darvon-N	**Tab:** 100mg			100mg q4h prn.	600mg/day.	Relief of mild to moderate pain.	Schedule IV
Propoxyphene napsylate/ Acetaminophen	Darvocet-N 50	**Tab:** 50mg/325mg			100mg propoxyphene napsylate/650mg APAP q4h prn.	600mg propoxyphene napsylate/day. Acetaminophen: 4g/day.	Relief of mild to moderate pain.	Schedule IV
	Darvocet-N 100	**Tab:** 100mg/650mg						
	Darvocet-A 500	**Tab:** 100mg/500mg						
Tramadol	Ultram	**Tab:** 50mg; **Tab, ER:** 100mg, 200mg, 300mg			Tab: 50-100mg q4-6h prn. Tab, ER: 100mg/day. Titrate: 100mg q 5 days.	Tab: 400mg/day. Tab, ER: 300mg/day.	Management of moderate to moderately severe pain.	Rx only
Morphine sulfate	Astramorph PF	**Inj:** 0.5mg/mL, 1mg/mL	40-60mg.	10mg.	IV: 2-10mg/70kg of body weight. Epidural: 2-4mg/ 24 hrs. IT: 0.2-1mg/24 hrs.		Management of pain where use of an opioid analgesic by PCA is appropriate.	Schedule II
	Duramorph	**Inj:** 0.5mg/mL, 1mg/mL			IV: 2-10mg/70kg of body weight. Epidural: 2-4mg/ 24 hrs. IT: 0.2-1mg/24 hrs.		Management of pain where use of an opioid analgesic by PCA is appropriate.	
	Avinza	**Cap, ER:** 30mg, 60mg, 90mg, 120mg			30mg q24h.	1600mg/day.	Relief of moderate to severe pain requiring continuous opioid therapy for an extended period of time.	
	Infumorph	**Inj:** 0.5mg/mL (5mg), 1mg/mL (10mg), 10mg/mL (200mg), 25mg/mL (500mg)			1-10mg/day		Treatment of intractable chronic pain in microinfusion devices.	

GENERIC	BRAND	DOSAGE FORMS	ORAL EQUI-ANALGESIC DOSE	EQUI-ANALGESIC DOSE	USUAL ADULT DOSE	MAX DOSE	INDICATION	DEA SCHEDULE
	Kadian	**Cap, ER:** 10mg, 20mg, 30mg, 50mg, 60mg, 80mg, 100mg, 200mg			Give 50% of daily oral morphine dose q12h or give 100% oral morphine dose q24h.	Do not give more frequently than q12h.	Management of moderate to severe pain.	
	MS Contin	**Tab, ER:** 15mg, 30mg, 60mg, 100mg, 200mg			Give 50% of pts 24-hr requirement q12h or ¹⁄₃ of pts 24-hr requirement q8h.		Relief of moderate to severe pain for patients who require repeated dosing with potent opioid analgesics over periods of more than a few days.	
	Oramorph SR	**Tab, ER:** 15mg, 30mg, 60mg, 100mg			Single dose is 1/2 of daily morphine requirement q12h.		Relief of pain in patients who require opioid analgesics for more than a few days.	
Hydromorphone HCl	Dilaudid, Dilaudid-HP	**Tab:** 8mg; **Sol:** 5mg/5mL; **HP:** 10mg/mL, 50mg/5mL, 500mg/50mL; **Pow:** 250mg	6.5-7.5mg.	1.3-2mg.	Tab: 2-4mg, PO every 4 to 6 hours. Sol: 2.5-10mL q3-6h as directed. HP: Individualized for each patient.		Management of pain. (HP) Relief of moderate to severe pain in opioid-tolerant patients who require larger than usual doses of opioids to provide adequate pain relief.	Schedule II
Methadone HCl	Dolophine	**Tab:** 5mg, 10mg; **Inj:** 10mg/mL	10-20mg.	10mg.	Dolophine: 2.5mg to 10mg every 8 to 12 hrs, slowly titrated to effect. Detox: Titrate to a total daily dose of about 40mg in divided doses. Inj: 2.5-10mg q8-12h.	21 days. May not repeat earlier than 4 weeks after completing previous course.	Detoxification and temporary maintenance treatment of narcotic addiction (heroin or other morphine-like drugs). Relief of severe pain.	Schedule II
	Methadose	**Concentrate:** 10mg/mL; **Tab:** 5mg, 10mg; **Tab, Dispersible:** 40mg			Methadose: 2.5mg to 10mg every 3-4 hrs.			

(Continued)

GENERIC	BRAND	DOSAGE FORMS	ORAL EQUI-ANALGESIC DOSE	EQUI-ANALGESIC DOSE	USUAL ADULT DOSE	MAX DOSE	INDICATION	DEA SCHEDULE
Fentanyl	Duragesic	**Patch:** 12.5mcg/hr, 25mcg/hr, 50mcg/hr, 75mcg/hr, 100mcg/hr			Initial: 25mcg/hr for 72 hrs. Individualize dose.		Management of moderate to severe chronic pain when continuous opioid analgesia is required and cannot be managed by lesser means.	Schedule II
Fentanyl citrate	Actiq	**Loz:** 200mcg, 400mcg, 600mcg, 800mcg, 1200mcg, 1600mcg	1000mcg/hr.	0.1mg.	Six 200mcg units. Individually titrate.	4 units/day.	Management of breakthrough cancer pain in patients with malignancies who are already receiving and are tolerant to opioid therapy for their underlying persistent cancer pain.	Schedule II
	Fentora	**Tab, Buccal:** 100mcg, 200mcg, 400mcg, 600mcg, 800mcg			Initial:100mcg.	Not more than 4 tabs simultaneously.	Management of breakthrough pain in patients with cancer who are already receiving and who are tolerant to opioid therapy for their underlying persistent cancer pain.	

ORAL ANTICONVULSANTS

DRUG (BRAND)	INDICATIONS	USUAL ADULT DOSE*	THERAPEUTIC SERUM LEVELS
BARBITURATES			
Mephobarbital (Mebaral)	Grand mal and petit mal epilepsy	400-600mg/day	NA
Phenobarbital	Cortical focal, tonic-clonic	60-250mg/day	10-40mcg/mL
Primidone (Mysoline)	Tonic-clonic, psychomotor, focal	750-2000mg/day	5-12mcg/mL
BENZODIAZEPINES			
Clonazepam (Klonopin, Klonopin Wafers)	Absence, myoclonic, akinetic, Lennox-Gastaut syndrome	1.5-20mg/day	NA
Clorazepate dipotassium (Tranxene-SD)	Partial	22.5-90mg/day	NA
Diazepam (Valium)	Convulsive disorders, all forms	4-40mg/day	NA
Diazepam (Diastat)	Refractory patients with epilepsy who require intermittent use to control bouts of increased seizure activity.	0.2mg/kg rectally	NA
HYDANTOIN			
Phenytoin (Dilantin, Phenytek)	Tonic-clonic, psychomotor	300-600mg/day	10-20mcg/mL
SUCCINIMIDES			
Ethosuximide (Zarontin)	Absence	20-30mg/kg/day	40-100mcg/mL
Methsuximide (Celontin)	Absence	300-1200mg/day	10-40mcg/mL
Zonisamide (Zonegran)	Partial	100-400mg/day	NA
MISCELLANEOUS			
Carbamazepine (Carbatrol, Tegretol)	Tonic-clonic, mixed, psychomotor	800-1200mg/day	4-12mcg/mL
Divalproex sodium (Depakote, Depakote ER) **Valproic acid** (Depakene)	Absence, partial	10-60mg/kg/day	50-100mcg/mL
Felbamate (Felbatol)	Partial (adults), partial/generalized with Lennox-Gastaut syndrome (pediatrics)	2400mg/day	NA
Gabapentin (Neurontin)	Partial with and without secondary generalization (adults), partial (pediatrics)	900-1800mg/day	NA
Lamotrigine (Lamictal, Lamictal CD)	Partial (adults), partial/generalized with Lennox-Gastaut syndrome (pediatrics)	100-400mg/day	NA
Levetiracetam (Keppra)	Partial	1000-3000mg/day	NA
Oxcarbazepine (Trileptal)	Partial	600-2400mg/day	NA
Pregabalin (Lyrica)	Partial	150-600mg/day	NA
Tiagabine (Gabitril)	Partial	32-56mg/day	NA
Topiramate (Topamax)	Partial, tonic-clonic, Lennox-Gastaut syndrome (pediatrics)	200-400mg/day	NA
Zonisamide (Zonegran)	Partial	100-400mg/day	NA

*Please refer to complete monograph for pediatric dosing.   NA = Not Available.

TRIPTANS FOR ACUTE MIGRAINE

DRUG	BRAND	HOW SUPPLIED	INITIAL & (MAX) DOSE*	HEPATIC/RENAL DOSE ADJUSTMENT*
Almotriptan malate	Axert	Tab: 6.25mg, 12.5mg	6.25-12.5mg. May repeat after 2 hours. (2 doses/24 hours)	Initial: 6.25mg. Max: 12.5mg/24 hours.
Eletriptan hydrobromide	Relpax	Tab: 20mg, 40mg	20-40mg. May repeat after 2 hours. (40mg/dose or 80mg/day)	Severe Hepatic Impairment: Avoid use.
Frovatriptan succinate	Frova	Tab: 2.5mg	2.5mg. May repeat after 2 hours. (7.5mg/day)	No adjustment.
Naratriptan hydrochloride	Amerge	Tab: 1mg, 2.5mg	1-2.5mg. May repeat after 4 hours. (5mg/24 hours)	Severe Renal/Hepatic Impairment: Avoid use. Mild-Moderate Renal/ Hepatic Impairment: Use lower dose. Max: 2.5mg/24 hours.
Rizatriptan benzoate	Maxalt	Tab: 5mg, 10mg	5-10mg. May repeat after 2 hours. (30mg/24 hours)	No adjustment.
	Maxalt MLT	Tab, Disintegrating: 5mg, 10mg	5-10mg. May repeat after 2 hours. (30mg/24 hours)	No adjustment.
Sumatriptan	Imitrex	Inj**: 6mg/0.5mL	6mg SQ. May repeat after 1 hour. (12mg/24 hours)	Severe Hepatic Impairment: Avoid use.
		Nasal Spray: 5mg, 20mg	5mg, 10mg, or 20mg. May repeat after 2 hours. (40mg/24 hours)	Severe Hepatic Impairment: Avoid use.
		Tab: 25mg, 50mg, 100mg	25-100mg. May repeat after 2 hours. (200mg/24 hours)	Severe Hepatic Impairment: Avoid use. Hepatic Disease: Max: 50mg/single dose.
Zolmitriptan	Zomig	Nasal Spray: 5mg	5mg. May repeat after 2 hours. (10mg/24 hours)	Hepatic Impairment: Use lower dose.
		Tab: 2.5mg, 5mg	2.5mg or lower. May repeat after 2 hours. (10mg/24 hours)	Hepatic Impairment: Use lower dose.
	Zomig-ZMT	Tab, Disintegrating: 2.5mg, 5mg	2.5mg or lower. May repeat after 2 hours. (10mg/24 hours)	Hepatic Impairment: Use lower dose.

* Dosages shown are for adults ≥18 yrs. For more detailed information, refer to the individual monograph listings or the drug's FDA-approved labeling.

** Also indicated for acute treatment of cluster headaches.

FERTILITY AGENTS

DRUG (BRAND)	INDICATIONS	HOW SUPPLIED	DOSAGE
Cetrorelix acetate (Cetrotide)	For inhibition of premature LH surges in women undergoing controlled ovarian stimulation.	Inj: 0.25mg, 3mg	Multiple-Dose Regimen: 0.25mg SQ qd; start on day 5 (AM or PM) or day 6 (AM). Continue until hCG administration. Single-Dose Regimen: 3mg SQ single dose when estradiol level indicates appropriate stimulation response, usually on Day 7. If hCG not given within 4 days, then give 0.25mg SQ qd until day of hCG administration.
Choriogonadotropin alfa (Ovidrel)	For induction of final follicular maturation and early luteinization in infertile women who have undergone pituitary desensitization and have been appropriately pretreated with follicle stimulating hormone in an Assisted Reproductive Technology program. To induce ovulation and pregnancy in anovulatory, infertile women in whom anovulation is not due to primary ovarian failure.	Inj: 250mcg/0.5mL	250mcg SQ 1 day following the last dose of follicle stimulating agent. Withhold if excessive ovarian response.
Chorionic gonadotropin (Novarel)	To induce ovulation (OI) and pregnancy in anovulatory, infertile women in whom anovulation is not due to primary ovarian failure and pretreated with human menotropins.	Inj: 10,000 U	OI: 5000-10,000 U IM 1 day after last dose of menotropins.
Chorionic gonadotropin (Pregnyl)	To induce ovulation (OI) and pregnancy in anovulatory, infertile women in whom anovulation is not due to primary ovarian failure and pretreated with human menotropins.	Inj: 10,000 U	OI: 5000-10,000 U IM 1 day after last dose of menotropins.
Clomiphene citrate (Clomid)	Treatment of ovulatory dysfunction in women desiring pregnancy.	Tab: 50mg* **scored	Initial: 50mg/day for 5 days. Start any time if no recent uterine bleeding. If progestin-induced bleeding is intended, or if spontaneous uterine bleeding occurs, start on the 5th day of the cycle. If ovulation does not occur, increase to 100mg qd for 5 days, 30 days after the 1st course. Max: 100mg qd for 5 days and 3 courses of therapy.
Clomiphene citrate (Serophene)	Treatment of ovulatory dysfunction in women desiring pregnancy.	Tab: 50mg	Initial: 50mg/day for 5 days. Start any time if no recent uterine bleeding. If progestin-induced bleeding is intended, or if spontaneous uterine bleeding occurs, start on the 5th day of the cycle. If ovulation does not occur, increase to 100mg qd for 5 days, 30 days after the 1st course. Max: 100mg qd for 5 days and 3 courses of therapy.

DRUG (BRAND)	INDICATIONS	HOW SUPPLIED	DOSAGE
Follitropin alfa (Gonal-F)	For development of multiple follicles in ovulatory patients participating in Assisted Reproductive Technology (ART). For the induction of ovulation and pregnancy in anovulatory infertile patients in whom the cause of infertility is functional and not due to primary ovarian failure. (Men) For induction of spermatogenesis in primary and secondary hypogonadotropic hypogonadism not due to primary testicular failure.	Inj: 75 IU, 450 IU, 300 IU/0.5mL, 450 IU/0.75mL, 900 IU/1.5mL	Individualize dose. Oligo-Anovulation: Initial: 75 IU/day SQ. Titrate: Increase up to 37.5 IU/day after 14 days and further increase after 7 days if needed. Give hCG 5000 U 1 day after last dose. Do not exceed 35 days of therapy unless an E2 rise indicates imminent follicular development. Max: 300 IU/day. ART: Initial: 150 IU/day SQ on cycle Day 2 or 3 (early follicular phase). If gonadotropins suppressed, initiate at 225 IU/day. Titrate: Adjust after 5 days if needed, then at intervals no less than 3-5 days and not exceeding 75-150 IU/adjustment. Max: 450 IU/day. Once follicular development is evident, give hCG 5000-10,000 U. Hypogonadotropic Hypogonadism: Pretreat with hCG 1000-2250 U 2-3x/week to achieve normal serum testosterone levels. When normal, give 150 IU SQ and hCG 1000 U 3x/week. Max: 300 IU 3x/week.
Follitropin beta (Follistim AQ)	For the development of multiple follicles in ovulatory patients participating in Assisted Reproductive Technology (ART). For the induction of ovulation and pregnancy in anovulatory infertile patients in whom the cause of infertility is functional and not due to primary ovarian failure.	Cartridge: 150 IU, 300 IU, 600 IU, 900 IU. Inj: 75 IU, 150 IU	Ovulation Induction: Cartridge: 75 IU for 7 days. Titrate: Increase by 25-50 IU at weekly intervals. Max: 175 IU daily. Inj: 75 IU for 14 days. Titrate: increase by 37.5 IU weekly. Administer hCG 5000-10,000 U when pre-ovulatory conditions are equivalent to or greater than a normal individual. ART: Initial 150 to 225 IU for 5 days (cartridge) or 4 days (inj). Titrate: Adjust based upon ovarian response. Administer hCG 5000-10,000 U when a sufficient number of follicles of adequate size are present.
Ganirelix acetate	For inhibition of premature LH surges in women undergoing controlled ovarian stimulation.	Inj: 250mcg/0.5mL	250mcg SQ qd during the mid to late follicular phase. Continue until hCG administration.
Lutropin alfa (Luveris)	Used in combination with Gonal-F (follitropin alfa) for stimulation of follicular development in infertile hypogonadotropic hypogonadal women with profound luteinizing hormone deficiency (LH<1.2 IU/L).	Inj: 75 IU	Initial: 75 IU with 75-150 IU of Gonal-F qd SQ as two separate injections. Give hCG 1 day after last dose. Do not exceed 14 days of therapy unless signs of imminent follicular development. Do not exceed 225 IU/day of Gonal-F.
Menotropins (Repronex)	With hCG, for multiple follicular development and ovulation in women who received pituitary suppression.	Inj: (FSH-LH) 75 IU-75 IU	Oligo-Anovulation: Individualize dose. Initial: 150 IU SQ/IM qd for 5 days. Adjust subsequent dose to individual response at intervals no less than every 2 days and not exceeding 75-150 IU/adjustment. Max: 450 IU/day. Dosing >12 days is not recommended. If adequate response, give 5000-10,000 U hCG. May repeat course if inadequate response. ART: Initial: 225 IU SQ/IM. Adjust subsequent dose to individual response at intervals no less than every 2 days and not exceeding 75-150 IU/ adjustment. Max: 450 IU/day. Dosing >12 days is not recommended. If adequate response, give 5000-10,000 U hCG.
Menotropins (Menopur)	Development of multiple follicles and pregnancy in the ovulatory patients participating in an ART program.	Inj: (FSH-LH) 75 IU-75 IU	Initial: 225 IU SQ. Titrate: Adjust subsequent dosing to individual response at intervals no less than every 2 days and not exceeding 150 IU/adjustment. Max: 450 IU/day. Dosing >20 days is not recommended. If adequate response, administer hCG. Withhold hCG if ovaries abnormally enlarged last day of therapy.

(Continued)

DRUG (BRAND)	INDICATIONS	HOW SUPPLIED	DOSAGE
Progesterone (Crinone)	(4%) Treatment of secondary amenorrhea. (8%) Progesterone replacement or supplementation in Assisted Reproductive Technology (ART).	Gel: (Crinone, Prochieve) 4% [45mg, 6s], (Crinone, Prochieve) 8% [90mg, 6s 18s]	ART: 90mg of 8% intravaginally qd if require progesterone supplementation. 90mg of 8% intravaginally bid with partial or complete ovarian failure requiring progesterone replacement. If pregnancy occurs, continue until placental autonomy is achieved, up to 10-12 weeks.
Progesterone (Endometrin)	To support embryo implantation and early pregnancy by supplementation of corpus luteal function as part of an Assisted Reproductive Technology (ART) treatment program for infertile women.	Vaginal Insert: 100mg [21s]	100mg vaginally bid or tid starting at oocyte retrieval and continuing for up to 10 weeks.
Urofollitropin (Bravelle)	With hCG, to induce ovulation in patients who previously received pituitary suppression. With hCG, for multiple follicular development (controlled ovarian stimulation) during assisted reproductive technologies (ART) cycles in patients who previously received pituitary suppression.	Inj: 75 IU	Ovulation Induction: Initial: 150 IU SQ/IM qd for 1st 5 days. Adjust subsequent dose to individual response at intervals no less than every 2 days and not exceeding 75-150 IU/adjustment. Max: 450 IU/day. Dosing >12 days is not recommended. If adequate response, give 5000–10,000 U hCG 1 day following last dose. May repeat course if inadequate follicle development or ovulation without pregnancy occurs. ART: 225 IU SQ qd for 1st 5 days. Adjust subsequent dose to individual response at intervals no less than every 2 days and not exceeding 75-150 IU/adjustment. Max: 450 IU/day. Dosing >12 days is not recommended. If adequate follicular development, give 5000–10,000 U hCG to induce final follicular maturation in preparation for oocyte retrieval.

GYNECOLOGICAL ANTI-INFECTIVES

DRUG	CLASS	FORMULATION	ROUTE	RECOMMENDED DOSAGE
ANTIBACTERIALS				
Clindamycin Cleocin Vaginal, Clindamax	RX	**Cream:** 2%	Vaginal	**Bacterial Vaginosis: Adults:** 1 applicatorful qhs x 3-7 days (non-pregnant) or x 7 days (2nd or 3rd trimester).
Cleocin Vaginal Ovules	RX	**Supp:** 100mg	Vaginal	**Bacterial Vaginosis: Adults:** 1 sup qhs x 3 days.
Clindesse	RX	**Cream:** 2%	Vaginal	**Bacterial Vaginosis: Adults:** 1 applicatorful qd (non-pregnant).
Metronidazole Flagyl	RX	**Cap:** 375mg **Tab:** 250mg, 500mg	Oral	**Trichomoniasis: Adults:** 375mg bid or 250mg tid x 7 days. **Alternate Regimen (Tab):** If non-pregnant, 2g as single or divided dose. Contraindicated in 1st trimester.
Flagyl ER	RX	**Tab, ER:** 750mg	Oral	**Bacterial Vaginosis: Adults:** 750mg qd x 7 days. Contraindicated in 1st trimester.
MetroGel Vaginal	RX	**Gel:** 0.75%	Vaginal	**Bacterial Vaginosis: Adults:** 1 applicatorful qd-bid x 5 days.
Vandazole	RX	**Gel:** 0.75%	Vaginal	**Adults:** 1 applicatorful qd-bid x 5 days.
Sulfanilamide AVC	RX	**Cream:** 15%	Vaginal	**Candidiasis: Adults:** 1 applicatorful qd-bid x 30 days.
ANTIFUNGALS: CANDIDIASIS TREATMENT				
Butoconazole Gynazole-1	RX	**Cream:** 2%	Vaginal	**Adults:** 1 applicatorful single dose.
Clotrimazole Mycelex-3	OTC	**Cream:** 2%	Vaginal	**Adults/Pediatrics ≥12 yrs:** 1 applicatorful qhs x 3 days.
Mycelex-7	OTC	**Cream:** 1%	Vaginal	**Adults/Pediatrics ≥12 yrs:** 1 applicatorful qhs x 7 days.
Mycelex-7 Combination Pack	OTC	**Cream:** 1% + **Sup:** 100mg	Vaginal	**Adults/Pediatrics ≥12 yrs:**1 sup qhs x 7 days. Apply cream externally qd-bid up to 7 days prn.
Gyne-Lotrimin 3	OTC	**Cream:** 2% + **Sup:** 200mg	Vaginal	**Adults/Pediatrics ≥12 yrs:** 1 applicatorful or 1 sup qhs x 3 days.
Gyne-Lotrimin 3 Combination Pack	OTC	**Cream:** 1% + **Sup:** 200mg	Vaginal	**Adults/Pediatrics ≥12 yrs:**1 sup qhs x 3 days. Apply cream externally qd-bid prn.
Gyne-Lotrimin Combination Pack	OTC	**Cream:** 1% + **Sup:** 100mg	Vaginal	**Adults/Pediatrics ≥12 yrs:** 1 sup qhs x 7 days. Apply cream externally qd-bid prn.
Fluconazole Diflucan	RX	**Tab:** 150mg	Oral	**Adults:** 150mg single dose.
Miconazole Monistat 1 Combination Pack	OTC	**Cream:** 2% + **Sup:** 1200mg	Vaginal	**Adults/Pediatrics ≥12 yrs:** 1 sup single dose. Apply cream externally bid up to 7 days prn.
Monistat 3	OTC	**Cream:** 4%	Vaginal	**Adults/Pediatrics ≥12 yrs:** 1 applicatorful qhs x 3 days.
Monistat 3 Combination Pack	OTC	**Cream:** 2% + **Sup:** 200mg	Vaginal	**Adults/Pediatrics ≥12 yrs:** 1 applicatorful qhs x 3 days. Apply cream bid externally prn x 7 days.

(Continued)

DRUG	CLASS	FORMULATION	ROUTE	RECOMMENDED DOSAGE
ANTIFUNGALS: CANDIDIASIS TREATMENT *(Continued)*				
Monistat 7	OTC	**Cream:** 2%	Vaginal	**Adults/Pediatrics** ≥**12 yrs:** 1 applicatorful qhs x 7 days.
Monistat 7 Combination Pack	OTC	**Cream:** 2% **Sup:** 100mg	Vaginal	**Adults/Pediatrics** ≥**12 yrs:** 1 sup qhs x 7 days. Apply cream bid externally x 7 days.
Nystatin	RX	**Tab, Vaginal:** 100,000U	Vaginal	**Adults:** 1 tablet daily x 14 days.
Terconazole Terazol 3	RX	**Cream:** 0.8% **Supp:** 80mg	Vaginal	**Adults:** 1 applicatorful or 1 sup qhs x 3 days.
Terazol 7	RX	**Cream:** 0.4%	Vaginal	**Adults:** 1 applicatorful qhs x 7 days.
Tioconazole Monistat 1, Vagistat 1	OTC	**Oint:** 6.5%	Vaginal	**Adults/Pediatrics** ≥**12 yrs:** 1 applicatorful single dose hs.

HORMONE THERAPY

DRUG	BRAND	DOSAGE (mg)		
INTRAMUSCULAR ESTROGEN PRODUCTS				
Estradiol valerate	Delestrogen	**(mg/mL)** 10mg/mL, 20mg/mL, 40mg/mL		
Estradiol cypionate	Depo-Estradiol	5mg/mL		
ORAL ESTROGEN PRODUCTS				
Conjugated equine estrogens	Premarin	0.3, 0.45, 0.625, 0.9, 1.25		
	Enjuvia	0.3, 0.45, 0.625, 0.9, 1.25		
Estradiol	Gynodiol	0.5, 1, 1.5, 2		
Estradiol acetate	Femtrace	0.45, 0.9, 1.8		
Synthetic conjugated estrogens	Cenestin	0.3, 0.45, 0.625, 0.9, 1.25		
Esterified estrogens	Menest	0.3, 0.625, 1.25, 2.5		
Micronized 17ß-estradiol	Estrace	0.5, 1, 2		
Estropipate (piperazine estrone sulfate)	Ortho-Est	0.75, 1.5		
	Ogen	0.625, 1.25, 2.5, 5		
TRANSDERMAL ESTROGEN PRODUCTS				
Estradiol gel transdermal	Divigel	0.1% (0.25, 0.5, 1g/packet)		
17ß-estradiol matrix patch	Alora	**RELEASE RATE (mg/day)** 0.025, 0.05, 0.075, 0.1		
	Climara	0.025, 0.0375, 0.05, 0.06, 0.075, 0.1		
	Vivelle, Vivelle-Dot	0.025, 0.0375, 0.05, 0.075, 0.1		
17ß-estradiol reservoir patch	Estraderm	0.05, 0.1		
VAGINAL ESTROGEN PRODUCTS				
Vaginal Creams 17ß-estradiol	Estrace Vaginal Cream	2-4g/day x 1-2 wks, reduce to 1-2g/day x 1-2 wks, then 1g/day x 1-3x/wk		
Conjugated equine estrogens	Premarin Vaginal Cream	0.5-2g/day x 3 wks on 1 wk off		
Vaginal Ring 17ß-estradiol	Estring	Releases 0.0075mg/day x 90 days		
	Femring	Releases 0.05-0.1mg/day x 90 days		
Vaginal Tablet Estradiol hemihydrate	Vagifem	25mcg/day x 2 wks then 25mcg BIW		
PROGESTOGEN ONLY PRODUCTS				
Medroxyprogesterone acetate	Provera	2.5, 5, 10		
Norethindrone acetate	Aygestin	5		
Progesterone USP (in peanut oil)	Prometrium	100, 200		
ESTROGEN + PROGESTOGEN COMBINATIONS				
Oral continuous-cyclic regimen Conjugated equine estrogens (E) + Medroxyprogesterone acetate (P)	Premphase	0.625mg (E), 5mg (P) [E alone for days 1-14, followed by E+P on days 15-28]		
Oral continuous-combined regimen Conjugated equine estrogens (E) + Medroxyprogesterone (P)	Prempro	0.3mg (E) + 1.5mg (P)	0.45mg + 1.5mg	0.625mg + 2.5 or 5mg
Ethinyl estradiol (E) + Norethindrone acetate (P)	femhrt	2.5mcg (E) + 0.5mg (P); 5mcg (E) + 1mg (P)		
17ß-estradiol (E) + Norethindrone acetate (P)	Activella	1mg (E) + 0.5mg (P); 0.5mg (E) + 0.1mg (P)		

(Continued)

DRUG	BRAND	DOSAGE (mg)
ESTROGEN + PROGESTOGEN COMBINATIONS *(Continued)*		
Transdermal continuous-cyclic or continuous-combined regimen 17ß-estradiol (E) + Norethindrone acetate (P)	CombiPatch	0.05mg/day (E) + 0.14 or 0.25mg/day (P)
Estradiol (E) + Levonorgestrel (P)	Climara Pro	0.045mg/day (E) + 0.015mg/day (P)
ESTROGEN + ANDROGEN COMBINATIONS		
Oral cyclic regimen Esterified estrogens (E) +	Estratest	1.25 (E) + 2.5 (A)
Methyltestosterone (A)	Estratest H.S.	0.625 (E) + 1.25 (A)

NOTE: This list is not inclusive of all estrogen and progestogen products available. Indications vary among the different products. For more detailed information please refer to the individual monograph listings or the drug's FDA-approved labeling. Unopposed estrogen replacement therapy (ERT) is for use in women without an intact uterus. For women with an intact uterus, progestin must be added to the estrogen (HRT) for protection against estrogen-induced endometrial cancer. As with any therapy, the lowest possible effective dosage should be used. Re-evaluate periodically.

ORAL CONTRACEPTIVES

DRUG	ESTROGEN	PROGESTIN	STRENGTH (ESTROGEN/PROGESTIN)
MONOPHASIC			
Alesse, Levlite	Ethinyl Estradiol	Levonorgestrel	20mcg/0.1mg
Brevicon, Modicon	Ethinyl Estradiol	Norethindrone	35mcg/0.5mg
Demulen 1/35	Ethinyl Estradiol	Ethynodiol Diacetate	35mcg/1mg
Demulen 1/50	Ethinyl Estradiol	Ethynodiol Diacetate	50mcg/1mg
Desogen, Ortho-Cept	Ethinyl Estradiol	Desogestrel	30mcg/0.15mg
Levlen, Nordette-28	Ethinyl Estradiol	Levonorgestrel	30mcg/0.15mg
Loestrin 21 1/20, Loestrin Fe 1/20	Ethinyl Estradiol	Norethindrone Acetate	20mcg/1mg
Loestrin 21 1.5/30, Loestrin Fe 1.5/30	Ethinyl Estradiol	Norethindrone Acetate	30mcg/1.5mg
Lo/Ovral	Ethinyl Estradiol	Norgestrel	30mcg/0.3mg
Lybrel	Ethinyl Estradiol	Levonorgestrel	20mcg/90mcg
Modicon	Ethinyl Estradiol	Norethindrone	0.035mg/0.5mg
Norinyl 1/35, Ortho-Novum 1/35	Ethinyl Estradiol	Norethindrone	35mcg/1mg
Norinyl 1/50, Ortho-Novum 1/50	Mestranol	Norethindrone	50mcg/1mg
Ortho-Cept	Ethinyl Estradiol	Desogestrel	0.03mg/0.15mg
Ortho-Cyclen	Ethinyl Estradiol	Norgestimate	35mcg/0.25mg
Ovcon 35	Ethinyl Estradiol	Norethindrone	35mcg/0.4mg
Ovcon 50	Ethinyl Estradiol	Norethindrone	50mcg/1mg
Seasonale	Ethinyl Estradiol	Levonorgestrel	30mcg/0.15mg
Seasonique	Ethinyl Estradiol	Levonorgestrel	0.01mg, 0.15mg/0.03mg
Yasmin	Ethinyl Estradiol	Drospirenone	30mcg/3mg
YAZ	Ethinyl Estradiol	Drospirenone	0.02mg/3mg
BIPHASIC			
Ortho-Novum 10/11	Ethinyl Estradiol	Norethindrone	**Phase 1:** 35mcg/0.5mg **Phase 2:** 35mcg/1mg
Mircette	Ethinyl Estradiol	Desogestrel	**Phase 1:** 20mcg/0.15mg **Phase 2:** 10mcg/NONE
TRIPHASIC			
Cyclessa	Ethinyl Estradiol	Desogestrel	**Phase 1:** 25mcg/0.1mg **Phase 2:** 25mcg/0.125mg **Phase 3:** 25mcg/0.15mg
Estrostep Fe	Ethinyl Estradiol	Norethindrone Acetate	**Phase 1:** 20mcg/1mg **Phase 2:** 30mcg/1mg **Phase 3:** 35mcg/1mg
Ortho-Novum 7/7/7	Ethinyl Estradiol	Norethindrone	**Phase 1:** 35mcg/0.5mg **Phase 2:** 35mcg/0.75mg **Phase 3:** 35mcg/1mg
Ortho Tri-Cyclen	Ethinyl Estradiol	Norgestimate	**Phase 1:** 35mcg/0.18mg **Phase 2:** 35mcg/0.215mg **Phase 3:** 35mcg/0.25mg
Ortho Tri-Cyclen Lo	Ethinyl Estradiol	Norgestimate	**Phase 1:** 25mcg/0.18mg **Phase 2:** 25mcg/0.215mg **Phase 3:** 25mcg/0.25mg

(Continued)

DRUG	ESTROGEN	PROGESTIN	STRENGTH (ESTROGEN/PROGESTIN)
TRIPHASIC (Continued)			
Tri-Levlen, Triphasil, Trivora 28	Ethinyl Estradiol	Levonorgestrel	**Phase 1:** 30mcg/0.05mg **Phase 2:** 40mcg/0.075mg **Phase 3:** 30mcg/0.125mg
Tri-Norinyl	Ethinyl Estradiol	Norethindrone	**Phase 1:** 35mcg/0.5mg **Phase 2:** 35mcg/1mg **Phase 3:** 35mcg/0.5mg
PROGESTIN ONLY			
Nor-Q.D., Ortho-Micronor		Norethindrone	0.35mg

COMMON OB/GYN ICD-9 CODES

WOMEN

BREAST DISEASES
Breast disease, unspec.	611.9
Breast lump	611.72
Benign Dysplasia	
Diffuse cystic mastopathy	610.1
Fibroadenosis	610.3
Solitary cyst	610.0
Benign mammary dysplasia, unspecified	610.9
Fibroadenosis	610.2
Fibrocystic disease	610.1
Galactorrhea	611.6
Gynecomastia	611.1
Mammogram, abnormal, unspec.	793.80
Mastitis, unspec.	611.0
Mastodynia	611.71

CONTRACEPTION
Counseling/Management	
Emerg contraceptive counsel	V25.03
Fitting, diaphragm	V25.02
Prescription, oral	V25.01
Prescription, vaginal agents	V25.02
Procreative, general	V26.49
Follow-up	
Implantable subdermal	V25.43
IUD††	V25.42
Oral agent prescript	V25.41
Insertion	
Implantable subdermal	V25.5
IUD††	V25.1
Sterilization	V25.2

DISORDERS OF MENSTRUATION
Amenorrhea	626.0
Bleeding, postmenopausal	627.1
Hormone replacement, postmenopausal	V07.4
Menopausal disorders, unspec.	627.9
Menopausal state, asymptomatic	V49.81
Menopausal state, symptomatic	627.2
Menstruation, excessive/frequent	626.2
Menstruation, painful	625.3
Metrorrhagia	626.6
Mittelschmerz	625.2
Premenstrual tension syndrome	625.4
Vaginitis, postmenopausal atrophic	627.3

ECTOPIC PREGNANCY
Abdominal w/o IUP†	633.0
Abdominal w/IUP†	633.01
Other ectopic, w/o IUP†	633.8
Other ectopic, w/IUP†	633.81
Ovarian, w/o IUP†	633.2
Ovarian, w/IUP†	633.21
Tubal, w/o IUP†	633.1
Tubal, w/IUP†	633.11

EXAMS/SCREENING
Amniotic Test	
Alpha-fetoprotein levels	V28.1
Chromosomal anomalies	V28.0
Supervision/Exam	
Exam after delivery	V24.0
Normal first pregnancy	V22.0
Other normal pregnancy	V22.1
Postpartum follow-up	V24.2
Preg w/hx of pre-term labor	V23.41
Preg w/other poor OB hx	V23.49
Ultrasound	
Fetal growth retardation	V28.4
Fetal malformation	V28.3
Other specified	V28.8

Other Exam
Fertility testing	V26.21
Follow-up pap smear after surgery	V67.01
Mammogram, high risk	V76.11
Preg exam, negative	V72.41
Preg exam, positive	V72.42
Preg exam, unconfirmed	V72.40
Preoperative, NOS	V72.84
Rape victim	V71.5
Routine gynecological	V72.31
Smear to confirm recent normal following abnormal smear	V72.32

Screening
Chlamydial disease, specified	V73.88
Genetic disease carrier status	V26.31
Neoplasm, breast exam, other	V76.19
Neoplasm, cervix, malignant	V76.2
Neoplasm, intestine	V76.50
Neoplasm, ovary	V76.46
Neoplasm, vagina	V76.47
Thyroid disorders	V77.0
Venereal disease	V74.5

FEMALE GENITAL ORGAN DISEASES
Adhesions, pelvic peritoneal	614.6
Atrophy, vulva	624.1
Bartholin abscess	616.3
Bartholin cyst	616.2
Cervical polyp, unspec.	622.7
Cervicitis	616.0
Corpus luteum cyst	620.1
Cyst of ovary, follicular	620.0
Cystocele/rectocele/prolapse, unspec.	618.9
Dyspareunia	625.0
Dysplasia, cervix	622.1
Dysplasia, vagina	623.0
Endometrial hyperplasia, unspec.	621.30
Endometriosis, unspec.	617.9
Female disease, other, unspec.	625.9
Leukorrhea, unspec.	623.5
Ovarian failure, other	256.39
Ovarian failure, postablative	256.2
Ovaries, polycystic	256.4
Pelvic inflammatory disease, unspec.	614.9
Prolapse, uterine	618.1
Salpingitis, oophoritis, acute	614.0
Stenosis, cervix	622.4
Stress incontinence, female	625.6
Uterus, hypertrophy	621.2
Uterus, malposition	621.6
Vaginismus	625.1
Vaginitis/vulvovaginitis, unspec.	616.10

FERTILITY PROBLEMS
Infertility, female, unspec.	628.9
Infertility, male, unspec.	606.9
Abnormality in fetal heart rate/rhythm	659.70
Abortion, induced, w/o complication, complete	635.92
Abortion, missed	632
Abortion, spontaneous, w/o complication, complete	634.92
Abortion, spontaneous, w/o complication, incomplete	634.91
Abortion, threatened, antepartum	640.03
Abscess of breast, postpartum	675.14
Complicated delivery/labor, unspec.	669.90
Cord around neck, unspec.	663.10
Cord entanglement, other and unspec.	663.30
Eclampsia, unspec.	642.60
Ectopic, pregnancy, tubal, w/o intrauterine pregnancy	633.10

COMMON OB/GYN ICD-9 CODES

Ectopic pregnancy w/o intrauterine pregnancy, unspec.	633.90
Endometritis, postpartum	670.04
Engorgement of breasts, postpartum	676.24
Fetal distress, delivered	656.31
Fetal movements, decreased, antepartum	655.73
Forceps/vacuum extractor delivery, delivered	669.51
Gestational diabetes, antepartum	648.83
Gestational hypertension, antepartum	642.33
Hemorrhage in pregnancy, unspec.	641.90
Hemorrhage, other immediate postpartum	666.14
Hemorrhage, 3rd stage, postpartum	666.04
Hydatidiform mole	630
Hyperemesis gravidarum, mild	643.03
Hyperemesis gravidarum, w/metabolic disturbance, antepartum	643.13
Induction of labor, failed	659.10
Infectious conditions, complicating pregnancy	647.93
Labor, precipitate, unspec.	661.30
Labor, prolonged, unspec.	662.10
Laceration of cervix, unspec.	665.30
Laceration, perineal, 1st deg., postpartum	664.04
Laceration, perineal, 2nd deg., postpartum	664.14
Laceration, perineal, 3rd deg., postpartum	664.24
Laceration, perineal, 4th deg., postpartum	664.34
Large-for-dates, delivered	656.61
Normal delivery	650
Obstruction, bony pelvis, delivered	660.11
Obstruction, malposition, delivered	660.01
Oligohydramnios, antepartum	658.03
Placenta previa, w/bleeding, unspec.	641.10
Placenta previa, w/o bleeding, unspec.	641.00
Polyhydramnios, antepartum	657.03
Postpartum follow-up, routine	V24.2
Post-term pregnancy, antepartum	645.03
Post-term pregnancy, delivered	645.01
Pre-eclampsia, unspec.	642.40
Pregnancy, other complications, unspec.	646.90
Pregnant state, incidental	V22.2
Premature labor, delivered	644.21
Premature labor, threatened, undelivered	644.03
Premature rupture of membranes, unspec.	658.10
Prenatal care, high risk, unspec.	V23.9
Prenatal care, normal, first pregnancy	V22.0
Prenatal care, normal, other pregnancy	V22.1
Puerperium/postpartum, complications, unspec.	674.84
Rhesus isoimmunization, delivered	656.11
Shoulder dystocia, delivered	660.41
Small-for-dates, antepartum	656.53
Thrombophlebitis, postpartum	671.44
Trial of labor, failed, delivered	660.61
Twins, unspec.	651.00
Urinary tract infection, antepartum	646.63
Uterine inertia, primary, unspec.	661.00
Uterine inertia, secondary, unspec.	661.10
Vomiting of pregnancy, unspec.	643.90

NEOPLASM

Benign	
Breast	217
Fallopian tube	221.0
Ovary	220
Vagina	221.1
Vulva	221.2
Carcinoma in situ	
Breast	233.0
Cervix uteri	233.1
Genitalia, NOS	233.3
Uterus, NOS	233.2
Malignant	
Breast, axillary tail	174.6
Breast, contiguous/other	174.8
Breast, upper, outer	174.4
Cervix, other site	180.8
Cervix, uteri, NOS	180.9
Corpus uteri, except isthmus	182.0
Endocervix	180.0
Exocervix	180.1
Fallopian tube	183.2
Isthmus	182.1
Labia majora	184.1
Labia minora	184.2
Ovary	183.0
Uterine body, other spec	182.8
Vagina	184.0
Vulva, NOS	184.4
Uterine leiomyoma	
Intramural	218.1
Submucous	218.0
Subserous	218.2

OSTEOARTHROSIS

Ankle/foot	715.17
Forearm	715.13
Hand	715.14
Lower leg	715.16
Pelvic region/thigh	715.15
Shoulder region	715.11
Upper arm	715.12

OSTEOPOROSIS

Disuse	733.03
Idiopathic	733.02
Other	733.09
Senile	733.01
Unspecified	733.00

INFANTS/PERINATAL

CONGENITAL ANOMALIES

Anomaly, unspec.	759.9
Arteriovenous malformation of brain	747.81
Arteriovenous malformation, unspec.	747.60
Atresia, auditory canal (external)	744.02
Atrial septal defect	745.5
Birthmarks	757.32
Branchial cleft sinus/fistula	744.41
Cervical rib	756.2
Cleft lip, unspec.	749.10
Cleft palate, unspec.	749.00
Cleft palate w/cleft lip	749.20
Dislocation of hip, unilateral	754.30
Down's syndrome	758.0
Heart anomaly, unspec.	746.9
Hirschsprung's disease	751.3
Hydrocephalus	742.3
Hypospadias	752.61
Imperforate anus	751.2
Imperforate hymen	752.42
Limb anomaly, unspec.	755.9
Marfan syndrome	759.82
Meckel's diverticulum	751.0
Microcephalus	742.1
Osteogenesis imperfecta	756.51
Pectus excavatum	754.81
Polycystic kidney, unspec.	753.12
Polydactyly, fingers	755.01
Pyloric stenosis	750.5
Spina bifida, lumbar, uncomplicated	741.93
Spina bifida occulta	756.17
Spondylolisthesis	756.12
Supernumerary nipple	757.6
Talipes equinovarus	754.51
Tear duct, blocked	743.65
Tongue tie	750.0

Torticollis, sternomastoid	754.1
Undescended testis	752.51
Ventricular septal defect	745.4

PERINATAL (INFANT)

Birth asphyxia, severe	768.5
Birth asphyxia, unspec.	768.9
Birth trauma, fracture of clavicle	767.2
Birth trauma, unspec.	767.9
Breast engorgement in newborn	778.7
Circumcision, routine	V50.2
Drug withdrawal syndrome in newborn	779.5
Exceptionally large baby, ≥4,500g	766.0
Exposure to alcohol, via placenta or breast milk	760.71
Exposure to cocaine, via placenta or breast milk	760.75
Exposure to narcotics, via placenta or breast milk	760.72
Feeding problem, newborn	779.3
Fetal distress, during labor, in infant	768.3
Fetal distress, unspec. time of onset	768.4
Hemolytic disease, ABO isoimmunization	773.1
Hemolytic disease, RH isoimmunization	773.0
Hypocalcemia	775.4
Hypoglycemia, neonatal	775.6
Infant of diabetic mother syndrome	775.0
Jaundice, newborn, prematurity	774.2
Jaundice, newborn, unspec.	774.30
Meconium aspiration syndrome w/o respiratory symptoms	770.11
Meconium aspiration syndrome w/respiratory symptoms	770.12
Necrotizing enterocolitis	777.5
Newborn affected by Premature rupture of membranes	761.1
Newborn, light-for-dates, weight unspec.	764.00
Post-term infant	766.21
Preterm infant, weight unspec.	765.10
Prolonged gestation of infant	766.22

Respiratory distress syndrome	769
Respiratory problem, other, unspec.	770.9
Sepsis, neonatal	771.81
Skin/temperature problem	778.9
Sudden infant death syndrome	798.0
Well newborn, in-hospital birth, c-section	V30.01
Well newborn, in-hospital birth, vaginal	V30.00

SYMPTOMS ASSOCIATED WITH OB/GYN DISORDERS

Abnormal loss of weight	783.21
Abnormal weight gain	783.1
Abnormal mammogram	793.8
Abnormal pap smear	
ASC-US* favor benign	795.01
ASC-US* favor dysplasia	795.02
HGSIL**	795.04
LGSIL***	795.03
Nonspecific, unspec.	795.00
Anorexia	783.0
Crying, infant, excessive	780.92
Decreased libido	799.81
Incontinence urge	788.31
Incontinence/enuresis, unspec.	788.30
Jaundice	782.4
Insomnia w/sleep apnea, unspec.	780.51
Insomnia, unspec.	780.52
Lack of normal physiologic dvlpmt., unspec.	783.40
Loss of height	781.91
Nausea, alone	787.02
Nausea w/vomiting	787.01
Underweight	783.22
Urgency of urination	788.63
Urinary frequency	788.41
Urinary hesitancy	788.64
Varicose veins of the lower extremities	
Asymptomatic	454.9
w/inflammation	454.1
w/ulcer	454.0
w/ulcer, inflammation	454.2
Vomiting, alone	787.03

NOS = not specified.

* ASC-US: atypical squamous cells of undetermined significance.

** HGSIL: high-grade squamous intraepithelial lesion.

*** LGSIL: low-grade squamous intraepithelial lesion.

† IUP: intrauterine pregnancy.

†† IUD: intrauterine device.

BREAST CANCER TREATMENT OPTIONS

DRUG (BRAND)	INDICATIONS	HOW SUPPLIED	DOSAGE
ANDROGEN			
Fluoxymesterone (Halotestin)	Palliation of androgen-responsive recurrent mammary cancer in females who are >1 to <5 yrs post-menopausal or who have a hormone-dependent tumor as shown by previous beneficial response to castration.	Tab: 2mg*, 5mg*, 10mg* *scored	10-40mg/day in divided doses tid-qid. Continue therapy for at least 1 month for satisfactory subjective response, and for 2-3 months for objective response.
Methyltestosterone (Testred)	Secondary treatment of advancing inoperable metastatic (skeletal) breast cancer in females 1-5 yrs postmenopausal.	Cap: 10mg	50-200mg/day.
Testosterone (Delatestryl)	May also be used secondarily in females with advancing inoperable metastatic (skeletal) mammary cancer who are 1-5 years postmenopausal.	Inj: 200mg/mL	200-400mg every 2-4 weeks.
ANTIESTROGEN			
Faslodex (Fulvestrant)	Treatment of hormone receptor positive metastatic breast cancer in postmenopausal women with disease progression following anti-estrogen therapy.	Inj: 50mg/mL [2.5mL, 5mL]	250mg IM into buttock once monthly as either a single 5mL injection or two concurrent 2.5mL injections. Administer slowly.
ESTROGEN			
Estrace (Estradiol)	Palliative treatment of metastatic breast cancer.	Tab: 0.5mg*, 1mg*, 2mg* *scored	10mg tid for at least 3 months.
Gynodiol (Estradiol)	Palliative treatment of breast cancer in patients with metastatic disease.	Tab: 0.5mg*, 1mg*, 1.5mg*, 2mg* *scored	10mg tid for at least 3 months.
Menest (Esterified estrogens)	Palliative therapy for metastatic breast cancer in selected men and women.	Tab: 0.3mg, 0.625mg, 1.25mg, 2.5mg	10mg tid for at least 3 months.
Premarin Tablets (Conjugated estrogens)	Palliative treatment of breast cancer in patients with metastatic disease.	Tab: 0.3mg, 0.45mg, 0.625mg, 0.9mg, 1.25mg	10mg tid for minimum 3 months.
LHRH AGONIST			
Zoladex 1-Month (Goserelin)	Palliative treatment of advanced breast cancer in pre-and perimenopausal women.	Implant: 3.6mg	Inject SQ into anterior abdominal wall below navel line. 3.6mg every 28 days.
PROGESTIN			
Megestrol (Megestrol)	Palliative treatment of advanced breast carcinoma (eg, recurrent, inoperable or metastatic disease).	Tab: 20mg*, 40mg* *scored	40mg qid for a minimum of 2 months. Elderly: Start at lower end of dosing range.
SELECTIVE ESTROGEN RECEPTOR MODULATORS			
Raloxifene (Evista)	Reduction in risk of invasive breast cancer in post-menopausal women with osteoporosis or at high risk for invasive breast cancer.	Tab: 60mg	60mg qd.

BREAST CANCER TREATMENT OPTIONS

DRUG (BRAND)	INDICATIONS	HOW SUPPLIED	DOSAGE
SELECTIVE ESTROGEN RECEPTOR MODULATORS *(continued)*			
Tamoxifen (Soltamox)	Treatment of metastatic breast cancer in women and men. Treatment of node-positive and axillary node-negative breast cancer in women following mastectomy, axillary dissection and breast irradiation. To reduce risk of invasive breast cancer in women with DCIS. Reduction of breast cancer incidence in high risk women. Use for up to 5 yrs.	Sol: 10mg/5mL	Treatment: 20-40mg qd. Divide dosages >20mg into AM and PM doses. Risk Reduction/DCIS: 20mg qd for 5 yrs.
Tamoxifen (Tamoxifen)	Treatment of metastatic breast cancer in women and men. Treatment of node-positive and axillary node-negative breast cancer in women following mastectomy, axillary dissection and breast irradiation. To reduce risk of invasive breast cancer in women with DCIS. Reduction of breast cancer incidence in high risk women. Use for up to 5 yrs.	Tab: 10mg, 20mg	Treatment: 20-40mg qd. Divide dosages >20mg into AM and PM doses. Risk Reduction/DCIS: 20mg qd for 5 yrs.
Toremifene (Fareston)	Treatment of metastatic breast cancer in post-menopausal women with estrogen-receptor positive or unknown tumors.	Tab: 60mg	60mg qd. Treat until disease progression is evident.
SELECTIVE NONSTEROIDAL AROMATASE INHIBITORS (POSTMENOPAUSAL WOMEN ONLY)			
Anastrozole (Arimidex)	Adjuvant treatment of post-menopausal women with hormone-receptor positive early breast cancer. First-line treatment of post-menopausal women with hormone-receptor positive or hormone-receptor unknown locally advanced or metastatic breast cancer. Treatment of advanced breast cancer in post-menopausal women with disease progression following tamoxifen therapy. Patients with ER-negative disease and patients who did not respond to previous tamoxifen therapy rarely respond.	Tab: 1mg	1mg qd. Continue until tumor progression with advanced breast cancer.
Letrozole (Femara)	First-line treatment of hormone-receptor positive or hormone-receptor unknown locally advanced or metastatic breast cancer in postmenopausal women. Treatment of advanced breast cancer with disease progression following antiestrogen therapy in postmenopausal women.	Tab: 2.5mg	2.5mg qd. Continue until tumor progression is evident. Cirrhosis/Severe Liver Dysfunction: 2.5mg every other day.

DRUG (BRAND)	INDICATIONS	HOW SUPPLIED	DOSAGE
CHEMOTHERAPY AGENTS			
ANTHRACYCLINES			
Epirubicin (Ellence)	Adjuvant treatment of primary breast cancer with axillary node tumor involvement following resection of primary breast cancer.	Inj: 2mg/mL [25mL, 100mL]	Initial: 100-120mg/m² IV infusion, repeat at 3-4 week cycles. May give total dose on Day 1 of each cycle or divide equally on Days 1 and 8. Bone Marrow Dysfunction: Initial: 75-90mg/m². Hepatic Dysfunction: Bilirubin 1.2-3mg/dL or AST 2-4X ULN: Give 1/2 of initial dose. Bilirubin >3mg/dL or AST 4X ULN: Give 1/4 of initial dose. Severe Renal Dysfunction: Serum Creatinine >5mg/dL: Lower dose. Give prophylactic therapy with SMZ-TMP or fluoroquinolone with 120mg/m² regimen. Consider pretreatment with antiemetics. Adjust dose after 1st treatment cycle based on hematologic and nonhematologic toxicities (see PI).
Doxorubicin	To produce regression in disseminated neoplastic conditions such as breast carcinoma. Adjuvant therapy in women with evidence of axillary lymph node involvement following resection of primary breast cancer.	Inj: (2mg/mL) 10mg, 20mg, 50mg	Monotherapy: 60-75mg/m² IV every 21 days. Use the lower dose with inadequate bone marrow reserves due to old age, prior therapy, or neoplastic marrow infiltration. Concomitant Chemotherapy: 40-60mg/m² IV every 21-28 days. Hyperbilirubinemia: Reduce dose by 50% if 1.2-3mg/dL; reduce dose by 75% if 3.1-5mg/dL. See PI for pediatric dosing.
ANTIMICROTUBULE AGENT			
Ixempra (Ixabepilone)	In combination with capecitabine for treatment of patients with metastatic or locally advanced breast cancer resistant to treatment with an anthracycline and a taxane, or whose cancer is taxane resistant and for whom further anthracycline therapy is contraindicated. As monotherapy for treatment of metastatic or locally advanced breast cancer in patients whose tumors are resistant or refractory to anthracyclines, taxanes, and capecitabine.	Inj: 15mg, 45mg	40mg/m² IV infusion over 3 hrs every 3 weeks. Adjust dose based on toxicities (see PI). Premedicate with H1-antagonist (eg, diphenhydramine 50mg PO) and H2-antagonist (eg, ranitidine 150-300mg PO) approximately 1hr before infusion. Also premedicate with corticosteroid (eg, dexamethasone 20mg, IV 30 min before infusion or PO 60 min before infusion) if prior hypersensitivity reaction to ixabepilone. Hepatic Impairment: Monotherapy: Mild: AST and ALT ≤2.5x ULN and Bilirubin ≤1x ULN: 40mg/m². AST or ALT ≤10x ULN and Bilirubin ≤1.5x ULN: 32mg/m². Moderate (AST and ALT ≤10x ULN and Bilirubin >1.5 to ≤3x ULN): 20-30mg/m². Strong CYP3A4 Inhibitors: Avoid or reduce dose to 20mg/m².
KINASE INHIBITOR			
Tykerb (Lepatinib)	Treatment of patients with advanced or metastatic breast cancer, in combination with capecitabine, whose tumors overexpress HER2 and received prior therapy including an anthracycline, a taxane, and trastuzumab.	Tab: 250mg	Usual: 1250mg qd on Days 1-21 continuously with capecitabine 2000mg/m²/day (administered orally in 2 doses 12 hrs apart) on Days 1-14 in a repeating 21-day cycle. Give at least 1 hr before or after a meal (however, give capecitabine with food). ≥ Grade 2 LVEF: D/C dose. If LVEF recovers and asymptomatic after 2 weeks,

BREAST CANCER TREATMENT OPTIONS

DRUG (BRAND)	INDICATIONS	HOW SUPPLIED	DOSAGE
KINASE INHIBITOR (continued)			
			restart at 1000mg/day. Hepatic Impairment (Child-Pugh Class C): Consider dose reduction to 750mg/day. Concomitant Strong CYP3A4 Inhibitors: Avoid use. Concomitant Strong CYP3A4 Inducers: Avoid use and if must coadminister titrate gradually from 1250mg/day up to 4500mg/day based on tolerability. ≥ Grade 2 NCI CTC Toxicity: D/C or interrupt dose and restart with 1250mg/day when toxicity <Grade 1. Restart at 1000mg/day if toxicity recurs.
MISCELLANEOUS			
Capecitabine (Xeloda)	Treatment of metastatic breast cancer in combination with docetaxel after failure of prior anthracycline-containing chemotherapy. Treatment of metastatic breast cancer in patients resistant to paclitaxel and anthracycline-containing chemotherapy or resistant to paclitaxel and for whom further anthracycline therapy is not indicated.	Tab: 150mg, 500mg	Take with water within 30 min after meals. Usual/Concomitantly w/ docetaxel: 1250mg/m² bid for 2 weeks, then 1 week off. Give as 3-week cycles. CrCl 30-50mL/min: Reduce to 75% of starting dose. Interrupt and/or reduce dose if toxicity occurs. Readjust according to adverse effects (see PI for details).
Cytoxan (Cyclophosphamide)	Treatment of breast carcinoma.	Inj (Lyophilized): 500mg, 1g, 2g; Tab: 25mg, 50mg	Malignant Diseases (Without Hematologic Deficiency): Monotherapy: Initial: 40-50mg/kg IV in divided doses over 2-5 days, or 10-15mg/kg IV given every 7-10 days, or 3-5mg/kg twice weekly. Oral Dosing: Initial/Maint: 1-5mg/kg/day PO. Adjust dose according to antitumor activity and/or leukopenia. May need to reduce dose when combined with other cytotoxic drugs. See PI for pediatric dosing.
Dexrazoxane (Zinecard)	To reduce the incidence and severity of cardiomyopathy associated with doxorubicin in women with metastatic breast cancer who received a cumulative doxorubicin dose of 300mg/m² and who will continue doxorubicin therapy.	Inj: 250mg, 500mg	IV: 10:1 ratio of dexrazoxane: doxorubicin (eg, 500mg/m² dexrazoxane: 50mg/m² doxorubicin). Hepatic Impairment: Reduce dose proportionally. Give by slow IV push or rapid IV infusion. Give doxorubicin within 30 min after start of infusion.
Fluorouracil	Palliative management of colon, rectum, breast, stomach, and pancreatic carcinomas.	Inj: 50mg/mL, [10mL, 50mL, 100mL]	12mg/kg IV qd for 4 days. Max: 800mg/day. If no toxicity, give 6mg/kg IV on 6th, 8th, 10th, and 12th days. Skip Days 5, 7, 9, and 11. Inadequate Nutritional State: 6mg/kg IV for 3 days. If no toxicity, give 3mg/kg IV on 5th, 7th, and 9th days. Max: 400mg/day. Skip Days 4, 6, and 8. Maint (Use Schedule 1 or Schedule 2): Schedule 1: If no toxicity, repeat 1st course every 30 days after last day of previous course. Schedule 2: When toxic signs from initial course subside, give 10-15mg/kg/week IV single dose; do not exceed 1g/week.

DRUG (BRAND)	INDICATIONS	HOW SUPPLIED	DOSAGE
MISCELLANEOUS (continued)			
Methotrexate (Methotrexate)	(Inj/PO) Treatment of neoplastic diseases, eg, acute lymphocytic leukemia, gestational choriocarcinoma, chorioadenoma destruens, hydatidiform mole, breast cancer, epidermoid cancer of the head and neck, advanced mycosis fungoides, lung cancer, advanced stage non-Hodgkin's lymphoma.	Inj: (Generic) (Methotrexate Sodium) 25mg/mL, 1g; Tab: (Generic) (Methotrexate) 2.5mg*; Tab: (Rheumatrex) (Methotrexate) 2.5mg* [Dose Pack 15mg, 4 x 6 tabs; 12.5mg, 4 x 5 tabs; 10mg, 4 x 4 tabs; 7.5mg, 4 x 3 tabs; 5mg, 4 x 2 tabs] *scored	Choriocarcinoma/Trophoblastic Disease: 15-30mg qd PO/IM for 5 days. May repeat 3-5 times as required with rest period of ≥ 1 week. Leukemia: Induction: 3.3mg/m² with prednisone 60mg/m² qd. Remission Maintenance: 15mg/m² PO/IM twice weekly or 2.5mg/kg IV every 14 days. Burkitt's Tumor: Stages Stages I-II: 10-25mg/day PO for 4-8 days. Administer several courses with rest periods of 7-10 days in between. Lymphosarcoma: Stage III: 0.625-2.5mg/kg/day with other antitumor agents.
MONOCLONAL ANTIBODY/HER2 BLOCKER			
Transtuzumab (Herceptin)	Part of treatment regimen containing doxorubicin, cyclophosphamide, and either paclitaxel or docetaxel or with docetaxel and carboplatin for adjuvant treatment of HER2-over-expressing breast cancer. Single agent for adjuvant treatment of HER2-over-expressing breast cancer in patients who received 1 or more chemotherapy regimens for metastatic disease.	Inj: 440mg	Adjuvant Treatment: Following Anthracycline/Concurrently With Paclitaxel for First 12 Weeks: IV infusion: Initial: 4mg/kg over 90 min. Maint: 2mg/kg/week over 30 min for total 52 doses. Following Completion of All Chemotherapy: IV Infusion: Initial: 8mg/kg. Maint: 6mg/kg every 3 weeks for total of 17 doses; give doses ≥4mg/kg over 90 min. Metastatic Breast Cancer: IV Infusion: Alone or With Paclitaxel: Initial: 4mg/kg over 90 min. Maint: 2mg/kg/week over 30 min until disease progression.
NUCLEOSIDE ANALOGUE/ANTIMETABOLITE			
Gemcitabine (Gemzar)	Adjunct with paclitaxel for 1st-line treatment of metastatic breast cancer after failure of prior anthracycline-containing adjuvant chemotherapy, unless anthracyclines were clinically contraindicated.	Inj: 200mg, 1g	1250mg/m² IV on Days 1 and 8 of each 21-day cycle. Give paclitaxel 175mg/m² IV on Day 1 before gemcitabine. All IV infusions given over 30 min. Adjust dose based on hematologic toxicity.
TAXANES			
Docetaxel (Taxotere)	Treatment of locally advanced or metastatic breast cancer after failure of prior chemotherapy. In combination with doxorubicin and cyclophosphamide for the adjuvant treatment of operable, node-positive breast cancer.	Inj: 20mg/0.5mL, 80mg/2mL	Premedicate with oral corticosteroids. Adjust dose based on febrile neutropenia, neutrophil count, cutaneous reactions, peripheral neuropathy, neurosensory signs/symptoms, or GI toxicities (see PI). Breast Cancer: 60-100mg/m² IV over 1 hr every 3 weeks. Adjuvant Treatment Operable Node-Positive Breast CA: 75mg/m² 1 hr after doxorubicin 50mg/m² and cyclophosphamide 500mg/m² every 3 weeks for 6 courses. Administer every 3 weeks for 3 cycles.
Paclitaxel (Taxol)	Treatment of breast cancer after failure with combination chemotherapy for metastatic disease or relapse within 6 months of adjuvant chemotherapy. Adjuvant treatment of node-positive breast cancer administered sequentially to doxorubicin-containing chemotherapy.	Inj: 6mg/mL	IV: Breast Cancer: 175mg/m² over 3 hrs every 3 weeks for 4 courses. Non-Small Cell Lung Cancer: 135mg/m² over 24 hrs every 3 weeks followed by cisplatin. Reduce dose of subsequent courses by 20% if neutrophils <500 cells/mm³ for ≥1 week or severe peripheral neuropathy occurs. Premedicate prior to administration with appropriate medications; see PI for additional information.

DRUG (BRAND)	INDICATIONS	HOW SUPPLIED	DOSAGE
TAXANES *(continued)*			
Paclitaxel protein-bound particle for injectable suspension (Abraxane)	Treatment of breast cancer after failure of combination chemotherapy for metastatic disease or relapse within 6 months of adjuvant chemotherapy. Prior therapy should have included an anthracyline unless clinically contraindicated.	Inj: 100mg	260mg/m² IV over 30 min every 3 weeks. Severe neutropenia (neutrophil <500 cells/mm³ for week or longer) or severe sensory neuropathy (Grade 3 or 4): Hold dose until neutrophil >1500 cells/mm³ or sensory neuropathy resolves to Grade 1 or 2. Reduce subsequent courses to 220mg/m², if recurrence reduce subsequent courses to 180mg/m².
VASCULAR ENDOTHELIAL GROWTH INHIBITOR			
Bevacizumab (Avastin)	Treatment of patients who have not received chemotherapy for metastatic HER2 negative breast cancer, in combination with paclitaxel.	Inj: 25mg/mL [4mL, 16mL]	10mg/kg every 2 weeks. Give as IV infusion over 90 min, if 1st infusion is well tolerated, give 2nd infusion over 60 min and subsequent doses over 30 min.
VINCA ALKALOID			
Vinblastine	Palliative treatment of unresponsive breast carcinoma.	Inj: 1mg/mL [10mL]	Dose at intervals of ≤7 days. 1st Dose: 3.7mg/m². 2nd Dose: 5.5mg/m². 3rd Dose: 7.4mg/m². 4th Dose: 9.25mg/m². 5th Dose: 11.1mg/m². Max: 18.5mg/m². Do not increase dose after that dose which reduces WBC to 3000 cells/mm³. Maint: Use dose of 1 increment smaller than this dose at weekly intervals. Reduce to 50% dose if direct serum bilirubin >3mg/100mL. Only dose if WBC ≥4000 cells/mm³.

BREAST CANCER RISK FACTORS

Unmodifiable risk factors	
Gender	Women > men
Age	1 out of 8 breast cancer diagnoses are among women <45 yrs, while about 2 out of 3 occur in women >55 yrs
Genetic	BRCA1 and BRCA2, ATM gene, CHEK2 gene, p53 tumor suppressor gene, PTEN gene mutations
Race	Whites > African Americans
Family history	Having a first-degree relative with breast cancer doubles risk; having 2 first-degree relatives increases risk about 5-fold
Personal history of breast cancer	Women with cancer in one breast have 3- to 4-fold increased risk of developing a new cancer in another area of the same breast or in the opposite breast
Abnormal breast biopsy	Nonproliferative lesions, proliferative lesions with or without atypia
Early menarche	Women who started menstruating at an early age (<12 yrs)
Age at menopause	Women who went through menopause at a late age (>55 yrs)
Personal history of breast abnormalities	Two breast tissue abnormalities–ductal carcinoma in situ (DCIS) and lobular carcinoma in situ (LCIS)–are associated with increased risk for developing invasive breast cancer
Earlier breast radiation exposure	Women who had radiation therapy to the chest area as treatment for another cancer
Breast density	Women with a higher proportion of dense breast tissue (eg, connective and milk duct tissue)

Lifestyle factors associated with increased risk of breast cancer

- Alcohol (2 drinks/day)
- High body mass index
- Not having children or having them when >30 yrs

Drugs associated with increased risk of breast cancer

- Birth control pills
- DES (diethylstilbestrol)
- Postmenopausal hormone therapy or hormone replacement therapy

Uncertain risk factors

- High-fat diets
- Miscarriages
- Night work
- Pollution
- Smoking (active or passive)

Sources: American Cancer Society and National Cancer Institute.

ANTIDEPRESSANTS

DRUG (BRAND)	HOW SUPPLIED	DAILY DOSE Initial (I), Usual (U), Max (M)	TITRATE
AMINOKETONE			
Bupropion (Wellbutrin)	**Tab:** 75mg, 100mg	(I)200mg (U)300mg (M)450mg	Increase by 100mg/d q3d.
(Wellbutrin SR)	**Tab, SR:** 100mg, 150mg, 200mg	(I)150mg (U)300mg (M)400mg	Increase by 150mg/d q4d.
(Wellbutrin XL)	**Tab, ER:** 150mg, 300mg	(I)150mg (U)300mg (M)450mg	Increase by 150mg/d q4d.
Bupropion HBr (Aplenzin)	**Tab, Extended-Release:** 174mg, 348mg, 522mg	(I)174mg (U)348mg (M)522mg	Increase by 174mg/d q4d.
MONOAMINE OXIDASE INHIBITORS			
Phenelzine (Nardil)	**Tab:** 15mg	(I)45mg (U)15mg qd or qod	Increase rapidly to 60-90mg/d then decrease to maintenance dose.
Tranylcypromine (Parnate)	**Tab:** 10mg	(I,U)30mg (M)60mg	Increase by 10mg/d q1-3 weeks.
PHENYLETHYLAMINE			
Venlafaxine (Effexor)	**Tab:** 25mg*, 37.5mg*, 50mg*, 75mg*, 100mg*	(I)75mg (U)150-225mg (M)375mg	Increase by 75mg/d q4d.
(Effexor XR)	**Cap, ER:** 37.5mg, 75mg, 150mg	(I)37.5-75mg (U)75-225mg (M)225mg	Increase by 75mg/d q4d.
Selegeline (Emsam)	**Patch:** 6mg/24hrs, 9mg/24hrs, 12mg/24hrs	(I)6mg/24hrs (U)6mg/24hrs (M)12mg/24hrs	Increase by 3mg/24hrs.
PHENYLPIPERAZINE			
Nefazodone	**Tab:** 50mg, 100mg*, 150mg*, 200mg, 250mg	(I)200mg (U)300-600mg (M)600mg	Increase by 100-200mg/d in no less than 1 week.
SELECTIVE SEROTONIN NOREPINEPHRINE REUPTAKE INHIBITOR			
Duloxetine (Cymbalta)	**Cap:** 20mg, 30mg, 60mg	(I,U)40-60mg (M)60mg	N/A
Desvenlafaxine (Pristiq)	**Tab, Extended-Release:** 50mg, 100mg	(I)50mg (M)400mg	N/A
SELECTIVE SEROTONIN REUPTAKE INHIBITORS			
Citalopram (Celexa)	**Sol:** 10mg/5mL; **Tab:** 10mg, 20mg*, 40mg*	(I)20mg (U)40mg (M)60mg	Increase by 20mg/d q week.
Escitalopram (Lexapro)	**Sol:** 5mg/5mL; **Tab:** 5mg, 10mg*, 20mg*	(I)10mg (U)10-20mg	Increase to 20mg/d after 1 week.
Fluoxetine (Prozac)	**Cap:** 10mg, 20mg, 40mg; **Sol:** 20mg/5mL; **Tab:** 10mg*	(I)20mg (M)80mg	Consider after several weeks of therapy.
Paroxetine (Paxil)	**Sus:** 10mg/5mL; **Tab:** 10mg*, 20mg*, 30mg, 40mg	(I)20mg (M)50mg	Increase by 10mg/d.
(Paxil CR)	**Tab, CR:** 12.5mg, 25mg, 37.5mg	(I)25mg (M)62.5mg	Increase by 12.5mg/d.
(Pexeva)	**Tab:** 10mg, 20mg, 30mg, 40mg	(I)20mg (M)50mg	Increase by 10mg/d.
Sertraline (Zoloft)	**Sol:** 20mg/mL; **Tab:** 25mg*, 50mg*, 100mg*	(I)50mg (M)200mg	Increase at 1-week intervals.

(Continued)

ANTIDEPRESSANTS

DRUG (BRAND)	HOW SUPPLIED	DAILY DOSE Initial (I), Usual (U), Max (M)	TITRATE
TETRACYCLIC			
Mirtazapine (Remeron)	**Tab:** 15mg*, 30mg*, 45mg; **Tab, Disintegrating:** 15mg, 30mg, 45mg	**(I)**15mg **(M)**45mg	Increase q 1-2 weeks.
TRIAZOLOPYRIDINE			
Trazodone (Desyrel)	**Tab:** 50mg*, 100mg*, 150mg*, 300mg*	**(I)**150mg **(M)**400-600mg	Increase by 50mg/d q3-4d.
TRICYCLICS			
Amitriptyline	**Inj:** 10mg/mL; **Tab:** 10mg, 25mg, 50mg, 75mg, 100mg, 150mg	**(I)**OP: 50-100mg, IP: 100mg **(U)**50-100mg **(M)**OP: 150mg, IP: 300mg	OP: Increase by 25-50mg/d. IP: Increase to 200mg/d.
Amoxapine	**Tab:** 25mg*, 50mg*, 100mg*, 150mg*	**(I)**100-150mg **(U)**200-300mg **(M)**OP: 400mg IP: 600mg	Increase to 100mg bid-tid by end of first week.
Clomipramine (Anafranil)	**Cap:** 25mg, 50mg, 75mg	**(I)**25mg **(U)**100-250mg **(M)**250mg	Increase to 100mg/d in 2 weeks, then increase gradually.
Desipramine (Norpramin)	**Tab:** 10mg, 25mg, 50mg, 75mg, 100mg, 150mg	**(I,U)**100-200mg **(M)**300mg	N/A
Doxepin (Sinequan)	**Cap:** 10mg, 25mg, 50mg, 75mg, 100mg, 150mg; **Sol:** 10mg/mL	**(I)**75mg **(U)**75-150mg **(M)**300mg	Increase gradually.
Imipramine (Tofranil PM)	**Cap:** 75mg, 100mg, 125mg, 150mg	**(I)**OP: 75mg, IP: 100mg **(U)**75-150mg **(M)**OP: 200mg, IP: 250-300mg	OP: Increase to 150mg/d. IP: Increase to 200mg/d.
(Tofranil)	**Tab:** 10mg, 25mg, 50mg	**(I)**OP: 75mg, IP: 100mg **(U)**50-150mg **(M)**OP: 200mg, IP: 250-300mg	OP: Increase to 150mg/d. IP: Increase to 200mg/d.
Nortriptyline (Pamelor, Aventyl)	**Cap:** 10mg, 25mg, 50mg, 75mg; **Sol:**10mg/5mL	**(I,U)**75-100mg **(M)**150mg	N/A
Protriptyline (Vivactil)	**Tab:** 5mg, 10mg	**(U)**15-40mg **(M)**60mg	Titrate morning dose.
Trimipramine (Surmontil)	**Cap:** 25mg, 50mg, 100mg	**(I)**OP: 75mg, IP: 100mg **(U)**50-150mg, IP: 200mg **(M)**OP: 200mg, IP: 250-300mg	OP: Increase to 150mg/d. IP: Increase to 200mg/d.

Abbreviations: IP=Inpatient; OP=Outpatient   *Scored.

ANTIPSYCHOTIC AGENTS

DRUG (BRAND)	HOW SUPPLIED (mg)*	INITIAL & (MAX) DOSE**	USUAL DOSE RANGE**
ATYPICAL			
Aripiprazole (Abilify)	**Tab:** 2, 5, 10, 15, 20, 30 **Sol:** 1mg/mL; **Inj:** 7.5mg/mL	10-15mg qd (30mg/day)	10-15mg qd
(Abilify Discmelt)	**Tab, Orally Disintegrating:** (Discmelt) 10, 15, 20, 30	10-15mg qd (30mg/day)	10-15mg qd
Clozapine (Clozaril)	**Tab:** 12.5†, 25, 100	12.5mg qd-bid (900mg/day)	100-900mg/day given tid
(Fazaclo)	**Tab, Orally Disintegrating:** 12.5, 25*, 50, 100**scored	12.5mg qd-bid (900mg/day)	100-900mg/day given tid
Olanzapine (Zyprexa, Zyprexa Zydis)	**Tab:** 2.5, 5, 7.5, 10, 15, 20 **Tab, Orally Disintegrating:** 5, 10, 15, 20	Schizophrenia: 5-10mg qd Bipolar Mania: 10-15mg qd (20mg/day for both)	Schizophrenia: 10-15mg qd Bipolar Mania: 5-20mg qd
(Zyprexa IntraMuscular)	**Inj:** 10mg	Agitation: 10mg IM (3 doses)	Agitation: 2.5-10mg IM
Paliperidone (Invega)	**Tab, Extended-Release:** 3, 6, 9	6mg qd (12mg/day)	3-12mg/day
Quetiapine fumarate (Seroquel)	**Tab:** 25, 100, 200, 300	Schizophrenia: 25mg bid Bipolar Mania: 50mg bid (800mg/day for both)	Schizophrenia: 150-750mg/day Bipolar Mania: 400-800mg/day
(Seroquel XR)	**Tab, Extended-Release:** 200, 300, 400	Initial: 300mg/day	400-800mg/day
Risperidone (Risperdal)	**Sol:** 1mg/mL **Tab:** 0.25, 0.5, 1, 2, 3, 4	Schizophrenia: 1mg bid (16mg/day)	Schizophrenia: 4-8mg/day Bipolar Mania: 1-6mg/day
(Risperdal M-Tab)	**Tab, Orally Disintegrating:** 0.5, 1, 2 (6mg/day)	Bipolar Mania: 2-3mg qd	
(Risperdal Consta)	**Inj:** 25, 37.5, 50	Schizophrenia: 25mg IM	Schizophrenia: 25-50mg IM q2wks (50mg/dose) q2wks
Ziprasidone HCl (Geodon)	**Cap:** 20, 40, 60, 80	20mg bid (160mg/day)	20-80mg bid
Ziprasidone mesylate (Geodon) for Injection)	**Inj:** 20mg/mL	10mg IM q2h or 20mg IM q4h (40mg/day)	Switch to oral for long-term therapy
CONVENTIONAL			
Chlorpromazine	**Cap, Extended-Release:** 30, 75, 150; **Inj:** 25mg/mL; **Sup:** 25, 100; **Syrup:** 10mg/5mL; **Tab:** 10, 25, 50, 100, 200	10-25mg PO bid-qid or 25mg IM (1000mg/day PO)	PO: 10-800mg/day IM: 25-50mg IM q4-6h‡ Switch to PO when controlled
Fluphenazine HCl (Prolixin)	**Elixir:** 2.5mg/5mL **Sol, Conc:** 5mg/mL **Tab:** 1†, 2.5, 5, 10 **Inj:** 2.5mg/mL	2.5mg-10mg/day in divided doses (40mg/day) 1.25mg IM q6-8h (10mg/day)	1-5mg qd
Fluphenazine decanoate (Prolixin Decanoate)	**Inj:** 25mg/mL	12.5-25mg IM/SQ q4-6 wks (100mg/dose)	2.5-10mg/day in divided doses

(Continued)

DRUG (BRAND)	HOW SUPPLIED (mg)*	INITIAL & (MAX) DOSE**	USUAL DOSE RANGE**
CONVENTIONAL (*Continued*)			
Haloperidol	**Sol, Conc:** 2mg/mL **Tab:** 0.5, 1, 2, 5, 10, 20	Moderate: 0.5-2mg bid-tid Sev/Resist: 3-5mg bid-tid (100mg/day)	2-20mg/day
Haloperidol lactate (Haldol)	**Inj:** 5mg/mL	2-5mg IM q4-8h or hourly if needed (100mg/day)	Switch to PO 12-24 hours after last injection
Haloperidol decanoate (Haldol Decanoate)	**Inj:** 50mg/mL, 100mg/mL	10-20x daily oral dose up to 100mg/dose (450mg/month)	10-15x daily oral dose
Loxapine succinate (Loxitane)	**Cap:** 5, 10, 25, 50	10mg bid, up to 50mg/day (250mg/day)©	60-100mg/day
Molindone (Moban)	**Tab:** 5, 10, 25, 50	50-75mg/day (225mg/day)	5-25mg tid/qid
Perphenazine	**Tab:** 2, 4, 8, 16	Non-hospitalized: 4-8mg tid Hospitalized: 8-16mg (64mg/day)	Reduce dose as soon as possible to minimum effective dose.
Prochlorperazine maleate	**Tab:** 5, 10	5-10mg tid-qid	Moderate/Severe: 50-75mg/day Severe: 100-150mg/day
Thioridazine HCl (Mellaril)	**Sol, Conc:** 30mg/mL, 100mg/mL **Tab:** 10†, 15, 25†, 50†, 100, 150†, 200	50-100mg tid (800mg/day)	200-800mg/day given bid-qid
Thiothixene (Navane)	**Cap:** 1, 2, 5, 10, 20	Mild: 2mg tid Severe: 5mg bid (60mg/day)	20-30mg/day
Trifluoperazine HCl	**Tab:** 1, 2, 5, 10	2-5mg bid (40mg/day or higher if needed)	15-20mg/day

Note: This list is not inclusive of all antipsychotic agents. Indications may vary among the different products.

* Unless otherwise indicated.

** Doses shown are for adults. For pediatric dosing and additional information please refer to the individual monograph listings or the drug's FDA-approved labeling. Dosages need to be adjusted by titration to individual patient needs and may need to be reduced in the elderly, debilitated, or with renal/hepatic impairment. Periodically reassess to determine the need for maintenance treatment.

† Available only in generic forms.

‡ Severe cases may require up to 2g/day or 400mg/dose IM.

BIPOLAR DISORDER PHARMACOTHERAPY

DRUG	BRAND	HOW SUPPLIED	USUAL DOSE	COMMENTS
MOOD STABILIZER				
Lithium	Various	**Cap:** 150mg, 300mg, 600mg; **Tab:** 300mg; **Tab, Extended-Release:** 450mg	**Adults/Pediatrics:** ≥12 yrs: Acute Mania: 600mg tid to achieve effective serum levels of 1-1.5mEq/L; monitor levels twice a week until stabilized. Maintenance Therapy: 300mg tid-qid or (ER) 450mg bid to maintain serum levels of 0.6-1.2 mEq/L; monitor levels every 2 months.	Treatment of manic episodes of bipolar disorder and maintenance treatment of bipolar disorder.
ANTICONVULSANTS				
Carbamazepine	Equetro	**Cap, Extended-Release:** 100mg, 200mg, 300mg	**Adults:** Initial: 400mg/day, given in divided doses, bid. Titrate: 200mg qd. **Max:**1600mg/day. Do not crush or chew.	Treatment of acute manic and mixed episodes associated with bipolar I disorder.
Divalproex sodium	Depakote ER	**Tab, Extended-Release:** 250mg, 500mg	**Adults:** Mania: Initial: 25mg/kg/day given once daily. Titrate: Increase dose rapidly to clinical effect. **Max:** 60mg/kg/day. Conversion from Depakote: Administer Depakote ER qd using a dose 8-20% higher than the total daily dose of Depakote. If cannot directly convert to Depakote ER, consider increasing to next higher Depakote total daily dose before converting to appropriate total daily Depakote ER dose. Elderly: Give lower initial dose and titrate slowly. Decrease dose or discontinue if decreased food or fluid intake or if excessive somnolence occurs. Swallow whole; do not crush or chew.	Acute manic or mixed episodes associated with bipolar I disorder.
	Depakote	**Tab, Delayed-Release:** 125mg, 250mg, 500mg	**Adults:** Mania: 750mg daily in divided doses. Titrate: Increase dose rapidly to clinical effect. **Max:** 60mg/kg/day. Decrease dose or discontinue if decreased food or fluid intake or if excessive somnolence occurs.	Treatment of mania associated with bipolar disorder.
Lamotrigine	Lamictal	**Tab:** 25mg*, 100mg*, 150mg*, 200mg*; **Tab, Chewable:** (Lamictal CD) 2mg, 5mg, 25mg *scored	**Adults:** Bipolar Disorder: Patients not taking carbamazepine, other enzyme-inducing drugs (EIDs) or VPA: **Weeks 1 and 2:** 25mg qd. **Weeks 3 and 4:** 50mg qd. **Week 5:** 100mg qd. **Weeks 6 and 7:** 200mg qd. Patients taking VPA: **Weeks 1 and 2:** 25mg every other day. **Weeks 3 and 4:** 25mg qd. **Week 5:** 50mg qd. **Weeks 6 and 7:** 100mg qd. Patients taking carbamazepine (or other EIDs) and not taking VPA: **Weeks 1 and 2:** 50mg qd. **Weeks 3 and 4:** 100mg qd (divided doses). **Week 5:** 200mg qd (divided doses). **Week 6:** 300mg qd (divided doses). **Week 7:** Up to 400mg qd (divided doses). After discontinuation of psychotropic drugs excluding VPA, carbamazepine, or other EIDs: Maintain current dose. After discontinuation of VPA and current lamotrigine dose of 100mg qd: **Week 1:** 150mg qd. Week 2 and onward: 200mg qd. After discontinuation of carbamazepine or other EIDs and current lamotrigine dose of 400mg qd: **Week 1:** 400mg qd. **Week 2:** 300mg qd. **Week 3 and onward:** 200mg	Maintenance treatment of bipolar I disorder to delay the time to occurrence of mood episodes (depression, mania, hypomania, mixed episodes) in patients treated for mood episodes with standard therapy.

(Continued)

DRUG	BRAND	HOW SUPPLIED	USUAL DOSE	COMMENTS
CONVENTIONAL ANTIPSYCHOTIC				
Chlorpromazine HCl	Thorazine	**Cap, Extended-Release:** 30mg, 75mg, 150mg; **Inj:** 25mg/mL; **Sup:** 25mg, 100mg; **Syrup:** 10mg/5mL; **Tab:** 10mg, 50mg, 100mg, 200mg	**Adults:** Inpatient: Acute Schizophrenic/ Manic State: 25mg IM, then 25-50mg IM in 1 hr if needed. Titrate: Increase over several days up to 400mg q4-6h until controlled then switch to PO. Usual: 500mg/day PO. **Max:** 1000mg/day PO. Less acutely disturbed: 25mg PO tid. Titrate: Increase gradually to 400mg/day. Outpatient: 10mg PO tid-qid or 25mg PO bid-tid. More Severe: 25mg PO tid. Titrate: After 1-2 days, increase by 20-50mg twice weekly until calm. Prompt control of severe symptoms: 25mg IM, may repeat in 1 hr then 25-50mg PO tid.	Control manifestations of manic type of manic-depressive illness.
ATYPICAL ANTIPSYCHOTICS				
Aripiprazole	Abilify	**Tab:** 2mg, 5mg, 10mg, 15mg, 20mg, 30mg; **Tab, Disintegrating:** 10mg, 15mg, (Discmelt) 10mg, 15mg; **Sol:** 1mg/mL [50mL, 150mL, 480mL]. **Inj:** 7.5mg/mL	**Adults:** (PO) Bipolar Disorder (Monotherapy or Adjunct): Initial/Target: 15mg/day. Max: 30mg/day. (Inj) Agitation: 9.75mg IM. Range: 5.25-15mg IM. Max: 30mg/day; initiate PO therapy as soon as possible. **Pediatrics:** Bipolar Disorder (Monotherapy or Adjunct) (10-17 yrs): Initial: 2mg/day. Titrate: 5mg after 2 days. May adjust dose in 5mg/day increments. Recommended: 10mg/day. Max: 30mg/day. Periodically reassess need for maintenance therapy. Oral sol can be given on mg-per-mg basis up to 25mg. Patients receiving 30mg tabs should receive 25mg of oral sol. Concomitant Strong CYP3A4 Inhibitors (eg, ketoconazole, clarithromycin): Reduce usual aripiprazole dose by 50%. Concomitant CYP2D6 Inhibitors (eg, quinidine, fluoxetine, paroxetine): Reduce usual aripiprazole dose by 50%. Concomitant CYP3A4 Inducers (eg, carbamazepine): Double aripiprazole dose.	(PO) Acute and maintenance treatment of manic and mixed episodes associated with bipolar I disorder with or without psychotic features in adults and pediatrics aged 10-17 yrs. Adjunctive therapy to either lithium or valproate for the acute treatment of manic and mixed episodes associated with bipolar I disorder with or without psychotic features in adults and pediatrics aged 10-17 yrs. (Inj) Acute treatment of agitation associated with schizophrenia or bipolar disorder, manic or mixed, in adults.
Olanzapine	Zyprexa, Zyprexa Zydis	**Inj:** 10mg; **Tab:** 2.5mg, 5mg, 7.5mg, 10mg, 15mg, 20mg; **Tab, Disintegrating:** (Zydis) 5mg, 10mg, 15mg, 20mg	**Adults:** Bipolar Mania: Initial: 10-15mg qd. Titrate: Increase/decrease by 5mg daily. **Max:** 20mg/day. With Lithium or Valproate: Initial/Usual: 10mg qd. Max: 20mg/day. Debilitated/ Hypotension risk/slow metabolizers/ sensitivity to olanzapine effects: Initial: 5mg qd. Titrate: Increase cautiously. (IM) Agitation: Initial: 10mg IM. Usual: 2.5-10mg IM. **Max:** 3 doses of 10mg q 2-4h. Elderly: 5mg IM. Debilitated/Hypotension risk/ sensitivity to olanzapine effects: 2.5mg IM. May initiate PO therapy when clinically appropriate.	(PO) Treatment of acute mixed or manic episodes in bipolar I disorder. Short-term treatment of acute manic episodes associated with bipolar I disorder in combination with lithium or valproate. (Inj) Agitation associated with schizophrenia, bipolar I mania.
Olanzapine-fluoxetine	Symbyax	**Cap:** (Olanzapine-Fluoxetine): 6-25mg, 6-50mg, 12-25mg, 12-50mg	**Adults:** ≥18 yrs: Initial: 6-25mg cap qpm. Titrate: Adjust dose based on efficacy and tolerability. **Max:** 18mg/75mg. Hypotension risk/ hepatic impairment/metabolizers: Initial: 6-25mg cap qpm. Titrate: Increase cautiously. Re-evaluate periodically.	Treatment of depressive episodes associated with bipolar disorder.

(Continued)

DRUG	BRAND	HOW SUPPLIED	USUAL DOSE	COMMENTS
ATYPICAL ANTIPSYCHOTICS *(Continued)*				
Quetiapine	**Seroquel**	**Tab:** 25mg, 50mg, 100mg, 200mg, 300mg, 400mg	**Adults:** Bipolar Depressive Episodes: Give once daily hs. Day 1: 50mg/day. Day 2: 100mg/day. Day 3: 200mg/day. Day 4: 300mg/day. Bipolar Mania: Monotherapy/Adjunctive: Give bid. Initial: 100mg/day on Day 1. Titrate: Increase to 400mg/day on Day 4 in increments of up to 100mg/day in bid divided doses. Adjust doses up to 800mg/day by Day 6 in increments ≤200mg/day. Max: 800mg/day. Maintenance for Bipolar I Disorder: Give bid. 400-800mg/day. Hepatic Impairment: Initial: 25mg/day. Titrate: Increase by 25-50mg/day to effective dose. Elderly/Debilitated/Predisposition to Hypotension: Consider slower rate of dose titration and lower target dose.	Treatment of depressive episodes associated with bipolar disorder. Treatment of acute manic episodes associated with bipolar I disorder, as monotherapy or adjunct therapy to lithium or divalproex. Maintenance treatment of bipolar I disorder as adjunct therapy to lithium or divalproex.
Risperidone	**Risperdal**	**Sol:** 1mg/mL [30mL]; **Tab:** 0.25mg, 0.5mg, 1mg, 2mg, 3mg, 4mg; **Tab, Disintegrating:** (M-Tab) 0.5mg, 1mg, 2mg, 3mg, 4mg	**Adults:** Bipolar Mania: Initial: 2-3mg qd. Titrate: Adjust dose at intervals no <24hrs and in increments/decrements of 1mg/day. Range: 1-6mg/day. **Max:** 6mg/day. **Pediatrics:** 10-17 yrs: Bipolar Mania: Initial: 0.5mg qd in morning or evening. Titrate: Adjust dose, if needed, in increments of 0.5 or 1mg/day and at intervals not <24hrs, as tolerated, to recommended dose of 2.5mg/day. **Max:** 6mg/day. Elderly/Debilitated/Hypotension/Severe Renal or Hepatic Impairment: Initial: 0.5mg bid. Titrate: Adjust dose in increments not >0.5mg bid. Increases to doses >1.5mg bid should occur at intervals of ≥1 week. Periodically reassess to determine maintenance treatment.	Short-term treatment of acute manic or mixed episodes associated with bipolar I disorder as monotherapy (Adults and Adolescents 10-17 yrs) or in combination with lithium or valproate (Adults).
Ziprasidone	**Geodon**	**Cap:** (HCl) 20mg, 40mg, 60mg, 80mg	**Adults:** Bipolar Mania: Initial: 40mg bid with food. Titrate: Increase to 60-80mg bid on 2nd day of treatment. Maint: 40-80mg bid.	Treatment of acute manic or mixed episodes associated with bipolar disorder, with or without psychotic features.

Source: FDA approved labeling.

ASTHMA MANAGEMENT

DRUG (BRAND)	DOSAGE FORM	ADULT DOSE	CHILD DOSE*
ANTICHOLINERGIC			
Ipratropium (Atrovent HFA)	**MDI:** 0.017mg/inh [12.9g]	2 inh qid	
Tiotropium (Spiriva)	**Cap, Inhalation:** 18mcg	1 cap qd	
SYSTEMIC CORTICOSTEROIDS			
Methylprednisolone	**Tab:** 2, 4, 8, 16, 32mg	7.5-60mg qd in a single dose or qod prn for control. Short course "burst": 40-60 mg/day as single dose or 2 divided doses for 3-10 days.	0.25-2mg/kg qd in a single dose or qod prn for control. Short course "burst": 1-2mg/kg/day. **Max:** 60mg/day for 3-10 days.
Prednisolone	**Tab:** 5mg; **Liq:** 5mg/5mL, 15mg/5mL		
Prednisone	**Tab:** 1, 2.5, 5, 10, 20, 50mg **Liq:** 5mg/mL, 5mg/5mL		
CROMOLYN & NEDOCROMIL			
Cromolyn (Intal)	**MDI:** 800mcg/puff	2 puffs qid	1-2 puffs tid-qid
Nedocromil (Tilade)	**MDI:** 1.75mg/puff	2-4 puffs bid-qid	1-2 puffs bid-qid
SHORT-ACTING β₂-AGONISTS			
Albuterol	**MDI:** 0.09mg/inh; **Sol (neb):** 0.083%, 0.5%; **Syrup:** 2mg/5mL; **Tab:** 2mg*, 4mg*; **Tab, Extended-Release (Repetabs):** 4mg *scored	2 inh q4-6h or 1 inh q4h. **(Repetabs) Initial:** 4-8mg q12h. **Max:** 32mg/day. **(Sol)** 2.5mg tid-qid by nebulizer. **(Syrup, Tabs)** 2-4mg tid qid. **Max:** 32mg/day (8mg qid).	**(Syrup) Initial:** 2-4mg tid-qid. **Max:** 8mg (Aerosol) 2 inh q4-6h or 1 inh q4h. **(Sol)** 2.5mcg tid-qid by nebulizer. **(Tabs) Initial:** 2-4mg tid-qid.
Albuterol Sulfate (ProAir HFA, Proventil HFA, Ventolin HFA)	**MDI:** 90mcg/inh	2 inh q4-6h or 1 inh q4h	2 inh q4-6h or 1 inh q4h
Aformoterol (Brovana)	**Sol, Inhalation:** 15mcg/2mL	5mcg bid	
Levalbuterol (Xopenex, Xopenex HFA)	**Sol:** 0.31mg/3mL, 0.63mg/3mL, 1.25mg/3mL (HFA) 45mcg/inh	0.63mg tid, q6-8h (HFA) 2 inh (90mcg) q4-6h or 1 inh (45mcg) q4h	0.63mg tid, q6-8h (HFA) 2 inh (90mcg) q4-6h or 1 inh (45mcg) q4h
Pirbuterol (Maxair)	**Autohaler:** 0.2mg/inh; **MDI:** 0.2mg/inh [14g]	1-2 inh q4-6h	1-2 inh q4-6h
LONG-ACTING β₂-AGONISTS			
Salmeterol (Serevent)	**DPI:** 50mcg/blister	1 blister q 12 hours	1 blister q 12 hours
Formoterol (Foradil)	**DPI:** 12mcg	1 cap q 12 hours	1 cap q 12 hours
COMBINATION AGENTS			
Ipratropium/Albuterol (Combivent)	**MDI:** (Albuterol-Ipratropium) 0.09mg-0.018mg/inh [14.7g]	2 inh qid.	
Ipratropium/Albuterol (Duoneb)	**Sol, Inhalation:** (Albuterol-Ipratropium) 3mg-0.5mg/3mL	3mL qid via nebulizer	
Fluticasone/ Salmeterol (Advair)	**DPI:** 100, 250, 500mcg/50mcg	1 puff bid	(100mcg/50mcg) 1 puff bid
Fluticasone/ Salmeterol (Advair HFA)	**MDI:** (45/21) 0.045mg-0.021mg/inh, (115/21) 0.115mg-0.021mg/inh, (230/21) 0.230mg-0.021mg/inh	Initial: 2 inh of 45/21 bid or 1 inh of 115/21 bid. **Max:** 2 inh of 230/21 bid.	Initial: 2 inh of 45/21 bid or 1 inh of 115/21 bid. **Max:** 2 inh of 230-21 bid.
Budesonide/Formoterol (Symbicort)	**MDI:** (Budesonide-Formoterol) 80mcg-4.5mcg/inh, 160mcg-4.5mcg/inh [10.2g]	2 puff bid of 80/4.5 or 160/4.5 depending on asthma severity. **Max:** 640mcg/18mcg (2 puff bid of 160/4.5).	2 inh bid of 80/4.5 or 160/4.5 depending on asthma severity. **Max:** 640mcg/18mcg (2 inh of 160/4.5).

(Continued)

DRUG (BRAND)	DOSAGE FORM	ADULT DOSE	CHILD DOSE*
METHYLXANTHINE			
Theophylline	Elixir; Caps & Tabs, Extended-Release	**Initial:** 10mg/kg/day up to 300mg max. **Usual Max:** 800mg/day.	**Initial:** 10mg/kg/day. **Usual Max:** <1 yr: 0.2 x age in weeks + 5 = mg/kg/day. 1 yr: 16mg/kg/day.
LEUKOTRIENE MODIFIERS			
Montelukast (Singulair)	Tab: 10mg; Tab, Chewable: 4mg, 5mg	10mg qhs	2-5 yrs: 4mg qhs. 6-14 yrs: 5mg qhs. 15 yrs: 10mg qhs.
Zafirlukast (Accolate)	Tab: 10mg, 20mg	20mg bid	≥12 yrs: 20mg bid. 5-11 yrs: 10mg bid.
Zileuton (Zyflo)	Tab: 600mg	600mg qid	≥12 yr: 600mg qid

ESTIMATED COMPARATIVE DAILY DOSAGES FOR INHALED CORTICOSTEROIDS					
	LOW DAILY DOSE		MEDIUM DAILY DOSE		HIGH DAILY DOSE
DRUG	ADULT	CHILD*	ADULT	CHILD*	ADULT	CHILD*
Beclomethasone HFA 40, 80mcg/puff (QVAR)	80-240mcg	80-160mcg	240-480mcg	160-320mcg	>480mcg	>320mcg
Budesonide DPI 200mcg/inhalation (Pulmicort Turbuhaler)	200-600mcg	200-400mcg	600-1200mcg	400-800mcg	>1200mcg	>800mcg
Budesonide Neb Sol: 0.25, 0.5mg/2mL (Pulmicort Respules)	N/A	0.5mg	N/A	1.0mg	N/A	2mg
Flunisolide 250mcg/puff (Aerobid)	500-1000mcg	500-750mcg	1000-2000mcg	1000-1250mcg	>2000mcg	>1250mcg
Fluticasone MDI 44, 110, or 220mcg/puff (Flovent HFA)	88-264mcg	88-176mcg	264-660mcg	176-440mcg	>660mcg	>440mcg
Mometasone Twisthaler 110mcg/inh, 220mcg/inh (Asmanex)	220-440mcg	220-440mcg	N/A	N/A	>880mcg	>880mcg
Triamcinolone acetonide 100mcg/puff (Azmacort)	400-1000mcg	400-800mcg	1000-2000mcg	800-1200mcg	>2000mcg	>1200mcg

*Children ≤12 yrs unless otherwise noted. MDI: metered-dose inhaler; DPI: dry powder inhaler.
Adopted from: The NAEPP Expert Panel Report: Guidelines for the Diagnosis and Management of Asthma– Update on Selected Topics 2002. http://www.nhlbi.nih.gov/guidelines/asthma/asthsumm.htm

ASTHMA TREATMENT PLAN

CLASSIFICATION	LUNG FUNCTION	STEPWISE APPROACH TO THERAPY IN PATIENTS >12 YEARS OF AGE
Intermittent • Symptoms ≤2 days a week • Short-acting β2-agonist use for symptom control ≤2 days a week • Nighttime awakenings ≤2 times/month • Interference with normal activity - none	• Normal FEV_1 b/w exacerbations • FEV_1 ≥80% predicted • FEV_1/FVC - normal	**Step 1** • **Short-acting inhaled β2-agonists as needed (2-4 puffs prn).** • Severe exacerbations may occur, separated by long periods of normal lung function and no symptoms; a course of systemic corticosteroids is recommended.
Mild persistent • Symptoms >2 days/week but not daily • Short-acting β2-agonist use for symptom control >2days/wk but not daily, and not more than 1x on any day • Nighttime awakenings 3-4x/month • Interference with normal activity - minor limitation	• FEV_1 ≥80% predicted • FEV_1/FVC - normal	**Step 2** • **Low-dose inhaled corticosteroids.** • **Short-acting inhaled β2-agonists as needed (2-4 puffs prn).** ALTERNATIVE TREATMENT: • Cromolyn, leukotriene modifier, nedocromil OR theophylline
Moderate persistent • Daily symptoms • Short-acting β2-agonist use for symptom control daily • Nighttime awakenings >1x/wk but not nightly • Interference with normal activity - some limitation	• FEV_1 >60% but <80% predicted • FEV_1/FVC reduced 5%	**Step 3** • **Low- to medium-dose inhaled corticosteroids** AND • **Long-acting inhaled β2-agonists.** • **Short-acting inhaled β2-agonists as needed (2-4 puffs prn).** ALTERNATIVE TREATMENT: • Low-dose ICS + either LTRA, theophylline, OR Zileuton
Severe persistent • Symptoms throughout the day • Short-acting β2-agonist use for symptom several times per day • Nighttime awakenings often >7x/week • Interference with normal activity - extreme limitation	• FEV_1 ≤60% predicted • FEV_1/FVC reduced >5%	**Step 4 or Step 5** • **Medium-dose ICS + LABA OR** • **High-dose ICS + LABA** AND • Consider Omalizumab for patients who have allergies • **Short-acting inhaled β2-agonists as needed (2-4 puffs prn).** ALTERNATIVE TREATMENT: • Medium-dose ICS + either LTRA, Theophylline, OR Zileuton

Note: Preferred treatments are in bold.
Key Points:

• Stepwise approach presents general guidelines. Review treatment every 1 to 6 months; a gradual stepwise reduction in treatment may be possible. If control is not maintained, consider step up.

• The presence of one of the features of severity is sufficient to place a patient in that category. An individual should be assigned to the most severe grade in which any feature occurs (PEF is % of personal best; FEV is % predicted).

• Intensity of treatment will depend on severity of exacerbation; up to 3 treatments at 20-minute intervals or a single nebulizer treatment as needed. Course of systemic corticosteroids may be needed.

• Use of short-acting beta2-agonists >2 days/week for a symptom relief generally indicates inadequate control and the need to step up treatment

• Airflow obstruction is indicated by reduced FEV_1 and FEV_1/FVC values relative to reference or predicted values.

• Abnormalities of lung function are categorized as restrictive and obstructive defects. A reduced ratio of FEV_1/FVC (eg, <65%) indicates obstruction to the flow of air from the lungs, whereas a reduced FVC with a normal FEV_1/FVC ratio suggests a restrictive pattern.

Abbreviations: FEV_1: Forced expiratory volume in one second. FVC: Forced vital capacity.

*Adapted from the Full Report 2007 *Guidelines for the Diagnosis and Management of Asthma*. NAEPP Expert Panel Report III.

ASTHMA TREATMENT PLAN

CLASSIFICATION	LUNG FUNCTION	STEPWISE APPROACH TO THERAPY IN PATIENTS >12 YEARS OF AGE
Intermittent • Symptoms ≤2 days/week • Short-acting β-agonist use for symptom control ≤2 days a week • Nighttime awakenings ≤2 times/month • Interference with normal activity – none	• Normal FEV₁ b/w exacerbations • FEV₁ ≥80% predicted • FEV₁/FVC – normal	**Step 1** • Short-acting inhaled β₂-agonists as needed (2-4 puffs prn) • Severe exacerbations may occur, separated by long periods of normal lung function and no symptoms • A course of systemic corticosteroids is recommended
Mild persistent • Symptoms >2 days/week but not daily • Short-acting β₂-agonist use for symptom control >2 days/week but not daily, and not more than 1x on any day • Nighttime awakenings 3-4x/month • Activity – minor limitation	• FEV₁ ≥80% predicted • FEV₁/FVC – normal	**Step 2** • Low-dose inhaled corticosteroids • Short-acting inhaled β₂-agonists as needed (2-4 puffs prn) ALTERNATIVE TREATMENT • Cromolyn, leukotriene modifier, nedocromil OR theophylline
Moderate persistent • Daily symptoms • Short-acting β₂-agonist use for symptom control daily • Nighttime awakenings >1x/week but not nightly • Interference with normal activity – some limitation	• FEV₁ >60% but <80% predicted • FEV₁/FVC reduced 5%	**Step 3** • Low- to medium-dose inhaled corticosteroids AND • Long-acting inhaled β₂-agonists • Short-acting inhaled β₂-agonists as needed (2-4 puffs prn) ALTERNATIVE TREATMENT • Combinations: ICS/LABA, LTR, theophylline OR zileuton
Severe persistent • Symptoms throughout the day • Short-acting β₂-agonist use for symptom several times/day • Nighttime awakenings often • Interference with normal activity – extreme limitation	• FEV₁ <60% predicted • FEV₁/FVC reduced >5%	**Step 5 or Step 6** • Medium-dose ICS + LABA OR • High-dose ICS + LABA AND • Consider Omalizumab for patients who have allergies • Short-acting inhaled β₂-agonists as needed (2-4 puffs prn) ALTERNATIVE TREATMENT • Medium-dose ICS + either LTR, theophylline OR zileuton

Note: Preferred treatments are in bold.

Key Points:

• Stepwise therapy: Decrease dosage gradually once asthma is controlled and maintain lowest dosage that provides adequate control.

ADMINISTRATION GUIDELINES FOR METERED-DOSE INHALERS

General Guidelines

1. Remove dust cap and hold inhaler upright.

2. Shake canister well before each use.

3. Tilt head back slightly and breathe out slowly and completely.

4. For **closed mouth** technique: Place mouthpiece in mouth and close lips tightly around (not recommended for steroid inhaler). For **open mouth** technique: Hold inhaler 1 to 2 inches from open mouth (about the width of 2 fingers).

5. Inhale slowly and deeply, and press down on the inhaler to release the medication. (The slower the breath, the greater the likelihood that the drug will reach the smaller airways.) **NOTE:** If needed, a spacer or holding chamber can be used in children or elderly patients having difficulty with coordination of technique. If using a spacer, put the mouthpiece of the spacer between teeth, and into mouth. Then, close mouth around the spacer. With the device in place, actuate the inhaler once and inhale the medication immediately after actuating the aerosol.

6. Breathe in slowly and hold breath for about 10 seconds to allow the medication to go into lungs.

7. Breathe out slowly and wait about 30 seconds to 1 minute before administering second inhalation. **NOTE:** Expect relief of symptoms within 5 to 15 minutes. Seek medical attention if symptomatic relief takes longer than 20 minutes (this should occur with short-acting medications like albuterol).

8. If using a steroid inhaler, rinse mouth with water after use. **NOTE:** Spit out the water after last puff; do not swallow.

Counseling Tips:

- Rinse only the inhaler mouthpiece and cap with warm running water and air dry. Do not wash the canister or immerse in water.

- Keep the dust cap over the mouthpiece of the inhaler when not in use.

- Do not puncture the canister. The contents are under pressure.

- Store the canister at room temperature (15°C to 30°C), away from heat (>48.9°F) or open flames.

Guidelines for Specific Products

Advair Diskus Administration

1. Hold the Diskus in one hand. Then, push the thumbgrip back as far as it will go, until the mouthpiece appears and snaps into position.

2. Hold the Diskus in a level, flat position with the mouthpiece towards.

3. Slide the lever away as far as it will go until it clicks.

4. Breathe out completely while holding the Diskus level.

5. Put the mouthpiece between the lips. Breathe in quickly and deeply through the Diskus. **NOTE:** Do not breathe in through the nose.

6. Remove the Diskus from the mouth.

7. Hold breathe for about 10 seconds. Then, breathe out slowly.

8. Close the Diskus by sliding the thumbgrip back as far as it will go.

9. Rinse the mouth with water after each use and spit out. Without swallowing.

Counseling Tips:

- Never breathe into the Diskus.

- Never take the Diskus apart.

- Use the Diskus in a level, flat position.

- Do not use with a spacer device.

- Rinse mouth with water after use. **NOTE:** Spit out the water after last puff and do not swallow the water.

- Never wash the mouthpiece or any part of the Diskus.

- Keep the Diskus in a dry place, away from heat.

Source: Advair Diskus Prescribing Information, http://us.gsk.com/products/assets/us_advair.pdf.

(Continued)

Pulmicort Flexhaler Administration

Loading a dose:

1. Turn the cover and lift it off.
2. Hold the Flexhaler upright, with mouthpiece up.
3. Twist the brown grip fully in one direction as far as it will go and twist back again in the opposite direction as far as it will go.

Inhaling the dose:

1. Twist the cover and lift it off. Hold the Flexhaler upright (mouthpiece up).
2. Twist the brown grip to the right as far as it will go, then back to the left until it clicks.
3. Turn your head away from the Flexhaler and breathe out completely. **NOTE:** Do not shake the inhaler after loading it.
4. Put the mouthpiece between the lips and inhale deeply and forcefully.
5. Remove the Flexhaler from the mouth and breathe out. **NOTE:** Do not blow into the mouthpiece.
6. Replace the cover and twist shut when finished.
7. Rinse mouth with water after each use. Spit out the water after last puff and do not swallow the water.

Counseling Tips:

- A new Flexhaler needs to be primed once before its first use. No further priming is indicated, even if it has been put aside for a long time.
- Flexhaler will deliver only one dose at a time, regardless of number of times you click the brown grip. **NOTE:** The dose indicator will continue to advance.
- Do not repeat inhalations even if you do not feel the sensation of medication when inhaling.
- Do not use with a spacer device.
- Do not chew or bite on the mouthpiece.
- Do not use Flexhaler if it has been damaged or if the mouthpiece has become detached.
- Wipe the outside of the mouthpiece once a week with a tissue.
- Keep the Flexhaler in a dry place, away from heat.

Source: Pulmicort Prescribing Information.

UROLOGICAL THERAPIES

OVERACTIVE BLADDER AGENTS

DRUG	BRAND	HOW SUPPLIED	DOSING	COMMENTS
Darifenacin	Enablex	**Tab, ER:** 7.5mg, 15mg	**Initial:** 7.5mg qd. **Max:** 15mg qd.	Swallow whole. Moderate Hepatic Impairment/ Concomitant Potent CYP3A4 Inhibitors: Do not exceed 7.5mg/d. Severe Hepatic Impairment: Avoid use.
Oxybutynin	Ditropan	**Syrup:** 5mg/5mL **Tab:** 5mg	**Usual:** 5mg bid-tid. **Max:** 5mg qid.	A lower starting dose of 2.5mg bid-tid is recommended for elderly patients.
	Ditropan XL	**Tab, ER:** 5mg, 10mg, 15mg	**Initial:** 5mg or 10mg qd. **Max:** 30mg/day.	Swallow whole. Increase dose by 5mg weekly if needed.
	Oxytrol	**Patch:** 3.9mg/day	**Usual:** Apply twice weekly.	Rotate site of application.
Solifenacin	VESIcare	**Tab:** 5mg, 10mg	**Usual:** 5mg qd. **Max:** 10mg qd.	Renal (CrCl <30mL/min)/Hepatic (Child Pugh B)/Concomitant Potent CYP3A4 Inhibitors: Do not exceed 5mg/d. Hepatic (Child Pugh C): Avoid use.
Tolterodine	Detrol	**Tab:** 1mg, 2mg	**Initial:** 2mg bid.	Decrease dose to 1mg bid if needed. Significant Hepatic/Renal Dysfunction/Concomitant CYP3A4 Inhibitors: 1mg bid.
	Detrol LA	**Cap, ER:** 2mg, 4mg	**Initial:** 4mg qd.	Swallow whole. Decrease dose to 2mg qd if needed. Significant Hepatic/ Renal Dysfunction/ Concomitant CYP3A4 Inhibitors: 2mg qd.
Trospium	Sanctura	**Tab:** 20mg	**Usual:** 20mg bid.	CrCl <30mL/min: 20mg qhs. Elderly ≥75 yrs: May titrate to 20mg qd based upon tolerability.
	Sanctura XR	**Cap, ER:** 60mg	**Usual:** 60mg qd.	CrCl <30mL/min: 20mg qhs. Elderly ≥75 yrs: May titrate to 20mg qd based upon tolerability.

BENIGN PROSTATIC HYPERTROPHY AGENTS

DRUG	BRAND	HOW SUPPLIED	DOSING	COMMENTS
ALPHA-BLOCKERS				
Alfuzosin	Uroxatral	**Tab, ER:** 10mg	**Usual:** 10mg qd.	Take dose immediately after the same meal each day. Swallow whole.
Doxazosin	Cardura	**Tab:** 1mg, 2mg, 4mg, 8mg	**Initial:** 1mg qd. **Max:** 8mg/day.	Double dose every two weeks if needed.
	Cardura XL	**Tab, ER:** 4mg, 8mg	**Initial:** 4mg qd. **Max:** 8mg qd.	Take with breakfast. Swallow whole.
Tamsulosin	Flomax	**Cap:** 0.4mg	**Initial:** 0.4mg qd. **Max:** 0.8mg qd.	Take dose ½ hour after the same meal each day. Titrate after 2-4 weeks if needed. Restart at initial dose if therapy is interrupted.
Terazosin	Hytrin	**Cap:** 1mg, 2mg, 5mg, 10mg	**Initial:** 1mg qhs. **Usual:** 10mg/day. **Max:** 20mg/day.	Increase stepwise as needed. Restart at initial dose if therapy is interrupted.
5-ALPHA-REDUCTASE INHIBITORS				
Dutasteride	Avodart	**Cap:** 0.5mg	**Usual:** 0.5mg qd.	Swallow whole.
Finasteride	Proscar	**Tab:** 5mg	**Usual:** 5mg qd.	May be administered with doxazosin.

RECOMMENDED IMMUNIZATION SCHEDULE FOR PERSONS AGED 0-6 YEARS

Vaccine ▼ Age ▶	Birth	1 month	2 months	4 months	6 months	12 months	15 months	18 months	19–23 months	2–3 years	4–6 years
Hepatitis B[1]	HepB	HepB		see footnote 1		HepB					
Rotavirus[2]			Rota	Rota	Rota						
Diphtheria, Tetanus, Pertussis[3]			DTaP	DTaP	DTaP	see footnote 3	DTaP				DTaP
Haemophilus influenzae type b[4]			Hib	Hib	Hib[4]	Hib					
Pneumococcal[5]			PCV	PCV	PCV	PCV				PPV	
Inactivated Poliovirus			IPV	IPV		IPV					IPV
Influenza[6]						Influenza (Yearly)					
Measles, Mumps, Rubella[7]						MMR					MMR
Varicella[8]						Varicella					Varicella
Hepatitis A[9]						HepA (2 doses)				HepA Series	
Meningococcal[10]										MCV4	

Range of recommended ages   Certain high-risk groups

This schedule indicates the recommended ages for routine administration of currently licensed childhood vaccines, as of December 1, 2007, for children aged 0 through 6 years. Additional information is available at www.cdc.gov/vaccines/recs/schedules. Any dose not administered at the recommended age should be administered at any subsequent visit, when indicated and feasible. Additional vaccines may be licensed and recommended during the year. Licensed combination vaccines may be used whenever any components of the combination are indicated and other components of the vaccine are not contraindicated and if approved by the Food and Drug Administration for that dose of the series. Providers should consult the respective Advisory Committee on Immunization Practices statement for detailed recommendations, including for **high-risk conditions: http://www.cdc.gov/pubs/ACIP-list.htm**. Clinically significant adverse events that follow immunization should be reported to the Vaccine Adverse Event Reporting System (VAERS). Guidance about how to obtain and complete a VAERS form is available at **http://www.vaers.hhs.gov** or by telephone, **800-822-7967**.

1. **Hepatitis B vaccine (HepB).** *(Minimum age: birth)*
   At birth:
   - Administer monovalent HepB to all newborns prior to hospital discharge.
   - If mother is hepatitis B surface antigen (HBsAg) positive, administer HepB and 0.5 mL of hepatitis B immune globulin (HBIG) within 12 hours of birth.
   - If mother's HBsAg status is unknown, administer HepB within 12 hours of birth. Determine the HBsAg status as soon as possible and if HBsAg positive, administer HBIG (no later than age 1 week).
   - If mother is HBsAg negative, the birth dose can be delayed, in rare cases, with a provider's order and a copy of the mother's negative HBsAg laboratory report in the infant's medical record.

   After the birth dose:
   - The HepB series should be completed with either monovalent HepB or a combination vaccine containing HepB. The second dose should be administered at age 1–2 months. The final dose should be administered no earlier than age 24 weeks. Infants born to HBsAg-positive mothers should be tested for HBsAg and antibody to HBsAg after completion of at least 3 doses of a licensed HepB series, at age 9–18 months (generally at the next well-child visit).

   4-month dose:
   - It is permissible to administer 4 doses of HepB when combination vaccines are administered after the birth dose. If monovalent HepB is used for doses after the birth dose, a dose at age 4 months is not needed.

2. **Rotavirus vaccine (Rota).** *(Minimum age: 6 weeks)*
   - Administer the first dose at age 6–12 weeks.
   - Do not start the series later than age 12 weeks.
   - Administer the final dose in the series by age 32 weeks. Do not administer any dose later than age 32 weeks.
   - Data on safety and efficacy outside of these age ranges are insufficient.

3. **Diphtheria and tetanus toxoids and acellular pertussis vaccine (DTaP).** *(Minimum age: 6 weeks)*
   - The fourth dose of DTaP may be administered as early as age 12 months, provided 6 months have elapsed since the third dose.
   - Administer the final dose in the series at age 4–6 years.

4. **Haemophilus influenzae type b conjugate vaccine (Hib).** *(Minimum age: 6 weeks)*
   - If PRP-OMP (PedvaxHIB® or ComVax® [Merck]) is administered at ages 2 and 4 months, a dose at age 6 months is not required.
   - TriHIBit® (DTaP/Hib) combination products should not be used for primary immunization but can be used as boosters following any Hib vaccine in children age 12 months or older.

(Continued)

5. **Pneumococcal vaccine.** *(Minimum age: 6 weeks for pneumococcal conjugate vaccine [PCV]; 2 years for pneumococcal polysaccharide vaccine [PPV])*

   • Administer one dose of PCV to all healthy children aged 24–59 months having any incomplete schedule.

   • Administer PPV to children aged 2 years and older with underlying medical conditions.

6. **Influenza vaccine.** *(Minimum age: 6 months for trivalent inactivated influenza vaccine [TIV]; 2 years for live, attenuated influenza vaccine [LAIV])*

   • Administer annually to children aged 6–59 months and to all eligible close contacts of children aged 0–59 months.

   • Administer annually to children 5 years of age and older with certain risk factors, to other persons (including household members) in close contact with persons in groups at higher risk, and to any child whose parents request vaccination.

   • For healthy persons (those who do not have under-lying medical conditions that predispose them to influenza complications) ages 2–49 years, either LAIV or TIV may be used.

   • Children receiving TIV should receive 0.25 mL if age 6–35 months or 0.5 mL if age 3 years or older.

   • Administer 2 doses (separated by 4 weeks or longer) to children younger than 9 years who are receiving influenza vaccine for the first time or who were vaccinated for the first time last season but only received one dose.

7. **Measles, mumps, and rubella vaccine (MMR).** *(Minimum age: 12 months)*

   • Administer the second dose of MMR at age 4–6 years. MMR may be administered before age 4–6 years, provided 4 weeks or more have elapsed since the first dose.

8. **Varicella vaccine.** *(Minimum age: 12 months)*

   • Administer second dose at age 4–6 years; may be administered 3 months or more after first dose.

   • Do not repeat second dose if administered 28 days or more after first dose.

9. **Hepatitis A vaccine (HepA).** *(Minimum age: 12 months)*

   • Administer to all children aged 1 year (i.e., aged 12–23 months). Administer the 2 doses in the series at least 6 months apart.

   • Children not fully vaccinated by age 2 years can be vaccinated at subsequent visits.

   • HepA is recommended for certain other groups of children, including in areas where vaccination programs target older children.

10. **Meningococcal vaccine.** *(Minimum age: 2 years for meningococcal conjugate vaccine (MCV4) and for meningococcal polysaccharide vaccine (MPSV4))*

   • Administer MCV4 to children aged 2–10 years with terminal complement deficiencies or anatomic or functional asplenia and certain other high-risk groups. MPSV4 is also acceptable.

   • Administer MCV4 to persons who received MPSV4 3 or more years previously and remain at increased risk for meningococcal disease.

The Recommended Immunization Schedules for Persons Aged 0–18 Years are approved by the Advisory Committee on Immunization Practices **(http://www.cdc.gov/vaccines/recs/acip)**, the American Academy of Pediatrics **(http://www.aap.org)**, and the American Academy of Family Physicians **(http://www.aafp.org)**.

RECOMMENDED IMMUNIZATION SCHEDULE FOR PERSONS AGED 7-18 YEARS

Vaccine ▼ Age ►	7–10 years	11–12 years	13–18 years
Diphtheria, Tetanus, Pertussis[1]	see footnote 1	Tdap	Tdap
Human Papillomavirus[2]	see footnote 2	HPV (3 doses)	HPV Series
Meningococcal[3]	MCV4	MCV4	MCV4
Pneumococcal[4]	PPV		
Influenza[5]	Influenza (Yearly)		
Hepatitis A[6]	HepA Series		
Hepatitis B[7]	HepB Series		
Inactivated Poliovirus[8]	IPV Series		
Measles, Mumps, Rubella[9]	MMR Series		
Varicella[10]	Varicella Series		

☐ Range of recommended ages   ☐ Catch-up immunization   ☐ Certain high-risk groups

This schedule indicates the recommended ages for routine administration of currently licensed childhood vaccines, as of December 1, 2007, for children aged 7–18 years. Additional information is available at **www.cdc.gov/ vaccines/recs/schedules**. Any dose not administered at the recommended age should be administered at any subsequent visit, when indicated and feasible. Additional vaccines may be licensed and recommended during the year. Licensed combination vaccines may be used whenever any components of the combination are indicated and other components of the vaccine are not contraindicated and if approved by the Food and Drug Administration for that dose of the series. Providers should consult the respective Advisory Committee on Immunization Practices statement for detailed recommendations, including for high risk conditions: **http://www.cdc.gov/vaccines/pubs/ ACIP-list.htm**. Clinically significant adverse events that follow immunization should be reported to the Vaccine Adverse Event Reporting System (VAERS). Guidance about how to obtain and complete a VAERS form is available at **www.vaers.hhs.gov** or by telephone, **800-822-7967**.

1. **Tetanus and diphtheria toxoids and acellular pertussis vaccine (Tdap).** *(Minimum age: 10 years for BOOSTRIX® and 11 years for ADACEL™)*

   - Administer at age 11–12 years for those who have completed the recommended childhood DTP/DTaP vaccination series and have not received a tetanus and diphtheria toxoids (Td) booster dose.
   - 13–18-year-olds who missed the 11–12 year Tdap or received Td only are encouraged to receive one dose of Tdap 5 years after the last Td/DTaP dose.

2. **Human papillomavirus vaccine (HPV).** *(Minimum age: 9 years)*

   - Administer the first dose of the HPV vaccine series to females at age 11–12 years.
   - Administer the second dose 2 months after the first dose and the third dose 6 months after the first dose.
   - Administer the HPV vaccine series to females at age 13–18 years if not previously vaccinated.

3. **Meningococcal vaccine.**

   - Administer MCV4 at age 11–12 years and at age 13–18 years if not previously vaccinated. MPSV4 is an acceptable alternative.
   - Administer MCV4 to previously unvaccinated college freshmen living in dormitories.
   - MCV4 is recommended for children aged 2–10 years with terminal complement deficiencies or anatomic or functional asplenia and certain other high-risk groups.

   - Persons who received MPSV 3 or more years previously and remain at increased risk for meningococcal disease should be vaccinated with MCV4.

4. **Pneumococcal polysaccharide vaccine (PPV).**

   - Administer PPV to certain high-risk groups.

5. **Influenza vaccine.**

   - Administer annually to all close contacts of children aged 0–59 months.
   - Administer annually to persons with certain risk factors, health-care workers, and other persons (including household members) in close contact with persons in groups at higher risk.
   - Administer 2 doses (separated by 4 weeks or longer) to children younger than 9 years who are receiving influenza vaccine for the first time or who were vaccinated for the first time last season but only received one dose.
   - For healthy nonpregnant persons (those who do not have underlying medical conditions that predispose them to influenza complications) ages 2–49 years, either LAIV or TIV may be used.

6. **Hepatitis A vaccine (HepA).**

   - Administer the 2 doses in the series at least 6 months apart.
   - HepA is recommended for certain other groups of children, including in areas where vaccination programs target older children.

(Continued)

7. Hepatitis B vaccine (HepB).

- Administer the 3-dose series to those who were not previously vaccinated.
- A 2-dose series of Recombivax HB® is licensed for children aged 11–15 years.

8. Inactivated poliovirus vaccine (IPV).

- For children who received an all-IPV or all-oral poliovirus (OPV) series, a fourth dose is not necessary if the third dose was administered at age 4 years or older.
- If both OPV and IPV were administered as part of a series, a total of 4 doses should be administered, regardless of the child's current age.

9. Measles, mumps, and rubella vaccine (MMR).

- If not previously vaccinated, administer 2 doses of MMR during any visit, with 4 or more weeks between the doses.

10. Varicella vaccine.

- Administer 2 doses of varicella vaccine to persons younger than 13 years of age at least 3 months apart. Do not repeat the second dose if administered 28 or more days following the first dose.
- Administer 2 doses of varicella vaccine to persons aged 13 years or older at least 4 weeks apart.

The Recommended Immunization Schedules for Persons Aged 0–18 Years are approved by the Advisory Committee on Immunization Practices **(http://www.cdc.gov/)**, the American Academy of Pediatrics **(http://www.aap.org)**, and the American Academy of Family Physicians **(http://www.aafp.org)**.

CATCH-UP IMMUNIZATION SCHEDULE FOR PERSONS AGED 4 MONTHS-18 YEARS WHO START LATE OR WHO ARE MORE THAN 1 MONTH BEHIND

Vaccine	Minimum Age for Dose 1	Dose 1 to Dose 2	Dose 2 to Dose 3	Dose 3 to Dose 4	Dose 4 to Dose 5
CATCH-UP SCHEDULE FOR PERSONS AGED 4 MONTHS–6 YEARS		**Minimum Interval Between Doses**			
Hepatitis B[1]	Birth	4 weeks	8 weeks (and 16 weeks after first dose)		
Rotavirus[2]	6 wks	4 weeks	4 weeks		
Diphtheria, Tetanus, Pertussis[3]	6 wks	4 weeks	4 weeks	6 months	6 months[3]
Haemophilus influenzae type b[4]	6 wks	4 weeks if first dose administered at younger than 12 months of age; 8 weeks (as final dose) if first dose administered at age 12-14 months; No further doses needed if first dose administered at 15 months of age or older	4 weeks[4] if current age is younger than 12 months; 8 weeks (as final dose)[4] if current age is 12 months or older and second dose administered at younger than 15 months of age; No further doses needed if previous dose administered at age 15 months or older	8 weeks (as final dose) This dose only necessary for children aged 12 months-5 years who received 3 doses before age 12 months	
Pneumococcal[5]	6 wks	4 weeks if first dose administered at younger than 12 months of age; 8 weeks (as final dose) if first dose administered at age 12 months or older or current age 24-59 months; No further doses needed for healthy children if first dose administered at age 24 months or older	4 weeks if current age is younger than 12 months; 8 weeks (as final dose) if current age is 12 months or older; No further doses needed for healthy children if previous dose administered at age 24 months or older	8 weeks (as final dose) This dose only necessary for children aged 12 months-5 years who received 3 doses before age 12 months	
Inactivated Poliovirus[6]	6 wks	4 weeks	4 weeks	4 weeks[6]	
Measles, Mumps, Rubella[7]	12 mos	4 weeks			
Varicella[8]	12 mos	3 months			
Hepatitis A[9]	12 mos	6 months			
CATCH-UP SCHEDULE FOR PERSONS AGED 7–18 YEARS					
Tetanus, Diphtheria/ Tetanus, Diphtheria, Pertussis[10]	7 yrs[10]	4 weeks	4 weeks if first dose administered at younger than 12 months of age; 6 months if first dose administered at age 12 months or older	6 months if first dose administered at younger than 12 months of age	
Human Papillomavirus[11]	9 yrs	4 weeks	12 weeks (and 24 weeks after the first dose)		
Hepatitis A[9]	12 mos	6 months			
Hepatitis B[1]	Birth	4 weeks	8 weeks (and 16 weeks after first dose)		
Inactivated Poliovirus[6]	6 wks	4 weeks	4 weeks	4 weeks[6]	
Measles, Mumps, Rubella[7]	12 mos	4 weeks			
Varicella[8]	12 mos	4 weeks if first dose administered at age 13 years or older; 3 months if first dose administered at younger than 13 years of age			

The table above provides catch-up schedules and minimum intervals between doses for children whose vaccinations have been delayed. A vaccine series does not need to be restarted, regardless of the time that has elapsed between doses. Use the section appropriate for the child's age.

---

1. Hepatitis B vaccine (HepB).

- Administer the 3-dose series to those who were not previously vaccinated.
- A 2-dose series of Recombivax HB® is licensed for children aged 11–15 years.

2. Rotavirus vaccine (Rota).

- Do not start the series later than age 12 weeks.
- Administer the final dose in the series by age 32 weeks.
- Do not administer a dose later than age 32 weeks.
- Data on safety and efficacy outside of these age ranges are insufficient.

3. Diphtheria and tetanus toxoids and acellular pertussis vaccine (DTaP).

- The fifth dose is not necessary if the fourth dose was administered at age 4 years or older.
- DTaP is not indicated for persons aged 7 years or older.

4. Haemophilus influenzae type b conjugate vaccine (Hib).

- Vaccine is not generally recommended for children aged 5 years or older.
- If current age is younger than 12 months and the first 2 doses were PRP-OMP (PedvaxHIB® or ComVax® [Merck]), the third (and final) dose should be administered at age 12–15 months and at least 8 weeks after the second dose.
- If first dose was administered at age 7–11 months, administer 2 doses separated by 4 weeks plus a booster at age 12–15 months.

5. Pneumococcal conjugate vaccine (PCV).

- Administer one dose of PCV to all healthy children aged 24–59 months having any incomplete schedule.
- For children with underlying medical conditions, administer 2 doses of PCV at least 8 weeks apart if previously received less than 3 doses, or 1 dose of PCV if previously received 3 doses.

(Continued)

6. Inactivated poliovirus vaccine (IPV).

- For children who received an all-IPV or all-oral poliovirus (OPV) series, a fourth dose is not necessary if third dose was administered at age 4 years or older.
- If both OPV and IPV were administered as part of a series, a total of 4 doses should be administered, regardless of the child's current age.
- IPV is not routinely recommended for persons aged 18 years and older.

7. Measles, mumps, and rubella vaccine (MMR).

- The second dose of MMR is recommended routinely at age 4–6 years but may be administered earlier if desired.
- If not previously vaccinated, administer 2 doses of MMR during any visit with 4 or more weeks between the doses.

8. Varicella vaccine.

- The second dose of varicella vaccine is recommended routinely at age 4–6 years but may be administered earlier if desired.
- Do not repeat the second dose in persons younger than 13 years of age if administered 28 or more days after the first dose.

9. Hepatitis A vaccine (HepA).

- HepA is recommended for certain groups of children, including in areas where vaccination programs target older children. See *MMWR* 2006;55 (No. RR-7):1–23.

10. Tetanus and diphtheria toxoids vaccine (Td) and tetanus and diphtheria toxoids and acellular pertussis vaccine (Tdap).

- Tdap should be substituted for a single dose of Td in the primary catch-up series or as a booster if age appropriate; use Td for other doses.
- A 5-year interval from the last Td dose is encouraged when Tdap is used as a booster dose. A booster (fourth) dose is needed if any of the previous doses were administered at younger than 12 months of age. Refer to ACIP recommendations for further information. See *MMWR* 2006;55(No. RR-3).

11. Human papillomavirus vaccine (HPV).

- Administer the HPV vaccine series to females at age 13–18 years if not previously vaccinated.

Information about reporting reactions after immunization is available online at **http://www.vaers.hhs.gov** or by telephone via the 24-hour national toll-free information line 800-822-7967. Suspected cases of vaccine-preventable diseases should be reported to the state or local health department. Additional information, including precautions and contraindications for immunization, is available from the National Center for Immunization and Respiratory Diseases at **http://www.cdc.gov/vaccines** or telephone, **800-CDC-INFO (800-232-4636).**

RECOMMENDED ADULT IMMUNIZATION SCHEDULE, BY VACCINE AND AGE GROUP

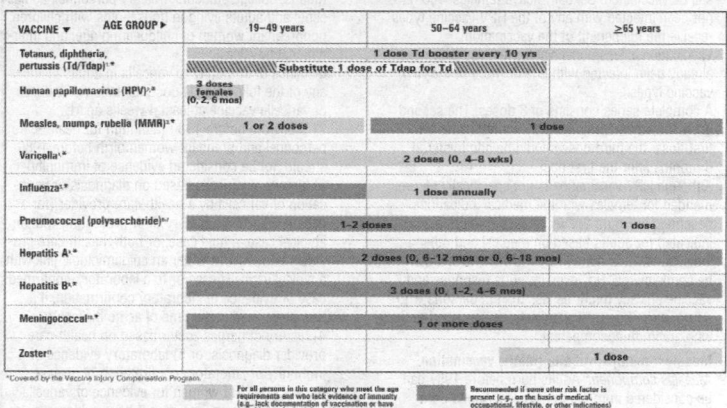

VACCINE ▼ AGE GROUP ▶	19–49 years	50–64 years	≥65 years
Tetanus, diphtheria, pertussis (Td/Tdap)¹·*	1 dose Td booster every 10 yrs		
	Substitute 1 dose of Tdap for Td		
Human papillomavirus (HPV)²·*	3 doses females (0, 2, 6 mos)		
Measles, mumps, rubella (MMR)³·*	1 or 2 doses	1 dose	
Varicella⁴·*	2 doses (0, 4–8 wks)		
Influenza⁵·*	1 dose annually		
Pneumococcal (polysaccharide)⁶·⁷	1–2 doses		1 dose
Hepatitis A⁸·*	2 doses (0, 6–12 mos or 0, 6–18 mos)		
Hepatitis B⁹·*	3 doses (0, 1–2, 4–6 mos)		
Meningococcal¹⁰·*	1 or more doses		
Zoster¹¹		1 dose	

*Covered by the Vaccine Injury Compensation Program.

For all persons in this category who meet the age requirements and who lack evidence of immunity (e.g., lack documentation of vaccination or have no evidence of prior infection)

Recommended if some other risk factor is present (e.g., on the basis of medical, occupational, lifestyle, or other indications)

Report all clinically significant postvaccination reactions to the Vaccine Adverse Event Reporting System (VAERS). Reporting forms and instructions on filing a VAERS report are available at **www.vaers.hhs.gov** or by telephone, 800-822-7967.

Information on how to file a Vaccine Injury Compensation Program claim is available at **www.hrsa.gov/vaccine compensation** or by telephone, 800-338-2382. To file a claim for vaccine injury, contact the U.S. Court of Federal Claims, 717 Madison Place, N.W., Washington, D.C. 20005; telephone, 202-357-6400.

Additional information about the vaccines in this schedule, extent of available data, and contraindications for vaccination is also available at **www.cdc.gov/vaccines** or from the CDC-INFO Contact Center at 800-CDC-INFO (800-232-4636) in English and Spanish, 24 hours a day, 7 days a week.

Use of trade names and commercial sources is for identification only and does not imply endorsement by the U.S. Department of Health and Human Services.

This schedule indicates the recommended age groups for which administration of currently licensed vaccines is commonly indicated for adults ages 19 years and older, as of October 1, 2007. Licensed combination vaccines may be used whenever any components of the combination are indicated and when the vaccine's other components are not contraindicated. For detailed recommendations on all vaccines, including those used primarily for travelers or that are issued during the year, consult the manufacturers' package inserts and the complete statements from the Advisory Committee on Immunization Practices (**www.cdc.gov/vaccines/pubs/acip-list.htm**).

1. **Tetanus, diphtheria, and acellular pertussis (Td/Tdap) vaccination.** Tdap should replace a single dose of Td for adults aged <65 years who have not previously received a dose of Tdap. Only one of two Tdap products (Adacel® [sanofi pasteur]) is licensed for use in adults.

   Adults with uncertain histories of a complete primary vaccination series with tetanus and diphtheria toxoid–containing vaccines should begin or complete a primary vaccination series. A primary series for adults is 3 doses of tetanus and diphtheria toxoid–containing vaccines; administer the first 2 doses at least 4 weeks apart and the third dose 6–12 months after the second. However, Td can substitute for any one of the doses of Td in the 3-dose primary series. The booster dose of tetanus and diphtheria toxoid–containing vaccine should be administered to adults who have completed a primary series and if the last vaccination was received ≥10 years previously. Tdap or Td vaccine may be used, as indicated.

   If the person is pregnant and received the last Td vaccination ≥10 years previously, administer Td during the second or third trimester; if the person received the last Td vaccination in <10 years, administer Tdap during the immediate postpartum period. A one-time administration of 1 dose of Tdap with an interval as short as 2 years from a previous Td vaccination is recommended for postpartum women, close contacts of infants aged <12 months, and all health-care workers with direct patient contact. In certain situations, Td can be deferred during pregnancy and Tdap substituted in the immediate postpartum period, or Tdap can be administered instead of Td to a pregnant woman after an informed discussion with the woman. Consult the ACIP statement for recommendations for administering Td as prophylaxis in wound management.

2. **Human papillomavirus (HPV) vaccination.** HPV vaccination is recommended for all females aged ≤26 years who have not completed the vaccine series. History of genital warts, abnormal Papanicolaou test, or positive HPV DNA test is not evidence of prior infection with all vaccine HPV types; HPV vaccination is still recommended for these persons.

(Continued)

Ideally, vaccine should be administered before potential exposure to HPV through sexual activity; however, females who are sexually active should still be vaccinated. Sexually active females who have not been infected with any of the HPV vaccine types receive the full benefit of the vaccination. Vaccination is less beneficial for females who have already been infected with one or more of the HPV vaccine types.

A complete series consists of 3 doses. The second dose should be administered 2 months after the first dose; the third dose should be administered 6 months after the first dose.

Although HPV vaccination is not specifically recommended for females with the medical indications described in Figure 2, "Vaccines that might be indicated for adults based on medical and other indications," it is not a live-virus vaccine and can be administered. However, immune response and vaccine efficacy might be less than in persons who do not have the medical indications described or who are immunocompetent.

3. **Measles, mumps, rubella (MMR) vaccination.**
Measles component: Adults born before 1957 can be considered immune to measles. Adults born during or after 1957 should receive ≥1 dose of MMR unless they have a medical contraindication, documentation of ≥1 dose, history of measles based on health-care provider diagnosis, or laboratory evidence of immunity.

A second dose of MMR is recommended for adults who 1) have been recently exposed to measles or are in an outbreak setting; 2) have been previously vaccinated with killed measles vaccine; 3) have been vaccinated with an unknown type of measles vaccine during 1963–1967; 4) are students in postsecondary educational institutions; 5) work in a health-care facility; or 6) plan to travel internationally.
Mumps component: Adults born before 1957 can generally be considered immune to mumps. Adults born during or after 1957 should receive 1 dose of MMR unless they have a medical contraindication, history of mumps based on health-care provider diagnosis, or laboratory evidence of immunity.

A second dose of MMR is recommended for adults who 1) are in an age group that is affected during a mumps outbreak; 2) are students in postsecondary educational institutions; 3) work in a health-care facility; or 4) plan to travel internationally. For unvaccinated health-care workers born before 1957 who do not have other evidence of mumps immunity, consider administering 1 dose on a routine basis and strongly consider administering a second dose during an outbreak.
Rubella component: Administer 1 dose of MMR vaccine to women whose rubella vaccination history is unreliable or who lack laboratory evidence of immunity. For women of childbearing age, regardless of birth year, routinely determine rubella immunity and counsel women regarding congenital rubella syndrome. Women who do not have evidence of immunity should receive MMR vaccine upon completion or termination of pregnancy and before discharge from the health-care facility.

4. **Varicella vaccination.** All adults without evidence of immunity to varicella should receive 2 doses of single-antigen varicella vaccine unless they have a medical contraindication. Special consideration should be given to those who 1) have close contact with persons at high risk for severe disease (e.g., health-care personnel and family contacts of immunocompromised persons) or 2) are at high risk for exposure or transmission (e.g., teachers; child care employees; residents and staff members of institutional settings, including correctional institutions; college students; military personnel; adolescents and adults living in households with children; nonpregnant women of childbearing age; and international travelers).

Evidence of immunity to varicella in adults includes any of the following: 1) documentation of 2 doses of varicella vaccine at least 4 weeks apart; 2) U.S.-born before 1980 (although for health-care personnel and pregnant women birth before 1980 should not be considered evidence of immunity); 3) history of varicella based on diagnosis or verification of varicella by a health-care provider (for a patient reporting a history of or presenting with an atypical case, a mild case, or both, health-care providers should seek either an epidemiologic link with a typical varicella case or to a laboratory-confirmed case or evidence of laboratory confirmation, if it was performed at the time of acute disease); 4) history of herpes zoster based on health-care provider diagnosis; or 5) laboratory evidence of immunity or laboratory confirmation of disease. Assess pregnant women for evidence of varicella immunity. Women who do not have evidence of immunity should receive the first dose of varicella vaccine upon completion or termination of pregnancy and before discharge from the health-care facility. The second dose should be administered 4–8 weeks after the first dose.

5. **Influenza vaccination.** *Medical indications:* Chronic disorders of the cardiovascular or pulmonary systems, including asthma; chronic metabolic diseases, including diabetes mellitus, renal or hepatic dysfunction, hemoglobinopathies, or immunosuppression (including immunosuppression caused by medications or human immunodeficiency virus [HIV]); any condition that compromises respiratory function or the handling of respiratory secretions or that can increase the risk of aspiration (e.g., cognitive dysfunction, spinal cord injury, or seizure disorder or other neuromuscular disorder); and pregnancy during the influenza season. No data exist on the risk for severe or complicated influenza disease among persons with asplenia; however, influenza is a risk factor for secondary bacterial infections that can cause severe disease among persons with asplenia.
Occupational indications: Health-care personnel and employees of long-term care and assisted-living facilities.
Other indications: Residents of nursing homes and other long-term care and assisted-living facilities; persons likely to transmit influenza to persons at high risk (e.g., in-home household contacts and caregivers of children aged 0–59 months, or persons of all ages with high-risk conditions); and anyone who would like to be vaccinated. Healthy, nonpregnant adults aged ≤49 years without high-risk medical conditions who are not contacts of severely immunocompromised persons in special care units can receive either intranasally administered live, attenuated influenza vaccine (FluMist®) or inactivated vaccine. Other persons should receive the inactivated vaccine.

6. **Pneumococcal polysaccharide vaccination.**
Medical indications: Chronic pulmonary disease (excluding asthma); chronic cardiovascular diseases; diabetes mellitus; chronic liver diseases, including liver disease as a result of alcohol abuse (e.g., cirrhosis); chronic alcoholism, chronic renal

(Continued)

failure or nephrotic syndrome; functional or anatomic asplenia (e.g., sickle cell disease or splenectomy [if elective splenectomy is planned, vaccinate at least 2 weeks before surgery]); immunosuppressive conditions; and cochlear implants and cerebrospinal fluid leaks. Vaccinate as close to HIV diagnosis as possible.

Other indications: Alaska Natives and certain American Indian populations and residents of nursing homes or other long-term care facilities.

7. **Revaccination with pneumococcal polysaccharide vaccine.** One-time revaccination after 5 years for persons with chronic renal failure or nephrotic syndrome; functional or anatomic asplenia (e.g., sickle cell disease or splenectomy); or immunosuppressive conditions. For persons aged ≥65 years, one-time revaccination if they were vaccinated ≥5 years previously and were aged <65 years at the time of primary vaccination.

8. **Hepatitis A vaccination.** *Medical indications:* Persons with chronic liver disease and persons who receive clotting factor concentrates.

Behavioral indications: Men who have sex with men and persons who use illegal drugs.

Occupational indications: Persons working with hepatitis A virus (HAV)–infected primates or with HAV in a research laboratory setting.

Other indications: Persons traveling to or working in countries that have high or intermediate endemicity of hepatitis A (a list of countries is available at **wwww.cdc.gov/travel/contentdiseases.aspx**) and any person seeking protection from HAV infection. Single-antigen vaccine formulations should be administered in a 2-dose schedule at either 0 and 6–12 months (Havrix®), or 0 and 6–18 months (Vaqta®). If the combined hepatitis A and hepatitis B vaccine (Twinrix®) is used, administer 3 doses at 0, 1, and 6 months.

9. **Hepatitis B vaccination.** *Medical indications:* Persons with end-stage renal disease, including patients receiving hemodialysis; persons seeking evaluation or treatment for a sexually transmitted disease (STD); persons with HIV infection; and persons with chronic liver disease.

Occupational indications: Health-care personnel and public-safety workers who are exposed to blood or other potentially infectious body fluids.

Behavioral indications: Sexually active persons who are not in a long-term, mutually monogamous relationship (e.g., persons with more than 1 sex partner during the previous 6 months); current or recent injection-drug users; and men who have sex with men.

Other indications: Household contacts and sex partners of persons with chronic hepatitis B virus (HBV) infection; clients and staff members of institutions for persons with developmental disabilities; international travelers to countries with high or intermediate prevalence of chronic HBV infection (a list of countries is available at **www.cdc.gov/travel/contentdiseases.aspx**); and any adult seeking protection from HBV infection.

Settings where hepatitis B vaccination is recommended for all adults: STD treatment facilities; HIV testing and treatment facilities; facilities providing drug-abuse treatment and prevention services; health-care settings targeting services to injection-drug users or men who have sex with men; correctional facilities; end-stage renal disease programs and facilities for chronic hemodialysis patients; and institutions and nonresidential daycare facilities for persons with developmental disabilities.

Special formulation indications: For adult patients receiving hemodialysis and other immunocompromised adults, 1 dose of 40 µg/mL (Recombivax HB®), or 2 doses of 20 µg/mL (Engerix-B®) administered simultaneously.

10. **Meningococcal vaccination.** *Medical indications:* Adults with anatomic or functional asplenia, or terminal complement component deficiencies.

Other indications: First-year college students living in dormitories; microbiologists who are routinely exposed to isolates of Neisseria meningitidis; military recruits; and persons who travel to or live in countries in which meningococcal disease is hyperendemic or epidemic (e.g., the "meningitis belt" of sub-Saharan Africa during the dry season [December–June]), particularly if their contact with local populations will be prolonged. Vaccination is required by the government of Saudi Arabia for all travelers to Mecca during the annual Hajj. Meningococcal conjugate vaccine is preferred for adults with any of the preceding indications who are aged ≤55 years, although meningococcal polysaccharide vaccine (MPSV4) is an acceptable alternative. Revaccination after 3–5 years might be indicated for adults previously vaccinated with MPSV4 who remain at increased risk for infection (e.g., persons residing in areas in which disease is epidemic).

11. **Herpes zoster vaccination.** A single dose of zoster vaccine is recommended for adults aged ≥60 years regardless of whether they report a prior episode of herpes zoster. Persons with chronic medical conditions may be vaccinated unless a contraindication or precaution exists for their condition.

12. **Selected conditions for which *Haemophilus influenzae* type b (Hib) vaccine may be used.** Hib conjugate vaccines are licensed for children aged 6 weeks–71 months. No efficacy data are available on which to base a recommendation concerning use of Hib vaccine for older children and adults with the chronic conditions associated with an increased risk for Hib disease. However, studies suggest good immunogenicity in patients who have sickle cell disease, leukemia, or HIV infection or who have had splenectomies; administering vaccine to these patients is not contraindicated.

13. **Immunocompromising conditions.** Inactivated vaccines are generally acceptable (e.g., pneumococcal, meningococcal, and influenza [trivalent inactivated influenza vaccine]), and live vaccines generally are avoided in persons with immune deficiencies or immune suppressive conditions. Information on specific conditions is available at **www.cdc.gov/vaccines/pubs/acip-list.htm**.

RECOMMENDED ADULT IMMUNIZATION SCHEDULE, BY VACCINE AND MEDICAL AND OTHER INDICATIONS

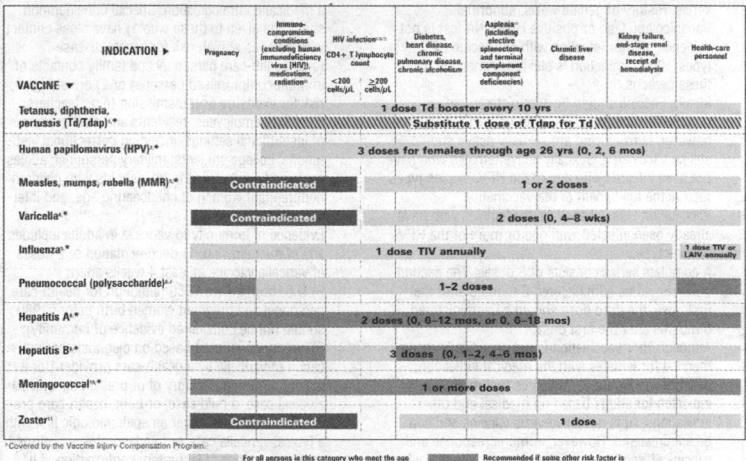

INDICATION ▶ VACCINE ▼	Pregnancy	Immuno-compromising conditions (excluding human immunodeficiency virus [HIV], medications, radiation)	HIV infection CD4+ T lymphocyte count < 200 cells/µL	HIV infection CD4+ T lymphocyte count ≥ 200 cells/µL	Diabetes, heart disease, chronic pulmonary disease, chronic alcoholism	Asplenia (including elective splenectomy and terminal complement component deficiencies)	Chronic liver disease	Kidney failure, end-stage renal disease, receipt of hemodialysis	Health-care personnel
Tetanus, diphtheria, pertussis (Td/Tdap)		1 dose Td booster every 10 yrs							
		Substitute 1 dose of Tdap for Td							
Human papillomavirus (HPV)		3 doses for females through age 26 yrs (0, 2, 6 mos)							
Measles, mumps, rubella (MMR)	Contraindicated				1 or 2 doses				
Varicella	Contraindicated				2 doses (0, 4–8 wks)				
Influenza		1 dose TIV annually							1 dose TIV or LAIV annually
Pneumococcal (polysaccharide)		1–2 doses							
Hepatitis A		2 doses (0, 6–12 mos, or 0, 6–18 mos)							
Hepatitis B		3 doses (0, 1–2, 4–6 mos)							
Meningococcal		1 or more doses							
Zoster	Contraindicated				1 dose				

*Covered by the Vaccine Injury Compensation Program.

For all persons in this category who meet the age requirements and who lack evidence of immunity (e.g., lack documentation of vaccination or have no evidence of prior infection)

Recommended if some other risk factor is present (e.g., on the basis of medical, occupational, lifestyle, or other indications)

Report all clinically significant postvaccination reactions to the Vaccine Adverse Event Reporting System (VAERS). Reporting forms and instructions on filing a VAERS report are available at **www.vaers.hhs.gov** or by telephone, 800-822-7967.

Information on how to file a Vaccine Injury Compensation Program claim is available at **www.hrsa.gov/vaccine compensation** or by telephone, 800-338-2382. To file a claim for vaccine injury, contact the U.S. Court of Federal Claims, 717 Madison Place, N.W., Washington, D.C. 20005; telephone, 202-357-6400.

Additional information about the vaccines in this schedule, extent of available data, and contraindications for vaccination is also available at **www.cdc.gov/vaccines** or from the CDC-INFO Contact Center at 800-CDC-INFO (800-232-4636) in English and Spanish, 24 hours a day, 7 days a week.

Use of trade names and commercial sources is for identification only and does not imply endorsement by the U.S. Department of Health and Human Services.

This schedule indicates the recommended medical indications for which administration of currently licensed vaccines is commonly indicated for adults ages 19 years and older, as of October 1, 2007. Licensed combination vaccines may be used whenever any components of the combination are indicated and when the vaccine's other components are not contraindicated. For detailed recommendations on all vaccines, including those used primarily for travelers or that are issued during the year, consult the manufacturers' package inserts and the complete statements from the Advisory Committee on Immunization Practices (**www.cdc.gov/vaccines/pubs/acip-list.htm**).

1. **Tetanus, diphtheria, and acellular pertussis (Td/Tdap) vaccination.** Tdap should replace a single dose of Td for adults aged <65 years who have not previously received a dose of Tdap. Only one of two Tdap products (Adacel® [sanofi pasteur]) is licensed for use in adults.
Adults with uncertain histories of a complete primary vaccination series with tetanus and diphtheria toxoid–containing vaccines should begin or complete a primary vaccination series. A primary series for adults is 3 doses of tetanus and diphtheria toxoid–containing vaccines; administer the first 2 doses at least 4 weeks apart and the third dose 6–12 months after the second. However, Td can substitute for any one of the doses of Td in the 3-dose primary series. The booster dose of tetanus and diphtheria toxoid–containing vaccine should be administered to adults who have completed a primary series and if the last vaccination was received ≥10 years previously. Tdap or Td vaccine may be used, as indicated.
If the person is pregnant and received the last Td vaccination ≥10 years previously, administer Td during the second or third trimester; if the person received the last Td vaccination in <10 years, administer Tdap during the immediate postpartum period. A one-time administration of 1 dose of Tdap with an interval as short as 2 years from a previous Td vaccination is recommended for postpartum women, close contacts of infants aged <12 months, and all health-care workers with direct patient contact. In certain situations, Td can be deferred during pregnancy and Tdap substituted in the immediate postpartum period, or Tdap can be administered instead of Td to a pregnant woman after an informed discussion with the woman.

(Continued)

Consult the ACIP statement for recommendations for administering Td as prophylaxis in wound management.

2. **Human papillomavirus (HPV) vaccination.** HPV vaccination is recommended for all females aged ≤26 years who have not completed the vaccine series. History of genital warts, abnormal Papanicolaou test, or positive HPV DNA test is not evidence of prior infection with all vaccine HPV types; HPV vaccination is still recommended for these persons.

Ideally, vaccine should be administered before potential exposure to HPV through sexual activity; however, females who are sexually active should still be vaccinated. Sexually active females who have not been infected with any of the HPV vaccine types receive the full benefit of the vaccination. Vaccination is less beneficial for females who have already been infected with one or more of the HPV vaccine types.

A complete series consists of 3 doses. The second dose should be administered 2 months after the first dose; the third dose should be administered 6 months after the first dose.

Although HPV vaccination is not specifically recommended for females with the medical indications described in Figure 2, "Vaccines that might be indicated for adults based on medical and other indications," it is not a live-virus vaccine and can be administered. However, immune response and vaccine efficacy might be less than in persons who do not have the medical indications described or who are immunocompetent.

3. **Measles, mumps, rubella (MMR) vaccination.**
Measles component: Adults born before 1957 can be considered immune to measles. Adults born during or after 1957 should receive ≥1 dose of MMR unless they have a medical contraindication, documentation of ≥1 dose, history of measles based on health-care provider diagnosis, or laboratory evidence of immunity.

A second dose of MMR is recommended for adults who 1) have been recently exposed to measles or are in an outbreak setting; 2) have been previously vaccinated with killed measles vaccine; 3) have been vaccinated with an unknown type of measles vaccine during 1963–1967; 4) are students in postsecondary educational institutions; 5) work in a health-care facility; or 6) plan to travel internationally.
Mumps component: Adults born before 1957 can generally be considered immune to mumps. Adults born during or after 1957 should receive 1 dose of MMR unless they have a medical contraindication, history of mumps based on health-care provider diagnosis, or laboratory evidence of immunity.

A second dose of MMR is recommended for adults who 1) are in an age group that is affected during a mumps outbreak; 2) are students in postsecondary educational institutions; 3) work in a health-care facility; or 4) plan to travel internationally. For unvaccinated health-care workers born before 1957 who do not have other evidence of mumps immunity, consider administering 1 dose on a routine basis and strongly consider administering a second dose during an outbreak.
Rubella component: Administer 1 dose of MMR vaccine to women whose rubella vaccination history is unreliable or who lack laboratory evidence of immunity. For women of childbearing age, regardless of birth year, routinely determine rubella immunity and counsel women regarding congenital rubella syndrome. Women who do not have evidence of

immunity should receive MMR vaccine upon completion or termination of pregnancy and before discharge from the health-care facility.

4. **Varicella vaccination.** All adults without evidence of immunity to varicella should receive 2 doses of single-antigen varicella vaccine unless they have a medical contraindication. Special consideration should be given to those who 1) have close contact with persons at high risk for severe disease (e.g., health-care personnel and family contacts of immunocompromised persons) or 2) are at high risk for exposure or transmission (e.g., teachers; child care employees; residents and staff members of institutional settings, including correctional institutions; college students; military personnel; adolescents and adults living in households with children; nonpregnant women of childbearing age; and international travelers).

Evidence of immunity to varicella in adults includes any of the following: 1) documentation of 2 doses of varicella vaccine at least 4 weeks apart; 2) U.S.-born before 1980 (although for health-care personnel and pregnant women birth before 1980 should not be considered evidence of immunity); 3) history of varicella based on diagnosis or verification of varicella by a health-care provider (for a patient reporting a history of or presenting with an atypical case, a mild case, or both, health-care providers should seek either an epidemiologic link with a typical varicella case or to a laboratory-confirmed case or evidence of laboratory confirmation, if it was performed at the time of acute disease); 4) history of herpes zoster based on health-care provider diagnosis; or 5) laboratory evidence of immunity or laboratory confirmation of disease. Assess pregnant women for evidence of varicella immunity. Women who do not have evidence of immunity should receive the first dose of varicella vaccine upon completion or termination of pregnancy and before discharge from the health-care facility. The second dose should be administered 4–8 weeks after the first dose.

5. **Influenza vaccination.** *Medical indications:* Chronic disorders of the cardiovascular or pulmonary systems, including asthma; chronic metabolic diseases, including diabetes mellitus, renal or hepatic dysfunction, hemoglobinopathies, or immunosuppression (including immunosuppression caused by medications or human immunodeficiency virus [HIV]); any condition that compromises respiratory function or the handling of respiratory secretions or that can increase the risk of aspiration (e.g., cognitive dysfunction, spinal cord injury, or seizure disorder or other neuromuscular disorder); and pregnancy during the influenza season. No data exist on the risk for severe or complicated influenza disease among persons with asplenia; however, influenza is a risk factor for secondary bacterial infections that can cause severe disease among persons with asplenia.
Occupational indications: Health-care personnel and employees of long-term care and assisted-living facilities.
Other indications: Residents of nursing homes and other long-term care and assisted-living facilities; persons likely to transmit influenza to persons at high risk (e.g., in-home household contacts and caregivers of children aged 0–59 months, or persons of all ages with high-risk conditions); and anyone who would like to be vaccinated. Healthy, nonpregnant adults aged ≤49 years without high-risk medical conditions who are not contacts of

(Continued)

severely immunocompromised persons in special care units can receive either intranasally administered live, attenuated influenza vaccine (FluMist®) or inactivated vaccine. Other persons should receive the inactivated vaccine.

6. **Pneumococcal polysaccharide vaccination.**
Medical indications: Chronic pulmonary disease (excluding asthma); chronic cardiovascular diseases; diabetes mellitus; chronic liver diseases, including liver disease as a result of alcohol abuse (e.g., cirrhosis); chronic alcoholism, chronic renal failure or nephrotic syndrome; functional or anatomic asplenia (e.g., sickle cell disease or splenectomy [if elective splenectomy is planned, vaccinate at least 2 weeks before surgery]); immunosuppressive conditions; and cochlear implants and cerebrospinal fluid leaks. Vaccinate as close to HIV diagnosis as possible.
Other indications: Alaska Natives and certain American Indian populations and residents of nursing homes or other long-term care facilities.

7. **Revaccination with pneumococcal polysaccharide vaccine.** One-time revaccination after 5 years for persons with chronic renal failure or nephrotic syndrome; functional or anatomic asplenia (e.g., sickle cell disease or splenectomy); or immunosuppressive conditions. For persons aged ≥65 years, one-time revaccination if they were vaccinated ≥5 years previously and were aged <65 years at the time of primary vaccination.

8. **Hepatitis A vaccination.** *Medical indications:* Persons with chronic liver disease and persons who receive clotting factor concentrates.
Behavioral indications: Men who have sex with men and persons who use illegal drugs.
Occupational indications: Persons working with hepatitis A virus (HAV)–infected primates or with HAV in a research laboratory setting.
Other indications: Persons traveling to or working in countries that have high or intermediate endemicity of hepatitis A (a list of countries is available at **wwwn.cdc.gov/travel/contentdiseases.aspx**) and any person seeking protection from HAV infection. Single-antigen vaccine formulations should be administered in a 2-dose schedule at either 0 and 6–12 months (Havrix®), or 0 and 6–18 months (Vaqta®). If the combined hepatitis A and hepatitis B vaccine (Twinrix®) is used, administer 3 doses at 0, 1, and 6 months.

9. **Hepatitis B vaccination.** *Medical indications:* Persons with end-stage renal disease, including patients receiving hemodialysis; persons seeking evaluation or treatment for a sexually transmitted disease (STD); persons with HIV infection; and persons with chronic liver disease.
Occupational indications: Health-care personnel and public-safety workers who are exposed to blood or other potentially infectious body fluids.
Behavioral indications: Sexually active persons who are not in a long-term, mutually monogamous relationship (e.g., persons with more than 1 sex partner during the previous 6 months); current or recent injection-drug users; and men who have sex with men.
Other indications: Household contacts and sex partners of persons with chronic hepatitis B virus (HBV) infection; clients and staff members of institutions for persons with developmental disabilities; international travelers to countries with high or intermediate prevalence of chronic HBV infection (a list of countries is available at **wwwn.cdc.gov/travel/contentdiseases.aspx**); and any adult seeking protection from HBV infection.
Settings where hepatitis B vaccination is recommended for all adults: STD treatment facilities; HIV testing and treatment facilities; facilities providing drug-abuse treatment and prevention services; health-care settings targeting services to injection-drug users or men who have sex with men; correctional facilities; end-stage renal disease programs and facilities for chronic hemodialysis patients; and institutions and nonresidential daycare facilities for persons with developmental disabilities.
Special formulation indications: For adult patients receiving hemodialysis and other immunocompromised adults, 1 dose of 40 µg/mL (Recombivax HB®), or 2 doses of 20 µg/mL (Engerix-B®) administered simultaneously.

10. **Meningococcal vaccination.** *Medical indications:* Adults with anatomic or functional asplenia, or terminal complement component deficiencies.
Other indications: First-year college students living in dormitories; microbiologists who are routinely exposed to isolates of Neisseria meningitidis; military recruits; and persons who travel to or live in countries in which meningococcal disease is hyperendemic or epidemic (e.g., the "meningitis belt" of sub-Saharan Africa during the dry season [December–June]), particularly if their contact with local populations will be prolonged. Vaccination is required by the government of Saudi Arabia for all travelers to Mecca during the annual Hajj. Meningococcal conjugate vaccine is preferred for adults with any of the preceding indications who are aged ≤55 years, although meningococcal polysaccharide vaccine (MPSV4) is an acceptable alternative. Revaccination after 3–5 years might be indicated for adults previously vaccinated with MPSV4 who remain at increased risk for infection (e.g., persons residing in areas in which disease is epidemic).

11. **Herpes zoster vaccination.** A single dose of zoster vaccine is recommended for adults aged ≥60 years regardless of whether they report a prior episode of herpes zoster. Persons with chronic medical conditions may be vaccinated unless a contraindication or precaution exists for their condition.

12. **Selected conditions for which *Haemophilus influenzae* type b (Hib) vaccine may be used.** Hib conjugate vaccines are licensed for children aged 6 weeks–71 months. No efficacy data are available on which to base a recommendation concerning use of Hib vaccine for older children and adults with the chronic conditions associated with an increased risk for Hib disease. However, studies suggest good immunogenicity in patients who have sickle cell disease, leukemia, or HIV infection or who have had splenectomies; administering vaccine to these patients is not contraindicated.

13. **Immunocompromising conditions.** Inactivated vaccines are generally acceptable (e.g., pneumococcal, meningococcal, and influenza [trivalent inactivated influenza vaccine]), and live vaccines generally are avoided in persons with immune deficiencies or immune suppressive conditions. Information on specific conditions is available at **www.cdc.gov/vaccines/pubs/acip-list.htm**.

DRUGS EXCRETED IN BREAST MILK

The following list is not comprehensive; generic forms and alternate brands of some products may be available. When recommending drugs to pregnant or nursing patients, always check product labeling for specific precautions.

Accolate	Cardizem	Diastat	Hydrocortone
Accuretic	Cataflam	Diflucan	HydroDIURIL
Aciphex	Catapres	Digitek	Iberet-Folic
Actiq	Ceclor	Dilacor	Ifex
Activella	Cefizox	Dilantin	Imitrex
Actonel	Cefobid	Dilaudid	Imuran
Actonel with Calcium	Cefotan	Diovan	Inderal
ActoPlus Met	Ceftin	Diprivan	Inderide
Actos	Celebrex	Diuril	Indocin
Adalat	Celexa	Dolobid	INFeD
Adderall	Cerebyx	Dolophine	Inspra
Advicor	Ceredase	Doral	Invanz
Aggrenox	Cipro	Doryx	Inversine
Aldactazide	Ciprodex	Droxia	Isoptin
Aldactone	Claforan	Duraclon	Kadian
Aldomet	Clarinex	Duragesic	Keflex
Aldoril	Claritin	Duramorph	Keppra
Alesse	Claritin-D	Duratuss	Kerlone
Alfenta	Cleocin	Duricef	Ketek
Allegra-D	Climara	Dyazide	Klonopin
Aloprim	Clozaril	Dyrenium	Kronofed-A
Altace	Codeine	E.E.S.	Kutrase
Ambien	CombiPatch	EC-Naprosyn	Lamictal
Anaprox	Combipres	Ecotrin	Lamisil
Androderm	Combivir	Effexor	Lamprene
Antara	Combunox	Elestat	Lanoxicaps
Apresoline	Compazine	EMLA	Lanoxin
Aralen	Cordarone	Enduron	Lariam
Arthrotec	Corgard	Epzicom	Lescol
Asacol	Cortisporin	Equetro	Levbid
Ativan	Corzide	ERYC	Levitra
Augmentin	Cosopt	EryPed	Levlen
Avalide	Coumadin	Ery-Tab	Levlite
Avandia	Covera-HS	Erythrocin	Levora
Avelox	Cozaar	Erythromycin	Levothroid
Axid	Crestor	Esgic-plus	Levoxyl
Axocet	Crinone	Eskalith	Levsin
Azactam	Cyclessa	Estrogel	Levsinex
Azasan	Cymbalta	Estrostep	Lexapro
Azathioprine	Cystospaz	Evista	Lexiva
Azulfidine	Cytomel	FazaClo	Lialda
Bactrim	Cytotec	Felbatol	Lindane
Baraclude	Cytoxan	Feldene	Lioresal
Benadryl	Dapsone	femhrt	Lipitor
Bentyl	Daraprim	Fiorinal	Lithium
Betapace	Darvon	Flagyl	Lithobid
Bextra	Darvon-N	Floxin	Lo/Ovral
Bexxar	Decadron	Foradil	Loestrin
Bicillin	Deconsal II	Fortamet	Lomotil
Blocadren	Demerol	Fortaz	Loniten
Boniva	Demulen	Fosamax Plus D	Lopressor
Brethine	Depacon	Furosemide	Lortab
Brevicon	Depakene	Gabitril	Lotensin
Brontex	Depakote	Galzin	Lotrel
Byetta	DepoDur	Garamycin	Luminal
Caduet	Depo-Provera	Glucophage	Luvox
Cafergot	Desogen	Glyset	Lyrica
Calan	Desoxyn	Guaifed	Macrobid
Campral	Desyrel	Halcion	Macrodantin
Capoten	Dexedrine	Haldol	Marinol
Capozide	DextroStat	Helidac	Maxipime
Captopril	D.H.E. 45	Hycamtin	Maxzide
Carbatrol	Diabinese	Hydrocet	Mefoxin

Menostar	OxyFast	Rozerem	Triphasil
Methergine	OxyIR	Sanctura	Trivora
Methotrexate	Pacerone	Sanctura XR	Trizivir
MetroCream/Gel/Lotion	Pamelor	Sandimmune	Trovan
Mexitil	Pancrease	Sarafem	Truvada
Micronor	Paxil	Seconal	Tygacil
Microzide	PCE	Sectral	Tylenol
Migranal	Pediapred	Semprex-D	Tylenol with Codeine
Miltown	Pediazole	Septra	Ultane
Minizide	Pediotic	Seroquel	Ultram
Minocin	Pentasa	Seroquel XR	Unasyn
Mirapex	Pepcid	Sinequan	Uniphyl
Mircette	Periostat	Slo-bid	Uniretic
M-M-R II	Persantine	Soma	Unithroid
Mobic	Pfizerpen	Sonata	Urimax
Modicon	Phenergan	Spiriva	Valium
Moduretic	Phenobarbital	Sprycel	Valtrex
Monodox	Phrenilin	Stadol	Vanceril
Monopril	Pipracil	Streptomycin	Vancocin
Morphine	Plan B	Stromectol	Vantin
MS Contin	Ponstel	Symbyax	Vascor
MSIR	Pravachol	Symmetrel	Vaseretic
Myambutol	Premphase	Synthroid	Vasotec
Mycamine	Prempro	Tagamet	Ventavis
Mysoline	Prevacid	Tambocor	Verelan
Namenda	Prevacid NapraPAC	Tapazole	Vermox
Naprelan	PREVPAC	Tarka	Versed
Naprosyn	Prinzide	Tasigna	Vibramycin
Nascobal	Prograf	Tavist	Vibra-Tabs
Necon	Proloprim	Tazicef	Vicodin
NegGram	Prometrium	Tazidime	Vigamox
Nembutal	Pronestyl	Tegretol	Viramune
Neoral	Propofol	Tenoretic	Voltaren
Niaspan	Prosed/DS	Tenormin	Vytorin
Nicotrol	Protonix	Tenuate	Wellbutrin
Niravam	Provera	Testoderm	Xanax
Nizoral	Prozac	Thalitone	Xolair
Norco	Pseudoephedrine	Theo-24	Zantac
Nor-QD	Pulmicort	Theo-Dur	Zarontin
Nordette	Pyrazinamide	Thorazine	Zaroxolyn
Norinyl	Quinidex	Tiazac	Zegerid
Noritate	Quinine	Timolide	Zemplar
Normodyne	Raptiva	Timoptic	Zestoretic
Norpace	Reglan	Tindamax	Zetia
Norplant	Relpax	Tobi	Ziac
Novantrone	Renese	Tofranil	Zinacef
Nubain	Requip	Tolectin	Zithromax
Nucofed	Reserpine	Toprol-XL	Zocor
Nydrazid	Restoril	Toradol	Zomig
Oramorph	Retrovir	Trandate	Zonalon
Oretic	Rifadin	Tranxene	Zonegran
Ortho-Cept	Rifamate	Trental	Zosyn
Ortho-Cyclen	Rifater	Tricor	Zovia
Ortho-Novum	Rimactane	Triglide	Zovirax
Ortho Tri-Cyclen	Risperdal	Trilafon	Zyban
Orudis	Rocaltrol	Trileptal	Zydone
Ovcon	Rocephin	Tri-Levlen	Zyloprim
Oxistat	Roferon A	Tri-Norinyl	Zyprexa
OxyContin	Roxanol	Triostat	Zyrtec

DRUGS THAT MAY CAUSE PHOTOSENSITIVITY

The drugs in this table are known to cause photosensitivity in some individuals. Effects can range from itching, scaling, rash, and swelling to skin cancer, premature skin aging, skin and eye burns, cataracts, reduced immunity, blood vessel damage, and allergic reactions. The list is not all-inclusive, and shows only representative brands of each generic. When in doubt, always check specific product labeling. Individuals should be advised to wear protective clothing and to apply sunscreens while taking the medications listed below.

GENERIC	BRAND
Acamprosate	Campral
Acetazolamide	Diamox
Acitretin	Soriatane
Acyclovir	Zovirax
Alendronate	Fosamax
Alitretinoin	Panretin
Almotriptan	Axert
Amiloride/ hydrochlorothiazide	Moduretic
Aminolevulinic acid	Levulan Kerastick
Amiodarone	Cordarone, Pacerone
Amitriptyline	Elavil
Amitriptyline/ chlordiazepoxide	Etrafon, Limbitrol
Amitriptyline/perphenazine	
Amlodipine/atorvastatin	Caduet
Amoxapine	
Amphetamine aspartate/ amphetamine sulfate/ dextroamphetamine saccharate/ dextroamphetamine sulfate	Adderall XR
Anagrelide	Agrylin
Aripiprazole	Abilify
Atazanavir	Reyataz
Atenolol/chlorthalidone	Tenoretic
Atorvastatin	Lipitor
Atovaquone/proguanil	Malarone
Azatadine/ pseudoephedrine	Rynatan, Trinalin
Azithromycin	Zithromax, Zmag
Benazepril	Lotensin
Benazepril/ hydrochlorothiazide	Lotensin HCT
Bendroflumethiazide/ nadolol	Corzide
Bexarotene	Targretin
Bismuth/metronidazole/ tetracycline	Helidac
Bismuth subcitrate potassium/ metronidazole/tetracycline	Pylera
Bisoprolol/ hydrochlorothiazide	Ziac
Brompheniramine/ dextromethorphan/ phenylephrine	Alacol DM, Dimetane DX
Brompheniramine/ dextromethorphan/ pseudoephedrine	Bromfed-DM
Buffered aspirin/ pravastatin	Pravigard PAC
Bupropion	Wellbutrin, Zyban
Candesartan/ hydrochlorothiazide	Atacand HCT
Capecitabine	Xeloda
Captopril	Capoten
Captopril/ hydrochlorothiazide	Capozide
Carbamazepine	Carbatrol, Equetro, Tegretol, Tegretol-XR
Carbinoxamine/ pseudoephedrine	Palgic-D, Palgic-DS, Pediatex-D

GENERIC	BRAND
Carvedilol	Coreg
Carvedilol phosphate	Coreg CR
Celecoxib	Celebrex
Cetirizine	Zyrtec
Cetirizine/pseudoephedrine	Zyrtec-D
Cevimeline	Evoxac
Chlorhexidine gluconate	Hibistat
Chloroquine	Aralen
Chlorothiazide sodium	Diuril I.V.
Chlorpheniramine/ hydrocodone/ pseudoephedrine	Tussend
Chlorpheniramine/ phenylephrine/pyrilamine	Rynatan
Chlorpromazine	Thorazine
Chlorpropamide	Diabinese
Chlorthalidone	Thalitone
Chlorthalidone/clonidine	Clorpres
Cidofovir	Vistide
Ciprofloxacin	Cipro, Cipro XR
Citalopram	Celexa
Clemastine	Tavist
Clindamycin phosphate	Clindagel
Clonidine/chlorthalidone	Clorpres
Clozapine	Clozaril, Fazaclo
Coagulation Factor IX (recombinant)	BeneFIX
Cromolyn sodium	Gastrocrom
Cyclobenzaprine	Flexeril
Cyproheptadine	Cyproheptadine
Dacarbazine	DTIC-Dome
Dantrolene	Dantrium
Demeclocycline	Declomycin
Desipramine	Norpramin
Diclofenac potassium	Cataflam
Diclofenac sodium	Voltaren
Diclofenac sodium/ misoprostol	Arthrotec
Diflunisal	Dolobid
Dihydroergotamine	D.H.E. 45
Diltiazem	Cardizem, Tiazac
Diphenhydramine	Benadryl
Divalproex	Depakote
Doxepin	Sinequan
Doxycycline hyclate	Doryx, Periostat, Vibra-Tabs, Vibramycin
Doxycycline monohydrate	Monodox
Duloxetine	Cymbalta
Efalizumab	Raptiva
Enalapril	Vasotec
Enalapril/felodipine	
Enalapril/ hydrochlorothiazide	Vaseretic
Enalaprilat (injection)	Vasotec I.V.
Epirubicin	Ellence
Eprosartan mesylate/ hydrochlorothiazide	Teveten HCT
Erythromycin/ sulfisoxazole	Pediazole
Escitalopram oxalate	Lexapro
Esomeprazole	Nexium
Estazolam	

GENERIC	BRAND	GENERIC	BRAND
Estradiol	Gynodiol, Estrogel	Hydroxocobalamin	Cyanokit Antidote
Eszopiclone	Lunesta	Hydroxychloroquine	Plaquenil
Ethionamide	Trecator-SC	Hypericum	Kira, St. John's wort
Etodolac	Lodine	Hypericum/vitamin B_1/	One-A-Day Tension
Felbamate	Felbatol	vitamin C/kava-kava	& Mood
Fenofibrate	Lofibra, Tricor, Triglide	Ibuprofen	Motrin
		Imatinib Mesylate	Gleevec
Floxuridine	Sterile FUDR	Imipramine	Tofranil
Flucytosine	Ancobon	Imiquimod	Aldara
Fluorouracil	Efudex	Indapamide	Lozol
Fluoxetine	Prozac, Sarafem	Interferon alfa-2b,	Intron A
Fluphenazine	Prolixin	recombinant	
Flutamide	Eulexin	Interferon alfa-n3	Alferon-N
Fluvastatin	Lescol	(human leukocyte derived)	
Fluvoxamine	Luvox	Interferon beta-1a	Avonex
Fosinopril	Monopril	Interferon beta-1b	Betaseron
Fosphenytoin	Cerebyx	Irbesartan/hydrochlorothiazide	Avalide
Furosemide	Lasix	Isocarboxazid	Marplan
Gabapentin	Neurontin	Isoniazid/pyrazinamide/	Rifater
Gatifloxacin	Tequin	rifampin	
Gemfibrozil	Lopid	Isotretinoin	Accutane, Amnesteem
Gemifloxacin mesylate	Factive		
Gentamicin	Garamycin	Itraconazole	Sporanox
Glatiramer acetate	Copaxone	Ketoprofen	Orudis, Oruvail
Glimepiride	Amaryl	Lamotrigine	Lamictal
Glimepiride/pioglitazone hydrochloride	Duetact	Leuprolide acetate	Lupron, Lupron Depot
Glimepiride/ rosiglitazone maleate	Avandaryl	Levamisole	Levamisole
		Levofloxacin	Levaquin
Glipizide	Glucotrol	Levofloxacin/5% dextrose	Levaquin Injection
Glyburide	DiaBeta, Glynase, Micronase	Lisinopril	Zestril
		Lisinopril/ hydrochlorothiazide	Prinivil, Zestoretic
Glyburide/metformin HCl	Glucovance		
Griseofulvin	Fulvicin P/G, Grifulvin, Gris-PEG	Lomefloxacin	Maxaquin
		Loratadine	Claritin
Haloperidol	Haldol	Loratadine/ pseudoephedrine	Claritin-D
Hexachlorophene	pHisoHex		
Hydralazine/ hydrochlorothiazide	Hydra-zide	Losartan	Cozaar
		Losartan/ hydrochlorothiazide	Hyzaar
Hydrochlorothiazide	HydroDIURIL, Microzide, Oretic		
		Lovastatin	Altoprev, Mevacor
Hydrochlorothiazide/ fosinopril	Monopril HCT		
		Lovastatin/niacin	Advicor
Hydrochlorothiazide/ irbesartan	Avalide	Maprotiline	Maprotiline
		Mefenamic acid	Ponstel
Hydrochlorothiazide/ lisinopril	Prinzide, Zestoretic	Meloxicam	Mobic
		Mesalamine	Pentasa
Hydrochlorothiazide/ losartan potassium	Hyzaar	Methazolamide	
		Methotrexate	Trexall
Hydrochlorothiazide/ methyldopa	Aldoril	Methoxsalen	Uvadex, Oxsoralen, 8-MOP
Hydroclorothiazide/ metoprolol tartrate	Lopressor HCT	Methyclothiazide	Enduron
		Methyldopa/ hydrochlorothiazide	Aldoril
Hydrochlorothiazide/ moexipril	Uniretic		
		Metolazone	Mykrox, Zaroxolyn
Hydrochlorothiazide/ propranolol	Inderide		
		Metoprolol succinate	Toprol-XL
Hydrochlorothiazide/ quinapril	Accuretic	Metoprolol tartrate	Lopressor
		Minocycline	Dynacin, Minocin, Solodyn
Hydrochlorothiazide/ spironolactone	Aldactazide		
		Mirtazapine	Remeron
Hydrochlorothiazide/ telmisartan	Micardis HCT	Moexipril	Univasc
		Moexipril/ hydrochlorothiazide	Uniretic
Hydrochlorothiazide/timolol	Timolide		
Hydrochlorothiazide/ triamterene	Dyazide, Maxzide	Moxifloxacin	Avelox
		Nabilone	Cesamet
Hydrochlorothiazide/ valsartan	Diovan HCT	Nabumetone	Relafen
		Nadolol/ bendroflumethiazide	Corzide
Hydroflumethiazide	Hydroflumethiazide		

GENERIC	BRAND	GENERIC	BRAND
Nalidixic acid	Nalidixic acid	Rizatriptan	Maxalt, Maxalt-MLT
Naproxen	Naprosyn, EC-Naprosyn	Ropinirole	Requip
		Rosuvastatin	Crestor
Naproxen sodium	Anaprox, Anaprox DS, Naprelan	Ruta graveolens	Rue
		Saquinavir mesylate	Invirase
Naratriptan	Amerge	Selegiline	Eldepryl, Emsam
Nefazodone	Serzone	Sertraline	Zoloft
Nifedipine	Adalat CC, Procardia	Sibutramine	Meridia
Nisoldipine	Sular	Sildenafil	Viagra
Norfloxacin	Noroxin	Simvastatin	Zocor
Nortriptyline	Pamelor	Simvastatin/ezetimibe	Vytorin
Ofloxacin	Floxin	Sirolimus	Rapamune
Olanzapine	Zyprexa	Somatropin	Serostim
Olanzapine/fluoxetine	Symbyax	Sotalol	Betapace, Betapace AF
Olmesartan medoxomil/ hydrochlorothiazide	Benicar HCT	Sulfamethoxazole/ trimethoprim	Bactrim, Septra
Olsalazine	Dipentum	Sulfasalazine	Azulfidine
Omeprazole/ sodium bicarbonate	Zegerid	Sulfisoxazole acetyl	Gantrisin Pediatric
Oxaprozin	Daypro	Sulindac	Clinoril
Oxcarbazepine	Trileptal	Sumatriptan	Imitrex
Oxycodone	Roxicodone	Tacrolimus	Prograf, Protopic
Oxytetracycline	Terramycin	Tazarotene	Tazorac
Panitumumab	Vectibix	Telmisartan/ hydrochlorothiazide	Micardis HCT
Pantoprazole	Protonix	Tetracycline	Sumycin
Paroxetine hydrochloride	Paxil	Thalidomide	Thalomid
Paroxetine mesylate	Pexeva	Thiothixene	Navane
Pastinaca sativa	Parsnip	Tiagabine	Gabitril
Pentosan polysulfate	Elmiron	Tigecycline	Tygacil
Pentostatin	Nipent	Tolazamide	Tolazamide
Perphenazine	Perphenazine	Tolbutamide	Tolbutamide
Pilocarpine	Salagen	Topiramate	Topamax
Piroxicam	Feldene	Tretinoin	Retin-A
Polymyxin B sulfate/ trimethopim sulfate	Polytrim	Triamcinolone acetonide	Azmacort Inhalation
Polythiazide	Renese	Triamterene	Dyrenium
Polythiazide/prazosin	Minizide	Triamterene/ hydrochlorothiazide	Dyazide, Maxzide
Porfimer sodium	Photofrin	Trifluoperazine	Trifluoperazine
Pramipexole dihydrochloride	Mirapex	Trimipramine	Surmontil
Pravastatin	Pravachol	Trovafloxacin	Trovan
Pregabalin	Lyrica	Valacyclovir	Valtrex
Prochlorperazine	Compazine, Compro	Valdecoxib	Bextra
Promethazine	Phenergan	Valproate	Depacon
Protriptyline	Vivactil	Valproic acid	Depakene
Pyrimethamine/sulfadoxine	Fansidar	Valsartan/ hydrochlorothiazide	Diovan HCT
Pyrazinamide	Pyrazinamide	Vardenafil	Levitra
Quetiapine	Seroquel	Varenicline tartrate	Chantix
Quinapril	Accupril	Venlafaxine	Effexor
Quinapril/ hydrochlorothiazide	Accuretic	Verteporfin	Visudyne
Quinidine gluconate	Quinidine	Vinblastine	Vinblastine
Quinidine sulfate	Quinidex	Voriconazole	Vfend
Rabeprazole sodium	Aciphex	Zalcitabine	Hivid
Ramipril	Altace	Zaleplon	Sonata
Rasagiline mesylate	Azilect	Ziprasidone	Geodon
Riluzole	Rilutek	Zolmitriptan	Zomig
Risperidone	Risperdal, Risperdal Consta	Zolpidem	Ambien, Ambien CR
Ritonavir	Norvir		

DRUGS THAT MAY CAUSE QT PROLONGATION

BRAND NAME	GENERIC NAME	BRAND NAME	GENERIC NAME
Abilify	Aripiprazole	Norpace	Disopyramide phosphate
AcipHex	Rabeprazole sodium	Norpramin	Desipramine
Advair	Fluticasone propionate/ salmeterol xinafoate	Noxafil	Posaconazole
		Orap	Pimozide
Advair HFA	Fluticasone propionate/ salmeterol xinafoate	OsmoPrep	Sodium phosphate mono-basic monohydrate/ sodium phosphate dibasic anhydrous
Aloxi Injection	Palonosetron HCl		
Amerge	Naratriptan HCl	Pacerone	Amiodarone HCl
Amitriptyline	Amitriptyline	PCE	Erythromycin particles
Anzemet	Dolasetron mesylate	Perforomist	Formoterol fumarate
Apokyn	Apomorphine HCl	Plenaxis*	Abarelix
Avelox	Moxifloxacin HCl	Pletal	Cilostazol
Betapace	Sotalol HCl	PREVPAC	Lansoprazole/amoxicillin/ clarithromycin
Betapace AF	Sotalol HCl		
Biaxin	Clarithromycin	Procainamide	Procainamide
Brovana	Arformoterol tartrate	Prograf	Tacrolimus
Celexa	Citalopram HBr	Prozac	Fluoxetine
Cipro	Ciprofloxacin	Quinidine gluconate	Quinidine gluconate
Cipro XR	Ciprofloxacin	Quinidine sulfate	Quinidine sulfate
Cordarone	Amiodarone HCl	Ranexa	Ranolazine
Corvert	Ibutilide fumarate	Raxar*	Grepafloxacin
Detrol LA	Tolterodine tartrate	Razadyne	Galantamine HBr
Dolophine	Methadone HCl	Risperdal Consta	Risperidone
Doxepin	Doxepin	Rythmol SR	Propafenone HCl
E.E.S.	Erythromycin ethylsuccinate	Serentil*	Mesoridazine besylate
		Serevent	Salmeterol
Effexor XR	Venlafaxine HCl	Seroquel	Quetiapine fumarate
Eraxis	Anidulafungin	Sporanox	Itraconazole
ERYC	Erythromycin	Sprycel	Dasatinib
EryPed	Erythromycin ethylsuccinate	Strattera	Atomoxetine HCl
		Sutent	Sunitinib malate
Erythrocin stearate	Erythromycin stearate	Symbicort	Budesonide/formoterol fumarate dihydrate
Erythromycin Base Filmtab	Erythromycin		
		Symbyax	Olanzapine/fluoxetine HCl
Erythromycin Delayed-Release	Erythromycin		
		Tambocor	Flecainide acetate
Exelon Patch	Rivastigmine	Tasigna	Nilotinib
Factive	Gemifloxacin mesylate	Tequin*	Gatifloxacin
Fleet Enema/Enema Extra/ Enema for Children	Monobasic sodium phosphate/dibasic sodium phosphate	Thioridazine HCl	Thioridazine HCl
		Tikosyn	Dofetilide
		Tofranil, Tofranil-PM	Imipramine
Foradil	Formoterol	Trisenox Injection	Arsenic trioxide
Geodon	Ziprasidone HCl	Tykerb	Lapatinib
Haldol	Haloperidol	Uroxatral	Alfuzosin HCl
Halfan*	Halofantrine HCl	Vascor*	Bepridil HCl
Imitrex Injection	Sumatriptan succinate	VFEND	Voriconazole
Inapsine	Droperidol	Viracept	Nelfinavir mesylate
Invega	Paliperidone	Visicol	Sodium phosphate
Ketek	Telithromycin	Zagam*	Sparfloxacin
Levaquin	Levofloxacin	Zanaflex	Tizanidine
Levitra	Vardenafil HCl	Zmax	Azithromycin
Lexapro	Escitalopram oxalate	Zofran	Ondansetron HCl
Maxaquin	Lomefloxacin HCl	Zolinza	Vorinostat
Methadose	Methadone HCl	Zoloft	Sertraline HCl
Namenda	Memantine HCl	Zomig	Zolmitriptan
Nizoral	Ketoconazole	Zomig-ZMT	Zolmitriptan
Noroxin	Norfloxacin		

* Drug no longer available in the U.S.
NOTE: This list does not include all of the drugs that may cause QT disturbance. For more information, please refer to the specific product's full Prescribing Information.

DRUGS THAT MAY CAUSE STEVENS-JOHNSON SYNDROME AND TEN*

BRAND NAME	GENERIC NAME	BRAND NAME	GENERIC NAME
ACAM2000	Smallpox vaccine, live	Covera-HS	Verapamil HCl
AcipHex	Rabeprazole sodium	Crixivan	Indinavir sulfate
Adderall XR	Dextroamphetamine sulfate/dextroamphetamine saccharate/amphetamine sulfate/amphetamine aspartate	Cymbalta	Duloxetine HCl
		Daraprim	Pyrimethamine
		Daypro	Oxaprozin
		Depakote ER	Divalproex sodium
		Diamox	Acetazolamide
Advicor	Niacin/lovastatin	Didronel	Etidronate disodium
Agenerase	Amprenavir	Dilantin	Phenytoin sodium
Aggrenox	Aspirin/dipyridamole	Diovan HCT	Valsartan/ hydrochlorothiazide
Albenza	Albendazole		
Aldoril	Methyldopa/ hydrochlorothiazide	Diuril	Chlorothiazide
		Dolobid	Diflunisal
Aloprim	Allopurinol sodium	Donnatal Extentabs	Phenobarbital
Altace	Ramipril	Duac Topical Gel	Clindamycin, 1%/benzoyl peroxide, 5%
Amoxil	Amoxicillin		
Anaprox	Naproxen	Dynacin	Minocycline HCl
Ancobon	Flucytosine	EC-Naprosyn	Naproxen
Ansaid	Flurbiprofen	E.E.S.	Erythromycin ethylsuccinate
Arava	Leflunomide	Effexor XR	Venlafaxine HCl
Arimidex	Anastrozole	Emend	Aprepitant
Arthrotec	Diclofenac sodium/ misoprostol	Engerix-B Vaccine	Hepatitis B vaccine (recombinant)
Atacand HCT	Candesartan cilexetil/ hydrochlorothiazide	Epzicom	Abacavir sulfate/lamivudine
		Equetro	Carbamazepine
Atripla	Efavirenz/emtricitabine/ tenofovir disoproxil fumarate	EryPed	Erythromycin ethylsuccinate
		Ethyol	Amifostine
		Etodolac	Etodolac
Attenuvax	Measles virus vaccine, live	Exelon	Rivastigmine tartrate
Augmentin	Amoxicillin/clavulanate potassium	Fansidar	Sulfadoxine/pyrimethamine
		Feldene	Piroxicam
Avalide	Irbesartan/ hydrochlorothiazide	Flebogamma 5%	Immune globulin intravenous (human)
Avandamet	Rosiglitazone maleate/ metformin HCl	Flector	Diclofenac epolamine topical patch
Avandia	Rosiglitazone maleate	Fluarix	Influenza virus vaccine
Avelox	Moxifloxacin HCl	Fortaz	Ceftazidime for injection
Azulfidine	Sulfasalazine	Fosamax	Alendronate sodium
Bactrim	Sulfamethoxazole/ trimethoprim	Fosamax Plus D	Alendronate sodium/ cholecalciferol
Betagan	Levobunolol HCl	Furadantin	Nitrofurantoin
Betoptic S	Betaxolol HCl	Gammagard	Immune globulin intravenous (human)
Biaxin	Clarithromycin		
Bleph-10	Sulfacetamide sodium	Gamunex	Immune globulin intravenous (human), 10% caprylate/ chromatography purified
Blephamide	Sulfacetamide sodium/ prednisolone acetate		
Caduet	Amlodipine besylate/ atorvastatin calcium		
		Gantrisin	Acetyl sulfisoxazole
Capoten	Captopril	Gleevec	Imatinib mesylate
Carbatrol	Carbamazepine	Hyzaar	Losartan potassium/ hydrochlorothiazide
Cataflam	Diclofenac potassium		
Ceftin	Cefuroxime axetil	Inderal LA	Propranolol HCl
Celebrex	Celecoxib	Intelence	Etravirine
Cialis	Tadalafil	Intron A	Interferon alfa-2b
Cimzia	Certolizumab pegol	Lozol	Indapamide
Cipro	Ciprofloxacin	Indocin	Indomethacin
Cleocin vaginal ovules	Clindamycin phosphate vaginal suppositories	Lamictal	Lamotrigine
		Lamisil	Terbinafine HCl
Clinoril	Sulindac	Lariam	Mefloquine HCl
Clorpres	Clonidine HCl/chlorthalidone	Lescol	Fluvastatin sodium
Clozaril	Clozapine	Leukeran	Chlorambucil
Combivir	Lamivudine/zidovudine	Leustatin	Cladribine
Combunox	Oxycodone HCl/ibuprofen	Levaquin	Levofloxacin
Comvax	Haemophilus b conjugate (meningococcal protein conjugate)/ hepatitis B (recombinant) vaccine	Lexapro	Escitalopram oxalate
		Lexiva	Fosamprenavir calcium
		Lipitor	Atorvastatin calcium
		Lyrica	Pregabalin

Drugs That May Cause Stevens-Johnson Syndrome and TEN*

BRAND NAME	GENERIC NAME	BRAND NAME	GENERIC NAME
Malarone	Atovaquone/proguanil HCl	Relafen	Nabumetone
Maxalt	Rizatriptan benzoate	Remicade for IV Injection	Infliximab
Mefoxin	Cefoxitin injection		
Merrem	Meropenem for injection	Rescriptor	Delavirdine mesylate
Meruvax II	Rubella virus vaccine, live	Retrovir	Zidovudine
Mevacor	Lovastatin	Reyataz	Atazanavir sulfate
Micardis HCT	Telmisartan/ hydrochlorothiazide	Rituxan	Rituximab
		Rosula NS	Sodium sulfacetamide
Minocin	Minocycline HCl	Septra	Trimethoprim/ sulfamethoxazole
Mintezol	Thiabendazole		
M-M-R II	Measles, mumps, and rubella virus vaccine, live	Seroquel	Quetiapine fumarate
		Solodyn	Minocycline HCl
Mobic	Meloxicam	Stromectol	Ivermectin
Moduretic	Amiloride HCl/ hydrochlorothiazide	Suprax	Cefixime for oral suspension
Motrin	Ibuprofen	Sustiva	Efavirenz
Mumpsvax	Mumps virus vaccine, live	Tamiflu	Oseltamivir phosphate
Nalfon	Fenoprofen calcium	Tarka	Trandolapril/verapamil HCl
Namenda	Memantine HCl	Taxotere	Docetaxel
Naprelan	Naproxen sodium	Tegretol	Carbamazepine
Naprosyn	Naproxen	Teveten HCT	Eprosartan mesylate/ hydrochlorothiazide
Neurontin	Gabapentin		
Nexium	Esomeprazole magnesium	Thalomid	Thalidomide
		Tiazac	Diltiazem HCl
Niravam	Alprazolam orally disintegrating	Ticlid	Ticlopidine HCl
		Timentin	Ticarcillin disodium/ clavulanate potassium
Noroxin	Norfloxacin		
Norvir	Ritonavir	Timolide	Timolol maleate/ hydrochlorothiazide
Nuvigil	Armodafinil		
Nystatin Oral	Nystatin	Tindamax	Tinidazole
Omnicef	Cefdinir	Topamax	Topiramate
Orthoclone OKT3 Sterile Solution	Muromonab-CD3	Tricor	Fenofibrate
		Trileptal	Oxcarbazepine
Ovace	Sodium sulfacetamide	Trizivir	Abacavir sulfate/ lamivudine/zidovudine
Paxil	Paroxetine HCl		
PCE	Erythromycin particles in tablets	Trusopt	Dorzolamide HCl
		Twinrix	Hepatitis A inactivated/ hepatitis B (recombinant) vaccine
PegIntron	Peginterferon alfa-2b		
Pepcid	Famotidine		
Phenytek	Phenytoin sodium	Vancocin	Vancomycin HCl
Plavix	Clopidogrel bisulfate	Varivax	Varicella virus vaccine, live
Pletal	Cilostazol	VFEND	Voriconazole
Ponstel	Mefenamic acid	Viramune	Nevirapine
Prevacid NapraPAC	Lansoprazole/naproxen	Voltaren	Diclofenac sodium
PREVPAC	Lansoprazole/ amoxicillin/clarithromycin	VoSpire ER	Albuterol sulfate
		Vytorin	Ezetimibe/simvastatin
Prezista	Darunavir	Vyvanse	Lisdexamfetamine dimesylate
Primaxin I.M./I.V.	Imipenem/cilastatin		
Prinivil	Lisinopril	Wellbutrin	Bupropion HCl
Prinzide	Lisinopril/ hydrochlorothiazide	Zegerid	Omeprazole/sodium bicarbonate
Prograf	Tacrolimus	Ziagen	Abacavir sulfate
Proleukin	Aldesleukin	Zinacef	Cefuroxime for injection
ProQuad	Measles, mumps, rubella and varicella virus vaccine, live	Zmax	Azithromycin extended release for oral suspension
Protonix	Pantoprazole sodium	Zocor	Simvastatin
Provigil	Modafinil	Zoloft	Sertraline HCl
Prozac	Fluoxetine	Zonegran	Zonisamide
Raniclor	Cefaclor	Zosyn	Piperacillin/tazobactam
Raptiva	Efalizumab	Zovirax	Acyclovir
Recombivax HB	Hepatitis B vaccine (recombinant)	Zyban	Bupropion HCl
		Zyvox	Linezolid

*TEN = toxic epidermal necrolysis.
Note: This list is not comprehensive. For more information, refer to the specific product's full Prescribing Information.

DRUGS THAT SHOULD NOT BE CRUSHED

Listed below are various slow-release as well as enteric-coated products that should not be crushed or chewed. Slow-release (sr) represents products that are controlled-release, extended-release, long-acting, or timed-release. Enteric-coated (ec) represents products that are delayed-release.

In general, capsules containing slow-release or enteric-coated particles may be opened and their contents administered on a spoonful of soft food. Instruct patients not to chew the particles, though. (Patients should, in fact, be discouraged from chewing any medication unless it is specifically formulated for that purpose.)

This list should not be considered all-inclusive. Generic and alternate brands of some products may exist. Tablets intended for sublingual or buccal administration (not included in this list) should also be administered only as intended, in an intact form.

DRUG	FORM	DRUG	FORM	DRUG	FORM
Abletex LA	sr	Ascriptin Enteric	ec	Claritin-D 24 Hour	sr
Aciphex	ec	Atrohist Pediatric	sr	Coldamine	sr
Adalat CC	sr	Augmentin XR	sr	Coldex-A	sr
Adderall XR	sr	Avinza	sr	Concerta	sr
Advicor	sr	Azulfidine Entabs	ec	Contac 12-Hour	sr
Aerohist	sr	Bayer Aspirin Regimen	ec	Correctol	ec
Aerohist Plus	sr	Biaxin XL	sr	Coreg CR	sr
Afeditab CR	sr	Bidex-A	sr	Cotazym-S	ec
Aggrenox	sr	Bidhist	sr	Covera-HS	sr
Ala-Hist	sr	Bidhist-D	sr	CPM 8/PE 20/MSC 1.25	sr
Ala-Hist D	sr	Bisac-Evac	ec	CPM-12	sr
Aleve Cold & Sinus	sr	Biscolax	ec	Creon 5	ec
Aleve Sinus & Headache	sr	Blanex-A	sr	Creon 10	ec
Allegra-D 12 Hour	sr	Bontril Slow-Release	sr	Creon 20	ec
Allegra-D 24 Hour	sr	Bromfed	sr	Cymbalta	sr
Allerx	sr	Bromfed-PD	sr	Dairycare	ec
Allerx-D	sr	Bromfenex	sr	Dallergy	sr
Allfen	sr	Bromfenex PD	sr	Dallergy-Jr	sr
Allfen-DM	sr	Bromfenex PE	sr	Deconamine SR	sr
Alophen	ec	Bromfenex PE Pediatric	sr	Deconex	sr
Altoprev	sr	Budeprion SR	sr	Deconsal II	sr
Ambi 45/800	sr	Budeprion XL	sr	Deconex DM	sr
Ambi 45/800/30	sr	Buproban	sr	Depakote	ec
Ambi 60/580	sr	Calan SR	sr	Depakote ER	sr
Ambi 60/580/30	sr	Campral	ec	Depakote Sprinkles	ec
Ambi 80/700	sr	Carbatrol	sr	Despec SR	sr
Ambi 80/700/40	sr	Cardene SR	sr	Detrol LA	sr
Ambi 1000/55	sr	Cardizem CD	sr	Dexedrine Spansules	sr
Ambien CR	sr	Cardizem LA	sr	D-Feda II	sr
Ambifed-G	sr	Cardura XL	sr	D-Hist D	sr
Ambifed-G DM	sr	Carox Plus	sr	Diabetes Trio	sr
Amdry-C	sr	Cartia XT	sr	Diamox Sequels	sr
Amdry-D	sr	Cemill 500	sr	Dilacor XR	sr
Amibid LA	sr	Cemill 1000	sr	Dilantin	sr
Amrix	sr	Certuss-D	sr	Dilantin Kapseals	sr
Anextuss	sr	Cevi-Bid	sr	Dilatrate-SR	sr
Anti-tussive	sr	Chlorex-A	sr	Diltia XT	sr
Aquabid-DM	sr	Chlor-Phen	sr	Dilt-CD	sr
Aquatab C	sr	Chlor-Trimeton Allergy	sr	Dilt-XR	sr
Aquatab D	sr	Chlor-Trimeton Allergy	sr	Dimetane Extentabs	sr
Aquatab DM	sr	Decongestant		Disophrol Chronotab	sr
Arthrotec	ec	Cipro XR	sr	Ditropan XL	sr
Asacol	ec	Clarinex-D 24 Hour	sr	Donnatal Extentabs	sr
Ascocid-500-D	sr	Claritin-D	sr	Doryx	ec
Ascocid-1000	sr	Claritin-D 12 Hour	sr	D-Phen 1000	sr

Enteric-coated= ec   Slow-release = sr

DRUG	FORM	DRUG	FORM	DRUG	FORM
Drexophed SR	sr	Fero-Grad-500	sr	Klor-Con 10	sr
Drihist SR	sr	Ferro-Sequels	sr	Klor-Con M10	sr
Drixoral	sr	Ferrous Fumarate DS	sr	Klor-Con M15	sr
Drixoral Plus	sr	Fetrin	sr	Klor-Con M20	sr
Drixoral Sinus	sr	Flagyl ER	sr	Klotrix	sr
Drize-R	sr	Fleet Bisacodyl	ec	K-Tab	sr
Drysec	sr	Focalin XR	sr	K-Tan	sr
D-Tab	sr	Folitab 500	sr	Lescol XL	sr
Dulcolax	ec	Fortamet	sr	Levall G	sr
Duomax	sr	Fumatinic	sr	Levsinex	sr
Durahist	sr	G/P 1200/75	sr	Lexxel	sr
Durahist D	sr	Genacote	ec	Lialda	ec
Durahist PE	sr	GFN 500/DM 30	sr	Lipram 4500	ec
Duratuss	sr	GFN 550/PSE 60	sr	Lipram-PN10	ec
Duratuss CS	sr	GFN 550/PSE 60/DM 30	sr	Lipram-PN16	ec
Duratuss DA	sr	GFN 595/PSE 48	sr	Lipram-PN20	ec
Duratuss GP	sr	GFN 595/PSE 48/DM 32	sr	Liquibid-D	sr
Dynacirc CR	sr	GFN 1000/DM 50	sr	Liquibid-D 1200	sr
Dynahist-ER Pediatric	sr	GFN 1200/DM 60/PSE 60	sr	Liquibid-PD	sr
Dynex LA	sr	GFN 1200/Phenylephrine 40	sr	Lithobid	sr
Dynex VR	sr	GFN 1200/PSE 50	sr	Lodrane-12 Hour	sr
Dytan-CS	sr	Gilphex TR	sr	Lodrane-12D	sr
Easprin	ec	Giltuss TR	sr	Lodrane 24	sr
EC Naprosyn	ec	Glucophage XR	sr	Lodrane 24D	sr
Ecotrin	ec	Glucotrol XL	sr	Lohist-12	sr
Ecotrin Adult Low Strength	ec	Glumetza	sr	Lohist-12D	sr
Ecotrin Maximum Strength	ec	Guaifenex DM	sr	Lusonex	sr
Ecpirin	ec	Guaifenex GP	sr	Mag Delay	ec
Ed A-Hist	sr	Guaifenex PSE 60	sr	Mag64	ec
Effexor-XR	sr	Guaifenex PSE 80	sr	Mag-SR Plus Calcium	sr
Efidac 24 Chlorpheniramine	sr	Guaifenex PSE 120	sr	Mag-Tab SR	sr
Efidac 24 Pseudoephedrine	sr	H 9600 SR	sr	Maxifed	sr
Enablex	sr	Halfprin	ec	Maxifed DM	sr
Endal	sr	Hemax	sr	Maxifed DMX	sr
Entab-DM	sr	Histacol LA	sr	Maxifed-G	sr
Entercote	ec	Hista-Vent DA	sr	Maxiphen DM	sr
Entex LA	sr	Hista-Vent PSE	sr	Medent DM	sr
Entex PSE	sr	Humavent LA	sr	Medent PE	sr
Entocort EC	ec	Humibid	sr	Mega-C	sr
Equetro	sr	Humibid DM	sr	Melfiat	sr
Ery-Tab	ec	Humibid LA	sr	Menopause Trio	sr
Eskalith-CR	sr	Iberet-500	sr	Mestinon Timespan	sr
Execof	sr	Iberet-Folic-500	sr	Metadate CD	sr
Exefen-DM	sr	Icar-C Plus SR	sr	Metadate ER	sr
Exefen-DMX	sr	Imdur	sr	Methylin ER	sr
Exefen-PD	sr	Inderal LA	sr	Micro-K	sr
Extendryl Jr	sr	Indocin SR	sr	Micro-K 10	sr
Extendryl SR	sr	Innopran XL	sr	Mild-C	sr
Extress-30	sr	Invega	sr	Mindal DM	sr
Exetuss-DM	sr	Isochron	sr	Montephen	sr
Extendryl G	sr	Isopro	sr	MS Contin	sr
Extress-60	sr	Isoptin SR	sr	Mucinex	sr
Feen-A-Mint	ec	Kadian	sr	Mucinex D	sr
Femilax	ec	Kaon-Cl 10	sr	Mucinex DM	sr
Fero-Folic-500	sr	Klor-Con 8	sr	Multi-Ferrous Folic	sr

DRUG	FORM	DRUG	FORM	DRUG	FORM
Multiret Folic-500	sr	Paxil CR	sr	Respa-PE	sr
Mydex	sr	PCE Dispertab	sr	Respahist	sr
Mydocs	sr	PCM LA	sr	Respahist-II	sr
Myfortic	ec	Pendex	sr	Respaire-60 SR	sr
Nacon	sr	Pentasa	sr	Respaire-120 SR	sr
Nalex-A	sr	Pentopak	sr	Rhinacon A	sr
Naprelan	sr	Pentoxil	sr	Risperdal Consta	sr
Nasatab LA	sr	Phenabid	sr	Ritalin LA	sr
New Ami-Tex LA	sr	Phenabid DM	sr	Ritalin-SR	sr
Nexium	ec	Phenavent	sr	Rodex Forte	sr
Niaspan	sr	Phenavent D	sr	Rondec-TR	sr
Nicomide\	sr	Phenavent LA	sr	Ru-Tuss	sr
Nifediac CC	sr	Phenavent PED	sr	Ryneze	sr
Nifedical XL	sr	Phendiet-105	sr	Rythmol SR	sr
Nitrocot	sr	Phenytek	sr	SAM-e	ec
Nitro-Time	sr	Phlemex-PE	sr	Sanctura XR	sr
Nohist	sr	Plendil	sr	Scopohist-PE	sr
Nohist-Plus	sr	Poly Hist Forte	sr	Seroquel XR	sr
Nohist-Plus Jr	sr	Poly-Vent	sr	Simuc-GP	sr
Norel SR	sr	Poly-Vent Jr	sr	Sinemet CR	sr
Norpace CR	sr	Prehist D	sr	Sinutuss DM	sr
Obstetrix EC	ec	Prevacid	ec	Sinuvent PE	sr
Omnihist LA	sr	Prilosec	ec	Slo-Niacin	sr
Opana ER	sr	Prilosec OTC	sr	Slow Fe	sr
Oramorph SR	sr	Procanbid	sr	Slow Fe With Folic Acid	sr
Oracea	sr	Procardia XL	sr	Slow-Mag	ec
Oruvail	sr	Prolex PD	sr	Solodyn	sr
Oxycontin	sr	Prolex-D	sr	St. Joseph Pain Reliever	ec
Palcaps 10	ec	Pronestyl-SR	sr	Stahist	sr
Palcaps 20	ec	Proquin XR	sr	Sudafed 12 Hour	sr
Pancrease	ec	Prosed EC	ec	Sudafed 24 Hour	sr
Pancrease MT 10	ec	Proset-D	sr	Sudahist	sr
Pancrease MT 16	ec	Protid	sr	Sudal DM	sr
Pancrease MT 20	ec	Protonix	ec	Sudal SR	sr
Pancrecarb MS-16	ec	Prozac Weekly	ec	Sudatex-DM	sr
Pancrecarb MS-4	ec	Pseubrom	sr	Sudatex-G	sr
Pancrecarb MS-8	ec	Pseubrom-PD	sr	Sudatrate	sr
Pancrelipase 4500	ec	Pseudocot-C	sr	Sudex Tab	sr
Pangestyme CN-10	ec	Pseudocot-G	sr	Sular	sr
Pangestyme CN-20	ec	Pseudovent	sr	Sulfazine EC	ec
Pangestyme EC	ec	Pseudovent 400	sr	Symax Duotab	sr
Pangestyme MT16	ec	Pseudovent DM	sr	Symax-SR	sr
Pangestyme UL12	ec	Pseudovent PED	sr	Tarka	sr
Pangestyme UL18	ec	Quibron-T/SR	sr	Taztia XT	sr
Pangestyme UL20	ec	Quindal	sr	Tegretol-XR	sr
Panmist DM	sr	Ralix	sr	Tenuate Dospan	sr
Panmist Jr	sr	Ranexa	sr	Theo-24	sr
Panmist LA	sr	Razadyne ER	sr	Theochron	sr
Panocaps	ec	Reliable Gentle Laxative	ec	Theo-Time	sr
Panocaps MT 16	ec	Rescon-Jr	sr	Tiazac	sr
Panocaps MT 20	ec	Rescon-MX	sr	Time-Hist	sr
Papacon	sr	Respa-1ST	sr	Toprol XL	sr
Para-Time SR	sr	Respa-AR	sr	Totalday	sr
Paser	sr	Respa-BR	sr	Touro Allergy	sr
Pavacot	sr	Respa-DM	sr	Touro CC	sr

Enteric-coated= ec   **Slow-release = sr**

DRUGS THAT SHOULD NOT BE CRUSHED

DRUG	FORM	DRUG	FORM	DRUG	FORM
Touro CC-LD	sr	Ultrase	ec	We Mist II LA	sr
Touro DM	sr	Ultrase MT12	ec	Wellbid-D	sr
Touro HC	sr	Ultrase MT18	ec	Wellbid-D 1200	sr
Touro LA	sr	Ultrase MT20	ec	Wellbutrin SR	sr
Touro LA-LD	sr	Uniphyl	sr	Wellbutrin XL	sr
Tranxene-SD	sr	Uni-Tex	sr	Wobenzym N	ec
Trental	sr	Urimax	ec	Woman's Wellbeing Menopause Relief	ec
Trikof-D	sr	Uritact-EC	ec		
Trinalin Repetabs	sr	Urocit-K 5	sr	Xanax XR	sr
Trituss-ER	sr	Urocit-K 10	sr	Xedec II	sr
Tussafed-LA	sr	Uroxatral	sr	Xiral	sr
Tussall-ER	sr	Utira	sr	Xpect-AT	sr
Tussi-Bid	sr	Veracolate	ec	Xpect-HC	sr
Tussicaps	sr	Verelan	sr	Zephrex LA	sr
Tusso-DM	sr	Verelan PM	sr	Zmax	sr
Tusso-HC	sr	Videx EC	ec	Zorprin	sr
Tylenol Arthritis	sr	Vivotif Berna	ec	Zotex-12D	sr
Ultrabrom	sr	Voltaren	ec	Zyban	sr
Ultrabrom PD	sr	Voltaren-XR	sr	Zymase	ec
Ultracaps MT 20	ec	Vospire	sr	Zyrtec-D	sr
Ultram ER	sr	We Mist LA	sr		

Enteric-coated = ec   Slow-release = sr

A262 PDR® Concise Drug Guide

ADMINISTRATION GUIDELINES FOR EAR DROPS

1. Wash hands thoroughly with soap and water.
2. Carefully wash and dry outside of the ear, taking care not to get water into the ear canal.
3. Warm ear drops to body temperature by holding the container in the palm of your hand for a few minutes.
4. Tilt head to the side, or lie down with the affected ear up. Use gentle restraint for an infant or a young child.
5. Position the dropper tip near, but not inside, the ear canal opening. **NOTE:** To prevent contamination and avoid injuring the ear, do not allow the dropper to touch the ear.
6. Pull ear backward and upward to open the ear canal and place the proper number of drops into the ear canal. Replace the cap on the container.
7. Gently press the small, flat skin flap over the ear canal opening to force out air bubbles and to push the drops down the ear canal.
8. Stay in the same position for the length of time indicated on the product instructions, or gently place a clean piece of cotton into the ear to prevent draining of medication. Do not leave it in the ear longer than one hour.
9. Repeat the procedure in the other ear, if needed.
10. Gently wipe the medication off the outside of the ear, using caution to avoid getting moisture in the ear canal.
11. Do not rinse the dropper after use. Wipe the tip of the dropper with a clean tissue and keep the container tightly closed.
12. Wash hands.

Counseling tips:
- If the drops are a suspension or if the label indicates, shake well before using.
- Do not warm the eardrop container in warm water. Hot ear drops can cause ear pain, nausea, and dizziness.
- Avoid contaminating applicator tip to preserve the sterility of the dropper.

ADMINISTRATION GUIDELINES FOR EYE DROPS & OINTMENT

Administration guidelines for eye drops:

1. Wash hands thoroughly.
2. Tilt head back.
3. Gently pull the lower eyelid away from the eye to create a pocket.
4. Hold the bottle upside down and look up just before applying a single drop. **NOTE:** To prevent contamination, do not let the tip of the eye drop applicator touch any surface (including the eye or eyelid). When not in use, keep the container tightly closed.
5. After applying the drop, look down for several seconds (still holding the eyelid away from the eye).
6. Slowly release the eyelid and close the eyes for 1 to 2 minutes. Do not blink.
7. Gently press on the inside corner of the eye (where the eyelid meets the nose) with a finger.
8. Blot excessive solution from around the eye with a tissue.

Administration guidelines for eye ointment:

1. Wash hands thoroughly.
2. Tilt head back.
3. Gently grasp lower outer eyelid below lashes, and pull eyelid away from the eye.
4. Place ointment tube over eye by directly looking at it. With a sweeping motion, place ¼ to ½-inch of ointment inside the lower eyelid by gently squeezing the tube. **NOTE:** To prevent contamination, do not let the tip of the tube touch any surface (including the eye or eyelid). When not in use, keep the tube tightly closed.
5. Slowly release eyelid and close eyes for 1 to 2 minutes.
6. Blot excessive ointment from around the eye with a tissue.
7. Vision may be temporarily blurred. Until vision clears, avoid activities requiring good visual ability.

Counseling tips:

- If having difficulty determining whether an eye dropper has touched the eye surface, keep the dropper in a refrigerator (not in a freezer).
- If more than one drop is needed, wait at least 5 minutes before instilling the next drop to prevent flushing away or diluting the first drop.
- If both eye drop and ointment therapy are needed, instill the eye drop at least 10 minutes before the ointment.

USE-IN-PREGNANCY RATINGS

The U.S. Food and Drug Administration's Use-in-Pregnancy rating system weighs the degree to which available information has ruled out risk to the fetus against the drug's potential benefit to the patient. Below is a listing of drugs (by generic name) for which ratings are available.

X

Contraindicated in pregnancy

Studies in animals or humans, or investigational or postmarketing reports, have demonstrated fetal risk which clearly outweighs any possible benefit to the patient.

Acetohydroxamic Acid
Acitretin
Ambrisentan
Amlodipine Besylate/
  Atorvastatin Calcium
Anisindione
Atorvastatin Calcium
Bexarotene
Bicalutamide
Bosentan
Cetrorelix Acetate
Clomiphene Citrate
Desogestrel/Ethinyl Estradiol
Diclofenac Sodium/Misoprostol
Dihydroergotamine Mesylate
Dutasteride
Estazolam
Estradiol
Estradiol Acetate
Estradiol Cypionate/
  Medroxyprogesterone Acetate
Estradiol Valerate
Estradiol/Levonorgestrel
Estradiol/Norethindrone Acetate
Estrogens, Conjugated
Estrogens, Conjugated, Synthetic A
Estrogens, Conjugated/
  Medroxyprogesterone Acetate
Estrogens, Esterified
Estrogens, Esterified/
  Methyltestosterone
Estropipate
Ethinyl Estradiol/Drospirenone
Ethinyl Estradiol/
  Ethynodiol Diacetate
Ethinyl Estradiol/Etonogestrel
Ethinyl Estradiol/Ferrous
  Fumarate/Norethindrone Acetate
Ethinyl Estradiol/
  Levonorgestrel
Ethinyl Estradiol/Norelgestromin
Ethinyl Estradiol/Norethindrone
Ethinyl Estradiol/Norethindrone
  Acetate

Ethinyl Estradiol/
  Norgestimate
Ethinyl Estradiol/Norgestrel
Ezetimibe/Simvastatin
Finasteride
Fluorouracil
Fluoxymesterone
Flurazepam Hydrochloride
Fluvastatin Sodium
Follitropin Alfa
Follitropin Beta
Ganirelix Acetate
Goserelin Acetate
Histrelin Acetate
Hydromorphone Hydrochloride
Interferon Alfa-2B,
  Recombinant/Ribavirin
Iodine I 131 Tositumomab/
  Tositumomab
Isotretinoin
Leflunomide
Leuprolide Acetate
Levonorgestrel
Lovastatin
Lovastatin/Niacin
Medroxyprogesterone Acetate
Megestrol Acetate
Menotropins
Mequinol/Tretinoin
Mestranol/Norethindrone
Methotrexate Sodium
Methyltestosterone
Miglustat
Misoprostol
Nafarelin Acetate
Norethindrone
Norethindrone Acetate
Norgestrel
Oxandrolone
Oxymetholone
Plicamycin
Pravastatin Sodium
Pravastatin Sodium/
  Aspirin Buffered
Raloxifene Hydrochloride
Ribavirin
Rosuvastatin Calcium
Simvastatin
Tazarotene
Testosterone
Testosterone Enanthate
Thalidomide
Tositumomab
Triptorelin Pamoate
Warfarin Sodium

D

Positive evidence of risk

Investigational or postmarketing data show risk to the fetus. Nevertheless, potential benefits may outweigh the potential risk.

Alitretinoin
Alprazolam
Altretamine
Amiodarone Hydrochloride
Amlodipine Besylate/
  Benazepril Hydrochloride
Amlodipine Besylate/Olmesartan
  Medoxomil
Amlodipine Besylate/Valsartan*
Anastrozole
Arsenic Trioxide
Aspirin Buffered/
  Pravastatin Sodium
Aspirin/Dipyridamole
Atenolol
Azathioprine
Azathioprine Sodium
Benazepril Hydrochloride*
Benazepril Hydrochloride/
  Hydrochlorothiazide*
Bortezomib
Busulfan
Candesartan Cilexetil*
Candesartan Cilexetil/
  Hydrochlorothiazide*
Capecitabine
Captopril*
Carbamazepine
Carboplatin
Carmustine (BiCNU)
Chlorambucil
Cladribine
Clofarabine
Clonazepam
Cytarabine Liposome
Dactinomycin
Daunorubicin Citrate Liposome
Daunorubicin Hydrochloride
Demeclocycline Hydrochloride
Dexrazoxane Hydrochloride
Diazepam
Divalproex Sodium
Docetaxel
Doxorubicin Hydrochloride
Doxorubicin Hydrochloride Liposome
Doxycycline

---

* Category C or D depending on the trimester the drug is given.

Doxycycline Calcium
Doxycycline Hyclate
Doxycycline Monohydrate
Efavirenz
Enalapril Maleate*
Enalapril Maleate/
    Hydrochlorothiazide*
Epirubicin Hydrochloride
Eprosartan Mesylate
Erlotinib
Exemestane
Floxuridine
Fludarabine Phosphate
Flutamide
Fosinopril Sodium*
Fosinopril Sodium/
    Hydrochlorothiazide*
Fosphenytoin Sodium
Fulvestrant
Gefitinib
Gemcitabine Hydrochloride
Gemtuzumab Ozogamicin
Genistein/Zinc Chelazome/
    Cholecalciferol
Goserelin Acetate
Ibritumomab Tiuxetan
Idarubicin Hydrochloride
Ifosfamide
Imatinib Mesylate
Irbesartan*
Irbesartan/Hydrochlorothiazide*
Irinotecan Hydrochloride
Ixabepilone
Letrozole
Lisinopril*
Lisinopril/Hydrochlorothiazide*
Lithium Carbonate
Losartan Potassium*
Losartan Potassium/
    Hydrochlorothiazide*
Mechlorethamine Hydrochloride
Melphalan
Melphalan Hydrochloride
Mephobarbital
Mercaptopurine
Methimazole
Midazolam Hydrochloride
Minocycline Hydrochloride
Mitoxantrone Hydrochloride
Moexipril Hydrochloride*
Moexipril Hydrochloride/
    Hydrochlorothiazide*
Nelarabine
Neomycin Sulfate/
    Polymyxin B Sulfate
Nicotine
Nilotinib Hydrochloride Monohydrate
Olmesartan Medoxomil
Oxaliplatin
Pamidronate Disodium
Pemetrexed
Penicillamine
Pentobarbital Sodium
Pentostatin

Perindopril Erbumine*
Phenytoin
Procarbazine Hydrochloride
Quinapril Hydrochloride*
Quinapril Hydrochloride/
    Hydrochlorothiazide*
Ramipril*
Sorafenib
Streptomycin Sulfate
Sunitinib
Tamoxifen Citrate
Telmisartan
Telmisartan/
    Hydrochlorothiazide
Temozolomide
Temsirolimus
Thioguanine
Tigecycline
Tobramycin
Topotecan Hydrochloride
Toremifene Citrate
Trandolapril*
Trandolapril/Verapamil
    Hydrochloride*
Tretinoin
Valproate Sodium
Valproic Acid
Valsartan*
Valsartan/Hydrochlorothiazide*
Vinorelbine Tartrate
Voriconazole
Zoledronic Acid

C

Risk cannot be ruled out

Human studies are lacking, and animal studies are either positive for risk or are lacking as well. However, potential benefits may outweigh the potential risk.

Abacavir Sulfate
Abacavir Sulfate/Lamivudine
Abacavir Sulfate/
    Lamivudine/Zidovudine
Abciximab
Acamprosate Calcium
Acetaminophen
Acetaminophen/
    Butalbital/Caffeine
Acetaminophen/Caffeine/
    Chlorpheniramine
    Maleate/Hydrocodone
    Bitartrate/Phenylephrine
    Hydrochloride
Acetazolamide
Acetazolamide Sodium
Acyclovir
Adapalene
Adefovir Dipivoxil

Adenosine
Alatrofloxacin Mesylate
Albendazole
Albumin (Human)
Albuterol
Albuterol Sulfate
Albuterol Sulfate/
    Ipratropium Bromide
Alclometasone Dipropionate
Aldesleukin
Alemtuzumab
Alendronate Sodium
Alendronate Sodium/
    Cholecalciferol
Allopurinol Sodium
Almotriptan Malate
Alpha1-Proteinase Inhibitor (Human)
Alprostadil
Alteplase
Amantadine Hydrochloride
Amifostine
Aminocaproic Acid
Aminohippurate Sodium
Aminolevulinic Acid Hydrochloride
Aminosalicylic Acid
Amlodipine Besylate
Amlodipine Besylate/Benazepril
    Hydrochloride
Amlodipine Besylate/
    Olmesartan Medoxomil*
Amlodipine Besylate/Valsartan*
Amoxicillin/Clarithromycin/
    Lansoprazole
Amphetamine Aspartate/
    Amphetamine Sulfate/
    Dextroamphetamine Saccharate/
    Dextroamphetamine Sulfate
Amprenavir
Anagrelide Hydrochloride
Anthralin
Antihemophilic Factor (Human)
Antihemophilic Factor (Recombinant)
Anti-Inhibitor Coagulant Complex
Anti-Thymocyte Globulin
Apomorphine Hydrochloride
Aripiprazole
Armodafinil
Arnica Montana/Herbals,
    Multiple/Sulfur
Asparaginase
Atomoxetine Hydrochloride
Atovaquone
Atovaquone/Proguanil Hydrochloride
Atropine Sulfate/Benzoic
    Acid/Hyoscyamine
    Sulfate/Methenamine/
    Methylene Blue/Phenyl Salicylate
Atropine Sulfate/Hyoscyamine
    Sulfate/Scopolamine
    Hydrobromide
Azelastine Hydrochloride
Bacitracin Zinc/Neomycin
    Sulfate/Polymyxin B Sulfate
Baclofen

BCG, Live (Intravesical)
Becaplermin
Beclomethasone Dipropionate
Beclomethasone Dipropionate
  Monohydrate
Benazepril Hydrochloride*
Benazepril Hydrochloride/
  Hydrochlorothiazide*
Bendroflumethiazide
Benzocaine
Benzonatate
Benzoyl Peroxide
Benzoyl Peroxide/Clindamycin
Benzoyl Peroxide/Erythromycin
Betamethasone Dipropionate
Betamethasone
  Dipropionate/Clotrimazole
Betamethasone Valerate
Betaxolol Hydrochloride
Bethanechol Chloride
Bevacizumab
Bimatoprost
Bisacodyl/Polyethylene
  Glycol/Potassium Chloride/Sodium
  Bicarbonate/Sodium Chloride
Bisoprolol Fumarate
Bisoprolol Fumarate/
  Hydrochlorothiazide
Bitolterol Mesylate
Black Widow Spider
  Antivenin (Equine)
Botulinum Toxin Type A
Botulinum Toxin Type B
Brimonidine Tartrate/Timolol Maleate
Brinzolamide
Brompheniramine
  Maleate/Dextromethorphan
  Hydrobromide/Phenylephrine
  Hydrochloride
Budesonide
Bupivacaine Hydrochloride
Bupivacaine Hydrochloride/
  Epinephrine Bitartrate
Buprenorphine Hydrochloride
Buprenorphine
  Hydrochloride/Naloxone
  Hydrochloride
Butabarbital/Hyoscyamine
  Hydrobromide/ Phenazopyridine
  Hydrochloride
Butalbital/Acetaminophen
Butenafine Hydrochloride
Butoconazole Nitrate
Butorphanol Tartrate
Caffeine Citrate
Calcipotriene
Calcitonin-Salmon
Calcitriol
Calcium Acetate
Candesartan Cilexetil*
Candesartan Cilexetil/
  Hydrochlorothiazide*
Capreomycin Sulfate

Captopril*
Carbetapentane
  Tannate/Chlorpheniramine Tannate
Carbetapentane
  Tannate/Chlorpheniramine
  Tannate/Ephedrine
  Tannate/Phenylephrine Tannate
Carbidopa/Entacapone/
  Levodopa
Carbidopa/Levodopa
Carbinoxamine Maleate/
  Dextromethorphan Hydrobromide/
  Pseudoephedrine Hydrochloride
Carteolol Hydrochloride
Carvedilol
Caspofungin Acetate
Celecoxib
Cetirizine Hydrochloride
Cetuximab
Cevimeline Hydrochloride
Chloramphenicol
Chloroprocaine Hydrochloride
Chlorothiazide
Chlorothiazide Sodium
Chlorpheniramine Maleate/
  Methscopolamine Nitrate/
  Phenylephrine Hydrochloride
Chlorpheniramine Maleate/
  Pseudoephedrine Hydrochloride
Chlorpheniramine
  Polistirex/Hydrocodone Polistirex
Chlorpheniramine
  Tannate/Phenylephrine Tannate
Chlorpropamide
Chlorthalidone/Clonidine
  Hydrochloride
Choline Magnesium Trisalicylate
Cidofovir
Cilostazol
Cinacalcet Hydrochloride
Ciprofloxacin Hydrochloride
Ciprofloxacin Hydrochloride/
  Hydrocortisone
Ciprofloxacin/Dexamethasone
Citalopram Hydrobromide
Clarithromycin
Clobetasol Propionate
Clonidine
Clonidine Hydrochloride
Codeine Phosphate/
  Acetaminophen
Colistimethate Sodium
Colistin Sulfate/Hydrocortisone
  Acetate/Neomycin Sulfate/
  Thonzonium Bromide
Corticorelin Ovine Triflutate
Cyanocobalamin
Cycloserine
Cyclosporine
Cytomegalovirus Immune Globulin
Dacarbazine
Daclizumab
Dantrolene Sodium

Dapsone
Darbepoetin Alfa
Darifenacin
Deferoxamine Mesylate
Delavirdine Mesylate
Denileukin Diftitox
Desloratadine
Desloratadine/Pseudoephedrine
  Sulfate
Desoximetasone
Dexamethasone
Dexamethasone Sodium Phosphate
Dexmethylphenidate Hydrochloride
Dexrazoxane
Dextroamphetamine Sulfate
Diazoxide
Dichlorphenamide
Diclofenac Potassium
Diclofenac Sodium
Diflorasone Diacetate
Diflunisal
Digoxin
Digoxin Immune Fab (Ovine)
Diltiazem Hydrochloride
Dimethyl Sulfoxide
Dinoprostone
Diphtheria & Tetanus Toxoids and
  Acellular Pertussis Vaccine
  Adsorbed
Diphtheria & Tetanus Toxoids and
  Acellular Pertussis Vaccine
  Adsorbed/Hepatitis B Vaccine,
  Recombinant/Poliovirus Vaccine
  Inactivated
Dirithromycin
Dofetilide
Donepezil Hydrochloride
Dorzolamide Hydrochloride
Dorzolamide Hydrochloride/Timolol
  Maleate
Doxazosin Mesylate
Dronabinol
Drotrecogin Alfa (Activated)
Duloxetine Hydrochloride
Echothiophate Iodide
Econazole Nitrate
Efalizumab
Eflornithine Hydrochloride
Eletriptan Hydrobromide
Enalapril Maleate*
Enalapril Maleate/Felodipine*
Enalapril Maleate/
  Hydrochlorothiazide*
Entacapone
Entecavir
Epinastine Hydrochloride
Epinephrine
Epoetin Alfa
Eprosartan Mesylate
Erythromycin Ethylsuccinate/
  Sulfisoxazole Acetyl
Escitalopram Oxalate
Eszopiclone

* Category C or D depending on the trimester the drug is given.

Ethionamide
Ethotoin
Etidronate Disodium
Exenatide
Ezetimibe
Factor IX Complex
Felodipine
Fenofibrate
Fentanyl
Fentanyl Citrate
Fentanyl Hydrochloride
Ferrous Fumarate/Folic Acid/
  Intrinsic Factor Concentrate/
  Liver Preparations/
  Vitamin B12/Vitamin C/
  Vitamins with Iron
Fexofenadine Hydrochloride
Fexofenadine Hydrochloride/
  Pseudoephedrine Hydrochloride
Filgrastim
Flecainide Acetate
Fluconazole
Flucytosine
Fludrocortisone Acetate
Flumazenil
Flunisolide
Fluocinolone Acetonide
Fluocinolone Acetonide/
  Hydroquinone/Tretinoin
Fluocinonide
Fluorometholone
Fluorometholone/Sulfacetamide
  Sodium
Fluoxetine Hydrochloride
Fluoxetine Hydrochloride/
  Olanzapine
Flurandrenolide
Flurbiprofen Sodium
Fluticasone Furoate
Fluticasone Propionate
Fluticasone Propionate HFA
Fluticasone Propionate/Salmeterol
  Xinafoate
Fomivirsen Sodium
Formoterol Fumarate
Fosamprenavir Calcium
Foscarnet Sodium*
Fosinopril Sodium*
Fosinopril Sodium/
  Hydrochlorothiazide*
Frovatriptan Succinate
Furosemide
Gabapentin
Gallium Nitrate
Ganciclovir
Ganciclovir Sodium
Gatifloxacin
Gemfibrozil
Gemifloxacin Mesylate
Gentamicin Sulfate
Gentamicin Sulfate/
  Prednisolone Acetate
Glimepiride
Glipizide

Glipizide/Metformin Hydrochloride
Globulin, Immune (Human)
Globulin, Immune (Human)/
  Rho (D) Immune Globulin
  (Human)
Glyburide
Gramicidin/Neomycin Sulfate/
  Polymyxin B Sulfate
Guaifenesin/Hydrocodone Bitartrate
Haemophilus B Conjugate Vaccine
Haemophilus B Conjugate
  Vaccine/Hepatitis B Vaccine,
  Recombinant
Halobetasol Propionate
Haloperidol Decanoate
Hemin
Heparin Sodium
Hepatitis A Vaccine, Inactivated
Hepatitis A Vaccine,
  Inactivated/Hepatitis B Vaccine,
  Recombinant
Hepatitis B Immune Globulin
  (Human)
Hepatitis B Vaccine, Recombinant
Homatropine
  Methylbromide/Hydrocodone
  Bitartrate
Homeopathic Formulations
Hydralazine Hydrochloride/Isosorbide
  Dinitrate
Hydrochlorothiazide
Hydrocodone Bitartrate
Hydrocodone
  Bitartrate/Acetaminophen
Hydrocodone Bitartrate/Ibuprofen
Hydrocortisone
Hydrocortisone Acetate
Hydrocortisone Acetate/Neomycin
  Sulfate/Polymyxin B Sulfate
Hydrocortisone Acetate/Pramoxine
  Hydrochloride
Hydrocortisone Butyrate
Hydrocortisone Probutate
Hydrocortisone/Neomycin
  Sulfate/Polymyxin B Sulfate
Hydromorphone Hydrochloride
Hydroquinone
Hyoscyamine Sulfate
Ibandronate Sodium
Ibutilide Fumarate
Iloprost
Imiglucerase
Imipenem/Cilastatin
Imiquimod
Immune Globulin Intravenous
  (Human)
Indinavir Sulfate
Indocyanine Green
Influenza Virus Vaccine
Insulin Aspart
Insulin Aspart Protamine,
  Human/Insulin Aspart, Human
Insulin Glargine
Insulin Glulisine

Interferon Alfa-2B, Recombinant
Interferon Alfacon-1
Interferon Alfa-N3
  (Human Leukocyte Derived)
Interferon Beta-1A
Interferon Beta-1B
Interferon Gamma-1B
Iodoquinol/Hydrocortisone
Irbesartan*
Irbesartan/Hydrochlorothiazide*
Iron Dextran
Isoniazid/
  Pyrazinamide/Rifampin
Isosorbide Mononitrate
Isradipine
Itraconazole
Ivermectin
Ketoconazole
Ketorolac Tromethamine
Ketotifen Fumarate
Labetalol Hydrochloride
Lamivudine
Lamivudine/Zidovudine
Lamotrigine
Lanreotide Acetate
Lanthanum Carbonate
Latanoprost
Levalbuterol Hydrochloride
Levalbuterol Tartrate
Levamisole Hydrochloride
Levetiracetam
Levobunolol Hydrochloride
Levofloxacin
Linezolid
Lisinopril*
Lisinopril/Hydrochlorothiazide*
Lopinavir/Ritonavir
Losartan Potassium*
Losartan Potassium/
  Hydrochlorothiazide*
Loteprednol Etabonate
Mafenide Acetate
Magnesium Salicylate Tetrahydrate
Measles Virus Vaccine, Live
Measles, Mumps & Rubella Virus
  Vaccine, Live
Mebendazole
Mecamylamine Hydrochloride
Mecasermin [rDNA Origin]
Medrysone
Mefenamic Acid
Mefloquine Hydrochloride
Meloxicam
Meningococcal Polysaccharide
  Diphtheria Toxoid Conjugate
  Vaccine
Meningococcal Polysaccharide
  Vaccine
Meperidine Hydrochloride
Mepivacaine Hydrochloride
Metaproterenol Sulfate
Metaraminol Bitartrate
Metformin Hydrochloride/Pioglitazone
  Hydrochloride

Metformin Hydrochloride/
    Rosiglitazone Maleate
Methamphetamine Hydrochloride
Methazolamide
Methenamine Mandelate/
    Sodium Acid Phosphate
Methocarbamol
Methoxsalen
Methoxy Polyethylene Glycol/
    Epoetin Beta
Methscopolamine Nitrate/
    Pseudoephedrine Hydrochloride
Methyldopa/Chlorothiazide
Methyldopa/Hydrochlorothiazide
Methylphenidate Hydrochloride
Metipranolol
Metoprolol Succinate
Metoprolol Tartrate
Metoprolol
    Tartrate/Hydrochlorothiazide
Metyrosine
Mexiletine Hydrochloride
Micafungin Sodium
Midodrine Hydrochloride
Mivacurium Chloride
Modafinil
Moexipril Hydrochloride*
Moexipril Hydrochloride/
    Hydrochlorothiazide*
Mometasone Furoate
Mometasone Furoate Monohydrate
Morphine Sulfate
Morphine Sulfate, Liposomal
Moxifloxacin Hydrochloride
Mumps Virus Vaccine, Live
Muromonab-CD3
Mycophenolate Mofetil
Mycophenolate Mofetil Hydrochloride
Mycophenolic Acid
Nabumetone
Nadolol
Nadolol/Bendroflumethiazide
Naloxone Hydrochloride/
    Pentazocine Hydrochloride
Naltrexone Hydrochloride
Naphazoline Hydrochloride
Naproxen
Naproxen Sodium
Naratriptan Hydrochloride
Natamycin
Nateglinide
Nebivolol
Nefazodone Hydrochloride
Neomycin Sulfate/Dexamethasone
    Sodium Phosphate
Neomycin Sulfate/Polymyxin B
    Sulfate/Prednisolone Acetate
Nesiritide
Nevirapine
Niacin
Nicardipine Hydrochloride
Nifedipine
Nilutamide
Nimodipine

Nisoldipine
Nitroglycerin
Norfloxacin
Ofloxacin
Olanzapine
Olmesartan Medoxomil/
    Hydrochlorothiazide
Olopatadine Hydrochloride
Olsalazine Sodium
Omega-3-Acid Ethyl Esters
Omeprazole
Oprelvekin
Orphenadrine Citrate
Oseltamivir Phosphate
Oxcarbazepine
Oxycodone Hydrochloride/
    Acetaminophen
Oxycodone Hydrochloride/ Ibuprofen
Oxymorphone Hydrochloride
Palifermin
Palivizumab
Pancrelipase
Paricalcitol
Paroxetine Hydrochloride
Paroxetine Mesylate
Peg-3350/Potassium Chloride/
    Sodium Bicarbonate/
    Sodium Chloride
Pegademase Bovine
Pegaspargase
Pegfilgrastim
Peginterferon Alfa-2A
Peginterferon Alfa-2B
Pemirolast Potassium
Pentazocine Hydrochloride/
    Acetaminophen
Pentoxifylline
Perindopril Erbumine*
Phenoxybenzamine Hydrochloride
Phentermine Hydrochloride
Pilocarpine Hydrochloride
Pimecrolimus
Pimozide
Pioglitazone Hydrochloride
Pirbuterol Acetate
Piroxicam
Plasma Fractions, Human/
    Rabies Immune Globulin (Human)
Plasma Protein Fraction (Human)
Pneumococcal Vaccine, Diphtheria
    Conjugate
Pneumococcal Vaccine, Polyvalent
Podofilox
Polyethylene Glycol
Polyethylene Glycol/
    Potassium Chloride/Sodium
    Bicarbonate/Sodium Chloride
Polyethylene Glycol/Potassium
    Chloride/Sodium
    Bicarbonate/Sodium
    Chloride/Sodium Sulfate
Polymyxin B Sulfate/
    Trimethoprim Sulfate
Polythiazide/Prazosin Hydrochloride

Porfimer Sodium
Potassium Acid Phosphate
Potassium Chloride
Potassium Citrate
Potassium Phosphate/
    Sodium Phosphate
Pralidoxime Chloride
Pramipexole Dihydrochloride
Pramlintide Acetate
Pramoxine Hydrochloride/
    Hydrocortisone Acetate
Prazosin Hydrochloride
Prednisolone Acetate
Prednisolone Acetate/
    Sulfacetamide Sodium
Prednisolone Sodium Phosphate
Pregabalin
Promethazine Hydrochloride
Propafenone Hydrochloride
Proparacaine Hydrochloride
Propranolol Hydrochloride
Pseudoephedrine Hydrochloride
Pyrimethamine
Quetiapine Fumarate
Quinapril Hydrochloride*
Quinidine Sulfate
Rabies Vaccine
Raltegravir Potassium
Ramelteon
Ramipril*
Rasburicase
Remifentanil Hydrochloride
Repaglinide
Reteplase
Rho (D) Immune Globulin (Human)
Rifampin
Rifapentine
Rifaximin
Riluzole
Rimantadine Hydrochloride
Risedronate Sodium
Risedronate Sodium/
    Calcium Carbonate
Risperidone
Rituximab
Rizatriptan Benzoate
Rocuronium Bromide
Rofecoxib
Ropinirole Hydrochloride
Rosiglitazone Maleate
Rotigotine
Rubella Virus Vaccine, Live
Salmeterol Xinafoate
Sapropterin Dihydrochloride
Sargramostim
Scopolamine
Selegiline Hydrochloride
Selenium Sulfide
Sertaconazole Nitrate
Sertraline Hydrochloride
Sevelamer Carbonate
Sevelamer Hydrochloride
Sibutramine Hydrochloride
    Monohydrate

* Category C or D depending on the trimester the drug is given.

Sirolimus
Sodium Benzoate/
    Sodium Phenylacelate
Sodium Phenylbutyrate
Sodium Polystyrene Sulfonate
Sodium Sulfacetamide/Sulfur
Solifenacin Succinate
Somatropin
Somatropin (rDNA Origin)
Stavudine
Streptokinase
Succimer
Sulfacetamide Sodium
Sulfamethoxazole/Trimethoprim
Sulfanilamide
Sumatriptan
Sumatriptan Succinate
Tacrine Hydrochloride
Tacrolimus
Telithromycin
Telmisartan*
Telmisartan/
    Hydrochlorothiazide*
Tenecteplase
Terazosin Hydrochloride
Teriparatide
Tetanus & Diphtheria Toxoids
    Adsorbed
Tetanus Immune Globulin (Human)
Theophylline
Theophylline Anhydrous
Thiabendazole
Thrombin
Thyrotropin Alfa
Tiagabine Hydrochloride
Tiludronate Disodium
Timolol Hemihydrate
Timolol Maleate
Timolol Maleate/
    Hydrochlorothiazide
Tinidazole
Tiotropium Bromide
Tipranavir
Tizanidine Hydrochloride
Tobramycin/Dexamethasone
Tobramycin/Loteprednol Etabonate
Tolcapone
Tolterodine Tartrate
Topiramate
Tramadol Hydrochloride
Tramadol Hydrochloride/
    Acetaminophen
Trandolapril*
Trandolapril/Verapamil
    Hydrochloride*
Travoprost
Tretinoin
Triamcinolone Acetonide
Triamterene
Triamterene/Hydrochlorothiazide
Trientine Hydrochloride
Triethanolamine Polypeptide Oleate-
    Condensate

Trifluridine
Trimethoprim Hydrochloride
Trimipramine Maleate
Tropicamide/
    Hydroxyamphetamine
    Hydrobromide
Trospium Chloride
Trovafloxacin Mesylate
Tuberculin Purified Protein
    Derivative, Diluted
Typhoid Vaccine Live Oral Ty21a
Unoprostone Isopropyl
Urea
Valdecoxib
Valganciclovir Hydrochloride
Valsartan*
Valsartan/Hydrochlorothiazide*
Varicella Virus Vaccine, Live
Venlafaxine Hydrochloride
Verapamil Hydrochloride
Verteporfin
Vitamin K$_1$
Yellow Fever Vaccine
Zalcitabine
Zaleplon
Zanamivir
Zidovudine
Ziprasidone Mesylate
Zolmitriptan
Zolpidem Tartrate
Zonisamide

B

No evidence of risk in humans

*Either animal findings show risk
while human findings do not, or, if no
adequate human studies have been
done, animal findings are negative.*

Acarbose
Acrivastine
Acyclovir
Acyclovir Sodium
Adalimumab
Agalsidase Beta
Alefacept
Alfuzosin Hydrochloride
Alosetron Hydrochloride
Amiloride Hydrochloride
Amiloride Hydrochloride/
    Hydrochlorothiazide
Amoxicillin
Amoxicillin/Clavulanate Potassium
Amphotericin B
Amphotericin B Lipid Complex
Amphotericin B, Liposomal
Amphotericin B/Cholesteryl Sulfate
    Complex
Ampicillin Sodium/
    Sulbactam Sodium

Anakinra
Antithrombin III
Aprepitant
Aprotinin
Argatroban
Arginine Hydrochloride
Atazanavir Sulfate
Azelaic Acid
Azithromycin
Azithromycin Dihydrate
Aztreonam
Balsalazide Disodium
Basiliximab
Bivalirudin
Brimonidine Tartrate
Budesonide
Bupropion Hydrochloride
Cabergoline
Carbenicillin Indanyl Sodium
Cefaclor
Cefazolin Sodium
Cefdinir
Cefditoren Pivoxil
Cefepime Hydrochloride
Cefixime
Cefoperazone Sodium
Cefotaxime Sodium
Cefotetan Disodium
Cefoxitin Sodium
Cefpodoxime Proxetil
Cefprozil
Ceftazidime Sodium
Ceftibuten Dihydrate
Ceftizoxime Sodium
Ceftriaxone Sodium
Cefuroxime
Cefuroxime Axetil
Cephalexin
Cetirizine Hydrochloride
Ciclopirox
Ciclopirox Olamine
Cimetidine
Cimetidine Hydrochloride
Cisatracurium Besylate
Clindamycin
    Hydrochloride/Clindamycin
    Phosphate
Clindamycin Palmitate Hydrochloride
Clindamycin Phosphate
Clopidogrel Bisulfate
Clotrimazole
Clozapine
Colesevelam Hydrochloride
Cromolyn Sodium
Cyclobenzaprine Hydrochloride
Cyproheptadine Hydrochloride
Dalfopristin/Quinupristin
Dalteparin Sodium
Dapiprazole Hydrochloride
Daptomycin
Desflurane
Desmopressin Acetate
Dicyclomine Hydrochloride

Didanosine
Diphenhydramine Hydrochloride
Dipivefrin Hydrochloride
Dipyridamole
Dolasetron Mesylate
Doripenem
Dornase Alfa
Doxapram Hydrochloride
Doxepin Hydrochloride
Doxercalciferol
Edetate Calcium Disodium
Emtricitabine
Emtricitabine/Tenofovir Disoproxil
    Fumarate
Enfuvirtide
Enoxaparin Sodium
Eplerenone
Epoprostenol Sodium
Ertapenem
Erythromycin
Erythromycin Ethylsuccinate
Erythromycin Stearate
Esomeprazole Magnesium
Esomeprazole Sodium
Etanercept
Ethacrynate Sodium
Ethacrynic Acid
Famciclovir
Famotidine
Fenoldopam Mesylate
Fondaparinux Sodium
Galantamine Hydrobromide
Glatiramer Acetate
Glucagon
Glyburide/Metformin Hydrochloride
Granisetron Hydrochloride
Hydrochlorothiazide
Ibuprofen
Indapamide
Infliximab
Insulin Lispro Protamine,
    Human/Insulin Lispro, Human
Insulin Lispro, Human
Ipratropium Bromide
Iron Sucrose
Isosorbide Mononitrate
Lactulose
Lansoprazole
Lansoprazole/Naproxen
Laronidase
Lepirudin
Levocarnitine
Levocetirizine Dihydrochloride
Lidocaine
Lidocaine Hydrochloride
Lidocaine/Prilocaine

Lindane
Loperamide Hydrochloride
Loracarbef
Loratadine
Malathion
Meclizine Hydrochloride
Memantine Hydrochloride
Meropenem
Mesalamine
Metformin Hydrochloride
Metformin Hydrochloride/
    Sitagliptin Phosphate
Methohexital Sodium
Methyldopa
Metolazone
Metronidazole
Miglitol
Montelukast Sodium
Mupirocin
Mupirocin Calcium
Naftifine Hydrochloride
Nalbuphine Hydrochloride
Nalmefene Hydrochloride
Naloxone Hydrochloride
Naproxen Sodium
Nedocromil Sodium
Nelfinavir Mesylate
Nitazoxanide
Nitrofurantoin Macrocrystals
Nitrofurantoin Macrocrystals/
    Nitrofurantoin Monohydrate
Nizatidine
Octreotide Acetate
Omalizumab
Ondansetron
Ondansetron Hydrochloride
Orlistat
Oxiconazole Nitrate
Oxybutynin
Oxybutynin Chloride
Oxycodone Hydrochloride
Palonosetron Hydrochloride
Pancrelipase
Pantoprazole Sodium
Pegvisomant
Pemoline
Penciclovir
Penicillin G Benzathine
Penicillin G Benzathine/
    Penicillin G Procaine
Penicillin G Potassium
Pentosan Polysulfate Sodium
Permethrin
Piperacillin Sodium
Piperacillin Sodium/
    Tazobactam Sodium

Praziquantel
Progesterone
Propofol
Pseudoephedrine Hydrochloride
Pseudoephedrine Sulfate
Psyllium Preparations
Rabeprazole Sodium
Ranitidine Hydrochloride
Retapamulin
Rifabutin
Ritonavir
Rivastigmine Tartrate
Ropivacaine Hydrochloride
Saquinavir Mesylate
Sevoflurane
Sildenafil Citrate
Silver Sulfadiazine
Sodium Ferric Gluconate
Somatropin
Sotalol Hydrochloride
Sucralfate
Sulfasalazine
Tadalafil
Tamsulosin Hydrochloride
Tenofovir Disoproxil Fumarate
Terbinafine Hydrochloride
Ticarcillin Disodium/
    Clavulanate Potassium
Ticlopidine Hydrochloride
Tirofiban Hydrochloride
Torsemide
Trastuzumab
Treprostinil Sodium
Urokinase
Ursodiol
Valacyclovir Hydrochloride
Vancomycin Hydrochloride
Vardenafil Hydrochloride
Zafirlukast

Controlled studies show no risk

*Adequate, well-controlled studies in
pregnant women have failed to
demonstrate risk to the fetus.*

Liothyronine Sodium
Liotrix
Nystatin

* Category C or D depending on the trimester the drug is given.